| midazolam HCl | morphine sulfate | nalbuphine HCl | pentazocine lactate | pentobarbital Na | perphenazine | phenobarbital Na | prochlorperazine edisylate | promazine HCl | promethazine HCl | ranitidine HCl | scopolamine HBr | secobarbital Na | sodium bicarbonate | thiethylperazine maleate | thiopental Na | |
|---|---|---|---|---|---|---|---|---|---|---|---|---|---|---|---|---|
| Y | P | Y | P | P | Y |  | P | P | P | Y | P |  |  |  |  | atropine sulfate |
| Y | Y |  | Y | N | Y |  | Y |  | Y |  | Y |  |  | Y |  | butorphanol tartrate |
| Y | P |  | P | N | Y |  | P | P | P | N* | P |  |  |  | N | chlorpromazine HCl |
| Y | Y | Y | Y | N | Y |  | Y | Y | Y |  | Y | N |  |  |  | cimetidine HCl |
|  |  |  |  |  |  |  |  |  |  |  |  |  |  |  |  | codeine phosphate |
|  |  |  |  |  |  |  |  |  | Y |  |  |  |  |  |  | dexamethasone sodium phosphate |
| N | P |  | P | N | Y |  | N | N | N | Y | P |  |  |  | N | dimenhydrinate |
| Y | P | Y | P | N | Y |  | P | P | P | Y | P |  |  |  | N | diphenhydramine HCl |
| Y | P | Y | P | N | Y |  | P | P | P |  | P |  |  |  |  | droperidol |
| Y | P |  | P | N | Y |  | P | P | P | Y | P |  |  |  |  | fentanyl citrate |
| Y | Y | Y | N | N |  |  | Y | Y | Y | Y | Y | N | N |  | N | glycopyrrolate |
|  | N* |  | N |  |  | P(5) |  | N |  |  |  |  |  |  |  | heparin Na |
| Y |  |  | Y | Y |  | N | N* |  | Y | Y | Y |  |  | Y |  | hydromorphone HCl |
| Y | P | Y | P | N | Y |  | P | P | P | N | P |  |  |  |  | hydroxyzine HCl |
| Y | N |  | P | N | Y |  | P | P | P | Y | P |  |  |  | N | meperidine HCl |
| Y | P |  | P |  | P* |  | P | P | P* | Y | P |  | N |  |  | metoclopramide HCl |
|  | Y | Y |  | N | N |  | N | Y | N | N | Y |  |  | Y |  | midazolam HCl |
| Y |  |  | P | N* | Y |  | P* | P | P* | Y | P |  |  |  | N | morphine sulfate |
| Y |  |  |  | N |  |  | Y |  | N* | Y | Y |  |  | Y |  | nalbuphine HCl |
|  | P |  |  | N | Y |  | P | P* | P* | Y | P |  |  |  |  | pentazocine lactate |
| N | N* | N | N |  |  |  | N | N | N | N | P |  | Y |  | Y | pentobarbital Na |
| N | Y |  | Y | N |  |  | Y |  | Y | Y | Y |  | N |  |  | perphenazine |
|  |  |  |  |  |  |  |  |  |  | N |  |  |  |  |  | phenobarbital Na |
| N | P* | Y | P | N | Y |  |  | P | P | Y | P |  |  |  | N | prochlorperazine edisylate |
| Y | P |  | P* | N |  |  | P |  | P |  | P |  |  |  |  | promazine HCl |
| Y | P* | N* | P* | N | Y |  | P | P |  | Y | P |  |  |  | N | promethazine HCl |
| N | Y | Y | Y | N | Y | N | Y |  | Y |  | Y |  |  | Y |  | ranitidine HCl |
| Y | P | Y | P | P | Y |  | P | P | P | Y |  |  |  |  | Y | scopolamine HBr |
|  |  |  |  |  |  |  |  |  |  |  |  |  |  |  |  | secobarbital Na |
|  |  |  | Y |  |  |  |  |  |  |  |  |  |  |  | N | sodium bicarbonate |
| Y |  | Y |  |  | N |  |  |  |  | Y |  |  |  |  |  | thiethylperazine maleate |
|  | N |  |  | Y |  |  | N |  | N |  | Y |  | N |  |  | thiopental Na |

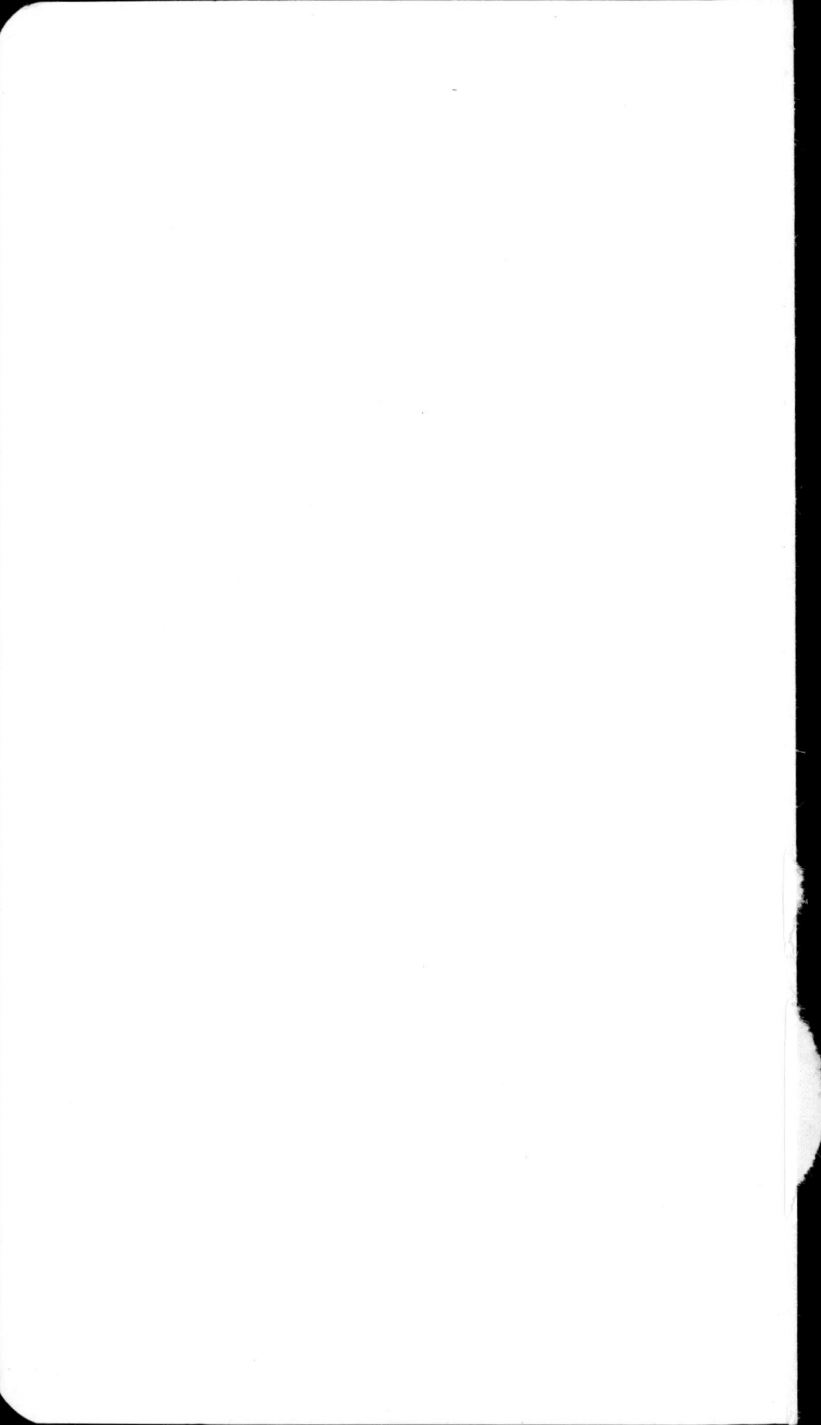

# 25th Anniversary Edition

# Nursing2005

# DRUG HANDBOOK®

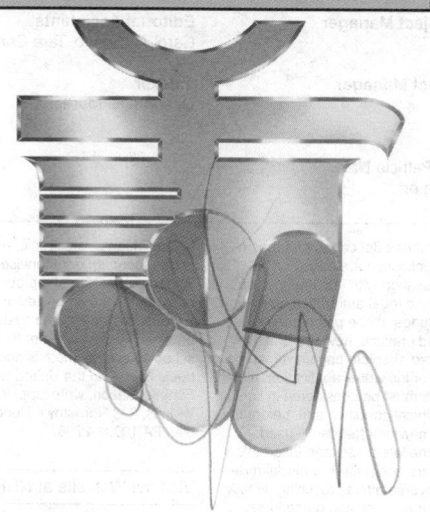

## LIPPINCOTT WILLIAMS & WILKINS
### A **Wolters Kluwer** Company

Philadelphia • Baltimore • New York • London
Buenos Aires • Hong Kong • Sydney • Tokyo

## Staff

**Executive Publisher**
Judith A. Schilling McCann, RN, MSN

**Editorial Director**
William J. Kelly

**Clinical Director**
Joan M. Robinson, RN, MSN

**Senior Art Director**
Arlene Putterman

**Art Director**
Elaine Kasmer

**Clinical Manager**
Eileen Cassin Gallen, RN, BSN

**Drug Information Editor**
Melissa M. Devlin, PharmD

**Electronic Project Manager**
John Macalino

**Editorial Project Manager**
Ann E. Houska

**Editors**
Rita M. Doyle, Patricia Nale, Carol A. Turkington

**Clinical Editors**
Lisa M. Bonsall, RN, MSN, CRNP; Shari A. Cammon, RN, MSN, CCRN; Christine M. Damico, RN, MSN, CPNP; Kimberly A. Zalewski, RN, MSN

**Copy Editors**
Michael P. Anello, Leslie Dworkin, Laura M. Healy, Caryl Knutsen, Louise Quinn, Jane Smith, Patricia Turkington, Jenifer F. Walker, Doris Weinstock

**Digital Composition Services**
Diane Paluba (manager), Joyce Rossi Biletz, Donald G. Knauss

**Manufacturing**
Patricia K. Dorshaw (director), Beth J. Welsh

**Editorial Assistants**
Carol A. Caputo, Tara Carter-Bell

**Indexer**
Deborah K. Tourtlotte

---

The clinical procedures described and recommended in this publication are based on research and consultation with nursing, medical, pharmaceutical, and legal authorities. To the best of our knowledge, these procedures reflect currently accepted practice; nevertheless, they can't be considered absolute and universal recommendations. For individual application, all recommendations must be considered in light of the patient's clinical condition and, before the administration of new or infrequently used drugs, in light of the latest package-insert information. The authors and publisher disclaim responsibility for adverse effects resulting directly or indirectly from the suggested procedures, from undetected errors, or from the reader's misunderstanding of the text.


For information, write Lippincott Williams & Wilkins, 323 Norristown Road, Suite 200, Ambler, PA 19002-2758.

Visit our Web site at NDHnow.com

NDH-D N O S A J J
06 05 04 10 9 8 7 6 5 4 3 2 1
ISSN 0273-320X
ISBN 1-58255-322-X

# Contents

## Topical Drugs

## Nutritional Drugs

## Miscellaneous Categories

## Appendices and Index

# Contributors and consultants

*At the time of publication, the contributors and consultants held the following positions.*

**Steven R. Abel, RPh, PharmD**
Professor and Head, Department of
    Pharmacy Practice
Purdue University School of Pharmacy
    and Pharmacal Sciences
Indianapolis, Ind.

**Jane Bliss-Holtz, DNSc, RC**
Nurse Researcher
Ann May Center for Nursing
Jersey Shore Medical Center
Neptune, N.J.

**Rosanne Burke, RN, MSN, CCRC**
Research Coordinator
National Institutes of Health
Bethesda, Md.

**Michael J. Burman, RPh**
Product Information Specialist III
Wyeth
St. Davids, Pa.

**Lawrence Carey, PharmD**
Assistant Professor, Physician Assistant
    Studies
Philadelphia University
Philadelphia, Pa.

**Susan M. Carver, RN, BSN, DNC**
Dermatology Nurse
Minneapolis VA Medical Center
Minneapolis, Minn.

**Jill C. Chappell, PharmD**
Independent Consultant
Noblesville, Ind.

**Michele A. Danish, RPh, PharmD**
Pharmacy Clinical Manager
St. Joseph Health Services
N. Providence, R.I.

**Linda Dean, MSN, CRNP, ACRN**
Director, Clinical Education, HIV/AIDS
    Medicine Division
MCP Hahnemann University
Philadelphia, Pa.

**Sarah M. Dunn, PharmD**
Purdue University School of Pharmacy
    and Pharmacal Sciences
Indianapolis, Ind.

**Patricia L. Eells, RN, MS, CPNP**
The Children's Hospital
Denver, Colo.

**S. Kim Genovese, RNC, MSN, MSA, CARN**
Associate Professor of Nursing
Purdue University, N.C.
Westville, Ind.

**Erin Jaynes, RN, MSN**
Administrative Nurse Specialist
Medical College of Ohio
Toledo, Ohio

**Mary Jo Gerlach, RN, MSN Ed**
Assistant Professor, Adult Nursing
    (Retired)
Medical College of Georgia
School of Nursing
Athens, Ga.

**Jennifer Justice Gorrell, PharmD**
Clinical Coordinator
Boone Memorial Hospital
Pharmacy Management & Consulting
    Services
Madison, W. Va.

**Tatyana Gurvich, PharmD**
Clinical Pharmacologist
Glendale Adventist Family Practice
    Residency Program
Glendale, Calif.

**Charles M. Karnack, PharmD, BCNSP**
Clinical Pharmacy Specialist
Mercy Hospital of Pittsburgh
Pittsburgh, Pa.

**Mary Kate Kelly, RPh, PharmD**
Publications Director
Institute for Safe Medication Practices
Huntingdon Valley, Pa.

**Julia Kleckner, PharmD**
Pharmacy Manager
Option Care
Upper Darby, Pa.

**Nancy L. Kranzley, RN, MS**
Pulmonary Clinical Nurse Specialist
Cincinnati Therapy Centers
Cincinnati, Ohio

**Lisa M. Kutney, RPh, PharmD**
Freelance Medical Writer
Ivyland, Pa.

**Thomas E. Lackner, PharmD, CGP, FASCP**
Professor, College of Pharmacy
University of Minnesota
Minneapolis, Minn.

**Kristi L. Lenz, PharmD**
Oncology Clinical Pharmacy Specialist
Medical University of South Carolina
Charleston, S.C.

**John S. Markowitz, PharmD, BCPP**
Associate Professor
Department of Pharmaceutical Sciences
Medical University of South Carolina
Charleston, S.C.

**George Melko, RPh, PharmD**
Manager, Regulatory Affairs
AstraZeneca Pharmaceuticals
Wayne, Pa.

**Zoe-Lina Ngo, RPh, PharmD**
Clinical Oncology Pharmacist
Assistant Clinical Professor
UCSF Comprehensive Cancer Center
San Francisco, Calif.

**William O'Hara, PharmD**
Clinical Team Leader
Thomas Jefferson University Hospital
Philadelphia, PA

**Christine K. O'Neil, PharmD, BCPS**
Associate Professor
Duquesne University
Pittsburgh, Pa.

**Jeffrey B. Purcell, PharmD**
Clinical Lead Pharmacist
Harborview Medical Center
Clinical Associate Professor
University of Washington School of
    Pharmacy
Seattle, Wash.

**Mary Clare A. Schafer, RN, BSN, MS, ONC**
Orthopaedic Specialist
Infection Control Coordinator
Osteoporosis Program Coordinator
Rehabilitation Hospital of South Jersey
Vineland, N.J.

**Elizabeth J. Scharman, PharmD, DABAT, BCPS, FAACT**
Director, West Virginia Poison Center
Professor, West Virginia University School
    of Pharmacy
Charleston, W. Va.

**Wendy J. Smith, RN, MSN, ACNP, AOCN**
The West Clinic
Memphis, Tenn.

**Kathleen Speer, RN, PhD, PNP-C**
Pediatric Nurse Practitioner
Children's Medical Center
Dallas, Tex.

**Erin M. Templin, PharmD**
Purdue University School of Pharmacy
    and Pharmacal Sciences
Indianapolis, Ind.

**Catherine Ultrino, RN, MS, OCN**
Staff Nurse
Kindred Care Hospital Tampa
Tampa, Fla.

**Eva M. Vasquez, PharmD, FCCP, BCPS**
Associate Professor
University of Illinois at Chicago
Chicago, Ill.

**Connie J. Webb, RPh**
Pharmacist
Hospital of the Florida Suncoast
Largo, Fla.

**Barbara J. Wiggins, PharmD, BCPS**
Pharmacy Clinical Specialist—Cardiology
University of Virginia Health System
Charlottesville, Va.

**Laurie Willhite, PharmD, RPh, CSPI**
Clinical Associate Professor
University of Minnesota College of
    Pharmacy
Minneapolis, Minn.

# How to use *Nursing2005 Drug Handbook*

*Nursing2005 Drug Handbook* was created by pharmacists and nurses to give the nursing profession drug information that pinpoints exactly what nurses need to know. *Nursing2005 Drug Handbook* focuses on that goal by emphasizing clinical aspects of drugs without trying to replace detailed pharmacology texts. The book is also designed to make the content readily accessible and applicable in any clinical setting.

## Features in this edition

The 25th anniversary edition contains several features to enhance nursing knowledge and skills:

- New monographs for 29 new FDA-approved drugs.
- A new symbol in the drug monographs indicating that a drug is pictured in the color photoguide.
- A symbol that indicates off-label uses at a glance.
- An "I.V. administration" section that provides step-by-step guidance on preparing and giving I.V. drugs.
- "Adjust-a-dose" logos that draw attention to dosage adjustments that may be needed in specific patient populations.
- Tables that show the route, onset, peak, and duration of each drug.
- An "Alert" logo that signals cautionary tips to help you avoid common medication errors, such as confusing one drug for another with a similar name.
- An "Effects on lab test results" section in every monograph.
- An "Interactions" section now highlighting drugs that cause a rapid-onset interaction.
- A guide to abbreviations in the front of the book that lists common abbreviations used throughout.
- A new appendix on drugs that affect the QTc interval, as well as appendices on herbal medicines, sound-alike and look-alike drugs, pain management drugs, and adverse reactions misinterpreted as age-related changes.
- Free NDH2005*Plus!* CD-ROM (inside the back cover) that lets you view and print complete drug monographs and customizable patient-teaching instructions for 200 commonly used drugs.
- A link from NDH2005*Plus!* to NDHnow.com, the *Nursing2005 Drug Handbook* Web site that provides monthly drug updates, important drug news, patient-teaching aids, 10 continuing-education tests, and more.

## Introductory chapters

Chapter 1 explains generally how drugs work. It includes drug actions, interactions, and reactions. Chapter 2 gives general guidelines about drug use in pregnancy and the presence of drugs in breast milk; it also covers the unique problems of giving drugs to children and elderly patients and offers suggestions to minimize problems in these areas. Chapter 3 discusses techniques and provides guidelines for safe drug administration.

## Therapeutic class chapters

Chapters 4 to 95 classify all drugs according to their approved therapeutic uses. Drugs with more than one therapeutic use are classified according to their most common use; they are also listed (with a cross-reference to the major drug entry) in drug groups that share their secondary applications. For example, nadolol, a beta blocker, is described in the chapter that covers antianginals because its major therapeutic application is the management of angina pectoris. Less commonly, nadolol is used to treat hypertension, so it's also listed among the generic drugs grouped as antihypertensives, with a cross-reference to Chapter 20, Antianginals.

Such classification by therapeutic use offers several advantages. It helps you identify an unknown drug by its clinical application alone. It also identifies all other drugs that share the same use and provides easy comparison of their dosages and effects. In this way, it quickly identifies potential pharmacotherapeutic alternatives for patients who can't tolerate or fail to respond to a particular drug.

Each chapter, representing a major therapeutic use, begins with an alphabetical list of the generic drugs described in

## Pregnancy risk categories

• A: Adequate studies in pregnant women have failed to show a risk to the fetus.
• B: Animal studies haven't shown a risk to the fetus, but controlled studies haven't been conducted in pregnant women; or animal studies have shown an adverse effect on the fetus, but adequate studies in pregnant women haven't shown a risk to the fetus.
• C: Animal studies have shown an adverse effect on the fetus, but adequate studies haven't been conducted in humans. The benefits from use in pregnant women may be acceptable despite potential risks.
• D: The drug may cause risk to the fetus, but the potential benefits of use in pregnant women may be acceptable despite the risks (such as in a life-threatening situation or a serious disease for which safer drugs can't be used or are ineffective).
• X: Studies in animals or humans show fetal abnormalities, or adverse reaction reports indicate evidence of fetal risk. The risks involved clearly outweigh potential benefits.
• NR: Not rated.

the chapter. This is followed by a list of selected combination products in which these drugs are found. Specific information on each drug is arranged under the following headings: *Pregnancy risk category, Controlled substance schedule* (when applicable), *Available forms, Indications & dosages, I.V. administration* (when applicable), *Action, Adverse reactions, Interactions, Effects on lab test results, Contraindications & cautions, Nursing considerations,* and *Patient teaching.* (See *Pregnancy risk categories* and *Controlled substance schedules.*)

In each drug entry, the generic name is followed by an alphabetized list of its brand names. A brand name followed by an open diamond ( ◊ ) indicates an OTC drug. Canadian brands are designated with a dagger (†); and Australian brands are followed by a double dagger (‡). Brand names that appear in the Photoguide to Tablets and Capsules are highlighted with

a capsule symbol (✐). A brand name with no symbol is available in the United States, Canada, and possibly Australia. The mention of a brand name in no way implies endorsement of that product or guarantees its legality.

**Alcohol content**

Many liquid drug preparations for oral use contain alcohol. Although the slight sedative effect that alcohol produces isn't harmful in most patients—and can sometimes be beneficial—alcohol ingestion can be undesirable and even dangerous. Oral drugs that contain alcohol should be given cautiously, if at all, to certain patients:
• Those who also take potent CNS depressants such as barbiturates
• Those who take drugs that may produce a disulfiram-type reaction (such as chlorpropamide or metronidazole)
• Those who take disulfiram as part of a treatment program for their alcoholism. When these patients ingest alcohol, they develop a severe reaction that may include blurred vision, confusion, dyspnea, flushing, sweating, and tachycardia.

To help prevent inadvertent exposure to alcohol, the text signals alcohol content with a single asterisk (*) after each brand name of a liquid preparation that may contain it. In many of the preparations so marked, the alcohol content is small. Nevertheless, these drugs should be avoided by patients susceptible to adverse effects after exposure to alcohol.

**Available forms**

This section lists the preparations available for each drug (for example, tablets, capsules, solutions for injection) and specifies available dosage forms and strengths. Dosage strengths specifically available in Canada are designated with a dagger (†), and those in Australia with a double dagger (‡). Preparations that don't require a prescription are marked with an open diamond ( ◊ ).

**Indications & dosages**

This section lists general dosage information for adults, children, and elderly patients, as applicable. Dosage instructions reflect current clinical trends in therapeutics and can't be considered absolute or universal recommendations. For individual application, dosage instructions must be considered in light of the patient's clinical condition.

Indications for dosages that aren't approved by the FDA are followed by a closed diamond ( ♦ ). The logo for "Adjust-a-dose" indicates dosage adjustments for certain patients, such as those with renal impairment.

## I.V. administration
This section provides guidelines for reconstituting and mixing I.V. drugs, giving them safely, and storing them properly.

## Action
This section succinctly describes the mechanism of action—that is, how the drug provides its therapeutic effect. For example, although all antihypertensives lower blood pressure, they don't all do so by the same pharmacologic process.

Also included, in table form, are the onset, peak (described in terms of effect or peak blood level), and duration of drug action for each route of administration, if data are available or applicable. Values listed are for patients with normal renal function, unless specified otherwise.

## Adverse reactions
This section lists adverse reactions to each drug by body system. The most common adverse reactions (those experienced by at least 10% of people taking the drug in clinical trials) appear in *italic* type; less common reactions are in roman type; life-threatening reactions are in ***bold italic*** type; and reactions that are common *and* life-threatening are in BOLD CAPITAL LETTERS.

## Interactions
This section lists each drug's confirmed, clinically significant interactions with other drugs (additive effects, potentiated effects, and antagonistic effects); herbs; foods; and lifestyle behaviors. Rapid-onset interactions, new to this edition, are highlighted in color in this section.

Drug interactions are listed under the drug that is adversely affected. For example, magnesium trisilicate, an ingredient in antacids, interacts with tetracycline to de-

---

## Controlled substance schedules

● Schedule I (C-I): High abuse potential and no accepted medical use. Examples include heroin, marijuana, and LSD.
● Schedule II (C-II): High abuse potential with severe dependence liability. Examples include opioids, amphetamines, and some barbiturates.
● Schedule III (C-III): Less abuse potential than schedule II drugs and moderate dependence liability. Examples include nonbarbiturate sedatives, nonamphetamine stimulants, anabolic steroids, and limited amounts of certain opioids.
● Schedule IV (C-IV): Less abuse potential than schedule III drugs and limited dependence liability. Examples include some sedatives, anxiolytics, and nonopioid analgesics.
● Schedule V (C-V): Limited abuse potential. This category includes mainly small amounts of opioids, such as codeine, used as antitussives or antidiarrheals. Under federal law, limited quantities of certain C-V drugs may be purchased without a prescription directly from a pharmacist if allowed under specific state statutes. The purchaser must be at least age 18 and must furnish suitable identification. All such transactions must be recorded by the dispensing pharmacist.

---

crease tetracycline absorption. Therefore, this interaction is listed under tetracycline. To check on the possible effects of using two or more drugs simultaneously, refer to the interaction entry for each of the drugs in question.

## Effects on lab test results
This section lists increased and decreased levels, counts, and other values in laboratory test results, which may be caused by the drug's systemic effects. It also indicates false-positive, false-negative, and otherwise altered results of laboratory tests a drug may cause.

## Contraindications & cautions
This section lists any conditions, especially diseases, in which the use of the drug is

undesirable, as well as those for which the drug should be given with caution.

**Nursing considerations**
This section provides information useful to nurses, such as monitoring techniques and suggestions for prevention and treatment of adverse reactions. Also included are suggestions for ensuring patient comfort and for preparing, giving, and storing the drug.

An "Alert" logo provides cautionary tips to avoid medication errors, such as those that may occur when drug names that sound or look alike are confused.

**Patient teaching**
This section gives the nurse guidelines on teaching the patient about each drug. It includes instructions for explaining the drug's purpose, promoting compliance, ensuring proper use and storage of the drug, and preventing or minimizing adverse reactions.

## Photoguide to tablets and capsules

To make drug identification easier and to enhance patient safety, *Nursing2005 Drug Handbook* offers a 32-page full-color photoguide to the most commonly prescribed tablets and capsules. Shown in actual size, the drugs are arranged alphabetically for quick reference, along with their most common dosage strengths. Below the name of each drug, you'll find a cross-reference to information on the drug. Brand names of drugs that appear in the photoguide are shown in the text with a special capsule symbol (✔). Page references to the drug photos appear in boldface type in the index (for example, **C12**).

# Guide to abbreviations

| | | | |
|---|---|---|---|
| ACE | angiotensin-converting enzyme | GGT | gamma-glutamyltransferase |
| ADH | antidiuretic hormone | GI | gastrointestinal |
| AIDS | acquired immunodeficiency syndrome | gtt | drops |
| | | GU | genitourinary |
| ALT | alanine transaminase | G6PD | glucose-6-phosphate dehydrogenase |
| AST | aspartate transaminase | $H_1$ | histamine$_1$ |
| AV | atrioventricular | $H_2$ | histamine$_2$ |
| b.i.d. | twice daily | HDL | high-density lipoprotein |
| BPH | benign prostatic hypertrophy | HIV | human immunodeficiency virus |
| BSA | body surface area | HMG-CoA | 3-hydroxy-3-methylglutaryl coenzyme A |
| BUN | blood urea nitrogen | | |
| cAMP | cyclic 3', 5' adenosine monophosphate | h.s. | at bedtime |
| | | I.D. | intradermal |
| CBC | complete blood count | I.M. | intramuscular |
| CK | creatine kinase | INR | International Normalized Ratio |
| CMV | cytomegalovirus | | |
| CNS | central nervous system | IPPB | intermittent positive-pressure breathing |
| COPD | chronic obstructive pulmonary disease | IU | international unit |
| CSF | cerebrospinal fluid | I.V. | intravenous |
| CV | cardiovascular | kg | kilogram |
| CVA | cerebrovascular accident | L | liter |
| $D_5W$ | dextrose 5% in water | lb | pound |
| DIC | disseminated intravascular coagulation | LDH | lactate dehydrogenase |
| | | LDL | low-density lipoprotein |
| dl | deciliter | M | molar |
| DNA | deoxyribonucleic acid | $m^2$ | square meter |
| ECG | electrocardiogram | MAO | monoamine oxidase |
| EEG | electroencephalogram | mcg | microgram |
| EENT | eyes, ears, nose, throat | mEq | milliequivalent |
| FDA | Food and Drug Administration | mg | milligram |
| | | MI | myocardial infarction |
| g | gram | min | minute |
| G | gauge | ml | milliliter |
| GFR | glomerular filtration rate | | |

| | |
|---|---|
| mm³ | cubic millimeter |
| msec | millisecond |
| NSAID | nonsteroidal anti-inflammatory drug |
| OTC | over-the-counter |
| PABA | para-aminobenzoic acid |
| PCA | patient-controlled analgesia |
| P.O. | by mouth |
| P.R. | by rectum |
| p.r.n. | as needed |
| PT | prothrombin time |
| PTT | partial thromboplastin time |
| PVC | premature ventricular contraction |
| q | every |
| q.i.d. | four times daily |
| RBC | red blood cell |
| RDA | recommended daily allowance |
| REM | rapid eye movement |
| RNA | ribonucleic acid |
| RSV | respiratory syncytial virus |
| SA | sinoatrial |
| S.C. | subcutaneous |
| sec | second |
| SIADH | syndrome of inappropriate antidiuretic hormone |
| S.L. | sublingual |
| SSRI | selective serotonin reuptake inhibitor |
| $T_3$ | triiodothyronine |
| $T_4$ | thyroxine |
| t.i.d. | three times daily |
| tsp | teaspoon |
| USP | United States Pharmacopeia |
| UTI | urinary tract infection |
| WBC | white blood cell |
| wk | week |

# 1

## Drug actions, interactions, and reactions

Any drug a patient takes causes a series of physicochemical events in his body. The first event, when a drug combines with cellular drug receptors, is the drug action. What happens next is the drug effect. Depending on the type of cellular drug receptors affected by a given drug, an effect can be local, systemic, or both. A systemic drug effect can follow a local effect. For example, when you apply a drug to the skin, it causes a local effect. But transdermal absorption of that drug can then produce a systemic effect. A local effect can also follow systemic absorption. For example, the peptic ulcer drug cimetidine produces a local effect after it's swallowed by blocking histamine receptors in the stomach's parietal cells. Diphenhydramine, on the other hand, brings about a systemic effect by blocking histamine receptors in widespread areas of the body.

### Drug properties

Drug absorption, distribution, metabolism, and excretion make up a drug's pharmacokinetic profile. This branch of pharmacology also describes a drug's onset of action, peak level, duration of action, and bioavailability.

### Absorption

Before a drug can act in the body, it must be absorbed into the bloodstream—usually after oral administration, the most common route. Before a drug contained in a tablet or capsule can be absorbed, the dosage form must disintegrate into particles small enough to dissolve in gastric juices. Only after dissolving can a drug be absorbed. Most absorption of orally given drugs occurs in the small intestine, where the mucosal villi provide extensive surface area. Once absorbed and circulated in the bloodstream, the drug is bioavailable, or ready to produce a drug effect. The speed of absorption and whether absorption is complete or partial depend on the drug's physicochemical effects, dosage form, administration route, interactions with other substances in the GI tract, and various pa-

tient characteristics. Oral solutions and elixirs, which bypass the need for disintegration and dissolution, are usually absorbed faster. Some tablets have enteric coatings to prevent disintegration in the acidic environment of the stomach; others have coatings of varying thickness that simply delay release of the drug.

Drugs given I.M. must first be absorbed through the muscle into the bloodstream. Rectal suppositories must dissolve to be absorbed through the rectal mucosa. Drugs given I.V., which are injected directly into the bloodstream, are bioavailable completely and immediately.

### Distribution

After absorption, a drug moves from the bloodstream into various fluids and tissues in the body, a movement known as distribution. The total area to which a drug is distributed is known as volume of distribution. Individual patient variations can change the amount of drug distributed throughout the body. For example, in an edematous patient, a given dose must be distributed to a larger volume than in a nonedematous patient. Occasionally, a dose is increased to account for this difference. In this case, the dose should be decreased after the edema is corrected. Conversely, a dose given to a dehydrated patient must be decreased to allow for its distribution to a much smaller volume. Patients who are particularly obese may present another problem when considering drug distribution. Some drugs—such as digoxin, gentamicin, and tobramycin—aren't well distributed to fatty tissue. Sometimes, dosing based on actual body weight may lead to overdose and serious toxicity. In these cases, dosing must be based on lean body weight, or adjusted body weight, which may be estimated from actuarial tables that give average weight range for height.

### Metabolism

Most drugs are metabolized in the liver. Hepatic diseases may affect the liver's metabolic functions and may increase or decrease a drug's usual metabolism. Closely monitor all patients with hepatic disease for drug effect and toxicity.

The rate at which a drug is metabolized varies from person to person. Some patients metabolize drugs so quickly that the drug levels in their blood and tissues prove therapeutically inadequate. In other patients, the rate of metabolism is so slow that ordinary doses can produce toxic results.

## Excretion
The body eliminates drugs by metabolism (usually hepatic) and excretion (usually renal). Drug excretion refers to the movement of a drug or its metabolites from the tissues back into circulation and from the circulation into the organs of excretion, where they are removed from the body. Although most drugs are excreted by the kidneys, some drugs can be eliminated via the lungs, exocrine glands (sweat, salivary, or mammary), liver, skin, and intestinal tract. Drugs may also be removed artificially by direct mechanical intervention, such as peritoneal dialysis or hemodialysis.

## Other modifying factors
An important factor influencing a drug's action and effect is its binding to plasma proteins, especially albumin, and other tissue components. Because only a free, unbound drug can act in the body, such binding greatly influences amount and duration of effect. Malnutrition, renal failure, and other protein-bound drugs can influence protein-binding. When protein-binding changes, drug dose may need to be changed also.

The patient's age is another important factor. Elderly patients usually have decreased hepatic function, less muscle mass, diminished renal function, and lower serum albumin levels. These patients need lower doses and sometimes longer dosage intervals to avoid toxicity. Neonates have underdeveloped metabolic enzyme systems and inadequate renal function. They need highly individualized dosages and careful monitoring.

Underlying disease can also affect drug action and effect. For example, acidosis may cause insulin resistance. Genetic diseases, such as G6PD deficiency and hepatic porphyria, may turn drugs into toxins with serious consequences. Patients with G6PD deficiency may develop hemolytic anemia when given certain drugs, such as sulfonamides. A genetically susceptible patient can develop acute porphyria if given a barbiturate. Also, a patient with a highly active hepatic enzyme system, such as a rapid acetylator, can develop hepatitis when treated with isoniazid because of the rapid intrahepatic buildup of a toxic metabolite.

## Drug administration issues
Factors related to the administration of a drug can also influence a drug's action in the body. The dosage form of a drug is important. Some tablets and capsules are too large to be easily swallowed by sick patients. An oral solution may be substituted, but it will produce higher drug blood levels than a tablet because the liquid is more easily and completely absorbed. When a potentially toxic drug (such as digoxin) is given, the increased amount that is absorbed could cause toxicity. Sometimes a change in dosage form also requires a change in dosage.

Routes of administration aren't therapeutically interchangeable. For example, diazepam is readily absorbed orally but is slowly and erratically absorbed I.M. On the other hand, gentamicin must be given parenterally because oral administration results in blood levels insufficient to treat systemic infections.

Improper storage can alter a drug's potency. Store most drugs in tight containers protected from direct sunlight and extremes in temperature and humidity that can cause them to deteriorate. Some may require special storage conditions, such as refrigeration. Caution patients not to store drugs in a bathroom because of the constantly changing environment.

The timing of drug administration can be important. Sometimes, giving an oral drug during or shortly after mealtime decreases the amount of drug absorbed. This isn't clinically significant with most drugs and may be desirable with irritating drugs such as aspirin. But penicillins and tetracyclines shouldn't be taken at mealtimes because certain foods can inactivate them. If in doubt about the effect of food on a certain drug, check with a pharmacist.

Consider the patient's age, height, and weight. The prescriber will need this information when calculating the dosage for many drugs. Record all information accurately on the patient's chart. The chart should also include all current laboratory data, especially renal and liver function studies, so the prescriber can adjust the dosage, as needed.

Watch for metabolic changes and physiologic changes (depressed respiratory function, acidosis, or alkalosis) that might alter drug effect.

Know the patient's medical history. Whenever possible, obtain a comprehensive family history from the patient or his family. Ask about past reactions to drugs, possible genetic traits that might affect drug response, and the current use of other drugs. Multiple drug therapy can cause serious and fatal drug interactions and dramatically change many drugs' effects.

## Drug interactions

A drug interaction occurs when one drug given with or shortly after another drug alters the effect of one or both drugs. Usually the effect of one drug is increased or decreased. For instance, one drug may inhibit or stimulate the metabolism or excretion of the other, or free it for further action by releasing the drug from plasma protein-binding sites.

Combination therapy is based on drug interaction. One drug may be given to complement the effects of another. Probenecid, which blocks the excretion of penicillin, is sometimes given with penicillin to maintain an adequate blood level of penicillin for a longer time. In many cases, two drugs with similar actions are given together precisely because of the additive effect. For instance, aspirin and codeine are commonly given in combination because together they provide greater pain relief than if either was given alone.

Drug interactions are sometimes used to prevent or antagonize certain adverse reactions. The diuretics hydrochlorothiazide and spironolactone are often given together because the former is potassi-

um-depleting, whereas the latter is potassium-sparing.

Not all drug interactions are beneficial. Multiple drugs can interact to produce effects that are undesirable and sometimes hazardous. Harmful drug interactions decrease efficacy or increase toxicity. For example, in a patient taking both a diuretic and lithium, the diuretic may cause an increase in the lithium level, resulting in lithium toxicity. This drug effect is known as antagonism. Avoid drug combinations that produce these effects, if possible. Another kind of inhibiting effect occurs when a tetracycline is given with calcium- or magnesium-containing drugs or foods (such as antacids or milk). These bind with tetracycline in the GI tract and cause its absorption to be inadequate.

## Adverse reactions

Drugs cause adverse effects; patients experience adverse reactions. An adverse reaction may be tolerated to obtain a therapeutic effect, or it may be hazardous and unacceptable. Some adverse reactions subside with continued use. For example, the drowsiness caused by paroxetine and the orthostatic hypotension caused by prazosin usually subside after several days as the patient develops tolerance. But many adverse reactions are dosage related and lessen or disappear only if the dosage is reduced. Most adverse reactions aren't therapeutically desirable, but a few can be put to clinical use. An outstanding example of this is the drowsiness caused by diphenhydramine, which makes it clinically useful as a mild sedative.

Hypersensitivity, a term sometimes used interchangeably with "drug allergy," is the result of an antigen-antibody immune reaction that occurs in the body when a drug is given to a susceptible patient. One of the most dangerous of all drug hypersensitivities is penicillin allergy. In its most severe form, penicillin anaphylaxis can become rapidly fatal.

Rarely, idiosyncratic reactions occur. These reactions are highly unpredictable and unusual. One of the best-known idiosyncratic adverse reactions is the aplastic anemia caused by the antibiotic chloramphenicol. This reaction appears in only 1 of 40,000 patients, but when it does occur, it can be fatal. A more common idiosyncratic reaction is extreme sensitivity to very low doses of a drug, or insensitivity to higher-than-normal doses.

To deal with adverse reactions correctly, you need to be alert to even minor changes in the patient's clinical status. Such minor changes may be an early warning of pending toxicity. Listen to the patient's complaints about his reactions to a drug, and consider each objectively. You may be able to reduce adverse reactions in several ways. Obviously, dosage reduction can help. But, in many cases, so does a simple rescheduling of the same dose. For example, pseudoephedrine may produce stimulation that will be no problem if it's given early in the day. Similarly, the drowsiness that occurs with antihistamines or tranquilizers can be harmless if given at bedtime. Most important, your patient needs to be told which adverse reactions to expect so that he won't become worried or even stop taking the drug on his own. Always advise the patient to report adverse reactions to the prescriber immediately.

Your ability to recognize signs and symptoms of drug allergies or serious idiosyncratic reactions may save your patient's life. Ask each patient about the drugs he is taking or has taken in the past and whether he experienced any unusual reactions from taking them. If a patient claims to be allergic to a drug, ask him to tell you exactly what happens when he takes it. He may be calling a harmless adverse reaction such as upset stomach an allergic reaction, or he may have a true tendency toward anaphylaxis. In either case, you and the prescriber need to know this. Of course, you must record and report clinical changes throughout the patient's hospital stay. If you suspect a severe adverse reaction, withhold the drug until you can check with the pharmacist and the prescriber.

## Toxic reactions

Chronic drug toxicities are usually caused by the cumulative effect and resulting buildup of the drug in the body. These effects may be extensions of the desired therapeutic effect. For example, glyburide will normalize blood sugar when given in usual doses but can produce undesired hypoglycemia when given in higher doses.

Drug toxicities occur when drug blood levels rise as a result of impaired metabolism or excretion. For example, blood levels of theophylline rise when hepatic dysfunction impairs metabolism of the drug. Similarly, impaired renal function may cause digoxin toxicity because digoxin is eliminated from the body almost exclusively by the kidneys. Of course, excessive dosage can cause toxic blood levels. For instance, tinnitus is usually a sign that the safe dose of aspirin has been exceeded.

Most drug toxicities are predictable and dosage related. They are reversible once the dosage is adjusted. So, be sure to monitor patients carefully for physiologic changes that might alter drug effect. Watch especially for impaired hepatic and renal function. Warn the patient about signs of pending toxicity, and tell him what to do if a toxic reaction occurs. Also, be sure to emphasize the importance of taking a drug exactly as prescribed. Warn the patient about serious problems that could arise if he changes the dose or the schedule or if he stops taking the drug without his prescriber's knowledge.

# Drug therapy across the lifespan

Drug therapy is a fact of life for millions of people of all ages, and certain aspects of a patient's life, such as age, growth, and development, can affect drug therapy.

## Drugs and pregnancy

Drug administration during pregnancy has been a source of serious medical concern and controversy since the thalidomide tragedy of the late 1950s, when thousands of malformed infants were born after their mothers were given this mild sedative-hypnotic while pregnant. To identify drugs that may cause such teratogenic effects, preclinical drug studies always include tests on pregnant laboratory animals. These studies may reveal gross teratogenicity, but they don't establish absolute safety. This is because different animal species react to drugs in different ways. Consequently, animal studies can't reveal all possible teratogenic effects in humans. For example, the preliminary studies on thalidomide gave no warning of teratogenic effects, and it was subsequently released for general use in Europe.

What about the placental barrier? Once thought to protect the fetus from drug effects, the placenta isn't much of a barrier at all. Almost every drug a pregnant woman takes crosses the placenta and enters the fetal circulation, except for drugs with exceptionally large molecular structure, such as heparin, the injectable anticoagulant. By this standard, heparin could be used in a pregnant woman without fear of harming the fetus. However, even heparin carries a warning for cautious use during pregnancy. Conversely, just because a drug crosses the placenta doesn't necessarily mean it's harmful to the fetus.

Actually, only one factor—stage of fetal development—seems clearly related to exaggerated risk during pregnancy. During the first and third trimesters of pregnancy, the fetus is especially vulnerable to damage from maternal use of drugs. During these times, give *all* drugs with extreme caution.

Organogenesis—when fetal organs differentiate—occurs during the first trimester. This is the most sensitive period for drug-induced fetal malformation. Withhold all drugs except those in category A or B during this time, unless this would jeopardize the mother's health. So, strongly advise your patient to avoid *all* self-prescribed drugs during early pregnancy.

Fetal sensitivity to drugs is also of special concern during the last trimester. At birth, when separated from his mother, the neonate must rely on his own metabolism to eliminate any remaining drug. Because his detoxifying systems aren't fully developed, any residual drug may take a long time to be metabolized, and thus may induce prolonged toxic reactions. For this reason, use drugs only when absolutely necessary during the last 3 months of pregnancy.

Of course, in many circumstances, pregnant women must continue to take certain drugs. For example, a woman with a seizure disorder that is well controlled with an anticonvulsant should continue the drug during pregnancy. Similarly, a pregnant woman with a bacterial infection must receive antibiotics. In such cases, the potential risk to the fetus is outweighed by the mother's medical needs. The relative risk to the fetus is expressed by the drug's pregnancy risk category (see *Pregnancy risk categories,* page 6).

Complying with these general guidelines can prevent indiscriminate and harmful use of drugs in pregnancy:

● Before a drug is prescribed for a woman of childbearing age, ask the date of her last menstrual period and whether she may be pregnant. If a drug is a known teratogen (for example, isotretinoin), some manufacturers may recommend special precautions to ensure that the drug is not given to a woman of childbearing age until pregnancy is ruled out and that contraceptives are used throughout the course of therapy.

## Pregnancy risk categories

The FDA has assigned a pregnancy risk category to each systemically absorbed drug based on available clinical and preclinical information. The five categories (A, B, C, D, and X) reflect a drug's potential to cause birth defects. Although drugs are best avoided during pregnancy, this rating system permits rapid assessment of the risk-benefit ratio should drug administration to a pregnant woman become necessary. Drugs in category A are generally considered safe to use in pregnancy; drugs in category X are generally contraindicated.

- A: Adequate studies in pregnant women have failed to show a risk to the fetus.
- B: Animal studies haven't shown a risk to the fetus, but controlled studies haven't been conducted in pregnant women; or animal studies have shown an adverse effect on the fetus, but adequate studies in pregnant women haven't shown a risk to the fetus.
- C: Animal studies have shown an adverse effect on the fetus, but adequate studies haven't been conducted in humans. The benefits from use in pregnant women may be acceptable despite potential risks.
- D: The drug may cause risk to the fetus, but the potential benefits of use in pregnant women may be acceptable despite the risks (such as in a life-threatening situation or a serious disease for which safer drugs can't be used or are ineffective).
- X: Studies in animals or humans show fetal abnormalities, or adverse reaction reports indicate evidence of fetal risk. The risks involved clearly outweigh potential benefits.
- NR: Not rated.

- Caution the pregnant patient to avoid all drugs except those essential to maintain the pregnancy or maternal health—especially during the first and third trimesters.
- Topical drugs are subject to the same warning against use during pregnancy. Many topically applied drugs can be absorbed in large enough amounts to be harmful to the fetus.

- When a pregnant patient needs a drug, the prescriber should order the safest drug in the lowest possible dose to minimize any harmful effect to the fetus.
- Instruct pregnant patients to check with their prescribers before taking any drug.

## Drugs and breast-feeding

Most drugs a breast-feeding mother takes appear in breast milk. Drug levels in breast milk tend to be high when drug levels in the blood are high—especially right after each dose. Therefore, advise the mother to breast-feed *before* taking each drug dose, not *after.*

A mother who wants to breast-feed usually may continue to do so with her prescriber's permission. However, breast-feeding should be temporarily interrupted and replaced with bottle-feeding when the mother must take tetracycline, chloramphenicol, a sulfonamide (during the first 2 weeks postpartum), an oral anticoagulant, a drug that contains iodine, or an antineoplastic.

Caution the breast-feeding patient to protect her infant by not taking drugs indiscriminately. Instruct the mother to first check with her prescriber to be sure she's taking the safest drug at the lowest dose. Also instruct her to provide a list of any and all drugs and herbs she is currently taking.

## Drug therapy in children

Providing drug therapy to infants, children, and adolescents is challenging. Physiologic differences between children and adults, including those in vital organ maturity and body composition, significantly influence a drug's effectiveness.

### Physiologic changes affecting drug action

A child's absorption, distribution (including drug binding to plasma proteins), metabolism, and excretion processes undergo profound changes that affect drug dosage. To ensure optimal drug effect and minimal toxicity, consider these factors when giving drugs to a child.

### *Absorption*

Drug absorption in children depends on the form of the drug, its physical properties, simultaneous ingestion of other drugs or food, physiologic changes, and concurrent disease.

The pH of neonatal gastric fluid is neutral or slightly acidic; it becomes more acidic as the infant matures, which affects drug absorption. For example, nafcillin and penicillin G are better absorbed in an infant than in an adult because of low gastric acidity.

Various infant formulas or milk products may increase gastric pH and impede absorption of acidic drugs. If possible, give a child oral drugs on an empty stomach.

Gastric emptying time and transit time through the small intestine—which is longer in children than in adults—can affect absorption. Also, intestinal hypermotility (as occurs in patients with diarrhea) can diminish the drug's absorption.

A child's comparatively thin epidermis allows increased absorption of topical drugs.

## Distribution

As with absorption, changes in body weight and physiology during childhood can significantly influence a drug's distribution and effects. In a premature infant, body fluid makes up about 85% of total body weight; in a full-term infant, it makes up 55% to 70%; in an adult, 50% to 55%. Extracellular fluid (mostly blood) constitutes 40% of a neonate's body weight, compared with 20% in an adult. Intracellular fluid remains fairly constant throughout life and has little effect on drug dosage.

Extracellular fluid volume influences a water-soluble drug's concentration and effect because most drugs travel through extracellular fluid to reach their receptors. Children have a larger proportion of fluid to solid body weight, so their distribution area is proportionately greater.

Because the proportion of fat to lean body mass increases with age, the distribution of fat-soluble drugs is more limited in children than adults. As a result, a drug's fat or water solubility affects the dosage for a child.

## Binding to plasma proteins

A decrease in albumin concentration or intermolecular attraction between drug and plasma protein causes many drugs to be less bound to plasma proteins in infants than in adults.

Drugs that strongly bind to plasma proteins may displace endogenous compounds, such as bilirubin or free fatty acids. Conversely, an endogenous compound may displace a weakly bound drug. For example, displacement of bound bilirubin can increase unbound bilirubin, which can lead to increased risk of kernicterus at normal bilirubin levels.

Because only an unbound (free) drug has a pharmacologic effect, a change in ratio of a protein-bound to an unbound active drug can greatly influence its effect.

Several diseases and disorders (such as nephrotic syndrome and malnutrition) can decrease plasma protein and increase the concentration of an unbound drug, which can either intensify the drug's effect or produce toxicity.

## Metabolism

A neonate's ability to metabolize a drug depends on the integrity of the hepatic enzyme system, intrauterine exposure to the drug, and the nature of the drug itself.

Certain metabolic mechanisms are underdeveloped in neonates. Glucuronidation is a metabolic process that renders most drugs more water soluble, facilitating renal excretion. This process isn't developed enough to permit full pediatric doses until the infant is 1 month old. The use of chloramphenicol in a neonate may cause gray baby syndrome because the infant can't metabolize the drug in his immature liver, and toxic levels accumulate in the blood. Thus, you should reduce the drug dosage in a neonate and periodically monitor his blood levels.

Conversely, intrauterine exposure to drugs may induce precocious development of hepatic enzyme mechanisms, increasing the infant's capacity to metabolize potentially harmful substances.

Older children can metabolize some drugs (theophylline, for example) more rapidly than adults can. This ability may come from their increased hepatic metabolic activity. Doses larger than those recommended for adults may be required.

Also, preparations given concurrently to a child may alter hepatic metabolism and induce production of hepatic enzymes. Phenobarbital, for example, causes hepatic enzyme production and accelerates the metabolism of drugs taken with it.

## Excretion

Renal excretion of a drug is the net result of glomerular filtration, active tubular secretion, and passive tubular reabsorption. Because so many drugs are excreted in the urine, the degree of renal development or presence of renal disease can greatly affect a child's dosage requirements. If a child can't excrete a drug renally, drug accumulation and toxicity may result unless the dosage is reduced.

Physiologically, an infant's kidneys differ from an adult's because they have a high resistance to blood flow and receive a smaller proportion of cardiac output. Infants have incomplete glomerular and tubular development and short, incomplete loops of Henle (a child's GFR reaches adult values between ages 2½ and 5 months; his tubular secretion rate may reach adult values between ages 7 and 12 months). Infants are also less able to concentrate urine or reabsorb certain filtered compounds. The proximal tubules in infants also are less able to secrete organic acids.

Children and adults have diurnal variations in urine pH that correlate with sleep-awake patterns.

## Special administration considerations

Biochemically, a drug displays the same mechanisms of action in all people. But the response to a drug can be affected by a child's age and size as well as the maturity of the target organ. To ensure optimal drug effect and minimal toxicity, consider the following factors when giving drugs to children.

## Adjusting dosages for children

When calculating children's dosages, don't use formulas that just modify adult dosages. Base pediatric dosages on either body weight (mg/kg) or body surface area ($mg/m^2$). A child isn't a scaled-down version of an adult.

Reevaluate dosages at regular intervals to ensure necessary adjustments as the child develops. Although body surface area provides a useful standard for adults and older children, use the body weight method instead in premature or full-term infants. Don't exceed the maximum adult dosage when calculating amounts per kilogram of body weight (except with certain drugs such as theophylline, if indicated).

Obtain an accurate maternal drug history, including prescription and nonprescription drugs, vitamins, herbs, or other health foods taken during pregnancy. Drugs passed into breast milk can also have adverse effects on the breast-feeding infant. Before a drug is prescribed for a breast-feeding mother, investigate the potential effects on the infant.

For example, a sulfonamide given to a breast-feeding mother for a urinary tract infection appears in breast milk and may cause kernicterus in an infant with low levels of unconjugated bilirubin. Also, high levels of isoniazid appear in the breast milk of a mother taking this drug. Because this drug is metabolized by the liver, the infant's immature hepatic enzyme mechanisms can't metabolize the drug, and he may develop CNS toxicity.

## Giving oral drugs

Remember the following when giving oral drugs to a child.

*If the patient is an infant,* give drug in liquid form, if possible. For accuracy, measure and give the preparation by oral syringe. It's very important to remove the syringe cap to prevent the infant from aspirating it and instruct parents to do the same. Never use a vial or cup. Lift the patient's head to prevent aspiration of the drug, and press down on his chin to prevent choking. You may also place the drug in a nipple and allow the infant to suck the contents.

*If the patient is a toddler,* explain how you're going to give him the drug. If possible, have the parents enlist the child's cooperation. Don't mix the drug with food or call it "candy," even if it has a pleasant taste. Let the child drink liquid drug from a calibrated medication cup rather than a spoon. It's easier and more accurate. If the preparation is available only in tablet form, crush and mix it with syrup. (Have the pharmacist verify that the tablet can be crushed without compromising its effectiveness.)

*If the patient is an older child* who can swallow a tablet or capsule by himself, have him place the drug on the back of his tongue and swallow it with water or nonacidic fruit juice because milk and milk products may interfere with drug absorption.

### Giving I.V. infusions

In infants, use a peripheral vein or a scalp vein in the temporal region for I.V. infusions. The scalp vein is safe because the needle isn't likely to dislodge, but the head must be shaved around the site. However, the needle and infiltrated fluids may cause temporary disfigurement. For these reasons, the scalp veins aren't used as commonly today as they were in the past.

The arms and legs are the most accessible insertion sites, but because patients tend to move about, take these precautions:
● Protect the insertion site to keep the catheter or needle from being dislodged.
● Use a padded arm board to reduce the risk of dislodgment. Remove the arm board during range-of-motion exercises.
● Place the clamp out of the child's reach. If extension tubing is used to allow the child greater mobility, securely tape the connection.
● Explain in simple terms to the child why he must be restrained while asleep, to alleviate anxiety and maintain trust.

During an I.V. infusion, monitor flow rates and check the child's condition and insertion site at least every hour. Titrate the flow rate only while the patient is composed; crying and emotional upset can constrict blood vessels. Flow rate may vary if a pump isn't used. Flow should be adequate because some drugs (calcium, for example) can be irritating at low flow rates. Infants, small children, and children with compromised cardiopulmonary status particularly are vulnerable to fluid overload with I.V. drug administration. To prevent this problem and help ensure that a limited amount of fluid is infused in a controlled manner, use a volume-control device in the I.V. tubing and an infusion pump or a syringe. Don't place more than 2 hours of I.V. fluid at a time in the volume-control set.

### Giving I.M. injections

I.M. injections are preferred when a drug can't be given by other parenteral routes and rapid absorption is necessary.

The vastus lateralis muscle is the preferred injection site in children younger than age 2. The ventrogluteal area or gluteus medius muscle can be used in older children. To select the correct needle size, consider the patient's age, muscle mass, nutritional status, and drug viscosity. Record and rotate injection sites. Explain to the patient that the injection will hurt but that the drug will help him. Restrain him during the injection, if needed, and comfort him afterward.

### Giving topical drugs and inhalants

When you give a child a topical drug or inhalant, consider the following:

Use eardrops warmed to room temperature. Cold drops can cause considerable pain and vertigo. To give drops, turn the patient on his side, with the affected ear up. If he's younger than age 3, pull the pinna down and back; if age 3 or older, pull the pinna up and back.

Avoid using inhalants in young children because it's difficult to get them to cooperate. Before you try to give a drug to an older child through a metered-dose nebulizer, explain the inhaler to him. Then have him hold the nebulizer upside down and close his lips around the mouthpiece. Have him exhale and pinch his nostrils shut. When he starts to inhale, release one dose of the drug into his mouth. Tell the patient to continue inhaling until his lungs feel full; then he can breathe normally and unpinch his nostrils. Most inhaled drugs aren't useful if taken orally—if you doubt the patient's ability to use the inhalant correctly, don't use it. Such devices as spacers or assist devices may help. Check with a pharmacist, the prescriber, or a respiratory therapist.

Use topical corticosteroids cautiously because prolonged use in children may delay growth. When you apply topical corticosteroids to the diaper area of infants, avoid covering the area with plastic or rubber pants, which act as an occlusive dressing and may enhance systemic absorption.

### Giving parenteral nutrition

Give I.V. nutrition to patients who can't or won't take adequate food orally and to patients with hypermetabolic conditions who need supplementation. The latter group includes premature infants and children with burns or other major trauma, intractable diarrhea, malabsorption syndromes, GI abnormalities, emotional disorders (such as anorexia nervosa), and congenital abnormalities.

Before giving fat emulsions to infants and children, weigh the potential benefits against any possible risks. Fats—supplied as 10% or 20% emulsions—are given both peripherally and centrally. Their use is limited by the child's ability to metabolize them. For example, an infant or child with a diseased liver can't efficiently metabolize fats.

Some fats, however, must be supplied both to prevent essential fatty acid deficiency and to permit normal growth and development. A minimum of calories (2% to 4%) must be supplied as linoleic acid— an essential fatty acid found in lipids. In infants, fats are essential for normal neurologic development.

Nevertheless, fat solutions may decrease oxygen perfusion and may adversely affect children with pulmonary disease. This risk can be minimized by supplying only the minimum fat needed for essential fatty acid requirements and not the usual intake of 40% to 50% of the child's total calories.

Fatty acids can also displace bilirubin bound to albumin, causing a rise in free, unconjugated bilirubin and an increased risk of kernicterus. But fat solutions may interfere with some bilirubin assays and cause falsely elevated levels. To avoid this complication, draw a blood sample 4 hours after infusion of the lipid emulsion; or if the emulsion is introduced over 24 hours, centrifuge the blood sample before the assay is performed.

## Drug therapy in elderly patients

If you're giving drugs to elderly patients, you'll want to understand the physiologic and pharmacokinetic changes that may affect appropriate drug dosage, cause common adverse reactions, or create compliance problems.

### Physiologic changes affecting drug action

As a person ages, gradual physiologic changes occur. Some of these age-related changes may alter the therapeutic and toxic effects of drugs.

### Body composition

Proportions of fat, lean tissue, and water in the body change with age. Total body mass and lean body mass tend to decrease, while the proportion of body fat tends to increase.

Body composition varies from person to person, and these changes in body composition affect the relationship between a drug's concentration and distribution in the body.

For example, a water-soluble drug such as gentamicin isn't distributed to fat. Because there's relatively less lean tissue in an elderly person, more drug remains in the blood.

### Gastrointestinal function

In elderly patients, decreases in gastric acid secretion and GI motility slow the emptying of stomach contents and movement through the entire intestinal tract. Also, research suggests that elderly patients may have more difficulty absorbing drugs than younger patients. This is an especially significant problem with drugs that have a narrow therapeutic range, such as digoxin, in which any change in absorption can be crucial.

### Hepatic function

The liver's ability to metabolize certain drugs decreases with age. This decrease is caused by diminished blood flow to the liver, which results from an age-related decrease in cardiac output, and from the lessened activity of certain liver enzymes. When an elderly patient takes a sleep medication such as flurazepam, for example, the liver's reduced ability to metabolize the drug can produce a hangover effect the next morning.

Decreased hepatic function may result in more intense drug effects caused by higher blood levels, longer-lasting drug effects because of prolonged blood levels, and a greater risk of drug toxicity.

### Renal function

An elderly person's renal function is usually sufficient to eliminate excess body fluid and waste, but their ability to eliminate some drugs may be reduced by 50% or more.

Many drugs commonly used by elderly patients, such as digoxin, are excreted primarily through the kidneys. If the kidneys' ability to excrete the drug is decreased, high blood levels may result. Digoxin toxicity can be relatively common in elderly patients who don't receive a reduced digoxin dosage to accommodate decreased renal function.

Drug dosages can be modified to compensate for age-related decreases in renal function. Aided by laboratory tests such as BUN and serum creatinine, prescribers may adjust drug dosages so the patient receives therapeutic benefits without the risk of toxicity. Also, observe the patient for signs and symptoms of toxicity. A patient taking digoxin, for example, may experience anorexia, nausea, vomiting, or confusion.

## Special administration considerations

Aging is usually accompanied by a decline in organ function that can affect drug distribution and clearance. This physiologic decline is likely to be exacerbated by a disease or a chronic disorder. Together, these factors can significantly increase the risk of adverse reactions and drug toxicity, as well as noncompliance. Be aware of these changes when giving a drug to an elderly patient.

### Adverse reactions

Compared with younger people, elderly patients experience twice as many adverse drug reactions, relating to greater drug use, poor compliance, and physiologic changes.

Signs and symptoms of adverse drug reactions—confusion, weakness, agitation, and lethargy—are often mistakenly attributed to senility or disease. If the adverse reaction isn't identified, the patient may continue to receive the drug. Furthermore, he may receive unnecessary additional drugs to treat complications caused by the original drug. This regimen can sometimes result in a pattern of inappropriate and excessive drug use.

Although any drug can cause adverse reactions, most of the serious reactions in the elderly are caused by relatively few drugs. Be particularly alert for toxicities resulting from diuretics, antihypertensives, digoxin, corticosteroids, anticoagulants, sleeping aids, and OTC drugs.

### Diuretic toxicity

Because total body water content decreases with age, a normal dosage of a potassium-wasting diuretic such as hydrochlorothiazide or furosemide may result in fluid loss and even dehydration in an elderly patient.

These diuretics may deplete a patient's potassium level, making him feel weak, and they may raise blood uric acid and glucose levels, complicating gout and diabetes mellitus.

### Antihypertensive toxicity

Many elderly people experience lightheadedness or fainting when taking antihypertensives, partly in response to atherosclerosis and decreased elasticity of the blood vessels. Antihypertensives can lower blood pressure too rapidly, resulting in insufficient blood flow to the brain, which can cause dizziness, fainting, or even a CVA.

Consequently, dosages of antihypertensives must be carefully individualized. In elderly patients, aggressive treatment of high blood pressure may be harmful. Treatment goals should be reasonable. Reducing blood pressure to 135/90 mm Hg is appropriate, but it needs to be done more slowly in elderly than in younger patients.

**Digoxin toxicity**
As the body's renal function and rate of excretion decline, the digoxin level in the blood of an elderly person taking this drug may increase to the point of causing nausea, vomiting, diarrhea, and, most seriously, cardiac arrhythmias. Try to prevent severe toxicity by monitoring the patient's digoxin level and observing him for early signs and symptoms of inotropic toxicity, such as appetite loss, confusion, or depression.

**Corticosteroid toxicity**
Elderly patients taking a corticosteroid may experience short-term effects, including fluid retention and psychological effects ranging from mild euphoria to acute psychotic reactions. Long-term toxic effects, such as osteoporosis, can be especially severe in elderly patients who have been taking prednisone or related steroidal compounds for months or even years. To prevent serious toxicity, carefully monitor patients on long-term regimens. Observe them for subtle changes in appearance, mood, and mobility; for impaired healing; and for fluid and electrolyte disturbances.

**Anticoagulant effects**
Elderly patients taking an anticoagulant have an increased risk of bleeding, especially when they take NSAIDs at the same time, which is common. They're also at increased risk of bleeding and bruising because older patients are more likely to fall. Observe the patient's INR carefully, and monitor him for bruising and other signs of bleeding.

**Sleeping aid toxicity**
Sedatives and sleeping aids such as flurazepam may cause excessive sedation or drowsiness. Keep in mind that consuming alcohol may increase depressant effects, even if the sleeping aid was taken the previous evening. Use these drugs sparingly in elderly patients.

**Over-the-counter drug toxicity**
Toxicity is minimal when aspirin, aspirin-containing analgesics, and other OTC NSAIDs (such as ibuprofen, ketoprofen, and naproxen) are used in moderation. But prolonged ingestion may cause GI irritation—even ulcers—and gradual blood loss resulting in severe anemia. Prescription NSAIDs may cause similar problems. Anemia from prolonged aspirin consumption can affect all age groups, but elderly patients may be less able to compensate because of their already reduced iron stores.

Laxatives may cause diarrhea in elderly patients, who are extremely sensitive to drugs such as bisacodyl. Long-term oral use of mineral oil as a lubricating laxative may result in lipid pneumonia from aspiration of small residual oil droplets in the patient's mouth.

*Noncompliance*
Poor compliance can be a problem with patients of any age. Many hospitalizations result from noncompliance with a medical regimen. In elderly patients, factors linked to aging, such as diminished visual acuity, hearing loss, forgetfulness, the need for multiple drug therapy, and socioeconomic factors, can combine to make compliance a special problem. About one-third of elderly patients fail to comply with their prescribed drug therapy. They may fail to take prescribed doses or to follow the correct schedule. They may take drugs prescribed for previous disorders, stop drugs prematurely, or indiscriminately use drugs that are to be taken "as needed." Elderly patients may also have multiple prescriptions for the same drug and inadvertently take an overdose.

Review the patient's drug regimen with him. Make sure he understands the dose amount, the time and frequency of doses, and why he's taking the drug. Also, explain in detail if a drug is to be taken with food, with water, or separate from other drugs.

Help the patient avoid drug therapy problems by suggesting that he use drug calendars, pill sorters, or other aids to help him comply. Refer him to the prescriber, pharmacist, or social services if he needs further information or assistance with his drug therapy.

# Safe drug administration

In the state where you practice nursing, a number of different health care professionals, including doctors, nurse practitioners, dentists, podiatrists, and optometrists, may be legally permitted to prescribe, dispense, and give drugs. Most often, however, doctors prescribe drugs, pharmacists dispense them, and nurses give them.

That means you're almost always on the front line when it comes to patients and their drugs. It also means you bear a major share of the responsibility for avoiding drug errors. Besides following your institution's administration policies, you can help prevent drug mistakes by reviewing the common errors outlined below and ways to prevent them.

Also included in this chapter is a section on important points to teach your patients so they may take their drugs safely at home.

## Drug orders
Prescribing and filling drug orders must be done carefully to avoid potential problems.

### Pharmacy computer systems
*Error:* The Institute for Safe Medication Practices (ISMP) performed a field test on 307 pharmacy computer systems; only four detected all of the unsafe orders. Many didn't detect potentially lethal orders, including doses that exceeded safe limits, drug ingredient duplications, and orders to give oral solutions I.V.
*Best practice or prevention:* Don't rely on the pharmacy computer system to detect all unsafe orders. Before you give a drug, understand the correct dosage, indications, and adverse effects. If necessary, check a current drug reference guide.

### Confusing drug names
*Error:* The approval of Lantus (insulin glargine [rDNA origin]) raises concerns that this drug will be confused with Lente insulin. This mix-up could easily happen with either a verbal or written order.

*Best practice or prevention:* Be aware of the drugs your patient takes regularly, and question any deviations from his regular routine. As with any drug, take your time and read the label carefully.

### Abbreviations
*Error:* Abbreviating drug names is risky. A cancer patient with anemia may receive epoetin alfa, commonly abbreviated EPO, to stimulate RBC production. In one case, when a cancer patient was admitted to a hospital, the doctor wrote, "May take own supply of EPO." But the patient wasn't anemic. Sensing that something was wrong, the pharmacist interviewed the patient, who confirmed that he was taking "EPO"—evening primrose oil—to lower his cholesterol level.
*Best practice or prevention:* Ask all prescribers to spell out drug names.

### Unclear orders
*Error:* A patient was supposed to receive one dose of the antineoplastic lomustine to treat brain cancer. (Lomustine is typically given as a single oral dose once every 6 weeks.) The doctor's order read "Administer h.s." Because this was misinterpreted to mean every night, the patient received nine daily doses, developed severe thrombocytopenia and leukopenia, and died.
*Best practice or prevention:* If you're unfamiliar with a drug, check a drug reference before giving it. If a prescriber uses "h.s." but doesn't specify the frequency of administration, clarify the order. When documenting orders, note "h.s. nightly" or "h.s.—one dose today."

### Misinterpretation of orders
*Error:* Several reports to the ISMP involved errors related to insulin orders. In one case, an order was written as "add 10U of regular insulin to each TPN bag," and the pharmacist preparing the solution misinterpreted the dose as 100 units. In another case, a pharmacy technician entering orders misinterpreted a sliding scale

when the insulin order used "u" for units, an error that could have caused a 10-fold overdose if a nurse hadn't caught it. Yet another report involved a nurse who received a verbal order to resume an insulin drip but wrote "resume heparin drip." Fortunately, the pharmacist caught the error.

*Best practice or prevention:* Before you give a drug such as insulin or heparin, which are ordered in units, always check the prescriber's written order against the provided dose. Never abbreviate "units." If you must accept a verbal order, have another nurse listen in; then transcribe that order directly onto an order form and repeat it to ensure that you've transcribed it correctly.

### Inadvertent overdose

*Error:* The inadvertent prescribing of harmful acetaminophen doses has become a disturbing trend. To relieve pain, prescribers may write orders for combined acetaminophen and opioid analgesic tablets (Lortab, Tylox, Darvocet-N) without realizing that the total acetaminophen dose could be toxic.

Consider this order: "Tylox, 1 to 2 tablets every 4 hours, as needed, for pain." By taking the higher dose, the patient would receive 1,000 mg of acetaminophen every 4 hours, exceeding the maximum recommended dose of 4 g/day.

*Best practice or prevention:* To prevent an acetaminophen overdose from combined analgesics, note the amount of acetaminophen in each drug. Beware of substitutions by the pharmacy because the amount of acetaminophen may vary.

### Lipid-based drugs

*Error:* Serious drug errors, some fatal, have occurred because of confusion between certain lipid-based (liposomal) drugs and their conventional counterparts. The drugs involved include:
- lipid-based amphotericin B (Abelcet, Amphotec, AmBisome) and conventional amphotericin B for injection (available generically and as Fungizone)
- the pegylated liposomal form of doxorubicin (Doxil) and its conventional form, doxorubicin hydrochloride (Adriamycin, Rubex)

- a liposomal form of daunorubicin (DaunoXome, daunorubicin citrate liposomal) and conventional daunorubicin hydrochloride (Cerubidine).

*Best practice or prevention:* Lipid-based products have different dosages than their conventional counterparts. Check the original order and labels carefully to avoid confusion.

## Drug preparation

When preparing to give a drug, be alert for potential problems.

### Syringe tip caps and children

*Error:* A syringe tip cap poses a potential choking hazard to a small child: If you forget to remove the cap from an oral syringe before you give a drug, the cap could blow off into the child's mouth when you press the plunger. If a cap from an oral or a hypodermic syringe gets lost in the linens, the child may find it later and swallow or aspirate it.

*Best practice or prevention:* Remove and discard the cap in a secure sharps container before you give the drug; don't place it in a trash can where the child may find it later.

Teach parents about the potential danger of syringe tip caps. Tell them to store a capped syringe where children can't reach it and to remove the cap before giving the drug.

### Inattentiveness

*Error:* When a hospital pharmacy received an order for Fludara (fludarabine), a pharmacy technician asked the pharmacist if Navelbine (vinorelbine) was the same as Fludara (both are antineoplastics). The preoccupied pharmacist said "yes." The technician prepared the Navelbine, but labeled it as Fludara. The pharmacist checked the preparation but didn't notice the error, and the patient received the wrong drug.

*Best practice or prevention:* To prevent errors of this type, the hospital posted tables of antineoplastics and their dosing guidelines in the pharmacy. As an added safeguard, the pharmacy now sends the empty drug vial or box top with the prepared solution for the nurse to double-check before infusing the drug.

### Injectable solution color changes

*Error:* In two cases, alert nurses noticed that antineoplastics prepared in the pharmacy didn't look the way they should.

In the first error, a 6-year-old child was to receive 12 mg of methotrexate intrathecally. In the pharmacy, a 1-g vial was mistakenly selected instead of a 20-mg vial, and the drug was reconstituted with 10 ml of normal saline solution. The vial containing 100 mg/ml was incorrectly labeled as containing 2 mg/ml, and 6 ml of the solution was drawn into a syringe. Although the syringe label indicated 12 mg of drug, the syringe actually contained 600 mg of drug.

When the nurse received the syringe and noted that the drug's color didn't appear right, she returned it to the pharmacy for verification. The pharmacist retrieved the vial used to prepare the dose and drew the remaining solution into another syringe. The solutions in both syringes matched, and no one noticed the vial's 1-g label. The pharmacist concluded that a manufacturing change caused the color difference.

The child received the 600-mg dose and experienced seizures 45 minutes later. A pharmacist responding to the emergency detected the error. The child received an antidote and recovered.

In the second error, a 20-year-old patient with leukemia received mitomycin instead of mitoxantrone. The nurse had questioned the drug's unusual bluish tint, but the pharmacist had assured her that the color difference was the result of a change in manufacturer. Fortunately, the patient didn't suffer any harm.

*Best practice or prevention:* If a familiar drug has an unfamiliar appearance, find out why. If the pharmacist cites a manufacturing change, ask him to double-check whether he has received verification from the manufacturer. Document the appearance discrepancy, your actions, and the pharmacist's response in the patient record.

### Dropper confusion

*Error:* Ordering drugs such as liquid ferrous sulfate by the dropperful is a dangerous practice. One person might correctly consider the dropper full when the liquid meets the upper calibration mark; another might incorrectly fill the entire length of the dropper. Also, parents giving the drug at home may use a different dropper, which could significantly change the dose given.

*Best practice or prevention:* Dosing directions for liquid drugs should always be expressed as weight per volume, such as 15 mg/0.6 ml. Verify the correct dose and teach parents to use only the dropper provided. Show them the mark on the dropper that indicates a full dose and ask them to demonstrate the proper technique.

### Incorrect allergy history

*Error:* After a patient was admitted to the hospital, a nurse faxed a list of the patient's allergies to the pharmacy. The pharmacist couldn't read it, so he accessed the files from the patient's previous admission. However, these records didn't reflect an allergy to the anti-infective cefazolin that the patient had recently developed.

A consulting doctor ordered cefazolin, and the pharmacy processed the order. The medication administration record (MAR) generated by the pharmacy's database didn't indicate the allergy, and the nurse didn't know about it either.

The patient received cefazolin and became hypotensive and unresponsive. The nurse immediately notified the doctor and gave the antihistamine diphenhydramine. The patient recovered and was discharged the next day.

*Best practice or prevention:* Obtain a new allergy history with each admission. If the patient's history must be faxed, name the drugs, note how many are included, and follow the facility's faxing safeguards. If the pharmacy also adheres to strict guidelines, the computer-generated MAR should be accurate.

## Giving drugs

When you give a drug, be careful to avoid the following potential problems.

### Misidentifying patients

*Error:* Two common errors for nurses who are giving drugs are inadvertently failing to check the patient's identification and confusing patients with similar names. Using a tactic that helps prevent wrong-site surgery—involving the patient in the identification process—could also help prevent these drug errors.

*Best practice or prevention:* Urge the patient to clearly state his full name, even without being asked, at admission and before accepting drugs, procedures, or treatments. Teach him to offer his identification bracelet for inspection when anyone arrives with drugs and to insist on having it replaced if it's removed.

## Herbal remedies

*Error:* Surveys suggest that about one-third of Americans use herbs as medicine. Some people take them with conventional drugs; others use them as replacements. Herbs are available without a prescription. Because government quality assurance standards don't apply to herbs' manufacturing and labeling, their ingredients may be misrepresented or contaminated.

Research on the effects of herbs is limited. Because these products may contain a mixture of chemicals, their use carries risks.

*Best practice or prevention:* Ask the patient about his use of alternative therapies, including herbs, and record your findings in his medical record. Monitor the patient carefully and report unusual events. Ask the patient to keep a diary of all therapies he uses and to take the diary for review each time he visits a health care professional.

## Calculation errors

*Error:* A physician assistant wrote the following order for a woman being admitted to the hospital for neck surgery: "methylprednisolone 10.6 g (30 mg/kg) over 1 hour IVPB before surgery" to minimize inflammation. The patient weighed 154 lb (70 kg), so the dose should have been 2.1 g, and not 10.6 g. Because neither the pharmacist nor the nurse independently checked the calculation, the patient received an overdose. She developed significant hyperglycemia and hypokalemia but recovered without injury.

*Best practice or prevention:* Writing the mg/kg or mg/m$^2$ dose and the calculated dose provides a safeguard against calculation errors. Whenever a prescriber provides the calculation, double-check it and document that the dose was verified.

## Eyedrops for two or more

*Error:* Using one bottle of eyedrops to treat several patients may seem like a good way to prevent waste, control cost, and save time. Some facilities, for example, give shared eyedrops to multiple patients undergoing outpatient cataract surgery. But this practice has risks.

Eyedrops contain preservatives to prevent bacterial growth, but contaminants may remain on the bottle top's inner surfaces or outer grooves. The dropper can also become contaminated if it accidentally touches an infected eye. (Cross-infections have been reported.)

Giving the wrong drug or wrong concentration is more likely when containers are shared because patient names don't appear on the containers. A patient may receive the wrong drops because the nurse can't check the bottle label against the patient's identification.

*Best practice or prevention:* Just as sharing any drug is poor practice, eyedrops shouldn't be used for more than one patient. If unit doses aren't available for surgical patients, each patient should fill his prescriptions before admission and bring his drugs with him.

## Trouble with liquids

*Error:* Liquid drugs may be more error-prone than solid drugs because of the calculations and dosage measurements needed. Here are a few examples: A 5-year-old boy who was receiving imipramine to treat his enuresis was given a 5-fold overdose because of an incorrectly compounded suspension. A prescription of Augmentin was dispensed with the instruction to take 2½ tsp instead of 2½ ml. In another case, a mother who misunderstood the written directions gave her child 7 ml instead of 0.7 ml of a liquid drug.

*Best practice or prevention:* Don't assume that liquid drugs are less likely to cause harm than other forms, including parenteral ones. Pediatric and geriatric patients often receive liquid drugs and may be especially sensitive to the effects of an inaccurate dose. If a unit-dose form isn't available, calculate carefully, and double-check your math and the drug label.

## Celexa, Celebrex, and Cerebyx confusion

*Error:* An 80-year-old woman mistakenly received 20 mg of Celexa (citalopram), a selective serotonin reuptake inhibitor (SSRI), b.i.d. for 1 month for arthritis pain. She should have received 100 mg of Celebrex (celecoxib), an NSAID. A member of the pharmacy staff had confused the drug names when pulling the product from the shelf. The patient wasn't harmed, but the potential for harm was great because she was already taking an SSRI.

*Best practice or prevention:* Help prevent errors related to Celebrex, Celexa, and the anticonvulsant Cerebyx (fosphenytoin) by asking prescribers to use the generic name and by confirming the drug's indication if the order doesn't clearly state it. For verbal orders, repeat the drug name and your understanding of its indication to the prescriber.

## Labels and toxicity

*Error:* A container of 5% acetic acid, used to clean tracheostomy tubing, was left near nebulization equipment in the room of a 10-month-old infant. A respiratory therapist mistook the liquid for normal saline solution and used it to dilute albuterol for the child's nebulizer treatment. During treatment, the child experienced bronchospasm, hypercapnic dyspnea, tachypnea, and tachycardia.

*Best practice or prevention:* Leaving potentially dangerous chemicals near patients is extremely risky, especially when the container labels don't indicate toxicity. To prevent such problems, read the label on every drug you prepare and never give anything that isn't labeled.

## Dosage equations

*Error:* A 13-month study at Albany (NY) Medical Center examined 200 prescribing errors arising from the use of dosage equations. Almost 70% involved pediatric patients, for whom dosage equations are commonly used. Mistakes in decimal point placement, mathematical calculation, or expression of the regimen accounted for more than 50% of the errors.

Examples include prescribing the entire day's drug as a single dose instead of at intervals and using an entire day's dose at each interval. Use of dosage equations invites drug errors.

*Best practice or prevention:* Alternatives to dosage equations include using preestablished ranges or tables, incorporating a calculator into a computer order entry system, and requiring both the calculated dose and dosage equation on orders to facilitate independent checks.

After you calculate a drug dosage, always have another nurse calculate it independently to double-check your results. If doubts or questions remain or if the calculations don't match, ask a pharmacist to calculate the dose before you give the drug.

## Misreading orders

*Error:* Two reports concerned incorrect dosing of the tricyclic antidepressant nortriptyline (Pamelor, Aventyl, or, in Australia, Allegron) when ordered for neuropathic pain syndromes. The cases involved 10-mg and 20-mg orders that were misread as 100 mg and 200 mg, respectively. One patient who received an incorrect dose required hospitalization; the other developed sedation and orthostatic hypotension after two doses, which led to recognition of the error.

*Best practice or prevention:* Nortriptyline and other tricyclic antidepressants aren't prescribed as frequently as they once were. To make sure you're familiar with recommended dosages, refer to a drug handbook and then ask a pharmacist, if necessary.

## Air bubbles in pump tubing

*Error:* After starting an I.V. drip to give insulin, 2 units/hour, to a 9-year-old patient, a nurse noted air bubbles in the tubing and pump chamber. To remove them and promote proper flow, she disconnected the tubing and increased the pump rate to 200 ml/hour. When the bubbles were cleared, she reconnected the tubing and restarted the infusion without resetting the rate. The child received about 50 units of insulin before the error was detected. Fortunately, the child wasn't harmed.

*Best practice or prevention:* To clear bubbles from I.V. tubing, never increase the pump's flow rate to flush the line. Instead, remove the tubing from the pump, disconnect it from the patient, and use the flow-control clamp to establish gravity flow. When the bubbles have been removed, return the tubing to the pump, restart the infusion, and recheck the flow rate.

## Misplacing decimals

*Error:* A patient in the intensive care unit was to receive the opioid fentanyl, 12.5 to 25 mcg I.V. every 4 to 6 hours, as needed, for pain. Unit stock consisted of 5-ml ampules of fentanyl 0.05 mg/ml, so each ampule contained 0.25 mg (250 mcg). A nurse preparing a dose confused the volume needed when she converted from milligrams to micrograms and gave 5 ml, thinking it contained 25 mcg. The patient suffered respiratory arrest but was resuscitated.

*Best practice or prevention:* Numerous serious fentanyl errors have been reported, and a misplaced decimal point caused many of them. A safer alternative for intermittent dosing is I.V. morphine. Fentanyl doses are best prepared in the pharmacy rather than in the unit. If a fentanyl dose must be prepared, refer to dosing charts, follow the facility's protocols, and ask another nurse to check your calculations.

## Incorrect administration route

*Error:* A nurse was caring for a patient who had a jejunostomy tube for oral drugs and a central I.V. line for hyperalimentation and I.V. drugs. At the bedside was a stock bottle of digoxin elixir. After checking the concentration, the nurse used a syringe to withdraw 2.5 ml of elixir for a 0.125-mg dose. She then mistakenly gave the elixir through the central line rather than the jejunostomy tube.

Using an incorrect route put the patient at risk for overdose and secondary infection from unsterile I.V. administration. Fortunately, he was receiving antibiotics for a preexisting infection and suffered no adverse reactions.

*Best practice or prevention:* This case emphasizes the need to ensure that the right route is being used to give any drug.

When the patient has multiple lines, label the distal end of each line. Using a parenteral syringe to prepare oral liquid drugs increases the chance for error because the syringe tip fits easily into I.V. ports. To safely give an oral drug through a feeding tube, use a dose prepared by the pharmacy and a syringe with the appropriate tip.

## Stress

*Error:* A nurse-anesthetist gave the sedative midazolam (Versed) to the wrong patient. When she discovered the error, she grabbed what she thought was a vial of the antidote flumazenil (Romazicon), withdrew 2.5 ml, and gave it. When the patient didn't respond, she realized she'd grabbed a vial of ondansetron (Zofran), an antiemetic, instead. Another practitioner assisted with proper I.V. administration of flumazenil, and the patient recovered without harm.

*Best practice or prevention:* Committing a serious error can cause enormous stress and cloud your judgment. If you're involved in a drug error, ask another professional to give the antidote.

## Patient teaching

Patients being discharged from an acute care setting may be at a greater risk for adverse drug reactions arising from drug-drug interactions. Changes are frequently made to a patient's regular drug regimen before discharge, either by altering the dose or adding one or more new drugs. Adverse effects may go unnoticed by the practitioner or unreported when the patient is at home. Carefully review the patient's drugs upon discharge, inform him of any potential adverse drug effects to be aware of, and tell him to call the prescriber if adverse effects become bothersome.

The following general guidelines will help to ensure that the patient receives the maximum therapeutic benefit and avoids adverse reactions, accidental overdose, and harmful changes in effectiveness.

• Instruct the patient to learn the brand and generic names of all drugs he is taking and to inform his regular prescriber about their use. Before you give a patient a drug, ask him to report unusual reactions

experienced in the past, allergies to foods and other substances, special medical problems, and drugs taken over the last few weeks, including OTC drugs or herbs.
● Advise the patient to always read the label before taking a drug, to take it exactly as prescribed, and never to share prescription drugs.
● Warn the patient not to change brands of a drug without consulting his prescriber, to avoid harmful changes in effectiveness. Certain generic preparations aren't equivalent in effect to brand-name preparations of the same drug.
● Tell the patient to check the expiration date before taking a drug.
● Instruct the patient to safely discard drugs that are outdated or no longer needed and to keep discarded drugs out of the reach of children and pets.
● Tell the patient to store each drug in its original container, at room temperature (unless directed otherwise), and in places that aren't accessible to children or exposed to sunlight. Avoid storage in the bathroom medicine cabinet, in the kitchen close to heat, or in the glove compartment or trunk of an automobile, where extremes of temperature and humidity will cause deterioration.
● Caution the patient about mixing different drugs in a single container, removing a drug from its original container, or removing the label. Relying on memory to identify a drug and specific directions for its use is dangerous.
● If the patient must remove pills from their original container to use a daily or weekly "medication planner" as a reminder, tell him to keep an index card with the planner with the drug's name, strength, dosing instructions, and physical description written on the card. This is particularly important when he is taking more than one prescription.
● Stress how important it is for the patient to tell the prescriber about adverse reactions he experiences during drug therapy.
● Advise the patient to have all prescriptions filled at the same pharmacy so that the pharmacist can identify and warn against potentially harmful drug interactions. Also, tell the patient to inform the pharmacist and prescriber about any OTC drugs or herbs he takes.

● Instruct the patient to call the prescriber, poison control center, or pharmacist immediately if he or someone else has taken an overdose. The National Poison Control Center phone number to call is 1-800-222-1222. Tell the patient to keep this and other emergency telephone numbers handy at all times.
● Advise the patient to inform medical personnel about use of drugs before undergoing surgery (including dental surgery).
● Tell the patient to have a sufficient supply of drugs when traveling. He should carry them with him in their original containers and not pack them in his luggage. Also, recommend that a patient who travels abroad should carry a letter from his prescriber authorizing the use of the drug, especially if the drug is a controlled substance.

**atovaquone**
**chloroquine hydrochloride**
   (See Chapter 7, ANTIMALARIALS.)
**chloroquine phosphate**
   (See Chapter 7, ANTIMALARIALS.)
**metronidazole**
**metronidazole hydrochloride**
**nitazoxanide**
**pentamidine isethionate**

### COMBINATION PRODUCTS
HELIDAC: metronidazole 250 mg (with povidone), tetracycline 500 mg, bismuth subsalicylate 262.4 mg (with povidone).

---

## atovaquone
Mepron

*Pregnancy risk category C*

---

### AVAILABLE FORMS
*Suspension:* 750 mg/5 ml

### INDICATIONS & DOSAGES
➤ **Acute, mild to moderate *Pneumocystis carinii* pneumonia in patients who can't tolerate co-trimoxazole**
*Adults and adolescents ages 13 to 16:*
750 mg P.O. b.i.d. with food for 21 days.
➤ **To prevent *P. carinii* pneumonia in patients who can't tolerate co-trimoxazole**
*Adults and adolescents ages 13 to 16:*
1,500 mg (10 ml) P.O. daily with food.

### ACTION
Unknown. Appears to interfere with electron transport in protozoal mitochondria, inhibiting enzymes needed for the synthesis of nucleic acids and adenosine triphosphate.

| Route | Onset | Peak | Duration |
|-------|-------|------|----------|
| P.O. | Unknown | Unknown | Unknown |

### ADVERSE REACTIONS
**CNS:** *headache, insomnia, fever, pain,* asthenia, anxiety, dizziness.
**CV:** hypotension.
**EENT:** sinusitis, rhinitis.
**GI:** *nausea, diarrhea, vomiting,* constipation, *abdominal pain,* anorexia, dyspepsia, *oral candidiasis,* taste perversion.
**Hematologic:** anemia, *neutropenia.*
**Metabolic:** *hypoglycemia,* hyponatremia.
**Respiratory:** *cough.*
**Skin:** *rash,* pruritus, *diaphoresis.*

### INTERACTIONS
**Drug-drug.** *Rifabutin, rifampin:* May decrease atovaquone's steady-state level. Avoid using together.

### EFFECTS ON LAB TEST RESULTS
● May increase alkaline phosphatase, ALT, and AST levels. May decrease sodium and glucose levels.
● May decrease hemoglobin and neutrophil count.

### CONTRAINDICATIONS & CAUTIONS
● Contraindicated in patients hypersensitive to drug.
● Use cautiously in breast-feeding patients because drug appears in breast milk.
● Use cautiously with other highly protein-bound drugs, and assess patient for toxicity when used together.

### NURSING CONSIDERATIONS
● *Alert:* Monitor patient closely during therapy because of risk of concurrent pulmonary infections.

### PATIENT TEACHING
● Instruct patient to take drug with meals because food significantly enhances absorption.

---

Reactions may be *common,* uncommon, *life-threatening*, or COMMON AND LIFE-THREATENING.

# metronidazole
Apo-Metronidazole†, Flagyl, Flagyl 375, Flagyl ER, Metrogyl‡, Novo-Nidazol†, Protostat, Trikacide†

# metronidazole hydrochloride
Flagyl IV RTU, Novo-Nidazol†

*Pregnancy risk category B*

## AVAILABLE FORMS
*Capsules:* 375 mg
*Injection:* 500 mg/100 ml ready-to-use
*Oral suspension (benzoyl metronidazole):* 200 mg/5 ml‡
*Powder for injection:* 500-mg single-dose vials
*Tablets:* 200 mg‡, 250 mg, 400 mg‡, 500 mg
*Tablets (extended-release):* 750 mg

## INDICATIONS & DOSAGES
➤ **Amebic liver abscess**
*Adults:* 500 to 750 mg P.O. t.i.d. for 5 to 10 days; or 2.4 g P.O. once daily for 1 to 2 days. Or, 500 mg I.V. q 6 hours for 10 days if patient can't tolerate P.O. dosing.
*Children:* 30 to 50 mg/kg daily in three divided doses for 10 days. Maximum 750 mg/dose.
➤ **Intestinal amebiasis**
*Adults:* 750 mg P.O. t.i.d. for 5 to 10 days; then treat with a luminal amebicide, such as iodoquinol or paromomycin.
*Children:* 30 to 50 mg/kg daily in three divided doses for 10 days; then treat with a luminal amebicide, such as iodoquinol or paromomycin.
➤ **Trichomoniasis**
*Adults:* 250 mg P.O. t.i.d. for 7 days or 2 g P.O. in single dose. May give the 2-g dose in two 1-g doses, each on the same day; 4 to 6 weeks should elapse between courses of therapy.
*Children:* 5 mg/kg P.O. t.i.d. for 7 days.
➤ **Refractory trichomoniasis**
*Adults:* 250 mg P.O. b.i.d. for 10 days. Or, 500 mg P.O. b.i.d. for 7 days.
➤ **Bacterial infections caused by anaerobic microorganisms**
*Adults:* Loading dose is 15 mg/kg I.V. infused over 1 hour. Maintenance dose is 7.5 mg/kg I.V. or P.O. q 6 hours. Give first

Maintenance dose 6 hours after loading dose. Maximum dose shouldn't exceed 4 g daily.
➤ **To prevent postoperative infection in contaminated or potentially contaminated colorectal surgery**
*Adults:* 15 mg/kg I.V. infused over 30 to 60 minutes and completed about 1 hour before surgery. Then, 7.5 mg/kg I.V. infused over 30 to 60 minutes at 6 and 12 hours after first dose.
➤ **Bacterial vaginosis (Flagyl ER only)**
*Adults:* 750 mg (extended-release) P.O. daily for 7 days.
➤ **Clostridium difficile–associated diarrhea and colitis ◆**
*Adults:* Usual dosages are 250 mg P.O. q.i.d. or 500 mg P.O. t.i.d. for 10 days. Or, 500 mg to 750 mg I.V. q 6 to 8 hours when P.O. route isn't practical.
*Children:* 30 to 50 mg/kg/day P.O. given in three to four equally divided doses for 7 to 10 days. Don't exceed adult dose.
➤ **Pelvic inflammatory disease (PID) ◆**
*Adults:* 500 mg I.V. q 8 hours with ofloxacin or with ciprofloxacin and doxycycline. For PID in ambulatory patients, 500 mg P.O. b.i.d. in addition to ofloxacin for 14 days.
➤ **Bacterial vaginosis ◆**
*Nonpregnant women:* 500 mg b.i.d. for 7 days. Or, 2 g P.O. as a single dose, or 250 mg P.O. t.i.d. for 7 days.
*Pregnant women:* 250 mg P.O. t.i.d. for 7 days or 2 g P.O. as a single dose.

## I.V. ADMINISTRATION
● Flagyl IV ready-to-use (RTU) needs no preparation.
● To prepare lyophilized vials of metronidazole, add 4.4 ml of sterile water for injection, bacteriostatic water for injection, sterile normal saline solution for injection, or bacteriostatic normal saline solution for injection. Reconstituted drug contains 100 mg/ml.
● Add contents of vial to 100 ml of $D_5W$, lactated Ringer's injection, or normal saline solution to yield 5 mg/ml. The resulting highly acidic solution must be neutralized before administering.
● Carefully add 5 mEq sodium bicarbonate for each 500 mg metronidazole; carbon dioxide gas will form and may need to be vented.

---

• Don't use equipment containing aluminum (needles, hubs) to reconstitute the drug or to transfer reconstituted medication. Equipment that contains aluminum will turn the solution orange; the potency isn't affected.
• *Alert:* Infuse drug over at least 1 hour. Don't give by I.V. push.
• Don't refrigerate the neutralized diluted solution; precipitation may occur. If Flagyl IV RTU is refrigerated, crystals may form. These disappear after the solution warms to room temperature.

## ACTION
A direct-acting trichomonacide and amebicide that works at both intestinal and extraintestinal sites. It's thought to enter the cells of microorganisms that contain nitroreductase. Unstable compounds are then formed that bind to DNA and inhibit synthesis, causing cell death.

| Route | Onset | Peak | Duration |
|-------|-------|------|----------|
| P.O. | Unknown | 2 hr | Unknown |
| I.V. | Immediate | 1 hr | Unknown |

## ADVERSE REACTIONS
**CNS:** fever, vertigo, *headache,* ataxia, dizziness, syncope, incoordination, confusion, irritability, depression, weakness, insomnia, *seizures,* peripheral neuropathy.
**CV:** flattened T wave, edema, flushing, thrombophlebitis after I.V. infusion.
**EENT:** rhinitis, sinusitis, pharyngitis.
**GI:** abdominal cramping or pain, stomatitis, epigastric distress, *nausea,* vomiting, anorexia, diarrhea, constipation, proctitis, dry mouth, metallic taste.
**GU:** darkened urine, polyuria, dysuria, cystitis, dyspareunia, dryness of vagina and vulva, vaginal candidiasis, *vaginitis,* genital pruritus.
**Hematologic:** *transient leukopenia, neutropenia.*
**Musculoskeletal:** fleeting joint pains.
**Respiratory:** upper respiratory tract infection.
**Skin:** rash.
**Other:** decreased libido, overgrowth of nonsusceptible organisms, especially *Candida.*

## INTERACTIONS
**Drug-drug.** *Cimetidine:* May increase risk of metronidazole toxicity because drugs inhibit hepatic metabolism. Monitor patient for toxicity.
*Disulfiram:* May cause acute psychoses and confused states. Avoid using metronidazole within 2 weeks of disulfiram.
*Lithium:* May increase lithium level, which may cause toxicity. Monitor lithium level.
*Oral anticoagulants:* May increase anticoagulant effects. Monitor PT and INR periodically.
*Phenobarbital, phenytoin:* May decrease metronidazole effectiveness; may reduce total phenytoin clearance. Monitor patient.
**Drug-lifestyle.** *Alcohol use:* May cause disulfiram-like reaction, including nausea, vomiting, headache, cramps, and flushing. Warn patient to avoid alcohol during and for 3 days after completion of drug therapy.

## EFFECTS ON LAB TEST RESULTS
• May decrease WBC and neutrophil counts.
• May falsely decrease triglyceride and aminotransferase levels.

## CONTRAINDICATIONS & CAUTIONS
• Contraindicated in patients hypersensitive to drug or other nitroimidazole derivatives and in patients in first trimester of pregnancy.
• *Alert:* Drug is contraindicated in the first trimester of pregnancy. But, if pregnant patient must take drug for trichomoniasis, the 7-day regimen is preferred over the 2-g, single-dose regimen because the 2-g dose produces a high serum level that's more likely to reach the fetal circulation.
• Use cautiously in patients with history of blood dyscrasia or CNS disorder and in those with retinal or visual field changes. Also use cautiously in patients with hepatic disease or alcoholism and in those who take hepatotoxic drugs.

## NURSING CONSIDERATIONS
• Monitor liver function test results carefully in elderly patients.
• Give oral form with meals.

• Observe patient for edema, especially if receiving corticosteroids; Flagyl IV RTU may cause sodium retention.
• Record number and character of stools when drug is used to treat amebiasis. Use metronidazole only after *Trichomonas vaginalis* infection has been confirmed by wet smear or culture or *Entamoeba histolytica* has been identified. Asymptomatic sexual partners of patients being treated for *T. vaginalis* infection need to be treated simultaneously to avoid reinfection.

**PATIENT TEACHING**
• Instruct patient to take oral form with food to minimize GI upset, but tell him to take extended-release tablets at least 1 hour before or 2 hours after meals.
• Inform patient of need for sexual partners to be treated simultaneously to avoid reinfection.
• Instruct patient in proper hygiene.
• Tell patient to avoid alcohol or alcohol-containing drugs during and for at least 3 days after treatment course.
• Tell patient he may experience a metallic taste and have dark or red-brown urine.
• Tell patient to report symptoms of candidal overgrowth.
• Tell patient to report any neurological symptoms (seizures, peripheral neuropathy) to their health care provider immediately.

✳ *NEW DRUG*

## nitazoxanide
Alinia

*Pregnancy risk category B*

**AVAILABLE FORMS**
*Oral suspension:* 100 mg/5 ml

**INDICATIONS & DOSAGES**
➤ Diarrhea caused by *Cryptosporidium parvum* or *Giardia lamblia*
*Children ages 4 to 11:* 10 ml (200 mg) P.O. with food q 12 hours for 3 days.
*Children ages 1 to 4:* 5 ml (100 mg) P.O. with food q 12 hours for 3 days.

**ACTION**
Thought to interfere with an enzyme-dependent electron transfer reaction, essential for anaerobic energy metabolism.

| Route | Onset | Peak | Duration |
|-------|-------|------|----------|
| P.O. | Rapid | 1-4 hr | Unknown |

**ADVERSE REACTIONS**
**CNS:** headache.
**GI:** abdominal pain, diarrhea, vomiting.

**INTERACTIONS**
**Drug-drug.** *Drugs that are highly protein-bound:* May compete for binding sites. Use together cautiously.

**EFFECTS ON LAB TEST RESULTS**
• May increase creatinine and glutamate pyruvate transaminase levels.

**CONTRAINDICATIONS & CAUTIONS**
• Contraindicated in patients hypersensitive to nitazoxanide.
• Use cautiously in patients with renal or hepatic dysfunction. Safety and efficacy haven't been established in HIV-positive patients, immunodeficient patients, adults, or children younger than age 1 or older than age 11.

**NURSING CONSIDERATIONS**
• Give drug with food.
• Monitor glucose level in child with diabetes.
• Store suspension and powder at 77° F (25° C).

**PATIENT TEACHING**
• Tell caregiver to give drug with food.
• Instruct caregiver to keep container tightly closed and to shake it well before each use.
• Advise caregiver to discard suspension after 7 days.
• Inform caregiver of diabetic patient that the suspension contains 1.48 g of sucrose per 5 ml.

## pentamidine isethionate
NebuPent, Pentam 300

*Pregnancy risk category C*

### AVAILABLE FORMS
*Aerosol, injection, powder for injection:*
300-mg vial

### INDICATIONS & DOSAGES
➤ *Pneumocystis carinii* **pneumonia**
*Adults and children:* 3 to 4 mg/kg I.V. or
I.M. once daily for 14 to 21 days.
➤ **To prevent** *P. carinii* **pneumonia in high-risk patients**
*Adults:* 300 mg by inhalation using a
Respirgard II nebulizer once q 4 weeks.

### I.V. ADMINISTRATION
● Reconstitute drug with 3 ml sterile water
for injection; then dilute in 50 to 250 ml
$D_5W$. Infuse over at least 60 minutes.
● *Alert:* To minimize risk of hypotension,
infuse drug slowly with patient lying
down. Closely monitor blood pressure.

### ACTION
Unknown. Believed to interfere with
biosynthesis of DNA, RNA, phospholipids, and proteins in susceptible organisms.

| Route | Onset | Peak | Duration |
|-------|-------|------|----------|
| I.V. | Unknown | 1 hr | Unknown |
| I.M., inhalation | Unknown | 30 min | Unknown |

### ADVERSE REACTIONS
**CNS:** confusion, hallucinations, *fatigue,
dizziness,* headache.
**CV:** *severe hypotension, ventricular
tachycardia, chest pain,* edema.
**EENT:** burning in throat (with inhaled
form), *pharyngitis.*
**GI:** *nausea, metallic taste, decreased ap-
petite, vomiting,* diarrhea, abdominal pain,
anorexia, *pancreatitis.*
**GU:** *acute renal failure.*
**Hematologic:** *leukopenia, thrombocy-
topenia,* anemia.
**Metabolic:** *hypoglycemia,* hyperglycemia,
hypocalcemia.
**Musculoskeletal:** myalgia.

**Respiratory:** *cough, bronchospasm,
shortness of breath,* pneumothorax, *congestion.*
**Skin:** rash, *Stevens-Johnson syndrome.*
**Other:** *night sweats, chills, sterile abscess, pain, induration at injection site.*

### INTERACTIONS
**Drug-drug.** *Aminoglycosides, amphotericin B, capreomycin, cisplatin,
methoxyflurane, polymyxin B, vancomycin:* May increase risk of nephrotoxicity. Monitor renal function test results
closely.
*Antineoplastics:* May cause additive bone
marrow suppression. Use together cautiously, and monitor hematologic study results.

### EFFECTS ON LAB TEST RESULTS
● May increase BUN, creatinine, and
potassium levels. May increase or decrease glucose levels.
● May decrease WBC and platelet counts,
hemoglobin, and hematocrit.

### CONTRAINDICATIONS & CAUTIONS
● Contraindicated in patients with history
of anaphylactic reaction to drug.
● Use cautiously in patients with hypertension, hypotension, hypoglycemia, hypocalcemia, leukopenia, thrombocytopenia,
anemia, diabetes, pancreatitis, Stevens-
Johnson syndrome, or hepatic or renal
dysfunction.
● It's unknown if drug appears in breast
milk. Use cautiously in breast-feeding
women.

### NURSING CONSIDERATIONS
● Give aerosol form only by Respirgard II
nebulizer. Dosage recommendations are
based on particle size and delivery rate of
this device. To give aerosol, mix contents
of one vial in 6 ml sterile water for injection. Don't use normal saline solution.
Don't mix with other drugs.
● Don't use low-pressure (less than
20 pounds per square inch [psi]) com-
pressors. The flow rate should be 5 to 7 L/
minute from a 40- to 50-psi air or oxygen
source.
● For I.M. injection, reconstitute drug with
3 ml sterile water for a solution containing
100 mg/ml; administer deeply. Expect pa-

tient to report pain and induration at injection site. Rotate injection sites.

• *Alert:* Monitor glucose, calcium, creatinine, and BUN levels daily. After parenteral administration, glucose level may decrease initially; hypoglycemia may be severe in 5% to 10% of patients. After several months of therapy, this may be followed by hyperglycemia and type 1 diabetes mellitus, which may be permanent because of pancreatic cell damage.

• In patients with AIDS, pentamidine may produce less severe adverse reactions than co-trimoxazole.

**PATIENT TEACHING**
• Instruct patient to use the aerosol device until the chamber is empty, which may take up to 45 minutes.
• Warn patient that I.M. injection is painful.
• Instruct patient to complete the full course of pentamidine therapy, even if he is feeling better.

# 5
# Anthelmintics

**mebendazole**
**pyrantel pamoate**

**COMBINATION PRODUCTS**
None.

---

## mebendazole
Vermox

*Pregnancy risk category C*

---

**AVAILABLE FORMS**
*Tablets (chewable):* 100 mg

**INDICATIONS & DOSAGES**
➤ **Pinworm**
*Adults and children older than age 2:*
100 mg P.O. as a single dose; repeat if infestation persists 2 to 3 weeks later.
➤ **Roundworm, whipworm, and hookworm**
*Adults and children older than age 2:*
100 mg P.O. b.i.d. for 3 days; repeat if infestation persists 3 weeks later.
➤ **Trichinosis ◆**
*Adults:* 200 to 400 mg P.O. t.i.d. for 3 days; then 400 to 500 mg t.i.d. for 10 days.
➤ **Capillariasis ◆**
*Adults and children:* 200 mg P.O. b.i.d. for 20 days.
➤ **Dracunculiasis ◆**
*Adults:* 400 to 800 mg P.O. daily for 6 days.

**ACTION**
Selectively and irreversibly inhibits uptake of glucose and other nutrients in susceptible helminths.

| Route | Onset | Peak | Duration |
|-------|-------|------|----------|
| P.O. | Unknown | 2-4 hr | Variable |

**ADVERSE REACTIONS**
**CNS:** *seizures,* fever.
**GI:** occasional, transient abdominal pain and diarrhea in massive infestation and during expulsion of worms.
**Skin:** urticaria.

**INTERACTIONS**
**Drug-drug.** *Carbamazepine, hydantoins:* May reduce plasma mebendazole levels, which may decrease drug's effect. Monitor patient for clinical effect.
*Cimetidine:* May increase plasma mebendazole levels. Monitor patient for increased adverse effects if used together.

**EFFECTS ON LAB TEST RESULTS**
None reported.

**CONTRAINDICATIONS & CAUTIONS**
● Contraindicated in patients hypersensitive to drug.
● Safe use in children younger than age 2 hasn't been established.

**NURSING CONSIDERATIONS**
● Tablets may be chewed, swallowed whole, or crushed and mixed with food.
● Give drug to all family members, as prescribed, to decrease risk of spreading the infestation.
● Dietary restrictions, laxatives, or enemas aren't necessary.

**PATIENT TEACHING**
● Teach patient about personal hygiene, especially good hand-washing technique. Advise him to refrain from preparing food for others.
● To avoid reinfestation, teach patient to wash perianal area daily, change undergarments and bedclothes daily, and wash hands and clean fingernails before meals and after bowel movements.

---

## pyrantel pamoate
Antiminth ◇ , Combantrin†, Pin-Rid ◇ , Pin-X ◇ , Reese's Pinworm ◇

*Pregnancy risk category C*

**AVAILABLE FORMS**
*Liquid:* 50 mg/ml
*Oral suspension:* 50 mg/ml
*Soft-gel capsules:* 62.5 mg (as base)

---

Reactions may be *common*, uncommon, ***life-threatening***, or COMMON AND LIFE-THREATENING.

## INDICATIONS & DOSAGES
### ➤ Roundworm and pinworm
*Adults and children age 2 and older:*
11 mg/kg P.O. as a single dose. Maximum
dose, 1 g. For pinworm, repeat dose in
2 weeks.

## ACTION
Blocks neuromuscular action, paralyzing
the worm and causing its expulsion by
normal peristalsis.

| Route | Onset | Peak | Duration |
|-------|-------|------|----------|
| P.O. | Variable | 1-3 hr | Variable |

## ADVERSE REACTIONS
**CNS:** headache, fever, dizziness, drowsi-
ness, insomnia, weakness.
**GI:** anorexia, nausea, vomiting, gastralgia,
abdominal cramps, diarrhea, tenesmus.
**Skin:** rash.

## INTERACTIONS
**Drug-drug.** *Piperazine salts:* May antagonize drug effects. Avoid using together.

## EFFECTS ON LAB TEST RESULTS
● May increase AST level.

## CONTRAINDICATIONS & CAUTIONS
● Contraindicated in patients hypersensitive to drug.
● Use cautiously in patients with severe
malnutrition or anemia and in those with
hepatic dysfunction.

## NURSING CONSIDERATIONS
● No dietary restrictions, laxatives, or ene-
mas are needed.
● Give drug to all family members.

## PATIENT TEACHING
● Inform patient that pyrantel may be tak-
en with food, milk, or fruit juices. Tell him
to shake suspension well.
● Teach patient about personal hygiene,
especially good hand-washing technique.
To avoid reinfestation, teach patient to
wash perianal area daily, to change undergarments and bedclothes daily, and to
wash hands and clean fingernails before
meals and after bowel movements.
● Advise patient not to prepare food for
others.

● Tell patient to take entire dosage as prescribed.

amphotericin B cholesteryl
  sulfate complex
amphotericin B desoxycholate
amphotericin B lipid complex
amphotericin B liposomal
caspofungin acetate
fluconazole
flucytosine
itraconazole
ketoconazole
nystatin
terbinafine hydrochloride
voriconazole

**COMBINATION PRODUCTS**
None.

## amphotericin B cholesteryl sulfate complex
Amphotec

*Pregnancy risk category B*

**AVAILABLE FORMS**
*Injection:* 50 mg/20 ml, 100 mg/50 ml

**INDICATIONS & DOSAGES**
➤ **Invasive aspergillosis in patients for whom renal impairment or unacceptable toxicity precludes use of amphotericin B deoxycholate in effective doses or for whom prior amphotericin B deoxycholate therapy has failed**
*Adults and children:* 3 to 4 mg/kg/day I.V. Dilute in $D_5W$ and give by continuous infusion at 1 mg/kg/hour. Perform a test dose before beginning new course of treatment; infuse 10 ml of final preparation containing 1.6 to 8.3 mg of drug over 15 to 30 minutes and monitor patient for next 30 minutes. May shorten infusion time to 2 hours or lengthen infusion time based on patient's tolerance.
➤ ***Candida* or *Cryptococcus* infections in patients who can't tolerate conventional amphotericin B or who failed to respond to conventional I.V. amphotericin B ♦**
*Adults:* 3 to 6 mg/kg/day. Dosages up to 7.5 mg/kg/day have been used for invasive fungal infections in bone marrow transplant patients.

**I.V. ADMINISTRATION**
● Reconstitute 50-mg vial with rapid addition of 10 ml of sterile water for injection, and 100-mg vial with rapid addition of 20 ml sterile water for injection. Shake vial gently. Don't use diluent other than sterile water for injection. Don't give undiluted drug.
● For infusion, add to bag of $D_5W$ to about 0.6 mg/ml. Don't reconstitute lyophilized powder with saline or dextrose solutions or mix reconstituted liquid with saline solution or electrolytes. The presence of a bacteriostatic product in the solution may cause precipitation of drug. Don't use a filter, including an in-line filter, and don't freeze.
● Infuse drug over at least 2 hours. Don't mix with other drugs. If given through an existing I.V. line, flush line with $D_5W$ before infusion or use a separate line.
● Store unopened vials at room temperature.
● Reconstituted drug is clear or opalescent liquid and is stable for 24 hours when refrigerated. Discard partially used vials.

**ACTION**
Binds to sterols of fungal cell membranes, altering cell permeability and causing cell death.

| Route | Onset | Peak | Duration |
|-------|-------|------|----------|
| I.V. | Unknown | 3 hr | Unknown |

**ADVERSE REACTIONS**
**CNS:** *fever,* abnormal thinking, anxiety, agitation, confusion, depression, dizziness, hallucinations, headache, hypertonia, neuropathy, nervousness, paresthesia, psychosis, ***seizures,*** somnolence, speech disorder, stupor, asthenia, syncope.

**CV:** *arrhythmias,* atrial fibrillation, *bradycardia, cardiac arrest, heart failure, hemorrhage,* hypertension, hypotension, phlebitis, chest pain, orthostatic hypotension, *shock, supraventricular tachycardia,* tachycardia, vasodilation, *ventricular extrasystoles,* edema.
**EENT:** amblyopia, deafness, epistaxis, eye hemorrhage, pharyngitis, tinnitus, rhinitis, sinusitis.
**GI:** anorexia, diarrhea, dry mouth, *GI hemorrhage,* gingivitis, glossitis, hematemesis, melena, mouth ulceration, *nausea,* oral candidiasis, stomatitis, *vomiting,* abdominal pain.
**GU:** albuminuria, dysuria, glycosuria, hematuria, oliguria, urinary incontinence or urine retention, *renal failure.*
**Hematologic:** anemia, coagulation disorders, ecchymosis, hypochromic anemia, leukocytosis, *leukopenia,* petechiae, *thrombocytopenia.*
**Hepatic:** *hyperbilirubinemia,* jaundice, *hepatic failure.*
**Metabolic:** weight changes, acidosis, dehydration, *hypokalemia,* hypocalcemia, *hypoglycemia,* hypoproteinemia, hyperglycemia, hypervolemia, hypophosphatemia, hyponatremia, *hyperkalemia,* hyperlipemia, hypernatremia, hypomagnesemia.
**Musculoskeletal:** arthralgia, myalgia, neck or back pain.
**Respiratory:** *apnea,* asthma, dyspnea, hemoptysis, hyperventilation, hypoxia, increased cough, lung or respiratory tract disorders, pleural effusion, pulmonary edema.
**Skin:** acne, alopecia, pruritus, rash, sweating, skin discoloration, nodules, ulcers, urticaria, pain or reaction at injection site.
**Other:** allergic reaction, *anaphylaxis, chills,* peripheral or facial edema, infection, mucous membrane disorder, *sepsis.*

**INTERACTIONS**
**Drug-drug.** *Antineoplastics:* May enhance renal toxicity, bronchospasm, and hypotension. Use together cautiously.
*Cardiac glycosides:* May enhance potassium excretion and increase digitalis toxicity. Monitor potassium level closely.
*Corticosteroids:* May enhance potassium depletion, which could predispose patient to cardiac dysfunction. Monitor electrolyte levels.

*Cyclosporine, tacrolimus:* May increase creatinine level. Monitor renal function.
*Flucytosine:* May increase toxicity by amphotericin. Use together cautiously.
*Imidazoles (clotrimazole, fluconazole, ketoconazole, miconazole):* May antagonize effects of amphotericin, although significance hasn't been determined. Monitor patient closely.
*Leukocyte transfusions:* May increase risk of pulmonary reactions, such as acute dyspnea, tachypnea, hypoxemia, hemoptysis, and interstitial infiltrates. Use together cautiously; separate doses as much as possible and monitor pulmonary function if drugs are used together.
*Nephrotoxic drugs (such as aminoglycosides, pentamidine):* May enhance renal toxicity. Monitor renal function closely.
*Skeletal muscle relaxants:* Amphotericin B-induced hypokalemia may enhance effects of skeletal muscle relaxants. Monitor potassium level closely.

**EFFECTS ON LAB TEST RESULTS**
• May increase BUN, creatinine, alkaline phosphatase, ALT, AST, bilirubin, GGT, and LDH levels. May decrease calcium, phosphate, magnesium, and protein levels. May increase or decrease glucose, sodium, and potassium levels.
• May decrease hemoglobin, platelet count, and INR. May increase or decrease WBC count and PT.

**CONTRAINDICATIONS & CAUTIONS**
• Contraindicated in patients hypersensitive to drug or its components, unless the benefits outweigh the risks.
• It's unknown if drug appears in breast milk. Because of the potential for serious adverse reactions in breast-fed infants, encourage the decision to either stop breast-feeding or stop treatment, taking into account importance of drug to the mother.

**NURSING CONSIDERATIONS**
• *Alert:* Different amphotericin B preparations aren't interchangeable, so dosages will vary. Confusing the preparations may cause permanent damage or death.
• *Alert:* Monitor vital signs every 30 minutes during initial therapy. Acute infusion-related reactions, including fever, chills, hypotension, nausea, and tachycardia, usu-

ally occur 1 to 3 hours after starting I.V. infusion. These reactions are usually more severe after initial doses and usually diminish with subsequent doses. If severe respiratory distress occurs, stop infusion immediately and don't treat further with drug.

• Reduce acute infusion-related reactions by pretreating with antihistamines, antipyretics, and corticosteroids; reducing infusion rate; and maintaining sodium balance.

• Reduce risk of nephrotoxicity by hydrating patient before infusion.

• Monitor intake and output; report changes in urine appearance or volume.

• Monitor renal and hepatic function test results, electrolyte levels (especially potassium, magnesium, and calcium), CBC, and PT.

**PATIENT TEACHING**
• Instruct patient to immediately report symptoms of hypersensitivity.

• Warn patient of possible discomfort at I.V. site.

• Advise patient of potential adverse reactions, such as fever, chills, nausea, and vomiting. Tell patient that these can be severe with first dose but usually subside with repeated doses.

---

## amphotericin B desoxycholate
Amphocin, Amphotericin B for Injection

*Pregnancy risk category B*

---

**AVAILABLE FORMS**
*Powder for injection:* 50 mg

**INDICATIONS & DOSAGES**
➤ **Systemic fungal infection (histoplasmosis, coccidioidomycosis, blastomycosis, cryptococcosis, disseminated candidiasis, aspergillosis, phycomycosis, zygomycosis) or meningitis**
*Adults:* Initially, test dose of 1 mg in 20 ml of $D_5W$ infused I.V. over 20 to 30 minutes. If that dosage is tolerated, daily dose is then started at 0.25 to 0.3 mg/kg by slow I.V. infusion (0.1 mg/ml) over 2 to 6 hours. Daily dose is gradually increased to maximum of 1.5 mg/kg in patients with poten-

tially fatal infections. If drug is stopped for 1 week or longer, it's resumed with initial dose and increased gradually.
➤ **To prevent fungal infection in bone marrow transplant patients ♦**
*Adults:* 0.1 mg/kg/day as I.V. infusion.

**I.V. ADMINISTRATION**
• Reconstitute amphotericin B with 10 ml of sterile water. To avoid precipitation, don't mix with solutions containing sodium chloride, other electrolytes, or bacteriostatic products such as benzyl alcohol. Don't use if solution contains precipitate or foreign matter.

• Use an infusion pump and in-line filter with mean pore diameter larger than 1 micron. Rapid infusion may cause CV collapse.

• Choose I.V. sites in distal veins. If veins become thrombosed, alternate administration sites.

• After giving test dose, monitor patient's pulse, respiratory rate, temperature, and blood pressure for at least 4 hours.

• Monitor vital signs every 30 minutes; fever, shaking chills, and hypotension may appear 1 to 2 hours after start of I.V. infusion and should subside within 4 hours of stopping drug.

• Give antibiotics separately; don't mix or piggyback them with amphotericin B.

• Amphotericin B appears to be compatible with limited amounts of heparin sodium, hydrocortisone sodium succinate, and methylprednisolone sodium succinate.

• Store the dry form at 36° to 46° F (2° to 8° C). Protect from light.

• Reconstituted solution is stable for 1 week under refrigeration or 24 hours at room temperature. It's stable for 8 hours in room light.

**ACTION**
Binds to sterols of fungal cell membranes, altering cell permeability and causing cell death.

| Route | Onset | Peak | Duration |
|-------|-------|------|----------|
| I.V. | Immediate | Unknown | Unknown |

**ADVERSE REACTIONS**
**CNS:** *headache, fever,* peripheral neuropathy, transient vertigo, *malaise,* **seizures.**

---

**CV:** hypotension, *arrhythmias, asystole,* hypertension, tachycardia, flushing, *phlebitis, thrombophlebitis.*

**EENT:** hearing loss, tinnitus, blurred vision, diplopia.

**GI:** *anorexia, nausea, vomiting, dyspepsia, diarrhea, epigastric pain, cramping,* melena, steatorrhea, *hemorrhagic gastroenteritis.*

**GU:** *abnormal renal function with azotemia, hyposthenuria, renal tubular acidosis, nephrocalcinosis; permanent renal impairment;* anuria; oliguria.

**Hematologic:** *normochromic anemia, normocytic anemia, thrombocytopenia, leukopenia, agranulocytosis,* eosinophilia, leukocytosis.

**Hepatic:** *hepatitis,* jaundice, *acute liver failure.*

**Metabolic:** *weight loss, hypokalemia, hypoglycemia,* hyperglycemia, hyperuricemia, hypomagnesemia.

**Musculoskeletal:** arthralgia, myalgia.

**Respiratory:** dyspnea, tachypnea, *bronchospasm,* wheezing.

**Skin:** *maculopapular rash,* pruritus, tissue damage with extravasation, *pain at injection site.*

**Other:** *chills, generalized pain, anaphylactoid reaction.*

**INTERACTIONS**

**Drug-drug.** *Antineoplastics (such as mechlorethamine):* May cause renal toxicity, bronchospasm, and hypotension. Use together cautiously.

*Cardiac glycosides:* May increase risk of digitalis toxicity in potassium-depleted patients. Monitor digoxin level closely.

*Corticosteroids:* May increase potassium depletion. Monitor potassium level.

*Flucytosine:* May have synergistic effect; may cause increased toxicity of flucytosine. Monitor patient closely for toxicity.

*Leukocyte transfusions:* May increase risk of pulmonary reactions, such as acute dyspnea, tachypnea, hypoxemia, hemoptysis, and interstitial infiltrates. Use together cautiously; separate doses as much as possible and monitor pulmonary function if drugs are used together.

*Nephrotoxic drugs such as antibiotics, pentamidine:* May cause additive renal toxicity. Use together cautiously and monitor renal function studies.

*Thiazides:* May intensify depletion of electrolytes, especially potassium. Monitor patient for hypokalemia.

**Drug-herb.** *Gossypol:* May increase risk of renal toxicity. Discourage use together.

**EFFECTS ON LAB TEST RESULTS**

● May increase urine urea, uric acid, BUN, creatinine, alkaline phosphatase, ALT, AST, GGT, LDH, and bilirubin levels. May decrease potassium and magnesium levels. May increase or decrease glucose level.

● May decrease hemoglobin and platelet and granulocyte counts. May increase or decrease WBC and eosinophil counts.

**CONTRAINDICATIONS & CAUTIONS**

● Contraindicated in patients hypersensitive to drug.

● Use cautiously in patients with impaired renal function.

**NURSING CONSIDERATIONS**

● Because of drug's dangerous adverse effects, it's used primarily to treat patients with progressive and potentially fatal fungal infections.

● Infusion-related reactions, including fever, shaking chills, hypotension, anorexia, nausea, vomiting, headache, dyspnea, and tachypnea, may occur 1 to 3 hours after starting infusion.

● *Alert:* Different amphotericin B preparations aren't interchangeable, so dosages will vary. Confusing the preparations may cause permanent damage or death.

● *Alert:* To reduce severe adverse effects, patient may receive premedication with antipyretics, antihistamines, antiemetics, or small doses of corticosteroids given on an alternate-day schedule. For severe reactions, stop drug and notify prescriber.

● Infusion-related reactions occur most frequently with initial doses and usually lessen with subsequent doses.

● Monitor fluid intake and output; report change in urine appearance or volume. Monitor BUN and creatinine levels or creatinine clearance at least weekly. Kidney damage may be reversible if drug is stopped at first sign of renal dysfunction.

● Hydration before infusion may reduce risk of nephrotoxicity.

• Obtain hepatic and renal function studies weekly, if ordered. Drug may be stopped if alkaline phosphatase or bilirubin level increases. If BUN level exceeds 40 mg/ 100 ml or if creatinine level exceeds 3 mg/ 100 ml, prescriber may reduce or stop drug until renal function improves. Monitor CBC weekly.
• Monitor potassium level closely, and report signs of hypokalemia. Hypokalemia occurs commonly and can be life-threatening. Potassium supplementation may be needed.
• Check calcium and magnesium levels twice weekly.
• Drug is potentially ototoxic. Report evidence of hearing loss, tinnitus, vertigo, or unsteady gait.

**PATIENT TEACHING**
• Warn patient of possible discomfort at I.V. site and of other potential adverse reactions. Instruct patient to report signs and symptoms of hypersensitivity immediately.
• Inform patient that therapy may take several months. Stress importance of compliance and follow-up.

## amphotericin B lipid complex
Abelcet

*Pregnancy risk category B*

**AVAILABLE FORMS**
*Suspension for injection:* 100 mg/20-ml vial

**INDICATIONS & DOSAGES**
➤ **Invasive fungal infections, including** *Aspergillus* **and** *Candida* **species, in patients who are refractory to or intolerant of conventional amphotericin B therapy**
*Adults and children:* 5 mg/kg daily I.V. as a single infusion given at rate of 2.5 mg/ kg/hour.

**I.V. ADMINISTRATION**
• To prepare, shake vial gently until there is no yellow sediment. Using aseptic technique, withdraw calculated dose into one or more 20-ml syringes, using an 18-gauge needle. More than one vial will be needed. Attach a 5-micron filter needle to syringe and inject dose into I.V. bag of $D_5W$. One filter needle can be used for up to four vials of amphotericin B lipid complex. Volume of $D_5W$ should be sufficient to yield 1 mg/ml.
• For children and patients with CV disease, dilute to 2 mg/ml.
• Don't mix with saline solution or infuse in same I.V. line as other drugs. Don't use an in-line filter.
• Use an infusion pump and give by continuous infusion at rate of 2.5 mg/kg/hour. If infusion time exceeds 2 hours, mix contents by shaking infusion bag every 2 hours.
• If infusing through an existing I.V. line, flush first with $D_5W$.
• If severe respiratory distress occurs, stop infusion, provide supportive therapy for anaphylaxis, and notify prescriber. Don't reinstitute drug.
• Monitor vital signs closely. Fever, shaking chills, and hypotension may appear within 2 hours of starting infusion. Slowing infusion rate may decrease risk of infusion-related reactions.
• Reconstituted drug is stable for up to 48 hours if refrigerated (36° to 46° F [2° to 8° C]) and up to 6 hours at room temperature.
• Discard any unused drug because drug doesn't contain a preservative.

**ACTION**
Binds to sterols of fungal cell membranes, altering cell permeability and causing cell death.

| Route | Onset | Peak | Duration |
|-------|-------|------|----------|
| I.V. | Unknown | Unknown | Unknown |

**ADVERSE REACTIONS**
**CNS:** *fever,* headache, pain.
**CV:** chest pain, ***cardiac arrest,*** hypertension, hypotension.
**GI:** abdominal pain, diarrhea, ***GI hemorrhage,*** nausea, vomiting.
**GU:** *renal failure.*
**Hematologic:** anemia, ***leukopenia, thrombocytopenia.***
**Hepatic:** bilirubinemia.
**Metabolic:** hypokalemia.
**Respiratory:** dyspnea, respiratory disorder, ***respiratory failure.***

Reactions may be *common,* uncommon, ***life-threatening,*** or COMMON AND LIFE-THREATENING.

**Skin:** rash.
**Other:** *chills,* infection, MULTIPLE
ORGAN FAILURE, *sepsis.*

## INTERACTIONS
**Drug-drug.** *Antineoplastics:* May increase risk of renal toxicity, bronchospasm, and hypotension. Use together cautiously.
*Cardiac glycosides:* May increase risk of
digitalis toxicity from amphotericin B-induced hypokalemia. Monitor potassium
level closely.
*Clotrimazole, fluconazole, itraconazole,
ketoconazole, miconazole:* May antagonize amphotericin B. Monitor patient
closely.
*Corticosteroids, corticotropin:* May enhance hypokalemia, which could lead to
cardiac toxicity. Monitor electrolyte levels
and cardiac function.
*Cyclosporine:* May increase renal toxicity.
Monitor renal function test results closely.
*Flucytosine:* May increase risk of flucytosine toxicity from increased cellular uptake or impaired renal excretion. Use together cautiously.
*Leukocyte transfusions:* Risk of pulmonary reactions such as acute dyspnea,
tachypnea, hypoxemia, hemoptysis, and
interstitial infiltrates. Use together cautiously; separate doses as much as possible, and monitor pulmonary function if
drugs are used together.
*Nephrotoxic drugs (such as aminoglyco-
sides, pentamidine):* May increase risk of
renal toxicity. Use together cautiously, and
monitor renal function closely.
*Skeletal muscle relaxants:* May enhance
skeletal muscle relaxant effects of amphotericin B-induced hypokalemia. Monitor
potassium level closely.
*Zidovudine:* May increase myelotoxicity
and nephrotoxicity. Monitor renal and
hematologic function.

## EFFECTS ON LAB TEST RESULTS
• May increase BUN, creatinine, alkaline
phosphatase, ALT, AST, bilirubin, GGT,
and LDH levels. May decrease potassium
level.
• May decrease hemoglobin and WBC and
platelet counts.

## CONTRAINDICATIONS & CAUTIONS
• Contraindicated in patients hypersensitive to amphotericin B or its components.
• Use cautiously in patients with renal impairment. Base the need for dosage adjustment on overall clinical status of patient.
Renal toxicity is more common at higher
dosages.
• It's unknown if drug appears in breast
milk. Encourage the decision to either
stop breast-feeding or stop treatment.

## NURSING CONSIDERATIONS
• *Alert:* Different amphotericin B preparations aren't interchangeable, so dosages
will vary. Confusing the preparations may
cause permanent damage or death.
• Premedicate patient with acetaminophen, antihistamines, or corticosteroids to prevent or lessen severity of infusion-related reactions such as fever, chills,
nausea, and vomiting, which occur 1 to
2 hours after start of infusion.
• Hydration before infusion may reduce
risk of nephrotoxicity.
• Monitor creatinine and electrolyte levels
(especially magnesium and potassium),
liver function, and CBC during therapy.

## PATIENT TEACHING
• Inform patient that fever, chills, nausea,
and vomiting may occur during infusion
and that these reactions usually subside
with subsequent doses.
• Instruct patient to report any redness or
pain at infusion site.
• Teach patient to recognize and report
signs or symptoms of acute hypersensitivity such as respiratory distress.
• Warn patient that therapy may take several months.
• Tell patient to expect frequent laboratory
testing to monitor kidney and liver function.

## amphotericin B liposomal
AmBisome

*Pregnancy risk category B*

## AVAILABLE FORMS
*Powder for injection:* 50-mg vial

---

## INDICATIONS & DOSAGES

➤ **Empirical therapy for presumed fungal infection in febrile, neutropenic patients**
*Adults and children:* 3 mg/kg I.V. infusion over 2 hours daily.

➤ **Systemic fungal infections caused by** *Aspergillus* **species,** *Candida* **species, or** *Cryptococcus* **species refractory to amphotericin B deoxycholate or in patients for whom renal impairment or unacceptable toxicity precludes use of amphotericin B deoxycholate**
*Adults and children:* 3 to 5 mg/kg I.V. infusion over 2 hours daily.

➤ **Visceral leishmaniasis in immunocompetent patients**
*Adults and children:* 3 mg/kg I.V. infusion over 2 hours daily on days 1 to 5, 14, and 21. A repeat course of therapy may be beneficial if initial treatment fails to clear parasites.

➤ **Visceral leishmaniasis in immunocompromised patients**
*Adults and children:* 4 mg/kg I.V. infusion over 2 hours daily on days 1 to 5, 10, 17, 24, 31, and 38. Refer patient for expert advice regarding further treatment if initial therapy fails or patient relapses.

➤ **Cryptococcal meningitis in HIV-infected patients**
*Adults and children:* 6 mg/kg/day I.V. infusion over 2 hours. Reduce infusion time to 1 hour if treatment is well tolerated, and increase infusion time if discomfort occurs.

## I.V. ADMINISTRATION

● Reconstitute each 50-mg vial of amphotericin B liposomal with 12 ml of sterile water for injection to yield a solution of 4 mg amphotericin B per milliliter.
● *Alert:* Don't reconstitute with bacteriostatic water for injection, and don't allow bacteriostatic product in solution. Don't reconstitute with saline solution, add saline solution to reconstituted concentration, or mix with other drugs.
● After reconstitution, shake vial vigorously for 30 seconds or until particulate matter disperses.
● Withdraw calculated amount of reconstituted solution into a sterile syringe, and inject through a 5-micron filter into appropriate amount of $D_5W$ to further dilute to

1 to 2 mg/ml. Concentrations of 0.2 to 0.5 mg/ml may provide sufficient volume of infusion for children.
● Flush existing I.V. line with $D_5W$ before infusing drug. If this isn't feasible, give drug through separate line.
● Use a controlled infusion device and an in-line filter with a mean pore diameter 1 micron or larger. Initially, infuse drug over at least 2 hours. Reduce infusion time to 1 hour if treatment is well tolerated, and increase infusion time if discomfort occurs.
● Store unopened vial at 36° to 46° F (2° to 8° C). Store reconstituted drug for up to 24 hours at 36° to 46° F. Don't freeze.

## ACTION

Binds to sterols of fungal cell membranes, altering cell permeability and causing cell death.

| Route | Onset | Peak | Duration |
|-------|-------|------|----------|
| I.V. | Unknown | Unknown | Unknown |

## ADVERSE REACTIONS

**CNS:** *fever, anxiety, confusion, headache, insomnia, asthenia, pain.*
**CV:** *chest pain, hypotension, tachycardia, hypertension, edema, flushing.*
**EENT:** *epistaxis, rhinitis.*
**GI:** *nausea, vomiting, abdominal pain, diarrhea,* **GI hemorrhage.**
**GU:** *hematuria.*
**Hepatic:** *bilirubinemia.*
**Metabolic:** *hyperglycemia,* hypernatremia, *hypocalcemia, hypokalemia, hypomagnesemia.*
**Musculoskeletal:** *back pain.*
**Respiratory:** *increased cough, dyspnea,* hypoxia, *pleural effusion, lung disorder,* hyperventilation.
**Skin:** *pruritus, rash, sweating.*
**Other:** *chills, infection,* **anaphylaxis, sepsis,** *blood product infusion reaction.*

## INTERACTIONS

**Drug-drug.** *Antineoplastics:* May enhance potential for renal toxicity, bronchospasm, and hypotension. Use together cautiously.
*Cardiac glycosides:* May increase risk of digitalis toxicity caused by amphotericin

B-induced hypokalemia. Monitor potassium level closely.

*Clotrimazole, fluconazole, ketoconazole, miconazole:* May induce fungal resistance to amphotericin B. Use together cautiously.

*Corticosteroids, corticotropin:* May increase potassium depletion, which could cause cardiac dysfunction. Monitor electrolyte levels and cardiac function.

*Flucytosine:* May increase flucytosine toxicity by increasing cellular reuptake or impairing renal excretion of flucytosine. Use together cautiously.

*Leukocyte transfusions:* May increase risk of pulmonary reactions, such as acute dyspnea, tachypnea, hypoxemia, hemoptysis, and interstitial infiltrates. Use together cautiously; separate doses as much as possible and monitor pulmonary function.

*Other nephrotoxic drugs, such as antibiotics and antineoplastics:* May cause additive nephrotoxicity. Use together cautiously; monitor renal function closely.

*Skeletal muscle relaxants:* May enhance effects of skeletal muscle relaxants resulting from amphotericin B-induced hypokalemia. Monitor potassium level.

### EFFECTS ON LAB TEST RESULTS
● May increase BUN, creatinine, glucose, sodium, alkaline phosphatase, ALT, AST, bilirubin, GGT, and LDH levels. May decrease potassium, calcium, and magnesium levels.

### CONTRAINDICATIONS & CAUTIONS
● Contraindicated in patients hypersensitive to drug or its components.
● Use cautiously in patients with impaired renal function, in elderly patients, and in pregnant women.
● It's unknown if drug appears in breast milk. Because of potential for serious adverse reactions in breast-fed infants, encourage the decision to either stop breast-feeding or stop treatment, taking into account importance of drug to mother.

### NURSING CONSIDERATIONS
● Patients also receiving chemotherapy or bone marrow transplantation are at greater risk for additional adverse reactions, including seizures, arrhythmias, and thrombocytopenia.

● *Alert:* Different amphotericin B preparations aren't interchangeable, so dosages will vary. Confusing the preparations may cause permanent damage or death.
● Premedicate patient with antipyretics, antihistamines, antiemetics, or corticosteroids.
● Hydration before infusion may reduce the risk of nephrotoxicity.
● Monitor BUN and creatinine and electrolyte levels (particularly magnesium and potassium), liver function, and CBC.
● Watch for signs and symptoms of hypokalemia (ECG changes, muscle weakness, cramping, drowsiness).
● Patients treated with amphotericin B liposomal have a lower risk of chills, elevated BUN level, hypokalemia, hypertension, and vomiting than patients treated with conventional amphotericin B.
● Therapy may take several weeks to months.
● Observe patient closely for adverse reactions during infusion. If anaphylaxis occurs, stop infusion immediately, provide supportive therapy, and notify prescriber.

### PATIENT TEACHING
● Teach patient signs and symptoms of hypersensitivity, and stress importance of reporting them immediately.
● Warn patient that therapy may take several months; teach personal hygiene and other measures to prevent spread and recurrence of lesions.
● Instruct patient to report any adverse reactions that occur while receiving drug.
● Tell patient to watch for and report signs and symptoms of low levels of potassium in the blood (muscle weakness, cramping, drowsiness).
● Advise patient that frequent laboratory testing will be needed.

## caspofungin acetate
Cancidas

*Pregnancy risk category C*

### AVAILABLE FORMS
*Lyophilized powder for injection:* 50-mg, 70-mg single-use vials

---

## INDICATIONS & DOSAGES
➤ **Invasive aspergillosis in patients who are refractory to or intolerant of other therapies (amphotericin B, lipid formulations of amphotericin B, or itraconazole)**
*Adults:* Single 70-mg I.V. loading dose on day 1, followed by 50 mg/day I.V. over about 1 hour. Base treatment duration on severity of patient's underlying disease, recovery from immunosuppression, and clinical response.
*Adjust-a-dose:* For patients with Child-Pugh score 7 to 9, after initial 70-mg loading dose, give 35 mg/day. No experience exists for dosage adjustment in patients with Child-Pugh score exceeding 9.

## I.V. ADMINISTRATION
• Allow refrigerated vial to warm to room temperature.
• For most patients, dilute 70-mg, 50-mg, and 35-mg doses of drug in 250 ml normal saline solution. For patients on fluid restriction, dilute the 50-mg and 35-mg doses may be diluted in 100 ml normal saline solution.
• Don't use diluents containing dextrose.
• Don't mix or infuse with other drugs.
• Give drug by slow I.V. infusion over about 1 hour.
• Use reconstituted vials within 1 hour or discard. The final product for infusion (solution in I.V. bag or bottle) can be stored at room temperature for 24 hours.

## ACTION
Inhibits synthesis of beta (1,3)-D-glucan in susceptible *Aspergillus* species. Drug is extensively distributed and has a prolonged half-life.

| Route | Onset | Peak | Duration |
|---|---|---|---|
| I.V. | Unknown | Unknown | Unknown |

## ADVERSE REACTIONS
**CNS:** fever, headache, *paresthesia.*
**CV:** *tachycardia,* phlebitis, infused vein complications.
**GI:** nausea, vomiting, diarrhea, abdominal pain, *anorexia.*
**GU:** proteinuria, hematuria.
**Hematologic:** eosinophilia, *anemia.*
**Metabolic:** hypokalemia.
**Musculoskeletal:** *pain, myalgia.*

**Respiratory:** *tachypnea.*
**Skin:** histamine-mediated symptoms including rash, facial swelling, pruritus, sensation of warmth.
**Other:** *chills, sweating.*

## INTERACTIONS
**Drug-drug.** *Cyclosporine:* May increase caspofungin level. Because of increased risk of elevated alanine transaminase levels, avoid using together unless potential benefit outweighs potential risk.
*Inducers of drug clearance or mixed inducer-inhibitors (carbamazepine, dexamethasone, efavirenz, nelfinavir, nevirapine, phenytoin, rifampin):* May reduce caspofungin level. May need to adjust dosage.
*Tacrolimus:* May reduce tacrolimus level. Monitor tacrolimus level. May need to adjust dosage.

## EFFECTS ON LAB TEST RESULTS
• May increase alkaline phosphatase level. May decrease potassium level.
• May increase eosinophil count. May decrease hemoglobin.

## CONTRAINDICATIONS & CAUTIONS
• Contraindicated in patients hypersensitive to drug or its components.
• Safety and efficacy in patients younger than age 18 aren't known.
• It's unknown if drug appears in breast milk. Use cautiously in breast-feeding women.

## NURSING CONSIDERATIONS
• The efficacy of a 70-mg-dose regimen in patients who aren't responding to the 50-mg daily dose isn't known. Limited safety data suggest that an increase in dosage to 70 mg daily is well tolerated. Safety and efficacy of doses above 70 mg haven't been adequately studied.
• Safety information on treatment lasting longer than 2 weeks is limited, but available data suggest that drug continues to be well tolerated with longer courses of therapy.
• Monitor I.V. site carefully for phlebitis.
• Observe patients for histamine-mediated reactions, including rash, facial swelling, pruritus, and a sensation of warmth.

## PATIENT TEACHING
• Instruct patient to report signs and symptoms of phlebitis.

---

# fluconazole
Diflucan✔

*Pregnancy risk category C*

## AVAILABLE FORMS
*Injection:* 200 mg/100 ml, 400 mg/200 ml
*Powder for oral suspension:* 10 mg/ml, 40 mg/ml
*Tablets:* 50 mg, 100 mg, 150 mg, 200 mg

## INDICATIONS & DOSAGES
➤ **Oropharyngeal candidiasis**
*Adults:* 200 mg P.O. or I.V. on first day, then 100 mg once daily for at least 2 weeks.
*Children:* 6 mg/kg P.O. or I.V. on first day, then 3 mg/kg daily for 2 weeks.
➤ **Esophageal candidiasis**
*Adults:* 200 mg P.O. or I.V. on first day, then 100 mg once daily. Up to 400 mg daily has been used, depending on patient's condition and tolerance of treatment. Patients should receive drug for at least 3 weeks and for 2 weeks after symptoms resolve.
*Children:* 6 mg/kg P.O. or I.V. on first day, then 3 mg/kg daily for at least 3 weeks, and for at least 2 weeks after symptoms resolve. Maximum daily dose 12 mg/kg.
➤ **Vulvovaginal candidiasis**
*Adults:* 150 mg P.O. for one dose only.
➤ **Systemic candidiasis**
*Adults:* 400 mg P.O. or I.V. on first day, then 200 mg daily for at least 4 weeks and for 2 weeks after symptoms resolve. Doses up to 400 mg/day may be used.
*Children:* 6 to 12 mg/kg/day P.O. or I.V.
➤ **Cryptococcal meningitis**
*Adults:* 400 mg P.O. or I.V. on first day, then 200 mg once daily for 10 to 12 weeks after CSF culture result is negative. Doses up to 400 mg/day may be used.
*Children:* 12 mg/kg/day P.O. or I.V. on first day, then 6 mg/kg/day for 10 to 12 weeks after CSF culture result is negative.

➤ **To prevent candidiasis in bone marrow transplant**
*Adults:* 400 mg P.O. or I.V. once daily. Start treatment several days before anticipated agranulocytosis, and continue for 7 days after neutrophil count exceeds 1,000 cells/mm³.
➤ **To suppress relapse of cryptococcal meningitis in patients with AIDS**
*Adults:* 200 mg P.O. or I.V. daily.
*Children:* 3 to 6 mg/kg/day P.O. or I.V.
*Adjust-a-dose:* For renally impaired patients, if creatinine clearance is 11 to 50 ml/minute, reduce dosage by 50%. Patients receiving regular hemodialysis treatment should receive usual dose after each dialysis session.

## I.V. ADMINISTRATION
• Don't remove protective overwrap from I.V. bags until just before use to ensure product sterility. The plastic container may show some opacity from moisture absorbed during sterilization. This doesn't affect drug and diminishes over time. Don't add other drugs to I.V. bag.
• *Alert:* Give by continuous infusion at rate not exceeding 200 mg/hour. Use an infusion pump. To prevent air embolism, don't connect in series with other infusions.

## ACTION
Inhibits fungal cytochrome P-450 (responsible for fungal sterol synthesis); weakens fungal cell walls.

| Route | Onset | Peak | Duration |
|-------|-------|------|----------|
| P.O. | Unknown | 1-2 hr | 30 hr |
| I.V. | Immediate | Immediate | Unknown |

## ADVERSE REACTIONS
**CNS:** *headache,* dizziness.
**GI:** nausea, vomiting, abdominal pain, diarrhea, dyspepsia, taste perversion.
**Hematologic:** *leukopenia, thrombocytopenia.*
**Skin:** rash.
**Other:** *anaphylaxis.*

## INTERACTIONS
**Drug-drug.** *Alprazolam, chlordiazepoxide, clonazepam, clorazepate, diazepam, estazolam, flurazepam, midazolam, quazepam, triazolam:* May increase and

prolong levels of these drugs, CNS depression, and psychomotor impairment. Avoid using together.

*Cimetidine:* May decrease fluconazole level. Monitor patient response to fluconazole.

*Cyclosporine, phenytoin, theophylline:* May increase levels of these drugs. Monitor cyclosporine, theophylline, and phenytoin levels.

*HMG-CoA reductase inhibitors atorvastatin, fluvastatin, lovastatin, pravastatin, simvastatin:* May increase levels and adverse effects of these drugs. Avoid using together, or reduce dosage of HMG-CoA reductase inhibitor.

*Isoniazid, oral sulfonylureas, phenytoin, rifampin, valproic acid:* May elevate hepatic transaminase levels. Monitor liver function test results closely.

*Oral sulfonylureas (such as glipizide, glyburide, tolbutamide):* May increase levels of these drugs. Monitor patient for enhanced hypoglycemic effect.

*Rifampin:* May enhance fluconazole metabolism. Monitor patient for lack of response.

*Warfarin:* May increase risk of bleeding. Monitor PT and INR.

*Zidovudine:* May increase zidovudine activity. Monitor patient closely.

**EFFECTS ON LAB TEST RESULTS**
• May increase alkaline phosphatase, ALT, AST, bilirubin, and GGT levels.
• May decrease WBC and platelet counts.

**CONTRAINDICATIONS & CAUTIONS**
• Contraindicated in patients hypersensitive to drug and breast-feeding patients.
• Use cautiously in patients hypersensitive to other antifungal azole compounds.

**NURSING CONSIDERATIONS**
• Serious hepatotoxicity has occurred in patients with underlying medical conditions.
• Periodically monitor liver function during prolonged therapy.
• If patient develops mild rash, monitor him closely. Stop drug if lesions progress, and notify prescriber.
• Risk of adverse reactions appears to be greater in HIV-infected patients.

**PATIENT TEACHING**
• Tell patient to take drug as directed, even after he feels better.
• Instruct patient to report adverse reactions promptly.

---

# flucytosine (5-FC, 5-fluorocytosine)
Ancobon, Ancotil‡

*Pregnancy risk category C*

**AVAILABLE FORMS**
*Capsules:* 250 mg, 500 mg

**INDICATIONS & DOSAGES**
➤ **Severe fungal infections caused by susceptible strains of *Candida* species, including septicemia, endocarditis, urinary tract and pulmonary infections, and of *Cryptococcus* species, including meningitis and urinary tract and pulmonary infections**
*Adults:* 50 to 150 mg/kg daily P.O. in four equally divided doses q 6 hours.

**ACTION**
Unknown. Appears to penetrate fungal cells and cause defective protein synthesis.

| Route | Onset | Peak | Duration |
|-------|-------|------|----------|
| P.O. | Unknown | 1-2 hr | Unknown |

**ADVERSE REACTIONS**
**CNS:** headache, vertigo, sedation, fatigue, weakness, confusion, hallucinations, psychosis, ataxia, hearing loss, paresthesia, parkinsonism, peripheral neuropathy.
**CV:** *cardiac arrest,* chest pain.
**GI:** nausea, vomiting, diarrhea, *hemorrhage,* abdominal pain, dry mouth, duodenal ulcer, ulcerative colitis, anorexia.
**GU:** azotemia, crystalluria, *renal failure.*
**Hematologic:** anemia, *leukopenia, bone marrow suppression, thrombocytopenia,* eosinophilia, *agranulocytosis, aplastic anemia.*
**Hepatic:** jaundice.
**Metabolic:** *hypoglycemia,* hypokalemia.
**Respiratory:** *respiratory arrest,* dyspnea.
**Skin:** occasional rash, pruritus, urticaria, photosensitivity.

---

Reactions may be *common,* uncommon, *life-threatening,* or COMMON AND LIFE-THREATENING.

## INTERACTIONS
**Drug-drug.** *Amphotericin B:* May cause synergistic effects and may enhance toxicity. Monitor patient for increased adverse reactions and toxicity.

## EFFECTS ON LAB TEST RESULTS
● May increase urine urea, alkaline phosphatase, ALT, AST, bilirubin, creatinine, and BUN levels. May decrease glucose and potassium levels.
● May increase eosinophil count. May decrease hemoglobin and WBC, platelet, and granulocyte counts.

## CONTRAINDICATIONS & CAUTIONS
● Contraindicated in patients hypersensitive to drug.
● Use with extreme caution in patients with impaired hepatic or renal function or bone marrow suppression.

## NURSING CONSIDERATIONS
● Patient should take capsules over 15 minutes to reduce adverse GI reactions.
● Monitor blood, liver, and renal function studies frequently during therapy; obtain susceptibility tests weekly to monitor drug resistance.
● If possible, regularly perform blood level assays of drug, to maintain therapeutic flucytosine level of 40 to 60 mcg/ml. Blood levels of drug above 100 mcg/ml may be toxic.
● Monitor fluid intake and output; report marked changes.

## PATIENT TEACHING
● Tell patient that therapeutic response may take weeks or months.
● Advise patient to report adverse reactions promptly.
● Instruct patient to take capsules over 15 minutes to reduce adverse GI reactions.

## itraconazole
Sporanox

*Pregnancy risk category C*

## AVAILABLE FORMS
*Capsules:* 100 mg
*Injection:* 10 mg/ml
*Oral solution:* 10 mg/ml

## INDICATIONS & DOSAGES
➤ **Pulmonary and extrapulmonary blastomycosis, nonmeningeal histoplasmosis**
*Adults:* 200 mg P.O. daily; increase as needed and tolerated by 100 mg to maximum of 400 mg daily. Give dosages exceeding 200 mg daily in two divided doses. Or, give 200 mg I.V. b.i.d. over 1 hour for four doses, followed by 200 mg I.V. daily for up to 14 days; then change to P.O. form. Treatment should continue for at least 3 months. In life-threatening illness, give a loading dose of 200 mg P.O. t.i.d. for 3 days.
➤ **Aspergillosis**
*Adults:* 200 to 400 mg P.O. daily. Or, 200 mg I.V. b.i.d. over 1 hour for four doses, followed by 200 mg I.V. daily for up to 14 days; then change to P.O. form.
➤ **Onychomycosis of the toenail (with or without fingernail involvement)**
*Adults:* 200 mg P.O. b.i.d. for 1 week, followed by 3 weeks drug free. Repeat cycle twice, for a total of three cycles.
➤ **Onychomycosis of the fingernail**
*Adults:* 200 mg P.O. b.i.d. for 1 week, followed by 3 weeks drug free. Repeat dosage.
➤ **Oropharyngeal candidiasis**
*Adults:* 200 mg oral solution swished in mouth vigorously and swallowed daily, for 1 to 2 weeks.
➤ **Oropharyngeal candidiasis in patients unresponsive to fluconazole tablets**
*Adults:* 100 mg oral solution swished in mouth vigorously and swallowed b.i.d., for 2 to 4 weeks.
➤ **Esophageal candidiasis**
*Adults:* 100 to 200 mg oral solution swished in mouth vigorously and swallowed daily, for at least 3 weeks. Treatment should continue for 2 weeks after symptoms resolve.

## I.V. ADMINISTRATION
● Use only components provided in the infusion kit. Don't substitute.
● Dilute contents of 250-mg ampule in 50-ml bag of normal saline solution to provide 75 ml of a solution containing 3.33 mg itraconazole per milliliter.

- Give by I.V. infusion over 1 hour, using infusion set provided and a controlled infusion device.
- Don't mix with other drugs or give through same I.V. line as other drugs.
- Flush infusion set via the 2-way stopcock with 15 to 20 ml of normal saline solution injection over 30 seconds to 15 minutes; then discard I.V. line.
- Store diluted injection at 36° to 46° F (2° to 8° C) or at 59° to 77° F (15° to 25° C) for up to 48 hours when protected from light.

## ACTION
Interferes with fungal cell-wall synthesis by inhibiting ergosterol formation and increasing cell-wall permeability, leading to osmotic instability.

| Route | Onset | Peak | Duration |
|---|---|---|---|
| P.O. | Unknown | 3-4 hr | Unknown |
| I.V. | Unknown | Unknown | Unknown |

## ADVERSE REACTIONS
**CNS:** fever, *headache,* dizziness, somnolence, fatigue, malaise, asthenia, pain, tremor, abnormal dreams, anxiety, depression.
**CV:** hypertension, edema, orthostatic hypotension, *heart failure.*
**EENT:** rhinitis, sinusitis, pharyngitis.
**GI:** *nausea,* vomiting, diarrhea, abdominal pain, anorexia, dyspepsia, flatulence, increased appetite, constipation, gastritis, gastroenteritis, ulcerative stomatitis, gingivitis.
**GU:** albuminuria, impotence, cystitis, UTI.
**Hematologic:** *neutropenia.*
**Hepatic:** impaired hepatic function, *hepatotoxicity, liver failure.*
**Metabolic:** hypokalemia, hypertriglyceridemia.
**Musculoskeletal:** myalgia.
**Respiratory:** upper respiratory tract infection, *pulmonary edema.*
**Skin:** rash, pruritus.
**Other:** decreased libido, injury, herpes zoster, *hypersensitivity reactions (urticaria, angioedema, Stevens-Johnson syndrome).*

## INTERACTIONS
**Drug-drug.** *Alprazolam, midazolam, triazolam:* May increase and prolong drug levels, CNS depression, and psychomotor impairment. Avoid using together.
*Antacids, H₂-receptor antagonists, phenytoin, rifampin:* May decrease itraconazole level. Avoid using together.
*Chlordiazepoxide, clonazepam, clorazepate, diazepam, estazolam, flurazepam, quazepam:* May increase and prolong drug levels, CNS depression, and psychomotor impairment. Avoid using together.
*Cyclosporine, digoxin, tacrolimus:* May increase levels of these drugs. Monitor drug levels.
*Dofetilide, pimozide, quinidine:* May increase levels of these drugs by CYP 3A4 metabolism, causing serious CV events, including torsades de pointes, QT interval prolongation, ventricular tachycardia, cardiac arrest, and sudden death. Avoid using together.
*HMG-CoA reductase inhibitors atorvastatin, fluvastatin, lovastatin, pravastatin, simvastatin:* May increase levels and adverse effects of these drugs. Avoid using together, or reduce dose of HMG-CoA reductase inhibitor.
*Isoniazid:* May decrease itraconazole level. Monitor patient for therapeutic effect.
*Oral anticoagulants:* May enhance anticoagulant effect. Monitor PT and INR.
*Oral antidiabetics:* May cause hypoglycemia, similar to effect of other antifungals. Monitor glucose level. Avoid using together.
**Drug-food.** *Grapefruit and orange juice:* May decrease itraconazole level and therapeutic effect. Take with liquid other than grapefruit or orange juice.

## EFFECTS ON LAB TEST RESULTS
- May increase alkaline phosphatase, ALT, AST, bilirubin, triglyceride, and GGT levels. May decrease potassium level.

## CONTRAINDICATIONS & CAUTIONS
- Contraindicated in patients hypersensitive to drug or those receiving alprazolam, triazolam, midazolam, pimozide, quinidine, or dofetilide; in those with ventricular dysfunction or a history of heart failure; and in those who are breast-feeding.

---

Reactions may be *common,* uncommon, ***life-threatening,*** or COMMON AND LIFE-THREATENING.

If signs and symptoms of heart failure occur, stop itraconazole.
• Use cautiously in patients with hypochlorhydria; they may not absorb drug readily.
• Use cautiously in HIV-infected patients because hypochlorhydria can accompany HIV infection.
• Use cautiously in patients receiving other highly bound drugs.

**NURSING CONSIDERATIONS**
• *Alert:* Capsules and oral solution aren't interchangeable.
• Confirm the diagnosis of onychomycosis before starting therapy, by having nail specimens undergo appropriate laboratory testing.
• Perform baseline liver function tests, and monitor results periodically. Unless the patient's condition is life threatening, avoid therapy in patients with baseline hepatic impairment. If liver dysfunction occurs during therapy, notify prescriber immediately.

**PATIENT TEACHING**
• Teach patient to recognize and report signs and symptoms of liver disease (anorexia, dark urine, pale stools, unusual fatigue, and jaundice).
• Instruct patient not to use oral solution interchangeably with capsules.
• Tell patient to use 10 ml of the oral solution at a time.
• Advise patient to take solution without food and to take capsules with a full meal.
• Urge patient to tell prescriber about all drugs he's taking to avoid potential drug interactions.
• Advise women of childbearing potential that an effective form of contraception must be used during therapy and for two menstrual cycles (2 months) after stopping therapy with itraconazole capsules.

## ketoconazole
Nizoral

*Pregnancy risk category C*

**AVAILABLE FORMS**
*Oral suspension:* 100 mg/5 ml†
*Tablets:* 200 mg

**INDICATIONS & DOSAGES**
➤ Systemic candidiasis, chronic mucocandidiasis, oral candidiasis, candiduria, coccidioidomycosis, blastomycosis, histoplasmosis, chromomycosis, and paracoccidioidomycosis; severe cutaneous dermatophyte infections resistant to therapy with topical or oral griseofulvin
*Adults and children weighing more than 40 kg (88 lb):* Initially, 200 mg P.O. daily in a single dose. Dosage may be increased to 400 mg once daily in patients who don't respond.
*Children age 2 and older:* 3.3 to 6.6 mg/kg P.O. daily in a single dose.
➤ Onychomycosis (caused by *Trichophyton* and *Candida* species); pityriasis versicolor (tinea versicolor); tinea pedis, tinea corporis, and tinea cruris ♦
*Adults:* 200 to 400 mg P.O. daily.
➤ Tinea capitis ♦
*Adults:* 3.3 to 6.6 mg/kg P.O. daily.

**ACTION**
Interferes with fungal cell-wall synthesis by inhibiting formation of ergosterol and increasing cell-wall permeability that makes the fungus susceptible to osmotic instability.

| Route | Onset | Peak | Duration |
|-------|-------|------|----------|
| P.O. | Unknown | 1-2 hr | Unknown |

**ADVERSE REACTIONS**
**CNS:** fever, headache, nervousness, dizziness, somnolence, *suicidal tendencies,* severe depression.
**EENT:** photophobia.
**GI:** *nausea, vomiting,* abdominal pain, diarrhea.
**GU:** impotence.
**Hematologic:** *thrombocytopenia,* hemolytic anemia, *leukopenia.*
**Hepatic:** *fatal hepatotoxicity.*
**Metabolic:** hyperlipidemia.
**Skin:** pruritus.
**Other:** gynecomastia with tenderness, chills.

**INTERACTIONS**
**Drug-drug.** *Alprazolam, triazolam:* May increase and prolong levels of these drugs. May cause CNS depression and psy-

chomotor impairment. Avoid using together.

*Antacids, anticholinergics, H₂-receptor antagonists:* May decrease absorption of ketoconazole. Wait at least 2 hours after ketoconazole dose before giving these drugs.

*Chlordiazepoxide, clonazepam, clorazepate, diazepam, estazolam, flurazepam, midazolam, quazepam:* May increase and prolong levels of these drugs. May cause CNS depression and psychomotor impairment. Avoid using together.

*Cyclosporine:* May increase cyclosporine level. Monitor cyclosporine level.

*Isoniazid, rifampin:* May increase ketoconazole metabolism. Monitor patient for decreased antifungal effect.

*HMG-CoA reductase inhibitors atorvastatin, fluvastatin, lovastatin, pravastatin, simvastatin:* May increase levels and adverse effects of these drugs. Avoid using together, or reduce dose of HMG-CoA reductase inhibitor.

*Paclitaxel:* May inhibit metabolism. Use together cautiously.

*Theophylline:* May decrease theophylline level. Monitor theophylline level.

*Warfarin:* May enhance effects of anticoagulant. Monitor INR, PT, and PTT and adjust dosage, as needed.

*Drug-herb. Yew:* May inhibit ketoconazole metabolism. Discourage use together.

**EFFECTS ON LAB TEST RESULTS**
● May increase lipid, alkaline phosphatase, ALT, and AST levels.
● May decrease hemoglobin and platelet and WBC counts.

**CONTRAINDICATIONS & CAUTIONS**
● Contraindicated in patients hypersensitive to drug and in those taking alprazolam or oral triazolam.
● Use cautiously in patients with hepatic disease and in those taking other hepatotoxic drugs.

**NURSING CONSIDERATIONS**
● *Alert:* Because of potential for hepatotoxicity, ketoconazole shouldn't be used for less serious conditions, such as fungal infections of skin or nails.
● Monitor patient for signs and symptoms of hepatotoxicity, including elevated liver

enzyme levels, nausea that doesn't subside, and unusual fatigue, jaundice, dark urine, or pale stool.
● Doses up to 800 mg/day can be used to treat fungal meningitis and intracerebral fungal lesions.

**PATIENT TEACHING**
● Instruct patient with achlorhydria to dissolve each tablet in 4 ml aqueous solution of 0.2 N hydrochloric acid, sip mixture through a glass or plastic straw, and then drink a glass of water because ketoconazole needs gastric acidity for dissolution and absorption.
● Instruct patient to wait at least 2 hours after dose before taking antacids.
● Make sure patient understands that treatment should continue until all tests indicate that active fungal infection has subsided. If drug is stopped too soon, infection will recur. Minimum treatment for candidiasis is 7 to 14 days; for other systemic fungal infections, 6 months; for resistant dermatophyte infections, at least 4 weeks.
● Reassure patient that nausea, which is common early in therapy, will subside. To minimize nausea, instruct patient to divide daily amount into two doses or take drug with meals.

---

**nystatin**
Mycostatin*, Nadostine†, Nilstat, Nystex

*Pregnancy risk category C*

**AVAILABLE FORMS**
*Lozenges:* 200,000 units
*Oral suspension:* 100,000 units/ml*
*Powder:* 50, 150, or 500 million units; 1, 2, or 5 billion units
*Tablets:* 500,000 units
*Vaginal tablets:* 100,000 units

**INDICATIONS & DOSAGES**
➤ **Intestinal candidiasis**
*Adults:* 500,000 to 1 million units as oral tablets t.i.d.
➤ **Oral candidiasis (thrush)**
*Adults and children:* 400,000 to 600,000 units oral suspension q.i.d. or

200,000 to 400,000 units lozenges four to
five times daily for up to 14 days.
*Infants:* 200,000 units oral suspension
q.i.d.
*Neonates and premature infants:*
100,000 units oral suspension q.i.d.
➤ **Vaginal candidiasis**
*Adults:* 100,000 units, as vaginal tablets,
inserted high into vagina, daily at h.s. or
b.i.d. for 14 days.

**ACTION**
Unknown. Probably binds to sterols in
fungal cell membrane, altering cell permeability and allowing leakage of intracellular components.

| Route | Onset | Peak | Duration |
|-------|-------|------|----------|
| P.O., topical | Unknown | Unknown | Unknown |

**ADVERSE REACTIONS**
**GI:** transient nausea, vomiting, diarrhea.
**GU:** irritation, sensitization, vulvovaginal
burning (vaginal form).
**Skin:** rash.

**INTERACTIONS**
None significant.

**EFFECTS ON LAB TEST RESULTS**
None reported.

**CONTRAINDICATIONS & CAUTIONS**
● Contraindicated in patients hypersensitive to drug.

**NURSING CONSIDERATIONS**
● Nystatin isn't effective against systemic
infections.
● Vaginal tablets can be used by pregnant
patients up to 6 weeks before term to treat
maternal infection that may cause oral
candidiasis in neonates.
● To treat oral candidiasis, after the patient's mouth is clean of food debris, have
him hold suspension in mouth for several
minutes before swallowing. When treating
infants, swab medication on oral mucosa.
Prescriber may instruct immunosuppressed patients to suck on vaginal tablets
(100,000 units) because this provides prolonged contact with oral mucosa.

**PATIENT TEACHING**
● Instruct patient not to chew or swallow
lozenge but to allow it to dissolve slowly
in mouth.
● Advise patient to continue taking drug
for at least 2 days after signs and symptoms disappear. Consult prescriber for exact length of therapy.
● Instruct patient to continue therapy during menstruation.
● Explain that factors predisposing patient
to vaginal infection include use of antibiotics, oral contraceptives, and corticosteroids; diabetes; reinfection by sexual partner; and tight-fitting pantyhose.
Encourage patient to use cotton underwear.
● Instruct women in careful hygiene for
affected areas, including cleaning perineal
area from front to back.
● Advise patient to report redness,
swelling, or irritation.
● Tell patient, especially an older patient,
that overusing mouthwash or wearing
poorly fitting dentures may promote infection.

## terbinafine hydrochloride
Lamisil

*Pregnancy risk category B*

**AVAILABLE FORMS**
*Tablets:* 250 mg

**INDICATIONS & DOSAGES**
➤ **Fingernail onychomycosis caused by
dermatophytes (tinea unguium)**
*Adults:* 250 mg P.O. once daily for 6
weeks.
➤ **Toenail onychomycosis caused by
dermatophytes (tinea unguium)**
*Adults:* 250 mg P.O. once daily for 12
weeks.

**ACTION**
Inhibits squalene epoxidase, a key enzyme
in sterol biosynthesis of fungi, leading to
ergosterol deficiency and a corresponding
accumulation of sterol within the fungal
cell.

| Route | Onset | Peak | Duration |
|-------|-------|------|----------|
| P.O. | Unknown | 2 hr | Unknown |

## ADVERSE REACTIONS
**CNS:** *headache.*
**EENT:** visual disturbances.
**GI:** taste disturbances, diarrhea, dyspepsia, abdominal pain, nausea, flatulence.
**Hematologic:** *neutropenia.*
**Hepatic:** hepatobiliary dysfunction, including cholestatic jaundice.
**Skin:** rash, pruritus, urticaria, *Stevens-Johnson syndrome, toxic epidermal necrolysis.*
**Other:** hypersensitivity reactions, *anaphylaxis.*

## INTERACTIONS
**Drug-drug.** *Caffeine:* May decrease I.V. caffeine clearance. Use cautiously together.
*Cimetidine:* May decrease clearance of terbinafine by one-third. Avoid using together.
*Cyclosporine:* May increase cyclosporine clearance. Monitor cyclosporine level.
*Rifampin:* May increase terbinafine clearance by 100%. Monitor response to therapy.

## EFFECTS ON LAB TEST RESULTS
● May increase AST and ALT levels.
● May decrease neutrophil and lymphocyte counts.

## CONTRAINDICATIONS & CAUTIONS
● Contraindicated in patients hypersensitive to drug, pregnant or breast-feeding patients, those with liver disease, or those with creatinine clearance below 50 ml/minute.

## NURSING CONSIDERATIONS
● *Alert:* Rarely, patients with and without preexisting liver disease may suffer liver failure, which can lead either to death or to liver transplant.
● Obtain pretreatment transaminase levels for all patients taking terbinafine. Tablets aren't recommended for patients with acute or chronic liver disease.
● Monitor CBC and hepatic enzyme levels in patients receiving drug for longer than 6 weeks. Stop drug if hepatobiliary dysfunction or cholestatic hepatitis develops.
● *Alert:* Don't confuse terbinafine with terbutaline or Lamictal with Lamisil.

## PATIENT TEACHING
● Inform patient that successful treatment may take 10 weeks for toenail infections and 4 weeks for fingernail infections.
● Tell patient to report visual disturbances immediately; changes in the ocular lens and retina have occurred. Patient should also immediately report persistent nausea, anorexia, fatigue, vomiting, right upper quadrant pain, jaundice, dark urine, or pale stools.

## voriconazole
Vfend

*Pregnancy risk category D*

## AVAILABLE FORMS
*Powder for injection:* 200 mg
*Tablets:* 50 mg, 200 mg

## INDICATIONS & DOSAGES
➤ **Invasive aspergillosis; serious infections caused by *Fusarium* species and *Scedosporium apiospermum* in patients intolerant of or refractory to other therapy**
*Adults:* Initially, 6 mg/kg I.V. q 12 hours for two doses; then maintenance dose of 4 mg/kg I.V. q 12 hours. Switch to P.O. form as tolerated, using the maintenance dosages shown here:
*Adults weighing more than 40 kg (88 lb):* 200 mg P.O. q 12 hours. May increase to 300 mg P.O. q 12 hours, if necessary.
*Adults weighing less than 40 kg:* 100 mg P.O. q 12 hours. May increase to 150 mg P.O. q 12 hours, if necessary.
*Adjust-a-dose:* In patients with Child-Pugh class A or B, decrease the maintenance dosage by 50%.

## I.V. ADMINISTRATION
● Reconstitute the powder with 19 ml of water for injection to obtain a volume of 20 ml of clear concentrate containing 10 mg/ml of voriconazole. Discard the vial if a vacuum doesn't pull the diluent into the vial. Shake the vial until all the powder is dissolved.
● Further dilute the 10-mg/ml solution to 5 mg/ml or less. Follow the manufacturer's instructions for diluting.

---

• Use the reconstituted solution immediately.
• Infuse over 1 to 2 hours at 5 mg/ml or less and a maximum hourly rate of 3 mg/kg.
• Don't infuse in the same I.V. line with other drugs, blood products, or electrolyte supplementation.

## ACTION

Inhibits the cytochrome P-450 dependent synthesis of ergosterol, a vital component of fungal cell membranes.

| Route | Onset | Peak | Duration |
|-------|-------|------|----------|
| P.O., I.V. | Immediate | 1-2 hr | 12 hr |

## ADVERSE REACTIONS

**CNS:** fever, headache, hallucinations, dizziness.
**CV:** tachycardia, hypertension, hypotension, vasodilatation.
**EENT:** abnormal vision, photophobia, chromatopsia, dry mouth.
**GI:** abdominal pain, nausea, vomiting, diarrhea.
**Hepatic:** cholestatic jaundice.
**Metabolic:** hypokalemia, hypomagnesemia.
**Skin:** rash, pruritus.
**Other:** chills, peripheral edema.

## INTERACTIONS

**Drug-drug.** *Benzodiazepines, calcium channel blockers, lovastatin, omeprazole, sulfonylureas, vinca alkaloids:* May increase levels of these drugs. Adjust dosages of these drugs, and monitor patient for adverse reactions.
*Carbamazepine, long-acting barbiturates, rifabutin, rifampin:* May decrease voriconazole level. Avoid using together.
*Coumarin anticoagulants, warfarin:* May significantly increase PT. Monitor PT and other appropriate anticoagulant test results.
*Cyclosporine, tacrolimus:* May increase levels of these drugs. Adjust dosages and monitor levels of these drugs.
*Ergot alkaloids (such as ergotamine), sirolimus:* May increase levels of these drugs. Avoid using together.
*HIV protease inhibitors (amprenavir, nelfinavir, saquinavir), nonnucleoside reverse transcriptase inhibitors (delavirdine, efavirenz):* May increase levels of both drugs. Monitor patient for adverse reactions.
*Phenytoin:* May decrease voriconazole level and increase phenytoin level. Increase voriconazole maintenance dose, and monitor phenytoin level.
*Pimozide, quinidine:* May increase levels of these drugs, possibly leading to QT interval prolongation and torsades de pointes. Avoid using together.
**Drug-lifestyle.** *Sun exposure:* May cause photosensitivity. Advise patient to avoid excessive sunlight exposure.

## EFFECTS ON LAB TEST RESULTS

• May increase AST, ALT, bilirubin, alkaline phosphatase, and creatinine levels. May decrease potassium level.
• May decrease hemoglobin, hematocrit, and platelet, WBC, and RBC counts.

## CONTRAINDICATIONS & CAUTIONS

• Contraindicated in patients hypersensitive to drug or its components; in those with rare hereditary problems of galactose intolerance, Lapp lactase deficiency, or glucose-galactose malabsorption; and in those taking rifampin, carbamazepine, a long-acting barbiturate, sirolimus, rifabutin, an ergot alkaloid, pimozide, or quinidine.
• Use cautiously in patients hypersensitive to other azoles. Use I.V. form cautiously in patients with creatinine clearance less than 50 ml/minute.
• *Alert:* Drug may harm fetus. If drug is used during pregnancy or if the patient becomes pregnant while taking the drug, inform patient of the potential hazard to the fetus.

## NURSING CONSIDERATIONS

• Infusion reactions, including flushing, fever, sweating, tachycardia, chest tightness, dyspnea, faintness, nausea, pruritus, and rash, may occur as soon as infusion is started. Notify prescriber if reaction occurs. Infusion may need to be stopped.
• Monitor liver function test results at the start of and during therapy. Monitor patients who develop abnormal liver function test results for more severe hepatic injury. Drug may need to be stopped if

patient develops signs and symptoms of liver disease.
• Monitor renal function during treatment. Patients with creatinine clearance less than 50 ml/minute may benefit more from oral formulation of drug.
• Visual changes may occur if treatment lasts longer than 28 days.

## PATIENT TEACHING
• Tell patient to take oral form at least 1 hour before or 1 hour after a meal.
• Advise patient to avoid driving or operating machinery while taking drug, especially at night, because vision changes, including blurring and photophobia, may occur.
• Tell patient to avoid strong, direct sunlight during therapy.
• Advise patient to avoid becoming pregnant during drug therapy because of potential fetal harm.

**7**

# Antimalarials

**atovaquone and proguanil hydrochloride**
**chloroquine hydrochloride**
**chloroquine phosphate**
**doxycycline**
(See Chapter 12, TETRACYCLINES.)
**hydroxychloroquine sulfate**
**mefloquine hydrochloride**
**primaquine phosphate**
**pyrimethamine**
**pyrimethamine with sulfadoxine**

**COMBINATION PRODUCTS**
None.

---

## atovaquone and proguanil hydrochloride
Malarone, Malarone Pediatric

*Pregnancy risk category C*

---

**AVAILABLE FORMS**
*Tablets:* 62.5 mg atovaquone and 25 mg proguanil hydrochloride (pediatric); 250 mg atovaquone and 100 mg proguanil hydrochloride

**INDICATIONS & DOSAGES**
➤ **To prevent *Plasmodium falciparum* malaria, including where chloroquine resistance has been reported**
*Adults and children weighing more than 40 kg (88 lb):* 1 adult-strength (250 mg atovaquone and 100 mg proguanil hydrochloride) tablet P.O. once daily with food or milk, beginning 1 or 2 days before entering a malaria-endemic area. Continue prophylactic treatment during stay and for 7 days after return.
*Children weighing 31 to 40 kg (68 to 88 lb):* 3 pediatric-strength (62.5 mg atovaquone and 25 mg proguanil hydrochloride) tablets P.O. once daily with food or milk, beginning 1 or 2 days before entering endemic area. Total daily dose is 187.5 mg atovaquone and 75 mg proguanil hydrochloride. Continue prophylactic treatment during stay and for 7 days after return.

*Children weighing 21 to 30 kg (46 to 66 lb):* 2 pediatric-strength tablets P.O. once daily with food or milk, beginning 1 or 2 days before entering endemic area. Total daily dose is 125 mg atovaquone and 50 mg proguanil hydrochloride. Continue prophylactic treatment during stay and for 7 days after return.
*Children weighing 11 to 20 kg (24 to 44 lb):* 1 pediatric-strength tablet P.O. daily with food or milk, beginning 1 or 2 days before entering endemic area. Total daily dose is 62.5 mg atovaquone and 25 mg proguanil hydrochloride. Continue prophylactic treatment during stay and for 7 days after return.
➤ **Acute, uncomplicated *P. falciparum* malaria**
*Adults and children weighing more than 40 kg (88 lb):* 4 adult-strength tablets (total daily dose 1 g atovaquone and 400 mg proguanil hydrochloride) P.O. once daily, with food or milk, for 3 consecutive days.
*Children weighing 31 to 40 kg (68 to 88 lb):* 3 adult-strength tablets P.O. once daily, with food or milk, for 3 consecutive days. Total daily dose is 750 mg atovaquone and 300 mg proguanil hydrochloride.
*Children weighing 21 to 30 kg (46 to 66 lb):* 2 adult-strength tablets P.O. once daily, with food or milk, for 3 consecutive days. Total daily dose is 500 mg atovaquone and 200 mg proguanil hydrochloride.
*Children weighing 11 to 20 kg (24 to 44 lb):* 1 adult-strength tablet P.O. once daily, with food or milk, for 3 consecutive days.

**ACTION**
Thought to interfere with nucleic acid replication in the malarial parasite by inhibiting the biosynthesis of pyrimidine compounds. Atovaquone selectively inhibits mitochondrial electron transport in the parasite. Cycloguanil, an active metabolite of proguanil hydrochloride, disrupts deoxythymidylate synthesis through inhibition of dihydrofolate reductase. Ato-

---

*Rapid onset* †Canada ‡Australia ◇OTC ♦Off-label use ✐Photoguide *Liquid contains alcohol.

vaquone and cycloguanil are active against the erythrocytic and exoerythrocytic stages of *Plasmodium* species.

| Route | Onset | Peak | Duration |
|-------|-------|------|----------|
| P.O. | Unknown | Unknown | Unknown |

## ADVERSE REACTIONS
**CNS:** fever, asthenia, dizziness, *headache*, dreams, insomnia.
**GI:** *abdominal pain,* diarrhea, anorexia, dyspepsia, gastritis, *nausea, vomiting,* oral ulcers.
**Respiratory:** cough.
**Skin:** pruritus.

## INTERACTIONS
**Drug-drug.** *Metoclopramide:* May decrease atovaquone bioavailability. Consider alternative antiemetics.
*Rifampin:* May decrease atovaquone level by about 50%. Avoid using together.
*Tetracycline:* May decrease atovaquone level by about 40%. Monitor patient with parasitemia closely.

## EFFECTS ON LAB TEST RESULTS
• May increase alkaline phosphatase, ALT, and AST levels.
• May decrease hemoglobin, hematocrit, and WBC count.

## CONTRAINDICATIONS & CAUTIONS
• Contraindicated in patients hypersensitive to atovaquone, proguanil hydrochloride, or any component of the formulation.
• Use cautiously in patients with severe renal impairment and in those who are vomiting.
• It isn't known if elderly patients respond differently to drug than younger patients. Use cautiously in elderly patients because they have a greater frequency of decreased renal, hepatic, and cardiac function.
• It isn't known if atovaquone appears in breast milk, but proguanil hydrochloride does appear in breast milk in small amounts, so use combination cautiously in breast-feeding patients.
• Safety and efficacy haven't been established in children weighing less than 11 kg.

## NURSING CONSIDERATIONS
• Atovaquone absorption may be decreased by persistent diarrhea or vomiting. Patients with persistent diarrhea or vomiting may need alternative antimalarial therapy.
• Atovaquone and proguanil hydrochloride haven't been studied for treatment of cerebral malaria or other forms of complicated malaria.
• If malaria treatment or prevention using this drug fails, use another antimalarial.
• Give atovaquone and proguanil hydrochloride at the same time each day with food or milk.
• Store tablets at controlled room temperature 59° to 86° F (15° to 30° C).

## PATIENT TEACHING
• Tell patient to take dose at the same time each day.
• Advise patient to take drug with food or milk.
• If patient vomits within 1 hour after taking a dose, tell him to repeat dose.
• Advise patient to notify prescriber if he can't complete the course of therapy as prescribed.
• Instruct patient to supplement preventive malarial with use of protective clothing, bed nets, and insect repellents.

# chloroquine hydrochloride
Aralen HCl, Chlorquin‡

# chloroquine phosphate
Aralen Phosphate, Chlorquin‡

*Pregnancy risk category C*

## AVAILABLE FORMS
**chloroquine hydrochloride**
*Injection:* 40 mg/ml base
**chloroquine phosphate**
*Tablets:* 250 mg (equivalent to 150 mg base), 500 mg (equivalent to 300 mg base)

## INDICATIONS & DOSAGES
➤ **Acute malarial attacks caused by** *Plasmodium vivax, P. malariae, P. ovale,* **and susceptible strains of** *P. falciparum*
*Adults:* Initially, 600 mg base P.O.; then 300 mg base at 6, 24, and 48 hours. Or, initially, 160 to 200 mg base I.M., repeat-

ed in 6 hours, p.r.n. Switch patient to oral therapy as soon as possible.
*Children:* Initially, 10 mg/kg base P.O.; then 5 mg/kg base at 6, 24, and 48 hours. Don't exceed adult dose. Or, initially, 5 mg/kg base I.M., repeated in 6 hours, p.r.n. Don't exceed 10 mg/kg base in 24 hours. Switch patient to oral therapy as soon as possible.

➤ **To prevent malaria**
*Adults:* 300 mg base P.O. once weekly on the same day each week, for 1 to 2 weeks before entering a malaria-endemic area and continued for 4 weeks after leaving the area. If treatment begins after exposure, give 600 mg P.O. initially, in two divided doses 6 hours apart, followed by the usual dosing regimen.
*Children:* 5 mg/kg base P.O. once weekly on the same day each week, for 1 to 2 weeks before entering a malaria-endemic area and continued for 4 weeks after leaving the area. Don't exceed 300 mg. If treatment begins after exposure, give 10 mg/kg base P.O. initially, in two divided doses 6 hours apart, followed by the usual dosing regimen.

➤ **Extraintestinal amebiasis**
*Adults:* 600 mg base P.O. once daily for 2 days; then 300 mg base daily for 2 to 3 weeks. Treatment is usually combined with an intestinal amebicide. When oral therapy isn't feasible, give 160 to 200 mg base I.M. daily for 10 to 12 days. Resume oral therapy as soon as possible.
*Children:* 10 mg/kg base P.O. once daily for 2 to 3 weeks. Maximum dose is 300 mg base daily.

## ACTION

Unknown. May bind to and alter the properties of DNA in susceptible parasites.

| Route | Onset | Peak | Duration |
|-------|---------|--------|----------|
| P.O. | Unknown | 1-3 hr | Unknown |
| I.M. | Unknown | 30 min | Unknown |

## ADVERSE REACTIONS

**CNS:** mild and transient headache, psychic stimulation, *seizures,* dizziness, neuropathy.
**CV:** hypotension, ECG changes.
**EENT:** blurred vision; difficulty in focusing; reversible corneal changes; typically irreversible, sometimes progressive or delayed retinal changes such as narrowing of arterioles, macular lesions, pallor of optic disk, optic atrophy, patchy retinal pigmentation, typically leading to blindness; ototoxicity; nerve deafness; vertigo; tinnitus.
**GI:** anorexia, abdominal cramps, diarrhea, nausea, vomiting, stomatitis.
**Hematologic:** *agranulocytosis, aplastic anemia,* hemolytic anemia, *thrombocytopenia.*
**Skin:** pruritus, lichen planus eruptions, skin and mucosal pigmentary changes, pleomorphic skin eruptions.

## INTERACTIONS

**Drug-drug.** *Cimetidine:* May decrease hepatic metabolism of chloroquine. Monitor patient for toxicity.
*Kaolin, magnesium, and aluminum salts:* May decrease GI absorption. Separate dose times.
**Drug-lifestyle.** *Sun exposure:* May worsen drug-induced dermatoses. Advise patient to avoid excessive sun exposure.

## EFFECTS ON LAB TEST RESULTS

● May decrease hemoglobin and granulocyte and platelet counts.

## CONTRAINDICATIONS & CAUTIONS

● Contraindicated in patients hypersensitive to drug and in those with retinal or visual field changes or porphyria.
● Use cautiously in patients with severe GI, neurologic, or blood disorders; in those with hepatic disease or alcoholism; and in those with G6PD deficiency or psoriasis.

## NURSING CONSIDERATIONS

● *Alert:* Drug dosage may be discussed in mg or mg base; be aware of the difference.
● Ensure that baseline and periodic ophthalmic examinations are performed. Check periodically for ocular muscle weakness after long-term use.
● Assist patient with obtaining audiometric examinations before, during, and after therapy, especially if therapy is long-term.
● Monitor CBC and liver function studies periodically during long-term therapy. If a severe blood disorder not attributable to the disease develops, drug may need to be discontinued.

---

• *Alert:* Monitor patient for overdose, which can quickly lead to toxic symptoms: headache, drowsiness, visual disturbances, CV collapse, and seizures, then cardiopulmonary arrest. Children are extremely susceptible to toxicity; avoid long-term treatment.

## PATIENT TEACHING
• Advise patient to take drug immediately before or after a meal on the same day each week, to improve compliance when using drug for prevention.
• Instruct patient to avoid excessive sun exposure to prevent worsening of drug-induced dermatoses.
• Tell patient to report adverse reactions promptly, especially blurred vision, increased sensitivity to light, tinnitus, hearing loss, or muscle weakness.
• Instruct patient to keep drug out of reach of children. Overdose may be fatal.

---

# hydroxychloroquine sulfate
Plaquenil Sulfate

*Pregnancy risk category C*

## AVAILABLE FORMS
*Tablets:* 200 mg (equivalent to 155 mg base)

## INDICATIONS & DOSAGES
➤ **Suppressive prophylaxis of malaria attacks caused by *Plasmodium vivax, P. malariae, P. ovale*, and susceptible strains of *P. falciparum***
*Adults:* 310 mg base P.O. weekly on the same day each week, beginning 1 to 2 weeks before entering malaria-endemic area and continuing for 4 weeks after leaving area. If not started before exposure, double initial dose to 620 mg base in two divided doses 6 hours apart.
*Children:* 5 mg/kg base P.O. weekly on the same day each week, beginning 1 to 2 weeks before entering malaria-endemic area and continuing for 4 weeks after leaving area. Don't exceed adult dose. If not started before exposure, double initial dose to 10 mg/kg base in two divided doses, 6 hours apart.

➤ **Acute malarial attacks**
*Adults:* Initially, 620 mg base P.O.; then 310 mg base 6 to 8 hours after initial dose; then 310 mg base daily for 2 days.
*Children:* Initially, 10 mg/kg base P.O.; then 5 mg/kg base at 6, 24, and 48 hours after the initial dose.
➤ **Lupus erythematosus**
*Adults:* 310 mg base P.O. daily or b.i.d., continued for several weeks or months, depending on response. For prolonged maintenance dose, 155 to 310 mg base daily.
➤ **Rheumatoid arthritis**
*Adults:* Initially, 310 to 465 mg base P.O. daily. When good response occurs, usually in 4 to 12 weeks, cut dosage in half.

## ACTION
Unknown. May bind to and alter the properties of DNA in susceptible organisms.

| Route | Onset | Peak | Duration |
|-------|-------|------|----------|
| P.O. | Unknown | 2-4½ hr | Unknown |

## ADVERSE REACTIONS
**CNS:** irritability, nightmares, ataxia, *seizures,* psychosis, vertigo, dizziness, hypoactive deep tendon reflexes, lassitude, headache.
**CV:** T-wave inversion or depression, widening of QRS complex.
**EENT:** blurred vision; difficulty in focusing; reversible corneal changes; nystagmus; typically irreversible, sometimes progressive or delayed retinal changes such as narrowing of arterioles, macular lesions, pallor of optic disk, optic atrophy, visual field defects, patchy retinal pigmentation, commonly leading to blindness; ototoxicity.
**GI:** anorexia, abdominal cramps, diarrhea, nausea, vomiting.
**Hematologic:** *agranulocytosis, leukopenia, thrombocytopenia, hemolysis in patients with G6PD deficiency, aplastic anemia.*
**Metabolic:** weight loss.
**Musculoskeletal:** skeletal muscle weakness.
**Skin:** pruritus, lichen planus eruptions, skin and mucosal pigmentary changes, pleomorphic skin eruptions, worsened psoriasis, alopecia, bleaching of hair.

---

## INTERACTIONS
**Drug-drug.** *Cimetidine:* May decrease hepatic metabolism of hydroxychloroquine. Monitor patient for toxicity.
*Kaolin, aluminum salts, magnesium:* May decrease GI absorption. Separate dose times.

## EFFECTS ON LAB TEST RESULTS
● May decrease hemoglobin and granulocyte, WBC, and platelet counts.

## CONTRAINDICATIONS & CAUTIONS
● Contraindicated in patients hypersensitive to drug and in those with retinal or visual field changes or porphyria.
● Contraindicated as long-term therapy for children.
● Use with extreme caution in patients with severe GI, neurologic, or blood disorders.
● Use cautiously in patients with hepatic disease or alcoholism because drug concentrates in liver. Also use cautiously in those with G6PD deficiency or psoriasis because drug may worsen these conditions.

## NURSING CONSIDERATIONS
● *Alert:* Drug dosage may be discussed in mg or mg base; be aware of the difference.
● Ensure that baseline and periodic ophthalmic examinations are performed. Check periodically for ocular muscle weakness after long-term use.
● Assist patient with obtaining audiometric examinations before, during, and after therapy, especially if therapy is long-term.
● Monitor CBC and liver function studies periodically during long-term therapy; if severe blood disorder not attributable to disease develops, drug may need to be discontinued.
● *Alert:* Monitor patient for possible overdose, which can quickly lead to toxic signs or symptoms: headache, drowsiness, visual disturbances, CV collapse, and seizures, then cardiopulmonary arrest. Children are extremely susceptible to toxicity; avoid long-term treatment.

## PATIENT TEACHING
● Advise patient to take drug immediately before or after a meal on the same day each week, to improve compliance when using drug for prevention.
● Instruct patient to report adverse reactions promptly.

---

## mefloquine hydrochloride
Lariam

*Pregnancy risk category C*

## AVAILABLE FORMS
*Tablets:* 250 mg

## INDICATIONS & DOSAGES
➤ **Acute malaria infections caused by mefloquine-sensitive strains of *Plasmodium falciparum* or *P. vivax***
*Adults:* 1,250 mg (5 tablets) P.O. as a single dose with food and at least 8 ounces of water. Patients with *P. vivax* infections should receive subsequent therapy with primaquine or after 8-aminoquinolines to avoid relapse after treatment of the initial infection.
*Children:* 20 to 25 mg/kg P.O. as a single dose with food and at least 8 ounces of water. Maximum dose 1,250 mg. Dosage may be divided into two doses given 6 to 8 hours apart to reduce the incidence and severity of adverse effects. Patients with *P. vivax* infections should receive subsequent therapy with primaquine or other 8-aminoquinolines to avoid relapse after treatment of the initial infection.
➤ **To prevent malaria**
*Adults and children weighing more than 45 kg (99 lb):* 250 mg P.O. once weekly. Prevention therapy should start 1 week before entering endemic area and continue for 4 weeks after returning. If patient returns to an area without malaria after a prolonged stay in an endemic area, prevention therapy should end after three doses.
*Children weighing 31 to 45 kg (68 to 99 lb):* 187.5 mg (¾ of a 250-mg tablet) P.O. once weekly.
*Children weighing 20 to 30 kg (44 to 66 lb):* 125 mg (½ of a 250-mg tablet) P.O. once weekly.
*Children weighing 15 to 19 kg (33 to 42 lb):* 62.5 mg (¼ of a 250-mg tablet) P.O. once weekly.

---

*Children weighing less than 15 kg (33 lb):*
5 mg/kg P.O. once weekly.

## ACTION
Unknown. Antimalarial action may be related to drug's ability to form complexes with hemin; may also act by raising intravesicular pH in parasite acid vesicles.

| Route | Onset | Peak | Duration |
|-------|-------|------|----------|
| P.O. | Unknown | 7-24 hr | Unknown |

## ADVERSE REACTIONS
**CNS:** fever, dizziness, syncope, headache, psychotic changes, hallucinations, confusion, anxiety, fatigue, vertigo, depression, *seizures,* tremor, ataxia, mood changes, panic attacks, *suicide.*
**CV:** chest pain, edema.
**EENT:** tinnitus, visual disturbances.
**GI:** anorexia, vomiting, *nausea,* loose stools, diarrhea, abdominal discomfort or pain, dyspepsia.
**Hematologic:** *leukopenia, thrombocytopenia.*
**Musculoskeletal:** myalgia.
**Skin:** rash.
**Other:** chills.

## INTERACTIONS
**Drug-drug.** *Beta blockers, quinidine, quinine:* May cause ECG abnormalities and cardiac arrest. Avoid using together.
*Chloroquine, quinine:* May increase risk of seizures. Avoid using together.
*Valproic acid:* May decrease valproic acid level and loss of seizure control at start of mefloquine therapy. Monitor anticonvulsant level.

## EFFECTS ON LAB TEST RESULTS
• May increase transaminase levels.
• May decrease hematocrit and WBC and platelet counts.

## CONTRAINDICATIONS & CAUTIONS
• Contraindicated in patients hypersensitive to mefloquine or related compounds. Also contraindicated to prevent malaria in patients with a history of seizures or an active or recent history of depression, generalized anxiety disorder, psychosis, schizophrenia, or other major psychiatric disorders.
• Use cautiously in patients with cardiac disease or seizure disorders.

## NURSING CONSIDERATIONS
• Because giving quinine and mefloquine together poses a health risk, mefloquine therapy shouldn't begin sooner than 12 hours after the last dose of quinine or quinidine.
• Patients with *P. vivax* infections are at high risk for relapse because drug doesn't eliminate the hepatic-phase exoerythrocytic parasites. Follow-up therapy with primaquine is advisable.
• Monitor liver function test results periodically.
• If overdose is suspected, induce vomiting or perform gastric lavage as appropriate because of potential for cardiotoxicity. Mefloquine has produced cardiac actions similar to quinidine and quinine.
• *Alert:* When drug is used preventatively, psychiatric symptoms (acute anxiety, depression, restlessness, confusion) that occur may precede onset of a more serious event. Replace drug with alternate therapy.

## PATIENT TEACHING
• Advise patient to take drug immediately before or after a meal on the same day each week, to improve compliance when using drug for prevention.
• Tell patient not to take drug on an empty stomach and always to take it with at least 8 ounces of water.
• Advise patient to use caution when performing activities that require alertness and coordination because dizziness, disturbed sense of balance, and neuropsychiatric reactions may occur.
• Instruct patient taking mefloquine prophylactically to stop drug and notify prescriber if signs or symptoms of impending toxicity, such as unexplained anxiety, depression, confusion, or restlessness occur.
• Advise patient undergoing long-term therapy to have periodic ophthalmic examinations because drug may cause ocular lesions.
• Advise women of childbearing age to use reliable contraception during treatment.

---

Reactions may be *common*, uncommon, *life-threatening*, or COMMON AND LIFE-THREATENING.

# primaquine phosphate

*Pregnancy risk category C*

## AVAILABLE FORMS
*Tablets:* 26.3 mg (equivalent to 15 mg base)

## INDICATIONS & DOSAGES
➤ **Radical cure of relapsing vivax malaria, eliminating symptoms and infection completely; prevention of relapse**
*Adults:* 15 mg base P.O. daily for 14 days. Begin therapy during the last 2 weeks of, or after, a course of suppression with chloroquine or comparable drug.
*Children:* 0.3 mg/kg/day base P.O. for 14 days. Maximum 15 mg base/dose. Begin therapy during the last 2 weeks of, or after, a course of suppression with chloroquine or comparable drug.

## ACTION
Unknown. May bind to and alter the properties of DNA in susceptible parasites.

| Route | Onset | Peak | Duration |
| --- | --- | --- | --- |
| P.O. | Unknown | 1-3 hr | Unknown |

## ADVERSE REACTIONS
**GI:** nausea, vomiting, epigastric distress, abdominal cramps.
**Hematologic:** *hemolytic anemia* in G6PD deficiency, methemoglobinemia in nicotinamide-adenine-dinucleotide (NADH) methemoglobin reductase deficiency.

## INTERACTIONS
**Drug-drug.** *Magnesium and aluminum salts:* Decreases GI absorption. Separate dose times.

## EFFECTS ON LAB TEST RESULTS
• May decrease RBC count and hemoglobin. May increase or decrease WBC count.

## CONTRAINDICATIONS & CAUTIONS
• Contraindicated in patients with systemic diseases in which agranulocytosis may develop, such as lupus erythematosus or rheumatoid arthritis, and in those taking a bone marrow suppressant, quinacrine, or a potentially hemolytic drug.
• Use cautiously in patients with previous idiosyncratic reaction, involving hemolytic anemia, methemoglobinemia, or leukopenia; in those with a family or personal history of favism; and in those with erythrocytic G6PD or NADH methemoglobin reductase deficiency.

## NURSING CONSIDERATIONS
• *Alert:* Drug dosage may be discussed in mg or mg base, so be aware of the difference.
• Give drug with meals.
• Drug is used along with a fast-acting antimalarial such as chloroquine, to reduce possibility of drug-resistant strains.
• Obtain frequent blood studies and urinalysis, in light-skinned patients taking more than 30 mg base daily, dark-skinned patients taking more than 15 mg base daily, and patients with severe anemia or suspected sensitivity.
• Monitor patient for markedly darkened urine and for suddenly reduced hemoglobin level or erythrocyte or leukocyte count, which suggest impending hemolytic reactions. Stop drug immediately and notify prescriber.

## PATIENT TEACHING
• Instruct patient to take drug with meals to minimize stomach upset. If nausea, vomiting, or stomach pain persists, tell patient to notify prescriber.
• Tell patient to report chills, fever, chest pain, and bluish skin discoloration; these signs and symptoms may suggest a hemolytic reaction.
• Tell patient to stop drug and notify prescriber immediately if urine darkens markedly.
• Stress importance of completing full course of therapy.

## pyrimethamine
Daraprim

## pyrimethamine with sulfadoxine
Fansidar

*Pregnancy risk category C*

### AVAILABLE FORMS
**pyrimethamine**
*Tablets:* 25 mg
**pyrimethamine with sulfadoxine**
*Tablets:* pyrimethamine 25 mg, sulfadoxine 500 mg

### INDICATIONS & DOSAGES
➤ **To prevent and control transmission of malaria**
*pyrimethamine*
*Adults and children age 10 and older:*
25 mg P.O. weekly for 6 to 10 weeks or longer after leaving malaria-endemic areas.
*Children ages 4 to 10:* 12.5 mg P.O. weekly continued for 6 to 10 weeks or longer after leaving malaria-endemic areas.
*Children younger than age 4:* 6.25 mg P.O. weekly continued for 6 to 10 weeks or longer after leaving endemic areas.
*pyrimethamine with sulfadoxine*
*Adults and children age 14 and older:*
1 tablet weekly, or 2 tablets q 2 weeks during exposure and for 4 to 6 weeks after exposure.
*Children ages 9 to 14:* ¾ tablet weekly, or 1½ tablets q 2 weeks during exposure and for 4 to 6 weeks after exposure.
*Children ages 4 to 8:* ½ tablet weekly, or 1 tablet q 2 weeks during exposure and for 4 to 6 weeks after exposure.
*Children younger than age 4:* ¼ tablet weekly, or ½ tablet q 2 weeks during exposure and for 4 to 6 weeks after exposure.
➤ **Acute attacks of malaria**
*pyrimethamine*
*Adults:* 50 mg P.O. daily for 2 days, then 25 mg once weekly for at least 10 weeks.
*Children ages 4 to 10:* 25 mg P.O. once daily for 2 days, then 12.5 mg once weekly for at least 10 weeks.

*pyrimethamine with sulfadoxine*
*Adults and children age 14 and older:* 3 tablets as a single dose, given on the last day of quinine therapy.
*Children ages 9 to 14:* 2 tablets as a single dose, given on the last day of quinine therapy.
*Children ages 4 to 8:* 1 tablet as a single dose, given on the last day of quinine therapy.
*Children ages 1 to 3:* ½ tablet as a single dose, given on the last day of quinine therapy.
*Children ages 2 to 11 months:* ¼ tablet as a single dose, given on the last day of quinine therapy.
➤ **Toxoplasmosis**
*pyrimethamine*
*Adults:* Initially, 50 to 75 mg P.O. with 1 to 4 g sulfadiazine; continue for 1 to 3 weeks. After 3 weeks, reduce dosage by half and continue for 4 to 5 weeks.
*Children:* Initially, 1 mg/kg/day P.O. in two equally divided doses for 2 to 4 days; then 0.5 mg/kg daily for 4 weeks, along with 100 mg sulfadiazine/kg P.O. daily, divided q 6 hours. Don't exceed 100 mg.

### ACTION
Inhibits the enzyme dihydrofolate reductase, thereby impeding reduction of dihydrofolic acid to tetrahydrofolic acid. Sulfadoxine competitively inhibits use of PABA.

| Route | Onset | Peak | Duration |
|-------|-------|------|----------|
| P.O. | Unknown | 1½-8 hr | 2 wk |

### ADVERSE REACTIONS
**CNS:** headache, peripheral neuritis, mental depression, *seizures,* ataxia, hallucinations, fatigue.
**CV:** *arrhythmias,* allergic myocarditis.
**EENT:** scleral irritation, periorbital edema.
**GI:** anorexia, vomiting, atrophic glossitis.
**Hematologic:** *agranulocytosis, aplastic anemia,* megaloblastic anemia, *leukopenia, thrombocytopenia, pancytopenia.*
**Skin:** *Stevens-Johnson syndrome,* generalized skin eruptions, urticaria, pruritus, photosensitivity.

## INTERACTIONS

**Drug-drug.** *Co-trimoxazole, methotrexate, sulfonamides:* May increase risk of bone marrow suppression. Avoid using together.

*Lorazepam:* May increase risk of hepatotoxicity. Avoid using together.

*PABA:* May decrease antitoxoplasmic effects. May need to adjust dosage.

## EFFECTS ON LAB TEST RESULTS

● May decrease hemoglobin and granulocyte, WBC, platelet, and RBC counts.

## CONTRAINDICATIONS & CAUTIONS

● Pyrimethamine is contraindicated in patients hypersensitive to drug and in those with megaloblastic anemia from folic acid deficiency. Pyrimethamine with sulfadoxine is contraindicated in patients with porphyria.

● Repeated use of pyrimethamine with sulfadoxine is contraindicated in patients with severe renal insufficiency, marked parenchymal damage to the liver, blood dyscrasias, hypersensitivity to pyrimethamine or sulfonamides, or documented megaloblastic anemia from folate deficiency. Also contraindicated in infants younger than age 2 months and in pregnant (at term) and breast-feeding women.

● Use cautiously after treatment with chloroquine and in patients with impaired hepatic or renal function, severe allergy or bronchial asthma, G6PD deficiency, or seizure disorders (smaller doses may be needed).

## NURSING CONSIDERATIONS

● Pyrimethamine alone isn't recommended for treatment of malaria in nonimmune patients. Use drug with fasteracting antimalarials such as chloroquine for 2 days to start transmission control and suppressive cure.

● Obtain twice-weekly blood counts, including platelets, for the patient with toxoplasmosis because usual dosages approach toxic levels. If signs of folic acid or folinic acid deficiency develop, expect to reduce dosage or stop drug while patient receives parenteral folinic acid (leucovorin) until blood counts return to normal.

● Adverse drug reactions related to sulfadiazine are similar to those related to sulfonamides.

● When used to treat toxoplasmosis in patients with AIDS, therapy may be lifelong.

● Use pyrimethamine with sulfadoxine only in areas where chloroquine-resistant malaria is prevalent and only if the traveler plans to stay longer than 3 weeks.

## PATIENT TEACHING

● Instruct patient to take drug with meals.

● Inform patient with toxoplasmosis of importance of frequent laboratory studies and compliance with therapy. Tell patient he may need long-term therapy.

● Warn patient taking pyrimethamine with sulfadoxine to stop drug and notify prescriber at first sign of rash, sore throat, or glossitis.

● Tell patient to take first preventive dose 1 to 2 days before traveling.

# 8

## Antituberculotics and antileprotics

clofazimine
cycloserine
dapsone
ethambutol hydrochloride
isoniazid
pyrazinamide
rifabutin
rifampin
rifapentine
streptomycin sulfate
    (See Chapter 9, AMINOGLYCOSIDES.)

**COMBINATION PRODUCTS**
RIFAMATE: isoniazid 150 mg and rifampin 300 mg.
RIFATER: isoniazid 50 mg, rifampin 120 mg, and pyrazinamide 300 mg.

---

## clofazimine
Lamprene

*Pregnancy risk category C*

---

**AVAILABLE FORMS**
*Capsules:* 50 mg

**INDICATIONS & DOSAGES**
➤ **Dapsone-resistant leprosy (Hansen's disease)**
*Adults:* 100 mg P.O. daily, combined with one or more other antileprotics, for 3 years; then, 100 mg daily, clofazimine alone.
➤ **Dapsone-sensitive multibacillary leprosy**
*Adults:* 50 mg P.O. once daily (with an additional 300-mg dose once monthly), combined with two other antileprotics, for at least 1 year, until skin smears are negative. Patients showing evidence of worsening disease should receive an additional 12 months of treatment.
➤ **Erythema nodosum leprosum**
*Adults:* 100 to 200 mg P.O. daily in divided doses for up to 3 months. When treatment is prolonged, combine with corticosteroids. Taper dosage to 100 mg daily as soon as possible. Maximum dosage is 200 mg daily.

➤ *Mycobacterium avium* **complex (MAC) infection** ♦
*Adults:* 100 mg P.O. one to three times daily, usually combined with several other antileprotics.

**ACTION**
Unknown. Thought to inhibit mycobacterial growth by binding preferentially to mycobacterial DNA. Also, anti-inflammatory effects suppress skin reactions of erythema nodosum leprosum.

| Route | Onset | Peak | Duration |
|-------|-------|------|----------|
| P.O. | Unknown | 1-6 hr | Unknown |

**ADVERSE REACTIONS**
**EENT:** *conjunctival and corneal pigmentation, dryness, burning, itching, irritation.*
**GI:** *epigastric pain, diarrhea, nausea, vomiting, GI intolerance,* **bowel obstruction, bleeding.**
**Hematologic:** eosinophilia.
**Metabolic:** hypokalemia, hyperglycemia.
**Skin:** *pink to brownish black pigmentation, ichthyosis, dryness,* rash, pruritus.
**Other:** *splenic infarction,* discolored body fluids and excrement.

**INTERACTIONS**
**Drug-drug.** *Dapsone:* May inhibit anti-inflammatory effects of clofazimine. No intervention is needed.
*Isoniazid:* May decrease level of clofazimine in skin and increase levels in serum and urine. Monitor patient for decreased effectiveness.
*Rifampin:* May decrease rifampin bioavailability. Monitor patient for decreased effectiveness.

**EFFECTS ON LAB TEST RESULTS**
● May increase albumin, bilirubin, and AST levels. May decrease potassium and glucose levels.
● May increase eosinophil count.

**CONTRAINDICATIONS & CAUTIONS**
● No known contraindications.

● Use cautiously in patients with GI dysfunction, such as abdominal pain and diarrhea.

**NURSING CONSIDERATIONS**
● Give dosages exceeding 100 mg daily for as short a period as possible and only under close medical supervision.
● If patient complains of colic, burning abdominal pain, or other GI symptoms, notify prescriber, who may reduce dose or increase interval between doses.

**PATIENT TEACHING**
● Advise patient to take drug with meals or milk.
● Warn patient that clofazimine may discolor skin, body fluids, and excrement. The color ranges from pink to brownish black. Reassure patient that the unsightly skin discoloration is reversible but may not disappear until several months or years after drug treatment ends.
● Tell patient to apply skin oil or cream to help reverse skin dryness or ichthyosis (dry, rough, scaling skin).

---

# cycloserine
Seromycin

*Pregnancy risk category C*

---

**AVAILABLE FORMS**
*Capsules:* 250 mg

**INDICATIONS & DOSAGES**
➤ **Adjunctive treatment for pulmonary or extrapulmonary tuberculosis**
*Adults:* Initially, 250 mg P.O. q 12 hours for 2 weeks; then, if blood levels are below 25 to 30 mcg/ml and no toxicity has developed, increase dosage to 250 mg q 8 hours for 2 weeks. If optimum blood levels still aren't achieved and no toxicity has developed, then increase dosage to 250 mg q 6 hours. Maximum dosage is 1 g/day. If CNS toxicity occurs, stop drug for 1 week, then resume at 250 mg daily for 2 weeks. If no serious toxic effects occur, increase dosage by 250-mg increments q 10 days until blood level of 25 to 30 mcg/ml is obtained.

*Children:* 10 to 20 mg/kg/day P.O. in two divided doses. Maximum dosage is 0.75 to 1 g/day.
➤ **Acute urinary tract infections**
*Adults:* 250 mg P.O. q 12 hours for 2 weeks.

**ACTION**
Inhibits cell-wall biosynthesis by interfering with the bacterial use of amino acids. Bacteriostatic or bactericidal, depending on the drug level attained at the site of infection and the susceptibility of the infecting organism.

| Route | Onset | Peak | Duration |
|-------|-------|------|----------|
| P.O. | Unknown | 4-8 hr | Unknown |

**ADVERSE REACTIONS**
**CNS:** *seizures,* drowsiness, somnolence, headache, tremor, dysarthria, vertigo, confusion, loss of memory, *possible suicidal tendencies,* psychosis, hyperirritability, paresthesia, paresis, hyperreflexia, *coma.*
**CV:** *sudden heart failure.*
**Other:** *hypersensitivity reactions.*

**INTERACTIONS**
**Drug-drug.** *Ethionamide:* May potentiate neurotoxic adverse reactions. Monitor patient closely.
*Isoniazid:* May increase risk of CNS toxicity, including dizziness or drowsiness. Monitor patient closely.
**Drug-lifestyle.** *Alcohol use:* May increase risk of CNS toxicity, including seizures. Discourage use together.

**EFFECTS ON LAB TEST RESULTS**
● May increase transaminase level.

**CONTRAINDICATIONS & CAUTIONS**
● Contraindicated in patients hypersensitive to drug, in those who use alcohol excessively, and in those with seizure disorders, depression, severe anxiety, psychosis, or severe renal insufficiency.
● Use cautiously in patients with impaired renal function; these patients need reduced dosage.

**NURSING CONSIDERATIONS**
● Obtain specimen for culture and sensitivity tests before therapy begins and then periodically to detect possible resistance.

---

• Cycloserine is considered a second-line drug in tuberculosis treatment and should always be given with other antituberculotics to prevent the development of resistant organisms.

• Use cycloserine to treat UTIs only when better alternatives are contraindicated and susceptibility to cycloserine is confirmed.

• Monitor cycloserine level periodically, especially in patients receiving high dosages (more than 500 mg daily) because toxic reactions may occur with blood levels above 30 mcg/ml.

• Observe patient receiving dosages of more than 500 mg daily for signs and symptoms of CNS toxicity, such as seizures, anxiety, and tremor.

• Monitor results of hematologic tests and renal and liver function tests.

• Observe patient for psychotic symptoms, hallucinations, and possible suicidal tendencies.

• Monitor patient for hypersensitivity reactions, such as allergic dermatitis.

• Give anticonvulsant, tranquilizer, or sedative to relieve adverse reactions.

**PATIENT TEACHING**
• Warn patient to avoid alcohol, which may cause serious neurologic reactions.

• Advise patient not to perform hazardous activities if drowsiness occurs.

• Tell patient to report adverse reactions promptly; dosage may need to be adjusted or other drugs prescribed to relieve adverse reactions.

---

**dapsone**
Avlosulfon†, Dapsone 100‡

*Pregnancy risk category C*

**AVAILABLE FORMS**
*Tablets:* 25 mg, 100 mg

**INDICATIONS & DOSAGES**
➤ **Multibacillary leprosy**
*Adults and children older than age 14:* 100 mg P.O. daily for 12 months, given with one or more antileprotics.
*Children ages 10 to 14:* 50 mg P.O. daily for 12 months, given with one or more antileprotics.

*Children younger than age 10:* 25 mg P.O. daily for 12 months, given with one or more antileprotics.
➤ **Paucibacillary leprosy**
*Adults and children older than age 14:* 100 mg P.O. daily with rifampin 600 mg once monthly for 6 months.
*Children ages 10 to 14:* 50 mg P.O. daily with rifampin 450 mg once monthly for 6 months.
*Children younger than age 10:* 25 mg P.O. daily with rifampin 300 mg once monthly for 6 months.
➤ **Dermatitis herpetiformis**
*Adults:* Initially, 50 mg P.O. daily; usual maintenance dosage in adults ranges from 25 to 400 mg daily.

**ACTION**
Unknown. May inhibit folic acid biosynthesis in susceptible organisms.

| Route | Onset | Peak | Duration |
|-------|-------|------|----------|
| P.O. | Unknown | 4-8 hr | Unknown |

**ADVERSE REACTIONS**
**CNS:** insomnia, psychosis, paresthesia, peripheral neuropathy, headache, vertigo, fever.
**CV:** tachycardia.
**EENT:** tinnitus, blurred vision.
**GI:** anorexia, abdominal pain, nausea, vomiting, *pancreatitis.*
**GU:** albuminuria, nephrotic syndrome, renal papillary necrosis, male infertility.
**Hematologic:** *hemolytic anemia, agranulocytosis, aplastic anemia.*
**Respiratory:** pulmonary eosinophilia.
**Skin:** lupus erythematosus, phototoxicity, exfoliative dermatitis, *toxic erythema, erythema multiforme, toxic epidermal necrolysis,* morbilliform and scarlatiniform reactions, urticaria, *erythema nodosum.*
**Other:** infectious mononucleosis–like syndrome, *sulfone syndrome.*

**INTERACTIONS**
**Drug-drug.** *Activated charcoal:* May decrease dapsone's GI absorption and enterohepatic recycling. Monitor patient.
*Didanosine:* May cause therapeutic failure of dapsone, leading to increased infection. Avoid using together.

---

*Folic acid antagonists such as methotrexate:* May increase risk of adverse hematologic reactions. Avoid using together.

*PABA:* May antagonize effect of dapsone by interfering with primary mechanism of action. Monitor patient for lack of efficacy.

*Probenecid:* May reduce urinary excretion of dapsone metabolites, increasing plasma levels. Monitor patient for increased adverse effects.

*Rifampin:* May increase hepatic metabolism of dapsone. Monitor patient for lack of efficacy.

*Trimethoprim:* May increase levels of both drugs, possibly increasing pharmacologic and toxic effects of each drug. Monitor patient.

**Drug-lifestyle.** *Sun exposure:* May cause photosensitivity. Advise patient to avoid excessive sunlight exposure.

**EFFECTS ON LAB TEST RESULTS**
● May decrease hemoglobin and granulocyte count.

**CONTRAINDICATIONS & CAUTIONS**
● Contraindicated in patients hypersensitive to drug.
● Contraindicated in breast-feeding women because of risk of tumorigenicity.
● Use cautiously in patients with chronic renal, hepatic, or CV disease; refractory types of anemia; and G6PD deficiency.

**NURSING CONSIDERATIONS**
● Obtain baseline CBC. Monitor CBC weekly for first month, monthly for 6 months, and then semiannually.
● Reduce or temporarily stop dapsone if hemoglobin falls below 9 g/dl, WBC count falls below 5,000/mm³, or RBC count falls below 2.5 million/mm³ or remains low.
● If generalized diffuse dermatitis occurs, notify prescriber and prepare to interrupt therapy.
● Give antihistamines to combat allergic dermatitis.
● Watch for signs and symptoms of erythema nodosum reaction, such as malaise, fever, painful inflammatory induration in skin and mucosa, iritis, and neuritis, which may occur during therapy as a result of *Mycobacterium leprae* bacilli. In

severe cases, stop therapy and give glucocorticoids cautiously.
● Watch for and report signs and symptoms of sulfone syndrome, including fever, malaise, jaundice with hepatic necrosis, lymphadenopathy, methemoglobinemia, and hemolytic anemia.

**PATIENT TEACHING**
● *Alert:* Instruct breast-feeding patient to immediately notify prescriber if bluish skin discoloration occurs in infant.
● Inform patient of need for long-term therapy. Stress importance of compliance with drug therapy.
● Advise patient to avoid unprotected exposure to sunlight or sunlamps.

---

# ethambutol hydrochloride
Etibi†, Myambutol

*Pregnancy risk category B*

**AVAILABLE FORMS**
*Tablets:* 100 mg, 400 mg

**INDICATIONS & DOSAGES**
➤ **Adjunctive treatment in pulmonary tuberculosis**
*Adults and children older than age 13:* In patients who haven't received previous antitubercular therapy, 15 mg/kg P.O. as a single daily dose.

Retreatment: 25 mg/kg P.O. daily as a single dose for 60 days (or until bacteriologic smears and cultures become negative) with at least one other antituberculotic; then decreased to 15 mg/kg/day as a single dose.

**ACTION**
Unknown. Appears to interfere with the synthesis of one or more metabolites of susceptible bacteria, altering cellular metabolism during cell division (bacteriostatic).

| Route | Onset | Peak | Duration |
|-------|-------|------|----------|
| P.O. | Unknown | 2-4 hr | Unknown |

**ADVERSE REACTIONS**
**CNS:** headache, dizziness, fever, mental confusion, hallucinations, malaise, peripheral neuritis.

**EENT:** optic neuritis.
**GI:** anorexia, nausea, vomiting, abdominal pain, GI upset.
**Hematologic:** *thrombocytopenia.*
**Metabolic:** hyperuricemia.
**Musculoskeletal:** joint pain.
**Respiratory:** bloody sputum.
**Skin:** dermatitis, pruritus, *toxic epidermal necrolysis.*
**Other:** *anaphylactoid reactions,* precipitation of acute gout.

**INTERACTIONS**
**Drug-drug.** *Aluminum salts:* May delay and reduce absorption of ethambutol. Separate doses by several hours.

**EFFECTS ON LAB TEST RESULTS**
• May increase ALT, AST, bilirubin, and uric acid levels. May decrease glucose level.

**CONTRAINDICATIONS & CAUTIONS**
• Contraindicated in children younger than age 13, patients hypersensitive to drug, and patients with optic neuritis.
• Use cautiously in patients with impaired renal function, cataracts, recurrent eye inflammation, gout, or diabetic retinopathy.

**NURSING CONSIDERATIONS**
• Perform visual acuity and color discrimination tests before and during therapy.
• Ensure that any changes in vision don't result from an underlying condition.
• Obtain AST and ALT levels before therapy, and monitor these levels every 3 to 4 weeks.
• Anticipate dosage reduction in patients with impaired renal function.
• Always give ethambutol with other antituberculotics to prevent development of resistant organisms.
• Monitor uric acid level; observe patient for signs and symptoms of gout.

**PATIENT TEACHING**
• Reassure patient that visual disturbances usually disappear several weeks to months after drug is stopped. Inflammation of the optic nerve is related to dosage and duration of treatment.
• Inform patient that drug is given with other antituberculotics.

• Stress importance of compliance with drug therapy.

---

# isoniazid (INH, isonicotinic acid hydrazide)
Isotamine†, Nydrazid, PMS-Isoniazid†

*Pregnancy risk category C*

**AVAILABLE FORMS**
*Injection:* 100 mg/ml
*Oral solution:* 50 mg/5 ml
*Tablets:* 100 mg, 300 mg

**INDICATIONS & DOSAGES**
➤ **Actively growing tubercle bacilli**
*Adults:* 5 to 10 mg/kg P.O. or I.M. daily in a single dose, up to 300 mg/day, with other drugs, continued for 6 months to 2 years.
*Infants and children:* 10 to 20 mg/kg P.O. or I.M. daily in a single dose, up to 300 mg/day, continued long enough to prevent relapse. Give with at least one other antituberculotic.
➤ **To prevent tubercle bacilli in those exposed to tuberculosis or those with positive skin test results whose chest X-rays and bacteriologic study results indicate nonprogressive tuberculosis**
*Adults:* 300 mg P.O. daily in a single dose, continued for 6 months to 1 year.
*Infants and children:* 10 mg/kg P.O. daily in a single dose, up to 300 mg/day, continued for up to 1 year.

**ACTION**
Unknown. Appears to inhibit cell-wall biosynthesis by interfering with lipid and DNA synthesis (bactericidal).

| Route | Onset | Peak | Duration |
|-------|-------|------|----------|
| P.O., I.M. | Unknown | 1-2 hr | Unknown |

**ADVERSE REACTIONS**
**CNS:** *peripheral neuropathy, seizures, toxic encephalopathy,* memory impairment, toxic psychosis.
**EENT:** optic neuritis and atrophy.
**GI:** nausea, vomiting, epigastric distress.
**Hematologic:** *agranulocytosis,* hemolytic anemia, *aplastic anemia,* eosinophilia, *thrombocytopenia,* sideroblastic anemia.

---

Reactions may be *common,* uncommon, *life-threatening,* or COMMON AND LIFE-THREATENING.

**Hepatic:** *hepatitis,* jaundice, bilirubine-mia.
**Metabolic:** hyperglycemia, metabolic acidosis, hypocalcemia, hypophosphatemia.
**Skin:** irritation at I.M. injection site.
**Other:** rheumatic and lupuslike syndromes, hypersensitivity reactions, pyridoxine deficiency, gynecomastia.

## INTERACTIONS
**Drug-drug.** *Antacids and laxatives containing aluminum:* May decrease isoniazid absorption. Give isoniazid at least 1 hour before antacid or laxative.
*Benzodiazepines such as diazepam, triazolam:* May inhibit metabolic clearance of benzodiazepines that undergo oxidative metabolism, possibly increasing benzodiazepine activity. Monitor patient for adverse reactions.
*Carbamazepine, phenytoin:* May increase levels of these drugs. Monitor plasma levels closely.
*Cycloserine:* May increase CNS adverse reactions. Institute safety precautions.
*Disulfiram:* May cause neurologic symptoms, including changes in behavior and coordination. Avoid using together.
*Enflurane:* In rapid acetylators of isoniazid, may cause high-output renal failure because of nephrotoxic levels of inorganic fluoride. Monitor renal function.
*Ketoconazole:* May decrease ketoconazole level. Monitor patient for lack of efficacy.
*Meperidine:* May increase CNS adverse reactions and hypotension. Institute safety precautions.
*Oral anticoagulants:* May enhance anticoagulant activity. Monitor PT and INR.
*Phenytoin:* May inhibit phenytoin metabolism and increase phenytoin level. Monitor patient for phenytoin toxicity.
**Drug-food.** *Foods containing tyramine:* May cause hypertensive crisis. Tell patient to avoid such foods or eat in small quantities.
**Drug-lifestyle.** *Alcohol use:* May increase risk of isoniazid-related hepatitis. Discourage use of alcohol.

## EFFECTS ON LAB TEST RESULTS
● May increase transaminase, glucose, and bilirubin levels. May decrease calcium and phosphate levels.

● May increase eosinophil count. May decrease hemoglobin and granulocyte and platelet counts.
● May alter result of urine glucose tests that use cupric sulfate method such as Benedict's reagent or Diastix.

## CONTRAINDICATIONS & CAUTIONS
● Contraindicated in patients with acute hepatic disease or isoniazid-related liver damage.
● Use cautiously in elderly patients, in those with chronic non–isoniazid-related liver disease or chronic alcoholism, in those with seizure disorders (especially those taking phenytoin), and in those with severe renal impairment.

## NURSING CONSIDERATIONS
● Always give isoniazid with other antituberculotics to prevent development of resistant organisms.
● Isoniazid pharmacokinetics may vary among patients because drug is metabolized in the liver by genetically controlled acetylation. Fast acetylators metabolize drug up to five times as fast as slow acetylators. About 50% of blacks and whites are slow acetylators; more than 80% of Chinese, Japanese, and Inuits are fast acetylators.
● Peripheral neuropathy is more common in patients who are slow acetylators or who are malnourished, alcoholic, or diabetic.
● Monitor hepatic function closely for changes. Elevated liver function study results occur in about 15% of patients; most abnormalities are mild and transient, but some may persist throughout treatment.
● *Alert:* Severe and sometimes fatal hepatitis may develop, even after many months of treatment. Risk increases with age. Monitor liver studies closely.
● Give pyridoxine to prevent peripheral neuropathy, especially in malnourished patients.

## PATIENT TEACHING
● Instruct patient to take drug exactly as prescribed; warn against stopping drug without prescriber's consent.
● Advise patient to take drug 1 hour before or 2 hours after meals.

---

• Tell patient to notify prescriber immediately if signs and symptoms of liver impairment occur, such as appetite loss, fatigue, malaise, yellow skin or eye discoloration, and dark urine.

• Advise patient to avoid alcoholic beverages while taking drug. Also tell him to avoid certain foods (fish such as skipjack and tuna; and products containing tyramine, such as aged cheese, beer, and chocolate) because drug has some MAO inhibitor activity.

• Encourage patient to comply fully with treatment, which may take months or years.

## pyrazinamide
Tebrazid†, Zinamide‡

*Pregnancy risk category C*

### AVAILABLE FORMS
*Tablets:* 500 mg

### INDICATIONS & DOSAGES
➤ **Alternative treatment of tuberculosis when primary and secondary antituberculotics can't be used or have failed**
*Adults:* 15 to 30 mg/kg P.O. once daily. Maximum dosage is 3 g daily. Or, when compliance is a problem, 50 to 70 mg/kg based on lean body mass P.O. twice weekly.

### ACTION
Unknown.

| Route | Onset | Peak | Duration |
|-------|-------|------|----------|
| P.O. | Unknown | 1-2 hr | Unknown |

### ADVERSE REACTIONS
**CNS:** malaise, fever.
**GI:** anorexia, nausea, vomiting.
**GU:** dysuria, interstitial nephritis.
**Hematologic:** sideroblastic anemia, *thrombocytopenia.*
**Hepatic:** *hepatotoxicity, hepatitis.*
**Metabolic:** hyperuricemia.
**Musculoskeletal:** *arthralgia, myalgia.*
**Skin:** rash, urticaria, pruritus, photosensitivity.
**Other:** gout, porphyria.

### INTERACTIONS
None significant.

### EFFECTS ON LAB TEST RESULTS
• May increase uric acid and protein-bound iodine and urate levels. May decrease 17-ketosteroid levels.
• May decrease platelet count and hemoglobin.
• May interfere with urine ketone determinations.

### CONTRAINDICATIONS & CAUTIONS
• Contraindicated in patients hypersensitive to drug and in those with severe hepatic disease or acute gout.
• Use cautiously in patients with diabetes mellitus, renal failure, or gout.

### NURSING CONSIDERATIONS
• Always give pyrazinamide with other antituberculotics to prevent the development of resistant organisms.
• Drug is given for the first 2 months of a 6-month or longer treatment regimen for drug-susceptible patients. Patients with HIV infection may need longer courses of therapy.
• Doses that exceed 35 mg/kg may damage the liver.
• Obtain baseline uric acid level and liver function test results before treatment.
• Monitor hematopoietic studies and uric acid levels.
• Monitor liver function test results; assess patient for jaundice and liver tenderness or enlargement before and frequently during therapy.
• *Alert:* Immediately report signs and symptoms of gout and liver impairment, such as anorexia, fatigue, malaise, jaundice, dark urine, and liver tenderness.
• When used with surgical management of tuberculosis, start pyrazinamide 1 to 2 weeks before surgery and continue for 4 to 6 weeks after surgery.

### PATIENT TEACHING
• Inform patient that he must take drug with other antituberculotics.
• Tell patient to report adverse reactions promptly, especially fever, malaise, appetite loss, nausea, vomiting, dark urine, yellow skin or eye discoloration, and pain or swelling of the joints.

- Stress importance of compliance with drug therapy. If daily therapy poses a problem, tell patient to ask prescriber about twice-weekly dosing.

## rifabutin
Mycobutin

*Pregnancy risk category B*

### AVAILABLE FORMS
*Capsules:* 150 mg

### INDICATIONS & DOSAGES
➤ To prevent disseminated *Mycobacterium avium* complex in patients with advanced HIV infection
*Adults:* 300 mg P.O. daily as a single dose or divided b.i.d.

### ACTION
Inhibits DNA-dependent RNA polymerase in susceptible bacteria, blocking bacterial protein synthesis.

| Route | Onset | Peak | Duration |
|-------|-------|------|----------|
| P.O. | Unknown | 2-4 hr | Unknown |

### ADVERSE REACTIONS
**CNS:** headache, fever.
**GI:** dyspepsia, eructation, flatulence, diarrhea, nausea, vomiting, abdominal pain, anorexia, taste perversion.
**GU:** discolored urine.
**Hematologic:** *neutropenia, leukopenia, thrombocytopenia,* eosinophilia.
**Musculoskeletal:** myalgia.
**Skin:** *rash.*

### INTERACTIONS
**Drug-drug.** *Azole antifungals, benzodiazepines, beta blockers, buspirone, corticosteroids, cyclosporine, delavirdine, doxycycline, hydantoins, indinavir, losartan, macrolides, methadone, morphine, nelfinavir, quinidine, quinine, theophylline, tricyclic antidepressants, zolpidem:* May decrease effectiveness of these drugs. Monitor patient for drug effects.
*Hormonal contraceptives:* May decrease contraceptive effectiveness. Tell patient to use alternate form of birth control.
*Indinavir:* May increase rifabutin level. Decrease rifabutin dosage by 50%.

*Warfarin:* May decrease effectiveness of warfarin. May require higher dosages of anticoagulants. Monitor PT and INR.
**Drug-food.** *High-fat foods:* May reduce rate but not extent of absorption. Discourage use together.

### EFFECTS ON LAB TEST RESULTS
- May increase aminotransferase level.
- May decrease neutrophil, WBC, and platelet counts.

### CONTRAINDICATIONS & CAUTIONS
- Contraindicated in patients hypersensitive to drug or other rifamycin derivatives such as rifampin and in patients with active tuberculosis because single-drug therapy with rifabutin increases risk of inducing bacterial resistance to both rifabutin and rifampin.
- Use cautiously in patients with neutropenia and thrombocytopenia.

### NURSING CONSIDERATIONS
- In patients with neutropenia or thrombocytopenia, obtain baseline hematologic studies and repeat periodically.
- Mix drug with soft foods such as applesauce for patients who have difficulty swallowing.
- Dosage may be divided to take twice daily to decrease GI adverse effects. Drug may also be taken with food to avoid GI upset.
- *Alert:* Don't confuse rifabutin with rifampin or rifapentine.

### PATIENT TEACHING
- Instruct patient to take drug for as long as prescribed, exactly as directed, even after feeling better.
- Tell patient that drug or its metabolites may cause brownish orange staining of urine, feces, sputum, saliva, tears, and skin. Tell him to avoid wearing soft contact lenses because they may be permanently stained.
- Instruct patient to report sensitivity to light, excessive tears, or eye pain immediately; drug may rarely cause eye inflammation.
- Advise patient to report tingling and joint stiffness, swelling, or tenderness.

# rifampin (rifampicin)
Rifadin, Rimactane, Rimycin‡, Rofact†

*Pregnancy risk category C*

## AVAILABLE FORMS
*Capsules:* 150 mg, 300 mg
*Powder for injection:* 600 mg

## INDICATIONS & DOSAGES
➤ **Pulmonary tuberculosis**
*Adults:* 600 mg P.O. or I.V. daily in single dose. Give oral doses 1 hour before or 2 hours after meals.
*Children older than age 5:* 10 to 20 mg/kg P.O. or I.V. daily in single dose. Give oral doses 1 hour before or 2 hours after meals. Maximum daily dose is 600 mg. Give with other antituberculotics.
➤ **Meningococcal carriers**
*Adults:* 600 mg P.O. or I.V. q 12 hours for 2 days; or 600 mg P.O. or I.V. once daily for 4 days.
*Children ages 1 month to 12 years:* 10 mg/kg P.O. or I.V. q 12 hours for 2 days, not to exceed 600 mg/day; or 20 mg/kg once daily for 4 days.
*Neonates:* 5 mg/kg P.O. or I.V. q 12 hours for 2 days.

## I.V. ADMINISTRATION
● Reconstitute drug with 10 ml of sterile water for injection to yield 60 mg/ml.
● Add to 100 ml of $D_5W$ and infuse over 30 minutes, or add to 500 ml of $D_5W$ and infuse over 3 hours.
● When dextrose is contraindicated, drug may be diluted with normal saline solution for injection. Don't use other I.V. solutions.
● Once prepared, dilutions in $D_5W$ are stable for up to 4 hours and dilutions in normal saline solution are stable for up to 24 hours at room temperature.

## ACTION
Inhibits DNA-dependent RNA polymerase, which impairs RNA synthesis (bactericidal).

| Route | Onset | Peak | Duration |
|-------|-------|------|----------|
| P.O. | Unknown | 2-4 hr | Unknown |
| I.V. | Unknown | Unknown | Unknown |

## ADVERSE REACTIONS
**CNS:** headache, fatigue, drowsiness, behavioral changes, dizziness, mental confusion, generalized numbness, ataxia.
**CV:** *shock.*
**EENT:** visual disturbances, exudative conjunctivitis.
**GI:** epigastric distress, anorexia, nausea, vomiting, abdominal pain, diarrhea, flatulence, sore mouth and tongue, *pseudomembranous colitis, pancreatitis.*
**GU:** hemoglobinuria, hematuria, *acute renal failure,* menstrual disturbances.
**Hematologic:** eosinophilia, *thrombocytopenia, transient leukopenia,* hemolytic anemia.
**Hepatic:** *hepatotoxicity.*
**Metabolic:** hyperuricemia.
**Musculoskeletal:** osteomalacia.
**Respiratory:** shortness of breath, wheezing.
**Skin:** pruritus, urticaria, rash.
**Other:** flulike syndrome, discoloration of body fluids, porphyria exacerbation.

## INTERACTIONS
**Drug-drug.** *Acetaminophen, analgesics, anticonvulsants, barbiturates, beta blockers, cardiac glycosides, chloramphenicol, clofibrate, corticosteroids, cyclosporine, dapsone, diazepam, disopyramide, hormonal contraceptives, methadone, mexiletine, opioids, progestins, quinidine, sulfonylureas, theophylline, verapamil:* May decrease effectiveness of these drugs. Monitor patient for clinical effects.
*Anticoagulants:* May increase requirements for anticoagulant. Monitor PT and INR closely and adjust dosage of anticoagulant as needed.
*Halothane:* May increase risk of hepatotoxicity. Monitor liver function test results.
*Isoniazid:* May increase risk of hepatotoxicity. Monitor liver function test results.
*Ketoconazole, para-aminosalicylate sodium:* May interfere with absorption of rifampin. Separate doses by 8 to 12 hours.
*Probenecid:* May increase rifampin levels. Use together cautiously.
**Drug-lifestyle.** *Alcohol use:* May increase risk of hepatotoxicity. Discourage use together.

---

**EFFECTS ON LAB TEST RESULTS**
- May increase ALT, AST, alkaline phosphatase, bilirubin, and uric acid levels.
- May increase eosinophil counts. May decrease hemoglobin and platelet and WBC counts.
- May alter standard folate and vitamin $B_{12}$ assay results.

**CONTRAINDICATIONS & CAUTIONS**
- Contraindicated in patients hypersensitive to rifampin or related drugs.
- Use cautiously in patients with liver disease.

**NURSING CONSIDERATIONS**
- Give drug with at least one other antituberculotic.
- Give P.O. doses 1 hour before or 2 hours after meals for optimal absorption; if GI irritation occurs, may give with meals.
- Monitor hepatic function, hematopoietic studies, and uric acid levels. Drug's systemic effects may cause asymptomatic elevation of liver function test results and uric acid level.
- Watch for and report to prescriber signs and symptoms of hepatic impairment.
- Drug may cause hemorrhage in neonates of rifampin-treated mothers.
- *Alert:* Don't confuse rifampin with rifabutin or rifapentine.

**PATIENT TEACHING**
- Instruct patient who develops drug-induced GI upset to take drug with meals.
- Warn patient that he may feel drowsy and that urine, feces, saliva, sweat, sputum, and tears may turn red-orange. Use of drug may also permanently stain soft contact lenses.
- Advise patient to avoid alcohol during drug therapy.

---

**rifapentine**
Priftin

*Pregnancy risk category C*

---

**AVAILABLE FORMS**
*Tablets (film-coated):* 150 mg

**INDICATIONS & DOSAGES**
➤ **Pulmonary tuberculosis, with at least one other antituberculotic to which the isolate is susceptible**
*Adults:* During intensive phase of short-course therapy, 600 mg P.O. twice weekly for 2 months, with an interval between doses of at least 3 days (72 hours).
   During continuation phase of short-course therapy, 600 mg P.O. once weekly for 4 months, combined with isoniazid or another drug to which the isolate is susceptible.

**ACTION**
Inhibits DNA-dependent RNA polymerase in susceptible strains of *Mycobacterium tuberculosis*. Demonstrates bactericidal activity against the organism both intracellularly and extracellularly.

| Route | Onset | Peak | Duration |
|-------|-------|------|----------|
| P.O. | Unknown | 5-6 hr | Unknown |

**ADVERSE REACTIONS**
**CNS:** headache, dizziness, pain.
**CV:** hypertension.
**GI:** anorexia, nausea, vomiting, dyspepsia, diarrhea.
**GU:** pyuria, proteinuria, hematuria, urinary casts.
**Hematologic:** *neutropenia,* lymphopenia, anemia, *leukopenia,* thrombocytosis.
**Metabolic:** *hyperuricemia.*
**Musculoskeletal:** arthralgia.
**Respiratory:** hemoptysis.
**Skin:** rash, pruritus, acne, maculopapular rash.

**INTERACTIONS**
**Drug-drug.** *Antiarrhythmics (disopyramide, mexiletine, quinidine, tocainide), antibiotics (chloramphenicol, clarithromycin, dapsone, doxycycline, fluoroquinolones), anticonvulsants (phenytoin), antifungals (fluconazole, itraconazole, ketoconazole), barbiturates, benzodiazepines (diazepam), beta blockers, calcium channel blockers (diltiazem, nifedipine, verapamil), cardiac glycosides, clofibrate, corticosteroids, haloperidol, HIV protease inhibitors (indinavir, nelfinavir, ritonavir, saquinavir), immunosuppressants (cyclosporine, tacrolimus), levothyroxine, opioid analgesics (methadone), oral anti-*

---

coagulants (warfarin), oral hypoglycemics (sulfonylureas), oral or other systemic hormonal contraceptives, progestins, quinine, reverse transcriptase inhibitors (delavirdine, zidovudine), sildenafil, theophylline, tricyclic antidepressants (amitriptyline, nortriptyline): May decrease activity of these drugs because of P-450 enzyme metabolism. May need to adjust dosage.

**EFFECTS ON LAB TEST RESULTS**
● May increase uric acid, ALT, and AST levels.
● May increase platelet count. May decrease hemoglobin and neutrophil and WBC counts.
● May alter folate and vitamin $B_{12}$ assay results.

**CONTRAINDICATIONS & CAUTIONS**
● Contraindicated in patients hypersensitive to rifamycins (rifapentine, rifampin, or rifabutin).
● Use drug cautiously and with frequent monitoring in patients with liver disease.

**NURSING CONSIDERATIONS**
● Rifamycin antibiotics may cause hepatotoxicity. Obtain baseline liver function test results before therapy starts.
● Give drug with pyridoxine (vitamin $B_6$) in malnourished patients; in those predisposed to neuropathy, such as alcoholics and diabetics; and in adolescents.
● *Alert:* Give drug with appropriate daily companion drugs. Compliance with all drug regimens, especially with daily companion drugs on the days when rifapentine isn't given, is crucial for early sputum conversion and protection from relapse of tuberculosis.
● If used during the last 2 weeks of pregnancy, drug may lead to postnatal hemorrhage in mother or infant. Monitor clotting parameters closely if drug is used at that time.
● *Alert:* Don't confuse rifapentine with rifabutin or rifampin.

**PATIENT TEACHING**
● Stress importance of strict compliance with this drug regimen and that of daily companion drugs, as well as necessary follow-up visits and laboratory tests.

● Advise a woman to use nonhormonal methods of birth control.
● Tell patient to take drug with food if nausea, vomiting, or GI upset occurs.
● Instruct patient to report to prescriber fever, loss of appetite, malaise, nausea, vomiting, darkened urine, yellowish discoloration of skin and eyes, pain or swelling of the joints, or excessive loose stools or diarrhea.
● Instruct patient to protect pills from excessive heat.
● Tell patient that rifapentine can turn body fluids red-orange and permanently stain contact lenses.

amikacin sulfate
gentamicin sulfate
neomycin sulfate
streptomycin sulfate
tobramycin sulfate

**COMBINATION PRODUCTS**
NEOSPORIN G.U. IRRIGANT: 40 mg
neomycin sulfate and 200,000 units
polymyxin B sulfate/ml.

---

### amikacin sulfate
Amikin

*Pregnancy risk category D*

**AVAILABLE FORMS**
*Injection:* 50 mg/ml (pediatric), 250 mg/ml

**INDICATIONS & DOSAGES**
➤ **Serious infections caused by sensitive strains of *Pseudomonas aeruginosa, Escherichia coli, Proteus, Klebsiella, Serratia, Enterobacter, Acinetobacter, Providencia, Citrobacter,* or *Staphylococcus***
*Adults and children:* 15 mg/kg/day I.M. or I.V. infusion, in divided doses q 8 to 12 hours.
*Neonates:* Initially, loading dose of 10 mg/kg I.V.; then 7.5 mg/kg q 12 hours.
➤ **Uncomplicated UTI caused by organisms not susceptible to less toxic drugs**
*Adults:* 250 mg I.M. or I.V. b.i.d.
➤ ***Mycobacterium avium* complex (MAC) infection ♦**
*Adults:* 15 mg/kg/day I.V. in divided doses q 8 to 12 hours as part of a multiple-drug regimen.
*Adjust-a-dose:* For adult patients with impaired renal function, initially, 7.5 mg/kg I.M. or I.V. Subsequent doses and frequency determined by amikacin levels and renal function studies. For adults undergoing hemodialysis, give supplemental doses of 50% to 75% of initial loading dose at end of each dialysis session. Monitor drug levels and adjust dosage accordingly.

**I.V. ADMINISTRATION**
● Dilute I.V. drug in 100 to 200 ml of $D_5W$ or normal saline solution, and infuse over 30 to 60 minutes.
● After I.V. infusion, flush line with normal saline solution or $D_5W$.

**ACTION**
Generally bactericidal. Inhibits protein synthesis by binding directly to the 30S ribosomal subunit.

| Route | Onset | Peak | Duration |
|-------|-------|------|----------|
| I.V. | Immediate | 30 min | 8-12 hr |
| I.M. | Unknown | 1 hr | 8-12 hr |

**ADVERSE REACTIONS**
**CNS:** *neuromuscular blockade.*
**EENT:** *ototoxicity.*
**GU:** *azotemia, nephrotoxicity,* possible increase in urinary excretion of casts.
**Musculoskeletal:** arthralgia.
**Respiratory:** *apnea.*

**INTERACTIONS**
**Drug-drug.** *Acyclovir, amphotericin B, cephalosporins, cisplatin, methoxyflurane, vancomycin, other aminoglycosides:* May increase nephrotoxicity. Use together cautiously, and monitor renal function test results.
*Atracurium, doxacurium, mivacurium, pancuronium, rocuronium, tubocurarine, vecuronium:* May increase effects of nondepolarizing muscle relaxants, including prolonged respiratory depression. Use together only when necessary, and expect to reduce dosage of nondepolarizing muscle relaxant.
*Dimenhydrinate:* May mask ototoxicity symptoms. Monitor patient's hearing.
*General anesthetics:* May increase neuromuscular blockade. Monitor patient for increased effects.
*Indomethacin:* May increase trough and peak amikacin levels. Monitor amikacin level.
*I.V. loop diuretics (such as furosemide):* May increase ototoxicity. Use together cautiously, and monitor patient's hearing.

---

*Parenteral penicillins (such as ticarcillin):* May inactivate amikacin in vitro. Don't mix.

**EFFECTS ON LAB TEST RESULTS**
• May increase BUN, creatinine, nonprotein nitrogen, and urine urea levels.

**CONTRAINDICATIONS & CAUTIONS**
• Contraindicated in patients hypersensitive to drug or other aminoglycosides.
• Use cautiously in patients with impaired renal function or neuromuscular disorders, in neonates and infants, and in elderly patients.

**NURSING CONSIDERATIONS**
• Obtain specimen for culture and sensitivity tests before giving first dose. Therapy may begin pending results.
• Evaluate patient's hearing before and during therapy if patient will be receiving drug for longer than 2 weeks. Notify prescriber if patient has tinnitus, vertigo, or hearing loss.
• Weigh patient and review renal function studies before therapy begins.
• Correct dehydration before therapy, as dehydration increases risk of toxicity.
• Obtain blood for peak amikacin level 1 hour after I.M. injection and 30 minutes to 1 hour after I.V. infusion ends; for trough levels, draw blood just before next dose. Don't collect blood in a heparinized tube; heparin is incompatible with aminoglycosides.
• Peak drug levels more than 35 mcg/ml and trough levels more than 10 mcg/ml may be linked to a higher risk of toxicity.
• Monitor renal function: urine output, specific gravity, urinalysis, BUN and creatinine levels, and creatinine clearance. Report to prescriber evidence of declining renal function.
• Watch for signs and symptoms of superinfection (especially of upper respiratory tract), such as continued fever, chills, and increased pulse rate.
• Therapy usually continues for 7 to 10 days. If no response occurs after 3 to 5 days, stop therapy and obtain new specimens for culture and sensitivity testing.
• **Alert:** Don't confuse Amikin with Amicar. Don't confuse amikacin (Amikin) with anakinra (Kineret).

**PATIENT TEACHING**
• Instruct patient to promptly report adverse reactions to prescriber.
• Encourage patient to maintain adequate fluid intake.

---

**gentamicin sulfate**
Cidomycin†, Garamycin

*Pregnancy risk category D*

**AVAILABLE FORMS**
*Injection:* 40 mg/ml (adults), 10 mg/ml (children)
*I.V. infusion (premixed):* 40 mg, 60 mg, 70 mg, 80 mg, 90 mg, 100 mg, 120 mg, in normal saline solution

**INDICATIONS & DOSAGES**
➤ **Serious infections caused by sensitive strains of** *Pseudomonas aeruginosa, Escherichia coli, Proteus, Klebsiella, Serratia, Enterobacter, Citrobacter,* **or** *Staphylococcus*
*Adults:* 3 mg/kg daily in three divided doses I.M. or I.V. infusion q 8 hours. For life-threatening infections, patient may receive up to 5 mg/kg daily in three to four divided doses; reduce dose to 3 mg/kg daily as soon as clinically indicated.
*Children:* 2 to 2.5 mg/kg q 8 hours I.M. or by I.V. infusion.
*Neonates older than 1 week and infants:* 2.5 mg/kg q 8 hours I.M. or by I.V. infusion.
*Neonates younger than 1 week and preterm infants:* 2.5 mg/kg q 12 hours I.M. or by I.V. infusion.
➤ **To prevent endocarditis for GI or GU procedure or surgery**
*Adults:* 1.5 mg/kg I.M. or I.V. 30 minutes before procedure or surgery. Maximum dose is 80 mg. Give with ampicillin (vancomycin in penicillin-allergic patients).
*Children:* 2 mg/kg I.M. or I.V. 30 minutes before procedure or surgery. Maximum dose is 80 mg. Give with ampicillin (vancomycin in penicillin-allergic patients).
*Adjust-a-dose:* For adults with impaired renal function, doses and frequency are determined by gentamicin levels and renal function. After hemodialysis to maintain therapeutic blood levels, adults should receive 1 to 1.7 mg/kg I.M. or by I.V. infu-

---

sion after each dialysis, and children should receive 2 to 2.5 mg/kg I.M. or by I.V. infusion after each dialysis.

### I.V. ADMINISTRATION
● When giving by intermittent I.V. infusion, dilute with 50 to 200 ml of $D_5W$ or normal saline solution for injection and infuse over 30 minutes to 2 hours.
● After completing I.V. infusion, flush the line with normal saline solution or $D_5W$.

### ACTION
Generally bactericidal. Inhibits protein synthesis by binding directly to the 30S ribosomal subunit.

| Route | Onset | Peak | Duration |
|-------|-------|------|----------|
| I.V. | Immediate | 30-90 min | Unknown |
| I.M. | Unknown | 30-90 min | Unknown |

### ADVERSE REACTIONS
**CNS:** fever, headache, lethargy, *encephalopathy,* confusion, dizziness, *seizures,* numbness, peripheral neuropathy, vertigo, ataxia, tingling.
**CV:** hypotension.
**EENT:** *ototoxicity,* blurred vision, tinnitus.
**GI:** vomiting, nausea.
**GU:** *nephrotoxicity,* possible increase in urinary excretion of casts.
**Hematologic:** anemia, eosinophilia, *leukopenia, thrombocytopenia, agranulocytosis.*
**Musculoskeletal:** muscle twitching, myasthenia gravis–like syndrome.
**Respiratory:** *apnea.*
**Skin:** rash, urticaria, pruritus, injection site pain.
**Other:** *anaphylaxis.*

### INTERACTIONS
**Drug-drug.** *Acyclovir, amphotericin B, cephalosporins, cisplatin, methoxyflurane, vancomycin, other aminoglycosides:* May increase ototoxicity and nephrotoxicity. Monitor hearing and renal function test results.
*Atracurium, doxacurium, mivacurium, pancuronium, rocuronium, tubocurarine, vecuronium:* May increase effects of nondepolarizing muscle relaxants, including prolonged respiratory depression. Use together only when necessary, and expect to reduce dosage of nondepolarizing muscle relaxant.
*Dimenhydrinate:* May mask ototoxicity symptoms. Monitor patient's hearing.
*General anesthetics:* May increase neuromuscular blockade. Monitor patient closely.
*Indomethacin:* May increase peak and trough levels of gentamicin. Monitor gentamicin level.
*I.V. loop diuretics (such as furosemide):* May increase risk of ototoxicity. Monitor patient's hearing.
*Parenteral penicillins (such as ampicillin and ticarcillin):* May inactivate gentamicin in vitro. Don't mix.

### EFFECTS ON LAB TEST RESULTS
● May increase BUN, creatinine, nonprotein nitrogen, ALT, AST, bilirubin, and LDH levels.
● May increase eosinophil count. May decrease hemoglobin and WBC, platelet, and granulocyte counts.

### CONTRAINDICATIONS & CAUTIONS
● Contraindicated in patients hypersensitive to drug or other aminoglycosides.
● Use cautiously in neonates, infants, elderly patients, and patients with impaired renal function or neuromuscular disorders.

### NURSING CONSIDERATIONS
● Obtain specimen for culture and sensitivity tests before giving first dose. Therapy may begin pending results.
● Evaluate patient's hearing before and during therapy. Notify prescriber if patient complains of tinnitus, vertigo, or hearing loss.
● Weigh patient and review renal function studies before therapy begins.
● *Alert:* Use preservative-free formulations of gentamicin when intrathecal route is ordered.
● Obtain blood for peak gentamicin level 1 hour after I.M. injection or 30 minutes after I.V. infusion finishes; for trough levels, draw blood just before next dose. Don't collect blood in a heparinized tube; heparin is incompatible with aminoglycosides.
● Maintain peak levels at 4 to 12 mcg/ml and trough levels at 1 to 2 mcg/ml. The maximum peak level is usually 8 mcg/ml,

except in patients with cystic fibrosis, who need increased lung penetration. Prolonged peak levels of 10 to 12 mcg/ml or prolonged trough levels greater than 2 mcg/ml may increase risk of toxicity.

• Monitor renal function: urine output, specific gravity, urinalysis, BUN and creatinine levels, and creatinine clearance. Report to prescriber evidence of declining renal function.

• Hemodialysis for 8 hours may remove up to 50% of drug from blood.

• Watch for signs and symptoms of superinfection (especially of upper respiratory tract), such as continued fever, chills, and increased pulse rate.

• Therapy usually continues for 7 to 10 days. If no response occurs in 3 to 5 days, stop therapy and obtain new specimens for culture and sensitivity testing.

**PATIENT TEACHING**
• Instruct patient to promptly report adverse reactions, such as dizziness, vertigo, unsteady gait, ringing in the ears, hearing loss, numbness, tingling, or muscle twitching.

• Encourage patient to drink plenty of fluids.

• Warn patient to avoid hazardous activities if adverse central nervous system reactions occur.

---

## neomycin sulfate
Mycifradin†, Neo-fradin, Neosulf‡, Neo-Tabs

*Pregnancy risk category D*

### AVAILABLE FORMS
*Oral solution:* 125 mg/5 ml
*Tablets:* 500 mg

### INDICATIONS & DOSAGES
➤ **Infectious diarrhea caused by enteropathogenic *Escherichia coli***
*Adults:* 50 mg/kg daily P.O. in four divided doses for 2 to 3 days; maximum of 3 g/day.
*Children:* 50 to 100 mg/kg daily P.O. in divided doses q 4 to 6 hours for 2 to 3 days.

➤ **To suppress intestinal bacteria before surgery**
*Adults:* Following saline cathartic, 1 g P.O. q hour for four doses; then 1 g q 4 hours for the balance of the 24 hours. Or, 88 mg/kg in six equally divided doses q 4 hours. Or, 1 g neomycin with 1 g erythromycin base at 1 p.m., 2 p.m., and 11 p.m. on day before 8 a.m. surgery.
*Children:* Following saline cathartic, 40 to 100 mg/kg daily P.O. in divided doses q 4 to 6 hours. Or, 88 mg/kg in six equally divided doses q 4 hours.

➤ **Adjunctive treatment for hepatic coma**
*Adults:* 1 to 3 g P.O. q.i.d. for 5 to 6 days; or 200 ml of 1% solution or 100 ml of 2% solution as enema retained for 20 to 60 minutes q 6 hours. For patients with chronic hepatic insufficiency, 4 g/day indefinitely may be needed.
*Children:* 50 to 100 mg/kg/day P.O. in divided doses for 5 to 6 days.

### ACTION
Generally bactericidal. Inhibits protein synthesis by binding directly to the 30S ribosomal subunit.

| Route | Onset | Peak | Duration |
|-------|-------|------|----------|
| P.O. | Unknown | 1-4 hr | 8 hr |

### ADVERSE REACTIONS
**EENT:** *ototoxicity.*
**GI:** nausea, vomiting, diarrhea, malabsorption syndrome, *Clostridium difficile*–related colitis.
**GU:** *nephrotoxicity,* possible increase in urinary excretion of casts.

### INTERACTIONS
**Drug-drug.** *Acyclovir, amphotericin B, cephalosporins, cisplatin, methoxyflurane, vancomycin, other aminoglycosides:* May increase nephrotoxicity. Monitor renal function test results.
*Atracurium, doxacurium, mivacurium, pancuronium, rocuronium, tubocurarine, vecuronium:* May increase effects of nondepolarizing muscle relaxants, including prolonged respiratory depression. Use together only when necessary, and expect to reduce dosage of nondepolarizing muscle relaxants.

---

*Digoxin:* May decrease digoxin absorption. Monitor digoxin level.
*I.V. loop diuretics (such as furosemide):* May increase ototoxicity. Monitor patient's hearing.
*Oral anticoagulants:* May inhibit vitamin K–producing bacteria; may increase anticoagulant effect. Monitor PT and INR.

**EFFECTS ON LAB TEST RESULTS**
• May increase BUN, creatinine, and nonprotein nitrogen levels.

**CONTRAINDICATIONS & CAUTIONS**
• Contraindicated in patients hypersensitive to other aminoglycosides and in those with intestinal obstruction.
• Use cautiously in elderly patients and in those with impaired renal function, neuromuscular disorders, or ulcerative bowel lesions.

**NURSING CONSIDERATIONS**
• Monitor renal function: urine output, specific gravity, urinalysis, BUN and creatinine levels, and creatinine clearance. Report to prescriber evidence of declining renal function.
• Evaluate patient's hearing before and during prolonged therapy. Notify prescriber if patient has tinnitus, vertigo, or hearing loss. Deafness may start several weeks after drug is stopped.
• Watch for signs and symptoms of superinfection, such as fever, chills, and increased pulse rate.
• When using drug as adjunctive treatment for hepatic coma, decrease patient's dietary protein and assess neurologic status frequently during therapy.
• When using drug for preoperative disinfection, provide a low-residue diet and a cathartic immediately before therapy.
• The ototoxic and nephrotoxic properties of neomycin limit its usefulness.

**PATIENT TEACHING**
• Instruct patient to report adverse reactions promptly.
• Encourage patient to maintain adequate fluid intake.

## streptomycin sulfate

*Pregnancy risk category D*

**AVAILABLE FORMS**
*Injection:* 1-g/2.5-ml ampules

**INDICATIONS & DOSAGES**
➤ **Streptococcal endocarditis**
*Adults:* 1 g q 12 hours I.M. for 1 week; then 500 mg I.M. q 12 hours for 1 week, given with penicillin.
*Adjust-a-dose:* In patients older than age 60, give 500 mg I.M. q 12 hours for entire 2 weeks, with penicillin.
➤ **Primary and adjunctive treatment in tuberculosis**
*Adults:* 15 mg/kg (maximum of 1 g) I.M. daily for 2 to 3 months; then 1 g I.M. two or three times weekly.
*Children:* 20 to 40 mg/kg (maximum of 1 g) I.M. daily in divided doses q 6 to 12 hours injected deeply into large muscle mass. Give with other antituberculotics, but not with capreomycin; continue until sputum test result becomes negative.
*Adjust-a-dose:* In elderly patients, give 10 mg/kg I.M. daily.
➤ **Enterococcal endocarditis**
*Adults:* 1 g I.M. q 12 hours for 2 weeks; then 500 mg I.M. q 12 hours for 4 weeks, given with penicillin.
➤ **Tularemia**
*Adults:* 1 to 2 g I.M. daily in divided doses injected deeply into upper outer quadrant of buttocks; continued for 7 to 14 days or until patient is afebrile for 5 to 7 days.

**ACTION**
Generally bactericidal. Inhibits protein synthesis by binding directly to the 30S ribosomal subunit.

| Route | Onset | Peak | Duration |
|-------|---------|--------|----------|
| I.M. | Unknown | 1-2 hr | Unknown |

**ADVERSE REACTIONS**
**CNS:** *neuromuscular blockade,* vertigo, facial paresthesia.
**EENT:** *ototoxicity.*
**GI:** vomiting, nausea.
**GU:** *nephrotoxicity,* increase in urinary excretion of casts.

**Hematologic:** eosinophilia, *leukopenia, thrombocytopenia, hemolytic anemia.*
**Respiratory:** *apnea.*
**Skin:** exfoliative dermatitis.
**Other:** hypersensitivity reactions, *anaphylaxis.*

## INTERACTIONS

**Drug-drug.** *Acyclovir, amphotericin B, cephalosporins, cisplatin, methoxyflurane, vancomycin, other aminoglycosides:* May increase nephrotoxicity. Monitor renal function test results.
*Atracurium, doxacurium, mivacurium, pancuronium, rocuronium, tubocurarine, vecuronium:* May increase effects of nondepolarizing muscle relaxants, including prolonged respiratory depression. Use together only when necessary, and expect to reduce dosage of nondepolarizing muscle relaxant.
*General anesthetics:* May increase neuromuscular blockade. Monitor patient closely.
*I.V. loop diuretics (such as furosemide):* May increase ototoxicity. Monitor patient's hearing.

## EFFECTS ON LAB TEST RESULTS

• May increase BUN, creatinine, and nonprotein nitrogen levels.
• May increase eosinophil count. May decrease WBC and platelet counts and hemoglobin.
• May cause false-positive reaction in copper sulfate tests for urine glucose such as Benedict's reagent or Diastix.

## CONTRAINDICATIONS & CAUTIONS

• Contraindicated in patients hypersensitive to drug or other aminoglycosides.
• Use cautiously in elderly patients and in patients with impaired renal function or neuromuscular disorders.

## NURSING CONSIDERATIONS

• Obtain specimen for culture and sensitivity tests before giving first dose except when treating tuberculosis. Therapy may begin pending results.
• Evaluate patient's hearing before therapy and for 6 months afterward. Notify prescriber if patient has hearing loss, feels fullness in ears, or hears roaring noises.

• Protect hands when preparing drug to avoid irritation.
• When giving I.M., inject deeply into upper outer quadrant of buttocks or midlateral thigh. Rotate injection sites.
• In children, give I.M. injection in midlateral thigh if possible, to minimize possibility of damaging sciatic nerve.
• Obtain blood for peak streptomycin level 1 to 2 hours after I.M. injection; obtain blood for trough level just before next dose. Don't use a heparinized tube; heparin is incompatible with aminoglycosides.
• Drug has been given as I.V. infusion over 30 to 60 minutes without unusual adverse effects in patients unable to tolerate I.M. injections.
• Watch for signs and symptoms of superinfection, such as continued fever, chills, and increased pulse rate.
• Nephrotoxicity occurs less frequently with streptomycin than with other aminoglycosides.
• When drug is used for primary treatment of tuberculosis, stop therapy when sputum test result becomes negative.

## PATIENT TEACHING

• Instruct patient to report adverse reactions promptly.
• Encourage patient to maintain adequate fluid intake.
• Emphasize need for blood tests to monitor streptomycin levels and determine effectiveness of therapy.

## tobramycin sulfate
Nebcin, TOBI

*Pregnancy risk category D*

## AVAILABLE FORMS

*Multidose vials:* 80-mg/2-ml, 20-mg/2-ml (children)
*Nebulizer solution (for inhalation):* 300-mg/5-ml
*Premixed parenteral injection for I.V. infusion:* 60 mg or 80 mg in normal saline solution

## INDICATIONS & DOSAGES

➤ **Serious infections caused by sensitive strains of *Escherichia coli, Proteus, Klebsiella, Enterobacter, Serratia, Mor-***

*ganella morganii, Staphylococcus aureus, Citrobacter, Pseudomonas,* or *Providencia*

*Adults:* 3 mg/kg/day I.M. or I.V. in divided doses. For life-threatening infections, give up to 5 mg/kg/day in divided doses q 6 to 8 hours; reduce to 3 mg/kg daily as soon as clinically indicated.

*Children:* 6 to 7.5 mg/kg/day I.M. or I.V. in three or four divided doses.

*Neonates younger than age 1 week or premature infants:* Up to 4 mg/kg/day I.V. or I.M. in two equal doses q 12 hours.

*Adjust-a-dose:* For patients with renal impairment, give loading dose of 1 mg/kg; then give decreased doses at 8-hour intervals or same dose at prolonged intervals. For patients with severe cystic fibrosis, initial dose is 10 mg/kg/day I.V. or I.M. in four divided doses.

➤ **To manage cystic fibrosis patients with *Pseudomonas aeruginosa***

*Adults and children age 6 and older:* 300 mg via nebulizer q 12 hours for 28 days. Continue cycle of 28 days on drug and 28 days off.

## I.V. ADMINISTRATION

● For adults, dilute in 50 to 100 ml of normal saline solution or $D_5W$; use a smaller volume for children.

● Infuse over 20 to 60 minutes.

● After I.V. infusion, flush line with normal saline solution or $D_5W$.

## ACTION

Generally bactericidal. Inhibits protein synthesis by binding directly to the 30S ribosomal subunit.

| Route | Onset | Peak | Duration |
|---|---|---|---|
| I.V. | Immediate | 30 min | 8 hr |
| I.M. | Unknown | 30-60 min | 8 hr |
| Inhalation | Unknown | Unknown | Unknown |

## ADVERSE REACTIONS

**CNS:** headache, lethargy, confusion, disorientation, fever, *seizures.*

**EENT:** *ototoxicity, hoarseness, pharyngitis.*

**GI:** vomiting, nausea, diarrhea.

**GU:** *nephrotoxicity,* possible increase in urinary excretion of casts.

**Hematologic:** anemia, eosinophilia, *leukopenia, thrombocytopenia, agranulocytosis.*

**Metabolic:** electrolyte imbalances.

**Musculoskeletal:** muscle twitching.

**Respiratory:** *bronchospasm.*

**Skin:** rash, urticaria, pruritus.

## INTERACTIONS

**Drug-drug.** *Acyclovir, amphotericin B, cephalosporins, cisplatin, methoxyflurane, other aminoglycosides, vancomycin:* May increase nephrotoxicity. Monitor renal function test results.

*Atracurium, doxacurium, mivacurium, pancuronium, rocuronium, tubocurarine, vecuronium:* May increase effects of nondepolarizing muscle relaxants, including prolonged respiratory depression. Use together only when necessary, and expect to reduce dosage of nondepolarizing muscle relaxant.

*Dimenhydrinate:* May mask symptoms of ototoxicity. Monitor patient's hearing.

*General anesthetics:* May increase neuromuscular blockade. Monitor patient for increased clinical effects.

*I.V. loop diuretics (such as furosemide):* May increase ototoxicity. Monitor patient's hearing.

*Parenteral penicillins (such as ticarcillin):* May inactivate tobramycin in vitro. Don't mix.

## EFFECTS ON LAB TEST RESULTS

● May increase BUN, creatinine, nonprotein nitrogen, and urine urea levels. May decrease calcium, magnesium, and potassium levels.

● May increase eosinophil count. May decrease WBC, platelet, and granulocyte counts.

## CONTRAINDICATIONS & CAUTIONS

● Contraindicated in patients hypersensitive to drug or other aminoglycosides.

● Use cautiously in patients with impaired renal function or neuromuscular disorders and in elderly patients.

## NURSING CONSIDERATIONS

● Obtain specimen for culture and sensitivity tests before giving first dose. Therapy may begin pending results.

- Weigh patient and review renal function studies before therapy.
- Evaluate patient's hearing before and during therapy. Notify prescriber if patient complains of tinnitus, vertigo, or hearing loss.
- Don't dilute or mix tobramycin sulfate with dornase alpha in the nebulizer.
- Unrefrigerated tobramycin sulfate, which is normally slightly yellow, may darken with age. This change doesn't indicate a change in product quality.
- Avoid exposing tobramycin sulfate ampules to intense light.
- Give nebulizer solution over 10 to 15 minutes using handheld Pari LC Plus reusable nebulizer with DeVilbiss Pulmo-Aide compressor.
- Obtain blood for peak level 1 hour after I.M. injection or ½ hour after infusion stops; draw blood for trough level just before next dose. Don't collect blood in a heparinized tube; heparin is incompatible with aminoglycosides.
- *Alert:* Peak blood levels over 12 mcg/ml and trough levels over 2 mcg/ml may increase the risk of toxicity. Reserve higher peak levels for cystic fibrosis patients, who need a greater lung penetration.
- Monitor renal function: urine output, specific gravity, urinalysis, creatinine clearance, and BUN and creatinine levels. Notify prescriber about signs and symptoms of decreasing renal function.
- Watch for signs and symptoms of superinfection, such as continued fever, chills, and increased pulse rate.
- If no response occurs in 3 to 5 days, therapy may be stopped and new specimens obtained for culture and sensitivity testing.
- *Alert:* Don't confuse tobramycin with Trobicin.

**PATIENT TEACHING**
- Instruct patient to report adverse reactions promptly.
- Caution patient not to perform hazardous activities if adverse CNS reactions occur.
- Encourage patient to maintain adequate fluid intake.
- Teach patient how to use and maintain nebulizer.

- Tell patient using multiple inhaled therapies to use tobramycin sulfate last.
- Instruct patient not to use tobramycin sulfate if it's cloudy, if there are particles in the solution, or if it has been stored at room temperature for longer than 28 days.

---

Reactions may be *common*, uncommon, *life-threatening*, or COMMON AND LIFE-THREATENING.

**amoxicillin and clavulanate
  potassium**
**amoxicillin trihydrate**
**ampicillin**
**ampicillin sodium**
**ampicillin sodium and sulbactam
  sodium**
**ampicillin trihydrate**
**nafcillin sodium**
**penicillin G benzathine**
**penicillin G potassium**
**penicillin G procaine**
**penicillin G sodium**
**penicillin V potassium**
**piperacillin sodium**
**piperacillin sodium and
  tazobactam sodium**
**ticarcillin disodium**
**ticarcillin disodium and
  clavulanate potassium**

## COMBINATION PRODUCTS
BICILLIN C-R: *Injection:* 300,000 units/
ml, 600,000 units/ml, 1.2 million units/
2 ml, 2.4 million units/4 ml, containing
equal volumes of penicillin G benzathine
and procaine.
BICILLIN C-R 900/300: *Injection:* 1.2 million units/2 ml, each ml contains
450,000 units penicillin G benzathine
and 150,000 million units penicillin G
procaine.

---

## amoxicillin and clavulanate
potassium (amoxycillin and
clavulanate potassium)
Augmentin♥, Augmentin ES-600,
Augmentin XR, Clavulin†

*Pregnancy risk category B*

## AVAILABLE FORMS
*Oral suspension:* 125 mg amoxicillin trihydrate and 31.25 mg clavulanic acid/5 ml
(after reconstitution); 200 mg amoxicillin
trihydrate and 28.5 mg clavulanic acid/
5 ml (after reconstitution); 250 mg amoxicillin trihydrate and 62.5 mg clavulanic
acid/5 ml (after reconstitution); 400 mg

amoxicillin trihydrate and 57 mg clavulanic acid/5 ml (after reconstitution); 600 mg
amoxicillin trihydrate and 42.9 mg clavulanic acid/5 ml after reconstitution
*Tablets (chewable):* 125 mg amoxicillin
trihydrate, 31.25 mg clavulanic acid;
200 mg amoxicillin trihydrate, 28.5 mg
clavulanic acid; 250 mg amoxicillin trihydrate, 62.5 mg clavulanic acid; 400 mg
amoxicillin trihydrate, 57 mg clavulanic
acid
*Tablets (extended-release):* 1,000 mg
amoxicillin trihydrate, 62.5 mg clavulanic
acid
*Tablets (film-coated):* 250 mg amoxicillin
trihydrate, 125 mg clavulanic acid;
500 mg amoxicillin trihydrate, 125 mg
clavulanic acid; 875 mg amoxicillin trihydrate, 125 mg clavulanic acid

## INDICATIONS & DOSAGES
➤ **Recurrent or persistent acute otitis
media caused by *Streptococcus pneumoniae*, *Haemophilus influenzae*, or
*Moraxella catarrhalis* in patients exposed to antibiotics within the last 3
months, who are 2 years old or younger
or in day-care facilities**
*Children age 3 months and older:* 90 mg/
kg/day Augmentin ES-600 P.O., based on
amoxicillin component, q 12 hours for
10 days.
➤ **Lower respiratory tract infections,
otitis media, sinusitis, skin and skin-
structure infections, and UTIs caused
by susceptible strains of gram-positive
and gram-negative organisms**
*Adults and children weighing 40 kg
(88 lb) or more:* 250 mg P.O., based on
amoxicillin component, q 8 hours; or
500 mg q 12 hours. For more severe infections, 500 mg q 8 hours or 875 mg q
12 hours.
*Children age 3 months and older and
weighing less than 40 kg:* 20 to 45 mg/kg
P.O., based on amoxicillin component and
severity of infection, daily in divided doses q 8 to 12 hours.
*Children younger than age 3 months:*
30 mg/kg/day P.O., based on amoxicillin

---

component of the 125-mg/5-ml oral suspension, in divided doses q 12 hours.
*Adjust-a-dose:* Don't give the 875-mg tablet to patients with renal impairment and creatinine clearance less than 30 ml/minute. If clearance is 10 to 30 ml/minute, give 250 to 500 mg P.O. q 12 hours. If clearance is less than 10 ml/minute, give 250 to 500 mg P.O. q 24 hours. Give hemodialysis patients 250 to 500 mg P.O. q 24 hours with an additional dose both during and after dialysis.

➤ **Community-acquired pneumonia or acute bacterial sinusitis caused by *H. influenzae, M. catarrhalis, H. parainfluenzae, Klebsiella pneumoniae,* methicillin-susceptible *Staphylococcus aureus,* or *S. pneumoniae* with reduced susceptibility to penicillin**
*Adults and children age 16 and older:* 2,000 mg/125 mg Augmentin XR tablets q 12 hours for 7 to 10 days for pneumonia; 10 days for sinusitis.
*Adjust-a-dose:* In patients with creatinine clearance less than 30 ml/minute and hemodialysis patients, don't use Augmentin XR.

## ACTION

Prevents bacterial cell-wall synthesis during replication. Increases amoxicillin effectiveness by inactivating beta-lactamases, which destroy amoxicillin.

| Route | Onset | Peak | Duration |
|---|---|---|---|
| P.O. | Unknown | 1-2½ hr | 6-8 hr |
| P.O. (Augmentin ES-600) | Unknown | 1-4 hr | Unknown |
| P.O. (Augmentin XR) | Unknown | 1-6 hr | Unknown |

## ADVERSE REACTIONS

**CNS:** agitation, anxiety, insomnia, confusion, behavioral changes, dizziness.
**GI:** nausea, vomiting, *diarrhea,* indigestion, gastritis, stomatitis, glossitis, black hairy tongue, enterocolitis, *pseudomembranous colitis,* mucocutaneous candidiasis, abdominal pain.
**GU:** vaginitis, vaginal candidiasis.
**Hematologic:** anemia, *thrombocytopenia, thrombocytopenic purpura,* eosinophilia, *leukopenia, agranulocytosis.*

**Other:** hypersensitivity reactions *(anaphylaxis,* rash, urticaria, pruritus, *angioedema)* overgrowth of nonsusceptible organisms, serum sickness–like reaction.

## INTERACTIONS

**Drug-drug.** *Allopurinol:* May increase risk of rash. Monitor patient for rash.
*Hormonal contraceptives:* May decrease hormonal contraceptive effectiveness. Recommend additional form of contraception during penicillin therapy.
*Probenecid:* May increase levels of amoxicillin and other penicillins. Probenecid may be used for this purpose.
**Drug-herb.** *Khat:* May decrease antimicrobial effect of certain penicillins. Discourage khat chewing, or tell patient to take amoxicillin 2 hours after khat chewing.

## EFFECTS ON LAB TEST RESULTS

● May increase eosinophil count.
● May falsely decrease aminoglycoside level. May alter results of urine glucose tests that use cupric sulfate, such as Benedict's reagent or Clinitest.

## CONTRAINDICATIONS & CAUTIONS

● Contraindicated in patients hypersensitive to drug or other penicillins and in those with a history of amoxicillin-related cholestatic jaundice or hepatic dysfunction.
● Contraindicated in patients on hemodialysis and those with creatinine clearance less than 30 ml/minute.
● Use cautiously in patients with other drug allergies (especially to cephalosporins) because of possible cross-sensitivity and in those with mononucleosis because of high risk of maculopapular rash.
● Use cautiously in breast-feeding women; drug appears in breast milk.
● Use cautiously in hepatically impaired patients, and monitor the hepatic function of these patients.

## NURSING CONSIDERATIONS

● Before giving drug, ask patient about allergic reactions to penicillin. However, a negative history of penicillin allergy is no guarantee against an allergic reaction.

• Obtain specimen for culture and sensitivity tests before giving first dose. Therapy may begin pending results.
• Give drug at least 1 hour before a bacteriostatic antibiotic.
• Each Augmentin XR tablet contains 29.3 mg (1.27 mEq) of sodium.
• Augmentin XR isn't indicated for the treatment of infections caused by *S. pneumoniae* with penicillin MIC 4 mcg/ml or greater.
• If large doses are given or therapy is prolonged, bacterial or fungal superinfection may occur, especially in elderly, debilitated, or immunosuppressed patients.
• *Alert:* Don't interchange the oral suspensions because of varying clavulanic acid contents.
• Augmentin ES-600 is intended for pediatric patients age 3 months to 12 years with persistent or recurrent acute otitis media only.
• Avoid use of 250-mg tablet in children weighing less than 40 kg (88 lb). Use chewable form instead.
• *Alert:* Both 250- and 500-mg film-coated tablets contain the same amount of clavulanic acid (125 mg). Therefore, two 250-mg tablets aren't equivalent to one 500-mg tablet. Regular tablets aren't equivalent to Augmentin XR.
• This drug combination is particularly useful in clinical settings with a high prevalence of amoxicillin-resistant organisms.
• After reconstitution, refrigerate the oral suspension; discard after 10 days.
• *Alert:* Don't confuse amoxicillin with amoxapine.

**PATIENT TEACHING**
• Tell patient to take entire quantity of drug exactly as prescribed, even after feeling better.
• Instruct patient to take drug with food to prevent GI upset. If he's taking the oral suspension, tell him to keep drug refrigerated, to shake it well before administration, and to discard remaining drug after 10 days.
• Tell patient to call prescriber if a rash occurs because rash is a sign of an allergic reaction.

# amoxicillin trihydrate (amoxycillin trihydrate)
Alphamox‡, Amoxil⌀, Apo-Amoxi†, Cilamox‡, Moxacin‡, Novamoxin†, Nu-Amoxi†, Trimox

*Pregnancy risk category B*

## AVAILABLE FORMS
*Capsules:* 250 mg, 500 mg
*Oral suspension:* 50 mg/ml (pediatric drops), 125 mg/5 ml, 200 mg/5 ml, 250 mg/5 ml, 400 mg/5 ml (after reconstitution)
*Tablets (chewable):* 125 mg, 200 mg, 250 mg, 400 mg
*Tablets (film-coated):* 500 mg, 875 mg

## INDICATIONS & DOSAGES
➤ **Systemic infections, acute and chronic UTIs caused by susceptible strains of gram-positive and gram-negative organisms**
*Adults and children weighing 20 kg (44 lb) or more:* 250 to 500 mg P.O. q 8 hours.
*Children weighing less than 20 kg:* 20 mg/kg P.O. daily in divided doses q 8 hours; in severe infection, 40 mg/kg P.O. daily in divided doses q 8 hours or 500 mg to 1 g/m$^2$ P.O. in divided doses q 8 hours.
➤ **Uncomplicated gonorrhea**
*Adults and children weighing more than 45 kg (99 lb):* 3 g P.O. with 1 g probenecid given as a single dose.
*Children age 2 and older weighing less than 45 kg:* 50 mg/kg to a maximum of 3 g P.O. with 25 mg/kg to a maximum of 1 g of probenecid as a single dose. Don't give probenecid to children younger than age 2.
➤ **To prevent endocarditis in patients having dental, GI, and GU procedures**
*Adults:* 2 g P.O. 1 hour before procedure.
*Children:* 50 mg/kg P.O. 1 hour before procedure.
➤ **To prevent penicillin-susceptible anthrax after exposure**
*Adults and children older than age 9:* 500 mg P.O. t.i.d. for 60 days.
*Children younger than age 9:* 80 mg/kg daily P.O., divided t.i.d. for 60 days.

---

*Rapid onset*   †Canada   ‡Australia   ◇OTC   ◆Off-label use   ⌀Photoguide   *Liquid contains alcohol.

## ACTION
Inhibits cell-wall synthesis during bacterial multiplication.

| Route | Onset | Peak | Duration |
|-------|-------|------|----------|
| P.O. | Unknown | 1-2 hr | 6-8 hr |

## ADVERSE REACTIONS
**CNS:** lethargy, hallucinations, *seizures,* anxiety, confusion, agitation, depression, dizziness, fatigue.
**GI:** *nausea,* vomiting, *diarrhea,* glossitis, stomatitis, gastritis, enterocolitis, abdominal pain, *pseudomembranous colitis,* black hairy tongue.
**GU:** interstitial nephritis, nephropathy, vaginitis.
**Hematologic:** anemia, *thrombocytopenia, thrombocytopenic purpura,* eosinophilia, *leukopenia,* hemolytic anemia, *agranulocytosis.*
**Other:** hypersensitivity reactions, *anaphylaxis,* overgrowth of nonsusceptible organisms.

## INTERACTIONS
**Drug-drug.** *Allopurinol:* May increase risk of rash. Monitor patient for rash.
*Hormonal contraceptives:* May decrease hormonal contraceptive effectiveness. Recommend additional form of contraception during penicillin therapy.
*Probenecid:* May increase levels of amoxicillin and other penicillins. Probenecid may be used for this purpose.
**Drug-herb.** *Khat:* May decrease antimicrobial effect of certain penicillins. Discourage khat chewing, or tell patient to take amoxicillin 2 hours after khat chewing.

## EFFECTS ON LAB TEST RESULTS
• May increase eosinophil count. May decrease hemoglobin and granulocyte, platelet, and WBC counts.
• May falsely decrease aminoglycoside level. May alter results of urine glucose tests that use cupric sulfate such as Benedict's reagent or Clinitest.

## CONTRAINDICATIONS & CAUTIONS
• Contraindicated in patients hypersensitive to drug or other penicillins.

• Use cautiously in patients with other drug allergies (especially to cephalosporins) because of possible cross-sensitivity.
• Use cautiously in those with mononucleosis because of high risk of maculopapular rash.

## NURSING CONSIDERATIONS
• Obtain specimen for culture and sensitivity tests before giving first dose. Therapy may begin pending results.
• Before giving, ask patient about allergic reactions to penicillin. A negative history of penicillin allergy is no guarantee against allergic reaction.
• If large doses are given or if therapy is prolonged, bacterial or fungal superinfection may occur, especially in elderly, debilitated, or immunosuppressed patients.
• Store Trimox oral suspension in refrigerator, if possible. It also may be stored at room temperature for up to 2 weeks. Be sure to check individual product labels for storage information.
• Amoxicillin usually causes fewer cases of diarrhea than does ampicillin.
• *Alert:* Don't confuse amoxicillin with amoxapine.

## PATIENT TEACHING
• Tell patient to take entire quantity of drug exactly as prescribed, even after he feels better.
• Instruct patient to take drug with or without food.
• Tell patient to notify prescriber if rash, fever, or chills develop. A rash is the most common allergic reaction, especially if allopurinol is also being taken.
• Tell parent to place pediatric drops directly on child's tongue for swallowing or add to formula, milk, fruit juice, water, ginger ale, or a cold drink; patient should take immediately and consume entirely.

# ampicillin
Apo-Ampi†, Novo Ampicillin†,
Nu-Ampi†

# ampicillin sodium
Ampicin†, Ampicyn‡, Penbritin†

# ampicillin trihydrate
Penbritin†, Principen

*Pregnancy risk category B*

## AVAILABLE FORMS
*Capsules:* 250 mg, 500 mg
*Injection:* 250 mg, 500 mg, 1 g, 2 g
*Oral suspension:* 125 mg/5 ml, 250 mg/
5 ml

## INDICATIONS & DOSAGES
➤ **Respiratory tract or skin and skin-structure infections**
*Adults and children weighing 40 kg
(88 lb) or more:* 250 to 500 mg P.O. q
6 hours.
*Children weighing less than 40 kg:* 25 to
50 mg/kg/day P.O. in equally divided doses q 6 hours. Pediatric dosages shouldn't
exceed recommended adult dosages.
➤ **GI infections or UTIs**
*Adults and children weighing 40 kg
(88 lb) or more:* 500 mg P.O. q 6 hours.
For severe infections, larger doses may be
needed.
*Children weighing less than 40 kg:* 50 to
100 mg/kg/day P.O. in equally divided
doses q 6 hours.
➤ **Bacterial meningitis or septicemia**
*Adults:* 150 to 200 mg/kg/day I.V. in divided doses q 3 to 4 hours. May be given
I.M. after 3 days of I.V. therapy. Maximum
recommended daily dose is 14 g.
*Children:* 100 to 200 mg/kg I.V. daily in
divided doses q 3 to 4 hours. Give I.V. for
3 days; then give I.M.
➤ **Uncomplicated gonorrhea**
*Adults and children weighing more than
45 kg (99 lb):* 3.5 g P.O. with 1 g
probenecid given as a single dose.
➤ **To prevent endocarditis in patients
having dental, GI, and GU procedures**
*Adults:* 2 g I.M. or I.V. within 30 minutes
before procedure. For high risk patients,
also give 1.5 mg/kg gentamicin 30 minutes before the procedure; 6 hours later,
ampicillin 1 g I.M. or I.V. or amoxicillin
1 g P.O.
*Children:* 50 mg/kg I.M. or I.V. within
30 minutes before procedure. For high risk
patients, also give 1.5 mg/kg gentamicin
30 minutes before the procedure; 6 hours
later, ampicillin 25 mg/kg I.M. or I.V. or
amoxicillin 25 mg/kg P.O.
*Adjust-a-dose:* In patients who have severe renal impairment, increase drug interval to 12 hours. Use same dose.

## I.V. ADMINISTRATION
● For I.V. injection, reconstitute with bacteriostatic water for injection. Use 5 ml for
the 250-mg, or 500-mg vials; 7.4 ml for
the 1-g vials; or 14.8 ml for the 2-g vials.
Give direct I.V. injections over 10 to 15
minutes to avoid the possibility of seizures. Don't exceed 100 mg/minute.
● For intermittent infusion, dilute in 50 to
100 ml of normal saline solution for injection and give over 15 to 30 minutes.
● *Alert:* Don't mix with solutions containing dextrose or fructose; these substances
promote rapid breakdown of ampicillin.
● Use first dilution within 1 hour. Follow
manufacturer's directions for stability data
when ampicillin is further diluted for I.V.
infusion.
● Give I.V. intermittently to prevent vein
irritation. Change site every 48 hours.

## ACTION
Inhibits cell-wall synthesis during bacterial multiplication.

| Route | Onset | Peak | Duration |
|-------|-------|------|----------|
| P.O. | Unknown | 2 hr | 6-8 hr |
| I.V. | Immediate | Immediate | Unknown |
| I.M. | Unknown | 1 hr | Unknown |

## ADVERSE REACTIONS
**CNS:** lethargy, hallucinations, *seizures,*
anxiety, confusion, agitation, depression,
dizziness, fatigue.
**CV:** vein irritation, thrombophlebitis.
**GI:** *nausea,* vomiting, *diarrhea,* glossitis,
stomatitis, gastritis, abdominal pain, enterocolitis, *pseudomembranous colitis,*
black hairy tongue.
**GU:** interstitial nephritis, nephropathy,
vaginitis.
**Hematologic:** anemia, *thrombocytopenia,
thrombocytopenia purpura,* eosinophilia,

*leukopenia,* hemolytic anemia, *agranulocytosis.*
**Skin:** pain at injection site.
**Other:** hypersensitivity reactions, overgrowth of nonsusceptible organisms.

## INTERACTIONS
**Drug-drug.** *Allopurinol:* May increase risk of rash. Monitor patient for rash.
*Hormonal contraceptives:* May decrease hormonal contraceptive effectiveness. Recommend additional form of contraception during penicillin therapy.
*Probenecid:* May increase levels of ampicillin and other penicillins. Probenecid may be used for this purpose.

## EFFECTS ON LAB TEST RESULTS
● May increase eosinophil count. May decrease hemoglobin and platelet, WBC, and granulocyte counts.
● May falsely decrease aminoglycoside level. May alter results of urine glucose tests that use cupric sulfate such as Benedict's reagent or Clinitest.

## CONTRAINDICATIONS & CAUTIONS
● Contraindicated in patients hypersensitive to drug or other penicillins.
● Use cautiously in patients with other drug allergies (especially to cephalosporins) because of possible cross-sensitivity and in those with mononucleosis because of high risk of maculopapular rash.

## NURSING CONSIDERATIONS
● Before giving drug, ask patient about allergic reactions to penicillin. A negative history of penicillin allergy is no guarantee against a future allergic reaction.
● Obtain specimen for culture and sensitivity tests before giving first dose. Therapy may begin pending results.
● Give drug I.M. or I.V. only if prescribed and the infection is severe or if patient can't take oral dose.
● Give drug 1 to 2 hours before or 2 to 3 hours after meals. When given orally, drug may cause GI disturbances. Food may interfere with absorption.
● Monitor sodium level because each gram of ampicillin contains 2.9 mEq of sodium.
● If large doses are given or if therapy is prolonged, bacterial or fungal superinfec-

tion may occur, especially in elderly, debilitated, or immunosuppressed patients.
● Watch for signs and symptoms of hypersensitivity, such as erythematous maculopapular rash, urticaria, and anaphylaxis.
● Decrease dosage in patients with impaired renal function.
● In pediatric meningitis, ampicillin may be given with parenteral chloramphenicol for 24 hours pending cultures.
● To prevent bacterial endocarditis in patients at high risk, give drug with gentamicin.

## PATIENT TEACHING
● Tell patient to take entire quantity of drug exactly as prescribed, even after he feels better.
● Instruct patient to take oral form on an empty stomach 1 hour before or 2 hours after meals.
● Inform patient to notify prescriber if rash, fever, or chills develop. A rash is the most common allergic reaction, especially if allopurinol is also being taken.
● Advise patient to report discomfort at I.V. injection site.

# ampicillin sodium and sulbactam sodium
Unasyn

*Pregnancy risk category B*

## AVAILABLE FORMS
*Injection:* Vials and piggyback vials containing 1.5 g (1 g ampicillin sodium with 0.5 g sulbactam sodium), 3 g (2 g ampicillin sodium with 1 g sulbactam sodium).

## INDICATIONS & DOSAGES
➤ **Intra-abdominal, gynecologic, and skin-structure infections caused by susceptible strains**
*Adults and children weighing more than 40 kg (88 lb):* 1.5 to 3 g I.M. or I.V. q 6 hours. Maximum daily dose is 12 g.
*Children age 1 and older weighing less than 40 kg:* 300 mg/kg daily I.V. in divided doses q 6 hours. Don't exceed 4 g daily.
*Adjust-a-dose:* For renally impaired patients with creatinine clearance of 15 to 29 ml/minute, give 1.5 to 3 g q 12 hours;

if clearance is 5 to 14 ml/minute, give 1.5 to 3 g q 24 hours.

## I.V. ADMINISTRATION
• When preparing I.V. injection, reconstitute powder with one of the following diluents: normal saline solution, sterile water for injection, $D_5W$, lactated Ringer's injection, 1/6 M sodium lactate, dextrose 5% in half-normal saline solution for injection, and 10% invert sugar. Stability varies with diluent, temperature, and concentration of solution.
• After reconstitution, let vials stand for a few minutes to allow foam to dissipate. This will permit visual inspection of contents for particles.
• When giving I.V., don't add or mix with other drugs because they might be incompatible.
• Give drug at least 1 hour before a bacteriostatic antibiotic.
• *Alert:* Give I.V. dose by slow injection over 10 to 15 minutes or dilute in 50 to 100 ml of a compatible diluent, and infuse over 15 to 30 minutes. If permitted, give intermittently to prevent vein irritation. Change site every 48 hours.

## ACTION
Inhibits cell-wall synthesis during bacterial multiplication.

| Route | Onset | Peak | Duration |
|---|---|---|---|
| I.V. | Immediate | 15 min | Unknown |
| I.M. | Unknown | Unknown | Unknown |

## ADVERSE REACTIONS
**CV:** thrombophlebitis, vein irritation.
**GI:** *nausea,* vomiting, *diarrhea,* glossitis, stomatitis, gastritis, black hairy tongue, enterocolitis, ***pseudomembranous colitis.***
**Hematologic:** anemia, ***thrombocytopenia, thrombocytopenic purpura,*** eosinophilia, ***leukopenia, agranulocytosis.***
**Skin:** *pain at injection site.*
**Other:** hypersensitivity reactions, ***anaphylaxis,*** overgrowth of nonsusceptible organisms.

## INTERACTIONS
**Drug-drug.** *Allopurinol:* May increase risk of rash. Monitor patient for rash.
*Hormonal contraceptives:* May decrease hormonal contraceptive effectiveness.

Recommend additional form of contraception during penicillin therapy.
*Probenecid:* May increase ampicillin level. Probenecid may be used for this purpose.

## EFFECTS ON LAB TEST RESULTS
• May increase BUN, creatinine, ALT, AST, alkaline phosphatase, bilirubin, LDH, CK, and GGT levels. May transiently decrease estradiol, conjugated estrone, conjugated estriol, and estriol glucuronide levels in pregnant women.
• May increase eosinophil count. May decrease hemoglobin and platelet, WBC, and granulocyte counts.
• May alter results of urine glucose tests that use cupric sulfate, such as Benedict's reagent or Clinitest.

## CONTRAINDICATIONS & CAUTIONS
• Contraindicated in patients hypersensitive to drug or other penicillins.
• Use cautiously in patients with other drug allergies (especially to cephalosporins) because of possible cross-sensitivity and in those with mononucleosis because of high risk of maculopapular rash.

## NURSING CONSIDERATIONS
• Before giving drug, ask patient about allergic reactions to penicillin. However, a negative history of penicillin allergy is no guarantee against future allergic reaction.
• Obtain specimen for culture and sensitivity tests before giving first dose. Therapy may begin pending results.
• Dosage is expressed as total drug. Each 1.5-g vial contains 1 g ampicillin sodium and 0.5 g sulbactam sodium.
• Decrease dosage in patients with impaired renal function.
• For I.M. injection, reconstitute with sterile water for injection or 0.5% or 2% lidocaine hydrochloride injection. Add 3.2 ml to a 1.5-g vial (or 6.4 ml to a 3-g vial) to yield a concentration of 375 mg/ml. Give deeply.
• Don't use I.M. route in children.
• Monitor liver function test results during therapy, especially in patients with impaired liver function.
• If large doses are given or if therapy is prolonged, bacterial or fungal superinfec-

tion may occur, especially in elderly, debilitated, or immunosuppressed patients.

**PATIENT TEACHING**
● Tell patient to report rash, fever, or chills. A rash is the most common allergic reaction.
● Advise patient to report discomfort at I.V. insertion site.
● Warn patient that I.M. injection may cause pain at injection site.

---

## nafcillin sodium

*Pregnancy risk category B*

**AVAILABLE FORMS**
*I.V. infusion:* 1 g, 2 g

**INDICATIONS & DOSAGES**
➤ **Systemic infections caused by susceptible organisms (methicillin-sensitive *Staphylococcus aureus*)**
*Adults:* 500 mg to 1 g I.V. q 4 hours, depending on severity of infection.
*Infants and children older than age 1 month:* 50 to 200 mg/kg I.V. daily in divided doses q 4 to 6 hours, depending on severity of infection.
*Neonates older than 7 days weighing more than 2 kg (4.4 lb):* 25 mg/kg I.V. q 6 hours.
*Neonates older than 7 days weighing less than 2 kg:* 25 mg/kg I.V. q 8 hours.
*Neonates age 7 days or younger weighing more than 2 kg:* 25 mg/kg I.V. q 8 hours.
*Neonates age 7 days or younger weighing less than 2 kg:* 25 mg/kg I.V. q 12 hours.
➤ **Meningitis**
*Adults:* 100 to 200 mg/kg/day I.V. in divided doses q 4 to 6 hours.
*Neonates older than 7 days weighing more than 2 kg (4.4 lb):* 50 mg/kg I.V. q 6 hours.
*Neonates older than 7 days weighing less than 2 kg:* 50 mg/kg I.V. q 8 hours.
*Neonates age 7 days or younger weighing more than 2 kg:* 50 mg/kg I.V. q 8 hours.
*Neonates age 7 days or younger weighing less than 2 kg:* 50 mg/kg I.V. q 12 hours.
➤ **Acute or chronic osteomyelitis caused by susceptible organism**
*Adults:* 1 to 2 g I.V. q 4 hours for 4 to 8 weeks.

*Children older than age 1 month:* 100 to 200 mg/kg/day in equally divided doses q 4 to 6 hours for 4 to 8 weeks.
➤ **Native valve endocarditis caused by susceptible organism**
*Adults:* 2 g I.V. q 4 hours for 4 to 6 weeks, combined with gentamicin.
*Children older than age 1 month:* 100 to 200 mg/kg/day in equally divided doses q 4 to 6 hours for 4 to 8 weeks in combination with gentamicin.

**I.V. ADMINISTRATION**
● Check container for leaks, cloudiness, or precipitate before use. Discard if present.
● Give over 30 to 60 minutes.
● Change site every 48 hours to prevent vein irritation.

**ACTION**
Inhibits cell-wall synthesis during bacterial multiplication.

| Route | Onset | Peak | Duration |
|-------|-------|------|----------|
| I.V. | Immediate | Immediate | Unknown |

**ADVERSE REACTIONS**
**CV:** thrombophlebitis, vein irritation.
**GI:** *nausea*, vomiting, diarrhea.
**Hematologic:** *neutropenia, agranulocytosis, thrombocytopenia.*
**Other:** hypersensitivity reactions, *anaphylaxis.*

**INTERACTIONS**
**Drug-drug.** *Aminoglycosides:* May have synergistic effect; drugs are chemically and physically incompatible. Don't combine in same I.V. solution.
*Hormonal contraceptives:* May decrease hormonal contraceptive effectiveness. Recommend additional form of contraception during penicillin therapy.
*Probenecid:* May increase nafcillin level. Probenecid may be used for this purpose.
*Rifampin:* May cause dose-dependent antagonism. Monitor patient closely.
*Warfarin:* May increase risk of bleeding when used with nafcillin. Monitor PT and INR closely.

**EFFECTS ON LAB TEST RESULTS**
● May decrease neutrophil, granulocyte, and platelet counts.

---

## CONTRAINDICATIONS & CAUTIONS
● Contraindicated in patients hypersensitive to drug or other penicillins.
● Use cautiously in patients with GI distress and in those with other drug allergies (especially to cephalosporins) because of possible cross-sensitivity.

## NURSING CONSIDERATIONS
● Before giving drug, ask patient about allergic reactions to penicillin.
● Obtain specimen for culture and sensitivity tests before giving first dose. Therapy may begin pending results.
● If large doses are given or if therapy is prolonged, bacterial or fungal superinfection may occur, especially in elderly, debilitated, or immunosuppressed patients.
● Monitor sodium level because each gram of nafcillin contains 2.9 mEq of sodium.
● Monitor WBC counts twice weekly in patients receiving nafcillin for longer than 2 weeks. Neutropenia commonly occurs in the third week.
● An abnormal urinalysis result may indicate drug-induced interstitial nephritis.

## PATIENT TEACHING
● Tell patient to report burning or irritation at the I.V. site.

---

## penicillin G benzathine
## (benzathine benzylpenicillin)
Bicillin L-A, Permapen

*Pregnancy risk category B*

## AVAILABLE FORMS
*Injection:* 600,000 units/ml, 1,200,000 units/2 ml, 2,400,000 units/4 ml

## INDICATIONS & DOSAGES
➤ **Congenital syphilis**
*Children younger than age 2:* 50,000 units/kg I.M. as a single dose.
➤ **Group A streptococcal upper respiratory tract infections**
*Adults:* 1.2 million units I.M. as a single injection.
*Children weighing 27 kg (59.5 lb) or more:* 900,000 units I.M. as a single injection.

*Children weighing less than 27 kg:* 300,000 to 600,000 units I.M. as a single injection.
➤ **To prevent poststreptococcal rheumatic fever**
*Adults and children:* 1.2 million units I.M. once monthly or 600,000 units I.M. q 2 weeks.
➤ **Syphilis of less than 1 year's duration**
*Adults:* 2.4 million units I.M. as a single dose.
*Children:* 50,000 units/kg I.M. as a single dose. Don't exceed adult dosage.
➤ **Syphilis of more than 1 year's duration**
*Adults:* 2.4 million units I.M. weekly for 3 weeks.
*Children:* 50,000 units/kg I.M. weekly for 3 weeks.

## ACTION
Inhibits cell-wall synthesis during bacterial multiplication.

| Route | Onset | Peak | Duration |
|-------|-------|------|----------|
| I.M. | Unknown | 13-24 hr | 1-4 wk |

## ADVERSE REACTIONS
**CNS:** neuropathy, *seizures,* lethargy, hallucinations, anxiety, confusion, agitation, depression, dizziness, fatigue.
**GI:** nausea, vomiting, enterocolitis, *pseudomembranous colitis.*
**GU:** interstitial nephritis, nephropathy.
**Hematologic:** eosinophilia, hemolytic anemia, *thrombocytopenia, leukopenia,* anemia, *agranulocytosis.*
**Skin:** maculopapular rash, exfoliative dermatitis.
**Other:** hypersensitivity reactions, *anaphylaxis,* pain, sterile abscess at injection site.

## INTERACTIONS
**Drug-drug.** *Aminoglycosides:* Physical and chemical incompatibility. Give separately.
*Colestipol:* May decrease penicillin G benzathine level. Give penicillin G benzathine 1 hour before or 4 hours after colestipol.
*Hormonal contraceptives:* May decrease hormonal contraceptive effectiveness.

---

Recommend additional form of contraception during penicillin therapy.
*Probenecid:* May increase penicillin level. Probenecid may be used for this purpose.
*Tetracycline:* May antagonize penicillin G benzathine effects. Avoid using together.

**EFFECTS ON LAB TEST RESULTS**
● May increase eosinophil count. May decrease hemoglobin and platelet, WBC, and granulocyte counts. May cause positive Coombs' test results.
● May falsely decrease aminoglycoside level. May cause false-positive CSF protein test results. May alter urine glucose testing using cupric sulfate (Benedict's reagent).

**CONTRAINDICATIONS & CAUTIONS**
● Contraindicated in patients hypersensitive to drug or other penicillins.
● Use cautiously in patients allergic to other drugs, especially to cephalosporins, because of possible cross-sensitivity.

**NURSING CONSIDERATIONS**
● Before giving drug, ask patient about allergic reactions to penicillin.
● Obtain specimen for culture and sensitivity tests before giving first dose. Therapy may begin pending results.
● Shake well before injection.
● **Alert:** Never give by I.V. route. Inadvertent I.V. administration has caused cardiac arrest and death.
● Inject deeply into upper outer quadrant of buttocks in adults and in midlateral thigh in infants and small children. Rotate injection sites. Avoid injection into or near major nerves or blood vessels to prevent permanent neurovascular damage.
● Give drug at least 1 hour before a bacteriostatic antibiotic.
● Drug's extremely slow absorption time makes allergic reactions difficult to treat.
● If large doses are given or if therapy is prolonged, bacterial or fungal superinfection may occur, especially in elderly, debilitated, or immunosuppressed patients.
● **Alert:** Don't confuse drug with Polycillin, penicillamine, or the various types of penicillin.

**PATIENT TEACHING**
● Tell patient to report adverse reactions promptly.
● Inform patient that fever and increased WBC count are the most common reactions.
● Warn patient that I.M. injection may be painful but that ice applied to the site may ease discomfort.

━━━━━━━━━━━━━━━━━━━━━

# penicillin G potassium (benzylpenicillin potassium)
Megacillin†, Pfizerpen

*Pregnancy risk category B*

**AVAILABLE FORMS**
*Injection:* 1 million units, 5 million units, 20 million units
*Oral suspension:* 250,000 units†, 500,000 units†
*Premixed injection:* 1 million units/50 ml, 2 million units/50 ml, 3 million units/50 ml
*Tablets:* 500,000 units†

**INDICATIONS & DOSAGES**
➤ **Moderate to severe systemic infection**
*Adults and children age 12 and older:* Highly individualized; 1.6 to 3.2 million units P.O. daily in divided doses q 6 hours; 1.2 to 24 million units I.M. or I.V. daily in divided doses q 4 to 6 hours.
*Children younger than age 12:* 25,000 to 100,000 units/kg P.O. daily in divided doses q 6 hours; or 25,000 to 400,000 units/kg I.M. or I.V. daily in divided doses q 4 to 6 hours.
➤ **Anthrax**
*Adults:* 5 to 20 million units I.V. daily in divided doses q 4 to 6 hours, for at least 14 days after symptoms abate. Or, 80,000 units/kg in the first hour, followed by a maintenance dose of 320,000 units/kg/day. The average adult dosage is 4 million units q 4 hours or 2 million units q 2 hours.
*Children:* 100,000 to 150,000 units/kg/day I.V. in divided doses q 4 to 6 hours for at least 14 days after symptoms abate.
**Adjust-a-dose:** For patients with renal impairment, refer to the table on the next page. If patient is uremic and creatinine

clearance is more than 10 ml/minute, give full loading dose, then half the loading dose q 4 to 5 hours for additional doses.

| Creatinine clearance (ml/min) | Dosage (after full loading dose) |
|---|---|
| 10-50 | Usual dose q 8-12 hr |
| < 10 | 50% of usual dose q 8-10 hr; or, give usual dose q 12-18 hr |

## I.V. ADMINISTRATION
● Reconstitute drug with sterile water for injection, $D_5W$, or normal saline solution for injection. Volume of diluent varies with manufacturer.
● For intermittent I.V. infusion, give drug over 1 to 2 hours.
● For continuous I.V. infusion, add reconstituted solution of drug to 1 to 2 L of compatible I.V. solution. Determine the volume of fluid and rate of administration required by the patient in a 24-hour period, and add the ordered drug dose to this fluid.

## ACTION
Inhibits cell-wall synthesis during bacterial multiplication.

| Route | Onset | Peak | Duration |
|---|---|---|---|
| P.O. | Unknown | 30-60 min | Unknown |
| I.V. | Immediate | Immediate | Unknown |
| I.M. | Unknown | 15-30 min | Unknown |

## ADVERSE REACTIONS
**CNS:** neuropathy, *seizures,* lethargy, hallucinations, anxiety, confusion, agitation, depression, dizziness, fatigue.
**CV:** thrombophlebitis.
**GI:** nausea, vomiting, enterocolitis, *pseudomembranous colitis.*
**GU:** interstitial nephritis, nephropathy.
**Hematologic:** hemolytic anemia, *leukopenia, thrombocytopenia,* anemia, eosinophilia, *agranulocytosis.*
**Metabolic:** *possible severe potassium poisoning.*
**Skin:** maculopapular eruptions, exfoliative dermatitis, pain at injection site.
**Other:** hypersensitivity reactions, *anaphylaxis,* overgrowth of nonsusceptible organisms.

## INTERACTIONS
**Drug-drug.** *Aminoglycosides:* Physically and chemically incompatible. Give separately.
*Colestipol:* May decrease penicillin G potassium level. Give penicillin G potassium 1 hour before or 4 hours after colestipol.
*Hormonal contraceptives:* May decrease hormonal contraceptive effectiveness. Recommend additional form of contraception during penicillin therapy.
*Potassium-sparing diuretics:* May increase risk of hyperkalemia. Avoid using together.
*Probenecid:* May increase penicillin level. Probenecid may be used for this purpose.

## EFFECTS ON LAB TEST RESULTS
● May increase potassium level.
● May increase eosinophil count. May decrease hemoglobin and platelet, WBC, and granulocyte counts. May cause positive Coombs' test result.
● May falsely decrease aminoglycoside levels. May cause false-positive CSF protein test result. May alter urine glucose testing using cupric sulfate (Benedict's reagent).

## CONTRAINDICATIONS & CAUTIONS
● Contraindicated in patients hypersensitive to drug or other penicillins.
● Use cautiously in patients with other drug allergies, especially to cephalosporins, because of possible cross-sensitivity.

## NURSING CONSIDERATIONS
● Before giving drug, ask patient about allergic reactions to penicillin.
● Obtain specimen for culture and sensitivity tests before giving first dose. Therapy may begin pending results.
● For I.M. injection, give deeply into large muscle; may be extremely painful.
● Give P.O. formulation 1 to 2 hours before or 2 to 3 hours after meals. When given orally, drug may cause GI disturbances. Food may interfere with absorption.
● Monitor renal function closely. Patients with poor renal function are predisposed to high blood levels of drug.

• Monitor potassium and sodium levels closely in patients receiving more than 10 million units I.V. daily.
• Observe patient closely. With large doses and prolonged therapy, bacterial or fungal superinfection may occur, especially in elderly, debilitated, or immunosuppressed patients.
• *Alert:* Don't confuse drug with Polycillin, penicillamine, or the various types of penicillin.

## PATIENT TEACHING
• Tell patient taking oral form to take entire amount exactly as prescribed, even after he feels better.
• Instruct patient to take oral drug on empty stomach.
• Tell patient to notify prescriber if rash, fever, or chills develop. A rash is the most common allergic reaction.
• Warn patient that I.M. injection may be painful but that ice applied to the site may help alleviate discomfort.

---

# penicillin G procaine (benzylpenicillin procaine)
Ayercillin†, Wycillin

*Pregnancy risk category B*

## AVAILABLE FORMS
*Injection:* 600,000 units/ml, 1,200,000 units/ml

## INDICATIONS & DOSAGES
➤ **Moderate to severe systemic infection**
*Adults:* 600,000 to 1.2 million units I.M. daily for a minimum of 10 days.
*Children older than age 1 month:* 25,000 to 50,000 units/kg I.M. daily in a single dose.
➤ **Uncomplicated gonorrhea**
*Adults:* 1 g probenecid P.O.; after 30 minutes, 4.8 million units of penicillin G procaine I.M. divided between two injection sites as a single dose.
➤ **Anthrax caused by *Bacillus anthracis*, including inhalation anthrax after exposure**
*Adults:* 1,200,000 units I.M. q 12 hours.
*Children:* 25,000 units/kg I.M.; not to exceed 1,200,000 units q 12 hours.

➤ **Cutaneous anthrax**
*Adults:* 600,000 to 1,000,000 units I.M. daily.

## ACTION
Inhibits cell-wall synthesis during bacterial multiplication.

| Route | Onset | Peak | Duration |
|-------|-------|------|----------|
| I.M. | Unknown | 1-4 hr | 1-5 days |

## ADVERSE REACTIONS
**CNS:** *seizures,* lethargy, hallucinations, anxiety, confusion, agitation, depression, dizziness, fatigue.
**GI:** nausea, vomiting, enterocolitis, *pseudomembranous colitis.*
**GU:** interstitial nephritis, nephropathy.
**Hematologic:** *thrombocytopenia, hemolytic anemia, leukopenia,* anemia, eosinophilia, *agranulocytosis.*
**Musculoskeletal:** arthralgia.
**Other:** hypersensitivity reactions, *anaphylaxis,* overgrowth of nonsusceptible organisms.

## INTERACTIONS
**Drug-drug.** *Aminoglycosides:* Physically and chemically incompatible. Give separately.
*Colestipol:* May decrease penicillin G procaine level. Give penicillin G procaine 1 hour before or 4 hours after colestipol.
*Hormonal contraceptives:* May decrease hormonal contraceptive effectiveness. Recommend additional form of contraception during penicillin therapy.
*Probenecid:* May increase penicillin level. Probenecid may be used for this purpose.

## EFFECTS ON LAB TEST RESULTS
• May increase eosinophil count. May decrease hemoglobin and platelet, WBC, and granulocyte counts.

## CONTRAINDICATIONS & CAUTIONS
• Contraindicated in patients hypersensitive to drug or other penicillins.
• Use cautiously in patients with other drug allergies, especially to cephalosporins, because of possible cross-sensitivity. Some formulations contain sulfites, which may cause allergic reactions in sensitive people.

---

Reactions may be *common,* uncommon, *life-threatening,* or COMMON AND LIFE-THREATENING.

## NURSING CONSIDERATIONS
● Before giving drug, ask patient about allergic reactions to penicillin.
● Obtain specimen for culture and sensitivity tests before giving first dose. Therapy may begin pending results.
● Give deep I.M. in upper outer quadrant of buttocks in adults; in midlateral thigh in small children. Rotate injection sites. Don't give S.C. Don't massage injection site. Avoid injection near major nerves or blood vessels to prevent permanent neurovascular damage.
● *Alert:* Continue postexposure treatment for inhalation anthrax for 60 days. Prescriber should consider the risk-benefit ratio of continuing penicillin longer than 2 weeks, compared with switching to an effective alternate drug.
● *Alert:* Never give by I.V. route. Inadvertent I.V. administration has resulted in death from CNS toxicity.
● Allergic reactions are hard to treat because of drug's slow absorption rate.
● Monitor renal and hematopoietic function periodically.
● If large doses are given or if therapy is prolonged, bacterial or fungal superinfection may occur, especially in elderly, debilitated, or immunosuppressed patients.
● Treatment duration depends on site and cause of infection.
● *Alert:* Don't confuse drug with Polycillin, penicillamine, or the various types of penicillin.

## PATIENT TEACHING
● Tell patient to report adverse reactions promptly. A rash is the most common allergic reaction.
● Warn patient that I.M. injection may be painful but that ice applied to the site may help alleviate discomfort.

---

## penicillin G sodium (benzylpenicillin sodium)
Crystapen†

*Pregnancy risk category B*

---

### AVAILABLE FORMS
*Injection:* 5 million-unit vial

## INDICATIONS & DOSAGES
➤ **Moderate to severe systemic infection**
*Adults and children age 12 and older:* 1.2 to 24 million units daily I.M. or I.V. in divided doses q 4 to 6 hours.
*Children younger than age 12:* 25,000 to 400,000 units/kg daily I.M. or I.V. in divided doses q 4 to 6 hours.
➤ **Neurosyphilis**
*Adults:* 18 to 24 million units I.V. daily in divided doses q 4 hours for 10 to 14 days.
*Adjust-a-dose:* For patients with renal impairment, refer to table below. If patient is uremic and creatinine clearance is more than 10 ml/minute, give full loading dose, then half the loading dose q 4 to 5 hours for additional doses.

| Creatinine clearance (ml/min) | Dosage (after full loading dose) |
|---|---|
| 10-50 | Usual dose q 8-12 hr |
| < 10 | 50% of usual dose q 8-10 hr; or, give usual dose q 12-18 hr |

## I.V. ADMINISTRATION
● Reconstitute drug with sterile water for injection, normal saline solution for injection, or $D_5W$. Check manufacturer's instructions for volume of diluent necessary to produce desired drug level.
● Give by intermittent I.V. infusion: Dilute drug in 50 to 100 ml, and give over 30 minutes to 2 hours q 4 to 6 hours.
● In neonates and children, give divided doses over 15 to 30 minutes.

## ACTION
Inhibits cell-wall synthesis during bacterial multiplication.

| Route | Onset | Peak | Duration |
|---|---|---|---|
| I.V. | Immediate | Immediate | Unknown |
| I.M. | Unknown | 15-30 min | Unknown |

## ADVERSE REACTIONS
**CNS:** neuropathy, *seizures,* lethargy, hallucinations, anxiety, confusion, agitation, depression, dizziness, fatigue.
**CV:** *heart failure,* thrombophlebitis.
**GI:** nausea, vomiting, enterocolitis, *pseudomembranous colitis.*
**GU:** interstitial colitis, nephropathy.

---

**Hematologic:** hemolytic anemia, *leukopenia, thrombocytopenia, agranulocytosis,* anemia, eosinophilia.
**Musculoskeletal:** arthralgia.
**Other:** hypersensitivity reactions, *anaphylaxis,* overgrowth of nonsusceptible organisms, pain at injection site, vein irritation.

## INTERACTIONS
**Drug-drug.** *Aminoglycosides:* Physically and chemically incompatible. Give separately.
*Colestipol:* May decrease penicillin G sodium level. Give penicillin G sodium 1 hour before or 4 hours after colestipol.
*Hormonal contraceptives:* May decrease hormonal contraceptive effectiveness. Recommend additional form of contraception during penicillin therapy.
*Probenecid:* May increase penicillin level. Probenecid may be used for this purpose.

## EFFECTS ON LAB TEST RESULTS
● May increase eosinophil count. May decrease hemoglobin and platelet, WBC, and granulocyte counts. May cause positive Coombs' test result.
● May falsely decrease aminoglycoside level. May cause false-positive CSF protein test result. May alter urine glucose testing using cupric sulfate (Benedict's reagent).

## CONTRAINDICATIONS & CAUTIONS
● Contraindicated in patients hypersensitive to drug or other penicillins and in those on sodium-restricted diets.
● Use cautiously in patients with other drug allergies, especially to cephalosporins, because of possible cross-allergenicity.

## NURSING CONSIDERATIONS
● Before giving drug, ask patient about allergic reactions to penicillin.
● Obtain specimen for culture and sensitivity tests before giving first dose. Therapy may begin pending results.
● Observe patient closely. With large doses and prolonged therapy, bacterial or fungal superinfection may occur, especially in elderly, debilitated, or immunosuppressed patients.

● *Alert:* Don't confuse drug with Polycillin, penicillamine, or the various types of penicillin.

## PATIENT TEACHING
● Tell patient to report adverse reactions promptly.
● Instruct patient to report discomfort at I.V. site.
● Warn patient receiving I.M. injection that the injection may be painful but that ice applied to site may help alleviate discomfort.

---

# penicillin V potassium (phenoxymethylpenicillin potassium)
Abbocillin VK‡, Apo-Pen VK†, Cilicaine VK‡, Nadopen-V 200†, Nadopen-V 400†, Novo-Pen-VK†, Nu-Pen-VK†, Pen-Vee†, PVF K†, Veetids

*Pregnancy risk category B*

## AVAILABLE FORMS
*Capsules:* 250 mg‡
*Oral suspension:* 125 mg/5 ml, 250 mg/5 ml (after reconstitution)
*Tablets:* 250 mg, 500 mg
*Tablets (film-coated):* 250 mg, 500 mg

## INDICATIONS & DOSAGES
➤ **Mild to moderate systemic infections**
*Adults and children age 12 and older:* 125 to 500 mg or P.O. q 6 hours.
*Children younger than age 12:* 15 to 62.5 mg/kg P.O. daily in divided doses q 6 to 8 hours.
➤ **To prevent recurrent rheumatic fever**
*Adults and children:* 250 mg P.O. b.i.d.
➤ **Erythema chronica migrans in Lyme disease ♦**
*Adults:* 250 to 500 mg P.O. q.i.d. for 10 to 20 days.
*Children younger than age 2:* 50 mg/kg/day (up to 2 g/day) P.O. in four divided doses for 10 to 20 days.
➤ **To prevent inhalation anthrax after possible exposure ♦**
*Adults:* 7.5 mg/kg P.O. q.i.d. Continue treatment until exposure is ruled out. If exposure is confirmed, anthrax vaccine

may be indicated. Continue treatment for 60 days.
*Children younger than age 9:* 50 mg/kg P.O. daily given in four divided doses. Continue treatment until exposure is ruled out. If exposure is confirmed, anthrax vaccine may be indicated. Continue treatment for 60 days.

## ACTION
Inhibits cell-wall synthesis during bacterial multiplication.

| Route | Onset | Peak | Duration |
|-------|-------|------|----------|
| P.O. | Unknown | 30-60 min | Unknown |

## ADVERSE REACTIONS
**CNS:** neuropathy.
**GI:** *epigastric distress,* vomiting, diarrhea, *nausea,* black hairy tongue.
**GU:** nephropathy.
**Hematologic:** eosinophilia, hemolytic anemia, *leukopenia, thrombocytopenia.*
**Other:** hypersensitivity reactions, *anaphylaxis,* overgrowth of nonsusceptible organisms.

## INTERACTIONS
**Drug-drug.** *Hormonal contraceptives:* May decrease hormonal contraceptive effectiveness. Recommend additional form of contraception during penicillin therapy. *Probenecid:* May increase penicillin level. Probenecid may be used for this purpose.

## EFFECTS ON LAB TEST RESULTS
• May increase eosinophil count. May decrease hemoglobin and platelet, WBC, and granulocyte counts.
• May alter results of turbidimetric test methods using sulfosalicylic acid, acetic acid, trichloroacetic acid, and nitric acid.

## CONTRAINDICATIONS & CAUTIONS
• Contraindicated in patients hypersensitive to drug or other penicillins.
• Use cautiously in patients with GI disturbances and in those with other drug allergies, especially to cephalosporins, because of possible cross-sensitivity.

## NURSING CONSIDERATIONS
• Before giving drug, ask patient about allergic reactions to penicillins.

• Obtain specimen for culture and sensitivity tests before giving first dose. Therapy may begin pending results.
• Periodically assess renal and hematopoietic function in patients receiving long-term therapy.
• If large doses are given or if therapy is prolonged, bacterial or fungal superinfection may occur, especially in elderly, debilitated, or immunosuppressed patients.
• The American Heart Association considers amoxicillin the preferred drug to prevent endocarditis because GI absorption is better and drug levels are sustained longer. Penicillin V is considered an alternative drug.
• *Alert:* Don't confuse drug with Polycillin, penicillamine, or the various types of penicillin.

## PATIENT TEACHING
• Instruct patient to take entire quantity of drug exactly as prescribed, even after he feels better.
• Tell patient to take drug with food if stomach upset occurs.
• Advise patient to notify prescriber if rash, fever, or chills develop. A rash is the most common allergic reaction.

# piperacillin sodium
Pipracil, Pipril‡

*Pregnancy risk category B*

## AVAILABLE FORMS
*Injection:* 2 g, 3 g, 4 g

## INDICATIONS & DOSAGES
➤ **Systemic infections from susceptible strains of gram-positive and especially gram-negative organisms including *Proteus species* and *Pseudomonas aeruginosa***
*Adults and children older than age 12:* 100 to 300 mg/kg I.V. or I.M. daily in divided doses q 4 to 6 hours, not to exceed 24 g daily. Patients with cystic fibrosis may receive up to 600 mg/kg/day.
➤ **To prevent surgical infections**
*Adults:* 2 g I.V., given 30 to 60 minutes before surgery. May repeat during surgery and once or twice more after surgery.

*Adjust-a-dose:* For patients with creatinine clearance of 20 to 40 ml/minute, 3 to 4 g I.V. q 8 hours; if clearance is less than 20 ml/minute, 3 to 4 g I.V. q 12 hours, depending on severity of infection.

## I.V. ADMINISTRATION
• For injection, reconstitute each gram of drug with 5 ml of diluent, such as sterile or bacteriostatic water for injection, normal saline solution for injection (with or without preservative), $D_5W$, or dextrose 5% in normal saline solution for injection. Shake until dissolved. Inject reconstituted solution directly into a vein or into the tubing of a free-flowing I.V. solution over 3 to 5 minutes.
• For intermittent infusion, dilute with at least 50 ml of a compatible I.V. solution, and give over 30 minutes.
• Avoid continuous infusions to prevent vein irritation. Change site every 48 hours.
• Aminoglycoside antibiotics, such as gentamicin and tobramycin, are chemically incompatible with piperacillin. Don't mix in the same I.V. container.

## ACTION
Inhibits cell-wall synthesis during bacterial multiplication.

| Route | Onset | Peak | Duration |
|-------|-------|------|----------|
| I.V. | Immediate | Immediate | Unknown |
| I.M. | Unknown | 30-50 min | Unknown |

## ADVERSE REACTIONS
**CNS:** *seizures,* headache, dizziness, fatigue.
**CV:** phlebitis, vein irritation.
**GI:** nausea, diarrhea, *pseudomembranous colitis,* vomiting.
**GU:** interstitial nephritis.
**Hematologic:** *neutropenia,* eosinophilia, *leukopenia, thrombocytopenia, bleeding.*
**Metabolic:** *hypokalemia,* hypernatremia.
**Musculoskeletal:** prolonged muscle relaxation.
**Skin:** pain at injection site.
**Other:** hypersensitivity reactions, *anaphylaxis,* overgrowth of nonsusceptible organisms.

## INTERACTIONS
**Drug-drug.** *Hormonal contraceptives:* May decrease hormonal contraceptive effectiveness. Recommend additional form of contraception during penicillin therapy.
*Probenecid:* May increase piperacillin. Probenecid may be used for this purpose.
*Vecuronium:* May prolong neuromuscular blockade. Avoid using together.

## EFFECTS ON LAB TEST RESULTS
• May increase ALT, AST, alkaline phosphatase, LDH, and sodium levels. May decrease potassium level.
• May increase eosinophil count. May decrease hemoglobin and platelet, WBC, and granulocyte counts. May cause positive Coombs' test result.
• May falsely decrease aminoglycoside level.

## CONTRAINDICATIONS & CAUTIONS
• Contraindicated in patients hypersensitive to drug or other penicillins.
• Use cautiously in patients with bleeding tendencies, uremia, hypokalemia, and other drug allergies, especially to cephalosporins, because of possible cross-sensitivity.

## NURSING CONSIDERATIONS
• Before giving drug, ask patient about allergic reactions to penicillin.
• Obtain specimen for culture and sensitivity tests before giving first dose. Therapy may begin pending results.
• For I.M. injection, reconstitute with sterile or bacteriostatic water for injection, normal saline solution for injection (with or without preservative), or 0.5% to 1% lidocaine hydrochloride. Add 2 ml of diluent for each gram of drug. Final solution will contain 1 g/2.5 ml. The manufacturer states to limit injections to 2 g per site, preferably in the upper outer buttocks.
• Check CBC and platelet counts frequently. Drug may cause thrombocytopenia.
• Monitor potassium and sodium levels.
• Monitor INR in patients receiving warfarin therapy because drug may prolong PT.
• If large doses are given or if therapy is prolonged, bacterial or fungal superinfection may occur, especially in elderly, debilitated, or immunosuppressed patients.
• Patients with cystic fibrosis tend to be most susceptible to fever or rash.

Reactions may be *common,* uncommon, *life-threatening,* or COMMON AND LIFE-THREATENING.

• Drug may be better suited for patients on sodium-free diets than ticarcillin (piperacillin contains 1.85 mEq of sodium/g).

• Piperacillin is typically used with another antibiotic such as gentamicin, but don't mix in same container.

### PATIENT TEACHING

• Tell patient to report adverse reactions promptly.

• Instruct patient receiving drug I.V. to report discomfort at I.V. site.

• Advise patient to limit salt intake during therapy because drug contains 1.85 mEq of sodium/g.

---

## piperacillin sodium and tazobactam sodium
Zosyn

*Pregnancy risk category B*

---

### AVAILABLE FORMS

*Powder for injection:* 2 g piperacillin and 0.25 g tazobactam per vial, 3 g piperacillin and 0.375 g tazobactam per vial, 4 g piperacillin and 0.5 g tazobactam per vial

### INDICATIONS & DOSAGES

➤ **Moderate to severe infections caused by piperacillin-resistant, piperacillin/ tazobactam-susceptible, beta-lactamase–producing strains of microorganisms in appendicitis (complicated by rupture or abscess) and peritonitis caused by *Escherichia coli, Bacteroides fragilis, B. ovatus, B. thetaiotaomicron, B. vulgatus;* skin and skin-structure infections caused by *Staphylococcus aureus;* postpartum endometritis or pelvic inflammatory disease caused by *E. coli;* moderately severe community-acquired pneumonia caused by *Haemophilus influenzae***

*Adults:* 3.375 g (3 g piperacillin/0.375 g tazobactam) q 6 hours as a 30-minute I.V. infusion. Duration of treatment is usually 7 to 10 days.

*Adjust-a-dose:* If creatinine clearance is 20 to 40 ml/minute, give 2.25 g (2 g piperacillin/0.25 g tazobactam) q 6 hours; if less than 20 ml/minute, give 2.25 g (2 g

piperacillin/0.25 g tazobactam) q 8 hours. In continuous ambulatory peritoneal dialysis (CAPD) patients, give 2.25 g (2 g piperacillin/0.25 g tazobactam) q 12 hours. In hemodialysis patients, give 2.25 g (2 g piperacillin/0.25 g tazobactam) q 12 hours with a supplemental dose of 0.75 g (0.67 g piperacillin/0.08 g tazobactam) after each dialysis period.

✴ *NEW INDICATION:* **Moderate to severe nosocomial pneumonia caused by piperacillin-resistant, beta-lactamase–producing strains of *Staphylococcus aureus* and by piperacillin/tazobactam-susceptible *Acinetobacter baumanii, Haemophilus influenzae, Klebsiella pneumoniae,* and *Pseudomonas aeruginosa***

*Adults:* 4.5 g (4 g piperacillin/0.5 g tazobactam) q 6 hours with aminoglycoside. Patients with *P. aeruginosa* should continue aminoglycoside treatment; if *P. aeruginosa* is not isolated, aminoglycoside treatment may be stopped. Duration of treatment is usually 7 to 14 days.

*Adjust-a-dose:* If creatinine clearance is 20 to 40 ml/minute, give 3.375 g (3 g piperacillin/0.375 g tazobactam) q 6 hours; if less than 20 ml/minute, give 2.25 g (2 g piperacillin/0.25 g tazobactam) q 6 hours. In CAPD patients, give 2.25 g (2 g piperacillin/0.25 g tazobactam) q 8 hours. In hemodialysis patients, give 2.25 g (2 g piperacillin/0.25 g tazobactam) q 8 hours with a supplemental dose of 0.75 g (0.67 g piperacillin/0.08 g tazobactam) after each dialysis period.

### I.V. ADMINISTRATION

• Reconstitute each gram of piperacillin with 5 ml of diluent, such as sterile or bacteriostatic water for injection, normal saline solution for injection, bacteriostatic normal saline solution for injection, $D_5W$, dextrose 5% in normal saline solution for injection, or dextran 6% in normal saline solution for injection.

• Don't use lactated Ringer's injection. Shake until dissolved. Further dilute to a final volume of 50 ml before infusion.

• Infuse over at least 30 minutes. Stop any primary infusion during administration, if possible. Don't mix with other drugs. Aminoglycoside antibiotics, such as amikacin, gentamicin, and tobramycin, are

---

chemically incompatible with this drug. Don't mix in the same I.V. container.
• Use drug immediately after reconstitution. Discard unused drug after 24 hours if stored at room temperature or 48 hours if refrigerated. Once diluted, drug is stable in I.V. bags for 24 hours at room temperature or 1 week if refrigerated.
• Change I.V. site every 48 hours.

## ACTION
Inhibits cell-wall synthesis during bacterial multiplication.

| Route | Onset | Peak | Duration |
|-------|-------|------|----------|
| I.V. | Immediate | Immediate | Unknown |

## ADVERSE REACTIONS
**CNS:** fever, *headache, insomnia,* agitation, dizziness, anxiety, *seizures.*
**CV:** hypertension, tachycardia, chest pain, edema.
**EENT:** rhinitis.
**GI:** *diarrhea, nausea, constipation,* vomiting, dyspepsia, stool changes, abdominal pain.
**GU:** interstitial nephritis, candidiasis.
**Hematologic:** *leukopenia,* anemia, eosinophilia, *thrombocytopenia.*
**Respiratory:** dyspnea.
**Skin:** rash, pruritus.
**Other:** pain, *anaphylaxis,* inflammation, phlebitis at I.V. site, hypersensitivity reactions.

## INTERACTIONS
**Drug-drug.** *Hormonal contraceptives:* May decrease hormonal contraceptive effectiveness. Recommend additional form of contraception during penicillin therapy. *Oral anticoagulants:* May prolong effectiveness. Monitor PT and INR closely. *Probenecid:* May increase piperacillin level. Probenecid may be used for this purpose.
*Vecuronium:* May prolong neuromuscular blockade. Monitor patient closely.

## EFFECTS ON LAB TEST RESULTS
• May increase eosinophil count. May decrease hemoglobin and WBC and platelet counts.
• May cause false-positive result for urine glucose tests using copper reduction method (such as Clinitest).

## CONTRAINDICATIONS & CAUTIONS
• Contraindicated in patients hypersensitive to drug or other penicillins.
• Use cautiously in patients with bleeding tendencies, uremia, hypokalemia, and other drug allergies, especially to cephalosporins, because of possible cross-sensitivity.

## NURSING CONSIDERATIONS
• Obtain specimen for culture and sensitivity tests before giving first dose. Therapy may begin pending results.
• Because peritoneal dialysis removes 6% of the piperacillin dose and 21% of the tazobactam dose, and hemodialysis removes 30% to 40% of a dose in 4 hours, additional dosing may be needed after each dialysis period.
• If large doses are given or if therapy is prolonged, bacterial or fungal superinfection may occur, especially in elderly, debilitated, or immunosuppressed patients.
• Drug contains 2.35 mEq sodium/g of piperacillin. Monitor patient's sodium intake.
• Patients with cystic fibrosis may have a higher rate of fever and rash. Monitor these patients closely.

## PATIENT TEACHING
• Tell patient to report adverse reactions promptly.
• Advise patient to alert nurse if discomfort occurs at I.V. site.

# ticarcillin disodium
Ticar

*Pregnancy risk category B*

## AVAILABLE FORMS
*Injection:* 3 g

## INDICATIONS & DOSAGES
➤ **Severe systemic infections caused by susceptible strains of gram-positive and especially gram-negative organisms, including *Pseudomonas* and *Proteus* species**
*Adults and children older than age 1 month:* 200 to 300 mg/kg I.V. daily in divided doses q 4 to 6 hours.

➤**UTIs**
*Adults and children weighing at least
40 kg (88 lb):* 1 g I.M. or I.V. q 6 hours.
For complicated infections, 150 to
200 mg/kg I.V. infusion daily in divided
doses q 4 to 6 hours.
*Infants and children older than age 1
month, weighing less than 40 kg:* 50 to
100 mg/kg I.M. or I.V. daily in divided
doses q 6 to 8 hours. For complicated infections, 150 to 200 mg/kg I.V. infusion
daily in divided doses q 4 to 6 hours.
*Adjust-a-dose:* For patients with renal impairment, if creatinine clearance is 30 to
60 ml/minute, dosage is 2 g I.V. q 4 hours;
if clearance is 10 to 29 ml/minute, 2 g I.V.
q 8 hours; and if below 10 ml/minute, 2 g
I.V. q 12 hours or 1 g I.M. q 6 hours.

## I.V. ADMINISTRATION
● For injection, reconstitute drug using
D₅W, normal saline solution for injection,
sterile water for injection, or other compatible solution. Add 4 ml of diluent for
each gram of drug.
● Further dilute to a maximum concentration of 50 mg/ml, and inject slowly directly into a vein or into the tubing of a free-
flowing I.V. solution.
● For intermittent infusion, dilute to a concentration of 10 to 100 mg/ml, and give
over 30 to 120 minutes in adults or 10 to
20 minutes in neonates.
● Aminoglycoside antibiotics, such as
amikacin, gentamicin, and tobramycin, are
chemically incompatible with this drug.
Don't mix in the same I.V. container.
● Avoid continuous infusion, to prevent
vein irritation. Change site every 48 hours.

## ACTION
Inhibits cell-wall synthesis during bacterial multiplication.

| Route | Onset | Peak | Duration |
|---|---|---|---|
| I.V. | Immediate | Immediate | Unknown |
| I.M. | Unknown | 30-75 min | Unknown |

## ADVERSE REACTIONS
**CNS:** neuromuscular excitability,
*seizures.*
**CV:** phlebitis, vein irritation.
**GI:** nausea, diarrhea, vomiting,
*pseudomembranous colitis.*

**Hematologic:** *leukopenia, neutropenia,*
eosinophilia, *thrombocytopenia,* hemolytic anemia.
**Metabolic:** hypokalemia, hypernatremia.
**Skin:** pain at injection site.
**Other:** hypersensitivity reactions, *anaphylaxis,* overgrowth of nonsusceptible organisms.

## INTERACTIONS
**Drug-drug.** *Hormonal contraceptives:*
May decrease hormonal contraceptive effectiveness. Recommend additional form
of contraception during penicillin therapy.
*Lithium:* May alter renal elimination of
lithium. Monitor lithium level closely.
*Probenecid:* May increase levels of ticarcillin and other penicillins. Probenecid
may be used for this purpose.

## EFFECTS ON LAB TEST RESULTS
● May increase ALT, AST, alkaline phosphatase, LDH, and sodium levels. May decrease potassium level.
● May increase eosinophil count. May decrease hemoglobin and platelet, WBC, and
granulocyte counts. May cause positive
Coombs' test result.
● May falsely decrease aminoglycoside
level. May alter turbidimetric test methods
that use sulfosalicylic acid, trichloroacetic
acid, acetic acid, or nitric acid.

## CONTRAINDICATIONS & CAUTIONS
● Contraindicated in patients hypersensitive to drug or other penicillins.
● Use cautiously in patients with other
drug allergies, especially to cephalosporins, because of possible cross-sensitivity,
and in those with impaired renal function,
hemorrhagic conditions, hypokalemia, or
sodium restrictions. Drug contains 5.2 to
6.5 mEq sodium/g.

## NURSING CONSIDERATIONS
● Before giving drug, ask patient about allergic reactions to penicillin.
● Obtain specimen for culture and sensitivity tests before giving first dose. Therapy may begin pending results.
● Give ticarcillin at least 1 hour before a
bacteriostatic antibiotic.
● For I.M. injection, reconstitute drug using sterile water for injection, normal
saline solution for injection, or lidocaine

1% (without epinephrine). Use 2 ml diluent for each gram of drug. Use only the 1-g vial for I.M. administration. Give deeply I.M. into large muscle. Don't exceed 2 g per injection.
• Monitor potassium and sodium levels.
• Check CBC and platelet counts frequently. Drug may cause thrombocytopenia.
• Ticarcillin is typically used with another antibiotic such as gentamicin.
• If large doses are given or if therapy is prolonged, bacterial or fungal superinfection may occur, especially in elderly, debilitated, or immunosuppressed patients.
• Monitor INR in patients receiving warfarin therapy because drug may prolong PT.
• Give patients receiving hemodialysis a 3-g dose after each dialysis session.

PATIENT TEACHING
• Tell patient to report adverse reactions promptly.
• Advise patient to report discomfort at I.V. insertion site.

## ticarcillin disodium and clavulanate potassium
Timentin

*Pregnancy risk category B*

AVAILABLE FORMS
*Injection:* 3 g ticarcillin and 100 mg clavulanic acid in 3.1-g vials
*Premixed:* 3.1 g/100 ml

INDICATIONS & DOSAGES
➤ **Lower respiratory tract, urinary tract, bone and joint, intra-abdominal, gynecologic, and skin and skin-structure infections and septicemia caused by beta-lactamase–producing strains of bacteria or by ticarcillin-susceptible organisms**
*Adults and children weighing more than 60 kg (132 lb):* 3 g ticarcillin and 100 mg clavulanic acid, given by I.V. infusion q 4 to 6 hours.
*Adults and children ages 3 months to 16 years weighing less than 60 kg:* 200 mg ticarcillin/kg I.V. daily in divided doses q 6 hours. For severe infections, 300 mg

ticarcillin/kg I.V. daily in divided doses q 4 hours.
*Adjust-a-dose:* For renally impaired patients, if creatinine clearance is 30 to 60 ml/minute, dosage is 2 g I.V. q 4 hours; if clearance is 10 to 29 ml/minute, 2 g I.V. q 8 hours; and if clearance is less than 10 ml/minute, 2 g I.V. q 12 hours.

I.V. ADMINISTRATION
• Reconstitute drug with 13 ml of sterile water for injection or normal saline solution for injection. Further dilute to a maximum of 10 to 100 mg/ml (based on ticarcillin component), and give by I.V. infusion over 30 minutes. In fluid-restricted patients, dilute to a maximum of 48 mg/ml if using $D_5W$, 43 mg/ml if using normal saline solution for injection, or 86 mg/ml if using sterile water for injection.
• Drug is chemically incompatible with aminoglycoside antibiotics (amikacin, gentamicin, tobramycin). Don't mix in the same I.V. container.

ACTION
Inhibits cell-wall synthesis during bacterial multiplication.

| Route | Onset | Peak | Duration |
|-------|-------|------|----------|
| I.V. | Immediate | Immediate | Unknown |

ADVERSE REACTIONS
**CNS:** neuromuscular excitability, headache, *seizures,* giddiness.
**CV:** phlebitis, vein irritation.
**EENT:** taste and smell disturbances.
**GI:** nausea, diarrhea, stomatitis, vomiting, epigastric pain, flatulence, *pseudomembranous colitis.*
**Hematologic:** *leukopenia, neutropenia,* eosinophilia, *thrombocytopenia,* hemolytic anemia, anemia.
**Metabolic:** hypokalemia, hypernatremia.
**Skin:** pain at injection site.
**Other:** hypersensitivity reactions, *anaphylaxis,* overgrowth of nonsusceptible organisms.

EFFECTS ON LAB TEST RESULTS
• May increase ALT, AST, alkaline phosphatase, LDH, and sodium levels. May decrease potassium level.

● May increase eosinophil count. May decrease hemoglobin, and platelet, WBC, and granulocyte counts.
● May alter results of turbidimetric test methods that use sulfosalicylic acid, trichloroacetic acid, acetic acid, or nitric acid.

**INTERACTIONS**
**Drug-drug.** *Hormonal contraceptives:* May decrease hormonal contraceptive effectiveness. Recommend additional form of contraception during penicillin therapy.
*Probenecid:* May increase ticarcillin level. Probenecid may be used for this purpose.

**CONTRAINDICATIONS & CAUTIONS**
● Contraindicated in patients hypersensitive to drug or other penicillins.
● Use cautiously in patients with other drug allergies, especially to cephalosporins, because of possible cross-sensitivity, and in those with impaired renal function, hemorrhagic conditions, hypokalemia, or sodium restrictions. Drug contains 4.5 mEq sodium/g.

**NURSING CONSIDERATIONS**
● Before giving drug, ask patient about allergic reactions to penicillin.
● Obtain specimen for culture and sensitivity tests before giving first dose. Therapy may begin pending results.
● Give drug at least 1 hour before a bacteriostatic antibiotic.
● Check CBC and platelet counts frequently. Drug may cause thrombocytopenia.
● Monitor potassium and sodium levels.
● If large doses are given or if therapy is prolonged, bacterial or fungal superinfection may occur, especially in elderly, debilitated, or immunosuppressed patients.
● Patients on hemodialysis should receive an additional 3.1 g dose after each dialysis session.

**PATIENT TEACHING**
● Tell patient to report adverse reactions promptly.
● Instruct patient to report discomfort at I.V. site.
● Advise patient to limit salt intake during drug therapy because of high sodium content.

---

*Rapid onset    †Canada    ‡Australia    ◇ OTC    ◆ Off-label use    ✐Photoguide    *Liquid contains alcohol.*

cefaclor
cefadroxil
cefazolin sodium
cefdinir
cefditoren pivoxil
cefepime hydrochloride
cefoperazone sodium
cefotaxime sodium
cefotetan disodium
cefoxitin sodium
cefpodoxime proxetil
cefprozil
ceftazidime
ceftizoxime sodium
ceftriaxone sodium
cefuroxime axetil
cefuroxime sodium
cephalexin hydrochloride
cephalexin monohydrate
cephradine
loracarbef

**COMBINATION PRODUCTS**
None.

---

## cefaclor
Ceclor, Ceclor CD

*Pregnancy risk category B*

---

### AVAILABLE FORMS
*Capsules:* 250 mg, 500 mg
*Oral suspension:* 125 mg/5 ml, 187 mg/5 ml, 250 mg/5 ml, 375 mg/5 ml
*Tablets (extended-release):* 375 mg, 500 mg

### INDICATIONS & DOSAGES
➤ **Respiratory tract infections, UTIs, skin and soft-tissue infections, and otitis media caused by** *Haemophilus influenzae, Streptococcus pneumoniae, S. pyogenes, Escherichia coli, Proteus mirabilis, Klebsiella* **species, and staphylococci**
*Adults:* 250 to 500 mg P.O. q 8 hours. For pharyngitis or otitis media, daily dose may be given in two equally divided doses q 12 hours. For extended-release forms,

500 mg P.O. q 12 hours for 7 days for bronchitis; for pharyngitis or skin and skin-structure infections, 375 mg P.O. q 12 hours for 10 days and 7 to 10 days, respectively.
*Children:* 20 mg/kg daily P.O. in divided doses q 8 hours. For pharyngitis or otitis media, daily dose may be given in two equally divided doses q 12 hours. In more serious infections, 40 mg/kg daily are recommended, not to exceed 1 g daily.

### ACTION
Second-generation cephalosporin that inhibits cell-wall synthesis, promoting osmotic instability; usually bactericidal.

| Route | Onset | Peak | Duration |
|---|---|---|---|
| P.O. | Unknown | 30-60 min | Unknown |
| P.O. (extended) | Unknown | 1½-2½ hr | Unknown |

### ADVERSE REACTIONS
**CNS:** fever, dizziness, headache, somnolence, malaise.
**GI:** *nausea,* vomiting, *diarrhea,* anorexia, dyspepsia, abdominal cramps, ***pseudomembranous colitis,*** oral candidiasis.
**GU:** vaginal candidiasis, vaginitis.
**Hematologic:** *transient leukopenia,* anemia, eosinophilia, ***thrombocytopenia,*** lymphocytosis.
**Skin:** *maculopapular rash,* dermatitis, pruritus.
**Other:** hypersensitivity reactions, serum sickness, ***anaphylaxis.***

### INTERACTIONS
**Drug-drug.** *Aminoglycosides:* May increase risk of nephrotoxicity. Avoid using together.
*Antacids:* May decrease absorption of extended-release cefaclor if taken within 1 hour. Separate doses by 1 hour.
*Anticoagulants:* May increase anticoagulant effects. Monitor PT and INR.
*Chloramphenicol:* May cause antagonistic effect. Avoid using together.

---

Reactions may be *common,* uncommon, ***life-threatening,*** or **COMMON AND LIFE-THREATENING.**

*Probenecid:* May inhibit excretion and increase cefaclor level. Monitor patient for increased adverse reactions.

**EFFECTS ON LAB TEST RESULTS**
● May increase ALT, AST, alkaline phosphatase, bilirubin, GGT, and LDH levels.
● May increase eosinophil count. May decrease hemoglobin and WBC and platelet counts.
● May falsely elevate serum or urine creatinine level in tests using Jaffe reaction. May cause false-positive results of Coombs' test and urine glucose tests using cupric sulfate (Benedict's reagent or Clinitest).

**CONTRAINDICATIONS & CAUTIONS**
● Contraindicated in patients hypersensitive to drug or other cephalosporins.
● Use cautiously in patients hypersensitive to penicillin because of the possibility of cross-sensitivity with other beta-lactam antibiotics.
● Use cautiously in breast-feeding women and in patients with a history of colitis and renal insufficiency.

**NURSING CONSIDERATIONS**
● Obtain specimen for culture and sensitivity tests before giving first dose. Therapy may begin pending results.
● If large doses are given, therapy is prolonged, or patient is at high risk, monitor patient for signs and symptoms of superinfection.
● Store reconstituted suspension in refrigerator. Suspension is stable for 14 days if refrigerated. Shake well before use.
● *Alert:* Don't confuse drug with other cephalosporins that sound alike.

**PATIENT TEACHING**
● Tell patient to take entire amount of drug exactly as prescribed, even after he feels better.
● Tell patient that drug may be taken with meals. If suspension is used, instruct him to shake container well before measuring dose and to keep the drug refrigerated.
● Advise patient to notify prescriber if rash develops or signs and symptoms of superinfection appear.
● Inform patient not to crush, cut, or chew extended-release tablets.

# cefadroxil
Duricef◊

*Pregnancy risk category B*

**AVAILABLE FORMS**
*Capsules:* 500 mg
*Oral suspension:* 125 mg/5 ml, 250 mg/5 ml, 500 mg/5 ml
*Tablets:* 1 g

**INDICATIONS & DOSAGES**
➤ **UTIs caused by** *Escherichia coli,* ***Proteus mirabilis,*** **and** *Klebsiella* **species; skin and soft-tissue infections caused by staphylococci and streptococci; pharyngitis or tonsillitis caused by group A beta-hemolytic streptococci**
*Adults:* 1 to 2 g P.O. daily, depending on infection being treated. Usually given once daily or in two divided doses.
*Children:* 30 mg/kg P.O. daily in two divided doses q 12 hours.
*Adjust-a-dose:* If creatinine clearance is 25 to 50 ml/minute, give 1 g P.O. then 500 mg q 12 hours. If clearance is between 10 and 24 ml/minute, give 1 g P.O. then 500 mg q 24 hours; if clearance is less than 10 ml/minute, give 1 g P.O. then 500 mg q 36 hours.

**ACTION**
First-generation cephalosporin that inhibits cell-wall synthesis, promoting osmotic instability; usually bactericidal.

| Route | Onset | Peak | Duration |
|-------|-------|------|----------|
| P.O. | Unknown | 1-2 hr | Unknown |

**ADVERSE REACTIONS**
**CNS:** fever, *seizures,* dizziness, headache.
**GI:** *pseudomembranous colitis, nausea,* vomiting, *diarrhea,* glossitis, abdominal cramps, oral candidiasis.
**GU:** genital pruritus, candidiasis, vaginitis, renal dysfunction.
**Hematologic:** *transient neutropenia,* eosinophilia, *leukopenia,* anemia, *agranulocytosis, thrombocytopenia.*
**Respiratory:** dyspnea.
**Skin:** *maculopapular and erythematous rashes,* urticaria.

**Other:** hypersensitivity reactions, *anaphylaxis, angioedema.*

## INTERACTIONS
**Drug-drug.** *Aminoglycosides:* May increase risk of nephrotoxicity. Avoid using together.
*Probenecid:* May inhibit excretion and increase cefadroxil level. Use together cautiously.

## EFFECTS ON LAB TEST RESULTS
● May increase ALT, AST, alkaline phosphatase, bilirubin, GGT, and LDH levels.
● May increase eosinophil count. May decrease hemoglobin and neutrophil, WBC, granulocyte, and platelet counts.
● May falsely elevate serum or urine creatinine level in tests using Jaffe reaction. May cause false-positive results of Coombs' test and urine glucose tests using cupric sulfate (Benedict's reagent or Clinitest).

## CONTRAINDICATIONS & CAUTIONS
● Contraindicated in patients hypersensitive to drug or other cephalosporins.
● Use cautiously in patients with a history of sensitivity to penicillin and in breast-feeding women.
● Use cautiously in patients with impaired renal function; dosage adjustments may be necessary.

## NURSING CONSIDERATIONS
● Obtain specimen for culture and sensitivity tests before giving first dose. Therapy may begin pending results.
● If creatinine clearance is below 50 ml/minute, lengthen dosage interval so drug doesn't accumulate. Monitor renal function in patients with renal dysfunction.
● If large doses are given, therapy is prolonged, or patient is high risk, monitor patient for superinfection.
● **Alert:** Don't confuse drug with other cephalosporins that sound alike.

## PATIENT TEACHING
● Instruct patient to take drug with food or milk to lessen GI discomfort.
● Tell patient to take entire amount of drug exactly as prescribed, even after he feels better.
● Advise patient to notify prescriber if rash develops or if signs and symptoms of

superinfection appear, such as recurring fever, chills, and malaise.

# cefazolin sodium
Ancef

*Pregnancy risk category B*

## AVAILABLE FORMS
*Infusion:* 500 mg/50-ml vial, 1 g/50-ml vial
*Injection (parenteral):* 250 mg, 500 mg, 1 g

## INDICATIONS & DOSAGES
➤ **Perioperative prevention in contaminated surgery**
*Adults:* 1 g I.M. or I.V. 30 to 60 minutes before surgery; then 0.5 to 1 g I.M. or I.V. q 6 to 8 hours for 24 hours. In operations lasting longer than 2 hours, give another 0.5- to 1-g dose I.M. or I.V. intraoperatively. Continue treatment for 3 to 5 days if life-threatening infection is likely.
➤ **Infections of respiratory, biliary, and GU tracts; skin, soft-tissue, bone, and joint infections; septicemia; endocarditis caused by *Escherichia coli*, *Enterobacteriaceae*, gonococci, *Haemophilus influenzae*, *Klebsiella* species, *Proteus mirabilis*, *Staphylococcus aureus*, *Streptococcus pneumoniae*, and group A beta-hemolytic streptococci**
*Adults:* 250 mg to 500 mg I.M. or I.V. q 8 hours for mild infections or 500 mg to 1.5 g I.M. or I.V. q 6 to 8 hours for moderate to severe or life-threatening infections. Maximum 12 g/day in life-threatening situations.
*Children older than age 1 month:* 25 to 50 mg/kg/day I.M. or I.V. in three or four divided doses. In severe infections, dose may be increased to 100 mg/kg/day.
**Adjust-a-dose:** For patients with creatinine clearance 35 to 54 ml/minute, give full dose q 8 hours; if clearance is 11 to 34 ml/minute, give 50% usual dose q 12 hours; if clearance is below 10 ml/minute, give 50% of usual dose q 18 to 24 hours.

## I.V. ADMINISTRATION
● Reconstitute drug with sterile water, bacteriostatic water, or normal saline solu-

tion as follows: 2 ml to 500-mg vial or 2.5 ml to 1-g vial. Shake well until dissolved. Resulting concentration: 225 mg/ml or 330 mg/ml, respectively.

• Reconstituted cefazolin is stable for 24 hours at room temperature or 96 hours under refrigeration.

• For direct injection, further dilute with 5 ml of sterile water for injection. Inject into a large vein or into the tubing of a free-flowing I.V. solution over 3 to 5 minutes. For intermittent infusion, add reconstituted drug to 50 to 100 ml of compatible solution or use premixed solution. Give commercially available frozen solutions of cefazolin in $D_5W$ only by intermittent or continuous I.V. infusion.

• Alternate injection sites if I.V. therapy lasts longer than 3 days. Use of small I.V. needles in larger available veins may be preferable.

## ACTION

First-generation cephalosporin that inhibits cell-wall synthesis, promoting osmotic instability; usually bactericidal.

| Route | Onset | Peak | Duration |
|-------|-------|------|----------|
| I.V. | Immediate | Immediate | Unknown |
| I.M. | Unknown | 1-2 hr | Unknown |

## ADVERSE REACTIONS

**CNS:** confusion, *seizures.*
**CV:** *phlebitis, thrombophlebitis with I.V. injection.*
**GI:** *pseudomembranous colitis,* nausea, anorexia, vomiting, *diarrhea,* glossitis, dyspepsia, abdominal cramps, anal pruritus, oral candidiasis.
**GU:** genital pruritus, candidiasis, vaginitis.
**Hematologic:** *neutropenia, leukopenia,* eosinophilia, *thrombocytopenia.*
**Skin:** *maculopapular and erythematous rashes, urticaria, pruritus, pain, induration, sterile abscesses, tissue sloughing at injection site, Stevens-Johnson syndrome.*
**Other:** hypersensitivity reactions, serum sickness, *anaphylaxis,* drug fever.

## INTERACTIONS

**Drug-drug.** *Aminoglycosides:* May increase risk of nephrotoxicity. Avoid using together.

*Probenecid:* May inhibit excretion and increase cefazolin level. Use together cautiously.

## EFFECTS ON LAB TEST RESULTS

• May increase ALT, AST, alkaline phosphatase, bilirubin, GGT, and LDH levels.
• May increase eosinophil count. May decrease neutrophil, WBC, and platelet counts.
• May falsely elevate serum or urine creatinine level in tests using Jaffe reaction. May cause false-positive results of Coombs' test and urine glucose tests using cupric sulfate (Benedict's reagent or Clinitest).

## CONTRAINDICATIONS & CAUTIONS

• Contraindicated in patients hypersensitive to drug or other cephalosporins.
• Use cautiously in patients hypersensitive to penicillin because of the possibility of cross-sensitivity with other beta-lactam antibiotics.
• Use cautiously in breast-feeding women and in patients with a history of colitis and renal insufficiency.

## NURSING CONSIDERATIONS

• Obtain specimen for culture and sensitivity tests before giving first dose. Therapy may begin pending results.
• Expect to adjust dosage and dosing interval if creatinine clearance falls below 55 ml/minute.
• After reconstitution, inject drug I.M. without further dilution. This drug isn't as painful as other cephalosporins. Give injection deeply into a large muscle, such as the gluteus maximus or lateral aspect of the thigh.
• If large doses are given, therapy is prolonged, or patient is at high risk, monitor patient for signs and symptoms of superinfection.
• *Alert:* Don't confuse drug with other cephalosporins that sound alike.

## PATIENT TEACHING

• Instruct patient to report adverse reactions promptly.
• Tell patient to report discomfort at I.V. injection site.

## cefdinir
Omnicef

*Pregnancy risk category B*

| Route | Onset | Peak | Duration |
|-------|-------|------|----------|
| P.O. | Unknown | 2-4 hr | Unknown |

### AVAILABLE FORMS
*Capsules:* 300 mg
*Suspension:* 125 mg/5 ml

### INDICATIONS & DOSAGES
➤ Mild to moderate infections caused by susceptible strains of microorganisms for conditions of community-acquired pneumonia, acute worsening of chronic bronchitis, acute maxillary sinusitis, acute bacterial otitis media, and uncomplicated skin and skin-structure infections
*Adults and children age 12 and older:* 300 mg P.O. q 12 hours; or 600 mg P.O. q 24 hours, for 10 days. Give q 12 hours for pneumonia and skin infections.
*Children ages 6 months to 12 years:* 7 mg/kg P.O. q 12 hours or 14 mg/kg P.O. q 24 hours, for 10 days, up to maximum dose of 600 mg daily. Give q 12 hours for skin infections.
➤ Pharyngitis, tonsillitis
*Adults and children age 12 and older:* 300 mg P.O. q 12 hours for 5 to 10 days; or 600 mg P.O. q 24 hours, for 10 days.
*Children ages 6 months to 12 years:* 7 mg/kg P.O. q 12 hours for 5 to 10 days; or 14 mg/kg P.O. q 24 hours, for 10 days.
*Adjust-a-dose:* If creatinine clearance is below 30 ml/minute, reduce dosage to 300 mg P.O. once daily for adults and 7 mg/kg up to 300 mg P.O. once daily for children. In patients receiving long-term hemodialysis, give 300 mg or 7 mg/kg P.O. at end of each dialysis session and subsequently every other day.

### ACTION
Third-generation cephalosporin that inhibits cell-wall synthesis, promoting osmotic instability; usually bactericidal. Some microorganisms resistant to penicillins and cephalosporins are susceptible to cefdinir. Active against a broad range of gram-positive and gram-negative aerobic microorganisms.

### ADVERSE REACTIONS
**CNS:** headache.
**GI:** abdominal pain, *diarrhea,* nausea, vomiting, ***pseudomembranous colitis.***
**GU:** vaginal candidiasis, vaginitis, increased urine proteins and RBCs.
**Skin:** rash, cutaneous candidiasis.

### INTERACTIONS
**Drug-drug.** *Aminoglycosides:* May increase risk of nephrotoxicity. Avoid using together.
*Antacids containing aluminum and magnesium, iron supplements, multivitamins containing iron:* May decrease cefdinir rate of absorption and bioavailability. Give such preparations 2 hours before or after cefdinir.
*Probenecid:* May inhibit renal excretion of cefdinir. Monitor patient for adverse reactions.

### EFFECTS ON LAB TEST RESULTS
● May increase GGT and alkaline phosphatase levels.
● May falsely elevate serum or urine creatinine level in tests using Jaffe reaction. May cause false-positive results of Coombs' test and urine glucose tests using cupric sulfate (Benedict's reagent or Clinitest).

### CONTRAINDICATIONS & CAUTIONS
● Contraindicated in patients hypersensitive to drug or other cephalosporins.
● Use cautiously in patients hypersensitive to penicillin because of the possibility of cross-sensitivity with other beta-lactam antibiotics.
● Use cautiously in patients with history of colitis and renal insufficiency.

### NURSING CONSIDERATIONS
● Prolonged drug treatment may result in emergence and overgrowth of resistant organisms. Monitor patient for signs and symptoms of superinfection.
● Pseudomembranous colitis has been reported with cefdinir and should be considered in patients with diarrhea after antibiotic therapy and in those with history of colitis.

---

Reactions may be *common,* uncommon, *life-threatening,* or COMMON AND LIFE-THREATENING.

● **Alert:** Don't confuse drug with other cephalosporins that sound alike.

| Route | Onset | Peak | Duration |
|---|---|---|---|
| P.O. | Unknown | 1½-3 hr | Unknown |

## PATIENT TEACHING
● Instruct patient to take antacids and iron supplements 2 hours before or after a dose of cefdinir.
● Inform diabetic patient that each teaspoon of suspension contains 2.86 g of sucrose.
● Tell patient that drug may be taken without regard to meals.
● Advise patient to report severe diarrhea or diarrhea accompanied by abdominal pain.
● Tell patient to report adverse reactions or signs and symptoms of superinfection promptly.

---

## cefditoren pivoxil
Spectracef

*Pregnancy risk category B*

---

## AVAILABLE FORMS
*Tablets:* 200 mg

## INDICATIONS & DOSAGES
➤ **Acute bacterial worsening of chronic bronchitis caused by *Haemophilus influenzae, H. parainfluenzae, Streptococcus pneumoniae,* or *Moraxella catarrhalis***
*Adults and adolescents age 12 and older:* 400 mg P.O. b.i.d. with meals for 10 days.
➤ **Pharyngitis or tonsillitis caused by S. pyogenes**
*Adults and adolescents age 12 and older:* 200 mg P.O. b.i.d. with meals for 10 days.
➤ **Uncomplicated skin and skin structure infections caused by *S. pyogenes***
*Adults and adolescents age 12 and older:* 200 mg P.O. b.i.d. with meals for 10 days.
*Adjust-a-dose:* For patients with creatinine clearance 30 to 49 ml/minute, don't exceed 200 mg b.i.d. For patients with clearance less than 30 ml/minute, give 200 mg daily.

## ACTION
Adheres to bacterial penicillin-binding proteins, inhibiting cell-wall synthesis. Active against many gram-positive and gram-negative organisms.

## ADVERSE REACTIONS
**CNS:** headache.
**GI:** abdominal pain, dyspepsia, *diarrhea,* nausea, vomiting.
**GU:** vaginal candidiasis, hematuria.
**Metabolic:** hyperglycemia.

## INTERACTIONS
**Drug-drug.** *$H_2$-receptor antagonists, magnesium and aluminum antacids:* May decrease cefditoren absorption. Avoid using together.
*Probenecid:* May increase cefditoren level. Avoid using together.
**Drug-food.** *Moderate- or high-fat meal:* May increase cefditoren bioavailability. Advise patient to take drug with meals.

## EFFECTS ON LAB TEST RESULTS
● May decrease glucose level.
● May increase WBC count in urine. May decrease hematocrit.
● May cause a false-positive direct Coombs' test result and a false-positive reaction for glucose in the urine in copper reduction tests (using Benedict's or Fehling's solution or Clinitest tablets).

## CONTRAINDICATIONS & CAUTIONS
● Contraindicated in patients hypersensitive to drug or other cephalosporins.
● Contraindicated in patients with carnitine deficiency or inborn errors of metabolism that may result in clinically significant carnitine deficiency.
● Because cefditoren tablets contain sodium caseinate, a milk protein, don't give drug to patients hypersensitive to milk protein (as distinct from those with lactose intolerance).
● Use cautiously in breast-feeding women because cephalosporins appear in breast milk, and safe use hasn't been established.
● Use cautiously in patients with impaired renal function or penicillin allergy.

## NURSING CONSIDERATIONS
● Give drug with a fatty meal to increase its bioavailability.

---

• If patient develops diarrhea after receiving cefditoren, keep in mind that this drug may cause pseudomembranous colitis.

• Don't use this drug if patient needs prolonged treatment.

• Monitor patient for overgrowth of resistant organisms.

• Patients with renal or hepatic impairment, in poor nutritional state, receiving a protracted course of antibiotics, or previously stabilized on anticoagulants may be at risk for decreased prothrombin activity. Monitor PT in these patients.

**PATIENT TEACHING**

• Instruct patient to take medication exactly as prescribed.

• Tell patient to take drug with food to increase its absorption.

• Caution patient not to take drug with an $H_2$ antagonist or an antacid because they may reduce cefditoren absorption.

• Instruct patient not to stop drug before completing treatment and to immediately call prescriber if he experiences any unpleasant adverse reactions.

• Instruct patient to contact prescriber if signs and symptoms of infection don't improve after several days of therapy.

• Inform patient of potential adverse reactions.

• Urge patient not to miss any doses. However, if he does, tell him to take the missed dose as soon as possible unless it's within 4 hours of the next scheduled dose. In that case, tell him to skip the missed dose and go back to the regular dosing schedule. Tell him not to double the dose.

---

## cefepime hydrochloride
Maxipime

*Pregnancy risk category B*

**AVAILABLE FORMS**
*Injection:* 500-mg vial, 1-g/100-ml piggyback bottle, 1-g ADD-Vantage vial, 1-g vial, 2-g/100-ml piggyback bottle, 2-g vial

**INDICATIONS & DOSAGES**
➤ **Mild to moderate UTIs caused by** *Escherichia coli, Klebsiella pneumoniae,* **or** *Proteus mirabilis,* **including concur-**rent bacteremia with these microorganisms
*Adults and children age 12 and older:*
0.5 to 1 g I.M. or I.V. infused over 30 minutes q 12 hours for 7 to 10 days. I.M. route used only for *E. coli* infections.

➤ **Severe UTIs, including pyelonephritis, caused by** *E. coli* **or** *K. pneumoniae*
*Adults and children age 12 and older:* 2 g I.V. infused over 30 minutes q 12 hours for 10 days.

➤ **Moderate to severe pneumonia caused by** *Streptococcus pneumoniae, Pseudomonas aeruginosa, K. pneumoniae,* **or** *Enterobacter* **species**
*Adults and children age 12 and older:* 1 to 2 g I.V. infused over 30 minutes q 12 hours for 10 days.

➤ **Moderate to severe skin infections, uncomplicated skin infections, and skin-structure infections caused by** *S. pyogenes* **or methicillin-susceptible strains of** *Staphylococcus aureus*
*Adults and children age 12 and older:* 2 g I.V. infused over 30 minutes q 12 hours for 10 days.

➤ **Complicated intra-abdominal infections caused by** *E. coli,* **viridans group** *streptococci, P. aeruginosa, K. pneumoniae, Enterobacter* **species, or B. fragilis**
*Adults:* 2 g I.V. infused over 30 minutes q 12 hours for 7 to 10 days. Use with metronidazole.

➤ **Empiric therapy for febrile neutropenia**
*Adults:* 2 g I.V. q 8 hours for 7 days or until neutropenia resolves.

➤ **Uncomplicated and complicated UTIs (including pyelonephritis), uncomplicated skin and skin-structure infections, pneumonia; as empiric therapy for febrile neutropenic children**
*Children ages 2 months to 16 years, weighing up to 40 kg (88 lb):* 50 mg/kg/dose I.V. infused over 30 minutes q 12 hours, or q 8 hours for febrile neutropenia, for 7 to 10 days. Don't exceed 2 g/dose.
*Adjust-a-dose:* For patients on hemodialysis, about 68% of drug is removed after a 3-hour dialysis session. Give a repeat dose, equivalent to the first dose, at the completion of dialysis.

For patients on continuous ambulatory peritoneal dialysis, give normal dosage q 48 hours.

---

## Dosage adjustments for renal impairment

| Creatinine clearance (ml/min) | If normal dosage would be | | | |
| --- | --- | --- | --- | --- |
| | 500 mg q 12 hr | 1 g q 12 hr | 2 g q 12 hr | 2 g q 8 hr |
| 30-60 | 500 mg q 24 hr | 1 g q 24 hr | 2 g q 24 hr | 2 g q 12 hr |
| 11-29 | 500 mg q 24 hr | 500 mg q 24 hr | 1 g q 24 hr | 2 g q 24 hr |
| < 11 | 250 mg q 24 hr | 250 mg q 24 hr | 500 mg q 24 hr | 1 g q 24 hr |

## I.V. ADMINISTRATION
- Follow manufacturer's guidelines closely when reconstituting drug. Variations occur in reconstituting drug for administration, depending on concentration of drug ordered and how drug is packaged (piggyback vial, ADD-Vantage vial, or regular vial).
- The type of diluent used for reconstitution varies, depending on the product used. Use only solutions recommended by the manufacturer. Give the resulting solution over about 30 minutes.
- Intermittent I.V. infusion with a Y-type administration set can be accomplished with compatible solutions. However, during infusion of a solution containing cefepime, discontinuing the other solution is recommended.

## ACTION
Fourth-generation cephalosporin that inhibits bacterial cell-wall synthesis, promotes osmotic instability, and destroys bacteria.

| Route | Onset | Peak | Duration |
| --- | --- | --- | --- |
| I.V., I.M. | 30 min | 1-2 hr | Unknown |

## ADVERSE REACTIONS
**CNS:** fever, headache.
**CV:** phlebitis.
**GI:** colitis, diarrhea, nausea, vomiting, oral candidiasis.
**GU:** vaginitis.
**Skin:** rash, pruritus, urticaria.
**Other:** pain, inflammation, hypersensitivity reactions, *anaphylaxis.*

## INTERACTIONS
**Drug-drug.** *Aminoglycosides:* May increase risk of nephrotoxicity. Monitor renal function closely.

*Potent diuretics:* May increase risk of nephrotoxicity. Monitor renal function closely.
*Probenecid:* May inhibit renal excretion of cefepime. Monitor patient for adverse reactions.

## EFFECTS ON LAB TEST RESULTS
- May falsely elevate serum or urine creatinine level in tests using Jaffe reaction. May cause false-positive results of Coombs' test and urine glucose tests using cupric sulfate (Benedict's reagent or Clinitest).

## CONTRAINDICATIONS & CAUTIONS
- Contraindicated in patients hypersensitive to drug, cephalosporins, beta-lactam antibiotics, or penicillins.
- Use cautiously in patients hypersensitive to penicillin because of possibility of cross-sensitivity with other beta-lactam antibiotics.
- Use cautiously in breast-feeding women and in patients with history of colitis and renal insufficiency.

## NURSING CONSIDERATIONS
- Obtain culture and sensitivity tests before giving first dose. Therapy may begin pending results.
- Dosage adjustment is necessary in patients with impaired renal function. Serious adverse reactions, including encephalopathy, myoclonus, seizures, and renal failure, may occur when dosage isn't adjusted.
- For I.M. administration, reconstitute drug using sterile water for injection, normal saline solution for injection, $D_5W$ injection, 0.5% or 1% lidocaine hydrochloride, or bacteriostatic water for injection with parabens or benzyl alcohol. Follow manufacturer's guidelines for quantity of diluent to use.

• Inspect solution for particulate matter before use. The powder and its solutions tend to darken, depending on storage conditions. Product potency isn't adversely affected when stored as recommended.
• Monitor patient for superinfection. Drug may cause overgrowth of nonsusceptible bacteria or fungi.
• Drug may reduce PT activity. Patients at risk include those with renal or hepatic impairment or poor nutrition and those receiving prolonged cefepime therapy. Monitor PT and INR in these patients, as ordered. Give exogenous vitamin K, as indicated.
• *Alert:* Don't confuse drug with other cephalosporins that sound alike.

**PATIENT TEACHING**
• Warn patient receiving drug I.M. that pain may occur at injection site.
• Instruct patient to report signs and symptoms of superinfection or GI disturbance.

---

**cefoperazone sodium**
Cefobid

*Pregnancy risk category B*

**AVAILABLE FORMS**
*Infusion:* 1 g, 2 g piggyback
*Parenteral:* 1-g, 2-g vials; 1 g, 2 g premixed

**INDICATIONS & DOSAGES**
➤ Serious respiratory tract infections; intra-abdominal, gynecologic, and skin infections; bacteremia; septicemia caused by susceptible microorganisms (*Streptococcus pneumoniae* and *S. pyogenes; Staphylococcus aureus* [penicillinase- and non–penicillinase-producing] and *S. epidermidis;* enterococci; *Escherichia coli; Haemophilus influenzae; Enterobacter, Citrobacter, Klebsiella,* and *Proteus* species; some *Pseudomonas species,* including *P. aeruginosa;* and *Bacteroides fragilis*)
*Adults:* Usual dosage is 1 to 2 g q 12 hours I.M. or I.V. In severe infections or in infections caused by less sensitive organisms, total daily dose or frequency may be increased to 16 g/day.

*Adjust-a-dose:* For patients with hepatic or biliary obstruction, don't exceed total dose of 4 g/day. For patients with hepatic and substantial renal impairment, don't exceed total dose of 2 g/day. Hemodialysis reduces drug's half-life; schedule dosing to follow a dialysis session.

**I.V. ADMINISTRATION**
• Reconstitute drug in 1- or 2-g vial with a minimum of 2.8 ml of compatible I.V. solution; manufacturer recommends using 5 ml/g.
• Give by direct injection into a large vein or into tubing of a free-flowing I.V. solution over 3 to 5 minutes.
• When giving by intermittent infusion, add reconstituted drug to 20 to 40 ml of a compatible I.V. solution and infuse over 15 to 30 minutes.

**ACTION**
Third-generation cephalosporin that inhibits cell-wall synthesis, promoting osmotic instability; usually bactericidal.

| Route | Onset | Peak | Duration |
|-------|-------|------|----------|
| I.V. | Immediate | Immediate | Unknown |
| I.M. | Unknown | 1-2 hr | Unknown |

**ADVERSE REACTIONS**
**CNS:** fever.
**CV:** *phlebitis, thrombophlebitis.*
**GI:** *pseudomembranous colitis,* nausea, vomiting, *diarrhea.*
**Hematologic:** *transient neutropenia,* eosinophilia, anemia, hypoprothrombinemia, bleeding.
**Skin:** *maculopapular and erythematous rashes, urticaria, pain, induration, sterile abscesses, temperature elevation, tissue sloughing at I.M. injection site.*
**Other:** hypersensitivity reactions, serum sickness, *anaphylaxis.*

**INTERACTIONS**
**Drug-drug.** *Aminoglycosides:* May increase risk of nephrotoxicity. Monitor renal function.
*Probenecid:* May inhibit excretion and increase cefoperazone level. Use together cautiously.
**Drug-lifestyle.** *Alcohol use:* May cause a disulfiram-like reaction. Warn patient not

---

to drink alcohol for several days after stopping cefoperazone.

**EFFECTS ON LAB TEST RESULTS**
• May increase ALT, AST, alkaline phosphatase, bilirubin, GGT, and LDH levels.
• May increase INR and eosinophil count. May decrease hemoglobin and neutrophil count. May increase or decrease PT.
• May falsely elevate serum or urine creatinine level in tests using Jaffe reaction. May cause false-positive results of Coombs' test and urine glucose tests using cupric sulfate (Benedict's reagent or Clinitest).

**CONTRAINDICATIONS & CAUTIONS**
• Contraindicated in patients hypersensitive to drug or other cephalosporins.
• Use cautiously in patients hypersensitive to penicillin because of possibility of cross-sensitivity with other beta-lactam antibiotics.
• Use cautiously in breast-feeding women and in patients with history of colitis and renal insufficiency.
• Give doses of 4 g/day cautiously to patients with hepatic disease or biliary obstruction. Higher dosages require monitoring of drug level.

**NURSING CONSIDERATIONS**
• Periodically monitor liver and renal function and compare to baseline.
• Obtain specimen for culture and sensitivity tests before giving first dose. Therapy may begin pending results.
• To prepare drug for I.M. injection using the 1-g vial, dissolve drug with 2 ml of sterile water for injection; then add 0.6 ml of 2% lidocaine hydrochloride for final concentration of 333 mg/ml. Or, dissolve drug with 2.6 ml of sterile water for injection; then add 1 ml of 2% lidocaine hydrochloride for final concentration of 250 mg/ml.
• To prepare drug for I.M. injection using the 2-g vial, dissolve drug with 3.8 ml of sterile water for injection; then add 1.2 ml of 2% lidocaine hydrochloride for final concentration of 333 mg/ml. Or, dissolve drug with 5.4 ml of sterile water for injection; then add 1.8 ml of 2% lidocaine hydrochloride for final concentration of 250 mg/ml.

• For I.M. administration, inject deeply into a large muscle, such as the gluteus maximus or the lateral aspect of the thigh.
• If large doses are given, therapy is prolonged, or patient is at high risk, monitor him for signs or symptoms of superinfection.
• Monitor PT and INR regularly. The drug's chemical structure has the methylthiotetrazole side chain that may cause bleeding disorders. Vitamin K promptly reverses bleeding if it occurs.
• *Alert:* Don't confuse drug with other cephalosporins that sound alike.

**PATIENT TEACHING**
• Tell patient to report adverse reactions and signs and symptoms of superinfection promptly.
• Instruct patient to report discomfort at I.V. insertion site.

---

## cefotaxime sodium
Claforan

*Pregnancy risk category B*

---

**AVAILABLE FORMS**
*Infusion:* 1-g, 2-g premixed package
*Injection:* 500-mg, 1-g, 2-g vials

**INDICATIONS & DOSAGES**
➤ **Perioperative prevention in contaminated surgery**
*Adults:* 1 g I.M. or I.V. 30 to 90 minutes before surgery. In patients undergoing bowel surgery, provide preoperative mechanical bowel cleansing and give a nonabsorbable anti-infective drug such as neomycin. In patients undergoing cesarean delivery, give 1 g I.M. or I.V. as soon as the umbilical cord is clamped; then 1 g I.M. or I.V. 6 and 12 hours later.
➤ **Uncomplicated gonorrhea caused by penicillinase-producing strains of *Neisseria gonorrhoeae* or non–penicillinase-producing strains of the organism**
*Adults and adolescents:* 500 mg I.M. as a single dose.
➤ **Rectal gonorrhea**
*Men:* 1 g I.M. as a single dose.
*Women:* 500 mg I.M. as a single dose.
➤ **Serious infections of the lower respiratory and urinary tracts, CNS, skin,**

---

*Rapid onset*   †Canada   ‡Australia   ◇OTC   ◆Off-label use   ✒Photoguide   *Liquid contains alcohol.

bone, and joints; gynecologic and intra-abdominal infections; bacteremia; septicemia caused by susceptible microorganisms, such as *streptococci* (including *Streptococcus pneumoniae* and *S. pyogenes*), *Staphylococcus aureus* (penicillinase- and non–penicillinase-producing) and *S. epidermidis, Escherichia coli, Klebsiella, Haemophilus influenzae, Serratia marcescens,* and species of *Pseudomonas* (including *P. aeruginosa*), *Enterobacter, Proteus,* and *Peptostreptococcus*

*Adults and children weighing 50 kg (110 lb) or more:* Usual dose is 1 g I.V. or I.M. q 6 to 8 hours. Up to 12 g daily can be given in life-threatening infections.

*Children ages 1 month to 12 years weighing less than 50 kg:* 50 to 180 mg/kg/day I.M. or I.V. in four to six divided doses.

*Neonates ages 1 to 4 weeks:* 50 mg/kg I.V. q 8 hours.

*Neonates to age 1 week:* 50 mg/kg I.V. q 12 hours.

***Adjust-a-dose:*** For patients with creatinine clearance below 20 ml/minute, give half usual dose at usual interval.

## I.V. ADMINISTRATION
● For direct injection, reconstitute drug in 500-mg, 1-g, or 2-g vials with 10 ml of sterile water for injection. Solutions containing 1 g/14 ml are isotonic. Inject drug into a large vein or into the tubing of a free-flowing I.V. solution over 3 to 5 minutes.
● For I.V. infusion, reconstitute drug in infusion vials with 50 to 100 ml of $D_5W$ or normal saline solution. Infuse drug over 20 to 30 minutes. Interrupt flow of primary I.V. solution during infusion.

## ACTION
Third-generation cephalosporin that inhibits cell-wall synthesis, promoting osmotic instability; usually bactericidal.

| Route | Onset | Peak | Duration |
|-------|-------|------|----------|
| I.V. | Immediate | Immediate | Unknown |
| I.M. | Unknown | 30 min | Unknown |

## ADVERSE REACTIONS
**CNS:** fever, headache, dizziness.
**CV:** *phlebitis, thrombophlebitis.*

**GI:** *pseudomembranous colitis,* nausea, vomiting, *diarrhea.*
**GU:** vaginitis, candidiasis, interstitial nephritis.
**Hematologic:** *transient neutropenia,* eosinophilia, hemolytic anemia, ***thrombocytopenia, agranulocytosis.***
**Skin:** *maculopapular and erythematous rashes, urticaria, pain, induration, sterile abscesses, temperature elevation, tissue sloughing at I.M. injection site.*
**Other:** hypersensitivity reactions, serum sickness, ***anaphylaxis.***

## INTERACTIONS
**Drug-drug.** *Aminoglycosides:* May increase risk of nephrotoxicity. Monitor patient's renal function tests.
*Probenecid:* May inhibit excretion and increase cefotaxime. Use together cautiously.

## EFFECTS ON LAB TEST RESULTS
● May increase ALT, AST, alkaline phosphatase, bilirubin, GGT, and LDH levels.
● May increase eosinophil count. May decrease hemoglobin and neutrophil, platelet, and granulocyte counts.
● May cause positive Coombs' test results.

## CONTRAINDICATIONS & CAUTIONS
● Contraindicated in patients hypersensitive to drug or other cephalosporins.
● Use cautiously in patients hypersensitive to penicillin because of possibility of cross-sensitivity with other beta-lactam antibiotics.
● Use cautiously in breast-feeding women and in patients with history of colitis and renal insufficiency.

## NURSING CONSIDERATIONS
● Obtain specimen for culture and sensitivity tests before giving first dose. Therapy may begin pending results.
● For I.M. administration, inject deeply into a large muscle, such as the gluteus maximus or the lateral aspect of the thigh.
● For I.M. doses of 2 g, divide the dose and give at different sites.
● If large doses are given, therapy is prolonged, or patient is at high risk, monitor patient for superinfection.
● ***Alert:*** Don't confuse drug with other cephalosporins that sound alike.

---

## PATIENT TEACHING
● Tell patient to report adverse reactions and signs and symptoms of superinfection promptly.
● Instruct patient to report discomfort at I.V. insertion site.

---

## cefotetan disodium
Cefotan

*Pregnancy risk category B*

### AVAILABLE FORMS
*Infusion:* 1 g, 2 g piggyback and pre-mixed
*Injection:* 1 g, 2 g

### INDICATIONS & DOSAGES
➤ **Serious UTIs, lower respiratory tract infections, and gynecologic, skin and skin-structure, intra-abdominal, and bone and joint infections caused by susceptible streptococci, penicillinase- and non–penicillinase-producing *Staphylococcus aureus* and *S. epidermidis, Escherichia coli, Haemophilus influenzae, Neisseria gonorrhoeae,* and species of *Proteus, Klebsiella, Enterobacter,* and *Bacteroides,* including *B. fragilis***
*Adults:* 1 to 2 g I.V. or I.M. q 12 hours for 5 to 10 days. Up to 6 g daily in life-threatening infections.
➤ **Perioperative prevention**
*Adults:* 1 to 2 g I.V. given once 30 to 60 minutes before surgery. In cesarean section, give dose as soon as umbilical cord is clamped.
*Adjust-a-dose:* In patients with creatinine clearance 10 to 30 ml/minute, give usual dose q 24 hours; if clearance is less than 10 ml/minute, give usual dose q 48 hours.

### I.V. ADMINISTRATION
● Reconstitute drug with sterile water for injection. Drug may then be mixed with 50 to 100 ml of D₅W or normal saline solution. Interrupt flow of primary I.V. solution during cefotetan infusion.
● Infuse over 20 to 60 minutes.

### ACTION
Second-generation cephalosporin that inhibits cell-wall synthesis, promoting osmotic instability; usually bactericidal.

| Route | Onset | Peak | Duration |
|-------|-------|------|----------|
| I.V. | Immediate | Immediate | Unknown |
| I.M. | Unknown | 1½-3 hr | Unknown |

### ADVERSE REACTIONS
**CNS:** fever.
**CV:** *phlebitis, thrombophlebitis.*
**GI:** *pseudomembranous colitis,* nausea, diarrhea.
**GU:** *nephrotoxicity.*
**Hematologic:** *transient neutropenia,* eosinophilia, hemolytic anemia, hypoprothrombinemia, bleeding, thrombocytosis, *agranulocytosis, thrombocytopenia.*
**Skin:** *maculopapular and erythematous rashes, urticaria, pain, induration, sterile abscesses, tissue sloughing at injection site.*
**Other:** hypersensitivity reactions, serum sickness, *anaphylaxis.*

### INTERACTIONS
**Drug-drug.** *Aminoglycosides:* May cause synergistic effect and increased risk of nephrotoxicity. Monitor renal function tests.
*Probenecid:* May inhibit excretion and increase cefotetan level. May use together for this effect.
**Drug-lifestyle.** *Alcohol:* May cause a disulfiram-like reaction. Strongly discourage use together and for several days after stopping drug.

### EFFECTS ON LAB TEST RESULTS
● May increase ALT, AST, alkaline phosphatase, bilirubin, and LDH levels.
● May increase PT and INR and eosinophil count. May decrease hemoglobin and neutrophil and granulocyte counts. May increase or decrease platelet count.
● May falsely elevate serum or urine creatinine level in tests using Jaffe reaction. May cause false-positive results of Coombs' test and urine glucose tests using cupric sulfate (Benedict's reagent or Clinitest).

### CONTRAINDICATIONS & CAUTIONS
● Contraindicated in patients hypersensitive to drug or other cephalosporins.
● Use cautiously in patients hypersensitive to penicillin because of possibility of cross-sensitivity with other beta-lactam antibiotics.

---

*Rapid onset* †Canada ‡Australia ◇OTC ◆Off-label use ✐Photoguide *Liquid contains alcohol.

• Use cautiously in breast-feeding women and in patients with history of colitis and renal insufficiency.

**NURSING CONSIDERATIONS**
• Obtain specimen for culture and sensitivity tests before giving first dose. Therapy may begin pending results.
• Reconstitute for I.M. injection with sterile water or bacteriostatic water for injection, normal saline solution for injection, or 0.5% or 1% lidocaine hydrochloride. Shake to dissolve and let stand until clear.
• Give I.M. injection deep into the body of a large muscle.
• Reconstituted solution is stable for 24 hours at room temperature or 96 hours refrigerated.
• Patients with renal or hepatic impairment, in poor nutritional state, receiving a protracted course of antibiotics, or previously stabilized on anticoagulants may be at risk for decreased prothrombin activity. Monitor PT in these patients.
• If large doses are given, therapy is prolonged, or patient is at high risk, monitor patient for signs and symptoms of superinfection.
• *Alert:* Don't confuse drug with other cephalosporins that sound alike.

**PATIENT TEACHING**
• Tell patient to report adverse reactions and signs and symptoms of superinfection promptly.
• Instruct patient to report discomfort at I.V. site.
• Tell patient to notify prescriber about loose stools or diarrhea.

## cefoxitin sodium
Mefoxin

*Pregnancy risk category B*

**AVAILABLE FORMS**
*Infusion:* 1 g, 2 g in 50-ml or 100-ml container
*Injection:* 1 g, 2 g

**INDICATIONS & DOSAGES**
➤ **Serious infections of the respiratory and GU tracts; skin, soft-tissue, bone, and joint infections; bloodstream and intra-abdominal infections caused by susceptible organisms (such as *Escherichia coli* and other coliform bacteria, penicillinase- and non–penicillinase-producing *Staphylococcus aureus*, *S. epidermidis, streptococci, Klebsiella, Haemophilus influenzae,* and *Bacteroides,* including *B. fragilis*)**
*Adults:* 1 to 2 g I.V. or I.M. q 6 to 8 hours for uncomplicated infections. Up to 12 g daily in life-threatening infections.
*Children older than age 3 months:* 80 to 160 mg/kg daily I.V. or I.M., given in four to six equally divided doses. Maximum daily dose is 12 g.
➤ **Uncomplicated gonorrhea**
*Adults:* 2 g I.M. with 1 g probenecid P.O. as a single dose. Give probenecid within 30 minutes before cefoxitin dose.
➤ **Perioperative prevention**
*Adults:* 2 g I.M. or I.V. 30 to 60 minutes before surgery, then 2 g I.M. or I.V. q 6 hours for up to 24 hours. For transurethral prostatectomy, give 1 g I.M. or I.V. before surgery, then continue giving 1 g q 8 hours for up to 5 days.
*Children age 3 months and older:* 30 to 40 mg/kg I.M. or I.V. 30 to 60 minutes before surgery, then 30 to 40 mg/kg q 6 hours for up to 24 hours.
*Adjust-a-dose:* For patients with creatinine clearance 30 to 50 ml/minute, give 1 to 2 g q 8 to 12 hours; if clearance is 10 to 29 ml/minute, give 1 to 2 g q 12 to 24 hours; if clearance is 5 to 9 ml/minute, give 0.5 to 1 g q 12 to 24 hours; and if clearance is less than 5 ml/minute, give 0.5 to 1 g q 24 to 48 hours.

**I.V. ADMINISTRATION**
• Reconstitute 1 g with at least 10 ml of sterile water for injection and 2 g with 10 to 20 ml of sterile water for injection. Solutions of $D_5W$ and normal saline solution for injection can also be used.
• For direct injection, inject drug into a large vein or into the tubing of a free-flowing I.V. solution over 3 to 5 minutes. For intermittent infusion, add reconstituted drug to 50 or 100 ml of $D_5W$ or dextrose 10% in water or normal saline solution for injection. Interrupt flow of primary I.V. solution during infusion.

● Assess I.V. site frequently. Such use has been linked to development of thrombophlebitis.

## ACTION
Second-generation cephalosporin that inhibits cell-wall synthesis, promoting osmotic instability; usually bactericidal.

| Route | Onset | Peak | Duration |
|-------|-------|------|----------|
| I.V. | Immediate | Immediate | Unknown |
| I.M. | Unknown | 20-30 min | Unknown |

## ADVERSE REACTIONS
**CNS:** fever.
**CV:** hypotension, *phlebitis, thrombophlebitis.*
**GI:** *pseudomembranous colitis,* nausea, vomiting, *diarrhea.*
**GU:** *acute renal failure.*
**Hematologic:** *transient neutropenia,* eosinophilia, hemolytic anemia, anemia, *thrombocytopenia.*
**Respiratory:** dyspnea.
**Skin:** *maculopapular and erythematous rashes, urticaria,* exfoliative dermatitis, *pain, induration, sterile abscesses, tissue sloughing at injection site.*
**Other:** hypersensitivity reactions, serum sickness, *anaphylaxis.*

## INTERACTIONS
**Drug-drug.** *Aminoglycosides:* May increase risk of nephrotoxicity. Monitor patient's renal function tests.
*Probenecid:* May inhibit excretion and increase cefoxitin level. Probenecid may be used for this effect.

## EFFECTS ON LAB TEST RESULTS
● May increase ALT, AST, alkaline phosphatase, bilirubin, and LDH levels.
● May increase eosinophil count. May decrease hemoglobin and neutrophil and platelet counts.
● May falsely elevate serum or urine creatinine level in tests using Jaffe reaction. May cause false-positive results of Coombs' test and urine glucose tests using cupric sulfate (Benedict's reagent or Clinitest).

## CONTRAINDICATIONS & CAUTIONS
● Contraindicated in patients hypersensitive to drug or other cephalosporins.

● Use cautiously in patients hypersensitive to penicillin because of possibility of cross-sensitivity with other beta-lactam antibiotics.
● Use cautiously in breast-feeding women and in patients with history of colitis and renal insufficiency.

## NURSING CONSIDERATIONS
● Obtain specimen for culture and sensitivity tests before giving first dose. Therapy may begin pending results.
● *Alert:* Mefoxin in Galaxy containers is for I.V. use only.
● For I.M. use, reconstitute each 1 g of drug with 2 ml of sterile water for injection or 0.5% or 1% lidocaine hydrochloride (without epinephrine) to minimize pain. Inject deeply into a large muscle, such as the gluteus maximus or the lateral aspect of the thigh.
● After reconstitution, store for 24 hours at room temperature or 1 week under refrigeration.
● If large doses are given, therapy is prolonged, or patient is at high risk, monitor patient for signs and symptoms of superinfection.
● *Alert:* Don't confuse drug with other cephalosporins that sound alike.

## PATIENT TEACHING
● Tell patient to report adverse reactions and signs and symptoms of superinfection promptly.
● Instruct patient to report discomfort at I.V. site.
● Advise patient to notify prescriber about loose stools or diarrhea.

## cefpodoxime proxetil
Vantin

*Pregnancy risk category B*

## AVAILABLE FORMS
*Oral suspension:* 50 mg/5 ml or 100 mg/5 ml in 100-ml bottles
*Tablets (film-coated):* 100 mg, 200 mg

## INDICATIONS & DOSAGES
➤ **Acute, community-acquired pneumonia caused by strains of** *Haemophi-*

*lus influenzae* or *Streptococcus pneumoniae*
*Adults and children age 12 and older:*
200 mg P.O. q 12 hours for 14 days.
➤ **Acute bacterial worsening of chronic bronchitis caused by** *S. pneumoniae* or *H. influenzae* **(strains that don't produce beta-lactamase only), or** *Moraxella catarrhalis*
*Adults and children age 12 and older:*
200 mg P.O. q 12 hours for 10 days.
➤ **Uncomplicated gonorrhea in men and women; rectal gonococcal infections in women**
*Adults and children age 12 and older:*
200 mg P.O. as a single dose. Follow with doxycycline 100 mg P.O. b.i.d. for 7 days.
➤ **Uncomplicated skin and skin-structure infections caused by** *Staphylococcus aureus* **or** *S. pyogenes*
*Adults and children age 12 and older:*
400 mg P.O. q 12 hours for 7 to 14 days.
➤ **Acute otitis media caused by** *S. pneumoniae* **(penicillin-susceptible strains only),** *S. pyogenes, H. influenzae,* **or** *M. catarrhalis*
*Children age 2 months to 12 years:* 5 mg/kg P.O. q 12 hours for 5 days. Don't exceed 200 mg per dose.
➤ **Pharyngitis or tonsillitis caused by** *S. pyogenes*
*Adults:* 100 mg P.O. q 12 hours for 5 to 10 days.
*Children age 2 months to 11 years:* 5 mg/kg P.O. q 12 hours for 5 to 10 days. Don't exceed 100 mg per dose.
➤ **Uncomplicated UTIs caused by** *Escherichia coli, Klebsiella pneumoniae, Proteus mirabilis,* **or** *S. saprophyticus*
*Adults:* 100 mg P.O. q 12 hours for 7 days.
➤ **Mild to moderate acute maxillary sinusitis caused by** *H. influenzae, S. pneumoniae,* **or** *M. catarrhalis*
*Adults and adolescents age 12 and older:*
200 mg P.O. q 12 hours for 10 days.
*Children ages 2 months to 11 years:* 5 mg/kg P.O. q 12 hours for 10 days; maximum is 200 mg/dose.
*Adjust-a-dose:* For patients with creatinine clearance below 30 ml/minute, increase dosage interval to q 24 hours. Give to dialysis patients three times weekly after dialysis.

## ACTION
Third-generation cephalosporin that inhibits cell-wall synthesis, promoting osmotic instability; usually bactericidal.

| Route | Onset | Peak | Duration |
|-------|-------|------|----------|
| P.O. | Unknown | 2-3 hr | Unknown |

## ADVERSE REACTIONS
**CNS:** headache.
**GI:** *diarrhea,* nausea, vomiting, abdominal pain, *pseudomembranous colitis.*
**GU:** vaginal fungal infections.
**Skin:** rash.
**Other:** hypersensitivity reactions, *anaphylaxis.*

## INTERACTIONS
**Drug-drug.** *Aminoglycosides:* May increase risk of nephrotoxicity. Monitor renal function tests closely.
*Antacids, $H_2$-receptor antagonists:* May decrease absorption of cefpodoxime. Avoid using together.
*Probenecid:* May decrease excretion of cefpodoxime. Monitor patient for toxicity.
**Drug-food.** *Any food:* May increase absorption. Give tablets with food to enhance absorption. Oral suspension may be given without regard to food.

## EFFECTS ON LAB TEST RESULTS
• May falsely elevate serum or urine creatinine level in tests using Jaffe reaction. May cause false-positive results of Coombs' test and urine glucose tests using cupric sulfate (Benedict's reagent or Clinitest).

## CONTRAINDICATIONS & CAUTIONS
• Contraindicated in patients hypersensitive to drug or other cephalosporins.
• Use cautiously in patients with a history of penicillin hypersensitivity because of risk of cross-sensitivity.
• Use cautiously in patients receiving nephrotoxic drugs because other cephalosporins have been shown to have nephrotoxic potential.
• Use cautiously in breast-feeding women because drug appears in breast milk.

## NURSING CONSIDERATIONS
• Monitor renal function and compare with baseline.

---

Reactions may be *common,* uncommon, *life-threatening,* or COMMON AND LIFE-THREATENING.

- Obtain specimen for culture and sensitivity tests before giving first dose. Therapy may begin pending results.
- Give drug with food to enhance absorption. Shake suspension well before using.
- Store suspension in the refrigerator (36° to 46° F [2° to 8° C]). Discard unused portion after 14 days.
- Monitor patient for superinfection. Drug may cause overgrowth of nonsusceptible bacteria or fungi.
- *Alert:* Don't confuse drug with other cephalosporins that sound alike.

**PATIENT TEACHING**
- Tell patient to take drug as prescribed, even after he feels better.
- Instruct patient to take drug with food. If patient is using suspension, tell him to shake container before measuring dose and to keep container refrigerated.
- Tell patient to call prescriber if rash or signs and symptoms of superinfection occur.
- Instruct patient to notify prescriber about loose stools or diarrhea.

---

## cefprozil
Cefzil✔

*Pregnancy risk category B*

**AVAILABLE FORMS**
*Oral suspension:* 125 mg/5 ml, 250 mg/5 ml
*Tablets:* 250 mg, 500 mg

**INDICATIONS & DOSAGES**
➤ **Pharyngitis or tonsillitis caused by** *Streptococcus pyogenes*
*Adults and children age 13 and older:* 500 mg P.O. daily for at least 10 days.
➤ **Otitis media caused by** *S. pneumoniae, Haemophilus influenzae,* **and** *Moraxella catarrhalis*
*Infants and children ages 6 months to 12 years:* 15 mg/kg P.O. q 12 hours for 10 days.
➤ **Secondary bacterial infections of acute bronchitis and acute bacterial worsening of chronic bronchitis caused by** *S. pneumoniae, H. influenzae,* **and** *M. catarrhalis*
*Adults and children age 13 and older:* 500 mg P.O. q 12 hours for 10 days.
➤ **Uncomplicated skin and skin-structure infections caused by** *Staphylococcus aureus* **and** *S. pyogenes*
*Adults and children age 13 and older:* 250 or 500 mg P.O. q 12 hours or 500 mg daily for 10 days.
➤ **Acute sinusitis caused by** *S. pneumoniae, H. influenzae* **(beta-lactamase–positive and negative strains), and** *M. catarrhalis* **(including beta-lactamase–producing strains)**
*Adults and children age 13 and older:* 250 mg P.O. q 12 hours for 10 days; for moderate to severe infection, 500 mg P.O. q 12 hours for 10 days.
*Children ages 6 months to 12 years:* 7.5 mg/kg P.O. q 12 hours for 10 days; for moderate to severe infections, 15 mg/kg P.O. q 12 hours for 10 days.
*Adjust-a-dose:* For renally impaired patients, if creatinine clearance is less than 30 ml/minute, give 50% of usual dose. Give after hemodialysis treatment is completed; drug is removed by hemodialysis.

**ACTION**
Second-generation cephalosporin that inhibits cell-wall synthesis, promoting osmotic instability; usually bactericidal.

| Route | Onset | Peak | Duration |
|-------|-------|------|----------|
| P.O. | Unknown | 1½ hr | Unknown |

**ADVERSE REACTIONS**
**CNS:** dizziness, hyperactivity, headache, nervousness, insomnia, confusion, somnolence.
**GI:** diarrhea, nausea, vomiting, abdominal pain.
**GU:** genital pruritus, vaginitis.
**Hematologic:** eosinophilia.
**Skin:** rash, urticaria, diaper rash.
**Other:** superinfection, hypersensitivity reactions, serum sickness, *anaphylaxis.*

**INTERACTIONS**
**Drug-drug.** *Aminoglycosides:* May increase risk of nephrotoxicity. Monitor renal function tests closely.

---

*Probenecid:* May inhibit excretion and increase cefprozil level. Use together cautiously.

**EFFECTS ON LAB TEST RESULTS**
● May increase BUN, creatinine, ALT, AST, alkaline phosphatase, bilirubin, and LDH levels.
● May increase eosinophil count. May decrease WBC, leukocyte, and platelet counts.
● May falsely elevate serum or urine creatinine level in tests using Jaffe reaction. May cause false-positive results of Coombs' test and urine glucose tests using cupric sulfate (Benedict's reagent or Clinitest).

**CONTRAINDICATIONS & CAUTIONS**
● Contraindicated in patients hypersensitive to drug or other cephalosporins.
● Use cautiously in patients hypersensitive to penicillin because of possibility of cross-sensitivity with other beta-lactam antibiotics.
● Use cautiously in breast-feeding women and in patients with history of colitis and renal insufficiency.

**NURSING CONSIDERATIONS**
● Monitor renal function and liver function test results.
● Obtain specimen for culture and sensitivity tests before giving first dose. Therapy may begin pending results.
● Monitor patient for superinfection. May cause overgrowth of nonsusceptible bacteria or fungi.
● *Alert:* Don't confuse drug with other cephalosporins that sound alike.

**PATIENT TEACHING**
● Advise patient to take drug as prescribed, even after he feels better.
● Tell patient to shake suspension well before measuring dose.
● Inform patient or parent that oral suspensions contain the drug in a bubble gum-flavored form to improve palatability and promote compliance in children. Tell him to refrigerate reconstituted suspension and to discard unused drug after 14 days.
● Instruct patient to notify prescriber if rash or signs and symptoms of superinfection occur.

# ceftazidime
Ceptaz, Fortaz, Tazicef, Tazidime

*Pregnancy risk category B*

**AVAILABLE FORMS**
*Infusion:* 1 g, 2 g in 50-ml and 100-ml vials (premixed)
*Injection (with arginine):* 1 g, 2 g
*Injection (with sodium carbonate):* 500 mg, 1 g, 2 g

**INDICATIONS & DOSAGES**
➤ **Serious UTIs and lower respiratory tract infections; skin, gynecologic, intra-abdominal, and CNS infections; bacteremia; and septicemia caused by susceptible microorganisms, such as streptococci (including *Streptococcus pneumoniae* and *S. pyogenes*), penicillinase- and non–penicillinase-producing *Staphylococcus aureus*, *Escherichia coli*, *Klebsiella*, Proteus, Enterobacter, Haemophilus influenzae, Pseudomonas, and some strains of *Bacteroides***
*Adults and children age 12 and older:* 1 to 2 g I.V. or I.M. q 8 to 12 hours; up to 6 g daily in life-threatening infections.
*Children ages 1 month to 11 years:* 25 to 50 mg/kg I.V. q 8 hours. Maximum dose is 6 g/day. Use sodium carbonate formulation.
*Neonates up to age 4 weeks:* 30 mg/kg I.V. q 12 hours. Use sodium carbonate formulation.
➤ **Uncomplicated UTIs**
*Adults:* 250 mg I.V. or I.M. q 12 hours.
➤ **Complicated UTIs**
*Adults and children age 12 and older:* 500 mg to 1 g I.V. or I.M. q 8 to 12 hours.
*Adjust-a-dose:* For renally impaired patients, if creatinine clearance is 31 to 50 ml/minute, give 1 g q 12 hours; if clearance is 16 to 30 ml/minute, give 1 g q 24 hours; if clearance is 6 to 15 ml/minute, give 500 mg q 24 hours; if clearance is less than 5 ml/minute, give 500 mg q 48 hours. Ceftazidime is removed by hemodialysis; give a supplemental dose of drug after each dialysis treatment.

---

## I.V. ADMINISTRATION

● Each brand of ceftazidime includes specific instructions for reconstitution. Read and follow them carefully.
● Reconstitute solutions containing sodium carbonate with sterile water for injection. Add 5 ml to a 500-mg vial, or add 10 ml to a 1-g or 2-g vial. Shake well to dissolve drug.
● Carbon dioxide is released during dissolution, and positive pressure will develop in vial.
● Reconstitute solutions containing arginine with 10 ml of sterile water for injection. This formulation won't release gas bubbles.
● Infuse drug over 15 to 30 minutes.

## ACTION

Third-generation cephalosporin that inhibits cell-wall synthesis, promoting osmotic instability; usually bactericidal.

| Route | Onset | Peak | Duration |
|-------|-------|------|----------|
| I.V. | Immediate | Immediate | Unknown |
| I.M. | Unknown | 1 hr | Unknown |

## ADVERSE REACTIONS

**CNS:** headache, dizziness, paresthesia, *seizures.*
**CV:** *phlebitis, thrombophlebitis.*
**GI:** *pseudomembranous colitis,* nausea, vomiting, diarrhea, abdominal cramps.
**GU:** vaginitis, candidiasis.
**Hematologic:** eosinophilia; thrombocytosis, *leukopenia,* hemolytic anemia, *agranulocytosis, thrombocytopenia.*
**Skin:** *maculopapular and erythematous rashes, urticaria, pain, induration, sterile abscesses, tissue sloughing at injection site.*
**Other:** hypersensitivity reactions, serum sickness, *anaphylaxis.*

## INTERACTIONS

**Drug-drug.** *Aminoglycosides:* May cause additive or synergistic effect against some strains of *Pseudomonas aeruginosa* and *Enterobacteriaceae;* increased risk of nephrotoxicity. Monitor patient for effects and monitor renal function.
*Chloramphenicol:* May cause antagonistic effect. Avoid using together.

## EFFECTS ON LAB TEST RESULTS

● May increase ALT, AST, alkaline phosphatase, bilirubin, and LDH levels.
● May increase eosinophil count. May decrease hemoglobin and WBC and granulocyte counts. May increase or decrease platelet count.
● May falsely elevate serum or urine creatinine level in tests using Jaffe reaction. May cause false-positive results of Coombs' test and urine glucose tests using cupric sulfate (Benedict's reagent or Clinitest).

## CONTRAINDICATIONS & CAUTIONS

● Contraindicated in patients hypersensitive to drug or other cephalosporins.
● Use cautiously in patients hypersensitive to penicillin because of possibility of cross-sensitivity with other beta-lactam antibiotics.
● Use cautiously in breast-feeding women and in patients with history of colitis and renal insufficiency.

## NURSING CONSIDERATIONS

● Obtain specimen for culture and sensitivity tests before giving first dose. Therapy may begin pending results.
● For I.M. administration, inject deeply into a large muscle, such as the gluteus maximus or the lateral aspect of the thigh.
● If large doses are given, therapy is prolonged, or patient is at high risk, monitor patient for signs and symptoms of superinfection.
● *Alert:* Commercially available preparations contain either sodium carbonate (Fortaz, Tazicef, Tazidime) or arginine (Ceptaz) to facilitate dissolution of drug. Safety and efficacy of solutions containing arginine in children younger than age 12 haven't been established.
● *Alert:* Don't confuse drug with other cephalosporins that sound alike.

## PATIENT TEACHING

● Tell patient to report adverse reactions or signs and symptoms of superinfection promptly.
● Instruct patient to report discomfort at I.V. insertion site.
● Advise patient to notify prescriber about loose stools or diarrhea.

---

*Rapid onset*   †Canada   ‡Australia   ◊ OTC   ♦ Off-label use   ✍Photoguide   *Liquid contains alcohol.

## ceftizoxime sodium
Cefizox

*Pregnancy risk category B*

### AVAILABLE FORMS
*Infusion:* 1 g, 2 g in 100-ml vials or in 50 ml of $D_5W$
*Injection:* 500 mg, 1 g, 2 g

### INDICATIONS & DOSAGES
➤ **Serious UTIs, lower respiratory tract infections, gynecologic infections, bacteremia, septicemia, meningitis, intra-abdominal infections, bone and joint infections, and skin infections caused by susceptible microorganisms, such as streptococci (including *Streptococcus pneumoniae* and *S. pyogenes*), *Staphylococcus aureus*, *S. epidermidis*, *Escherichia coli*, *Haemophilus influenzae*, and *Klebsiella*, *Enterobacter*, *Proteus*, *Peptostreptococcus*, and some *Pseudomonas* species**
*Adults:* Usual dosage is 1 to 2 g I.V. or I.M. q 8 to 12 hours. In life-threatening infections, give up to 2 g q 4 hours.
*Children older than age 6 months:* 50 mg/kg I.V. q 6 to 8 hours. For serious infections, up to 200 mg/kg/day in divided doses may be used. Don't exceed 12 g/day.
➤ **Uncomplicated gonorrhea**
*Adults:* 1 g I.M. as a single dose.
***Adjust-a-dose:*** For renally impaired patients, if creatinine clearance is 50 to 79 ml/minute, give 500 mg to 1.5 g q 8 hours; if clearance is 5 to 49 ml/minute, give 250 mg to 1 g q 12 hours; if clearance is below 5 ml/minute or patient undergoes hemodialysis, give 500 mg to 1 g q 48 hours, or 250 to 500 mg q 24 hours.

### I.V. ADMINISTRATION
● To reconstitute powder, add 5 ml of sterile water to a 500-mg vial, 10 ml to a 1-g vial, or 20 ml to a 2-g vial.
● Reconstitute drug in piggyback vials with 50 to 100 ml of normal saline solution or $D_5W$. Shake well.
● Inject directly into vein over 3 to 5 minutes or slowly into I.V. tubing with free-flowing compatible solution.
● Infuse drug over 15 to 30 minutes.

### ACTION
Third-generation cephalosporin that inhibits cell-wall synthesis, promoting osmotic instability; usually bactericidal.

| Route | Onset | Peak | Duration |
|---|---|---|---|
| I.V. | Immediate | Immediate | Unknown |
| I.M. | Unknown | 30-90 min | Unknown |

### ADVERSE REACTIONS
**CNS:** fever.
**CV:** *phlebitis, thrombophlebitis.*
**GI:** *pseudomembranous colitis,* nausea, anorexia, vomiting, *diarrhea.*
**GU:** vaginitis.
**Hematologic:** *transient neutropenia,* eosinophilia, hemolytic anemia, ***thrombocytosis,*** anemia, ***thrombocytopenia.***
**Respiratory:** dyspnea.
**Skin:** *maculopapular and erythematous rashes, urticaria, pain, induration, sterile abscesses, tissue sloughing at injection site.*
**Other:** hypersensitivity reactions, serum sickness, ***anaphylaxis.***

### INTERACTIONS
**Drug-drug.** *Aminoglycosides:* May increase nephrotoxicity. Monitor renal function.
*Probenecid:* May inhibit excretion and increase ceftizoxime level. Probenecid may be used for this effect.

### EFFECTS ON LAB TEST RESULTS
● May increase BUN, creatinine, ALT, AST, alkaline phosphatase, bilirubin, GGT, and LDH levels. May decrease albumin and protein levels.
● May decrease hemoglobin and PT and RBC, WBC, platelet, granulocyte, and neutrophil counts.
● May falsely elevate serum or urine creatinine level in tests using Jaffe reaction. May cause false-positive results of Coombs' test and urine glucose tests using cupric sulfate (Benedict's reagent or Clinitest).

### CONTRAINDICATIONS & CAUTIONS
● Contraindicated in patients hypersensitive to drug or other cephalosporins.
● Use cautiously in patients hypersensitive to penicillin because of possibility of cross-sensitivity with other beta-lactam antibiotics.

---

Reactions may be *common*, uncommon, *life-threatening*, or COMMON AND LIFE-THREATENING.

• Use cautiously in breast-feeding women and in patients with history of colitis and renal insufficiency.

**NURSING CONSIDERATIONS**
• Obtain specimen for culture and sensitivity tests before giving first dose. Therapy may begin pending results.
• To prepare I.M. injection, mix 1.5 ml of diluent per 500 mg of drug. For I.M. administration, inject deeply into a large muscle, such as the gluteus maximus or the lateral aspect of the thigh. Divide larger doses (2 g) and give at two separate sites.
• If large doses are given, therapy is prolonged, or patient is at high risk, monitor patient for signs or symptoms of superinfection.
• *Alert:* Don't confuse drug with other cephalosporins that sound alike.

**PATIENT TEACHING**
• Tell patient to report adverse reactions and signs and symptoms of superinfection promptly.
• Instruct patient to report discomfort at I.V. site.
• Tell patient to notify prescriber about loose stools or diarrhea.

## ceftriaxone sodium
Rocephin

*Pregnancy risk category B*

**AVAILABLE FORMS**
*Infusion:* 1 g, 2 g piggyback; 1 g, 2 g/ 50 ml premixed
*Injection:* 250 mg, 500 mg, 1 g, 2 g

**INDICATIONS & DOSAGES**
➤ **Uncomplicated gonococcal vulvovaginitis**
*Adults:* 125 mg I.M. as a single dose, plus azithromycin 1 g P.O. as a single dose or doxycycline 100 mg P.O. b.i.d. for 7 days.
➤ **Most infections caused by susceptible organisms; serious UTIs and lower respiratory tract infections; gynecologic, bone and joint, intra-abdominal, and skin infections; bacteremia; septicemia; and Lyme disease caused by such sus-**ceptible microorganisms as streptococci (including *Streptococcus pneumoniae* and *S. pyogenes*); penicillinase- and non–penicillinase-producing *Staphylococcus aureus, S. epidermidis, Escherichia coli, Haemophilus influenzae, Neisseria meningitidis, N. gonorrhoeae, Serratia marcescens,* and *Enterobacter, Klebsiella, Proteus, Peptostreptococcus,* and *Pseudomonas* species**
*Adults and children older than age 12:* 1 to 2 g I.M. or I.V. daily or in equally divided doses q 12 hours. Total daily dose shouldn't exceed 4 g.
*Children age 12 and younger:* 50 to 75 mg/kg I.M. or I.V., not to exceed 2 g/ day, given in divided doses q 12 hours.
➤ **Meningitis**
*Adults and children:* Initially, 100 mg/kg I.M. or I.V. Don't exceed 4 g; then 100 mg/kg I.M. or I.V., given once daily or in divided doses q 12 hours, not to exceed 4 g, for 7 to 14 days.
➤ **Perioperative prevention**
*Adults:* 1 g I.V. as a single dose 30 minutes to 2 hours before surgery.
➤ **Acute bacterial otitis media**
*Children:* 50 mg/kg I.M. as a single dose. Don't exceed 1 g.
➤ **Neurologic complications, carditis, and arthritis from penicillin G–refractory Lyme disease ◆**
*Adults:* 2 g I.V. daily for 14 to 28 days.

**I.V. ADMINISTRATION**
• Reconstitute drug with sterile water for injection, normal saline solution for injection, $D_5W$ or dextrose 10% in water injection, or a combination of normal saline solution and dextrose injection and other compatible solutions.
• Reconstitute by adding 2.4 ml of diluent to the 250-mg vial, 4.8 ml to the 500-mg vial, 9.6 ml to the 1-g vial, and 19.2 ml to the 2-g vial. All reconstituted solutions yield a concentration that averages 100 mg/ml.
• After reconstitution, dilute further for intermittent infusion to desired concentration. I.V. dilutions are stable for 24 hours at room temperature.

## ACTION
Third-generation cephalosporin that inhibits cell-wall synthesis, promoting osmotic instability; usually bactericidal.

| Route | Onset | Peak | Duration |
|-------|-------|------|----------|
| I.V. | Immediate | Immediate | Unknown |
| I.M. | Unknown | 1½-4 hr | Unknown |

## ADVERSE REACTIONS
**CNS:** fever, headache, dizziness.
**CV:** phlebitis.
**GI:** *pseudomembranous colitis,* diarrhea.
**GU:** genital pruritus, candidiasis.
**Hematologic:** eosinophilia, thrombocytosis, *leukopenia.*
**Skin:** pain, induration, tenderness at injection site, *rash,* pruritus.
**Other:** hypersensitivity reactions, serum sickness, *anaphylaxis,* chills.

## INTERACTIONS
**Drug-drug.** *Aminoglycosides:* May cause synergistic effect against some strains of *P. aeruginosa* and *Enterobacteriaceae* species. Monitor patient.
*Probenecid:* High doses (1 g or 2 g daily) may enhance hepatic clearance of ceftriaxone and shorten its half-life. Avoid using together.

## EFFECTS ON LAB TEST RESULTS
- May increase BUN, ALT, AST, alkaline phosphatase, bilirubin, and LDH levels.
- May increase eosinophil and platelet counts. May decrease WBC count.
- May falsely elevate serum or urine creatinine level in tests using Jaffe reaction. May cause false-positive results of Coombs' test and urine glucose tests using cupric sulfate (Benedict's reagent or Clinitest).

## CONTRAINDICATIONS & CAUTIONS
- Contraindicated in patients hypersensitive to drug or other cephalosporins.
- Use cautiously in patients hypersensitive to penicillin because of possibility of cross-sensitivity with other beta-lactam antibiotics.
- Use cautiously in breast-feeding women and in patients with history of colitis and renal insufficiency.

## NURSING CONSIDERATIONS
- Obtain specimen for culture and sensitivity tests before giving first dose. Therapy may begin pending results.
- A commercially available I.M. kit containing 1% lidocaine as a diluent is available from the manufacturer.
- For I.M. administration, inject deeply into a large muscle, such as the gluteus maximus or the lateral aspect of the thigh.
- If large doses are given, therapy is prolonged, or patient is at high risk, monitor patient for signs and symptoms of superinfection.
- Monitor PT and INR in patients with impaired vitamin K synthesis or low vitamin K stores. Vitamin K therapy may be needed.
- Drug is commonly used in home antibiotic programs for outpatient treatment of serious infections such as osteomyelitis and community-acquired pneumonia.
- **Alert:** Don't confuse drug with other cephalosporins that sound alike.

## PATIENT TEACHING
- Tell patient to report adverse reactions promptly.
- Instruct patient to report discomfort at I.V. insertion site.
- Teach patient and family receiving home care how to prepare and give drug.
- If home care patient is diabetic and is testing his urine for glucose, tell him drug may affect results of cupric sulfate tests; he should use an enzymatic test instead.
- Tell patient to notify prescriber about loose stools or diarrhea.

---

# cefuroxime axetil
Ceftin*◊*

# cefuroxime sodium
Zinacef

*Pregnancy risk category B*

## AVAILABLE FORMS
**cefuroxime axetil**
*Suspension:* 125 mg/5 ml, 250 mg/5 ml
*Tablets:* 125 mg, 250 mg, 500 mg

---

**cefuroxime sodium**
*Infusion:* 750 mg, 1.5-g premixed, frozen solution
*Injection:* 750 mg, 1.5 g

**INDICATIONS & DOSAGES**
➤ **Pharyngitis, tonsillitis, infections of the urinary and lower respiratory tracts, and skin and skin-structure infections caused by *Streptococcus pneumoniae* and *S. pyogenes, Haemophilus influenzae, Staphylococcus aureus, Escherichia coli, Moraxella catarrhalis* (including beta-lactamase–producing strains), *Neisseria gonorrhoeae,* and *Klebsiella* and *Enterobacter* species**
*Adults and children age 12 and older:*
250 mg cefuroxime axetil P.O. q 12 hours. For severe infections, increase dosage to 500 mg q 12 hours.
➤ **Serious lower respiratory tract infections, UTIs, skin and skin-structure infections, bone and joint infections, septicemia, meningitis, and gonorrhea**
*Adults and children age 12 and older:*
750 mg to 1.5 g cefuroxime sodium I.M. or I.V. q 8 hours for 5 to 10 days. For life-threatening infections and infections caused by less susceptible organisms, 1.5 g I.M. or I.V. q 6 hours; for bacterial meningitis, up to 3 g I.V. q 8 hours.
*Children and infants older than age 3 months:* 50 to 100 mg/kg/day cefuroxime sodium I.M. or I.V. in equally divided doses q 6 to 8 hours. Use higher dosage of 100 mg/kg/day, not to exceed maximum adult dosage, for more severe or serious infections. For bacterial meningitis, 200 to 240 mg/kg cefuroxime sodium I.V. in divided doses q 6 to 8 hours.
➤ **Uncomplicated UTIs**
*Adults:* 125 to 250 mg P.O. q 12 hours for 7 to 10 days.
➤ **Otitis media**
*Children ages 3 months to 12 years:*
250 mg P.O. q 12 hours for 10 days for children who can swallow tablets whole. Or, 30 mg/kg/day of oral suspension P.O. in 2 divided doses for 10 days for children who can't swallow tablets.
➤ **Pharyngitis and tonsillitis**
*Children ages 3 months to 12 years:*
125 mg P.O. q 12 hours for 10 days, in children who can swallow tablets whole.

Or, 20 mg/kg daily of oral suspension in two divided doses for 10 days, in children who can't swallow tablets.
➤ **Perioperative prevention**
*Adults:* 1.5 g I.V. 30 to 60 minutes before surgery; in lengthy operations, 750 mg I.V. or I.M. q 8 hours. For open-heart surgery, 1.5 g I.V. at induction of anesthesia and then q 12 hours for a total dose of 6 g.
➤ **Early Lyme disease (erythema migrans) caused by *Borrelia burgdorferi***
*Adults and children age 13 and older:*
500 mg P.O. b.i.d. for 20 days.
➤ **Secondary bacterial infection of acute bronchitis**
*Adults:* 250 to 500 mg tablets P.O. b.i.d. for 5 to 10 days.
➤ **Uncomplicated gonorrhea**
*Adults:* 1.5 g I.M. with 1 g probenecid P.O. for one dose. Alternatively, 1 g P.O. as a single dose.
➤ **Acute bacterial maxillary sinusitis caused by *Streptococcus pneumoniae* or *Haemophilus influenzae* (only strains that don't produce beta-lactamase)**
*Adults and children age 13 and older:*
250-mg tablet P.O. b.i.d. for 10 days.
*Children ages 3 months to 12 years:*
30 mg/kg/day oral suspension P.O. in two divided doses for 10 days.
***Adjust-a-dose:*** In patients with creatinine clearance 10 to 20 ml/minute, give 750 mg I.M. or I.V. q 12 hours; if clearance is less than 10 ml/minute, give 750 mg I.M. or I.V. q 24 hours.

**I.V. ADMINISTRATION**
● Reconstitute each 750-mg vial with 8 ml of sterile water for injection; for each 1.5-g vial, reconstitute with 16 ml. Withdraw entire contents of vial for a dose.
● For direct injection, inject into a large vein or into the tubing of a free-flowing I.V. solution over 3 to 5 minutes.
● For intermittent infusion, add reconstituted drug to 100 ml $D_5W$, normal saline solution for injection, or other compatible I.V. solution. Infuse over 15 to 60 minutes.

## ACTION
Second-generation cephalosporin that inhibits cell-wall synthesis, promoting osmotic instability; usually bactericidal.

| Route | Onset | Peak | Duration |
|-------|-------|------|----------|
| P.O. | Unknown | 15-60 min | Unknown |
| I.V. | Immediate | Immediate | Unknown |
| I.M. | Unknown | 2 hr | Unknown |

## ADVERSE REACTIONS
**CV:** *phlebitis, thrombophlebitis.*
**GI:** ***pseudomembranous colitis,*** nausea, anorexia, vomiting, *diarrhea.*
**Hematologic:** *transient neutropenia,* eosinophilia, *hemolytic anemia,* **thrombocytopenia.**
**Skin:** *maculopapular and erythematous rashes, urticaria, pain, induration, sterile abscesses, temperature elevation, tissue sloughing at I.M. injection site.*
**Other:** hypersensitivity reactions, serum sickness, **anaphylaxis.**

## INTERACTIONS
**Drug-drug.** *Aminoglycosides:* May cause synergistic activity against some organisms; may increase nephrotoxicity. Monitor patient's renal function closely.
*Loop diuretics:* May increase risk of adverse renal reactions. Monitor renal function test results closely.
*Probenecid:* May inhibit excretion and increase cefuroxime level. Probenecid may be used for this effect.
**Drug-food.** *Any food:* May increase absorption. Give drug with food.

## EFFECTS ON LAB TEST RESULTS
• May increase ALT, AST, alkaline phosphatase, bilirubin, and LDH levels.
• May increase PT and INR and eosinophil count. May decrease hemoglobin, hematocrit, and neutrophil and platelet counts.
• May falsely elevate serum or urine creatinine level in tests using Jaffe reaction. May cause false-positive results of Coombs' test and urine glucose tests using cupric sulfate (Benedict's reagent or Clinitest).

## CONTRAINDICATIONS & CAUTIONS
• Contraindicated in patients hypersensitive to drug or other cephalosporins.

• Use cautiously in patients hypersensitive to penicillin because of possibility of cross-sensitivity with other beta-lactam antibiotics.
• Use cautiously in breast-feeding women and in patients with history of colitis and renal insufficiency.

## NURSING CONSIDERATIONS
• Obtain specimen for culture and sensitivity tests before giving first dose. Therapy may begin pending results.
• For I.M. administration, inject deeply into a large muscle mass, such as the gluteus maximus or the lateral aspect of the thigh.
• Absorption of cefuroxime axetil is enhanced by food.
• Cefuroxime axetil tablets may be crushed, if absolutely necessary, for patients who can't swallow tablets. Tablets may be dissolved in small amounts of apple, orange, or grape juice or chocolate milk. However, the drug has a bitter taste that is difficult to mask, even with food.
• *Alert:* Cefuroxime axetil film-coated tablet and oral suspension aren't bioequivalent. Don't substitute on a mg/mg basis.
• If large doses are given, therapy is prolonged, or patient is at high risk, monitor patient for signs and symptoms of superinfection.
• *Alert:* Don't confuse drug with other cephalosporins that sound alike.

## PATIENT TEACHING
• Tell patient to take drug as prescribed, even after he feels better.
• Instruct patient to take oral form with food.
• If patient has difficulty swallowing tablets, show him how to dissolve or crush tablets but warn him that the bitter taste is hard to mask, even with food.
• If suspension is being used, tell patient to shake container well before measuring dose.
• Instruct patient to notify prescriber about rash or evidence of superinfection.
• Advise patient receiving drug I.V. to report discomfort at I.V. insertion site.
• Tell patient to notify prescriber about loose stools or diarrhea.

---

Reactions may be *common*, uncommon, *life-threatening*, or COMMON AND LIFE-THREATENING.

## cephalexin hydrochloride
Keftab

## cephalexin monohydrate
Apo-Cephalex†, Biocef, Keflex,
Novo-Lexin†, Nu-Cephalex†

*Pregnancy risk category B*

## AVAILABLE FORMS
**cephalexin hydrochloride**
*Tablets:* 500 mg
**cephalexin monohydrate**
*Capsules:* 250 mg, 500 mg
*Oral suspension:* 125 mg/5 ml, 250 mg/5 ml
*Tablets:* 250 mg, 500 mg, 1 g

## INDICATIONS & DOSAGES
➤ **Respiratory tract, GI tract, skin, soft-tissue, bone, and joint infections and otitis media caused by** *Escherichia coli* **and other coliform bacteria, group A beta-hemolytic streptococci,** *Klebsiella species, Proteus mirabilis, Streptococcus pneumoniae,* **and staphylococci**
*Adults:* 250 mg to 1 g P.O. q 6 hours or 500 mg q 12 hours. Maximum 4 g daily.
*Children:* 25 to 50 mg/kg/day P.O. in two to four equally divided doses. In severe infections, dose can be doubled.
*Adjust-a-dose:* For adults with impaired renal function, initial dose is the same. For subsequent dosing in those with creatinine clearance less than 5 ml/minute, give 250 mg P.O. q 12 to 24 hours; for clearance of 5 to 10 ml/minute, give 250 mg P.O. q 12 hours; and for clearance of 11 to 40 ml/minute, give 500 mg P.O. q 8 to 12 hours.

## ACTION
First-generation cephalosporin that inhibits cell-wall synthesis, promoting osmotic instability; usually bactericidal.

| Route | Onset | Peak | Duration |
|-------|-------|------|----------|
| P.O. | Unknown | 1 hr | Unknown |

## ADVERSE REACTIONS
**CNS:** dizziness, headache, fatigue, agitation, confusion, hallucinations.
**GI:** *pseudomembranous colitis,* nausea, anorexia, vomiting, *diarrhea,* gastritis, glossitis, dyspepsia, abdominal pain, anal pruritus, tenesmus, oral candidiasis.
**GU:** genital pruritus, candidiasis, vaginitis, interstitial nephritis.
**Hematologic:** *neutropenia,* eosinophilia, anemia, *thrombocytopenia.*
**Musculoskeletal:** arthritis, arthralgia, joint pain.
**Skin:** *maculopapular and erythematous rashes, urticaria.*
**Other:** hypersensitivity reactions, serum sickness, *anaphylaxis.*

## INTERACTIONS
**Drug-drug.** *Aminoglycosides:* May increase risk of nephrotoxicity. Avoid using together.
*Probenecid:* May increase cephalosporin level. Probenecid may be used for this effect.

## EFFECTS ON LAB TEST RESULTS
● May increase ALT, AST, alkaline phosphatase, bilirubin, and LDH levels.
● May increase eosinophil count. May decrease hemoglobin and neutrophil and platelet counts.
● May falsely elevate serum or urine creatinine level in tests using Jaffe reaction. May cause false-positive results of Coombs' test and urine glucose tests using cupric sulfate (Benedict's reagent or Clinitest).

## CONTRAINDICATIONS & CAUTIONS
● Contraindicated in patients hypersensitive to cephalosporins.
● Use cautiously in patients hypersensitive to penicillin because of possibility of cross-sensitivity with other beta-lactam antibiotics.
● Use cautiously in breast-feeding women and in patients with history of colitis and renal insufficiency.

## NURSING CONSIDERATIONS
● Ask patient about past reaction to cephalosporin or penicillin therapy before giving first dose.
● Obtain specimen for culture and sensitivity tests before giving first dose. Therapy may begin pending results.
● To prepare oral suspension: Add required amount of water to powder in two portions. Shake well after each addition. After mixing, store in refrigerator. Mix-

ture will remain stable for 14 days. Keep tightly closed and shake well before using.
● If large doses are given or if therapy is prolonged, monitor patient for superinfection, especially if patient is high risk.
● Treat group A beta-hemolytic streptococcal infections for a minimum of 10 days.
● *Alert:* Don't confuse drug with other cephalosporins that sound alike.

**PATIENT TEACHING**
● Tell patient to take drug exactly as prescribed, even after he feels better.
● Instruct patient to take drug with food or milk to lessen GI discomfort. If patient is taking suspension form, instruct him to shake container well before measuring dose and to store in refrigerator.
● Tell patient to notify prescriber if rash or signs and symptoms of superinfection develop.

## cephradine
Velosef

*Pregnancy risk category B*

**AVAILABLE FORMS**
*Capsules:* 250 mg, 500 mg
*Oral suspension:* 125 mg/5 ml, 250 mg/5 ml

**INDICATIONS & DOSAGES**
➤ **Serious infections of respiratory, GU, or GI tract; skin and soft-tissue infections; bone and joint infections; septicemia; endocarditis; and otitis media caused by such susceptible organisms as *Escherichia coli* and other coliform bacteria, group A beta-hemolytic streptococci, *Klebsiella, Proteus mirabilis, Staphylococcus aureus, Streptococcus pneumoniae, S. viridans,* and staphylococci; perioperative prevention**
*Adults:* 250 to 500 mg P.O. q 6 hours or 500 mg to 1 g P.O. q 12 hours. For severe or chronic infections, may give up to 1 g q 6 hours.
*Children older than age 9 months:* 25 to 50 mg/kg P.O. daily in divided doses q 6 to 12 hours. For severe or chronic infections, may give up to 1 g q 6 hours.

➤ **Otitis media**
*Children:* 75 to 100 mg/kg P.O. daily in equally divided doses q 6 to 12 hours. Don't exceed 4 g daily.
*Adjust-a-dose:* For patients with creatinine clearance of 20 ml/minute or more, give 500 mg q 6 hours; for clearance of 5 to 20 ml/minute, give 250 mg q 6 hours; for clearance of less than 5 ml/minute, give 250 mg q 12 hours. In hemodialysis patients, initially 250 mg at the start of dialysis, then 250 mg 12 hours later and 250 mg 36 to 48 hours later.

**ACTION**
First-generation cephalosporin that inhibits cell-wall synthesis, promoting osmotic instability; usually bactericidal.

| Route | Onset | Peak | Duration |
|-------|---------|------|----------|
| P.O. | Unknown | 1 hr | Unknown |

**ADVERSE REACTIONS**
**CNS:** dizziness, headache, malaise, paresthesia.
**GI:** *pseudomembranous colitis, nausea, anorexia,* vomiting, heartburn, abdominal cramps, *diarrhea,* oral candidiasis.
**GU:** genital pruritus, candidiasis, vaginitis.
**Hematologic:** *transient neutropenia,* eosinophilia, *thrombocytopenia.*
**Skin:** *maculopapular and erythematous rashes, urticaria.*
**Other:** hypersensitivity reactions, serum sickness, *anaphylaxis.*

**INTERACTIONS**
**Drug-drug.** *Aminoglycosides:* May increase risk of nephrotoxicity. Avoid using together.
*Probenecid:* May increase level of cephalosporin. Probenecid may be used for this effect.

**EFFECTS ON LAB TEST RESULTS**
● May increase ALT, AST, alkaline phosphatase, bilirubin, and LDH levels.
● May increase eosinophil count. May decrease neutrophil and platelet counts.
● May falsely elevate serum or urine creatinine level in tests using Jaffe reaction. May cause false-positive results of Coombs' test and urine glucose tests using cupric sulfate (Benedict's reagent or Clinitest).

## CONTRAINDICATIONS & CAUTIONS
• Contraindicated in patients hypersensitive to drug and to other cephalosporins.
• Use cautiously in patients hypersensitive to penicillin because of possibility of cross-sensitivity with other beta-lactam antibiotics.
• Use cautiously in breast-feeding women and in patients with history of colitis and renal insufficiency.

## NURSING CONSIDERATIONS
• Monitor renal function.
• Obtain specimen for culture and sensitivity tests before giving first dose. Therapy may begin pending results.
• Treat group A beta-hemolytic streptococcal infections for a minimum of 10 days.
• If large doses are given, therapy is prolonged, or patient is at high risk, monitor patient for signs and symptoms of superinfection.
• *Alert:* Don't confuse drug with other cephalosporins that sound alike.

## PATIENT TEACHING
• Instruct patient to take drug as prescribed, even after he feels better.
• Advise patient to take drug with food or milk to lessen GI discomfort. If patient is taking suspension form, tell him to shake it well before measuring dose.
• Tell patient to notify prescriber if rash or signs and symptoms of superinfection occur.
• Instruct patient to notify prescriber about loose stools or diarrhea.

---

# loracarbef
Lorabid

*Pregnancy risk category B*

## AVAILABLE FORMS
*Capsules:* 200 mg, 400 mg
*Powder for oral suspension:* 100 mg/5 ml, 200 mg/5 ml in 50-ml, 75-ml, and 100-ml bottles

## INDICATIONS & DOSAGES
➤ **Secondary bacterial infections of acute bronchitis**
*Adults:* 200 to 400 mg P.O. q 12 hours for 7 days.

➤ **Acute bacterial worsening of chronic bronchitis**
*Adults:* 400 mg P.O. q 12 hours for 7 days.
➤ **Pneumonia**
*Adults:* 400 mg P.O. q 12 hours for 14 days.
➤ **Pharyngitis, sinusitis, tonsillitis**
*Adults:* 200 to 400 mg P.O. q 12 hours for 10 days.
*Children ages 6 months to 12 years:* 15 mg/kg P.O. daily in divided doses q 12 hours for 10 days.
➤ **Acute otitis media**
*Children ages 6 months to 12 years:* 30 mg/kg oral suspension P.O. daily in divided doses q 12 hours for 10 days.
➤ **Uncomplicated skin and skin-structure infections**
*Adults:* 200 mg P.O. q 12 hours for 7 days.
➤ **Impetigo**
*Children ages 6 months to 12 years:* 15 mg/kg P.O. daily in divided doses q 12 hours for 7 days.
➤ **Uncomplicated cystitis**
*Adults:* 200 mg P.O. daily for 7 days.
➤ **Uncomplicated pyelonephritis**
*Adults:* 400 mg P.O. q 12 hours for 14 days.
*Adjust-a-dose:* For patients with creatinine clearance of 10 to 49 ml/minute, give half usual dose at same interval; if clearance is less than 10 ml/minute, give usual dose q 3 to 5 days. Hemodialysis patients require an additional dose after dialysis.

## ACTION
Synthetic beta-lactam antibiotic of the carbacephem class that inhibits cell-wall synthesis, promoting osmotic instability; usually bactericidal.

| Route | Onset | Peak | Duration |
|-------|-------|------|----------|
| P.O. | Unknown | 30-60 min | Unknown |

## ADVERSE REACTIONS
**CNS:** headache, somnolence, nervousness, insomnia, dizziness.
**CV:** vasodilation.
**GI:** diarrhea, nausea, vomiting, abdominal pain, anorexia, *pseudomembranous colitis.*
**GU:** vaginal candidiasis.

**Hematologic:** *transient thrombocytopenia, leukopenia,* eosinophilia, *pancytopenia, neutropenia.*
**Skin:** rash, urticaria, pruritus, *erythema multiforme.*
**Other:** hypersensitivity reactions, *anaphylaxis.*

## INTERACTIONS
**Drug-drug.** *Probenecid:* May decrease excretion of loracarbef, causing increased drug levels. Monitor patient for toxicity.
**Drug-food.** *Any food:* May decrease absorption. Have patient take drug on empty stomach at least 1 hour before or 2 hours after a meal.

## EFFECTS ON LAB TEST RESULTS
● May increase BUN, creatinine, ALT, AST, and alkaline phosphatase levels.
● May increase PT and INR and eosinophil count. May decrease platelet, WBC, RBC, and neutrophil counts.

## CONTRAINDICATIONS & CAUTIONS
● Contraindicated in patients hypersensitive to drug or other cephalosporins.
● Use cautiously in patients hypersensitive to penicillin because of possibility of cross-sensitivity with other beta-lactam antibiotics.
● Use cautiously in breast-feeding women and in patients with history of colitis and renal insufficiency.
● Safety and efficacy of drug haven't been established in infants younger than age 6 months.

## NURSING CONSIDERATIONS
● Obtain specimen for culture and sensitivity tests before giving first dose. Therapy may begin pending results.
● To reconstitute powder for oral suspension, add 30 ml of water in two portions to the 50-ml bottle, 45 ml of water in two portions to the 75-ml bottle, or 60 ml of water in two portions to the 100-ml bottle; shake after each addition.
● After reconstitution, store oral suspension for 14 days at 59° to 86° F (15° to 30° C).
● Monitor patient for superinfection. Drug may cause overgrowth of nonsusceptible bacteria or fungi.
● Monitor renal function.

● For otitis media, the more rapidly absorbed oral suspension produces higher peak drug levels than do capsules.
● *Alert:* Don't confuse Lorabid with Lortab.

## PATIENT TEACHING
● Instruct patient to take drug prescribed, even after he feels better.
● Tell patient to take drug on an empty stomach, at least 1 hour before or 2 hours after meals. Tell him to shake container of suspension well before measuring dose.
● Advise patient to discard unused portion after 14 days.
● Instruct patient to notify prescriber if rash or signs and symptoms of superinfection appear.
● Instruct patient to notify prescriber if loose stools or diarrhea occurs.

doxycycline calcium
doxycycline hyclate
doxycycline hydrochloride
doxycycline monohydrate
minocycline hydrochloride
tetracycline hydrochloride

## COMBINATION PRODUCTS

HELIDAC: tetracycline 500 mg, bismuth salicylate 262.4 mg, and metronidazole 250 mg.

### doxycycline calcium
Vibramycin

### doxycycline hyclate
Apo-Doxy†, Doryx, Doxy 100, Doxy 200, Doxycin†, Doxytec† Novo-Doxylin†, Nu-Doxycycline†, Periostat, Vibramycin, Vibra-Tabs

### doxycycline hydrochloride‡
Doryx‡, Doxsig‡ Doxylin‡, Doxy Tablets‡ Vibramycin‡, Vibra-Tabs 50‡

### doxycycline monohydrate
Adoxa, Monodox, Vibramycin

*Pregnancy risk category D*

## AVAILABLE FORMS
**doxycycline calcium**
*Syrup:* 50 mg/5 ml
**doxycycline hyclate**
*Capsules:* 20 mg, 50 mg, 100 mg
*Capsules (coated pellets):* 75 mg, 100 mg
*Injection:* 100 mg, 200 mg
*Tablets:* 20 mg, 100 mg
**doxycycline hydrochloride‡**
*Capsules:* 50 mg‡, 100 mg‡
*Tablets:* 50 mg‡, 100 mg‡
**doxycycline monohydrate**
*Capsules:* 50 mg, 100 mg
*Oral suspension:* 25 mg/5 ml
*Tablets:* 50 mg, 75 mg, 100 mg

## INDICATIONS & DOSAGES
➤ **Infections caused by susceptible gram-positive and gram-negative organisms (including *Haemophilus ducreyi*, *Yersinia pestis*, and *Campylobacter fetus*), *Rickettsiae* species, *Mycoplasma pneumoniae*, *Chlamydia trachomatis*, and *Borrelia burgdorferi* (Lyme disease); psittacosis; granuloma inguinale**
*Adults and children older than age 8, weighing at least 45 kg (99 lb):* 100 mg P.O. q 12 hours on first day; then 100 mg P.O. daily. Or, 200 mg I.V. on first day in one or two infusions; then 100 to 200 mg I.V. daily.
*Children older than age 8, weighing less than 45 kg:* 4.4 mg/kg P.O. or I.V. daily, in divided doses q 12 hours on first day; then 2.2 to 4.4 mg/kg daily in one or two divided doses.
   Give I.V. infusion slowly (minimum 1 hour). Infusion must be completed within 12 hours (within 6 hours in lactated Ringer's solution or dextrose 5% in lactated Ringer's solution).
➤ **Gonorrhea in patients allergic to penicillin**
*Adults:* 100 mg P.O. b.i.d. for 7 days. Use for 10 days for epididymitis.
➤ **Primary or secondary syphilis in patients allergic to penicillin**
*Adults:* 300 mg P.O. daily in divided doses for at least 10 days.
➤ **Uncomplicated urethral, endocervical, or rectal infections caused by *C. trachomatis* or *Ureaplasma urealyticum***
*Adults:* 100 mg P.O. b.i.d. for at least 7 days. In those with epididymitis, treat for 10 days.
➤ **To prevent malaria**
*Adults:* 100 mg P.O. daily beginning 1 to 2 days before travel to endemic area and continued for 4 weeks after travel.
*Children older than age 8:* 2 mg/kg P.O. once daily beginning 1 to 2 days before travel to endemic area and continued for 4 weeks after travel. Don't exceed daily dose of 100 mg.

➤ **Pelvic inflammatory disease**
*Adults:* 100 mg I.V. q 12 hours with cefoxitin or cefotetan and continued for at least 2 days after symptomatic improvement; then 100 mg P.O. q 12 hours for a total course of 14 days.

➤ **Adjunct to other antibiotics for inhalation, GI, and oropharyngeal anthrax**
*Adults:* 100 mg q 12 hours I.V. initially until susceptibility test results are known. Switch to 100 mg P.O. b.i.d. when appropriate. Treat for 60 days total.
*Children older than age 8, weighing more than 45 kg (99 lb):* 100 mg q 12 hours I.V., then switch to 100 mg P.O. b.i.d. when appropriate. Treat for 60 days total.
*Children older than age 8, weighing 45 kg or less:* 2.2 mg/kg q 12 hours I.V., then switch to 2.2 mg/kg P.O. b.i.d. when appropriate. Treat for 60 days total.
*Children age 8 and younger:* 2.2 mg/kg q 12 hours I.V., then switch to 2.2 mg/kg P.O. b.i.d. when appropriate. Treat for 60 days total.

➤ **Cutaneous anthrax**
*Adults:* 100 mg P.O. q 12 hours for 60 days.
*Children older than age 8, weighing more than 45 kg (99 lb):* 100 mg P.O. q 12 hours for 60 days.
*Children older than age 8, weighing 45 kg or less:* 2.2 mg/kg q 12 hours P.O. for 60 days.
*Children age 8 and younger:* 2.2 mg/kg P.O. q 12 hours for 60 days.

➤ **Adjunct to scaling and root planing to improve attachment and reduce pocket depth in patients with adult periodontitis**
*Adults:* 20 mg P.O. Periostat b.i.d., more than 1 hour before or 2 hours after the morning and evening meals and after scaling and root planing. Effective for 9 months.

➤ **Adjunctive treatment for severe acne**
*Adults:* 200 mg Adoxa P.O. on the first day of treatment (100 mg given q 12 hours or 50 mg q 6 hours), followed by a maintenance dose of 100 mg/day in single or divided doses.

➤ **To prevent traveler's diarrhea caused by E. coli ◆**
*Adults:* 100 mg P.O. daily.

**I.V. ADMINISTRATION**
● Reconstitute powder for injection with sterile water for injection. Use 10 ml in 100-mg vial and 20 ml in 200-mg vial. Dilute solution to 100 to 1,000 ml for I.V. infusion.
● Don't infuse solutions with concentrations greater than 1 mg/ml.
● Infusion time varies with dose but usually ranges from 1 to 4 hours. Infusion must be completed within 12 hours.
● Monitor I.V. infusion site for signs and symptoms of thrombophlebitis, which may occur with I.V. administration.
● Don't expose drug to light or heat. Protect it from sunlight during infusion.
● Reconstituted injectable solution is stable for 72 hours if refrigerated and protected from light.

**ACTION**
Unknown. Thought to exert bacteriostatic effect by binding to the 30S and possibly 50S ribosomal subunits of microorganisms, thus inhibiting protein synthesis. May also alter the cytoplasmic membrane of susceptible microorganisms.

| Route | Onset | Peak | Duration |
|-------|-------|------|----------|
| P.O. | Unknown | 1½-4 hr | Unknown |
| I.V. | Immediate | Unknown | Unknown |

**ADVERSE REACTIONS**
**CNS:** *intracranial hypertension.*
**CV:** pericarditis, thrombophlebitis.
**GI:** anorexia, glossitis, dysphagia, *epigastric distress, nausea,* vomiting, *diarrhea,* oral candidiasis, enterocolitis, anogenital inflammation.
**Hematologic:** *neutropenia,* eosinophilia, *thrombocytopenia,* hemolytic anemia.
**Musculoskeletal:** bone growth retardation in children younger than age 8.
**Skin:** *maculopapular and erythematous rashes, photosensitivity, increased pigmentation, urticaria.*
**Other:** hypersensitivity reactions, ***anaphylaxis,*** superinfection; permanent discoloration of teeth, enamel defects.

**INTERACTIONS**
**Drug-drug.** *Antacids (including sodium bicarbonate) and laxatives containing aluminum, magnesium, or calcium; antidiarrheals:* May decrease antibiotic ab-

sorption. Give antibiotic 1 hour before or 2 hours after any of these drugs.

*Carbamazepine, phenobarbital:* May decrease antibiotic effect. Avoid using together.

*Ferrous sulfate and other iron products, zinc:* May decrease antibiotic absorption. Give drug 2 hours before or 3 hours after iron administration.

*Hormonal contraceptives:* May decrease contraceptive effectiveness and increase risk of breakthrough bleeding. Advise use of a nonhormonal contraceptive.

*Methoxyflurane:* May cause nephrotoxicity with tetracyclines. Avoid using together.

*Oral anticoagulants:* May increase anticoagulant effect. Monitor PT and INR, and adjust dosage.

*Penicillins:* May interfere with bactericidal action of penicillins. Avoid using together.

**Drug-lifestyle.** *Alcohol use:* May decrease antibiotic effect. Discourage use together.

*Sun exposure:* May cause photosensitivity reactions. Advise patient to avoid excessive sunlight exposure.

**EFFECTS ON LAB TEST RESULTS**
• May increase BUN and liver enzyme levels.
• May increase eosinophil count. May decrease hemoglobin and platelet, neutrophil, and WBC counts.
• May falsely elevate fluorometric tests for urine catecholamines. May cause false-negative results in urine glucose tests using glucose oxidase reagent (Diastix or Chemstrip uG). Parenteral form may cause false-positive Clinitest results.

**CONTRAINDICATIONS & CAUTIONS**
• Contraindicated in patients hypersensitive to drug or other tetracyclines.
• Use cautiously in patients with impaired renal or hepatic function. Use of these drugs during last half of pregnancy and in children younger than age 8 may cause permanent discoloration of teeth, enamel defects, and bone growth retardation in children.

**NURSING CONSIDERATIONS**
• Obtain specimen for culture and sensitivity tests before giving first dose. Therapy may begin pending test results.

• *Alert:* Check expiration date. Outdated or deteriorated tetracyclines have been linked to reversible nephrotoxicity (Fanconi's syndrome).
• Give drug with milk or food if adverse GI reactions occur.
• If large doses are given, therapy is prolonged, or patient is at high risk, monitor patient for signs and symptoms of superinfection.
• Cutaneous anthrax with signs of systemic involvement, extensive edema, or lesions on the head or neck requires I.V. therapy and a multidrug approach.
• Additional antimicrobials for anthrax multidrug regimens may include rifampin, vancomycin, penicillin, ampicillin, chloramphenicol, imipenem, clindamycin, and clarithromycin.
• Steroids may be considered as adjunctive therapy for anthrax patients with severe edema and for meningitis, based on experience with bacterial meningitis of other etiologies.
• If meningitis is suspected, doxycycline would be less optimal because of poor CNS penetration.
• Ciprofloxacin or doxycycline is the first-line therapy for anthrax. Amoxicillin 500 mg P.O. t.i.d. for adults and 80 mg/kg/day in divided doses every 8 hours for children is an option for completion of therapy after clinical improvement.
• Give pregnant women and immunocompromised patients the usual dosage schedule used for anthrax. In pregnant women, adverse effects on developing teeth and bones are dose-limited; therefore, doxycycline might be used for a short time (7 to 14 days) before 6 months of gestation.
• Check patient's tongue for signs of fungal infection. Stress good oral hygiene.
• Photosensitivity reactions may occur within a few minutes to several hours after exposure. Photosensitivity lasts after therapy ends.
• *Alert:* Don't confuse doxycycline, doxylamine, and dicyclomine.

**PATIENT TEACHING**
• Tell patient to take entire amount of drug exactly as prescribed, even after he feels better.

• Instruct patient to report adverse reactions promptly. If drug is being given I.V., tell him to report discomfort at I.V site.
• Advise patient to take oral form of drug with food or milk if stomach upset occurs.
• Advise patient to increase fluid intake and not to take oral tablets or capsules within 1 hour of bedtime because of possible esophageal irritation or ulceration.
• Advise parent giving drug to a child that tablets may be crushed and mixed with low-fat milk, chocolate milk, chocolate pudding, or apple juice mixed equally with sugar. Tell parent to store mixtures in refrigerator (except apple juice mixture, which can be stored at room temperature) and to discard after 24 hours.
• Warn patient to avoid direct sunlight and ultraviolet light, wear protective clothing, and use sunscreen.
• Tell patient to report signs and symptoms of superinfection to prescriber.

## minocycline hydrochloride
Akamin‡, Alti-Minocycline†, Apo-Minocycline†, Dynacin, Minocin, Minomycin‡, Novo-Minocycline†, PMS-Minocycline†

*Pregnancy risk category D*

### AVAILABLE FORMS
*Capsules:* 50 mg, 75 mg, 100 mg
*Capsules (pellet-filled):* 50 mg, 100 mg
*Injection:* 100 mg/vial
*Tablets:* 50 mg, 75 mg, 100 mg

### INDICATIONS & DOSAGES
➤ **Infections caused by susceptible gram-negative and gram-positive organisms (including *Haemophilus ducreyi*, *Yersinia pestis*, and *Campylobacter fetus*), *Rickettsiae* species, *Mycoplasma pneumoniae*, and *Chlamydia trachomatis*; psittacosis; granuloma inguinale**
*Adults:* Initially, 200 mg I.V.; then 100 mg I.V. q 12 hours. Don't exceed 400 mg/day. Or, 200 mg P.O. initially; then 100 mg P.O. q 12 hours. May use 100 or 200 mg P.O. initially; then 50 mg q.i.d.
*Children older than age 8:* Initially, 4 mg/kg P.O. or I.V.; then 2 mg/kg q 12 hours.

Give I.V. in 500-ml to 1,000-ml solution without calcium, over 6 hours.
➤ **Gonorrhea in patients allergic to penicillin**
*Adults:* Initially, 200 mg P.O.; then 100 mg q 12 hours for at least 4 days. Obtain samples for follow-up cultures within 2 to 3 days after treatment is finished.
➤ **Syphilis in patients allergic to penicillin**
*Adults:* Initially, 200 mg P.O.; then 100 mg q 12 hours for 10 to 15 days.
➤ **Meningococcal carrier state**
*Adults:* 100 mg P.O. q 12 hours for 5 days.
➤ **Uncomplicated urethral, endocervical, or rectal infection caused by *C. trachomatis* or *Ureaplasma urealyticum***
*Adults:* 100 mg P.O. b.i.d. for at least 7 days.
➤ **Uncomplicated gonococcal urethritis in men**
*Adults:* 100 mg P.O. b.i.d. for 5 days.

### I.V. ADMINISTRATION
• Reconstitute 100 mg of powder with 5 ml of sterile water for injection, with further dilution to 500 to 1,000 ml for I.V. infusion. Although reconstituted solution is stable for 24 hours at room temperature, use as soon as possible.
• Infusions are usually given over 6 hours.
• Patient may develop thrombophlebitis with I.V. administration. Switch to oral therapy as soon as possible.

### ACTION
Unknown. Thought to exert bacteriostatic effect by binding to the 30S and possibly 50S ribosomal subunits of microorganisms, thus inhibiting protein synthesis. May also alter the cytoplasmic membrane of susceptible microorganisms.

| Route | Onset | Peak | Duration |
|-------|-------|------|----------|
| P.O. | Unknown | 1-4 hr | Unknown |
| I.V. | Immediate | Immediate | Unknown |

### ADVERSE REACTIONS
**CNS:** headache, *intracranial hypertension,* light-headedness, dizziness, vertigo.
**CV:** pericarditis, *thrombophlebitis.*
**GI:** *anorexia,* dysphagia, glossitis, epigastric distress, oral candidiasis, *nausea,* vomiting, *diarrhea,* enterocolitis, inflammatory lesions in anogenital region.

**Hematologic:** *neutropenia,* eosinophilia, *thrombocytopenia,* hemolytic anemia.

**Musculoskeletal:** bone growth retardation in children younger than age 8.

**Skin:** *maculopapular and erythematous rashes, photosensitivity, increased pigmentation, urticaria.*

**Other:** hypersensitivity reactions, *anaphylaxis,* superinfection; permanent discoloration of teeth, enamel defects.

## INTERACTIONS

**Drug-drug.** *Antacids (including sodium bicarbonate) and laxatives containing aluminum, magnesium, or calcium; antidiarrheals:* May decrease antibiotic absorption. Give antibiotic 1 hour before or 2 hours after any of these drugs.

*Ferrous sulfate and other iron products, zinc:* May decrease antibiotic absorption. Give drug 2 hours before or 3 hours after iron administration.

*Hormonal contraceptives:* May decrease contraceptive effectiveness and increase risk of breakthrough bleeding. Advise patient to use nonhormonal contraceptive.

*Methoxyflurane:* May cause nephrotoxicity when given with tetracyclines. Avoid using together.

*Oral anticoagulants:* May increase anticoagulant effect. Monitor PT and INR, and adjust dosage.

*Penicillins:* May disrupt bactericidal action of penicillins. Avoid using together.

**Drug-lifestyle.** *Sun exposure:* May cause photosensitivity reactions. Advise patient to avoid excessive sunlight exposure.

## EFFECTS ON LAB TEST RESULTS

- May increase BUN and liver enzyme levels.
- May increase eosinophil count. May decrease hemoglobin and platelet and neutrophil counts.
- May falsely elevate fluorometric test results for urine catecholamines. May cause false-negative results in urine glucose tests using glucose oxidase reagent (Diastix or Chemstrip uG). Parenteral form may cause false-positive results of copper sulfate test (Clinitest).

## CONTRAINDICATIONS & CAUTIONS

- Contraindicated in patients hypersensitive to drug or other tetracyclines.

- Use cautiously in patients with impaired renal or hepatic function. Use of these drugs during last half of pregnancy and in children younger than age 8 may cause permanent discoloration of teeth, enamel defects, and bone growth retardation.

## NURSING CONSIDERATIONS

- Monitor renal and liver function test results.
- Obtain specimen for culture and sensitivity tests before first dose. Therapy may begin pending test results.
- *Alert:* Check expiration date. Outdated or deteriorated tetracyclines may cause reversible nephrotoxicity (Fanconi's syndrome).
- Don't expose drug to light or heat. Keep cap tightly closed.
- If large doses are given, therapy is prolonged, or patient is at high risk, monitor patient for signs and symptoms of superinfection.
- Check patient's tongue for signs of candidal infection. Stress good oral hygiene.
- Drug may discolor teeth in young adults. Watch for brown pigmentation, and notify prescriber if it occurs.
- Don't use drug to treat neurosyphilis.
- Photosensitivity reactions may occur within a few minutes to several hours after exposure. Photosensitivity lasts after therapy ends.
- *Alert:* Don't confuse Minocin, niacin, and Mithracin.

## PATIENT TEACHING

- Tell patient to take entire amount of drug exactly as prescribed, even after he feels better.
- Instruct patient to take oral form of drug with a full glass of water. Drug may be taken with food. Tell patient not to take within 1 hour of bedtime, to avoid esophageal irritation or ulceration.
- Warn patient to avoid driving or other hazardous tasks because of possible adverse CNS effects.
- Caution patient to avoid direct sunlight and ultraviolet light, wear protective clothing, and use sunscreen.

## tetracycline hydrochloride
Achromycin, Apo-Tetra†, Novo-
Tetra†, Nu-Tetra†, Sumycin,
Tetrex‡

*Pregnancy risk category D*

### AVAILABLE FORMS
*Capsules:* 250 mg, 500 mg
*Oral suspension:* 125 mg/5 ml

### INDICATIONS & DOSAGES
➤ **Infections caused by susceptible gram-negative and -positive organisms (including *Haemophilus ducreyi*, *Yersinia pestis*, and *Campylobacter fetus*), *Rickettsiae* species, *Mycoplasma pneumoniae*, and *Chlamydia trachomatis*; psittacosis; granuloma inguinale**
*Adults:* 250 to 500 mg P.O. q 6 hours.
*Children older than age 8:* 25 to 50 mg/kg P.O. daily, in divided doses q 6 hours.
➤ **Uncomplicated urethral, endocervical, or rectal infections caused by *C. trachomatis***
*Adults:* 500 mg P.O. q.i.d. for at least 7 days, 10 days for epididymitis, and for at least 14 days for lymphogranuloma venereum.
➤ **Brucellosis**
*Adults:* 500 mg P.O. q 6 hours for 3 weeks with 1 g of streptomycin I.M. q 12 hours for first week; once daily for second week.
➤ **Gonorrhea in patients allergic to penicillin**
*Adults:* Initially, 1.5 g P.O.; then 500 mg P.O. q 6 hours for total dose of 9 g. For epididymitis, 500 mg P.O. q 6 hours for 7 days.
➤ **Syphilis in patients allergic to penicillin**
*Adults and adolescents:* 500 mg P.O. q.i.d. for 2 weeks. If infection has lasted 1 year or longer, treat for 4 weeks.
➤ **Acne**
*Adults and adolescents:* Initially, 250 mg P.O. q 6 hours; then 125 to 500 mg daily or every other day.
➤ ***Helicobacter pylori* infection**
*Adults:* 500 mg P.O. q 6 hours for 10 to 14 days with other drugs, such as metronidazole, bismuth subsalicylate, amoxicillin, or omeprazole.
➤ **Cholera**
*Adults:* 500 mg P.O. q 6 hours for 48 to 72 hours.
➤ **Malaria caused by *Plasmodium falciparum***
*Adults:* 250 to 500 mg P.O. daily for 7 days with quinine sulfate 650 mg P.O. q 8 hours for 3 to 7 days.
➤ **To prevent infection in rape victims**
*Adults:* 500 mg P.O. q.i.d. for 7 days.

### ACTION
Unknown. Thought to exert bacteriostatic effect by binding to the 30S and possibly 50S ribosomal subunits of microorganisms, thus inhibiting protein synthesis. May also alter the cytoplasmic membrane of susceptible microorganisms.

| Route | Onset | Peak | Duration |
|-------|-------|------|----------|
| P.O. | Unknown | 1-4 hr | Unknown |

### ADVERSE REACTIONS
**CNS:** dizziness, headache, *intracranial hypertension.*
**CV:** pericarditis.
**EENT:** sore throat.
**GI:** anorexia, dysphagia, glossitis, *epigastric distress, nausea,* vomiting, *diarrhea,* esophagitis, stomatitis, enterocolitis, oral candidiasis.
**GU:** inflammatory lesions in anogenital region.
**Hematologic:** *neutropenia,* eosinophilia, *thrombocytopenia.*
**Musculoskeletal:** *bone growth retardation in children younger than age 8.*
**Skin:** *candidal superinfection, maculopapular and erythematous rash, urticaria, photosensitivity, increased pigmentation.*
**Other:** hypersensitivity reactions, permanent discoloration of teeth, enamel defects.

### INTERACTIONS
**Drug-drug.** *Antacids (including sodium bicarbonate) and laxatives containing aluminum, magnesium, or calcium; antidiarrheals containing kaolin, pectin, or bismuth subsalicylate:* May decrease antibiotic absorption. Give antibiotic 1 hour before or 2 hours after these drugs.
*Ferrous sulfate and other iron products, zinc:* May decrease antibiotic absorption.

Give tetracycline 2 hours before or 3 hours after these products.

*Hormonal contraceptives:* May decrease contraceptive effectiveness and increase risk of breakthrough bleeding. Advise patient to use nonhormonal contraceptive.

*Methoxyflurane:* May cause severe nephrotoxicity. Avoid using together.

*Oral anticoagulants:* May increase anticoagulant effects. Monitor PT and INR, and adjust anticoagulant dosage.

*Penicillins:* May interfere with bactericidal action of penicillins. Avoid using together.

**Drug-food.** *Dairy products, other foods:* May decrease antibiotic absorption. Give antibiotic 1 hour before or 2 hours after any of these products.

**Drug-lifestyle.** *Sun exposure:* May cause photosensitivity reactions. Advise patient to avoid excessive sunlight exposure.

### EFFECTS ON LAB TEST RESULTS

- May increase BUN and liver enzyme levels.
- May increase eosinophil counts. May decrease platelet and neutrophil counts.
- May falsely elevate fluorometric test results for urine catecholamines. May cause false-negative results in urine glucose tests using glucose oxidase reagent (Diastix or Chemstrip uG).

### CONTRAINDICATIONS & CAUTIONS

- Contraindicated in patients hypersensitive to drug or other tetracyclines.
- Use cautiously in patients with renal or hepatic impairment. Avoid using or use cautiously during last half of pregnancy and in children younger than age 8 because drug may cause permanent discoloration of teeth, enamel defects, and bone growth retardation.

### NURSING CONSIDERATIONS

- Obtain specimen for culture and sensitivity tests before giving first dose. Therapy may begin pending test results.
- *Alert:* Check expiration date. Outdated or deteriorated tetracyclines have been linked to reversible nephrotoxicity (Fanconi's syndrome).
- Don't expose drug to light or heat.
- If large doses are given, therapy is prolonged, or patient is at high risk, monitor patient for signs and symptoms of superinfection.
- In patients with renal or hepatic impairment, monitor renal and liver function test results if drug is used.
- Check patient's tongue for signs of candidal infection. Stress good oral hygiene.
- Drug isn't indicated for treatment of neurosyphilis.
- Photosensitivity reactions may occur within a few minutes to several hours after sun exposure. Photosensitivity lasts after therapy ends.
- Panmycin may contain tartrazine.

### PATIENT TEACHING

- Tell patient to take drug exactly as prescribed, even after he feels better, and to take entire amount prescribed.
- Explain that effectiveness is reduced when drug is taken with milk or other dairy products, food, antacids, or iron products. Tell patient to take each dose with a full glass of water on an empty stomach, at least 1 hour before or 2 hours after meals. Also tell him to take it at least 1 hour before bedtime to prevent esophageal irritation or ulceration.
- Warn patient to avoid direct sunlight and ultraviolet light, wear protective clothing, and use sunscreen.

# 13

## Sulfonamides

co-trimoxazole
sulfadiazine
sulfisoxazole
sulfisoxazole acetyl

### COMBINATION PRODUCTS

Azo-Sulfisoxazole tablets (film-coated): sulfisoxazole 500 mg and phenazopyridine hydrochloride 50 mg.
Eryzole, Pediazole: sulfisoxazole 600 mg and erythromycin ethylsuccinate 200 mg/5 ml.

---

## co-trimoxazole
## (sulfamethoxazole and trimethoprim)

Apo-Sulfatrim†, Apo-Sulfatrim DS†, Bactrim*, Bactrim DS✲, Bactrim IV, Cotrim, Cotrim D.S., Cotrim Pediatric*, Novo-Trimel†, Novo-Trimel DS†, Nu-Cotrimox†, Resprim‡, Roubac†, Septra*, Septra DS, Septra IV, Septrin‡, Sulfatrim

*Pregnancy risk category C*

---

### AVAILABLE FORMS

*Injection:* trimethoprim 16 mg/ml and sulfamethoxazole 80 mg/ml in 5-ml, 10-ml, 20-ml, and 30-ml vials
*Oral suspension:* trimethoprim 40 mg and sulfamethoxazole 200 mg/5 ml*
*Tablets (double-strength):* trimethoprim 160 mg and sulfamethoxazole 800 mg
*Tablets (single-strength):* trimethoprim 80 mg and sulfamethoxazole 400 mg

### INDICATIONS & DOSAGES

➤ **Shigellosis or UTIs caused by susceptible strains of *Escherichia coli*, *Proteus* (indole positive or negative), *Klebsiella*, or *Enterobacter* species**
*Adults:* 160 mg trimethoprim/800 mg sulfamethoxazole, one double-strength tablet, P.O. q 12 hours for 10 to 14 days in UTIs and for 5 days in shigellosis. If indicated, I.V. infusion is given: 8 to 10 mg/kg/day based on trimethoprim component in two

to four divided doses q 6, 8, or 12 hours for 5 days for shigellosis or up to 14 days for severe UTIs. Maximum daily dose is 960 mg trimethoprim (as co-trimoxazole).
*Children age 2 months and older:* 8 mg/kg/day based on trimethoprim component P.O., in two divided doses q 12 hours for 10 days for UTIs and 5 days for shigellosis. If indicated, I.V. infusion is given: 8 to 10 mg/kg/day based on trimethoprim component, in two to four divided doses q 6, 8, or 12 hours. Don't exceed adult dose.
➤ **Otitis media in patients with penicillin allergy or penicillin-resistant infection**
*Children age 2 months and older:* 8 mg/kg/day based on trimethoprim component P.O., in two divided doses q 12 hours for 10 to 14 days.
➤ **Chronic bronchitis, upper respiratory tract infections**
*Adults:* 160 mg trimethoprim and 800 mg sulfamethoxazole P.O. q 12 hours for 10 to 14 days.
➤ **Traveler's diarrhea**
*Adults:* 160 mg trimethoprim and 800 mg sulfamethoxazole P.O. b.i.d. for 3 to 5 days. Some patients may only need up to 2 days of therapy.
➤ **To prevent *Pneumocystis carinii* pneumonia**
*Adults:* 160 mg of trimethoprim and 800 mg sulfamethoxazole P.O. daily; or 80 mg trimethoprim/400 mg sulfamethoxazole P.O. three times weekly.
*Children age 2 months and older:* 150 mg/m² trimethoprim/750 mg/m² sulfamethoxazole P.O. daily in two divided doses on 3 consecutive days each week.
➤ **P. carinii pneumonia**
*Adults and children older than age 2 months:* 15 to 20 mg/kg/day based on trimethoprim I.V. or P.O. in three or four divided doses for 14 to 21 days.
**Adjust-a-dose:** For patients with creatinine clearance 15 to 30 ml/minute, reduce daily dose by 50%. Don't give to patients with creatinine clearance below 15 ml/minute.

---

## I.V. ADMINISTRATION

● Dilute each 5 ml of concentrate for I.V. infusion in 75 to 125 ml of $D_5W$ before administration. Don't mix with other drugs or solutions.

● Infuse slowly over 60 to 90 minutes. Don't give by rapid infusion or bolus injection.

● Don't refrigerate; use within 6 hours if diluted in 125 ml and within 2 hours if diluted in 75 ml. Discard solution if cloudiness or crystallization is noted after mixing.

## ACTION

Sulfamethoxazole inhibits formation of dihydrofolic acid from PABA; trimethoprim inhibits dihydrofolate reductase formation. Both decrease bacterial folic acid synthesis; bactericidal.

| Route | Onset | Peak | Duration |
|-------|-------|------|----------|
| P.O. | Unknown | 1-4 hr | Unknown |
| I.V. | Immediate | 1-1½ hr | Unknown |

## ADVERSE REACTIONS

**CNS:** headache, depression, aseptic meningitis, tinnitus, apathy, *seizures,* hallucinations, ataxia, nervousness, fatigue, vertigo, insomnia.
**CV:** thrombophlebitis.
**GI:** *nausea, vomiting, diarrhea,* abdominal pain, anorexia, stomatitis, *pancreatitis, pseudomembranous colitis.*
**GU:** *toxic nephrosis with oliguria and anuria,* crystalluria, hematuria, interstitial nephritis.
**Hematologic:** *agranulocytosis, aplastic anemia,* megaloblastic anemia, *thrombocytopenia, leukopenia,* hemolytic anemia.
**Hepatic:** jaundice, *hepatic necrosis.*
**Musculoskeletal:** arthralgia, myalgia, muscle weakness.
**Respiratory:** pulmonary infiltrates.
**Skin:** *erythema multiforme, Stevens-Johnson syndrome,* generalized skin eruption, *toxic epidermal necrolysis,* exfoliative dermatitis, photosensitivity, urticaria, pruritus.
**Other:** hypersensitivity reactions, serum sickness, drug fever, *anaphylaxis.*

## INTERACTIONS

**Drug-drug.** *Cyclosporine:* May decrease cyclosporine level and increase nephrotoxicity risk. Avoid using together.

*Dofetilide:* May increase dofetilide level and effects. May increase risk of prolonged QT syndrome and fatal ventricular arrhythmias. Avoid using together.
*Hormonal contraceptives:* May decrease contraceptive effectiveness and increase risk of breakthrough bleeding. Advise patient to use a nonhormonal contraceptive.
*Methotrexate:* May increase methotrexate level. Monitor methotrexate level.
*Oral anticoagulants:* May increase anticoagulant effect. Monitor patient for bleeding; monitor PT and INR.
*Oral antidiabetics:* May increase hypoglycemic effect. Monitor glucose level.
*Phenytoin:* May inhibit hepatic metabolism of phenytoin. Monitor phenytoin level.
**Drug-herb.** *Dong quai, St. John's wort:* May cause photosensitivity reactions. Advise patient to avoid excessive sunlight exposure.
**Drug-lifestyle.** *Sun exposure:* May cause photosensitivity reactions. Advise patient to avoid excessive sunlight exposure.

## EFFECTS ON LAB TEST RESULTS

● May increase BUN, creatinine, aminotransferase, and bilirubin levels.
● May decrease hemoglobin and granulocyte, platelet, and WBC counts.

## CONTRAINDICATIONS & CAUTIONS

● Contraindicated in patients hypersensitive to trimethoprim or sulfonamides.
● Contraindicated in those with creatinine clearance less than 15 ml/minute, porphyria, or megaloblastic anemia from folate deficiency.
● Contraindicated in pregnant women at term, in breast-feeding women, and in infants younger than age 2 months.
● Use cautiously and in reduced dosages in patients with creatinine clearance 15 to 30 ml/minute, severe allergy or bronchial asthma, G6PD deficiency, and blood dyscrasia.

## NURSING CONSIDERATIONS

● Obtain specimen for culture and sensitivity tests before first dose. Therapy may begin pending results.
● *Alert:* Double-check dosage, which may be written as trimethoprim component.
● *Alert:* "DS" product means "double strength."

---

*Rapid onset    †Canada    ‡Australia    ◊OTC    ◆ Off-label use    ⦿Photoguide    *Liquid contains alcohol.*

• Never give drug I.M.
• Monitor renal and liver function test results.
• Promptly report rash, sore throat, fever, cough, mouth sores, or iris lesions—early signs and symptoms of erythema multiforme, which may progress to Stevens-Johnson syndrome, which is sometimes fatal. These symptoms may also represent early signs of blood dyscrasias.
• Watch for signs and symptoms of superinfection, such as fever, chills, and increased pulse.
• *Alert:* Adverse reactions, especially hypersensitivity reactions, rash, and fever, occur much more frequently in patients with AIDS.

**PATIENT TEACHING**
• Tell patient to take drug as prescribed, even if he feels better.
• Encourage patient to drink plenty of fluids.
• Tell patient to report adverse reactions promptly.
• Instruct patient receiving drug I.V. to report discomfort at I.V. insertion site.
• Advise patient to avoid prolonged sun exposure, wear protective clothing, and use sunscreen.
• Instruct patient to take oral form with 8 ounces (240 ml) of water on an empty stomach.

---

## sulfadiazine
Coptin†

*Pregnancy risk category C*

**AVAILABLE FORMS**
*Tablets:* 500 mg

**INDICATIONS & DOSAGES**
➤ **Asymptomatic meningococcal carrier**
*Adults:* 1 g P.O. q 12 hours for 2 days.
*Children ages 1 to 12:* 500 mg P.O. q 12 hours for 2 days.
*Children ages 2 to 12 months:* 500 mg P.O. daily for 2 days.
➤ **Rheumatic fever prevention, as an alternative to penicillin**
*Children weighing more than 30 kg (66 lb):* 1 g P.O. daily.

*Children weighing less than 30 kg:* 500 mg P.O. daily.
➤ **Adjunctive treatment for toxoplasmosis**
*Adults:* 4 to 6 g P.O. daily divided q 6 hours for 6 to 8 weeks or until improvement occurs. Usually given with pyrimethamine.
*Children:* 100 to 200 mg/kg P.O. daily divided q 6 hours for 6 to 8 weeks or until improvement occurs. Maximum 6 g daily. Usually given with pyrimethamine.
➤ **Nocardiosis**
*Adults:* 4 to 8 g P.O. daily given in divided doses for at least 6 weeks.

**ACTION**
Inhibits formation of dihydrofolic acid from PABA, decreasing bacterial folic acid synthesis; bacteriostatic.

| Route | Onset | Peak | Duration |
|-------|--------|--------|----------|
| P.O. | Unknown | 4-6 hr | Unknown |

**ADVERSE REACTIONS**
**CNS:** headache, depression, *seizures,* hallucinations.
**GI:** *nausea, vomiting, diarrhea,* abdominal pain, anorexia, stomatitis.
**GU:** *toxic nephrosis with oliguria and anuria,* crystalluria, hematuria.
**Hematologic:** *agranulocytosis, aplastic anemia,* megaloblastic anemia, *thrombocytopenia, leukopenia,* hemolytic anemia.
**Hepatic:** jaundice.
**Skin:** *erythema multiforme, Stevens-Johnson syndrome, generalized skin eruption, toxic epidermal necrolysis,* exfoliative dermatitis, photosensitivity, urticaria, pruritus.
**Other:** hypersensitivity reactions, serum sickness, drug fever, *anaphylaxis.*

**INTERACTIONS**
**Drug-drug.** *Hormonal contraceptives:* May decrease contraceptive effectiveness. Increased risk of breakthrough bleeding. Advise patient to use a nonhormonal contraceptive.
*Methotrexate:* May increase methotrexate level. Monitor methotrexate level.
*Oral anticoagulants:* May increase anticoagulant effect. Monitor patient for bleeding; monitor PT and INR.

Reactions may be *common,* uncommon, *life-threatening,* or COMMON AND LIFE-THREATENING.

*Oral antidiabetics:* May increase hypoglycemic effect. Monitor glucose level.
*PABA-containing drugs:* May inhibit antibacterial action. Avoid using together.
**Drug-herb.** *Dong quai, St. John's wort:* May cause photosensitivity reaction. Advise patient to avoid excessive sunlight exposure.
**Drug-lifestyle.** *Sun exposure:* May cause photosensitivity reaction. Advise patient to avoid excessive sunlight exposure.

## EFFECTS ON LAB TEST RESULTS
● May increase BUN, creatinine, transaminase, and bilirubin levels.
● May increase eosinophil count. May decrease hemoglobin and PT and fibrinogen, granulocyte, platelet, and WBC counts.
● May alter results of urine glucose tests using cupric sulfate (Benedict's reagent or Chemstrip uG).

## CONTRAINDICATIONS & CAUTIONS
● Contraindicated in patients hypersensitive to sulfonamides, in those with porphyria, in infants younger than age 2 months (except in congenital toxoplasmosis), in pregnant women at term, and in breast-feeding women.
● Use cautiously and in reduced doses in patients with impaired hepatic or renal function, bronchial asthma, history of multiple allergies, G6PD deficiency, and blood dyscrasia.

## NURSING CONSIDERATIONS
● Give drug on schedule to maintain constant blood level.
● Monitor patient for signs and symptoms of blood dyscrasia (purpura, ecchymoses, sore throat, fever, and pallor) and report to prescriber immediately.
● Promptly report rash, sore throat, fever, cough, mouth sores, or iris lesions—early signs and symptoms of erythema multiforme, which may progress to the sometimes-fatal Stevens-Johnson syndrome.
● Monitor urine cultures, CBCs, and urinalyses before and during therapy.
● Monitor renal and liver function test results.
● Watch for signs and symptoms of superinfection, such as fever, chills, and increased pulse.

● Folic or folinic acid may be used during rest periods in toxoplasmosis therapy to reverse hematopoietic depression or anemia caused by pyrimethamine and sulfadiazine.
● Monitor fluid intake and output. Maintain intake between 3,000 and 4,000 ml daily for adults to produce output of 1,500 ml daily. If fluid intake isn't adequate to prevent crystalluria, sodium bicarbonate may be given to alkalinize urine. Monitor urine pH daily.
● *Alert:* Don't confuse sulfadiazine with sulfasalazine. Don't confuse sulfonamide drugs.

## PATIENT TEACHING
● Tell patient to take drug as prescribed, even if he feels better.
● Urge patient to drink a glass of water with each dose, plus plenty of water each day to prevent urine crystals.
● Instruct patient to report adverse reactions promptly.
● Warn patient to avoid prolonged exposure to sunlight, wear protective clothing, and use sunscreen.

---

# sulfisoxazole (sulfafurazole, sulphafurazole)
Novo-Soxazole†

# sulfisoxazole acetyl
Gantrisin

*Pregnancy risk category C*

---

## AVAILABLE FORMS
**sulfisoxazole**
*Tablets:* 500 mg
**sulfisoxazole acetyl**
*Liquid:* 500 mg/5 ml*

## INDICATIONS & DOSAGES
➤ **UTIs and systemic infections**
*Adults:* Initially, 2 to 4 g P.O.; then 4 to 8 g daily divided in four to six doses.
*Children older than age 2 months:* Initially, 75 mg/kg P.O. daily or 2 g/m² P.O.; then 150 mg/kg or 4 g/m² P.O. daily in divided doses q 6 hours. Don't exceed total daily dose of 6 g.
*Adjust-a-dose:* For patients with renal impairment, use normal dose at longer inter-

vals. If creatinine clearance is 10 to 50 ml/ minute, give q 8 to12 hours; if clearance is less than 10 ml/minute, give q 12 to 24 hours.

## ACTION
Inhibits formation of dihydrofolic acid from PABA, decreasing bacterial folic acid synthesis; bacteriostatic.

| Route | Onset | Peak | Duration |
|-------|-------|------|----------|
| P.O. | Unknown | 1-4 hr | Unknown |

## ADVERSE REACTIONS
**CNS:** headache, depression, *seizures,* hallucinations, syncope, dizziness.
**CV:** tachycardia, palpitations, cyanosis.
**GI:** *nausea, vomiting, diarrhea,* abdominal pain, anorexia, stomatitis, *pseudomembranous colitis.*
**GU:** *toxic nephrosis with oliguria and anuria,* crystalluria, hematuria, *acute renal failure.*
**Hematologic:** *agranulocytosis, aplastic anemia,* megaloblastic anemia, *thrombocytopenia, leukopenia,* hemolytic anemia.
**Hepatic:** jaundice, *hepatitis.*
**Skin:** *erythema multiforme,* generalized skin eruption, *toxic epidermal necrolysis,* exfoliative dermatitis, photosensitivity, urticaria, pruritus.
**Other:** hypersensitivity reactions, serum sickness, drug fever, *anaphylaxis.*

## INTERACTIONS
**Drug-drug.** *Hormonal contraceptives:* May decrease contraceptive effectiveness and increase risk of breakthrough bleeding. Advise patient to use a nonhormonal contraceptive.
*Methotrexate:* May increase methotrexate level. Monitor methotrexate level.
*Oral anticoagulants:* May increase anticoagulant effect. Monitor patient for bleeding; monitor PT and INR.
*Oral antidiabetics:* May increase hypoglycemic effect. Monitor glucose level.
**Drug-herb.** *Dong quai, St. John's wort:* May cause photosensitivity reactions. Advise patient to avoid excessive sunlight exposure.
**Drug-lifestyle.** *Sun exposure:* May cause photosensitivity reactions. Advise patient to avoid excessive sunlight exposure.

## EFFECTS ON LAB TEST RESULTS
● May increase BUN, creatinine, aminotransferase, and bilirubin levels.
● May increase eosinophil count. May decrease hemoglobin and PT and fibrinogen, granulocyte, platelet, and WBC counts.
● May alter results of urine glucose tests using cupric sulfate (Benedict's reagent or Chemstrip uG).

## CONTRAINDICATIONS & CAUTIONS
● Contraindicated in patients hypersensitive to sulfonamides, in infants younger than age 2 months (except in congenital toxoplasmosis), in pregnant women at term, and in breast-feeding women.
● Use cautiously in patients with impaired hepatic or renal function, severe allergy or bronchial asthma, and G6PD deficiency.

## NURSING CONSIDERATIONS
● Obtain specimen for culture and sensitivity tests before giving first dose. Therapy may begin pending results.
● Monitor urine cultures, CBC, PT, INR, and urinalyses before and during therapy.
● Monitor renal and liver function test results.
● Report moderate to severe diarrhea to prescriber.
● Watch for signs and symptoms of superinfection, such as fever, chills, and increased pulse.
● Monitor fluid intake and output. Maintain intake between 3,000 and 4,000 ml daily for adults to produce output of 1,500 ml daily. If fluid intake isn't adequate to prevent crystalluria, sodium bicarbonate may be given to alkalinize urine. Monitor urine pH daily.
● *Alert:* Don't confuse sulfisoxazole with sulfasalazine. Don't confuse the combination products with sulfisoxazole alone.

## PATIENT TEACHING
● Tell patient to take drug as prescribed, even if he feels better.
● Instruct patient to drink a glass of water with each dose, plus plenty of water each day to prevent urine crystals.
● Advise patient to report rash, sore throat, fever, pallor, or yellowed skin or eyes immediately.

---

Reactions may be *common,* uncommon, *life-threatening,* or COMMON AND LIFE-THREATENING.

# 14
## Fluoroquinolones

ciprofloxacin
gatifloxacin
gemifloxacin mesylate
levofloxacin
moxifloxacin hydrochloride
norfloxacin
ofloxacin

**COMBINATION PRODUCTS**
None.

## ciprofloxacin
Cipro✐, Cipro I.V., Cipro XR, Ciproxin‡

*Pregnancy risk category C*

**AVAILABLE FORMS**
*Infusion (premixed):* 200 mg in 100 ml $D_5W$, 400 mg in 200 ml $D_5W$
*Injection:* 200 mg, 400 mg
*Suspension (oral):* 5 g/100 ml (5%), 10 g/100 ml (10%)
*Tablets (extended-release, film-coated):* 500 mg
*Tablets (film-coated):* 100 mg, 250 mg, 500 mg, 750 mg

**INDICATIONS & DOSAGES**
➤ **Mild to moderate UTIs caused by** *Escherichia coli, Klebsiella pneumoniae, Enterobacter cloacae, Serratia marcescens, Proteus mirabilis, Providencia rettgeri, Morganella morgani, Citrobacter diversus, C. freundii, Pseudomonas aeruginosa, Staphylococcus epidermidis,* **and** *Enterococcus faecalis*
*Adults:* 250 mg P.O. or 200 mg I.V. q 12 hours.
➤ **Severe or complicated UTIs; mild to moderate bone and joint infections caused by** *E. cloacae, P. aeruginosa,* **and** *S. marcescens;* **mild to moderate respiratory infections caused by** *E. coli, K. pneumoniae, E. cloacae, P. mirabilis, P. aeruginosa, Haemophilus influenzae,* **and** *H. parainfluenzae;* **mild to moderate skin and skin-structure infections caused by** *E. coli, K. pneumoniae, E.*

*cloacae, P. mirabilis, P. vulgaris, Providencia stuartii, M. morganii, C. freundii, Streptococcus pyogenes, P. aeruginosa, Staphylococcus aureus,* **and** *S. epidermidis;* **infectious diarrhea caused by** *E. coli, Campylobacter jejuni, Shigella flexneri,* **and** *S. sonnei;* **typhoid fever**
*Adults:* 500 mg P.O. or 400 mg I.V. q 12 hours.
➤ **Severe or complicated bone or joint infections, severe respiratory tract infections, severe skin and skin-structure infections**
*Adults:* 750 mg P.O. q 12 hours or 400 mg I.V. q 8 to 12 hours.
➤ **Chronic bacterial prostatitis caused by** *E. coli* **or** *P. mirabilis*
*Adults:* 500 mg P.O. q 12 hours or 400 mg I.V. q 12 hours for 28 days.
➤ **Complicated intra-abdominal infections caused by** *E. coli, P. aeruginosa, P. mirabilis, K. pneumoniae,* **or** *Bacteroides fragilis*
*Adults:* 500 mg P.O. or 400 mg I.V. q 12 hours for 7 to 14 days. Give with metronidazole.
➤ **Acute uncomplicated cystitis**
*Adults:* 100 mg or 250 mg P.O. q 12 hours for 3 days.
➤ **Uncomplicated UTI**
*Adults:* 500 mg extended-release tablet P.O. once daily for 3 days.
➤ **Mild to moderate acute sinusitis caused by** *H. influenzae, Streptococcus pneumoniae,* **or** *Moraxella catarrhalis*
*Adults:* 500 mg P.O. or 400 mg I.V. q 12 hours for 10 days.
➤ **Empirical therapy in febrile neutropenic patients**
*Adults:* 400 mg I.V. q 8 hours used with piperacillin 50 mg/kg I.V. q 4 hours (not to exceed 24 g/day maximum).
➤ **Inhalation anthrax (postexposure)**
*Adults:* 400 mg I.V. q 12 hours initially until susceptibility test results are known, then 500 mg P.O. b.i.d.
*Children:* 10 mg/kg I.V. q 12 hours, then 15 mg/kg P.O. q 12 hours. Don't exceed 800 mg/day I.V. or 1,000 mg/day P.O.

---

*Rapid onset*   †Canada   ‡Australia   ◇OTC   ♦ Off-label use   ✐Photoguide   *Liquid contains alcohol.

*For all patients:* Give drug with one or two additional antimicrobials. Switch to oral therapy when appropriate. Treat for 60 days (I.V. and P.O. combined).

➤ **Cutaneous anthrax ◆**
*Adults:* 500 mg P.O. b.i.d. for 60 days.
*Children:* 10 to 15 mg/kg q 12 hours. Don't exceed 1,000 mg/day. Treat for 60 days.

**Adjust-a-dose:** For patients with creatinine clearance 30 to 50 ml/minute, give 250 to 500 mg P.O. q 12 hours or the usual I.V. dose; if clearance is 5 to 29 ml/minute, give 250 to 500 mg P.O. q 18 hours or 200 to 400 mg I.V. q 18 to 24 hours. If patient is on hemodialysis, give 250 to 500 mg P.O. q 24 hours after dialysis.

## I.V. ADMINISTRATION
● Dilute drug using $D_5W$ or normal saline solution for injection to 1 to 2 mg/ml. Infuse over 1 hour into a large vein to minimize discomfort and venous irritation.
● If giving drug through a Y-type set, stop the other I.V. solution during ciprofloxacin infusion.

## ACTION
Inhibits bacterial DNA synthesis, mainly by blocking DNA gyrase; bactericidal.

| Route | Onset | Peak | Duration |
|-------|-------|------|----------|
| P.O. | Unknown | 30-120 min | Unknown |
| P.O. (Cipro XR) | Unknown | 1-4 hr | Unknown |
| I.V. | Unknown | Immediate | Unknown |

## ADVERSE REACTIONS
**CNS:** headache, restlessness, tremor, dizziness, fatigue, drowsiness, insomnia, depression, light-headedness, confusion, hallucinations, *seizures,* paresthesia.
**CV:** thrombophlebitis, edema, chest pain.
**GI:** *nausea, diarrhea,* vomiting, abdominal pain or discomfort, oral candidiasis, *pseudomembranous colitis,* dyspepsia, flatulence, constipation.
**GU:** crystalluria, interstitial nephritis.
**Hematologic:** eosinophilia, *leukopenia, neutropenia, thrombocytopenia.*
**Musculoskeletal:** arthralgia, arthropathy, joint or back pain, joint inflammation, joint stiffness, tendon rupture, aching, neck pain.

**Skin:** *rash,* photosensitivity, *Stevens-Johnson syndrome, toxic epidermal necrolysis,* exfoliative dermatitis, burning, pruritus, erythema.
**Other:** hypersensitivity reactions.

## INTERACTIONS
**Drug-drug.** *Aluminum hydroxide, aluminum-magnesium hydroxide, calcium carbonate, didanosine (chewable tablets, buffered tablets, or pediatric powder for oral solution), magnesium hydroxide, products containing zinc:* May decrease ciprofloxacin absorption and effects. Give ciprofloxacin 2 hours before or 6 hours after these drugs.
*Iron salts:* May decrease absorption of ciprofloxacin, reducing anti-infective response. Give at least 2 hours apart.
*NSAIDs:* May increase risk of CNS stimulation. Monitor patient closely.
*Probenecid:* May elevate level of ciprofloxacin. Monitor patient for toxicity.
*Sucralfate:* May decrease absorption of the ciprofloxacin reducing anti-infective response. If use together can't be avoided, give at least 6 hours apart.
*Theophylline:* May increase theophylline level and prolong theophylline half-life. Monitor level of theophylline and observe for adverse effects.
*Warfarin:* May increase anticoagulant effects. Monitor PT and INR closely.
**Drug-herb.** *Dong quai, St. John's wort:* May cause photosensitivity. Advise patient to avoid excessive sunlight exposure.
*Yerba maté:* May decrease clearance of yerba maté's methylxanthines and cause toxicity. Discourage use together.
**Drug-food.** *Caffeine:* May increase effect of caffeine. Monitor patient closely.
*Dairy products, other foods:* Delays peak drug levels. Advise patient to take drug on an empty stomach.
*Orange juice fortified with calcium:* May decrease GI absorption of drug, thereby reducing effects. Advise patient to avoid taking drug with calcium-fortified orange juice.
**Drug-lifestyle.** *Sun exposure:* May cause photosensitivity reactions. Advise patient to avoid excessive sunlight exposure.

---

Reactions may be *common,* uncommon, *life-threatening*, or COMMON AND LIFE-THREATENING.

## EFFECTS ON LAB TEST RESULTS
• May increase BUN, creatinine, ALT, AST, alkaline phosphatase, bilirubin, LDH, and GGT levels.
• May increase eosinophil count. May decrease WBC, neutrophil, and platelet counts.

## CONTRAINDICATIONS & CAUTIONS
• Contraindicated in patients sensitive to fluoroquinolones.
• Use cautiously in patients with CNS disorders, such as severe cerebral arteriosclerosis or seizure disorders, and in those at risk for seizures. Drug may cause CNS stimulation.
• Safety in children younger than age 18 hasn't been established; however, drug may be used as recommended by the CDC for inhalational or cutaneous anthrax, as indicated. Drug may cause cartilage erosion.

## NURSING CONSIDERATIONS
• Obtain specimen for culture and sensitivity tests before giving first dose. Therapy may begin pending results.
• Be aware of drug interactions. Some require waiting up to 6 hours after ciprofloxacin administration before giving another drug to avoid decreasing drug's effects. Food doesn't affect absorption but may delay peak drug levels.
• Monitor patient's intake and output and observe for signs of crystalluria.
• Tendon rupture may occur in patients receiving quinolones. Stop drug if pain, inflammation, or tendon rupture occurs.
• Long-term therapy may result in overgrowth of organisms resistant to ciprofloxacin.
• Cutaneous anthrax patients with signs of systemic involvement, extensive edema, or lesions on the head or neck need I.V. therapy and a multidrug approach.
• Additional antimicrobials for anthrax multidrug regimens can include rifampin, vancomycin, penicillin, ampicillin, chloramphenicol, imipenem, clindamycin, and clarithromycin.
• Steroids may be considered as adjunctive therapy for anthrax patients with severe edema and for meningitis, based on experience with bacterial meningitis of other etiologies.
• Ciprofloxacin or doxycycline is a first-line therapy for anthrax. Amoxicillin 500 mg P.O. t.i.d. for adults and 80 mg/kg daily in divided doses every 8 hours for children is an option for completion of therapy after clinical improvement.
• Follow current CDC recommendations for anthrax.
• Pregnant women and immunocompromised patients should receive the usual doses and regimens for anthrax.

## PATIENT TEACHING
• Tell patient to take drug as prescribed, even after he feels better.
• Advise patient to drink plenty of fluids to reduce risk of urine crystals.
• Advise patient not to crush, split, or chew the extended-release tablets.
• Warn patient to avoid hazardous tasks that require alertness, such as driving, until effects of drug are known.
• Instruct patient to avoid caffeine while taking drug because of potential for increased caffeine effects.
• Advise patient that hypersensitivity reactions may occur even after first dose. If a rash or other allergic reaction occurs, tell him to stop drug immediately and notify prescriber.
• Tell patient to report pain, inflammation, or tendon rupture immediately.
• Tell patient to avoid excessive sunlight or artificial ultraviolet light during therapy and to stop drug and call prescriber if phototoxicity occurs.
• Because drug appears in breast milk, advise woman to stop breast-feeding during treatment or to consider treatment with another drug.

---

# gatifloxacin
Tequin

*Pregnancy risk category C*

## AVAILABLE FORMS
*Injection:* 200 mg/20-ml vial, 400 mg/40-ml vial; 200 mg in 100 ml $D_5W$, 400 mg in 200 ml $D_5W$
*Tablets:* 200 mg, 400 mg

## INDICATIONS & DOSAGES

➤ **Acute bacterial worsening of chronic bronchitis caused by** *Streptococcus pneumoniae, Haemophilus influenzae, H. parainfluenzae, Moraxella catarrhalis,* **or** *Staphylococcus aureus;* **complicated UTI caused by** *Escherichia coli, Klebsiella pneumoniae,* **or** *Proteus mirabilis;* **acute pyelonephritis caused by** *E. coli*

*Adults:* 400 mg I.V. or P.O. daily for 7 to 10 days for acute pyelonephritis and complicated UTIs and 5 days for chronic bronchitis.

➤ **Uncomplicated skin and skin structure infections caused by** *S. pyogenes* **or methicillin-susceptible** *S. aureus*

*Adults:* 400 mg I.V. or P.O. daily for 7 to 10 days.

➤ **Acute sinusitis caused by** *S. pneumoniae* **or** *H. influenzae*

*Adults:* 400 mg I.V. or P.O. daily for 10 days.

➤ **Community-acquired pneumonia caused by** *S. pneumoniae, H. influenzae, H. parainfluenzae, M. catarrhalis, S. aureus, Mycoplasma pneumoniae, Chlamydia pneumoniae,* **or** *Legionella pneumophila*

*Adults:* 400 mg I.V. or P.O. daily for 7 to 14 days.

*Adjust-a-dose:* For patients with creatinine clearance less than 40 ml/minute, those on hemodialysis, and those on continuous peritoneal dialysis, first dose is 400 mg I.V. or P.O. daily, and subsequent doses are 200 mg I.V. or P.O. daily. For patients on hemodialysis, give after hemodialysis session ends.

➤ **Uncomplicated urethral gonorrhea in men and cervical gonorrhea or acute uncomplicated rectal infections in women caused by** *Neisseria gonorrhoeae*

*Adults:* 400 mg P.O. as single dose.

➤ **Uncomplicated UTIs caused by** *E. coli, K. pneumoniae,* **or** *P. mirabilis*

*Adults:* 400 mg I.V. or P.O. as single dose, or 200 mg I.V. or P.O. daily for 3 days.

## I.V. ADMINISTRATION

● Dilute drug in single-use vials with D₅W or normal saline solution to 2 mg/ml before giving. Diluted solutions are stable for 14 days at room temperature or refrigerated.

● Frozen solutions are stable for up to 6 months except for 5% sodium bicarbonate solutions. Thaw at room temperature. Thawed solutions are stable for 14 days after being removed from the freezer, when stored at room temperature or under refrigeration.

● Don't mix with other drugs.

● Infuse over 60 minutes.

● Discard any unused portion of the single-dose vials.

## ACTION

Inhibits DNA gyrase and topoisomerase, preventing cell replication and division.

| Route | Onset | Peak | Duration |
|-------|---------|---------|----------|
| P.O. | Unknown | 1-2 hr | Unknown |
| I.V. | Unknown | Unknown | Unknown |

## ADVERSE REACTIONS

**CNS:** headache, dizziness, abnormal dreams, insomnia, fever, paresthesia, tremor, vertigo.
**CV:** palpitations, chest pain, peripheral edema.
**EENT:** tinnitus, abnormal vision, pharyngitis.
**GI:** nausea, diarrhea, abdominal pain, constipation, dyspepsia, oral candidiasis, glossitis, stomatitis, mouth ulcer, vomiting, taste perversion.
**GU:** dysuria, hematuria, vaginitis.
**Musculoskeletal:** arthralgia, myalgia, back pain.
**Respiratory:** dyspnea.
**Skin:** redness at injection site, rash, sweating.
**Other:** *anaphylaxis*, chills.

## INTERACTIONS

**Drug-drug.** *Aluminum hydroxide, didanosine buffered solution, tablets, or buffered powder, aluminum-magnesium hydroxide, calcium carbonate, magnesium hydroxide, products containing zinc:* May decrease effects of gatifloxacin. Give drug at least 6 hours before or 2 hours after gatifloxacin.
*Antidiabetics (glyburide, insulin):* May cause symptomatic hypoglycemia or hyperglycemia. Monitor glucose level.
*Antipsychotics, erythromycin, tricyclic antidepressants:* May prolong QTc interval. Use together cautiously.

---

*Class IA antiarrhythmics (procainamide, quinidine), class III antiarrhythmics (amiodarone, dofetilide, sotalol):* May prolong QTc interval. Avoid using together.

*Digoxin:* May increase digoxin level. Watch for signs of digoxin toxicity.

*NSAIDs:* May increase risk of CNS stimulation and seizures. Use together cautiously.

*Probenecid:* May increase gatifloxacin levels and prolongs its half-life. Monitor patient closely.

*Warfarin:* May enhance effects of warfarin. Monitor PT and INR.

**Drug-herb.** *Dong quai, St. John's wort:* May cause photosensitivity. Advise patient to avoid excessive sunlight exposure.

**Drug-lifestyle.** *Sun exposure:* May cause photosensitivity. Advise patient to avoid excessive sunlight exposure.

**EFFECTS ON LAB TEST RESULTS**
None reported.

**CONTRAINDICATIONS & CAUTIONS**
• Contraindicated in patients hypersensitive to fluoroquinolones.
• Don't use in patients with prolonged QTc interval or uncorrected hypokalemia.
• Use cautiously in patients with clinically significant bradycardia, acute myocardial ischemia, known or suspected CNS disorders, or renal insufficiency.

**NURSING CONSIDERATIONS**
• Monitor glucose level in patients with diabetes.
• Monitor patients also receiving digoxin for signs and symptoms of digoxin toxicity.
• Monitor kidney function in patients with renal insufficiency.
• Stop drug if patient experiences seizures, increased intracranial pressure, psychosis, or CNS stimulation leading to tremors, restlessness, light-headedness, confusion, hallucinations, paranoia, depression, nightmares, or insomnia.
• Stop drug if rash or other sign of hypersensitivity occurs.
• Stop drug if patient experiences pain, inflammation, or rupture of a tendon.
• In patients being treated for gonorrhea, test for syphilis at time of diagnosis.

**PATIENT TEACHING**
• Tell patient to take drug as prescribed and to finish it, even if symptoms disappear.
• Advise patient to appropriately space products containing aluminum, magnesium, zinc, or iron when taking drug.
• Advise patient to use sunscreen and protective clothing when exposed to excessive sunlight.
• Warn patient to avoid hazardous tasks until adverse effects of drug are known.
• Advise diabetic patient to monitor blood sugar levels and notify prescriber if low blood sugar occurs.
• Advise patient to immediately report palpitations, fainting spells, rash, hives, difficulty swallowing or breathing, tightness in throat, hoarseness, swelling of lips, tongue, or face or other symptoms of allergic reaction.
• Advise patient to stop drug, refrain from exercise, and notify prescriber if pain, inflammation, or rupture of a tendon occurs.

✳ *NEW DRUG*

## gemifloxacin mesylate
Factive

*Pregnancy risk category C*

**AVAILABLE FORMS**
*Tablets:* 320 mg

**INDICATIONS & DOSAGES**
➤ **Acute bacterial worsening of chronic bronchitis caused by *Streptococcus pneumoniae, Haemophilus influenzae, H. parainfluenzae,* or *Moraxella catarrhalis***
*Adults:* 320 mg P.O. once daily for 5 days.
➤ **Mild to moderate community-acquired pneumonia caused by *S. pneumoniae* (including multi-drug resistant strains), *H. influenzae, M. catarrhalis, Mycoplasma pneumoniae, Chlamydia pneumoniae,* or *Klebsiella pneumoniae***
*Adults:* 320 mg P.O. once daily for 7 days.
*Adjust-a-dose:* If patient's creatinine clearance is 40 ml/minute or less or if he receives routine hemodialysis or continuous ambulatory peritoneal dialysis, reduce dosage to 160 mg P.O. once daily.

## ACTION
Prevents cell growth by inhibiting DNA gyrase and topoisomerase IV, which interferes with DNA synthesis.

| Route | Onset | Peak | Duration |
|-------|-------|------|----------|
| P.O. | Unknown | ½-2 hr | Unknown |

## ADVERSE REACTIONS
**CNS:** headache.
**GI:** diarrhea, nausea.
**Musculoskeletal:** ruptured tendons.
**Skin:** rash.
**Other:** hypersensitivity reactions.

## INTERACTIONS
**Drug-drug.** *Antacids (magnesium or aluminum), didanosine (chewable tablets, buffered tablets, or pediatric powder for oral solution), ferrous sulfate, multivitamins containing metal cations (such as zinc):* May decrease gemifloxacin level. Give these drugs at least 3 hours before or 2 hours after gemifloxacin.
*Antiarrhythmics of class IA (procainamide, quinidine) or class III (amiodarone, sotalol):* May increase risk of prolonged QTc interval. Avoid using together.
*Antipsychotics, erythromycin, tricyclic antidepressants:* May increase risk of prolonged QTc interval. Use together cautiously.
*Probenecid:* May increase gemifloxacin level. May use with probenecid for this reason.
*Sucralfate:* May decrease gemifloxacin level. Use together cautiously.
*Warfarin:* May increase anticoagulation effect. Monitor PT and INR.
**Drug-lifestyle.** *Sun exposure:* May increase risk of photosensitivity. Advise patient to avoid excessive sunlight exposure.

## EFFECTS ON LAB TEST RESULTS
● May increase ALT, AST, creatine phosphokinase, potassium, GGT, alkaline phosphatase, bilirubin, BUN, and creatinine levels. May decrease sodium, albumin, and protein levels. May increase or decrease calcium levels.
● May increase or decrease hemoglobin, hematocrit, and platelet, neutrophil, and RBC counts.

## CONTRAINDICATIONS & CAUTIONS
● Contraindicated in patients hypersensitive to fluoroquinolones, gemifloxacin, or their components.
● Contraindicated in patients with a history of prolonged QTc interval, those with uncorrected electrolyte disorders (such as hypokalemia or hypomagnesemia), and those taking a drug that could prolong the QTc interval.
● Use cautiously in patients with a proarrhythmic condition (such as bradycardia or acute myocardial ischemia), epilepsy, or a predisposition to seizures.
● Safety and efficacy haven't been established for children younger than age 18. Don't use drug in children.

## NURSING CONSIDERATIONS
● Use drug only for infections caused by susceptible bacteria.
● *Alert:* Don't exceed recommended dosage because of increased risk of prolonging the QTc interval.
● Mild to moderate maculopapular rash may appear, usually 8 to 10 days after therapy starts. It's more likely in women younger than age 40, especially those taking hormone therapy. Stop drug if rash appears.
● *Alert:* Serious, occasionally fatal, hypersensitivity reactions may occur. Stop drug immediately if hypersensitivity reaction occurs.
● Fluoroquinolones occasionally cause tendon rupture, arthropathy, or osteochondrosis; stop drug if patient reports pain, inflammation, or rupture.
● Stop drug if patient has a photosensitivity reaction.
● Fluoroquinolones may cause CNS effects, such as tremors and anxiety. Monitor patient carefully.
● Serious diarrhea may reflect pseudomembranous colitis; drug may need to be stopped.
● Keep patient adequately hydrated to avoid concentration of urine.

## PATIENT TEACHING
● Urge patient to finish full course of treatment, even if symptoms improve.
● Tell patient that drug may be taken with or without food, but that it shouldn't be

taken within 3 hours after or 2 hours before an antacid.
● Tell patient to stop drug and seek medical care if evidence of hypersensitivity reaction develops.
● Instruct patient to drink fluids liberally during treatment.
● Warn patient against taking OTC medications or dietary supplements with this drug without consulting a health care provider.
● Tell patient to avoid excessive exposure to sunlight or ultraviolet light.
● Urge patient to report pain, inflammation, or rupture of tendons.
● Warn patient to avoid driving or other hazardous activities until effects of drug are known.

---

## levofloxacin
Levaquin🔗

*Pregnancy risk category C*

---

**AVAILABLE FORMS**
*Infusion (premixed):* 250 mg in 50 ml
$D_5W$, 500 mg in 100 ml $D_5W$, 750 mg in
150 ml $D_5W$
*Single-use vials:* 500 mg, 750 mg
*Tablets:* 250 mg, 500 mg, 750 mg

**INDICATIONS & DOSAGES**
➤ **Acute maxillary sinusitis caused by susceptible strains of *Streptococcus pneumoniae, Moraxella catarrhalis,* or *Haemophilus influenzae;* mild to moderate skin and skin-structure infections caused by *Staphylococcus aureus* or *S. pyogenes***
*Adults:* 500 mg P.O. or I.V. daily for 10 to 14 days.
➤ **Acute bacterial worsening of chronic bronchitis caused by *S. aureus, S. pneumoniae, M. catarrhalis, H. influenzae,* or *Haemophilus parainfluenzae***
*Adults:* 500 mg P.O. or I.V. daily for 7 days.
➤ **Community-acquired pneumonia caused by *S. aureus, S. pneumoniae (including penicillin-resistant strains), M. catarrhalis, H. influenzae, H. parainfluenzae, Klebsiella pneumoniae, Chlamydia pneumoniae, Legionella***

*pneumophila,* or *Mycoplasma pneumoniae*
*Adults:* 500 mg P.O. or I.V. infusion over 60 minutes once daily for 7 to 14 days.
✹ *NEW INDICATION:* **Chronic bacterial prostatitis caused by *Escherichia coli, Enterococcus faecalis,* or *Staphylococcus epidermidis***
*Adults:* 500 mg P.O. or I.V. daily for 28 days.
*Adjust-a-dose:* In patients with creatinine clearance 20 to 49 ml/minute, give first dose of 500 mg, then 250 mg daily. If clearance is 10 to 19 ml/minute, give first dose of 500 mg, then 250 mg q 48 hours. For patients on dialysis or chronic ambulatory peritoneal dialysis, give first dose of 500 mg, then 250 mg q 48 hours.
➤ **Complicated skin and skin-structure infections caused by methicillin-sensitive *S. aureus, E. faecalis, S. pyogenes,* or *Proteus mirabilis***
*Adults:* 750 mg P.O. or I.V. infusion over 90 minutes q 24 hours for 7 to 14 days.
➤ **Nosocomial pneumonia caused by methicillin-susceptible *S. aureus, Pseudomonas aeruginosa, Serratia marcescens, E. coli, K. pneumoniae, H. influenzae,* or *S. pneumoniae***
*Adults:* 750 mg P.O. or I.V. daily for 7 to 14 days.
*Adjust-a-dose:* If creatinine clearance is 20 to 49 ml/minute, give 750 mg initially, then 750 mg q 48 hours; if clearance is 10 to 19 ml/minute, or patient is receiving hemodialysis or chronic ambulatory peritoneal dialysis, give 750 mg initially, then 500 mg q 48 hours.
➤ **Mild to moderate UTI caused by *E. faecalis, Enterobacter cloacae, E. coli, K. pneumoniae, P. mirabilis,* or *P. aeruginosa;* mild to moderate acute pyelonephritis caused by *E. coli***
*Adults:* 250 mg P.O. or I.V. daily for 10 days.
*Adjust-a-dose:* If creatinine clearance is 10 to 19 ml/minute, increase dosage interval to q 48 hours.
➤ **Mild to moderate uncomplicated UTI caused by *E. coli, K. pneumoniae,* or *Staphylococcus saprophyticus***
*Adults:* 250 mg P.O. daily for 3 days.
➤ **Traveler's diarrhea** ◆
*Adults:* 500 mg P.O. daily for up to 3 days.

➤ **To prevent traveler's diarrhea** ♦
*Adults:* 500 mg P.O. once daily during period of risk, for up to 3 weeks.
➤ **Uncomplicated cervical, urethral, or rectal gonorrhea** ♦
*Adults:* 250 mg P.O. as a single dose.
➤ **Disseminated gonococcal infection** ♦
*Adults:* 250 mg I.V. once daily and continued for 24 to 48 hours after patient starts to improve. Therapy may be switched to 500 mg P.O. daily to complete at least 1 week of therapy.
➤ **Nongonococcal urethritis** ♦ **; urogenital chlamydial infections** ♦
*Adults:* 500 mg P.O. once daily for 7 days.
➤ **Acute pelvic inflammatory disease** ♦
*Adults:* 500 mg I.V. once daily with or without metronidazole 500 mg q 8 hours. Stop parenteral therapy 24 hours after patient improves; then begin doxycycline 100 mg P.O. b.i.d. to complete 14 days of treatment. Or, 500 mg P.O. once daily for 14 days with or without metronidazole 500 mg b.i.d. for 14 days.

## I.V. ADMINISTRATION
● Give levofloxacin injection only by I.V. infusion.
● Dilute drug in single-use vials, according to manufacturer's instructions, with $D_5W$ or normal saline solution for injection to a final concentration of 5 mg/ml.
● Infuse over 60 minutes.
● Reconstituted solution should be clear, slightly yellow, and free of particulate matter.
● Reconstituted drug is stable for 72 hours at room temperature, for 14 days when refrigerated in plastic containers, and for 6 months when frozen.
● Thaw at room temperature or in refrigerator.
● Don't mix with other drugs.

## ACTION
Inhibits bacterial DNA gyrase and prevents DNA replication, transcription, repair, and recombination in susceptible bacteria.

| Route | Onset | Peak | Duration |
|---|---|---|---|
| P.O., I.V. | Unknown | 1-2 hr | Unknown |

## ADVERSE REACTIONS
**CNS:** headache, insomnia, pain, dizziness, *encephalopathy*, paresthesia, *seizures.*
**CV:** chest pain, palpitations, vasodilation.
**GI:** nausea, diarrhea, constipation, vomiting, abdominal pain, dyspepsia, flatulence, *pseudomembranous colitis.*
**GU:** vaginitis.
**Hematologic:** eosinophilia, hemolytic anemia, *lymphopenia.*
**Metabolic:** *hypoglycemia.*
**Musculoskeletal:** back pain, tendon rupture.
**Respiratory:** allergic pneumonitis.
**Skin:** rash, photosensitivity, pruritus, *erythema multiforme, Stevens-Johnson syndrome.*
**Other:** hypersensitivity reactions, *anaphylaxis, multisystem organ failure.*

## INTERACTIONS
**Drug-drug.** *Aluminum hydroxide, aluminum–magnesium hydroxide, calcium carbonate, didanosine, magnesium hydroxide, products containing zinc, sucralfate:* May interfere with GI absorption of levofloxacin. Take levofloxacin 2 hours before or 6 hours after these products.
*Antidiabetics:* May alter glucose level. Monitor glucose level closely.
*Iron salts:* May decrease absorption of levofloxacin, reducing anti-infective response. Separate doses by at least 2 hours.
*NSAIDs:* May increase CNS stimulation. Monitor patient for seizure activity.
*Theophylline:* May decrease clearance of theophylline. Monitor theophylline level.
*Warfarin and derivatives:* May increase effect of oral anticoagulant. Monitor PT and INR.
**Drug-herb.** *Dong quai, St. John's wort:* May cause photosensitivity reactions. Advise patient to avoid excessive sunlight exposure.
**Drug-lifestyle.** *Sun exposure:* May cause photosensitivity reactions. Advise patient to avoid excessive sunlight exposure.

## EFFECTS ON LAB TEST RESULTS
● May decrease glucose level.
● May increase eosinophil count. May decrease hemoglobin and WBC count.
● May produce false-positive opiate assay results.

---

Reactions may be *common*, uncommon, *life-threatening*, or COMMON AND LIFE-THREATENING.

## CONTRAINDICATIONS & CAUTIONS
• Contraindicated in patients hypersensitive to drug, its components, or other fluoroquinolones.
• Safety and efficacy of drug in children younger than age 18 and in pregnant and breast-feeding women haven't been established.
• Use cautiously in patients with history of seizure disorders or other CNS diseases, such as cerebral arteriosclerosis.
• Use cautiously and with dosage adjustment in patients with renal impairment.

## NURSING CONSIDERATIONS
• If patient experiences symptoms of excessive CNS stimulation (restlessness, tremor, confusion, hallucinations), stop drug and notify prescriber. Begin seizure precautions.
• Patients with acute hypersensitivity reactions may need treatment with epinephrine, oxygen, I.V. fluids, antihistamines, corticosteroids, pressor amines, and airway management.
• Most antibacterial drugs can cause pseudomembranous colitis. Notify prescriber if diarrhea occurs. Drug may be stopped.
• Drug may cause an abnormal ECG.
• Obtain specimen for culture and sensitivity tests before starting therapy and as needed to determine if bacterial resistance has occurred.
• **Alert:** If *P. aeruginosa* is a confirmed or suspected pathogen, use combination therapy with a beta-lactam.
• Monitor glucose and renal, hepatic, and hematopoietic blood studies.

## PATIENT TEACHING
• Tell patient to take drug as prescribed, even if signs and symptoms disappear.
• Advise patient to take drug with plenty of fluids and to appropriately space antacids, sucralfate, and products containing iron or zinc after each dose of levofloxacin.
• Warn patient to avoid hazardous tasks until adverse effects of drug are known.
• Advise patient to avoid excessive sunlight, use sunscreen, and wear protective clothing when outdoors.

• Instruct patient to stop drug and notify prescriber if rash or other signs or symptoms of hypersensitivity develop.
• Tell patient that tendon rupture can occur with drug and to notify prescriber if he experiences pain or inflammation.
• Instruct diabetic patient to monitor glucose levels and notify prescriber if low glucose reaction occurs.
• Instruct patient to notify prescriber if he has loose stools or diarrhea.

---

# moxifloxacin hydrochloride
Avelox, Avelox I.V.

*Pregnancy risk category C*

## AVAILABLE FORMS
*Injection:* 400 mg/250 ml
*Tablets (film-coated):* 400 mg

## INDICATIONS & DOSAGES
➤ **Acute bacterial sinusitis caused by** *Streptococcus pneumoniae, Haemophilus influenzae,* **or** *Moraxella catarrhalis*
*Adults:* 400 mg P.O. or I.V. once daily for 10 days.
➤ **Mild to moderate community-acquired pneumonia caused by** *S. pneumoniae, H. influenzae, Mycoplasma pneumoniae, Chlamydia pneumoniae,* **or** *M. catarrhalis*
*Adults:* 400 mg P.O. or I.V. once daily for 7 to 14 days.
➤ **Acute bacterial worsening of chronic bronchitis caused by** *S. pneumoniae, H. influenzae, H. parainfluenzae, Klebsiella pneumoniae, Staphylococcus aureus,* **or** *M. catarrhalis*
*Adults:* 400 mg P.O. or I.V. once daily for 5 days.
➤ **Uncomplicated skin and skin-structure infections caused by** *Staphylococcus aureus* **or** *S. pyogenes*
*Adults:* 400 mg P.O. or I.V. once daily for 7 days.

## I.V. ADMINISTRATION
• Give only by I.V. infusion over 1 hour.
• Avoid rapid or bolus infusion.
• Don't mix with other drugs.
• Flush I.V. line with a compatible solution such as $D_5W$, normal saline, or

---

Ringer's lactate solution before and after use.
● Don't use if particulate matter is visible.

## ACTION
Interferes with action of enzymes necessary for bacterial replication. Inhibits topoisomerases I (DNA gyrase) and IV, thereby impairing processes of bacterial DNA replication, transcription, repair, and recombination.

| Route | Onset | Peak | Duration |
|---|---|---|---|
| P.O., I.V. | Unknown | 1-3 hr | Unknown |

## ADVERSE REACTIONS
**CNS:** dizziness, headache, asthenia, pain, malaise, insomnia, nervousness, anxiety, confusion, somnolence, tremor, vertigo, paresthesia.
**CV:** *prolongation of QT interval,* chest pain, palpitations, tachycardia, hypertension, peripheral edema.
**GI:** *pseudomembranous colitis,* nausea, diarrhea, abdominal pain, vomiting, dyspepsia, dry mouth, constipation, oral candidiasis, anorexia, stomatitis, glossitis, flatulence, GI disorder, taste perversion.
**GU:** vaginitis, vaginal candidiasis.
**Hematologic:** *thrombocytosis, thrombocytopenia, leukopenia,* eosinophilia.
**Hepatic:** abnormal liver function, cholestatic jaundice.
**Musculoskeletal:** leg pain, back pain, arthralgia, myalgia, tendon rupture.
**Respiratory:** dyspnea.
**Skin:** injection site reaction, rash (maculopapular, purpuric, pustular), pruritus, sweating.
**Other:** candidiasis, allergic reaction.

## INTERACTIONS
**Drug-drug.** *Aluminum hydroxide, aluminum–magnesium hydroxide, calcium carbonate, didanosine, magnesium hydroxide, multivitamins, products containing zinc:* May interfere with GI absorption of moxifloxacin. Take moxifloxacin 4 hours before or 8 hours after these products.
*Class IA antiarrhythmics (such as procainamide, quinidine), class III antiarrhythmics (such as amiodarone, sotalol):* May increase risk of cardiac arrhythmias. Avoid using together.

*Drugs known to prolong QT interval, such as antipsychotics, erythromycin, tricyclic antidepressants:* May have additive effect. Avoid using together.
*NSAIDs:* May increase risk of CNS stimulation and seizures. Avoid using together.
*Sucralfate:* May decrease absorption of the moxifloxacin reducing anti-infective response. If use together can't be avoided, give at least 6 hours apart.
*Warfarin:* May increase anticoagulant effects. Monitor PT/INR closely.
**Drug-lifestyle.** *Sun exposure:* May cause photosensitivity reactions. Advise patient to avoid excessive sunlight exposure.

## EFFECTS ON LAB TEST RESULTS
● May increase GGT, amylase, and LDH levels.
● May increase eosinophil count. May decrease PT and WBC count. May increase or decrease platelet count.

## CONTRAINDICATIONS & CAUTIONS
● Contraindicated in patients hypersensitive to drug or other fluoroquinolones and in those with prolonged QT interval or uncorrected hypokalemia.
● Use cautiously in patients with ongoing proarrhythmic conditions, such as clinically significant bradycardia or acute myocardial ischemia.
● Use cautiously in patients who may have CNS disorders and in those with other risk factors that may lower the seizure threshold or predispose them to seizures.
● Safety and efficacy in children, adolescents younger than age 18, and pregnant or breast-feeding women haven't been established.

## NURSING CONSIDERATIONS
● Drug may be given without regard to meals. Give at same time each day.
● *Alert:* Monitor patient for adverse CNS effects, including seizures, dizziness, confusion, tremors, hallucinations, depression, and suicidal thoughts or acts. If these effects occur, stop drug and institute appropriate measures.
● Serious hypersensitivity reactions, including anaphylaxis, have occurred in patients receiving fluoroquinolones. Stop drug and institute supportive measures, as indicated.

Reactions may be *common*, uncommon, *life-threatening*, or COMMON AND LIFE-THREATENING.

• Consider the possibility of pseudomembranous colitis if diarrhea develops after therapy begins.
• Rupture of the Achilles and other tendons has been linked to fluoroquinolones. If pain, inflammation, or rupture of a tendon occurs, stop drug.
• Store drug at controlled room temperature.

**PATIENT TEACHING**
• Instruct patient to take drug once daily, at the same time each day, without regard to meals.
• Tell patient to finish entire course of therapy, even if symptoms are relieved.
• Advise patient to drink plenty of fluids.
• Tell patient to appropriately space antacids, sucralfate, multivitamins, and products containing aluminum, magnesium, iron, and zinc to avoid decreasing drug's therapeutic effects.
• Instruct patient to contact prescriber and stop drug if he experiences allergic reaction, rash, heart palpitations, fainting, or persistent diarrhea.
• Direct patient to contact prescriber, stop drug, rest, and refrain from exercise if he experiences pain, inflammation, or rupture of a tendon.
• Warn patient that drug may cause dizziness and light-headedness. Tell patient to avoid hazardous activities, such as driving or operating machinery, until effects of drug are known.
• Instruct patient to avoid excessive sunlight exposure and ultraviolet light and to report photosensitivity reactions to prescriber.

---

## norfloxacin
Noroxin

*Pregnancy risk category C*

---

**AVAILABLE FORMS**
*Tablets (film-coated):* 400 mg

**INDICATIONS & DOSAGES**
➤ Complicated or uncomplicated UTI from susceptible strains of *Enterococcus faecalis, Escherichia coli, Klebsiella pneumoniae, Enterobacter aerogenes, E. cloacae, Proteus mirabilis, P. vulgaris,*

*Pseudomonas aeruginosa, Citrobacter freundii, Staphylococcus agalactiae, S. aureus, S. epidermidis, S. saprophyticus,* or *Serratia marcescens*
*Adults:* 400 mg P.O. q 12 hours for 7 to 10 days (uncomplicated infection). Or, 400 mg P.O. q 12 hours for 10 to 21 days (complicated infection).
➤ Prostatitis
*Adults:* 400 mg P.O. q 12 hours for 28 days.
➤ Cystitis caused by *E. coli, K. pneumoniae,* or *P. mirabilis*
*Adults:* 400 mg P.O. q 12 hours for 3 days.
*Adjust-a-dose:* For adult patients with creatinine clearance of 30 ml/minute or less, give 400 mg once daily for above indications.
➤ Acute, uncomplicated urethral and cervical gonorrhea
*Adults:* 800 mg P.O. as a single dose, then doxycycline therapy to treat any coexisting chlamydial infection.

**ACTION**
Inhibits bacterial DNA synthesis, mainly by blocking DNA gyrase; bactericidal.

| Route | Onset | Peak | Duration |
|-------|-------|------|----------|
| P.O. | Unknown | 30-120 min | Unknown |

**ADVERSE REACTIONS**
**CNS:** fatigue, somnolence, headache, dizziness, *seizures,* depression, insomnia, fever.
**GI:** anorexia, nausea, constipation, flatulence, heartburn, dry mouth, abdominal pain, diarrhea, vomiting.
**GU:** crystalluria.
**Hematologic:** eosinophilia, *neutropenia.*
**Musculoskeletal:** back pain.
**Skin:** rash, photosensitivity, hyperhidrosis.
**Other:** hypersensitivity reactions, *anaphylaxis.*

**INTERACTIONS**
**Drug-drug.** *Aluminum hydroxide, aluminum–magnesium hydroxide, calcium carbonate, magnesium hydroxide:* May decrease norfloxacin level. Give antacid at least 6 hours before or 2 hours after norfloxacin.

---

*Iron salts:* May decrease absorption of norfloxacin, reducing anti-infective response. Give at least 2 hours apart.
*Cyclosporine:* May increase cyclosporine level. Monitor cyclosporine level.
*Nitrofurantoin:* May antagonize norfloxacin effect. Monitor patient closely.
*Oral anticoagulants:* May increase anticoagulant effect. Monitor PT and INR.
*Probenecid:* May increase norfloxacin level by decreasing its excretion. May give probenecid for this reason, but monitor high-risk patient for toxicity.
*Sucralfate:* May decrease absorption of the norfloxacin reducing anti-infective response. If use together can't be avoided, give at least 6 hours apart.
*Theophylline:* May impair theophylline metabolism, increasing drug level and risk of toxicity. Monitor patient closely.
**Drug-herb.** *Dong quai, St. John's wort:* May cause photosensitivity reactions. Advise patient to avoid excessive sunlight exposure.

**EFFECTS ON LAB TEST RESULTS**
• May increase BUN, creatinine, ALT, AST, and alkaline phosphatase levels.
• May increase eosinophil count. May decrease hematocrit and neutrophil count.

**CONTRAINDICATIONS & CAUTIONS**
• Contraindicated in patients hypersensitive to drug or other fluoroquinolones.
• Use cautiously in patients with conditions such as cerebral arteriosclerosis that may predispose them to seizure disorders.
• Use cautiously and monitor renal function in those with renal impairment.
• Safety in children younger than age 18 hasn't been established.

**NURSING CONSIDERATIONS**
• Obtain specimen for culture and sensitivity testing before starting therapy.
• Tendon rupture has occurred in patients receiving quinolones. Stop drug if pain, inflammation, or rupture of a tendon occurs.
• *Alert:* Don't confuse Noroxin (norfloxacin) for Neurontin (gabapentin) or Floxin (ofloxacin).

**PATIENT TEACHING**
• Tell patient to take drug as prescribed, even after he feels better.
• Advise patient to take drug 1 hour before or 2 hours after meals because food may hinder absorption.
• Advise patient to appropriately space iron products and antacids when taking norfloxacin.
• Warn patient not to exceed the recommended dosages and to drink several glasses of water throughout the day to maintain hydration and adequate urine output.
• Warn patient to avoid hazardous tasks that require alertness until effects of drug are known.
• Instruct patient to avoid exposure to sunlight, wear protective clothing, and use sunscreen while outdoors.
• Tell patient to report pain, inflammation, or tendon rupture, and to refrain from exercise until diagnosis of rupture or tendonitis is excluded.

## ofloxacin
Floxin✱, Floxin I.V.

*Pregnancy risk category C*

**AVAILABLE FORMS**
*Injection:* 20 mg/ml, 40 mg/ml; 200 mg premixed in $D_5W$; 400 mg premixed in $D_5W$
*Tablets:* 200 mg, 300 mg, 400 mg

**INDICATIONS AND DOSAGES**
➤ **Acute bacterial worsening of chronic bronchitis, uncomplicated skin and skin-structure infections, and community-acquired pneumonia**
*Adults:* 400 mg P.O. or I.V. q 12 hours for 10 days.
➤ **Sexually transmitted diseases, such as acute uncomplicated urethral and cervical gonorrhea, nongonococcal urethritis and cervicitis, and mixed infections of urethra and cervix**
*Adults:* For acute uncomplicated gonorrhea, 400 mg P.O. or I.V. once as a single dose; for cervicitis and urethritis, 300 mg P.O. or I.V. q 12 hours for 7 days.

➤**Cystitis from *Escherichia coli, Klebsiella pneumoniae,* or other organisms**
*Adults:* 200 mg P.O. or I.V. q 12 hours for 3 days (*E. coli* or *K. pneumoniae*), 200 mg P.O. or I.V. q 12 hours for 7 days (other organisms).
➤**Complicated UTI**
*Adults:* 200 mg P.O. or I.V. q 12 hours for 10 days.
➤**Prostatitis**
*Adults:* 300 mg P.O. or I.V. q 12 hours for 6 weeks. Switch from I.V. to P.O. after 10 days.
➤**Pelvic inflammatory disease**
*Adults:* 400 mg P.O. or I.V. q 12 hours with metronidazole for 10 to 14 days.
➤**To prevent inhalation anthrax ♦**
*Adults:* 400 mg P.O. or I.V. b.i.d. Give first doses I.V. if signs and symptoms of disease exist. Switch to P.O. after patient's condition improves. Continue therapy for 60 days if no vaccine is available. If vaccine is available, continue for 28 to 45 days and until three doses of the vaccine have been given.
➤**Traveler's diarrhea**
*Adults:* 300 mg P.O. b.i.d. for 3 days.
***Adjust-a-dose:*** For patients with creatinine clearance less than 20 ml/minute, give first dose as recommended, then give subsequent doses at 50% of recommended dose q 24 hours. For patients with hepatic impairment, don't exceed 400 mg/day.

**I.V. ADMINISTRATION**
• The injection concentrate in 20- or 40-mg/ml vials must be diluted to a maximum of 4 mg/ml.
• Compatible with most common I.V. solutions, including D₅W injection, normal saline injection, dextrose 5% in normal saline injection, dextrose 5% in 0.45% saline injection, and 5% dextrose in lactated Ringer's solution. Give over at least 60 minutes and avoid rapid or bolus injection.
• If giving infusion at a Y-site, stop the flow of the other solution.

**ACTION**
Interferes with DNA gyrase, which is needed for synthesis of bacterial DNA. Spectrum of action includes many gram-positive and gram-negative aerobic bacteria including *Enterobacteriaceae* and *Pseudomonas aeruginosa.*

| Route | Onset | Peak | Duration |
|-------|-------|------|----------|
| P.O. | Unknown | 15-120 min | Unknown |
| I.V. | Unknown | Immediate | Unknown |

**ADVERSE REACTIONS**
**CNS:** dizziness; headache, fever, fatigue, lethargy, malaise, drowsiness, sleep disorders, nervousness, insomnia, visual disturbances, *seizures.*
**CV:** phlebitis, chest pain.
**GI:** *nausea, pseudomembranous colitis,* anorexia, abdominal pain or discomfort, diarrhea, vomiting, constipation, dry mouth, flatulence, dysgeusia.
**GU:** hematuria, glucosuria, proteinuria, vaginitis, vaginal discharge, genital pruritus.
**Hematologic:** eosinophilia, *leukopenia, neutropenia,* anemia, leukocytosis.
**Metabolic:** hyperglycemia, *hypoglycemia.*
**Musculoskeletal:** body pain.
**Skin:** rash, pruritus, photosensitivity.
**Other:** hypersensitivity reactions, *anaphylactoid reaction.*

**INTERACTIONS**
**Drug-drug.** *Aluminum hydroxide, aluminum–magnesium hydroxide, calcium carbonate, magnesium hydroxide:* May decrease effects of ofloxacin. Give antacid at least 6 hours before or 2 hours after ofloxacin.
*Antidiabetics:* May affect glucose level, causing hypoglycemia or hyperglycemia. Monitor patient closely.
*Didanosine (chewable or buffered tablets or pediatric powder for oral solution):* May interfere with GI absorption of ofloxacin. Separate doses by 2 hours.
*Iron salts:* May decrease absorption of ofloxacin, reducing anti-infective response. Separate doses by at least 2 hours.
*Sucralfate:* May decrease absorption of ofloxacin, reducing anti-infective response. If use together can't be avoided, separate doses by at least 6 hours.
*Theophylline:* May increase theophylline level. Monitor patient closely and adjust theophylline dosage as needed.
*Warfarin:* May prolong PT and INR. Monitor PT and INR.

**Drug-lifestyle.** *Sun exposure:* May cause photosensitivity reactions. Advise patient to avoid excessive sunlight exposure.

## EFFECTS ON LAB TEST RESULTS
• May increase BUN, creatinine, and liver enzyme levels. May increase or decrease glucose levels.
• May increase erythrocyte sedimentation rate and eosinophil count. May decrease hemoglobin, hematocrit, and neutrophil count. May increase or decrease WBC count.
• May produce false-positive opiate assay results.

## CONTRAINDICATIONS & CAUTIONS
• Contraindicated in patients hypersensitive to drug or other fluoroquinolones.
• Use cautiously in pregnant patients and in patients with seizure disorders, CNS diseases such as cerebral arteriosclerosis, hepatic disorders, or renal impairment.
• Ofloxacin appears in breast milk in levels similar to those found in plasma. Safety hasn't been established in breast-feeding women.
• Safety and efficacy in children younger than age 18 haven't been established.

## NURSING CONSIDERATIONS
• Give drug I.V. for no longer than 10 days; after 10 days, change I.V. to P.O.
• *Alert:* Patients treated for gonorrhea should have a serologic test for syphilis. Drug isn't effective against syphilis, and treatment of gonorrhea may mask or delay symptoms of syphilis.
• Periodically assess organ system functions during prolonged therapy.
• Monitor patient for overgrowth of non-susceptible organisms.
• Monitor renal and hepatic studies and CBC in prolonged therapy.

## PATIENT TEACHING
• Tell patient to drink plenty of fluids during drug therapy and to finish the entire prescription even if he starts feeling better.
• Tell patient drug may be taken without regard to meals, but he shouldn't take antacids and vitamins at the same time as ofloxacin.
• Warn patient that dizziness and light-headedness may occur. Advise caution when driving or operating hazardous machinery until effects of drug are known.
• Warn patient that hypersensitivity reactions may follow first dose; he should stop drug at first sign of rash or other allergic reaction and call prescriber immediately.
• Advise patient to avoid prolonged exposure to direct sunlight and to use a sunscreen when outdoors.

abacavir sulfate
acyclovir
acyclovir sodium
adefovir dipivoxil
amantadine hydrochloride
amprenavir
atazanavir sulfate
cidofovir
delavirdine mesylate
didanosine
efavirenz
emtricitabine
enfuvirtide
famciclovir
fomivirsen sodium
fosamprenavir
foscarnet sodium
ganciclovir
indinavir sulfate
lamivudine
lamivudine and zidovudine
lopinavir and ritonavir
nelfinavir mesylate
nevirapine
oseltamivir phosphate
ribavirin
rimantadine hydrochloride
ritonavir
saquinavir
saquinavir mesylate
stavudine
tenofovir disoproxil fumarate
valacyclovir hydrochloride
valganciclovir
zalcitabine
zanamivir
zidovudine

**COMBINATION PRODUCTS**
None.

## abacavir sulfate
Ziagen

*Pregnancy risk category C*

**AVAILABLE FORMS**
*Oral solution:* 20 mg/ml
*Tablets:* 300 mg

**INDICATIONS & DOSAGES**
➤ **HIV-1 infection**
*Adults:* 300 mg P.O. b.i.d. with other anti-retrovirals.
*Children ages 3 months to 16 years:* 8 mg/kg P.O. b.i.d., up to maximum of 300 mg P.O. b.i.d., with other antiretrovirals.

**ACTION**
Converted intracellularly to the active metabolite carbovir triphosphate, which inhibits activity of HIV-1 reverse transcriptase, terminating viral DNA growth.

| Route | Onset | Peak | Duration |
|-------|-------|------|----------|
| P.O. | Unknown | Unknown | Unknown |

**ADVERSE REACTIONS**
**CNS:** insomnia and sleep disorders, fever, headache.
**GI:** *nausea, vomiting, diarrhea, anorexia.*
**Skin:** rash.
**Other:** hypersensitivity reaction.

**INTERACTIONS**
**Drug-lifestyle.** *Alcohol use:* May decrease elimination of abacavir, increasing overall exposure to drug. Monitor alcohol consumption. Discourage use together.

**EFFECTS ON LAB TEST RESULTS**
• May increase GGT, glucose, and triglyceride levels.

**CONTRAINDICATIONS & CAUTIONS**
• Contraindicated in patients hypersensitive to drug or its components.
• Use cautiously when giving drug to patients at risk for liver disease. Lactic acidosis and severe hepatomegaly with steatosis, including fatal cases, have been reported with the use of nucleoside analogues alone or in combination, including abacavir and other antiretrovirals. Stop treatment with drug if events occur.
• Use cautiously in pregnant women because no adequate studies of the effects of abacavir on pregnancy exist. Use during pregnancy only if the potential benefits

outweigh the risk. Register pregnant women taking abacavir with the Antiretroviral Pregnancy Registry at 1-800-258-4263.

**NURSING CONSIDERATIONS**
● Women are more likely than men to experience lactic acidosis and severe hepatomegaly with steatosis. Obesity and prolonged nucleoside exposure may be risk factors.
● *Alert:* Abacavir can cause fatal hypersensitivity reactions; as soon as patient develops signs or symptoms of hypersensitivity (such as fever, rash, fatigue, nausea, vomiting, diarrhea, or abdominal pain), stop drug and seek medical attention immediately.
● *Alert:* Don't restart drug after a hypersensitivity reaction because severe signs and symptoms will recur within hours and may include life-threatening hypotension and death. To facilitate reporting of hypersensitivity reactions, register patients with the Abacavir Hypersensitivity Reaction Registry at 1-800-270-0425.
● Always give drug with other antiretrovirals, and never alone.
● Because of a high rate of early virologic resistance, triple antiretroviral therapy with abacavir, lamivudine, and tenofovir shouldn't be used as new treatment regimen for naive or pretreated patients. Monitor patients currently controlled with this combination and those who use this combination in addition to other antiretrovirals, and consider modification of therapy.
● Drug may mildly elevate glucose level.
● *Alert:* Don't confuse abacavir with amprenavir.

**PATIENT TEACHING**
● Inform patient that abacavir can cause a life-threatening hypersensitivity reaction. Warn patient who develops signs or symptoms of hypersensitivity (such as fever, rash, severe tiredness, achiness, a generally ill feeling, nausea, vomiting, diarrhea, or stomach pain) to stop taking drug and notify prescriber immediately.
● Include information leaflet about drug with each new prescription and refill. Patient also should receive, and be instructed to carry, a warning card summarizing signs and symptoms of abacavir hypersensitivity reaction.
● Inform patient that this drug doesn't cure HIV infection. Tell patient that drug hasn't been shown to reduce the risk of transmission of HIV to others through sexual contact or blood contamination and that its long-term effects are unknown.
● Tell patient to take drug exactly as prescribed.
● Inform patient that drug can be taken with or without food.

---

## acyclovir
Acihexal‡, Acyclo-V‡, Avirax†, Lovir ‡, Zovirax✔

## acyclovir sodium
Aciclovir‡, Acihexal ‡, Avirax†, Zovirax

*Pregnancy risk category C*

**AVAILABLE FORMS**
*Capsules:* 200 mg
*Injection:* 500 mg/vial, 1 g/vial
*Suspension:* 200 mg/5 ml
*Tablets:* 400 mg, 800 mg

**INDICATIONS & DOSAGES**
➤ **First and recurrent episodes of mucocutaneous herpes simplex virus (HSV-1 and HSV-2) infections in immunocompromised patients; severe first episodes of genital herpes in patients who aren't immunocompromised**
*Adults and children age 12 and older:* 5 mg/kg given I.V. over 1 hour q 8 hours for 7 days. Give for 5 to 7 days for severe first episode of genital herpes.
*Children younger than age 12:* 10 mg/kg given I.V. over 1 hour q 8 hours for 7 days.
➤ **First genital herpes episode**
*Adults:* 200 mg P.O. q 4 hours while awake five times daily; or 400 mg P.O. q 8 hours. Continue for 7 to 10 days for treatment of first genital herpes episodes.
➤ **Intermittent therapy for recurrent genital herpes**
*Adults:* 200 mg P.O. q 4 hours while awake for total of five capsules daily. Treatment should continue for 5 days. Begin therapy at first sign of recurrence.

---

➤ **Long-term suppressive therapy for recurrent genital herpes**
*Adults:* 400 mg P.O. b.i.d. for up to 12 months. Or, 200 mg P.O. three to five times daily for up to 12 months.

➤ **Varicella (chickenpox) infections in immunocompromised patients**
*Adults and children age 12 and older:* 10 mg/kg I.V. over 1 hour q 8 hours for 7 days. Dosage for obese patients is 10 mg/kg based on ideal body weight q 8 hours for 7 days. Don't exceed maximum dosage equivalent of 20 mg/kg q 8 hours.
*Children younger than age 12:* 20 mg/kg I.V. over 1 hour q 8 hours for 7 days.

➤ **Varicella infection in immunocompetent patients**
*Adults and children weighing more than 40 kg (88 lb):* 800 mg P.O. q.i.d. for 5 days.
*Children age 2 and older, weighing less than 40 kg:* 20 mg/kg (maximum 800 mg/ dose) P.O. q.i.d. for 5 days. Start therapy as soon as symptoms appear.

➤ **Acute herpes zoster infection in immunocompetent patients**
*Adults and children age 12 and older:* 800 mg P.O. q 4 hours five times daily for 7 to 10 days.

➤ **Herpes simplex encephalitis**
*Adults and children age 12 and older:* 10 mg/kg I.V. over 1 hour q 8 hours for 10 days.
*Children ages 3 months to 12 years:* 20 mg/kg I.V. over 1 hour q 8 hours for 10 days.

➤ **Neonatal herpes simplex virus infection**
*Neonates to 3 months old:* 10 mg/kg I.V. over 1 hour q 8 hours for 10 days.
*Adjust-a-dose:* For patients receiving the I.V. form, if creatinine clearance is 25 to 50 ml/minute, give 100% of dose q 12 hours; if clearance is 10 to 24 ml/minute, 100% of dose q 24 hours; if clearance is less than 10 ml/minute, 50% of dose q 24 hours.
For patients receiving the P.O. form, if normal dose is 200 mg q 4 hours five times daily and creatinine clearance is less than 10 ml/minute, give 200 mg P.O. q 12 hours. If normal dose is 400 mg q 12 hours and clearance is less than 10 ml/ minute, 200 mg q 12 hours. If normal dose is 800 mg q 4 hours five times daily and if clearance is 10 to 25 ml/minute, 800 mg q 8 hours; if clearance is less than 10 ml/minute, 800 mg q 12 hours.

**I.V. ADMINISTRATION**
● Give I.V. infusion over at least 1 hour to prevent renal tubular damage. Don't give by bolus injection. Bolus injection, dehydration (decreased urine output), renal disease, and use together with other nephrotoxic drugs increase the risk of renal toxicity.
● Solutions concentrated at 7 mg/ml or more may cause a higher risk of phlebitis.
● Encourage fluid intake because patient must be adequately hydrated during acyclovir infusion. Monitor intake and output, especially within the first 2 hours after I.V. administration.

**ACTION**
Interferes with DNA synthesis and inhibits viral multiplication.

| Route | Onset | Peak | Duration |
|-------|-------|------|----------|
| P.O. | Unknown | 2½ hr | Unknown |
| I.V. | Immediate | Immediate | Unknown |

**ADVERSE REACTIONS**
**CNS:** *malaise, headache, **encephalopathic changes*** (including lethargy, obtundation, tremor, confusion, hallucinations, agitation, *seizures, coma*).
**GI:** *nausea, vomiting,* diarrhea.
**GU:** hematuria, *acute renal failure.*
**Hematologic:** *thrombocytopenia, leukopenia,* thrombocytosis.
**Skin:** rash, itching, urticaria, *inflammation or phlebitis at injection site.*

**INTERACTIONS**
**Drug-drug.** *Interferon:* May have synergistic effect. Monitor patient closely.
*Probenecid:* May increase acyclovir level. Monitor patient for possible toxicity.
*Zidovudine:* May cause drowsiness or lethargy. Use together cautiously.

**EFFECTS ON LAB TEST RESULTS**
● May increase BUN and creatinine levels.
● May decrease WBC count. May increase or decrease platelet count.

## CONTRAINDICATIONS & CAUTIONS
• Contraindicated in patients hypersensitive to drug.
• Use cautiously in patients with neurologic problems, renal disease, or dehydration and in those receiving other nephrotoxic drugs. Monitor renal function.
• Because no adequate studies have been done in pregnant women, give acyclovir during pregnancy only if potential benefits outweigh risks to fetus.

## NURSING CONSIDERATIONS
• *Alert:* Don't give I.M. or S.C.
• Encephalopathic changes are more likely to occur in patients with neurologic disorders or in those who have had neurologic reactions to cytotoxic drugs.
• *Alert:* Don't confuse acyclovir sodium (Zovirax) with acetazolamide sodium (Diamox) vials, which may look alike.
• *Alert:* Don't confuse Zovirax with Zyvox (linezolid); both come in 400-mg strength.

## PATIENT TEACHING
• Tell patient to take drug as prescribed, even after he feels better.
• Tell patient drug is effective in managing herpes infection but doesn't eliminate or cure it. Warn patient that acyclovir won't prevent spread of infection to others.
• Tell patient to avoid sexual contact while visible lesions are present.
• Teach patient about early signs and symptoms of herpes infection (such as tingling, itching, or pain).
• Tell him to notify prescriber and get a prescription for acyclovir before the infection fully develops. Early treatment is most effective.

---

# adefovir dipivoxil
Hepsera

*Pregnancy risk category C*

## AVAILABLE FORMS
*Tablets:* 10 mg

## INDICATIONS & DOSAGES
➤ **Chronic hepatitis B infection**
*Adults:* 10 mg P.O. once daily.
*Adjust-a-dose:* In patients with creatinine clearance 20 to 49 ml/minute, give 10 mg P.O. q 48 hours. In patients with clearance 10 to 19 ml/minute, give 10 mg P.O. q 72 hours. In patients receiving hemodialysis, give 10 mg P.O. q 7 days, after dialysis session.

## ACTION
An acyclic nucleotide analogue that inhibits hepatitis B virus reverse transcription via viral DNA chain termination.

| Route | Onset | Peak | Duration |
|---|---|---|---|
| P.O. | Unknown | 1-4 hr | Unknown |

## ADVERSE REACTIONS
**CNS:** *asthenia,* headache, fever.
**EENT:** pharyngitis, sinusitis.
**GI:** abdominal pain, diarrhea, dyspepsia, flatulence, nausea, vomiting.
**GU:** *renal failure, renal insufficiency, hematuria,* glycosuria.
**Hepatic:** *hepatomegaly with steatosis, hepatic failure.*
**Metabolic:** *lactic acidosis.*
**Respiratory:** cough.
**Skin:** pruritus, rash.

## INTERACTIONS
**Drug-drug.** *Ibuprofen:* May increase adefovir bioavailability. Monitor patient for adverse effects.
*Nephrotoxic drugs (aminoglycosides, cyclosporine, NSAIDs, tacrolimus, vancomycin):* May increase risk of nephrotoxicity. Use together cautiously.

## EFFECTS ON LAB TEST RESULTS
• May increase ALT, amylase, AST, creatine kinase, creatinine, and lactate levels.

## CONTRAINDICATIONS & CAUTIONS
• Contraindicated in patients hypersensitive to any component of the drug.
• Use cautiously in patients with renal dysfunction, in those receiving nephrotoxic drugs, and in those with known risk factors for hepatic disease.
• Use cautiously in elderly patients because they're more likely to have decreased renal and cardiac function.
• Pregnant women exposed to drug may call the Antiretroviral Pregnancy Registry at 1-800-258-4263 to monitor fetal outcome.

---

• Safety and efficacy in children haven't been established.

## NURSING CONSIDERATIONS
• Monitor renal function, especially in patients with renal dysfunction or concurrent treatment with nephrotoxic drugs.
• *Alert:* Patients may develop lactic acidosis and severe hepatomegaly with steatosis during treatment. Risk factors include female gender, obesity, and concurrent antiretroviral therapy.
• Monitor hepatic function. Notify prescriber if patient develops signs or symptoms of lactic acidosis and severe hepatomegaly with steatosis. Treatment may have to be stopped.
• Severe exacerbations of hepatitis may result from discontinuation of adefovir. Monitor hepatic function closely in patients who stop anti-hepatitis B therapy.
• The optimal duration of treatment with adefovir hasn't been established.
• Offer HIV antibody testing to patients receiving adefovir. Adefovir may promote resistance to antiretrovirals in patients with unrecognized or untreated HIV infection.

## PATIENT TEACHING
• Inform the patient that adefovir may be taken without regard to meals.
• Tell patient to immediately report weakness, muscle pain, trouble breathing, stomach pain with nausea and vomiting, dizziness, light-headedness, fast or irregular heartbeat, and feeling cold, especially in arms and legs.
• Warn patient not to stop taking this drug unless directed because it could cause hepatitis to become worse.
• Instruct woman to tell her prescriber if she becomes pregnant or is breast-feeding. It's unknown if drug appears in breast milk. Use cautiously in breast-feeding women.

---

## amantadine hydrochloride
Symmetrel

*Pregnancy risk category C*

## AVAILABLE FORMS
*Capsules:* 100 mg

*Syrup:* 50 mg/5 ml
*Tablets:* 100 mg

## INDICATIONS & DOSAGES
➤ **To prevent or treat symptoms of influenza type A virus and respiratory tract illnesses**
*Adults up to age 65 with normal renal function:* 200 mg P.O. daily in a single dose or 100 mg P.O. b.i.d.
*Children ages 9 to 12:* 100 mg P.O. b.i.d.
*Children ages 1 to 9 or weighing less than 45 kg (99 lb):* 4.4 to 8.8 mg/kg P.O. as a total daily dose given once daily or divided equally b.i.d. Maximum daily dose is 150 mg.
*Elderly patients:* 100 mg P.O. once daily in patients older than age 65 with normal renal function.

Begin treatment within 24 to 48 hours after symptoms appear and continue for 24 to 48 hours after symptoms disappear (usually 2 to 7 days). Start prophylaxis as soon as possible after exposure and continue for at least 10 days after exposure. May continue prophylactic treatment up to 90 days for repeated or suspected exposures if influenza vaccine is unavailable. If used with influenza vaccine, continue dose for 2 to 3 weeks until antibody response to vaccine has developed.
*Adjust-a-dose:* For patients with creatinine clearance 30 to 50 ml/minute, give 200 mg the first day and 100 mg thereafter; if clearance is 15 to 29 ml/minute, give 200 mg the first day, then 100 mg on alternate days; if clearance is below 15 ml/minute or if patient is on hemodialysis, give 200 mg q 7 days.

## ACTION
Unknown. Possibly inhibits the uncoating of the influenza A virus, preventing release of infection's viral nucleic acid into the host cell.

| Route | Onset | Peak | Duration |
|-------|-------|------|----------|
| P.O. | Unknown | 1-4 hr | Unknown |

## ADVERSE REACTIONS
**CNS:** depression, fatigue, confusion, *dizziness,* hallucinations, anxiety, *irritability,* ataxia, *insomnia,* headache, *light-headedness.*

**CV:** peripheral edema, orthostatic hypotension, *heart failure.*
**EENT:** blurred vision.
**GI:** anorexia, *nausea,* constipation, vomiting, dry mouth.
**Skin:** livedo reticularis.

**INTERACTIONS**
**Drug-drug.** *Anticholinergics:* May increase anticholinergic effects. Use together cautiously; reduce dosage of anticholinergic before starting amantadine.
*CNS stimulants:* May increase CNS stimulation. Use together cautiously.
**Drug-herb.** *Jimsonweed:* May adversely affect CV function. Discourage use together.
**Drug-lifestyle.** *Alcohol use:* May increase CNS effects. Discourage use together.

**EFFECTS ON LAB TEST RESULTS**
None reported.

**CONTRAINDICATIONS & CAUTIONS**
• Contraindicated in patients hypersensitive to drug.
• Use cautiously in elderly patients and in patients with seizure disorders, heart failure, peripheral edema, hepatic disease, mental illness, eczematoid rash, renal impairment, orthostatic hypotension, and CV disease. Monitor renal and liver function tests.

**NURSING CONSIDERATIONS**
• Begin treatment within 24 to 48 hours after symptoms appear and continue for 24 to 48 hours after symptoms disappear (usually 2 to 7 days of therapy).
• Start prophylaxis as soon as possible after first exposure and continue for at least 10 days after exposure. For repeated or suspected exposures, if influenza vaccine is unavailable, may continue prophylaxis for up to 90 days. If used with influenza vaccine, continue dose for 2 to 3 weeks until antibody response to vaccine has developed.
• *Alert:* Elderly patients are more susceptible to adverse neurologic effects. Monitor patient for mental status changes.
• Suicidal ideation and attempts have been reported in patients both with and without prior psychiatric problems.

• Drug can worsen mental problems in patients with a history of psychiatric disorders or substance abuse.
• *Alert:* Don't confuse amantadine with rimantadine.

**PATIENT TEACHING**
• Tell patient to take drug exactly as prescribed. Taking more than prescribed can result in serious adverse reactions or death.
• If insomnia occurs, tell patient to take drug several hours before bedtime.
• If dizziness upon standing up occurs, instruct patient not to stand or change positions too quickly.
• Instruct patient to notify prescriber of adverse reactions, especially dizziness, depression, anxiety, nausea, and urine retention.
• Caution patient to avoid activities that require mental alertness until effects of drug are known.
• Advise patient to avoid alcohol while taking drug.

# amprenavir
Agenerase

*Pregnancy risk category C*

**AVAILABLE FORMS**
*Capsules:* 50 mg, 150 mg
*Oral solution:* 15 mg/ml

**INDICATIONS & DOSAGES**
➤ **HIV-1 infection (with other antiretrovirals)**
*Adults and children ages 13 to 16, weighing 50 kg (110 lb) or more:* 1,200 mg (eight 150-mg capsules) P.O. b.i.d. with other antiretrovirals.
*Children ages 4 to 12, or ages 13 to 16 and weighing less than 50 kg (110 lb):*
For capsules, give 20 mg/kg P.O. b.i.d. or 15 mg/kg P.O. t.i.d., to maximum daily dose of 2,400 mg with other antiretrovirals.
For oral solution, give 22.5 mg/kg (1.5 ml/kg) P.O. b.i.d. or 17 mg/kg (1.1 ml/kg) P.O. t.i.d., to maximum daily dose of 2,800 mg with other antiretrovirals.

*Adjust-a-dose:* For patients with hepatic impairment and a Child-Pugh score from 5 to 8, reduce dose for capsules to 450 mg P.O. b.i.d. For patients with a Child-Pugh score from 9 to 12, reduce dose for capsules to 300 mg P.O. b.i.d.

## ACTION
Inhibits HIV-1 protease by binding to the active site of HIV-1 protease, which causes immature noninfectious viral particles to form.

| Route | Onset | Peak | Duration |
|-------|-------|------|----------|
| P.O. | Unknown | 1-2 hr | Unknown |

## ADVERSE REACTIONS
**CNS:** *oral and perioral paresthesia,* depression or mood disorders.
**GI:** *nausea, vomiting, diarrhea or loose stools,* taste disorders.
**Metabolic:** *hyperglycemia, hypertriglyceridemia,* hypercholesterolemia.
**Skin:** *rash,* **Stevens-Johnson syndrome.**

## INTERACTIONS
**Drug-drug.** *Antacids:* May decrease amprenavir absorption. Separate doses by at least 1 hour.
*Antiarrhythmics such as amiodarone, lidocaine (systemic), quinidine; anticoagulants such as warfarin; tricyclic antidepressants:* May alter levels of these drugs. Monitor patient closely.
*Dihydroergotamine, midazolam, rifampin, triazolam:* May cause serious and life-threatening interactions. Avoid using together.
*Efavirenz:* May decrease amprenavir exposure. May need to increase dose.
*Ethinyl estradiol and norethindrone:* May cause loss of virologic response and possible resistance to amprenavir. Advise the use of nonhormonal contraception.
*HMG-CoA reductase inhibitors, such as atorvastatin, lovastatin, simvastatin:* May increase levels of these drugs; may increase risk of myopathy, including rhabdomyolysis. Avoid using together.
*Indinavir, nelfinavir, ritonavir:* May increase amprenavir level. Monitor patient closely for adverse reactions.
*Ketoconazole:* May increase levels of both drugs. Monitor patient closely for adverse reactions.

*Macrolides:* May increase amprenavir level. Don't adjust dosage.
*Methadone:* May decrease amprenavir level. Consider alternative antiretroviral or pain therapy. May need to increase methadone dosage if used together.
*Psychotherapeutic agents:* May increase CNS effects. Monitor patient closely.
*Rifabutin:* May decrease amprenavir exposure. May increase rifabutin level by 200%. May need to decrease rifabutin dose to 150 mg daily or 300 mg two to three times a week.
*Saquinavir:* May decrease amprenavir exposure. Monitor patient closely.
*Sildenafil:* May increase sildenafil level, which may increase sildenafil-associated effects, including hypotension, visual changes, and priapism. Don't exceed 25 mg of sildenafil in 48 hours.
**Drug-herb.** *St. John's wort:* May decrease amprenavir level. Discourage use together.
**Drug-food.** *Grapefruit juice:* May affect amprenavir level. Monitor patient closely.
*High-fat meals:* May decrease drug absorption. Advise patient to avoid taking drug with a high-fat meal.

## EFFECTS ON LAB TEST RESULTS
● May increase glucose, triglyceride, and cholesterol levels.

## CONTRAINDICATIONS & CAUTIONS
● Contraindicated in patients hypersensitive to drug or its components. Contraindicated in infants, children younger than age 4, pregnant women, patients with liver or kidney failure, and patients treated with disulfiram (Antabuse) or metronidazole (Flagyl).
● Use cautiously in patients with moderate or severe hepatic impairment, diabetes mellitus, a known sulfonamide allergy, or hemophilia A or B.
● Use cautiously in pregnant women because no adequate studies exist regarding the effects of amprenavir when given during pregnancy. Use during pregnancy only if the potential benefits outweigh the risks. Register pregnant woman taking amprenavir with the Antiretroviral Pregnancy Registry by calling 1-800-258-4263.

## NURSING CONSIDERATIONS

● *Alert:* Drug can cause severe or life-threatening rash, including Stevens-Johnson syndrome. Stop therapy if patient develops a severe or life-threatening rash or a moderate rash accompanied by systemic signs and symptoms.

● *Alert:* Because amprenavir may interact with many drugs, obtain patient's complete drug history. Ask patient to show you the drugs he's taking.

● Patient shouldn't take drug with high-fat foods because they may decrease absorption of amprenavir.

● Amprenavir oral solution should only be used when the capsules and other protease inhibitor formulations are not therapeutic options.

● Monitor patient for adverse reactions. A patient taking a protease inhibitor may experience a redistribution of body fat, including central obesity, dorsocervical fat enlargement (buffalo hump), peripheral wasting, breast enlargement, and cushingoid appearance. The mechanism and long-term consequences of these effects are unknown.

● Drug provides high daily doses of vitamin E, which may worsen coagulopathy caused by vitamin K deficiency.

● Protease inhibitors have caused spontaneous bleeding in some patients with hemophilia A or B. In some patients, additional factor VIII was needed. In many of the reported cases, treatment with protease inhibitors was continued or restarted.

● Advise patient receiving sildenafil of increased adverse reactions. Don't exceed 25 mg of sildenafil in a 48-hour period.

● Amprenavir capsules aren't interchangeable with amprenavir oral solution on a milligram-per-milligram basis.

● *Alert:* Don't confuse amprenavir with abacavir.

## PATIENT TEACHING

● Advise patient that drug doesn't cure HIV infection; patient may continue to develop opportunistic infections and other complications from the disease. Also, tell patient that drug doesn't reduce risk of HIV transmission through sexual contact.

● Tell patient that although drug can be taken without regard to food, he shouldn't take it with a high-fat meal because of decreased drug absorption.

● Tell patient to report adverse reactions, especially rash.

● Advise patient to take drug daily, as prescribed, with other antiretrovirals. Dosage must not be altered or stopped without prescriber's approval.

● Inform patient to take an antacid 1 hour before or after amprenavir to prevent a decrease in amprenavir absorption.

● If a dose is missed by more than 4 hours, advise patient to wait and take the next dose at the regularly scheduled time. If a dose is missed by less than 4 hours, advise him to take the dose as soon as possible and then take the next dose at the regularly scheduled time. If a dose is skipped, patient shouldn't double the dose.

● Advise patient using hormonal contraception to use another contraceptive method during drug therapy.

● Advise patient to notify prescriber if pregnancy occurs during therapy.

● Advise patient not to take supplemental vitamin E because drug contains a significant amount of the vitamin.

✳ *NEW DRUG*

## atazanavir sulfate
Reyataz◆

*Pregnancy risk category B*

### AVAILABLE FORMS
*Capsules:* 100 mg, 150 mg, 200 mg

### INDICATIONS & DOSAGES
➤ **HIV-1 infection, with other antiretrovirals**
*Adults:* 400 mg P.O. once daily with food. When drug is given with efavirenz, patient should receive atazanavir 300 mg, ritonavir 100 mg, and efavirenz 600 mg as a single daily dose with food.
*Adjust-a-dose:* In patients with Child-Pugh class B hepatic insufficiency, reduce dosage to 300 mg P.O. once daily.

## ACTION
Inhibits viral maturation in HIV-1–infected cells, resulting in the formation of immature noninfectious viral particles.

| Route | Onset | Peak | Duration |
|-------|-------|------|----------|
| P.O. | Unknown | 2½ hr | Unknown |

## ADVERSE REACTIONS
**CNS:** depression, dizziness, fatigue, fever, *headache,* insomnia, peripheral neurologic symptoms.
**EENT:** scleral yellowing.
**GI:** *abdominal pain, diarrhea, nausea,* vomiting.
**Hepatic:** jaundice.
**Metabolic:** lipodystrophy.
**Musculoskeletal:** arthralgia, back pain.
**Respiratory:** increased cough.
**Skin:** *rash.*
**Other:** pain.

## INTERACTIONS
**Drug-drug.** *Amiodarone, lidocaine (systemic), quinidine, tricyclic antidepressants:* May increase levels of these drugs. Monitor drug levels.
*Antacids, buffered drugs, didanosine:* May decrease atazanavir level. Give atazanavir 2 hours before or 1 hour after these drugs.
*Atorvastatin:* May increase atorvastatin levels increasing the risk of myopathy and rhabdomyolysis. Use cautiously together.
*Clarithromycin:* May increase clarithromycin level and prolong QTc interval. Decrease clarithromycin by 50% when using together.
*Clarithromycin:* May reduce clarithromycin metabolite. Avoid using together, except to treat *Mycobacterium avium* complex infection.
*Cyclosporine, sirolimus, tacrolimus:* May increase immunosuppressant level. Monitor immunosuppressant level.
*Diltiazem, felodipine, nicardipine, nifedipine, verapamil:* May increase calcium channel blocker level. Use together cautiously, with close ECG monitoring. Adjust calcium channel blocker dosage as needed. Decrease diltiazem dose by 50%.
*Efavirenz:* May alter atazanavir level. Reduce atazanavir dosage.
*Ergot derivatives, pimozide:* May cause serious or life-threatening reactions. Avoid using together.

*Ethinyl estradiol and norethindrone:* May increase ethinyl estradiol and norethindrone levels. Use cautiously together, and give the lowest effective dose of hormonal contraceptive.
*H₂-receptor antagonists:* May decrease atazanavir level, reducing therapeutic effect. Separate doses by at least 12 hours.
*Indinavir:* May increase risk of indirect (unconjugated) hyperbilirubinemia. Avoid using together.
*Irinotecan:* May interfere with irinotecan metabolism and increase irinotecan toxicity. Avoid using together.
*Lovastatin, simvastatin:* May cause myopathy and rhabdomyolysis. Avoid using together.
*Midazolam, triazolam:* May cause prolonged or increased sedation or respiratory depression. Avoid using together.
*Proton-pump inhibitors, rifampin:* May significantly reduce atazanavir level. Avoid using together.
*Rifabutin:* May increase rifabutin level. Reduce rifabutin dose up to 75%.
*Ritonavir:* May increase atazanavir level. Decrease atazanavir dose to 300 mg.
*Saquinavir (soft gelatin capsules):* May increase saquinavir level. Avoid using together.
*Sildenafil:* May increase sildenafil level, causing hypotension, visual changes, and priapism. Use together cautiously, and reduce dose to 25 mg q 48 hours; watch for adverse events.
*Warfarin:* May increase warfarin level, which may cause life-threatening bleeding. Monitor INR.
**Drug-herb.** *St. John's wort:* May decrease atazanavir level, reducing therapeutic effect and causing drug resistance. Discourage use together.
**Drug-food.** *Any food:* May increase bioavailability of drug. Tell patient to take drug with food.

## EFFECTS ON LAB TEST RESULTS
● May increase AST, ALT, bilirubin, amylase, and lipase levels.
● May decrease hemoglobin and neutrophil count.

## CONTRAINDICATIONS & CAUTIONS
● Contraindicated in patients hypersensitive to atazanavir or its ingredients.

• Contraindicated in patients taking drugs cleared mainly by CYP 3A4 or drugs that can cause serious or life-threatening reactions at high levels (dihydroergotamine, ergonovine, ergotamine, midazolam, methylergonovine, pimozide, triazolam).
• Use cautiously in patients with conduction system disease or hepatic impairment.
• Use cautiously in elderly patients because of the increased likelihood of other disease, additional drug therapy, and decreased hepatic, renal, or cardiac function.

**NURSING CONSIDERATIONS**
• *Alert:* Atazanavir may prolong the PR interval.
• Monitor the patient for hyperglycemia and new-onset diabetes or worsened diabetes. Insulin and oral hypoglycemic dosages may need adjustment.
• Monitor a patient with hepatitis B or C for elevated liver enzymes or hepatic decompensation.
• Watch for lactic acidosis syndrome (sometimes fatal) or symptomatic hyperlactatemia, especially in women and obese patients.
• If the patient has hemophilia, watch for bleeding.
• Most patients have an asymptomatic increase in indirect bilirubin, possibly with yellowed skin or sclerae. This hyperbilirubinemia will resolve when atazanavir therapy stops.
• Although cross resistance occurs among protease inhibitors, resistance to atazanavir doesn't preclude use of other protease inhibitors.
• Give drug to a pregnant woman only if the potential benefit justifies the potential risk to the fetus.
• To monitor maternal-fetal outcomes among pregnant women who receive atazanavir, an Antiretroviral Pregnancy Registry has been formed. Patients can be registered by calling 1-800-258-4263.

**PATIENT TEACHING**
• Urge patient to take atazanavir with food every day and to take other antiretrovirals as prescribed.
• Explain that atazanavir doesn't cure HIV infection and that the patient may develop opportunistic infections and other complications of HIV disease.

• Caution the patient that atazanavir doesn't reduce the risk of transmitting the HIV virus to others.
• Tell patient drug may cause altered or increased body fat, central obesity, buffalo hump, peripheral wasting, facial wasting, breast enlargement, and a cushingoid appearance.
• Tell patient to report yellowed skin or sclerae, dizziness, or light-headedness.
• Caution patient not to take other prescription, OTC, or herbal remedies without first consulting his prescriber.

## cidofovir
Vistide

*Pregnancy risk category C*

**AVAILABLE FORMS**
*Injection:* 75 mg/ml in 5-ml vial

**INDICATIONS & DOSAGES**
➤ **CMV retinitis in patients with AIDS**
*Adults:* Initially, 5 mg/kg I.V. infused over 1 hour once weekly for 2 consecutive weeks; then maintenance dose of 5 mg/kg I.V. infused over 1 hour once q 2 weeks. Give probenecid and prehydration with normal saline solution I.V. concomitantly; may reduce potential for nephrotoxicity.
*Adjust-a-dose:* For patients with creatinine level 0.3 to 0.4 mg/dl above baseline, reduce dosage to 3 mg/kg at same rate and frequency. If creatinine level reaches 0.5 mg/dl or more above baseline, stop drug.

**I.V. ADMINISTRATION**
• Because of the mutagenic properties of cidofovir, prepare drug in a class II laminar flow biological safety cabinet. Personnel preparing drug should wear surgical gloves and a closed-front surgical gown with knit cuffs.
• Using a syringe, withdraw prescribed dose and add it to an I.V. bag containing 100 ml of normal saline solution. Discard any partially used vials. Infuse over 1 hour using an infusion pump.
• Because of the potential for increased nephrotoxicity, don't exceed recommended dosages or frequency or rate of infusion.

---

Reactions may be *common*, uncommon, *life-threatening*, or COMMON AND LIFE-THREATENING.

• If drug contacts the skin, wash and flush thoroughly with water. Place excess drug and all other materials used in the preparation and administration in a leak-proof, puncture-proof container.
• Give within 24 hours of preparation. Admixture may be refrigerated at 36° to 46° F (2° to 8° C) for up to 24 hours. Allow cidofovir to reach room temperature before use.
• Don't add other drugs or supplements to admixture. Compatibility with Ringer's, lactated Ringer's, or bacteriostatic solutions hasn't been evaluated.

## ACTION
A nucleotide analogue that suppresses CMV replication by selective inhibition of viral DNA synthesis.

| Route | Onset | Peak | Duration |
|-------|-------|------|----------|
| I.V. | Unknown | Unknown | Unknown |

## ADVERSE REACTIONS
**CNS:** *asthenia, headache,* amnesia, anxiety, confusion, *fever, seizures,* depression, dizziness, abnormal gait, hallucinations, insomnia, neuropathy, paresthesia, somnolence, malaise.
**CV:** hypotension, orthostatic hypotension, pallor, syncope, tachycardia, vasodilation.
**EENT:** amblyopia, conjunctivitis, pharyngitis, eye disorders, *ocular hypotony,* iritis, retinal detachment, uveitis, abnormal vision, rhinitis, sinusitis.
**GI:** *nausea, vomiting, diarrhea, anorexia, abdominal pain,* dry mouth, colitis, constipation, tongue discoloration, dyspepsia, dysphagia, flatulence, gastritis, melena, oral candidiasis, rectal disorders, stomatitis, aphthous stomatitis, mouth ulcerations, taste perversion.
**GU:** *nephrotoxicity, proteinuria,* glycosuria, hematuria, urinary incontinence, UTI.
**Hematologic:** *neutropenia, anemia, thrombocytopenia.*
**Hepatic:** hepatomegaly.
**Metabolic:** weight loss, fluid imbalance, hyperglycemia, hyperlipemia, hypocalcemia, hypokalemia.
**Musculoskeletal:** arthralgia; myasthenia; myalgia; pain in back, chest, or neck.

**Respiratory:** asthma, bronchitis, coughing, *dyspnea,* hiccups, increased sputum, lung disorders, pneumonia.
**Skin:** *rash, alopecia,* acne, skin discoloration, dry skin, pruritus, sweating, urticaria.
**Other:** *infections, chills,* allergic reactions, herpes simplex, facial edema, *sarcoma, sepsis.*

## INTERACTIONS
**Drug-drug.** *Nephrotoxic drugs (such as aminoglycosides, amphotericin B, foscarnet, I.V. pentamidine):* May increase nephrotoxicity. Avoid using together.

## EFFECTS ON LAB TEST RESULTS
• May increase BUN, creatinine, alkaline phosphatase, ALT, AST, and LDH levels. May decrease creatinine clearance and bicarbonate level.
• May decrease hemoglobin and neutrophil and platelet counts.

## CONTRAINDICATIONS & CAUTIONS
• Contraindicated in patients hypersensitive to drug or to probenecid or other sulfa-containing drugs.
• Contraindicated in patients receiving drugs with nephrotoxic potential (stop such drugs at least 7 days before starting cidofovir therapy) and in those with creatinine level exceeding 1.5 mg/dl, creatinine clearance of 55 ml/minute or less, or urine protein level of 100 mg/dl or more (equivalent to 2+ proteinuria or more).
• Safety and effectiveness in children haven't been established.
• It's unknown if cidofovir appears in breast milk.
• Use cautiously in patients with renal impairment. Monitor renal function tests and patient's fluid balance.

## NURSING CONSIDERATIONS
• Don't give as a direct intraocular injection because this may decrease intraocular pressure and impair vision.
• Cidofovir is indicated only for the treatment of CMV retinitis in patients with AIDS. Safety and efficacy of drug haven't been established for treating other CMV infections, congenital or neonatal CMV disease, or CMV disease in patients not infected with HIV.

---

*Rapid onset* †Canada ‡Australia ◇OTC ♦ Off-label use ✐Photoguide *Liquid contains alcohol.

- Give 1 L normal saline solution I.V. usually over 1- to 2-hour period, immediately before cidofovir infusion.
- Give probenecid with cidofovir.
- Monitor creatinine and urine protein levels and WBC counts with differential before each dose.
- Drug may cause Fanconi's syndrome and decreased bicarbonate level with renal tubular damage. Monitor patient closely.
- Drug may cause granulocytopenia.
- Stop zidovudine therapy or reduce dosage by 50% on the days when cidofovir is given; probenecid reduces metabolic clearance of zidovudine.

**PATIENT TEACHING**
- Inform patient that drug doesn't cure CMV retinitis and that regular ophthalmologic follow-up examinations are needed.
- Alert patient taking zidovudine that he'll need to obtain dosage guidelines on days cidofovir is given.
- Tell patient that close monitoring of kidney function will be needed and that abnormalities may require a change in cidofovir therapy.
- Stress importance of completing a full course of probenecid with each cidofovir dose. Tell patient to take probenecid after a meal to decrease nausea.
- Patients with AIDS should use effective contraception, especially during and for 1 month after treatment with cidofovir.
- Advise man to practice barrier contraception during and for 3 months after treatment with drug.

---

**delavirdine mesylate**
Rescriptor

*Pregnancy risk category C*

**AVAILABLE FORMS**
*Tablets:* 100 mg, 200 mg

**INDICATIONS & DOSAGES**
➤ **HIV-1 infection when therapy is warranted**
*Adults:* 400 mg P.O. t.i.d. with other appropriate antiretrovirals.

**ACTION**
A nonnucleoside reverse-transcriptase inhibitor of HIV-1. Drug binds directly to reverse transcriptase and blocks RNA- and DNA-dependent DNA polymerase activities.

| Route | Onset | Peak | Duration |
|-------|-------|------|----------|
| P.O. | Unknown | 1 hr | Unknown |

**ADVERSE REACTIONS**
**CNS:** pain, fever, depression, *fatigue, headache,* insomnia, *asthenia.*
**EENT:** pharyngitis, sinusitis.
**GI:** diarrhea, *nausea,* vomiting, abdominal cramps, distention, or pain.
**GU:** epididymitis, hematuria, hemospermia, impotence, renal calculi, renal pain, metrorrhagia, nocturia, polyuria, proteinuria, vaginal candidiasis.
**Respiratory:** bronchitis, cough, upper respiratory tract infection.
**Skin:** *rash.*
**Other:** flu syndrome.

**INTERACTIONS**
**Drug-drug.** *Amphetamines, nonsedating antihistamines, benzodiazepines, calcium channel blockers, clarithromycin, dapsone, ergot alkaloid preparations, indinavir, quinidine, rifabutin, sedative hypnotics, warfarin:* May increase or prolong therapeutic and adverse effects of these drugs. Avoid using together, or, if use together is unavoidable, reduce doses of indinavir and clarithromycin.
*Antacids:* May reduce absorption of delavirdine. Separate doses by at least 1 hour.
*Carbamazepine, phenobarbital, phenytoin:* May decrease delavirdine level. Use together cautiously.
*Clarithromycin, fluoxetine, ketoconazole:* May cause a 50% increase in delavirdine bioavailability. Monitor patient and reduce dose of clarithromycin.
*Didanosine:* May decrease absorption of both drugs by 20%. Separate doses by at least 1 hour.
*H₂-receptor antagonists:* May increase gastric pH and reduces absorption of delavirdine. Long-term use together isn't recommended.
*HMG-CoA reductase inhibitors, such as atorvastatin, lovastatin, simvastatin:* May

increase levels of these drugs, which increases risk of myopathy, including rhabdomyolysis. Avoid using together.
*Rifabutin, rifampin:* May decrease delavirdine level. May increase rifabutin level by 100%. Avoid using together.
*Saquinavir:* May increase bioavailability of saquinavir fivefold. Monitor AST and ALT levels frequently when used together.
*Sildenafil:* May increase sildenafil level and may increase sildenafil-linked adverse events, including hypotension, visual changes, and priapism. Don't exceed 25 mg of sildenafil in 48 hours.
**Drug-herb.** *St. John's wort:* May decrease delavirdine level. Discourage use together.

### EFFECTS ON LAB TEST RESULTS
● May increase ALT, AST, gamma glutamyl transpeptidase, lipase, alkaline phosphatase, amylase, CK, and creatinine levels. May decrease glucose level.
● May increase PTT, PT, and eosinophil count. May decrease hemoglobin, hematocrit, and granulocyte, neutrophil, WBC, RBC, and platelet counts.

### CONTRAINDICATIONS & CAUTIONS
● Contraindicated in patients hypersensitive to drug or its components.
● Use cautiously in patients with impaired hepatic function.

### NURSING CONSIDERATIONS
● Because drug's effects in patients with hepatic or renal impairment haven't been studied, monitor renal and liver function test results carefully.
● Drug-induced diffuse, maculopapular, erythematous, pruritic rash occurs most commonly on upper body and arms of patients with lower CD4+ cell counts, usually within first 3 weeks of treatment. Dosage adjustment doesn't seem to affect rash. Treat symptoms with diphenhydramine, hydroxyzine, or topical corticosteroids.
● Drug doesn't reduce risk of transmission of HIV-1.
● Because resistance develops rapidly when used as monotherapy, always use drug with appropriate antiretrovirals.
● Monitor patient's fluid balance and weight.

### PATIENT TEACHING
● Tell patient to stop drug and call prescriber if severe rash or such symptoms as fever, fatigue, headache, nausea, abdominal pain, or cough occur.
● Inform patient that drug doesn't cure HIV-1 infection and that he may continue to acquire illnesses related to HIV-1 infection, including opportunistic infections. Therapy hasn't been shown to reduce the risk or frequency of such illnesses. Drug hasn't been shown to reduce transmission of HIV.
● Advise patient to remain under medical supervision when taking drug because the long-term effects aren't known.
● Tell patient to take drug as prescribed and not to alter doses without prescriber's approval. If a dose is missed, tell patient to take the next dose as soon as possible; he shouldn't double the next dose.
● Inform patient that drug may be dispersed in water before ingestion. Add tablets to at least 5 ounces (148 ml) of water, allow to stand for a few minutes, and stir until a uniform dispersion occurs. Tell patient to drink dispersion promptly, rinse glass, and swallow the rinse to ensure that entire dose is consumed.
● Tell patient that drug may be taken without regard to food.
● Instruct patient with absence of hydrochloric acid in the stomach to take drug with an acidic beverage, such as orange or cranberry juice.
● Instruct patient to take drug and antacids at least 1 hour apart.
● Advise patient to report use of other prescription or nonprescription drugs, including herbal remedies.
● Advise patient receiving sildenafil of an increased risk of sildenafil-associated adverse events, including low blood pressure, visual changes, and painful penile erection, and to promptly report any symptoms to his prescriber. Tell patient not to exceed 25 mg of sildenafil in a 48-hour period.

# didanosine (ddl)
Videx, Videx EC

*Pregnancy risk category B*

## AVAILABLE FORMS
*Delayed-release capsules:* 125 mg,
200 mg, 250 mg, 400 mg
*Powder for oral solution (buffered):*
100 mg/packet, 167 mg/packet, 250 mg/
packet
*Powder for oral solution (pediatric):*
4-ounce, 8-ounce glass bottles containing
2 g and 4 g of Videx, respectively
*Tablets (buffered, chewable):* 25 mg,
50 mg, 100 mg, 150 mg, 200 mg

## INDICATIONS & DOSAGES
➤ **HIV infection when antiretroviral
therapy is warranted**
*Adults weighing 60 kg (132 lb) or more:*
200 mg tablets P.O. q 12 hours or 400 mg
P.O. once daily; or 250 mg buffered powder P.O. q 12 hours; or 400 mg capsule
P.O. daily.
*Adults weighing less than 60 kg:* 125 mg
tablets P.O. q 12 hours or 250 mg P.O. once
daily; or 167 mg buffered powder P.O. q
12 hours; or 250 mg capsule P.O. daily.
*Children:* 120 mg/m² P.O. q 12 hours;
Videx EC has not been studied in children.
*Adjust-a-dose:* Dialysis patients should
receive 25% of usual dose once daily
(Videx). If patient weighs 60 kg or more,
give 125 mg (Videx EC) once daily. Don't
use in patients who weigh less than 60 kg.
If creatinine clearance is less than 10 ml/
minute, don't give a supplemental dose after hemodialysis for either drug.

In adults who weigh 60 kg or more
with creatinine clearance of 30 to 59 ml/
minute, give 100-mg tablet b.i.d., 200-mg
tablet or 200-mg capsule once daily, or
100-mg buffered powder b.i.d.; for clearance of 10 to 29 ml/minute, give 150-mg
tablet, 125-mg capsule, or 167-mg buffered powder once daily; for clearance less
than 10 ml/minute, give 100-mg tablet,
125-mg capsule, or 100-mg buffered powder once daily.

In adults who weigh less than 60 kg
and have a clearance of 30 to 59 ml/
minute, give 75-mg tablet b.i.d., 150-mg
tablet or 125-mg capsule once daily, or
100-mg buffered powder b.i.d.; for clearance of 10 to 29 ml/minute, give 100-mg
tablet, 125-mg capsule, or 100-mg buffered powder once daily. For clearance less
than 10 ml/minute, give 75-mg tablet or
100-mg buffered powder once daily; capsule not indicated for these patients.

## ACTION
Inhibits the enzyme HIV-RNA–dependent
DNA polymerase (reverse transcriptase)
and terminates DNA chain growth.

| Route | Onset | Peak | Duration |
|-------|-------|------|----------|
| P.O. | Unknown | 30-60 min | Unknown |

## ADVERSE REACTIONS
**CNS:** *headache, seizures,* confusion, anx-
iety, pain, *fever,* nervousness, abnormal
thinking, twitching, depression, *peripheral
neuropathy, dizziness,* asthenia, insomnia.
**CV:** hypertension, edema, **heart failure.**
**EENT:** retinal changes, optic neuritis.
**GI:** *diarrhea, nausea, vomiting, abdomi-
nal pain, pancreatitis,* anorexia, dry
mouth.
**Hematologic:** *leukopenia,* granulocytosis,
*thrombocytopenia,* anemia.
**Hepatic:** *hepatic failure.*
**Metabolic:** hyperuricemia.
**Musculoskeletal:** myopathy.
**Respiratory:** dyspnea, pneumonia.
**Skin:** rash, pruritus, alopecia.
**Other:** infection, *sarcoma,* allergic reac-
tions, *chills.*

## INTERACTIONS
**Drug-drug.** *Amprenavir, delavirdine, indinavir, nelfinavir, ritonavir, saquinavir:*
May alter pharmacokinetics of didanosine
or these drugs. Separate dosage times.
*Antacids containing magnesium or alu-
minum hydroxides:* May enhance adverse
effects of the antacid component (including diarrhea or constipation) when given
with didanosine tablets or pediatric suspension. Avoid using together.
*Co-trimoxazole, pentamidine, other drugs
linked to pancreatitis:* May increase risk
of pancreatic toxicity. Use together cautiously; consider temporarily stopping didanosine during administration of these
drugs.
*Dapsone, drugs that require gastric acid
for adequate absorption, ketoconazole:*

May decrease absorption from buffering action. Give these drugs 2 hours before didanosine.

*Fluoroquinolones, tetracyclines:* May decrease absorption from buffering products in didanosine tablets or antacids in pediatric suspension. Separate dosage times by at least 2 hours.

*Itraconazole:* May decrease itraconazole level. Avoid using together.

**Drug-herb.** *St. John's wort:* May decrease drug level, decreasing therapeutic effects. Discourage use together.

**Drug-food.** *Any food:* May decrease rate of absorption. Advise patient to take drug on an empty stomach at least 30 minutes before a meal.

## EFFECTS ON LAB TEST RESULTS
● May increase uric acid, AST, ALT, alkaline phosphatase, and bilirubin levels.
● May decrease hemoglobin and WBC, granulocyte, and platelet counts.

## CONTRAINDICATIONS & CAUTIONS
● Contraindicated in patients hypersensitive to drug or its components.
● Use cautiously in patients with history of pancreatitis; deaths have occurred. Also use cautiously in patients with peripheral neuropathy, renal or hepatic impairment, or hyperuricemia. Monitor liver and renal function tests.

## NURSING CONSIDERATIONS
● Give didanosine on an empty stomach, at least 30 minutes or 2 hours after eating, regardless of dosage form used; giving drug with meals can decrease absorption by 50%.
● To give single-dose packets containing buffered powder for oral solution, pour contents into 4 ounces (120 ml) of water. Don't use fruit juice or other beverages that may be acidic. Stir for 2 or 3 minutes until the powder dissolves completely. Give immediately.
● The powder for oral solution may cause diarrhea. The manufacturer suggests switching to the tablet formulation if diarrhea is a problem.
● *Alert:* The pediatric powder for oral solution must be prepared by a pharmacist before dispensing. It must be constituted with purified USP water and then diluted

with an antacid (either Mylanta Double Strength Liquid, Extra Strength Maalox Plus Suspension, or Maalox TC Suspension) to a final concentration of 10 mg/ml. The admixture is stable for 30 days at 36° to 46° F (2° to 8° C). Shake the solution well before measuring dose.
● *Alert:* Don't confuse drug with other antivirals that use abbreviations for identification.

## PATIENT TEACHING
● Instruct patient to take drug on an empty stomach, 30 minutes before or 2 hours after eating.
● Because the tablets contain buffers that raise stomach pH to levels that prevent degradation of the active drug, instruct patient to chew tablets thoroughly before swallowing and drink at least 1 ounce (30 ml) of water with each dose. Teach patient how to prepare crushed tablets or buffered powder form for ingestion, if appropriate.
● To reduce the risk of GI adverse effects from excess antacid, advise patient to take no more than 4 didanosine buffered tablets at each dose.
● Inform patient on a sodium-restricted diet that each 2-tablet dose of didanosine contains 529 mg of sodium; each single packet of buffered powder for oral solution contains 1.38 g of sodium.
● Tell patient to report symptoms of inflammation of the pancreas, such as abdominal pain, nausea, vomiting, diarrhea, or symptoms of peripheral neuropathy.

---

# efavirenz
Sustiva

*Pregnancy risk category C*

---

## AVAILABLE FORMS
*Capsules:* 50 mg, 100 mg, 200 mg
*Tablets:* 600 mg

## INDICATIONS & DOSAGES
➤ **HIV-1 infection, with a protease inhibitor or nucleoside analogue reverse transcriptase inhibitors**
*Adults and children age 3 and older, weighing 40 kg (88 lb) or more:* 600 mg (three 200-mg capsules or one 600-mg

tablet) P.O. once daily on an empty stomach, preferably h.s.

*Children age 3 and older, weighing 33 to less than 40 kg (72 to under 88 lb):*
400 mg P.O. once daily on an empty stomach, preferably h.s.

*Children age 3 and older, weighing 25 to less than 33 kg (55 to under 72 lb):*
350 mg P.O. once daily on an empty stomach, preferably h.s.

*Children age 3 and older, weighing 20 to less than 25 kg (44 to under 55 lb):*
300 mg P.O. once daily on an empty stomach, preferably h.s.

*Children age 3 and older, weighing 15 to less than 20 kg (33 to under 44 lb):*
250 mg P.O. once daily on an empty stomach, preferably h.s.

*Children age 3 and older, weighing 10 to less than 15 kg (22 to under 33 lb):*
200 mg P.O. once daily on an empty stomach, preferably h.s.

## ACTION

A nonnucleoside, reverse transcriptase inhibitor that inhibits the transcription of HIV-1 RNA to DNA, a critical step in the viral replication process.

| Route | Onset | Peak | Duration |
|-------|-------|------|----------|
| P.O. | Unknown | 3-5 hr | Unknown |

## ADVERSE REACTIONS

**CNS:** abnormal dreams or thinking, agitation, amnesia, confusion, depersonalization, depression, *dizziness,* euphoria, fever, fatigue, hallucinations, headache, hypoesthesia, impaired concentration, insomnia, somnolence, nervousness.
**GI:** abdominal pain, anorexia, *diarrhea,* dyspepsia, flatulence, *nausea,* vomiting.
**GU:** hematuria, kidney stones.
**Skin:** increased sweating, ***erythema multiforme, Stevens-Johnson syndrome, toxic epidermal necrolysis,*** rash, pruritus.

## INTERACTIONS

**Drug-drug.** *Amprenavir, clarithromycin, indinavir, lopinavir:* May decrease levels of these drugs. Consider alternative therapy or dosage adjustment.
*Drugs that induce the cytochrome P-450 enzyme system (such as phenobarbital, rifampin):* May increase clearance of efavirenz, resulting in lower drug level. Avoid using together.
*Ergot derivatives, midazolam, triazolam:* May inhibit metabolism of these drugs and cause serious or life-threatening adverse events (such as arrhythmias, prolonged sedation, or respiratory depression). Avoid using together.
*Estrogens, ritonavir:* May increase drug levels. Monitor patient.
*Hormonal contraceptives:* May increase ethinyl estradiol level; no data on progesterone component. Advise use of a reliable method of barrier contraception in addition to use of hormonal contraceptives.
*Psychoactive drugs:* May cause additive CNS effects. Avoid using together.
*Rifabutin:* May decrease rifabutin concentrations. Increase rifabutin dosage to 450 to 600 mg once daily or 600 mg two to three times a week.
*Ritonavir:* May increase levels of both drugs. Monitor patient and liver function closely.
*Saquinavir:* May decrease saquinavir level. Don't use with saquinavir as sole protease inhibitor. Use of saquinavir also decreases efavirenz exposure to the body by 12% to 13%.
*Warfarin:* May increase or decrease level and effects of warfarin. Monitor INR.
**Drug-herb.** *St. John's wort:* May decrease efavirenz level. Discourage use together.
**Drug-food.** *High-fat meals:* May increase absorption of drug. Instruct patient to maintain a proper low-fat diet.
**Drug-lifestyle.** *Alcohol use:* May enhance CNS effects. Discourage use together.

## EFFECTS ON LAB TEST RESULTS

● May increase ALT, AST, and cholesterol levels.
● May cause false-positive urine cannabinoid test results.

## CONTRAINDICATIONS & CAUTIONS

● Contraindicated in patients hypersensitive to drug or its components.
● Use cautiously in patients with hepatic impairment and in those receiving hepatotoxic drugs. Monitor liver function test results in patients with history of hepatitis B or C and in those taking ritonavir.

---

## NURSING CONSIDERATIONS
- Monitor cholesterol level.
- **Alert:** Drug shouldn't be used as monotherapy or added on as a single drug to a failing regimen caused by virus resistance.
- Using drug with ritonavir may increase adverse effects (such as dizziness, nausea, paresthesia) and laboratory abnormalities (elevated liver enzyme levels).
- Give drug at bedtime to decrease CNS adverse effects.
- Pregnancy must be ruled out before starting therapy in women of childbearing age.
- Children may be more prone to adverse reactions, especially diarrhea, nausea, vomiting, and rash.

## PATIENT TEACHING
- Instruct patient to take drug with water, preferably at bedtime and on an empty stomach.
- Inform patient about need for scheduled blood tests to monitor liver function and cholesterol level.
- Tell patient to use a reliable method of barrier contraception in addition to hormonal contraceptives and to notify prescriber immediately if pregnancy is suspected.
- Inform patient that drug doesn't cure HIV infection, that opportunistic infections and other complications of HIV infection may continue to occur, and that transmission of HIV to others through sexual contact or blood contamination is still possible.
- Instruct patient to take drug at the same time daily and always with other antiretrovirals.
- Tell patient to take drug exactly as prescribed and not to stop it without medical approval. Also instruct patient to report adverse reactions.
- Inform patient that rash is the most common adverse effect. Tell patient to report rash immediately because it may be serious (in rare cases).
- Advise patient to report use of other drugs.
- Advise patient that dizziness, difficulty sleeping or concentrating, drowsiness, or unusual dreams may occur during the first few days of therapy. Reassure him that

these symptoms typically resolve after 2 to 4 weeks and may be less problematic if drug is taken at bedtime.
- Tell patient to avoid alcohol, driving, or operating machinery until the drug's effects are known.

✷ **NEW DRUG**

## emtricitabine
Emtriva

*Pregnancy risk category B*

## AVAILABLE FORMS
*Capsules:* 200 mg

## INDICATIONS & DOSAGES
➤ **HIV-1 infection, with other antiretrovirals—**
*Adults:* 200 mg P.O. once daily.
**Adjust-a-dose:** In patients with creatinine clearance 30 to 49 ml/minute, give 200 mg P.O. q 48 hours; if clearance is 15 to 29 ml/minute, give 200 mg P.O. q 72 hours; if clearance is less than 15 ml/minute or patient is on dialysis, give 200 mg P.O. q 96 hours. If dose is due on dialysis day, give after dialysis session ends.

## ACTION
Inhibits replication of HIV by blocking viral DNA synthesis. Also inhibits reverse transcriptase by acting as an alternative for the enzyme's substrate, deoxycytidine triphosphate.

| Route | Onset | Peak | Duration |
|-------|-------|------|----------|
| P.O. | Unknown | 1-2 hr | Unknown |

## ADVERSE REACTIONS
**CNS:** *abnormal dreams, asthenia,* depressive disorders, *dizziness, headache, insomnia,* neuritis, paresthesia, peripheral neuropathy.
**EENT:** *rhinitis.*
**GI:** *abdominal pain, diarrhea,* dyspepsia, *nausea,* vomiting.
**Musculoskeletal:** arthralgia, myalgia.
**Respiratory:** *increased cough.*
**Skin:** *allergic skin reaction, discoloration, maculopapular rash, pruritus, urticarial and purpuric lesions, vesiculobullous rash.*

## INTERACTIONS
None reported.

## EFFECTS ON LAB TEST RESULTS
• May increase ALT, AST, bilirubin, triglycerides, amylase, lipase, creatine kinase, and serum glucose levels.
• May decrease neutrophil count.

## CONTRAINDICATIONS & CAUTIONS
• Contraindicated in patients hypersensitive to drug or its ingredients.
• Don't use drug for treating chronic hepatitis B virus (HBV); safety and efficacy haven't been established in patients infected with both HBV and HIV.
• Use cautiously in elderly patients because of the increased likelihood of concurrent disease or drug therapy, and decreased hepatic, renal, or cardiac function.
• Use cautiously in patients with impaired renal function.

## NURSING CONSIDERATIONS
• Test all patients for HBV before starting drug.
• Hepatitis B may worsen after emtricitabine therapy stops. Patients with both HIV and HBV need close clinical and laboratory follow-up for several months or longer after stopping drug.
• Like other antiretrovirals, emtricitabine may cause changes or increases in body fat, including central obesity, buffalo hump, peripheral wasting, facial wasting, breast enlargement, and a cushingoid appearance.
*Alert:* Notify prescriber immediately if lactic acidosis or pronounced hepatotoxicity occurs.
• Use drug only if clearly needed in pregnant women.

## PATIENT TEACHING
• Explain that drug doesn't cure HIV infection.
• Remind patient that anti-HIV medicine must be taken for life.
• Caution patient that drug doesn't reduce the risk of transmitting HIV to others.
• Explain possible adverse reactions, including lactic acidosis, hepatotoxicity, and changes or increases in body fat.
• Tell patient to notify prescriber immediately if she is or could be pregnant.

• Inform patient the drug may be taken with or without food.

✴ *NEW DRUG*

# enfuvirtide
Fuzeon

*Pregnancy risk category B*

## AVAILABLE FORMS
*Powder for injection:* 108-mg single-use vials (90 mg/1 ml after reconstitution)

## INDICATIONS & DOSAGES
➤ **To help control HIV-1 infection, with other antiretrovirals, in patients who have continued HIV-1 replication despite antiretroviral therapy**
*Adults:* 90 mg/1 ml S.C. b.i.d., injected into the upper arm, anterior thigh, or abdomen.
*Children ages 6 to 16:* 2 mg/kg S.C. b.i.d.; maximum 90 mg per dose.

## ACTION
Interferes with entry of HIV-1 into cells by inhibiting fusion of HIV-1 to cell membranes.

| Route | Onset | Peak | Duration |
|-------|-------|------|----------|
| S.C. | Unknown | 4-8 hr | Unknown |

## ADVERSE REACTIONS
**CNS:** anxiety, asthenia, depression, *fatigue, insomnia,* peripheral neuropathy.
**EENT:** conjunctivitis, sinusitis, taste disturbance.
**GI:** abdominal pain, constipation, *diarrhea, nausea,* **pancreatitis.**
**Metabolic:** anorexia, weight decrease.
**Musculoskeletal:** myalgia.
**Respiratory:** *bacterial pneumonia,* cough.
**Skin:** *injection site reactions,* pruritus, skin papilloma.
**Other:** herpes simplex, influenza, influenza-like illness, lymphadenopathy.

## INTERACTIONS
None reported.

## EFFECTS ON LAB TEST RESULTS
• May increase triglyceride, amylase, lipase, ALT, AST, CPK, and GGT levels.

---

Reactions may be *common,* uncommon, *life-threatening,* or COMMON AND LIFE-THREATENING.

• May decrease hemoglobin and eosinophil count.

## CONTRAINDICATIONS & CAUTIONS
• Contraindicated in patients hypersensitive to drug and in those not infected with HIV.
• Use in pregnant patients only if clearly needed. Pregnant patients can be registered in the Antiretroviral Pregnancy Registry by phoning 1-800-258-4263.
• Safety and efficacy haven't been established in patients younger than age 6.

## NURSING CONSIDERATIONS
• *Alert:* Drug is available only through a progressive distribution program. Information may be obtained by calling 866-694-6670.
• For S.C. administration, reconstitute vial with 1.1 ml sterile water for injection. Tap vial for 10 seconds and then gently roll to prevent foaming. Let drug stand for up to 45 minutes to ensure reconstitution. Or, gently roll vial between hands until product is completely dissolved. Then draw up correct dose and inject drug.
• If you won't be using drug immediately after reconstitution, refrigerate in original vial and use within 24 hours. Don't inject drug until it's at room temperature.
• Store unreconstituted vials at room temperature.
• Vial is for single use; discard unused portion.
• Rotate injection sites. Don't inject into the same site for two consecutive doses, and don't inject into moles, scar tissue, bruises, or the navel.
• Injection site reactions (pain, discomfort, induration, erythema, pruritus, nodules, cysts, ecchymosis) are common and may require analgesics or rest.
• *Alert:* Monitor patient closely for evidence of bacterial pneumonia. Patients at high risk include those with a low initial CD4 count or high initial viral load, those who use I.V. drugs or smoke, and those with history of lung disease.
• Hypersensitivity may occur with the first dose or later doses. If symptoms occur, stop drug.

## PATIENT TEACHING
• Teach patient how to prepare and give drug and how to safely dispose of used needles and syringes.
• Tell patient to rotate injection sites and to watch for cellulitis or local infection.
• Urge patient to immediately report evidence of pneumonia, such as cough with fever, rapid breathing, or shortness of breath.
• Tell patient to stop taking drug and seek medical attention if evidence of hypersensitivity develops, such as rash, fever, nausea, vomiting, chills, rigors, and hypotension.
• Teach patient that drug doesn't cure HIV infection and that it must be taken with other antiretroviral drugs.
• Tell patient to inform prescriber if she's pregnant, plans to become pregnant, or is breast-feeding while taking this drug. Because HIV could be transmitted to the infant, HIV-infected mothers shouldn't breast-feed.
• Tell patient that drug may impair the ability to drive or operate machinery.

# famciclovir
Famvir

*Pregnancy risk category B*

## AVAILABLE FORMS
*Tablets:* 125 mg, 250 mg, 500 mg

## INDICATIONS & DOSAGES
➤ **Acute herpes zoster infection (shingles)**
*Adults:* 500 mg P.O. q 8 hours for 7 days.
*Adjust-a-dose:* For patients with creatinine clearance 40 to 59 ml/minute, give 500 mg P.O. q 12 hours; if clearance is 20 to 39 ml/minute, give 500 mg P.O. q 24 hours; and if it's below 20 ml/minute, give 250 mg P.O. q 24 hours. For hemodialysis patients, 250 mg P.O. after each hemodialysis session.
➤ **Recurrent genital herpes**
*Adults:* 125 mg P.O. b.i.d. for 5 days. Begin therapy as soon as symptoms occur.
*Adjust-a-dose:* For patients with creatinine clearance 20 to 39 ml/minute, give 125 mg P.O. q 24 hours; if clearance is below 20 ml/minute, give 125 mg P.O. q

48 hours. For hemodialysis patients, give 125 mg P.O. after each hemodialysis session.

➤ **Recurrent mucocutaneous herpes simplex infections in HIV-infected patients**
*Adults:* 500 mg P.O. b.i.d. for 7 days.
*Adjust-a-dose:* For patients with creatinine clearance 20 to 39 ml/minute, give 500 mg P.O. q 24 hours; if clearance is below 20 ml/minute, give 250 mg P.O. q 24 hours. For hemodialysis patients, give 250 mg P.O. after each hemodialysis session.

## ACTION
A guanosine nucleoside that is converted to penciclovir, which enters viral cells and inhibits DNA polymerase and viral DNA synthesis.

| Route | Onset | Peak | Duration |
|-------|-------|------|----------|
| P.O. | Unknown | 1 hr | Unknown |

## ADVERSE REACTIONS
**CNS:** *headache,* fatigue, fever, dizziness, paresthesia, somnolence.
**EENT:** pharyngitis, sinusitis.
**GI:** diarrhea, *nausea,* vomiting, constipation, anorexia, abdominal pain.
**Musculoskeletal:** back pain, arthralgia.
**Skin:** pruritus.
**Other:** zoster-related signs, symptoms, and complications.

## INTERACTIONS
**Drug-drug.** *Probenecid:* May increase level of penciclovir, the active metabolite of famciclovir. Monitor patient for increased adverse reactions.

## EFFECTS ON LAB TEST RESULTS
None reported.

## CONTRAINDICATIONS & CAUTIONS
● Contraindicated in patients hypersensitive to drug.
● Use cautiously in patients with renal or hepatic impairment.

## NURSING CONSIDERATIONS
● Drug may be taken without regard to meals.
● Dosage adjustment may be needed in patients with renal or hepatic impairment.

● Monitor renal and liver function tests in these patients.

## PATIENT TEACHING
● Inform patient that drug doesn't cure genital herpes but can decrease the length and severity of symptoms.
● Teach patient how to avoid spreading infection to others.
● Urge patient to recognize the early signs and symptoms of herpes infection, such as tingling, itching, and pain, and to report them. Treatment is more effective if therapy is started within 48 hours of rash onset.

---

# fomivirsen sodium
Vitravene

*Pregnancy risk category C*

## AVAILABLE FORMS
*Intravitreal injection:* Preservative-free, 0.25-ml, single-use vials containing 6.6 mg/ml

## INDICATIONS & DOSAGES
➤ **Local treatment of CMV retinitis in patients with AIDS who have intolerance or a contraindication to other treatments or who didn't respond to previous treatment**
*Adults:* Induction dose is 330 mcg (0.05 ml) by intravitreal injection every other week for two doses. Subsequent maintenance dose is 330 mcg (0.05 ml) by intravitreal injection once q 4 weeks after induction.

## ACTION
A phosphorothioate oligonucleotide that inhibits human cytomegalovirus (CMV) replication by binding to the target mRNA and subsequently inhibiting virus replication.

| Route | Onset | Peak | Duration |
|-------|-------|------|----------|
| Intravitreal | Unknown | Unknown | Unknown |

## ADVERSE REACTIONS
**CNS:** asthenia, headache, fever, abnormal thinking, depression, dizziness, neuropathy, pain.
**CV:** chest pain.

---

Reactions may be *common,* uncommon, *life-threatening,* or COMMON AND LIFE-THREATENING.

**EENT:** abnormal or blurred vision, anterior chamber inflammation, cataract, conjunctival hemorrhage, decreased visual acuity, desaturation of color vision, eye pain, floaters, increased intraocular pressure, photophobia, retinal detachment, retinal edema, retinal hemorrhage, retinal pigment changes, *uveitis, vitreitis,* application site reaction, conjunctival hyperemia, conjunctivitis, corneal edema, decreased peripheral vision, eye irritation, hypotony, keratic precipitates, optic neuritis, photopsia, retinal vascular disease, visual field defect, vitreous hemorrhage, vitreous opacity, sinusitis.

**GI:** abdominal pain, anorexia, diarrhea, nausea, vomiting, oral candidiasis, *pancreatitis.*

**GU:** catheter infection, *renal failure.*

**Hematologic:** anemia, lymphoma-like reaction, *neutropenia, thrombocytopenia.*

**Metabolic:** dehydration, weight loss.

**Musculoskeletal:** back pain.

**Respiratory:** bronchitis, dyspnea, increased cough, pneumonia.

**Skin:** rash, sweating.

**Other:** allergic reactions, cachexia, flu syndrome, infection, *sepsis,* systemic CMV.

**INTERACTIONS**
None significant.

**EFFECTS ON LAB TEST RESULTS**
• May increase ALT, AST, GGT, and alkaline phosphatase levels.
• May decrease hemoglobin and neutrophil and platelet counts.

**CONTRAINDICATIONS & CAUTIONS**
• Contraindicated in patients hypersensitive to drug or its components and in those who have recently (within 2 to 4 weeks) been treated with either I.V. or intravitreal cidofovir because of an increased risk of exaggerated ocular inflammation.

**NURSING CONSIDERATIONS**
• *Alert:* Drug is for ophthalmic use by intravitreal injection only.
• Drug provides localized therapy limited to the treated eye and doesn't provide treatment for systemic CMV disease. Monitor patient for extraocular CMV disease or disease in the other eye.

• Ocular inflammation (uveitis) is more common during induction dosing.
• Monitor light perception and optic nerve head perfusion postinjection.
• Watch for intraocular pressure. This is usually transient and returns to normal without treatment or with temporary use of topical drugs.

**PATIENT TEACHING**
• Inform patient that drug doesn't cure CMV retinitis, and that some patients experience worsening of retinal inflammation during and after treatment.
• Tell patient that drug treats only the eye in which it has been injected and that CMV may also exist in the body. Stress importance of follow-up visits to monitor progress and to check for additional infections.
• Instruct patient to also have regular eye care follow-up examinations.
• Advise HIV-infected patient to continue taking antiretroviral therapy, as indicated.

※ *NEW DRUG*

**fosamprenavir calcium**
Lexiva

*Pregnancy risk category C*

**AVAILABLE FORMS**
*Tablets:* 700 mg

**INDICATIONS & DOSAGES**
➤ **HIV infection, with other antiretrovirals**
*Adults:* In patients not previously treated, 1,400 mg P.O. b.i.d. (without ritonavir). Or, 1,400 mg P.O. once daily and ritonavir 200 mg P.O. once daily. Or, 700 mg P.O. b.i.d. and ritonavir 100 mg P.O. b.i.d. In patients previously treated with a protease inhibitor, 700 mg P.O. b.i.d. plus ritonavir 100 mg P.O. b.i.d.
*Adjust-a-dose:* If the patient receives efavirenz, fosamprenavir, and ritonavir once daily, give an additional 100 mg/day of ritonavir (300 mg total).
  If the patient has mild or moderate hepatic impairment and takes fosamprenavir without ritonavir, reduce the dosage to 700 mg P.O. b.i.d.

---

*Rapid onset*  †Canada  ‡Australia  ◇OTC  ◆Off-label use  ✎Photoguide  *Liquid contains alcohol.

## ACTION

Converts rapidly to amprenavir, which binds to the active site of HIV-1 protease and forms immature noninfectious viral particles.

| Route | Onset | Peak | Duration |
|---|---|---|---|
| P.O. | Unknown | 1½-4 hr | Unknown |

## ADVERSE REACTIONS

**CNS:** *depression, fatigue, headache, oral paresthesia.*
**GI:** *abdominal pain, diarrhea, nausea, vomiting.*
**Skin:** pruritus, *rash.*

## INTERACTIONS

**Drug-drug.** *Amitriptyline, cyclosporine, imipramine, rapamycin, tacrolimus:* May increase levels of these drugs. Monitor drug levels.
*Antiarrhythmics (amiodarone, systemic lidocaine, quinidine):* May increase antiarrhythmic level. Use together cautiously, and monitor antiarrhythmic levels.
*Atorvastatin:* May increase atorvastatin level. Give 20 mg/day or less of atorvastatin, and monitor patient carefully. Or, consider other HMG-CoA reductase inhibitors, such as fluvastatin, pravastatin, or rosuvastatin.
*Benzodiazepines (alprazolam, clorazepate, diazepam, flurazepam):* May increase benzodiazepine level. Decrease benzodiazepine dosage as needed.
*Bepridil:* May increase bepridil level, possibly leading to arrhythmias. Use together cautiously.
*Calcium channel blockers (amlodipine, diltiazem, felodipine, isradipine, nifedipine, nicardipine, nimodipine, nisoldipine, verapamil):* May increase calcium channel blocker level. Use together cautiously.
*Carbamazepine, dexamethasone, H₂-receptor antagonists, phenobarbital, phenytoin, proton-pump inhibitors:* May decrease amprenavir level. Use together cautiously.
*Delavirdine:* May cause loss of virologic response and resistance to delavirdine. Avoid using together.
*Dihydroergotamine, ergonovine, ergotamine, flecainide, methylergonovine, midazolam, pimozide, propafenone, triazolam:* May cause serious adverse reactions. Avoid using together.
*Efavirenz, nevirapine, saquinavir:* May decrease amprenavir level. Appropriate combination doses haven't been established.
*Efavirenz with ritonavir:* May decrease amprenavir level. Increase ritonavir by 100 mg/day (300 mg total) when giving efavirenz, fosamprenavir, and ritonavir once daily. No change needed in ritonavir when giving efavirenz, fosamprenavir, and ritonavir twice daily.
*Ethinyl estradiol and norethindrone:* May increase ethinyl estradiol and norethindrone levels. Recommend nonhormonal contraception.
*Indinavir, nelfinavir:* May increase amprenavir level. Appropriate combination doses haven't been established.
*Ketoconazole, itraconazole:* May increase ketoconazole and itraconazole levels. Reduce ketoconazole or itraconazole dosage as needed if patient receives more than 400 mg/day. (More than 200 mg/day isn't recommended.)
*Lopinavir with ritonavir:* May decrease amprenavir and lopinavir levels. Appropriate combination doses haven't been established.
*Lovastatin, simvastatin:* May increase risk of myopathy, including rhabdomyolysis. Avoid using together.
*Methadone:* May decrease methadone level. Increase methadone dosage as needed.
*Rifabutin:* May increase rifabutin level. Obtain CBC weekly to watch for neutropenia, and decrease rifabutin dosage by at least half. If patient receives ritonavir, decrease dosage by at least 75% from the usual 300 mg/day. (Maximum, 150 mg every other day or three times weekly.)
*Rifampin:* May decrease amprenavir level and drug effect. Avoid using together.
*Sildenafil, vardenafil:* May increase sildenafil and vardenafil levels. Recommend cautious use of sildenafil at 25 mg every 48 hours or vardenafil at no more than 2.5 mg every 24 hours. If patient receives ritonavir, advise no more than 2.5 mg vardenafil every 72 hours, and tell patient to report adverse events.
*Warfarin:* May alter warfarin level. Monitor INR.

Reactions may be *common*, uncommon, *life-threatening*, or COMMON AND LIFE-THREATENING.

**Drug-herb.** *St. John's wort:* May cause loss of virologic response and resistance to fosamprenavir or its class of protease inhibitors. Discourage use together.

**EFFECTS ON LAB TEST RESULTS**
• May increase glucose, lipase, triglyceride, AST, and ALT levels.
• May decrease neutrophil count.

**CONTRAINDICATIONS & CAUTIONS**
• Contraindicated in patients hypersensitive to amprenavir or its components.
• Contraindicated with dihydroergotamine, ergonovine, ergotamine, flecainide, methylergonovine, midazolam, pimozide, propafenone, and triazolam.
• Avoid use in patients with severe hepatic impairment.
• Use cautiously in patients allergic to sulfonamides and those with mild to moderate hepatic impairment.
• Use in pregnant patient only when benefit to mother justifies risk to fetus.
• Tell patient not to breast-feed during fosamprenavir therapy.

**NURSING CONSIDERATIONS**
• Patients with hepatitis B or C or marked increase in transaminases before treatment may have increased risk of transaminase elevation. Monitor patient closely during treatment.
• Monitor triglyceride, lipase, ALT, AST, and glucose levels before starting therapy and periodically throughout treatment.
• Ask patient if he's allergic to sulfa drugs.
• Monitor patient with hemophilia for spontaneous bleeding.
• During first treatment, monitor patient for such opportunistic infections as mycobacterium avium complex, cytomegalovirus, *Pneumocystis carinii* pneumonia, and tuberculosis.
• Assess patient for redistribution or accumulation of body fat, as in central obesity, dorsocervical fat enlargement (buffalo hump), peripheral wasting, facial wasting, breast enlargement, and a cushingoid appearance.

**PATIENT TEACHING**
• Tell patient that fosamprenavir doesn't reduce the risk of transmitting HIV to others.

• Inform patient that the drug may reduce the risk of progression to AIDS.
• Explain that fosamprenavir must be used with other antiretrovirals.
• Tell patient not to alter the dose or stop taking fosamprenavir without consulting his prescriber.
• Because fosamprenavir interacts with many drugs, urge patient to tell prescriber about any prescription drugs, OTC drugs, or herbs he's taking (especially St. John's wort).
• Explain that body fat may redistribute or accumulate.

# foscarnet sodium (phosphonoformic acid)
Foscavir

*Pregnancy risk category C*

**AVAILABLE FORMS**
*Injection:* 24 mg/ml in 250- and 500-ml bottles

**INDICATIONS & DOSAGES**
➤ **CMV retinitis in patients with AIDS**
*Adults:* Initially, for induction, 60 mg/kg I.V. q 8 hours or 90 mg/kg I.V. q 12 hours for 2 to 3 weeks, depending on patient response. Follow with a maintenance infusion of 90 to 120 mg/kg daily.
➤ **Acyclovir-resistant herpes simplex virus infections**
*Adults:* 40 mg/kg I.V. over 1 hour q 8 to 12 hours for 2 to 3 weeks or until healed.
***Adjust-a-dose:*** Adjust dosage when creatinine clearance is less than 1.5 ml/kg/minute. If clearance falls below 0.4 ml/kg/minute, stop drug.

**I.V. ADMINISTRATION**
• Drug may be infused via a central or peripheral vein that has adequate blood flow for rapid distribution and dilution into circulation.
• Don't dilute the commercially available form (24 mg/ml) when infusing in a central vein, but further dilute to 12 mg/ml with $D_5W$ or normal saline solution before giving into a peripheral vein, to decrease risk of local irritation.
• Use an infusion pump to give foscarnet. To minimize renal toxicity, make sure pa-

tient is adequately hydrated before and during the infusion.

• Give induction treatment over 1 hour; maintenance infusions over 2 hours.

• *Alert:* Don't exceed the recommended dosage, infusion rate, or frequency of administration. All doses must be individualized according to patient's renal function.

## ACTION

Inhibits all known herpes viruses in vitro by blocking the pyrophosphate-binding site on DNA polymerases and reverse transcriptases.

| Route | Onset | Peak | Duration |
|-------|-------|------|----------|
| I.V. | Unknown | Immediate | Unknown |

## ADVERSE REACTIONS

**CNS:** cerebrovascular disorder, *headache, seizures,* fatigue, malaise, asthenia, paresthesia, dizziness, *hypoesthesia, neuropathy,* pain, tremor, ataxia, generalized spasms, dementia, stupor, sensory disturbances, meningitis, *fever,* aphasia, abnormal coordination, EEG abnormalities, depression, confusion, aggression, anxiety, insomnia, somnolence, nervousness, amnesia, agitation, hallucinations.

**CV:** *hypertension, palpitations, ECG abnormalities, sinus tachycardia, firstdegree AV block, hypotension, flushing,* edema, chest pain.

**EENT:** visual disturbances, eye pain, conjunctivitis, sinusitis, pharyngitis, rhinitis.

**GI:** taste perversion, *nausea, diarrhea, vomiting, abdominal pain, anorexia,* constipation, dysphagia, rectal hemorrhage, dry mouth, dyspepsia, melena, flatulence, ulcerative stomatitis, *pancreatitis.*

**GU:** *abnormal renal function,* albuminuria, dysuria, polyuria, urethral disorder, urine retention, UTI, *acute renal failure,* candidiasis.

**Hematologic:** *anemia, granulocytopenia, leukopenia, bone marrow suppression, thrombocytopenia,* thrombocytosis.

**Hepatic:** abnormal hepatic function.

**Metabolic:** *hypokalemia, hypomagnesemia, hypophosphatemia, hyperphosphatemia, hypocalcemia, hyponatremia.*

**Musculoskeletal:** leg cramps, arthralgia, myalgia, back pain.

**Respiratory:** *cough, dyspnea,* pneumonitis, respiratory insufficiency, pulmonary infiltration, stridor, pneumothorax, *bronchospasm,* hemoptysis.

**Skin:** *rash, diaphoresis,* pruritus, skin ulceration, erythematous rash, seborrhea, skin discoloration, facial edema.

**Other:** lymphadenopathy, *sepsis,* rigors, inflammation and pain at infusion site, lymphoma-like disorder, *sarcoma,* bacterial or fungal infections, abscess, flulike symptoms.

## INTERACTIONS

**Drug-drug.** *Nephrotoxic drugs (such as aminoglycosides, amphotericin B):* May increase risk of nephrotoxicity. Avoid using together.

*Pentamidine:* May increase risk of nephrotoxicity; severe hypocalcemia also has been reported. Monitor renal function tests and electrolytes.

*Zidovudine:* May increase risk or severity of anemia. Monitor blood counts.

## EFFECTS ON LAB TEST RESULTS

• May increase creatinine, phosphate, ALT, AST, alkaline phosphatase, and bilirubin levels. May decrease calcium, magnesium, phosphate, potassium, and sodium levels.

• May increase platelet count. May decrease hemoglobin and granulocyte, WBC, and platelet counts.

## CONTRAINDICATIONS & CAUTIONS

• Contraindicated in patients hypersensitive to drug.

• Use cautiously and at reduced dosage in patients with abnormal renal function. Because drug is nephrotoxic, it can worsen renal impairment. Some degree of nephrotoxicity occurs in most patients treated with drug.

## NURSING CONSIDERATIONS

• Because drug is highly toxic and toxicity is probably dose-related, always use the lowest effective maintenance dose during therapy.

• Monitor creatinine clearance frequently during therapy because of drug's adverse effects on renal function. A baseline 24-hour creatinine clearance is recommended; then regular determinations two to three times weekly during induction

and at least once every 1 to 2 weeks during maintenance.
• Because drug can alter electrolyte levels, monitor levels using a schedule similar to that established for creatinine clearance. Assess patient for tetany and seizures caused by abnormal electrolyte levels.
• Monitor patient's hemoglobin and hematocrit. Anemia occurs in up to 33% of patients treated with drug. It may be severe enough to require transfusions.
• Drug may cause a dose-related transient decrease in ionized calcium, which may not always be reflected in patient's laboratory values.

**PATIENT TEACHING**
• Explain the importance of adequate hydration throughout therapy.
• Advise patient to report tingling around the mouth, numbness in the arms and legs, and pins-and-needles sensations.
• Tell patient to alert nurse if discomfort occurs at I.V. insertion site.

---

## ganciclovir
Cytovene

*Pregnancy risk category C*

**AVAILABLE FORMS**
*Capsules:* 250 mg, 500 mg
*Injection:* 500 mg/vial

**INDICATIONS & DOSAGES**
➤ **CMV retinitis in immunocompromised patients, including those with AIDS and normal renal function**
*Adults and children older than age 3 months:* Induction treatment is 5 mg/kg I.V. q 12 hours for 14 to 21 days. Maintenance treatment is 5 mg/kg daily or 6 mg/kg daily 5 times weekly. Or, for maintenance therapy, give 1,000 mg P.O. t.i.d. with food or 500 mg P.O. q 3 hours while awake (6 times daily).
➤ **To prevent CMV disease in patients with advanced HIV infection and normal renal function**
*Adults:* 1,000 mg P.O. t.i.d. with food.

➤ **To prevent CMV disease in transplant recipients with normal renal function**
*Adults:* 5 mg/kg I.V. (given at a constant rate over 1 hour) q 12 hours for 7 to 14 days; then 5 mg/kg daily or 6 mg/kg daily 5 times weekly. Duration of therapy depends on degree of immunosuppression.
***Adjust-a-dose:*** Adjust dosage in patients with renal impairment according to the table below. If patient is receiving hemodialysis, first I.V. dosage is 1.25 mg/kg 3 times weekly, given shortly after hemodialysis session is complete; maintenance I.V. dosage is 0.625 mg/kg 3 times weekly; and P.O. dosage is 500 mg 3 times weekly.

**First I.V. therapy**

| Creatinine clearance (ml/min) | Dose (mg/kg) | Interval |
|---|---|---|
| 50-69 | 2.5 | 12 hr |
| 25-49 | 2.5 | 24 hr |
| 10-24 | 1.25 | 24 hr |
| < 10 | 1.25 | 3 times weekly |

**Maintenance I.V. therapy**

| Creatinine clearance (ml/min) | Dose (mg/kg) | Interval |
|---|---|---|
| 50-69 | 2.5 | 24 hr |
| 25-49 | 1.25 | 24 hr |
| 10-24 | 0.625 | 24 hr |
| < 10 | 0.625 | 3 times weekly |

**P.O. therapy**

| Creatinine clearance (ml/min) | Dose (mg) | Interval |
|---|---|---|
| 50-69 | 1,500 | 24 hr |
|  | 500 | 8 hr |
| 25-49 | 1,000 | 24 hr |
|  | 500 | 12 hr |
| 10-24 | 500 | 24 hr |
| < 10 | 500 | 3 times weekly |

**I.V. ADMINISTRATION**
• Reconstitute by adding 10 ml of sterile water for injection to vial containing 500 mg ganciclovir. Shake vial well to dissolve drug. Further dilute in 50 to 250 ml (usually 100 ml) of compatible I.V. solu-

tion. If fluids are being restricted, dilute to no more than 10 mg/ml.
● Using an infusion pump, give infusion over at least 1 hour; too-rapid infusions are toxic. Don't give as I.V. bolus.

### ACTION
Inhibits binding of deoxyguanosine triphosphate to DNA polymerase, resulting in inhibition of DNA synthesis.

| Route | Onset | Peak | Duration |
|-------|-------|------|----------|
| P.O. | Unknown | 2-3 hr | Unknown |
| I.V. | Unknown | Immediate | Unknown |

### ADVERSE REACTIONS
**CNS:** altered dreams, *fever,* confusion, ataxia, headache, *seizures, coma,* dizziness, somnolence, tremor, abnormal thinking, agitation, amnesia, anxiety, neuropathy, paresthesia, asthenia.
**EENT:** retinal detachment in CMV retinitis patients.
**GI:** *nausea, vomiting, diarrhea, anorexia, abdominal pain,* flatulence, dyspepsia, dry mouth.
**Hematologic:** *agranulocytosis, thrombocytopenia, leukopenia,* anemia.
**Respiratory:** pneumonia.
**Skin:** *rash; sweating;* pruritus; inflammation, pain, and phlebitis at injection site.
**Other:** infection, chills, *sepsis.*

### INTERACTIONS
**Drug-drug.** *Amphotericin B, cyclosporine, other nephrotoxic drugs:* May increase risk of nephrotoxicity. Monitor renal function.
*Cilastatin, imipenem:* May increase seizure activity. Use together only if potential benefits outweigh risks.
*Cytotoxic drugs:* May increase toxic effects, especially hematologic effects and stomatitis. Monitor patient closely.
*Immunosuppressants (such as azathioprine, corticosteroids, cyclosporine):* May enhance immune and bone marrow suppression. Use together cautiously.
*Probenecid:* May increase ganciclovir level. Monitor patient closely.
*Zidovudine:* May increase incidence of agranulocytosis. Use together cautiously; monitor hematologic function closely.

### EFFECTS ON LAB TEST RESULTS
● May increase creatinine, ALT, AST, GGT, and alkaline phosphatase levels.
● May decrease hemoglobin and granulocyte, platelet, neutrophil, and WBC counts.

### CONTRAINDICATIONS & CAUTIONS
● Contraindicated in patients hypersensitive to drug or acyclovir and in those with an absolute neutrophil count below 500/mm³ or a platelet count below 25,000/mm³.
● Use cautiously and reduce dosage in patients with renal dysfunction. Monitor renal function tests.

### NURSING CONSIDERATIONS
● Use caution when preparing ganciclovir solution, which is alkaline.
● *Alert:* Don't give S.C. or I.M.
● Because of the frequency of agranulocytosis and thrombocytopenia, obtain neutrophil and platelet counts every 2 days during twice-daily ganciclovir dosing and at least weekly thereafter.

### PATIENT TEACHING
● Explain importance of drinking plenty of fluids during therapy.
● Instruct patient to report adverse reactions promptly.
● Tell patient to report discomfort at I.V. insertion site.
● Advise patient that drug causes birth defects. Instruct women to use effective birth control methods during treatment; men should use barrier contraception during and for at least 90 days after treatment with ganciclovir.

---

## indinavir sulfate
Crixivan◈

*Pregnancy risk category C*

### AVAILABLE FORMS
*Capsules:* 100 mg, 200 mg, 333 mg, 400 mg

### INDICATIONS & DOSAGES
➤ **HIV infection, with other antiretrovirals when antiretroviral therapy is warranted**
*Adults:* 800 mg P.O. q 8 hours.

---

*Adjust-a-dose:* For patients with mild to moderate hepatic insufficiency from cirrhosis, reduce dosage to 600 mg P.O. q 8 hours.

## ACTION

Inhibits HIV protease, enzyme required for the proteolytic cleavage of viral polyprotein precursors into individual functional proteins found in infectious HIV. Indinavir binds to the protease active site and inhibits activity of the enzyme, preventing cleavage of the viral polyproteins and resulting in formation of immature noninfectious viral particles.

| Route | Onset | Peak | Duration |
|-------|-------|------|----------|
| P.O. | Unknown | < 1 hr | Unknown |

## ADVERSE REACTIONS

**CNS:** headache, insomnia, dizziness, somnolence, asthenia, malaise, fatigue.
**CV:** chest pain, palpitations.
**EENT:** blurred vision, eye pain or swelling.
**GI:** abdominal pain, *nausea,* diarrhea, vomiting, acid regurgitation, anorexia, dry mouth, taste perversion.
**GU:** nephrolithiasis, hematuria.
**Hematologic:** *neutropenia, thrombocytopenia,* anemia.
**Metabolic:** *hyperbilirubinemia,* hyperglycemia.
**Musculoskeletal:** back pain.
**Other:** flank pain.

## INTERACTIONS

**Drug-drug.** *Amprenavir, saquinavir:* May increase levels of these drugs. Dosage adjustments not necessary.
*Carbamazepine:* May decrease indinavir exposure to the body. Consider an alternative drug.
*Clarithromycin:* May alter clarithromycin level. Dosage adjustments not necessary.
*Didanosine:* May alter absorption of indinavir. Separate doses by 1 hour on an empty stomach.
*Efavirenz, nevirapine:* May decrease indinavir level. Increase indinavir to 1,000 mg q 8 hours.
*HMG-CoA reductase inhibitors:* May increase levels of these drugs and increase risk of myopathy and rhabdomyolysis. Avoid using together.

*Ketoconazole, itraconazole, delavirdine:* May increase indinavir level. Consider reducing indinavir to 600 mg q 8 hours.
*Lopinavir and ritonavir combination:* May increase indinavir level. Adjust indinavir dosage to 600 mg b.i.d.
*Midazolam, triazolam:* May inhibit metabolism of these drugs, which may cause serious or life-threatening events, such as arrhythmias or prolonged sedation. Avoid using together.
*Nelfinavir:* May increase indinavir level by 50% and nelfinavir by 80%. May need to adjust dosage to indinavir 1,200 mg b.i.d. and nelfinavir 1,250 mg b.i.d. Monitor patient closely.
*Rifabutin:* May increase rifabutin level and decrease indinavir level. Give indinavir 1,000 mg q 8 hours and decrease the rifabutin dose to either 150 mg daily or 300 mg two to three times a week.
*Rifampin:* May decrease indinavir level. Avoid using together.
*Ritonavir:* May increase indinavir level twofold to fivefold. Adjust dosage to indinavir 400 mg b.i.d. and ritonavir 400 mg b.i.d., or indinavir 800 mg b.i.d. and ritonavir 100 to 200 mg b.i.d.
*Sildenafil:* May increase sildenafil level and increase adverse effects (hypotension, visual changes, and priapism). Don't exceed 25 mg of sildenafil in 48 hours.
**Drug-herb.** *St. John's wort:* May reduce indinavir level by more than 50%. Discourage use together.
**Drug-food.** *Grapefruit and grapefruit juice:* May decrease level and therapeutic effect of indinavir. Discourage use together.

## EFFECTS ON LAB TEST RESULTS

- May increase ALT, AST, bilirubin, amylase, and glucose levels.
- May decrease hemoglobin and neutrophil and platelet counts.

## CONTRAINDICATIONS & CAUTIONS

- Contraindicated in patients hypersensitive to drug or its components.
- Use cautiously in patients with hepatic insufficiency from cirrhosis.
- Safety and effectiveness in children haven't been established. Don't use drug in children.

## NURSING CONSIDERATIONS
● Drug must be taken at 8-hour intervals.
● Drug may cause nephrolithiasis. If signs and symptoms of nephrolithiasis occur, prescriber may stop drug for 1 to 3 days during acute phases.
● To prevent nephrolithiasis, patient should maintain adequate hydration (at least 48 ounces or 1.5 L of fluids q 24 hours while taking indinavir).

## PATIENT TEACHING
● Tell patient that drug doesn't cure HIV infection and that he may continue to develop opportunistic infections and other complications of HIV infection. Drug hasn't been shown to reduce the risk of HIV transmission.
● Advise patient to use barrier protection during sexual intercourse.
● Caution patient not to adjust dosage or stop indinavir therapy without first consulting prescriber.
● Advise patient that if a dose of indinavir is missed, he should take the next dose at the regularly scheduled time and shouldn't double the dose.
● Instruct patient to take drug on an empty stomach with water 1 hour before or 2 hours after a meal. Or, he may take it with other liquids (such as skim milk, juice, coffee, or tea) or a light meal. Inform patient that a meal high in fat, calories, and protein reduces absorption of drug.
● Instruct patient to store and use capsules in the original container and to keep desiccant in the bottle; capsules are sensitive to moisture.
● Tell patient to drink at least 48 ounces (1.5 L) of fluid daily.
● Advise woman to avoid breast-feeding because indinavir may appear in breast milk. Also, to prevent transmitting virus to infant, advise an HIV-positive woman not to breast-feed.
● Advise patient receiving sildenafil that he may be at higher risk of sildenafil-associated adverse events including low blood pressure, visual changes, and painful erections, and to promptly report any symptoms to his prescriber. Patient shouldn't take more than 25 mg of sildenafil in a 48-hour period.

# lamivudine
Epivir, Epivir-HBV

*Pregnancy risk category C*

## AVAILABLE FORMS
**Epivir**
*Oral solution:* 10 mg/ml
*Tablets:* 150 mg, 300 mg
**Epivir-HBV**
*Oral solution:* 5 mg/ml
*Tablets:* 100 mg

## INDICATIONS & DOSAGES
➤ **HIV infection, with other antiretrovirals**
*Adults and children older than age 16:*
300 mg Epivir P.O. once daily or 150 mg P.O. b.i.d.
*Children ages 3 months to 16 years:*
4 mg/kg Epivir P.O. b.i.d. Maximum dose is 150 mg b.i.d.
*Neonates age 30 days and younger ◆ :*
2 mg/kg Epivir P.O. b.i.d.
***Adjust-a-dose:*** For patients with creatinine clearance 30 to 49 ml/minute, give 150 mg Epivir P.O. daily. If clearance is 15 to 29 ml/minute, 150 mg P.O. on day 1, then 100 mg daily; if 5 to 14 ml/minute, 150 mg on day 1, then 50 mg daily; if less than 5 ml/minute, 50 mg on day 1, then 25 mg daily.
➤ **Chronic hepatitis B with evidence of hepatitis B viral replication and active liver inflammation**
*Epivir-HBV*
*Adults:* 100 mg Epivir-HBV P.O. once daily.
*Children ages 2 to 17:* 3 mg/kg Epivir-HBV P.O. once daily, up to a maximum dose of 100 mg daily. Optimum duration of treatment isn't known; safety and efficacy of treatment beyond 1 year haven't been established.
***Adjust-a-dose:*** For adult patients with creatinine clearance 30 to 49 ml/minute, give first dose of 100 mg Epivir-HBV; then 50 mg P.O. once daily. If clearance is 15 to 29 ml/minute, first dose of 100 mg; then 25 mg P.O. once daily. If clearance is 5 to 14 ml/minute, first dose of 35 mg; then 15 mg P.O. once daily. If clearance is less than 5 ml/minute, first dose of 35 mg; then 10 mg P.O. once daily.

## ACTION
A synthetic nucleoside analogue that inhibits HIV and HBV reverse transcription via viral DNA chain termination. RNA- and DNA-dependent DNA polymerase activities.

| Route | Onset | Peak | Duration |
|-------|-------|------|----------|
| P.O. | Unknown | 1-3 hr | Unknown |

## ADVERSE REACTIONS
Adverse reactions pertain to the combination therapy of lamivudine and zidovudine.
**CNS:** *headache, fatigue, fever, neuropathy, malaise, dizziness, insomnia and other sleep disorders,* depressive disorders.
**EENT:** *nasal symptoms.*
**GI:** *nausea, diarrhea, vomiting, anorexia,* abdominal pain, abdominal cramps, dyspepsia, *pancreatitis.*
**Hematologic:** *neutropenia,* anemia, *thrombocytopenia.*
**Musculoskeletal:** *musculoskeletal pain,* myalgia, arthralgia.
**Respiratory:** *cough.*
**Skin:** rash.
**Other:** *chills.*

## INTERACTIONS
**Drug-drug.** *Trimethoprim and sulfamethoxazole:* May increase lamivudine level because of decreased clearance of drug. Monitor patient for toxicity.
*Zalcitabine:* May inhibit activation of both drugs. Avoid using together.
*Zidovudine:* May increase zidovudine level. Monitor patient closely for adverse reactions.

## EFFECTS ON LAB TEST RESULTS
• May increase ALT and bilirubin levels.
• May decrease hemoglobin and neutrophil and platelet counts.

## CONTRAINDICATIONS & CAUTIONS
• Contraindicated in patients hypersensitive to drug.
• Use cautiously in patients with renal impairment.
• **Alert:** Use drug cautiously, if at all, in children with history of pancreatitis or other significant risk factors for development of pancreatitis.

• An Antiretroviral Pregnancy Registry monitors maternal-fetal outcomes of pregnant women exposed to lamivudine. To register a pregnant patient, the prescriber can call the Antiretroviral Pregnancy Registry at 1-800-258-4263.

## NURSING CONSIDERATIONS
• **Alert:** Stop lamivudine treatment immediately and notify prescriber if clinical signs, symptoms, or laboratory abnormalities suggest pancreatitis. Monitor amylase level.
• **Alert:** Lactic acidosis and hepatotoxicity have been reported. Notify prescriber if signs of lactic acidosis or hepatotoxicity occurs.
• Hepatitis may recur in some patients with chronic hepatitis B virus when they stop taking drug.
• Safety and effectiveness of treatment with Epivir-HBV for longer than 1 year haven't been established; optimum duration of treatment isn't known. Test patients for HIV before starting treatment and during therapy because formulation and dosage of lamivudine in Epivir-HBV aren't appropriate for those infected with both hepatitis B virus and HIV. If lamivudine is given to patients with hepatitis B virus and HIV, use the higher dosage indicated for HIV therapy as part of an appropriate combination regimen.
• Because of a high rate of early virologic resistance, triple antiretroviral therapy with abacavir, lamivudine, and tenofovir shouldn't be used as new treatment regimen for naive or pretreated patients. Monitor patients currently controlled with this combination and those who use this combination in addition to other antiretrovirals, and consider modification of therapy.
• Monitor patient's CBC, platelet count, and renal and liver function studies. Report abnormalities.

## PATIENT TEACHING
• Inform patient that long-term effects of lamivudine are unknown.
• Stress importance of taking lamivudine exactly as prescribed.
• Teach parents or guardians the signs and symptoms of inflammation of the pancreas (pancreatitis). Advise them to report signs and symptoms immediately.

---

*Rapid onset*   †Canada   ‡Australia   ◊OTC   ♦Off-label use   ✐Photoguide   *Liquid contains alcohol.

# lamivudine and zidovudine
Combivir✐

*Pregnancy risk category C*

## AVAILABLE FORMS
*Tablets:* 150 mg lamivudine and 300 mg
zidovudine

## INDICATIONS & DOSAGES
➤ **HIV infection**
*Adults and children age 12 and older,
weighing more than 50 kg (110 lb):* 1 tablet P.O. b.i.d.

## ACTION
Inhibit reverse transcriptase via DNA
chain termination. Both drugs are also
weak inhibitors of DNA polymerase.
Together, they have synergistic antiretroviral activity. Combination therapy with
lamivudine and zidovudine is targeted at
suppressing or delaying the emergence of
resistant strains that can occur with retro-
viral monotherapy because dual resistance
requires multiple mutations.

| Route | Onset | Peak | Duration |
|-------|-------|------|----------|
| P.O. | Unknown | Unknown | Unknown |

## ADVERSE REACTIONS
**CNS:** *headache, malaise, fatigue, insom-
nia, dizziness, neuropathy,* depression,
fever.
**EENT:** *nasal signs and symptoms.*
**GI:** *nausea, diarrhea, vomiting, anorexia,*
abdominal pain, abdominal cramps, dys-
pepsia.
**Hematologic:** ***neutropenia,*** anemia.
**Musculoskeletal:** *musculoskeletal pain,*
myalgia, arthralgia.
**Respiratory:** *cough.*
**Skin:** *rash.*
**Other:** *chills.*

## INTERACTIONS
**Drug-drug.** *Atovaquone, fluconazole,
methadone, probenecid, and valproic
acid:* May increase bioavailability of
zidovudine. Dosage modification isn't
needed.
*Co-trimoxazole or nelfinavir:* May increase bioavailability of lamivudine.
Dosage modification isn't needed.

*Doxorubicin, ribavirin, stavudine:* May
have antagonistic effects when used with
zidovudine Avoid using together.
*Ganciclovir, interferon alpha, and other
bone marrow suppressive or cytotoxic
agents:* May increase hematologic toxicity
of zidovudine. Use together cautiously.
*Nelfinavir, ritonavir:* May decrease bioavailability of zidovudine. Dosage modification isn't needed.
*Zalcitabine:* Zalcitabine and lamivudine
may inhibit intracellular phosphorylation
of one another. Use together isn't recommended.

## EFFECTS ON LAB TEST RESULTS
● May increase ALT, AST, and amylase
levels.
● May decrease hemoglobin, hematocrit,
and neutrophil count.

## CONTRAINDICATIONS & CAUTIONS
● Contraindicated in patients hypersensitive to drug or its components and in those
who are younger than age 12, who weigh
less than 50 kg, or who have creatinine
clearance below 50 ml/minute. Also contraindicated in patients experiencing dose-
limiting adverse effects.
● Use combination cautiously in patients
with bone marrow suppression as evidenced by granulocyte count below
1,000 cells/mm³ or hemoglobin level below 9.5 g/dl.
● An Antiretroviral Pregnancy Registry
monitors maternal-fetal outcomes of pregnant women exposed to Combivir. To register a pregnant patient, prescriber can call
the Antiretroviral Pregnancy Registry at
1-800-258-4263.

## NURSING CONSIDERATIONS
● Some patients with chronic hepatitis B
virus (HBV) may experience recurrence
of hepatitis if lamivudine is discontinued.
Patients with liver disease may have more
severe consequences. Patients with liver
disease and HBV should have periodic
monitoring of both liver function tests and
markers of HBV replication.
● Safety and efficacy of lamivudine hasn't
been established for treatment of HBV in
patients infected with both HIV and HBV.
Emergence of lamivudine-resistant HBV
variants has been reported in patients

---

Reactions may be *common*, uncommon, ***life-threatening***, or COMMON AND LIFE-THREATENING.

with HBV and HIV who have received lamivudine-containing antiretroviral regimens.

● Lactic acidosis and severe hepatomegaly with steatosis have been reported in patients receiving lamivudine and zidovudine either alone or as adjunctive therapy. Notify prescriber if signs and symptoms of lactic acidosis or hepatotoxicity (abdominal pain, jaundice) develop.

● *Alert:* Monitor patient for bone marrow toxicity with frequent blood counts, particularly in patients with advanced HIV infection. Monitor patients for signs and symptoms of lactic acidosis and hepatotoxicity.

● Assess patient's fine motor skills and peripheral sensation for evidence of peripheral neuropathies. Assess patient for myopathy and myositis.

● *Alert:* Don't confuse Combivir with Combivent.

**PATIENT TEACHING**
● Tell patient that the lamivudine-zidovudine combination therapy doesn't cure HIV infection and that he may continue to experience illness, including opportunistic infections.

● Warn patient that HIV transmission can still occur with drug therapy.

● Educate patient about using condoms when engaging in sexual activities to prevent disease transmission.

● Teach patient signs and symptoms of drop in white blood cells count and hemoglobin (fever, chills, infection, fatigue) and instruct him to report such occurrences.

● Tell patient to have blood counts followed closely while on drug, especially if he has advanced disease.

● Advise patient to consult prescriber before taking other drugs.

● Warn patient to report abdominal pain immediately.

● Instruct patient to report signs and symptoms of muscle disease (myopathy or myositis), including muscle inflammation, pain, weakness, decrease in muscle size.

● Stress importance of taking combination drug therapy exactly as prescribed, to reduce the development of resistance.

● Tell patient he may take drug combination with or without food.

● Inform woman that breast-feeding is contraindicated in HIV infection and during drug therapy.

# lopinavir and ritonavir
Kaletra🖉

*Pregnancy risk category C*

**AVAILABLE FORMS**
*Capsules:* lopinavir 133.3 mg and ritonavir 33.3 mg
*Solution:* lopinavir 400 mg and ritonavir 100 mg/5 ml (80 mg and 20 mg/ml)

**INDICATIONS & DOSAGES**
➤ **HIV infection, with other antiretrovirals**
*Adults and children older than age 12:* 400 mg lopinavir and 100 mg ritonavir (3 capsules or 5 ml) P.O. b.i.d. with food.
*Adjust-a-dose:* In treatment-experienced patient also taking efavirenz or nevirapine, when reduced susceptibility to lopinavir is suspected, consider dosage of 533 mg lopinavir and 133 mg ritonavir (4 capsules or 6.5 ml) P.O. b.i.d. with food.
*Children ages 6 months to 12 years, weighing 15 to 40 kg (33 to 88 lb):* 10 mg/kg (lopinavir content) P.O. b.i.d. with food up to a maximum of 400 mg lopinavir and 100 mg ritonavir in children weighing more than 40 kg.
*Adjust-a-dose:* In treatment-experienced patient also taking efavirenz or nevirapine who weighs 15 to 50 kg (33 to 110 lb), when reduced susceptibility to lopinavir is suspected, consider dosage of 11 mg/kg (lopinavir content) P.O. b.i.d. Treatment-experienced children weighing more than 50 kg can receive adult dosage.
*Children ages 6 months to 12 years, weighing 7 to 15 kg (15 to 33 lb):* 12 mg/kg (lopinavir content) P.O. b.i.d. with food.
*Adjust-a-dose:* In treatment-experienced patient also taking efavirenz or nevirapine, when reduced susceptibility to lopinavir is suspected, consider dosage of 13 mg/kg (lopinavir content) P.O. b.i.d. with food.

**ACTION**
Lopinavir is an HIV protease inhibitor. Inhibition of HIV protease results in the pro-

duction of immature, noninfectious viral particles. Ritonavir, also an HIV protease inhibitor, inhibits the metabolism of lopinavir, thereby increasing lopinavir level.

| Route | Onset | Peak | Duration |
|-------|-------|------|----------|
| P.O. | Unknown | 4 hr | 5-6 hr |

## ADVERSE REACTIONS

**CNS:** asthenia, headache, pain, insomnia, malaise, fever, abnormal dreams, agitation, amnesia, anxiety, ataxia, confusion, depression, dizziness, dyskinesia, emotional lability, *encephalopathy,* hypertonia, nervousness, neuropathy, paresthesia, peripheral neuritis, somnolence, abnormal thinking, tremors.
**CV:** chest pain, deep vein thrombosis, hypertension, palpitations, thrombophlebitis, vasculitis, edema.
**EENT:** sinusitis, abnormal vision, eye disorder, otitis media, tinnitus.
**GI:** abdominal pain, abnormal stools, *diarrhea, nausea,* vomiting, anorexia, cholecystitis, constipation, dry mouth, dyspepsia, dysphagia, enterocolitis, eructation, esophagitis, fecal incontinence, flatulence, gastritis, gastroenteritis, GI disorder, *hemorrhagic colitis, pancreatitis,* inflammation of the salivary glands, stomatitis, ulcerative stomatitis, taste perversion.
**GU:** abnormal ejaculation, hypogonadism, renal calculus, urine abnormality.
**Hematologic:** anemia, *leukopenia, neutropenia; thrombocytopenia in children.*
**Hepatic:** hyperbilirubinemia in children.
**Metabolic:** Cushing's syndrome, hypothyroidism, dehydration, decreased glucose tolerance, lactic acidosis, weight loss, hyperglycemia, hyperuricemia, hyponatremia in children.
**Musculoskeletal:** back pain, arthralgia, arthrosis, myalgia.
**Respiratory:** bronchitis, dyspnea, lung edema.
**Skin:** rash, acne, alopecia, dry skin, exfoliative dermatitis, furunculosis, nail disorder, pruritus, benign skin neoplasm, skin discoloration, sweating.
**Other:** gynecomastia, chills, facial edema, flu syndrome, viral infection, lymphadenopathy, peripheral edema, decreased libido.

## INTERACTIONS

**Drug-drug.** *Amiodarone, bepridil, lidocaine, quinidine:* May increase antiarrhythmic level. Use together cautiously. Monitor levels of these drugs, if possible.
*Amprenavir, indinavir, saquinavir:* May increase levels of these drugs. Avoid using together.
*Antiarrhythmics (flecainide, propafenone), pimozide:* May increase risk of cardiac arrhythmias. Avoid using together.
*Atorvastatin:* May increase level of this drug. Use lowest possible dose and monitor patient carefully.
*Atovaquone, methadone:* May decrease levels of these drugs. Consider increasing doses of these drugs.
*Carbamazepine, dexamethasone, phenobarbital, phenytoin:* May decrease lopinavir level. Use together cautiously.
*Clarithromycin:* May increase clarithromycin level in patients with renal impairment. Adjust clarithromycin dosage.
*Cyclosporine, rapamycin, tacrolimus:* May increase levels of these drugs. Monitor therapeutic levels.
*Delavirdine:* May increase lopinavir level. Avoid using together.
*Didanosine:* May decrease absorption of didanosine because lopinavir-ritonavir combination is taken with food. Give didanosine 1 hour before or 2 hours after lopinavir-ritonavir combination.
*Dihydroergotamine, ergonovine, ergotamine, methylergonovine:* May increase risk of ergot toxicity characterized by peripheral vasospasm and ischemia. Avoid using together.
*Disulfiram, metronidazole:* May cause disulfiram-like reaction. Avoid using together.
*Efavirenz, nevirapine:* May decrease lopinavir concentrations. Consider increasing dose of lopinavir-ritonavir combination.
*Felodipine, nicardipine, nifedipine:* May increase levels of these drugs. Use together cautiously.
*Hormonal contraceptives (ethinyl estradiol):* May decrease effectiveness of contraceptives. Recommend alternative contraception measures.
*Itraconazole, ketoconazole:* May increase levels of these drugs. Don't give more than 200 mg/day of these drugs.

Reactions may be *common,* uncommon, *life-threatening,* or COMMON AND LIFE-THREATENING.

*Lovastatin, simvastatin:* May increase risk of adverse reactions, such as myopathy, rhabdomyolysis. Avoid using together.

*Midazolam, triazolam:* May cause prolonged or increased sedation or respiratory depression. Avoid using together.

*Rifabutin:* May increase rifabutin level. Decrease rifabutin dose by 75%. Monitor patient for adverse effects.

*Rifampin:* May decrease effectiveness of lopinavir-ritonavir combination. Avoid using together.

*Sildenafil:* May increase sildenafil level and adverse effects, such as hypotension and priapism. Warn patient not to take more than 25 mg of sildenafil in 48 hours.

*Warfarin:* May affect warfarin concentration. Monitor PT and INR.

**Drug-herb.** *St. John's wort:* Loss of virologic response and possible resistance to lopinavir and ritonavir. Discourage use together.

**Drug-food.** *Any food:* May increase absorption of drug. Tell patient to take with food.

**EFFECTS ON LAB TEST RESULTS**
● May increase amylase, cholesterol, and triglyceride levels.
● May decrease hemoglobin, hematocrit, and RBC, WBC, neutrophil, and platelet counts.

**CONTRAINDICATIONS & CAUTIONS**
● Contraindicated in patients hypersensitive to drug or any of its components.
● Use cautiously in patients with a history of pancreatitis or with hepatic impairment, hepatitis B or C, marked elevations in liver enzyme levels, or hemophilia.
● Use cautiously in elderly patients.
● The Antiretroviral Pregnancy Registry monitors maternal-fetal outcomes of pregnant women exposed to lopinavir-ritonavir combination. Health care providers are encouraged to enroll patients by calling 1-800-258-4263.

**NURSING CONSIDERATIONS**
● *Alert:* Many drug interactions are possible. Review all drugs patient is taking.
● Give drug with food.
● Refrigerated drug remains stable until expiration date on package. If stored at room temperature, use drug within 2 months.
● Monitor patient for signs of fat redistribution, including central obesity, buffalo hump, peripheral wasting, breast enlargement, and cushingoid appearance.
● Monitor total cholesterol and triglycerides before starting therapy and periodically thereafter.
● Monitor patient for signs and symptoms of pancreatitis (nausea, vomiting, abdominal pain, or increased lipase and amylase values).
● Monitor patient for signs and symptoms of bleeding (hypotension, rapid heart rate).
● *Alert:* Don't confuse Kaletra with Keppra.

**PATIENT TEACHING**
● Tell patient to take drug with food.
● Tell patient also taking didanosine to take it 1 hour before or 2 hours after lopinavir-ritonavir combination.
● Advise patient to report side effects to prescriber.
● Tell patient to immediately report severe nausea, vomiting, or abdominal pain.
● Advise patient receiving sildenafil of an increased risk of sildenafil-associated adverse events, including low blood pressure, visual changes, and painful erections, and to promptly report any symptoms to his prescriber. Tell him not to take more than 25 mg of sildenafil in 48 hours.
● Warn patient to tell prescriber about any other prescription or nonprescription medicine that he's taking, including herbal supplements.
● Tell patient that drug doesn't cure HIV.

# nelfinavir mesylate
Viracept

*Pregnancy risk category B*

**AVAILABLE FORMS**
*Powder:* 50 mg/g powder in 144-g bottle
*Tablets:* 250 mg, 625 mg

**INDICATIONS & DOSAGES**
➤ **HIV infection when antiretroviral therapy is warranted**
*Adults:* 1,250 mg b.i.d. or 750 mg P.O. t.i.d. with meals or light snack.

*Children ages 2 to 13:* 20 to 30 mg/kg/
dose P.O. t.i.d. with meals or light snack;
don't exceed 750 mg t.i.d.

➤ **To prevent infection after occupational exposure to HIV ♦**
*Adults:* 750 mg P.O. t.i.d. in combination
with two other antiretrovirals (zidovudine
and lamivudine, lamivudine and stavudine, or didanosine and stavudine) for 4
weeks.

## ACTION
An HIV-1 protease inhibitor, thereby preventing cleavage of the viral polyprotein,
resulting in the production of immature,
noninfectious virus.

| Route | Onset | Peak | Duration |
|-------|-------|------|----------|
| P.O. | Unknown | 2-4 hr | Unknown |

## ADVERSE REACTIONS
**CNS:** *seizures, suicidal ideation.*
**GI:** nausea, *diarrhea,* flatulence, *pancre-
atitis.*
**Hematologic:** *leukopenia, thrombocy-
topenia.*
**Hepatic:** *hepatitis.*
**Metabolic:** dehydration, diabetes mellitus,
hyperlipidemia, hyperuricemia, *hypogly-
cemia.*
**Skin:** rash.
**Other:** redistribution or accumulation of
body fat.

## INTERACTIONS
**Drug-drug.** *Amiodarone, ergot derivatives, lovastatin, midazolam, pimozide,
quinidine, simvastatin, or triazolam:* May
increase levels of these drugs, causing increased risk of serious or life-threatening
adverse events. Avoid using together.
*Atorvastatin:* May increase atorvastatin
level. Use lowest possible dose or consider
using pravastatin or fluvastatin instead.
*Azithromycin:* May increase azithromycin
level. Monitor patient for liver impairment.
*Carbamazepine, phenobarbital:* May reduce the effectiveness of nelfinavir. Use
together cautiously.
*Cyclosporine, sirolimus, tacrolimus:* May
increase levels of these immunosuppressants. Use cautiously together.
*Delavirdine, HIV protease inhibitors (in-
dinavir or saquinavir), nevirapine:* May

increase levels of protease inhibitors. Use
together cautiously.
*Didanosine:* May decrease didanosine absorption. Take nelfinavir with food at least
2 hours before or 1 hour after didanosine.
*Ethinyl estradiol:* May decrease contraceptive level and effectiveness. Advise patient to use alternative contraceptive measures during therapy.
*Methadone, phenytoin:* May decrease levels of these drugs. Adjust dosage of these
drugs accordingly.
*Rifabutin:* May increase rifabutin level,
and decreases nelfinavir level. Reduce
dosage of rifabutin to half the usual dose
and increase nelfinavir to 1,250 mg b.i.d.
*Sildenafil:* May increase adverse effects of
sildenafil. Use together cautiously. Don't
exceed 25 mg of sildenafil in a 48-hour
period.
**Drug-herb.** *St. John's wort:* May decrease
nelfinavir level. Discourage use together.

## EFFECTS ON LAB TEST RESULTS
● May increase ALT, AST, alkaline phosphatase, bilirubin, GGT, amylase, CPK,
and lipid levels. May increase or decrease
glucose level.
● May decrease hemoglobin and WBC and
platelet counts.

## CONTRAINDICATIONS & CAUTIONS
● Contraindicated in patients hypersensitive to drug or its components. Drug is
also contraindicated in patients receiving
concomitant amiodarone, ergot derivatives, lovastatin, midazolam, pimozide,
quinidine, simvastatin, or triazolam.
● Use cautiously in patients with hepatic
dysfunction or hemophilia types A and B.
Monitor liver function test results.
● It's not known if drug appears in breast
milk. Because safety hasn't been established, advise HIV-infected women not to
breast-feed, to avoid transmitting virus to
the infant.

## NURSING CONSIDERATIONS
● Drug dosage is the same whether used
alone or with other antiretrovirals.
● Give oral powder in children unable to
take tablets. May mix oral powder with
small amount of water, milk, formula, soy
formula, soy milk, or dietary supplements.
Patient should consume entire contents.

- Don't reconstitute with water in its original container.
- Use reconstituted powder within 6 hours.
- Mixing with acidic foods or juice isn't recommended because of bitter taste.
- *Alert:* Don't confuse nelfinavir with nevirapine.

## PATIENT TEACHING
- Advise patient to take drug with food.
- Inform patient that drug doesn't cure HIV infection.
- Tell patient that long-term effects of drug are unknown and that there are no data stating that nelfinavir reduces risk of HIV transmission.
- Advise patient to take drug daily as prescribed and not to alter dose or stop drug without medical approval.
- If patient misses a dose, tell him to take it as soon as possible and then return to his normal schedule. Advise patient not to double the dose.
- Tell patient that diarrhea is the most common adverse effect and that it can be controlled with loperamide, if necessary.
- Instruct patient taking hormonal contraceptives to use alternative or additional contraceptive measures while taking nelfinavir.
- Advise patient receiving sildenafil of an increased risk of sildenafil-associated adverse events including low blood pressure, visual changes, and painful erections, and that he should promptly report any symptoms. Tell him not to exceed 25 mg of sildenafil in a 48-hour period.
- Warn patient with phenylketonuria that powder contains 11.2 mg phenylalanine/g.
- Advise patient to report use of other prescribed or OTC drugs because of possible drug interactions.

---

## nevirapine
Viramune

*Pregnancy risk category C*

---

## AVAILABLE FORMS
*Oral suspension:* 50 mg/5 ml
*Tablets:* 200 mg

## INDICATIONS & DOSAGES
➤ **Adjunct treatment in patients with HIV-1 infection who have experienced clinical or immunologic deterioration**
*Adults:* 200 mg P.O. daily for the first 14 days, then 200 mg P.O. b.i.d. Used with nucleoside analogue antiretrovirals.
➤ **Adjunct treatment in children infected with HIV-1**
*Children age 8 and older:* 4 mg/kg P.O. once daily for first 14 days; then 4 mg/kg P.O. b.i.d. thereafter. Maximum daily dose is 400 mg.
*Children ages 2 months to 8 years:* 4 mg/kg P.O. once daily for first 14 days, then 7 mg/kg P.O. b.i.d. thereafter. Maximum daily dose is 400 mg.

## ACTION
A nonnucleoside reverse transcriptase inhibitor that binds directly to reverse transcriptase and blocks RNA-dependent and DNA-dependent DNA polymerase activities by causing a disruption of the enzyme's catalytic site.

| Route | Onset | Peak | Duration |
|-------|-------|------|----------|
| P.O. | Unknown | 4 hr | Unknown |

## ADVERSE REACTIONS
**CNS:** headache, *fever,* paresthesia.
**GI:** *nausea,* diarrhea, abdominal pain, ulcerative stomatitis.
**Hematologic:** *neutropenia.*
**Hepatic:** *hepatitis.*
**Musculoskeletal:** myalgia.
**Skin:** *rash, blistering, Stevens-Johnson syndrome.*

## INTERACTIONS
**Drug-drug.** *Drugs extensively metabolized by P-450 CYP3A:* May lower levels of these drugs. Dosage adjustment of these drugs may be required.
*Ketoconazole:* May decrease ketoconazole level. Avoid using together.
*Protease inhibitors or hormonal contraceptives:* May decrease levels of these drugs. Use together cautiously.
*Rifabutin, rifampin:* Dosage adjustment may be needed. Monitor patient closely.
**Drug-herb.** *St. John's wort:* May decrease nevirapine level. Discourage use together.

---

## EFFECTS ON LAB TEST RESULTS
• May increase ALT, AST, GGT, and bilirubin levels.
• May decrease hemoglobin and neutrophil count.

## CONTRAINDICATIONS & CAUTIONS
• Contraindicated in patients hypersensitive to drug.
• Use cautiously in patients with impaired renal and hepatic function; pharmacokinetics haven't been evaluated in those patients.
• Safety and effectiveness in children haven't been established. Don't use drug in children.
• Nevirapine appears in breast milk. Don't use drug in breast-feeding patients.

## NURSING CONSIDERATIONS
• Perform clinical chemistry tests, including renal and liver function tests, before starting drug therapy and regularly throughout therapy.
• Use drug with at least one other antiretroviral.
• **Alert:** Monitor patient for blistering, oral lesions, conjunctivitis, muscle or joint aches, or general malaise. Be especially alert for a severe rash or rash accompanied by fever. Report such signs and symptoms to prescriber. Patients who experience a rash during the first 14 days of therapy shouldn't have the dosage increased until the rash has resolved. Most rashes occur within the first 6 weeks of therapy.
• **Alert:** Moderate and severe liver function test abnormalities and hepatotoxicity may warrant temporarily stopping therapy; drug may be restarted at half the previous dose level.
• Patients who have nevirapine therapy interrupted for longer than 7 days should restart therapy as if receiving drug for the first time.
• Antiretroviral therapy may be changed if disease progresses while patient is receiving nevirapine.
• **Alert:** Don't confuse nevirapine with nelfinavir.

## PATIENT TEACHING
• Inform patient that nevirapine doesn't cure HIV and that illnesses associated with advanced HIV-1 infection still may occur. Explain that drug doesn't reduce risk of HIV-1 transmission.
• Instruct patient to report rash immediately and to stop drug until told to resume.
• Stress importance of taking drug exactly as prescribed. If a dose is missed, tell patient to take the next dose as soon as possible. Patient shouldn't double next dose.
• Tell patient not to use other drugs unless approved by prescriber.
• Advise woman of childbearing age that hormonal contraceptives and other hormonal methods of birth control shouldn't be used with nevirapine.
• Advise woman to avoid breast-feeding during drug therapy to reduce risk of postnatal HIV transmission.

# oseltamivir phosphate
Tamiflu

*Pregnancy risk category C*

## AVAILABLE FORMS
*Capsules:* 75 mg
*Oral suspension:* 12 mg/ml after reconstitution

## INDICATIONS & DOSAGES
➤ **Uncomplicated, acute illness caused by influenza infection in patients who have had symptoms for 2 days or less**
*Adults:* 75 mg P.O. b.i.d. for 5 days.
*Adjust-a-dose:* For patients with creatinine clearance of 10 to 30 ml/minute, reduce dosage to 75 mg P.O. once daily for 5 days.
➤ **To prevent influenza after close contact with infected person**
*Adults and adolescents age 13 and older:* 75 mg P.O. once daily, beginning within 2 days of exposure, for at least 7 days.
➤ **To prevent influenza during a community outbreak**
*Adults and adolescents age 13 and older:* 75 mg P.O. once daily for up to 6 weeks.
➤ **Influenza in children age 1 and older**
*Children age 1 and older, weighing more than 40 kg (88 lb):* 75 mg oral suspension P.O. b.i.d.
*Children age 1 and older, weighing 23 to 40 kg (51 to 88 lb):* 60 mg oral suspension P.O. b.i.d.

*Children age 1 and older, weighing 15 to
23 kg (33 to 51 lb):* 45 mg oral suspension
P.O. b.i.d.
*Children age 1 and older, weighing 15 kg
(33 lb) or less:* 30 mg oral suspension P.O.
b.i.d.

## ACTION
Inhibits influenza A and B virus enzyme
neuraminidase, which is thought to play a
role in viral particle aggregation and release from the host cell. Neuraminidase
inhibition, therefore, appears to interfere
with viral replication.

| Route | Onset | Peak | Duration |
|-------|-------|------|----------|
| P.O. | Unknown | Unknown | Unknown |

## ADVERSE REACTIONS
**CNS:** dizziness, insomnia, headache, ver-
tigo, fatigue.
**GI:** abdominal pain, diarrhea, nausea,
vomiting.
**Respiratory:** bronchitis, cough.

## INTERACTIONS
None significant.

## EFFECTS ON LAB TEST RESULTS
None reported.

## CONTRAINDICATIONS & CAUTIONS
• Contraindicated in patients hypersensitive to drug or its components.
• Use cautiously in patients with chronic
cardiac or respiratory diseases, or any
medical condition that may require imminent hospitalization. Also use cautiously
in patients with renal failure.
• It's unknown if drug or its metabolite appears in breast milk. Use only if benefits
to patient outweigh risks to infant.

## NURSING CONSIDERATIONS
• No evidence supports drug use to treat
viral infections other than influenza virus
types A and B.
• Drug must be given within 2 days of onset of symptoms.
• Drug isn't a replacement for the annual
influenza vaccination. Patients for whom
vaccine is indicated should continue to receive the vaccine each fall.
• Safety and efficacy of repeated treatment
courses haven't been established.

• Drug may be given with meals to decrease GI adverse effects.
• Store at controlled room temperature
(59° to 86° F [15° to 30° C]).

## PATIENT TEACHING
• Instruct patient to begin treatment as
soon as possible after appearance of flu
symptoms.
• Inform patient that drug may be taken
with or without meals. If nausea or vomiting occurs, he can take drug with food or
milk.
• Tell patient that, if a dose is missed, to
take it as soon as possible. He should skip
missed dose, however, if next dose is due
within 2 hours, and take the next dose on
schedule.
• Advise patient to complete the full 5
days of treatment, even if symptoms resolve.
• Alert patient that drug isn't a replacement for the annual influenza vaccination.
Patients for whom vaccine is indicated
should continue to receive the vaccine
each fall.

## ribavirin
Virazole

*Pregnancy risk category X*

## AVAILABLE FORMS
*Powder to be reconstituted for inhalation:*
6 g in 100-ml glass vial

## INDICATIONS & DOSAGES
➤ **Hospitalized infants and young children infected by RSV**
*Infants and young children:* Solution in
concentration of 20 mg/ml delivered via
the Viratek Small Particle Aerosol Gener-
ator (SPAG-2) and mechanical ventilator
or oxygen hood, face mask, or oxygen tent
at a rate of about 12.5 L of mist/minute.
Treatment is given for 12 to 18 hours/day
for at least 3 days, and no longer than 7
days.

## ACTION
Inhibits viral activity by an unknown
mechanism, possibly by inhibiting RNA

and DNA synthesis by depleting intracellular nucleotide pools.

| Route | Onset | Peak | Duration |
|---|---|---|---|
| Inhalation | Unknown | Unknown | Unknown |

**ADVERSE REACTIONS**
**CV:** *cardiac arrest,* hypotension, *bradycardia.*
**EENT:** conjunctivitis, rash or erythema of eyelids.
**Hematologic:** anemia, reticulocytosis.
**Respiratory:** *bronchospasm,* pulmonary edema, worsening respiratory state, *apnea,* bacterial pneumonia, pneumothorax.

**INTERACTIONS**
None significant.

**EFFECTS ON LAB TEST RESULTS**
● May increase ALT, AST, and bilirubin levels.
● May increase reticulocyte count. May decrease hemoglobin.

**CONTRAINDICATIONS & CAUTIONS**
● Contraindicated in patients hypersensitive to drug. Although drug is used in children, manufacturer states that it's contraindicated in women who are or may become pregnant during treatment.

**NURSING CONSIDERATIONS**
● Give ribavirin aerosol by the Viratek SPAG-2 only. Don't use any other aerosol-generating device.
● Use sterile USP water for injection, not bacteriostatic water. Water used to reconstitute this drug must not contain any antimicrobial product.
● Discard solutions placed in the SPAG-2 unit at least every 24 hours before adding newly reconstituted solution.
● *Alert:* The most frequent adverse effects reported in health care personnel exposed to aerosolized ribavirin include eye irritation and headache. Advise pregnant personnel of these effects.
● *Alert:* Monitor ventilator function frequently. Ribavirin may precipitate in ventilator apparatus, causing equipment malfunction with serious consequences.
● Store reconstituted solutions at room temperature for 24 hours.

● Ribavirin aerosol is indicated only for severe lower respiratory tract infection caused by RSV. Although treatment may begin while awaiting diagnostic test results, existence of RSV infection must be documented eventually.
● Most infants and children with RSV infection don't require treatment with antivirals because the disease is commonly mild and self-limiting. Premature infants or those with cardiopulmonary disease experience RSV in its severest form and benefit most from treatment with ribavirin aerosol.

**PATIENT TEACHING**
● Inform parents of need for drug, and answer any questions.
● Encourage parents to immediately report any subtle change in child.

---

**rimantadine hydrochloride**
Flumadine

*Pregnancy risk category C*

**AVAILABLE FORMS**
*Syrup:* 50 mg/5 ml
*Tablets (film-coated):* 100 mg

**INDICATIONS & DOSAGES**
➤ **To prevent influenza A**
*Adults and children age 10 and older:*
100 mg P.O. b.i.d. beginning as soon as possible after first exposure and continued through course of influenza A outbreak.
*Children younger than age 10:* 5 mg/kg P.O. once daily. Maximum daily dose 150 mg.
*Elderly patients:* 100 mg P.O. daily beginning as soon as possible after first exposure and continued through course of influenza A outbreak.
➤ **Influenza A**
*Adults:* 100 mg P.O. b.i.d. initiated within 24 to 48 hours after onset of symptoms and continued for 48 hours after symptoms disappear (usually 7-day total course).
*Adjust-a-dose:* For patients with severe hepatic or renal dysfunction or those experiencing adverse effects with normal dosage, 100 mg P.O. daily.

---

## ACTION

Unknown. Appears to prevent viral uncoating, an early step in virus reproductive cycle.

| Route | Onset | Peak | Duration |
|-------|-------|------|----------|
| P.O. | Unknown | 6 hr | Unknown |

## ADVERSE REACTIONS

**CNS:** insomnia, headache, dizziness, nervousness, fatigue, asthenia.
**GI:** nausea, vomiting, anorexia, dry mouth, abdominal pain.

## INTERACTIONS

**Drug-drug.** *Acetaminophen, aspirin:* May reduce level of rimantadine. Monitor patient for decreased effectiveness of rimantadine.
*Cimetidine:* May decrease clearance of rimantadine. Monitor patient for adverse reactions.

## EFFECTS ON LAB TEST RESULTS

None reported.

## CONTRAINDICATIONS & CAUTIONS

● Contraindicated in patients hypersensitive to drug or amantadine.
● Use cautiously in patients with renal or hepatic impairment and in patients with a history of seizures. Pregnant patients should consider the risks versus benefits before taking drug.

## NURSING CONSIDERATIONS

● Elderly patients are more likely to experience adverse effects than younger patients, mainly adverse CNS or GI effects.
● Monitor patients with a history of seizures for an increased incidence of seizure-like activity.
● Safety of therapy lasting longer than 6 weeks hasn't been established.
● Use drug for prevention in children up to 6 weeks after first dose of influenza vaccine or until 2 weeks after second dose of vaccine.
● Consider the risk to contacts of treated patients who may get sick with the influenza A virus. Influenza A–resistant strains can emerge during therapy. Patients taking drug may still be able to spread the disease.

● *Alert:* Don't confuse rimantadine with amantadine.

## PATIENT TEACHING

● Instruct patient to take drug several hours before bedtime to prevent insomnia.
● Inform patient that he may still be able to infect others with influenza A and to take infection-control precautions.
● Inform patient that drug may be used in children for prevention only. Safety and effectiveness for treatment of influenza A has not been established.
● Advise patient to complete the full course of treatment and to take the drug at evenly spaced time intervals. If he misses a dose, he should take the missed dose as soon as possible unless it's almost time for the next dose. He should not take a double dose to catch up.
● Advise patient to use caution when driving a car or performing other potentially hazardous activities if dizziness or other adverse CNS effects occur.
● Tell patient to contact prescriber if there is no improvement within a few days.
● Tell patient or caregiver using the syrup formulation, to use a specially marked oral syringe or measuring spoon to measure the correct dose. An average household teaspoon may not provide the correct amount of the drug.
● It's unknown if drug appears in breast milk. Use cautiously in breast-feeding women.

## ritonavir
Norvir

*Pregnancy risk category B*

## AVAILABLE FORMS

*Capsules:* 100 mg
*Oral solution:* 80 mg/ml

## INDICATIONS & DOSAGES

➤ **HIV infection, with other antiretrovirals, when antiretroviral therapy is warranted**
*Adults:* 600 mg P.O. b.i.d with meals. If nausea occurs, gradually increasing dose may provide some relief: 300 mg b.i.d. for 1 day, 400 mg b.i.d. for 2 days, 500 mg

b.i.d. for 1 day, and then 600 mg b.i.d. thereafter.
*Children age 2 and older:* 400 mg/m² P.O. b.i.d.; Don't exceed 600 mg P.O. b.i.d. Initially, may start with 250 mg/m² b.i.d. and increase by 50 mg/m² P.O. q 12 hours at 2- to 3-day intervals. If children can't reach b.i.d. doses of 400 mg/m² because of adverse effects, consider alternative therapy.

## ACTION

An HIV protease inhibitor with activity against HIV-1 and HIV-2 proteases. HIV protease is an enzyme required for the proteolytic cleavage of viral polyprotein precursors into the individual functional proteins in infectious HIV. Ritonavir binds to the protease active site and inhibits activity of the enzyme, preventing cleavage of the viral polyproteins and resulting in the formation of immature, noninfectious viral particles.

| Route | Onset | Peak | Duration |
|-------|-------|------|----------|
| P.O. | Unknown | 2-4 hr | Unknown |

## ADVERSE REACTIONS

**CNS:** *asthenia,* fever, headache, malaise, circumoral paresthesia, dizziness, insomnia, paresthesia, peripheral paresthesia, somnolence, thinking abnormality, migraine headache.
**CV:** vasodilation.
**EENT:** local throat irritation, blepharitis, diplopia, pharyngitis, photophobia.
**GI:** abdominal pain, anorexia, constipation, *diarrhea, nausea, vomiting,* dyspepsia, flatulence, cramping, *taste perversion.*
**GU:** dysuria, hematuria, nocturia, polyuria, pyelonephritis, urethritis.
**Hematologic:** *leukopenia, thrombocytopenia.*
**Hepatic:** jaundice.
**Metabolic:** hyperlipidemia, hyperglycemia, *hyperkalemia,* hyperuricemia.
**Musculoskeletal:** myalgia.
**Skin:** rash, sweating, urticaria.

## INTERACTIONS

**Drug-drug.** *Alprazolam, clorazepate, diazepam, estazolam, flurazepam, midazolam, triazolam, zolpidem:* May cause extreme sedation and respiratory depression from these agents. Avoid using together.

*Alprazolam, methadone:* May decrease levels of these drugs. Use together cautiously.
*Amiodarone, bupropion, clozapine, encainide, flecainide, meperidine, piroxicam, propafenone, propoxyphene, quinidine, rifabutin:* May significantly increase levels of these drugs, increasing risk of arrhythmias, hematologic abnormalities, or seizures. Use together is contraindicated.
*Amprenavir:* May increase amprenavir exposure. May adjust dose of amprenavir 600 to 1,200 mg b.i.d. and ritonavir 100 to 200 mg b.i.d.
*Clarithromycin:* May increase clarithromycin level. In patients with creatinine clearance 30 to 60 ml/minute receiving drug with ritonavir, reduce clarithromycin dose by 50% reduction; if clearance is below 30 ml/minute, reduce dose by 75%.
*Delavirdine, nevirapine:* May alter ritonavir level. No dosage adjustment is necessary.
*Desipramine:* May increase desipramine level. May require dosage adjustment.
*Disopyramide:* May cause cardiac and neurologic events. Use together cautiously.
*Disulfiram or other drugs that produce disulfiram-like reactions, such as metronidazole:* May increase risk of disulfiram-like reactions. Monitor patient.
*Drugs that increase CYP3A activity, such as carbamazepine, dexamethasone, phenobarbital, phenytoin, rifabutin, and rifampin:* May increase ritonavir clearance, resulting in decreased ritonavir level. Monitor anticonvulsant level. May reduce rifabutin dosage if necessary.
*Efavirenz:* May increase levels of both drugs. Leave the dose at 600 mg b.i.d., or may reduce dosage of ritonavir to 500 mg b.i.d. if intolerance develops.
*Glucuronosyltransferases, including oral anticoagulants or immunosuppressants:* May cause loss of therapeutic effects. May need to adjust dosage, monitor drug levels and effects. A dosage reduction greater than 50% may be required for those drugs extensively metabolized by CYP3A.
*HMG-CoA reductase inhibitors:* May increase statin levels, causing myopathy. Avoid using together.
*Hormonal contraceptives:* May decrease contraceptive effectiveness. May require a dosage increase in the hormonal contra-

---

Reactions may be *common,* uncommon, *life-threatening,* or COMMON AND LIFE-THREATENING.

ceptive or alternate contraceptive measures.

*Ketoconazole:* May increase levels of both drugs. Use together cautiously and monitor patient carefully.

*Nelfinavir:* May increase nelfinavir level. Adjust dosage by taking ritonavir 400 mg b.i.d. and nelfinavir 500 to 750 mg b.i.d.

*Theophylline:* May decrease theophylline level. May need to increase dosage.

*Saquinavir:* May increase saquinavir level. Adjust dosage by taking saquinavir 400 mg b.i.d. and ritonavir 400 mg b.i.d.

*Sildenafil:* May increase sildenafil level. Use together cautiously. Don't exceed 25 mg of sildenafil in 48 hours.

**Drug-herb.** *St. John's wort:* May reduce drug levels, causing loss of therapeutic effects. Discourage use together.

**Drug-food.** *Any food:* May increase absorption. Advise patient to take drug with food.

**EFFECTS ON LAB TEST RESULTS**
● May increase ALT, AST, alkaline phosphatase, GGT, bilirubin, glucose, triglycerides, lipids, potassium, CK, and uric acid levels.
● May increase PT and INR. May decrease hemoglobin, hematocrit, and WBC, platelet, neutrophil, and eosinophil counts.

**CONTRAINDICATIONS & CAUTIONS**
● Contraindicated in patients hypersensitive to drug or its components.
● Use cautiously in patients with hepatic insufficiency.
● Safety and effectiveness in children younger than age 12 haven't been established.
● It's unknown if ritonavir appears in breast milk. Use cautiously in breast-feeding women.

**NURSING CONSIDERATIONS**
● Patients beginning combination regimens with ritonavir and nucleosides may improve GI tolerance by starting ritonavir alone and subsequently adding nucleosides before completing 2 weeks of ritonavir.
● **Alert:** Don't confuse Norvir with Norvasc.

**PATIENT TEACHING**
● Inform patient that drug doesn't cure HIV infection. He may continue to develop opportunistic infections and other complications of HIV infection. Drug hasn't been shown to reduce the risk of transmitting HIV to others through sexual contact or blood contamination.
● Caution patient to take drug as prescribed and not to adjust dosage or stop therapy without first consulting prescriber.
● Tell patient that taste of ritonavir oral solution may be improved by mixing it with chocolate milk, Ensure, or Advera within 1 hour of the scheduled dose.
● Instruct patient to take drug with a meal to improve absorption.
● Tell patient that if a dose is missed, he should take the next dose as soon as possible. If a dose is skipped, he shouldn't double the next dose.
● Advise patient receiving sildenafil of an increased risk of sildenafil-associated adverse events, including low blood pressure, visual changes, and painful erections, and they should promptly report any symptoms to their prescribers. Tell patient not to exceed 25 mg of sildenafil in a 48-hour period.
● Advise patient to report use of other drugs, including OTC drugs; ritonavir interacts with many drugs.
● Advise woman not to breast-feed to prevent transmission of infection.

# saquinavir
Fortovase

# saquinavir mesylate
Invirase

*Pregnancy risk category B*

**AVAILABLE FORMS**
**saquinavir**
*Capsules (soft gelatin):* 200 mg
**saquinavir mesylate**
*Capsules (hard gelatin):* 200 mg

**INDICATIONS & DOSAGES**
➤ **Adjunct treatment of advanced HIV infection in selected patients**
*Adults:* 600 mg (Invirase) or 1,200 mg (Fortovase) P.O. t.i.d. taken within 2 hours

after a full meal and with a nucleoside analogue such as zalcitabine at a dose of 0.75 mg P.O. t.i.d. or zidovudine at a dose of 200 mg P.O. t.i.d.

## ACTION
Inhibits the activity of HIV protease and prevents the cleavage of HIV polyproteins, which are essential for HIV maturation.

| Route | Onset | Peak | Duration |
|-------|-------|------|----------|
| P.O. | Unknown | Unknown | Unknown |

## ADVERSE REACTIONS
**CNS:** paresthesia, headache, dizziness, asthenia, numbness, depression, insomnia, anxiety.
**CV:** chest pain.
**GI:** *diarrhea,* ulcerated buccal mucosa, abdominal pain, *nausea,* dyspepsia, ***pancreatitis,*** flatulence, vomiting, altered taste, constipation.
**Hematologic:** ***pancytopenia, thrombocytopenia.***
**Musculoskeletal:** musculoskeletal pain.
**Respiratory:** bronchitis, cough.
**Skin:** rash.

## INTERACTIONS
**Drug-drug.** *Amprenavir:* May decrease amprenavir level. Use together cautiously.
*Carbamazepine, phenobarbital, phenytoin:* May decrease saquinavir level. Avoid using together.
*Delavirdine:* May increase saquinavir level. Use cautiously and monitor hepatic enzymes. Decrease dose when used together.
*Dexamethasone:* May decrease saquinavir level. Avoid using together.
*Efavirenz:* May decrease levels of both drugs. Avoid using together.
*HMG-CoA reductase inhibitors:* May increase levels of these drugs, which increases risk of myopathy, including rhabdomyolysis. Avoid using together.
*Indinavir, lopinavir and ritonavir combination, nelfinavir, ritonavir:* May increase saquinavir level. Use together cautiously.
*Ketoconazole:* May increase saquinavir level. Don't adjust dosage.
*Macrolide antibiotics, such as clarithromycin:* May increase levels of both drugs. Use together cautiously.
*Nevirapine:* May decrease saquinavir level. Monitor patient.

*Rifabutin, rifampin:* May decrease saquinavir level. Use with rifabutin cautiously. Don't use with rifampin.
*Sildenafil:* May increase peak level and exposure of sildenafil to the body. Reduce first dose of sildenafil to 25 mg when giving with saquinavir.
**Drug-herb.** *Garlic supplements:* May decrease saquinavir level by about 50%. Discourage use together.
*St. John's wort:* May substantially reduce drug level, which could cause loss of therapeutic effects. Discourage use together.
**Drug-food.** *Any food:* May increase drug absorption. Advise patient to take drug with food.
*Grapefruit juice:* May increase drug level. Take with liquid other than grapefruit juice.

## EFFECTS ON LAB TEST RESULTS
● May decrease WBC, RBC, and platelet counts.

## CONTRAINDICATIONS & CAUTIONS
● Contraindicated in patients hypersensitive to drug or its components.
● Safety of drug hasn't been established in pregnant or breast-feeding women or in children younger than age 16. Use cautiously in these patients.

## NURSING CONSIDERATIONS
● *Alert:* Don't confuse the two forms of this drug because dosages are different.
● Invirase will be phased out over time and completely replaced by Fortovase.
● Evaluate CBC, platelets, electrolytes, uric acid, liver enzymes, and bilirubin before therapy begins and at appropriate intervals throughout therapy.
● If serious toxicity occurs during treatment, stop drug until cause is identified or toxicity resolves. Drug may be resumed with no dosage modifications.
● Monitor patient's hydration if adverse GI reactions occur.
● Monitor patient for adverse reactions to adjunct therapy (zidovudine or zalcitabine).

## PATIENT TEACHING
● Advise patient to take drug with food or within 2 hours of a full meal to increase drug absorption.

---

Reactions may be *common,* uncommon, *life-threatening,* or COMMON AND LIFE-THREATENING.

• Inform patient that drug is usually given with other AIDS-related antivirals.
• Instruct patient to avoid missing any doses, to decrease the risk of developing HIV resistance.
• Inform patient to change from Invirase to Fortovase capsules only under prescriber's supervision.
• Advise patient receiving sildenafil of an increased risk of sildenafil-associated adverse events, including low blood pressure, visual changes, and painful erections, and to promptly report any symptoms to his prescriber. Tell patient not to exceed 25 mg of sildenafil in a 48-hour period.
• Tell patient to store Fortovase capsules in the refrigerator; Invirase capsules can be kept at room temperature.

---

## stavudine (2,3 didehydro-3-deoxythymidine, d4T)
Zerit, Zerit XR

*Pregnancy risk category C*

---

### AVAILABLE FORMS
*Capsules:* 15 mg, 20 mg, 30 mg, 40 mg
*Capsules (extended-release):* 37.5 mg, 50 mg, 75 mg, 100 mg
*Oral solution:* 1 mg/ml

### INDICATIONS & DOSAGES
➤ **HIV-infection in combination with other antiretrovirals**
*Adults weighing 60 kg (132 lb) or more:* 40 mg P.O. regular-release q 12 hours or 100 mg P.O. extended-release once daily.
*Adults weighing 30 kg (66 lb) to 60 kg:* 30 mg P.O. regular-release q 12 hours or 75 mg P.O. extended-release once daily.
*Children weighing 60 kg or more:* 40 mg P.O. regular-release q 12 hours.
*Children weighing 30 kg to 60 kg:* 30 mg P.O. regular-release q 12 hours.
*Children 14 days or older weighing less than 30 kg:* 1 mg/kg P.O. regular-release q 12 hours.
*Newborns 0 to 13 days old:* 0.5 mg/kg P.O. regular-release q 12 hours.
*Adjust-a-dose:* For patients experiencing peripheral neuropathy, withdraw temporarily, then resume therapy at 50% re-

commended dose. Consider discontinuing therapy if neuropathy recurs.
For patients with creatinine clearance 26 to 50 ml/minute, adjust dosage to 20 mg (if weight exceeds 60 kg) or 15 mg (if weight is less than 60 kg) P.O. q 12 hours; if clearance is 10 to 25 ml/minute, 20 mg (if weight exceeds 60 kg) or 15 mg (if weight is less than 60 kg) P.O. q 24 hours.
Don't use extended-release form in patients with creatinine clearance of 50 ml/minute or less.

### ACTION
A thymidine nucleoside analogue that prevents replication of retroviruses, including HIV, by inhibiting the enzyme reverse transcriptase and causing termination of DNA chain growth.

| Route | Onset | Peak | Duration |
|-------|-------|------|----------|
| P.O. | Unknown | 1 hr | Unknown |

### ADVERSE REACTIONS
**CNS:** peripheral neuropathy, *fever,* headache, malaise, insomnia, anxiety, *asthenia,* depression, nervousness, dizziness.
**CV:** chest pain.
**EENT:** conjunctivitis.
**GI:** *abdominal pain, diarrhea, nausea, vomiting, anorexia,* dyspepsia, constipation, *pancreatitis.*
**Hematologic:** *neutropenia, thrombocytopenia,* anemia.
**Hepatic:** *hepatotoxicity, severe hepatomegaly with steatosis.*
**Metabolic:** weight loss, *lactic acidosis.*
**Musculoskeletal:** *arthralgia, myalgia, back pain.*
**Respiratory:** *dyspnea.*
**Skin:** *rash, diaphoresis, pruritus,* maculopapular rash.
**Other:** *chills.*

### INTERACTIONS
**Drug-drug.** *Methadone:* May decrease stavudine absorption and concentration. Separate dosage times and monitor for clinical effect if drugs must be used together.
*Zidovudine:* May inhibit phosphorylation of stavudine. Avoid using together.

## EFFECTS ON LAB TEST RESULTS
● May increase ALT and AST levels.
● May decrease hemoglobin and neutrophil and platelet counts.

## CONTRAINDICATIONS & CAUTIONS
● Contraindicated in patients hypersensitive to drug.
● Use cautiously in patients with renal impairment or history of peripheral neuropathy. Adjust dosage for creatinine clearance below 50 ml/minute; adjust dosage or stop drug in patients with peripheral neuropathy.
● Use cautiously in pregnant women; fatal lactic acidosis has been reported in pregnant women who received stavudine and didanosine with other antiretrovirals.
● Safety and efficacy of extended-release form in children haven't been established. Don't give extended-release form to children.

## NURSING CONSIDERATIONS
● Monitor patient for signs and symptoms of pancreatitis, especially if he takes stavudine with didanosine or hydroxyurea. If patient has pancreatitis, reinstate drug cautiously.
● Monitor liver function test results.
● **Alert:** Motor weakness, mimicking the clinical presentation of Guillain-Barré syndrome (including respiratory failure) in HIV patients taking stavudine along with other antiretrovirals has been reported. Most of the cases were reported in the setting of lactic acidosis. Monitor patient for factors of lactic acidosis, including generalized fatigue, GI problems, tachypnea, or dyspnea. Symptoms may continue or worsen when drug is stopped. Patients with these symptoms should promptly interrupt antiretroviral therapy and rapidly receive a full medical work-up. Consider permanent discontinuation of stavudine.
● **Alert:** Peripheral neuropathy appears to be the major dose-limiting adverse effect of stavudine. It may or may not resolve after drug is stopped.
● Monitor CBC results and creatinine.

## PATIENT TEACHING
● Tell patient that drug may be taken without regard to meals.

● Warn patient not to take other drugs for HIV or AIDS unless prescriber has approved them.
● Teach patient signs and symptoms of peripheral neuropathy (pain, burning, aching, weakness, or pins and needles in the limbs) and tell him to report these immediately.
● Tell patient to report symptoms of lactic acidosis, including fatigue, GI problems, dyspnea, or tachypnea.
● Tell patient to report symptoms of pancreatitis, including abdominal pain, nausea, vomiting, weight loss, or fatty stools.
● Tell patient to monitor weight patterns and report weight loss or gain.
● Explain to patient who has difficulty swallowing that extended-release capsules can be opened and contents mixed with 2 tablespoons of yogurt or applesauce. Caution patient not to chew or crush the beads while swallowing.

# tenofovir disoproxil fumarate
Viread

*Pregnancy risk category B*

## AVAILABLE FORMS
*Tablets:* 300 mg as the fumarate salt (equivalent to 245 mg of tenofovir disoproxil)

## INDICATIONS & DOSAGES
➤ **HIV-1 infection, with other antiretrovirals**
*Adults:* 300 mg P.O. once daily with a meal. When given with didanosine, give 2 hours before or 1 hour after didanosine.

## ACTION
Hydrolyzed to produce tenofovir, a nucleoside analogue of adenosine monophosphate that yields tenofovir diphosphate. Tenofovir diphosphate inhibits HIV replication.

| Route | Onset | Peak | Duration |
|---|---|---|---|
| P.O. | Unknown | 1-2 hr | Unknown |

## ADVERSE REACTIONS
**CNS:** asthenia, headache.
**GI:** abdominal pain, anorexia, diarrhea, flatulence, *nausea,* vomiting.

**GU:** glycosuria.
**Hematologic:** *neutropenia.*
**Metabolic:** hyperglycemia.

### INTERACTIONS
**Drug-drug.** *Didanosine (buffered formulation):* May increase didanosine bioavailability. Monitor patient for didanosine-related adverse effects, such as bone marrow suppression, GI distress, and peripheral neuropathy. Give tenofovir 2 hours before or 1 hour after didanosine.
*Drugs that reduce renal function or compete for renal tubular secretion (acyclovir, cidofovir, ganciclovir, valacyclovir, valganciclovir):* May increase levels of tenofovir or other renally eliminated drugs. Monitor patient for adverse effects.

### EFFECTS ON LAB TEST RESULTS
• May increase amylase, AST, ALT, creatinine kinase, serum and urine glucose, creatinine, phosphaturia, and triglyceride levels.
• May decrease neutrophil count.

### CONTRAINDICATIONS & CAUTIONS
• Contraindicated in patients hypersensitive to any component of the drug. Don't use in patients with creatinine clearance less than 60 ml/minute.
• Use very cautiously in patients with risk factors for liver disease or with hepatic impairment.
• Because the effects of tenofovir on pregnant women aren't known, give this drug to pregnant women only if its benefits clearly outweigh the risks.
• It's unknown if tenofovir appears in breast milk. Use cautiously in breast-feeding women.
• Safety and efficacy haven't been studied in children. Don't use drug in children.

### NURSING CONSIDERATIONS
• *Alert:* Antiretrovirals, alone or combined, have been linked to lactic acidosis and severe (including fatal) hepatomegaly with steatosis. These effects may occur without elevated transaminase levels. Risk factors may include long-term antiretroviral use, obesity, and being female. Monitor all patients for hepatotoxicity, including lactic acidosis and hepatomegaly with steatosis.

• Antiretrovirals may cause body fat to accumulate and be redistributed, resulting in central obesity, peripheral wasting, and a buffalo hump. The long-term effects of these changes are unknown. Monitor patient for changes in body fat.
• Tenofovir may be linked to osteomalacia and decreased bone mineral density and increased creatinine and phosphaturia levels. Monitor patient carefully during long-term treatment.
• Drug may lead to decreased HIV-1 RNA level and CD4+ cell counts.
• The effects of tenofovir on the progression of HIV infection are unknown.
• Use tenofovir cautiously in elderly patients because these patients are more likely to have renal impairment and concurrent drug therapy.
• Because of a high rate of early virologic resistance, triple antiretroviral therapy with abacavir, lamivudine, and tenofovir shouldn't be used as new treatment regimen for naive or pretreated patient. Monitor patients currently controlled with this combination and those who use this combination in addition to other antiretrovirals, and consider modification of therapy.

### PATIENT TEACHING
• Instruct patient to take tenofovir with a meal to enhance bioavailability.
• If patient takes tenofovir and didanosine (buffered form), instruct him to take tenofovir 2 hours before or 1 hour after didanosine.
• Tell patient to report adverse effects, including nausea, vomiting, diarrhea, flatulence, and headache.

---

## valacyclovir hydrochloride
Valtrex

*Pregnancy risk category B*

---

### AVAILABLE FORMS
*Tablets:* 500 mg, 1,000 mg

### INDICATIONS & DOSAGES
➤ **Herpes zoster infection (shingles)**
*Adults:* 1 g P.O. t.i.d. for 7 days.
*Adjust-a-dose:* For patients with creatinine clearance 30 to 49 ml/minute, give 1 g P.O. q 12 hours; if clearance is 10 to

29 ml/minute, give 1 g P.O. q 24 hours; if clearance is less than 10 ml/minute, give 500 mg P.O. q 24 hours.

➤ **First episode of genital herpes**
*Adults:* 1 g P.O. b.i.d. for 10 days.
*Adjust-a-dose:* For patients with creatinine clearance 10 to 29 ml/minute, give 1 g P.O. q 24 hours; if clearance is below 10 ml/minute, give 500 mg P.O. q 24 hours.

➤ **Recurrent genital herpes in immunocompetent patients**
*Adults:* 500 mg P.O. b.i.d. for 3 days, given at the first sign or symptom of an episode.
*Adjust-a-dose:* For patients with creatinine clearance of 29 ml/minute or less, give 500 mg P.O. q 24 hours.

➤ **Long-term suppression of recurrent genital herpes**
*Adults:* 1 g P.O. once daily. In patients with a history of nine or fewer recurrences per year, use alternative dose of 500 mg once daily.
*Adjust-a-dose:* For patients with creatinine clearance of 29 ml/minute or less, 500 mg P.O. q 24 hours; q 48 hours if patient has nine or fewer occurrences per year.

➤ **Cold sores (herpes labialis)**
*Adults:* 2 g P.O. q 12 hours for 2 doses.
*Adjust-a-dose:* For patients with creatinine clearance of 30 to 49 ml/minute, give 1 g q 12 hours for two doses; if clearance is 10 to 29 ml/minute, give 500 mg q 12 hours for two doses; if clearance is less than 10 ml/minute, give 500 mg as a single dose.

✳ *NEW INDICATION:* **Long-term suppression of recurrent genital herpes in HIV-infected patients with CD4 cell count of 100 cells/mm³ or more**
*Adults:* 500 mg P.O. b.i.d. Safety and efficacy of therapy beyond 6 months hasn't been established.
*Adjust-a-dose:* For patients with creatinine clearance 29 ml/minute or less, give 500 mg P.O. q 24 hours.

✳ *NEW INDICATION:* **To reduce transmission of genital herpes in patients with history of nine or fewer occurrences per year**
*Adults:* 500 mg P.O. daily.

**ACTION**
Rapidly converts to acyclovir, which in turn becomes incorporated into viral DNA, thereby terminating growth of the DNA chain; inhibits viral DNA polymerase, causing inhibition of viral replication.

| Route | Onset | Peak | Duration |
|-------|-------|------|----------|
| P.O. | 30 min | Unknown | Unknown |

**ADVERSE REACTIONS**
**CNS:** *headache,* dizziness, depression.
**GI:** *nausea,* vomiting, diarrhea, abdominal pain.
**GU:** dysmenorrhea.
**Musculoskeletal:** arthralgia.

**INTERACTIONS**
**Drug-drug.** *Cimetidine, probenecid:* May reduce rate but not extent of conversion of valacyclovir to acyclovir and may decrease renal clearance of acyclovir, thus increasing acyclovir level. Monitor patient for acyclovir toxicity.

**EFFECTS ON LAB TEST RESULTS**
• May increase AST, ALT, alkaline phosphatase, and creatinine levels.
• May decrease hemoglobin and WBC and platelet counts.

**CONTRAINDICATIONS & CAUTIONS**
• Contraindicated in patients hypersensitive to or intolerant of valacyclovir, acyclovir, or components of the formulation.
• *Alert:* Valacyclovir isn't recommended for use in patients with HIV infection or in bone marrow or renal transplant recipients because of the occurrence of thrombotic thrombocytopenic purpura and hemolytic uremic syndrome in these patients at doses of 8 g/day.
• Use cautiously in elderly patients, those with renal impairment, and those receiving other nephrotoxic drugs. Monitor renal function test results.
• Consider use of drug during pregnancy only if the benefits outweigh the risks.
• If patient is breast-feeding, drug may need to be discontinued.
• Safety and efficacy in prepubertal children haven't been established.

---

Reactions may be *common*, uncommon, *life-threatening*, or COMMON AND LIFE-THREATENING.

## NURSING CONSIDERATIONS
● *Alert:* Don't confuse valacyclovir (Valtrex) with valganciclovir (Valcyte).
● Although there are no reports of overdose, precipitation of acyclovir in renal tubules may occur when solubility (2.5 mg/ml) is exceeded in the intratubular fluid. With acute renal failure and anuria, the patient may benefit from hemodialysis until renal function is restored.

## PATIENT TEACHING
● Inform patient that valacyclovir may be taken without regard to meals.
● Teach patient the signs and symptoms of herpes infection (rash, tingling, itching, and pain), and advise him to notify prescriber immediately if they occur. Treatment should begin as soon as possible after symptoms appear, preferably within 48 hours of the onset of zoster rash.
● Tell patient that valacyclovir isn't a cure for herpes but may decrease the length and severity of symptoms.

---

# valganciclovir
Valcyte

*Pregnancy risk category C*

---

## AVAILABLE FORMS
*Tablets:* 450 mg

## INDICATIONS & DOSAGES
➤ **Active CMV retinitis in patients with AIDS**
*Adults:* 900 mg (two 450-mg tablets) P.O. b.i.d. with food for 21 days; maintenance dose is 900 mg (two 450-mg tablets) P.O. daily with food.
➤ **Inactive CMV retinitis**
*Adults:* 900 mg (two 450-mg tablets) P.O. daily with food.
*Adjust-a-dose:* For patients with creatinine clearance 40 to 59 ml/minute, induction dose is 450 mg b.i.d.; maintenance dose is 450 mg daily. If clearance is 25 to 39 ml/minute, induction dose is 450 mg daily; maintenance dose is 450 mg q 2 days. If clearance is 10 to 24 ml/minute, induction dose is 450 mg q 2 days; maintenance dose is 450 mg twice weekly.

## ACTION
Drug is converted to the active drug ganciclovir, which inhibits replication of CMV.

| Route | Onset | Peak | Duration |
|-------|-------|------|----------|
| P.O. | Unknown | 1-3 hr | Unknown |

## ADVERSE REACTIONS
**CNS:** *headache, insomnia,* peripheral neuropathy, paresthesia, *pyrexia,* **seizures,** psychosis, hallucinations, confusion, agitation.
**EENT:** *retinal detachment.*
**GI:** *diarrhea, nausea, vomiting, abdominal pain.*
**Hematologic:** NEUTROPENIA, *anemia,* **thrombocytopenia, pancytopenia, bone marrow depression, aplastic anemia.**
**Other:** catheter-related infection, *sepsis,* local or systemic infections, hypersensitivity reactions.

## INTERACTIONS
**Drug-drug.** *Didanosine:* May increase absorption of didanosine. Monitor patient closely for didanosine toxicity.
*Immunosuppressants, zidovudine:* May enhance neutropenia, anemia, thrombocytopenia, and bone marrow depression. Monitor CBC results.
*Mycophenolate mofetil:* May increase levels of both drugs in renally impaired patients. Use together cautiously.
*Probenecid:* May decrease renal clearance of ganciclovir. Monitor patient for ganciclovir toxicity.
**Drug-food.** *Any food:* May increase absorption of drug. Give drug with food.

## EFFECTS ON LAB TEST RESULTS
● May decrease hemoglobin, hematocrit, and RBC, WBC, neutrophil, and platelet counts.

## CONTRAINDICATIONS & CAUTIONS
● Contraindicated in patients with hypersensitivity to valganciclovir or ganciclovir. Don't use in patients receiving hemodialysis.
● Use cautiously in patients with preexisting cytopenias and in those who have received immunosuppressants or radiation.

---

## NURSING CONSIDERATIONS
- Make sure to adhere to dosing guidelines for valganciclovir because ganciclovir and valganciclovir aren't interchangeable and overdose may occur.
- Clinical toxicities include severe leukopenia, neutropenia, anemia, pancytopenia, bone marrow depression, aplastic anemia, and thrombocytopenia. Don't use if patient's absolute neutrophil count is less than 500 cells/mm³, platelets are less than 25,000/mm³, or hemoglobin is less than 8 g/dl.
- Monitor CBC, platelet counts, and creatinine level or creatinine clearance values frequently during treatment.
- Cytopenia may occur at any time during treatment and increase with continued dosing. Cell counts usually recover 3 to 7 days after stopping drug.
- No drug interaction studies have been conducted with valganciclovir; however, because drug is converted to ganciclovir, it can be assumed that drug interactions would be similar.
- Drug may cause temporary or permanent inhibition of spermatogenesis.
- **Alert:** Don't confuse valganciclovir hydrochloride (Valcyte) with valacyclovir (Valtrex).

## PATIENT TEACHING
- Tell patient to take drug with food.
- Tell patient to follow dosing instructions precisely. Ganciclovir capsules and valganciclovir tablets are not interchangeable on a one-to-one basis.
- Advise patient that blood tests are needed during treatment. Doses may need to be adjusted based on blood counts.
- Tell woman of childbearing age to use contraception during treatment. Inform man that he should use barrier contraception during and for 90 days after treatment.
- Advise patient that ganciclovir is considered a potential carcinogen.
- Tell patient that CNS effects (seizures, ataxia, dizziness) can occur and to use care in driving or operating machinery.
- Advise patient that this drug isn't a cure for CMV retinitis and that the condition may recur. Tell patient to have ophthalmologic examinations at least every 4 to 6 weeks during treatment.

# zalcitabine (ddC, dideoxycytidine)
Hivid

*Pregnancy risk category C*

## AVAILABLE FORMS
*Tablets:* 0.375 mg, 0.75 mg

## INDICATIONS & DOSAGES
➤ **Treatment of HIV disease in combination with other antiretrovirals**
*Adults and adolescents age 13 and older:* 0.75 mg P.O. q 8 hours.
*Adjust-a-dose:* For patients with creatinine clearance 10 to 40 ml/minute, give 0.75 mg P.O. q 12 hours; if clearance is less than 10 ml/minute, give 0.75 mg P.O. q 24 hours. If patient has moderate discomfort and signs and symptoms of peripheral neuropathy, stop drug temporarily. If symptoms improve after stopping therapy, drug may be reintroduced at 0.375 mg P.O. q 8 hours.

## ACTION
Nucleoside reverse transcriptase inhibitor that inhibits replication of HIV by blocking viral DNA synthesis.

| Route | Onset | Peak | Duration |
|-------|-------|------|----------|
| P.O. | Unknown | 1-2 hr | Unknown |

## ADVERSE REACTIONS
**CNS:** *peripheral neuropathy, headache, fatigue,* dizziness, *fever,* confusion, *seizures,* impaired concentration, amnesia, insomnia, mental depression, tremor, hypertonia, anxiety.
**CV:** cardiomyopathy, *heart failure,* chest pain.
**EENT:** pharyngitis, ocular pain, abnormal vision, ototoxicity, nasal discharge.
**GI:** nausea, vomiting, diarrhea, abdominal pain, anorexia, constipation, stomatitis, esophageal ulcer, glossitis, *pancreatitis.*
**Hematologic:** anemia, *neutropenia, leukopenia, thrombocytopenia.*
**Metabolic:** *hypoglycemia.*
**Musculoskeletal:** myalgia, arthralgia.
**Respiratory:** cough.
**Skin:** pruritus; night sweats; *erythematous, maculopapular, or follicular rash;* urticaria.

## INTERACTIONS
**Drug-drug.** *Aminoglycosides, amphotericin B, foscarnet, other drugs that may impair renal function:* May increase risk of nephrotoxicity. Monitor renal function.
*Antacids containing aluminum or magnesium:* May decrease bioavailability of zalcitabine. Separate dosage times.
*Chloramphenicol, cisplatin, dapsone, didanosine, disulfiram, ethionamide, glutethimide, gold salts, hydralazine, iodoquinol, isoniazid, metronidazole, nitrofurantoin, other drugs that can cause peripheral neuropathy, phenytoin, ribavirin, stavudine, vincristine:* May increase risk of peripheral neuropathy. Avoid using together.
*Cimetidine, probenecid:* May increase zalcitabine level. Monitor patient closely.
*Pentamidine:* May increase risk of pancreatitis. Avoid using together.
**Drug-food.** *Any food:* May decrease rate of absorption. Give drug on an empty stomach.

## EFFECTS ON LAB TEST RESULTS
• May increase glucose, alkaline phosphatase, ALT, and AST levels.
• May decrease hemoglobin and neutrophil, WBC, and platelet counts.

## CONTRAINDICATIONS & CAUTIONS
• Contraindicated in patients hypersensitive to drug or its components.
• Use with extreme caution in patients with peripheral neuropathy.
• Use cautiously in patients with hepatic failure, history of pancreatitis or heart failure, or baseline cardiomyopathy. Monitor liver function test results and pancreatic enzymes.

## NURSING CONSIDERATIONS
• *Alert:* Occasionally fatal cases of lactic acidosis, severe hepatomegaly with steatosis, and hepatic failure have been reported. Monitor patient closely.
• Toxic effects of drug may cause abnormalities in several laboratory tests, including CBC, hemoglobin, leukocyte, reticulocyte, granulocyte, and platelet counts; and AST, ALT, and alkaline phosphatase levels.
• Don't give drug with food because it decreases the rate and extent of absorption.

• Assess patients for signs and symptoms of peripheral neuropathy, characterized by numbness and burning in the limbs, the drug's major toxic effects. If drug isn't withdrawn, peripheral neuropathy can progress to sharp shooting pain or severe continuous burning pain requiring opioid analgesics. The pain may or may not be reversible.
• *Alert:* Don't confuse drug with other antivirals identified by initials.

## PATIENT TEACHING
• Instruct patient to take drug on an empty stomach.
• Make sure patient understands that the drug doesn't cure HIV infection and that opportunistic infections may occur despite continued use. Review safe sex practices with patient.
• Inform patient that peripheral neuropathy is the major toxic condition associated with drug and that inflammation of the pancreas is the major life-threatening toxic reaction. Review the signs and symptoms of these adverse reactions, and tell patient to call prescriber promptly if any appear.
• Advise patient of childbearing age to use an effective contraceptive while taking drug.

## zanamivir
Relenza

*Pregnancy risk category C*

## AVAILABLE FORMS
*Powder for inhalation:* 5 mg/blister

## INDICATIONS & DOSAGES
➤ **Uncomplicated acute illness caused by influenza virus A and B in patients who have had symptoms for no longer than 2 days**
*Adults and children age 7 and older:* 2 oral inhalations (one 5-mg blister per inhalation for total dose of 10 mg) b.i.d. using the Diskhaler inhalation device for 5 days. Give two doses on first day of treatment, allowing at least 2 hours to elapse between doses. Give subsequent doses about 12 hours apart (in the morning and evening) at about the same time each day.

## ACTION
Likely exerts its antiviral action by inhibiting neuraminidase on the surface of the influenza virus, potentially altering virus particle aggregation and release.

| Route | Onset | Peak | Duration |
|-------|-------|------|----------|
| Inhalation | Unknown | 1-2 hr | Unknown |

## ADVERSE REACTIONS
**CNS:** headache, dizziness.
**EENT:** nasal signs and symptoms; sinusitis; ear, nose, and throat infections.
**GI:** diarrhea, nausea, vomiting.
**Respiratory:** bronchitis, cough.

## INTERACTIONS
None significant.

## EFFECTS ON LAB TEST RESULTS
• May increase liver enzyme and CK levels.
• May decrease lymphocyte and neutrophil counts.

## CONTRAINDICATIONS & CAUTIONS
• Contraindicated in patients hypersensitive to drug or its components.
• Use cautiously in patients with severe or decompensated COPD, asthma, or other underlying respiratory disease.

## NURSING CONSIDERATIONS
• Patients with underlying respiratory disease should have a fast-acting bronchodilator available in case of wheezing while taking zanamivir. Patients scheduled to use an inhaled bronchodilator for asthma should use their bronchodilator before taking zanamivir.
• Safety and efficacy of drug haven't been established in patients who begin treatment after 48 hours of symptoms.
• Safety and efficacy of drug haven't been established for influenza prophylaxis. Use of drug shouldn't affect evaluation of patient for annual influenza vaccination.
• Monitor patient for bronchospasm and decline in lung function. Stop drug in such situations.

## PATIENT TEACHING
• Tell patient to carefully read the instructions for the Diskhaler inhalation device to properly give drug.

• Advise patient to keep the Diskhaler level when loading and inhaling zanamivir. Tell him to always check inside the mouthpiece of the Diskhaler before each use to make sure it's free of foreign objects.
• Tell patient to exhale fully before putting the mouthpiece in his mouth; then, keeping the Diskhaler level, to close his lips around the mouthpiece and breathe in steadily and deeply. Advise patient to hold his breath for a few seconds after inhaling to help drug stay in the lungs.
• Advise patient with respiratory disease who is scheduled to use an inhaled bronchodilator to do so before taking zanamivir. Tell patient to have a fast-acting bronchodilator available in case of wheezing while taking zanamivir.
• Advise patient that it's important to finish the entire 5-day course of treatment even if he starts to feel better and symptoms improve before the fifth day.
• Advise patient that the use of zanamivir hasn't been shown to reduce the risk of transmission of influenza virus to others.

---

# zidovudine (azidothymidine, AZT)
Apo-Zidovudine†, Novo-AZT†, Retrovir🍁

*Pregnancy risk category C*

## AVAILABLE FORMS
*Capsules:* 100 mg
*Injection:* 10 mg/ml
*Syrup:* 50 mg/5 ml
*Tablets:* 300 mg

## INDICATIONS & DOSAGES
➤ **HIV infection in combination with other antiretrovirals**
*Adults:* 600 mg daily P.O. in divided doses. If patient unable to tolerate oral zidovudine, give 1 mg/kg I.V. over 1 hour five to six times daily.
*Children ages 6 weeks to 12 years:* 160 mg/m$^2$ q 8 hours (480 mg/m$^2$/day up to a maximum of 200 mg q 8 hours) in combination with other antiretrovirals. Some prescribers recommend 120 mg/m$^2$ I.V. q 6 hours, or 20 mg/m$^2$/hour continuous I.V. infusion.

➤ **To prevent maternal-fetal transmission of HIV**

*Pregnant women more than 14 weeks' gestation:* 100 mg P.O. five times daily until the start of labor. Then, 2 mg/kg I.V. over 1 hour followed by a continuous I.V. infusion of 1 mg/kg/hour until the umbilical cord is clamped.

*Neonates:* 2 mg/kg P.O. q 6 hours starting within 12 hours after birth and continuing until 6 weeks old. Or, give 1.5 mg/kg via I.V. infusion over 30 minutes q 6 hours.

*Adjust-a-dose:* In patients with significant anemia (hemoglobin less than 7.5 g/dl or more than 25% below baseline) or significant neutropenia (granulocyte count less than 750 cells/mm³ or more than 50% below baseline), interrupt therapy until evidence proves marrow has recovered.

In patients on hemodialysis or peritoneal dialysis, give 100 mg P.O. or 1 mg/kg I.V. q 6 to 8 hours.

For patients with mild to moderate hepatic dysfunction or liver cirrhosis, daily dose may need to be reduced.

## I.V. ADMINISTRATION
● Remove the calculated dose from the vial; add to D₅W to achieve a concentration no greater than 4 mg/ml.
● Infuse drug over 1 hour at a constant rate. Avoid rapid infusion or bolus injection. Don't add mixture to biological or colloidal fluids (such as blood products and protein solutions).
● Give by I.V. route only until oral therapy can be tolerated.
● Protect undiluted vials from light.

## ACTION
Nucleoside reverse transcriptase inhibitor that inhibits replication of HIV by blocking DNA synthesis.

| Route | Onset | Peak | Duration |
|-------|-------|------|----------|
| P.O., I.V. | Unknown | 30-90 min | Unknown |

## ADVERSE REACTIONS
**CNS:** *headache, seizures,* paresthesia, *malaise,* insomnia, *asthenia, dizziness,* somnolence, *fever.*
**GI:** nausea, anorexia, abdominal pain, vomiting, constipation, diarrhea, taste perversion, dyspepsia, *pancreatitis.*

**Hematologic:** *severe bone marrow suppression,* anemia, *agranulocytosis, thrombocytopenia.*
**Metabolic:** lactic acidosis.
**Musculoskeletal:** myalgia.
**Skin:** *rash,* diaphoresis.

## INTERACTIONS
**Drug-drug.** *Atovaquone, fluconazole, methadone, probenecid, valproic acid:* May increase bioavailability of zidovudine. May need to adjust dosage.
*Doxorubicin, ribavirin, stavudine:* May have antagonistic effects. Avoid using together.
*Ganciclovir, interferon alfa, other bone marrow suppressive or cytotoxic drugs:* May increase hematologic toxicity of zidovudine. Use together cautiously.
*Phenytoin:* May alter phenytoin level and decrease zidovudine clearance by 30%. Monitor patient closely.

## EFFECTS ON LAB TEST RESULTS
● May increase ALT, AST, alkaline phosphatase, and LDH levels.
● May decrease hemoglobin and granulocyte and platelet counts.

## CONTRAINDICATIONS & CAUTIONS
● Contraindicated in patients hypersensitive to drug.
● Use cautiously and with close monitoring in patients with advanced symptomatic HIV infection and in patients with severe bone marrow depression.
● Use with caution in patients with hepatomegaly, hepatitis, or other risk factors for liver disease and in those with renal insufficiency. Monitor renal and liver function tests.

## NURSING CONSIDERATIONS
● *Alert:* Although rare, lactic acidosis without hypoxemia may occur with the use of antiretroviral nucleoside analogues, including zidovudine. Notify prescriber if patient develops unexplained tachypnea, dyspnea, or a decrease in bicarbonate level. Drug therapy may need to be suspended until lactic acidosis is ruled out.
● Monitor blood studies every 2 weeks to detect anemia or agranulocytosis. Patients may need dosage reduction or temporary discontinuation of drug.

---

• Drug may temporarily decrease morbidity and mortality in certain patients with AIDS.

**PATIENT TEACHING**
• Tell patient to take drug exactly as directed and not to share it with others.
• Instruct patient to take drug on an empty stomach. To avoid esophageal irritation, tell patient to take drug while sitting upright and with adequate fluids.
• Remind patient to comply with the dosage schedule. Suggest ways to avoid missing doses, perhaps by using an alarm clock.
• Advise patient that blood transfusions may be needed during treatment. Zidovudine often causes a low RBC count.
• Tell patient that dosages vary among patients and not to change his dosing instructions unless directed to do so by his prescriber.
• Tell patient that his gums may bleed. Recommend good mouth care with a soft toothbrush.
• Warn patient not to take other drugs for AIDS unless prescriber has approved them.
• Advise pregnant, HIV-infected patient that drug therapy only reduces the risk of HIV transmission to her newborn. Long-term risks to infants are unknown.
• Advise patient that monotherapy isn't recommended and to discuss any questions with prescriber.
• Advise health care worker considering zidovudine prophylaxis after occupational exposure (such as needle-stick injury) that drug's safety or efficacy hasn't been established.
• Tell patient not to keep capsules in the kitchen, bathroom, or other places that may be damp or hot. Heat and moisture may cause the drug to break down and affect the intended results.

azithromycin
clarithromycin
erythromycin base
erythromycin estolate
erythromycin ethylsuccinate
erythromycin lactobionate
erythromycin stearate

**COMBINATION PRODUCTS**
ERYZOLE, PEDIAZOLE: erythromycin
(200 mg) and sulfisoxazole (600 mg)/
5 ml.

---

## azithromycin
Zithromax*⌖*

*Pregnancy risk category B*

**AVAILABLE FORMS**
*Injection:* 500 mg
*Powder for oral suspension:* 100 mg/5 ml,
200 mg/5 ml; 1,000 mg/packet
*Tablets:* 250 mg, 500 mg, 600 mg

**INDICATIONS & DOSAGES**
➤ **Acute bacterial worsening of COPD
caused by *Haemophilus influenzae,
Moraxella catarrhalis,* or *Streptococcus
pneumoniae;* uncomplicated skin and
skin structure infections caused by
*Staphylococcus aureus, Streptococcus
pyogenes,* or *Streptococcus agalactiae;*
second-line therapy for pharyngitis or
tonsillitis caused by *Staphylococcus
pyogenes***
*Adults and adolescents age 16 and older:*
Initially, 500 mg P.O. as a single dose on
day 1, followed by 250 mg daily on days
2 through 5. Total cumulative dose is
1.5 g. Or, for worsening COPD, 500 mg
P.O. daily for 3 days.
➤ **Community-acquired pneumonia
caused by *Chlamydia pneumoniae,
H. influenzae, Mycoplasma pneumoniae,*
or *S. pneumoniae;* or caused by *Legionella pneumophila, M. catarrhalis,*
or *S. aureus***
*Adults and adolescents age 16 and older:*
For mild infections, give 500 mg P.O. as a

single dose on day 1; then 250 mg P.O.
daily on days 2 through 5. Total dose is
1.5 g. For more severe infections or those
caused by *S. aureus,* give 500 mg I.V. as a
single daily dose for 2 days; then 500 mg
P.O. as a single daily dose to complete a
7- to 10-day course of therapy. Switch
from I.V. to P.O. therapy at the prescriber's
discretion and based on patient's clinical
response.
➤ **Community-acquired pneumonia
caused by *Chlamydia pneumoniae,
H. influenzae, Mycoplasma pneumoniae,
S. pneumoniae***
*Children 6 months and older:* 10 mg/kg
P.O. (maximum of 500 mg) as a single
dose on day 1, followed by 5 mg/kg
(maximum of 250 mg) daily on days 2
through 5.
➤ **Chancroid**
*Adults:* 1 g P.O. as a single dose.
*Infants and children ♦ :* 20 mg/kg (maximum of 1 g) P.O. as a single dose.
➤ **Nongonococcal urethritis or cervicitis caused by *C. trachomatis***
*Adults and adolescents age 16 and older:*
1 g P.O. as a single dose.
➤ **To prevent disseminated *Mycobacterium avium* complex in patients with
advanced HIV infection**
*Adults and adolescents:* 1.2 g P.O. once
weekly alone or in combination with rifabutin.
*Infants and children ♦ :* 20 mg/kg P.O.
(maximum of 1.2 g) weekly or 5 mg/kg
(maximum of 250 mg) can be given P.O.
daily. Children 6 years and older may also
receive rifabutin 300 mg P.O. daily.
➤ ***Mycobacterium avium* complex in patients with advanced HIV infection**
*Adults:* 600 mg P.O. daily with ethambutol
15 mg/kg daily.
➤ **Urethritis and cervicitis caused by
*Neisseria gonorrhoeae***
*Adults:* 2 g P.O. as a single dose.
➤ **Pelvic inflammatory disease caused
by *C. trachomatis, N. gonorrhoeae,* or**

---

*Mycoplasma hominis* in patients who need initial I.V. therapy
*Adults and adolescents age 16 and older:* 500 mg I.V. as a single daily dose for 1 to 2 days; then 250 mg P.O. daily to complete a 7-day course of therapy. Expect to switch from I.V. to P.O. therapy, based on patient's clinical response.

➤ **Otitis media**
*Children older than 6 months:* 30 mg/kg P.O. as a single dose; or, 10 mg/kg P.O. once daily for 3 days; or, 10 mg/kg P.O. on day 1, then 5 mg/kg once daily on days 2 to 5.

➤ **Pharyngitis, tonsillitis**
*Children age 2 and older:* 12 mg/kg (maximum 500 mg) P.O. daily for 5 days.

➤ **To prevent bacterial endocarditis in penicillin-allergic adults at moderate to high risk ◆**
*Adults:* 500 mg P.O. 1 hour before procedure.
*Children:* 15 mg/kg P.O. 1 hour before procedure. Don't exceed adult dose.

➤ **Chlamydial infections; uncomplicated gonococcal infections of the cervix, urethra, rectum, and pharynx; to prevent such infections after sexual assault ◆**
*Adults:* 1 g P.O. as a single dose, with other agents as recommended by the CDC.

## I.V. ADMINISTRATION
● Reconstitute drug in 500-mg vial with 4.8 ml of sterile water for injection, and shake well until all the drug is dissolved (yields 100 mg/ml).
● Dilute solution further in at least 250 ml of normal saline solution, half-normal saline solution, $D_5W$, or lactated Ringer's solution to yield 1 to 2 mg/ml.
● *Alert:* Infuse a 500-mg dose of azithromycin I.V. over 1 hour or longer. Never give it as a bolus or I.M. injection.

## ACTION
Binds to the 50S subunit of bacterial ribosomes, blocking protein synthesis; bacteriostatic or bactericidal, depending on concentration.

| Route | Onset | Peak | Duration |
|-------|-------|------|----------|
| P.O. | Unknown | 2-5 hr | Unknown |
| I.V. | Unknown | Unknown | Unknown |

## ADVERSE REACTIONS
**CNS:** dizziness, vertigo, headache, fatigue, somnolence.
**CV:** palpitations, chest pain.
**GI:** *nausea, vomiting, diarrhea, abdominal pain,* dyspepsia, flatulence, melena, *pseudomembranous colitis.*
**GU:** candidiasis, vaginitis, nephritis.
**Hepatic:** cholestatic jaundice.
**Skin:** rash, photosensitivity.
**Other:** *angioedema.*

## INTERACTIONS
**Drug-drug.** *Antacids containing aluminum and magnesium:* May lower peak azithromycin level. Separate doses by at least 2 hours.
*Carbamazepine, cyclosporine, phenytoin:* May increase levels of these drugs. Monitor drug levels.
*Digoxin:* May increase digoxin level. Monitor digoxin level.
*Ergotamine:* May cause acute ergotamine toxicity. Monitor patient closely.
*Pimozide:* May prolong QT interval and cause ventricular tachycardia. Monitor patient closely.
*Theophylline:* May increase theophylline level. Monitor theophylline level carefully.
*Triazolam:* May decrease triazolam clearance. Monitor patient closely.
*Warfarin:* May increase INR. Monitor INR carefully.
**Drug-food.** *Any food:* May decrease absorption of multidose oral suspension formulation. Advise patient to take drug on empty stomach.
**Drug-lifestyle.** *Sun exposure:* May cause photosensitivity reactions. Advise patient to avoid excessive sunlight exposure.

## EFFECTS ON LAB TEST RESULTS
None reported.

## CONTRAINDICATIONS & CAUTIONS
● Contraindicated in patients hypersensitive to erythromycin or other macrolides.
● Use cautiously in patients with impaired hepatic function.

## NURSING CONSIDERATIONS
● Obtain specimen for culture and sensitivity tests before giving first dose. Therapy may begin pending results.

---

Reactions may be *common,* uncommon, *life-threatening,* or COMMON AND LIFE-THREATENING.

● Give multidose oral suspension 1 hour before or 2 hours after meals; don't give with antacids. Tablets and single-dose packets for oral suspension can be taken with or without food.

● Monitor patient for superinfection. Drug may cause overgrowth of nonsusceptible bacteria or fungi.

● Reconstitute single-dose, 1-g packets for suspension with 2 ounces (60 ml) water, mixed, and given to patient. Patient should rinse glass with additional 2 ounces water and drink to ensure he has consumed entire dose. Packets aren't for pediatric use.

**PATIENT TEACHING**
● Tell patient that tablets or oral suspension may be taken with or without food.
● Tell patient to take drug as prescribed, even after he feels better.

## clarithromycin
Biaxin⦿, Biaxin XL⦿

*Pregnancy risk category C*

**AVAILABLE FORMS**
*Suspension:* 125 mg/5 ml, 250 mg/5 ml
*Tablets (extended-release):* 500 mg
*Tablets (film-coated):* 250 mg, 500 mg

**INDICATIONS & DOSAGES**
➤ **Pharyngitis or tonsillitis caused by**
*Streptococcus pyogenes*
*Adults:* 250 mg P.O. q 12 hours for 10 days.
*Children:* 15 mg/kg/day P.O. divided q 12 hours for 10 days.
➤ **Acute maxillary sinusitis caused by**
*S. pneumoniae, Haemophilus influenzae,*
*or Moraxella catarrhalis*
*Adults:* 500 mg P.O. q 12 hours for 14 days or two 500-mg extended-release tablets P.O. daily for 14 days.
*Children:* 15 mg/kg/day P.O. divided q 12 hours for 10 days.
➤ **Acute worsening of chronic bronchitis caused by** *M. catarrhalis, S. pneumoniae;* **community-acquired pneumonia caused by** *H. influenzae, S. pneumoniae, Mycoplasma pneumoniae,* **or** *Chlamydia pneumoniae*
*Adults:* 250 mg P.O. q 12 hours for 7 days (*H. influenzae*) or 7 to 14 days (others).

➤ **Acute worsening of chronic bronchitis caused by** *H. influenzae or H. parainfluenzae*
*Adults:* 500 mg P.O. q 12 hours for 7 days (*H. parainfluenzae*) or 7 to 14 days (*H. influenzae*).
➤ **Acute worsening of chronic bronchitis caused by** *M. catarrhalis, S. pneumoniae, H. parainfluenzae,* **or** *H. influenzae*
*Adults:* Two 500-mg P.O. extended-release tablets daily for 7 days.
➤ **Mild-to-moderate community-acquired pneumonia, caused by** *H. influenzae, H. parainfluenzae, M. catarrhalis, S. pneumoniae, C. pneumoniae,* **or** *M. pneumoniae*
*Adults:* Two 500-mg P.O. extended-release tablets daily for 7 days.
➤ **Community-acquired pneumonia caused by** *S. pneumoniae, C. pneumoniae,* **and** *M. pneumoniae*
*Children:* 15 mg/kg/day P.O. divided q 12 hours for 10 days.
➤ **Uncomplicated skin and skin structure infections caused by** *Staphylococcus aureus or S. pyogenes*
*Adults:* 250 mg P.O. q 12 hours for 7 to 14 days.
*Children:* 15 mg/kg/day P.O. divided q 12 hours for 10 days.
➤ **Acute otitis media caused by** *H. influenzae, M. catarrhalis, or S. pneumoniae*
*Children:* 15 mg/kg/day P.O. divided q 12 hours for 10 days.
➤ **To prevent and treat disseminated infection caused by** *Mycobacterium avium* **complex**
*Adults:* 500 mg P.O. b.i.d.
*Children:* 7.5 mg/kg P.O. b.i.d., up to 500 mg b.i.d.
➤ *Helicobacter pylori,* **to reduce risk of duodenal ulcer recurrence**
*Adults:* 500 mg clarithromycin with 30 mg lansoprazole and 1 g amoxicillin, all given q 12 hours for 10 to 14 days. Or, 500 mg clarithromycin with 20 mg omeprazole and 1 g amoxicillin, all given q 12 hours for 10 days. Or, 500 mg clarithromycin b.i.d., 20 mg rabeprazole b.i.d., and 1 g amoxicillin b.i.d., all for 7 days.

Or, two-drug regimen with 500 mg clarithromycin q 8 hours and 40 mg omeprazole once daily for 14 days. Continue omeprazole for 14 additional days.

*Adjust-a-dose:* In patients with creatinine clearance of less than 30 ml/minute, cut dose in half or double frequency interval.

## ACTION
Binds to the 50S subunit of bacterial ribosomes, blocking protein synthesis; bacteriostatic or bactericidal, depending on concentration.

| Route | Onset | Peak | Duration |
|-------|-------|------|----------|
| P.O. | Unknown | 2-4 hr | Unknown |
| P.O. (extended) | Unknown | 5-6 hr | Unknown |

## ADVERSE REACTIONS
**CNS:** headache.
**GI:** diarrhea, nausea, taste perversion, abdominal pain or discomfort, ***pseudomembranous colitis,*** vomiting (pediatric).
**Hematologic:** *leukopenia,* coagulation abnormalities.
**Skin:** rash (pediatric).

## INTERACTIONS
**Drug-drug.** *Alprazolam, midazolam, triazolam:* May decrease clearance of these drugs, causing adverse reactions. Use together cautiously.
*Carbamazepine:* May inhibit metabolism of carbamazepine, increasing carbamazepine level and risk of toxicity. Avoid using together.
*Digoxin:* May increase digoxin level. Monitor patient for digitalis toxicity.
*Dihydroergotamine, ergotamine:* May cause acute ergot toxicity. Avoid using together
*Disopyramide, pimozide, quinidine:* May cause torsades de pointes. Monitor ECG for QTc interval prolongation. Avoid using together.
*Fluconazole:* May increase clarithromycin level. Monitor patient closely.
*HMG-CoA reductase inhibitors:* May increase levels of these drugs; may rarely cause rhabdomyolysis. Use together cautiously.
*Ritonavir:* May prolong absorption of clarithromycin. No dosage adjustment in patients with normal renal function; if creatinine clearance is 30 to 60 ml/minute, give 50% of clarithromycin dose; if less than 30 ml/minute, give 25% of clarithromycin dose.

*Sildenafil:* May prolong absorption of sildenafil. May need to reduce sildenafil dosage.
*Theophylline:* May increase theophylline level. Monitor drug level.
*Warfarin:* May increase PT and INR. Monitor PT and INR carefully.
*Zidovudine:* May alter zidovudine level. Monitor patient closely.

## EFFECTS ON LAB TEST RESULTS
● May increase creatinine, BUN, ALT, AST, alkaline phosphatase, bilirubin, GGT, and LDH levels.
● May increase PT and INR. May decrease thrombocyte, neutrophil, and WBC counts.

## CONTRAINDICATIONS & CAUTIONS
● Contraindicated in patients hypersensitive to clarithromycin, erythromycin, or other macrolides and in those receiving pimozide or other drugs that cause prolonged QT interval or cardiac arrhythmias.
● Use cautiously in patients with hepatic or renal impairment.

## NURSING CONSIDERATIONS
● *Alert:* The safety and efficacy of the extended-release formulation haven't been established for treating other infections for which the original formulation has been approved.
● Obtain specimen for culture and sensitivity tests before giving first dose. Therapy may begin pending results.
● Monitor patient for superinfection. Drug may cause overgrowth of nonsusceptible bacteria or fungi.
● Drugs metabolized by CYP3A, hexobarbital, phenytoin, and valproate may interact with clarithromycin.

## PATIENT TEACHING
● Tell patient to take drug as prescribed, even after he feels better.
● Advise patient to report persistent adverse reactions.
● Inform patient that drug may be taken with or without food. Don't refrigerate the suspension form. Discard unused portion after 14 days.

## erythromycin base
Apo-Erythro Base†, E-Base,
EMU-V Tablets‡, E-Mycin⚕,
Erybid†, Eryc⚕, Ery-Tab⚕,
Erythromid†, Erythromycin
Filmtabs, Novo-rythro, PCE
Dispertab

## erythromycin estolate
Ilosone, Novo-rythro†

## erythromycin ethylsuccinate
Apo-Erythro-ES†, E.E.S., EES
Granules, EryPed, EryPed 200,
EryPed 400

## erythromycin lactobionate
Erythrocin, Erythromycin
Lactobionate

## erythromycin stearate
Apo-Erythro-S†, Erythrocin
Stearate, Novo-rythro†

*Pregnancy risk category B*

---

### AVAILABLE FORMS
**erythromycin base**
*Capsules (delayed-release):* 250 mg
*Tablets (enteric-coated):* 250 mg, 333 mg,
500 mg
*Tablets (filmtabs):* 250 mg, 500 mg
**erythromycin estolate**
*Capsules:* 250 mg
*Oral suspension:* 125 mg/5 ml, 250 mg/
5 ml
*Tablets:* 500 mg
**erythromycin ethylsuccinate**
*Oral suspension:* 100 mg/2.5 ml, 200 mg/
5 ml, 400 mg/5 ml
*Tablets (chewable):* 200 mg
*Tablets (film-coated):* 400 mg
**erythromycin lactobionate**
*Injection:* 500-mg, 1-g vials
**erythromycin stearate**
*Tablets (film-coated):* 250 mg, 500 mg

### INDICATIONS & DOSAGES
➤ **Acute pelvic inflammatory disease
caused by** *Neisseria gonorrhoeae*
*Adults:* 500 mg I.V. lactobionate q 6 hours
for 3 days; then 250 mg base or stearate or
400 mg ethylsuccinate P.O. q 6 hours for
7 days.

➤ **Intestinal amebiasis caused by** *Entamoeba histolytica*
*Adults:* 250 mg P.O. q.i.d. or 333 mg P.O.
q 8 hours, or 500 mg delayed-release
tablets P.O. q 12 hours for 10 to 14 days.
*Children:* 30 to 50 mg/kg P.O. daily, in divided doses, for 10 to 14 days.
➤ **Erythrasma**
*Adults:* 250 mg P.O. t.i.d. for 21 days.
➤ **To prevent rheumatic fever**
*Adults:* 250 mg P.O. q 12 hours.
➤ **Mild to moderately severe respiratory tract, skin, and soft-tissue infections caused by sensitive group A beta-
hemolytic streptococci,** *Streptococcus
pneumoniae, Mycoplasma pneumoniae,
Corynebacterium diphtheriae,* **or** *Borde-
tella pertussis*
*Adults:* 250 to 500 mg base, estolate, or
stearate P.O. q 6 hours; or 400 to 800 mg
ethylsuccinate P.O. q 6 hours; or 15 to
20 mg/kg I.V. daily, as continuous infusion
or in divided doses q 6 hours for 10 days
(3 weeks for *Mycoplasma* species infection).
*Children:* 30 to 50 mg/kg oral erythromycin salts P.O. daily, in divided doses q
6 hours; or 15 to 20 mg/kg I.V. daily, in
divided doses q 4 to 6 hours for 10 days
(3 weeks for *Mycoplasma* species infection).
➤ *Listeria monocytogenes* **infection**
*Adults:* 250 mg P.O. q 6 hours or 500 mg
P.O. q 12 hours.
➤ **Nongonococcal urethritis caused by**
*Ureaplasma urealyticum*
*Adults:* 500 mg P.O. q 6 hours for at least
7 days or 250 mg P.O. q.i.d. for 14 days if
patient can't tolerate higher doses.
➤ **Syphilis in patients allergic to penicillin**
*Adults:* 500 mg P.O. q.i.d. for 2 weeks.
➤ **Legionnaires' disease**
*Adults:* 1 to 4 g P.O. daily in divided doses
for 10 to 14 days alone or with rifampin.
I.V. route may be used initially in severe
cases.
➤ **Uncomplicated urethral, endocervi-
cal, or rectal infections caused by**
*Chlamydia trachomatis,* **when tetracyclines are contraindicated**
*Adults:* 500 mg base P.O. q.i.d. for at least
7 days or 666 mg P.O. q 8 hours for at
least 7 days or 250 mg P.O. q.i.d. for 14
days if patient can't tolerate higher doses.

---

➤ **Urogenital *C. trachomatis* infections during pregnancy**
*Adults:* 500 mg base, estolate, or stearate P.O. q.i.d. for at least 7 days or 250 mg base, estolate, or stearate or 400 mg ethylsuccinate P.O. q.i.d. for at least 14 days.

➤ **Conjunctivitis caused by *C. trachomatis* in neonates**
*Neonates:* 50 mg/kg base, estolate, or stearate P.O. daily in four divided doses for 14 days.

➤ **Pneumonia in infants caused by *C. trachomatis***
*Infants:* 50 mg/kg/day base, estolate, or stearate P.O. in four divided doses for 21 days or 15 to 20 mg/kg/day lactobionate I.V. as a continuous infusion or in four divided doses.

➤ **Chancroid caused by *Haemophilus ducreyi* ♦**
*Adults:* 500 mg base P.O. q.i.d. for 7 days.

➤ **Diarrhea caused by *Campylobacter jejuni enteriti* or enterocolitis**
*Adults:* 500 mg base P.O. q.i.d. for 7 days.

## I.V. ADMINISTRATION

● Reconstitute drug according to manufacturer's directions and dilute each 250 mg in at least 100 ml of normal saline solution. Infuse over 1 hour.
● *Alert:* Don't give erythromycin lactobionate with other drugs.

## ACTION

Inhibits bacterial protein synthesis by binding to the 50S subunit of the ribosome. Bacteriostatic or bactericidal, depending on concentration.

| Route | Onset | Peak | Duration |
|-------|-------|------|----------|
| P.O. | Unknown | 1½ hr | Unknown |
| I.V. | Immediate | 1½ hr | Unknown |

## ADVERSE REACTIONS

**CNS:** fever.
**CV:** *ventricular arrhythmias; vein irritation or thrombophlebitis after I.V. injection.*
**EENT:** hearing loss (with high I.V. doses).
**GI:** *abdominal pain and cramping, nausea, vomiting, diarrhea.*
**Hepatic:** cholestatic jaundice (with erythromycin estolate).
**Skin:** urticaria, rash, eczema.

**Other:** overgrowth of nonsusceptible bacteria or fungi, *anaphylaxis.*

## INTERACTIONS

**Drug-drug.** *Carbamazepine:* May inhibit metabolism of carbamazepine, increasing blood level and risk of toxicity. Avoid using together.
*Clindamycin, lincomycin:* May be antagonistic. Avoid using together.
*Cyclosporine:* May increase cyclosporine level. Monitor drug level.
*Digoxin:* May increase digoxin level. Monitor patient for digoxin toxicity.
*Disopyramide:* May increase disopyramide level, which may cause arrhythmias and prolonged QT intervals. Monitor ECG.
*Midazolam, triazolam:* May increase effects of these drugs. Monitor patient closely.
*Oral anticoagulants:* May increase anticoagulant effect. Monitor PT and INR closely.
*Theophylline:* May decrease erythromycin level and increase theophylline toxicity. Use together cautiously.
**Drug-herb.** *Pill-bearing spurge:* May inhibit CYP3A enzymes, affecting drug metabolism. Urge caution.

## EFFECTS ON LAB TEST RESULTS

● May increase alkaline phosphatase, ALT, AST, and bilirubin levels.
● May interfere with fluorometric determination of urine catecholamines and with colorimetric assays.

## CONTRAINDICATIONS & CAUTIONS

● Contraindicated in pregnant patients and those hypersensitive to drug or other macrolides.
● Erythromycin estolate is contraindicated in patients with hepatic disease.
● Use erythromycin salts cautiously in patients with impaired hepatic function. Monitor liver function test results.
● Erythromycin estolate isn't recommended during pregnancy because of the potential adverse effects on the mother and fetus.
● Drug appears in breast milk. Use cautiously in breast-feeding women.
● Don't use drug to treat neurosyphilis.

---

## NURSING CONSIDERATIONS
● Obtain urine specimen for culture and sensitivity tests before giving first dose. Therapy may begin pending results.
● When giving suspension, note the concentration.
● Monitor patient for superinfection. Drug may cause overgrowth of nonsusceptible bacteria or fungi.
● Monitor hepatic function. Erythromycin estolate may cause serious hepatotoxicity in adults (reversible cholestatic jaundice). Other erythromycin salts cause less serious hepatotoxicity.
● Ototoxicity may occur, especially in patients with renal or hepatic insufficiency and in those receiving high doses of drug.
● Coated tablets or encapsulated pellets cause less GI upset, so they may be better tolerated by patients who can't tolerate erythromycin.

## PATIENT TEACHING
● Tell patient to take drug as prescribed, even after he feels better.
● Instruct patient to take oral form of drug with full glass of water 1 hour before or 2 hours after meals for best absorption.
● Drug may be taken with food if GI upset occurs. Tell patient not to take drug with fruit juice or to swallow whole chewable erythromycin tablets.
● Instruct patient to report adverse reactions, especially nausea, abdominal pain, vomiting, and fever.

aztreonam
chloramphenicol sodium
    succinate
clindamycin hydrochloride
clindamycin palmitate
    hydrochloride
clindamycin phosphate
daptomycin
drotrecogin alfa (activated)
ertapenem sodium
imipenem and cilastatin sodium
linezolid
meropenem
nitrofurantoin macrocrystals
nitrofurantoin microcrystals
quinupristin and dalfopristin
trimethoprim
vancomycin hydrochloride

**COMBINATION PRODUCTS**
MACROBID: nitrofurantoin macrocrystals
25 mg and nitrofurantoin monohydrate
75 mg.

---

aztreonam
Azactam

*Pregnancy risk category B*

**AVAILABLE FORMS**
*Injection:* 500-mg vials, 1-g vials, 2-g
vials

**INDICATIONS & DOSAGES**
➤ UTIs; septicemia; infections of lower
respiratory tract, skin, and skin structures; intra-abdominal infections, surgical infections, and gynecologic infections caused by susceptible *Escherichia
coli, Klebsiella pneumoniae, Proteus
mirabilis, Pseudomonas aeruginosa, Enterobacter cloacae, K. oxytoca, Citrobacter* species, and *Serratia marcescens;*
respiratory infections caused by *Haemophilus influenzae*
*Adults:* 500 mg to 2 g I.V. or I.M. q 8 to
12 hours. For severe systemic or life-
threatening infections, 2 g q 6 to 8 hours.
Maximum dose is 8 g daily.

*Children ages 9 months to 15 years:*
30 mg/kg q 6 to 8 hours I.V. Maximum
dose is 120 mg/kg/day.
*Adjust-a-dose:* For adults with creatinine
clearance 10 to 30 ml/minute, give 1 to
2 g; then 50% of the usual dose at usual
interval. If clearance is less than 10 ml/
minute, give 500 mg to 2 g; then 25% of
the usual dose at usual interval. For adults
with alcoholic cirrhosis, decrease dose by
20% to 25%.

**I.V. ADMINISTRATION**
● For direct injection, reconstitute with
6 to 10 ml of sterile water for injection
and immediately shake vial vigorously.
● To give a bolus, inject drug over 3 to
5 minutes, directly into a vein or I.V. tubing.
● For infusion, reconstitute with a compatible I.V. solution to yield 20 mg/ml or less.
● Give thawed solutions only by I.V. infusion.
● Give infusions over 20 minutes to 1
hour.

**ACTION**
Inhibits bacterial cell-wall synthesis, ultimately causing cell-wall destruction; bactericidal.

| Route | Onset | Peak | Duration |
|-------|-------|------|----------|
| I.V. | Unknown | Immediate | Unknown |
| I.M. | Unknown | < 1 hr | Unknown |

**ADVERSE REACTIONS**
**CNS:** *seizures,* headache, insomnia, con-
fusion.
**CV:** hypotension, thrombophlebitis.
**GI:** diarrhea, nausea, vomiting,
*pseudomembranous colitis.*
**Hematologic:** *neutropenia,* anemia, *pan-
cytopenia, thrombocytopenia,* leukocyto-
sis, thrombocytosis.
**Skin:** discomfort and swelling at I.M. in-
jection site.
**Other:** hypersensitivity reactions.

## INTERACTIONS
**Drug-drug.** *Aminoglycosides:* May have synergistic nephrotoxic effects. Monitor renal function.
*Cefoxitin, imipenem:* May have antagonistic effect. Avoid using together.
*Probenecid:* May increase aztreonam level. Avoid using together.

## EFFECTS ON LAB TEST RESULTS
● May increase BUN, creatinine, ALT, AST, and LDH levels.
● May increase PT, PTT, and INR. May decrease hemoglobin and neutrophil and RBC counts. May increase or decrease WBC and platelet counts.
● May cause false-positive Coombs' test result. May alter urine glucose determinations using cupric sulfate (Clinitest or Benedict's reagent).

## CONTRAINDICATIONS & CAUTIONS
● Contraindicated in patients hypersensitive to drug or to any component of the formulation.
● Use cautiously in elderly patients and in those with impaired renal or hepatic function. Dosage adjustment may be needed. Monitor renal function tests.

## NURSING CONSIDERATIONS
● Obtain specimen for culture and sensitivity tests before giving first dose. Therapy may begin pending results.
● To prepare I.M. injection, add at least 3 ml of one of the following solutions per gram of aztreonam: sterile water for injection, bacteriostatic water for injection, normal saline solution, or bacteriostatic normal saline solution.
● Give I.M. injections deep into a large muscle, such as the upper outer quadrant of the gluteus maximus or the lateral aspect of the thigh. Give doses exceeding 1 g I.V.
● **Alert:** Don't give I.M. injection to children.
● Observe patient for signs and symptoms of superinfection.
● **Alert:** Because drug is ineffective against gram-positive and anaerobic organisms, anticipate combining it with other antibiotics for immediate treatment of life-threatening illnesses.

● **Alert:** Patients allergic to penicillins or cephalosporins may not be allergic to aztreonam. Monitor closely those who have had an immediate hypersensitivity reaction to these antibiotics, especially to ceftazidime.

## PATIENT TEACHING
● Warn patient receiving I.M. drug that pain and swelling may occur at injection site.
● Tell patient to report discomfort at I.V. insertion site.
● Instruct patient to report adverse reactions and signs and symptoms of superinfection promptly.

# chloramphenicol sodium succinate
Chloromycetin Sodium Succinate, Pentamycetin†

*Pregnancy risk category C*

## AVAILABLE FORMS
*Injection:* 1-g vial

## INDICATIONS & DOSAGES
➤ *Haemophilus influenzae* **meningitis, acute** *Salmonella typhi* **infection, and meningitis, bacteremia, or other severe infections caused by sensitive** *Salmonella* **species, rickettsia, lymphogranuloma, psittacosis, or various sensitive gram-negative organisms**
*Adults:* 50 to 100 mg/kg I.V. daily, divided q 6 hours. Maximum dose is 100 mg/kg daily.
*Full-term infants older than age 2 weeks with normal metabolic processes:* Up to 50 mg/kg I.V. daily, divided q 6 hours. May use up to 100 mg/kg/day in four divided doses for meningitis.
*Premature infants, neonates age 2 weeks and younger, and children and infants with immature metabolic processes:* 25 mg/kg I.V. once daily.

## I.V. ADMINISTRATION
● Reconstitute 1-g vial of powder for injection with 10 ml of sterile water for injection, to yield 100 mg/ml.

---

• Give I.V. slowly over at least 1 minute. Check injection site daily for phlebitis and irritation.
• Stable for 30 days at room temperature but should refrigerate. Don't use cloudy solutions.

## ACTION
Inhibits bacterial protein synthesis by binding to the 50S subunit of the ribosome; bacteriostatic.

| Route | Onset | Peak | Duration |
|-------|-------|------|----------|
| I.V. | Unknown | 1-3 hr | Unknown |

## ADVERSE REACTIONS
**CNS:** headache, mild depression, confusion, delirium, peripheral neuropathy with prolonged therapy.
**EENT:** optic neuritis in patients with cystic fibrosis, decreased visual acuity.
**GI:** nausea, vomiting, stomatitis, diarrhea, enterocolitis, glossitis.
**Hematologic:** *aplastic anemia, hypoplastic anemia, granulocytopenia, thrombocytopenia.*
**Hepatic:** jaundice.
**Other:** hypersensitivity reactions, *anaphylaxis, gray syndrome in neonates.*

## INTERACTIONS
**Drug-drug.** *Anticoagulants, barbiturates, hydantoins, iron salts, sulfonylureas:* May increase levels of these drugs. Monitor patient for toxicity.
*Penicillins:* May have synergistic or antagonistic effects. Monitor patient for change in effectiveness.
*Rifampin:* May reduce chloramphenicol level. Monitor patient for changes in effectiveness.
*Vitamin $B_{12}$:* May decrease response of vitamin B in patients with pernicious anemia. Monitor patient closely.

## EFFECTS ON LAB TEST RESULTS
• May decrease hemoglobin and granulocyte and platelet counts.
• May falsely elevate urine PABA levels if given during a bentiromide test for pancreatic function. May cause false-positive results of tests for urine glucose using cupric sulfate (Clinitest).

## CONTRAINDICATIONS & CAUTIONS
• Contraindicated in patients hypersensitive to drug.
• Use cautiously in patients with impaired hepatic or renal function, acute intermittent porphyria, and G6PD deficiency; also use cautiously in those taking other drugs that cause bone marrow suppression or blood disorders.
• *Alert:* Use cautiously in premature infants and newborns because potentially fatal gray syndrome may occur. Symptoms include abdominal distention, gray cyanosis, vasomotor collapse, respiratory distress, and death within a few hours of symptom onset.

## NURSING CONSIDERATIONS
• Obtain specimen for culture and sensitivity tests before giving first dose. Therapy may begin pending results.
• Obtain drug level measurement and maintain level at 5 to 20 mcg/ml.
• Monitor CBC, platelets, iron, and reticulocytes before and every 2 days during therapy. Stop drug and notify prescriber immediately if anemia, reticulocytopenia, leukopenia, or thrombocytopenia develops.
• Monitor patient for signs and symptoms of superinfection.

## PATIENT TEACHING
• Instruct patient to notify prescriber if adverse reactions occur, especially nausea, vomiting, diarrhea, fever, confusion, sore throat, or mouth sores.
• Tell patient receiving drug I.V. to report discomfort at I.V. insertion site.
• Instruct patient to report signs and symptoms of superinfection.

---

Reactions may be *common,* uncommon, *life-threatening,* or COMMON AND LIFE-THREATENING.

## clindamycin hydrochloride
Cleocin HCl, Dalacin C†‡

## clindamycin palmitate hydrochloride
Cleocin Pediatric, Dalacin C Flavored Granules†

## clindamycin phosphate
Cleocin Phosphate, Dalacin C Phosphate Sterile Solution†‡

*Pregnancy risk category B*

## AVAILABLE FORMS
**clindamycin hydrochloride**
*Capsules:* 75 mg, 150 mg, 300 mg
**clindamycin palmitate hydrochloride**
*Granules for oral solution:* 75 mg/5 ml
**clindamycin phosphate**
*Injectable infusion (in D₅W):* 300 mg (50 ml), 600 mg (50 ml), 900 mg (50 ml)
*Injection:* 150-mg base/ml, 300-mg base/ 2 ml, 600-mg base/4 ml, 900-mg base/6 ml

## INDICATIONS & DOSAGES
➤ **Infections caused by sensitive staphylococci, streptococci, pneumococci,** *Bacteroides, Fusobacterium, Clostridium perfringens,* **and other sensitive aerobic and anaerobic organisms**
*Adults:* 150 to 450 mg P.O. q 6 hours; or 300 to 600 mg I.M. or I.V. q 6, 8, or 12 hours.
*Children older than age 1 month:* 8 to 20 mg/kg P.O. daily, in divided doses q 6 to 8 hours; or 15 to 40 mg/kg I.M. or I.V. daily, in divided doses q 6 or 8 hours.
➤ **Pelvic inflammatory disease**
*Adults and adolescents:* 900 mg I.V. q 8 hours, with gentamicin. Continue at least 48 hours after symptoms improve; then switch to oral clindamycin 450 mg q.i.d. for total of 10 to 14 days or doxycycline 100 mg P.O. q 12 hours for total of 10 to 14 days.
➤ *Pneumocystis carinii* **pneumonia ♦**
*Adults:* 600 mg I.V. q 6 hours or 900 mg I.V. q 8 hours, with primaquine.
➤ **CNS toxoplasmosis in AIDS patients, as alternative to sulfonamides with pyrimethamine ♦**
*Adults:* 1,200 to 2,400 mg/day in divided doses.

## I.V. ADMINISTRATION
● For I.V. infusion, dilute each 300 mg in 50-ml solution, and give no faster than 30 mg/minute (over 10 to 60 minutes). Never give undiluted as a bolus.
● When giving I.V., check site daily for phlebitis and irritation.

## ACTION
Inhibits bacterial protein synthesis by binding to the 50S subunit of the ribosome.

| Route | Onset | Peak | Duration |
|-------|-------|------|----------|
| P.O. | Unknown | 45-60 min | Unknown |
| I.V. | Immediate | Immediate | Unknown |
| I.M. | Unknown | 3 hr | Unknown |

## ADVERSE REACTIONS
**CV:** thrombophlebitis.
**GI:** *nausea,* vomiting, abdominal pain, diarrhea, *pseudomembranous colitis.*
**Hematologic:** *transient leukopenia,* eosinophilia, *thrombocytopenia.*
**Hepatic:** jaundice.
**Skin:** maculopapular rash, urticaria.
**Other:** *anaphylaxis.*

## INTERACTIONS
**Drug-drug.** *Erythromycin:* May block access of clindamycin to its site of action. Avoid using together.
*Kaolin:* May decrease absorption of oral clindamycin. Separate dosage times.
*Neuromuscular blockers:* May increase neuromuscular blockade. Monitor patient closely.
**Drug-food.** *Diet foods with sodium cyclamate:* May decrease drug level. Discourage use together.

## EFFECTS ON LAB TEST RESULTS
● May increase bilirubin, AST, and alkaline phosphatase levels.
● May increase eosinophil count. May decrease WBC and platelet counts.

## CONTRAINDICATIONS & CAUTIONS
● Contraindicated in patients hypersensitive to drug or lincomycin.
● Use cautiously in neonates and patients with renal or hepatic disease, asthma, history of GI disease, or significant allergies.

---

*Rapid onset* †Canada ‡Australia ◇OTC ♦Off-label use ✐Photoguide *Liquid contains alcohol.

## NURSING CONSIDERATIONS
● Obtain specimen for culture and sensitivity tests before giving first dose. Therapy may begin pending results.
● For I.M. administration, inject deeply. Rotate sites. Don't exceed 600 mg per injection.
● I.M. injection may raise CK level in response to muscle irritation.
● Don't refrigerate reconstituted oral solution because it will thicken. Drug is stable for 2 weeks at room temperature.
● Monitor renal, hepatic, and hematopoietic functions during prolonged therapy.
● Observe patient for signs and symptoms of superinfection.
● *Alert:* Don't give opioid antidiarrheals to treat drug-induced diarrhea; they may prolong and worsen this condition.
● Drug doesn't penetrate blood-brain barrier.

## PATIENT TEACHING
● Advise patient to take capsule form with a full glass of water to prevent esophageal irritation.
● Warn patient that I.M. injection may be painful.
● Tell patient to report discomfort at I.V. insertion site.
● Instruct patient to notify prescriber of adverse reactions (especially diarrhea). Warn him not to treat such diarrhea himself because clindamycin therapy may cause severe, even life-threatening, colitis.

✻ NEW DRUG

---

# daptomycin
Cubicin

*Pregnancy risk category B*

---

## AVAILABLE FORMS
*Powder for injection:* 250-mg vial, 500-mg vial

## INDICATIONS & DOSAGES
➤ **Complicated skin and skin structure infections caused by susceptible strains of *Staphylococcus aureus* (including methicillin-resistant strains), *Streptococcus pyogenes, Streptococcus agalactiae, Streptococcus dysgalactiae,* and**

*Enterococcus faecalis* (vancomycin-susceptible strains only)
*Adults:* 4 mg/kg I.V. over 30 minutes q 24 hours for 7 to 14 days.
*Adjust-a-dose:* For patients with a creatinine clearance below 30 ml/minute, including those receiving hemodialysis or continuous ambulatory peritoneal dialysis, give 4 mg/kg I.V. q 48 hours. When possible, give drug after hemodialysis.

## I.V. ADMINISTRATION
● Reconstitute 250-mg vial with 5 ml and 500-mg vial with 10 ml of normal saline solution. Further dilute admixture with normal saline solution. Vials are for single use; discard excess.
● Drug is incompatible with dextrose solutions and other drugs. If an I.V. line is used for several drugs, flush the line with a compatible solution, such as normal saline solution or lactated Ringer's injection between drugs.
● Infuse over 30 minutes.
● Refrigerate vials at 36° to 46° F (2° to 8° C). Reconstituted and diluted solutions are stable 12 hours at room temperature or 48 hours at 36° to 46° F (2° to 8° C).

## ACTION
Binds to and depolarizes bacterial membranes to inhibit protein, DNA, and RNA synthesis, thus causing bacterial cell death.

| Route | Onset | Peak | Duration |
|-------|-------|------|----------|
| I.V. | Rapid | < 1 hr | Unknown |

## ADVERSE REACTIONS
**CNS:** anxiety, confusion, dizziness, fever, headache, insomnia.
**CV:** *cardiac failure,* chest pain, edema, hypertension, hypotension.
**EENT:** sore throat.
**GI:** abdominal pain, constipation, decreased appetite, diarrhea, nausea, *pseudomembranous colitis,* vomiting.
**GU:** *renal failure,* urinary tract infection.
**Hematologic:** anemia.
**Metabolic:** hyperglycemia, *hypoglycemia,* hypokalemia.
**Musculoskeletal:** limb and back pain.
**Respiratory:** cough, dyspnea.

---

**Skin:** cellulites, injection site reactions, pruritus, rash.
**Other:** fungal infections.

### INTERACTIONS
**Drug-drug.** *HMG-CoA reductase inhibitors:* May increase risk of myopathy. Consider stopping these drugs while giving daptomycin.
*Tobramycin:* May affect levels of both drugs. Use together cautiously.
*Warfarin:* May alter anticoagulant activity. Monitor PT and INR for the first several days of daptomycin therapy.

### EFFECTS ON LAB TEST RESULTS
• May increase CPK and alkaline phosphatase levels. May decrease potassium level. May increase or decrease glucose level.
• May increase liver function test values. May decrease hemoglobin and hematocrit.

### CONTRAINDICATIONS & CAUTIONS
• Contraindicated in patients hypersensitive to drug.
• Use cautiously in those with renal insufficiency and those who are older than age 65, pregnant, or breast-feeding.
• Safety and efficacy haven't been established in patients younger than age 18.

### NURSING CONSIDERATIONS
• Obtain specimen for culture and sensitivity tests before giving first dose.
• Monitor CBC and renal and liver function tests periodically.
• *Alert:* Because drug may increase the risk of myopathy, monitor CPK levels weekly. If CPK levels rise, monitor them more often. Stop drug in patients with evidence of myopathy and CPK levels over 1,000 units/L. Also stop drug in patients with CPK levels more than 10 times the upper limit of normal. Consider stopping all other drugs linked with myopathy (such as HMG-CoA reductase inhibitors) while giving daptomycin.
• Monitor patient for superinfection because drug may cause overgrowth of non-susceptible organisms.
• Watch for evidence of pseudomembranous colitis and treat accordingly.

### PATIENT TEACHING
• Advise patient to immediately report muscle weakness and infusion site irritation.
• Tell patient to report severe diarrhea, rash, and infection.
• Inform patient about possible adverse reactions.

## drotrecogin alfa (activated)
Xigris

*Pregnancy risk category C*

### AVAILABLE FORMS
*Injection:* 5-mg vial, 20-mg vial

### INDICATIONS AND DOSAGES
➤ **To reduce the risk of death in patients with severe sepsis from acute organ dysfunction**
*Adults:* 24 mcg/kg/hour I.V. infusion for a total of 96 hours.

### I.V. ADMINISTRATION
• Reconstitute 5- or 20-mg vial with 2.5 or 10 ml sterile water for injection respectively. Gently swirl each vial until powder is completely dissolved. Avoid inverting or shaking the vial.
• Use reconstituted solution immediately. If necessary, it may be stored at 59° to 86° F (15° to 30° C). for up to 3 hours.
• Further dilute with sterile normal saline for injection. Withdraw appropriate amount and add to infusion bag of sterile normal saline solution, directing the stream to the side of the bag to minimize agitation of the solution.
• Gently invert the infusion bag to mix. Don't transport the infusion bag between locations using mechanical delivery systems.
• Inspect for particle matter and discoloration before administration.
• I.V. administration must be completed within 12 hours after the I.V. solution is prepared.
• When using an I.V. pump, dilute drug to between 100 mcg/ml and 200 mcg/ml.
• When a syringe pump is used, dilute drug to between 100 mcg/ml and 1,000 mcg/ml. When drug is diluted to less than 200 mcg/ml and flow rate is less

than 5 ml/hour, prime the infusion set for about 15 minutes at 5 ml/hour.
• Give through a dedicated I.V. line or lumen of a multilumen central venous catheter. The only other solutions that can be given through the same line are normal saline solution, lactated Ringer's injection, D₅W, or dextrose in saline mixtures.
• Avoid exposing drug to heat or direct sunlight.
• Store in a refrigerator at 35° to 46° F (2° to 8° C). Don't freeze.

**ACTION**
Unknown. Thought to produce dose-dependent reductions in D-dimer and IL-6. Activated protein C exerts an antithrombotic effect by inhibiting factors Va and VIIIa.

| Route | Onset | Peak | Duration |
|-------|-------|------|----------|
| I.V. | Immediate | Unknown | Unknown |

**ADVERSE REACTIONS**
**Hematologic:** *hemorrhage.*

**INTERACTIONS**
**Drug-drug.** *Drugs that affect hemostasis:* May increase risk of bleeding. Use together cautiously.

**EFFECTS ON LAB TEST RESULTS**
• May prolong PTT and PT.

**CONTRAINDICATIONS & CAUTIONS**
• Contraindicated in patients hypersensitive to drug or any of its components, those with active internal bleeding, and those who have had hemorrhagic stroke in the past 3 months or intracranial or intraspinal surgery in the past 2 months; also contraindicated in patients with severe head trauma, trauma with increased risk of life-threatening bleeding, an epidural catheter, intracranial neoplasm or mass lesion, or cerebral herniation.
• Use cautiously with other drugs that affect hemostasis. Consider the increased risk of bleeding in patients taking heparin (at least 15 units/kg/hour) and in those with a platelet count less than 30,000 × 10⁶/L (even if the platelet count is increased after transfusions) or an INR greater than 3. The risk may also be in-

creased in patients who have had GI bleeding in the past 6 weeks, thrombolytic therapy in the past 3 days, oral anticoagulants or glycoprotein IIb/IIIa inhibitors in the past week, aspirin (more than 650 mg/day) or other platelet inhibitors in the past week, ischemic stroke in the past 3 months, intracranial arteriovenous malformation or aneurysm, bleeding diathesis, chronic severe hepatic disease, or any condition in which bleeding poses a significant hazard or would be difficult to manage because of its location.

**NURSING CONSIDERATIONS**
• Use aseptic technique during preparation.
• If the infusion is interrupted, restart at the 24-mcg/kg/hour infusion rate.
• Monitor patient closely for bleeding. Notify prescriber if bleeding occurs.
• Stop drug 2 hours before an invasive surgical procedure. After hemostasis has been achieved, drug may be restarted 12 hours after major invasive procedure or immediately after uncomplicated less invasive procedure.
• Because drug has minimal effect on the PT, this value can be used to monitor the patient's coagulopathy status.

**PATIENT TEACHING**
• Inform patient of the potential adverse reactions.
• Instruct patient to promptly report signs of bleeding.
• Advise patient that bleeding may occur for up to 28 days after treatment.

---

**ertapenem sodium**
Invanz

*Pregnancy risk category B*

**AVAILABLE FORMS**
*Injection:* 1 g

**INDICATIONS AND DOSAGES**
➤ **Complicated intra-abdominal infections caused by** *Escherichia coli, Clostridium clostridiiforme, Eubacterium lentum, Peptostreptococcus species, Bac-*

*teroides fragilis, B. distasonis, B. ovatus,
B. thetaiotaomicron,* or *B. uniformis*
*Adults:* 1 g I.V. or I.M. once daily for 5 to
14 days.
➤ **Complicated skin and skin structure
infections caused by** *Staphylococcus
aureus* **(methicillin-susceptible strains),**
*Streptococcus pyogenes, E. coli,* or *Peptostreptococcus* **species**
*Adults:* 1 g I.V. or I.M. once daily for 7 to
14 days.
➤ **Community-acquired pneumonia
caused by** *S. pneumoniae* **(penicillin-
susceptible strains),** *Haemophilus influenzae* **(beta-lactamase–negative
strains), or** *Moraxella catarrhalis;* **complicated UTIs, including pyelonephritis,
caused by** *E. coli* **or** *Klebsiella pneumoniae*
*Adults:* 1 g I.V. or I.M. once daily for 10 to
14 days. If patient improves after at least
3 days of treatment, use appropriate oral
therapy to complete the full course of therapy.
➤ **Acute pelvic infections including
postpartum endomyometritis, septic
abortion, and postsurgical gynecologic
infections caused by** *S. agalactiae,
E. coli, B. fragilis, Porphyromonas asac-
charolyticus, Peptostreptococcus* **species,
or** *Prevotella bivia*
*Adults:* 1 g I.V. or I.M. once daily for 3 to
10 days.
*Adjust-a-dose:* In patients with creatinine
clearance 30 ml/minute or less, give
500 mg/day.
   In hemodialysis patients receiving daily
500-mg dose fewer than 6 hours before
hemodialysis, give supplementary 150-mg
dose afterward. In hemodialysis patients
receiving dose 6 hours or more before hemodialysis, no supplementary dose is
needed.

**I.V. ADMINISTRATION**
● Reconstitute 1-g vial with 10 ml of sterile water for injection, normal saline for
injection, or bacteriostatic water for injection. Shake well to dissolve and immediately transfer contents to 50 ml of normal
saline solution. Infuse over 30 minutes.
Complete the infusion within 6 hours of
reconstitution.

● Don't mix or infuse ertapenem with other drugs. Don't use diluents containing
dextrose.

**ACTION**
Inhibits cell wall synthesis through
penicillin-binding proteins.

| Route | Onset | Peak | Duration |
|---|---|---|---|
| I.V. | Immediate | 30 min | 24 hr |
| I.M. | Unknown | 2 hr | 24 hr |

**ADVERSE REACTIONS**
**CNS:** fever, asthenia, fatigue, anxiety, altered mental status, dizziness, headache,
insomnia.
**CV:** edema, swelling, chest pain, hypertension, hypotension, tachycardia, infused
vein complication, phlebitis, throm-
bophlebitis.
**EENT:** pharyngitis.
**GI:** abdominal pain, acid regurgitation,
oral candidiasis, constipation, *diarrhea,*
dyspepsia, nausea, vomiting.
**GU:** vaginitis, renal dysfunction.
**Hematologic:** coagulation abnormalities,
eosinophilia, anemia, *neutropenia, leukopenia, thrombocytopenia,* thrombocytosis.
**Hepatic:** jaundice.
**Metabolic:** hyperglycemia, *hyperkalemia.*
**Musculoskeletal:** leg pain.
**Respiratory:** cough, dyspnea, rales,
rhonchi, respiratory distress.
**Skin:** erythema, pruritus, rash, extravasa-
tion.

**INTERACTIONS**
**Drug-drug.** *Probenecid:* May reduce renal clearance and increases half-life.
Don't give together with probenecid to extend half-life.

**EFFECTS ON LAB TEST RESULTS**
● May increase albumin, ALT, AST, alkaline phosphatase, creatinine, glucose,
potassium, and bilirubin levels.
● May increase PT, eosinophil count, and
urinary RBC or WBC counts. May decrease hemoglobin, hematocrit, and seg-
mented neutrophil and WBC counts. May
increase or decrease platelet count.

## CONTRAINDICATIONS & CAUTIONS
● Contraindicated in patients hypersensitive to any component of the drug or to other drugs in the same class and in patients who have had anaphylactic reactions to beta-lactams. I.M. use is contraindicated in patients hypersensitive to local anesthetics of the amide type (because of the diluent lidocaine hydrochloride).
● Use cautiously in patients with CNS disorders, compromised renal function, or both, as seizures may occur in these patients.

## NURSING CONSIDERATIONS
● Check for previous penicillin, cephalosporin, or other beta-lactam hypersensitivity before giving first dose.
● Check for hypersensitivity to local anesthetics of the amide type if giving dose I.M.
● Obtain specimens for culture and sensitivity testing before giving first dose. Therapy may start pending results.
● To give I.M., reconstitute 1-g vial with 3.2 ml of 1% lidocaine hydrochloride injection (without epinephrine). Shake vial thoroughly to form solution. Immediately withdraw the contents of the vial and give by deep I.M. injection into a large muscle, such as the gluteal muscles or lateral part of the thigh. Use the reconstituted I.M. solution within 1 hour after preparation. Don't give reconstituted solution I.V.
● Don't store lyophilized powder above 77° F (25° C). The reconstituted solution, immediately diluted in normal saline, may be stored at room temperature (25° C) and used within 6 hours or refrigerated for 24 hours at 41° F (5° C) and used within 4 hours after removal from refrigeration. Don't freeze solutions of ertapenem.
● If diarrhea persists during therapy, notify prescriber and collect stool specimen for culture to rule out pseudomembranous colitis.
● If allergic reaction occurs, stop drug immediately.
● Anaphylactic reactions require immediate emergency treatment with epinephrine, oxygen, I.V. steroids, and airway management.
● Anticonvulsants may continue in patients with seizure disorders. If focal tremors, myoclonus, or seizures occur, notify prescriber. The dosage of ertapenem may need to be decreased or stopped.
● Monitor renal, hepatic, and hematopoietic function during prolonged therapy.
● Methicillin-resistant staphylococci and *Enterococcus* species are resistant to ertapenem.
● *Alert:* Don't confuse Invanz (ertapenem) with Avinza (morphine sulfate)

## PATIENT TEACHING
● Inform patient of potential adverse reactions.
● Tell patient to alert nurse if discomfort occurs at injection site.

---

# imipenem and cilastatin sodium
Primaxin I.M., Primaxin I.V.

*Pregnancy risk category C*

## AVAILABLE FORMS
*Powder for injection:* 250 mg, 500 mg, 750 mg

## INDICATIONS & DOSAGES
➤ **Serious lower respiratory tract, bone, intra-abdominal, gynecologic, joint, skin, and soft-tissue infections; UTIs; endocarditis; and bacterial septicemia, caused by** *Acinetobacter, Enterococcus, Staphylococcus, Streptococcus, Escherichia coli, Haemophilus, Klebsiella, Morganella, Proteus, Enterobacter, Pseudomonas aeruginosa,* **and** *Bacteroides,* **including** *B. fragilis*
*Adults weighing more than 70 kg (154 lb):* 250 mg to 1 g by I.V. infusion q 6 to 8 hours. Maximum daily dose is 50 mg/kg/ day or 4 g/day, whichever is less. Or, 500 to 750 mg I.M. q 12 hours. Maximum I.M. daily dose is 1,500 mg.
*Children age 3 months and older (except for CNS infections):* 15 to 25 mg/kg I.V. q 6 hours. Maximum daily dose is 2 to 4 g.
*Infants ages 4 weeks to 3 months, weighing 1.5 kg (3.3 lb) or more (except for CNS infections):* 25 mg/kg I.V. q 6 hours.
*Neonates ages 1 to 4 weeks, weighing 1.5 kg or more (except for CNS infections):* 25 mg/kg I.V. q 8 hours.

*Neonates younger than age 1 week, weighing 1.5 kg or more (except for CNS infections):* 25 mg/kg I.V. q 12 hours.
***Adjust-a-dose:*** For patients with creatinine clearance below 70 ml/minute, adjust dosage and monitor renal function test results.

## I.V. ADMINISTRATION
● Reconstitute piggyback units with 100 ml of compatible I.V. solution to provide solution containing 2.5 to 5 mg/ml.
● When reconstituting powder, shake until the solution is clear. Solutions may range from colorless to yellow; variations of color or within this range don't affect drug's potency.
● After reconstitution, solution is stable for 4 hours at room temperature and for 24 hours when refrigerated.
● Don't give by direct I.V. bolus injection.
● For adults, give each 250- or 500-mg dose by I.V. infusion over 20 to 30 minutes. Infuse each 750-mg to 1-g dose over 40 to 60 minutes.
● For children, infuse doses of 500 mg or less over 15 to 30 minutes. Infuse doses greater than 500 mg over 40 to 60 minutes. If nausea occurs, the infusion may be slowed.

## ACTION
Inhibits bacterial cell-wall synthesis; enzymatic breakdown of drug in the kidneys causes adequate antibacterial levels of drug in the urine.

| Route | Onset | Peak | Duration |
|-------|-------|------|----------|
| I.V. | Immediate | Immediate | Unknown |
| I.M. | Unknown | 1-2 hr | Unknown |

## ADVERSE REACTIONS
**CNS:** *seizures,* dizziness, fever, somnolence.
**CV:** hypotension; thrombophlebitis.
**GI:** nausea, vomiting, diarrhea, *pseudomembranous colitis.*
**Hematologic:** eosinophilia, *thrombocytopenia, leukopenia.*
**Skin:** rash, urticaria, pruritus, injection site pain.
**Other:** hypersensitivity reactions, *anaphylaxis.*

## INTERACTIONS
**Drug-drug.** *Beta-lactam antibiotics:* May have antagonistic effect. Avoid using together.
*Ganciclovir:* May cause seizures. Avoid using together.
*Probenecid:* May increase cilastatin level. May be used together for this effect.

## EFFECTS ON LAB TEST RESULTS
● May increase BUN, creatinine, ALT, AST, alkaline phosphatase, bilirubin, and LDH levels.
● May increase eosinophil count. May decrease WBC and platelet counts.
● May interfere with glucose determination by Benedict's solution or Clinitest.

## CONTRAINDICATIONS & CAUTIONS
● Contraindicated in patients hypersensitive to drug, in those with a history of hypersensitivity to local anesthetics of the amide type, and in those with severe shock or heart block.
● Use cautiously in patients allergic to penicillins or cephalosporins because drug has similar properties.
● Use cautiously in patients with history of seizure disorders, especially if they also have compromised renal function.
● Use cautiously in children younger than age 3 months.

## NURSING CONSIDERATIONS
● *Alert:* Don't use for CNS infections in children because it increases the risk of seizures.
● Obtain specimen culture and sensitivity tests before giving first dose. Therapy may begin pending results.
● *Alert:* Don't give I.M. solution by I.V. route.
● *Alert:* If seizures develop and persist despite anticonvulsant therapy, stop drug and notify prescriber.
● Monitor patient for bacterial or fungal superinfections and resistant infections during and after therapy.

## PATIENT TEACHING
● Instruct patient to report adverse reactions promptly.
● Tell patient to report discomfort at I.V. insertion site.

---

• Urge patient to notify prescriber about loose stools or diarrhea.

---

# linezolid
Zyvox

*Pregnancy risk category C*

## AVAILABLE FORMS
*Injection:* 2 mg/ml
*Powder for oral suspension:* 100 mg/5 ml when reconstituted
*Tablets:* 400 mg, 600 mg

## INDICATIONS & DOSAGES
➤ **Vancomycin-resistant *Enterococcus faecium* infections, including those with concurrent bacteremia**
*Adults and children age 12 and older:* 600 mg I.V. or P.O. q 12 hours for 14 to 28 days.
*Neonates age 7 days or older and infants and children through age 11:* 10 mg/kg I.V. or P.O. q 8 hours for 14 to 28 days.
*Neonates younger than age 7 days:* 10 mg/kg I.V. or P.O. q 12 hours for 14 to 28 days. Increase to 10 mg/kg q 8 hours when patient is 7 days old. Consider this dosage increase if neonate has inadequate response.
➤ **Nosocomial pneumonia caused by *Staphylococcus aureus* (methicillin-susceptible [MSSA] and methicillin-resistant [MRSA] strains) or *Streptococcus pneumoniae* (penicillin-susceptible strains only); complicated skin and skin-structure infections caused by *S. aureus* (MSSA and MSRA), *S. pyogenes,* or *S. agalactiae;* community-acquired pneumonia caused by *S. pneumoniae* (penicillin-susceptible strains only), including those with concurrent bacteremia, or *S. aureus* (MSSA only)**
*Adults and children age 12 and older:* 600 mg I.V. or P.O. q 12 hours for 10 to 14 days.
*Neonates 7 days or older, infants and children through 11 years:* 10 mg/kg I.V. or P.O. q 8 hours for 10 to 14 days.
*Neonates younger than age 7 days:* 10 mg/kg I.V. or P.O. q 12 hours for 10 to 14 days. Increase to 10 mg/kg q 8 hours when patient is 7 days old. Consider this dosage increase if neonate has inadequate response.

➤ **Uncomplicated skin and skin-structure infections caused by *S. aureus* (MSSA only) or *S. pyogenes***
*Adults:* 400 mg P.O. q 12 hours for 10 to 14 days.
*Children ages 12 to 18:* 600 mg P.O. q 12 hours for 10 to 14 days.
*Children ages 5 to 11:* 10 mg/kg P.O. q 12 hours for 10 to 14 days.
*Neonates age 7 days or older and infants and children younger than age 5:* 10 mg/kg P.O. q 8 hours for 10 to 14 days.
*Neonates younger than age 7 days:* 10 mg/kg I.V. or P.O. q 12 hours for 10 to 14 days. Increase to 10 mg/kg q 8 hours when patient is 7 days old. Consider this dosage increase if neonate has inadequate response.

## I.V. ADMINISTRATION
• Inspect for particulate matter and leaks.
• Linezolid is compatible with $D_5W$ injection, normal saline solution for injection, and lactated Ringer's injection.
• Infuse over a period of 30 minutes to 2 hours. Don't infuse linezolid in a series connection.
• **Alert:** Don't inject additives into infusion bag. Give other I.V. drugs separately or via a separate I.V. line to avoid incompatibilities. If single I.V. line is used, flush line before and after linezolid infusion with a compatible solution.
• Store drug at room temperature in its protective overwrap. Solution may turn yellow over time but this doesn't affect drug's potency.

## ACTION
Prevents bacterial protein synthesis by interfering with DNA translation in the ribosomes. Also prevents formation of a functional 70S ribosomal subunit by binding to a site on the bacterial 50S ribosomal subunit.

| Route | Onset | Peak | Duration |
|-------|-------|------|----------|
| P.O. | Unknown | 1 hr | Unknown |
| I.V. | Unknown | 30 min | Unknown |

## ADVERSE REACTIONS
**CNS:** fever, *headache,* insomnia, dizziness.
**GI:** *diarrhea, nausea,* vomiting, constipation, altered taste, tongue discoloration,

---

oral candidiasis, *pseudomembranous colitis.*
**GU:** vaginal candidiasis.
**Hematologic:** anemia, *leukopenia, neutropenia, myelosuppression, thrombocytopenia.*
**Skin:** rash.
**Other:** fungal infection.

### INTERACTIONS
**Drug-drug.** *Adrenergic drugs (such as dopamine, epinephrine, pseudoephedrine):* May cause hypertension. Monitor blood pressure and heart rate; start continuous infusions of dopamine and epinephrine at lower doses and titrate to response.
*Serotoninergic drugs:* May cause serotonin syndrome, including confusion, delirium, restlessness, tremors, blushing, diaphoresis, and hyperpyrexia. If you note signs and symptoms of serotonin syndrome, notify prescriber immediately.
**Drug-food.** *Foods and beverages high in tyramine (such as aged cheeses, air-dried meats, red wines, sauerkraut, soy sauce, tap beers):* May increase blood pressure when linezolid is used with high-tyramine diet. Advise patient that tyramine content of meals shouldn't exceed 100 mg.

### EFFECTS ON LAB TEST RESULTS
• May increase ALT, AST, bilirubin, alkaline phosphatase, creatinine, amylase, lipase, and BUN levels.
• May decrease hemoglobin and WBC, neutrophil, and platelet counts.

### CONTRAINDICATIONS & CAUTIONS
• Contraindicated in patients hypersensitive to drug or its components.

### NURSING CONSIDERATIONS
• Obtain specimen for culture and sensitivity tests before linezolid therapy. Use sensitivity results to guide subsequent therapy.
• No dosage adjustment is needed when switching from I.V. to P.O. forms.
• Reconstitute oral suspension according to manufacturer's instructions. Store reconstituted suspension at room temperature and use within 21 days.
• *Alert:* Don't confuse Zyvox (linezolid) with Zovirax (acyclovir). Both come in a 400-mg strength.

• Drug may cause thrombocytopenia. Monitor platelet count in patients at increased risk for bleeding, in those with existing thrombocytopenia, in those taking other drugs that may cause thrombocytopenia, and in those receiving linezolid for longer than 14 days.
• Drug may lead to myelosuppression. Monitor CBC weekly in patients receiving linezolid.
• *Alert:* Pseudomembranous colitis or superinfection may occur. Consider these diagnoses and take appropriate measures in patients with persistent diarrhea or secondary infections.
• Inappropriate use of antibiotics may lead to development of resistant organisms; carefully consider alternative drugs before instituting linezolid therapy, especially in outpatient setting.
• *Alert:* Safety and efficacy of drug for longer than 28 days haven't been studied.

### PATIENT TEACHING
• Tell patient that tablets and oral suspension may be taken with or without meals.
• Stress importance of completing entire course of therapy, even if patient feels better.
• Tell patient to alert prescriber if he has high blood pressure, is taking cough or cold preparations, or is being treated with SSRIs or other antidepressants.
• Advise patient to avoid large quantities of tyramine-containing foods (such as aged cheeses, soy sauce, tap beers, red wine) while on linezolid.
• Inform patient with phenylketonuria that each 5 ml of linezolid oral suspension contains 20 mg of phenylalanine. Linezolid tablets and injection don't contain phenylalanine.

---

## meropenem
Merrem IV

*Pregnancy risk category B*

### AVAILABLE FORMS
*Powder for injection:* 500 mg, 1 g

### INDICATIONS & DOSAGES
➤ **Complicated appendicitis and peritonitis caused by viridans group strep-**

tococci, *Escherichia coli, Klebsiella pneumoniae, Pseudomonas aeruginosa, Bacteroides fragilis, B. thetaiotaomicron,* and *Peptostreptococcus* species; **bacterial meningitis (children only) caused by** *Streptococcus pneumoniae, Haemophilus influenzae,* and *Neisseria meningitidis*

*Adults:* 1 g I.V. q 8 hours over 15 to 30 minutes as I.V. infusion or over 3 to 5 minutes as I.V. bolus injection (5 to 20 ml).

*Children weighing 50 kg or more:* 1 g I.V. q 8 hours for intra-abdominal infections and 2 g I.V. q 8 hours for meningitis.

*Children age 3 months and older, weighing less than 50 kg (110 lb):* 20 mg/kg (intra-abdominal infection) or 40 mg/kg (bacterial meningitis) q 8 hours over 15 to 30 minutes as I.V. infusion or over 3 to 5 minutes as I.V. bolus injection (5 to 20 ml). Maximum dosage is 2 g I.V. q 8 hours.

*Adjust-a-dose:* For patients with creatinine clearance 26 to 50 ml/minute, give usual dose q 12 hours; if clearance is 10 to 25 ml/minute, give half the usual dose q 12 hours; and if clearance is below 10 ml/minute, give half the usual dose q 24 hours.

## I.V. ADMINISTRATION
● For I.V. bolus administration, add 10 ml of sterile water for injection to 500 mg/20-ml vial or 20 ml to 1 g/30-ml vial. Shake to dissolve, and let stand until clear.
● For I.V. infusion, an infusion vial (500 mg/100 ml or 1 g/100 ml) may be directly reconstituted with a compatible infusion fluid. Or, an injection vial may be reconstituted and the resulting solution added to an I.V. container and further diluted with an appropriate infusion fluid. Don't use ADD-Vantage vials for this purpose.
● For ADD-Vantage vials, constitute only with half-normal saline solution for injection, normal saline solution for injection, or D₅W in 50-, 100-, or 250-ml Abbott ADD-Vantage flexible diluent containers. Follow manufacturer's guidelines closely when using ADD-Vantage vials.
● Don't mix meropenem with solutions containing other drugs.
● Use freshly prepared solutions of drug immediately whenever possible. Stability

of drug varies with form of drug used (injection vial, infusion vial, or ADD-Vantage container).

## ACTION
Inhibits cell-wall synthesis in bacteria. It readily penetrates cell wall of most gram-positive and -negative bacteria to reach penicillin-binding-protein targets.

| Route | Onset | Peak | Duration |
|-------|-------|------|----------|
| I.V. | Unknown | 1 hr | Unknown |

## ADVERSE REACTIONS
**CNS:** *seizures,* headache.
**CV:** phlebitis, thrombophlebitis.
**GI:** diarrhea, nausea, vomiting, constipation, *pseudomembranous colitis,* oral candidiasis, glossitis.
**GU:** presence of RBCs in urine.
**Respiratory:** *apnea,* dyspnea.
**Skin:** rash, pruritus, injection site inflammation.
**Other:** hypersensitivity reactions, *anaphylaxis,* inflammation.

## INTERACTIONS
**Drug-drug.** *Probenecid:* May decrease renal excretion of meropenem; probenecid competes with meropenem for active tubular secretion, which significantly increases elimination half-life of meropenem and extent of systemic exposure. Avoid using together.

## EFFECTS ON LAB TEST RESULTS
● May increase ALT, AST, bilirubin, alkaline phosphatase, LDH, creatinine, and BUN levels.
● May increase eosinophil count. May decrease hemoglobin, hematocrit, and WBC count. May increase or decrease PT, PTT, and INR, and platelet count.

## CONTRAINDICATIONS & CAUTIONS
● Contraindicated in patients hypersensitive to components of drug or other drugs in same class and in patients who have had anaphylactic reactions to beta-lactams.
● Use cautiously in elderly patients and in those with a history of seizure disorders or impaired renal function.
● Safety and effectiveness of drug haven't been established for patients younger than

age 3 months. Don't use drug in these patients.
● It's unknown if meropenem appears in breast milk. Use drug cautiously in breast-feeding women.
● Drug isn't used to treat methicillin-resistant staphylococci.

**NURSING CONSIDERATIONS**
● Obtain specimen for culture and sensitivity tests before giving first dose. Therapy may begin pending test results.
● *Alert:* Serious and occasionally fatal hypersensitivity reactions may occur in patients receiving beta-lactams. Before therapy begins, determine if patient has had previous hypersensitivity reactions to penicillins, cephalosporins, other beta-lactams, or other allergens.
● Stop drug and notify prescriber if an allergic reaction occurs. Serious anaphylactic reactions require immediate emergency treatment.
● Drug may cause seizures and other CNS adverse reactions in patients with CNS disorders, bacterial meningitis, and compromised renal function.
● If seizures occur during drug therapy, stop infusion and notify prescriber. Dosage adjustment may be needed.
● Monitor patient for signs and symptoms of superinfection. Drug may cause overgrowth of nonsusceptible bacteria or fungi.
● Periodic assessment of organ system functions, including renal, hepatic, and hematopoietic function, is recommended during prolonged therapy.
● Monitor patient's fluid balance and weight carefully.

**PATIENT TEACHING**
● Advise breast-feeding woman about risk of transmitting drug to infant through breast milk.
● Instruct patient to report adverse reactions or signs and symptoms of superinfection.

## nitrofurantoin macrocrystals
Macrobid✐, Macrodantin

## nitrofurantoin microcrystals
Apo-Nitrofurantoin†, Furadantin, Novo-Furantoin†

*Pregnancy risk category B*

**AVAILABLE FORMS**
**nitrofurantoin macrocrystals**
*Capsules:* 25 mg, 50 mg, 100 mg
**nitrofurantoin microcrystals**
*Oral suspension:* 25 mg/5 ml

**INDICATIONS & DOSAGES**
➤ **UTIs caused by susceptible *Escherichia coli, Staphylococcus aureus, enterococci;* or certain strains of *Klebsiella* and *Enterobacter* species**
*Adults and children older than age 12:* 50 to 100 mg P.O. q.i.d. with meals and h.s. Or, 100 mg Macrobid P.O. q 12 hours for 7 days.
*Children ages 1 month to 12 years:* 5 to 7 mg/kg P.O. daily, divided q.i.d.
➤ **Long-term suppression therapy**
*Adults:* 50 to 100 mg P.O. daily h.s.
*Children:* 1 mg/kg P.O. daily in a single dose h.s. or divided into two doses given q 12 hours.

**ACTION**
Unknown. May interfere with bacterial enzyme systems and bacterial cell-wall formation.

| Route | Onset | Peak | Duration |
|-------|-------|------|----------|
| P.O. | Unknown | Unknown | Unknown |

**ADVERSE REACTIONS**
**CNS:** peripheral neuropathy, headache, dizziness, drowsiness, *ascending polyneuropathy with high doses or renal impairment.*
**GI:** *anorexia, nausea, vomiting,* abdominal pain, *diarrhea.*
**GU:** overgrowth of nonsusceptible organisms in urinary tract.
**Hematologic:** *hemolysis in patients with G6PD deficiency, agranulocytosis, thrombocytopenia.*
**Hepatic:** *hepatitis, hepatic necrosis.*
**Metabolic:** *hypoglycemia.*

**Respiratory:** *pulmonary sensitivity reactions, asthmatic attacks.*
**Skin:** maculopapular, erythematous, or eczematous eruption; transient alopecia; pruritus; urticaria; exfoliative dermatitis; *Stevens-Johnson syndrome.*
**Other:** hypersensitivity reactions, *anaphylaxis,* drug fever.

## INTERACTIONS
**Drug-drug.** *Antacids containing magnesium:* May decrease nitrofurantoin absorption. Separate dosage times by 1 hour.
*Probenecid, sulfinpyrazone:* May inhibit excretion of nitrofurantoin, increasing blood levels and risk of toxicity. The resulting decreased urinary levels could lessen antibacterial effects. Avoid using together.
**Drug-food.** *Any food:* May increase absorption. Advise patient to take drug with food or milk.

## EFFECTS ON LAB TEST RESULTS
● May increase bilirubin and alkaline phosphatase levels. May decrease glucose level.
● May decrease granulocyte and platelet counts.
● May cause false-positive results in urine glucose tests using cupric sulfate (such as Benedict's reagent, Fehling's solution, or Chemstrip Ug).

## CONTRAINDICATIONS & CAUTIONS
● Contraindicated in infants age 1 month and younger and in patients with anuria, oliguria, or creatinine clearance less than 60 ml/minute. Also contraindicated in pregnant patients at 38 to 42 weeks' gestation and during labor and delivery.
● Use cautiously in patients with renal impairment, asthma, anemia, diabetes mellitus, electrolyte abnormalities, vitamin B deficiency, debilitating disease, and G6PD deficiency.

## NURSING CONSIDERATIONS
● Obtain urine specimen for culture and sensitivity tests before giving first dose. Repeat as needed. Therapy may begin pending results.
● Give drug with food or milk to minimize GI distress and improve absorption.

● Drug may cause an asthma attack in patients with a history of asthma.
● Monitor fluid intake and output carefully. May turn urine brown or dark yellow.
● Monitor CBC and pulmonary status regularly.
● *Alert:* Monitor patient for signs and symptoms of superinfection. Use of nitrofurantoin may result in growth of nonsusceptible organisms, especially *Pseudomonas* species.
● Monitor patient for pulmonary sensitivity reactions, including cough, chest pain, fever, chills, dyspnea, and pulmonary infiltration with consolidation or effusions.
● *Alert:* Hypersensitivity may develop when drug is used for long-term therapy.
● Some patients may experience fewer adverse GI effects with nitrofurantoin macrocrystals.
● Dual-release capsules (25 mg nitrofurantoin macrocrystals combined with 75 mg nitrofurantoin monohydrate) enable patients to take drug only twice daily.
● Continue treatment for 3 days after sterile urine specimens have been obtained.
● Store drug in amber container. Keep away from metals other than stainless steel or aluminum to avoid precipitate formation.

## PATIENT TEACHING
● Instruct patient to take drug for as long as prescribed, exactly as directed, even after he feels better.
● Tell patient to take drug with food or milk to minimize stomach upset.
● Instruct patient to report adverse reactions, especially peripheral neuropathy, which can become severe or irreversible.
● Alert patient that drug may turn urine dark yellow or brown.
● Warn patient not to store drug in container made of metal other than stainless steel or aluminum.

# quinupristin and dalfopristin
Synercid

*Pregnancy risk category B*

## AVAILABLE FORMS
*Injection:* 500 mg/10 ml (150 mg quinupristin and 350 mg dalfopristin)

---

Reactions may be *common,* uncommon, *life-threatening,* or COMMON AND LIFE-THREATENING.

## INDICATIONS & DOSAGES

➤ **Serious or life-threatening infections with vancomycin-resistant *Enterococcus faecium* bacteremia**
*Adults and adolescents age 16 and older:*
7.5 mg/kg I.V. over 1 hour q 8 hours.
Length of treatment depends on site and severity of infection.

➤ **Complicated skin and skin-structure infections caused by methicillin-susceptible *Staphylococcus aureus* or *Streptococcus pyogenes***
*Adults and adolescents age 16 and older:*
7.5 mg/kg I.V. over 1 hour q 12 hours for at least 7 days.

## I.V. ADMINISTRATION

• Reconstitute powder for injection by adding 5 ml of either sterile water for injection or D$_5$W and gently swirling vial by manual rotation to ensure dissolution; avoid shaking to limit foaming. Reconstituted solutions must be further diluted within 30 minutes.
• Add appropriate dose of reconstituted solution to 250 ml of D$_5$W, according to patient's weight, to yield no more than 2 mg/ml. This diluted solution is stable for 5 hours at room temperature or 54 hours if refrigerated.
• Fluid-restricted patients with a central venous catheter may receive dose in 100 ml of D$_5$W. This concentration isn't recommended for peripheral venous administration.
• If moderate to severe peripheral venous irritation occurs, consider increasing infusion volume to 500 or 750 ml, changing injection site, or infusing by a central venous catheter.
• Give all doses by I.V. infusion over 1 hour. An infusion pump or device may be used to control infusion rate.
• *Alert:* Quinupristin and dalfopristin are incompatible with saline and heparin solutions. Don't dilute drug with solutions containing saline or infuse into lines that contain saline or heparin. Flush line with D$_5$W before and after each dose.

## ACTION

The two antibiotics work synergistically to inhibit or destroy susceptible bacteria through combined inhibition on protein synthesis in bacterial cells. Without the ability to manufacture new proteins, the bacterial cells are inactivated or die.

| Route | Onset | Peak | Duration |
|-------|-------|------|----------|
| I.V. | Unknown | Unknown | Unknown |

## ADVERSE REACTIONS

**CNS:** headache.
**CV:** thrombophlebitis.
**GI:** nausea, diarrhea, vomiting.
**Musculoskeletal:** arthralgia, myalgia.
**Skin:** rash; pruritus; *inflammation, pain, edema at infusion site; infusion site reaction.*

## INTERACTIONS

**Drug-drug.** *Cyclosporine:* May lower metabolism; may increase drug level. Monitor cyclosporine level.
*Drugs metabolized by cytochrome P-450 3A4 (such as carbamazepine, delavirdine, diazepam, diltiazem, disopyramide, docetaxel, indinavir, lidocaine, lovastatin, methylprednisolone, midazolam, nevirapine, nifedipine, paclitaxel, ritonavir, tacrolimus, verapamil, vinblastine):* May increase levels of these drugs, which could increase both their therapeutic effects and adverse reactions. Use together cautiously.
*Drugs metabolized by cytochrome P-450 3A4 that may prolong the QTc interval (such as quinidine):* May decrease metabolism of these drugs, prolonging QTc interval. Avoid using together.

## EFFECTS ON LAB TEST RESULTS

• May increase AST, ALT, and bilirubin levels.

## CONTRAINDICATIONS & CAUTIONS

• Contraindicated in patients hypersensitive to drug or other streptogramin antibiotics.

## NURSING CONSIDERATIONS

• Drug isn't active against *Enterococcus faecalis.* Appropriate blood cultures are needed to avoid misidentifying *E. faecalis* as *E. faecium.*
• Because drug may cause mild to life-threatening pseudomembranous colitis, consider this diagnosis in patient who develops diarrhea during or after therapy.

• Adverse reactions, such as arthralgia and myalgia, may be reduced by decreasing dosage interval to every 12 hours.
• Because overgrowth of nonsusceptible organisms may occur, monitor patient closely for signs and symptoms of super-infection.
• Monitor liver function tests during therapy.

**PATIENT TEACHING**
• Advise patient to immediately report irritation at I.V. site, pain in joints or muscles, and diarrhea.
• Tell patient about importance of reporting persistent or worsening signs and symptoms of infection, such as pain or redness.

---

**trimethoprim**
Primsol, Proloprim, Trimpex, Triprim‡

*Pregnancy risk category C*

**AVAILABLE FORMS**
*Oral solution:* 50 mg/5 ml
*Tablets:* 100 mg, 200 mg

**INDICATIONS & DOSAGES**
➤ **Uncomplicated UTIs caused by susceptible strains of** *Escherichia coli, Proteus mirabilis, Klebsiella pneumoniae, Enterobacter* **species, and coagulase-negative** *Staphylococcus,* **including** *S. saprophyticus*
*Adults:* 200 mg P.O. daily as a single dose (as tablet or solution) or in divided doses q 12 hours for 10 days.
*Adjust-a-dose:* For patients with creatinine clearance of 15 to 30 ml/minute, give 50 mg P.O. q 12 hours; if clearance is below 15 ml/minute, don't use drug.
➤ **Acute otitis media caused by susceptible strains of** *Streptococcus pneumoniae* **and** *Haemophilus influenzae*
*Children 6 months of age and older:* 10 mg/kg/day of Primsol, in divided doses q 12 hours for 10 days.

**ACTION**
Interferes with the action of dihydrofolate reductase, inhibiting bacterial synthesis of folic acid.

| Route | Onset | Peak | Duration |
|-------|-------|------|----------|
| P.O. | Unknown | 1-4 hr | Unknown |

**ADVERSE REACTIONS**
**CNS:** fever.
**GI:** *epigastric distress, nausea, vomiting,* glossitis.
**Hematologic:** *thrombocytopenia, leukopenia,* megaloblastic anemia, methemoglobinemia.
**Skin:** *rash, pruritus.*

**INTERACTIONS**
**Drug-drug.** *Phenytoin:* May decrease phenytoin metabolism and increase drug level. Monitor patient for toxicity.

**EFFECTS ON LAB TEST RESULTS**
• May increase BUN, creatinine, bilirubin, and aminotransferase levels.
• May decrease hemoglobin and platelet and WBC counts.

**CONTRAINDICATIONS & CAUTIONS**
• Contraindicated in patients hypersensitive to drug.
• Contraindicated in patients younger than age 12 and in those with megaloblastic anemia from folate deficiency.
• Use cautiously in patients with impaired hepatic or renal function.
• Use cautiously in patients with possible folate deficiency.

**NURSING CONSIDERATIONS**
• Obtain urine specimen for culture and sensitivity tests before giving first dose. Therapy may begin pending results.
• Monitor renal and liver function test results in patients who may have folate deficiency.
• Monitor CBC routinely. Sore throat, fever, pallor, or purpura may be early indications of serious blood disorders.
• Monitor patient's fluid balance.
• *Alert:* Prolonged use of trimethoprim at high doses may cause bone marrow suppression.
• Because resistance to trimethoprim develops rapidly when the drug is given alone, it's usually given with other drugs.
• *Alert:* Trimethoprim is also used with sulfamethoxazole; don't confuse the two products.

---

Reactions may be *common,* uncommon, *life-threatening,* or COMMON AND LIFE-THREATENING.

## PATIENT TEACHING
● Instruct patient to take entire amount of drug, as prescribed, even after he feels better.
● Tell patient to report adverse reactions promptly, especially signs of infection or unusual bruising.
● Inform patient of the need for drinking plenty of liquids during therapy (2 to 3 L/day).

## vancomycin hydrochloride
Vancocin, Vancoled

*Pregnancy risk category C*

### AVAILABLE FORMS
*Capsules:* 125 mg, 250 mg
*Powder for injection:* 500-mg vials, 1-g vials
*Powder for oral solution:* 1-g bottles, 10-g bottles

### INDICATIONS & DOSAGES
➤ **Serious or severe infections when other antibiotics are ineffective or contraindicated, including those caused by methicillin-resistant *Staphylococcus aureus*, *S. epidermidis*, or diphtheroid organisms**
*Adults:* 1 to 1.5 g I.V. q 12 hours.
*Children:* 10 mg/kg I.V. q 6 hours.
*Neonates and young infants:* 15 mg/kg I.V. loading dose, then 10 mg/kg I.V. q 12 hours if child is younger than age 1 week or 10 mg/kg I.V. q 8 hours if age is older than 1 week but younger than 1 month.
*Elderly patients:* 15 mg/kg I.V. loading dose. Subsequent doses are based on renal function and serum drug levels.
➤ **Antibiotic-related pseudomembranous (*Clostridium difficile*) and *S. enterocolitis***
*Adults:* 125 to 500 mg P.O. q 6 hours for 7 to 10 days.
*Children:* 40 mg/kg P.O. daily, in divided doses q 6 hours for 7 to 10 days. Maximum daily dose is 2 g.
➤ **Endocarditis prophylaxis for dental procedures**
*Adults:* 1 g I.V. slowly over 1 to 2 hours, completing infusion 30 minutes before procedure.

*Children:* 20 mg/kg I.V. over 1 to 2 hours, completing infusion 30 minutes before procedure.
**Adjust-a-dose:** In renal insufficiency, adjust dosage based on degree of renal impairment, drug level, severity of infection, and susceptibility of causative organism. Initially, give 15 mg/kg, and adjust subsequent doses, p.r.n.
One possible schedule is as follows: If creatinine level is less than 1.5 mg/dl, give 1 g q 12 hours. If creatinine level is 1.5 to 5 mg/dl, give 1 g q 3 to 6 days. If creatinine level is greater than 5 mg/dl, give 1 g q 10 to 14 days. Or, if GFR is 10 to 50 ml/minute, give usual dose q 3 to 10 days, and if GFR is less than 10 ml/minute, give usual dose q 10 days.

### I.V. ADMINISTRATION
● For I.V. infusion, dilute in 200 ml normal saline solution for injection or $D_5W$, and infuse over 60 minutes; if dose is greater than 1 g, infuse over 90 minutes.
● Check site daily for phlebitis and irritation. Severe irritation and necrosis can result from extravasation.
● Refrigerate I.V. solution after reconstitution and use within 14 days.

### ACTION
Hinders bacterial cell-wall synthesis, damaging the bacterial plasma membrane and making the cell more vulnerable to osmotic pressure. Also interferes with RNA synthesis.

| Route | Onset | Peak | Duration |
|---|---|---|---|
| P.O. | Unknown | Unknown | Unknown |
| I.V. | Immediate | Immediate | Unknown |

### ADVERSE REACTIONS
**CNS:** fever, pain.
**CV:** hypotension, thrombophlebitis at injection site.
**EENT:** tinnitus, ototoxicity.
**GI:** nausea, *pseudomembranous colitis.*
**GU:** *nephrotoxicity.*
**Hematologic:** *neutropenia, leukopenia,* eosinophilia.
**Respiratory:** wheezing, dyspnea.
**Skin:** red-man syndrome (with rapid I.V. infusion).
**Other:** chills, *anaphylaxis,* superinfection.

## INTERACTIONS
**Drug-drug.** *Aminoglycosides, amphotericin B, cisplatin, pentamidine:* May increase risk of nephrotoxicity and ototoxicity. Monitor renal function and hearing function tests.

## EFFECTS ON LAB TEST RESULTS
• May increase BUN and creatinine levels.
• May increase eosinophil counts. May decrease neutrophil and WBC counts.

## CONTRAINDICATIONS & CAUTIONS
• Contraindicated in patients hypersensitive to drug.

## NURSING CONSIDERATIONS
• Use cautiously in patients receiving other neurotoxic, nephrotoxic, or ototoxic drugs; in patients older than age 60; and in those with impaired hepatic or renal function, preexisting hearing loss, or allergies to other antibiotics. Patients with renal dysfunction need dosage adjustment. Monitor blood levels to adjust I.V. dosage. Normal therapeutic levels of vancomycin are peak, 30 to 40 mg/L (drawn 1 hour after infusion ends), and trough, 5 to 10 mg/L (drawn just before next dose is given).
• Obtain specimen for culture and sensitivity tests before giving first dose. Because of the emergence of vancomycin-resistant enterococci, reserve use of drug for treatment of serious infections caused by gram-positive bacteria resistant to beta-lactam anti-infectives.
• Obtain hearing evaluation and renal function studies before therapy.
• Monitor patient's fluid balance and watch for oliguria and cloudy urine.
• Monitor patient carefully for red-man syndrome, which can occur if drug is infused too rapidly. Signs and symptoms include maculopapular rash on face, neck, trunk, and limbs and pruritus and hypotension caused by histamine release. If wheezing, urticaria, or pain and muscle spasm of the chest and back occur, stop infusion and notify prescriber.
• Don't give drug I.M.
• *Alert:* Oral administration is ineffective for systemic infections, and I.V. administration is ineffective for pseudomembranous (*Clostridium difficile*) diarrhea.

• Oral preparation is stable for 2 weeks if refrigerated.
• Monitor renal function (BUN, creatinine, and creatinine clearance levels; urinalysis; and urine output) during therapy. Also monitor patient for signs and symptoms of superinfection.
• Have patient's hearing evaluated during prolonged therapy.
• When using drug to treat staphylococcal endocarditis, give for at least 4 weeks.

## PATIENT TEACHING
• Tell patient to take entire amount of drug exactly as directed, even after he feels better.
• Instruct patient receiving drug I.V. to report discomfort at I.V. insertion site.
• Tell patient to report ringing in ears.

# 18

## Inotropics

**digoxin**
**inamrinone lactate**
**milrinone lactate**

**COMBINATION PRODUCTS**
None.

## digoxin
Digitek, Digoxin, Lanoxicaps,
Lanoxin*✔

*Pregnancy risk category C*

**AVAILABLE FORMS**
*Capsules:* 0.05 mg, 0.1 mg, 0.2 mg
*Elixir:* 0.05 mg/ml
*Injection:* 0.05 mg/ml†, 0.1 mg/ml (pediatric), 0.25 mg/ml
*Tablets:* 0.125 mg, 0.25 mg

**INDICATIONS & DOSAGES**
➤ **Heart failure, paroxysmal supraventricular tachycardia, atrial fibrillation and flutter**
*Tablets, elixir*
*Adults:* For rapid digitalization, give 0.75 to 1.25 mg P.O. over 24 hours in two or more divided doses q 6 to 8 hours. For slow digitalization, give 0.125 to 0.5 mg daily for 5 to 7 days. Maintenance dose is 0.125 to 0.5 mg daily.
*Children age 10 and older:* 10 to 15 mcg/kg P.O. over 24 hours in two or more divided doses q 6 to 8 hours. Maintenance dose is 25% to 35% of total digitalizing dose.
*Children ages 5 to 10:* 20 to 35 mcg/kg P.O. over 24 hours in two or more divided doses q 6 to 8 hours. Maintenance dose is 25% to 35% of total digitalizing dose.
*Children ages 2 to 5:* 30 to 40 mcg/kg P.O. over 24 hours in two or more divided doses q 6 to 8 hours. Maintenance dose is 25% to 35% of total digitalizing dose.
*Infants ages 1 month to 2 years:* 35 to 60 mcg/kg P.O. over 24 hours in two or more divided doses q 6 to 8 hours. Maintenance dose is 25% to 35% of total digitalizing dose.

*Neonates:* 25 to 35 mcg/kg P.O. over 24 hours in two or more divided doses q 6 to 8 hours. Maintenance dose is 25% to 35% of total digitalizing dose.
*Premature infants:* 20 to 30 mcg/kg P.O. over 24 hours in two or more divided doses q 6 to 8 hours. Maintenance dose is 20% to 30% of total digitalizing dose.
*Capsules*
*Adults:* For rapid digitalization, give 0.4 to 0.6 mg P.O. initially, followed by 0.1 to 0.3 mg q 6 to 8 hours, as needed and tolerated, for 24 hours. For slow digitalization, give 0.05 to 0.35 mg daily in two divided doses for 7 to 22 days, p.r.n., until therapeutic levels are reached. Maintenance dose is 0.05 to 0.35 mg daily in one or two divided doses.
*Children:* Digitalizing dose is based on child's age and is given in three or more divided doses over the first 24 hours. First dose is 50% of the total dose; subsequent doses are given q 4 to 8 hours as needed and tolerated.
*Children age 10 and older:* For rapid digitalization, give 8 to 12 mcg/kg P.O. over 24 hours, divided as above. Maintenance dose is 25% to 35% of total digitalizing dose, given daily as a single dose.
*Children ages 5 to 10:* For rapid digitalization, give 15 to 30 mcg/kg P.O. over 24 hours, divided as above. Maintenance dose is 25% to 35% of total digitalizing dose, divided and given in two or three equal portions daily.
*Children ages 2 to 5:* For rapid digitalization, give 25 to 35 mcg/kg P.O. over 24 hours, divided as above. Maintenance dose is 25% to 35% of total digitalizing dose, divided and given in two or three equal portions daily.
*Injection*
*Adults:* For rapid digitalization, give 0.4 to 0.6 mg I.V. initially, followed by 0.1 to 0.3 mg I.V. q 4 to 8 hours, as needed and tolerated, for 24 hours. For slow digitalization, give appropriate daily maintenance dose for 7 to 22 days as needed until therapeutic levels are reached. Maintenance

dose is 0.125 to 0.5 mg I.V. daily in one or two divided doses.

*Children:* Digitalizing dose is based on child's age and is given in three or more divided doses over the first 24 hours. First dose is 50% of total dose; subsequent doses are given q 4 to 8 hours as needed and tolerated.

*Children age 10 and older:* For rapid digitalization, give 8 to 12 mcg/kg I.V. over 24 hours, divided as above. Maintenance dose is 25% to 35% of total digitalizing dose, given daily as a single dose.

*Children ages 5 to 10:* For rapid digitalization, give 15 to 30 mcg/kg I.V. over 24 hours, divided as above. Maintenance dose is 25% to 35% of total digitalizing dose, divided and given in two or three equal portions daily.

*Children ages 2 to 5:* For rapid digitalization, give 25 to 35 mcg/kg I.V. over 24 hours, divided as above. Maintenance dose is 25% to 35% of total digitalizing dose, divided and given in two or three equal portions daily.

*Infants ages 1 month to 2 years:* For rapid digitalization, give 30 to 50 mcg/kg I.V. over 24 hours, divided as above. Maintenance dose is 25% to 35% of total digitalizing dose, divided and given in two or three equal portions daily.

*Neonates:* For rapid digitalization, give 20 to 30 mcg/kg I.V. over 24 hours, divided as above. Maintenance dose is 25% to 35% of the total digitalizing dose, divided and given in two or three equal portions daily.

*Premature infants:* For rapid digitalization, give 15 to 25 mcg/kg I.V. over 24 hours, divided as above. Maintenance dose is 20% to 30% of the total digitalizing dose, divided and given in two or three equal portions daily.

*Adjust-a-dose:* Give smaller loading and maintenance doses to patients with impaired renal function.

## I.V. ADMINISTRATION

- Dilute fourfold with $D_5W$, normal saline solution, or sterile water for injection to reduce the chance of precipitation.
- Infuse drug slowly over at least 5 minutes.
- Protect preparations from light.

## ACTION

Inhibits sodium potassium–activated adenosine triphosphatase, promoting movement of calcium from extracellular to intracellular cytoplasm and strengthening myocardial contraction. Also acts on CNS to enhance vagal tone, slowing conduction through the SA and AV nodes and providing an antiarrhythmic effect.

| Route | Onset | Peak | Duration |
|-------|-------|------|----------|
| P.O. | 90-120 min | 2-6 hr | 3-4 days |
| I.V. | 5-30 min | 1-4 hr | 3-4 days |

## ADVERSE REACTIONS

**CNS:** *fatigue, generalized muscle weakness, agitation, hallucinations,* headache, malaise, dizziness, vertigo, stupor, paresthesia.

**CV:** *arrhythmias.*

**EENT:** yellow-green halos around visual images, blurred vision, light flashes, photophobia, diplopia.

**GI:** *anorexia, nausea,* vomiting, diarrhea.

## INTERACTIONS

**Drug-drug.** *Amiloride:* May decrease digoxin effect and increase digoxin excretion. Monitor patient for altered digoxin effect.

*Amiodarone, diltiazem, indomethacin, nifedipine, quinidine, verapamil:* May increase digoxin level. Monitor patient for toxicity.

*Amphotericin B, carbenicillin, corticosteroids, diuretics (such as chlorthalidone, loop diuretics, metolazone, thiazides), ticarcillin:* May cause hypokalemia, predisposing patient to digitalis toxicity. Monitor potassium level.

*Antacids, kaolin-pectin:* May decrease absorption of oral digoxin. Separate doses as much as possible.

*Antibiotics:* May increase risk of toxicity because of altered intestinal flora. Monitor patient for toxicity.

*Anticholinergics:* May increase digoxin absorption of oral digoxin tablets. Monitor drug level and observe for toxicity.

*Cholestyramine, colestipol, metoclopramide:* May decrease absorption of oral digoxin. Monitor patient for decreased digoxin effect and low drug level. Give digoxin 1½ hours before or 2 hours after other drugs.

---

Reactions may be *common,* uncommon, *life-threatening,* or **COMMON AND LIFE-THREATENING.**

*Parenteral calcium, thiazides:* May cause hypercalcemia and hypomagnesemia, predisposing patient to digitalis toxicity. Monitor calcium and magnesium levels.

**Drug-herb.** *Betel palm, fumitory, goldenseal, hawthorn, lily of the valley, motherwort, rue, shepherd's purse:* May increase cardiac effects. Discourage use together.

*Gossypol, horsetail, licorice, oleander, Siberian ginseng, squill:* May increase toxicity. Monitor patient closely.

*Plantain, St. John's wort:* May decrease effectiveness of digoxin. Discourage use together.

**EFFECTS ON LAB TEST RESULTS**
None reported.

**CONTRAINDICATIONS & CAUTIONS**
• Contraindicated in patients hypersensitive to drug and in those with digitalis-induced toxicity, ventricular fibrillation, or ventricular tachycardia unless caused by heart failure.
• Use with extreme caution in elderly patients and in those with acute MI, incomplete AV block, sinus bradycardia, PVCs, chronic constrictive pericarditis, hypertrophic cardiomyopathy, renal insufficiency, severe pulmonary disease, or hypothyroidism.

**NURSING CONSIDERATIONS**
• Drug-induced arrhythmias may increase the severity of heart failure and hypotension.
• In children, cardiac arrythmias, including sinus bradycardia, are usually early signs of toxicity.
• Patients with hypothyroidism are extremely sensitive to cardiac glycosides and may need lower doses.
• Before giving loading dose, obtain baseline data (heart rate and rhythm, blood pressure, and electrolytes) and ask patient about use of cardiac glycosides within the previous 2 to 3 weeks.
• Loading dose is usually divided over the first 24 hours.
• Before giving drug, take apical-radial pulse for 1 minute. Record and notify prescriber of significant changes (sudden increase or decrease in pulse rate, pulse deficit, irregular beats and, particularly,

regularization of a previously irregular rhythm). If these occur, check blood pressure and obtain a 12-lead ECG.
• Toxic effects on the heart may be life-threatening and require immediate attention.
• Absorption of digoxin from liquid-filled capsules is superior to absorption from tablets or elixir. Expect dosage reduction of 20% to 25% when changing from tablets or elixir to liquid-filled capsules or parenteral therapy.
• Monitor digoxin level. Therapeutic level ranges from 0.8 to 2 ng/ml. Obtain blood for digoxin level at least 6 to 8 hours after last oral dose, preferably just before next scheduled dose.
• *Alert:* Excessive slowing of the pulse rate (60 beats per minute or less) may be a sign of digitalis toxicity. Withhold drug and notify prescriber.
• Monitor potassium level carefully. Take corrective action before hypokalemia occurs.
• Reduce drug dose for 1 to 2 days before elective cardioversion. Adjust dosage after cardioversion.
• *Alert:* Don't confuse digoxin with doxepin.

**PATIENT TEACHING**
• Teach patient and a responsible family member about drug action, dosage regimen, how to take pulse, reportable signs, and follow-up care.
• Tell patient to report pulse below 60 beats/minute or above 110 beats/minute, or skipped beats or other rhythm changes.
• Instruct patient to report adverse reactions promptly. Nausea, vomiting, diarrhea, appetite loss, and visual disturbances may be early indicators of toxicity.
• Encourage patient to eat potassium-rich foods.
• Tell patient not to substitute one brand of digoxin for another.
• Advise patient to avoid the use of herbal medications or to consult his prescriber before taking one.

## inamrinone lactate

*Pregnancy risk category C*

### AVAILABLE FORMS
*Injection:* 5 mg/ml in 20-ml ampules

### INDICATIONS & DOSAGES
➤ **Short-term management of heart failure**
*Adults:* Initially, 0.75 mg/kg I.V. bolus over 2 to 3 minutes. Then begin maintenance infusion of 5 to 10 mcg/kg/minute. May give additional bolus of 0.75 mg/kg 30 minutes after starting therapy. Don't exceed total daily dose of 10 mg/kg.

### I.V. ADMINISTRATION
● Give drug with an infusion pump. Use drug as supplied, or dilute in half-normal saline solution or normal saline solution to a concentration of 1 to 3 mg/ml. Use diluted solution within 24 hours.
● Don't dilute with solutions containing dextrose because a slow chemical reaction occurs over 24 hours. Inamrinone can be injected into free-flowing dextrose infusions through a Y-connector or directly into tubing.
● *Alert:* Don't give furosemide or torsemide and inamrinone through the same I.V. line because precipitation occurs.
● Monitor blood pressure and heart rate throughout the infusion. If patient's blood pressure falls, slow or stop infusion and notify prescriber.

### ACTION
Produces inotropic action by increasing cellular levels of cAMP. Produces vasodilation through a direct relaxant effect on vascular smooth muscle.

| Route | Onset | Peak | Duration |
|-------|-------|------|----------|
| I.V. | 2-5 min | 10 min | 30-120 min |

### ADVERSE REACTIONS
**CNS:** fever.
**CV:** *arrhythmias,* hypotension, chest pain.
**GI:** nausea, vomiting, anorexia, abdominal pain.
**Hematologic:** *thrombocytopenia.*
**Metabolic:** hypokalemia.

**Skin:** burning at injection site.
**Other:** hypersensitivity reactions.

### INTERACTIONS
**Drug-drug.** *Cardiac glycosides:* May increase inotropic effect, which is a beneficial drug interaction. Monitor patient.
*Disopyramide:* May cause excessive hypotension. Monitor blood pressure.

### EFFECTS ON LAB TEST RESULTS
● May increase liver enzyme levels. May decrease potassium level.
● May decrease platelet count.

### CONTRAINDICATIONS & CAUTIONS
● Contraindicated in patients hypersensitive to inamrinone or bisulfites.
● Contraindicated in patients with severe aortic or pulmonic valvular disease in place of surgery or during acute phase of MI.
● Use cautiously in patients with hypertrophic cardiomyopathy.
● Safety and effectiveness haven't been established in children younger than age 18. Don't use drug in children.

### NURSING CONSIDERATIONS
● Inamrinone is prescribed primarily for patients who haven't responded to cardiac glycosides, diuretics, and vasodilators.
● Dosage depends on clinical response, including assessment of pulmonary wedge pressure and cardiac output.
● Anticipate that drug may be added to cardiac glycoside therapy in patients with atrial fibrillation and flutter because it slightly enhances AV conduction and increases ventricular response rate.
● Correct hypokalemia before or during therapy.
● Monitor platelet count. If it falls below 150,000/mm³, decrease dosage.
● Monitor patient for hypersensitivity reactions, such as pericarditis, ascites, myositis vasculitis, and pleuritis.
● Monitor intake and output and daily weight.
● Patients with end-stage cardiac disease may receive home treatment with an inamrinone drip while awaiting heart transplantation.

---

Reactions may be *common,* uncommon, *life-threatening*, or COMMON AND LIFE-THREATENING.

● *Alert:* Because of confusion with amiodarone, the generic name amrinone was changed to inamrinone.

## PATIENT TEACHING
● Warn patient that burning may occur at injection site.
● Instruct home care patient and family on drug administration; tell them to report adverse reactions promptly.

---

## milrinone lactate
Primacor

*Pregnancy risk category C*

## AVAILABLE FORMS
*Injection:* 1 mg/ml
*Injection (premixed):* 200 mcg/ml in $D_5W$

## INDICATIONS & DOSAGES
➤ Short-term treatment of heart failure
*Adults:* First loading dose is 50 mcg/kg I.V., given slowly over 10 minutes; then continuous I.V. infusion of 0.375 to 0.75 mcg/kg/minute. Titrate infusion dose based on clinical and hemodynamic responses.
*Adjust-a-dose:* For patients with creatinine clearance 50 ml/minute or less, adjust dosage to maximum clinical effect; don't exceed 1.13 mg/kg/day.

## I.V. ADMINISTRATION
● Prepare I.V. infusion solution using half-normal saline solution, normal saline solution, or $D_5W$. Prepare the 100-mcg/ml solution by adding 180 ml of diluent per 20-mg (20-ml) vial, the 150-mcg/ml solution by adding 113 ml of diluent per 20-mg (20-ml) vial, and the 200-mcg/ml solution by adding 80 ml of diluent per 20-mg (20-ml) vial.
● *Alert:* If furosemide or torsemide is given into an I.V. line that contains milrinone, a precipitate will form.

## ACTION
Produces inotropic action by increasing cellular levels of cAMP. Produces vasodilation by directly relaxing vascular smooth muscle.

| Route | Onset | Peak | Duration |
|-------|-------|------|----------|
| I.V. | 5-15 min | 1-2 hr | 3-6 hr |

## ADVERSE REACTIONS
**CNS:** headache.
**CV:** VENTRICULAR ARRHYTHMIAS, *ventricular ectopic activity,* nonsustained ventricular tachycardia, **sustained ventricular tachycardia, ventricular fibrillation.**

## INTERACTIONS
None significant.

## EFFECTS ON LAB TEST RESULTS
None reported.

## CONTRAINDICATIONS & CAUTIONS
● Contraindicated in patients hypersensitive to drug.
● Contraindicated for use in patients with severe aortic or pulmonic valvular disease in place of surgery and during acute phase of MI.
● Use cautiously in patients with atrial flutter or fibrillation because drug slightly shortens AV node conduction time and may increase ventricular response rate.

## NURSING CONSIDERATIONS
● Give a cardiac glycoside, if ordered, before beginning milrinone therapy.
● Drug is typically given with digoxin and diuretics.
● Improved cardiac output may increase urine output. Expect dosage reduction in patient's diuretic therapy as heart failure improves. Potassium loss may predispose patient to digitalis toxicity.
● Monitor fluid and electrolyte status, blood pressure, heart rate, and renal function during therapy. Excessive decrease in blood pressure requires stopping or slowing rate of infusion. Correct hypoxemia if it occurs during treatment.

## PATIENT TEACHING
● Instruct patient to report adverse reactions promptly, especially angina.
● Tell patient that drug may cause headache, which can be treated with analgesics.
● Tell patient to report discomfort at I.V. insertion site.

---

*Rapid onset*   †Canada   ‡Australia   ◇OTC   ♦Off-label use   ✐Photoguide   *Liquid contains alcohol.

# 19
## Antiarrhythmics

adenosine
amiodarone hydrochloride
atropine sulfate
diltiazem hydrochloride
    (See Chapter 20, ANTIANGINALS.)
disopyramide
disopyramide phosphate
dofetilide
esmolol hydrochloride
flecainide acetate
ibutilide fumarate
lidocaine hydrochloride
mexiletine hydrochloride
moricizine hydrochloride
phenytoin
    (See Chapter 28, ANTICONVULSANTS.)
phenytoin sodium
    (See Chapter 28, ANTICONVULSANTS.)
procainamide hydrochloride
propranolol hydrochloride
    (See Chapter 20, ANTIANGINALS.)
quinidine bisulfate
quinidine gluconate
quinidine sulfate
sotalol hydrochloride
tocainide hydrochloride
verapamil hydrochloride
    (See Chapter 20, ANTIANGINALS.)

**COMBINATION PRODUCTS**
None.

---

## adenosine
Adenocard

*Pregnancy risk category C*

**AVAILABLE FORMS**
*Injection:* 3 mg/ml in 2-ml and 5-ml vials
and syringes

**INDICATIONS & DOSAGES**
➤ **To convert paroxysmal supraventricular tachycardia (PSVT) to sinus
rhythm**
*Adults and children weighing 50 kg
(110 lb) or more:* 6 mg I.V. by rapid bolus
injection over 1 to 2 seconds. If PSVT
isn't eliminated in 1 to 2 minutes, give

12 mg by rapid I.V. push and repeat, if
needed.
*Children weighing less than 50 kg:* Initially, 0.05 to 0.1 mg/kg I.V. by rapid bolus
injection followed by a saline flush. If
PSVT isn't eliminated in 1 to 2 minutes,
give additional bolus injections, increasing
the amount given by 0.05- to 0.1-mg/kg
increments, followed by a saline flush.
Continue, p.r.n., until conversion or a
maximum single dose of 0.3 mg/kg is
given.

**I.V. ADMINISTRATION**
● Give by rapid I.V. injection to ensure
drug action.
● Give directly into a vein, if possible;
when giving through an I.V. line, use the
port closest to the patient.
● Flush immediately and rapidly with normal saline solution to ensure that drug
quickly reaches the systemic circulation.
● Don't give single doses exceeding
12 mg.
● In adult patients, avoid giving the drug
through a central line because more prolonged asystole may occur.

**ACTION**
A naturally occurring nucleoside that acts
on the AV node to slow conduction and inhibit reentry pathways. Adenosine is also
useful in treating PSVT, including those
with accessory bypass tracts (Wolff-
Parkinson-White syndrome).

| Route | Onset | Peak | Duration |
|-------|-------|------|----------|
| I.V. | Immediate | Immediate | Unknown |

**ADVERSE REACTIONS**
**CNS:** dizziness, light-headedness, numb-
ness, tingling in arms, headache.
**CV:** *facial flushing.*
**GI:** nausea.
**Respiratory:** chest pressure, *dyspnea,
shortness of breath.*

---

## INTERACTIONS

**Drug-drug.** *Carbamazepine:* May result in higher degrees of heart block. Use together cautiously.

*Digoxin, verapamil:* May cause ventricular fibrillation. Monitor ECG closely.

*Dipyridamole:* May increase adenosine's effects. Smaller doses may be needed. Use together cautiously.

*Methylxanthines (caffeine, theophylline):* May increase adenosine's effects. Patients receiving methylxanthines may require higher doses or may not respond to adenosine therapy.

**Drug-herb.** *Guarana:* May decrease response. Monitor patient.

## EFFECTS ON LAB TEST RESULTS
None reported.

## CONTRAINDICATIONS & CAUTIONS
• Contraindicated in patients hypersensitive to drug.
• Contraindicated in those with second- or third-degree heart block or sinus node disease (such as sick sinus syndrome and symptomatic bradycardia), except those with a pacemaker.
• Use cautiously in patients with asthma, emphysema, or bronchitis because bronchoconstriction may occur.

## NURSING CONSIDERATIONS
• Adenosine decreases conduction through the AV node and may produce first-, second-, or third-degree heart block. Patients who develop high-level heart block after a single dose of adenosine shouldn't receive additional doses.
• **Alert:** Because new arrhythmias, including heart block and transient asystole, may develop, monitor cardiac rhythm and be prepared to give appropriate therapy.
• Crystals may form if solution is cold. If crystals are visible, gently warm solution to room temperature. Don't use solutions that aren't clear.
• Discard unused drug; adenosine lacks preservatives.

## PATIENT TEACHING
• Instruct patient to report adverse reactions promptly.
• Tell patient to report discomfort at I.V. site.

• Inform patient that he may experience flushing or chest pain lasting 1 to 2 minutes.

# amiodarone hydrochloride
Aratac‡, Cordarone◊, Cordarone X‡, Pacerone

*Pregnancy risk category D*

## AVAILABLE FORMS
*Injection:* 50 mg/ml in 3-ml ampules, vials
*Tablets:* 100 mg‡, 200 mg, 400 mg

## INDICATIONS & DOSAGES
➤ **Life-threatening recurrent ventricular fibrillation or recurrent hemodynamically unstable ventricular tachycardia unresponsive to adequate doses of other antiarrhythmics or when alternative drugs can't be tolerated**
*Adults:* Give loading dose of 800 to 1,600 mg P.O. daily divided b.i.d. for 1 to 3 weeks until first therapeutic response occurs; then 600 to 800 mg P.O. daily for 1 month, followed by maintenance dose 200 to 600 mg P.O. daily.

Or, give loading dose of 150 mg I.V. over 10 minutes (15 mg/minute); then 360 mg I.V. over next 6 hours (1 mg/minute), followed by 540 mg I.V. over next 18 hours (0.5 mg/minute). After first 24 hours, continue with maintenance I.V. infusion of 720 mg/24 hours (0.5 mg/minute).
➤ **Cardiac arrest, pulseless ventricular tachycardia, or ventricular fibrillation**
*Adults:* 300 mg diluted in 20 to 30 ml of a compatible solution, as I.V. push.
➤ **Supraventricular arrhythmias** ◆
*Adults:* Give loading dose of 600 to 800 mg P.O. daily for 1 to 4 weeks or until SVT is controlled or adverse reactions occur. Reduce gradually to maintenance dose of 100 to 400 mg P.O. daily.
➤ **Ventricular and supraventricular arrhythmias** ◆
*Children:* Give loading dose of 10 to 15 mg/kg/day or 600 to 800 mg/1.73 m$^2$ P.O. daily for 4 to 14 days or until arrhythmia is controlled or adverse reactions occur. Reduce dosage to 5 mg/kg/day or 200 to 400 mg/1.73 m$^2$ for several weeks;

then reduce dosage to lowest effective level.

Or, give loading dose 5 mg/kg I.V. infused over several minutes to 1 hour. Give additional 5-mg/kg doses if needed, to a maximum of 15 mg/kg/day. Or, 5 mg/kg I.V. in five divided doses of 1 mg/kg over 5 to 10 minutes to minimize exposure to diethylhexyl phthalate (DEHP).

➤ **Short-term management of atrial fibrillation** ◆

*Adults:* 125 mg/hour I.V. for 24 hours (total 3,000 mg have been used).

➤ **Long-term management of recurrent atrial fibrillation** ◆

*Adults:* 10 mg/kg P.O. daily for 14 days; then 300 mg P.O. daily for 4 weeks; then maintenance dose of 200 mg P.O. daily.

➤ **Heart failure (impaired left ventricular ejection fraction, impaired exercise tolerance, and ventricular arrhythmias)** ◆

*Adults:* 200 mg P.O. daily.

## I.V. ADMINISTRATION

● Give drug I.V. only where continuous ECG monitoring and electrophysiologic techniques are available. Mix first dose of 150 mg in 100 ml of $D_5W$ solution. Drug is incompatible with normal saline solution. Mix infusions planned for administration over 2 hours or longer in glass or polyolefin bottles.

● Use an in-line filter with I.V. administration.

● Give I.V. amiodarone whenever possible through a central line dedicated to that purpose. If concentration is 2 mg/ml or more, use a central line.

● Continuously monitor cardiac status of patient receiving drug I.V. If hypotension occurs, reduce infusion rate.

● *Alert:* Cordarone I.V. leaches out plasticizers such as DEHP from I.V. tubing, which can adversely affect male reproductive tract development in fetuses, infants, and toddlers.

## ACTION

Effects result from blockade of potassium chloride leading to a prolongation of action potential duration.

| Route | Onset | Peak | Duration |
|-------|-------|------|----------|
| P.O. | Variable | 3-7 hr | Variable |
| I.V. | Unknown | Unknown | Variable |

## ADVERSE REACTIONS

**CNS:** peripheral neuropathy, ataxia, paresthesia, *tremor,* insomnia, sleep disturbances, headache, *malaise, fatigue.*

**CV:** *bradycardia,* hypotension, *arrhythmias, heart failure, heart block, sinus arrest,* edema.

**EENT:** *asymptomatic corneal microdeposits,* optic neuropathy or neuritis resulting in visual impairment, abnormal smell, *visual disturbances.*

**GI:** abnormal taste, anorexia, *nausea, vomiting,* constipation, abdominal pain.

**Hematologic:** *coagulation abnormalities.*

**Hepatic:** hepatic dysfunction, *hepatic failure.*

**Metabolic:** *hypothyroidism,* hyperthyroidism.

**Respiratory:** *acute respiratory distress syndrome,* SEVERE PULMONARY TOXICITY.

**Skin:** *photosensitivity,* solar dermatitis, blue-gray skin.

## INTERACTIONS

**Drug-drug.** *Antiarrhythmics:* May reduce hepatic or renal clearance of certain antiarrhythmics, especially flecainide, procainamide, and quinidine. Use of amiodarone with other antiarrhythmics, especially mexiletine, propafenone, disopyramide, and procainamide, may induce torsades de pointes. Avoid using together.

*Antihypertensives:* May increase hypotensive effect. Use together cautiously.

*Beta blockers, calcium channel blockers:* May increase cardiac depressant effects; may increase slowing of SA node and AV conduction. Use together cautiously.

*Cimetidine:* May increase amiodarone level. Use together cautiously.

*Cyclosporine:* May increase creatinine level. Creatinine level may remain elevated even after cyclosporine dosage is reduced. Monitor renal function.

*Digoxin:* May increase digoxin level 70% to 100%. Monitor digoxin level closely, and reduce digoxin dosage by half or stop

---

Reactions may be *common*, uncommon, *life-threatening*, or COMMON AND LIFE-THREATENING.

drug completely when starting amiodarone therapy.

*Fentanyl:* May cause hypotension, bradycardia, and decreased cardiac output. Monitor patient closely.

*Fluoroquinolones:* May increase risk of arrhythmias. Avoid using together.

*Methotrexate:* May impair methotrexate metabolism, causing toxicity. Use together cautiously.

*Phenytoin:* May decrease phenytoin metabolism and amiodarone level. Monitor phenytoin level and adjust dosages of drugs if necessary.

*Quinidine:* May increase quinidine level, causing life-threatening cardiac arrhythmias. Avoid using together, or monitor quinidine level closely if use together can't be avoided. Adjust quinidine dosage as needed.

*Rifamycins:* May decrease amiodarone level. Monitor patient closely.

*Ritonavir:* May increase amiodarone level. Avoid using together.

*Theophylline:* May increase theophylline level and cause toxicity. Monitor theophylline level.

*Warfarin:* May increase anticoagulant response with the potential for serious or fatal bleeding. Decrease warfarin dosage 33% to 50% when starting amiodarone. Monitor patient closely.

**Drug-herb.** *Pennyroyal:* May change the rate of formation of toxic metabolites of pennyroyal. Discourage use together.

**Drug-lifestyle.** *Sun exposure:* May cause photosensitivity reaction. Advise patient to avoid excessive sunlight exposure.

### EFFECTS ON LAB TEST RESULTS
- May increase ALT, AST, alkaline phosphatase, $T_4$, and GGT levels. May decrease $T_3$ level.
- May increase PT and INR.

### CONTRAINDICATIONS & CAUTIONS
- Contraindicated in patients hypersensitive to drug.
- Contraindicated in those with cardiogenic shock, second- or third-degree AV block, severe SA node disease resulting in bradycardia unless an artificial pacemaker is present, and in those for whom bradycardia has caused syncope.
- Use cautiously in patients receiving other antiarrhythmics.
- Use cautiously in patients with pulmonary, hepatic, or thyroid disease.

### NURSING CONSIDERATIONS
- Be aware of the high risk of adverse reactions.
- Obtain baseline pulmonary, liver, and thyroid function tests and baseline chest X-ray.
- Give loading doses in a hospital setting and with continuous ECG monitoring because of the slow onset of antiarrhythmic effect and the risk of life-threatening arrhythmias.
- Divide oral loading dose into two equal doses and give with meals to decrease GI intolerance. Maintenance dose may be given once daily or divided into two doses taken with meals if GI intolerance occurs.
- **Alert:** Drug poses major and potentially life-threatening management problems in patients at risk for sudden death. Use only in patients with documented, life-threatening, recurrent ventricular arrhythmias unresponsive to documented adequate doses of other antiarrhythmics or when alternative drugs can't be tolerated. Amiodarone can cause fatal toxicities, including hepatic and pulmonary toxicity.
- **Alert:** Amiodarone is a highly toxic drug. Watch carefully for pulmonary toxicity. Risk increases in patients receiving doses over 400 mg/day.
- Watch for evidence of pneumonitis exertional dyspnea, nonproductive cough, and pleuritic chest pain. Monitor pulmonary function tests and chest X-ray.
- Monitor liver and thyroid function tests and levels of electrolytes, particularly potassium and magnesium.
- Monitor PT and INR if patient takes warfarin and digoxin level if he takes digoxin.
- Instill methylcellulose ophthalmic solution during amiodarone therapy to minimize corneal microdeposits. About 1 to 4 months after starting amiodarone, most patients develop corneal microdeposits, although 10% or less have vision disturbances.
- Monitor blood pressure and heart rate and rhythm frequently. Perform continuous ECG monitoring when starting or

changing dosage. Notify prescriber of significant change in assessment results.
• Life-threatening gasping syndrome may occur in neonates given I.V. solutions containing benzyl alcohol.
• *Alert:* Don't confuse amiodarone with amiloride.

## PATIENT TEACHING
• Advise patient to wear sunscreen or protective clothing to prevent sensitivity reaction to the sun. Monitor patient for skin burning or tingling, followed by redness and blistering. Exposed skin may turn blue-gray.
• Tell patient to take oral drug with food if GI reactions occur.
• Inform patient that adverse effects of drug are more common at high doses and become more frequent with treatment lasting longer than 6 months but are generally reversible when drug is stopped. Resolution of adverse reactions may take up to 4 months.

---

## atropine sulfate
Sal-Tropine

*Pregnancy risk category C*

---

## AVAILABLE FORMS
*Injection:* 0.05 mg/ml, 0.1 mg/ml, 0.3 mg/ml, 0.4 mg/ml, 0.5 mg/ml, 0.8 mg/ml, 1 mg/ml
*Tablets:* 0.4 mg

## INDICATIONS & DOSAGES
➤ **Symptomatic bradycardia, bradyarrhythmia (junctional or escape rhythm)**
*Adults:* Usually 0.5 to 1 mg I.V. push, repeated q 3 to 5 minutes to maximum of 2 mg p.r.n.
*Children and adolescents:* 0.02 mg/kg I.V., with minimum dose of 0.1 mg and maximum single dose of 0.5 mg in children or 1 mg in adolescents. May repeat dose at 5-minute intervals to a maximum total dose of 1 mg in children or 2 mg in adolescents.
➤ **Antidote for anticholinesterase insecticide poisoning**
*Adults:* 2 to 3 mg I.V. repeated q 5 to 10 minutes until muscarinic signs and symptoms disappear or signs of atropine toxicity appear. Severe poisoning may require up to 6 mg hourly.
*Children:* 0.05 mg/kg I.M. or I.V. repeated q 10 to 30 minutes until muscarinic signs and symptoms disappear (may be repeated if they reappear) or until atropine toxicity occurs.
➤ **Preoperatively to diminish secretions and block cardiac vagal reflexes**
*Adults and children weighing 20 kg (44 lb) or more:* 0.4 to 0.6 mg I.M. or S.C. 30 to 60 minutes before anesthesia.
*Children weighing less than 20 kg:* 0.01 mg/kg I.M. or S.C. up to maximum dose of 0.4 mg 30 to 60 minutes before anesthesia.
*Infants weighing more than 5 kg (11 lb):* 0.03 mg/kg q 4 to 6 hours p.r.n.
*Infants weighing 5 kg or less:* 0.04 mg/kg q 4 to 6 hours p.r.n.
➤ **Adjunct treatment of peptic ulcer disease; functional GI disorders such as irritable bowel syndrome**
*Adults:* 0.4 to 0.6 mg P.O. q 4 to 6 hours.
*Children:* 0.01 mg/kg or 0.3 mg/m² P.O. (not to exceed 0.4 mg) q 4 to 6 hours.

## I.V. ADMINISTRATION
• Give I.V. into a large vein or into I.V. tubing over at least 1 minute.
• Slow I.V. administration may cause paradoxical slowing of the heart rate.

## ACTION
An anticholinergic that inhibits acetylcholine at the parasympathetic neuroeffector junction, blocking vagal effects on the SA and AV nodes, thereby enhancing conduction through the AV node and increasing the heart rate.

| Route | Onset | Peak | Duration |
|-------|-------|------|----------|
| P.O. | 30-120 min | 1-2 hr | 4 hr |
| I.V. | Immediate | 2-4 min | 4 hr |
| I.M. | 5-40 min | 20-60 min | 4 hr |
| S.C. | Unknown | Unknown | Unknown |

## ADVERSE REACTIONS
**CNS:** *headache, restlessness,* ataxia, disorientation, hallucinations, delirium, *insomnia, dizziness,* excitement, agitation, confusion.
**CV:** palpitations, ***bradycardia,*** tachycardia.

---

**EENT:** photophobia, *blurred vision, mydriasis,* cycloplegia, increased intraocular pressure.
**GI:** *dry mouth,* thirst, *constipation,* nausea, vomiting.
**GU:** urine retention, impotence.
**Other:** *anaphylaxis.*

### INTERACTIONS
**Drug-drug.** *Antacids:* May decrease absorption of oral anticholinergics. Separate doses by at least 1 hour.
*Anticholinergics, drugs with anticholinergic effects (amantadine, antiarrhythmics, antiparkinsonians, glutethimide, meperidine, phenothiazines, tricyclic antidepressants):* May increase anticholinergic effects. Use together cautiously.
*Ketoconazole, levodopa:* May decrease absorption. Avoid using together.
*Potassium chloride wax-matrix tablets:* May increase risk of mucosal lesions. Use together cautiously.
**Drug-herb.** *Jaborandi tree, pill-bearing spurge:* May decrease effectiveness of drug. Discourage use together.
*Jimsonweed:* May adversely affect CV function. Discourage use together.
*Squaw vine:* Tannic acid may decrease metabolic breakdown of drug. Monitor patient.

### EFFECTS ON LAB TEST RESULTS
None reported.

### CONTRAINDICATIONS & CAUTIONS
• Contraindicated in patients hypersensitive to drug.
• Contraindicated in those with acute angle-closure glaucoma, obstructive uropathy, obstructive disease of GI tract, paralytic ileus, toxic megacolon, intestinal atony, unstable CV status in acute hemorrhage, tachycardia, myocardial ischemia, asthma, or myasthenia gravis.
• Use cautiously in patients with Down syndrome because they may be more sensitive to drug.

### NURSING CONSIDERATIONS
• Many adverse reactions (such as dry mouth and constipation) vary with the dose.

• In adults, avoid doses less than 0.5 mg because of the risk of paradoxical bradycardia.
• **Alert:** Watch for tachycardia in cardiac patients because it may lead to ventricular fibrillation.
• Monitor fluid intake and urine output. Drug causes urine retention and urinary hesitancy.

### PATIENT TEACHING
• Teach patient receiving oral form of drug how to handle distressing anticholinergic effects.
• Instruct patient to report serious or persistent adverse reactions promptly.
• Tell patient about potential for sensitivity of the eyes to the sun and suggest use of sunglasses.

## disopyramide
Rythmodan†‡

## disopyramide phosphate
Norpace, Norpace CR, Rythmodan-LA†

*Pregnancy risk category C*

### AVAILABLE FORMS
**disopyramide**
*Capsules:* 100 mg†, 150 mg†
**disopyramide phosphate**
*Capsules:* 100 mg, 150 mg
*Capsules (controlled-release):* 100 mg, 150 mg
*Tablets (sustained-release):* 250 mg†

### INDICATIONS & DOSAGES
➤ **Ventricular tachycardia and life-threatening ventricular arrhythmias**
*Adults weighing more than 50 kg (110 lb):* 150 mg P.O. q 6 hours with regular-release formulation or 300 mg q 12 hours with extended-release preparations.
*Adults weighing 50 kg or less:* 100 mg P.O. q 6 hour with regular-release formulation or 200 mg P.O. q 12 hours with extended-release preparations.
*Children ages 12 to 18:* 6 to 15 mg/kg P.O. daily, divided into four doses (q 6 hours).
*Children ages 4 to 12:* 10 to 15 mg/kg P.O. daily, divided into four doses (q 6 hours).

*Children ages 1 to 4:* 10 to 20 mg/kg P.O. daily, divided into four doses (q 6 hours).
*Children younger than age 1:* 10 to 30 mg/kg P.O. daily, divided into four doses (q 6 hours).
**Adjust-a-dose:** If creatinine clearance is 30 to 40 ml/minute, give 100 mg q 8 hours; if clearance is 15 to 30 ml/minute, give 100 mg q 12 hours; if clearance is below 15 ml/minute, give 100 mg q 24 hours.

## ACTION

A class IA antiarrhythmic that depresses phase 0 and prolongs the action potential. All class I drugs have membrane-stabilizing effects.

| Route | Onset | Peak | Duration |
|-------|-------|------|----------|
| P.O. | ½-3½ hr | 2-2½ hr | 1½-8½ hr |

## ADVERSE REACTIONS

**CNS:** dizziness, *agitation,* depression, fatigue, headache, nervousness, acute psychosis, syncope.
**CV:** *hypotension, heart failure, heart block,* edema, *arrhythmias,* shortness of breath, chest pain.
**EENT:** blurred vision, dry eyes or nose.
**GI:** *dry mouth,* nausea, vomiting, anorexia, bloating, gas, weight gain, abdominal pain, *constipation,* diarrhea.
**GU:** *urinary hesitancy,* urinary retention, urinary frequency, urinary urgency, impotence.
**Hepatic:** cholestatic jaundice.
**Musculoskeletal:** muscle weakness, aches, pain.
**Skin:** rash, pruritus, dermatosis.

## INTERACTIONS

**Drug-drug.** *Antiarrhythmics:* May increase QRS complex or QT interval, which may lead to other arrhythmias. Monitor ECG closely.
*Clarithromycin, erythromycin:* May increase disopyramide level, resulting in arrhythmias. Monitor ECG closely.
*Phenytoin:* May increase metabolism of disopyramide. Watch for decreased antiarrhythmic effect.
*Rifampin:* May decrease disopyramide level. Monitor patient for lack of effect.

*Thioridazine:* May cause life-threatening arrhythmias including torsades de pointes. Avoid using together.
*Verapamil:* May cause additive effects and impairment of left ventricular function. Don't give disopyramide 48 hours before starting verapamil therapy or 24 hours after verapamil is stopped.
**Drug-herb.** *Jimsonweed:* May adversely affect CV function. Discourage use together.

## EFFECTS ON LAB TEST RESULTS

None reported.

## CONTRAINDICATIONS & CAUTIONS

● Contraindicated in patients hypersensitive to drug.
● Contraindicated in those with sick sinus syndrome, cardiogenic shock, congenital QT interval prolongation, or second- or third-degree heart block in the absence of an artificial pacemaker.
● Use with extreme caution or avoid, if possible, in patients with heart failure.
● Use cautiously in patients with underlying conduction abnormalities, urinary tract diseases (especially prostatic hyperplasia), hepatic or renal impairment, myasthenia gravis, or acute angle-closure glaucoma.

## NURSING CONSIDERATIONS

● Correct electrolyte abnormalities before starting therapy.
● Digitalize patients with atrial fibrillation or flutter before starting disopyramide because of the risk of enhancing AV conduction.
● Check apical pulse before giving drug. Notify prescriber if pulse rate is slower than 60 beats/minute or faster than 120 beats/minute.
● Don't use sustained- or controlled-release preparations to control ventricular arrhythmias when therapeutic drug level must be rapidly attained, in patients with cardiomyopathy or possible cardiac decompensation, or in those with severe renal impairment.
● *Alert:* Don't open the extended-release capsules.
● For use in young children, pharmacist may prepare disopyramide suspension using 100-mg capsules and cherry syrup.

Pharmacist should dispense suspension in amber glass bottles. Protect suspension from light.

• Watch for recurrence of arrhythmias and check for adverse reactions; notify prescriber if any occur.

• Stop drug if heart block develops, if QRS complex widens by more than 25%, or if QT interval lengthens by more than 25% above baseline.

• *Alert:* Don't confuse disopyramide with desipramine or dipyridamole.

## PATIENT TEACHING
• Teach patient importance of taking drug on time and exactly as prescribed. This may require use of an alarm clock for nighttime doses.

• When transferring patient from immediate-release to sustained-release capsules, advise him to take the first sustained-release capsule 6 hours after taking the last immediate-release capsule.

• Tell patient not to crush or chew sustained-release capsules or tablets.

• If not contraindicated, advise patient to chew gum or hard candy to relieve dry mouth and to increase fiber and fluid intake to relieve constipation.

---

## dofetilide
Tikosyn

*Pregnancy risk category C*

## AVAILABLE FORMS
*Capsules:* 125 mcg, 250 mcg, 500 mcg

## INDICATIONS & DOSAGES
➤ **To maintain normal sinus rhythm in patients with symptomatic atrial fibrillation or atrial flutter lasting longer than 1 week who have been converted to normal sinus rhythm; to convert atrial fibrillation and atrial flutter to normal sinus rhythm**
*Adults:* Individualized dosage based on creatinine clearance and baseline QTc interval (or QT interval if heart rate is below 60 beats/minute), determined before first dose; usually 500 mcg P.O. b.i.d. for patients with creatinine clearance greater than 60 ml/minute.

*Adjust-a-dose:* If creatinine clearance is 40 to 60 ml/minute, starting dose is 250 mcg P.O. b.i.d.; if clearance is 20 to 39 ml/minute, starting dose is 125 mcg P.O. b.i.d. Don't use drug at all if clearance is less than 20 ml/minute.

Determine QTc interval 2 to 3 hours after first dose. If QTc interval has increased by more than 15% above baseline or if it's more than 500 msec (550 msec in patients with ventricular conduction abnormalities), adjust dosage as follows: If starting dose based on creatinine clearance was 500 mcg P.O. b.i.d., give 250 mcg P.O. b.i.d. If starting dose based on clearance was 250 mcg b.i.d., give 125 mcg b.i.d. If starting dose based on clearance was 125 mcg b.i.d., give 125 mcg once a day.

Determine QTc interval 2 to 3 hours after each subsequent dose while patient is in hospital. If at any time after second dose the QTc interval is more than 500 msec (550 msec in patients with ventricular conduction abnormalities), stop drug.

## ACTION
Class III antiarrhythmic; prolongs repolarization without affecting conduction velocity. Drug doesn't affect sodium channels, alpha-adrenergic receptors, or beta-adrenergic receptors.

| Route | Onset | Peak | Duration |
|-------|-------|------|----------|
| P.O. | Unknown | 2-3 hr | Unknown |

## ADVERSE REACTIONS
**CNS:** *headache,* dizziness, insomnia, anxiety, migraine, cerebral ischemia, *CVA,* asthenia, paresthesia, syncope.
**CV:** *ventricular fibrillation, ventricular tachycardia, torsades de pointes, AV block,* bundle-branch block, *heart block,* chest pain, angina, atrial fibrillation, hypertension, palpitations, *bradycardia,* edema, *cardiac arrest, MI.*
**GI:** nausea, diarrhea, abdominal pain.
**GU:** urinary tract infection.
**Hepatic:** liver damage.
**Musculoskeletal:** back pain, arthralgia, facial paralysis.
**Respiratory:** respiratory tract infection, dyspnea, increased cough.
**Skin:** rash, sweating.

---

**Other:** flu syndrome, ***angioedema***, peripheral edema.

## INTERACTIONS
**Drug-drug.** *Antiarrhythmics (classes I and III):* May increase dofetilide level. Withhold other antiarrhythmics for at least three plasma half-lives before dofetilide dosing.
*Cimetidine, ketoconazole, trimethoprim with sulfamethoxazole, verapamil:* May increase dofetilide level. Avoid using together.
*Drugs that prolong QT interval:* No studies done with dofetilide. May increase risk of QT interval prolongation. Avoid using together.
*Inhibitors of CYP3A4 (amiodarone, azole antifungals, cannabinoids, diltiazem, macrolides, nefazodone, norfloxacin, protease inhibitors, quinine, SSRIs, zafirlukast):* May decrease metabolism and increase dofetilide level. Use together cautiously.
*Inhibitors of renal cationic secretion (amiloride, megestrol, metformin, prochlorperazine, triamterene):* May increase dofetilide level. Use together cautiously.
*Potassium-depleting diuretics:* May increase risk of hypokalemia or hypomagnesemia. Monitor potassium and magnesium levels.
**Drug-food.** *Grapefruit juice:* May decrease hepatic metabolism and increase drug level. Discourage use together.

## EFFECTS ON LAB TEST RESULTS
None reported.

## CONTRAINDICATIONS & CAUTIONS
• Contraindicated in patients hypersensitive to drug, in those with congenital or acquired long QT interval syndromes or with baseline QTc interval greater than 440 msec (500 msec in patients with ventricular conduction abnormalities), and in those with creatinine clearance less than 20 ml/minute.
• Use cautiously in patients with severe hepatic impairment.

## NURSING CONSIDERATIONS
• Provide continuous ECG monitoring for at least 3 days.

• Don't discharge patient within 12 hours of conversion to normal sinus rhythm.
• Monitor patient for prolonged diarrhea, sweating, and vomiting. Report these signs to prescriber because electrolyte imbalance may increase potential for arrhythmia development.
• Monitor renal function and QTc interval every 3 months.
• Use of potassium-depleting diuretics may cause hypokalemia and hypomagnesemia, increasing the risk of torsades de pointes. Give dofetilide after potassium level reaches and stays in normal range.
• If patient doesn't convert to normal sinus rhythm within 24 hours of starting dofetilide, consider electrical conversion.
• Before starting dofetilide, stop previous antiarrhythmics while carefully monitoring patient for a minimum of three plasma half-lives. Don't give drug after amiodarone therapy until amiodarone level falls below 0.3 mcg/ml or until amiodarone has been stopped for at least 3 months.
• If dofetilide must be stopped to allow dosing with interacting drugs, allow at least 2 days before starting other drug therapy.

## PATIENT TEACHING
• Tell patient to report any change in OTC or prescription drug use, or supplement or herb use.
• Inform patient that drug can be taken without regard to meals or antacid administration.
• Tell patient to immediately report excessive or prolonged diarrhea, sweating, vomiting, or loss of appetite or thirst.
• Advise patient not to take drug with grapefruit juice.
• Advise patient to use antacids such as Zantac 75 mg, Pepcid, Prilosec, Axid, or Prevacid if needed for ulcers or heartburn instead of OTC Tagamet HB.
• Instruct patient to tell prescriber if she becomes pregnant.
• Advise patient not to breast-feed while taking dofetilide because drug appears in breast milk.
• If a dose is missed, tell patient not to double a dose but to skip that dose and take the next regularly scheduled dose.

# esmolol hydrochloride
Brevibloc

*Pregnancy risk category C*

## AVAILABLE FORMS
*Injection:* 10 mg/ml in 10-ml vials,
250 mg/ml in 10-ml ampules

## INDICATIONS & DOSAGES
➤ **Supraventricular tachycardia; post-operative tachycardia or hypertension; noncompensatory sinus tachycardias**
*Adults:* 500 mcg/kg/minute as loading
dose by I.V. infusion over 1 minute; then
4-minute maintenance infusion of 50 mcg/
kg/minute. If adequate response doesn't
occur within 5 minutes, repeat loading
dose and follow with maintenance infusion of 100 mcg/kg/minute for 4 minutes.
Repeat loading dose and increase maintenance infusion by increments of 50 mcg/
kg/minute. Maximum maintenance infusion for tachycardia is 200 mcg/kg/
minute.
➤ **Intraoperative tachycardia or hyper-tension**
*Adults:* For intraoperative treatment of
tachycardia or hypertension, 80 mg (about
1 mg/kg) I.V. bolus over 30 seconds; then
150 mcg/kg/minute I.V. infusion, if needed. Titrate infusion rate, p.r.n., to maximum of 300 mcg/kg/minute.

## I.V. ADMINISTRATION
● Give esmolol using an infusion control
device rather than by I.V. push. Use the
10-mg/ml single-dose vials without diluting, but dilute the injection concentrate
(250 mg/ml) to maximum of 10 mg/ml before infusion. Remove and discard 20 ml
from 500-ml bag of D$_5$W, lactated Ringer's
solution, half-normal or normal saline solution, and add 2 ampules of esmolol (final
level 10 mg/ml) to the I.V. bag.
● Esmolol solutions are incompatible with
diazepam, furosemide, sodium bicarbonate, and thiopental sodium.
● Give concentrations greater than 10 mg/
ml through a central line.

## ACTION
A class II antiarrhythmic and ultrashort-
acting selective beta blocker that decreases heart rate, contractility, and blood pressure.

| Route | Onset | Peak | Duration |
|-------|-------|------|----------|
| I.V. | Immediate | 30 min | 30 min after infusion |

## ADVERSE REACTIONS
**CNS:** anxiety, depression, dizziness, som-
nolence, headache, agitation, fatigue, con-
fusion.
**CV:** HYPOTENSION, peripheral ischemia.
**GI:** nausea, vomiting.
**Skin:** inflammation or induration at infu-
sion site.

## INTERACTIONS
**Drug-drug.** *Digoxin:* May increase digoxin level by 10% to 20%. Monitor digoxin
level.
*Morphine:* May increase esmolol level.
Adjust esmolol dosage carefully.
*Prazosin:* May increase risk of orthostatic
hypotension. Help patient to stand slowly
until effects are known.
*Reserpine, other catecholamine-depleting
drugs:* May increase bradycardia and hypotension. Adjust esmolol dosage carefully.
*Succinylcholine:* May prolong neuromuscular blockade. Monitor patient closely.
*Verapamil:* May increase the effects of
both drugs. Monitor cardiac function
closely and decrease dosages as necessary.

## EFFECTS ON LAB TEST RESULTS
None reported.

## CONTRAINDICATIONS & CAUTIONS
● Contraindicated in patients with sinus
bradycardia, second- or third-degree heart
block, cardiogenic shock, or overt heart
failure.
● Use cautiously if patient has renal impairment, diabetes, or bronchospasm.

## NURSING CONSIDERATIONS
● Dosage for postoperative treatment of
tachycardia and hypertension is same as
for supraventricular tachycardia.
● *Alert:* Monitor ECG and blood pressure
continuously during infusion. Up to 50%
of all patients treated with esmolol develop hypotension. Diaphoresis and dizziness
may accompany hypotension. Monitor pa-

tient closely, especially if pretreatment blood pressure was low.
• Hypotension can usually be reversed within 30 minutes by decreasing the dose or, if needed, by stopping the infusion. Notify prescriber if this becomes necessary.
• If a local reaction develops at the infusion site, change to another site. Avoid using butterfly needles.
• Esmolol is recommended only for short-term use, no longer than 48 hours. Watch infusion site carefully for signs of extravasation; if they occur, stop infusion immediately and call prescriber.
• When patient's heart rate becomes stable, esmolol will be replaced by alternative (longer-acting) antiarrhythmics, such as propranolol, digoxin, or verapamil. A half-hour after the first dose of the alternative drug is given, reduce infusion rate by 50%. Monitor patient response and, if heart rate is controlled for 1 hour after administration of the second dose of the alternative drug, stop esmolol infusion.

**PATIENT TEACHING**
• Instruct patient to report adverse reactions promptly.
• Tell patient to report discomfort at I.V. site.

---

## flecainide acetate
Tambocor

*Pregnancy risk category C*

**AVAILABLE FORMS**
*Injection:* 10 mg/ml‡
*Tablets:* 50 mg, 100 mg, 150 mg

**INDICATIONS & DOSAGES**
➤ **Paroxysmal supraventricular tachycardia, including AV nodal re-entrant tachycardia and AV re-entrant tachycardia, paroxysmal atrial fibrillation or flutter in patients without structural heart disease; life-threatening ventricular arrhythmias such as sustained ventricular tachycardia**
*Adults:* For paroxysmal supraventricular tachycardia, 50 mg P.O. q 12 hours. In-

crease in increments of 50 mg b.i.d. q 4 days. Maximum dose is 300 mg/day.
For life-threatening ventricular arrhythmias, 100 mg P.O. q 12 hours. Increase in increments of 50 mg b.i.d. q 4 days until desired effect occurs. Maximum dose for most patients is 400 mg/day.
Or, where available for emergency treatment,‡ 2 mg/kg I.V. push over not less than 10 minutes to maximum dose of 150 mg; or dilute dose and give as an infusion over 10 to 30 minutes.
*Adjust-a-dose:* If creatinine clearance is 35 ml/minute or less, first dose is 100 mg P.O. once daily or 50 mg P.O. b.i.d.

**I.V. ADMINISTRATION‡**
• When giving by I.V. push, give over at least 10 minutes. For I.V. infusion, mix only with $D_5W$.
• Because of drug's long half-life, full therapeutic effect may take 3 to 5 days. Give together with I.V. lidocaine for first several days.

**ACTION**
A class IC antiarrhythmic that decreases excitability, conduction velocity, and automaticity as a result of slowed atrial, AV node, His-Purkinje system, and intraventricular conduction; causes a slight but significant prolongation of refractory periods in these tissues.

| Route | Onset | Peak | Duration |
|---|---|---|---|
| P.O. | Unknown | 2-3 hr | Unknown |
| I.V. | Immediate | Immediate | Unknown |

**ADVERSE REACTIONS**
**CNS:** *dizziness, headache,* fatigue, fever, tremor, anxiety, insomnia, depression, malaise, paresthesia, ataxia, vertigo, *lightheadedness, syncope,* asthenia.
**CV:** *new or worsened arrhythmias,* chest pain, **heart failure, cardiac arrest,** palpitations, edema, flushing.
**EENT:** eye pain, eye irritation, *blurred vision and other visual disturbances.*
**GI:** nausea, constipation, abdominal pain, dyspepsia, vomiting, diarrhea, anorexia.
**Respiratory:** *dyspnea.*
**Skin:** rash.

## INTERACTIONS

**Drug-drug.** *Amiodarone, cimetidine:* May increase level of flecainide. Watch for toxicity.

*Digoxin:* May increase digoxin level by 15% to 25%. Monitor digoxin level.

*Disopyramide, verapamil:* May increase negative inotropic properties. Avoid using together.

*Propranolol, other beta blockers:* May increase flecainide and propranolol levels by 20% to 30%. Watch for propranolol and flecainide toxicity.

*Urine-acidifying and urine-alkalinizing drugs:* May cause extremes of urine pH, which may alter flecainide excretion. Monitor patient for flecainide toxicity or decreased effectiveness.

**Drug-lifestyle.** *Smoking:* May decrease flecainide level. Monitor patient closely.

## EFFECTS ON LAB TEST RESULTS
None reported.

## CONTRAINDICATIONS & CAUTIONS
• Contraindicated in patients hypersensitive to drug and in those with second- or third-degree AV block or right bundle-branch block with a left hemiblock (in the absence of an artificial pacemaker), recent MI, or cardiogenic shock.
• Use cautiously in patients with heart failure, cardiomyopathy, severe renal or hepatic disease, prolonged QT interval, sick sinus syndrome, or blood dyscrasia.

## NURSING CONSIDERATIONS
• When used to prevent ventricular arrhythmias, reserve drug for patients with documented life-threatening arrhythmias.
• Check that pacing threshold was determined 1 week before and after starting therapy in a patient with a pacemaker; flecainide can alter endocardial pacing thresholds.
• Correct hypokalemia or hyperkalemia before giving flecainide because these electrolyte disturbances may alter drug's effect.
• Monitor ECG rhythm for proarrhythmic effects.
• Most patients can be adequately maintained on an every-12-hour dosing schedule, but some need to receive flecainide every 8 hours.

• Adjust dosage only once every 3 to 4 days.
• Monitor flecainide level, especially if patient has renal or heart failure. Therapeutic flecainide levels range from 0.2 to 1 mcg/ml. Risk of adverse effects increases when trough blood level exceeds 1 mcg/ml.

## PATIENT TEACHING
• Stress importance of taking drug exactly as prescribed.
• Instruct patient to report adverse reactions promptly and to limit fluid and sodium intake to minimize fluid retention.
• Tell patient receiving drug I.V. to report discomfort at insertion site.

---

# ibutilide fumarate
Corvert

*Pregnancy risk category C*

## AVAILABLE FORMS
*Injection:* 0.1 mg/ml in 10-ml vials

## INDICATIONS & DOSAGES
➤ **Rapid conversion of recent onset atrial fibrillation or atrial flutter to sinus rhythm**
*Adults weighing 60 kg (132 lb) or more:* 1 mg I.V. over 10 minutes.
*Adults weighing less than 60 kg:* 0.01 mg/kg I.V. over 10 minutes.

## I.V. ADMINISTRATION
• Give drug undiluted or diluted in 50 ml of diluent, and add to normal saline solution for injection or $D_5W$ before infusion. Add contents of 10-ml vial (0.1 mg/ml) to 50-ml infusion bag to form admixture of about 0.017 mg/ml ibutilide. Use drug with polyvinyl chloride plastic bags or polyolefin bags.
• Give drug over 10 minutes.
• *Alert:* Stop infusion if arrhythmia is terminated or patient develops ventricular tachycardia or marked prolongation of QT or QTc interval. If arrhythmia isn't terminated 10 minutes after infusion ends, may give a second 10-minute infusion of equal strength.
• Admixtures with approved diluents are stable for 24 hours at room temperature; 48 hours if refrigerated.

---

• Don't infuse parenteral products that contain particulate matter or are discolored.

## ACTION
Prolongs action potential in isolated cardiac myocyte and increases atrial and ventricular refractoriness, namely class III electrophysiologic effects.

| Route | Onset | Peak | Duration |
|-------|-------|------|----------|
| I.V. | Unknown | Unknown | Unknown |

## ADVERSE REACTIONS
**CNS:** headache.
**CV:** ventricular extrasystoles, nonsustained ventricular tachycardia, hypotension, bundle-branch block, *sustained polymorphic ventricular tachycardia, AV block, heart failure,* hypertension, prolonged QT interval, *bradycardia,* palpitations, tachycardia.
**GI:** nausea.

## INTERACTIONS
**Drug-drug.** *Class IA antiarrhythmics (disopyramide, procainamide, quinidine), other class III drugs (amiodarone, sotalol):* May increase potential for prolonged refractoriness. Don't give these drugs for at least five half-lives before and 4 hours after ibutilide dose.
*Digoxin:* Supraventricular arrhythmias may mask cardiotoxicity from excessive digoxin level. Use cautiously and monitor digoxin level.
*H₁-receptor antagonist antihistamines, phenothiazines, tetracyclic antidepressants, tricyclic antidepressants, other drugs that prolong QT interval:* May increase risk for proarrhythmia. Monitor patient closely.

## EFFECTS ON LAB TEST RESULTS
None reported.

## CONTRAINDICATIONS & CAUTIONS
• Contraindicated in patients hypersensitive to drug or its components.
• Contraindicated in patients with history of polymorphic ventricular tachycardia and in breast-feeding women.
• Use cautiously in patients with hepatic or renal dysfunction.

• Safety and effectiveness of drug haven't been established in children.

## NURSING CONSIDERATIONS
• Skilled personnel only should give drug. Cardiac monitor, intracardiac pacing, cardioverter or defibrillator, and drugs to treat sustained ventricular tachycardia must be available.
• Before therapy, correct hypokalemia and hypomagnesemia to reduce proarrhythmia potential. Patients with atrial fibrillation lasting longer than 2 to 3 days must be adequately anticoagulated, generally over at least 2 weeks.
• Monitor ECG continuously during administration and for at least 4 hours afterward or until QTc interval returns to baseline; drug can induce or worsen ventricular arrhythmias. Longer monitoring is required if ECG shows arrhythmia or patient has hepatic insufficiency.
• Don't give class IA or other class III antiarrhythmics with ibutilide infusion or for 4 hours afterward.

## PATIENT TEACHING
• Tell patient to report adverse reactions promptly.
• Instruct patient to alert nurse of discomfort at injection site.

## lidocaine hydrochloride (lignocaine hydrochloride)
LidoPen Auto-Injector, Xylocaine, Xylocard†‡

*Pregnancy risk category B*

## AVAILABLE FORMS
*Infusion (premixed):* 0.2% (2 mg/ml), 0.4% (4 mg/ml), 0.8% (8 mg/ml)
*Injection (for direct I.V. use):* 1% (10 mg/ml), 2% (20 mg/ml)
*Injection (for I.M. use):* 300 mg/3 ml automatic injection device
*Injection (for I.V. admixtures):* 4% (40 mg/ml), 10% (100 mg/ml), 20% (200 mg/ml)

## INDICATIONS & DOSAGES
➤ **Ventricular arrhythmias caused by MI, cardiac manipulation, or cardiac glycosides**
*Adults:* 50 to 100 mg (1 to 1.5 mg/kg) by I.V. bolus at 25 to 50 mg/minute. Bolus dose is repeated q 3 to 5 minutes until arrhythmias subside or adverse reactions develop. Don't exceed 300-mg total bolus during a 1-hour period. Simultaneously, constant infusion of 20 to 50 mcg/kg/minute (1 to 4 mg/minute) is begun. If single bolus has been given, smaller bolus dose may be repeated 15 to 20 minutes after start of infusion to maintain therapeutic level. Or, 200 to 300 mg I.M.; then second I.M. dose 60 to 90 minutes later, if needed.
*Children:* 1 mg/kg by I.V. or intraosseous bolus. If no response, start infusion of 20 to 50 mcg/kg/minute. Give an additional bolus dose of 0.5 to 1 mg/kg if delay of greater than 15 minutes between initial bolus and starting the infusion.
*Elderly patients:* Reduce dosage and rate of infusion by 50%.
*Adjust-a-dose:* For patients with heart failure, with renal or liver disease, or who weigh less than 50 kg (110 lb), use reduced dosage.

## I.V. ADMINISTRATION
• Lidocaine injections (additive syringes and single-use vials) containing 40, 100, or 200 mg/ml are for the preparation of I.V. infusion solutions only and must be diluted before use.
• Prepare I.V. infusion by adding 1 g of lidocaine hydrochloride (using 25 ml of 4% or 5 ml of 20% injection) to 1 L of $D_5W$ injection to provide a solution containing 1 mg/ml.
• Use a more concentrated solution of up to 8 mg/ml if patient is fluid restricted.
• Patients receiving infusions must be on a cardiac monitor and must be attended at all times. Use an infusion control device for giving infusion precisely. Don't exceed 4 mg/minute; faster rate greatly increases risk of toxicity.
• Avoid giving injections containing preservatives I.V.

## ACTION
A class IB antiarrhythmic that decreases the depolarization, automaticity, and excitability in the ventricles during the diastolic phase by direct action on the tissues, especially the Purkinje network.

| Route | Onset | Peak | Duration |
|-------|-------|------|----------|
| I.V. | Immediate | Immediate | 10-20 min |
| I.M. | 5-15 min | 10 min | 2 hr |

## ADVERSE REACTIONS
**CNS:** *confusion, tremor,* lethargy, somnolence, *stupor, restlessness,* anxiety, hallucinations, nervousness, *light-headedness,* paresthesia, muscle twitching, *seizures.*
**CV:** *hypotension,* **bradycardia, new or worsened arrhythmias, cardiac arrest.**
**EENT:** *tinnitus, blurred or double vision.*
**GI:** vomiting.
**Respiratory:** *respiratory depression and arrest.*
**Skin:** soreness at injection site.
**Other:** *anaphylaxis,* sensation of cold.

## INTERACTIONS
**Drug-drug.** *Atenolol, metoprolol, nadolol, pindolol, propranolol:* May reduce hepatic metabolism of lidocaine, increasing the risk of toxicity. Give bolus doses of lidocaine at a slower rate, and monitor lidocaine level closely.
*Beta blockers:* May decrease metabolism of lidocaine. Monitor patient for toxicity.
*Cimetidine:* May decrease clearance of lidocaine increasing the risk of toxicity. Consider using a different $H_2$ antagonist if possible. Monitor lidocaine level closely.
*Mexiletine, tocainide:* May increase pharmacologic effects. Avoid using together.
*Phenytoin, procainamide, propranolol, quinidine:* May increase cardiac depressant effects. Monitor patient closely.
*Succinylcholine:* May prolong neuromuscular blockade. Monitor patient closely.
**Drug-herb.** *Pareira:* May increase the effects of neuromuscular blockade. Discourage use together.
**Drug-lifestyle.** *Smoking:* May increase metabolism of lidocaine. Monitor patient closely.

## EFFECTS ON LAB TEST RESULTS
None reported.

## CONTRAINDICATIONS & CAUTIONS
• Contraindicated in patients hypersensitive to the amide-type local anesthetics.
• Contraindicated in those with Adams-Stokes syndrome, Wolff-Parkinson-White syndrome, and severe degrees of SA, AV, or intraventricular block in the absence of an artificial pacemaker.
• Use cautiously and at reduced dosages in patients with complete or second-degree heart block or sinus bradycardia, in elderly patients, in those with heart failure or renal or hepatic disease, and in those weighing less than 50 kg (110 lb).

## NURSING CONSIDERATIONS
• Give I.M. injections in the deltoid muscle only.
• Monitor isoenzymes when using I.M. drug for suspected MI. A patient who has received I.M. lidocaine will show a seven-fold increase in CK level. Such an increase originates in the skeletal muscle, not the heart.
• Monitor drug level. Therapeutic levels are 2 to 5 mcg/ml.
• *Alert:* Monitor patient for toxicity. In many severely ill patients, seizures may be the first sign of toxicity, but severe reactions are usually preceded by somnolence, confusion, tremors, and paresthesia.
• If signs of toxicity such as dizziness occur, stop drug at once and notify prescriber. Continuing could lead to seizures and coma. Give oxygen through a nasal cannula if not contraindicated. Keep oxygen and cardiopulmonary resuscitation equipment available.
• Monitor patient's response, especially blood pressure and electrolytes, BUN, and creatinine levels. Notify prescriber promptly if abnormalities develop.
• Stop infusion and notify prescriber if arrhythmias worsen or ECG changes, such as widening QRS complex or substantially prolonged PR interval, appear.

## PATIENT TEACHING
• Tell patient receiving lidocaine I.M. that drug may cause soreness at injection site. Tell him to report discomfort at the site.
• Tell patient to report adverse reactions promptly because toxicity can occur.

# mexiletine hydrochloride
Mexitil

*Pregnancy risk category C*

## AVAILABLE FORMS
*Capsules:* 50 mg‡, 100 mg†, 150 mg, 200 mg, 250 mg

## INDICATIONS & DOSAGES
➤ **Life-threatening ventricular arrhythmias, including ventricular tachycardia and PVCs**
*Adults:* Initially, 200 mg P.O. q 8 hours. If satisfactory control isn't obtained at this dosage, increase dosage by 50 to 100 mg q 2 to 3 days up to maximum of 400 mg q 8 hours. If rapid control of ventricular rate is desired, give a loading dose of 400 mg P.O., followed by 200 mg 8 hours later. Patients controlled on 300 mg or less q 8 hours can receive the total daily dose in evenly divided doses q 12 hours.

## ACTION
A class IB antiarrhythmic. Blocks the fast sodium channel in cardiac tissues, especially the Purkinje network, without involving the autonomic nervous system. Reduces rate of rise, amplitude and duration of action potential, and automaticity and effective refractory period in the Purkinje fibers.

| Route | Onset | Peak | Duration |
|---|---|---|---|
| P.O. | 30-120 min | 2-3 hr | Unknown |

## ADVERSE REACTIONS
**CNS:** *tremor, dizziness,* confusion, *lightheadedness, incoordination,* changes in sleep habits, paresthesia, weakness, fatigue, speech difficulties, depression, *nervousness,* headache.
**CV:** NEW OR WORSENED ARRHYTHMIAS, palpitations, chest pain, nonspecific edema, angina.
**EENT:** blurred vision, diplopia, tinnitus.
**GI:** *nausea, vomiting, upper GI distress, heartburn,* diarrhea, constipation, dry mouth, changes in appetite, abdominal pain.
**Skin:** rash.

---

Reactions may be *common,* uncommon, *life-threatening*, or COMMON AND LIFE-THREATENING.

## INTERACTIONS
**Drug-drug.** *Antacids, atropine, narcotics:* May slow mexiletine absorption. Monitor patient for effectiveness.
*Cimetidine:* May alter mexiletine level. Monitor patient.
*Methylxanthines (such as caffeine, theophylline):* May reduce methylxanthine clearance, which may cause toxicity. Monitor drug level.
*Metoclopramide:* May speed up mexiletine absorption. Monitor patient for toxicity.
*Phenobarbital, phenytoin, rifampin, urine acidifiers:* May decrease mexiletine level. Monitor patient for effectiveness.
*Urine alkalinizers:* May increase mexiletine level. Monitor patient for adverse reactions.

## EFFECTS ON LAB TEST RESULTS
• May increase AST level.

## CONTRAINDICATIONS & CAUTIONS
• Contraindicated in patients with cardiogenic shock or second- or third-degree AV block in the absence of an artificial pacemaker.
• Use cautiously in patients with first-degree heart block, a ventricular pacemaker, sinus node dysfunction, intraventricular conduction disturbances, hypotension, severe heart failure, or seizure disorder.

## NURSING CONSIDERATIONS
• When changing from lidocaine to mexiletine, stop the lidocaine infusion when the first mexiletine dose is given. But keep the infusion line open until the arrhythmia is satisfactorily controlled.
• Give oral dose with meals or antacids to lessen GI distress.
• If patient may be a good candidate for every-12-hour therapy, notify prescriber. Twice-daily dosage enhances compliance.
• Monitor therapeutic drug level, which may range from 0.5 to 2 mcg/ml.
• An early sign of mexiletine toxicity is tremor, usually a fine tremor of the hands, progressing to dizziness and then to ataxia and nystagmus as drug level in the blood increases. Watch for and ask patients about these symptoms.
• Monitor blood pressure and heart rate and rhythm frequently. Notify prescriber of significant change.

## PATIENT TEACHING
• Tell patient to take drug exactly as prescribed and to take with food or antacids if GI reactions occur.
• Instruct patient to report adverse reactions promptly.
• Advise patient to notify prescriber if he develops jaundice, fever, or general tiredness; these symptoms may indicate liver damage.

# moricizine hydrochloride
Ethmozine

*Pregnancy risk category B*

## AVAILABLE FORMS
*Tablets:* 200 mg, 250 mg, 300 mg

## INDICATIONS & DOSAGES
➤ **Life-threatening ventricular arrhythmias**
*Adults:* Individualized dosage is based on patient response and tolerance. Begin therapy in the hospital. Most patients respond to 600 to 900 mg P.O. daily in divided doses q 8 hours. Increase daily dose by 150 mg q 3 days until desired effect occurs.
➤ **Ventricular premature contractions, couplets, nonsustained ventricular tachycardia**
*Adults:* 600 to 900 mg P.O. daily.
*Adjust-a-dose:* For patients with hepatic or renal impairment, 600 mg or less P.O. daily.

## ACTION
A class I antiarrhythmic that reduces the fast inward current carried by sodium ions across myocardial cell membranes. Drug has potent local anesthetic activity and membrane-stabilizing effect.

| Route | Onset | Peak | Duration |
|---|---|---|---|
| P.O. | Unknown | 30-120 min | 10-24 hr |

## ADVERSE REACTIONS
**CNS:** *dizziness,* headache, fatigue, hyperesthesia, anxiety, asthenia, depression, nervousness, paresthesia, sleep disorders.
**CV:** *ventricular tachycardia, PVCs, supraventricular arrhythmias, ECG abnormalities including conduction defects, si-*

*nus pause, junctional rhythm, and AV block,* **heart failure,** palpitations, thrombophlebitis, chest pain, **cardiac death,** hypotension, hypertension, vasodilation, cerebrovascular events.
**EENT:** blurred vision.
**GI:** nausea, vomiting, abdominal pain, dyspepsia, diarrhea, dry mouth.
**GU:** urine retention, urinary frequency, dysuria.
**Musculoskeletal:** musculoskeletal pain.
**Respiratory:** dyspnea.
**Skin:** rash, diaphoresis.
**Other:** drug-induced fever.

### INTERACTIONS

**Drug-drug.** *Cimetidine:* May increase level and decreases clearance of moricizine. Begin moricizine at no more than 600 mg daily, and monitor drug level and therapeutic effect closely.
*Digoxin, propranolol:* May increase PR interval prolongation. Monitor patient closely.
*Theophylline:* May increase clearance and reduces level of theophylline. Monitor drug level and therapeutic response; adjust theophylline dosage, as needed.

### EFFECTS ON LAB TEST RESULTS
• May increase liver function test results.

### CONTRAINDICATIONS & CAUTIONS
• Contraindicated in patients hypersensitive to drug, cardiogenic shock, or second- or third-degree AV block or right bundle-branch block with left hemiblock (bifascicular block) unless an artificial pacemaker is present.
• Because drug appears in breast milk, the decision to stop breast-feeding or stop taking the drug depends on importance of drug to the mother.
• Use with extreme caution in patients with sick sinus syndrome because drug may cause sinus bradycardia or sinus arrest. Also use with extreme caution in patients with coronary artery disease and left ventricular dysfunction because these patients may be at risk for sudden death when treated with the drug.
• Patients with hepatic or renal dysfunction have decreased moricizine clearance. Give drug cautiously and monitor effects closely.

### NURSING CONSIDERATIONS
• Monitor patients with heart failure carefully for worsening of heart failure.
• When substituting moricizine for another antiarrhythmic, withdraw previous drug for one to two of the drug's half-lives before starting moricizine. During withdrawal and adjustment to moricizine, hospitalize patients who developed life-threatening arrhythmias after withdrawal of previous antiarrhythmic. Guidelines for when to start moricizine therapy are as follows: disopyramide, 6 to 12 hours after last dose; flecainide, 12 to 24 hours after last dose; mexiletine, 8 to 12 hours after last dose; procainamide, 3 to 6 hours after last dose; propafenone, 8 to 12 hours after last dose; quinidine, 6 to 12 hours after last dose; and tocainide, 8 to 12 hours after last dose.
• Determine electrolyte status and correct imbalances before therapy, as prescribed. Hypokalemia, hyperkalemia, and hypomagnesemia may alter drug's effects.
• **Alert:** Don't confuse Ethmozine with Erythrocin.

### PATIENT TEACHING
• Inform patient that he'll need to be hospitalized for start of therapy.
• Instruct patient to take drug exactly as prescribed and not to abruptly stop use.
• Tell patient to avoid hazardous activities if adverse CNS reactions or blurred vision occurs.
• Instruct patient to report persistent or serious adverse reactions promptly.

# procainamide hydrochloride
Procanbid, Pronestyl, Pronestyl Filmlok, Pronestyl-SR Filmlok

*Pregnancy risk category C*

### AVAILABLE FORMS
*Capsules:* 250 mg, 375 mg, 500 mg
*Injection:* 100 mg/ml, 500 mg/ml
*Tablets:* 250 mg, 375 mg, 500 mg
*Tablets (extended-release):* 250 mg, 500 mg, 750 mg, 1,000 mg

---

Reactions may be *common,* uncommon, **life-threatening,** or COMMON AND LIFE-THREATENING.

## INDICATIONS & DOSAGES
➤ **Symptomatic PVCs; life-threatening ventricular tachycardia**

*Adults:* 100 mg q 5 minutes by slow I.V. push, no faster than 25 to 50 mg/minute, until arrhythmias disappear, adverse effects develop, or 500 mg has been given. Usual effective loading dose is 500 to 600 mg. Or, give a loading dose of 500 to 600 mg I.V. infusion over 25 to 30 minutes. Maximum total dose is 1 g. When arrhythmias disappear, give continuous infusion of 2 to 6 mg/minute. Usual effective loading dose is 500 to 600 mg (maximum 1 g). If arrhythmias recur, repeat bolus as above and increase infusion rate.

For I.M. administration, give 50 mg/kg divided q 3 to 6 hours; if arrhythmias occur during surgery, give 100 to 500 mg I.M.

For oral therapy, start at 50 mg/kg/day of conventional formulation P.O. in divided doses q 3 hours until therapeutic level is reached. For maintenance, substitute extended-release form to deliver the total daily dose divided q 6 hours or, using Procanbid, to deliver total daily dose divided q 12 hours.

*Children ♦ :* Dosage not established. Recommendations include 2 to 5 mg/kg I.V., not exceeding 100 mg, repeated p.r.n. q 5 to 10 minutes, up to a total of 15 mg/kg in 24 hours or 500 mg in 30 minutes. Or, 15 mg/kg infused over 30 to 60 minutes; then maintenance infusion of 0.02 to 0.08 mg/kg/minute.

➤ **To convert atrial fibrillation or paroxysmal atrial tachycardia ♦**

*Adults:* 1.25 g P.O. If arrhythmias persist after 1 hour, give additional 750 mg. If no change occurs, give 500 mg to 1 g P.O. q 2 hours until arrhythmias disappear or adverse effects occur. Maintenance dose is 1 g q 6 hours.

*Children:* 15 to 50 mg/kg/day P.O. divided q 3 to 6 hours. Maximum dose 4 g daily. Or, 20 to 30 mg/kg/day I.M. Or, loading dose of 3 to 6 mg/kg I.V. over 5 minutes, up to 100 mg/dose; then maintenance dose 20 to 80 mcg/kg/minute as continuous I.V. infusion. Maximum daily dose is 2 g.

➤ **To maintain normal sinus rhythm after conversion of atrial flutter ♦**

*Adults:* 0.5 to 1 g P.O. q 4 to 6 hours.

➤ **Malignant hyperthermia ♦**

*Adults:* 200 to 900 mg I.V., followed by maintenance infusion.

***Adjust-a-dose:*** For patients with renal or hepatic dysfunction, decrease doses or increase dosing intervals, as needed.

## I.V. ADMINISTRATION
● Vials for I.V. injection contain 1 g of drug: 100 mg/ml (10 ml) or 500 mg/ml (2 ml).

● Dilute with compatible I.V. solution such as $D_5W$ injection, and give with the patient supine at a rate not exceeding 25 to 50 mg/minute. Keep patient supine during I.V. administration.

● Attend patient receiving infusion at all times. Use an infusion-control device to give infusion precisely.

● ***Alert:*** Monitor blood pressure and ECG continuously during I.V. administration. Watch for prolonged QTc intervals and QRS complexes, heart block, or increased arrhythmias. If such reactions occur, withhold drug, obtain rhythm strip, and notify prescriber immediately. If drug is given too rapidly, hypotension can occur. Watch closely for adverse reactions during infusion, and notify prescriber if they occur.

## ACTION
A class IA antiarrhythmic that decreases excitability, conduction velocity, automaticity, and membrane responsiveness with prolonged refractory period. Larger than usual doses may induce AV block.

| Route | Onset | Peak | Duration |
|-------|-------|------|----------|
| P.O. | Unknown | 90-120 min | Unknown |
| I.V. | Immediate | Immediate | Unknown |
| I.M. | 10-30 min | 15-60 min | Unknown |

## ADVERSE REACTIONS
**CNS:** *fever,* hallucinations, psychosis, giddiness, confusion, *seizures,* depression, dizziness.

**CV:** hypotension, ***bradycardia, AV block, ventricular fibrillation, ventricular asystole.***

**GI:** abdominal pain, nausea, vomiting, anorexia, diarrhea, bitter taste.

**Skin:** *maculopapular rash, urticaria, pruritus, flushing, angioneurotic edema.*

**Other:** *lupuslike syndrome.*

## INTERACTIONS

**Drug-drug.** *Amiodarone:* May increase procainamide level and toxicity; additive effects on QTc interval and QRS complex. Avoid using together.

*Anticholinergics:* May increase antivagal effects. Monitor patient closely.

*Anticholinesterases:* May decrease effect of anticholinesterases. Anticholinesterase dosage may need to be increased.

*Beta blockers, ranitidine, trimethoprim:* May increase procainamide level. Watch for toxicity.

*Cimetidine:* May increase procainamide level. Avoid this combination if possible. Monitor procainamide level closely and adjust the dosage as necessary.

*Neuromuscular blockers:* May increase skeletal muscle relaxant effect. Monitor patient closely.

**Drug-herb.** *Jimsonweed:* May adversely affect CV function. Discourage use together.

*Licorice:* May have additive effect and prolong QTc interval. Urge caution.

**Drug-lifestyle.** *Alcohol use:* May reduce drug level. Discourage use together.

## EFFECTS ON LAB TEST RESULTS

- May increase ALT, AST, alkaline phosphatase, LDH, and bilirubin levels.
- May cause positive antinuclear antibody (ANA) titers, positive direct antiglobulin (Coombs') tests, and ECG changes.

## CONTRAINDICATIONS & CAUTIONS

- Contraindicated in patients hypersensitive to procaine and related drugs.
- Contraindicated in those with complete, second-, or third-degree heart block in the absence of an artificial pacemaker. Also contraindicated in those with myasthenia gravis, systemic lupus erythematosus, or atypical ventricular tachycardia (torsades de pointes).
- Use with extreme caution in patients with ventricular tachycardia during coronary occlusion.
- Use cautiously in patients with heart failure or other conduction disturbances, such as bundle-branch heart block, sinus bradycardia, or digitalis intoxication, and in those with hepatic or renal insufficiency. Also use cautiously in patients with

blood dyscrasias or bone marrow suppression.

## NURSING CONSIDERATIONS

- Monitor level of procainamide and its active metabolite NAPA. To suppress ventricular arrhythmias, therapeutic levels of procainamide are 4 to 8 mcg/ml; therapeutic levels of NAPA are 10 to 30 mcg/ml.
- Monitor QTc interval closely. Dosage reduction may be necessary if QTc interval is prolonged more than 50% from baseline.
- Hypokalemia predisposes patient to arrhythmias. Monitor electrolytes, especially potassium level.
- Elderly patients may be more likely to develop hypotension. Monitor blood pressure carefully.
- Monitor CBC frequently during first 3 months of therapy.
- Positive ANA titer is common in about 60% of patients who don't have symptoms of lupuslike syndrome. This response seems to be related to prolonged use, not dosage. May progress to systemic lupus erythematosus if drug isn't stopped.
- *Alert:* Don't crush the extended-release tablets.
- The Filmlok formulation may contain tartrazine.
- *Alert:* Don't confuse Procanbid with probenecid.

## PATIENT TEACHING

- Stress importance of taking drug exactly as prescribed. This may require use of an alarm clock for nighttime doses.
- Instruct patient to report fever, rash, muscle pain, diarrhea, bleeding, bruises, or pleuritic chest pain.
- Tell patient not to crush or break extended-release tablets.
- Reassure patient who is taking extended-release form that a wax-matrix "ghost" from the tablet may be passed in stools. Drug is completely absorbed before this occurs.

---

Reactions may be *common*, uncommon, *life-threatening*, or COMMON AND LIFE-THREATENING.

## quinidine bisulfate
(66.4% quinidine base), Kinidin
Durules‡

## quinidine gluconate
(62% quinidine base) Quinaglute
Dura-Tabs, Quinate†

## quinidine sulfate
(83% quinidine base) Apo-
Quinidine†, Novoquinidin†,
Quinidex Extentabs

*Pregnancy risk category C*

### AVAILABLE FORMS
**quinidine bisulfate**
*Tablets (extended-release):* 250 mg‡
**quinidine gluconate**
*Injection:* 80 mg/ml
*Tablets (extended-release):* 324 mg,
325 mg†
**quinidine sulfate**
*Injection:* 200 mg/ml†
*Tablets:* 200 mg, 300 mg
*Tablets (extended-release):* 300 mg

### INDICATIONS & DOSAGES
➤ **Atrial flutter or fibrillation**
*Adults:* 300 to 400 mg quinidine sulfate or
equivalent base P.O. q 6 hours. Or, 200 mg
P.O. q 2 to 3 hours for five to eight doses,
increased daily until sinus rhythm is restored or toxic effects develop. Maximum,
3 to 4 g daily.
➤ **Paroxysmal supraventricular tachycardia**
*Adults:* 400 to 600 mg P.O. gluconate q
2 to 3 hours until toxic adverse reactions
develop or arrhythmia subsides.
➤ **Premature atrial and ventricular
contractions, paroxysmal AV junctional
rhythm, paroxysmal atrial tachycardia,
paroxysmal ventricular tachycardia,
maintenance after cardioversion of atrial fibrillation or flutter**
*Adults:* Test dose is 200 mg P.O. or I.M.
Quinidine sulfate or equivalent base
200 to 400 mg P.O. q 4 to 6 hours or
600 mg quinidine sulfate extended-release
q 8 to 12 hours; or quinidine gluconate
800 mg (10 ml of commercially available
solution) added to 40 ml of D₅W, infused
I.V. at 2.5 mg/kg/minute.

➤ **Severe *Plasmodium falciparum*
malaria**
*Adults:* 10 mg/kg gluconate I.V. diluted in
250 ml normal saline solution and infused
over 1 to 2 hours; then continuous infusion of 0.02 mg/kg/minute for 72 hours or
until parasitemia is reduced to less than
1% or oral therapy can be started.
*Children ◆ :* 30 mg/kg P.O. daily in five divided doses.
***Adjust-a-dose:*** Use reduced dosage for
patients with impaired hepatic function or
heart failure.

### I.V. ADMINISTRATION
● For quinidine gluconate infusion to treat
atrial fibrillation or flutter in adults, dilute
800 mg (10 ml of injection) with 40 ml
D₅W and infuse at up to 0.25 mg/kg/
minute.
● For quinidine gluconate infusion to treat
malaria, dilute in 5 ml/kg (usually 250 ml)
normal saline solution and infuse over 1 to
2 hours, followed by a continuous maintenance infusion.
● During infusion, continuously monitor
patient's blood pressure and ECG.
● Adjust rate so that the arrhythmia is corrected without disturbing the normal
mechanism of the heartbeat.

### ACTION
A class IA antiarrhythmic with direct and
indirect (anticholinergic) effects on cardiac tissue. Decreases automaticity, conduction velocity, and membrane responsiveness; prolongs effective refractory
period; and reduces vagal tone.

| Route | Onset | Peak | Duration |
|-------|-------|------|----------|
| P.O. | 1-3 hr | 1-6 hr | 6-8 hr |
| I.V. | Immediate | Immediate | Unknown |
| I.M. | 30-90 sec | Unknown | Unknown |

### ADVERSE REACTIONS
**CNS:** *vertigo, fever, headache,* ataxia,
*light-headedness,* confusion, depression,
dementia.
**CV:** *PVCs, ventricular tachycardia, atypical ventricular tachycardia,* hypotension,
***complete AV block,*** *tachycardia,* **aggravated heart failure,** *ECG changes.*
**EENT:** *tinnitus,* blurred vision, diplopia,
photophobia.

---

*Rapid onset*    \*Liquid contains alcohol    †Canada    ‡Australia    ◇ OTC    ◆ Off-label use    ✐Photoguide

**GI:** *diarrhea, nausea, vomiting,* anorexia, excessive salivation, abdominal pain.
**Hematologic:** hemolytic anemia, ***thrombocytopenia, agranulocytosis.***
**Hepatic:** *hepatotoxicity.*
**Respiratory:** *acute asthmatic attack, respiratory arrest.*
**Skin:** rash, petechial hemorrhage of buccal mucosa, pruritus, urticaria, photosensitivity.
**Other:** *angioedema, cinchonism,* lupus erythematosus.

### INTERACTIONS
**Drug-drug.** *Acetazolamide, antacids, sodium bicarbonate, thiazide diuretics:* May increase quinidine level. Monitor patient for increased effect.
*Amiodarone:* May increase quinidine level, producing life-threatening cardiac arrhythmias. Monitor quinidine level closely if use together can't be avoided. Adjust quinidine as needed.
*Barbiturates, phenytoin, rifampin:* May decrease quinidine level. Monitor patient for decreased effect.
*Cimetidine:* May increase quinidine level. Monitor patient for increased arrhythmias.
*Digoxin:* May increase digoxin level after starting quinidine therapy. Monitor digoxin level.
*Fluvoxamine, nefazodone, tricyclic antidepressants:* May increase antidepressant level, thus increasing its effect. Monitor patient for adverse reactions.
*Neuromuscular blockers:* May potentiate effects of these drugs. Avoid use of quinidine immediately after surgery.
*Nifedipine:* May decrease quinidine level. May need to adjust dosage.
*Other antiarrhythmics (such as lidocaine, procainamide, propranolol):* May increase risk of toxicity. Use together cautiously.
*Verapamil:* May decrease quinidine clearance and cause hypotension, bradycardia, AV block, or pulmonary edema. Monitor blood pressure and heart rate.
*Warfarin:* May increase anticoagulant effect. Monitor patient closely.
**Drug-herb.** *Grapefruit:* May delay absorption and onset of action of drug. Discourage use together.
*Jimsonweed:* May adversely affect CV function. Discourage use together.

*Licorice:* May have additive effect and prolong QT interval. Urge caution.

### EFFECTS ON LAB TEST RESULTS
● May decrease hemoglobin and platelet and granulocyte counts.

### CONTRAINDICATIONS & CAUTIONS
● Contraindicated in patients with idiosyncrasy or hypersensitivity to quinidine or related cinchona derivatives.
● Contraindicated in those with myasthenia gravis, intraventricular conduction defects, digitalis toxicity when AV conduction is grossly impaired, abnormal rhythms caused by escape mechanisms, and history of prolonged QT interval syndrome.
● Contraindicated in patients who developed thrombocytopenia after exposure to quinidine or quinine.
● Use cautiously in patients with asthma, muscle weakness, or infection accompanied by fever because hypersensitivity reactions to drug may be masked.
● Use cautiously in patients with hepatic or renal impairment because systemic accumulation may occur.

### NURSING CONSIDERATIONS
● Check apical pulse rate and blood pressure before therapy. If extremes in pulse rate are detected, withhold drug and notify prescriber at once.
● *Alert:* For atrial fibrillation or flutter, give quinidine only after AV node has been blocked with a beta blocker, digoxin, or a calcium channel blocker to avoid increasing AV conduction.
● Anticoagulant therapy is commonly advised before quinidine therapy in longstanding atrial fibrillation because restoration of normal sinus rhythm may result in thromboembolism caused by dislodgment of thrombi from atrial wall.
● Monitor patient for atypical ventricular tachycardia such as torsades de pointes and ECG changes, particularly widening of QRS complex, widened QT and PR intervals.
● *Alert:* When changing route of administration or oral salt form, prescriber should alter dosage to compensate for variations in quinidine base content.
● Never use discolored (brownish) quinidine solution.

---

Reactions may be *common,* uncommon, ***life-threatening***, or COMMON AND LIFE-THREATENING.

• Quinidine gluconate I.M. is no longer recommended for arrhythmias because of erratic absorption.

• *Alert:* Hospitalize patients with severe malaria in an intensive-care setting, with continuous monitoring. Decrease infusion rate if quinidine level exceeds 6 mcg/ml, uncorrected QT interval exceeds 0.6 second, or QRS complex widening exceeds 25% of baseline.

• Monitor liver function test results during first 4 to 8 weeks of therapy.

• Monitor quinidine level. Therapeutic levels for antiarrhythmic effects are 4 to 8 mcg/ml.

• Monitor patient response carefully. If adverse GI reactions occur, especially diarrhea, notify prescriber. Check quinidine level, which is increasingly toxic when greater than 10 mcg/ml. GI symptoms may be decreased by giving drug with meals or aluminum hydroxide antacids.

• Store drug away from heat and direct light.

• *Alert:* Don't crush the extended-release formulation.

• *Alert:* Don't confuse quinidine with quinine or clonidine.

**PATIENT TEACHING**
• Stress importance of taking drug exactly as prescribed and taking it with food if adverse GI reactions occur.

• Instruct patient not to crush or chew extended-release tablets.

• Tell patient to avoid grapefruit juice because it may delay drug absorption and inhibit drug metabolism.

• Advise patient to report persistent or serious adverse reactions promptly, especially signs and symptoms of quinidine toxicity (ringing in the ears, visual disturbances, dizziness, headache, nausea).

## sotalol hydrochloride
Betapace, Betapace AF,
Sotacor†‡

*Pregnancy risk category B*

**AVAILABLE FORMS**
**Betapace**
*Tablets:* 80 mg, 120 mg, 160 mg, 240 mg

**Betapace AF**
*Tablets:* 80 mg, 120 mg, 160 mg

**INDICATIONS & DOSAGES**
➤ **Documented, life-threatening ventricular arrhythmias**
*Adults:* Initially, 80 mg Betapace P.O. b.i.d. Increase dosage q 3 days as needed and tolerated. Most patients respond to 160 to 320 mg/day, although some patients with refractory arrhythmias need up to 640 mg/day.
*Adjust-a-dose:* For patients with creatinine clearance 30 to 60 ml/minute, increase dosage interval to q 24 hours; if clearance is 10 to 30 ml/minute, increase interval to q 36 to 48 hours; and if clearance is less than 10 ml/minute, individualize dosage.
➤ **To maintain normal sinus rhythm or to delay recurrence of atrial fibrillation or atrial flutter in patients with symptomatic atrial fibrillation or flutter who are currently in sinus rhythm**
*Adults:* 80 mg Betapace AF P.O. b.i.d. Increase dosage p.r.n. to 120 mg P.O. b.i.d. after 3 days if the QTc interval is less than 500 msec. Maximum dose is 160 mg P.O. b.i.d.
*Adjust-a-dose:* For patients with creatinine clearance 40 to 60 ml/minute, increase dosage interval to q 24 hours.

**ACTION**
A nonselective beta blocker that depresses sinus heart rate, slows AV conduction, decreases cardiac output, and lowers systolic and diastolic blood pressure.

| Route | Onset | Peak | Duration |
|-------|-------|------|----------|
| P.O. | Unknown | 2½-4 hr | Unknown |

**ADVERSE REACTIONS**
**CNS:** *asthenia, headache, dizziness, weakness, fatigue,* sleep problems, *lightheadedness.*
**CV:** *bradycardia, arrhythmias, heart failure, AV block, proarrhythmic events (including polymorphic ventricular tachycardia, PVCs, ventricular fibrillation),* edema, *palpitations, chest pain,* ECG abnormalities, hypotension.
**GI:** *nausea, vomiting,* diarrhea, dyspepsia.
**Metabolic:** hyperglycemia.
**Respiratory:** *dyspnea, bronchospasm.*

## INTERACTIONS

**Drug-drug.** *Antiarrhythmics:* May increase drug effects. Avoid using together.
*Antihypertensives, catecholamine-depleting drugs (such as guanethidine, reserpine):* May increase hypotensive effects. Monitor blood pressure closely.
*Calcium channel blockers:* May increase myocardial depression. Avoid using together.
*Clonidine:* May enhance rebound effect after withdrawal of clonidine. Stop sotalol several days before withdrawing clonidine.
*General anesthetics:* May increase myocardial depression. Monitor patient closely.
*Insulin, oral antidiabetics:* May cause hyperglycemia and may mask signs and symptoms of hypoglycemia. Adjust dosage accordingly.
*Prazosin:* May increase the risk of orthostatic hypotension. Assist patient to stand slowly until effects are known.
**Drug-food.** *Any food:* May decrease absorption by 20%. Advise patient to take on empty stomach.

## EFFECTS ON LAB TEST RESULTS

● May increase glucose level. May cause false-positive catecholamine level.

## CONTRAINDICATIONS & CAUTIONS

● Contraindicated in patients hypersensitive to drug.
● Contraindicated in those with severe sinus node dysfunction, sinus bradycardia, second- and third-degree AV block unless patient has a pacemaker, congenital or acquired long QT-interval syndrome, cardiogenic shock, uncontrolled heart failure, and bronchial asthma.
● Use cautiously in patients with renal impairment or diabetes mellitus (beta blockers may mask signs and symptoms of hypoglycemia).

## NURSING CONSIDERATIONS

● Because proarrhythmic events may occur at start of therapy and during dosage adjustments, hospitalize patient for a minimum of 3 days. Facilities and personnel should be available for cardiac rhythm monitoring and interpretation of ECG.

● Assess patient for new or worsened symptoms of heart failure.
● Although patients receiving I.V. lidocaine may start sotalol therapy without ill effect, withdraw other antiarrhythmics before therapy begins. Sotalol therapy typically is delayed until two or three half-lives of the withdrawn drug have elapsed. After withdrawing amiodarone, give sotalol only after QT interval normalizes.
● Adjust dosage slowly, allowing 3 days between dosage increments for adequate monitoring of QT intervals and for drug levels to reach a steady-state level.
● **Alert:** Don't substitute Betapace for Betapace AF.
● Monitor electrolytes regularly, especially if patient is receiving diuretics. Electrolyte imbalances, such as hypokalemia or hypomagnesemia, may enhance QT-interval prolongation and increase the risk of serious arrhythmias such as torsades de pointes.
● **Alert:** Don't confuse sotalol with Stadol.

## PATIENT TEACHING

● Explain to patient that he will need to be hospitalized for initiation of drug therapy.
● Stress need to take drug as prescribed, even when the patient is feeling well. Caution patient against stopping drug suddenly.
● Caution patient against using nonprescription drugs and decongestants while taking drug.
● Because food and antacids can interfere with absorption, tell patient to take drug on an empty stomach, 1 hour before or 2 hours after meals or antacids.

---

# tocainide hydrochloride
Tonocard

*Pregnancy risk category C*

## AVAILABLE FORMS
*Tablets:* 400 mg, 600 mg

## INDICATIONS & DOSAGES
➤ **Suppression of symptomatic life-threatening ventricular arrhythmias**
*Adults:* Initially, 400 mg P.O. q 8 hours. Usual dose is between 1,200 and 1,800 mg daily in three divided doses.

---

➤ **Myotonic dystrophy** ♦
*Adults:* 800 to 1,200 mg P.O. daily.
➤ **Trigeminal neuralgia** ♦
*Adults:* 20 mg/kg/day P.O. in three divided doses.
*Adjust-a-dose:* For patients with renal or hepatic impairment, a dose less than 1,200 mg daily may be adequate.

## ACTION
A class IB antiarrhythmic. Blocks the fast sodium channel in cardiac tissues, especially the Purkinje network, without involving the autonomic nervous system. Reduces rate of rise and duration and amplitude of action potential and decreases automaticity and effective refractory period in the Purkinje fibers.

| Route | Onset | Peak | Duration |
|---|---|---|---|
| P.O. | Unknown | 30-120 min | 8 hr |

## ADVERSE REACTIONS
**CNS:** ataxia, *light-headedness, tremor,* paresthesia, *dizziness, vertigo,* drowsiness, fatigue, confusion, headache.
**CV:** hypotension, *new or worsened arrhythmias, heart failure, bradycardia,* palpitations.
**EENT:** blurred vision, tinnitus.
**GI:** *nausea, vomiting,* diarrhea, anorexia.
**Hematologic:** *agranulocytosis, bone marrow depression, thrombocytopenia, aplastic anemia, neutropenia.*
**Hepatic:** *hepatitis.*
**Respiratory:** *pulmonary fibrosis,* pulmonary edema, interstitial pneumonitis, fibrosing alveolitis.
**Skin:** rash, diaphoresis.

## INTERACTIONS
**Drug-drug.** *Beta blockers:* May decrease myocardial contractility; may increase CNS toxicity. Monitor patient closely.
*Cimetidine:* May reduce tocainide level. Monitor tocainide effectiveness.
*Rifampin:* May increase clearance of tocainide. Monitor tocainide effectiveness.

## EFFECTS ON LAB TEST RESULTS
● May decrease hemoglobin, hematocrit, and platelet and granulocyte counts. May cause abnormal liver function test values.

## CONTRAINDICATIONS & CAUTIONS
● Contraindicated in patients hypersensitive to lidocaine or other amide-type local anesthetics and in those with second- or third-degree AV block in the absence of an artificial pacemaker.
● Use cautiously in patients with heart failure or diminished cardiac reserve and in those with hepatic or renal impairment. These patients often may be treated effectively with a lower dose.

## NURSING CONSIDERATIONS
● Drug may ease transition from I.V. lidocaine to oral antiarrhythmic. Monitor patient carefully.
● Correct potassium deficits. Drug may be ineffective in patients with hypokalemia.
● Monitor patient for tremor, which may indicate that maximum dosage has been reached.
● Notify prescriber if patient develops signs and symptoms of infection; perform a CBC immediately to rule out agranulocytosis.

## PATIENT TEACHING
● Instruct patient to report immediately unusual bruising or bleeding or signs or symptoms of infection. Severe blood cell deficiency and bone marrow suppression have been reported in patients taking usual doses of drug, typically within first 12 weeks of therapy.
● Advise patient to immediately report sudden onset of breathing problems, such as coughing, wheezing, or labored breathing after exertion. Drug may cause serious breathing problems.
● Tell elderly patient to take safety precautions to reduce the risk of dizziness and falling.

amlodipine besylate
diltiazem hydrochloride
isosorbide dinitrate
isosorbide mononitrate
nadolol
nicardipine hydrochloride
nifedipine
nitroglycerin
propranolol hydrochloride
verapamil hydrochloride

## COMBINATION PRODUCTS
LOTREL: amlodipine 2.5 mg and benazepril hydrochloride 10 mg, amlodipine 5 mg and benazepril hydrochloride 10 mg, amlodipine 5 mg and benazepril hydrochloride 20 mg; amlodipine 10 mg and benazepril hydrochloride 20 mg.

## amlodipine besylate
Norvasc⊘

*Pregnancy risk category C*

### AVAILABLE FORMS
*Tablets:* 2.5 mg, 5 mg, 10 mg

### INDICATIONS & DOSAGES
➤ **Chronic stable angina, vasospastic angina (Prinzmetal's or variant angina)**
*Adults:* Initially, 5 to 10 mg P.O. daily. Most patients need 10 mg daily.
*Elderly patients:* Initially, 5 mg P.O. daily.
*Adjust-a-dose:* For small, frail patients or those with hepatic insufficiency, initially 5 mg P.O. daily.
➤ **Hypertension**
*Adults:* Initially, 2.5 to 5 mg P.O. daily. Dosage adjusted according to patient response and tolerance. Maximum daily dose is 10 mg.
*Elderly patients:* Initially, 2.5 mg P.O. daily.
*Adjust-a-dose:* For small, frail patients, those currently receiving other antihypertensives, or those with hepatic insufficiency, initially 2.5 mg P.O. daily.

### ACTION
Inhibits calcium ion influx across cardiac and smooth-muscle cells, thus decreasing myocardial contractility and oxygen demand; also dilates coronary arteries and arterioles.

| Route | Onset | Peak | Duration |
|---|---|---|---|
| P.O. | Unknown | 6-12 hr | 24 hr |

### ADVERSE REACTIONS
**CNS:** headache, somnolence, fatigue, dizziness, light-headedness, paresthesia.
**CV:** *edema,* flushing, palpitations.
**GI:** nausea, abdominal pain.
**GU:** sexual difficulties.
**Musculoskeletal:** muscle pain.
**Respiratory:** dyspnea.
**Skin:** rash, pruritus.

### INTERACTIONS
**Drug-food.** *Grapefruit juice:* May increase drug level and adverse reactions. Discourage use together.

### EFFECTS ON LAB TEST RESULTS
None reported.

### CONTRAINDICATIONS & CAUTIONS
● Contraindicated in patients hypersensitive to drug.
● Use cautiously in patients receiving other peripheral vasodilators, especially those with severe aortic stenosis, and in those with heart failure. Because drug is metabolized by the liver, use cautiously and in reduced dosage in patients with severe hepatic disease.

### NURSING CONSIDERATIONS
● *Alert:* Monitor patient carefully. Some patients, especially those with severe obstructive coronary artery disease, have developed increased frequency, duration, or severity of angina or acute MI after initiation of calcium channel blocker therapy or at time of dosage increase.
● Monitor blood pressure frequently during initiation of therapy. Because drug-

induced vasodilation has a gradual onset, acute hypotension is rare.

• Notify prescriber if signs of heart failure occur, such as swelling of hands and feet or shortness of breath.

• *Alert:* Don't confuse amlodipine with amiloride.

### PATIENT TEACHING
• Caution patient to continue taking drug, even when feeling better.
• Tell patient S.L. nitroglycerin may be taken as needed when angina symptoms are acute. If patient continues nitrate therapy during adjustment of amlodipine dosage, urge continued compliance.

---

## diltiazem hydrochloride
Apo-Diltiaz†, Cardizem✒,
Cardizem CD✒, Cardizem LA✒,
Cardizem SR✒, CartiaXT, Dilacor
XR, Diltia XT, Tiazac

*Pregnancy risk category C*

### AVAILABLE FORMS
**Cardizem**
*Tablets:* 30 mg, 60 mg, 90 mg, 120 mg
*Injections:* 5 mg/ml (25 mg and 50 mg)
**Cardizem CD**
*Capsules (extended-release):* 120 mg, 180 mg, 240 mg, 300 mg, 360 mg
**Cardizem LA**
*Tablets (extended-release):* 120 mg, 180 mg, 240 mg, 300 mg, 360 mg, 420 mg
**Cardizem SR**
*Capsules (sustained-release):* 60 mg, 90 mg, 120 mg
**Cartia XT**
*Capsules (extended-release):* 120 mg, 180 mg, 240 mg, 300 mg
**Dilacor XR**
*Capsules (extended-release) containing multiple units of 60-mg:* 120 mg, 180 mg, 240 mg
**Diltia XT**
*Capsules (extended-release) containing multiple units of 60-mg:* 120 mg, 180 mg, 240 mg
**Tiazac**
*Capsules (extended-release):* 120 mg, 180 mg, 240 mg, 300 mg, 360 mg, 420 mg

### INDICATIONS & DOSAGES
➤ **To manage Prinzmetal's or variant angina or chronic stable angina pectoris**
*Adults:* 30 mg P.O. q.i.d. before meals and h.s. Increase dose gradually to maximum of 360 mg/day divided into three to four doses, as indicated. Or, give 120 or 180 mg (extended-release) P.O. once daily. Adjust over a 7- to 14-day period as needed and tolerated up to a maximum dose of 480 mg daily.
➤ **Hypertension**
*Adults:* 60 to 120 mg P.O. b.i.d. (sustained-release). Adjust up to maximum recommended dose of 360 mg/day, p.r.n. Or, give 180 to 240 mg (extended-release) P.O. once daily. Adjust dosage based on patient response to a maximum dose of 480 mg/day. Or 120 to 240 mg P.O. (Cardizem LA) once daily. Dosage can be adjusted about every 2 weeks to a maximum of 540 mg daily.
➤ **Atrial fibrillation or flutter; paroxysmal supraventricular tachycardia**
*Adults:* 0.25 mg/kg I.V. as a bolus injection over 2 minutes. Repeat after 15 minutes if response isn't adequate with a dose of 0.35 mg/kg I.V. over 2 minutes. Follow bolus with continuous I.V. infusion at 5 to 15 mg/hour (for up to 24 hours).

### I.V. ADMINISTRATION
• Reconstitute drug in Cardizem Monovials labeled as containing 100 mg according to manufacturer's directions.
• For direct I.V. injection, no dilution of 5 mg/ml injection is needed.
• For continuous I.V. infusion, add 5 mg/ml injection to 100, 200, or 500 ml of normal saline solution, $D_5W$, or 5% dextrose and half-normal saline solution to produce a final concentration of 1, 0.83, or 0.45 mg/ml.
• For direct injection or continuous infusion, give slowly while continuously monitoring ECG and blood pressure.
• Don't give infusions lasting longer than 24 hours.

### ACTION
A calcium channel blocker that inhibits calcium ion influx across cardiac and smooth-muscle cells, decreasing myocardial contractility and oxygen demand.

---

Also dilates coronary arteries and arterioles.

| Route | Onset | Peak | Duration |
|-------|-------|------|----------|
| P.O. | 30-60 min | 2-3 hr | 6-8 hr |
| P.O. (extended, sustained) | 2-3 hr | 10-14 hr | 12-24 hr |
| P.O. (Cardizem LA) | 3-4 hr | 11-18 hr | 6-9 hr |
| I.V. | Within 3 min | 2-7 min | 1-10 hr |

## ADVERSE REACTIONS

**CNS:** *headache,* dizziness, asthenia, somnolence.
**CV:** *edema,* **arrhythmias,** flushing, **bradycardia,** hypotension, conduction abnormalities, **heart failure, AV block,** abnormal ECG.
**GI:** nausea, constipation, abdominal discomfort.
**Hepatic:** *acute hepatic injury.*
**Skin:** rash.

## INTERACTIONS

**Drug-drug.** *Anesthetics:* May increase effects of anesthetics. Monitor patient.
*Carbamazepine:* May increase level of carbamazepine. Monitor carbamazepine level, and watch for signs and symptoms of toxicity.
*Cimetidine:* May inhibit diltiazem metabolism, increasing additive AV node conduction slowing. Monitor patient for toxicity.
*Cyclosporine:* May increase cyclosporine level, possibly by decreasing its metabolism, leading to increased risk of cyclosporine toxicity. Monitor cyclosporine level with each dosage change.
*Diazepam, midazolam, triazolam:* May increase CNS depression and prolonged effects of these drugs. Use lower dose of these benzodiazepines.
*Digoxin:* May increase digoxin level. Monitor patient for digoxin toxicity.
*Furosemide:* May form a precipitate when mixed with diltiazem injection. Give through separate I.V. lines.
*Propranolol, other beta blockers:* May precipitate heart failure or prolong conduction time. Use together cautiously.
*Sirolimus, tacrolimus:* May increase level of these drugs. Monitor drug level and patient for toxicity.

## EFFECTS ON LAB TEST RESULTS
None reported.

## CONTRAINDICATIONS & CAUTIONS
● Contraindicated in patients hypersensitive to drug and in those with sick sinus syndrome or second- or third-degree AV block in the absence of an artificial pacemaker, ventricular tachycardia, systolic blood pressure below 90 mm Hg, acute MI, or pulmonary congestion (documented by X-ray).
● I.V. preparations are contraindicated in patients who have atrial fibrillation or flutter with an accessory bypass tract, as in Wolff-Parkinson-White syndrome or short PR interval syndrome.
● Use cautiously in elderly patients and in those with heart failure or impaired hepatic or renal function.

## NURSING CONSIDERATIONS
● Patients controlled on diltiazem alone or in combination with other medications may be switched to Cardizem LA tablets once a day at the nearest equivalent total daily dose.
● Monitor blood pressure and heart rate when starting therapy and during dosage adjustments.
● Maximum antihypertensive effect may not be seen for 14 days.
● If systolic blood pressure is below 90 mm Hg or heart rate is below 60 beats/minute, withhold dose and notify prescriber.
● *Alert:* Don't confuse Cardizem SR with Cardene SR.

## PATIENT TEACHING
● Instruct patient to take medication as prescribed, even when feeling better.
● Advise patient to avoid hazardous activities during start of therapy.
● Stress patient compliance if nitrate therapy is prescribed during adjustment of diltiazem dosage. Tell patient that S.L. nitroglycerin may be taken with drug, as needed, when angina symptoms are acute.
● *Alert:* Tell patient to swallow extended-release capsules whole, and not to open, crush, or chew them.

---

Reactions may be *common,* uncommon, *life-threatening,* or COMMON AND LIFE-THREATENING.

# isosorbide dinitrate
Apo-ISDN†, Cedocard SR†,
Dilatrate-SR, Isordil, Isordil
Tembids, Isordil Titradose,
Sorbitrate

# isosorbide mononitrate
Imdur, ISMO, Isotrate ER,
Monoket

*Pregnancy risk category C*

## AVAILABLE FORMS
**isosorbide dinitrate**
*Capsules (sustained-release):* 40 mg
*Tablets:* 5 mg, 10 mg, 20 mg, 30 mg,
40 mg
*Tablets (chewable):* 5 mg, 10 mg
*Tablets (S.L.):* 2.5 mg, 5 mg, 10 mg
*Tablets (sustained-release):* 40 mg
**isosorbide mononitrate**
*Tablets:* 10 mg, 20 mg
*Tablets (extended-release):* 30 mg, 60 mg,
120 mg

## INDICATIONS & DOSAGES
➤ **Acute anginal attacks (S.L. and chewable tablets of isosorbide dinitrate only); for prevention in situations likely to cause anginal attacks**
*Adults:* 2.5 to 5 mg S.L. tablets for prompt relief of angina, repeated q 5 to 10 minutes (maximum of three doses for each 30-minute period). For prevention, 2.5 to 10 mg q 2 to 3 hours.
*Adults:* 5 to 10 mg chewable tablets, p.r.n., for acute attack or q 2 to 3 hours for prophylaxis, but only after initial test dose of 5 mg to determine risk of severe hypotension.
*Adults:* 5 to 40 mg isosorbide dinitrate P.O. b.i.d. or t.i.d. for prevention only (use smallest effective dose).
*Adults:* 30 to 60 mg isosorbide mononitrate using Imdur P.O. once daily on arising; increased to 120 mg once daily after several days, if needed.
*Adults:* 20 mg isosorbide mononitrate using ISMO or Monoket b.i.d. with the two doses given 7 hours apart.

## ACTION
Not completely known. Thought to reduce cardiac oxygen demand by decreasing preload and afterload. Drug also may increase blood flow through the collateral coronary vessels.

| Route | Onset | Peak | Duration |
|---|---|---|---|
| P.O. | 15-40 min | Unknown | 4-8 hr |
| P.O. (chewable) | 2-5 min | Unknown | 2-3 hr |
| P.O. (extended) | ½-4 hr | Unknown | 6-12 hr |
| P.O. (S.L.) | 2-5 min | Unknown | 1-4 hr |

## ADVERSE REACTIONS
**CNS:** *headache,* dizziness, weakness.
**CV:** *orthostatic hypotension, tachycardia, palpitations, ankle edema,* fainting, *flushing.*
**EENT:** S.L. burning.
**GI:** nausea, vomiting.
**Skin:** cutaneous vasodilation, rash.

## INTERACTIONS
**Drug-drug.** *Antihypertensives:* May increase hypotensive effects. Monitor patient closely during initial therapy.
*Sildenafil:* May cause severe hypotension. Use of nitrates in any form with sildenafil is contraindicated.
**Drug-lifestyle.** *Alcohol use:* May increase hypotension. Discourage use together.

## EFFECTS ON LAB TEST RESULTS
● May cause falsely reduced value in cholesterol tests using the Zlatkis-Zak color reaction.

## CONTRAINDICATIONS & CAUTIONS
● Contraindicated in patients with hypersensitivity or idiosyncrasy to nitrates and in those with severe hypotension, angle-closure glaucoma, increased intracranial pressure, shock, or acute MI with low left ventricular filling pressure.
● Use cautiously in patients with blood volume depletion (such as from diuretic therapy) or mild hypotension.

## NURSING CONSIDERATIONS
● To prevent tolerance, a nitrate-free interval of 8 to 12 hours per day is recommended. The regimen for isosorbide mononitrate (1 tablet on awakening with the second dose in 7 hours, or 1 extended-release tablet daily) is intended to mini-

mize nitrate tolerance by providing a substantial nitrate-free interval.
• Monitor blood pressure and intensity and duration of drug response.
• Drug may cause headaches, especially at beginning of therapy. Dosage may be reduced temporarily, but tolerance usually develops. Treat headache with aspirin or acetaminophen.
• Methemoglobinemia has been seen with nitrates. Symptoms are those of impaired oxygen delivery despite adequate cardiac output and adequate arterial partial pressure of oxygen.
• *Alert:* Don't confuse Isordil with Isuprel or Inderal.

**PATIENT TEACHING**
• Caution patient to take drug regularly, as prescribed, and to keep it accessible at all times.
• *Alert:* Advise patient that stopping drug abruptly may cause spasm of the coronary arteries with increased angina symptoms and potential risk of heart attack.
• Tell patient to take S.L. tablet at first sign of attack. He should wet tablet with saliva and place under his tongue until absorbed; the patient should sit down and rest. Dose may be repeated every 10 to 15 minutes for a maximum of three doses. If drug doesn't provide relief, tell patient to seek medical help promptly.
• Advise patient who complains of tingling sensation with S.L. drug to try holding tablet in cheek.
• Warn patient not to confuse S.L. with P.O. form.
• Advise patient taking P.O. form of isosorbide dinitrate to take oral tablet on an empty stomach either 30 minutes before or 1 to 2 hours after meals, to swallow oral tablets whole, and to chew chewable tablets thoroughly before swallowing.
• Tell patient to minimize dizziness upon standing up by changing to upright position slowly. Advise him to go up and down stairs carefully and to lie down at first sign of dizziness.
• Caution patient to avoid alcohol because it may worsen low blood pressure effects.
• Advise patient that use of sildenafil with any nitrate may cause severe low blood pressure. Patient should talk to his prescriber before using these drugs together.

• Instruct patient to store drug in a cool place, in a tightly closed container, and away from light.

---

# nadolol
Corgard

*Pregnancy risk category C*

**AVAILABLE FORMS**
*Tablets:* 20 mg, 40 mg, 80 mg, 120 mg, 160 mg

**INDICATIONS & DOSAGES**
▶ **Angina pectoris**
*Adults:* 40 mg P.O. once daily. Increase in 40- to 80-mg increments at 3- to 7-day intervals until optimum response occurs. Usual maintenance dose is 40 to 80 mg once daily; up to 240 mg once daily may be needed.
▶ **Hypertension**
*Adults:* 40 mg P.O. once daily. Increase in 40- to 80-mg increments until optimum response occurs. Usual maintenance dose is 40 to 80 mg once daily. Doses of 320 mg may be needed.
*Adjust-a-dose:* If creatinine clearance is 31 to 50 ml/minute, q 24 to 36 hours; if clearance is 10 to 30 ml/minute, q 24 to 48 hours; and if clearance is below 10 ml/minute, q 40 to 60 hours.

**ACTION**
A beta blocker that reduces cardiac oxygen demand by blocking catecholamine-induced increases in heart rate, blood pressure, and force of myocardial contraction. Depresses renin secretion.

| Route | Onset | Peak | Duration |
|-------|-------|------|----------|
| P.O. | Unknown | 2-4 hr | Unknown |

**ADVERSE REACTIONS**
**CNS:** fatigue, dizziness, fever.
**CV:** *bradycardia, hypotension, heart failure,* peripheral vascular disease, rhythm and conduction disturbances.
**GI:** nausea, vomiting, diarrhea, abdominal pain, constipation, anorexia.
**Respiratory:** *increased airway resistance.*
**Skin:** rash.

---

Reactions may be *common*, uncommon, *life-threatening*, or COMMON AND LIFE-THREATENING.

## INTERACTIONS
**Drug-drug.** *Antihypertensives:* May increase antihypertensive effect. Monitor blood pressure closely.
*Cardiac glycosides:* May cause excessive bradycardia and additive effects on AV conduction. Use together cautiously.
*Epinephrine:* May cause an initial hypertensive episode followed by bradycardia. Stop beta blocker 3 days before anticipated epinephrine use. Monitor patient closely.
*Insulin:* May mask symptoms of hypoglycemia, as a result of beta blockade (such as tachycardia). Use with extreme caution in patients with diabetes.
*I.V. lidocaine:* May reduce hepatic metabolism of lidocaine, increasing the risk of toxicity. Give bolus doses of lidocaine at a slower rate and monitor lidocaine level closely.
*NSAIDs:* May decrease antihypertensive effect. Monitor blood pressure and adjust dosage.
*Oral antidiabetics:* May alter dosage requirements in previously stabilized diabetic patients. Monitor glucose closely.
*Phenothiazines:* May increase hypotensive effects. Monitor blood pressure.
*Prazosin:* May increase risk of orthostatic hypotension in the early phases of use together. Assist patient to stand slowly until effects are known.
*Verapamil:* May increase effects of both drugs. Monitor cardiac function closely and decrease dosages as necessary.

## EFFECTS ON LAB TEST RESULTS
None reported.

## CONTRAINDICATIONS & CAUTIONS
• Contraindicated in patients with bronchial asthma, sinus bradycardia and greater than first-degree heart block, cardiogenic shock, and overt heart failure.
• Use cautiously in patients with heart failure, chronic bronchitis, emphysema, or renal or hepatic impairment and in patients undergoing major surgery involving general anesthesia.
• Use cautiously in diabetic patients because beta blockers may mask certain signs and symptoms of hypoglycemia.

## NURSING CONSIDERATIONS
• Check apical pulse before giving drug. If slower than 60 beats/minute, withhold drug and call prescriber.
• Monitor blood pressure frequently. If patient develops severe hypotension, give a vasopressor, as prescribed.
• **Alert:** Abrupt discontinuation can worsen angina and cause MI. Reduce dosage gradually over 1 to 2 weeks.
• Drug masks signs and symptoms of shock and hyperthyroidism.

## PATIENT TEACHING
• Explain importance of taking drug as prescribed, even when patient is feeling well.
• Teach patient how to check pulse rate and tell him to check it before each dose. If pulse rate is below 60 beats/minute, tell patient to notify prescriber.
• Warn patient not to stop drug suddenly.

---

## nicardipine hydrochloride
Cardene, Cardene I.V., Cardene SR

*Pregnancy risk category C*

## AVAILABLE FORMS
*Capsules:* 20 mg, 30 mg
*Capsules (sustained-release):* 30 mg, 45 mg, 60 mg
*Injection:* 2.5 mg/ml

## INDICATIONS & DOSAGES
➤ **Chronic stable angina (used alone or with other antianginals)**
*Adults:* Initially, 20 mg P.O. t.i.d. (immediate-release). Dosage adjusted based on patient response q 3 days. Usual range is 20 to 40 mg t.i.d.
➤ **Hypertension**
*Adults:* Initially, 20 mg P.O. t.i.d. (immediate-release); range, 20 to 40 mg t.i.d. Or, 30 mg b.i.d. (sustained-release); range, 30 to 60 mg b.i.d. Dosage increased based on patient response. Or, for patient unable to take oral nicardipine, 50 ml/hour (5 mg/hour) I.V. infusion initially; then increased by 25 ml/hour (2.5 mg/hour) q 15 minutes to maximum of 150 ml/hour (15 mg/hour).

## I.V. ADMINISTRATION

• Dilute with compatible I.V. solution before administration. The drug is compatible with $D_5W$, dextrose 5% in normal saline solution or half-normal saline solution, and normal saline solution or half-normal saline solution for 24 hours at room temperature.

• The drug is incompatible with sodium bicarbonate and lactated Ringer's solution.

• Give by slow I.V. infusion in a concentration of 0.1 mg/ml.

• Closely monitor blood pressure during and after completion of infusion.

• Titrate infusion rate if hypotension or tachycardia occurs.

• Change peripheral infusion site every 12 hours to minimize risk of venous irritation.

• When switching to oral therapy other than nicardipine, initiate therapy upon ending of infusion. If oral nicardipine is to be used, give first dose of t.i.d. regimen 1 hour before stopping infusion.

## ACTION

A calcium channel blocker that inhibits calcium ion influx across cardiac and smooth-muscle cells, decreasing myocardial contractility and oxygen demand. Also dilates coronary arteries and arterioles.

| Route | Onset | Peak | Duration |
|---|---|---|---|
| P.O. (immediate) | 30-90 sec | 1-2 hr | Unknown |
| P.O. (sustained) | 20 min | 1-4 hr | 12 hr |
| I.V. | Immediate | Immediate | Unknown |

## ADVERSE REACTIONS

**CNS:** dizziness, light-headedness, *headache*, asthenia.
**CV:** *peripheral edema, palpitations*, angina, tachycardia, *flushing*.
**GI:** nausea, abdominal discomfort, dry mouth.
**Skin:** rash.

## INTERACTIONS

**Drug-drug.** *Antihypertensives:* May increase antihypertensive effect. Monitor blood pressure closely.
*Beta blockers:* May increase cardiac depressant effects. Monitor patient closely.

*Cimetidine:* May decrease metabolism of calcium channel blockers. Monitor patient for increased pharmacologic effect.
*Cyclosporine:* May increase plasma level of cyclosporine. Monitor patient for toxicity.
*Theophylline:* May increase pharmacologic effects of theophylline. Monitor patient for toxicity.

## EFFECTS ON LAB TEST RESULTS

None reported.

## CONTRAINDICATIONS & CAUTIONS

• Contraindicated in patients hypersensitive to drug and in those with advanced aortic stenosis.

• Use cautiously in patients with hypotension, heart failure, or impaired hepatic and renal function.

## NURSING CONSIDERATIONS

• Measure blood pressure frequently during initial therapy. Maximum blood pressure response occurs about 1 hour after dosing with the immediate-release form and 2 to 4 hours afterward with the sustained-release form. Check for potential orthostatic hypotension. Because large swings in blood pressure may occur based on blood level of drug, assess adequacy of antihypertensive effect 8 hours after dosing.

• Extended-release form is preferred because of improved medication adherence, fewer fluctuations in blood pressure, and increased risk in mortality with short-acting drugs.

• **Alert:** Don't confuse Cardene with Cardura or codeine. Don't confuse Cardene SR with Cardizem SR.

## PATIENT TEACHING

• Tell patient to take oral form of drug exactly as prescribed.

• Advise patient to report chest pain immediately. Some patients may experience increased frequency, severity, or duration of chest pain at beginning of therapy or during dosage adjustments.

• Inform patient to get up from a sitting or lying position slowly to avoid dizziness caused by a decrease in blood pressure.

---

Reactions may be *common*, uncommon, *life-threatening*, or COMMON AND LIFE-THREATENING.

# nifedipine
Adalat, Adalat CC, Adalat PA†,
Adalat XL†, Apo-Nifed†, Nifedical
XL, Novo-Nifedin†, Nu-Nifed†,
Procardia◆, Procardia XL◆

*Pregnancy risk category C*

## AVAILABLE FORMS
*Capsules:* 10 mg, 20 mg
*Tablets (extended-release):* 30 mg, 60 mg,
90 mg

## INDICATIONS & DOSAGES
➤ **Vasospastic angina (Prinzmetal's or
variant angina), classic chronic stable
angina pectoris**
*Adults:* Initially, 10 mg P.O. t.i.d. Usual effective dosage range is 10 to 20 mg t.i.d.
Some patients may require up to 30 mg
q.i.d. Maximum daily dose is 180 mg. Adjust dosage over 7 to 14 days to evaluate
response.
➤ **Hypertension**
*Adults:* 30 or 60 mg P.O. (extended-
release) once daily. Adjusted over 7 to
14 days. Doses larger than 90 mg (Adalat
CC) and 120 mg (Procardia XL) aren't recommended.

## ACTION
Unknown. Thought to inhibit calcium ion
influx across cardiac and smooth-muscle
cells, decreasing contractility and oxygen
demand. Also may dilate coronary arteries
and arterioles.

| Route | Onset | Peak | Duration |
|-------|-------|------|----------|
| P.O. | 20 min | 30-60 min | 4-8 hr |
| P.O. (extended) | 20 min | 6 hr | 24 hr |

## ADVERSE REACTIONS
**CNS:** *dizziness, light-headedness,* somno-
lence, *headache, weakness,* syncope, ner-
vousness.
**CV:** *peripheral edema,* hypotension, pal-
pitations, **heart failure, MI,** *flushing.*
**EENT:** nasal congestion.
**GI:** *nausea,* diarrhea, constipation, ab-
dominal discomfort.
**Metabolic:** hypokalemia.
**Musculoskeletal:** muscle cramps.

**Respiratory:** dyspnea, pulmonary edema,
cough.
**Skin:** rash, pruritus.

## INTERACTIONS
**Drug-drug.** *Cimetidine, ranitidine:* May
decrease nifedipine metabolism. May
need to adjust dosage.
*Digoxin:* May cause elevated digoxin level. Monitor digoxin level.
*Fentanyl:* May cause severe hypotension.
Monitor blood pressure.
*Phenytoin:* May reduce phenytoin metabolism. Monitor phenytoin level.
*Propranolol, other beta blockers:* May
cause hypotension and heart failure. Use
together cautiously.
**Drug-herb.** *Dong quai:* May increase antihypertensive effect. Discourage use together.
*Ginkgo:* May increase effects of nifedipine. Discourage use together.
*Ginseng:* May increase nifedipine levels;
possible toxicity. Discourage use together.
*Melatonin:* May interfere with antihypertensive effect. Discourage use together.
**Drug-food.** *Grapefruit juice:* May increase bioavailability of nifedipine. Discourage use together.

## EFFECTS ON LAB TEST RESULTS
● May increase ALT, AST, alkaline phosphatase, and LDH levels. May decrease
potassium level.

## CONTRAINDICATIONS & CAUTIONS
● Contraindicated in patients hypersensitive to drug.
● Use cautiously in patients with heart failure or hypotension and in elderly patients.
Use extended-release tablets cautiously in
patients with severe GI narrowing.

## NURSING CONSIDERATIONS
● Don't give immediate-release form within 1 week of acute MI or in acute coronary
syndrome.
● *Alert:* Despite the previously widespread
S.L. use of nifedipine capsules (or the
"bite and swallow" method), avoid this
route of administration. Excessive hypotension, MI, and death may result.
● Monitor blood pressure regularly, especially in patients who take beta blockers or
antihypertensives.

---

• Watch for symptoms of heart failure.
• Although rebound effect hasn't been observed when drug is stopped, reduce dosage slowly under prescriber's supervision.
• **Alert:** Don't confuse nifedipine with nimodipine or nicardipine.

**PATIENT TEACHING**
• If patient is kept on nitrate therapy while nifedipine dosage is being adjusted, urge continued compliance. Patient may take S.L. nitroglycerin, as needed, for acute chest pain.
• Tell patient that chest pain may worsen briefly when beginning drug or when dosage is increased.
• Instruct patient to swallow extended-release tablets without breaking, crushing, or chewing them.
• Advise patient to avoid taking drug with grapefruit juice.
• Reassure patient taking the extended-release form that a wax-matrix "ghost" from the tablet may be passed in the stools. Drug is completely absorbed before this occurs.
• Warn patient not to switch brands. Procardia XL and Adalat CC aren't therapeutically equivalent because of major differences in the way the drug is metabolized in the body.
• Tell patient to protect capsules from direct light and moisture and to store at room temperature.

---

## nitroglycerin (glyceryl trinitrate)
Anginine‡, Deponit, Minitran, Nitradisc‡, Nitrek, Nitro-Bid, Nitro-Bid IV, Nitrodisc, Nitro-Dur, Nitrogard, Nitroglyn, Nitrolingual, Nitrong, NitroQuick, Nitrostat⌀, NitroTab, Nitro-Time, NTS, Transderm-Nitro, Transiderm-Nitro‡, Tridil

*Pregnancy risk category C*

---

**AVAILABLE FORMS**
*Aerosol (translingual):* 0.4-mg metered spray
*Capsules (sustained-release):* 2.5 mg, 6.5 mg, 9 mg, 13 mg
*Injection:* 0.5 mg/ml, 5 mg/ml
*Tablets (buccal):* 1 mg, 2 mg, 3 mg
*Tablets (S.L.):* 0.3 mg (¹⁄₂₀₀ grain), 0.4 mg (¹⁄₁₅₀ grain), 0.6 mg (¹⁄₁₀₀ grain)
*Tablets (sustained-release):* 2.6 mg, 6.5 mg, 9 mg, 13 mg
*Topical:* 2% ointment
*Transdermal:* 0.1 mg/hour, 0.2 mg/hour, 0.3 mg/hour, 0.4 mg/hour, 0.6 mg/hour, 0.8 mg/hour release rate

**INDICATIONS & DOSAGES**
➤ **Prophylaxis against chronic anginal attacks**
*Adults:* 2.5 or 2.6 mg sustained-release capsule or tablet q 8 to 12 hours, adjusted upward to an effective dose in 2.5- or 2.6-mg increments b.i.d. to q.i.d. Or, use 2% ointment: Start dosage with ½-inch ointment, increasing by ½-inch increments until desired results are achieved. Range of dosage with ointment is ½ to 5 inches. Usual dose is 1 to 2 inches. Or, transdermal disc or pad (Nitrodisc, Nitro-Dur, or Transderm-Nitro) 0.2 to 0.4 mg/hour once daily.
➤ **Acute angina pectoris, prophylaxis to prevent or minimize anginal attacks before stressful events**
*Adults:* 1 S.L. tablet (¹⁄₄₀₀ grain, ¹⁄₂₀₀ grain, ¹⁄₁₅₀ grain, ¹⁄₁₀₀ grain) dissolved under the tongue or in the buccal pouch as soon as angina begins. Repeat q 5 minutes, if needed, for 15 minutes. Or, using Nitrolingual spray, one or two sprays into mouth, preferably onto or under the tongue. Repeat q 3 to 5 minutes, if needed, to a maximum of three doses within a 15-minute period. Or, 1 to 3 mg transmucosally q 3 to 5 hours while awake.
➤ **Hypertension from surgery, heart failure after MI, angina pectoris in acute situations, to produce controlled hypotension during surgery (by I.V. infusion)**
*Adults:* Initially, infuse at 5 mcg/minute, increasing p.r.n. by 5 mcg/minute q 3 to 5 minutes until response occurs. If a 20-mcg/minute rate doesn't produce a response, increase dosage by as much as 20 mcg/minute q 3 to 5 minutes. Up to 100 mcg/minute may be needed.

---

## I.V. ADMINISTRATION
• Dilute with D₅W or normal saline solution for injection. Concentration shouldn't exceed 400 mcg/ml.
• Always give with an infusion control device and titrate to desired response.
• Always mix in glass bottles, and avoid use of I.V. filters because drug binds to plastic. Regular polyvinyl chloride tubing can bind up to 80% of drug, making it necessary to infuse higher dosages.
• A special nonabsorbent polyvinyl chloride tubing is available from the manufacturer; patients receive more drug when these infusion sets are used.
• Use the same type of infusion set when changing I.V. lines.
• When changing the concentration of infusion, flush the I.V. administration set with 15 to 20 ml of the new concentration before use. This will clear the line of the old drug solution.

## ACTION
A nitrate that reduces cardiac oxygen demand by decreasing left ventricular end-diastolic pressure (preload) and, to a lesser extent, systemic vascular resistance (afterload). Also increases blood flow through the collateral coronary vessels.

| Route | Onset | Peak | Duration |
|---|---|---|---|
| P.O. | 20-45 min | Unknown | 3-8 hr |
| I.V. | Immediate | Immediate | 3-5 min |
| Topical | 30 min | Unknown | 2-12 hr |
| Transdermal | 30 min | Unknown | 24 hr |
| S.L. | 1-3 min | Unknown | 30-60 min |
| Buccal | 3 min | Unknown | 3-5 hr |
| Translingual | 2-4 min | Unknown | 30-60 min |

## ADVERSE REACTIONS
**CNS:** *headache, dizziness,* weakness.
**CV:** *orthostatic hypotension, tachycardia, flushing, palpitations,* fainting.
**EENT:** S.L. burning.
**GI:** nausea, vomiting.
**Skin:** cutaneous vasodilation, contact dermatitis, rash.
**Other:** hypersensitivity reactions.

## INTERACTIONS
**Drug-drug.** *Alteplase:* May decrease tPA antigen concentrations. Avoid use togeth-

er. If concomitant use is unavoidable, use lowest effective dose of nitroglycerin.
*Antihypertensives:* May increase hypotensive effect. Monitor blood pressure closely.
*Heparin:* I.V. nitroglycerin may interfere with anticoagulant effect of heparin. Monitor PTT.
*Sildenafil:* May cause severe hypotension. Use of nitrates in any form with sildenafil is contraindicated.
**Drug-lifestyle.** *Alcohol use:* May increase hypotension. Discourage alcohol intake.

## EFFECTS ON LAB TEST RESULTS
• May falsely decrease values in cholesterol determination tests using the Zlatkis-Zak color reaction.

## CONTRAINDICATIONS & CAUTIONS
• Contraindicated in patients with early MI, severe anemia, increased intracranial pressure, angle-closure glaucoma, orthostatic hypotension, allergy to adhesives (transdermal), or hypersensitivity to nitrates. I.V. nitroglycerin is contraindicated in patients hypersensitive to I.V. form, cardiac tamponade, restrictive cardiomyopathy, or constrictive pericarditis.
• Use cautiously in patients with hypotension or volume depletion.

## NURSING CONSIDERATIONS
• Closely monitor vital signs during infusion, particularly blood pressure, especially in a patient with an MI. Excessive hypotension may worsen the MI.
• To apply ointment, measure the prescribed amount on the application paper; then place the paper on any nonhairy area. Don't rub in. Cover with plastic film to aid absorption and to protect clothing. Remove all excess ointment from previous site before applying the next dose. Avoid getting ointment on fingers.
• Transdermal dosage forms can be applied to any nonhairy part of the skin except distal parts of the arms or legs (absorption won't be maximal at distal sites). Patch may cause contact dermatitis.
• Remove transdermal patch before defibrillation. Because of the aluminum backing on the patch, the electric current may cause arcing that can damage the paddles and burn the patient.

• When stopping transdermal treatment of angina, gradually reduce the dosage and frequency of application over 4 to 6 weeks.

• Monitor blood pressure and intensity and duration of drug response.

• Drug may cause headaches, especially at beginning of therapy. Dosage may be reduced temporarily, but tolerance usually develops. Treat headache with aspirin or acetaminophen.

• Tolerance to drug can be minimized with a 10- to 12-hour nitrate-free interval. To achieve this, remove the transdermal system in the early evening and apply a new system the next morning or omit the last daily dose of a buccal, sustained-release, or ointment form. Check with the prescriber for alterations in dosage regimen if tolerance is suspected.

• *Alert:* Don't confuse Nitro-Bid with Nicobid or nitroglycerin with nitroprusside.

**PATIENT TEACHING**

• Caution patient to take nitroglycerin regularly, as prescribed, and to have it accessible at all times.

• *Alert:* Advise patient that stopping drug abruptly causes spasm of the coronary arteries.

• Teach patient how to give the prescribed form of nitroglycerin.

• Tell patient to take S.L. tablet at first sign of attack. Patient should wet the tablet with saliva and place under the tongue until absorbed, and he should sit down and rest. Dose may be repeated every 5 minutes for a maximum of three doses. If drug doesn't provide relief, medical help obtain promptly.

• Advise patient who complains of a tingling sensation with S.L. drug to try holding tablet in cheek.

• Tell patient to take oral tablets on an empty stomach either 30 minutes before or 1 to 2 hours after meals, to swallow oral tablets whole, and not to chew tablets.

• Remind patient using translingual aerosol form that he shouldn't inhale the spray, but should release it onto or under the tongue. Tell him to wait about 10 seconds or so before swallowing.

• Tell patient to place the buccal tablet between the lip and gum above the incisors or between the cheek and gum. Tablets shouldn't be swallowed or chewed.

• Tell patient to take an additional dose before anticipated stress or at bedtime if chest pain occurs at night.

• Instruct patient wearing skin patch to use caution when near a microwave oven. Leaking radiation may heat patch's metallic backing and cause burns.

• Urge patient using skin patches to dispose of them carefully because enough medication remains after normal use to be hazardous to children and pets.

• Advise patient to avoid alcohol.

• To minimize dizziness when standing up, tell patient to rise slowly. Advise him to go up and down stairs carefully and to lie down at the first sign of dizziness.

• Advise patient that use of sildenafil with any nitrate may cause severe low blood pressure. The patient should talk to his prescriber before considering use of these drugs together.

• Tell patient to store drug in cool, dark place in a tightly closed container. Tell him to remove cotton from container because it absorbs drug.

• Tell patient to store S.L. tablets in original container or other container specifically approved for this use and to carry the container in a jacket pocket or purse, not in a pocket close to the body.

---

**propranolol hydrochloride**
Apo-Propranolol†, Deralin‡, Inderal◆, Inderal LA◆, Novopranol†, pms Propranolol†

*Pregnancy risk category C*

**AVAILABLE FORMS**
*Capsules (extended-release):* 60 mg, 80 mg, 120 mg, 160 mg
*Injection:* 1 mg/ml
*Oral solution:* 4 mg/ml, 8 mg/ml, 80 mg/ml (concentrate)
*Tablets:* 10 mg, 20 mg, 40 mg, 60 mg, 80 mg, 90 mg

**INDICATIONS & DOSAGES**
➤ **Angina pectoris**
*Adults:* Total daily doses of 80 to 320 mg P.O. when given b.i.d., t.i.d., or q.i.d. Or,

one 80-mg extended-release capsule daily. Dosage increased at 3- to 7-day intervals.

➤ **To decrease risk of death after MI**
*Adults:* 180 to 240 mg P.O. daily in divided doses beginning 5 to 21 days after MI has occurred. Usually given t.i.d. or q.i.d.

➤ **Supraventricular, ventricular, and atrial arrhythmias; tachyarrhythmias caused by excessive catecholamine action during anesthesia, hyperthyroidism, or pheochromocytoma**
*Adults:* 0.5 to 3 mg by slow I.V. push, not to exceed 1 mg/minute. After 3 mg have been given, another dose may be given in 2 minutes; subsequent doses, no sooner than q 4 hours. May be diluted and infused slowly. Usual maintenance dose is 10 to 30 mg P.O. t.i.d. or q.i.d.

➤ **Hypertension**
*Adults:* Initially, 80 mg P.O. daily in two divided doses or extended-release form once daily. Increase at 3- to 7-day intervals to maximum daily dose of 640 mg. Usual maintenance dose is 120-240 mg daily or 120 to 160 mg daily as extended-release.

➤ **To prevent frequent, severe, uncontrollable, or disabling migraine or vascular headache**
*Adults:* Initially, 80 mg P.O. daily in divided doses or one extended-release capsule daily. Usual maintenance dose is 160 to 240 mg daily, t.i.d. or q.i.d.

➤ **Essential tremor**
*Adults:* 40 mg tablets or oral solution P.O. b.i.d. Usual maintenance dose is 120 to 320 mg daily in three divided doses.

➤ **Hypertrophic subaortic stenosis**
*Adults:* 20 to 40 mg P.O. t.i.d. or q.i.d.; or 80 to 160 mg extended-release capsules once daily.

➤ **Adjunct therapy in pheochromocytoma**
*Adults:* 60 mg P.O. daily in divided doses with an alpha blocker 3 days before surgery.

## I.V. ADMINISTRATION
● For direct injection, give into a large vessel or into the tubing of a free-flowing, compatible I.V. solution; don't give by continuous I.V. infusion.
● For intermittent infusion, dilute drug with normal saline solution and give over 10 to 15 minutes in 0.1- to 0.2-mg increments.
● Drug is compatible with $D_5W$, half-normal saline solution, normal saline solution, and lactated Ringer's solution.
● Infusion rate shouldn't exceed 1 mg/minute.
● Double-check dose and route. I.V. doses are much smaller than oral doses.
● Monitor blood pressure, ECG, central venous pressure, and heart rate and rhythm frequently, especially during I.V. administration. If patient develops severe hypotension, notify prescriber; a vasopressor may be prescribed.
● For overdose, give I.V. isoproterenol, I.V. atropine, or glucagon; refractory cases may require a pacemaker.

## ACTION
A nonselective beta blocker that reduces cardiac oxygen demand by blocking catecholamine-induced increases in heart rate, blood pressure, and force of myocardial contraction. Depresses renin secretion and prevents vasodilation of cerebral arteries.

| Route | Onset | Peak | Duration |
|-------|-------|------|----------|
| P.O. | 30 min | 60-90 min | 12 hr |
| I.V. | Immediate | 1 min | 5 min |

## ADVERSE REACTIONS
**CNS:** *fatigue, lethargy,* fever, vivid dreams, hallucinations, mental depression, light-headedness, insomnia.
**CV:** *bradycardia,* hypotension, *heart failure,* intermittent claudication, *intensification of AV block.*
**GI:** abdominal cramping, constipation, diarrhea, nausea, vomiting.
**Hematologic:** *agranulocytosis.*
**Respiratory:** *bronchospasm.*
**Skin:** rash.

## INTERACTIONS
**Drug-drug.** *Aminophylline:* May antagonize beta-blocking effects of propranolol. Use together cautiously.
*Cardiac glycosides, diltiazem, verapamil:* May cause hypotension, bradycardia, and increased depressant effect on myocardium. Use together cautiously.

---

*Rapid onset*   †Canada   ‡Australia   ◊OTC   ♦Off-label use   🖊Photoguide   *Liquid contains alcohol.

*Cimetidine:* May inhibit metabolism of propranolol. Watch for increased beta-blocking effect.

*Epinephrine:* May cause severe vasoconstriction. Monitor blood pressure and observe patient carefully.

*Glucagon, isoproterenol:* May antagonize propranolol effect. May be used therapeutically and in emergencies.

*Haloperidol:* May cause cardiac arrest. Avoid using together.

*Insulin, oral antidiabetics:* May alter requirements for these drugs in previously stabilized diabetics. Monitor patient for hypoglycemia.

*Phenothiazines, reserpine:* May cause additive effect. Use together cautiously.

**Drug-herb.** *Betel palm:* May decrease temperature-elevating effects and enhanced CNS effects. Discourage use together.

*Ma huang:* May decrease antihypertensive effects. Discourage use together.

**Drug-lifestyle.** *Cocaine use:* May increase angina-inducing potential of cocaine. Inform patient of this interaction.

**EFFECTS ON LAB TEST RESULTS**
● May increase BUN, transaminase, alkaline phosphatase, and LDH levels.
● May decrease granulocyte count.

**CONTRAINDICATIONS & CAUTIONS**
● Contraindicated in patients with bronchial asthma, sinus bradycardia and heart block greater than first-degree, cardiogenic shock, and heart failure (unless failure is secondary to a tachyarrhythmia that can be treated with propranolol).
● Use cautiously in patients with hepatic or renal impairment, nonallergic bronchospastic diseases, or hepatic disease and in those taking other antihypertensives.
● Because drug blocks some symptoms of hypoglycemia, use cautiously in patients who have diabetes mellitus.
● Use cautiously in patients with thyrotoxicosis because drug may mask some signs and symptoms of that disorder.
● Elderly patients may experience enhanced adverse reactions and may need dosage adjustment.

**NURSING CONSIDERATIONS**
● Always check patient's apical pulse before giving drug. If extremes in pulse rates occur, withhold drug and notify prescriber immediately.
● Give drug consistently with meals. Food may increase absorption of propranolol.
● Drug masks common signs and symptoms of shock and hypoglycemia.
● *Alert:* Don't discontinue drug before surgery for pheochromocytoma. Before any surgical procedure, tell anesthesiologist that patient is receiving propranolol.
● Compliance may be improved by giving drug twice daily or as extended-release capsules. Check with prescriber.
● *Alert:* Don't confuse propranolol with Pravachol. Don't confuse Inderal with Inderide, Isordil, Adderall, or Imuran.

**PATIENT TEACHING**
● Caution patient to continue taking this drug as prescribed, even when he's feeling well.
● Instruct patient to take drug with food.
● *Alert:* Tell patient not to stop drug suddenly because this can worsen chest pain and trigger a heart attack.

---

## verapamil hydrochloride
Anpec‡, Anpec SR‡, Apo-Verap†, Calan❖, Calan SR, Cordilox‡, Cordilox SR‡, Covera-HS, Isoptin‡, Isoptin SR❖, Novo-Veramil†, Nu-Verap†, Veracaps SR‡, Verahexal‡, Verelan❖, Verelan PM

*Pregnancy risk category C*

---

**AVAILABLE FORMS**
**verapamil**
*Tablets:* 40 mg, 80 mg, 120 mg
**verapamil hydrochloride**
*Capsules (extended-release):* 100 mg, 120 mg, 180 mg, 200 mg, 240 mg, 300 mg
*Capsules (sustained-release):* 120 mg, 160 mg‡, 180 mg, 240 mg, 360 mg
*Injection:* 2.5 mg/ml
*Tablets:* 40 mg, 80 mg, 120 mg, 160 mg‡
*Tablets (extended-release):* 100 mg, 120 mg, 180 mg, 200 mg, 240 mg

---

*Tablets (sustained-release):* 120 mg, 180 mg, 240 mg

## INDICATIONS & DOSAGES
➤ **Vasospastic angina (Prinzmetal's or variant angina); classic chronic, stable angina pectoris; chronic atrial fibrillation**
*Adults:* Starting dose is 80 to 120 mg P.O. t.i.d. Increase dosage at daily or weekly intervals, p.r.n. Some patients may require up to 480 mg daily.
➤ **To prevent paroxysmal supraventricular tachycardia**
*Adults:* 80 to 120 mg P.O. t.i.d. or q.i.d.
➤ **Supraventricular arrhythmias**
*Adults:* 0.075 to 0.15 mg/kg (5 to 10 mg) by I.V. push over 2 minutes with ECG and blood pressure monitoring. Repeat dose in 30 minutes if no response occurs.
*Children ages 1 to 15:* 0.1 to 0.3 mg/kg as I.V. bolus over 2 minutes; not to exceed 5 mg.
*Children younger than age 1:* 0.1 to 0.2 mg/kg as I.V. bolus over 2 minutes with continuous ECG monitoring. Repeat dose in 30 minutes if no response occurs.
➤ **Digitalized patients with chronic atrial fibrillation or flutter**
*Adults:* 240 to 320 mg P.O. daily, divided t.i.d. or q.i.d.
➤ **Hypertension**
*Adults:* 240 mg extended-release tablet P.O. once daily in the morning. If response isn't adequate, give an additional 120 mg in the evening or 240 mg q 12 hours, or an 80-mg immediate-release tablet t.i.d.

## I.V. ADMINISTRATION
● Give drug by direct injection into a vein or into the tubing of a free-flowing, compatible I.V. solution.
● Compatible solutions include $D_5W$, half-normal saline solution, normal saline solution, Ringer's solution, and lactated Ringer's solution. Drug is incompatible with sodium bicarbonate.
● Give I.V. doses over at least 2 minutes (3 minutes in elderly patients) to minimize the risk of adverse reactions.
● Monitor ECG and blood pressure continuously in patient receiving I.V. verapamil.

## ACTION
Not clearly defined. A calcium channel blocker that inhibits calcium ion influx across cardiac and smooth-muscle cells, thus decreasing myocardial contractility and oxygen demand; it also dilates coronary arteries and arterioles.

| Route | Onset | Peak | Duration |
|---|---|---|---|
| P.O. | 30 min | 1-2 hr | 8-10 hr |
| P.O. (extended) | 30 min | 5-9 hr | 24 hr |
| I.V. | Immediate | 1-5 min | 1-6 hr |

## ADVERSE REACTIONS
**CNS:** dizziness, headache, asthenia.
**CV:** *transient hypotension,* **heart failure,** pulmonary edema, **bradycardia, AV block, ventricular asystole, ventricular fibrillation,** peripheral edema.
**GI:** *constipation,* nausea.
**Skin:** rash.

## INTERACTIONS
**Drug-drug.** *Acebutolol, atenolol, betaxolol, carteolol, esmolol, metoprolol, nadolol, penbutolol, pindolol, propanolol, timolol:* May increase effects of both drugs. Monitor cardiac function closely and decrease doses as necessary.
*Antihypertensives, quinidine:* May cause hypotension. Monitor blood pressure.
*Carbamazepine, cardiac glycosides:* May increase levels of these drugs. Monitor patient for toxicity.
*Cyclosporine:* May increase cyclosporine level. Monitor cyclosporine level.
*Disopyramide, flecainide:* May cause heart failure. Use together cautiously.
*Lithium:* May decrease or increase lithium level. Monitor lithium level.
*Rifampin:* May decrease oral bioavailability of verapamil. Monitor patient for lack of effect.
**Drug-herb.** *Black catechu:* May cause additive effects. Discourage use together.
*Yerba maté:* May decrease clearance of yerba maté methylxanthines and cause toxicity. Urge caution.
**Drug-food.** *Any food:* May increase absorption. Advise patient to take drug with food.
*Grapefruit juice:* May increase levels of verapamil. Discourage use together.

**Drug-lifestyle.** *Alcohol use:* May enhance the effects of alcohol. Discourage use together.

## EFFECTS ON LAB TEST RESULTS
● May increase ALT, AST, alkaline phosphatase, and bilirubin levels.

## CONTRAINDICATIONS & CAUTIONS
● Contraindicated in patients hypersensitive to drug and in those with severe left ventricular dysfunction, cardiogenic shock, second- or third-degree AV block or sick sinus syndrome except in presence of functioning pacemaker, atrial flutter or fibrillation and accessory bypass tract syndrome, severe heart failure (unless secondary to verapamil therapy), and severe hypotension.
● I.V. verapamil is contraindicated in patients receiving I.V. beta blockers and in those with ventricular tachycardia.
● Use cautiously in elderly patients and in patients with increased intracranial pressure or hepatic or renal disease.

## NURSING CONSIDERATIONS
● Although drug should be taken with food, taking extended-release tablets with food may decrease rate and extent of absorption but allows smaller fluctuations of peak and trough blood levels.
● Pellet-filled capsules may be administered by carefully opening the capsule and sprinkling the pellets on a spoonful of applesauce. This should be swallowed immediately without chewing, followed by a glass of cool water to ensure all pellets are swallowed.
● Patients with severely compromised cardiac function or those receiving beta blockers should receive lower doses of verapamil. Monitor these patients closely.
● If verapamil is being used to terminate supraventricular tachycardia, prescriber may have the patient perform vagal maneuvers after receiving drug.
● Monitor blood pressure at the start of therapy and during dosage adjustments. Assist patient with walking because dizziness may occur.
● Notify prescriber if signs and symptoms of heart failure occur, such as swelling of hands and feet and shortness of breath.

● Monitor liver function test results during prolonged treatment.
● **Alert:** Don't confuse Verelan with Vivarin, Voltaren, or Virilon.

## PATIENT TEACHING
● Instruct patient to take oral form of drug exactly as prescribed.
● Tell patient that long-acting forms shouldn't be crushed or chewed.
● Advise patient to take drug with food.
● Caution patient against abruptly stopping drug.
● If patient is kept on nitrate therapy during adjustment of oral verapamil dosage, urge continued compliance. S.L. nitroglycerin may be taken, as needed, when chest pain symptoms are acute.
● Encourage patient to increase fluid and fiber intake to combat constipation. Give a stool softener.
● Advise patient to avoid or severely limit alcohol consumption. Verapamil significantly inhibits alcohol elimination.

# 21
## Antihypertensives

amlodipine besylate
  (See Chapter 20, ANTIANGINALS.)
atenolol
benazepril hydrochloride
betaxolol hydrochloride
candesartan cilexetil
captopril
carteolol hydrochloride
carvedilol
clonidine
clonidine hydrochloride
diazoxide
diltiazem hydrochloride
  (See Chapter 20, ANTIANGINALS.)
doxazosin mesylate
enalaprilat
enalapril maleate
eplerenone
eprosartan mesylate
felodipine
fosinopril sodium
hydralazine hydrochloride
irbesartan
labetalol hydrochloride
lisinopril
losartan potassium
methyldopa
methyldopate hydrochloride
metoprolol succinate
metoprolol tartrate
minoxidil
nadolol
  (See Chapter 20, ANTIANGINALS.)
nicardipine hydrochloride
  (See Chapter 20, ANTIANGINALS.)
nifedipine
  (See Chapter 20, ANTIANGINALS.)
nisoldipine
nitroprusside sodium
olmesartan medoxomil
perindopril erbumine
pindolol
prazosin hydrochloride
propranolol hydrochloride
  (See Chapter 20, ANTIANGINALS.)
quinapril hydrochloride
ramipril
telmisartan
terazosin hydrochloride
timolol maleate

trandolapril
valsartan
verapamil hydrochloride
  (See Chapter 20, ANTIANGINALS.)

## COMBINATION PRODUCTS

ALDOCLOR-150: chlorothiazide 150 mg and methyldopa 250 mg.
ALDOCLOR-250: chlorothiazide 250 mg and methyldopa 250 mg.
ALDORIL 15: hydrochlorothiazide 15 mg and methyldopa 250 mg.
ALDORIL 25: hydrochlorothiazide 25 mg and methyldopa 250 mg.
ALDORIL D30: hydrochlorothiazide 30 mg and methyldopa 500 mg.
ALDORIL D50: hydrochlorothiazide 50 mg and methyldopa 500 mg.
APRESAZIDE 25/25: hydrochlorothiazide 25 mg and hydralazine hydrochloride 25 mg.
APRESAZIDE 50/50: hydrochlorothiazide 50 mg and hydralazine hydrochloride 50 mg.
BENICAR HCT: olmesartan medoxomil 20 mg and hydrochlorothiazide 12.5 mg.
BENICAR HCT: olmesartan medoxomil 40 mg and hydrochlorothiazide 12.5 mg.
BENICAR HCT: olmesartan medoxomil 40 mg and hydrochlorothiazide 25 mg.
CAPOZIDE 25/15: hydrochlorothiazide 15 mg and captopril 25 mg.
CAPOZIDE 25/25: hydrochlorothiazide 25 mg and captopril 25 mg.
CAPOZIDE 50/15: hydrochlorothiazide 15 mg and captopril 50 mg.
CAPOZIDE 50/25: hydrochlorothiazide 25 mg and captopril 50 mg.
COMBIPRES 0.1: chlorthalidone 15 mg and clonidine hydrochloride 0.1 mg.
COMBIPRES 0.2: chlorthalidone 15 mg and clonidine hydrochloride 0.2 mg.
COMBIPRES 0.3: chlorthalidone 15 mg and clonidine hydrochloride 0.3 mg.
CORZIDE: nadolol 40 mg or 80 mg and bendroflumethiazide 5 mg.
DIOVAN HCT: 80 mg valsartan and 12.5 mg hydrochlorothiazide.
DIOVAN HCT: 160 mg valsartan and 12.5 mg hydrochlorothiazide.

---

*Rapid onset*   †Canada   ‡Australia   ◇OTC   ♦Off-label use   ⌀Photoguide   *Liquid contains alcohol.

DIOVAN HCT: 160 mg valsartan and 25 mg hydrochlorothiazide.

DIURIGEN WITH RESERPINE: chlorothiazide 250 mg and reserpine 0.125 mg.

DIUTENSEN-R: methyclothiazide 2.5 mg and reserpine 0.1 mg.

ENDURONYL: methyclothiazide 5 mg and deserpidine 0.25 mg.

ENDURONYL FORTE: methyclothiazide 5 mg and deserpidine 0.5 mg.

HYDROSERPINE: hydrochlorothiazide 25 or 50 mg and reserpine 0.125 mg.

HYZAAR: losartan 50 mg and hydrochlorothiazide 12.5 mg.

INDERIDE 40/25: propranolol hydrochloride 40 mg and hydrochlorothiazide 25 mg.

INDERIDE 80/25: propranolol hydrochloride 80 mg and hydrochlorothiazide 25 mg.

INDERIDE LA 80/50: propranolol hydrochloride 80 mg and hydrochlorothiazide 50 mg.

INDERIDE LA 120/50: propranolol hydrochloride 120 mg and hydrochlorothiazide 50 mg.

INDERIDE LA 160/50: propranolol hydrochloride 160 mg and hydrochlorothiazide 50 mg.

LEXXEL: enalapril maleate 5 mg and felodipine 5 mg.

LOPRESSOR HCT 50/25: metoprolol tartrate 50 mg and hydrochlorothiazide 25 mg.

LOPRESSOR HCT 100/25: metoprolol tartrate 100 mg and hydrochlorothiazide 25 mg.

LOPRESSOR HCT 100/50: metoprolol tartrate 100 mg and hydrochlorothiazide 50 mg.

MAXZIDE: triamterene 75 mg and hydrochlorothiazide 50 mg.

MINIZIDE 1: polythiazide 0.5 mg and prazosin hydrochloride 1 mg.

MINIZIDE 2: polythiazide 0.5 mg and prazosin hydrochloride 2 mg.

MINIZIDE 5: polythiazide 0.5 mg and prazosin hydrochloride 5 mg.

PRINZIDE 12.5: lisinopril 20 mg and hydrochlorothiazide 12.5 mg.

PRINZIDE 25: lisinopril 20 mg and hydrochlorothiazide 25 mg.

RAUZIDE*: bendroflumethiazide 4 mg and powdered rauwolfia serpentina 50 mg.

REGROTON: chlorthalidone 50 mg and reserpine 0.25 mg.

RENESE-R: polythiazide 2 mg and reserpine 0.25 mg.

SALUTENSIN-DEMI: hydroflumethiazide 25 mg and reserpine 0.125 mg.

SALUTENSIN TABLETS: hydroflumethiazide 50 mg and reserpine 0.125 mg.

Ser-Ap-Es: hydrochlorothiazide 15 mg, reserpine 0.1 mg, and hydralazine hydrochloride 25 mg.

Tenoretic 50: atenolol 50 mg and chlorthalidone 25 mg.

Tenoretic 100: atenolol 100 mg and chlorthalidone 25 mg.

Teveten HCT: 600 mg eprosartan mesylate and hydrochlorothiazide 12.5 mg

Teveten HCT: 600 mg eprosartan mesylate and hydrochlorothiazide 25 mg

Timolide 10-25: timolol maleate 10 mg and hydrochlorothiazide 25 mg.

Tri-Hydroserpine: hydrochlorothiazide 15 mg, hydralazine hydrochloride 25 mg, and reserpine 0.1 mg.

VASERETIC 10-25: enalapril maleate 10 mg and hydrochlorothiazide 25 mg.

ZESTORETIC: lisinopril 20 mg and hydrochlorothiazide 12.5 mg.

ZESTORETIC: lisinopril 20 mg and hydrochlorothiazide 25 mg.

ZIAC TABLETS: bisoprolol fumarate 2.5 mg, 5 mg, or 10 mg and hydrochlorothiazide 6.5 mg.

ZIAC TABLETS: bisoprolol fumarate 5 mg and hydrochlorothiazide 6.5 mg.

ZIAC TABLETS: bisoprolol fumarate 10 mg and hydrochlorothiazide 6.5 mg.

## atenolol
Anselol‡, Apo-Atenolol†, Noten‡, Tenormin◊, Tensig‡

*Pregnancy risk category D*

### AVAILABLE FORMS
*Injection:* 5 mg/10 ml
*Tablets:* 25 mg, 50 mg, 100 mg

### INDICATIONS & DOSAGES
➤ **Hypertension**
*Adults:* Initially, 50 mg P.O. daily alone or in combination with a diuretic as a single dose, increased to 100 mg once daily after 7 to 14 days. Dosages of more than

100 mg are unlikely to produce further benefit.

➤ **Angina pectoris**

*Adults:* 50 mg P.O. once daily, increased p.r.n. to 100 mg daily after 7 days for optimal effect. Maximum, 200 mg daily.

➤ **Reduce risk of CV-related death and reinfarction in patients with acute MI**

*Adults:* 5 mg I.V. over 5 minutes; then another 5 mg after 10 minutes. After another 10 minutes, give 50 mg P.O.; then give another 50 mg P.O. in 12 hours. Subsequently, give 100 mg P.O. daily (as a single dose or 50 mg b.i.d.) for at least 7 days.

*Adjust-a-dose:* For patients with creatinine clearance of 15 to 35 ml/minute, maximum dose is 50 mg/day; if clearance is below 15 ml/minute, maximum dose is 25 mg/day.

Hemodialysis patients need 25 to 50 mg after each dialysis session.

## I.V. ADMINISTRATION

● I.V. doses may be mixed with D₅W, normal saline, or dextrose and saline solutions. Solution is stable for 48 hours after mixing.

● Give by slow I.V. injection, not exceeding 1 mg/minute.

## ACTION

A beta blocker that selectively blocks beta-adrenergic receptors; decreases cardiac output, peripheral resistance, and cardiac oxygen consumption; and depresses renin secretion.

| Route | Onset | Peak | Duration |
|-------|-------|------|----------|
| P.O. | 1 hr | 2-4 hr | 24 hr |
| I.V. | 5 min | 5 min | 12 hr |

## ADVERSE REACTIONS

**CNS:** *fatigue,* lethargy, vertigo, drowsiness, *dizziness,* fever.

**CV:** *bradycardia, hypotension, heart failure,* intermittent claudication.

**GI:** nausea, diarrhea.

**Musculoskeletal:** leg pain.

**Respiratory:** dyspnea, *bronchospasm.*

**Skin:** rash.

## INTERACTIONS

**Drug-drug.** *Amiodarone:* May increase risk of bradycardia, AV block, and myo-

cardial depression. Monitor ECG and vital signs.

*Antihypertensives:* May increase hypotensive effect. Use together cautiously.

*Calcium-channel blockers, hydralazine, methyldopa:* May cause additive hypotensive effects. Adjust dosage as needed.

*Cardiac glycosides, diltiazem:* May cause excessive bradycardia and increased depressant effect on myocardium. Use together cautiously.

*Dolasetron:* May decrease clearance of dolasetron and increase risk of toxicity. Monitor patient for toxicity.

*Insulin, oral antidiabetics:* May alter dosage requirements in previously stabilized diabetic patient. Observe patient carefully.

*I.V. lidocaine:* May reduce hepatic metabolism of lidocaine, increasing risk of toxicity. Give bolus doses of lidocaine at a slower rate and monitor lidocaine level closely.

*NSAIDs:* May decrease antihypertensive effects. Monitor blood pressure.

*Prazosin:* May increase the risk of orthostatic hypotension in the early phases of use together. Help patient stand slowly until effects are known.

*Reserpine:* May cause hypotension. Use together cautiously.

*Verapamil:* May increase the effects of both drugs. Monitor cardiac function closely and decrease dosages as necessary.

## EFFECTS ON LAB TEST RESULTS

● May increase BUN, creatinine, potassium, uric acid, glucose, transaminase, alkaline phosphatase, and LDH levels. May decrease glucose level.

● May increase platelet count.

## CONTRAINDICATIONS & CAUTIONS

● Contraindicated in patients with sinus bradycardia, heart block greater than first degree, overt cardiac failure, or cardiogenic shock.

● Use cautiously in patients at risk for heart failure and in those with bronchospastic disease, diabetes, hyperthyroidism, and impaired renal or hepatic function.

## NURSING CONSIDERATIONS
• Check apical pulse before giving drug; if slower than 60 beats/minute, withhold drug and call prescriber.
• Monitor patient's blood pressure.
• Monitor hemodialysis patients closely because of hypotension risk.
• Beta blockers may mask tachycardia caused by hyperthyroidism. In patients with suspected thyrotoxicosis, withdraw beta blocker gradually to avoid thyroid storm.
• Drug may mask signs and symptoms of hypoglycemia in diabetic patients.
• Drug may cause changes in exercise tolerance and ECG.
• *Alert:* Withdraw drug gradually over 2 weeks to avoid serious adverse reactions.
• *Alert:* Don't confuse atenolol with timolol or albuterol.

## PATIENT TEACHING
• Instruct patient to take drug exactly as prescribed, at the same time every day.
• Caution patient not to stop drug suddenly, but to notify prescriber if unpleasant adverse reactions occur.
• Teach patient how to take his pulse. Tell him to withhold drug and call prescriber if pulse rate is below 60 beats/minute.
• Tell women to notify prescriber about planned, suspected, or known pregnancy. Drug will need to be stopped.
• Advise breast-feeding mother to contact prescriber; drug isn't recommended for breast-feeding women.
• Tell patient that drug may deplete body's stores of coenzyme Q10 and that he should discuss need for supplements with prescriber.

---

## benazepril hydrochloride
Lotensin♦

*Pregnancy risk category C; D in second and third trimesters*

### AVAILABLE FORMS
*Tablets:* 5 mg, 10 mg, 20 mg, 40 mg

### INDICATIONS & DOSAGES
➤ **Hypertension**
*Adults:* For patients not receiving a diuretic, 10 mg P.O. daily initially. Dosage adjusted p.r.n. and as tolerated; most patients take 20 to 40 mg daily in one or two divided doses. For patients receiving a diuretic, initially 5 mg P.O. daily.
*Adjust-a-dose:* For patients with creatinine clearance below 30 ml/minute, 5 mg P.O. daily. Dose may be adjusted up to 40 mg/day.

### ACTION
Drug and its active metabolite, benazeprilat, inhibit ACE, preventing conversion of angiotensin I to angiotensin II, a potent vasoconstrictor. Reduced formation of angiotensin II decreases peripheral arterial resistance, thus decreasing aldosterone secretion, which in turn reduces sodium and water retention and lowers blood pressure. Drug also exhibits antihypertensive activity in patients with low-renin hypertension.

| Route | Onset | Peak | Duration |
|-------|-------|------|----------|
| P.O. | 1 hr | 2-4 hr | 24 hr |

### ADVERSE REACTIONS
**CNS:** headache, dizziness, drowsiness, fatigue, somnolence.
**CV:** symptomatic hypotension.
**GI:** nausea.
**GU:** impotence.
**Metabolic:** *hyperkalemia.*
**Musculoskeletal:** arthralgia, arthritis, myalgia.
**Respiratory:** dry, persistent, nonproductive cough.
**Skin:** increased diaphoresis.
**Other:** hypersensitivity reactions.

### INTERACTIONS
**Drug-drug.** *Azathioprine:* May increase risk of anemia or leukopenia. Monitor hematologic studies if used together.
*Diuretics, other antihypertensives:* May cause excessive hypotension. Stop diuretic or lower dose of benazepril, as needed.
*Lithium:* May increase lithium level and lithium toxicity. Use together cautiously; monitor lithium level.
*Nesiritide:* May increase risk of hypotension. Monitor blood pressure.
*NSAIDs:* May decrease antihypertensive effects. Monitor blood pressure.
*Potassium-sparing diuretics, potassium supplements:* May cause risk of hyperkalemia. Monitor patient closely.

---

**Drug-herb.** *Capsaicin:* May cause cough. Discourage use together.
*Ma-huang:* May decrease antihypertensive effects. Discourage use together.
**Drug-food.** *Salt substitutes containing potassium:* May cause hyperkalemia. Monitor patient closely.

**EFFECTS ON LAB TEST RESULTS**
• May increase BUN, creatinine, and potassium levels.

**CONTRAINDICATIONS & CAUTIONS**
• Contraindicated in patients hypersensitive to ACE inhibitors.
• Use cautiously in patients with impaired hepatic or renal function.

**NURSING CONSIDERATIONS**
• Safety and efficacy of dosages of more than 80 mg/day haven't been established.
• Monitor patient for hypotension. Excessive hypotension can occur when drug is given with diuretics. If possible, diuretic therapy should be stopped 2 to 3 days before starting benazepril to decrease potential for excessive hypotensive response. If drug doesn't adequately control blood pressure, diuretic may be reinstituted with care.
• Although ACE inhibitors reduce blood pressure in all races studied, this response is less in blacks who receive the drug as monotherapy. Therapy with a thiazide diuretic produces a more favorable response.
• ACE inhibitors appear to increase risk of angioedema in black patients.
• Measure blood pressure when drug level is at peak (2 to 6 hours after administration) and at trough (just before a dose) to verify adequate blood pressure control.
• Assess renal and hepatic function before and periodically throughout therapy. Monitor potassium level.
• *Alert:* Don't confuse benazepril with Benadryl or Lotensin with Loniten or lovastatin.

**PATIENT TEACHING**
• Instruct patient to avoid salt substitutes; these products may contain potassium, which can cause high potassium level in patients taking drug.
• Inform patient that light-headedness can occur, especially during first few days of

therapy. Tell him to rise slowly to minimize this effect and to report dizziness to prescriber. If fainting occurs, he should stop drug and call prescriber immediately.
• Warn patient to use caution in hot weather and during exercise. Inadequate fluid intake, vomiting, diarrhea, and excessive perspiration can lead to light-headedness and fainting.
• Advise patient to report signs of infection, such as fever and sore throat. Tell him to call prescriber if the following signs or symptoms occur: easy bruising or bleeding; swelling of tongue, lips, face, eyes, mucous membranes, or extremities; difficulty swallowing or breathing; or hoarseness.
• Tell woman to notify prescriber if pregnancy occurs. Drug will need to be stopped.

# betaxolol hydrochloride
Kerlone

*Pregnancy risk category C*

**AVAILABLE FORMS**
*Tablets:* 10 mg, 20 mg

**INDICATIONS & DOSAGES**
➤ **Hypertension (used alone or with other antihypertensives)**
*Adults:* Initially, 10 mg P.O. once daily; if desired response doesn't occur in 7 to 14 days, 20 mg P.O. once daily. Maximum, 40 mg daily.
*Elderly patients:* First dose, 5 mg P.O. once daily.

**ACTION**
Unknown. A selective beta blocker that decreases blood pressure, possibly by slowing heart rate and decreasing cardiac output and peripheral resistance.

| Route | Onset | Peak | Duration |
|-------|-------|------|----------|
| P.O. | 3 hr | 2-4 hr | 24-48 hr |

**ADVERSE REACTIONS**
**CNS:** dizziness, fatigue, headache, insomnia, lethargy, anxiety.
**CV:** *bradycardia,* chest pain, *heart failure,* edema.
**EENT:** pharyngitis.

**GI:** nausea, diarrhea, dyspepsia.
**GU:** impotence.
**Musculoskeletal:** arthralgia.
**Respiratory:** dyspnea, *bronchospasm.*
**Skin:** rash.

## INTERACTIONS
**Drug-drug.** *Amiodarone:* May increase the risk of bradycardia, AV block, and myocardial depression. Monitor ECG and vital signs if used together.
*Antihypertensives:* May increase hypotensive effect. Monitor blood pressure.
*Calcium channel blockers:* May cause hypotension, left-sided heart failure, and AV conduction disturbances. Use I.V. calcium channel blockers with caution.
*Catecholamine-depleting drugs, reserpine:* May have an additive effect. Monitor patient closely.
*Digoxin:* May increase potential for AV block and bradycardia. Monitor ECG and vital signs.
*General anesthetics:* May cause hypotensive effects. Monitor patient carefully for excessive hypotension, bradycardia, or orthostatic hypotension.
*Lidocaine:* May increase lidocaine's effects. Monitor patient.
*NSAIDs:* May decrease antihypertensive effects. Monitor blood pressure.
*Prazosin:* May increase the risk of orthostatic hypotension in the early phases of use together. Help patient stand slowly until effects are known.
*Verapamil:* May increase effects of both drugs. Monitor cardiac function closely and decrease dosages as necessary.
**Drug-herb.** *Ma-huang:* May decrease antihypertensive effects. Discourage use together.

## EFFECTS ON LAB TEST RESULTS
None reported.

## CONTRAINDICATIONS & CAUTIONS
● Contraindicated in patients hypersensitive to drug; also contraindicated in those with severe bradycardia, greater than first-degree heart block, cardiogenic shock, or uncontrolled heart failure.
● Use cautiously in patients with heart failure controlled by cardiac glycosides and diuretics because these patients may exhibit signs of cardiac decompensation with beta-blocker therapy.

## NURSING CONSIDERATIONS
● When stopping drug, withdraw gradually over 2 weeks.
● Monitor blood pressure closely.
● Monitor glucose level regularly in patients with diabetes. Beta blockade may inhibit glycogenolysis as well as the signs and symptoms of hypoglycemia (such as tachycardia and blood pressure changes). Oral beta blockers may alter the results of glucose tolerance tests.
● Withdrawal of beta-blocker therapy before surgery is controversial. Withdrawal is sometimes advocated to prevent impairment of cardiac responsiveness to reflex stimuli and decreased responsiveness to administration of catecholamines. Advise anesthesiologist that patient is receiving a beta blocker so that isoproterenol or dobutamine can be readily available for reversal of drug's cardiac effects.
● Beta blockers may mask tachycardia caused by hyperthyroidism. In patients with suspected thyrotoxicosis, withdraw beta blocker gradually to avoid thyroid storm.

## PATIENT TEACHING
● Instruct patient to take drug exactly as prescribed.
● *Alert:* Advise patient that abrupt discontinuation may precipitate chest pain in patients with unrecognized coronary artery disease.
● Emphasize importance of promptly reporting signs and symptoms of heart failure, including shortness of breath or difficulty breathing, unusually fast heartbeat, cough, and fatigue with exertion.
● Advise patient not to drive or do other tasks that require mental alertness until effects of drug are known.
● Tell patient that drug may deplete body's stores of coenzyme Q10 and that he should discuss need for supplements with prescriber.

# candesartan cilexetil
Atacand

*Pregnancy risk category C; D in second and third trimesters*

## AVAILABLE FORMS
*Tablets:* 4 mg, 8 mg, 16 mg, 32 mg

## INDICATIONS & DOSAGES
➤ **Hypertension (used alone or with other antihypertensives)**
*Adults:* Initially, 16 mg P.O. once daily when used as monotherapy; usual range is 8 to 32 mg P.O. daily as a single dose or divided b.i.d.
*Adjust-a-dose:* For patients taking a diuretic, consider a lower starting dose.

## ACTION
Inhibits vasoconstrictive action of angiotensin II by blocking angiotensin II receptor on the surface of vascular smooth muscle and other tissue cells.

| Route | Onset | Peak | Duration |
|-------|-------|------|----------|
| P.O. | Unknown | 3-4 hr | 24 hr |

## ADVERSE REACTIONS
**CNS:** dizziness, fatigue, headache.
**CV:** chest pain, peripheral edema.
**EENT:** pharyngitis, rhinitis, sinusitis.
**GI:** abdominal pain, diarrhea, nausea, vomiting.
**GU:** albuminuria.
**Musculoskeletal:** arthralgia, back pain.
**Respiratory:** coughing, bronchitis, upper respiratory tract infection.

## INTERACTIONS
**Drug-drug.** *Potassium-sparing diuretics, potassium supplements:* May cause hyperkalemia. Monitor patient closely.
**Drug-herb.** *Ma-huang:* May decrease antihypertensive effects. Discourage use together.
**Drug-food.** *Salt substitutes containing potassium:* May cause hyperkalemia. Monitor patient closely.

## EFFECTS ON LAB TEST RESULTS
None reported.

## CONTRAINDICATIONS & CAUTIONS
• Contraindicated in patients hypersensitive to drug or its components.
• Use cautiously in patients whose renal function depends on the renin-angiotensin-aldosterone system (such as patients with heart failure) because of risk of oliguria and progressive azotemia with acute renal failure or death.
• Use cautiously in pregnant patients, especially in the second and third trimesters.
• Use cautiously in patients who are volume- or salt-depleted because of potential for symptomatic hypotension. Start therapy with a lower dosage range and monitor blood pressure carefully.

## NURSING CONSIDERATIONS
• Drugs such as candesartan that act directly on the renin-angiotensin system can cause fetal and neonatal illness and death when given to pregnant women. These problems haven't been detected when exposure has been limited to first trimester. If pregnancy is suspected, notify prescriber because drug should be stopped.
• If hypotension occurs after a dose of candesartan, place patient in the supine position and, if needed, give an I.V. infusion of normal saline solution.
• Most of drug's antihypertensive effect is present within 2 weeks. Maximal antihypertensive effect is obtained within 4 to 6 weeks. Diuretic may be added if blood pressure isn't controlled by drug alone.
• Carefully monitor therapeutic response and the occurrence of adverse reactions in elderly patients and in those with renal disease.

## PATIENT TEACHING
• Inform woman of childbearing age of the consequences of second and third trimester exposure to drug. Advise her to notify prescriber immediately if she thinks she's pregnant.
• Advise breast-feeding woman of the risk of adverse effects on the infant and the need to stop either breast-feeding or drug.
• Instruct patient to store drug at room temperature and to keep container tightly sealed.
• Inform patient to report adverse reactions without delay.

• Tell patient that drug may be taken without regard to meals.

## captopril
Acenorm‡, Capoten⃰, Enzace‡, Novo-Captoril†

*Pregnancy risk category C; D in second and third trimesters*

### AVAILABLE FORMS
*Tablets:* 12.5 mg, 25 mg, 50 mg, 100 mg

### INDICATIONS & DOSAGES
➤ **Hypertension**
*Adults:* Initially, 25 mg P.O. b.i.d. or t.i.d. If blood pressure isn't satisfactorily controlled in 1 or 2 weeks, increase dosage to 50 mg b.i.d. or t.i.d. If not satisfactorily controlled after another 1 or 2 weeks, expect a diuretic to be added. If further blood pressure reduction is needed, dosage may be raised to 150 mg t.i.d. while continuing diuretic. Maximum daily dose is 450 mg.
➤ **Diabetic nephropathy**
*Adults:* 25 mg P.O. t.i.d.
➤ **Heart failure**
*Adults:* Initially, 25 mg P.O. t.i.d. Can start with 6.25 or 12.5 mg P.O. t.i.d. in patients with normal or low blood pressure who have been vigorously treated with diuretics and who may be hyponatremic or hypovolemic; first dosage may be adjusted over several days. Gradually increase dose to 50 mg P.O. t.i.d. Once 50 mg t.i.d. has been reached, further increases in dosage should be delayed at least 2 weeks. Maximum dosage is 450 mg daily.
*Elderly patients:* Initially, 6.25 mg P.O. b.i.d. Increase gradually p.r.n.
➤ **Left ventricular dysfunction after acute myocardial infarction**
*Adults:* Start therapy as early as 3 days after myocardial infarction with 6.25 mg P.O. for one dose, followed by 12.5 mg P.O. t.i.d. Increase over several days to 25 mg P.O. t.i.d., followed by an increase to 50 mg P.O. t.i.d. over several weeks.

### ACTION
Thought to inhibit ACE, preventing conversion of angiotensin I to angiotensin II, a potent vasoconstrictor. Reduced formation of angiotensin II decreases peripheral arterial resistance, decreasing aldosterone secretion, which reduces sodium and water retention and lowers blood pressure.

| Route | Onset | Peak | Duration |
|---|---|---|---|
| P.O. | 15-60 min | 60-90 min | 6-12 hr |

### ADVERSE REACTIONS
**CNS:** dizziness, fainting, headache, malaise, fatigue, fever.
**CV:** tachycardia, hypotension, angina pectoris.
**GI:** abdominal pain, anorexia, constipation, diarrhea, dry mouth, dysgeusia, nausea, vomiting.
**Hematologic:** *leukopenia, agranulocytosis, pancytopenia,* anemia, *thrombocytopenia.*
**Metabolic:** *hyperkalemia.*
**Respiratory:** dyspnea; *dry, persistent, nonproductive cough.*
**Skin:** *urticarial rash, maculopapular rash,* pruritus, alopecia.
**Other:** *angioedema.*

### INTERACTIONS
**Drug-drug.** *Antacids:* May decrease captopril effect. Separate dosage times.
*Digoxin:* May increase digoxin level by 15% to 30%. Monitor patient.
*Diuretics, other antihypertensives:* May cause excessive hypotension. May need to stop diuretic or reduce captopril dosage.
*Insulin, oral antidiabetics:* May cause hypoglycemia when captopril therapy is started. Monitor patient closely.
*Lithium:* May increase lithium level and symptoms of toxicity possible. Monitor patient closely.
*NSAIDs:* May reduce antihypertensive effect. Monitor blood pressure.
*Potassium-sparing diuretics, potassium supplements:* May cause hyperkalemia. Avoid using together unless hypokalemia is confirmed.
**Drug-herb.** *Black catechu:* May cause additional hypotensive effect. Discourage use together.
*Capsaicin:* May worsen cough. Discourage use together.
**Drug-food.** *Salt substitutes containing potassium:* May cause hyperkalemia. Monitor patient closely.

---

Reactions may be *common,* uncommon, *life-threatening,* or **COMMON AND LIFE-THREATENING.**

**EFFECTS ON LAB TEST RESULTS**
• May increase alkaline phosphatase, bilirubin, and potassium levels.
• May decrease hemoglobin, hematocrit, and WBC, granulocyte, RBC, and platelet counts.
• May cause false-positive urinary acetone test results.

**CONTRAINDICATIONS & CAUTIONS**
• Contraindicated in patients hypersensitive to drug or other ACE inhibitors.
• Use cautiously in patients with impaired renal function or serious autoimmune disease, especially systemic lupus erythematosus, and in those who have been exposed to other drugs that affect WBC counts or immune response.

**NURSING CONSIDERATIONS**
• Monitor patient's blood pressure and pulse rate frequently.
• *Alert:* Elderly patients may be more sensitive to drug's hypotensive effects.
• Assess patient for signs of angioedema.
• Drug causes the most frequent occurrence of cough, compared with other ACE inhibitors.
• In patients with impaired renal function or collagen vascular disease, monitor WBC and differential counts before starting treatment, every 2 weeks for the first 3 months of therapy, and periodically thereafter.
• *Alert:* Don't confuse captopril with Capitrol.

**PATIENT TEACHING**
• Instruct patient to take drug 1 hour before meals; food in the GI tract may reduce absorption.
• Inform patient that light-headedness is possible, especially during first few days of therapy. Tell him to rise slowly to minimize this effect and to report occurrence to prescriber. If fainting occurs, he should stop drug and call prescriber immediately.
• Tell patient to use caution in hot weather and during exercise. Lack of fluids, vomiting, diarrhea, and excessive perspiration can lead to light-headedness and syncope.
• Advise patient to report signs and symptoms of infection, such as fever and sore throat.

• Tell woman to notify prescriber if pregnancy occurs. Drug will need to be stopped.
• Urge patient to promptly report swelling of the face, lips, or mouth, or difficulty breathing.

---

# carteolol hydrochloride
Cartrol

*Pregnancy risk category C*

**AVAILABLE FORMS**
*Tablets:* 2.5 mg, 5 mg

**INDICATIONS & DOSAGES**
➤ **Hypertension**
*Adults:* Initially, 2.5 mg P.O. as a single daily dose; gradually increased to 5 or 10 mg as a single daily dose, p.r.n. Doses that exceed 10 mg daily don't produce a greater response and may actually decrease it.
*Adjust-a-dose:* For patients with renal insufficiency, if creatinine clearance is between 20 and 60 ml/minute, dosage interval is 48 hours; if below 20 ml/minute, dosage interval is 72 hours.

**ACTION**
Unknown. A nonselective beta blocker with intrinsic sympathomimetic activity. Its antihypertensive effects are probably caused by decreased sympathetic outflow from the brain and decreased cardiac output. Drug doesn't have a consistent effect on renin output.

| Route | Onset | Peak | Duration |
|-------|---------|--------|----------|
| P.O. | Unknown | 1-3 hr | 24 hr |

**ADVERSE REACTIONS**
**CNS:** lassitude, fatigue, somnolence, *asthenia,* paresthesia.
**CV:** conduction disturbances, **bradycardia.**
**EENT:** nasal congestion.
**GI:** diarrhea, nausea, abdominal pain.
**Musculoskeletal:** *muscle cramps,* arthralgia.
**Skin:** sweating, rash.

---

## INTERACTIONS

**Drug-drug.** *Aminophylline, theophylline:* May act antagonistically, reducing effects of one or both drugs and inhibiting theophylline elimination. Monitor theophylline level and patient closely.

*Amiodarone:* May increase the risk of bradycardia, AV block, and myocardial depression. Monitor patient's ECG and vital signs.

*Diltiazem, verapamil:* May cause hypotension, left-sided heart failure, and AV conduction disturbances. Use together cautiously.

*Cardiac glycosides:* May produce additive effects on slowing AV node conduction. Avoid using together.

*Catecholamine-depleting drugs, reserpine:* May have an additive effect. Monitor patient closely.

*Epinephrine:* May cause a hypertensive episode followed by bradycardia. Stop beta blocker 3 days before anticipated epinephrine use. Monitor patient closely.

*General anesthetics:* May cause hypotension. Observe carefully for excessive hypotension, bradycardia, or orthostatic hypotension.

*Insulin:* May mask symptoms of hypoglycemia, such as tachycardia, as a result of beta blockade. Use with extreme caution in patients with diabetes.

*NSAIDs:* May decrease antihypertensive effects. Monitor blood pressure.

*Oral antidiabetics:* May alter hypoglycemic response. Adjust dosage, as needed.

*Prazosin:* May increase risk of orthostatic hypotension in the early phases of use together. Help patient stand slowly until effects are known.

*Verapamil:* May increase effects of both drugs. Monitor cardiac function closely and decrease dosages as necessary.

**Drug-herb.** *Ma-huang:* May decrease antihypertensive effects. Discourage use together.

## EFFECTS ON LAB TEST RESULTS
None reported.

## CONTRAINDICATIONS & CAUTIONS
● Contraindicated in patients with bronchial asthma, severe bradycardia, greater than first-degree heart block, cardiogenic shock, or uncontrolled heart failure.

● Use cautiously in patients with heart failure controlled by cardiac glycosides and diuretics because these patients may exhibit signs of cardiac decompensation with beta-blocker therapy.

## NURSING CONSIDERATIONS
● Monitor blood pressure frequently.
● Beta blockade may inhibit glycogenolysis and the signs and symptoms of hypoglycemia (such as tachycardia and blood pressure changes). It also may attenuate insulin release. Monitor glucose level frequently.
●*Alert:* Withdrawal of beta-blocker therapy before surgery is controversial. Although withdrawal may be advocated to prevent decreased cardiac responsiveness to reflex stimuli and to catecholamines, the beta-blocking effects of carteolol may persist for weeks and stopping the drug before surgery may be impractical. Advise anesthesiologist that patient is receiving a beta blocker so that isoproterenol or dobutamine can be readily available to reverse drug's cardiac effects.
● Beta blockers may mask tachycardia caused by hyperthyroidism. In patients with suspected thyrotoxicosis, gradually withdraw beta-blocker therapy to avoid thyroid storm.
●*Alert:* Patients with unrecognized coronary artery disease may exhibit signs of angina pectoris on withdrawal of drug. Monitor patient closely.

## PATIENT TEACHING
● Instruct patient to take drug exactly as prescribed.
● Tell patient not to stop drug suddenly but to notify prescriber and discuss unpleasant adverse reactions.
● Emphasize importance of reporting signs and symptoms of heart failure, including shortness of breath or difficulty breathing, unusually fast heartbeat, cough, or fatigue with exertion.

# carvedilol
Coreg◆

*Pregnancy risk category C*

## AVAILABLE FORMS
*Tablets:* 3.125 mg, 6.25 mg, 12.5 mg, 25 mg

## INDICATIONS & DOSAGES
➤ **Hypertension**
*Adults:* Dosage highly individualized. Initially, 6.25 mg P.O. b.i.d. Measure standing blood pressure 1 hour after first dose. If tolerated, continue dosage for 7 to 14 days. May increase to 12.5 mg P.O. b.i.d. for 7 to 14 days, following same blood pressure monitoring protocol as before. Maximum dose is 25 mg P.O. b.i.d. as tolerated.
➤ **Mild to severe heart failure**
*Adults:* Dosage highly individualized. Initially, 3.125 mg P.O. b.i.d. for 2 weeks; if tolerated, may increase to 6.25 mg P.O. b.i.d. Dosage may be doubled q 2 weeks as tolerated. Maximum dose for patients weighing less than 85 kg (187 lb) is 25 mg P.O. b.i.d.; for those weighing more than 85 kg, dose is 50 mg P.O. b.i.d.
*Adjust-a-dose:* In patient with pulse rate below 55 beats/minute, use reduced dosage.
➤ **Angina pectoris ◆**
*Adults:* 25 to 50 mg P.O. b.i.d.
➤ **Idiopathic cardiomyopathy ◆**
*Adults:* 6.25 to 25 mg P.O. b.i.d.
✹ *NEW INDICATION:* **Left ventricular dysfunction after MI**
*Adults:* Dosage individualized. Start therapy after patient is hemodynamically stable and fluid retention has been minimized. Initially, 6.25 mg P.O. b.i.d. Increase after 3 to 10 days to 12.5 mg b.i.d., then again to a target dose of 25 mg b.i.d. Or start with 3.25 mg b.i.d., or adjust dosage slower if indicated.

## ACTION
Nonselective beta blocker with alpha-blocking activity.

| Route | Onset | Peak | Duration |
|-------|-------|------|----------|
| P.O. | Unknown | 1-2 hr | 7-10 hr |

## ADVERSE REACTIONS
**CNS:** *asthenia, fatigue,* pain, *dizziness,* headache, malaise, fever, hypesthesia, paresthesia, vertigo, somnolence, ***cerebrovascular accident,*** depression, insomnia.
**CV:** *hypotension, postural hypertension,* edema, **bradycardia,** syncope, angina pectoris, peripheral edema, hypovolemia, fluid overload, *AV block,* hypertension, palpitation, peripheral vascular disorder, chest pain.
**EENT:** sinusitis, abnormal vision, blurred vision, pharyngitis, rhinitis.
**GI:** *diarrhea,* vomiting, nausea, melena, periodontitis, abdominal pain, dyspepsia.
**GU:** impotence, abnormal renal function, albuminuria, hematuria, UTI.
**Hematologic:** purpura, anemia, ***thrombocytopenia.***
**Metabolic:** *hyperglycemia, weight gain,* weight loss, hypercholesterolemia, hyperuricemia, hypoglycemia, hyponatremia, glycosuria, hypervolemia, diabetes mellitus, ***hyperkalemia,*** gout, hypertriglyceridemia.
**Musculoskeletal:** arthralgia, back pain, muscle cramps, hypotonia, arthritis.
**Respiratory:** bronchitis, *upper respiratory tract infection,* cough, rales, dyspnea, ***lung edema.***
**Other:** *hypersensitivity reactions,* infection, flulike syndrome, viral infection, injury.

## INTERACTIONS
**Drug-drug.** *Amiodarone:* May increase risk of bradycardia, AV block, and myocardial depression. Monitor patient's ECG and vital signs.
*Catecholamine-depleting drugs, such as MAO inhibitors, reserpine:* May cause bradycardia or severe hypotension. Monitor patient closely.
*Cimetidine:* May increase bioavailability of carvedilol. Monitor vital signs closely.
*Clonidine:* May increase blood pressure and heart rate lowering effects. Monitor vital signs closely.
*Cyclosporine:* May increase cyclosporine level. Monitor cyclosporine level.
*Digoxin:* May increase digoxin level by about 15% when given together. Monitor digoxin level.

*Diltiazem, verapamil:* May cause isolated conduction disturbances. Monitor patient's heart rhythm and blood pressure.

*Fluoxetine, paroxetine, propafenone, quinidine:* May increase level of R(+) enantiomer of carvedilol. Monitor patient for hypotension and dizziness.

*Insulin, oral antidiabetics:* May enhance hypoglycemic properties. Monitor glucose level.

*NSAIDs:* May decrease antihypertensive effects. Monitor blood pressure.

*Rifampin:* May reduce carvedilol level by 70%. Monitor vital signs closely.

**Drug-herb.** *Ma-huang:* May decrease antihypertensive effects. Discourage use together.

**Drug-food.** *Any food:* May delay rate of absorption of carvedilol with no change in bioavailability. Advise patient to take drug with food to minimize orthostatic effects.

### EFFECTS ON LAB TEST RESULTS

• May increase creatinine, BUN, ALT, AST, GGT, cholesterol, triglycerides, alkaline phosphatase, sodium, uric acid, potassium, and nonprotein nitrogen levels. May increase or decrease glucose level.

• May decrease PT, INR, and platelet count.

### CONTRAINDICATIONS & CAUTIONS

• Contraindicated in patients hypersensitive to drug and in those with New York Heart Association class IV decompensated cardiac failure requiring I.V. inotropic therapy.

• Contraindicated in those with bronchial asthma or related bronchospastic conditions, second- or third-degree AV block, sick sinus syndrome (unless a permanent pacemaker is in place), cardiogenic shock, severe bradycardia, or symptomatic hepatic impairment.

• Use cautiously in hypertensive patients with left-sided heart failure, perioperative patients who receive anesthetics that depress myocardial function (such as cyclopropane and trichloroethylene), and diabetic patients receiving insulin or oral antidiabetics, and in those subject to spontaneous hypoglycemia.

• Use with caution in patients with thyroid disease (may mask hyperthyroidism; withdrawal may precipitate thyroid storm or exacerbation of hyperthyroidism), pheochromocytoma, Prinzmetal's or variant angina, bronchospastic disease, or peripheral vascular disease (may precipitate or aggravate symptoms of arterial insufficiency).

• Use cautiously in breast-feeding women.

• Safety and efficacy in patients younger than age 18 haven't been established. Don't use drug in these patients.

### NURSING CONSIDERATIONS

• *Alert:* Patients receiving beta-blocker therapy who have a history of severe anaphylactic reaction to several allergens may be more reactive to repeated challenge (accidental, diagnostic, or therapeutic). They may be unresponsive to dosages of epinephrine typically used to treat allergic reactions.

• Mild hepatocellular injury may occur during therapy. At first sign of hepatic dysfunction, perform tests for hepatic injury or jaundice; if present, stop drug.

• If drug must be stopped, do so gradually over 1 to 2 weeks.

• Monitor patient with heart failure for worsened condition, renal dysfunction, or fluid retention; diuretics may need to be increased.

• Monitor diabetic patient closely; drug may mask signs of hypoglycemia, or hyperglycemia may be worsened.

• Observe patient for dizziness or lightheadedness for 1 hour after giving each new dosage.

• Before starting carvedilol, make sure dosages of digoxin, diuretics, and ACE inhibitors are stabilized.

• Monitor elderly patients carefully; drug levels are about 50% higher in elderly patients than in younger patients.

### PATIENT TEACHING

• Tell patient not to interrupt or stop drug without medical approval.

• Inform patient that improvement of heart failure symptoms might take several weeks of drug therapy.

• Advise patient with heart failure to call prescriber if weight gain or shortness of breath occurs.

• Inform patient that he may experience low blood pressure when standing. If dizziness or fainting (rare) occurs, advise him to sit or lie down and to notify prescriber if symptoms persist.

---

Reactions may be *common*, uncommon, *life-threatening*, or COMMON AND LIFE-THREATENING.

• Caution patient against performing hazardous tasks during start of therapy.
• Advise diabetic patient to promptly report changes in glucose level.
• Inform patient who wears contact lenses that his eyes may feel dry.

## clonidine
Catapres-TTS

## clonidine hydrochloride
Catapres, Dixarit†‡, Duracion, Duraclon

*Pregnancy risk category C*

### AVAILABLE FORMS
**clonidine**
*Transdermal:* TTS-1 (releases 0.1 mg/24 hours), TTS-2 (releases 0.2 mg/24 hours), TTS-3 (releases 0.3 mg/24 hours)
**clonidine hydrochloride**
*Injection for epidural use:* 100 mcg/ml
*Injection for epidural use, concentrate:* 500 mcg/ml
*Tablets:* 0.025 mg†‡, 0.1 mg, 0.2 mg, 0.3 mg

### INDICATIONS & DOSAGES
➤ **Essential and renal hypertension**
*Adults:* Initially, 0.1 mg P.O. b.i.d.; then increased by 0.1 to 0.2 mg daily on a weekly basis. Usual range is 0.2 to 0.6 mg daily in divided doses; infrequently, dosages as high as 2.4 mg daily are used.
Or, apply transdermal patch to nonhairy area of intact skin on upper arm or torso once q 7 days, starting with 0.1-mg system and adjusted with another 0.1-mg system or larger system.
*Children:* 50 to 400 mcg P.O. b.i.d.
➤ **Severe cancer pain that is unresponsive to epidural or spinal opiate analgesia or other more conventional methods of analgesia**
*Adults:* Initially, 30 mcg/hour by continuous epidural infusion. Experience with rates greater than 40 mcg/hour is limited.
*Children:* Initially, 0.5 mcg/kg/hour by epidural infusion. Dosage should be cautiously adjusted, based on response.
➤ **Pheochromocytoma diagnosis** ♦
*Adults:* 0.3 mg P.O. for a single dose.

➤ **Migraine prophylaxis** ♦
*Adults:* 0.025 mg P.O. two to four times daily or up to 0.15 mg P.O. daily in divided doses.
➤ **Dysmenorrhea** ♦
*Adults:* 0.025 mg P.O. b.i.d. for 14 days before and during menses.
➤ **Vasomotor symptoms of menopause** ♦
*Adults:* 0.025 to 0.2 mg P.O. b.i.d. or 0.1 mg/24 hours patch applied once q 7 days.
➤ **Opiate dependence** ♦
*Adults:* Initially, 0.005 or 0.006 mg/kg test dose, followed by 0.017 mg/kg P.O. daily in three or four divided doses for 10 days. Or, initially, 0.1 mg P.O. three or four times daily, with dosage adjusted by 0.1 to 0.2 mg/day. Dosage range is 0.3 to 1.2 mg P.O. daily. Stop drug gradually. Follow protocols.
➤ **Alcohol dependence** ♦
*Adults:* 0.5 mg P.O. b.i.d. to t.i.d.
➤ **Smoking cessation** ♦
*Adults:* Initially, 0.1 mg P.O. b.i.d., beginning on or shortly before the day of smoking cessation. Increase dosage q 7 days by 0.1 mg/day, if needed. Or, 0.1 mg/24 hours transdermal patch applied q 7 days. Therapy should begin on or shortly before the day of smoking cessation. Increase dosage by 0.1 mg/24 hours at weekly intervals, if needed.
➤ **Attention deficit hyperactivity disorder** ♦
*Children:* Initially, 0.05 mg P.O. h.s. May increase dosage cautiously over 2 to 4 weeks. Maintenance dosage is 0.05 to 0.4 mg P.O. daily.

### ACTION
Unknown. Thought to stimulate alpha$_2$-adrenergic receptors centrally and inhibit the central vasomotor centers, thereby decreasing sympathetic outflow to the heart, kidneys, and peripheral vasculature, resulting in decreased peripheral vascular resistance, systolic and diastolic blood pressure, and heart rate.

| Route | Onset | Peak | Duration |
|---|---|---|---|
| P.O. | 30-60 min | 2-4 hr | 12-24 hr |
| Trans-dermal | 2-3 days | 2-3 days | 7-8 days |
| Epidural | Unknown | 30-60 min | Unknown |

## ADVERSE REACTIONS

**CNS:** *drowsiness, dizziness,* fatigue, *sedation, weakness,* malaise, agitation, depression.
**CV:** orthostatic hypotension, ***bradycardia, severe rebound hypertension.***
**GI:** *constipation, dry mouth,* nausea, vomiting, anorexia.
**GU:** urine retention, impotence.
**Metabolic:** weight gain.
**Skin:** *pruritus, dermatitis with transdermal patch,* rash.
**Other:** loss of libido.

## INTERACTIONS

**Drug-drug.** *Amitriptyline, amoxapine, clomipramine, desipramine, doxepin, imipramine, nortriptyline, protriptyline, trimipramine:* May cause loss of blood pressure control with life-threatening elevations in blood pressure. Avoid using together.
*CNS depressants:* May increase CNS depression. Use together cautiously.
*Diuretics, other antihypertensives:* May increase hypotensive effect. Monitor patient closely.
*Levodopa:* May reduce effectiveness of levodopa. Monitor patient.
*MAO inhibitors, prazosin:* May decrease antihypertensive effect. Use together cautiously.
*Propranolol, other beta blockers:* May cause paradoxical hypertensive response. Monitor patient carefully.
*Verapamil:* May cause AV block and severe hypotension. Monitor patient.
**Drug-herb.** *Capsicum:* May reduce antihypertensive effectiveness. Discourage use together.
*Ma-huang:* May decrease antihypertensive effects. Discourage use together.

## EFFECTS ON LAB TEST RESULTS

● May decrease urinary excretion of vanillylmandelic acid and catecholamines.
● May cause a weakly positive Coombs' test result.

## CONTRAINDICATIONS & CAUTIONS

● Contraindicated in patients hypersensitive to drug.
● Transdermal form is contraindicated in patients hypersensitive to any component of the adhesive layer of transdermal system.
● Epidural form is contraindicated in patients receiving anticoagulant therapy, in those with bleeding diathesis, in those with an injection site infection, and in those who are hemodynamically unstable or have severe CV disease.
● Use cautiously in patients with severe coronary insufficiency, recent MI, cerebrovascular disease, chronic renal failure, or impaired liver function.

## NURSING CONSIDERATIONS

● Drug may be given to lower blood pressure rapidly in some hypertensive emergencies.
● Monitor blood pressure and pulse rate frequently. Dosage is usually adjusted to patient's blood pressure and tolerance.
● Elderly patients may be more sensitive than younger ones to drug's hypotensive effects.
● Observe patient for tolerance to drug's therapeutic effects, which may require increased dosage.
● Noticeable antihypertensive effects of transdermal clonidine may take 2 to 3 days. Oral antihypertensive therapy may have to be continued in the interim.
● *Alert:* Remove transdermal patch before defibrillation to prevent arcing.
● When stopping therapy in patients receiving both clonidine and a beta blocker, gradually withdraw the beta blocker first to minimize adverse reactions.
● Don't stop drug before surgery.
● *Alert:* Don't confuse clonidine with quinidine or clomiphene; or Catapres with Cetapred or Combipres.
● *Alert:* The injection form is for epidural use only.
● The injection form concentrate containing 500 mcg/ml must be diluted before use in normal saline injection to yield 100 mcg/ml.
● When drug is given epidurally, carefully monitor infusion pump and inspect catheter tubing for obstruction or dislodgment.

## PATIENT TEACHING

● Instruct patient to take drug exactly as prescribed.

---

Reactions may be *common,* uncommon, ***life-threatening***, or COMMON AND LIFE-THREATENING.

• Advise patient that stopping drug abruptly may cause severe rebound high blood pressure. Tell him dosage must be reduced gradually over 2 to 4 days as instructed by prescriber.

• Tell patient to take the last dose immediately before bedtime.

• Reassure patient that the transdermal patch usually remains attached despite showering and other routine daily activities. Instruct him on the use of the adhesive overlay to provide additional skin adherence, if needed. Also tell him to place patch at a different site each week.

• Caution patient that drug may cause drowsiness but that this adverse effect usually diminishes over 4 to 6 weeks.

• Inform patient that dizziness upon standing can be minimized by rising slowly from a sitting or lying position and avoiding sudden position changes.

## diazoxide
Hyperstat IV, Proglycem

*Pregnancy risk category C*

### AVAILABLE FORMS
*Injection:* 15 mg/ml in 20-ml ampules
*Oral suspension:* 50 mg/ml

### INDICATIONS & DOSAGES
➤ **Hypertensive crisis**
*Adults and children:* 1 to 3 mg/kg by I.V. bolus (to maximum of 150 mg) q 5 to 15 minutes until adequate response is seen (diastolic blood pressure less than 100 mm Hg). Repeat at 4- to 24-hour intervals, p.r.n.
➤ **Hypoglycemia caused by hyperinsulinemia**
*Adults and children:* Initially, 3 mg/kg P.O. daily, in three equal doses given q 8 hours. Usual maintenance dose is 3 to 8 mg/kg P.O. daily, in two or three divided doses at 12- or 8-hour intervals, respectively.
*Infants and neonates:* Initially, 10 mg/kg P.O. daily divided into three equal doses given q 8 hours. Usual maintenance dose is 8 to 15 mg/kg daily, in two or three equal doses given q 12 hours or q 8 hours, respectively.

### I.V. ADMINISTRATION
• Protect I.V. solutions from light. Darkened I.V. solutions of diazoxide are subpotent and shouldn't be used.
• Give drug through peripheral vein only. Don't give I.M., S.C., or into body cavities.
• Monitor blood pressure and ECG continuously. Place patient supine or in Trendelenburg's position during infusion and for 1 hour afterward.
• Notify prescriber immediately if severe hypotension develops. Keep norepinephrine available.

### ACTION
Unknown. Directly relaxes arteriolar smooth muscle and decreases peripheral vascular resistance.

| Route | Onset | Peak | Duration |
|-------|-------|------|----------|
| P.O. | 1 hr | 4 hr | 8 hr |
| I.V. | 1 min | 2-5 min | 2-12 hr |

### ADVERSE REACTIONS
**CNS:** *headache,* dizziness, light-headedness, weakness, *seizures, paralysis,* euphoria, *cerebral ischemia.*
**CV:** *sodium and water retention,* orthostatic hypotension, flushing, warmth, angina pectoris, myocardial ischemia, *arrhythmias,* ECG changes, *shock, MI.*
**EENT:** optic nerve damage.
**GI:** *nausea, vomiting,* abdominal discomfort, dry mouth, constipation, diarrhea.
**Metabolic:** *hyperglycemia,* hyperuricemia.
**Skin:** inflammation and pain resulting from extravasation, diaphoresis.

### INTERACTIONS
**Drug-drug.** *Antihypertensives such as beta blockers, hydralazine, methyldopa, minoxidil, nitrates, prazosin, reserpine:* May cause severe hypotension. Separate doses by 6 hours.
*Hydantoins:* May decrease hydantoin level, resulting in decreased anticonvulsant action. Monitor patient.
*Sulfonylureas:* May cause hyperglycemia. Monitor glucose level.
*Thiazide diuretics:* May increase diazoxide's effects. Use together cautiously.

### EFFECTS ON LAB TEST RESULTS
• May increase glucose, IgG, and uric acid levels; may decrease cortisol level.

---

• May increase renin secretion. May decrease glucose-stimulated insulin release.
• May cause false-negative insulin response to glucagon.

**CONTRAINDICATIONS & CAUTIONS**
• Contraindicated in patients hypersensitive to drug, other thiazides, or other sulfonamide-derived drugs.
• Contraindicated in those with compensatory hypertension (as caused by aortic coarctation or arteriovenous shunt).
• Use cautiously in patients with impaired cerebral or cardiac function or uremia.

**NURSING CONSIDERATIONS**
• Monitor patient's blood pressure frequently during bolus.
• Check patient's standing blood pressure before discontinuing close monitoring for hypotension.
• Monitor patient's fluid intake and output carefully. If fluid or sodium retention develops, prescriber may order diuretics.
• Weigh patient daily and notify prescriber of weight increase.
• Diazoxide may alter requirements for insulin, diet, or oral antidiabetics in patients with previously controlled diabetes. Monitor glucose level daily; watch for signs and symptoms of severe hyperglycemia or hyperosmolar hyperosmotic nonketotic syndrome. Insulin may be needed.
• Check uric acid level frequently and report abnormalities to prescriber.
• *Alert:* Don't confuse diazoxide with Dyazide or diazepam, or Hyperstat with Nitrostat, Hyper-Tet, or HyperHep.
• When drug is used to treat hypoglycemia, monitor glucose level until the patient's condition has stabilized.
• Don't use drug to manage functional hypoglycemia.

**PATIENT TEACHING**
• Inform patient that low blood pressure and dizziness upon standing can be minimized by rising slowly and avoiding sudden position changes. Tell patient to remain lying down for 60 minutes after injection.
• Tell patient to alert nurse if discomfort occurs at I.V. insertion site.

# doxazosin mesylate
Cardura✧, Carduran‡

*Pregnancy risk category C*

**AVAILABLE FORMS**
*Tablets:* 1 mg, 2 mg, 4 mg, 8 mg

**INDICATIONS & DOSAGES**
➤ **Essential hypertension**
*Adults:* Initially, 1 mg P.O. daily; determine effect on standing and supine blood pressure at 2 to 6 hours and 24 hours after dosing. May increase at 2-week intervals to 2 mg and, thereafter, 4 mg and 8 mg once daily, p.r.n. Maximum daily dose is 16 mg, but doses over 4 mg daily increase the risk of adverse reactions.
➤ **BPH**
*Adults:* Initially, 1 mg P.O. once daily in the morning or evening; may increase at 1- or 2-week intervals to 2 mg and, thereafter, 4 mg and 8 mg once daily, p.r.n.

**ACTION**
An alpha blocker that acts on the peripheral vasculature to reduce peripheral vascular resistance and produce vasodilation.

| Route | Onset | Peak | Duration |
|-------|-------|------|----------|
| P.O. | 1-2 hr | 2-3 hr | 24 hr |

**ADVERSE REACTIONS**
**CNS:** *dizziness,* vertigo, somnolence, drowsiness, *asthenia, headache,* pain.
**CV:** *orthostatic hypotension,* hypotension, edema, palpitations, *arrhythmias,* tachycardia.
**EENT:** rhinitis, pharyngitis, abnormal vision.
**GI:** nausea, vomiting, diarrhea, constipation.
**Hematologic:** *leukopenia, neutropenia.*
**Musculoskeletal:** arthralgia, myalgia.
**Respiratory:** dyspnea.
**Skin:** rash, pruritus.

**INTERACTIONS**
**Drug-drug.** *Midodrine:* May decrease the effectiveness of midodrine. Monitor patient for clinical effect.
**Drug-herb.** *Butcher's broom:* May decrease effect of doxazosin. Discourage use together.

---

Reactions may be *common,* uncommon, *life-threatening,* or COMMON AND LIFE-THREATENING.

*Ma-huang:* May decrease antihypertensive effects. Discourage use together.

**EFFECTS ON LAB TEST RESULTS**
● May decrease WBC and neutrophil counts.

**CONTRAINDICATIONS & CAUTIONS**
● Contraindicated in patients hypersensitive to drug and quinazoline derivatives (including prazosin and terazosin).
● Use cautiously in patients with impaired hepatic function.

**NURSING CONSIDERATIONS**
● Monitor blood pressure closely.
● If syncope occurs, place patient in a recumbent position and treat supportively. A transient hypotensive response isn't considered a contraindication to continued therapy.
● *Alert:* Don't confuse doxazosin with doxapram, doxorubicin, or doxepin.
● *Alert:* Don't confuse Cardura with Coumadin, K-Dur, Cardene, or Cordarone.

**PATIENT TEACHING**
● Instruct patient to take drug exactly as prescribed.
● *Alert:* Advise patient that he is susceptible to a first-dose effect (marked low blood pressure on standing up with dizziness or fainting) similar to that produced by other alpha blockers. This is most common after first dose but also can occur during dosage adjustment or interruption of therapy.
● Warn patient that dizziness or fainting may occur during therapy. Advise him to avoid driving and other hazardous activities until drug's effects on the CNS are known.

---

**enalaprilat**

**enalapril maleate**
Amprace‡, Renitec‡, Vasotec⁄

*Pregnancy risk category C; D in second and third trimesters*

---

**AVAILABLE FORMS**
enalaprilat
*Injection:* 1.25 mg/ml

**enalapril maleate**
*Tablets:* 2.5 mg, 5 mg, 10 mg, 20 mg

**INDICATIONS & DOSAGES**
➤ **Hypertension**
*Adults:* In patients not taking diuretics, initially, 5 mg P.O. once daily; then adjusted based on response. Usual dosage range is 10 to 40 mg daily as a single dose or two divided doses. Or, 1.25 mg I.V. infusion over 5 minutes q 6 hours.
*Adjust-a-dose:* For patients taking diuretics, initially, 2.5 mg P.O. once daily. Or 0.625 mg I.V. over 5 minutes, repeated in 1 hour, if needed; then 1.25 mg I.V. q 6 hours.
➤ **To convert from I.V. therapy to oral therapy**
*Adults:* Initially, 2.5 mg P.O. once daily; if patient was receiving 0.625 mg I.V. q 6 hours, then 2.5 mg P.O once daily. Dosage is adjusted based on response.
➤ **To convert from oral therapy to I.V. therapy**
*Adults:* 1.25 mg I.V. over 5 minutes q 6 hours. Higher dosages haven't shown greater efficacy.
*Adjust-a-dose:* For patients with creatinine level more than 1.6 mg/dl or sodium level below 130 mEq/L, start dosage at 2.5 mg P.O. daily and adjust slowly.
➤ **To manage symptomatic heart failure**
*Adults:* Initially, 2.5 mg P.O. daily or b.i.d., increased gradually over several weeks. Maintenance is 5 to 20 mg daily in two divided doses. Maximum daily dose is 40 mg in two divided doses.
➤ **Asymptomatic left ventricular dysfunction**
*Adults:* Initially, 2.5 mg P.O. b.i.d. Increase as tolerated to target daily dose of 20 mg P.O. in divided doses.

**I.V. ADMINISTRATION**
● Compatible solutions include $D_5W$, normal saline solution for injection, dextrose 5% in lactated Ringer's injection, dextrose 5% in normal saline solution for injection, and Isolyte E.
● Inject drug slowly over at least 5 minutes, or dilute in 50 ml of a compatible solution and infuse over 15 minutes.

## ACTION
Unknown. Thought to inhibit ACE, preventing conversion of angiotensin I to angiotensin II, a potent vasoconstrictor. Reduced formation of angiotensin II decreases peripheral arterial resistance, thus decreasing aldosterone secretion, thereby reducing sodium and water retention and lowering blood pressure.

| Route | Onset | Peak | Duration |
|-------|-------|------|----------|
| P.O. | 1 hr | 4-6 hr | 24 hr |
| I.V. | 15 min | 1-4 hr | 6 hr |

## ADVERSE REACTIONS
**CNS:** headache, dizziness, fatigue, vertigo, *asthenia,* syncope.
**CV:** hypotension, chest pain, angina pectoris.
**GI:** diarrhea, nausea, abdominal pain, vomiting.
**GU:** decreased renal function (in patients with bilateral renal artery stenosis or heart failure).
**Hematologic:** bone marrow depression.
**Respiratory:** dyspnea; *dry, persistent, tickling, nonproductive cough.*
**Skin:** rash.
**Other:** *angioedema.*

## INTERACTIONS
**Drug-drug.** *Azathioprine:* May increase risk of anemia or leukopenia. Monitor hematologic studies if used together.
*Diuretics:* May excessively reduce blood pressure. Use together cautiously.
*Insulin, oral antidiabetics:* May cause hypoglycemia, especially at start of enalapril therapy. Monitor patient closely.
*Lithium:* May cause lithium toxicity. Monitor lithium level.
*NSAIDs:* May reduce antihypertensive effect. Monitor blood pressure.
*Potassium-sparing diuretics, potassium supplements:* May cause hyperkalemia. Avoid using together unless hypokalemia is confirmed.
**Drug-herb.** *Capsaicin:* May cause cough. Discourage use together.
*Ma-huang:* May decrease antihypertensive effects. Discourage use together.
**Drug-food.** *Salt substitutes containing potassium:* May cause hyperkalemia. Monitor patient closely.

## EFFECTS ON LAB TEST RESULTS
● May increase BUN, creatinine, potassium, and bilirubin levels. May decrease sodium level.
● May increase liver function test values; may decrease hemoglobin and hematocrit.

## CONTRAINDICATIONS & CAUTIONS
● Contraindicated in patients hypersensitive to drug and in those with a history of angioedema related to previous treatment with an ACE inhibitor.
● Use cautiously in renally impaired patients or those with aortic stenosis or hypertrophic cardiomyopathy.

## NURSING CONSIDERATIONS
● Closely monitor blood pressure response to drug.
● *Alert:* Similar packaging and labeling of enalaprilat injection and pancuronium, a paralyzing drug, could result in a fatal medication error. Check all labeling carefully.
● Monitor CBC with differential counts before and during therapy.
● Diabetic patients, those with impaired renal function or heart failure, and those receiving drugs that can increase potassium level may develop hyperkalemia. Monitor potassium intake and potassium level.
● *Alert:* Don't confuse enalapril with Anafranil or Eldepryl.

## PATIENT TEACHING
● Instruct patient to report breathing difficulty or swelling of face, eyes, lips, or tongue. Swelling of the face and throat (including swelling of the larynx) may occur, especially after first dose.
● Advise patient to report signs of infection, such as fever and sore throat.
● Inform patient that light-headedness can occur, especially during first few days of therapy. Tell him to rise slowly to minimize this effect and to notify prescriber if symptoms develop. If he faints, he should stop taking drug and call prescriber immediately.
● Tell patient to use caution in hot weather and during exercise. Inadequate fluid intake, vomiting, diarrhea, and excessive perspiration can lead to light-headedness and fainting.

---

Reactions may be *common*, uncommon, *life-threatening*, or COMMON AND LIFE-THREATENING.

• Advise patient to avoid salt substitutes; these products may contain potassium, which can cause high potassium levels in patients taking this drug.
• Tell woman to notify prescriber if pregnancy occurs. Drug will need to be stopped.

## eplerenone
Inspra

*Pregnancy risk category B*

### AVAILABLE FORMS
*Tablets:* 25 mg, 50 mg, 100 mg

### INDICATIONS & DOSAGES
➤ **Hypertension**
*Adults:* 50 mg P.O. once daily. If response is inadequate after 4 weeks, increase dosage to 50 mg P.O. b.i.d. Maximum daily dose 100 mg.

### ACTION
Binds to mineralocorticoid receptors and blocks aldosterone, which increases blood pressure through induction of sodium reabsorption and possibly other mechanisms.

| Route | Onset | Peak | Duration |
|-------|-------|------|----------|
| P.O. | Unknown | 90 min | Unknown |

### ADVERSE REACTIONS
**CNS:** dizziness, fatigue.
**GI:** diarrhea, abdominal pain.
**GU:** albuminuria, abnormal vaginal bleeding.
**Respiratory:** cough.
**Metabolic:** *hyperkalemia.*
**Other:** flulike symptoms, gynecomastia.

### INTERACTIONS
**Drug-drug.** *ACE inhibitors, angiotensin II receptor antagonists:* May increase risk of hyperkalemia. Use together cautiously.
*Lithium:* May increase risk of lithium toxicity. Monitor lithium level.
*NSAIDs:* May reduce the antihypertensive effect and cause severe hyperkalemia in patients with impaired renal function. Monitor blood pressure and potassium level.
*Potassium supplements, potassium-sparing diuretics (amiloride, spironolactone, triamterene):* May increase risk of hyperkalemia and sometimes-fatal arrhythmias. Avoid using together.
*Strong CYP 3A4 inhibitors (itraconazole, ketoconazole):* May increase eplerenone level. Avoid using together.
*Weak CYP 3A4 inhibitors (erythromycin, fluconazole, saquinavir, verapamil):* May increase eplerenone level. Reduce eplerenone starting dose to 25 mg P.O. once daily.
**Drug-herb.** *St. John's wort:* May decrease eplerenone level over time. Discourage use together.

### EFFECTS ON LAB TEST RESULTS
• May increase potassium, creatinine, BUN, triglyceride, cholesterol, uric acid, ALT, and GGT levels. May decrease sodium level.

### CONTRAINDICATIONS & CAUTIONS
• Contraindicated in patients with potassium level greater than 5.5 mEq/L, type 2 diabetes with microalbuminuria, creatinine level greater than 2 mg/dl in men or greater than 1.8 mg/dl in women, or creatinine clearance less than 50 ml/minute. Also contraindicated in patients taking potassium supplements, potassium-sparing diuretics (amiloride, spironolactone, or triamterene), or strong CYP 3A4 inhibitors such as ketoconazole and itraconazole.
• Use cautiously in patient with mild-to-moderate hepatic impairment.
• Use in pregnant woman only if the potential benefits justify the potential risk to the fetus. It's unknown if drug appears in breast milk. Use cautiously in breast-feeding women.

### NURSING CONSIDERATIONS
• Drug may be used alone or with other antihypertensives.
• Full therapeutic effect of the drug occurs within 4 weeks.
• Monitor patient for signs and symptoms of hyperkalemia.

### PATIENT TEACHING
• Inform patient that drug may be taken with or without food.

- Advise patient to avoid potassium supplements and salt substitutes during treatment.
- Tell patient to report adverse reactions.

---

## eprosartan mesylate
Teveten

*Pregnancy risk category C; D in second and third trimesters*

### AVAILABLE FORMS
*Tablets:* 400 mg, 600 mg

### INDICATIONS & DOSAGES
➤ **Hypertension (alone or with other antihypertensives)**
*Adults:* Initially, 600 mg P.O. daily. Dosage ranges from 400 to 800 mg daily, given as single daily dose or two divided doses.

### ACTION
An angiotensin II receptor antagonist that reduces blood pressure by blocking the vasoconstrictor and aldosterone-secreting effects of angiotensin II. Eprosartan selectively blocks the binding of angiotensin II to its receptor sites found in many tissues, such as vascular smooth muscle and the adrenal gland.

| Route | Onset | Peak | Duration |
|-------|-------|------|----------|
| P.O. | 1-2 hr | 1-3 hr | 24 hr |

### ADVERSE REACTIONS
**CNS:** depression, fatigue, headache, dizziness.
**CV:** chest pain, dependent edema.
**EENT:** pharyngitis, rhinitis, sinusitis.
**GI:** abdominal pain, dyspepsia, diarrhea.
**GU:** UTI.
**Hematologic:** *neutropenia.*
**Musculoskeletal:** arthralgia, myalgia.
**Respiratory:** cough, upper respiratory tract infection, bronchitis.
**Other:** injury, viral infection.

### INTERACTIONS
**Drug-drug.** *NSAIDs:* May decrease antihypertensive effects. Monitor blood pressure.

**Drug-herb.** *Ma-huang:* May decrease antihypertensive effects. Discourage use together.

### EFFECTS ON LAB TEST RESULTS
- May increase BUN and triglyceride levels.
- May decrease neutrophil counts.

### CONTRAINDICATIONS & CAUTIONS
- Contraindicated in patients hypersensitive to eprosartan or its components.
- Use cautiously in patients with renal artery stenosis; in patients with an activated renin-angiotensin system, such as volume- or salt-depleted patients; and in patients whose renal function may depend on the activity of the renin-angiotensin-aldosterone system, such as those with severe heart failure.
- Safety and effectiveness in children haven't been established.

### NURSING CONSIDERATIONS
- Correct hypovolemia and hyponatremia before starting therapy to reduce the risk of symptomatic hypotension.
- Monitor blood pressure closely for 2 hours during start of treatment. If hypotension occurs, place patient in a supine position and, if needed, give an I.V. infusion of normal saline solution.
- A transient episode of hypotension isn't a contraindication to continued treatment. Drug may be restarted once patient's blood pressure has stabilized.
- Drug may be used alone or with other antihypertensives, such as diuretics and calcium channel blockers. Maximal blood pressure response may take 2 or 3 weeks.
- Monitor patient for facial or lip swelling because angioedema has occurred with other angiotensin II antagonists.
- Closely observe infants exposed to eprosartan in utero for hypotension, oliguria, and hyperkalemia.

### PATIENT TEACHING
- Advise woman of childbearing age to use a reliable form of contraception and to notify her prescriber immediately if pregnancy is suspected. Treatment may need to be stopped under medical supervision.

---

• Advise patient to report facial or lip swelling and signs and symptoms of infection, such as fever and sore throat.
• Tell patient to notify prescriber before taking OTC medication to treat a dry cough.
• Inform patient that drug may be taken without regard to meals.
• Advise breast-feeding woman of potential for serious adverse reactions in breast-fed infants. She should either stop therapy or stop breast-feeding.
• Tell patient to store drug at 68° to 77° F (20° to 25° C).

## felodipine
Agon SR‡, Plendil, Plendil ER‡, Renedil†

*Pregnancy risk category C*

### AVAILABLE FORMS
*Tablets (extended-release):* 2.5 mg, 5 mg, 10 mg

### INDICATIONS & DOSAGES
➤ **Hypertension**
*Adults:* Initially, 5 mg P.O. daily. Adjust dosage based on patient response, usually at intervals not less than 2 weeks. Usual dose is 2.5 to 10 mg daily; maximum dosage is 10 mg daily.
*Elderly patients:* 2.5 mg P.O. daily; adjust dosage as for adults. Maximum dosage is 10 mg daily.
*Adjust-a-dose:* For patients with impaired hepatic function, 2.5 mg P.O. daily; adjust dosage as for adults. Maximum daily dose is 10 mg.

### ACTION
Unknown. A dihydropyridine-derivative calcium channel blocker that prevents entry of calcium ions into vascular smooth-muscle and cardiac cells; shows some selectivity for smooth muscle compared with cardiac muscle.

| Route | Onset | Peak | Duration |
|-------|-------|------|----------|
| P.O. | 2-5 hr | 2½-5 hr | 24 hr |

### ADVERSE REACTIONS
**CNS:** *headache,* dizziness, paresthesia, asthenia.

**CV:** *peripheral edema,* chest pain, palpitations, flushing.
**EENT:** rhinorrhea, pharyngitis.
**GI:** abdominal pain, nausea, constipation, diarrhea.
**Musculoskeletal:** muscle cramps, back pain.
**Respiratory:** upper respiratory tract infection, cough.
**Skin:** rash.

### INTERACTIONS
**Drug-drug.** *Anticonvulsants:* May decrease felodipine level. Avoid using together.
*CYP 3A4 inhibitors such as azole antifungals, cimetidine, erythromycin:* May decrease clearance of felodipine. Reduce doses of felodipine; monitor patient for toxicity.
*Metoprolol:* May alter pharmacokinetics of metoprolol. Monitor patient for adverse reactions.
*NSAIDs:* May decrease antihypertensive effects. Monitor blood pressure.
*Theophylline:* May slightly decrease theophylline level. Monitor patient response closely.
**Drug-herb.** *Ma-huang:* May decrease antihypertensive effects. Discourage use together
**Drug-food.** *Grapefruit, lime:* May increase drug's level and adverse effects. Discourage use together.

### EFFECTS ON LAB TEST RESULTS
None reported.

### CONTRAINDICATIONS & CAUTIONS
• Contraindicated in patients hypersensitive to drug.
• Use cautiously in patients with heart failure, particularly those receiving beta blockers, and in patients with impaired hepatic function.

### NURSING CONSIDERATIONS
• Monitor blood pressure for response.
• Monitor patient for peripheral edema, which appears to be both dose- and age-related. It's more common in patients taking higher doses, especially those older than age 60.
• **Alert:** Don't confuse Plendil with pindolol.

## PATIENT TEACHING
- Tell patient to swallow tablets whole and not to crush or chew them.
- Tell patient to take drug without food or with a light meal.
- Advise patient not to take drug with grapefruit juice.
- Advise patient to continue taking drug even when he feels better, to watch his diet, and to check with prescriber or pharmacist before taking other drugs, including OTC drugs, nutritional supplements, or herbal remedies.
- Advise patient to observe good oral hygiene and to see a dentist regularly; use of drug may cause mild gum problems.

---

## fosinopril sodium
Monopril⬦

*Pregnancy risk category C; D in second and third trimesters*

### AVAILABLE FORMS
*Tablets:* 10 mg, 20 mg, 40 mg

### INDICATIONS & DOSAGES
➤ **Hypertension**
*Adults:* Initially, 10 mg P.O. daily; adjust dosage based on blood pressure response at peak and trough levels. Usual dosage is 20 to 40 mg daily; maximum is 80 mg daily. Dosage may be divided.
➤ **Heart failure**
*Adults:* Initially, 10 mg P.O. once daily. Increase dosage over several weeks to a maximum of 40 mg P.O. daily, if needed.
*Adjust-a-dose:* For patients with moderate to severe renal failure or vigorous diuresis, start with 5 mg P.O. once daily.

### ACTION
Antihypertensive action not clearly defined. Thought to inhibit ACE, preventing conversion of angiotensin I to angiotensin II, a potent vasoconstrictor. Reduced formation of angiotensin II decreases peripheral arterial resistance, thus decreasing aldosterone secretion, which reduces sodium and water retention and lowers blood pressure.

| Route | Onset | Peak | Duration |
|-------|-------|------|----------|
| P.O. | 1 hr | 3 hr | 24 hr |

## ADVERSE REACTIONS
**CNS:** *CVA,* headache, *dizziness,* fatigue, syncope, paresthesia, sleep disturbance.
**CV:** chest pain, angina pectoris, *MI,* rhythm disturbances, palpitations, hypotension, orthostatic hypotension.
**EENT:** tinnitus, sinusitis.
**GI:** nausea, vomiting, diarrhea, *pancreatitis,* dry mouth, abdominal distention, abdominal pain, constipation.
**GU:** sexual dysfunction, renal insufficiency.
**Hepatic:** *hepatitis.*
**Metabolic:** *hyperkalemia.*
**Musculoskeletal:** arthralgia, musculoskeletal pain, myalgia.
**Respiratory:** *bronchospasm; dry, persistent, tickling, nonproductive cough.*
**Skin:** urticaria, rash, photosensitivity reactions, pruritus.
**Other:** *angioedema,* decreased libido, gout.

## INTERACTIONS
**Drug-drug.** *Antacids:* May impair absorption. Separate dosage times by at least 2 hours.
*Azathioprine:* May increase risk of anemia or leukopenia. Monitor hematologic studies if used together.
*Diuretics, other antihypertensives:* May cause excessive hypotension. Diuretic may need to be stopped or fosinopril dosage lowered.
*Lithium:* May increase lithium level and lithium toxicity. Monitor lithium level.
*Nesiritide:* May increase hypotensive effects. Monitor blood pressure.
*NSAIDs:* May decrease antihypertensive effects. Monitor blood pressure.
*Potassium-sparing diuretics, potassium supplements:* May cause risk of hyperkalemia. Monitor patient closely.
**Drug-herb.** *Capsaicin:* May cause cough. Discourage use together.
*Ma-huang:* May decrease antihypertensive effects. Discourage use together.
**Drug-food.** *Salt substitutes containing potassium:* May cause hyperkalemia. Urge patient to avoid using together.

## EFFECTS ON LAB TEST RESULTS
- May increase liver function test values and BUN, creatinine, and potassium levels.

---

Reactions may be *common,* uncommon, *life-threatening,* or COMMON AND LIFE-THREATENING.

● May decrease hemoglobin and hematocrit.

● May cause falsely low digoxin level with the Digi-Tab radioimmunoassay kit for digoxin.

**CONTRAINDICATIONS & CAUTIONS**
● Contraindicated in patients hypersensitive to drug or other ACE inhibitors and in breast-feeding women.
● Use cautiously in patients with impaired renal or hepatic function.

**NURSING CONSIDERATIONS**
● Monitor blood pressure for effect.
● Although ACE inhibitors reduce blood pressure in all races studied, this response is less in black patients who receive the drug as monotherapy. Therapy with a thiazide diuretic produces a more favorable response.
● ACE inhibitors appear to cause a higher risk of angioedema in black patients.
● Monitor potassium intake and potassium level. Diabetic patients, those with impaired renal function, and those receiving drugs that can increase potassium level may develop hyperkalemia.
● Other ACE inhibitors may cause agranulocytosis and neutropenia. Monitor CBC with differential counts before therapy and periodically thereafter.
● Assess renal and hepatic function before and periodically throughout therapy.
● *Alert:* Don't confuse fosinopril with lisinopril.
● *Alert:* Don't confuse Monopril with Monurol.

**PATIENT TEACHING**
● Tell patient to avoid salt substitutes; these products may contain potassium, which can cause high potassium level in patients taking drug.
● Instruct patient to contact prescriber if light-headedness or fainting occurs.
● Advise patient to report evidence of infection, such as fever and sore throat.
● Instruct patient to call prescriber if the following signs or symptoms occur: easy bruising or bleeding; swelling of tongue, lips, face, eyes, mucous membranes, or limbs; difficulty swallowing or breathing; and hoarseness.

● Urge patient to use caution in hot weather and during exercise. Inadequate fluid intake, vomiting, diarrhea, and excessive perspiration can lead to light-headedness and fainting.
● Tell woman to notify prescriber if pregnancy occurs. Drug will need to be stopped.

---

# hydralazine hydrochloride
Alphapress‡, Apresoline, Novo-Hylazin†, Supres†

*Pregnancy risk category C*

**AVAILABLE FORMS**
*Injection:* 20 mg/ml
*Tablets:* 10 mg, 25 mg, 50 mg, 100 mg

**INDICATIONS & DOSAGES**
➤ **Essential hypertension (orally, alone, or with other antihypertensives), severe essential hypertension (parenterally, to lower blood pressure quickly)**
*Adults:* Initially, 10 mg P.O. q.i.d.; gradually increased to 50 mg q.i.d., p.r.n. Maximum recommended dose is 200 mg daily, but some patients may need 300 to 400 mg daily.
Or, give 10 to 20 mg I.V. slowly and repeat p.r.n.; switch to oral form as soon as possible.
Or, give 10 to 50 mg I.M., repeat p.r.n.; switch to oral form as soon as possible.
*Children:* Initially, 0.75 mg/kg daily P.O. divided into four doses; gradually increased over 3 to 4 weeks to maximum of 7.5 mg/kg or 200 mg daily. Maximum first P.O. dose is 25 mg.
Or, 0.1 to 0.2 mg/kg I.V. q 4 to 6 hours, p.r.n. Maximum first parenteral dose is 20 mg.
➤ **Preeclampsia, eclampsia**
*Adults:* Initially, 5 to 10 mg I.V., followed by 5 to 10 mg I.V. doses (range 5 to 20 mg) q 20 to 30 minutes, p.r.n. Or, 0.5 to 10 mg/hour I.V. infusion.
➤ **Heart failure ◆**
*Adults:* Initially, 50 to 75 mg P.O. daily. Maintenance doses range from 200 to 600 mg P.O. daily in divided doses q 6 to 12 hours.

---

## I.V. ADMINISTRATION
• Give drug slowly and repeat as needed, generally q 4 to 6 hours. Hydralazine undergoes color change in most infusion solutions; these color changes don't indicate loss of potency.
• Drug is compatible with normal saline, Ringer's, lactated Ringer's, and several other common I.V. solutions. Drug may react with dextrose. The manufacturer doesn't recommend mixing drug in infusion solutions. Check with pharmacist for additional compatibility information.
• Oral therapy should replace parenteral therapy as soon as possible.

## ACTION
Unknown. A direct-acting vasodilator that mainly relaxes arteriolar smooth muscle.

| Route | Onset | Peak | Duration |
|-------|-------|------|----------|
| P.O. | 20-30 min | 1-2 hr | 2-4 hr |
| I.V. | 5-20 min | 10-80 min | 2-6 hr |
| I.M. | 10-30 min | 1 hr | 2-6 hr |

## ADVERSE REACTIONS
**CNS:** peripheral neuritis, *headache,* dizziness.
**CV:** orthostatic hypotension, *tachycardia,* edema, *angina pectoris, palpitations.*
**EENT:** nasal congestion.
**GI:** *nausea, vomiting, diarrhea, anorexia,* constipation.
**Hematologic:** *neutropenia, leukopenia, agranulocytopenia, agranulocytosis, thrombocytopenia with or without purpura.*
**Skin:** rash.
**Other:** *lupuslike syndrome.*

## INTERACTIONS
**Drug-drug.** *Diazoxide, MAO inhibitors:* May cause severe hypotension. Use together cautiously.
*Diuretics, other hypotensive drugs:* May cause excessive hypotension. Dosage adjustment may be needed.
*Indomethacin:* May decrease effects of hydralazine. Monitor blood pressure.
*Metoprolol, propranolol:* May increase levels and effects of these beta blockers. Monitor patient closely. May need to adjust dosage of either drug.

## EFFECTS ON LAB TEST RESULTS
• May decrease hemoglobin and neutrophil, WBC, granulocyte, platelet, and RBC counts.

## CONTRAINDICATIONS & CAUTIONS
• Contraindicated in patients hypersensitive to drug
• Contraindicated in those with coronary artery disease or mitral valvular rheumatic heart disease.
• Use cautiously in patients with suspected cardiac disease, CVA, or severe renal impairment and in those taking other antihypertensives.

## NURSING CONSIDERATIONS
• Monitor patient's blood pressure, pulse rate, and body weight frequently. Hydralazine may be given with diuretics and beta blockers to decrease sodium retention and tachycardia and to prevent angina attacks.
• Elderly patients may be more sensitive to drug's hypotensive effects.
• Monitor CBC, lupus erythematosus cell preparation, and antinuclear antibody titer determination before therapy and periodically during long-term therapy.
• *Alert:* Monitor patient closely for signs and symptoms of lupuslike syndrome (sore throat, fever, muscle and joint aches, rash). Notify prescriber immediately if these develop.
• Improve patient compliance by giving drug b.i.d. Check with prescriber.
• *Alert:* Don't confuse hydralazine with hydroxyzine or Apresoline with Apresazide.
• Apresoline may contain tartrazine.

## PATIENT TEACHING
• Instruct patient to take oral form with meals to increase absorption.
• Inform patient that low blood pressure and dizziness upon standing can be minimized by rising slowly and avoiding sudden position changes.
• Tell woman to notify prescriber if she suspects pregnancy; tell her to stop taking drug.
• Advise patient that the body's stores of vitamin $B_6$ (pyridoxine) and coenzyme Q10 may be depleted and that he should discuss supplements with prescriber.

---

Reactions may be *common,* uncommon, *life-threatening,* or **COMMON AND LIFE-THREATENING.**

• Tell patient to notify prescriber of unexplained prolonged general tiredness or fever, muscle or joint aching, or chest pain.

## irbesartan
Avapro

*Pregnancy risk category C; D in second and third trimesters*

### AVAILABLE FORMS
*Tablets:* 75 mg, 150 mg, 300 mg

### INDICATIONS & DOSAGES
➤ **Hypertension**
*Adults and children age 13 and older:* Initially, 150 mg P.O. daily, increased to maximum of 300 mg daily, if needed.
*Children ages 6 to 12:* Initially, 75 mg P.O. once daily, increased to a maximum of 150 mg daily, if needed.
*Adjust-a-dose:* For volume- and salt-depleted patients, initially, 75 mg P.O. daily
➤ **Nephropathy in patients with type 2 diabetes**
*Adults:* 300 mg P.O. once daily.

### ACTION
Produces antihypertensive effect by competitive antagonist activity at the angiotensin II receptor.

| Route | Onset | Peak | Duration |
|-------|-------|------|----------|
| P.O. | Unknown | 1½-2 hr | 24 hr |

### ADVERSE REACTIONS
**CNS:** fatigue, anxiety, dizziness, headache.
**CV:** chest pain, edema, tachycardia.
**EENT:** pharyngitis, rhinitis, sinus abnormality.
**GI:** diarrhea, dyspepsia, abdominal pain, nausea, vomiting.
**GU:** UTI.
**Musculoskeletal:** musculoskeletal trauma or pain.
**Respiratory:** upper respiratory tract infection, cough.
**Skin:** rash.

### INTERACTIONS
**Drug-herb.** *Ma-huang:* May decrease antihypertensive effects. Discourage use together.

### EFFECTS ON LAB TEST RESULTS
None reported.

### CONTRAINDICATIONS & CAUTIONS
• Contraindicated in patients hypersensitive to drug or its components.
• Use cautiously in patients with impaired renal function, heart failure, and renal artery stenosis and in breast-feeding women.
• Use during pregnancy can cause injury and death to the developing fetus. When pregnancy is detected, stop drug as soon as possible.

### NURSING CONSIDERATIONS
• Drug may be given with a diuretic or other antihypertensive, if needed, for control of hypertension.
• Symptomatic hypotension may occur in volume- or salt-depleted patients (vigorous diuretic use or dialysis). Correct the cause of volume depletion before administration or before a lower dose is used.
• If hypotension occurs, place patient in a supine position and give an I.V. infusion of normal saline solution, if needed. Once blood pressure has stabilized after a transient hypotensive episode, drug may be continued.
• Dizziness and orthostatic hypotension may occur more frequently in patients with type 2 diabetes and renal disease.

### PATIENT TEACHING
• Warn woman of childbearing age of consequences of drug exposure to fetus. Tell her to call prescriber immediately if pregnancy is suspected.
• Tell patient that drug may be taken once daily without regard to food.

## labetalol hydrochloride
Normodyne, Presolol‡, Trandate

*Pregnancy risk category C*

### AVAILABLE FORMS
*Injection:* 5 mg/ml
*Tablets:* 100 mg, 200 mg, 300 mg

## INDICATIONS & DOSAGES
➤ **Hypertension**
*Adults:* 100 mg P.O. b.i.d. with or without a diuretic. If needed, dosage is increased to 200 mg b.i.d. after 2 days. Further increases may be made q 2 to 3 days until optimum response is reached. Usual maintenance dose is 200 to 400 mg b.i.d.
➤ **Severe hypertension, hypertensive emergencies**
*Adults:* 200 mg diluted in 160 ml of $D_5W$, infused at 2 mg/minute until satisfactory response is obtained; then infusion is stopped. May be repeated q 6 to 12 hours.

Or, give by repeated I.V. injection: initially, 20 mg I.V. slowly over 2 minutes. Repeat injections of 40 to 80 mg q 10 minutes until maximum dose of 300 mg is reached, p.r.n.

## I.V. ADMINISTRATION
• Drug may be given by slow, direct I.V. injection over 2 minutes at 10-minute intervals.
• For I.V. infusion, prepare by diluting with $D_5W$ or normal saline solutions; for example, 200 mg of drug to 160 ml $D_5W$ to yield 1 mg/ml.
• Give labetalol infusion with an infusion control device.
• Monitor blood pressure closely every 5 minutes for 30 minutes, then every 30 minutes for 2 hours, then hourly for 6 hours.
• Patient should remain supine for 3 hours after infusion. When given I.V. for hypertensive emergencies, drug produces a rapid, predictable fall in blood pressure within 5 to 10 minutes.

## ACTION
Unknown. May be related to reduced peripheral vascular resistance, as a result of alpha and beta blockade.

| Route | Onset | Peak | Duration |
|-------|-------|------|----------|
| P.O. | 20 min | 2-4 hr | 8-12 hr |
| I.V. | 2-5 min | 5 min | 2-4 hr |

## ADVERSE REACTIONS
**CNS:** vivid dreams, fatigue, headache, paresthesia, transient scalp tingling, *dizziness, syncope.*
**CV:** *orthostatic hypotension,* **ventricular arrhythmias.**

**EENT:** nasal congestion.
**GI:** nausea, vomiting.
**GU:** sexual dysfunction, urine retention.
**Respiratory:** dyspnea, ***bronchospasm.***
**Skin:** rash.

## INTERACTIONS
**Drug-drug.** *Beta-adrenergic agonists:* May blunt bronchodilator effect of these drugs in patients with bronchospasm. May need to increase dosages of these drugs.
*Cimetidine:* May enhance labetalol's effect. Use together cautiously.
*Halothane:* May increase hypotensive effect. Monitor blood pressure closely.
*Insulin, oral antidiabetics:* May alter dosage requirements in previously stabilized diabetic patient. Monitor patient closely.
*NSAIDs:* May decrease antihypertensive effects. Monitor blood pressure.
**Drug-herb.** *Ma-huang:* May decrease antihypertensive effects. Discourage use together.

## EFFECTS ON LAB TEST RESULTS
• May increase transaminase and urea levels.
• May cause a false-positive increase of urine free and total catecholamine levels when measured by a nonspecific trihydroxyindole fluorometric method.

## CONTRAINDICATIONS & CAUTIONS
• Contraindicated in patients hypersensitive to drug and in those with bronchial asthma, overt cardiac failure, greater than first-degree heart block, cardiogenic shock, severe bradycardia, and other conditions that may cause severe and prolonged hypotension.
• Use cautiously in patients with heart failure, hepatic failure, chronic bronchitis, emphysema, peripheral vascular disease, and pheochromocytoma.

## NURSING CONSIDERATIONS
• Monitor blood pressure frequently. Drug masks common signs and symptoms of shock.
• If dizziness occurs, ask prescriber if patient may take a dose at bedtime or take smaller doses t.i.d. to help minimize this adverse reaction.

---

• When switching from I.V. to P.O. form, begin P.O. regimen at 200 mg after blood pressure begins to rise; repeat dose with 200 to 400 mg in 6 to 12 hours. Adjust dosage according to blood pressure response.

• Monitor glucose level in diabetic patients closely because beta blockers may mask certain signs and symptoms of hypoglycemia.

• *Alert:* Don't confuse Trandate with Trental or Tridrate.

• *Alert:* Sodium bicarbonate injection is incompatible with I.V. labetalol.

## PATIENT TEACHING

• *Alert:* Tell patient that stopping drug abruptly can worsen chest pain and trigger an MI.

• Advise patient that dizziness is the most troublesome adverse reaction and tends to occur in the early stages of treatment, in patients also receiving diuretics, and in those receiving higher dosages. Inform patient that dizziness can be minimized by rising slowly and avoiding sudden position changes.

• Warn patient that occasional scalp tingling may occur, especially at start of therapy, but is harmless.

• Tell patient that drug may deplete body's stores of coenzyme Q10 and that he should discuss the need for supplements with prescriber.

---

## lisinopril
Prinivil⊘, Zestril⊘

*Pregnancy risk category C; D in second and third trimesters*

## AVAILABLE FORMS
*Tablets:* 2.5 mg, 5 mg, 10 mg, 20 mg, 40 mg

## INDICATIONS & DOSAGES
➤ **Hypertension**
*Adults:* Initially, 10 mg P.O. daily for patients not taking a diuretic. Most patients are well controlled on 20 to 40 mg daily as a single dose. For patients taking a diuretic, initially, 5 mg P.O. daily.
*Adjust-a-dose:* For patients with creatinine clearance 10 to 30 ml/minute, give 5 mg P.O. daily; if clearance is less than 10 ml/minute, give 2.5 mg P.O. daily.

➤ **Adjunct treatment (with diuretics and cardiac glycosides) for heart failure**
*Adults:* Initially, 5 mg P.O. daily; increased p.r.n. to maximum of 20 mg P.O. daily.
*Adjust-a-dose:* For patients with sodium level less than 130 mEq/L or creatinine clearance less than 30 ml/minute, start treatment at 2.5 mg daily.

➤ **Hemodynamically stable patients within 24 hours of acute MI to improve survival**
*Adults:* Initially, 5 mg P.O.; then 5 mg after 24 hours, 10 mg after 48 hours, followed by 10 mg once daily for 6 weeks.
*Adjust-a-dose:* For patients with systolic blood pressure 120 mm Hg or less when treatment is started or during first 3 days after an infarct, decrease dosage to 2.5 mg P.O. If systolic blood pressure drops to 100 mm Hg or less, reduce daily maintenance dose of 5 mg to 2.5 mg, if needed. If prolonged systolic blood pressure stays under 90 mm Hg for longer than 1 hour, withdraw drug.

## ACTION
Unknown. Thought to result primarily from suppression of the renin-angiotensin-aldosterone system.

| Route | Onset | Peak | Duration |
|-------|-------|------|----------|
| P.O. | 1 hr | 7 hr | 24 hr |

## ADVERSE REACTIONS
**CNS:** *dizziness,* headache, fatigue, paresthesia.
**CV:** hypotension, *orthostatic hypotension,* chest pain.
**EENT:** *nasal congestion.*
**GI:** *diarrhea,* nausea, dyspepsia.
**GU:** impaired renal function, impotence.
**Metabolic:** *hyperkalemia.*
**Respiratory:** dyspnea, dry, persistent, tickling, nonproductive cough.
**Skin:** rash.

## INTERACTIONS
**Drug-drug.** *Allopurinol:* May cause hypersensitivity reaction. Use together cautiously.
*Azathioprine:* May increase risk of anemia or leukopenia. Monitor hematologic studies if used together.

---

*Diuretics, thiazide diuretics:* May cause excessive hypotension with diuretics. Monitor blood pressure closely.

*Indomethacin, NSAIDs:* May reduce hypotensive effects of drug. Adjust dose as needed.

*Insulin, oral antidiabetics:* May cause hypoglycemia, especially at start of lisinopril therapy. Monitor glucose level.

*Phenothiazines:* May increase hypotensive effects. Monitor blood pressure closely.

*Potassium-sparing diuretics, potassium supplements:* May cause hyperkalemia. Monitor laboratory values.

**Drug-herb.** *Capsaicin:* May cause ACE inhibitor–induced cough. Discourage use together.

*Ma-huang:* May decrease antihypertensive effects. Discourage use together.

**Drug-food.** *Potassium-containing salt substitutes:* May cause hyperkalemia. Monitor laboratory values.

## EFFECTS ON LAB TEST RESULTS
• May increase BUN, creatinine, potassium, and bilirubin levels.
• May increase liver function test values.

## CONTRAINDICATIONS & CAUTIONS
• Contraindicated in patients hypersensitive to ACE inhibitors and in those with a history of angioedema related to previous treatment with ACE inhibitor.
• Use cautiously in patients with impaired renal function; dosage adjustment is needed.
• Use cautiously in patients at risk for hyperkalemia and in those with aortic stenosis or hypertrophic cardiomyopathy.

## NURSING CONSIDERATIONS
• When using drug in acute MI, give patient the appropriate and standard recommended treatment, such as thrombolytics, aspirin, and beta blockers.
• Although ACE inhibitors reduce blood pressure in all races studied, this response is less in black patients who receive the drug as monotherapy. Therapy with a thiazide diuretic produces a more favorable response.
• ACE inhibitors appear to increase risk of angioedema in black patients.

• Monitor blood pressure frequently. If drug doesn't adequately control blood pressure, diuretics may be added.
• Monitor WBC with differential counts before therapy, every 2 weeks for first 3 months of therapy, and periodically thereafter.
• *Alert:* Don't confuse lisinopril with fosinopril or Lioresal.
• *Alert:* Don't confuse Zestril with Zostrix.
• *Alert:* Don't confuse Prinivil with Proventil or Prilosec.

## PATIENT TEACHING
• *Alert:* Rarely, facial and throat swelling (including swelling of the larynx) may occur, especially after first dose. Advise patient to report signs or symptoms of breathing problems or swelling of face, eyes, lips, or tongue.
• Inform patient that light-headedness can occur, especially during first few days of therapy. Tell him to rise slowly to minimize this effect and to report symptoms to prescriber. If he faints, advise patient to stop taking drug and call prescriber immediately.
• If unpleasant adverse reactions occur, tell patient not to stop drug suddenly but to notify prescriber.
• Advise patient to report signs and symptoms of infection, such as fever and sore throat.
• Tell women to notify prescriber if pregnancy occurs. Drug will need to be stopped.
• Instruct patient not to use salt substitutes that contain potassium without first consulting prescriber.

---

# losartan potassium
Cozaar◊

*Pregnancy risk category C; D in second and third trimesters*

## AVAILABLE FORMS
*Tablets:* 25 mg, 50 mg, 100 mg

## INDICATIONS & DOSAGES
➤ **Hypertension**
*Adults:* Initially, 25 to 50 mg P.O. daily. Maximum daily dose is 100 mg in one or two divided doses.

---

Reactions may be *common*, uncommon, *life-threatening*, or COMMON AND LIFE-THREATENING.

*Adjust-a-dose:* For patients who are hepatically impaired or intravascularly volume-depleted (such as those taking diuretics), initially, 25 mg.

✷ *NEW INDICATION:* **Nephropathy in type 2 diabetic patients**

*Adults:* 50 mg P.O. once daily. Increase dosage to 100 mg once daily based on blood pressure response.

✷ *NEW INDICATION:* **To reduce risk of stroke in patients with hypertension and left ventricular hypertrophy**

*Adults:* Initially, 50 mg losartan P.O. once daily. Adjust dosage based on blood pressure response, adding hydrochlorothiazide 12.5 mg once daily, increasing losartan to 100 mg daily, or both. If further adjustments are required, may increase the daily dosage of hydrochlorothiazide to 25 mg.

**ACTION**
Inhibits vasoconstrictive and aldosterone-secreting action of angiotensin II by blocking angiotensin II receptor on the surface of vascular smooth muscle and other tissue cells.

| Route | Onset | Peak | Duration |
|-------|-------|------|----------|
| P.O. | Unknown | 1 hr | Unknown |

**ADVERSE REACTIONS**
**Patients with hypertension or left ventricular hypertrophy**
**CNS:** dizziness, asthenia, fatigue, headache, insomnia.
**CV:** edema, chest pain.
**EENT:** nasal congestion, sinusitis, pharyngitis, sinus disorder.
**GI:** abdominal pain, nausea, diarrhea, dyspepsia.
**Musculoskeletal:** muscle cramps, myalgia, back or leg pain.
**Respiratory:** cough, upper respiratory infection.
**Other:** *angioedema.*
**Nephropathy patients**
**CNS:** *asthenia, fatigue,* fever, hypesthesia.
**CV:** *chest pain,* hypotension, orthostatic hypotension.
**EENT:** sinusitis, cataract.
**GI:** *diarrhea,* dyspepsia, gastritis.
**GU:** *UTI.*
**Hematologic:** anemia.
**Metabolic:** *hyperkalemia, hypoglycemia,* weight gain.

**Musculoskeletal:** *back pain,* leg or knee pain, muscle weakness.
**Respiratory:** *cough, bronchitis.*
**Skin:** cellulitis.
**Other:** infection, *flulike syndrome,* trauma, diabetic neuropathy, ***diabetic vascular disease, angioedema.***

**INTERACTIONS**
**Drug-drug.** *Lithium:* May increase lithium level. Monitor lithium level and patient for toxicity.
*NSAIDs:* May decrease antihypertensive effects. Monitor blood pressure.
*Potassium-sparing diuretics, potassium supplements:* May cause hyperkalemia. Monitor patient closely.
**Drug-herb.** *Ma-huang:* May decrease antihypertensive effects. Discourage use together.
**Drug-food.** *Salt substitutes containing potassium:* May cause hyperkalemia. Monitor patient closely.

**EFFECTS ON LAB TEST RESULTS**
None reported.

**CONTRAINDICATIONS & CAUTIONS**
• Contraindicated in patients hypersensitive to drug. Breast-feeding isn't recommended during losartan therapy.
• Use cautiously in patients with impaired renal or hepatic function.
• Drugs that act directly on the renin-angiotensin system (such as losartan) can cause fetal and neonatal morbidity and death when given to women in the second or third trimester of pregnancy. These problems haven't been detected when exposure was limited to the first trimester. If pregnancy is suspected, notify prescriber because drug should be stopped.

**NURSING CONSIDERATIONS**
• Drug can be used alone or with other antihypertensives.
• If antihypertensive effect is inadequate as measured by the trough level of drug using once-daily dosing, a b.i.d. regimen using the same or increased total daily dose may give a more satisfactory response.
• Monitor patient's blood pressure closely to evaluate effectiveness of therapy. When losartan is used alone, the effect on blood

pressure is notably less in black patients than in patients of other races.

● Monitor patients who are also taking diuretics for symptomatic hypotension.

● Regularly assess the patient's renal function (via creatinine and BUN levels).

● Patients with severe heart failure whose renal function depends on the angiotensin-aldosterone system have experienced acute renal failure during ACE inhibitor therapy. Losartan's manufacturer states that drug would be expected to have the same effect. Closely monitor patient, especially during first few weeks of therapy.

● *Alert:* Don't confuse Cozaar with Zocor.

### PATIENT TEACHING

● Tell patient to avoid salt substitutes; these products may contain potassium, which can cause high potassium level in patients taking losartan.

● Inform woman of childbearing age about consequences of second- and third-trimester exposure to drug; instruct her to notify prescriber immediately if pregnancy is suspected.

● Advise patient to immediately report swelling of face, eyes, lips, or tongue or any breathing difficulty.

---

## methyldopa
Aldomet, Aldopren‡, Apo-Methyldopa†, Dopamet†, Hydopa‡, Novo-Medopa†, Nu-Medopa†

## methyldopate hydrochloride
Aldomet

*Pregnancy risk category B (P.O.) or C (I.V.)*

---

### AVAILABLE FORMS
**methyldopa**
*Oral suspension:* 250 mg/5 ml
*Tablets:* 125 mg, 250 mg, 500 mg
**methyldopate hydrochloride**
*Injection:* 250 mg/5 ml (50 mg/ml in 5-ml and 10-ml vials)

### INDICATIONS & DOSAGES
➤ **Hypertension, hypertensive crisis**
*Adults:* Initially, 250 mg P.O. b.i.d. to t.i.d. in first 48 hours. Increase, p.r.n., q 2 days.

May give entire daily dose in evening or h.s. Adjust dosages if other antihypertensives are added to or deleted from therapy. Maintenance dosage is 500 mg to 2 g daily in two to four divided doses. Maximum recommended dose is 3 g daily. Or, 250 to 500 mg I.V. q 6 hours. Maximum dosage is 1 g q 6 hours. Switch to oral antihypertensives as soon as possible.

*Children:* Initially, 10 mg/kg P.O. daily in two to four divided doses; or, 20 to 40 mg/kg I.V. daily in four divided doses. Increase dose daily until desired response occurs. Maximum daily dose is 65 mg/kg or 3 g, whichever is less.

### I.V. ADMINISTRATION
● Dilute appropriate dose in 100 ml $D_5W$. Infuse slowly over 30 to 60 minutes.

### ACTION
Unknown. Thought to inhibit the central vasomotor centers, thereby decreasing sympathetic outflow to the heart, kidneys, and peripheral vasculature.

| Route | Onset | Peak | Duration |
|-------|-------|------|----------|
| P.O. | 4-6 hr | Unknown | 12-48 hr |
| I.V. | 4-6 hr | Unknown | 10-16 hr |

### ADVERSE REACTIONS
**CNS:** *sedation, headache,* weakness, dizziness, *decreased mental acuity,* paresthesia, parkinsonism, involuntary choreoathetoid movements, psychic disturbances, depression, nightmares.
**CV:** *bradycardia, orthostatic hypotension,* aggravated angina, *myocarditis, edema.*
**EENT:** *nasal congestion.*
**GI:** nausea, vomiting, diarrhea, *pancreatitis, dry mouth,* constipation.
**GU:** galactorrhea.
**Hematologic:** hemolytic anemia, *thrombocytopenia, leukopenia, bone marrow depression.*
**Hepatic:** *hepatic necrosis, hepatitis.*
**Musculoskeletal:** arthralgia.
**Skin:** rash.
**Other:** drug-induced fever, gynecomastia.

### INTERACTIONS
**Drug-drug.** *Amphetamines, nonselective beta blockers, norepinephrine, phenothiazines, tricyclic antidepressants:* May

---

Reactions may be *common,* uncommon, ***life-threatening**,* or COMMON AND LIFE-THREATENING.

cause hypertensive effects. Monitor patient closely.
*Anesthetics:* May need lower doses of anesthetics. Use together cautiously.
*Barbiturates:* May decrease actions of methyldopa. Monitor patient closely.
*Haloperidol:* May cause psychomotor retardation, impaired memory, and difficulty concentrating in nonschizophrenic patients; increases sedation. Use together cautiously.
*Levodopa:* May increase hypotensive effects, which may increase adverse CNS reactions. Monitor patient closely.
*Lithium:* May increase lithium level. Watch for increased lithium level and signs and symptoms of toxicity.
*MAO inhibitors:* May cause excessive sympathetic stimulation. Avoid using together.
*Tolbutamide:* May impair metabolism of tolbutamide. Monitor patient for hypoglycemic effect.
**Drug-herb.** *Capsicum:* May reduce antihypertensive effectiveness. Discourage use together.

**EFFECTS ON LAB TEST RESULTS**
● May increase creatinine level.
● May increase liver function test values. May decrease hemoglobin, hematocrit, and platelet and WBC counts.
● May falsely increase urine catecholamine level, interfering with the diagnosis of pheochromocytoma.

**CONTRAINDICATIONS & CAUTIONS**
● Contraindicated in patients hypersensitive to drug and in those with active hepatic disease (such as acute hepatitis) or active cirrhosis.
● Contraindicated in those whose previous methyldopa therapy caused liver problems and in those taking MAO inhibitors.
● Use cautiously in patients with history of impaired hepatic function or sulfite sensitivity and in breast-feeding women.

**NURSING CONSIDERATIONS**
● Monitor patient's blood pressure regularly. Elderly patients are more likely than younger ones to experience hypotension and sedation.
● Occasionally tolerance may occur, usually between the second and third months of

therapy. The addition of a diuretic or a dosage adjustment may be needed. Notify prescriber if patient response changes significantly.
● After dialysis, monitor patient for hypertension and notify prescriber, if needed. Patient may need an extra dose of methyldopa.
● Monitor CBC with differential counts before therapy and periodically thereafter.
● Patients who need blood transfusions should have direct and indirect Coombs' tests to prevent crossmatching problems.
● Monitor patient's Coombs' test results. In patients who have received drug for several months, positive reaction to direct Coombs' test indicates hemolytic anemia.
● Observe for and report involuntary choreoathetoid movements. Drug may have to be stopped.
● **Alert:** Don't confuse Aldomet with Aldoril or Anzemet.

**PATIENT TEACHING**
● Tell patient not to suddenly stop taking drug, but to notify prescriber if unpleasant adverse reactions occur.
● Instruct patient to report signs and symptoms of infection.
● Tell patient to check his weight daily and to notify prescriber if he gains more than 5 lb. Sodium and water retention may occur but can be relieved with diuretics.
● Warn patient that drug may impair ability to perform tasks that require mental alertness, particularly at start of therapy. A once-daily dose at bedtime will minimize daytime drowsiness.
● Inform patient that low blood pressure and dizziness on standing can be minimized by rising slowly and avoiding sudden position changes. Dry mouth can be relieved by chewing gum or sucking on hard candy or ice chips.
● Tell patient that urine may turn dark if left standing in toilet bowl or if toilet bowl has been treated with bleach.

# metoprolol succinate
Toprol-XL✲

# metoprolol tartrate
Apo-Metoprolol†, Apo-Metoprolol (Type L)†, Betaloc†‡, Betaloc Durules†, Lopresor†, Lopresor SR†, Lopressor, Minax‡, Novo-Metoprol†, Nu-Metop†

*Pregnancy risk category C*

## AVAILABLE FORMS
**metoprolol succinate**
*Tablets (extended-release):* 25 mg, 50 mg, 100 mg, 200 mg
**metoprolol tartrate**
*Injection:* 1 mg/ml in 5-ml ampules
*Tablets:* 50 mg, 100 mg
*Tablets (extended-release):* 100 mg†, 200 mg†

## INDICATIONS & DOSAGES
➤ **Hypertension**
*Adults:* Initially, 50 mg P.O. b.i.d. or 100 mg P.O. once daily; then up to 100 to 450 mg daily in two or three divided doses. Or, 50 to 100 mg of extended-release tablets (tartrate equivalent) once daily. Adjust dosage as needed and tolerated at intervals of not less than 1 week to maximum of 400 mg daily.
➤ **Early intervention in acute MI**
*Adults:* 5 mg metoprolol tartrate I.V. bolus q 2 minutes for three doses. Then, 15 minutes after the last I.V. dose, give 25 to 50 mg P.O. q 6 hours for 48 hours. Maintenance dosage is 100 mg P.O. b.i.d.
➤ **Angina pectoris**
*Adults:* Initially, 100 mg P.O. daily as a single dose or in two equally divided doses; increased at weekly intervals until an adequate response or a pronounced decrease in heart rate is seen. Effects of daily dose beyond 400 mg aren't known. Or, give 100 mg of extended-release tablets (tartrate equivalent) once daily. Adjust dosage as needed and tolerated at intervals of not less than 1 week to maximum of 400 mg daily.
➤ **Stable symptomatic heart failure (New York Heart Association class II)**

**resulting from ischemia, hypertension, or cardiomyopathy**
*Adults:* 25 mg (Toprol-XL) P.O. once daily for 2 weeks. Double the dose q 2 weeks, as tolerated, to a maximum of 200 mg daily.
*Adjust-a-dose:* In patients with more severe heart failure, start with 12.5 mg (Toprol-XL) P.O. once daily for 2 weeks.

## I.V. ADMINISTRATION
● Give drug undiluted by direct injection.
● Although mixing with other drugs should be avoided, metoprolol is compatible when mixed with meperidine hydrochloride or morphine sulfate or when given with alteplase infusion at a Y-site connection.

## ACTION
Unknown. A selective beta blocker that selectively blocks $beta_1$-adrenergic receptors; decreases cardiac output, peripheral resistance, and cardiac oxygen consumption; and depresses renin secretion.

| Route | Onset | Peak | Duration |
|---|---|---|---|
| P.O. | 15 min | 1 hr | 6-12 hr |
| P.O. (extended-release) | 15 min | 6-12 hr | 24 hr |
| I.V. | 5 min | 20 min | 5-8 hr |

## ADVERSE REACTIONS
**CNS:** *fatigue, dizziness,* depression.
**CV:** **bradycardia,** hypotension, **heart failure, AV block.**
**GI:** nausea, diarrhea.
**Respiratory:** dyspnea.
**Skin:** rash.

## INTERACTIONS
**Drug-drug.** *Amobarbital, aprobarbital, butabarbital, butalbital, mephobarbital, pentobarbital, phenobarbital, primidone, secobarbital:* May reduce metoprolol effect. May need to increase beta-blocker dose.
*Cardiac glycosides, diltiazem:* May cause excessive bradycardia and increased depressant effect on myocardium. Use together cautiously.
*Catecholamine-depleting drugs such as $H_2$ antagonists, MAO inhibitors, reser-*

*pine:* May have additive effect. Monitor patient for hypotension and bradycardia.

*Chlorpromazine:* May decrease hepatic clearance. Watch for greater beta-blocking effect.

*Cimetidine:* May increase beta-blocker effects. Consider another $H_2$ agonist or decrease dose of beta blocker.

*Hydralazine:* May increase levels and effects of both drugs. Monitor patient closely. May need to adjust dosage.

*Indomethacin, NSAIDs:* May decrease antihypertensive effect. Monitor blood pressure and adjust dosage.

*Insulin, oral antidiabetics:* May alter dosage requirements in previously stabilized diabetic patients. Monitor patient closely.

*I.V. lidocaine:* May reduce hepatic metabolism of lidocaine, increasing risk of toxicity. Give bolus doses of lidocaine at a slower rate, and monitor lidocaine level closely.

*Prazosin:* May increase risk of orthostatic hypotension in the early phases of use together. Assist patient to stand slowly until effects are known.

*Propafenone:* May increase metoprolol level. Monitor vital signs.

*Rifampin:* May increase metoprolol metabolism. Watch for decreased effect.

*Terbutaline:* May antagonize bronchodilatory effects of terbutaline. Monitor patient.

*Verapamil:* May increase effects of both drugs. Monitor cardiac function closely, and decrease dosages as needed.

**Drug-herb.** *Ma-huang:* May decrease antihypertensive effects. Discourage use together.

**Drug-food.** *Any food:* May increase absorption. Encourage patient to take drug with food.

## EFFECTS ON LAB TEST RESULTS
● May increase transaminase, alkaline phosphatase, LDH, and uric acid levels.

## CONTRAINDICATIONS & CAUTIONS
● Contraindicated in patients hypersensitive to drug or other beta blockers.
● Contraindicated in patients with sinus bradycardia, greater than first-degree heart block, cardiogenic shock, or overt cardiac failure when used to treat hypertension or

angina. When used to treat MI, drug is contraindicated in patients with heart rate less than 45 beats/minute, greater than first-degree heart block, PR interval of 0.24 second or longer with first-degree heart block, systolic blood pressure less than 100 mm Hg, or moderate to severe cardiac failure.
● Use cautiously in patients with heart failure, diabetes, or respiratory or hepatic disease.

## NURSING CONSIDERATIONS
● Always check patient's apical pulse rate before giving drug. If it's slower than 60 beats/minute, withhold drug and call prescriber immediately.
● Monitor glucose level closely in diabetic patients because drug masks common signs and symptoms of hypoglycemia.
● Monitor blood pressure frequently; metoprolol masks common signs and symptoms of shock.
● Beta blockers may mask tachycardia caused by hyperthyroidism. In patients with suspected thyrotoxicosis, withdraw beta blocker gradually to avoid thyroid storm.
● When therapy is stopped, reduce dose gradually over 1 to 2 weeks.
● Store drug at room temperature and protect from light. Discard solution if it's discolored or contains particles.
● $Beta_1$ selectivity is lost at higher doses. Watch for peripheral side effects.
● *Alert:* Don't confuse metoprolol with metaproterenol or metolazone.
● *Alert:* Don't confuse Toprol with Topamax.

## PATIENT TEACHING
● Instruct patient to take drug exactly as prescribed and to take it with meals.
● Caution patient to avoid driving and other tasks requiring mental alertness until response to therapy has been established.
● Advise patient to inform dentist or prescriber about use of this drug before procedures or surgery.
● Tell patient to alert prescriber if shortness of breath occurs.
● Instruct patient not to stop drug suddenly but to notify prescriber about unpleasant adverse reactions. Inform him that

drug must be withdrawn gradually over 1 or 2 weeks.
• Inform patient that metoprolol isn't advised in breast-feeding women.
• Tell patient that drug may deplete body's stores of coenzyme Q10 and that he should discuss the need for supplements with prescriber.

## minoxidil
Loniten

*Pregnancy risk category C*

### AVAILABLE FORMS
*Tablets:* 2.5 mg, 10 mg

### INDICATIONS & DOSAGES
➤ **Severe hypertension**
*Adults:* Initially, 2.5 to 5 mg P.O. as a single dose. Effective dosage range is usually 10 to 40 mg daily. Maximum dose is 100 mg daily.
*Children younger than age 12:* 0.2 mg/kg P.O. (maximum 5 mg) as a single daily dose. Effective dosage range is usually 0.25 to 1 mg/kg daily. Maximum dose is 50 mg daily.

### ACTION
Unknown. Drug's predominant effect produces direct arteriolar vasodilation.

| Route | Onset | Peak | Duration |
|-------|-------|------|----------|
| P.O. | 30 min | 2-3 hr | 2-5 days |

### ADVERSE REACTIONS
**CV:** *edema, tachycardia, pericardial effusion and tamponade,* **heart failure,** ECG changes, rebound hypertension.
**GI:** *nausea, vomiting.*
**Metabolic:** weight gain.
**Skin:** rash, ***Stevens-Johnson syndrome.***
**Other:** *hypertrichosis,* breast tenderness.

### INTERACTIONS
**Drug-drug.** *Antihypertensives:* May cause severe orthostatic hypotension. Advise patient to stand up slowly.
*NSAIDs:* May decrease antihypertensive effects. Monitor blood pressure.
**Drug-herb.** *Ma-huang:* May decrease antihypertensive effects. Discourage use together.

### EFFECTS ON LAB TEST RESULTS
• May increase BUN, creatinine, and alkaline phosphatase levels.
• May decrease hemoglobin and hematocrit.

### CONTRAINDICATIONS & CAUTIONS
• Contraindicated in patients hypersensitive to drug and in those with pheochromocytoma. Also contraindicated in patients with acute MI or dissecting aortic aneurysm.
• Use cautiously in patients with impaired renal function and after recent MI (within past month).

### NURSING CONSIDERATIONS
• Closely monitor blood pressure and pulse rate at beginning of therapy.
• Elderly patients may be more sensitive to drug's hypotensive effects.
• Drug is removed by hemodialysis. Be sure to give dose after dialysis.
• Monitor fluid intake and urine output. Check for weight gain and edema.
• Monitor patient for elongated, thickened, and enhanced pigmentation of fine body hair.
• Minoxidil may elevate antinuclear antibody titers.
• *Alert:* Don't confuse Loniten with Lotensin.
• Because of drug may cause serious adverse reactions, don't use for milder forms of hypertension.

### PATIENT TEACHING
• Make sure patient receives and reads manufacturer's package insert that describes the drug and its adverse reactions. Also provide an oral explanation.
• Tell patient not to suddenly stop taking drug but to notify prescriber if unpleasant adverse effects occur.
• Make sure patient understands importance of compliance with total treatment regimen. Drug is usually prescribed with a beta blocker to control rapid heart rate and a diuretic to counteract fluid retention.
• Teach patient how to take his own pulse and to notify prescriber of increases of more than 20 beats/minute.
• Tell patient to weigh himself at least weekly and to report weight gain of more than 5 lb.

---

Reactions may be *common,* uncommon, *life-threatening,* or COMMON AND LIFE-THREATENING.

• About 8 of 10 patients experience elongation, thickening, and enhanced pigmentation of fine body hair within 3 to 6 weeks of beginning treatment. Shaving or using a depilatory can control unwanted hair. Assure patient that extra hair disappears within 1 to 6 months of stopping minoxidil. Advise patient not to stop drug without prescriber's approval.

• Advise women to discuss drug therapy with prescriber if considering pregnancy or currently breast-feeding.

# nisoldipine
Sular

*Pregnancy risk category C*

## AVAILABLE FORMS
*Tablets (extended-release):* 10 mg, 20 mg, 30 mg, 40 mg

## INDICATIONS & DOSAGES
➤ **Hypertension**
*Adults:* Initially, 20 mg P.O. once daily; increased by 10 mg/week or at longer intervals, p.r.n. Usual maintenance dose is 20 to 40 mg/day. Doses of more than 60 mg/day aren't recommended.
*Patients older than age 65:* Initially, 10 mg P.O. once daily; dosage is adjusted as for adults.
*Adjust-a-dose:* For patients with impaired liver function, initially, 10 mg P.O. once daily; dosage is adjusted as for adults.

## ACTION
Prevents calcium ions from entering vascular smooth-muscle cells, causing dilation of arterioles, which decreases peripheral vascular resistance.

| Route | Onset | Peak | Duration |
|-------|-------|------|----------|
| P.O. | Unknown | 6-12 hr | 24 hr |

## ADVERSE REACTIONS
**CNS:** *headache,* dizziness.
**CV:** vasodilation, palpitations, chest pain, *peripheral edema.*
**EENT:** sinusitis, pharyngitis.
**GI:** nausea.
**Skin:** rash.

## INTERACTIONS
**Drug-drug.** *Cimetidine:* May increase bioavailability and peak nisoldipine level. Monitor blood pressure closely.
*CYP 3A4 inducers such as phenytoin:* May decrease nisoldipine level. Avoid using together; consider alternative antihypertensive therapy.
*Quinidine:* May decrease bioavailability of nisoldipine. Adjust dosage accordingly.
**Drug-herb.** *Ma-huang:* May decrease antihypertensive effects. Discourage use together.
*Peppermint oil:* May decrease effect of nisoldipine. Discourage use together.
**Drug-food.** *Grapefruit, grapefruit juice:* May increase drug level, increasing adverse reactions. Discourage use together.
*High-fat foods:* May increase peak drug level. Discourage use together.

## EFFECTS ON LAB TEST RESULTS
None reported.

## CONTRAINDICATIONS & CAUTIONS
• Contraindicated in patients hypersensitive to dihydropyridine calcium channel blockers.
• Contraindicated in breast-feeding women.
• Use cautiously in patients with heart failure or compromised ventricular function, particularly those receiving beta blockers and those with severe hepatic dysfunction.

## NURSING CONSIDERATIONS
• Monitor patient carefully. Some patients, especially those with severe obstructive coronary artery disease, have developed increased frequency, duration, or severity of angina or even acute MI after starting calcium channel blocker therapy or at time of dosage increase.
• Monitor blood pressure regularly, especially when starting therapy and during dosage adjustment.

## PATIENT TEACHING
• Tell patient to take drug as prescribed, even if he feels better.
• Advise patient to swallow tablet whole and not to chew, divide, or crush it.
• Remind patient not to take drug with a high-fat meal or with grapefruit juice.

Both may increase drug level in the body beyond intended amount.

## nitroprusside sodium
Nipride†, Nitropress

*Pregnancy risk category C*

### AVAILABLE FORMS
*Injection:* 50 mg/vial in 2-ml and 5-ml vials

### INDICATIONS & DOSAGES
➤ **To lower blood pressure quickly in hypertensive emergencies, to produce controlled hypotension during anesthesia, to reduce preload and afterload in cardiac pump failure or cardiogenic shock (may be used with or without dopamine)**
*Adults and children:* Begin infusion at 0.25 to 0.3 mcg/kg/minute I.V. and gradually titrate q few minutes to a maximum infusion rate of 10 mcg/kg/minute.
***Adjust-a-dose:*** Patients taking other antihypertensives with nitroprusside are extremely sensitive to nitroprusside. Titrate dosage accordingly. Use with caution in patients with renal failure; reduce dosage as much as possible.

### I.V. ADMINISTRATION
● Don't use bacteriostatic water for injection or sterile saline solution for reconstitution.
● Prepare solution by dissolving 50 mg in 2 to 3 ml of $D_5W$ injection or according to manufacturer's instructions. Further dilute concentration in 250, 500, or 1,000 ml of $D_5W$ to provide solutions with 200, 100, or 50 mcg/ml, respectively. Reconstitute ADD-Vantage vials labeled as containing 50 mg of drug according to manufacturer's directions.
● Because drug is sensitive to light, wrap I.V. solution in foil or other opaque material; it's not necessary to wrap the tubing. Fresh solution should have faint brownish tint. Discard if highly discolored after 24 hours.
● Infuse with an infusion pump. Drug is best given via piggyback through a peripheral line with no other drug. Don't titrate rate of main I.V. line while drug is being infused. Even a small bolus of nitroprusside can cause severe hypotension.
● Check blood pressure every 5 minutes at start of infusion and every 15 minutes thereafter.
● If severe hypotension occurs, stop nitroprusside infusion—effects of drug quickly reverse. Notify prescriber.
● If possible, start an arterial pressure line. Regulate drug flow to desired blood pressure response.
● **Alert:** Excessive doses or infusion at a rate greater than 10 mcg/kg/minute can cause cyanide toxicity. If these factors are present, check thiocyanate level every 72 hours. Level higher than 100 mcg/ml may be toxic. If profound hypotension, metabolic acidosis, dyspnea, headache, loss of consciousness, ataxia, or vomiting occurs, stop drug immediately and notify prescriber.

### ACTION
Relaxes both arteriolar and venous smooth muscle.

| Route | Onset | Peak | Duration |
|-------|-------|------|----------|
| I.V. | Immediate | 1-2 min | 10 min |

### ADVERSE REACTIONS
**CNS:** *headache, dizziness,* loss of consciousness, apprehension, ***increased ICP,*** restlessness.
**CV:** ***bradycardia,*** hypotension, tachycardia, palpitations, ECG changes, flushing.
**GI:** *nausea, abdominal pain,* ileus.
**Hematologic:** ***methemoglobinemia.***
**Metabolic:** acidosis, hypothyroidism.
**Musculoskeletal:** *muscle twitching.*
**Skin:** pink color, rash, *diaphoresis.*
**Other:** ***thiocyanate toxicity, cyanide toxicity,*** venous streaking, irritation at infusion site.

### INTERACTIONS
**Drug-drug.** *Antihypertensives:* May cause sensitivity to nitroprusside. Adjust dosage. *Ganglionic blocking drugs, general anesthetics, negative inotropic drugs, other antihypertensives:* May cause additive effects. Monitor blood pressure closely. *Sildenafil, vardenafil:* May increase hypotensive effects. Monitor blood pressure.

**EFFECTS ON LAB TEST RESULTS**
• May increase creatinine level.
• May decrease RBC and WBC counts.

**CONTRAINDICATIONS & CAUTIONS**
• Contraindicated in patients hypersensitive to drug.
• Contraindicated in those with compensatory hypertension (such as in arteriovenous shunt or coarctation of the aorta), inadequate cerebral circulation, acute heart failure with reduced peripheral vascular resistance, congenital optic atrophy, or tobacco-induced amblyopia.
• Use with extreme caution in patients with increased intracranial pressure.
• Use cautiously in patients with hypothyroidism, hepatic or renal disease, hyponatremia, or low vitamin $B_{12}$ level.

**NURSING CONSIDERATIONS**
• Obtain baseline vital signs before giving drug; find out parameters prescriber wants to achieve.
• Keep patient in the supine position when starting therapy or titrating drug.
• *Alert:* Don't confuse nitroprusside with nitroglycerin.

**PATIENT TEACHING**
• Instruct patient to report adverse reactions promptly.
• Tell patient to alert nurse if discomfort occurs at I.V. insertion site.

---

**olmesartan medoxomil**
Benicar🕮

*Pregnancy risk category C; D in
second and third trimesters*

**AVAILABLE FORMS**
*Tablets:* 5 mg, 20 mg, 40 mg

**INDICATIONS AND DOSAGES**
➤ **Hypertension**
*Adults:* 20 mg P.O. once daily if patient has no volume depletion. May increase dosage to 40 mg P.O. once daily if blood pressure isn't reduced after 2 weeks of therapy.
*Adjust-a-dose:* In patients with possible depletion of intravascular volume (those with impaired renal function who are tak-

ing diuretics), consider using lower starting dose.

**ACTION**
Blocks the vasoconstrictor and aldosterone-secreting effects of angiotensin II by selectively blocking the binding of angiotensin II to the angiotensin I receptor in the vascular smooth muscle.

| Route | Onset | Peak | Duration |
|-------|-------|------|----------|
| P.O. | Rapid | 1-2 hr | 24 hr |

**ADVERSE REACTIONS**
**CNS:** headache.
**EENT:** pharyngitis, rhinitis, sinusitis.
**GI:** diarrhea.
**GU:** hematuria.
**Metabolic:** hyperglycemia, hypertriglyceridemia.
**Musculoskeletal:** back pain.
**Respiratory:** bronchitis, upper respiratory tract infection.
**Other:** flulike symptoms, accidental injury.

**INTERACTIONS**
**Drug-herb.** *Ma-huang:* May decrease antihypertensive effects. Discourage use together.

**EFFECTS ON LAB TEST RESULTS**
• May increase glucose, triglyceride, uric acid, liver enzyme, bilirubin, and creatine phosphokinase levels.
• May decrease hemoglobin and hematocrit.

**CONTRAINDICATIONS & CAUTIONS**
• Contraindicated in patients hypersensitive to the drug or any of its components and in patients who are pregnant.
• Use cautiously in patients who are volume- or salt-depleted, those whose renal function depends on the renin-angiotensin-aldosterone system (such as patients with severe heart failure), and those with unilateral and bilateral renal-artery stenosis.
• It's unknown if drug appears in breast milk. Patient should stop either breast-feeding or drug.
• Safety and efficacy in children haven't been established. Don't give drug to children.

---

## NURSING CONSIDERATIONS
- Symptomatic hypotension may occur in patients who are volume- or salt-depleted, especially those being treated with high doses of a diuretic. If hypotension occurs, place patient supine and treat supportively. Treatment may continue once blood pressure is stabilized.
- If blood pressure isn't adequately controlled, a diuretic or other antihypertensive drugs also may be prescribed.
- Overdose may cause hypotension and tachycardia, along with bradycardia from parasympathetic (vagal) stimulation. Treatment should be supportive.
- Closely monitor patients with heart failure for oliguria, azotemia, and acute renal failure.
- Monitor BUN and creatinine level in patients with unilateral or bilateral renal artery stenosis.
- Drugs that act on the renin-angiotensin system may cause fetal and neonatal complications and death when given to pregnant women after the first trimester. If patient taking drug becomes pregnant, stop drug immediately.

## PATIENT TEACHING
- Tell patient to take drug exactly as prescribed and not to stop taking it even if he feels better.
- Tell patient that drug may be taken without regard to meals.
- Tell patient to report to health care provider any adverse reactions promptly, especially light-headedness and fainting.
- Advise women of childbearing age to immediately report pregnancy to health care provider.
- Inform diabetic patients that glucose readings may rise and that the dosage of their diabetes drugs may need adjustment.
- Warn patients that inadequate fluid intake, excessive perspiration, diarrhea, or vomiting may lead to an excessive drop in blood pressure, light-headedness, and possibly fainting.
- Instruct patients that other antihypertensives can have additive effects. Patient should inform his prescriber of all medications he's taking, including OTC drugs.

# perindopril erbumine
Aceon

*Pregnancy risk category C; D in second and third trimesters*

## AVAILABLE FORMS
*Tablets:* 2 mg, 4 mg, 8 mg

## INDICATIONS & DOSAGES
➤ **Essential hypertension**
*Adults:* Initially, 4 mg P.O. once daily. Increase dosage until blood pressure is controlled or to maximum of 16 mg/day; usual maintenance dose is 4 to 8 mg once daily; may be given in two divided doses.
*Patients older than age 65:* Initially, 4 mg P.O. daily as one dose or in two divided doses. Dosage may be increased by more than 8 mg/day only under close medical supervision.
***Adjust-a-dose:*** For patients with renal insufficiency, initially 2 mg P.O. daily. Maximum daily maintenance dose is 8 mg. In patients taking diuretics, initially 2 to 4 mg P.O. daily as single dose or in two divided doses, with close medical supervision for several hours and until blood pressure has stabilized. Adjust dosage based on patient's blood pressure response.

## ACTION
A prodrug that is converted by the liver to the active metabolite perindoprilat, which inhibits ACE activity, thereby preventing conversion of angiotensin I to angiotensin II, a potent vasoconstrictor. Inhibition of ACE results in decreased vasoconstriction and decreased aldosterone activity, thus reducing sodium and water retention and lowering blood pressure.

| Route | Onset | Peak | Duration |
|-------|-------|------|----------|
| P.O. | Unknown | 1 hr | Unknown |

## ADVERSE REACTIONS
**CNS:** dizziness, asthenia, sleep disorder, paresthesia, depression, somnolence, nervousness, *headache*, fever.
**CV:** palpitations, edema, chest pain, abnormal ECG.
**EENT:** rhinitis, sinusitis, ear infection, pharyngitis, tinnitus.

**GI:** dyspepsia, diarrhea, abdominal pain, nausea, vomiting, flatulence.

**GU:** proteinuria, UTI, male sexual dysfunction, menstrual disorder.

**Musculoskeletal:** back pain, hypertonia, neck pain, joint pain, myalgia, arthritis, arm or leg pain.

**Respiratory:** *cough,* upper respiratory tract infection.

**Skin:** rash.

**Other:** viral infection, injury, seasonal allergy.

### INTERACTIONS

**Drug-drug.** *Diuretics:* May increase hypotensive effect. Monitor patient closely.

*Lithium:* May increase lithium level and risk of lithium toxicity. Use together cautiously; monitor lithium level.

*NSAIDs:* May decrease antihypertensive effects. Monitor blood pressure.

*Potassium-sparing diuretics (amiloride, spironolactone, triamterene), potassium supplements, other drugs capable of increasing potassium level (cyclosporine, heparin, indomethacin):* May increase hyperkalemic effect. Use together cautiously; monitor potassium level frequently.

**Drug-herb.** *Capsaicin:* May cause cough. Discourage use together.

*Ma-huang:* May decrease antihypertensive effects. Discourage use together.

**Drug-food.** *Salt substitutes containing potassium:* May cause hyperkalemia. Discourage use together.

### EFFECTS ON LAB TEST RESULTS

● May increase ALT and triglyceride levels.

### CONTRAINDICATIONS & CAUTIONS

● Contraindicated in patients hypersensitive to drug or other ACE inhibitors and in those with a history of angioedema secondary to ACE inhibitors.

● Contraindicated in pregnant women.

● Use cautiously in patients with a history of angioedema unrelated to ACE inhibitor therapy.

● Use cautiously in patients with renal impairment, heart failure, ischemic heart disease, cerebrovascular disease, or renal artery stenosis, and in those with collagen vascular disease, such as systemic lupus erythematosus or scleroderma.

### NURSING CONSIDERATIONS

● Although ACE inhibitors reduce blood pressure in all races studied, this response is less in black patients who receive the drug alone. Therapy with a thiazide diuretic produces a more favorable response.

● ACE inhibitors appear to increase risk of angioedema in black patients.

● *Alert:* Angioedema involving the face, extremities, lips, tongue, glottis, and larynx may occur. Stop drug and observe patient until swelling disappears. If swelling is confined to face and lips, it will probably resolve without treatment, but antihistamines may be useful in relieving symptoms. Angioedema of the tongue, glottis, or larynx may be fatal because of airway obstruction. Give appropriate therapy, such as S.C. epinephrine solution, promptly.

● Patients with a history of angioedema unrelated to ACE inhibitor therapy may be at increased risk for angioedema while receiving an ACE inhibitor.

● Other ACE inhibitors have caused agranulocytosis and neutropenia. Monitor CBC with differential before therapy, especially in renally impaired patients with systemic lupus erythematosus or scleroderma.

● Excessive hypotension can occur when drug is given with diuretics. If possible, stop diuretic 2 to 3 days before starting perindopril, to reduce the potential for excessive hypotensive response. If it isn't possible to stop the diuretic, consider starting perindopril with a lower dosage or decreasing dosage of diuretic.

● Monitor patient at risk for hypotension closely during initiation of therapy, for first 2 weeks of treatment, and whenever dosage of perindopril or concomitant diuretic is increased. If severe hypotension occurs, place patient in supine position and treat symptomatically.

● Hypotension can occur when starting therapy or adjusting dosage in patient who is volume- or salt-depleted from prolonged diuretic therapy, dietary salt restriction, dialysis, diarrhea, or vomiting. Correct volume and salt depletion before starting drug.

● ACE inhibitors rarely have been linked to a syndrome of cholestatic jaundice, fulminant hepatic necrosis, and death. Stop drug in patient who develops jaundice or

---

*Rapid onset* †Canada ‡Australia ◇OTC ◆ Off-label use ✐Photoguide *Liquid contains alcohol.

marked elevations of hepatic enzyme levels during therapy.
• Monitor renal function before and periodically throughout therapy. Don't use drug in patient with a creatinine clearance less than 30 ml/minute.
• Monitor potassium level closely.

**PATIENT TEACHING**
• Inform patient that throat and facial swelling, including swelling of the larynx, can occur during therapy, especially with the first dose. Advise patient to stop taking drug and immediately report any signs or symptoms of swelling of face, extremities, eyes, lips, or tongue; hoarseness; or difficulty in swallowing or breathing.
• Advise patient to report promptly any sign or symptom of infection (sore throat, fever) or jaundice (yellowing of eyes or skin).
• Advise patient to avoid salt substitutes containing potassium unless instructed otherwise by prescriber.
• Caution patient that light-headedness may occur, especially during first few days of therapy. Advise patient to report light-headedness and, if fainting occurs, to stop drug and consult prescriber promptly.
• Caution patient that inadequate fluid intake or excessive perspiration, diarrhea, or vomiting can lead to an excessive drop in blood pressure.
• Advise woman of childbearing age of the consequences of second- and third-trimester exposure to drug. Advise her to notify prescriber immediately if she suspects pregnancy.

# pindolol
Barbloc‡, Novo-Pindol†, Syn-Pindolol†, Visken

*Pregnancy risk category B*

**AVAILABLE FORMS**
*Tablets:* 5 mg, 10 mg, 15 mg‡

**INDICATIONS & DOSAGES**
➤ **Hypertension**
*Adults:* Initially, 5 mg P.O. b.i.d. Dosage may be increased as needed and tolerated, to maximum of 60 mg daily.

➤ **Chronic stable angina pectoris ◆**
*Adults:* 15 to 40 mg P.O. daily in three or four divided doses.

**ACTION**
Unknown. A nonselective beta blocker that has intrinsic sympathomimetic activity. Possible mechanisms include reduced cardiac output, decreased sympathetic outflow to peripheral vasculature, and inhibited renin release by the kidneys.

| Route | Onset | Peak | Duration |
|-------|-------|------|----------|
| P.O. | Unknown | 1-2 hr | 24 hr |

**ADVERSE REACTIONS**
**CNS:** *insomnia, fatigue, dizziness, nervousness,* vivid dreams, weakness, paresthesia.
**CV:** *edema, **bradycardia, heart failure,*** chest pain.
**GI:** *nausea,* abdominal discomfort.
**Musculoskeletal:** *muscle pain, joint pain.*
**Respiratory:** *increased airway resistance,* dyspnea.
**Skin:** rash, pruritus.

**INTERACTIONS**
**Drug-drug.** *Aminophylline, theophylline:* May act antagonistically, reducing the effects of one or both drugs. May reduce elimination of theophylline. Monitor theophylline level and patient closely.
*Cardiac glycosides, diltiazem:* May cause excessive bradycardia and increase depression of AV node. Use together cautiously.
*Catecholamine-depleting drugs such as reserpine:* May have additive effects. Monitor patient for hypotension and bradycardia.
*Epinephrine:* May cause an hypertensive episode followed by bradycardia. Stop beta blocker 3 days before anticipated epinephrine use. Monitor patient closely.
*Indomethacin, NSAIDs:* May decrease antihypertensive effect. Monitor blood pressure and adjust dosage.
*Insulin:* May mask symptoms of hypoglycemia as a result of beta blockade (such as tachycardia). Use together cautiously in patients with diabetes.
*I.V. lidocaine:* May reduce hepatic metabolism of lidocaine, increasing the risk of toxicity. Give bolus doses of lidocaine at a

slower rate, and monitor lidocaine level closely.

*Oral antidiabetics:* May alter requirements for these drugs in previously stabilized diabetic patients. Monitor patient for hypoglycemia.

*Prazosin:* May increase risk of orthostatic hypotension in the early phases of use together. Assist patient to stand slowly until effects are known.

*Thioridazine:* May prolong QTc interval and increase the risk of potentially fatal cardiac arrhythmias; may increase drug level. Avoid using together.

*Verapamil:* May increase effects of both drugs. Monitor cardiac function closely and decrease dosages as necessary.

**Drug-herb.** *Ma-huang:* May decrease antihypertensive effects. Discourage use together.

**EFFECTS ON LAB TEST RESULTS**
• May increase transaminase, alkaline phosphatase, LDH, AST, ALT, and uric acid levels.

**CONTRAINDICATIONS & CAUTIONS**
• Contraindicated in patients hypersensitive to drug and in those taking thioridazine.
• Contraindicated in those with bronchial asthma, severe bradycardia, greater than first-degree heart block, cardiogenic shock, or overt cardiac failure.
• Use cautiously in patients with heart failure, nonallergic bronchospastic disease, diabetes, hyperthyroidism, and impaired renal or hepatic function.

**NURSING CONSIDERATIONS**
• Always check patient's apical pulse rate before giving drug. If extremes in pulse rate are detected, withhold drug and call prescriber immediately.
• Monitor blood pressure frequently and notify prescriber if severe hypotension occurs. A vasopressor may be needed.
• Withdraw drug over 1 or 2 weeks after long-term therapy.
• Monitor glucose level in diabetic patients closely because drug masks certain signs and symptoms of hypoglycemia.
• Beta blockers may mask tachycardia caused by hyperthyroidism. In patients with suspected thyrotoxicosis, withdraw

beta blocker gradually to avoid thyroid storm.
• **Alert:** Don't confuse pindolol with Parlodel, Panadol, or Plendil.
• **Alert:** Don't confuse Visken with Visine.

**PATIENT TEACHING**
• Advise patient to take drug exactly as prescribed.
• Tell patient not to stop drug suddenly, but to notify prescriber to discuss unpleasant adverse drug reactions.
• Inform patient that drug may deplete body's stores of coenzyme Q10 and that he should discuss need for supplements with prescriber.

---

## prazosin hydrochloride
Minipress

*Pregnancy risk category C*

---

**AVAILABLE FORMS**
*Capsules:* 1 mg, 2 mg, 5 mg

**INDICATIONS & DOSAGES**
➤ **Mild to moderate hypertension, alone or with a diuretic or other antihypertensive**
*Adults:* Test dose is 1 mg P.O. h.s. to prevent first-dose syncope (severe syncope with loss of consciousness). First dosage is 1 mg P.O. b.i.d. or t.i.d. Dosage may be increased slowly. Maximum daily dose is 20 mg. Maintenance dosage is 6 to 15 mg daily in three divided doses. Some patients need larger dosages (up to 40 mg daily). If other antihypertensives or diuretics are added to therapy, decrease prazosin dosage to 1 to 2 mg t.i.d. and readjust to maintenance dosage.
➤ **Benign prostatic hyperplasia**
*Adults:* 2 mg P.O. b.i.d. Dose range is 1 to 9 mg P.O. daily.

**ACTION**
Unknown. Drug's alpha-blocking activity is thought to account primarily for its effects.

| Route | Onset | Peak | Duration |
|-------|-------|------|----------|
| P.O. | 30-90 min | 2-4 hr | 7-10 hr |

## ADVERSE REACTIONS
**CNS:** *dizziness,* headache, drowsiness, nervousness, paresthesia, weakness, *first-dose syncope,* depression, fever.
**CV:** orthostatic hypotension, palpitations, edema.
**EENT:** blurred vision, tinnitus, conjunctivitis, epistaxis, nasal congestion.
**GI:** vomiting, diarrhea, abdominal cramps, nausea.
**GU:** priapism, impotence, urinary frequency, incontinence.
**Musculoskeletal:** arthralgia, myalgia.
**Respiratory:** dyspnea.
**Skin:** pruritus.

## INTERACTIONS
**Drug-drug.** *Acebutolol, atenolol, betaxolol, carteolol, esmolol, metoprolol, nadolol, pindolol, propranolol, sotalol, timolol:* May increase the risk of orthostatic hypotension in the early phases of use together. Help patient stand slowly until effects are known.
*Diuretics:* May increase frequency of syncope with loss of consciousness. Advise patient to sit or lie down if dizziness occurs.
*Verapamil:* May increase prazosin level. Monitor patient closely.
**Drug-herb.** *Butcher's broom:* May reduce effect. Discourage use together.
*Ma-huang:* May decrease antihypertensive effects. Discourage use together.

## EFFECTS ON LAB TEST RESULTS
• May increase BUN and uric acid levels.
• May increase liver function test values.

## CONTRAINDICATIONS & CAUTIONS
• Contraindicated in patients hypersensitive to drug or other alpha blockers.
• Use cautiously in patients receiving other antihypertensives.

## NURSING CONSIDERATIONS
• Monitor patient's blood pressure and pulse rate frequently.
• Elderly patients may be more sensitive to drug's hypotensive effects.
• Compliance might be improved with twice-daily dosing. Discuss this dosing change with prescriber if compliance problems are suspected.

• Drug alters results of screening tests for pheochromocytoma and causes increases in levels of the urinary metabolite of nor-epinephrine and vanillylmandelic acid; it may cause positive antinuclear antibody titer.
• *Alert:* If first dose is more than 1 mg, first-dose syncope may occur.

## PATIENT TEACHING
• Warn patient that dizziness may occur with first dose. If he experiences dizziness, tell him to sit or lie down. Reassure him that this effect disappears with continued dosing.
• Caution patient to avoid driving or performing hazardous tasks for the first 24 hours after starting this drug or increasing the dose.
• Tell patient not to suddenly stop taking drug, but to notify prescriber if unpleasant adverse reactions occur.
• Advise patient to minimize low blood pressure and dizziness upon standing by rising slowly and avoiding sudden position changes. Dry mouth can be relieved by chewing gum or sucking on hard candy or ice chips.

---

# quinapril hydrochloride
Accupril✦, Asig‡

*Pregnancy risk category C; D in second and third trimesters*

## AVAILABLE FORMS
*Tablets:* 5 mg, 10 mg, 20 mg, 40 mg

## INDICATIONS & DOSAGES
➤ **Hypertension**
*Adults:* Initially, 10 to 20 mg P.O. daily. Dosage may be adjusted based on patient response at intervals of about 2 weeks. Most patients are controlled at 20, 40, or 80 mg daily as a single dose or in two divided doses. If patient is taking a diuretic, start therapy with 5 mg daily.
*Elderly patients:* For patients older than age 65, start therapy at 10 mg P.O. daily.
*Adjust-a-dose:* For adults with creatinine clearance over 60 ml/minute, initially, 10 mg maximum dose; for clearance 30 to 60 ml/minute, 5 mg; for clearance 10 to 30 ml/minute, 2.5 mg.

---

➤ **Heart failure**
*Adults:* Initially, 5 mg P.O. b.i.d. if patient is taking a diuretic and 10 to 20 mg P.O. b.i.d. if patient isn't taking a diuretic. Dosage may be increased at weekly intervals. Usual effective dose is 20 to 40 mg daily in two equally divided doses.
*Adjust-a-dose:* For patients with creatinine clearance over 30 ml/minute, first dose is 5 mg daily; if clearance is 10 to 30 ml/minute, 2.5 mg.

## ACTION
Unknown. Thought to be involved with inhibiting conversion of angiotensin I to angiotensin II, a potent vasoconstrictor. Reduced formation of angiotensin II decreases peripheral arterial resistance, thus decreasing aldosterone secretion.

| Route | Onset | Peak | Duration |
|-------|-------|------|----------|
| P.O. | 1 hr | 2-6 hr | 24 hr |

## ADVERSE REACTIONS
**CNS:** somnolence, vertigo, nervousness, headache, dizziness, fatigue, depression.
**CV:** palpitations, tachycardia, angina pectoris, *hypertensive crisis,* orthostatic hypotension, rhythm disturbances.
**GI:** dry mouth, abdominal pain, constipation, vomiting, nausea, *hemorrhage,* diarrhea.
**Metabolic:** *hyperkalemia.*
**Respiratory:** dry, persistent, tickling, nonproductive cough.
**Skin:** pruritus, photosensitivity reactions, diaphoresis.

## INTERACTIONS
**Drug-drug.** *Diuretics, other antihypertensives:* May cause excessive hypotension. Stop diuretic or reduce dose of quinapril, as needed.
*Lithium:* May increase lithium level and lithium toxicity. Monitor lithium level.
*NSAIDs:* May decrease antihypertensive effects. Monitor blood pressure.
*Potassium-sparing diuretics, potassium supplements:* May cause hyperkalemia. Monitor patient closely.
*Tetracycline:* May decrease absorption if taken with quinapril. Avoid using together.
**Drug-herb.** *Capsaicin:* May cause cough. Discourage use together.

*Ma-huang:* May decrease antihypertensive effects. Discourage use together.
**Drug-food.** *Salt substitutes containing potassium:* May cause hyperkalemia. Discourage use together.

## EFFECTS ON LAB TEST RESULTS
● May increase potassium level.
● May increase liver function test values.

## CONTRAINDICATIONS & CAUTIONS
● Contraindicated in patients hypersensitive to ACE inhibitors and in those with a history of angioedema related to treatment with an ACE inhibitor.
● Use cautiously in patients with impaired renal function.

## NURSING CONSIDERATIONS
● Assess renal and hepatic function before and periodically throughout therapy.
● Monitor blood pressure for effectiveness of therapy.
● Monitor potassium level. Risk factors for the development of hyperkalemia include renal insufficiency, diabetes, and concomitant use of drugs that raise potassium level.
● Although ACE inhibitors reduce blood pressure in all races studied, this response is less in black patients who receive the drug as monotherapy. Therapy with a thiazide diuretic produces a more favorable response.
● ACE inhibitors appear to increase risk of angioedema in black patients.
● Other ACE inhibitors have caused agranulocytosis and neutropenia. Monitor CBC with differential counts before therapy and periodically thereafter.

## PATIENT TEACHING
● Advise patient to report signs of infection, such as fever and sore throat.
● *Alert:* Facial and throat swelling (including swelling of the larynx) may occur, especially after first dose. Advise patient to report signs or symptoms of breathing difficulty or swelling of face, eyes, lips, or tongue.
● Light-headedness can occur, especially during first few days of therapy. Tell patient to rise slowly to minimize effect and to report signs and symptoms to prescriber.

---

If he faints, patient should stop taking drug and call prescriber immediately.

• Inform patient that inadequate fluid intake, vomiting, diarrhea, and excessive perspiration can lead to light-headedness and fainting. Tell him to use caution in hot weather and during exercise.

• Tell patient to avoid salt substitutes. These products may contain potassium, which can cause high potassium level in patients taking quinapril.

• Advise women to notify prescriber if pregnancy occurs. Drug will need to be stopped.

## ramipril
Altace, Ramace‡, Tritace‡

*Pregnancy risk category C; D in second and third trimesters*

### AVAILABLE FORMS
*Capsules:* 1.25 mg, 2.5 mg, 5 mg, 10 mg

### INDICATIONS & DOSAGES
➤ **Hypertension**
*Adults:* Initially, 2.5 mg P.O. once daily for patients not taking a diuretic, and 1.25 mg P.O. once daily for patients taking a diuretic. Increase dosage, p.r.n., based on patient response. Maintenance dose is 2.5 to 20 mg daily as a single dose or in divided doses.
*Adjust-a-dose:* For patients with creatinine clearance less than 40 ml/minute, give 1.25 mg P.O. daily. Adjust dosage gradually based on response. Maximum daily dose is 5 mg.
➤ **Heart failure**
*Adults:* Initially, 2.5 mg P.O. b.i.d. If hypotension occurs, decrease dosage to 1.25 mg P.O. b.i.d. Adjust as tolerated to target dosage of 5 mg P.O. twice daily.
*Adjust-a-dose:* For patients with creatinine clearance less than 40 ml/minute, give 1.25 mg P.O. daily. Adjust dosage gradually based on response; maximum 2.5 mg b.i.d.
➤ **To reduce risk of MI, stroke, and death from CV causes**
*Adults age 55 and older:* 2.5 mg P.O. once daily for 1 week, then 5 mg P.O. once daily for 3 weeks. Increase as tolerated to a

maintenance dose of 10 mg P.O. once daily.
*Adjust-a-dose:* In patients who are hypertensive or who have recently had an MI, daily dose may be divided.

### ACTION
Unknown. Thought to be involved with inhibiting conversion of angiotensin I to angiotensin II, a potent vasoconstrictor. Reduced formation of angiotensin II decreases peripheral arterial resistance, thus decreasing aldosterone secretion.

| Route | Onset | Peak | Duration |
|-------|-------|------|----------|
| P.O. | 1-2 hr | 1-3 hr | 24 hr |

### ADVERSE REACTIONS
**CNS:** headache, dizziness, fatigue, asthenia, malaise, light-headedness, anxiety, amnesia, depression, insomnia, nervousness, neuralgia, neuropathy, paresthesia, somnolence, tremor, vertigo, syncope.
**CV:** *heart failure, hypotension,* postural hypotension, angina pectoris, chest pain, palpitations, *MI,* edema.
**EENT:** epistaxis, tinnitus.
**GI:** nausea, vomiting, abdominal pain, anorexia, constipation, diarrhea, dyspepsia, dry mouth, gastroenteritis.
**GU:** impotence.
**Metabolic:** hyperglycemia, *hyperkalemia,* weight gain.
**Musculoskeletal:** arthralgia, arthritis, myalgia.
**Respiratory:** dyspnea; dry, persistent, tickling, nonproductive cough.
**Skin:** rash, dermatitis, pruritus, photosensitivity reactions, increased diaphoresis.
**Other:** hypersensitivity reactions.

### INTERACTIONS
**Drug-drug.** *Diuretics:* May cause excessive hypotension, especially at start of therapy. Stop diuretic at least 3 days before therapy begins, increase sodium intake, or reduce starting dose of ramipril.
*Insulin, oral antidiabetics:* May cause hypoglycemia, especially at start of ramipril therapy. Monitor patient closely.
*Lithium:* May increase lithium level. Use together cautiously and monitor lithium level.
*Nesiritide:* May increase hypotensive effects. Monitor blood pressure.

---

Reactions may be *common,* uncommon, *life-threatening,* or COMMON AND LIFE-THREATENING.

*NSAIDs:* May decrease antihypertensive effects. Monitor blood pressure.
*Potassium-sparing diuretics, potassium supplements:* May cause hyperkalemia; ramipril attenuates potassium loss. Monitor potassium level closely.
**Drug-herb.** *Capsaicin:* May cause cough. Discourage use together.
*Ma-huang:* May decrease antihypertensive effects. Discourage use together.
**Drug-food.** *Salt substitutes containing potassium:* May cause hyperkalemia; ramipril attenuates potassium loss. Discourage use of salt substitutes during therapy.

## EFFECTS ON LAB TEST RESULTS
● May increase BUN, creatinine, bilirubin, liver enzymes, glucose, and potassium levels.
● May decrease hemoglobin, hematocrit, and RBC and platelet counts.

## CONTRAINDICATIONS & CAUTIONS
● Contraindicated in patients hypersensitive to ACE inhibitors and in those with a history of angioedema related to treatment with an ACE inhibitor.
● Use cautiously in patients with renal impairment.

## NURSING CONSIDERATIONS
● Monitor blood pressure regularly for drug effectiveness.
● Closely assess renal function in patients during first few weeks of therapy. Regular assessment of renal function is advisable. Patients with severe heart failure whose renal function depends on the renin-angiotensin-aldosterone system have experienced acute renal failure during ACE inhibitor therapy. Hypertensive patients with renal artery stenosis also may show signs of worsening renal function during first few days of therapy.
● Although ACE inhibitors reduce blood pressure in all races studied, this response is less in black patients who receive the drug as monotherapy. Therapy with a thiazide diuretic produces a more favorable response.
● ACE inhibitors appear to increase risk of angioedema in black patients.
● Monitor CBC with differential counts before therapy and periodically thereafter.

Drug may reduce hemoglobin and WBC, RBC, and platelet counts, especially in patients with impaired renal function or collagen vascular diseases (systemic lupus erythematosus or scleroderma).
● Monitor potassium level. Risk factors for the development of hyperkalemia include renal insufficiency, diabetes, and concomitant use of drugs that raise potassium level.

## PATIENT TEACHING
● Tell patient to notify prescriber if any adverse reactions occur. Dosage adjustment or discontinuation of drug may be needed.
● *Alert:* Rarely, swelling of the face and throat (including swelling of the larynx) may occur, especially after first dose. Advise patient to report signs or symptoms of breathing difficulty or swelling of face, eyes, lips, or tongue.
● Inform patient that light-headedness can occur, especially during the first few days of therapy. Tell him to rise slowly to minimize this effect and to report signs and symptoms to prescriber. If he faints, patient should stop taking drug and call prescriber immediately.
● Tell patient that if he has difficulty swallowing capsules, he can open drug and sprinkle contents on a small amount of applesauce.
● Advise patient to report signs and symptoms of infection, such as fever and sore throat.
● Tell patient to avoid salt substitutes. These products may contain potassium, which can cause high potassium level in patients taking ramipril.
● Tell women to notify prescriber if pregnancy occurs. Drug will need to be stopped.

----

# telmisartan
Micardis

*Pregnancy risk category C; D in second and third trimesters*

## AVAILABLE FORMS
*Tablets:* 40 mg, 80 mg

----

## INDICATIONS & DOSAGES
➤ **Hypertension (used alone or with other antihypertensives)**
*Adults:* 40 mg P.O. daily. Blood pressure response is dose-related over a range of 20 to 80 mg daily.

## ACTION
Blocks the vasoconstricting and aldosterone-secreting effects of angiotensin II by selectively blocking the binding of angiotensin II to the angiotensin I receptor in many tissues, such as vascular smooth muscle and the adrenal gland.

| Route | Onset | Peak | Duration |
|-------|-------|------|----------|
| P.O. | Unknown | 30-60 min | 24 hr |

## ADVERSE REACTIONS
**CNS:** dizziness, pain, fatigue, headache.
**CV:** chest pain, hypertension, peripheral edema.
**EENT:** pharyngitis, sinusitis.
**GI:** abdominal pain, diarrhea, dyspepsia, *nausea.*
**GU:** UTI.
**Musculoskeletal:** back pain, myalgia.
**Respiratory:** cough, upper respiratory tract infection.
**Other:** flulike symptoms.

## INTERACTIONS
**Drug-drug.** *Digoxin:* May increase digoxin level. Monitor digoxin level closely.
*Warfarin:* May decrease warfarin level. Monitor INR.
**Drug-herb.** *Ma-huang:* May decrease antihypertensive effects. Discourage use together.
**Drug-food.** *Salt substitutes containing potassium:* May cause hyperkalemia. Discourage use together.

## EFFECTS ON LAB TEST RESULTS
● May increase liver enzyme levels.

## CONTRAINDICATIONS & CAUTIONS
● Contraindicated in patients hypersensitive to drug or its components.
● Use cautiously in patients with biliary obstruction disorders or renal and hepatic insufficiency and in those with an activated renin-angiotensin system, such as volume- or salt-depleted patients (for ex-

ample, those being treated with high doses of diuretics).
● Drugs such as telmisartan that act on the renin-angiotensin system can cause fetal and neonatal morbidity and death when given to pregnant women. These problems haven't been detected when exposure has been limited to the first trimester. If pregnancy is suspected, notify prescriber because drug should be stopped.

## NURSING CONSIDERATIONS
● Monitor patient for hypotension after starting drug. Place patient supine if hypotension occurs, and give I.V. normal saline, if needed.
● Most of the antihypertensive effect occurs within 2 weeks. Maximal blood pressure reduction is usually reached after 4 weeks. Diuretic may be added if blood pressure isn't controlled by drug alone.
● For patients whose renal function may depend on the activity of the renin-angiotensin-aldosterone system (such as those with severe heart failure), treatment with ACE inhibitors and angiotensin receptor antagonists has caused oliguria or progressive azotemia and (rarely) acute renal failure or death.
● Drug isn't removed by hemodialysis. Patients undergoing dialysis may develop orthostatic hypotension. Closely monitor blood pressure.

## PATIENT TEACHING
● Instruct patient to report suspected pregnancy to prescriber immediately.
● Inform woman of childbearing age of the consequences of second- and third-trimester exposure to drug.
● Advise breast-feeding woman about risk of adverse drug effects in infants and the need to stop either drug or breast-feeding.
● Tell patient that if he feels dizzy or has low blood pressure on standing, he should lie down, rise slowly from a lying to standing position, and climb stairs slowly.
● Tell patient that drug may be taken without regard to meals.
● Tell patient not to remove drug from blister-sealed packet until immediately before use.

## terazosin hydrochloride
Hytrin◆

*Pregnancy risk category C*

### AVAILABLE FORMS
*Capsules:* 1 mg, 2 mg, 5 mg, 10 mg
*Tablets:* 1 mg, 2 mg, 5 mg, 10 mg

### INDICATIONS & DOSAGES
➤ **Hypertension**
*Adults:* Initially, 1 mg P.O. h.s. Dosage may be increased gradually based on response. Usual dosage range is 1 to 5 mg daily. Maximum recommended dose is 20 mg daily.
➤ **Symptomatic BPH**
*Adults:* Initially, 1 mg P.O. h.s. Dosage may be increased in a stepwise fashion to 2, 5, or 10 mg once daily to achieve optimal response. Most patients need 10 mg daily for optimal response.

### ACTION
May decrease blood pressure by vasodilation produced in response to blockade of alpha-adrenergic receptors. It improves urine flow in patients with BPH by blocking alpha-adrenergic receptors in the smooth muscle of the bladder neck and prostate, thus relieving urethral pressure and reestablishing urine flow.

| Route | Onset | Peak | Duration |
|-------|-------|------|----------|
| P.O. | 15 min | 2-3 hr | 24 hr |

### ADVERSE REACTIONS
**CNS:** asthenia, *dizziness, headache,* nervousness, paresthesia, somnolence.
**CV:** palpitations, orthostatic hypotension, tachycardia, *peripheral edema,* atrial fibrillation.
**EENT:** *nasal congestion,* sinusitis, blurred vision.
**GI:** nausea.
**GU:** impotence, priapism.
**Hematologic:** *thrombocytopenia.*
**Musculoskeletal:** back pain, muscle pain.
**Respiratory:** dyspnea.

### INTERACTIONS
**Drug-drug.** *Antihypertensives:* May cause excessive hypotension. Use together cautiously.
*Clonidine:* May decrease clonidine's antihypertensive effect. Monitor patient.
**Drug-herb.** *Butcher's broom:* May cause diminished effect of drug. Discourage use together.
*Ma-huang:* May decrease antihypertensive effects. Discourage use together.

### EFFECTS ON LAB TEST RESULTS
● May decrease total protein and albumin levels.
● May decrease hematocrit, hemoglobin, and WBC and platelet counts.

### CONTRAINDICATIONS & CAUTIONS
● Contraindicated in patients hypersensitive to drug.

### NURSING CONSIDERATIONS
● Monitor blood pressure frequently.
● *Alert:* If terazosin is stopped for several days, readjust dosage using first dosing regimen (1 mg P.O. h.s.).

### PATIENT TEACHING
● Tell patient not to stop drug suddenly, but to notify prescriber if adverse reactions occur.
● Warn patient to avoid hazardous activities that require mental alertness, such as driving or operating heavy machinery, for 12 hours after first dose.
● Tell patient that light-headedness can occur, especially during the first few days of therapy. Advise him to rise slowly to minimize this effect and to report signs and symptoms to prescriber.

## timolol maleate
Apo-Timol†, Blocadren

*Pregnancy risk category C*

### AVAILABLE FORMS
*Tablets:* 5 mg, 10 mg, 20 mg

### INDICATIONS & DOSAGES
➤ **Hypertension**
*Adults:* Initially, 10 mg P.O. b.i.d. Usual daily maintenance dose is 20 to 40 mg. Maximum daily dose is 60 mg. Allow at least 7 days between increases in dosage.

➤ **Long-term prevention of MI in patients who have survived acute phase**
*Adults:* 10 mg P.O. b.i.d.

➤ **To prevent migraine headache**
*Adults:* Initially, 10 mg P.O. b.i.d. During maintenance therapy, the 20 mg daily dosage can be given as a single dose, rather than a divided dose. Increase dosage as needed and tolerated to maximum of 30 mg daily as a divided dose. Stop treatment if no response occurs after 6 to 8 weeks at maximum dose.

## ACTION
Unknown. In MI, drug may decrease myocardial oxygen requirements. For migraine headache prophylaxis, drug prevents arterial dilation through beta blockade.

| Route | Onset | Peak | Duration |
|-------|-------|------|----------|
| P.O. | 15-30 min | 1-2 hr | 6-12 hr |

## ADVERSE REACTIONS
**CNS:** fatigue, lethargy, dizziness.
**CV:** *bradycardia,* hypotension, *heart failure,* peripheral vascular disease, *arrhythmias.*
**GI:** nausea, vomiting, diarrhea.
**Metabolic:** *hyperkalemia,* hyperglycemia.
**Respiratory:** dyspnea, *bronchospasm, increased airway resistance, pulmonary edema.*
**Skin:** pruritus.

## INTERACTIONS
**Drug-drug.** *Aminophylline, theophylline:* May act antagonistically, reducing the effects of one or both drugs; may slow elimination of theophylline. Monitor theophylline level and patient closely.
*Amiodarone:* May increase risk of bradycardia, AV block, and myocardial depression. Monitor patient's ECG and vital signs.
*Cardiac glycosides, diltiazem:* May cause excessive bradycardia and increased depressant effect on myocardium. Use together cautiously.
*Catecholamine-depleting drugs such as reserpine:* May have additive effect when given with beta blockers. Watch for hypotension and bradycardia.
*Cimetidine:* May increase effects of beta blocker. Consider another $H_2$ agonist or decrease dose of beta blocker.

*Epinephrine:* May cause hypertensive episode, followed by bradycardia. Stop beta blocker 3 days before anticipated epinephrine use. Monitor patient closely.
*Indomethacin, NSAIDs:* May decrease antihypertensive effect. Monitor blood pressure and adjust dosage.
*Insulin:* May mask symptoms of hypoglycemia as a result of beta blockade (such as tachycardia). Use with extreme caution in patients with diabetes.
*Oral antidiabetics:* May alter requirements for these drugs in previously stabilized diabetic patients. Monitor patient for hypoglycemia.
*Prazosin:* May increase risk of orthostatic hypotension in early phases of use together. Help patient stand slowly until effects are known.
*Verapamil:* May increase effects of both drugs. Monitor cardiac function closely and decrease dosages as necessary.
**Drug-herb.** *Ma-huang:* May decrease antihypertensive effects. Discourage use together.

## EFFECTS ON LAB TEST RESULTS
● May increase BUN, potassium, uric acid, and glucose levels.

## CONTRAINDICATIONS & CAUTIONS
● Contraindicated in patients hypersensitive to drug and in those with bronchial asthma, severe COPD, sinus bradycardia, and heart block greater than first-degree or cardiogenic shock.
● Use cautiously in patients with hepatic, renal, or respiratory disease, diabetes, and hyperthyroidism.
● Although drug should be avoided in patient with overt heart failure, it may be used cautiously in patients with well-compensated heart failure.

## NURSING CONSIDERATIONS
● Check patient's apical pulse rate before giving drug. If extremes in pulse rates are detected, withhold drug and notify prescriber immediately.
● Monitor blood pressure frequently.
● Monitor glucose level in diabetic patients; drug can mask signs and symptoms of hypoglycemia.
● Beta blockers may mask tachycardia caused by hyperthyroidism. In patients

with suspected thyrotoxicosis, withdraw beta blocker gradually to avoid thyroid storm.
● **Alert:** Don't confuse timolol with atenolol.

**PATIENT TEACHING**
● Tell patient to take drug exactly as prescribed.
● Instruct patient not to stop drug suddenly, but to notify prescriber if adverse reactions occur. Tell patient to reduce dosage gradually over 1 or 2 weeks.
● Advise patient that drug may deplete body's stores of coenzyme Q10 and that he should discuss need for supplements with prescriber.

# trandolapril
Mavik

*Pregnancy risk category C; D in second and third trimesters*

**AVAILABLE FORMS**
*Tablets:* 1 mg, 2 mg, 4 mg

**INDICATIONS & DOSAGES**
➤ **Hypertension**
*Adults:* For patients not taking a diuretic, initially 2 mg P.O. for a black patient and 1 mg P.O. for all other races, once daily. If control isn't adequate, increase dosage at intervals of at least 1 week. Maintenance doses for most patients range from 2 to 4 mg daily. Some patients taking once-daily doses of 4 mg may need b.i.d. doses. For patients also taking a diuretic, initially, 0.5 mg P.O. once daily. Subsequent dosage adjustment is based on blood pressure response.
➤ **Heart failure or ventricular dysfunction after MI**
*Adults:* Initially, 1 mg P.O. daily, adjusted to 4 mg P.O. daily. If patient can't tolerate 4 mg, continue at highest tolerated dose.
*Adjust-a-dose:* For patients with creatinine clearance below 30 ml/minute, first dose is 0.5 mg daily.

**ACTION**
Unknown. Thought to result primarily from inhibition of circulating and tissue ACE activity, thereby reducing angio-

tensin II formation, decreasing vasoconstriction and aldosterone secretion, and increasing renin level. Decreased aldosterone secretion leads to diuresis, natriuresis, and a small increase in potassium. Drug is converted in the liver to the prodrug, trandolaprilat.

| Route | Onset | Peak | Duration |
|-------|-------|------|----------|
| P.O. | 4 hr | 1-10 hr | 24 hr |

**ADVERSE REACTIONS**
**CNS:** *dizziness,* headache, fatigue, drowsiness, insomnia, paresthesia, vertigo, anxiety.
**CV:** chest pain, first-degree AV block, *bradycardia,* edema, flushing, *hypotension,* palpitations.
**EENT:** epistaxis, throat irritation.
**GI:** diarrhea, dyspepsia, abdominal distention, abdominal pain or cramps, constipation, vomiting, *pancreatitis.*
**GU:** urinary frequency, impotence.
**Hematologic:** *neutropenia, leukopenia.*
**Metabolic:** *hyperkalemia,* hyponatremia.
**Respiratory:** dyspnea, *persistent, nonproductive cough;* upper respiratory tract infection.
**Skin:** rash, pruritus, pemphigus.
**Other:** decreased libido.

**INTERACTIONS**
**Drug-drug.** *Azathioprine:* May increase risk of anemia or leukopenia. Monitor hematologic studies if used together.
*Diuretics:* May cause excessive hypotension. Stop diuretic or reduce first dosage of trandolapril.
*Lithium:* May increase lithium level and lithium toxicity. Avoid using together; monitor lithium level.
*NSAIDs:* May decrease antihypertensive effects. Monitor blood pressure.
*Potassium-sparing diuretics, potassium supplements:* May cause hyperkalemia. Monitor potassium level closely.
**Drug-herb.** *Capsaicin:* May cause cough. Discourage use together.
*Ma-huang:* May decrease antihypertensive effects. Discourage use together.
**Drug-food.** *Salt substitutes containing potassium:* May cause hyperkalemia. Discourage use of salt substitutes.

## EFFECTS ON LAB TEST RESULTS
• May increase BUN, creatinine, potassium, and liver enzyme levels. May decrease sodium level.
• May decrease neutrophil and WBC counts.

## CONTRAINDICATIONS & CAUTIONS
• Contraindicated in patients hypersensitive to drug and in those with a history of angioedema related to previous treatment with an ACE inhibitor. Also contraindicated in pregnant patients.
• Safety and effectiveness of drug in children haven't been established. Don't give drug to children.
• It's unknown if drug appears in breast milk. Don't use drug in breast-feeding women.
• Use cautiously in patients with impaired renal function, heart failure, or renal artery stenosis.

## NURSING CONSIDERATIONS
• Monitor potassium level closely.
• Watch for hypotension. Excessive hypotension can occur when drug is given with diuretics. If possible, stop diuretic therapy 2 to 3 days before starting trandolapril to decrease potential for excessive hypotension response. If drug doesn't adequately control blood pressure, diuretic therapy may be started again cautiously.
• Assess patient's renal function before and periodically throughout therapy.
• Other ACE inhibitors have caused agranulocytosis and neutropenia. Monitor CBC with differential before therapy, especially in patients with collagen vascular disease and impaired renal function.
• Although ACE inhibitors reduce blood pressure in all races studied, this response is less in black patients who receive the drug as monotherapy. Therapy with a thiazide diuretic produces a more favorable response.
• *Alert:* Angioedema involving the tongue, glottis, or larynx may be fatal because of airway obstruction. Order appropriate therapy, including epinephrine 1:1,000 (0.3 to 0.5 ml) S.C.; have resuscitation equipment for maintaining a patent airway readily available. The risk of angioedema is higher in black patients.

• If patient develops jaundice, stop drug under prescriber's advice because, although rare, ACE inhibitors have been linked to a syndrome of cholestatic jaundice, fulminant hepatic necrosis, and death.

## PATIENT TEACHING
• Instruct patient to report yellowing of skin or eyes.
• Advise patient to report fever and sore throat (signs of infection), easy bruising or bleeding; swelling of the tongue, lips, face, eyes, mucous membranes, or extremities; difficulty swallowing or breathing; hoarseness; and nonproductive, persistent cough.
• Tell patient to avoid salt substitutes during drug therapy. These products may contain potassium, which can cause high potassium level in patients taking drug.
• Tell patient that light-headedness can occur, especially during first few days of therapy. Advise him to rise slowly to minimize this effect and to report it immediately.
• Advise patient to use caution in hot weather and during exercise. Inadequate fluid intake, vomiting, diarrhea, and excessive perspiration can lead to light-headedness and fainting.
• Tell woman to report suspected pregnancy immediately. Drug will need to be stopped.
• Advise patient planning to undergo surgery or receive anesthesia to inform prescriber that he is taking this drug.

---

# valsartan
Diovan

*Pregnancy risk category C; D in second and third trimesters*

## AVAILABLE FORMS
*Tablets:* 80 mg, 160 mg, 320 mg

## INDICATIONS & DOSAGES
➤ **Hypertension (used alone or with other antihypertensives)**
*Adults:* Initially, 80 mg P.O. once daily. Expect to see a reduction in blood pressure in 2 to 4 weeks. If additional antihypertensive effect is needed, dose may be

increased to 160 or 320 mg daily, or a diuretic may be added. (Addition of a diuretic has a greater effect than dosage increases beyond 80 mg.) Usual dosage range is 80 to 320 mg daily.

➤ **New York Heart Association class II to IV heart failure in patients intolerant of ACE inhibitors**
*Adults:* Initially, 40 mg P.O. b.i.d.; increase as tolerated to 80 mg b.i.d. Maximum dose is 160 mg b.i.d.

## ACTION

Blocks the binding of angiotensin II to receptor sites in vascular smooth muscle and the adrenal gland, which inhibits the pressor effects of the renin-angiotensin-aldosterone system.

| Route | Onset | Peak | Duration |
|-------|-------|------|----------|
| P.O. | 2 hr | 2-4 hr | 24 hr |

## ADVERSE REACTIONS

**CNS:** *dizziness,* headache, insomnia, fatigue, vertigo.
**CV:** edema, hypotension, orthostatic hypotension, syncope.
**EENT:** rhinitis, sinusitis, pharyngitis, blurred vision.
**GI:** abdominal pain, diarrhea, nausea, dyspepsia.
**GU:** renal impairment.
**Hematologic:** *neutropenia.*
**Metabolic:** *hyperkalemia.*
**Musculoskeletal:** arthralgia, back pain.
**Respiratory:** upper respiratory tract infection, cough.
**Other:** viral infection, *angioedema.*

## INTERACTIONS

**Drug-drug.** *Lithium:* May increase lithium level. Monitor lithium level and patient for toxicity.
*Potassium-sparing diuretics, potassium supplements, other angiotensin II blockers:* May increase potassium level. May also increase creatinine level in heart failure patients. Avoid using together.
**Drug-herb.** *Ma-huang:* May decrease antihypertensive effects. Discourage use together.
**Drug-food.** *Salt substitutes containing potassium:* May increase potassium level. May also increase creatinine level in heart failure patients. Avoid using together.

## EFFECTS ON LAB TEST RESULTS

• May increase potassium level.
• May decrease neutrophil count.

## CONTRAINDICATIONS & CAUTIONS

• Contraindicated in patients hypersensitive to drug.
• Drug can cause fetal or neonatal morbidity and death if given to a pregnant woman in the second or third trimester. Breast-feeding women shouldn't take drug.
• Safety and effectiveness of drug in children haven't been established. Don't give drug to children.
• Use cautiously in patients with renal or hepatic disease.

## NURSING CONSIDERATIONS

• Watch for hypotension. Excessive hypotension can occur when drug is given with high doses of diuretics.
• Correct volume and salt depletions before starting drug.

## PATIENT TEACHING

• Tell woman to notify prescriber if she becomes pregnant. Drug will need to be stopped.
• Advise patient that drug may be taken without regard to food.

# 22

## Antilipemics

atorvastatin calcium
cholestyramine
colesevelam hydrochloride
ezetimibe
fenofibrate (micronized)
fluvastatin sodium
gemfibrozil
lovastatin
niacin
   (See Chapter 89, VITAMINS AND
   MINERALS.)
pravastatin sodium
rosuvastatin
simvastatin

**COMBINATION PRODUCTS**
None

---

## atorvastatin calcium
Lipitor♦

*Pregnancy risk category X*

---

**AVAILABLE FORMS**
*Tablets:* 10 mg, 20 mg, 40 mg, 80 mg

**INDICATIONS & DOSAGES**
➤ **Adjunct to diet to reduce LDL cholesterol, total cholesterol, apolipoprotein B, and triglyceride levels and to increase HDL cholesterol levels in patients with primary hypercholesterolemia (heterozygous familial and nonfamilial) and mixed dyslipidemia (Fredrickson types IIa and IIb); adjunct to diet to reduce triglyceride level (Fredrickson type IV); primary dysbetalipoproteinemia (Fredrickson type III) in patients who don't respond adequately to diet**
*Adults:* Initially, 10 or 20 mg P.O. once daily. Patients who require a large reduction in LDL cholesterol (more than 45%) may be started at 40 mg once daily. Increase dose, p.r.n., to maximum of 80 mg daily as single dose. Dosage based on lipid levels drawn within 2 to 4 weeks after starting therapy.

➤ **Alone or as an adjunct to lipid-lowering treatments such as LDL apheresis to reduce total and LDL cholesterol in patients with homozygous familial hypercholesterolemia**
*Adults:* 10 to 80 mg P.O. once daily.
➤ **Heterozygous familial hypercholesterolemia**
*Children ages 10 to 17 (girls should be 1 year postmenarche):* Initially, 10 mg P.O. once daily. Adjustment intervals should be at least 4 weeks. Maximum daily dose is 20 mg.

**ACTION**
Inhibits 3-hydroxy-3-methylglutaryl-coenzyme A (HMG-CoA) reductase, which is an early (and rate-limiting) step in cholesterol biosynthesis.

| Route | Onset | Peak | Duration |
|-------|-------|------|----------|
| P.O. | Unknown | 1-2 hr | Unknown |

**ADVERSE REACTIONS**
**CNS:** *headache,* asthenia, insomnia.
**CV:** peripheral edema.
**EENT:** rhinitis, pharyngitis, sinusitis.
**GI:** abdominal pain, dyspepsia, flatulence, nausea, constipation, diarrhea.
**GU:** urinary tract infection.
**Musculoskeletal:** arthritis, arthralgia, myalgia.
**Respiratory:** bronchitis.
**Skin:** rash.
**Other:** infection, flulike syndrome, allergic reactions.

**INTERACTIONS**
**Drug-drug.** *Antacids:* May decrease drug level. Monitor patient.
*Azole antifungals, cyclosporine, erythromycin, fibric acid derivatives, niacin:* May increase risk of myopathy. Avoid using together.
*Colestipol, isradipine:* May decrease drug level. Monitor patient.
*Digoxin:* May increase digoxin level. Monitor digoxin level and patient for evidence of toxicity.

---

*Erythromycin:* May increase atorvastatin level. Monitor patient.

*Fluconazole, itraconazole, ketoconazole, voriconazole:* May increase atorvastatin level and adverse effects. Avoid using together, or, if they must be given together, reduce dose of atorvastatin.

*Hormonal contraceptives:* May increase levels of hormones. Consider when selecting a hormonal contraceptive.

**Drug-herb.** *Eucalyptus, jin bu huan, kava:* May increase risk of hepatotoxicity. Discourage use together.

*Red yeast rice:* May increase risk of adverse reactions because herb contains compounds similar to those of statin drugs. Discourage use together.

**Drug-food.** *Grapefruit juice:* Elevates levels of drug, increasing risk of adverse reactions. Advise patient to take with liquid other than grapefruit juice.

**EFFECTS ON LAB TEST RESULTS**
● May increase ALT and AST levels.

**CONTRAINDICATIONS & CAUTIONS**
● Contraindicated in patients hypersensitive to drug and in those with active liver disease or unexplained persistent elevations of transaminase levels.
● Contraindicated in pregnant and breast-feeding women and in women of childbearing potential.
● Use cautiously in patients with history of liver disease or heavy alcohol use.
● Withhold or stop drug in patients at risk for renal failure caused by rhabdomyolysis resulting from trauma; in serious, acute conditions that suggest myopathy; and in major surgery, severe acute infection, hypotension, uncontrolled seizures, or severe metabolic, endocrine, or electrolyte disorders.
● Use of atorvastatin in children has been limited to those older than age 9 with homozygous familial hypercholesterolemia.

**NURSING CONSIDERATIONS**
● Use only after diet and other nondrug therapies prove ineffective. Patient should follow a standard low-cholesterol diet before and during therapy.
● Before starting treatment, exclude secondary causes for hypercholesterolemia and do a baseline lipid profile. Obtain periodic liver function test results and lipid levels before starting treatment and at 6 and 12 weeks after initiation, or after an increase in dosage and periodically thereafter.
● Drug may be given as a single dose at any time of day, with or without food.
● Watch for signs of myositis.
● *Alert:* Don't confuse Lipitor with Levatol.

**PATIENT TEACHING**
● Teach patient about proper dietary management, weight control, and exercise. Explain their importance in controlling high fat levels.
● Warn patient to avoid alcohol.
● Tell patient to inform prescriber of adverse reactions, such as muscle pain, malaise, and fever.
● Advise patient that drug can be taken at any time of day, without regard to meals.
● Tell patient that drug may deplete the body's stores of coenzyme Q10; he should discuss the need for supplements with prescriber.
● *Alert:* Tell woman to stop drug and notify prescriber immediately if she is or may be pregnant or if she's breast-feeding.

---

# cholestyramine
LoCHOLEST, LoCHOLEST Light, Prevalite, Questran, Questran Light, Questran Lite‡

*Pregnancy risk category C*

**AVAILABLE FORMS**
*Powder:* 378-g cans, 9-g single-dose packets. Each scoop of powder or single-dose packet contains 4 g of cholestyramine resin.

**INDICATIONS & DOSAGES**
➤ **Primary hyperlipidemia or pruritus caused by partial bile obstruction, adjunct for reduction of elevated cholesterol levels in patients with primary hypercholesterolemia**
*Adults:* 4 g once or twice daily. Maintenance dose is 8 to 16 g daily divided into two doses. Maximum daily dose is 24 g.

## ACTION
A bile-acid sequestrant that combines with bile acid to form an insoluble compound that is excreted. The liver must synthesize new bile acid from cholesterol, which reduces LDL cholesterol levels.

| Route | Onset | Peak | Duration |
|-------|-------|------|----------|
| P.O. | Unknown | Unknown | 2-4 wk |

## ADVERSE REACTIONS
**CNS:** *headache,* anxiety, *vertigo, dizziness,* insomnia, fatigue, syncope, tinnitus.
**GI:** *constipation, fecal impaction,* hemorrhoids, *abdominal discomfort,* flatulence, *nausea,* vomiting, steatorrhea, GI bleeding, diarrhea, anorexia.
**GU:** hematuria, dysuria.
**Hematologic:** anemia, bleeding tendencies, ecchymoses.
**Metabolic:** hyperchloremic acidosis.
**Musculoskeletal:** backache, muscle and joint pains, osteoporosis.
**Skin:** *rash;* irritation of skin, tongue, and perianal area.
**Other:** *vitamin A, D, E, and K deficiencies from decreased absorption.*

## INTERACTIONS
**Drug-drug.** *Acetaminophen, beta blockers, cardiac glycosides, corticosteroids, estrogens, fat-soluble vitamins (A, D, E, and K), iron preparations, niacin, penicillin G, phenobarbital, progestins, tetracycline, thiazide diuretics, thyroid hormones, warfarin and other coumarin derivatives:* Absorption may be substantially decreased by cholestyramine. Give other drugs 1 hour before or 4 to 6 hours after cholestyramine.

## EFFECTS ON LAB TEST RESULTS
● May increase alkaline phosphatase level.
● May decrease hemoglobin and hematocrit.

## CONTRAINDICATIONS & CAUTIONS
● Contraindicated in patients hypersensitive to bile-acid sequestering resins and in those with complete biliary obstruction.
● Use cautiously in patients predisposed to constipation and in those with conditions aggravated by constipation, such as severe, symptomatic coronary artery disease.

## NURSING CONSIDERATIONS
● Monitor cholesterol and triglyceride levels regularly during therapy.
● Monitor levels of cardiac glycosides in patients receiving cardiac glycosides and cholestyramine together. If cholestyramine therapy is stopped, adjust dosage of cardiac glycosides to avoid toxicity.
● Monitor bowel habits. Encourage a diet high in fiber and fluids. If severe constipation develops, decrease dosage, add a stool softener, or stop drug.
● Watch for hyperchloremic acidosis with long-term use or very high doses.
● Long-term use may lead to deficiencies of vitamins A, D, E, and K, and folic acid.
● Cholecystography using iopanoic acid yields abnormal results because iopanoic acid is also bound by cholestyramine.
● *Alert:* Don't confuse Questran with Quarzan.

## PATIENT TEACHING
● *Alert:* Tell patient never to take drug in its dry form because it may irritate the esophagus or cause severe constipation.
● Tell patient to prepare drug in a large glass containing water, milk, or juice (especially pulpy fruit juice). Powder can be sprinkled on the surface of the preferred beverage; let the mixture stand for a few minutes, and then stir thoroughly. Avoid mixing with carbonated beverages because of excessive foaming. After drinking preparation, patients should swirl a small additional amount of liquid in the same glass and then drink again to make sure they have taken the entire dose.
● Advise patient to take at mealtime, if possible.
● Advise patient to take all other drugs at least 1 hour before or 4 to 6 hours after cholestyramine to avoid blocking their absorption.
● Teach patient about proper dietary management of fats. When appropriate, recommend weight control, exercise, and smoking cessation programs.
● Tell patient that drug may deplete body stores of vitamins A, D, E, and K and folic acid. Patient should discuss need for supplements with prescriber.

## colesevelam hydrochloride
Welchol

*Pregnancy risk category B*

### AVAILABLE FORMS
*Tablets:* 625 mg

### INDICATIONS & DOSAGES
➤ **Adjunct to diet and exercise, either alone or with an HMG-CoA reductase inhibitor, to reduce elevated LDL cholesterol in patients with primary hypercholesterolemia (Fredrickson type IIa)**
*Adults:* 3 tablets (1,875 mg) P.O. b.i.d. with meals and liquid, or 6 tablets (3,750 mg) once daily with a meal and liquid. Maximum dosage is 7 tablets (4,375 mg) daily.

### ACTION
Binds bile acids in the intestinal tract, impeding their absorption and causing their elimination in feces. In response to this bile acid depletion, LDL cholesterol levels decrease as the liver uses LDL cholesterol to replenish reduced bile acid stores.

| Route | Onset | Peak | Duration |
|-------|-------|------|----------|
| P.O. | Unknown | 2 wk | Unknown |

### ADVERSE REACTIONS
**CNS:** *headache,* pain, asthenia.
**EENT:** pharyngitis, rhinitis, sinusitis.
**GI:** abdominal pain, *constipation,* diarrhea, dyspepsia, *flatulence,* nausea.
**Musculoskeletal:** myalgia, back pain.
**Respiratory:** increased cough.
**Other:** accidental injury, *infection,* flulike syndrome.

### INTERACTIONS
None reported.

### EFFECTS ON LAB TEST RESULTS
None reported.

### CONTRAINDICATIONS & CAUTIONS
• Contraindicated in patients hypersensitive to drug or any of its components and in patients with bowel obstruction.
• Use cautiously in patients susceptible to vitamin K or fat-soluble vitamin deficiencies and in patients with dysphagia, swallowing disorders, severe GI motility disorders, or major GI tract surgery.
• Use cautiously in patients with triglyceride levels greater than 300 mg/dl.

### NURSING CONSIDERATIONS
• Rule out secondary causes of hypercholesterolemia before starting drug, such as poorly controlled diabetes, hypothyroidism, nephrotic syndrome, dysproteinemias, obstructive liver disease, other drug therapy, and alcoholism.
• Give drug with a meal and a liquid.
• Store tablets at room temperature and protect them from moisture.
• Monitor patient's bowel habits. If severe constipation develops, decrease dosage, add a stool softener, or stop drug.
• Monitor the effects of concurrent drug therapy to identify possible drug interactions.
• Monitor total and LDL cholesterol and triglyceride levels periodically during therapy.
• Use only when clearly needed in breast-feeding patients because it's not known if drug appears in breast milk.

### PATIENT TEACHING
• Instruct patient to take drug with a meal and a liquid.
• Teach patient to monitor bowel habits. Encourage a diet high in fiber and fluids. Instruct patient to notify prescriber promptly if severe constipation develops.
• Encourage patient to follow prescribed diet, exercise, and monitoring of cholesterol and triglyceride levels.
• Tell patient to notify prescriber if she is pregnant or breast-feeding.

## ezetimibe
Zetia✒

*Pregnancy risk category C*

### AVAILABLE FORMS
*Tablets:* 10 mg

### INDICATIONS & DOSAGES
➤ **Adjunct to diet and exercise to reduce total cholesterol, LDL cholesterol, and apolipoprotein-B levels in patients with primary hypercholesterol-**

emia, alone or combined with HMG-CoA reductase inhibitors (statins) or bile acid sequestrants; adjunct to other lipid-lowering drugs (combined with atorvastatin or simvastatin) in patients with homozygous familial hypercholesterolemia; adjunct to diet in patients with homozygous sitosterolemia to reduce sitosterol and campesterol levels
*Adults:* 10 mg/day P.O.

## ACTION
Inhibits absorption of cholesterol by the small intestine, unlike other drugs used for cholesterol reduction. This action reduces hepatic cholesterol stores and increases cholesterol clearance from the blood.

| Route | Onset | Peak | Duration |
|-------|-------|------|----------|
| P.O. | Unknown | 4-12 hr | Unknown |

## ADVERSE REACTIONS
**CNS:** dizziness, headache, fatigue.
**CV:** chest pain.
**EENT:** pharyngitis, sinusitis.
**GI:** abdominal pain, diarrhea.
**Musculoskeletal:** back pain, arthralgia, myalgia.
**Respiratory:** cough, *upper respiratory tract infection.*
**Other:** viral infection.

## INTERACTIONS
**Drug-drug.** *Bile acid sequestrant (cholestyramine):* May decrease ezetimibe level. Give ezetimibe at least 2 hours before or 4 hours after cholestyramine.
*Cyclosporine, fenofibrate, gemfibrozil:* May increase ezetimibe level. Monitor patient closely for adverse reactions.
*Fibrates:* May increase excretion of cholesterol into the gallbladder bile. Avoid using together.

## EFFECTS ON LAB TEST RESULTS
• May increase liver function test values.

## CONTRAINDICATIONS & CAUTIONS
• Contraindicated in patients allergic to any component of the drug. Use together with HMG-CoA reductase inhibitor is contraindicated in pregnant or breast-feeding patients and in patients with active

hepatic disease or unexplained increase in transaminase levels.
• Use cautiously in elderly patients.

## NURSING CONSIDERATIONS
• Before starting treatment, evaluate patient for secondary causes of dyslipidemia.
• Obtain baseline triglyceride and total, LDL, and HDL cholesterol levels.
• When ezetimibe is used with an HMG-CoA reductase inhibitor, check liver function test values at start of therapy and thereafter according to the recommendations of the HMG-CoA reductase inhibitor manufacturer.
• Use of ezetimibe with an HMG-CoA reductase inhibitor significantly reduces total and LDL cholesterol, apolipoprotein B, and triglyceride levels and (except with pravastatin) increases HDL cholesterol level more than use of an HMG-CoA reductase inhibitor alone.
• Patient should maintain a cholesterol-lowering diet during treatment.

## PATIENT TEACHING
• Emphasize importance of following a cholesterol-lowering diet.
• Tell patient he may take drug without regard to meals.
• Advise patient to notify prescriber of unexplained muscle pain, weakness, or tenderness.
• Urge patient to tell his prescriber about any herbal or dietary supplements he's taking.
• Advise patient to visit his prescriber for routine follow-up and blood tests.
• Tell patient to notify prescriber if she becomes pregnant.

---

# fenofibrate (micronized)
Lofibra, Tricor

*Pregnancy risk category C*

## AVAILABLE FORMS
*Capsules:* 67 mg, 134 mg, 200 mg
*Capsules (micronized):* 67 mg, 134 mg, 200 mg
*Tablets:* 54 mg, 160 mg

## INDICATIONS & DOSAGES

➤ **Adjunct to diet to reduce very high triglyceride levels (type IV and V hyperlipidemia) in patients at high risk for pancreatitis who don't respond adequately to diet alone**

*Adults:* 67- to 200-mg capsule or 54- to 160-mg tablet P.O. daily. Based on response, increase dose if necessary after repeating triglyceride level check at 4- to 8-week intervals to maximum dose of 200-mg capsule or 160-mg tablet daily.

*Adjust-a-dose:* Minimize dose in patients whose creatinine clearance is less than 50 ml/minute and in elderly patients. Start therapy at 67-mg capsule or 54-mg tablet daily and increase only after effects on renal function and triglyceride levels have been evaluated at this dose.

➤ **Adjunct to diet to reduce LDL and total cholesterol, triglyceride levels, and apolipoprotein B levels and to increase HDL cholesterol levels in patients with primary hypercholesterolemia or mixed dyslipidemia (Fredrickson types IIa and IIb)**

*Adults:* 200-mg capsule or 160-mg tablet P.O. daily.

*Adjust-a-dose:* In patients with creatinine clearance less than 50 ml/minute and in elderly patients, initially, give 67-mg capsule or 54-mg tablet daily and increase only after effects on renal function and triglyceride levels have been evaluated at this dose.

## ACTION

Unknown. Thought to lower triglyceride levels by inhibiting triglyceride synthesis, resulting in decreased very low density lipoproteins released into the circulation. Drug may stimulate breakdown of triglyceride-rich protein.

| Route | Onset | Peak | Duration |
|-------|---------|--------|----------|
| P.O. | Unknown | 6-8 hr | Unknown |

## ADVERSE REACTIONS

**CNS:** *dizziness,* localized pain, asthenia, fatigue, paresthesia, insomnia, increased appetite, *headache.*
**CV:** *arrhythmias.*
**EENT:** eye discomfort, eye floaters, earache, conjunctivitis, blurred vision, rhinitis, sinusitis.

**GI:** dyspepsia, eructation, flatulence, nausea, vomiting, abdominal pain, constipation, diarrhea.
**GU:** polyuria, vaginitis.
**Musculoskeletal:** arthralgia.
**Respiratory:** cough.
**Skin:** pruritus, rash.
**Other:** decreased libido, hypersensitivity reactions, *infection,* flulike syndrome.

## INTERACTIONS

**Drug-drug.** *Bile-acid sequestrants:* May bind and inhibit absorption of fenofibrate. Give drug 1 hour before or 4 to 6 hours after bile-acid sequestrants.
*Coumarin-type anticoagulants:* May potentiate anticoagulant effect, prolonging PT and INR. Monitor PT and INR closely. May need to reduce anticoagulant dosage.
*Cyclosporine, immunosuppressants, nephrotoxic drugs:* May induce renal dysfunction that may affect fenofibrate elimination. Use together cautiously.
*HMG-CoA reductase inhibitors:* May increase risk of adverse musculoskeletal effects. Avoid using together, unless potential benefit outweighs risk.
**Drug-food.** *Any food:* May increase absorption of fenofibrate. Advise patient to take drug with meals.
**Drug-lifestyle.** *Alcohol use:* May elevate triglyceride levels. Discourage use together.

## EFFECTS ON LAB TEST RESULTS

• May increase BUN, creatinine, ALT, and AST levels. May decrease uric acid levels.
• May decrease hemoglobin, hematocrit, and WBC count.

## CONTRAINDICATIONS & CAUTIONS

• Contraindicated in patients hypersensitive to drug and in those with gallbladder disease, hepatic dysfunction, primary biliary cirrhosis, severe renal dysfunction, or unexplained persistent liver function abnormalities.
• Use cautiously in patients with a history of pancreatitis.

## NURSING CONSIDERATIONS

• Obtain baseline lipid levels and liver function test results before starting therapy. Monitor liver function periodically for duration of drug therapy. Stop drug if

enzyme levels persist above three times normal limit.
• Watch for signs and symptoms of pancreatitis, myositis, rhabdomyolysis, cholelithiasis, and renal failure. Monitor patient for muscle pain, tenderness, or weakness, especially with malaise or fever.
• If an adequate response hasn't been obtained after 2 months of treatment with maximum daily dose, therapy must be stopped.
• Drug lowers uric acid levels in patients with or without hyperuricemia by increasing uric acid excretion.
• Beta blockers, estrogens, and thiazide diuretics may increase triglyceride levels; evaluate continued use of these drugs.
• Mild to moderate decreases in hemoglobin, hematocrit, and WBC count may occur when therapy starts, but they stabilize with long-term administration.

**PATIENT TEACHING**
• Inform patient that drug therapy doesn't reduce need for following a triglyceride-lowering diet.
• Advise patient to promptly report unexplained muscle weakness, pain, or tenderness, especially if accompanied by malaise or fever.
• Inform patient to take drug with meals for best drug absorption.
• Advise patient to continue weight control measures, including diet and exercise, and to drink less alcohol before starting drug therapy.
• Instruct patient who is also taking a bile-acid resin to take fenofibrate 1 hour before or 4 to 6 hours after taking resin.
• Advise patient about potential for tumor growth.
• Tell women that a decision must be made to stop either breast-feeding or drug.

# fluvastatin sodium
Lescol◆, Lescol XL

*Pregnancy risk category X*

## AVAILABLE FORMS
*Capsules:* 20 mg, 40 mg
*Tablets (extended-release):* 80 mg

## INDICATIONS & DOSAGES
➤ **To reduce LDL and total cholesterol levels in patients with primary hypercholesterolemia (types IIa and IIb); to slow progression of coronary atherosclerosis in patients with coronary artery disease; elevated triglyceride and apolipoprotein B levels in patients with primary hypercholesterolemia and mixed dyslipidemia whose response to dietary restriction and other nonpharmacologic measures has been inadequate**
*Adults:* Initially, 20 to 40 mg P.O. h.s., increasing p.r.n. to maximum of 80 mg daily in divided doses or 80 mg Lescol XL P.O. h.s.
✹ *NEW INDICATION:* **To reduce the risk of undergoing coronary revascularization procedures**
*Adults:* For patients who must reduce LDL cholesterol level by at least 25%, initially one 40-mg capsule, or one 80-mg extended-release tablet as a single dose in the evening, or 40-mg capsule P.O. b.i.d. For patients who must reduce LDL cholesterol level by less than 25%, initially 20 mg P.O. daily. Dosing range is 20 to 80 mg daily.

## ACTION
Inhibits HMG-CoA reductase, which is an early (and rate-limiting) step in the synthetic pathway of cholesterol.

| Route | Onset | Peak | Duration |
|-------|-------|------|----------|
| P.O. | Unknown | 1 hr | Unknown |

## ADVERSE REACTIONS
**CNS:** headache, fatigue, dizziness, insomnia.
**EENT:** sinusitis, rhinitis, pharyngitis.
**GI:** dyspepsia, diarrhea, nausea, vomiting, abdominal pain, constipation, flatulence.
**Hematologic:** *thrombocytopenia,* hemolytic anemia, *leukopenia.*
**Musculoskeletal:** arthralgia, back pain, myalgia.
**Respiratory:** *upper respiratory tract infection,* cough, bronchitis.
**Other:** hypersensitivity reactions.

## INTERACTIONS
**Drug-drug.** *Cholestyramine, colestipol:* May bind with fluvastatin in the GI tract

and decrease absorption. Separate doses by at least 4 hours.

*Cimetidine, omeprazole, ranitidine:* May decrease fluvastatin metabolism. Monitor patient for enhanced effects.

*Cyclosporine and other immunosuppressants, erythromycin, gemfibrozil, niacin:* May increase risk of polymyositis and rhabdomyolysis. Avoid using together.

*Digoxin:* May alter digoxin pharmacokinetics. Monitor digoxin level carefully.

*Fluconazole, itraconazole, ketoconazole:* May increase fluvastatin level and adverse effects. Avoid using together, or, if they must be given together, reduce dose of fluvastatin.

*Rifampin:* May enhance fluvastatin metabolism and decrease levels. Monitor patient for lack of effect.

*Warfarin:* May increase anticoagulant effect with bleeding. Monitor patient.

**Drug-herb.** *Eucalyptus, jin bu huan, kava:* May increase risk of hepatotoxicity. Discourage use together.

*Red yeast rice:* May increase risk of adverse reactions because herb contains compounds similar to those of statin drugs. Discourage use together.

**Drug-lifestyle.** *Alcohol use:* May increase risk of hepatotoxicity. Discourage use together.

**EFFECTS ON LAB TEST RESULTS**
• May increase ALT, AST, and CK levels.
• May decrease hemoglobin, hematocrit, and platelet and WBC counts.

**CONTRAINDICATIONS & CAUTIONS**
• Contraindicated in patients hypersensitive to drug and in those with active liver disease or unexplained persistent elevations of transaminase levels; also contraindicated in pregnant and breast-feeding women and in women of childbearing potential.
• Use cautiously in patients with severe renal impairment and history of liver disease or heavy alcohol use.

**NURSING CONSIDERATIONS**
• Use only after diet and other nondrug therapies prove ineffective. Patient should follow a standard low-cholesterol diet during therapy.

• Test liver function at start of therapy, at 12 weeks after start of therapy, 12 weeks after an increase in dose, and then periodically. Stop drug if there is a persistent increase in ALT or AST levels of at least three times the upper limit of normal.
• Watch for signs of myositis.
• *Alert:* Don't confuse fluvastatin with fluoxetine.

**PATIENT TEACHING**
• Tell patient that drug may be taken without regard to meals, but that drug will work better if it's taken in the evening.
• Advise the patient who is also taking a bile-acid resin such as cholestyramine to take fluvastatin at bedtime, at least 4 hours after taking the resin.
• Teach patient about proper dietary management, weight control, and exercise. Explain their importance in controlling elevated cholesterol and triglyceride levels.
• Warn patient to avoid alcohol.
• Tell patient to notify prescriber of adverse reactions, particularly muscle aches and pains.
• Advise patient that it may take up to 4 weeks for the drug to be completely effective.
• Tell patient that drug may deplete body's stores of coenzyme Q10 and that he should discuss need for supplements with prescriber.
• *Alert:* Tell woman to stop drug and notify prescriber immediately if she is or may be pregnant or if she's breast-feeding.

# gemfibrozil
Apo-Gemfibrozil†, Lopid*

*Pregnancy risk category C*

**AVAILABLE FORMS**
*Tablets:* 600 mg

**INDICATIONS & DOSAGES**
➤ **Types IV and V hyperlipidemia unresponsive to diet and other drugs; to reduce risk of coronary heart disease in patients with type IIb hyperlipidemia who can't tolerate or who are refractory**

**to treatment with bile-acid sequestrants or niacin**
*Adults:* 1,200 mg P.O. daily in two divided doses, 30 minutes before morning and evening meals.

## ACTION
Inhibits peripheral lipolysis and reduces triglyceride synthesis in the liver. Lowers triglyceride levels and increases HDL cholesterol levels.

| Route | Onset | Peak | Duration |
|-------|-------|------|----------|
| P.O. | 2-5 days | 4 wk | Unknown |

## ADVERSE REACTIONS
**CNS:** headache, fatigue, vertigo.
**CV:** atrial fibrillation.
**GI:** *abdominal and epigastric pain,* diarrhea, nausea, vomiting, *dyspepsia,* constipation, acute appendicitis.
**Hematologic:** anemia, *leukopenia,* eosinophilia, *thrombocytopenia.*
**Hepatic:** bile duct obstruction.
**Metabolic:** hypokalemia.
**Skin:** rash, dermatitis, pruritus, eczema.

## INTERACTIONS
**Drug-drug.** *Glyburide:* May increase hypoglycemic effects. Monitor glucose, and watch for signs of hypoglycemia.
*HMG-CoA reductase inhibitors:* May cause myopathy with rhabdomyolysis. Avoid using together.
*Oral anticoagulants:* May enhance effects of oral anticoagulants. Monitor patient closely.

## EFFECTS ON LAB TEST RESULTS
● May increase ALT, AST, and CK levels. May decrease potassium level.
● May decrease hemoglobin, hematocrit, and eosinophil, WBC, and platelet counts.

## CONTRAINDICATIONS & CAUTIONS
● Contraindicated in patients hypersensitive to drug and in those with hepatic or severe renal dysfunction (including primary biliary cirrhosis) or gallbladder disease.

## NURSING CONSIDERATIONS
● Check CBC and test liver function periodically during the first 12 months of therapy.

● If drug has no beneficial effects after 3 months of therapy, expect prescriber to stop drug.

## PATIENT TEACHING
● Instruct patient to take drug 30 minutes before breakfast and dinner.
● Teach patient about proper dietary management of cholesterol and triglycerides. When appropriate, recommend weight control, exercise, and smoking cessation programs.
● Because of possible dizziness and blurred vision, advise patient to avoid driving or other potentially hazardous activities until effects of drug are known.
● Tell patient to observe bowel movements and to report evidence of excess fat in feces or other signs of bile duct obstruction.

# lovastatin (mevinolin)
Altocor, Mevacor✿

*Pregnancy risk category X*

## AVAILABLE FORMS
*Tablets:* 10 mg, 20 mg, 40 mg
*Tablets (extended-release):* 10 mg, 20 mg, 40 mg, 60 mg

## INDICATIONS & DOSAGES
➤ **To prevent and treat coronary heart disease; hyperlipidemia**
*Adults:* Initially, 20 mg P.O. once daily with evening meal. Recommended range is 10 to 80 mg as a single dose or in two divided doses; the maximum daily recommended dosage is 80 mg.

Or, 20 to 60 mg extended-release tablets P.O. h.s. Starting dose of 10 mg can be used for patients requiring smaller reductions; usual dosage range is 10 to 60 mg daily.
➤ **Heterozygous familial hypercholesterolemia in adolescents**
*Adolescents ages 10 to 17:* 10 to 40 mg/day P.O. with evening meal. Patients requiring reductions in LDL cholesterol level of 20% or more should start with 20 mg/day.
***Adjust-a-dose:*** For patients also taking cyclosporine, give 10 mg P.O. daily, not to exceed 20 mg daily. Avoid use of lovastatin with fibrates or niacin; if combined

with either, the dose of lovastatin shouldn't exceed 20 mg/day. For patient with creatinine clearance less than 30 ml/minute, carefully consider dosage increase above 20 mg/day and implement cautiously if necessary.

## ACTION
Inhibits HMG-CoA reductase, which is an early (and rate-limiting) step in cholesterol biosynthesis.

| Route | Onset | Peak | Duration |
|-------|-------|------|----------|
| P.O. | Unknown | 2 hr | Unknown |
| P.O. (extended-release) | Unknown | 14 hr | Unknown |

## ADVERSE REACTIONS
**CNS:** *headache,* dizziness, peripheral neuropathy, insomnia.
**CV:** chest pain.
**EENT:** blurred vision.
**GI:** constipation, diarrhea, dyspepsia, flatulence, abdominal pain or cramps, heartburn, nausea, vomiting.
**Musculoskeletal:** muscle cramps, myalgia, myositis, *rhabdomyolysis.*
**Skin:** rash, pruritus, alopecia.

## INTERACTIONS
**Drug-drug.** *Azole antifungals, clarithromycin, cyclosporine or other immunosuppressants, erythromycin, gemfibrozil, nefazodone, niacin:* May cause polymyositis and rhabdomyolysis. Don't exceed 20 mg lovastatin daily.
*Fluconazole, itraconazole, ketoconazole:* May increase lovastatin level and adverse effects. Avoid using together, or, if they must be given together, reduce dose of lovastatin.
*Oral anticoagulants:* May enhance oral anticoagulant effect. Monitor patient closely.
**Drug-herb.** *Eucalyptus, jin bu huan, kava:* May increase risk of hepatotoxicity. Discourage use together.
*Pectin:* May decrease lovastatin effect. Discourage use together.
*Red yeast rice:* May increase risk of adverse reactions because herb contains compounds similar to those of statin drugs. Discourage use together.

**Drug-food.** *Grapefruit juice:* May increase drug level, increasing risk of side effects. Discourage use together.
**Drug-lifestyle.** *Alcohol use:* May increase risk of hepatotoxicity. Discourage use together.

## EFFECTS ON LAB TEST RESULTS
● May increase ALT, AST, and CK levels.

## CONTRAINDICATIONS & CAUTIONS
● Contraindicated in patients hypersensitive to drug and in those with active liver disease or unexplained persistent elevations of transaminase levels; also contraindicated in pregnant and breast-feeding women, in women of childbearing potential, and in patients taking mibefradil.
● Use cautiously in patients who consume substantial quantities of alcohol or have a history of liver disease.
● In patients with severe renal insufficiency, dosage shouldn't exceed 20 mg/day.

## NURSING CONSIDERATIONS
● Use only after diet and other nondrug therapies prove ineffective. Have patient follow a standard low-cholesterol diet during therapy.
● Obtain liver function test results at the start of therapy, at 6 and 12 weeks after the start of therapy, and when increasing dose; then monitor results periodically.
● Heterozygous familial hypercholesterolemia can be diagnosed in adolescent boys and in girls who are at least 1 year postmenarche and are 10 to 17 years old, if, after an adequate trial of diet therapy, LDL cholesterol level remains over 189 mg/dl or LDL cholesterol remains over 160 mg/dl and patient has a positive family history of premature CV disease or two or more other CV disease risk factors.
● *Alert:* Don't confuse lovastatin with Lotensin, Leustatin, or Livostin.
● *Alert:* Don't confuse Mevacor with Mivacron.
● *Alert:* Don't confuse Altocor (lovastatin, extended-release) with Advicor (niacin and lovastatin extended-release).

## PATIENT TEACHING
● Instruct patient to take drug with the evening meal, which will improve absorption and cholesterol biosynthesis.

- Teach patient about proper dietary management of cholesterol and triglycerides. When appropriate, recommend weight control, exercise, and smoking cessation programs.
- Advise patient to have periodic eye examinations; related compounds cause cataracts.
- Instruct patient to store tablets at room temperature in a light-resistant container.
- Advise patient to promptly report unexplained muscle pain, tenderness, or weakness, particularly when accompanied by malaise or fever.
- Tell patient that drug may deplete body's stores of coenzyme Q10 and that he should discuss need for supplements with prescriber.
- *Alert:* Tell woman to stop drug and notify prescriber immediately if she is or may be pregnant or if she's breast-feeding.
- *Alert:* Advise patient not to crush or chew extended-release tablets.

## pravastatin sodium (eptastatin)
Pravachol⌀

*Pregnancy risk category X*

### AVAILABLE FORMS
*Tablets:* 10 mg, 20 mg, 40 mg, 80 mg

### INDICATIONS & DOSAGES
➤ **Primary and secondary prevention of coronary events; hyperlipidemia**
*Adults:* Initially, 40 mg P.O. once daily at the same time each day, with or without food. Adjust dosage q 4 weeks based on patient tolerance and response; maximum daily dose is 80 mg.
✳ *NEW INDICATION:* **Heterozygous familial hypercholesterolemia**
*Adolescents ages 14 to 18:* 40 mg P.O. once daily.
*Children ages 8 to 13:* 20 mg P.O. once daily.
*Adjust-a-dose:* In patients with renal or hepatic dysfunction, start with 10 mg P.O. daily. In patients also taking immunosuppressants, begin with 10 mg P.O. at bedtime and adjust to higher dosages with caution. Most patients treated with the combination of immunosuppressants and

pravastatin receive a maximum daily dose of 20 mg.

### ACTION
Inhibits HMG-CoA reductase, which is an early (and rate-limiting) step in cholesterol biosynthesis.

| Route | Onset | Peak | Duration |
|-------|---------|----------|----------|
| P.O. | Unknown | 60-90 min | Unknown |

### ADVERSE REACTIONS
**CNS:** headache, dizziness, fatigue.
**CV:** chest pain.
**EENT:** rhinitis.
**GI:** vomiting, diarrhea, heartburn, abdominal pain, constipation, flatulence, *nausea.*
**GU:** *renal failure* caused by myoglobinuria, urinary abnormality.
**Musculoskeletal:** myositis, myopathy, *localized muscle pain,* myalgia, **rhabdomyolysis.**
**Respiratory:** cough, influenza, common cold.
**Skin:** rash.
**Other:** flulike symptoms.

### INTERACTIONS
**Drug-drug.** *Cholestyramine, colestipol:* May decrease plasma levels of pravastatin. Give pravastatin 1 hour before or 4 hours after these drugs.
*Drugs that decrease levels or activity of endogenous steroids (such as cimetidine, ketoconazole, spironolactone):* May cause endocrine dysfunction. No intervention is needed; obtain complete drug history in patients who develop endocrine dysfunction.
*Erythromycin, fibric acid derivatives (such as clofibrate, gemfibrozil), immunosuppressants (such as cyclosporine), high dosages (1 g or more daily) of niacin (nicotinic acid):* May cause rhabdomyolysis. Monitor patient closely if use together can't be avoided.
*Fluconazole, itraconazole, ketoconazole:* May increase pravastatin level and adverse effects. Avoid using together or, if they must be given together, reduce dose of pravastatin.
*Gemfibrozil:* May decrease protein-binding and urinary clearance of pravastatin. Avoid using together.

---

*Hepatotoxic drugs:* May increase risk of hepatotoxicity. Avoid using together.
**Drug-herb.** *Eucalyptus, jin bu huan, kava:* May increase the risk of hepatotoxicity. Discourage use together.
*Red yeast rice:* May increase risk of adverse reactions because herb contains compounds similar to those of statin drugs. Discourage use together.
**Drug-lifestyle.** *Alcohol use:* May increase risk of hepatotoxicity. Discourage use together.

### EFFECTS ON LAB TEST RESULTS
● May increase ALT, AST, CK, alkaline phosphatase, and bilirubin levels.
● May alter thyroid function test values.

### CONTRAINDICATIONS & CAUTIONS
● Contraindicated in patients hypersensitive to drug and in those with active liver disease or conditions that cause unexplained, persistent elevations of transaminase levels.
● Contraindicated in pregnant and breast-feeding women and in women of childbearing age.
● Safety and efficacy in children younger than age 8 haven't been established.
● Use cautiously in patients who consume large quantities of alcohol or have history of liver disease.

### NURSING CONSIDERATIONS
● Use only after diet and other nondrug therapies prove ineffective. Patients should follow a standard low-cholesterol diet during therapy.
● Use in children with heterozygous familial hypercholesterolemia if LDL cholesterol level is at least 190 mg/dl or if LDL cholesterol is at least 160 mg/dl and patient has either a positive family history of premature CV disease or two or more other CV disease risk factors.
● Obtain liver function test results at start of therapy and then periodically. A liver biopsy may be performed if elevated liver enzyme levels persist.
● *Alert:* Don't confuse Pravachol with Prevacid or propranolol.

### PATIENT TEACHING
● Tell patient to take the prescribed dose in the evening, preferably at bedtime.

● Advise patient who is also taking a bile-acid resin such as cholestyramine to take pravastatin at least 1 hour before or 4 hours after taking resin.
● Tell patient to notify prescriber of adverse reactions, particularly muscle aches and pains.
● Teach patient about proper dietary management of cholesterol and triglycerides. When appropriate, recommend weight control, exercise, and smoking cessation programs.
● Inform patient that it will take up to 4 weeks to achieve full therapeutic effect.
● *Alert:* Tell woman to stop drug and notify prescriber immediately if she is or may be pregnant or if she's breast-feeding.

✳ *NEW DRUG*

## rosuvastatin calcium
Crestor◆

*Pregnancy risk category X*

### AVAILABLE FORMS
*Tablets:* 5 mg, 10 mg, 20 mg, 40 mg

### INDICATIONS & DOSAGES
➤ **Adjunct to diet to reduce LDL cholesterol, total cholesterol, apolipoprotein B (ApoB), non-HDL cholesterol, and triglyceride (TG) levels and to increase HDL cholesterol level in patients with primary hypercholesterolemia (heterozygous familial and nonfamilial) and mixed dyslipidemia (Fredrickson types IIa and IIb); adjunct to diet to treat elevated TG level (Fredrickson type IV)**
*Adults:* Initially, 10 mg P.O. once daily. Patients requiring less aggressive LDL cholesterol level reduction or those predisposed to myopathy may start therapy at 5 mg once daily. For aggressive lipid lowering, starting dosage may be 20 mg once daily. Increase p.r.n. to maximum of 40 mg daily. Dosage may be increased q 2 to 4 weeks, based on lipid levels.
➤ **Adjunct to lipid-lowering therapies, to reduce LDL cholesterol, ApoB, and total cholesterol levels in homozygous familial hypercholesterolemia**
*Adults:* Initially, 20 mg P.O. once daily. Maximum, 40 mg once daily.

**Adjust-a-dose:** If patient's creatinine clearance is less than 30 ml/minute, start with 5 mg once daily; don't exceed 10 mg once daily.

## ACTION
Inhibits HMG-CoA reductase, increases LDL receptors on liver cells, and inhibits hepatic synthesis of very low–density lipoprotein (VLDL).

| Route | Onset | Peak | Duration |
|-------|-------|------|----------|
| P.O. | Unknown | 3-5 hr | Unknown |

## ADVERSE REACTIONS
**CNS:** anxiety, asthenia, depression, dizziness, headache, insomnia, neuralgia, paresthesia, vertigo.
**CV:** angina pectoris, chest pain, hypertension, palpitations, peripheral edema, vasodilation.
**EENT:** pharyngitis, rhinitis, sinusitis.
**GI:** abdominal pain, constipation, diarrhea, dyspepsia, flatulence, gastritis, gastroenteritis, nausea, periodontal abscess, vomiting.
**GU:** UTI.
**Hematologic:** anemia, ecchymosis.
**Metabolic:** diabetes mellitus.
**Musculoskeletal:** arthralgia, arthritis, back pain, hypertonia, myalgia, neck pain, pain, pathological fracture, pelvic pain.
**Respiratory:** asthma, bronchitis, dyspnea, increased cough, pneumonia.
**Skin:** pruritus, rash.
**Other:** accidental injury, flulike syndrome, infection.

## INTERACTIONS
**Drug-drug.** *Antacids:* May decrease rosuvastatin level. Give antacids at least 2 hours after rosuvastatin.
*Cimetidine, ketoconazole, spironolactone:* May decrease level or effect of endogenous steroid hormones. Use together cautiously.
*Cyclosporine:* May increase rosuvastatin level and risk of myopathy or rhabdomyolysis. Don't exceed 5 mg of rosuvastatin daily. Watch for evidence of toxicity.
*Gemfibrozil:* May increase rosuvastatin level and risk of myopathy or rhabdomyolysis. Don't exceed 10 mg of rosuvastatin once daily. Watch for evidence of toxicity.

*Hormonal contraceptives:* May increase ethinyl estradiol and norgestrel levels. Watch for adverse effects.
*Warfarin:* May increase INR and risk of bleeding. Monitor INR, and watch for evidence of increased bleeding.
**Drug-lifestyle.** *Alcohol use:* May increase risk of hepatotoxicity. Discourage use together.

## EFFECTS ON LAB TEST RESULTS
● May increase creatinine phosphokinase, transaminase, glucose, glutamyl transpeptidase, alkaline phosphatase, and bilirubin levels.
● May decrease hemoglobin and hematocrit. May cause thyroid function abnormalities, dipstick-positive proteinuria, and microscopic hematuria.

## CONTRAINDICATIONS & CAUTIONS
● Contraindicated in patients hypersensitive to rosuvastatin or its components, pregnant patients, patients with active liver disease, and patients with unexplained persistent increase in serum transaminases.
● Use cautiously in patients who drink substantial amounts of alcohol, patients with a history of liver disease, and patients at increased risk for myopathies, such as those with renal impairment, advanced age, or hypothyroidism.

## NURSING CONSIDERATIONS
● Before therapy starts, assess patient for secondary causes of hypercholesterolemia, including poorly controlled diabetes, hypothyroidism, nephrotic syndrome, dyslipoproteinemias, obstructive liver disease, other drug therapy, and alcoholism.
● Before therapy starts, patient should try to control hypercholesterolemia with diet, exercise, and weight reduction.
● Test liver function before therapy starts, 12 weeks afterward, 12 weeks after any increase in dosage, and twice a year routinely. If AST or ALT level persists at more than three times the upper limit of normal, decrease dose or stop drug.
● **Alert:** Rarely, rhabdomyolysis with acute renal failure has developed in patients tak-

ing drugs in this class, including rosuvastatin.
● Notify prescriber if CK level becomes markedly elevated or myopathy is suspected, or if routine urinalysis shows persistent proteinuria and patient is taking 40 mg daily.
● Withhold drug temporarily if anything occurs that predisposes patient to myopathy or rhabdomyolysis, such as sepsis, hypotension, major surgery, trauma, uncontrolled seizures, or severe metabolic, endocrine, or electrolyte disorders.

## PATIENT TEACHING
● Instruct patient to take drug exactly as prescribed.
● Teach patient about diet, exercise, and weight control.
● Tell patient to immediately report unexplained muscle pain, tenderness, or weakness, especially if accompanied by malaise or fever.
● Instruct patient to wait at least 2 hours after taking rosuvastatin before taking aluminum- or magnesium-containing antacids.

---

## simvastatin (synvinolin)
Lipex‡, Zocor✿

*Pregnancy risk category X*

## AVAILABLE FORMS
*Tablets:* 5 mg, 10 mg, 20 mg, 40 mg, 80 mg

## INDICATIONS & DOSAGES
➤ **To reduce risk of death from CV disease and CV events in patients at high-risk for coronary events**
*Adults:* Initially, 20 mg P.O. daily in evening. Adjust dosage q 4 weeks based on patient tolerance and response. Maximum, 80 mg daily.
➤ **To reduce total and LDL cholesterol levels in patients with homozygous familial hypercholesterolemia**
*Adults:* 40 mg daily in evening; or, 80 mg daily given in three divided doses of 20 mg in morning, 20 mg in afternoon, and 40 mg in evening.

✹ *NEW INDICATION:* **Heterozygous familial hypercholesterolemia**
*Children ages 10 to 17:* 10 mg P.O. once daily in the evening. Maximum, 40 mg daily.
*Adjust-a-dose:* For patients taking cyclosporine, begin with 5 mg P.O. simvastatin daily; don't exceed 10 mg P.O. simvastatin daily. In patients taking fibrates or niacin, maximum is 10 mg P.O. simvastatin daily. In patients taking amiodarone or verapamil, maximum is 20 mg P.O. simvastatin daily. In patients with severe renal insufficiency, start with 5 mg P.O. daily.

## ACTION
Inhibits HMG-CoA reductase, which is an early (and rate-limiting) step in cholesterol biosynthesis.

| Route | Onset | Peak | Duration |
|-------|-------|------|----------|
| P.O. | Unknown | 1-2 hr | Unknown |

## ADVERSE REACTIONS
**CNS:** headache, asthenia.
**GI:** abdominal pain, constipation, diarrhea, dyspepsia, flatulence, *nausea, vomiting.*
**Respiratory:** upper respiratory tract infection.

## INTERACTIONS
**Drug-drug.** *Amiodarone, verapamil:* May increase risk of myopathy and rhabdomyolysis. Don't exceed 20 mg simvastatin daily.
*Clarithromycin, erythromycin, HIV protease inhibitors, nefazodone:* May increase risk of myopathy and rhabdomyolysis. Avoid using together, or suspend therapy during treatment with clarithromycin or erythromycin.
*Cyclosporine, fibrates, niacin:* May increase risk of myopathy and rhabdomyolysis. Avoid using together, or, if combination can't be avoided, monitor patient closely and don't exceed 10 mg simvastatin daily.
*Digoxin:* May slightly elevate digoxin level. Closely monitor digoxin levels at the start of simvastatin therapy.
*Fluconazole, itraconazole, ketoconazole:* May increase simvastatin level and adverse effects. Avoid using together, or, if

combination can't be avoided, reduce dose of simvastatin.

*Hepatotoxic drugs:* May increase risk for hepatotoxicity. Avoid using together.

*Warfarin:* May slightly enhance anticoagulant effect. Monitor PT and INR when therapy starts and when dose is adjusted.

**Drug-herb.** *Eucalyptus, jin bu huan, kava:* May increase risk of hepatotoxicity. Discourage use together.

*Red yeast rice:* May increase risk of adverse events or toxicity because it contains similar components to those of statin drugs. Discourage use together.

**Drug-food.** *Grapefruit juice:* May increase drug levels, increasing risk of adverse effects including myopathy and rhabdomyolysis. Discourage use together.

**Drug-lifestyle.** *Alcohol use:* May increase risk of hepatotoxicity. Discourage use together.

**EFFECTS ON LAB TEST RESULTS**
● May increase ALT, AST, and CK levels.

**CONTRAINDICATIONS & CAUTIONS**
● Contraindicated in patients hypersensitive to drug and in those with active liver disease or conditions that cause unexplained persistent elevations of transaminase levels. Also contraindicated in pregnant and breast-feeding women and in women of childbearing potential.
● Use cautiously in patients who consume substantial quantities of alcohol or have a history of liver disease.

**NURSING CONSIDERATIONS**
● Use drug only after diet and other nondrug therapies prove ineffective. Patient should follow a standard low-cholesterol diet during therapy.
● Obtain liver function test results at start of therapy and then periodically. A liver biopsy may be performed if enzyme elevations persist.
● Simvastatin 40 mg daily significantly reduces death from coronary heart disease, nonfatal MIs, CVA, and revascularization procedures.
● **Alert:** Don't confuse Zocor with Cozaar.

**PATIENT TEACHING**
● Instruct patient to take drug with the evening meal, because absorption is enhanced and cholesterol biosynthesis is greater.
● Teach patient about proper dietary management of cholesterol and triglycerides. When appropriate, recommend weight control, exercise, and smoking cessation programs.
● Tell patient to inform prescriber if adverse reactions occur, particularly muscle aches and pains.
● Tell patient that drug may deplete body's stores of coenzyme Q10 and that he should discuss need for supplements with prescriber.
● **Alert:** Tell woman to stop drug and notify prescriber immediately if she is or may be pregnant or if she's breast-feeding.

abciximab
alprostadil
arbutamine hydrochloride
bosentan
cilostazol
clopidogrel bisulfate
dipyridamole
eptifibatide
nesiritide
pentoxifylline
ticlopidine hydrochloride
tirofiban hydrochloride
treprostinil sodium

**COMBINATION PRODUCTS**
None.

---

## abciximab
ReoPro

*Pregnancy risk category C*

**AVAILABLE FORMS**
*Injection:* 2 mg/ml

**INDICATIONS & DOSAGES**
➤ **Adjunct to percutaneous translumi-nal coronary angioplasty (PTCA) or atherectomy to prevent acute cardiac ischemic complications in patients at high risk for abrupt closure of treated coronary vessel**
*Adults:* 0.25 mg/kg as an I.V. bolus given 10 to 60 minutes before start of PTCA or atherectomy; then a continuous I.V. infu-sion of 0.125 mcg/kg/minute to a maxi-mum of 10 mcg/minute for 12 hours.
➤ **Unstable angina not responding to conventional medical therapy in pa-tients scheduled for percutaneous coro-nary intervention within 24 hours**
*Adults:* 0.25 mg/kg as an I.V. bolus; then an 18- to 24-hour infusion of 10 mcg/minute, concluding 1 hour after percuta-neous coronary intervention.

**I.V. ADMINISTRATION**
● Inspect solution for particulate matter before administration. If opaque particles are visible, discard solution and obtain new vial. Withdraw needed amount of drug for I.V. bolus through a sterile, non-pyogenic, low-protein-binding 0.2- or 0.22-micron filter into a syringe. Give I.V. bolus 10 to 60 minutes before procedure.
● Withdraw needed amount of drug for continuous I.V. infusion through a sterile, nonpyogenic, low-protein-binding 0.2- or 0.22-micron filter into a syringe. Inject into 250 ml of sterile normal saline solu-tion or $D_5W$, and infuse at 0.125 mcg/kg/minute to a maximum of 10 mcg/minute for 12 hours via a continuous infusion pump equipped with an in-line filter. Dis-card unused portion at end of 12-hour in-fusion.
● Give drug in a separate I.V. line whenev-er possible; add no other drug to the infu-sion solution.

**ACTION**
Binds to the glycoprotein IIb/IIIa (GPIIb/IIIa) receptor of human platelets and inhibits platelet aggregation.

| Route | Onset | Peak | Duration |
|-------|-------|------|----------|
| I.V. | Immediate | Immediate | 48 hr |

**ADVERSE REACTIONS**
**CNS:** hyperesthesia, hypoesthesia, confu-sion, headache, pain.
**CV:** *hypotension,* **bradycardia,** peripheral edema.
**EENT:** abnormal vision.
**GI:** *nausea,* vomiting, abdominal pain.
**Hematologic:** *bleeding, thrombocytope-nia,* anemia, leukocytosis.
**Respiratory:** pleural effusion, pleurisy, pneumonia.

**INTERACTIONS**
**Drug-drug.** *Antiplatelet drugs, dipyri-damole, heparin, NSAIDs, other anticoag-ulants, thrombolytics, ticlopidine:* May in-crease risk of bleeding. Monitor patient closely.

## EFFECTS ON LAB TEST RESULTS
• May decrease hemoglobin and platelet and WBC counts.

## CONTRAINDICATIONS & CAUTIONS
• Contraindicated in patients hypersensitive to drug, its ingredients, or murine proteins.
• Contraindicated in those with active internal bleeding, significant GI or GU bleeding within 6 weeks, CVA within past 2 years, significant residual neurologic deficit, bleeding diathesis, thrombocytopenia (platelet count under 100,000/mm$^3$), major surgery or trauma within 6 weeks, intracranial neoplasm, intracranial arteriovenous malformation, intracranial aneurysm, severe uncontrolled hypertension, or history of vasculitis.
• Contraindicated when oral anticoagulants have been given within past 7 days unless PT is 1.2 times control or less, or when I.V. dextran is used before PTCA.
• Use with caution in patients at increased risk for bleeding, including those weighing less than 165 lb (75 kg) or older than age 65, those who have a history of GI disease, and those who are receiving thrombolytics. Conditions that increase patient's risk of bleeding include PTCA within 12 hours of onset of symptoms for acute MI, prolonged PTCA (lasting longer than 70 minutes), or failed PTCA. Heparin used with drug also may contribute to the risk of bleeding.

## NURSING CONSIDERATIONS
• The risk of bleeding is reduced by using low-dose, weight-adjusted heparin, early sheath removal, and careful maintenance of access site immobility.
• Consider patients undergoing PTCA who have one or more of the following conditions as candidates for drug therapy: unstable angina or a non–Q-wave MI, acute Q-wave MI within 12 hours of onset of symptoms, presence of two type B lesions in the artery to be dilated, presence of one type B lesion in the artery to be dilated in women older than age 65 or in diabetic patients, presence of one type C lesion in the artery to be dilated, or angioplasty of an infarct-related lesion within 7 days of MI.

• Review and monitor concomitant drugs; drug is intended for use with aspirin and heparin.
• *Alert:* Keep epinephrine, dopamine, theophylline, antihistamines, and corticosteroids readily available in case of anaphylaxis.
• Monitor patient closely for bleeding at the arterial access site used for cardiac catheterization and internal bleeding involving the GI or GU tract or retroperitoneal sites.
• Institute bleeding precautions. Maintain patient on bed rest for 6 to 8 hours after sheath removal or end of drug infusion, whichever is later. Minimize or avoid, if possible, arterial and venous punctures; I.M. injections; use of urinary catheters, nasogastric tubes, or automatic blood pressure cuffs; and nasotracheal intubation.
• Sheath may be removed during abciximab infusion, but only after heparin has been stopped and its effects largely reversed.
• Obtain platelet counts before treatment, 2 to 4 hours after the bolus dose, and at 24 hours or before discharge, whichever is first.
• Anticipate stopping abciximab and giving platelets for severe bleeding or thrombocytopenia.
• *Alert:* Don't confuse abciximab with arcitumomab.

## PATIENT TEACHING
• Explain use and administration of drug to patient and family.
• Instruct patient to report adverse reactions immediately.

## alprostadil
Prostin VR Pediatric

*Pregnancy risk category NR*

## AVAILABLE FORMS
*Injection:* 500 mcg/ml

## INDICATIONS & DOSAGES
➤ **Palliative therapy for temporary maintenance of patency of ductus**

---

Reactions may be *common*, uncommon, *life-threatening*, or COMMON AND LIFE-THREATENING.

arteriosus until surgery can be performed

*Neonates:* 0.05 to 0.1 mcg/kg/minute by I.V. infusion. When therapeutic response is achieved, reduce infusion rate to lowest dose that will maintain response. Maximum dose is 0.4 mcg/kg/minute. Or, drug can be given through umbilical artery catheter placed at ductal opening.

### I.V. ADMINISTRATION
● Dilute drug before giving. Prepare fresh solution daily; discard solution after 24 hours.
● For infusion, dilute 1 ml of concentrate labeled as containing 500 mcg in normal saline solution or $D_5W$ injection to yield a solution containing 2 to 20 mcg/ml.
● When using a device with a volumetric infusion chamber, add appropriate volume of diluent to the chamber; then add 1 ml of alprostadil concentrate.
● During dilution, avoid direct contact between concentrate and wall of plastic volumetric infusion chamber because solution may become hazy. If this occurs, discard solution.
● Don't use diluents that contain benzyl alcohol. Fatal toxic syndrome may occur.
● Reduce infusion rate if fever or significant hypotension occurs.
● Drug isn't recommended for direct injection or intermittent infusion. Give by continuous infusion using an infusion pump. Infuse through a large peripheral or central vein or through an umbilical artery catheter placed at the level of the ductus arteriosus. If flushing from peripheral vasodilation occurs, reposition catheter.

### ACTION
A prostaglandin derivative that relaxes the smooth muscle of the ductus arteriosus.

| Route | Onset | Peak | Duration |
|---|---|---|---|
| I.V. | 20 min | 1-2 hr | Length of infusion |

### ADVERSE REACTIONS
**CNS:** *seizures,* fever.
**CV:** *bradycardia,* hypotension, tachycardia, *cardiac arrest,* edema, flushing.
**GI:** diarrhea.

**Hematologic:** *DIC.*
**Metabolic:** hypokalemia.
**Respiratory:** APNEA.
**Other:** *sepsis.*

### INTERACTIONS
None significant.

### EFFECTS ON LAB TEST RESULTS
● May decrease potassium level.

### CONTRAINDICATIONS & CAUTIONS
● Contraindicated before making differential diagnosis between respiratory distress syndrome and cyanotic heart disease and in neonates who have respiratory distress syndrome.
● Use cautiously in neonates with bleeding tendencies because drug inhibits platelet aggregation.

### NURSING CONSIDERATIONS
● Keep respiratory support available.
● In infants with restricted pulmonary blood flow, measure drug's effectiveness by monitoring blood oxygenation. In infants with restricted systemic blood flow, measure drug's effectiveness by monitoring systemic blood pressure and blood pH.
● Monitor arterial pressure by umbilical artery catheter, auscultation, or Doppler transducer. Slow rate of infusion if arterial pressure falls significantly.
● Carefully monitor neonates receiving drug at recommended doses for longer than 120 hours for gastric outlet obstruction and antral hyperplasia.
● *Alert:* Apnea is most often seen in neonates weighing less than 2 kg (4.5 lb) at birth and usually appears during the first hour of drug infusion. CV and CNS adverse reactions occur more often in infants weighing less than 2 kg and in those receiving infusions for longer than 48 hours.
● *Alert:* Apnea and bradycardia may reflect drug overdose; if either occurs, stop infusion immediately.
● *Alert:* Don't confuse alprostadil with alprazolam.

### PATIENT TEACHING
● Inform parents of the need for drug, and explain its use.

---

*Rapid onset*  †Canada  ‡Australia  ◇OTC  ♦Off-label use  ⌀Photoguide  *Liquid contains alcohol.

● Encourage parents to ask questions and express concerns.

---

# arbutamine hydrochloride
GenESA

*Pregnancy risk category B*

---

## AVAILABLE FORMS
*Injection:* 20-ml prefilled syringe containing 1 mg (0.05 mg/ml)

## INDICATIONS & DOSAGES
➤ **Single-dose diagnostic aid in patients with suspected coronary artery disease who can't exercise adequately**
*Adults:* 0.1 mcg/kg/minute for 1 minute via GenESA I.V. infusion system. The device adjusts dose until maximal heart rate limit (set by user) or maximal infusion rate of 0.8 mcg/kg/minute (maximum total dose, 10 mcg/kg) is achieved.

## I.V. ADMINISTRATION
● Drug is manufactured with a prefilled glass syringe and plunger rod.
● *Alert:* Don't dilute drug before use. Give drug only via the prefilled syringe using the GenESA system (a closed-loop, computer-controlled I.V. infusion device).
● Before administration, inspect syringe for evidence of particulate matter or discoloration.

## ACTION
A sympathomimetic that increases cardiac workload through both positive inotropic and chronotropic actions.

| Route | Onset | Peak | Duration |
|-------|-------|------|----------|
| I.V. | 1 min | Unknown | Variable |

## ADVERSE REACTIONS
**CNS:** anxiety, dizziness, fatigue, *headache,* hypoesthesia, paresthesia, *tremor.*
**CV:** *angina pectoris,* **ARRHYTHMIAS,** chest pain, flushing, hot flashes, hypotension, palpitations, vasodilation.
**GI:** dry mouth, taste perversion, nausea.
**Respiratory:** dyspnea.
**Skin:** increased sweating.
**Other:** pain.

## INTERACTIONS
**Drug-drug.** *Beta blockers:* May attenuate arbutamine's effects. Stop drug at least 48 hours before giving arbutamine.

## EFFECTS ON LAB TEST RESULTS
None reported.

## CONTRAINDICATIONS & CAUTIONS
● Contraindicated in patients hypersensitive to drug and in those with idiopathic hypertrophic subaortic stenosis, a history of recurrent sustained ventricular tachycardia, or New York Heart Association class III or IV.
● Contraindicated in patients who have an implanted cardiac pacemaker or automated cardioverter or defibrillator and in those receiving digoxin, atropine, other anticholinergic drugs, class I antiarrhythmics (such as quinidine, lidocaine, or flecainide), or tricyclic antidepressants.
● Contraindicated in patients with unstable angina, mechanical left ventricular outflow obstruction (such as severe valvular aortic stenosis), uncontrolled systemic hypertension, cardiac transplantation, history of cerebrovascular disease, peripheral vascular disorder resulting in cerebral or aortic aneurysm, angle-closure glaucoma, supraventricular tachyarrhythmias or ventricular arrhythmias, or uncontrolled hyperthyroidism.
● Use cautiously in patients allergic to sulfites. Arbutamine contains sodium metabisulfite, which may produce an allergic response in susceptible patients.
● Safety and efficacy of drug in patients who have had an MI within 30 days haven't been evaluated.

## NURSING CONSIDERATIONS
● Don't give atropine to enhance drug-induced chronotropic response; taking these drugs together may lead to tachyarrhythmia.
● *Alert:* Before using the GenESA system, read and understand the manufacturer's directions.
● Monitor blood pressure, heart rate, and continuous ECG throughout drug infusion.

---

Reactions may be *common,* uncommon, *life-threatening,* or COMMON AND LIFE-THREATENING.

• Make sure resuscitation equipment is available by the bedside during drug administration.
• Drug transiently prolongs the QTc interval, as measured from a surface ECG.
• Drug causes transient reductions in potassium level but rarely to the point of hypokalemia.

**PATIENT TEACHING**
• Instruct patient to stop beta blockers at least 48 hours before undergoing cardiac stress testing with arbutamine.
• Inform patient that drug will temporarily increase heart rate but that he will be closely monitored.
• Inform patient of potential adverse effects.

## bosentan
Tracleer

*Pregnancy risk category X*

**AVAILABLE FORMS**
*Tablets:* 62.5 mg, 125 mg

**INDICATIONS & DOSAGES**
➤ **Pulmonary arterial hypertension in patients with World Health Organization class III or IV symptoms, to improve exercise ability and decrease rate of clinical worsening**
*Adults:* 62.5 mg P.O. b.i.d. in the morning and evening for 4 weeks. Increase to maintenance dosage of 125 mg P.O. b.i.d. in the morning and evening.
*Adjust-a-dose:* For patients who develop ALT and AST abnormalities, the dose may need to be decreased or the therapy stopped until levels return to normal. If therapy is resumed, begin with initial dose. Test levels within 3 days; thereafter, give according to the recommendations shown in the table at the top of the next column. If liver function abnormalities are accompanied by symptoms of liver injury or if bilirubin level is at least twice the upper limit of normal (ULN), stop treatment and don't restart.

In patients weighing less than 40 kg, the initial and maintenance dosage is 62.5 mg b.i.d.

| ALT and AST levels | Treatment and monitoring recommendations |
|---|---|
| > 3 and < 5 × ULN | Confirm with repeat test; if confirmed, reduce dose or interrupt treatment and retest q 2 wk. Once levels return to pretreatment values, continue or reintroduce treatment at starting dose. |
| > 5 and < 8 × ULN | Confirm with repeat test; if confirmed, stop treatment and retest at least q 2 wk. Once levels return to pretreatment values, consider reintroduction of treatment. |
| > 8 × ULN | Stop treatment; don't consider restarting drug. |

**ACTION**
Specific and competitive antagonist for endothelin-1 (ET-1). ET-1 levels are elevated in patients with pulmonary arterial hypertension, suggesting a pathogenic role for ET-1 in this disease.

| Route | Onset | Peak | Duration |
|---|---|---|---|
| P.O. | Unknown | 3-5 hr | Unknown |

**ADVERSE REACTIONS**
**CNS:** *headache,* fatigue.
**CV:** hypotension, palpitations, flushing, edema.
**EENT:** *nasopharyngitis.*
**GI:** dyspepsia.
**Hematologic:** *anemia.*
**Hepatic:** HEPATOTOXICITY.
**Skin:** pruritus.
**Other:** leg edema.

**INTERACTIONS**
**Drug-drug.** *Cyclosporine:* May increase levels of bosentan and decrease levels of cyclosporine. Avoid using together.
*Glyburide:* May increase risk of elevated liver function test results and decrease levels of both drugs. Avoid using together.
*Hormonal contraceptives:* May cause contraceptive failure. Advise use of an additional method of birth control.
*Ketoconazole:* May increase effects of bosentan. Watch for adverse effects.
*Simvastatin, other statins:* May decrease levels of these drugs. Monitor cholesterol

levels to assess need for statin dose adjustment.

### EFFECTS ON LAB TEST RESULTS
• May increase liver aminotransferase levels.
• May decrease hemoglobin and hematocrit.

### CONTRAINDICATIONS & CAUTIONS
• Contraindicated in patients hypersensitive to drug, in pregnant patients, and in those taking cyclosporine or glyburide. Don't use in patients with moderate-to-severe liver impairment or in those with elevated aminotransferase levels greater than three times the ULN.
• Use cautiously in patients with mild liver impairment.
• Drug may harm the fetus. Be sure patient isn't pregnant before starting treatment. Hormonal contraceptives shouldn't be used as the sole means of contraception because failure may occur.
• Because it's unknown whether drug appears in breast milk, drug isn't recommended for breast-feeding women.
• Safety and effectiveness in children haven't been established.

### NURSING CONSIDERATIONS
• Serious liver injury may occur with therapy. Measure aminotransferase levels before treatment and monthly thereafter. Adjust dosage accordingly.
• AST and ALT level elevations may be dose dependent and reversible, so monitor these levels carefully. If elevations are accompanied by symptoms of liver injury (nausea, vomiting, fever, abdominal pain, jaundice, or unusual lethargy or fatigue) or bilirubin increases by greater than twice the ULN, notify prescriber immediately.
• Monitor hemoglobin after 1 and 3 months of therapy and then every 3 months thereafter.
• Gradual dose reduction is recommended before stopping drug.

### PATIENT TEACHING
• Advise patient to take doses in the morning and evening, with or without food.
• Warn patient to avoid becoming pregnant while taking this drug. Hormonal contraceptives, including oral, implant-

able, and injectable methods, may not be effective when used together with this drug. Advise patient to use a back-up method of contraception. A monthly pregnancy test must be performed.
• Advise patient to have liver function tests and blood counts performed regularly.

## cilostazol
Pletal⁄

*Pregnancy risk category C*

### AVAILABLE FORMS
*Tablets:* 50 mg, 100 mg

### INDICATIONS & DOSAGES
➤ **To reduce symptoms of intermittent claudication**
*Adults:* 100 mg P.O. b.i.d., at least 30 minutes before or 2 hours after breakfast and dinner.
*Adjust-a-dose:* Decrease dose to 50 mg P.O. b.i.d. when giving with drugs that may interact to cause an increase in cilostazol level.

### ACTION
A quinolinone derivative thought to inhibit the enzyme phosphodiesterase III, thus inhibiting platelet aggregation and causing vasodilation.

| Route | Onset | Peak | Duration |
|-------|-------|------|----------|
| P.O. | Unknown | 2-4 hr | Unknown |

### ADVERSE REACTIONS
**CNS:** *headache, dizziness,* vertigo.
**CV:** *palpitations,* tachycardia, peripheral edema.
**EENT:** *pharyngitis, rhinitis.*
**GI:** *abnormal stools, diarrhea,* dyspepsia, abdominal pain, flatulence, nausea.
**Musculoskeletal:** back pain, myalgia.
**Respiratory:** increased cough.
**Other:** *infection.*

### INTERACTIONS
**Drug-drug.** *Diltiazem:* May increase cilostazol level. Reduce cilostazol dosage to 50 mg b.i.d.
*Erythromycin, other macrolides:* May increase level of cilostazol and its metabo-

---

Reactions may be *common,* uncommon, *life-threatening,* or COMMON AND LIFE-THREATENING.

lites. Reduce cilostazol dosage to 50 mg b.i.d.
*Omeprazole:* May increase level of cilostazol metabolite. Reduce cilostazol dosage to 50 mg b.i.d.
*Strong inhibitors of CYP3A4 (such as fluconazole, fluoxetine, fluvoxamine, itraconazole, ketoconazole, miconazole, nefazodone, sertraline):* May increase level of cilostazol and its metabolites. Reduce cilostazol dosage to 50 mg b.i.d.
**Drug-food.** *Grapefruit juice:* May increase drug level. Discourage use together.
**Drug-lifestyle.** *Smoking:* May decrease drug exposure. Discourage smoking.

**EFFECTS ON LAB TEST RESULTS**
None reported.

**CONTRAINDICATIONS & CAUTIONS**
• Contraindicated in patients hypersensitive to drug or its components and in those with heart failure of any severity.
• Use cautiously in patients with severe underlying heart disease; also use cautiously with other drugs having antiplatelet activity.

**NURSING CONSIDERATIONS**
• Give drug at least 30 minutes before or 2 hours after breakfast and dinner.
• Beneficial effects may not be seen for up to 12 weeks after therapy starts.
• *Alert:* Cilostazol and similar drugs that inhibit the enzyme phosphodiesterase decrease the likelihood of survival in patients with class III and IV heart failure.
• *Alert:* CV risk is unknown in patients who use drug on long-term basis and in those with severe underlying heart disease.
• Dosage can be reduced or stopped without such rebound effects as platelet hyperaggregation.
• Drug may cause reduced triglyceride levels and increased HDL cholesterol level.

**PATIENT TEACHING**
• Instruct patient to take drug on an empty stomach, at least 30 minutes before or 2 hours after breakfast and dinner.
• Tell patient that beneficial effect of drug on cramping pain isn't likely to be noticed

for 2 to 4 weeks and that it may take as long as 12 weeks.
• Advise patient to avoid drinking grapefruit juice during drug therapy.
• Inform patient that CV risk is unknown in patients who use drug on a long-term basis and in those with severe underlying heart disease.
• Tell patient that drug may cause dizziness. Caution patient not to drive or perform other activities that require alertness until response to drug is known.

## clopidogrel bisulfate
Plavix

*Pregnancy risk category B*

**AVAILABLE FORMS**
*Tablets:* 75 mg

**INDICATIONS & DOSAGES**
➤ **To reduce thrombotic events in patients with atherosclerosis documented by recent CVA, MI, or peripheral arterial disease**
*Adults:* 75 mg P.O. daily.
➤ **To reduce thrombotic events in patients with acute coronary syndrome (unstable angina and non–Q-wave MI), including those receiving drugs and those having percutaneous coronary intervention (with or without stent) or coronary artery bypass graft (CABG)**
*Adults:* Initially, a single 300-mg P.O. loading dose, then 75 mg P.O. once daily. Start and continue aspirin (75 to 325 mg once daily) with clopidogrel.

**ACTION**
Hinders platelet aggregation by inhibiting the binding of adenosine diphosphate (ADP) to its platelet receptor, impeding ADP-mediated activation and subsequent platelet aggregation. Clopidogrel irreversibly modifies the platelet ADP receptor.

| Route | Onset | Peak | Duration |
|-------|-------|------|----------|
| P.O. | 2 hr | Unknown | 5 days |

**ADVERSE REACTIONS**
**CNS:** headache, dizziness, fatigue, depression, pain.

**CV:** edema, hypertension.
**EENT:** rhinitis, epistaxis.
**GI:** *hemorrhage,* abdominal pain, dyspepsia, gastritis, constipation, diarrhea, ulcers.
**GU:** UTI.
**Hematologic:** purpura.
**Musculoskeletal:** arthralgia.
**Respiratory:** bronchitis, coughing, dyspnea, upper respiratory tract infection.
**Skin:** *rash,* pruritus.
**Other:** flulike syndrome.

### INTERACTIONS
**Drug-drug.** *Aspirin, NSAIDs:* May increase risk of GI bleeding. Monitor patient.
*Heparin, warfarin:* Safety hasn't been established. Use together cautiously.
**Drug-herb.** *Red clover:* May increase risk of bleeding. Discourage use together.

### EFFECTS ON LAB TEST RESULTS
• May decrease platelet count.

### CONTRAINDICATIONS & CAUTIONS
• Contraindicated in patients hypersensitive to drug or its components and in those with pathologic bleeding (such as peptic ulcer or intracranial hemorrhage).
• Use cautiously in patients at risk for increased bleeding from trauma, surgery, or other pathologic conditions and in those with hepatic impairment.

### NURSING CONSIDERATIONS
• Platelet aggregation won't return to normal for at least 5 days after drug has been stopped.
• *Alert:* Don't confuse Plavix with Paxil.

### PATIENT TEACHING
• Advise patient it may take longer than usual to stop bleeding. Tell him to refrain from activities in which trauma and bleeding may occur, and encourage him to wear a seatbelt when in a car.
• Instruct patient to notify prescriber if unusual bleeding or bruising occurs.
• Tell patient to inform all health care providers, including dentists, before undergoing procedures or starting new drug therapy, that he is taking drug.
• Inform patient that drug may be taken without regard to meals.

# dipyridamole
Apo-Dipyridamole FC†, Novo-Dipiradol†, Persantin‡, Persantine

*Pregnancy risk category B*

### AVAILABLE FORMS
*Injection:* 5 mg/ml in 2- and 10-ml vials
*Tablets:* 25 mg, 50 mg, 75 mg

### INDICATIONS & DOSAGES
➤ **To inhibit platelet adhesion in prosthetic heart valves (given together with warfarin)**
*Adults:* 75 to 100 mg P.O. q.i.d.
➤ **Alternative to exercise in evaluation of coronary artery disease during thallium myocardial perfusion scintigraphy**
*Adults:* 0.57 mg/kg as an I.V. infusion at a constant rate over 4 minutes (0.142 mg/kg/minute).

### I.V. ADMINISTRATION
• If giving as a diagnostic drug, dilute in half-normal or normal saline solution or $D_5W$ in at least a 1:2 ratio for a total volume of 20 to 50 ml. Inject Tl-201 within 5 minutes after completing the 4-minute dipyridamole infusion.

### ACTION
Unknown. Possibly involves drug's ability to increase adenosine, which is a coronary vasodilator and platelet aggregation inhibitor.

| Route | Onset | Peak | Duration |
|-------|-------|------|----------|
| P.O. | Unknown | 75 min | Unknown |
| I.V. | Unknown | 2 min | Unknown |

### ADVERSE REACTIONS
**CNS:** *headache, dizziness,* syncope.
**CV:** flushing, hypotension, angina pectoris, chest pain, *ECG abnormalities,* blood pressure lability, hypertension.
**GI:** *nausea,* vomiting, diarrhea, abdominal distress.
**Skin:** rash, irritation, pruritus.

### INTERACTIONS
**Drug-drug.** *Heparin:* May increase risk of bleeding. Monitor patient closely.
*Theophylline:* May prevent coronary vasodilation by I.V. dipyridamole, causing a

false-negative thallium-imaging result. Avoid using together.

**EFFECTS ON LAB TEST RESULTS**
None reported.

**CONTRAINDICATIONS & CAUTIONS**
• Contraindicated in patients hypersensitive to drug.
• Use cautiously in patients with hypotension.

**NURSING CONSIDERATIONS**
• If GI distress develops, give drug 1 hour before meals or with meals.
• Observe for adverse reactions, especially with large doses. Monitor blood pressure.
• Observe for signs and symptoms of bleeding; note prolonged bleeding time (especially with large doses or long-term therapy).
• The value of dipyridamole as part of an antithrombotic regimen is controversial; its use may not provide significantly better results than aspirin alone.
• *Alert:* Don't confuse dipyridamole with disopyramide.
• *Alert:* Don't confuse Persantine with Periactin.
• Persantine may contain tartrazine.

**PATIENT TEACHING**
• Instruct patient to take drug exactly as prescribed.
• Tell patient to report adverse reactions promptly.
• Tell patient receiving drug I.V. to report discomfort at insertion site.

---

# eptifibatide
Integrilin

*Pregnancy risk category B*

**AVAILABLE FORMS**
*Injection:* 10-ml (2 mg/ml), 100-ml (0.75 mg/ml) vials

**INDICATIONS & DOSAGES**
➤ **Acute coronary syndrome (unstable angina or non–Q-wave MI) in patients receiving drug therapy and in those**
**having percutaneous coronary intervention (PCI)**
*Adults with creatinine level less than 2 mg/dl:* 180 mcg/kg I.V. bolus as soon as possible after diagnosis, followed by a continuous I.V. infusion at a rate of 2 mcg/kg/minute until hospital discharge or initiation of coronary artery bypass graft (CABG) surgery, for up to 72 hours. If patient is having PCI, continue infusion until hospital discharge or for 18 to 24 hours after the procedure, whichever comes first, for up to 96 hours. Patients weighing more than 121 kg (266 lb) should receive a bolus not to exceed 22.6 mg, followed by a maximum infusion rate of 15 mg/hour.
*Adults with creatinine level of 2 to 4 mg/dl:* 180 mcg/kg I.V. bolus as soon as possible after diagnosis, followed by a continuous I.V. infusion at a rate of 1 mcg/kg/minute. Patients weighing more than 121 kg should receive a bolus not to exceed 22.6 mg, followed by a maximum infusion rate of 7.5 mg/hour.
➤ **In patients having PCI**
*Adults with creatinine level less than 2 mg/dl, started at time of PCI:* 180 mcg/kg I.V. bolus given just before the procedure, immediately followed by an infusion of 2 mcg/kg/minute and a second I.V. bolus of 180 mcg/kg given 10 minutes after the first bolus. Continue infusion until hospital discharge or for 18 to 24 hours, whichever comes first; a minimum of 12 hours of eptifibatide infusion is recommended. Patients weighing more than 121 kg should receive a bolus not to exceed 22.6 mg, followed by a maximum infusion rate of 15 mg/hour.
*Adults with creatinine level of 2 to 4 mg/dl, started at time of PCI:* 180 mcg/kg given just before the procedure, immediately followed by an infusion of 1 mcg/kg/minute and a second bolus of 180 mcg/kg given 10 minutes after the first bolus. Patients weighing more than 121 kg should receive a bolus not to exceed 22.6 mg, followed by a maximum infusion rate of 7.5 mg/hour.

**I.V. ADMINISTRATION**
• Withdraw bolus dose from 10-ml vial into a syringe and give by I.V. push over 1 or 2 minutes. Give I.V. infusion undilut-

ed directly from 100-ml vial using an infusion pump.
• Inspect solution for particulate matter before use. If particles are visible, the sterility is suspect; discard solution.
• Drug may be given in same I.V. line as alteplase, atropine, dobutamine, heparin, lidocaine, meperidine, metoprolol, midazolam, morphine, nitroglycerin, or verapamil; and in the same I.V. line with normal saline or normal saline and D₅W. Main infusion may also contain up to 60 mEq/L of potassium chloride.
• *Alert:* Don't give drug in same I.V. line as furosemide.
• Store vials in refrigerator at 36° to 46° F (2° to 8° C). The drug may be stored at room temperature for no longer than 2 months before use. Vials must be discarded if unused after 2 months of room temperature storage. Protect from light until administration

**ACTION**
Reversibly binds to the glycoprotein IIb/IIIa (GP IIb/IIIa) receptor on human platelets and inhibits platelet aggregation.

| Route | Onset | Peak | Duration |
|-------|-------|------|----------|
| I.V. | Immediate | Immediate | 4-6 hr |

**ADVERSE REACTIONS**
**CV:** hypotension.
**GU:** hematuria.
**Hematologic:** *bleeding, thrombocytopenia.*
**Other:** bleeding at femoral artery access site.

**INTERACTIONS**
**Drug-drug.** *Clopidogrel, dipyridamole, NSAIDs, oral anticoagulants (warfarin), thrombolytics, ticlopidine:* May increase risk of bleeding. Monitor patient closely.
*Other inhibitors of platelet receptor IIb/IIIa:* May cause serious bleeding. Avoid using together.

**EFFECTS ON LAB TEST RESULTS**
• May decrease platelet count.

**CONTRAINDICATIONS & CAUTIONS**
• Contraindicated in patients hypersensitive to drug or its ingredients and in those with history of bleeding diathesis or evi-

dence of active abnormal bleeding within previous 30 days; severe hypertension (systolic blood pressure higher than 200 mm Hg or diastolic blood pressure higher than 110 mm Hg) not adequately controlled with antihypertensives; major surgery within previous 6 weeks; history of CVA within 30 days or history of hemorrhagic CVA; current or planned use of another parenteral GP IIb/IIIa inhibitor; or platelet count less than 100,000/mm³. Drug also is contraindicated in patients whose creatinine level is 4 mg/dl or higher and in patients who depend on renal dialysis.
• Use cautiously in patients at increased risk for bleeding, in those with platelet count less than 150,000/mm³, in patients with hemorrhagic retinopathy, and in those weighing more than 143 kg (315 lb).

**NURSING CONSIDERATIONS**
• Drug is intended for use with heparin and aspirin.
• Stop eptifibatide and heparin and achieve sheath hemostasis by standard compressive techniques at least 4 hours before hospital discharge.
• The sheath may be removed during eptifibatide infusion, but only after heparin has been stopped and its effects largely reversed.
• If patient is to undergo CABG surgery, stop infusion before surgery.
• Minimize use of arterial and venous punctures, I.M. injections, urinary catheters, and nasotracheal and nasogastric tubes.
• When obtaining I.V. access, avoid use of noncompressible sites (such as subclavian or jugular veins).
• Monitor patient for bleeding.
• *Alert:* If patient's platelet count is less than 100,000/mm³, stop eptifibatide and heparin.
• Perform baseline laboratory tests before start of drug therapy; also determine hemoglobin, hematocrit, PT, INR, APTT, platelet count, and creatinine level.

**PATIENT TEACHING**
• Explain that drug is a blood thinner used to prevent chest pain and heart attack.
• Explain that benefits of drug far outweigh risk of serious bleeding.

---

Reactions may be *common*, uncommon, *life-threatening*, or COMMON AND LIFE-THREATENING.

• Tell patient to report chest discomfort or other adverse effects immediately.

---

# nesiritide
Natrecor

*Pregnancy risk category C*

---

## AVAILABLE FORMS
*Injection:* Single-dose vials of 1.5 mg sterile, lyophilized powder

## INDICATIONS & DOSAGES
➤ **Acutely decompensated heart failure in patients with dyspnea at rest or with minimal activity**
*Adults:* 2 mcg/kg by I.V. bolus over 60 seconds followed by continuous infusion of 0.01 mcg/kg/minute.
*Adjust-a-dose:* If hypotension develops during administration, reduce dosage or stop drug. Drug may be restarted at a dosage reduced by 30% with no bolus doses.

## I.V. ADMINISTRATION
• Reconstitute one 1.5-mg vial with 5 ml of diluent (such as $D_5W$, normal saline solution, 5% dextrose and 0.2% saline solution injection, or 5% dextrose and half-normal saline solution) from a prefilled 250-ml I.V. bag.
• Gently rock (don't shake) vial until a clear, colorless solution results.
• Withdraw contents of vial and add back to the 250-ml I.V. bag to yield 6 mcg/ml. Invert the bag several times to ensure complete mixing, and use the solution within 24 hours.
• Use the formulas below to calculate bolus volume (2 mcg/kg) and infusion flow rate (0.01 mcg/kg/minute):

Bolus volume = 0.33 × patient weight
(ml)                              (kg)

Infusion flow rate = 0.1 × patient weight
(ml/hr)                            (kg)

• Before giving bolus dose, prime the I.V. tubing. Withdraw the bolus and give over 60 seconds through an I.V. port in the tubing.

• Immediately after giving bolus, infuse drug at 0.1 ml/kg/hr to deliver 0.01 mcg/kg/minute.
• Store drug at 68° to 77° F (20° to 25° C).

## ACTION
A human B-type natriuretic peptide that binds to receptors on vascular smooth muscle and endothelial cells, increasing cGMP level, relaxing smooth muscle, and dilating veins and arteries. Reduces pulmonary capillary wedge pressure and systemic arterial pressure in patients with heart failure.

| Route | Onset | Peak | Duration |
|-------|-------|------|----------|
| I.V. | 15 min | 1 hr | 3 hr |

## ADVERSE REACTIONS
**CNS:** headache, confusion, somnolence, insomnia, dizziness, anxiety, paresthesia, tremor, fever.
**CV:** *hypotension, ventricular tachycardia,* ventricular extrasystoles, angina, *bradycardia,* atrial fibrillation, AV node conduction abnormalities.
**GI:** nausea, vomiting, abdominal pain.
**Hematologic:** anemia, increased creatinine level.
**Musculoskeletal:** back pain, leg cramps.
**Respiratory:** *apnea,* cough.
**Skin:** injection site reactions, pain at the site, rash, sweating, pruritus.

## INTERACTIONS
**Drug-drug.** *ACE inhibitors:* May increase hypotension symptoms. Monitor blood pressure closely.

## EFFECTS ON LAB TEST RESULTS
• May increase creatinine level more than 0.5 mg/dl above baseline.
• May decrease hemoglobin and hematocrit.

## CONTRAINDICATIONS & CAUTIONS
• Contraindicated in patients hypersensitive to drug or its components.
• Contraindicated in patients with cardiogenic shock, systolic blood pressure below 90 mm Hg, low cardiac filling pressures, conditions in which cardiac output depends on venous return, or conditions that make vasodilators inappropriate, such as

valvular stenosis, restrictive or obstructive cardiomyopathy, constrictive pericarditis, or pericardial tamponade.

## NURSING CONSIDERATIONS
● Don't start drug at higher-than-recommended dosage because this may cause hypotension and may increase creatinine level.
● *Alert:* This drug may cause hypotension. Monitor patient's blood pressure closely, particularly if he also takes an ACE inhibitor.
● *Alert:* Natrecor binds heparin and could bind the heparin lining of a heparin-coated catheter, decreasing the amount of nesiritide delivered. Don't give nesiritide through a central heparin-coated catheter.
● *Alert:* Drug is incompatible with injectable forms of bumetanide, enalaprilat, ethacrynate sodium, furosemide, heparin, hydralazine, and insulin. These drugs shouldn't be given through the same line with nesiritide.
● *Alert:* The preservative sodium metabisulfite is incompatible with nesiritide. Don't give injectable drugs with this preservative in the same line as nesiritide.
● Nesiritide may affect renal function in some people. In patients with severe heart failure whose renal function depends on the renin-angiotensin-aldosterone system, treatment may lead to azotemia.
● Results of giving this drug for longer than 48 hours are unknown because experience is limited.

## PATIENT TEACHING
● Tell patient to report discomfort at I.V. site.
● Urge patient to report symptoms of hypotension, such as dizziness, light-headedness, blurred vision, or sweating.
● Tell patient to report other adverse effects promptly.

## pentoxifylline
Trental⌀

*Pregnancy risk category C*

## AVAILABLE FORMS
*Tablets (extended-release):* 400 mg

## INDICATIONS & DOSAGES
➤ **Intermittent claudication from chronic occlusive vascular disease**
*Adults:* 400 mg P.O. t.i.d. with meals. May decrease to 400 mg b.i.d. if GI and CNS adverse effects occur.

## ACTION
Unknown. Improves capillary blood flow, probably by increasing RBC flexibility and lowering blood viscosity.

| Route | Onset | Peak | Duration |
|-------|---------|------|----------|
| P.O. | Unknown | 1 hr | Unknown |

## ADVERSE REACTIONS
**CNS:** headache, dizziness.
**GI:** dyspepsia, nausea, vomiting.

## INTERACTIONS
**Drug-drug.** *Anticoagulants:* May increase anticoagulant effect. Adjust anticoagulant dosage.
*Antihypertensives:* May increase hypotensive effect. May need to adjust dosage.
*Theophylline:* May increase theophylline level. Monitor patient closely.
**Drug-lifestyle.** *Smoking:* May cause vasoconstriction. Advise patient to avoid smoking because it may worsen his condition.

## EFFECTS ON LAB TEST RESULTS
None reported.

## CONTRAINDICATIONS & CAUTIONS
● Contraindicated in patients intolerant to methylxanthines, such as caffeine, theophylline, and theobromine, and in those with recent cerebral or retinal hemorrhage.

## NURSING CONSIDERATIONS
● Drug is useful in patients who aren't good surgical candidates.
● Elderly patients may be more sensitive to drug's effects.
● *Alert:* Don't confuse Trental with Trandate.

## PATIENT TEACHING
● Advise patient to take drug with meals to minimize GI upset.
● Instruct patient to swallow tablet whole, without breaking, crushing, or chewing.

---

Reactions may be *common,* uncommon, *life-threatening,* or COMMON AND LIFE-THREATENING.

• Tell patient to report GI or CNS adverse reactions; prescriber may reduce dosage.
• Urge patient not to stop drug during the first 8 weeks of therapy unless directed by prescriber.

---

## ticlopidine hydrochloride
Ticlid🖊

*Pregnancy risk category B*

### AVAILABLE FORMS
*Tablets:* 250 mg

### INDICATIONS & DOSAGES
➤ **To reduce risk of thrombotic CVA in patients who have had a CVA or CVA precursors**
*Adults:* 250 mg P.O. b.i.d. with meals.
➤ **Adjunct to aspirin to prevent suba-cute stent thrombosis in patients having coronary stent placement**
*Adults:* 250 mg P.O. b.i.d., combined with antiplatelet doses of aspirin. Start therapy after stent placement and continue for 30 days.

### ACTION
Unknown. An antiplatelet that probably blocks adenosine diphosphate-induced platelet-to-fibrinogen and platelet-to-platelet binding.

| Route | Onset | Peak | Duration |
|-------|-------|------|----------|
| P.O. | Unknown | 2 hr | Unknown |

### ADVERSE REACTIONS
**CNS:** dizziness, peripheral neuropathy, *intracranial bleeding.*
**CV:** vasculitis.
**EENT:** conjunctival hemorrhage.
**GI:** *diarrhea,* nausea, dyspepsia, abdominal pain, anorexia, vomiting, flatulence, bleeding.
**GU:** hematuria, dark urine.
**Hematologic:** *neutropenia, pancytopenia, agranulocytosis, immune thrombocytopenia.*
**Musculoskeletal:** arthropathy, myositis.
**Respiratory:** *allergic pneumonitis.*
**Skin:** rash, pruritus, maculopapular rash, urticaria, *thrombocytopenic purpura,* ecchymoses.

**Other:** hypersensitivity reactions, postoperative bleeding.

### INTERACTIONS
**Drug-drug.** *Antacids:* May decrease ticlopidine level. Separate doses by at least 2 hours.
*Aspirin:* May increase effect of aspirin on platelets. Use together cautiously.
*Cimetidine:* May decrease clearance of ticlopidine and increase risk of toxicity. Avoid using together.
*Digoxin:* May decrease digoxin level. Monitor digoxin level.
*Phenytoin:* May increase phenytoin level. Monitor patient closely.
*Theophylline:* May decrease theophylline clearance and risk of toxicity. Monitor patient closely and adjust theophylline dosage.
**Drug-herb.** *Red clover:* May cause bleeding. Discourage use together.

### EFFECTS ON LAB TEST RESULTS
• May increase ALT, AST, and alkaline phosphatase levels.
• May decrease neutrophil, WBC, RBC, platelet, and granulocyte counts.

### CONTRAINDICATIONS & CAUTIONS
• Contraindicated in patients hypersensitive to drug and in those with severe hepatic impairment, hematopoietic disorders, active pathologic bleeding from peptic ulceration, or active intracranial bleeding.
• Use cautiously and with close monitoring of CBC and WBC differentials. Moderate to severe neutropenia and agranulocytosis have occurred in patients taking ticlopidine.

### NURSING CONSIDERATIONS
• Because of life-threatening adverse reactions, use drug only in patients who are allergic to, can't tolerate, or have failed aspirin therapy.
• Obtain baseline liver function test results before therapy.
• Determine CBC and WBC differentials at second week of therapy and repeat every 2 weeks until end of third month.
• Monitor liver function tests and repeat if dysfunction is suspected.

---

• Thrombocytopenia has occurred rarely. Stop drug in patients with platelet count of 80,000/mm³ or less. If needed, give methylprednisolone 20 mg I.V. to normalize bleeding time within 2 hours.
• When used preoperatively, drug may decrease risk of graft occlusion in patients receiving coronary artery bypass grafts and reduce severity of drop in platelet count in patients receiving extracorporeal hemoperfusion during open heart surgery.

**PATIENT TEACHING**
• Tell patient to take drug with meals.
• Warn patient to avoid aspirin and aspirin-containing products and to check with prescriber or pharmacist before taking OTC drugs.
• Explain that drug will prolong bleeding time and that patient should report unusual or prolonged bleeding. Advise patient to tell dentists and other health care providers that he takes ticlopidine.
• Stress importance of regular blood tests. Because neutropenia can result with increased risk of infection, tell patient to immediately report signs and symptoms of infection, such as fever, chills, or sore throat.
• If drug is being substituted for a fibrinolytic or anticoagulant, tell patient to stop those drugs before starting ticlopidine therapy.
• Advise patient to stop drug 10 to 14 days before undergoing elective surgery. Also tell patient to immediately report yellow skin or sclera, severe or persistent diarrhea, rashes, bleeding under the skin, light-colored stools, or dark urine.

---

## tirofiban hydrochloride
Aggrastat

*Pregnancy risk category B*

**AVAILABLE FORMS**
*Injection:* 25-ml and 50-ml vials (250 mcg/ml), 250-ml and 500-ml premixed vials (50 mcg/ml)

**INDICATIONS & DOSAGES**
➤ **Acute coronary syndrome, with heparin or aspirin, including patients who**
**are to be managed medically and those undergoing PTCA or atherectomy**
*Adults:* I.V. loading dose of 0.4 mcg/kg/minute for 30 minutes; then continuous I.V. infusion of 0.1 mcg/kg/minute. Continue infusion through angiography and for 12 to 24 hours after angioplasty or atherectomy.
*Adjust-a-dose:* For patients with creatinine clearance less than 30 ml/minute, use a loading dose of 0.2 mcg/kg/minute for 30 minutes; then continuous infusion of 0.05 mcg/kg/minute. Continue infusion through angiography and for 12 to 24 hours after angioplasty or atherectomy.

**I.V. ADMINISTRATION**
• Dilute injections of 250 mcg/ml to same strength as 500-ml premixed vials (50 mcg/ml) as follows: Withdraw and discard 100 ml from a 500-ml bag of sterile normal saline solution or $D_5W$ and replace this volume with 100 ml of tirofiban injection (from four 25-ml vials or two 50-ml vials); or withdraw 50 ml from a 250-ml bag of sterile normal saline solution or $D_5W$ and replace this volume with 50 ml of tirofiban injection (from two 25-ml vials or one 50-ml vial), to yield 50 mcg/ml.
• Inspect solution for particulate matter before administration, and check for leaks by squeezing the inner bag firmly. If particles are visible or leaks occur, discard solution.
• Give heparin and tirofiban through same I.V. catheter. Give tirofiban through same I.V. line as dopamine, lidocaine, potassium chloride, and famotidine. Don't give drug through the same I.V. line as diazepam.
• Discard unused solution 24 hours after the start of infusion.
• Store drug at room temperature. Protect from light.

**ACTION**
Reversibly binds to the glycoprotein IIb/IIIa (GP IIb/IIIa) receptor on human platelets and inhibits platelet aggregation.

| Route | Onset | Peak | Duration |
|-------|-------|------|----------|
| I.V. | Immediate | Immediate | 4-6 hr |

---

Reactions may be *common*, uncommon, *life-threatening*, or COMMON AND LIFE-THREATENING.

## ADVERSE REACTIONS
**CNS:** dizziness, headache, fever.
**CV: *bradycardia, coronary artery dissection,*** edema, vasovagal reaction.
**GI:** nausea, *occult bleeding.*
**Hematologic:** *bleeding, thrombocytopenia.*
**Musculoskeletal:** leg pain.
**Skin:** sweating.
**Other:** *bleeding at arterial access site,* pelvic pain.

## INTERACTIONS
**Drug-drug.** *Anticoagulants such as warfarin, clopidogrel, dipyridamole, heparin, NSAIDs, thrombolytics, ticlopidine:* May increase risk of bleeding. Monitor patient closely.
*Levothyroxine, omeprazole:* May increase tirofiban renal clearance. Monitor patient.

## EFFECTS ON LAB TEST RESULTS
● May decrease hemoglobin, hematocrit, and platelet count.

## CONTRAINDICATIONS & CAUTIONS
● Contraindicated in patients hypersensitive to drug or its components.
● Contraindicated in those with active internal bleeding or history of bleeding diathesis within the previous 30 days and in those with history of intracranial hemorrhage, intracranial neoplasm, arteriovenous malformation, aneurysm, thrombocytopenia after previous exposure to tirofiban, CVA within 30 days, or hemorrhagic CVA.
● Contraindicated in those with history, symptoms, or findings suggestive of aortic dissection; severe hypertension (systolic blood pressure higher than 180 mm Hg or diastolic blood pressure higher than 110 mm Hg); acute pericarditis; major surgical procedure or severe physical trauma within previous month; or concomitant use of another parenteral GP IIb/IIIa inhibitor.
● Use cautiously in patients with increased risk of bleeding, including those with hemorrhagic retinopathy or platelet count less than 150,000/mm³.
● Safety and effectiveness of drug haven't been studied in patients younger than age 18.

## NURSING CONSIDERATIONS
● Monitor hemoglobin level, hematocrit, and platelet counts before starting therapy, 6 hours after loading dose, and at least daily during therapy. Notify prescriber if thrombocytopenia occurs.
● Give drug with aspirin and heparin.
● Monitor patient for bleeding.
● *Alert:* The most common adverse effect is bleeding at the arterial access site for cardiac catheterization.
● The risk of bleeding may be decreased by early sheath removal and by keeping the access site immobile. The sheath may be removed during tirofiban infusion, but only after heparin has been stopped and its effects largely reversed.
● Minimize use of arterial and venous punctures, I.M. injections, urinary catheters, and nasotracheal and nasogastric tubes.
● When obtaining I.V. access, avoid use of noncompressible sites (such as subclavian or jugular veins).
● *Alert:* Don't confuse Aggrastat with argatroban.

## PATIENT TEACHING
● Explain that drug is a blood thinner used to prevent chest pain and heart attack.
● Explain that risk of serious bleeding is far outweighed by the benefits of drug.
● Instruct patient to report chest discomfort or other adverse effects immediately.
● Tell patient that frequent blood sampling may be needed to evaluate therapy.

# treprostinil sodium
Remodulin

*Pregnancy risk category B*

## AVAILABLE FORMS
*Injection:* 1 mg/ml, 2.5 mg/ml, 5 mg/ml, 10 mg/ml

## INDICATIONS & DOSAGES
➤ **To reduce symptoms caused by exercise in patients with New York Heart Association class II to IV pulmonary arterial hypertension**
*Adults:* Initially, 1.25 nanogram/kg/minute by continuous S.C. infusion. If patient doesn't tolerate initial dose, reduce infu-

sion rate to 0.625 nanogram/kg/minute. Increase by 1.25-nanogram/kg/minute increments each week for the first 4 weeks and then by no more than 2.5 nanogram/kg/minute each week for the remaining duration of infusion. Maximum infusion rate is 40 nanogram/kg/minute.

*Adjust-a-dose:* In patients with mild or moderate hepatic insufficiency, initially give 0.625 nanogram/kg ideal body weight per minute and increase cautiously.

## ACTION
Directly vasodilates pulmonary and systemic arterial vascular beds and inhibits platelet aggregation.

| Route | Onset | Peak | Duration |
|-------|-------|------|----------|
| S.C. | Unknown | Unknown | Unknown |

## ADVERSE REACTIONS
**CNS:** dizziness, *headache,* fatigue.
**CV:** *vasodilation,* hypotension, edema, chest pain, right ventricular **heart failure.**
**GI:** *diarrhea, nausea.*
**Musculoskeletal:** *jaw pain.*
**Respiratory:** dyspnea.
**Skin:** *infusion site pain, infusion site reaction, rash,* pruritus, pallor.

## INTERACTIONS
**Drug-drug.** *Antihypertensives, diuretics, vasodilators:* May exacerbate reduction in blood pressure. Monitor blood pressure.
*Anticoagulants:* May increase risk of bleeding. Monitor patient closely for bleeding.

## EFFECTS ON LAB TEST RESULTS
None reported.

## CONTRAINDICATIONS & CAUTIONS
• Contraindicated in patients hypersensitive to drug or structurally related compounds.
• Use cautiously in patients with hepatic or renal impairment and in elderly patients.

## NURSING CONSIDERATIONS
• Assess the patient's ability to accept, place, and care for an S.C. catheter and to use an infusion pump.
• Give only by continuous S.C. infusion via a self-inserted S.C. catheter, using an infusion pump designed for S.C. drug delivery. The infusion pump should be small and lightweight; adjustable to approximately 0.002 ml/hour; have occlusion/no delivery, low battery, programming error, and motor malfunction alarms; have delivery accuracy of ± 6% or better; and be positive-pressure driven. The reservoir should be made of polyvinyl chloride, polypropylene, or glass.
• During use, a single reservoir syringe can be given up to 72 hours at 98.6° F (37° C).
• Don't use a single vial longer than 14 days after the initial introduction to the vial.
• Inspect for particulate matter and discoloration before administration.
• Start treatment in setting where adequate monitoring and emergency care are available.
• Increase dose if patient doesn't improve or symptoms worsen, and decrease if drug effects become excessive or unacceptable infusion site symptoms develop.
• Avoid abrupt withdrawal or sudden large dose reductions because pulmonary arterial hypertension symptoms may worsen.

## PATIENT TEACHING
• Inform patient that he'll need to continue therapy for prolonged periods, possibly years.
• Tell patient that subsequent disease management may require the initiation of I.V. therapy.
• Inform patient that many side effects may be related to the underlying disease (labored breathing, fatigue, chest pain).
• Tell patient that the most common local reactions are pain, redness, tissue hardening, and rash at the infusion site.

**acetaminophen**
**aspirin**
**diflunisal**

### COMBINATION PRODUCTS

ALLEREST NO DROWSINESS ◇,
COLDRINE ◇, ORNEX CAPLETS ◇, SINUS-
RELIEF, SINUTAB MAXIMUM STRENGTH
WITHOUT DROWSINESS ◇: acetaminophen
325 mg and pseudoephedrine hydrochloride 30 mg.

ASCRIPTIN, MAGNAPRIN: aspirin 325 mg,
magnesium hydroxide 50 mg, aluminum
hydroxide 50 mg, and calcium carbonate
50 mg ◇.

ASCRIPTIN A/D, MAGNAPRIN ARTHRITIS
STRENGTH: aspirin 325 mg, magnesium
hydroxide 75 mg, aluminum hydroxide
75 mg, and calcium carbonate 75 mg ◇.

BUFFERIN AF NITE TIME ◇, EXCEDRIN
P.M. ◇: acetaminophen 500 mg and
diphenhydramine citrate 38 mg.

CAMA ARTHRITIS PAIN RELIEVER: aspirin
500 mg, magnesium oxide 150 mg, and
aluminum hydroxide 150 mg.

EXCEDRIN EXTRA STRENGTH ◇: aspirin
250 mg, acetaminophen 250 mg, and caffeine 65 mg.

EXCEDRIN MIGRAINE: acetaminophen
250 mg, aspirin 250 mg, and caffeine
65 mg.

FIORICET WITH CODEINE, ISOPAP, MEDI-
GESIC, REPAN, TRIAD: acetaminophen
325 mg, caffeine 40 mg, and butalbital
50 mg.

FIORINAL WITH CODEINE: aspirin 325 mg,
caffeine 40 mg, and butalbital 50 mg.

MIDOL MAXIMUM STRENGTH MENSTRUAL:
acetaminophen 500 mg, caffeine 60 mg,
and pyrilamine maleate 15 mg.

MIDRIN: isometheptene mucate 65 mg,
dichloralphenazone 100 mg, and acetaminophen 325 mg.

P-A-C ANALGESIC ◇: aspirin 400 mg and
caffeine 32 mg.

SINUS EXCEDRIN EXTRA STRENGTH ◇:
acetaminophen 500 mg and pseudoephedrine hydrochloride 30 mg.

SINUTAB ◇: acetaminophen 325 mg,
chlorpheniramine maleate 2 mg, and pseudoephedrine hydrochloride 30 mg.

SINUTAB MAXIMUM STRENGTH WITHOUT
DROWSINESS ◇: acetaminophen 500 mg,
pseudoephedrine hydrochloride 30 mg.

TECNAL†: aspirin 330 mg, caffeine 40 mg,
and butalbital 50 mg.

TYLENOL PM EXTRA STRENGTH ◇: acetaminophen 500 mg, and diphenhydramine
25 mg.

VANQUISH ◇: aspirin 227 mg, acetaminophen 194 mg, caffeine 33 mg, aluminum hydroxide 25 mg, and magnesium
hydroxide 50 mg.

---

## acetaminophen (APAP, paracetamol)

Abenol† ◇; Acephen; Aceta ◇;
Acetaminophen ◇; Actamin ◇;
Aminofen ◇; Apacet ◇; Apo-
Acetaminophen† ◇; Atasol† ◇;
Banesin ◇; Dapa ◇; Dymadon‡ ◇;
Dymadon P‡ ◇; Exdol†;
Feverall ◇; Genapap ◇; Genebs ◇;
Liquiprin ◇; Neopap ◇; Oraphen-
PD ◇; Panadol ◇; Panamax‡ ◇;
Paralgin‡ ◇; Redutemp ◇;
Robigesic† ◇; Rounox† ◇;
Snaplets-FR ◇; St. Joseph
Aspirin-Free Fever Reducer for
Children ◇; Suppap ◇; Tapanol ◇;
Tempra ◇; Tylenol ◇; Valorin ◇

*Pregnancy risk category B*

---

### AVAILABLE FORMS

*Caplets:* 160 mg, 500 mg
*Caplets (extended-release):* 650 mg ◇
*Capsules:* 325 mg ◇, 500 mg ◇
*Elixir:* 80 mg/2.5 ml, 80 mg/5 ml,
120 mg/5 ml, 160 mg/5 ml* ◇, 325 mg/
5 ml* ◇
*Gelcaps:* 500 mg ◇
*Oral liquid:* 160 mg/5 ml ◇, 500 mg/
15 ml ◇
*Oral solution:* 48 mg/ml ◇, 100 mg/ml ◇
*Oral suspension:* 80 mg/0.8 ml ◇,
120 mg/5 ml‡, 160 mg/5 ml ◇

---

*Oral syrup:* 16 mg/ml ◊
*Sprinkles:* 80 mg/capsule ◊, 160 mg/capsule ◊
*Suppositories:* 80 mg ◊, 120 mg ◊, 125 mg ◊, 300 mg ◊, 325 mg ◊, 650 mg ◊
*Tablets:* 160 mg ◊, 325 mg ◊, 500 mg ◊, 650 mg ◊
*Tablets (chewable):* 80 mg ◊

## INDICATIONS & DOSAGES
➤ **Mild pain or fever**
*P.O.*
*Adults:* 325 to 650 mg P.O. q 4 to 6 hours; or 1 g P.O. t.i.d. or q.i.d., p.r.n. Or, two extended-release caplets P.O. q 8 hours. Maximum, 4 g daily. For long-term therapy, don't exceed 2.6 g daily unless prescribed and monitored closely by health care provider.
*Children older than age 14:* 650 mg P.O. q 4 to 6 hours, p.r.n.
*Children ages 12 to 14:* 640 mg P.O. q 4 to 6 hours, p.r.n.
*Children age 11:* 480 mg P.O. q 4 to 6 hours, p.r.n.
*Children ages 9 to 10:* 400 mg P.O. q 4 to 6 hours, p.r.n.
*Children ages 6 to 8:* 320 mg P.O. q 4 to 6 hours, p.r.n.
*Children ages 4 to 5:* 240 mg P.O. q 4 to 6 hours, p.r.n.
*Children ages 2 to 3:* 160 mg P.O. q 4 to 6 hours, p.r.n.
*Children ages 12 to 23 months:* 120 mg P.O. q 4 to 6 hours, p.r.n.
*Children ages 4 to 11 months:* 80 mg P.O. q 4 to 6 hours, p.r.n.
*Children up to age 3 months:* 40 mg P.O. q 4 to 6 hours, p.r.n.
Or, 10 to 15 mg/kg/dose q 4 hours, p.r.n. Don't exceed five doses in 24 hours.
*P.R.*
*Adults:* 650 mg P.R. q 4 to 6 hours, p.r.n. Maximum, 4 g daily. For long-term therapy, don't exceed 2.6 g daily unless prescribed and monitored closely by health care provider.
*Children ages 6 to 12:* 325 mg P.R. q 4 to 6 hours, p.r.n.
*Children ages 3 to 6:* 120 to 125 mg P.R. q 4 to 6 hours, p.r.n.
*Children ages 1 to 3:* 80 mg P.R. q 4 to 6 hours, p.r.n.

*Children ages 3 to 11 months:* 80 mg P.R. q 6 hours, p.r.n.

## ACTION
Unknown. Thought to produce analgesia by blocking pain impulses, probably by inhibiting synthesis of prostaglandin in the CNS or of other substances that sensitize pain receptors to mechanical or chemical stimulation. It's thought to relieve fever by central action in the hypothalamic heat-regulating center.

| Route | Onset | Peak | Duration |
|-------|-------|------|----------|
| P.O., P.R. | Unknown | ½-2 hr | 3-4 hr |

## ADVERSE REACTIONS
**Hematologic:** hemolytic anemia, *neutropenia, leukopenia, pancytopenia.*
**Hepatic:** *liver damage,* jaundice.
**Metabolic:** *hypoglycemia.*
**Skin:** rash, urticaria.

## INTERACTIONS
**Drug-drug.** *Barbiturates, carbamazepine, hydantoins, rifampin, sulfinpyrazone:* High doses or long-term use of these drugs may reduce therapeutic effects and enhance hepatotoxic effects of acetaminophen. Avoid using together.
*Lamotrigine:* May decrease lamotrigine level. Monitor patient for therapeutic effects.
*Warfarin:* May increase hypoprothrombinemic effects with long-term use with high doses of acetaminophen. Monitor INR closely.
*Zidovudine:* May decrease zidovudine effects. Monitor patient closely.
**Drug-herb.** *Watercress:* May inhibit oxidative metabolism of acetaminophen. Discourage use together.
**Drug-food.** *Caffeine:* May enhance analgesic effects of acetaminophen. Products may combine caffeine and acetaminophen for therapeutic advantage.
**Drug-lifestyle.** *Alcohol use:* May increase risk of hepatic damage. Discourage use together.

## EFFECTS ON LAB TEST RESULTS
● May decrease glucose level.
● May decrease hemoglobin, hematocrit, and neutrophil, WBC, RBC, and platelet counts.

---

Reactions may be *common*, uncommon, *life-threatening*, or **COMMON AND LIFE-THREATENING**.

• May falsely decrease glucose level in home monitoring systems; may cause false-positive test result for urinary 5-hydroxyindoleacetic acid.

**CONTRAINDICATIONS & CAUTIONS**
• Contraindicated in patients hypersensitive to drug.
• Use cautiously in patients with long-term alcohol use because therapeutic doses cause hepatotoxicity in these patients.

**NURSING CONSIDERATIONS**
• *Alert:* Many OTC products contain acetaminophen; be aware of this when calculating total daily dose.
• Use liquid form for children and patients who have difficulty swallowing.
• In children, don't exceed five doses in 24 hours.

**PATIENT TEACHING**
• Tell parents to consult prescriber before giving drug to children younger than age 2.
• Advise patient that drug is only for short-term use and to consult prescriber if giving to children for longer than 5 days or adults for longer than 10 days.
• *Alert:* Advise patient or caregiver that many OTC products contain acetaminophen; be aware of this when calculating total daily dose.
• Tell patient not to use for marked fever (temperature higher than 103.1° F [39.5° C]), fever persisting longer than 3 days, or recurrent fever unless directed by prescriber.
• *Alert:* Warn patient that high doses or unsupervised long-term use can cause liver damage. Excessive alcohol use may increase the risk of liver damage. Caution long-term alcoholics to limit acetaminophen intake to less than or equal to 2 g/day.
• Tell breast-feeding woman that acetaminophen appears in breast milk in low levels (less than 1% of dose). Drug may be used safely if therapy is short-term and doesn't exceed recommended doses.

# aspirin (acetylsalicylic acid)
Artria S.R.◇, ASA◇, Aspergum◇, Aspro‡, Bayer Aspirin◇, Bex‡, Coryphen†◇, Easprin◇, Ecotrin◇, Empirin◇, Entrophen†◇, Halfprin, Norwich Extra-Strength◇, Novasen†◇, Solprin‡, Vincent's Powders‡, ZORprin◇

*Pregnancy risk category D*

**AVAILABLE FORMS**
*Chewing gum:* 227.5 mg◇
*Suppositories:* 120 mg◇, 200 mg◇, 300 mg◇, 600 mg◇
*Tablets:* 325 mg◇, 500 mg◇
*Tablets (chewable):* 81 mg◇
*Tablets (controlled-release):* 800 mg
*Tablets (enteric-coated):* 81 mg◇, 165 mg◇, 325 mg◇, 500 mg◇, 650 mg◇, 975 mg
*Tablets (timed-release):* 650 mg◇

**INDICATIONS & DOSAGES**
➤ **Rheumatoid arthritis, osteoarthritis, or other polyarthritic or inflammatory conditions**
*Adults:* Initially, 2.4 to 3.6 g P.O. daily in divided doses. Maintenance dosage is 3.2 to 6 g P.O. daily in divided doses.
➤ **Juvenile rheumatoid arthritis**
*Children:* 60 to 110 mg/kg daily P.O. divided q 6 to 8 hours.
➤ **Mild pain or fever**
*Adults and children older than age 11:* 325 to 650 mg P.O. or P.R. q 4 hours, p.r.n.
*Children ages 2 to 11:* 10 to 15 mg/kg/dose P.O. or P.R. q 4 hours up to 80 mg/kg daily.
➤ **To prevent thrombosis**
*Adults:* 1.3 g P.O. daily in two to four divided doses.
➤ **To reduce risk of MI in patients with previous MI or unstable angina**
*Adults:* 75 to 325 mg P.O. daily.
➤ **Kawasaki syndrome (mucocutaneous lymph node syndrome)**
*Adults:* 80 to 180 mg/kg P.O. daily in four divided doses during febrile phase. When fever subsides, decrease to 10 mg/kg once daily and adjust according to salicylate level.

---

*Rapid onset*   †Canada   ‡Australia   ◇OTC   ◆Off-label use   ⌀Photoguide   *Liquid contains alcohol.

➤ **Acute rheumatic fever**
*Adults:* 5 to 8 g P.O. daily.
*Children:* 100 mg/kg daily P.O. for 2 weeks; then 75 mg/kg daily P.O. for 4 to 6 weeks.
➤ **To reduce risk of recurrent transient ischemic attacks and stroke or death in patients at risk**
*Adults:* 50 to 325 mg P.O. daily.
➤ **Acute ischemic stroke**
*Adults:* 160 to 325 mg P.O. daily, started within 48 hours of stroke onset and continued for up to 2 to 4 weeks.
➤ **Acute pericarditis after MI**
*Adults:* 160 to 325 mg P.O. daily. Higher doses (650 mg P.O. q 4 to 6 hours) may be needed.

**ACTION**
Unknown. Thought to produce analgesia by blocking pain impulses, probably by inhibiting synthesis of prostaglandin in the CNS or of other substances that sensitize pain receptors to mechanical or chemical stimulation. It's thought to relieve fever by central action in the hypothalamic heat-regulating center. Exerts its anti-inflammatory effect by inhibiting prostaglandin synthesis and may inhibit the synthesis or action of other mediators of the inflammatory response as well. In low doses, aspirin also appears to impede clotting by blocking prostaglandin synthesis, which prevents formation of the platelet-aggregating substance, thromboxane $A_2$.

| Route | Onset | Peak | Duration |
|---|---|---|---|
| P.O. (buffered) | 5-30 min | 1-2 hr | 1-4 hr |
| P.O. (enteric-coated) | 5-30 min | Variable | 1-4 hr |
| P.O. (extended) | 5-30 min | 1-4 hr | 1-4 hr |
| P.O. (solution) | 5-30 min | 15-40 min | 1-4 hr |
| P.O. (tablet) | 5-30 min | 25-40 min | 1-4 hr |
| P.R. | Unknown | 3-4 hr | Unknown |

**ADVERSE REACTIONS**
**EENT:** *tinnitus, hearing loss.*
**GI:** nausea, GI distress, occult bleeding, dyspepsia, *GI bleeding.*
**Hematologic:** *leukopenia, thrombocytopenia,* prolonged bleeding time.

**Hepatic:** *hepatitis.*
**Skin:** *rash,* bruising, urticaria.
**Other:** *angioedema,* hypersensitivity reactions, *Reye's syndrome.*

**INTERACTIONS**
**Drug-drug.** *ACE inhibitors:* May decrease antihypertensive effects. Monitor blood pressure closely.
*Ammonium chloride, other urine acidifiers:* May increase levels of aspirin products. Watch for aspirin toxicity.
*Antacids in high doses, other urine alkalinizers:* May decrease levels of aspirin products. Watch for decreased aspirin effect.
*Anticoagulants:* May increase risk of bleeding. Use with extreme caution if must be used together.
*Beta blockers:* May decrease antihypertensive effect. Avoid long-term aspirin use if patient is taking antihypertensives.
*Corticosteroids:* May enhance salicylate elimination and decrease drug level. Watch for decreased aspirin effect.
*Heparin:* May increase risk of bleeding. Monitor coagulation studies and patient closely if used together.
*Methotrexate:* May increase risk of methotrexate toxicity. Avoid using together.
*Nizatidine:* May increase risk of salicylate toxicity in patients receiving high doses of aspirin. Monitor patient closely.
*NSAIDs:* May decrease NSAID level and increase risk of GI bleeding. Avoid using together.
*Oral antidiabetics:* May increase hypoglycemic effect. Monitor patient closely.
*Probenecid, sulfinpyrazone:* May decrease uricosuric effect. Avoid using together.
*Valproic acid:* May increase valproic acid level. Avoid using together.
**Drug-herb.** *Dong quai, feverfew, ginkgo, horse chestnut, kelpware, red clover:* May increase risk of bleeding. Monitor patient closely for increased effects. Discourage use together.
*White willow:* May increase risk of adverse effects. Discourage use together.
**Drug-food.** *Caffeine:* May increase the absorption of aspirin. Watch for increased effects.
**Drug-lifestyle.** *Alcohol use:* May increase risk of GI bleeding. Discourage use together.

Reactions may be *common,* uncommon, *life-threatening,* or COMMON AND LIFE-THREATENING.

## EFFECTS ON LAB TEST RESULTS
• May increase liver function test values. May decrease WBC and platelet counts.
• May falsely increase protein-bound iodine levels. May interfere with urinary glucose analysis performed with Diastix, Chemstrip uG, Clinitest, and Benedict's solution; with urinary 5-hydroxyindoleacetic acid and vanillylmandelic acid tests; and with Gerhardt's test for urine acetoacetic acid.

## CONTRAINDICATIONS & CAUTIONS
• Contraindicated in patients hypersensitive to drug and in those with NSAID-induced sensitivity reactions, G6PD deficiency, or bleeding disorders, such as hemophilia, von Willebrand's disease, or telangiectasia.
• Use cautiously in patients with GI lesions, impaired renal function, hypoprothrombinemia, vitamin K deficiency, thrombocytopenia, thrombotic thrombocytopenic purpura, or severe hepatic impairment.
• Oral and rectal OTC products containing aspirin and non-aspirin salicylates shouldn't be given to children or teenagers who have or are recovering from chickenpox or flulike symptoms because of the risk of developing Reye syndrome.

## NURSING CONSIDERATIONS
• For inflammatory conditions, rheumatic fever, and thrombosis, give aspirin on a schedule rather than p.r.n.
• Because enteric-coated and sustained-release tablets are slowly absorbed, they aren't suitable for rapid relief of acute pain, fever, or inflammation. They cause less GI bleeding and may be better suited for long-term therapy, such as treatment of arthritis.
• For patient with swallowing difficulties, crush nonenteric-coated aspirin and dissolve in soft food or liquid. Give liquid immediately after mixing because drug will break down rapidly.
• For patients who can't tolerate oral drugs, ask prescriber about using aspirin rectal suppositories. Watch for rectal mucosal irritation or bleeding.
• Febrile, dehydrated children can develop toxicity rapidly.

• Monitor elderly patients closely because they may be more susceptible to aspirin's toxic effects.
• Monitor salicylate level. Therapeutic salicylate level in arthritis is 150 to 300 mcg/ml. Tinnitus may occur at levels above 200 mcg/ml, but this isn't a reliable indicator of toxicity, especially in very young patients and those older than age 60. With long-term therapy, severe toxic effects may occur with levels exceeding 400 mcg/ml.
• During prolonged therapy, assess hematocrit, hemoglobin, PT, INR, and renal function periodically.
• Aspirin irreversibly inhibits platelet aggregation. Stop aspirin 5 to 7 days before elective surgery to allow time for production and release of new platelets.
• Monitor patient for hypersensitivity reactions such as anaphylaxis or asthma.
• *Alert:* Don't confuse aspirin with Asendin or Afrin.

## PATIENT TEACHING
• Tell patient who is allergic to tartrazine dye to avoid aspirin.
• Advise patient on a low-salt diet that 1 tablet of buffered aspirin contains 553 mg of sodium.
• Advise patient to take drug with food, milk, antacid, or large glass of water to reduce unpleasant GI reactions.
• Tell patient not to crush or chew sustained-release or enteric-coated forms but to swallow them whole.
• Instruct patient to discard aspirin tablets that have a strong vinegar-like odor.
• Tell patient to consult prescriber if giving drug to children for longer than 5 days or adults for longer than 10 days.
• Advise patient receiving prolonged treatment with large doses of aspirin to watch for small round red pinprick spots, bleeding gums, and signs of GI bleeding, and to drink plenty of fluids. Encourage use of a soft-bristled toothbrush.
• Because of many possible drug interactions involving aspirin, warn patient taking prescription drugs to check with prescriber or pharmacist before taking aspirin or OTC products containing aspirin.
• Urge pregnant woman to avoid aspirin during last trimester of pregnancy unless specifically directed by prescriber.

• Aspirin is a leading cause of poisoning in children. Caution parents to keep drug out of reach of children. Encourage use of child-resistant containers.

---

## diflunisal
Dolobid

*Pregnancy risk category C*

### AVAILABLE FORMS
*Tablets:* 250 mg, 500 mg

### INDICATIONS & DOSAGES
➤ **Osteoarthritis, rheumatoid arthritis**
*Adults:* 500 to 1,000 mg P.O. daily in two divided doses, usually q 12 hours. Maximum, 1,500 mg daily.
*Elderly patients:* In patients older than age 65, one-half usual adult dosage.
➤ **Mild to moderate pain**
*Adults:* 1 g P.O., then 500 mg q 8 to 12 hours. A lower dosage of 500 mg P.O., then 250 mg q 8 to 12 hours may be appropriate.

### ACTION
Unknown. Probably related to inhibition of prostaglandin synthesis.

| Route | Onset | Peak | Duration |
|-------|-------|------|----------|
| P.O. | 1 hr | 2-3 hr | 8-12 hr |

### ADVERSE REACTIONS
**CNS:** dizziness, somnolence, insomnia, headache, fatigue.
**EENT:** tinnitus.
**GI:** nausea, dyspepsia, GI pain, diarrhea, vomiting, constipation, flatulence, stomatitis.
**GU:** renal impairment, hematuria, *interstitial nephritis.*
**Skin:** rash, pruritus, sweating, *erythema multiforme, Stevens-Johnson syndrome.*

### INTERACTIONS
**Drug-drug.** *Acetaminophen, hydrochlorothiazide, indomethacin:* May substantially increase levels of these drugs, increasing risk of toxicity. Avoid using together.
*Antacids, aspirin:* May decrease diflunisal level. Monitor patient for reduced therapeutic effect.

*Anticoagulants, thrombolytics:* May enhance effects of these drugs. Use together cautiously.
*Cyclosporine:* May enhance the nephrotoxicity of cyclosporine. Avoid using together.
*Methotrexate:* May enhance the toxicity of methotrexate. Avoid using together.
*Sulindac:* May decrease level of sulindac's metabolite. Monitor patient for reduced effect.

### EFFECTS ON LAB TEST RESULTS
• May falsely elevate salicylate level.

### CONTRAINDICATIONS & CAUTIONS
• Contraindicated in patients hypersensitive to drug and in those for whom acute asthmatic attacks, urticaria, or rhinitis are precipitated by aspirin or other NSAIDs.
• Use cautiously in patients with GI bleeding, history of peptic ulcer disease, renal impairment, compromised cardiac function, hypertension, or other conditions predisposing patient to fluid retention.

### NURSING CONSIDERATIONS
• *Alert:* Because of the epidemiologic link to Reye's syndrome, the Centers for Disease Control and Prevention recommend not giving salicylates to children and teenagers with chickenpox or flulike illness.

### PATIENT TEACHING
• Advise patient to take with water, milk, or meals.
• Tell patient that tablets must be swallowed whole.
• Instruct patient to avoid aspirin or acetaminophen while using diflunisal, unless prescribed.
• Inform breast-feeding woman that drug appears in breast milk and that she should stop either breast-feeding or taking drug.

---

Reactions may be *common*, uncommon, *life-threatening*, or COMMON AND LIFE-THREATENING.

# 25

## Nonsteroidal anti-inflammatory drugs

celecoxib
diclofenac potassium
diclofenac sodium
etodolac
ibuprofen
indomethacin
indomethacin sodium trihydrate
ketoprofen
ketorolac tromethamine
meloxicam
nabumetone
naproxen
naproxen sodium
piroxicam
rofecoxib
sulindac
valdecoxib

### COMBINATION PRODUCTS

ADVIL COLD AND SINUS CAPLETS ◊,
DIMETAPP SINUS CAPLETS, DRISTAN
SINUS CAPLETS ◊, SINE-AID IB CAPLETS:
pseudoephedrine hydrochloride 30 mg and
ibuprofen 200 mg.
ARTHROTEC: diclofenac 50 mg and misoprostol 200 mcg; diclofenac 75 mg and
misoprostol 200 mcg.
CHILDREN'S ADVIL COLD: suspension:
ibuprofen 100 mg and pseudoephedrine
15 mg per 5 ml.

---

## celecoxib
Celebrex✐

*Pregnancy risk category C*

---

### AVAILABLE FORMS
*Capsules:* 100 mg, 200 mg

### INDICATIONS & DOSAGES
➤ **Relief from signs and symptoms of
osteoarthritis**
*Adults:* 200 mg P.O. daily as a single dose
or divided equally b.i.d.
➤ **Relief from signs and symptoms of
rheumatoid arthritis**
*Adults:* 100 to 200 mg P.O. b.i.d.
➤ **Adjunctive treatment for familial
adenomatous polyposis to reduce the

number of adenomatous colorectal
polyps**
*Adults:* 400 mg P.O. b.i.d. with food for up
to 6 months.
➤ **Acute pain and primary dysmenorrhea**
*Adults:* 400 mg P.O. initially, followed by
an additional 200-mg dose if needed. On
subsequent days, 200 mg P.O. b.i.d. p.r.n.
*Adjust-a-dose:* For patients weighing less
than 50 kg (110 lb), start at lowest recommended dosage. For patients with moderate hepatic impairment (Child-Pugh Class
II), start therapy with reduced dosage.

### ACTION
Thought to inhibit prostaglandin synthesis, primarily via inhibition of
cyclooxygenase-2 (COX-2), thereby producing anti-inflammatory, analgesic, and
antipyretic effects.

| Route | Onset | Peak | Duration |
|---|---|---|---|
| P.O. | Unknown | 3 hr | Unknown |

### ADVERSE REACTIONS
**CNS:** dizziness, *headache,* insomnia.
**CV:** peripheral edema.
**EENT:** pharyngitis, rhinitis, sinusitis.
**GI:** abdominal pain, diarrhea, dyspepsia,
flatulence, nausea.
**Metabolic:** hyperchloremia.
**Musculoskeletal:** back pain.
**Respiratory:** upper respiratory tract in-
fection.
**Skin:** rash.
**Other:** accidental injury.

### INTERACTIONS
**Drug-drug.** *ACE inhibitors:* May decrease antihypertensive effects. Monitor
patient's blood pressure.
*Aluminum- and magnesium-containing
antacids:* May decrease celecoxib level.
Separate doses.
*Aspirin:* May increase risk of ulcers; low
aspirin dosages can be used safely to reduce the risk of CV events. Monitor patient for signs and symptoms of GI bleeding.

---

*Fluconazole:* May increase celecoxib level. Reduce dosage of celecoxib to minimal effective dose.

*Furosemide, thiazides:* May reduce sodium excretion caused by diuretics, leading to sodium retention. Monitor patient for swelling and increased blood pressure.

*Lithium:* May increase lithium level. Monitor lithium level closely during treatment.

*Warfarin:* May increase PT and bleeding complications. Monitor PT and INR, and check for signs and symptoms of bleeding.

**Drug-herb.** *Dong quai, feverfew, garlic, ginger, horse chestnut, red clover:* May increase risk of bleeding. Discourage use together.

*White willow:* Herb contains components similar to those of aspirin. Discourage use together.

**Drug-lifestyle.** *Long-term alcohol use, smoking:* May cause GI irritation or bleeding. Check for signs and symptoms of bleeding.

**EFFECTS ON LAB TEST RESULTS**
● May increase BUN, ALT, AST, and chloride levels. May decrease phosphate level.

**CONTRAINDICATIONS & CAUTIONS**
● Contraindicated in patients hypersensitive to drug, sulfonamides, aspirin, or other NSAIDs.
● Contraindicated in those with severe hepatic impairment.
● Contraindicated in women in the third trimester of pregnancy.
● Use cautiously in patients with history of ulcers or GI bleeding, advanced renal disease, dehydration, anemia, symptomatic liver disease, hypertension, edema, heart failure, or asthma and in poor P-450 2C9 metabolizers.
● Use cautiously in elderly or debilitated patients.

**NURSING CONSIDERATIONS**
● *Alert:* Patients may be allergic to drug if they are allergic to or have had anaphylactic reactions to sulfonamides, aspirin, or other NSAIDs.
● Patient with history of ulcers or GI bleeding is at higher risk for GI bleeding while taking NSAIDs such as celecoxib.

Other risk factors for GI bleeding include treatment with corticosteroids or anticoagulants, longer duration of NSAID treatment, smoking, alcoholism, older age, and poor overall health.
● Although drug may be used with low aspirin dosages, the combination may increase risk of GI bleeding.
● Watch for signs and symptoms of overt and occult bleeding.
● NSAIDs such as celecoxib can cause fluid retention; monitor patient with hypertension, edema, or heart failure.
● Drug may be hepatotoxic; watch for signs and symptoms of liver toxicity.
● Before starting drug therapy, rehydrate patient who is dehydrated.
● Drug can be given without regard to meals, but food may decrease GI upset.
● *Alert:* Don't confuse Celebrex with Cerebyx or Celexa.

**PATIENT TEACHING**
● Tell patient to report history of allergic reactions to sulfonamides, aspirin, or other NSAIDs before starting therapy.
● Instruct patient to promptly report signs of GI bleeding such as blood in vomit, urine, or stool; or black, tarry stools.
● Advise patient to immediately report rash, unexplained weight gain, or swelling.
● Tell woman to notify prescriber if she becomes pregnant or is planning to become pregnant during drug therapy.
● Instruct patient to take drug with food if stomach upset occurs.
● Teach patient that all NSAIDs, including celecoxib, may harm the liver. Signs and symptoms of liver toxicity include nausea, fatigue, lethargy, itching, yellowing of skin or eyes, right upper quadrant tenderness, and flulike syndrome. Advise patient to stop therapy and seek immediate medical advice if he experiences these signs or symptoms.
● Inform patient that it may take several days before he feels consistent pain relief.

---

Reactions may be *common*, uncommon, *life-threatening*, or COMMON AND LIFE-THREATENING.

# diclofenac potassium
Cataflam

# diclofenac sodium
Fenac‡, Voltaren, Voltaren-XR,
Voltaren Rapide†, Voltaren SR†

*Pregnancy risk category B*

## AVAILABLE FORMS
**diclofenac potassium**
*Tablets:* 50 mg
**diclofenac sodium**
*Suppositories:* 50 mg†, 100 mg†
*Tablets (delayed-release):* 25 mg, 50 mg,
75 mg
*Tablets (extended-release):* 100 mg

## INDICATIONS & DOSAGES
➤ **Ankylosing spondylitis**
*Adults:* 25 mg delayed-release diclofenac
sodium P.O. q.i.d.; may add another 25-mg
dose h.s.
➤ **Osteoarthritis**
*Adults:* 50 mg P.O. b.i.d. or t.i.d., or 75 mg
P.O. b.i.d. diclofenac potassium or
delayed-release diclofenac sodium only.
Or, 100 mg P.O. daily or b.i.d. extended-
release diclofenac sodium only.
➤ **Rheumatoid arthritis**
*Adults:* 50 mg P.O. t.i.d. or q.i.d., or 75 mg
P.O. b.i.d. diclofenac potassium or
delayed-release diclofenac sodium only.
Or, 100 mg P.O. daily or b.i.d. extended-
release diclofenac sodium only, or 50 to
100 mg diclofenac sodium P.R. h.s., as
substitute for last P.O. dose of the day.
Don't exceed 150 mg daily.
➤ **Analgesia, primary dysmenorrhea**
*Adults:* 50 mg diclofenac potassium P.O.
t.i.d. For some patients, the first dose on
the first day may be 100 mg, followed by
50 mg for the second and third doses;
maximum dose for first day is 200 mg.
Don't exceed 150 mg/day after the first
day.

## ACTION
Unknown. Produces anti-inflammatory,
analgesic, and antipyretic effects, possibly
by inhibiting prostaglandin synthesis.

| Route | Onset | Peak | Duration |
|---|---|---|---|
| P.O. (delayed-release) | 30 min | 2-3 hr | 8 hr |
| P.O. (extended-release) | Unknown | 5-6 hr | Unknown |
| P.O., P.R. | 10 min | 1 hr | 8 hr |

## ADVERSE REACTIONS
**CNS:** anxiety, depression, dizziness,
drowsiness, insomnia, irritability, headache, *aseptic meningitis.*
**CV:** *heart failure,* hypertension, edema,
fluid retention.
**EENT:** tinnitus, *laryngeal edema,*
swelling of the lips and tongue, blurred
vision, eye pain, night blindness, epistaxis,
reversible hearing loss.
**GI:** abdominal pain or cramps, constipation, diarrhea, indigestion, nausea, abdominal distention, flatulence, taste disorder,
peptic ulceration, bleeding, melena,
bloody diarrhea, appetite change, colitis.
**GU:** proteinuria, *acute renal failure,* oliguria, interstitial nephritis, papillary
necrosis, *nephrotic syndrome,* fluid retention.
**Hepatic:** jaundice, *hepatitis, hepatotoxicity.*
**Metabolic:** *hypoglycemia,* hyperglycemia.
**Musculoskeletal:** back, leg, or joint pain.
**Respiratory:** asthma.
**Skin:** rash, pruritus, urticaria, eczema,
dermatitis, alopecia, photosensitivity reactions, bullous eruption, *Stevens-Johnson
syndrome,* allergic purpura.
**Other:** *anaphylaxis, anaphylactoid reactions, angioedema.*

## INTERACTIONS
**Drug-drug.** *Anticoagulants, including
warfarin:* May cause bleeding. Monitor
patient closely.
*Aspirin:* May decrease effectiveness of diclofenac and increase GI toxicity. Avoid
using together.
*Beta blockers:* May blunt antihypertensive
effects. Monitor patient closely.
*Cyclosporine, digoxin, lithium, methotrex-
ate:* May reduce renal clearance of these
drugs and increase risk of toxicity. Monitor patient closely.
*Diuretics:* May decrease effectiveness of
diuretics. Avoid using together.

*Insulin, oral antidiabetics:* May alter requirements for antidiabetics. Monitor patient closely.

*Potassium-sparing diuretics:* May enhance potassium retention and increase potassium level. Monitor potassium level.

**Drug-herb.** *Dong quai, feverfew, garlic, ginger, horse chestnut, red clover:* May cause bleeding based on the known effects or components. Discourage use together.

*White willow:* Herb contains components similar to those of aspirin. Discourage use together.

**Drug-lifestyle.** *Sun exposure:* May cause photosensitivity reactions. Advise patient to avoid excessive sunlight exposure.

## EFFECTS ON LAB TEST RESULTS
● May increase ALT, AST, BUN, creatinine, and bilirubin levels. May increase or decrease glucose level.

## CONTRAINDICATIONS & CAUTIONS
● Contraindicated in patients hypersensitive to drug and in those with hepatic porphyria or history of asthma, urticaria, or other allergic reactions after taking aspirin or other NSAIDs. Drug isn't recommended for use during late pregnancy or breast-feeding.
● Use cautiously in patients with history of peptic ulcer disease, hepatic dysfunction, cardiac disease, hypertension, fluid retention, or impaired renal function.

## NURSING CONSIDERATIONS
● Because NSAIDs impair the synthesis of renal prostaglandins, they can decrease renal blood flow and lead to reversible renal impairment, especially in patients with renal or heart failure or liver dysfunction, in elderly patients, and in those taking diuretics. Monitor these patients closely.
● Liver function test values may become elevated during therapy. Monitor transaminase, especially ALT levels, periodically in patients undergoing long-term therapy. Make first transaminase measurement no later than 8 weeks after therapy begins.
● Because of their antipyretic and anti-inflammatory actions, NSAIDs may mask the signs and symptoms of infection.
● Serious GI toxicity, including peptic ulcers and bleeding, can occur in patient taking NSAIDs, despite lack of symptoms.
● *Alert:* Don't confuse diclofenac with Diflucan or Duphalac.

## PATIENT TEACHING
● Tell patient to take drug with milk, meals, or antacids to minimize GI distress.
● Instruct patient not to crush, break, or chew enteric-coated tablets.
● Advise patient not to take this drug with any other diclofenac-containing products (such as Arthrotec).
● Teach patient signs and symptoms of GI bleeding, including blood in vomit, urine, or stool; coffee-ground vomit; and black, tarry stool. Tell him to notify prescriber immediately if any of these occurs.
● Teach patient the signs and symptoms of damage to the liver, including nausea, fatigue, lethargy, itching, yellowed skin or eyes, right upper quadrant tenderness, and flulike symptoms. Tell the patient to contact prescriber immediately if these symptoms occur.
● Advise patient to avoid consuming alcohol or aspirin during drug therapy.
● Tell patient to wear sunscreen or protective clothing because drug may cause sensitivity to sunlight.
● Warn patient to avoid hazardous activities that require alertness until it is known whether the drug causes CNS symptoms.
● Tell pregnant woman to avoid use of drug during last trimester.

## etodolac
Lodine, Lodine XL

*Pregnancy risk category C*

## AVAILABLE FORMS
*Capsules:* 200 mg, 300 mg
*Tablets:* 400 mg, 500 mg
*Tablets (extended-release):* 400 mg, 500 mg, 600 mg

## INDICATIONS & DOSAGES
➤ **Acute pain**
*Adults:* 200 to 400 mg P.O. q 6 to 8 hours, p.r.n., not to exceed 1,200 mg daily. In patients weighing 60 kg (132 lb) or less, don't exceed total daily dose of 20 mg/kg.

➤ **Short- and long-term management of osteoarthritis and rheumatoid arthritis**
*Adults:* 600 to 1,000 mg P.O. daily, divided into two or three doses. Maximum daily dose is 1,200 mg. For extended-release tablets, 400 to 1,000 mg P.O. daily. Maximum daily dose is 1,200 mg.

## ACTION
Unknown. Produces anti-inflammatory, analgesic, and antipyretic effects, possibly by inhibiting prostaglandin synthesis.

| Route | Onset | Peak | Duration |
|-------|-------|------|----------|
| P.O. | 30 min | 1-2 hr | 4-12 hr |
| P.O. (extended-release) | Unknown | 3-12 hr | 6-12 hr |

## ADVERSE REACTIONS
**CNS:** asthenia, malaise, dizziness, depression, drowsiness, nervousness, insomnia, syncope, fever.
**CV:** hypertension, *heart failure,* flushing, palpitations, edema, fluid retention.
**EENT:** blurred vision, tinnitus, photophobia.
**GI:** *dyspepsia,* flatulence, abdominal pain, diarrhea, nausea, constipation, gastritis, melena, vomiting, anorexia, *peptic ulceration with or without GI bleeding or perforation,* ulcerative stomatitis, thirst, dry mouth.
**GU:** dysuria, urinary frequency, *renal failure.*
**Hematologic:** anemia, *leukopenia,* hemolytic anemia.
**Hepatic:** *hepatitis.*
**Metabolic:** weight gain.
**Respiratory:** asthma.
**Skin:** pruritus, rash, cutaneous vasculitis, *Stevens-Johnson syndrome.*
**Other:** chills.

## INTERACTIONS
**Drug-drug.** *Antacids:* May decrease etodolac's peak level. Watch for decreased effect of etodolac.
*Aspirin:* May decrease protein-binding of etodolac without altering its clearance. May increase GI toxicity. Avoid using together.
*Beta blockers, diuretics:* May blunt effects of these drugs. Monitor patient closely.

*Cyclosporine:* May increase risk of nephrotoxicity. Avoid using together.
*Digoxin, lithium, methotrexate:* May impair elimination of these drugs, increasing risk of toxicity. Monitor drug levels.
*Phenylbutazone:* May increase etodolac level. Avoid using together.
*Phenytoin:* May increase phenytoin level. Monitor patient for toxicity.
*Warfarin:* May decrease the protein-binding of warfarin but doesn't change its clearance. Although no dosage adjustment is needed, monitor INR closely and watch for bleeding.
**Drug-herb.** *Dong quai, feverfew, garlic, ginger, horse chestnut, red clover:* May increase risk of bleeding. Discourage use together.
*White willow:* Herb contains components similar to those of aspirin. Advise patients to avoid use with NSAIDs.
**Drug-lifestyle.** *Alcohol use:* May increase risk of adverse effects. Discourage use together.
*Sun exposure:* May cause photosensitivity reactions. Advise patient to avoid excessive sunlight exposure.

## EFFECTS ON LAB TEST RESULTS
• May decrease uric acid level.
• May decrease hemoglobin, hematocrit, and WBC count.
• May cause a false-positive test result for urinary bilirubin, possibly from phenolic metabolites and ketone bodies.

## CONTRAINDICATIONS & CAUTIONS
• Contraindicated in patients hypersensitive to drug and in those with history of aspirin- or NSAID-induced asthma, rhinitis, urticaria, or other allergic reactions.
• Use cautiously in patients with history of renal or hepatic impairment, preexisting asthma, or GI bleeding, ulceration, and perforation.

## NURSING CONSIDERATIONS
• Because NSAIDs impair the synthesis of renal prostaglandins, they can decrease renal blood flow and lead to reversible renal impairment, especially in patients with renal or heart failure or liver dysfunction, in elderly patients, and in those taking diuretics. Monitor these patients closely.

• Serious GI toxicity, including peptic ulcers and bleeding, can occur in patient taking NSAIDs, despite lack of symptoms.
• *Alert:* Don't confuse Lodine with codeine, iodine, or Iopidine.

### PATIENT TEACHING
• Tell patient to take drug with milk or meals to minimize GI discomfort.
• Teach patient signs and symptoms of GI bleeding, including blood in vomit, urine, or stool; coffee-ground vomit; and black, tarry stool. Tell him to notify prescriber immediately if any of these occurs.
• Advise patient to avoid consuming alcohol or aspirin while taking drug.
• Warn patient to avoid hazardous activities that require alertness until harmful CNS effects of drug are known.
• Teach patient signs and symptoms of liver damage, including nausea, fatigue, lethargy, itching, yellowed skin or eyes, right upper quadrant tenderness, and flu-like symptoms. Tell him to contact prescriber immediately if any of these symptoms occur.
• Advise patient to use a sunblock, wear protective clothing, and avoid prolonged exposure to sunlight because of possible sensitivity to sunlight.
• Tell pregnant woman to avoid use of drug during last trimester.

## ibuprofen
ACT-3‡, Actiprofen‡, Advil◇, Apo-Ibuprofen†, Bayer Select Ibuprofen Pain Relief Formula, Brufen‡, Children's Advil, Children's Motrin◇, Excedrin IB◇, Genpril◇, Haltran◇, Ibu-Tab◇, Medipren◇, Menadol, Midol IB, Motrin℮◇, Novo-Profen†, Nuprin◇, Nurofen‡, Nurofen Junior‡, Pamprin-IB, Rafen‡, Rufen, Saleto-200, Trendar◇

*Pregnancy risk category B; D in 3rd trimester*

### AVAILABLE FORMS
*Capsules:* 200 mg◇
*Oral drops:* 40 mg/ml◇
*Oral suspension:* 100 mg/2.5 ml◇, 100 mg/5 ml◇

*Tablets:* 100 mg, 200 mg◇, 300 mg, 400 mg, 600 mg, 800 mg
*Tablets (chewable):* 50 mg◇, 100 mg◇

### INDICATIONS & DOSAGES
➤ **Rheumatoid arthritis, osteoarthritis, arthritis**
*Adults:* 300 to 800 mg P.O. t.i.d. or q.i.d., not to exceed 3.2 g daily.
➤ **Mild to moderate pain, dysmenorrhea**
*Adults:* 400 mg P.O. q 4 to 6 hours, p.r.n.
➤ **Fever**
*Adults:* 200 to 400 mg P.O. q 4 to 6 hours. Don't exceed 1.2 g daily or give longer than 3 days.
*Children ages 6 months to 12 years:* If child's temperature is below 102.5° F (39.2° C), give 5 mg/kg P.O. q 6 to 8 hours. Treat higher temperatures with 10 mg/kg q 6 to 8 hours. Don't exceed 40 mg/kg daily.
➤ **Juvenile arthritis**
*Children:* 30 to 40 mg/kg daily P.O. in three or four divided doses. Maximum daily dose is 50 mg/kg.

### ACTION
Unknown. Produces anti-inflammatory, analgesic, and antipyretic effects, possibly by inhibiting prostaglandin synthesis.

| Route | Onset | Peak | Duration |
|-------|-------|------|----------|
| P.O. | Variable | 1-2 hr | 4-6 hr |

### ADVERSE REACTIONS
**CNS:** headache, dizziness, nervousness, *aseptic meningitis.*
**CV:** peripheral edema, fluid retention, edema.
**EENT:** tinnitus.
**GI:** epigastric distress, nausea, occult blood loss, peptic ulceration, diarrhea, constipation, abdominal pain, bloating, GI fullness, dyspepsia, flatulence, heartburn, decreased appetite.
**GU:** *acute renal failure,* azotemia, cystitis, hematuria.
**Hematologic:** prolonged bleeding time, anemia, *neutropenia, pancytopenia, thrombocytopenia, aplastic anemia, leukopenia, agranulocytosis.*
**Metabolic:** *hypoglycemia, hyperkalemia.*
**Respiratory:** *bronchospasm.*

---

Reactions may be *common,* uncommon, *life-threatening,* or COMMON AND LIFE-THREATENING.

**Skin:** pruritus, rash, urticaria, *Stevens-Johnson syndrome.*

## INTERACTIONS
**Drug-drug.** *Antihypertensives, furosemide, thiazide diuretics:* May decrease the effectiveness of diuretics or antihypertensives. Monitor patient closely.
*Aspirin:* May decrease ibuprofen level. Avoid using together.
*Aspirin, corticosteroids:* May cause adverse GI reactions. Avoid using together.
*Bisphosphonates:* May increase risk of gastric ulceration. Monitor patient for signs of gastric irritation or bleeding.
*Cyclosporine:* May increase nephrotoxicity of both drugs. Avoid using together.
*Digoxin, lithium, oral anticoagulants:* May increase levels or effects of these drugs. Monitor patient toxicity.
*Methotrexate:* May decrease methotrexate clearance and increases toxicity. Use together cautiously.
**Drug-herb.** *Dong quai, feverfew, garlic, ginger, ginkgo biloba, horse chestnut, red clover:* May increase risk of bleeding, based on the known effects of components. Discourage use together.
*White willow:* Herb contains components similar to those of aspirin. Advise patients to avoid use with NSAIDs.
**Drug-lifestyle.** *Alcohol use:* May cause adverse GI reactions. Discourage use together.
*Sun exposure:* May cause photosensitivity reactions. Advise patient to avoid excessive sunlight exposure.

## EFFECTS ON LAB TEST RESULTS
● May increase BUN, creatinine, ALT, AST, and potassium levels. May decrease glucose level.
● May decrease hemoglobin, hematocrit, and neutrophil, WBC, RBC, platelet, and granulocyte counts.

## CONTRAINDICATIONS & CAUTIONS
● Contraindicated in patients hypersensitive to drug and in those with angioedema, syndrome of nasal polyps, or bronchospastic reaction to aspirin or other NSAIDs.
● Contraindicated in pregnant women.
● Use cautiously in patients with GI disorders, history of peptic ulcer disease, he-

patic or renal disease, cardiac decompensation, hypertension, preexisting asthma, or known intrinsic coagulation defects.

## NURSING CONSIDERATIONS
● Check renal and hepatic function periodically in patients on long-term therapy. Stop drug if abnormalities occur and notify prescriber.
● Because of their antipyretic and anti-inflammatory actions, NSAIDs may mask signs and symptoms of infection.
● Blurred or diminished vision and changes in color vision have occurred.
● It may take 1 or 2 weeks before full anti-inflammatory effects occur.
● Serious GI toxicity, including peptic ulcers and bleeding, can occur in patient taking NSAIDs, despite lack of symptoms.
● If patient consumes three or more alcoholic drinks per day, use of ibuprofen may lead to stomach bleeding.
● *Alert:* Don't confuse Trendar with Trandate.

## PATIENT TEACHING
● Tell patient to take with meals or milk to reduce adverse GI reactions.
● *Alert:* Drug is available OTC. Instruct patient not to exceed 1.2 g daily, give to children younger than age 12, or take for extended periods (longer than 3 days for fever or longer than 10 days for pain) without consulting prescriber.
● Tell patient that full therapeutic effect for arthritis may be delayed for 2 to 4 weeks. Although pain relief occurs at low dosage levels, inflammation doesn't improve at dosages less than 400 mg q.i.d.
● Caution patient that use with aspirin, alcohol, or corticosteroids may increase risk of GI adverse reactions.
● Teach patient signs and symptoms of GI bleeding, including blood in vomit, urine, or stool; coffee-ground vomit; and black, tarry stool. Tell him to notify prescriber immediately if any of these occurs.
● Tell patient to contact prescriber before using this drug if fluid intake hasn't been adequate or if fluids have been lost as a result of vomiting or diarrhea.
● Warn patient to avoid hazardous activities that require mental alertness until effects on CNS are known.

• Advise patient to wear sunscreen to avoid hypersensitivity to sunlight.

## indomethacin
Apo-Indomethacin†, Arthrexin‡, Indocid†‡, Indocid SR†, Indocin, Indocin SR, Novo-Methacin†

## indomethacin sodium trihydrate
Apo-Indomethacin†, Indocin I.V., Novo-Methacin†

*Pregnancy risk category B; D in 3rd trimester*

### AVAILABLE FORMS
**indomethacin**
*Capsules:* 25 mg, 50 mg
*Capsules (sustained-release):* 75 mg
*Oral suspension:* 25 mg/5 ml
*Suppositories:* 50 mg
**indomethacin sodium trihydrate**
*Injection:* 1-mg vials

### INDICATIONS & DOSAGES
➤ **Moderate to severe rheumatoid arthritis or osteoarthritis, ankylosing spondylitis**
*Adults:* 25 mg P.O. or P.R. b.i.d. or t.i.d. with food or antacids; increase daily dose by 25 or 50 mg q 7 days, up to 200 mg daily. Or, sustained-release capsules (75 mg): 75 mg P.O. to start, in morning or h.s., followed by 75 mg b.i.d. if needed.
➤ **Acute gouty arthritis**
*Adults:* 50 mg P.O. t.i.d. Reduce dose as soon as possible; then stop therapy. Don't use sustained-release form.
➤ **Acute painful shoulders (bursitis or tendinitis)**
*Adults:* 75 to 150 mg P.O. daily in divided doses t.i.d. or q.i.d. for 7 to 14 days.
➤ **To close a hemodynamically significant patent ductus arteriosus in premature neonates (I.V. form only)**
*Neonates older than age 7 days:* 0.2 mg/kg I.V.; then two doses of 0.25 mg/kg at 12- to 24-hour intervals.
*Neonates ages 2 to 7 days:* 0.2 mg/kg I.V.; then two doses of 0.2 mg/kg at 12- to 24-hour intervals.

*Neonates younger than age 48 hours:* 0.2 mg/kg I.V.; then two doses of 0.1 mg/kg at 12- to 24-hour intervals.

### I.V. ADMINISTRATION
• Reconstitute powder for injection with sterile water or normal saline solution. For each 1-mg vial, add 1 or 2 ml of diluent for a solution containing 1 mg/ml or 0.5 mg/ml, respectively. Give over 20 to 30 minutes.
• *Alert:* Use only preservative-free sterile saline solution or sterile water to prepare I.V. injection. Never use diluents containing benzyl alcohol because it has been linked to toxicity in newborns. Because injection contains no preservatives, reconstitute drug immediately before use, and discard unused solution.
• Withhold administration of second or third scheduled I.V. dose if anuria or marked oliguria is evident; notify prescriber.
• Watch carefully for bleeding and for reduced urine output with I.V. administration.

### ACTION
Unknown. Produces anti-inflammatory, analgesic, and antipyretic effects, possibly by inhibiting prostaglandin synthesis.

| Route | Onset | Peak | Duration |
|-------|-------|------|----------|
| P.O. | 30 min | 1-4 hr | 4-6 hr |
| I.V. | Immediate | Immediate | 4-6 hr |
| P.R. | Unknown | Unknown | 4-6 hr |

### ADVERSE REACTIONS
**P.O. and P.R.**
**CNS:** *headache,* dizziness, depression, drowsiness, confusion, somnolence, fatigue, peripheral neuropathy, psychic disturbances, syncope, vertigo.
**CV:** hypertension, edema.
**EENT:** hearing loss, tinnitus.
**GI:** nausea, anorexia, diarrhea, abdominal pain, peptic ulceration, GI bleeding, constipation, dyspepsia, *pancreatitis.*
**GU:** hematuria.
**Hematologic:** iron-deficiency anemia.
**Metabolic:** *hyperkalemia.*
**Skin:** pruritus, urticaria, ***Stevens-Johnson syndrome.***
**Other:** hypersensitivity reactions.

---

Reactions may be *common,* uncommon, *life-threatening,* or COMMON AND LIFE-THREATENING.

**I.V.**

**GU:** hematuria, proteinuria, interstitial nephritis.

**INTERACTIONS**

**Drug-drug.** *Aminoglycosides, cyclosporine, methotrexate:* May enhance toxicity of these drugs. Avoid using together.

*Anticoagulants:* May cause bleeding. Monitor patient closely.

*Antihypertensives:* May decrease antihypertensive effect. Monitor patient closely.

*Antihypertensives, furosemide, thiazide diuretics:* May impair response to both drugs. Avoid using together, if possible.

*Aspirin:* May decrease level of indomethacin. Avoid using together.

*Aspirin, corticosteroids:* May increase risk of GI toxicity. Avoid using together.

*Bisphosphonates:* May increase risk of gastric ulceration. Monitor patient for symptoms of gastric irritation or GI bleeding.

*Diflunisal, probenecid:* May decrease indomethacin excretion. Watch for increased indomethacin adverse reactions.

*Digoxin:* May prolong half-life of digoxin. Use together cautiously.

*Dipyridamole:* May enhance fluid retention. Avoid using together.

*Lithium:* May increase lithium level. Monitor patient for toxicity.

*Penicillamine:* May increase bioavailability of penicillamine. Monitor patient closely.

*Phenytoin:* May increase phenytoin level. Monitor patient closely.

*Triamterene:* May cause nephrotoxicity. Monitor patient closely.

**Drug-herb.** *Dong quai, feverfew, garlic, ginger, horse chestnut, red clover:* May cause bleeding. Discourage use together.

*Senna:* May inhibit diarrheal effects. Discourage use together.

*White willow:* Herb contains components similar to those of aspirin. Discourage use together.

**Drug-lifestyle.** *Alcohol use:* May cause GI toxicity. Discourage use together.

**EFFECTS ON LAB TEST RESULTS**

• May increase potassium level. May elevate liver function test results.

• May decrease hemoglobin and hematocrit.

**CONTRAINDICATIONS & CAUTIONS**

• Contraindicated in patients hypersensitive to drug and in those with a history of aspirin- or NSAID-induced asthma, rhinitis, or urticaria.

• Contraindicated in pregnant or breast-feeding women and in neonates with untreated infection, active bleeding, coagulation defects or thrombocytopenia, congenital heart disease needing patency of the ductus arteriosus, necrotizing enterocolitis, or significant renal impairment. Suppositories are contraindicated in patients with history of proctitis or recent rectal bleeding.

• Contraindicated in pregnant women.

• Use cautiously in patients with epilepsy, parkinsonism, hepatic or renal disease, CV disease, infection, and mental illness or depression. Also use cautiously in elderly patients and patients with history of GI disease.

**NURSING CONSIDERATIONS**

• Because of the high risk of adverse effects from long-term use, indomethacin shouldn't be used routinely as an analgesic or antipyretic.

• Sustained-release capsules shouldn't be used for treatment of acute gouty arthritis.

• Give oral dose with food, milk, or antacid to decrease GI upset.

• If ductus arteriosus reopens, a second course of one to three doses may be given. If ineffective, surgery may be needed.

• Watch for bleeding in patients receiving anticoagulants, patients with coagulation defects, and neonates.

• Because NSAIDs impair synthesis of renal prostaglandins, they can decrease renal blood flow and lead to reversible renal impairment, especially in patients with renal failure, heart failure, or liver dysfunction; in elderly patients; and in those taking diuretics. Monitor these patients closely.

• Drug causes sodium retention; watch for weight gain (especially in elderly patients) and increased blood pressure in patients with hypertension.

• Monitor patient for rash and respiratory distress, which may indicate a hypersensitivity reaction.

• Because of their antipyretic and anti-inflammatory actions, NSAIDs may mask signs and symptoms of infection.

• Serious GI toxicity (including peptic ulcers and bleeding) can occur in patient taking NSAIDs, despite lack of symptoms.

**PATIENT TEACHING**
• Tell patient to take oral drug with food, milk, or antacid to prevent GI upset.
• Alert patient that using oral form with aspirin, alcohol, or corticosteroids may increase risk of adverse GI reactions.
• Teach patient signs and symptoms of GI bleeding, including blood in vomit, urine, or stool; coffee-ground vomit; and black, tarry stool. Tell him to notify prescriber immediately if any of these occurs.
• Warn patient to avoid hazardous activities that require mental alertness until CNS effects are known.
• Tell patient to notify prescriber immediately if visual or hearing changes occur. Monitor patient on long-term oral therapy for toxicity by conducting regular eye examinations, hearing tests, complete blood counts, and kidney function tests.

---

# ketoprofen
Actron, Apo-Keto†, Apo-Keto-E†, Novo-Keto-EC†, Orudis, Orudis E†, Orudis KT, Orudis SR†‡, Oruvail, Rhodis†, Rhodis-EC†

*Pregnancy risk category B*

---

**AVAILABLE FORMS**
*Capsules:* 25 mg, 50 mg, 75 mg
*Capsules (extended-release):* 100 mg, 150 mg, 200 mg
*Suppositories:* 50 mg†, 100 mg†
*Tablets:* 12.5 mg◊
*Tablets (enteric-coated):* 50 mg†, 100 mg†
*Tablets (extended-release):* 200 mg†

**INDICATIONS & DOSAGES**
➤ **Rheumatoid arthritis, osteoarthritis**
*Adults:* 75 mg t.i.d. or 50 mg q.i.d., or 200 mg as an extended-release tablet once daily. Maximum dose is 300 mg daily, or 200 mg daily for extended-release capsules. Or, 50 or 100 mg P.R. b.i.d.; or one suppository h.s. (with oral ketoprofen during the day).
*Adults older than age 75:* 75 to 150 mg P.O. daily. Adjust dose according to patient's response and tolerance.

➤ **Mild to moderate pain, dysmenorrhea**
*Adults:* 25 to 50 mg P.O. q 6 to 8 hours, p.r.n. Maximum dose is 300 mg/day.
➤ **Minor aches and pain or fever**
*Adults:* 12.5 mg q 4 to 6 hours. Don't exceed 25 mg in 4 to 6 hours or 75 mg in 24 hours.
*Adjust-a-dose:* For elderly patients and those with impaired renal function, reduce first dose to between one-third and one-half of normal first dose.

**ACTION**
Unknown. Produces anti-inflammatory, analgesic, and antipyretic effects, possibly by inhibiting prostaglandin synthesis.

| Route | Onset | Peak | Duration |
|---|---|---|---|
| P.O. (extended-release) | 2-3 hr | 6-7 hr | Unknown |
| P.O., P.R. | 1-2 hr | 30-120 min | 3-4 hr |

**ADVERSE REACTIONS**
**CNS:** headache, dizziness, CNS excitation (insomnia, nervousness, dreams) or depression (somnolence, malaise, depression).
**CV:** peripheral edema.
**EENT:** tinnitus, visual disturbances.
**GI:** nausea, abdominal pain, diarrhea, constipation, flatulence, peptic ulceration, *dyspepsia,* anorexia, vomiting, stomatitis.
**GU:** *nephrotoxicity.*
**Hematologic:** prolonged bleeding time.
**Respiratory:** dyspnea.
**Skin:** rash, photosensitivity reactions.

**INTERACTIONS**
**Drug-drug.** *Aspirin, corticosteroids:* May increase risk of adverse GI reactions. Avoid using together.
*Aspirin, probenecid:* May increase ketoprofen level. Avoid using together.
*Cyclosporine:* May increase nephrotoxicity. Avoid using together.
*Hydrochlorothiazide, other diuretics:* May decrease diuretic effectiveness. Monitor patient for lack of effect.
*Lithium, methotrexate, phenytoin:* May increase levels of these drugs, leading to toxicity. Monitor patient closely.
*Warfarin:* May increase risk of bleeding. Monitor patient closely.

---

Reactions may be *common*, uncommon, *life-threatening*, or COMMON AND LIFE-THREATENING.

**Drug-herb.** *Dong quai, feverfew, garlic, ginger, horse chestnut, red clover:* May cause bleeding based on the known effects of components. Discourage use together. *White willow:* Herb contains components similar to those of aspirin. Advise patients to avoid use with NSAIDs.

**Drug-lifestyle.** *Alcohol use:* May cause GI toxicity. Discourage use together. *Sun exposure:* May cause photosensitivity reactions. Advise patient to avoid excessive sunlight exposure.

## EFFECTS ON LAB TEST RESULTS
• May increase creatinine, BUN, ALT, and AST levels.
• May increase bleeding time. May increase or decrease iron test results.
• May falsely increase bilirubin level.

## CONTRAINDICATIONS & CAUTIONS
• Contraindicated in patients hypersensitive to drug and in those with history of aspirin- or NSAID-induced asthma, urticaria, or other allergic reactions.
• Avoid use during last trimester of pregnancy.
• Drug isn't recommended for children or breast-feeding women.
• Use cautiously in patients with history or for patients in acute pain.

• Because NSAIDs impair synthesis of renal prostaglandins, they can decrease renal blood flow and lead to reversible renal impairment, especially in patients with renal or heart failure or liver dysfunction, in elderly patients, and in those taking diuretics. Monitor these patients closely.
• Check renal and hepatic function every 6 months or as indicated.
• Drug decreases platelet adhesion and aggregation, and can prolong bleeding time about 3 to 4 minutes from baseline.
• NSAIDs may mask signs and symptoms of infection because of their antipyretic and anti-inflammatory actions.
• Serious GI toxicity, including peptic ulcers and bleeding, can occur in patient

taking NSAIDs, despite lack of symptoms.

## PATIENT TEACHING
• **Alert:** Drug is available without prescription. Instruct patient not to exceed 75 mg/day.
• Tell patient to take drug 30 minutes before or 2 hours after meals with a full glass of water. If adverse GI reactions occur, patient may take drug with milk or meals.
• Tell patient not to crush delayed-release or extended-release tablets.
• Tell patient that full therapeutic effect may be delayed for 2 to 4 weeks.
• Teach patient signs and symptoms of GI bleeding, including blood in vomit, urine, or stool; coffee-ground vomit; and black, tarry stool. Tell him to notify prescriber immediately if any of these occurs.
• Alert patient that using with aspirin, alcohol, or corticosteroids may increase risk of adverse GI reactions.
• Warn patient to avoid hazardous activities that require mental alertness until CNS effects are known.
• Because of possibility of sensitivity to the sun, advise patient to use a sunblock, wear protective clothing, and avoid prolonged exposure to sunlight.
• Instruct patient to report problems with light and hearing immediately.
• Instruct patient to protect drug from direct and excessive heat and humidity.

## ketorolac tromethamine
Toradol

*Pregnancy risk category C*

### AVAILABLE FORMS
*Injection:* 15 mg/ml, 30 mg/ml
*Tablets:* 10 mg

### INDICATIONS & DOSAGES
► **Short-term management of moderately severe, acute pain for single-dose treatment**
*Adults:* For patients younger than age 65, 60 mg I.M. or 30 mg I.V.
*Elderly patients:* In patients age 65 and older, 30 mg I.M. or 15 mg I.V.

*Adjust-a-dose:* For renally impaired patients or those weighing less than 50 kg (110 lb), 30 mg I.M. or 15 mg I.V.

➤ **Short-term management of moderately severe, acute pain for multiple-dose treatment**

*Adults:* In patients younger than age 65, 30 mg I.M. or I.V. q 6 hours. Maximum daily dose is 120 mg.

*Elderly patients:* In patients age 65 and older, 15 mg I.M. or I.V. q 6 hours. Maximum daily dose is 60 mg.

*Adjust-a-dose:* For renally impaired patients or those weighing less than 50 kg, 15 mg I.M. or I.V. q 6 hours. Maximum daily dose is 60 mg.

➤ **Short-term management of moderately severe, acute pain when switching from parenteral to oral administration (oral therapy is indicated only as continuation of parenterally given drug and should never be given without patient first having received parenteral therapy)**

*Adults:* For patients younger than age 65, 20 mg P.O. as single dose; then 10 mg P.O. q 4 to 6 hours. Maximum daily dose is 40 mg.

*Elderly patients:* For patients age 65 and older, 10 mg P.O. as single dose; then 10 mg P.O. q 4 to 6 hours. Maximum daily dose is 40 mg.

*Adjust-a-dose:* For renally impaired patients or those weighing less than [...]
10 mg P.O. as single dose; then 10 mg P.O. q 4 to 6 hours. Maximum daily dose is 40 mg.

## I.V. ADMINISTRATION
- Don't mix with morphine sulfate, meperidine hydrochloride, promethazine hydrochloride, or hydroxyzine hydrochloride. Ketorolac will precipitate out in solution.
- Dilute with normal saline solution, D₅W, 5% dextrose and normal saline solution, Ringer's solution, lactated Ringer's solution, or Plasma-Lyte A.
- Give I.V. injection in no less than 15 seconds.

## ACTION
Unknown. Produces anti-inflammatory, analgesic, and antipyretic effects, possibly by inhibiting prostaglandin synthesis.

| Route | Onset | Peak | Duration |
|-------|-------|------|----------|
| P.O. | 30-60 min | 30-60 min | 6-8 hr |
| I.V. | Immediate | 1-3 min | 6-8 hr |
| I.M. | 10 min | 30-60 min | 6-8 hr |

## ADVERSE REACTIONS
**CNS:** drowsiness, sedation, dizziness, *headache.*
**CV:** edema, hypertension, palpitations, *arrhythmias.*
**GI:** *nausea, dyspepsia, GI pain,* diarrhea, peptic ulceration, vomiting, constipation, flatulence, stomatitis.
**Hematologic:** decreased platelet adhesion, purpura, prolonged bleeding time.
**Skin:** pruritus, rash, diaphoresis.
**Other:** pain at injection site.

## INTERACTIONS
**Drug-drug.** *ACE inhibitors:* May cause renal impairment, particularly in volume-depleted patients. Avoid using together in volume-depleted patients.
*Anticoagulants, salicylates:* May increase levels of free (unbound) salicylates or anticoagulants in the blood. Use together with extreme caution and monitor patient closely.
*Antihypertensives, diuretics:* May decrease effectiveness. Monitor patient closely.
*Lithium:* May increase lithium level. Monitor [...]
**Drug-herb.** *[...] ginger, horse chestnut [...]* [...] cause bleeding. Discourage [...]
*White willow:* Herb contains components similar to those of aspirin. Discourage use together.

## EFFECTS ON LAB TEST RESULTS
- May increase ALT and AST levels.
- May increase bleeding time.

## CONTRAINDICATIONS & CAUTIONS
- Contraindicated in patients hypersensitive to drug and in those with active peptic ulcer disease, recent GI bleeding or perforation, advanced renal impairment, cerebrovascular bleeding, hemorrhagic diathesis, or incomplete hemostasis, and those at [...]

Reactions may be common, uncommon, *life-threatening,* or **COMMON AND LIFE-THREATENING.**

risk for renal impairment from volume depletion or at risk of bleeding.
- Contraindicated in children and in patients with history of peptic ulcer disease or GI bleeding, past allergic reactions to aspirin or other NSAIDs, and during labor and delivery or breast-feeding.
- Contraindicated as prophylactic analgesic before major surgery or intraoperatively when hemostasis is critical; and in patients currently receiving aspirin, an NSAID, or probenecid.
- Use cautiously in patients with hepatic or renal impairment or cardiac decompensation.

## NURSING CONSIDERATIONS
- Correct hypovolemia before giving ketorolac.
- *Alert:* The maximum combined duration of therapy (parenteral and oral) is 5 days.
- I.M. administration may cause pain at injection site. Hold pressure over site for 15 to 30 seconds after injection to minimize local effects. Give by deep I.M. injection.
- Don't give drug epidurally or intrathecally because of alcohol content.
- Carefully observe patients with coagulopathies and those taking anticoagulants. Drug inhibits platelet aggregation and can prolong bleeding time. This effect disappears within 48 hours of stopping drug and doesn't alter platelet count, INR, PTT, or PT.
- NSAIDs may mask signs and symptoms of infection because of their antipyretic and anti-inflammatory actions.
- Serious GI toxicity, including peptic ulcers and bleeding, can occur in patient taking NSAIDs, despite lack of symptoms.
- *Alert:* Don't confuse Toradol with Tegretol or Foradil.

## PATIENT TEACHING
- Warn patient receiving drug I.M. that pain may occur at injection site.
- Teach patient signs and symptoms of GI bleeding, including blood in vomit, urine, or stool; coffee-ground vomit; and black, tarry stool. Tell him to notify prescriber immediately if any of these occurs.

# meloxicam
Mobic

*Pregnancy risk category C; D in 3rd trimester*

## AVAILABLE FORMS
*Tablets:* 7.5 mg

## INDICATIONS & DOSAGES
➤ **Relief from signs and symptoms of osteoarthritis**
*Adults:* 7.5 mg P.O. once daily. May increase p.r.n. to maximum dose of 15 mg daily.

## ACTION
Unknown. Produces anti-inflammatory, analgesic, and antipyretic effects, possibly by inhibiting prostaglandin synthesis.

| Route | Onset | Peak | Duration |
|-------|---------|--------|----------|
| P.O. | Unknown | 4-5 hr | Unknown |

## ADVERSE REACTIONS
**CNS:** dizziness, headache, insomnia, fatigue, *seizures*, paresthesia, tremor, vertigo, anxiety, confusion, depression, nervousness, somnolence, malaise, syncope, fever.
**CV:** *arrhythmias*, palpitations, tachycardia, angina pectoris, *heart failure*, hypertension, hypotension, *MI*, edema.
**EENT:** pharyngitis, abnormal vision, conjunctivitis, tinnitus, taste perversion.
**GI:** abdominal pain, diarrhea, dyspepsia, flatulence, nausea, constipation, colitis, dry mouth, duodenal ulcer, esophagitis, gastric ulcer, gastritis, gastroesophageal reflux, *hemorrhage, pancreatitis*, vomiting, increased appetite.
**GU:** albuminuria, hematuria, urinary frequency, *renal failure*, urinary tract infection.
**Hematologic:** anemia, *leukopenia*, purpura, *thrombocytopenia*.
**Hepatic:** *hepatitis*.
**Metabolic:** dehydration, weight increase or decrease.
**Musculoskeletal:** arthralgia, back pain.
**Respiratory:** upper respiratory tract infection, *asthma, bronchospasm*, dyspnea, coughing.

---

**Skin:** rash, pruritus, alopecia, bullous eruption, photosensitivity reactions, sweating, urticaria.
**Other:** accidental injury, allergic reaction, *angioedema,* flulike symptoms.

**INTERACTIONS**
**Drug-drug.** *ACE inhibitors:* May decrease antihypertensive effects. Monitor blood pressure.
*Aspirin:* May cause adverse effects. Avoid using together.
*Furosemide, thiazide diuretics:* May reduce sodium excretion caused by diuretics, leading to sodium retention. Monitor patient for edema and increased blood pressure.
*Lithium:* May increase lithium level. Monitor lithium level closely.
*Warfarin:* May increase PT and INR and increases risk of bleeding complications. Monitor PT and INR, and check for signs and symptoms of bleeding.
**Drug-lifestyle.** *Alcohol use:* May cause GI irritation and bleeding. Discourage use together.
*Smoking:* May cause GI irritation and bleeding. Discourage use together.

**EFFECTS ON LAB TEST RESULTS**
● May increase BUN, creatinine, ALT, AST, and bilirubin levels.
● May decrease hemoglobin, hematocrit, and WBC and platelet counts.

**CONTRAINDICATIONS & CAUTIONS**
● Contraindicated in patients hypersensitive to drug and in those who have experienced asthma, urticaria, or allergic reactions after taking aspirin or other NSAIDs.
● Contraindicated in patients late in pregnancy.
● Use with extreme caution in patients with history of ulcers, GI bleeding, or preexisting asthma. Use cautiously in patients with dehydration, anemia, hepatic disease, renal disease, hypertension, fluid retention, heart failure, or asthma. Also use cautiously in elderly and debilitated patients because of increased risk of fatal GI bleeding.

**NURSING CONSIDERATIONS**
● *Alert:* Patient may be allergic to meloxicam, and the drug can produce allergic reactions in those hypersensitive to aspirin and other NSAIDs.
● Patient with a history of ulcers or GI bleeding is at higher risk for GI bleeding while taking NSAIDs. Other risk factors for GI bleeding include treatment with corticosteroids or anticoagulants, longer duration of NSAID treatment, smoking, alcoholism, older age, and poor overall health.
● Watch for signs and symptoms of overt and occult bleeding.
● NSAIDs can cause fluid retention; closely monitor patients who have hypertension, edema, or heart failure.
● Drug may be hepatotoxic. Watch for elevated ALT and AST levels. If signs and symptoms of liver disease develop, or if systemic signs and symptoms such as eosinophilia rash occur, stop drug and call prescriber.
● Rehydrate patients who are dehydrated before starting drug.
● Monitor hemoglobin and hematocrit in patients on long-term therapy.

**PATIENT TEACHING**
● Tell patient to report history of allergic reactions to aspirin or other NSAIDs before starting therapy.
● Tell patient drug can be taken without regard to meals.
● Advise patient to report signs and symptoms of GI ulcers and bleeding, such as blood in vomit or stool, and black, tarry stools, and to contact prescriber if they occur.
● Instruct patient to report any skin rash, weight gain, or swelling.
● Advise patient to report warning signs of liver damage, such as nausea, fatigue, lethargy, itching, yellowed skin or eyes, right upper quadrant tenderness, and flulike symptoms.
● Warn patient with history of asthma that asthma may recur while taking drug. Tell him to stop drug and contact prescriber if asthma recurs.
● Tell woman to notify prescriber if she becomes pregnant or is planning to become pregnant while taking drug.
● Inform patient that it may take several days to achieve consistent pain relief.

# nabumetone
Relafen◈

*Pregnancy risk category C*

## AVAILABLE FORMS
*Tablets:* 500 mg, 750 mg

## INDICATIONS & DOSAGES
➤ **Rheumatoid arthritis, osteoarthritis**
*Adults:* Initially, 1,000 mg P.O. daily as a single dose or in divided doses b.i.d. Maximum, 2,000 mg daily.

## ACTION
Unknown. Produces anti-inflammatory, analgesic, and antipyretic effects, possibly by inhibiting prostaglandin synthesis.

| Route | Onset | Peak | Duration |
|-------|-------|------|----------|
| P.O. | Unknown | 9-12 hr | Unknown |

## ADVERSE REACTIONS
**CNS:** dizziness, headache, fatigue, insomnia, nervousness, somnolence.
**CV:** vasculitis, edema.
**EENT:** tinnitus.
**GI:** *diarrhea, dyspepsia, abdominal pain,* constipation, flatulence, nausea, dry mouth, gastritis, stomatitis, anorexia, vomiting, ***bleeding,*** ulceration.
**Respiratory:** dyspnea, pneumonitis.
**Skin:** pruritus, rash, increased diaphoresis.

## INTERACTIONS
**Drug-drug.** *Diuretics:* May decrease diuretic effectiveness. Monitor patient closely.
*Warfarin, other highly protein-bound drugs:* May cause adverse effects from displacement of drugs by nabumetone. Use together cautiously.
**Drug-herb.** *Dong quai, feverfew, garlic, ginger, horse chestnut, red clover:* May cause bleeding. Discourage use together.
*White willow:* Herb contains components similar to those of aspirin. Discourage use together.
**Drug-food.** *Any food:* May increase absorption. Advise patient to take drug with food.

**Drug-lifestyle.** *Alcohol use:* May increase risk of additive GI toxicity. Discourage use together.

## EFFECTS ON LAB TEST RESULTS
None reported.

## CONTRAINDICATIONS & CAUTIONS
• Contraindicated in patients with hypersensitivity reactions and history of aspirin- or NSAID-induced asthma, urticaria, or other allergic-type reactions.
• Contraindicated in children and in pregnant women during third trimester of pregnancy.
• Use cautiously in patients with renal or hepatic impairment; heart failure, hypertension, or other conditions that may predispose patient to fluid retention; or a history of peptic ulcer disease.

## NURSING CONSIDERATIONS
• Because NSAIDs impair synthesis of renal prostaglandins, they can decrease renal blood flow and lead to reversible renal impairment, especially in patients with renal or heart failure or liver dysfunction, in elderly patients, and in those taking diuretics. Monitor these patients closely.
• During long-term therapy, periodically monitor renal and liver function, CBC, and hematocrit; assess patients for signs and symptoms of GI bleeding.
• Serious GI toxicity, including peptic ulcers and bleeding, can occur in patient taking NSAIDs, despite lack of symptoms.

## PATIENT TEACHING
• Instruct patient to take drug with food, milk, or antacids. Drug is absorbed more rapidly when taken with food or milk.
• Advise patient to limit alcohol intake because using drug with alcohol increases the risk of GI problems.
• Teach patient signs and symptoms of GI bleeding, including blood in vomit, urine, or stool; coffee-ground vomit; and black, tarry stool. Tell him to notify prescriber immediately if any of these occurs.
• Warn patient against hazardous activities that require mental alertness until CNS effects are known.

# naproxen

Apo-Naproxen†, EC-Naprosyn, Naprosyn✐, Naprosyn-E†, Naprosyn-SR, Naxen†, Novo-Naprox†, Nu-Naprox†

## naproxen sodium

Aleve◊, Anaprox, Anaprox DS, Apo-Napro-Na†◊, Naprelan, Naprogesic‡, Novo-Naprox Sodium†, Synflex†

*Pregnancy risk category B*

## AVAILABLE FORMS

**naproxen**
*Oral suspension:* 125 mg/5 ml
*Suppositories:* 500 mg‡
*Tablets:* 250 mg, 375 mg, 500 mg
*Tablets (delayed-release):* 375 mg, 500 mg
*Tablets (extended-release):* 750 mg, 1,000 mg
**naproxen sodium**
*Tablets (controlled-release):* 412.5 mg, 550 mg
*Tablets (film-coated):* 220 mg◊, 275 mg, 550 mg
*Note:* 275 mg of naproxen sodium contains 250 mg of naproxen.

## INDICATIONS & DOSAGES

➤ **Rheumatoid arthritis, osteoarthritis, ankylosing spondylitis, pain, dysmenorrhea, tendinitis, bursitis**
*Adults:* 250 to 500 mg naproxen b.i.d.; maximum, 1.5 g daily for a limited time. Or, 375 to 500 mg delayed-release EC-Naprosyn b.i.d. Or, 750 to 1,000 mg controlled-release Naprelan daily. Or, 275 to 550 mg naproxen sodium b.i.d.
➤ **Juvenile arthritis**
*Children:* 10 mg/kg P.O. in two divided doses.
➤ **Acute gout**
*Adults:* 750 mg naproxen P.O.; then 250 mg q 8 hours until attack subsides. Or, 825 mg naproxen sodium; then 275 mg q 8 hours until attack subsides. Or, 1,000 to 1,500 mg/day controlled-release Naprelan on first day; then 1,000 mg daily until attack subsides.

➤ **Mild to moderate pain, primary dysmenorrhea**
*Adults:* 500 mg naproxen P.O.; then 250 mg q 6 to 8 hours up to 1.25 g/day. Or, 550 mg naproxen sodium; then 275 mg q 6 to 8 hours up to 1,375 mg/day. Or, 1,000 mg controlled-release Naprelan once daily.
*Elderly patients:* In patients older than age 65, don't exceed 400 mg/day.

## ACTION

Unknown. Produces anti-inflammatory, analgesic, and antipyretic effects, possibly by inhibiting prostaglandin synthesis.

| Route | Onset | Peak | Duration |
|-------|-------|------|----------|
| P.O. | 1 hr | 2-4 hr | 7 hr |
| P.R. | Unknown | Unknown | Unknown |

## ADVERSE REACTIONS

**CNS:** headache, drowsiness, dizziness, vertigo.
**CV:** edema, palpitations.
**EENT:** visual disturbances, *tinnitus,* auditory disturbances.
**GI:** epigastric pain, occult blood loss, abdominal pain, nausea, peptic ulceration, constipation, dyspepsia, heartburn, diarrhea, stomatitis, thirst.
**Hematologic:** increased bleeding time, ecchymoses.
**Metabolic:** *hyperkalemia.*
**Respiratory:** dyspnea.
**Skin:** pruritus, rash, urticaria, diaphoresis, purpura.

## INTERACTIONS

**Drug-drug.** *ACE inhibitors:* May cause renal impairment. Use together cautiously.
*Antihypertensives, diuretics:* May decrease effect of these drugs. Monitor patient closely.
*Aspirin, corticosteroids:* May cause adverse GI reactions. Avoid using together.
*Lithium:* May increase lithium level. Observe patient for toxicity and monitor level. Adjustment of lithium dosage may be required.
*Methotrexate:* May cause toxicity. Monitor patient closely.
*Oral anticoagulants, other sulfonylureas, highly protein-bound drugs:* May cause toxicity. Monitor patient closely.

*Probenecid:* May decrease elimination of naproxen. Monitor patient for toxicity.

**Drug-herb.** *Dong quai, feverfew, garlic, ginger, horse chestnut, red clover:* May cause bleeding, based on the known effects of components. Discourage use together.

*White willow:* Herb contains components similar to those of aspirin. Discourage use together.

**Drug-lifestyle.** *Alcohol use:* May cause adverse GI reactions. Discourage use together.

## EFFECTS ON LAB TEST RESULTS
● May increase BUN, creatinine, ALT, AST, and potassium levels.
● May increase bleeding time.
● May interfere with urinary 5-hydroxyindoleacetic acid and 17-hydroxycorticosteroid determinations.

## CONTRAINDICATIONS & CAUTIONS
● Contraindicated in patients hypersensitive to drug and in those with the syndrome of asthma, rhinitis, and nasal polyps.
● Patient should avoid drug during last trimester of pregnancy.
● Use cautiously in elderly patients and in patients with renal disease, CV disease, GI disorders, hepatic disease, or history of peptic ulcer disease.

## NURSING CONSIDERATIONS
● Because NSAIDs impair synthesis of renal prostaglandins, they can decrease renal blood flow and lead to reversible renal impairment, especially in patients with renal failure, heart failure, or liver dysfunction; in elderly patients; and in those taking diuretics. Monitor these patients closely.
● Monitor CBC and renal and hepatic function every 4 to 6 months during long-term therapy.
● Serious GI toxicity, including peptic ulcers and bleeding, can occur in patient taking NSAIDs, despite lack of symptoms.
● Because of their antipyretic and anti-inflammatory actions, NSAIDs may mask signs and symptoms of infection.
● Naproxen may have a heart benefit, similar to aspirin, in preventing blood clotting.

## PATIENT TEACHING
● *Alert:* Drug is available without prescription (naproxen sodium, 200 mg). Instruct patient not to take more than 600 mg in 24 hours. Dosage in patient older than age 65 shouldn't exceed 400 mg/day.
● Advise patient to take drug with food or milk to minimize GI upset. Tell him to take a full glass of water or other liquid with each dose.
● Tell patient taking prescription doses of naproxen for arthritis that full therapeutic effect may be delayed 2 to 4 weeks.
● Warn patient against taking naproxen and naproxen sodium at the same time.
● Teach patient signs and symptoms of GI bleeding, including blood in vomit, urine, or stool; coffee-ground vomit; and black, tarry stool. Tell him to notify prescriber immediately if any of these occurs.
● Caution patient that use with aspirin, alcohol, or corticosteroids may increase risk of adverse GI reactions.
● Warn patient against hazardous activities that require mental alertness until CNS effects are known.

---

# piroxicam
Apo-Piroxicam†, Feldene, Novo-Pirocam†, Pirox‡

*Pregnancy risk category B (D in third trimester or near delivery)*

## AVAILABLE FORMS
*Capsules:* 10 mg, 20 mg

## INDICATIONS & DOSAGES
➤ **Osteoarthritis, rheumatoid arthritis**
*Adults:* 20 mg P.O. daily. If desired, dose may be divided b.i.d.

## ACTION
Unknown. Produces anti-inflammatory, analgesic, and antipyretic effects, possibly by inhibiting prostaglandin synthesis.

| Route | Onset | Peak | Duration |
|---|---|---|---|
| P.O. | 1 hr | 3-5 hr | 48-72 hr |

## ADVERSE REACTIONS
**CNS:** *headache,* drowsiness, *dizziness,* somnolence, vertigo.
**CV:** peripheral edema.

**EENT:** auditory disturbances.
**GI:** epigastric distress, nausea, vomiting, occult blood loss, peptic ulceration, *severe GI bleeding,* diarrhea, constipation, abdominal pain, heart burn, dyspepsia, flatulence, anorexia, stomatitis.
**GU:** *nephrotoxicity.*
**Hematologic:** prolonged bleeding time, anemia, *leukopenia, agranulocytosis,* eosinophilia.
**Metabolic:** *hyperkalemia, hypoglycemia in diabetic patients.*
**Skin:** *pruritus, rash.*

## INTERACTIONS

**Drug-drug.** *Antihypertensives, diuretics:* May decrease effects. Avoid using together.
*Aspirin, corticosteroids:* May cause GI toxicity; may decrease level of piroxicam. Avoid using together.
*Cyclosporine, methotrexate:* May increase toxicity. Monitor patient closely.
*Lithium:* May increase lithium level. Monitor patient for toxicity.
*Oral anticoagulants, other highly protein-bound drugs:* May be toxic. Monitor patient closely.
*Oral antidiabetics:* May enhance antidiabetic effects. Monitor patient closely.
*Ritonavir:* May increase piroxicam level. Monitor patient for signs of toxicity.
**Drug-herb.** *Dong quai, feverfew, garlic, ginger, horse chestnut, red clover:* May cause bleeding. Discourage use together.
*St. John's wort:* May cause photosensitivity reaction. Advise patient to avoid excessive sunlight exposure.
*White willow:* Herb contains components similar to those of aspirin. Discourage use together.
**Drug-lifestyle.** *Alcohol use:* May cause GI toxicity, may decrease level of piroxicam. Discourage use together.
*Sun exposure:* May cause photosensitivity reaction. Advise patient to avoid excessive sunlight exposure.

## EFFECTS ON LAB TEST RESULTS

● May increase BUN, creatinine, liver enzyme, and potassium levels. May decrease glucose level.
● May decrease hemoglobin, hematocrit, and WBC, granulocyte, and eosinophil counts.

## CONTRAINDICATIONS & CAUTIONS

● Contraindicated in patients hypersensitive to drug and in those with bronchospasm or angioedema precipitated by aspirin or NSAIDs. Also contraindicated in pregnant or breast-feeding patients.
● Use cautiously in elderly patients and in patients with GI disorders, history of renal or peptic ulcer disease, cardiac disease, hypertension, or conditions predisposing to fluid retention.

## NURSING CONSIDERATIONS

● Because NSAIDs impair the synthesis of renal prostaglandins, they can decrease renal blood flow and lead to reversible renal impairment, especially in elderly patients, in patients taking diuretics, and in patients with renal failure, heart failure, or liver dysfunction. Monitor these patients closely.
● Check renal, hepatic, and auditory function and CBC periodically during prolonged therapy. Stop drug and notify prescriber if abnormalities occur.
● Serious GI toxicity, including peptic ulcers and bleeding, can occur in patient taking NSAIDs, despite lack of symptoms.
● NSAIDs may mask signs and symptoms of infection because of their antipyretic and anti-inflammatory actions.

## PATIENT TEACHING

● Tell patient to take drug with milk, antacids, or meals if adverse GI reactions occur.
● Inform patient that full therapeutic effects may be delayed for 2 to 4 weeks.
● Teach patient signs and symptoms of GI bleeding, including blood in vomit, urine, or stool; coffee-ground vomit; and black, tarry stool. Tell him to notify prescriber immediately if any of these occurs.
● Warn patient against hazardous activities that require mental alertness until CNS effects are known.
● Because drug causes adverse skin reactions more often than other drugs in its class, advise patient to use a sunblock, wear protective clothing, and avoid prolonged exposure to sunlight. Sensitivity to the sun is the most common reaction.

Reactions may be *common,* uncommon, *life-threatening*, or COMMON AND LIFE-THREATENING.

# rofecoxib
Vioxx✔

*Pregnancy risk category C*

## AVAILABLE FORMS
*Oral suspension:* 12.5 mg/5 ml, 25 mg/ 5 ml
*Tablets:* 12.5 mg, 25 mg, 50 mg

## INDICATIONS & DOSAGES
➤ **Relief from signs and symptoms of osteoarthritis**
*Adults:* Initially, 12.5 mg P.O. once daily, increased, p.r.n., to maximum of 25 mg P.O. once daily.
➤ **Acute pain, primary dysmenorrhea**
*Adults:* 50 mg P.O. once daily, p.r.n., for up to 5 days. Long-term use of 50 mg daily isn't recommended.
✴ *NEW INDICATION:* **Rheumatoid arthritis**
*Adults:* 25 mg P.O. once daily. Maximum recommended daily dose is 25 mg.

## ACTION
Unknown. Produces anti-inflammatory, analgesic, and antipyretic effects, possibly by inhibiting prostaglandin synthesis.

| Route | Onset | Peak | Duration |
|-------|-------|------|----------|
| P.O. | Unknown | 2-3 hr | Unknown |

## ADVERSE REACTIONS
**CNS:** headache, asthenia, fatigue, dizziness, *aseptic meningitis.*
**CV:** hypertension, leg edema.
**EENT:** sinusitis.
**GI:** diarrhea, dyspepsia, epigastric discomfort, heartburn, nausea, abdominal pain.
**GU:** urinary tract infection.
**Metabolic:** hyponatremia.
**Musculoskeletal:** back pain.
**Respiratory:** bronchitis, upper respiratory tract infection.
**Other:** flulike syndrome.

## INTERACTIONS
**Drug-drug.** *ACE inhibitors:* May decrease antihypertensive effects of ACE inhibitors. Monitor blood pressure closely.
*Aspirin:* May increase rate of GI ulceration and other complications. Avoid using together, if possible. If used together, monitor patient closely for GI bleeding.
*Furosemide, thiazide diuretics:* May decrease efficacy of these drugs. Monitor patient closely.
*Lithium:* May increase lithium level and decrease lithium clearance. Monitor patient for toxic reaction to lithium.
*Methotrexate:* May increase methotrexate level. Monitor patient closely for toxic reaction to methotrexate.
*Rifampin:* May decrease rofecoxib level by about 50%. Start therapy with a higher dosage of rofecoxib.
*Theophylline:* May increase theophylline level. Monitor level closely.
*Warfarin:* May increase effects of warfarin. Monitor INR more frequently in first few days after therapy is initiated or dosage is changed.
**Drug-herb.** *Dong quai, feverfew, garlic, ginger, horse chestnut, red clover:* May cause bleeding based on the known effects or components. Discourage use together.
*White willow:* Herb contains components similar to those of aspirin. Discourage use together.
**Drug-lifestyle.** *Long-term alcohol use, smoking:* May cause GI bleeding. Monitor patient closely.

## EFFECTS ON LAB TEST RESULTS
● May increase ALT and AST levels. May decrease sodium level.

## CONTRAINDICATIONS & CAUTIONS
● Contraindicated in patients hypersensitive to drug or its components and in those who have experienced asthma, urticaria, or allergic reactions after taking aspirin or other NSAIDs.
● Contraindicated in patients with advanced kidney disease or moderate or severe hepatic insufficiency, in breastfeeding women, and in pregnant women because drug may cause premature closure of ductus arteriosus.
● Use cautiously in patients with history of ulcer disease or GI bleeding and in those taking such drugs as oral corticosteroids and anticoagulants.
● Use cautiously in patients with conditions such as older age, alcoholism, poor

general health, and addiction to smoking that may increase risk of GI bleeding.
• Use cautiously in patients with fluid retention, hypertension, or heart failure.
• Use cautiously in dehydrated patients. Rehydrate before starting therapy.
• Use cautiously in patients with history of ischemic heart disease. Because of its lack of platelet effects, rofecoxib isn't a substitute for aspirin for preventing CV events, so don't stop antiplatelet therapy in patients taking rofecoxib

**NURSING CONSIDERATIONS**
• *Alert:* NSAIDs may cause serious GI toxicity. Signs and symptoms include bleeding, ulceration, and perforation of the stomach, small intestine, and large intestine. Such toxicity can occur any time, with or without warning. To minimize risk of an adverse GI event, use lowest effective dose for the shortest possible duration. Monitor patient for GI bleeding.
• In patients with fluid retention, hypertension, or heart failure, start at lowest dosage. Monitor blood pressure and check patient for fluid retention or worsening heart failure.
• In patient older than age 65, start therapy at the lowest recommended dosage.
• Patient may be allergic to drug if he has an allergy to aspirin or other NSAIDs.
• Monitor patient for signs and symptoms of hepatotoxicity. Stop drug if patient develops signs and symptoms of liver disease.
• Shake oral suspension well before giving it.
• Have hemoglobin and hematocrit checked in patient undergoing long-term treatment if he has signs or symptoms of anemia or blood loss.
• Vioxx may cause more than twice as many heart attacks, strokes, and other cardiac events as naproxen.
• The risk of GI toxicity with rofecoxib 50 mg once daily is significantly less than with naproxen 500 mg twice daily.
• Report prenatal exposure to the pregnancy registry at 1-800-986-8999.

**PATIENT TEACHING**
• Warn patient that he may experience signs and symptoms of GI bleeding, including blood in vomit, urine, and stool,

or black, tarry stools. Advise patient to call prescriber if these symptoms occur.
• Advise patient to report rash, unexplained weight gain, or swelling.
• Tell patient to avoid aspirin and aspirin-containing products unless prescriber has instructed him otherwise.
• Urge patient to avoid OTC anti-inflammatories such as ibuprofen unless prescriber has instructed him otherwise.
• Tell patient that all NSAIDs, including rofecoxib, may harm the liver. Signs and symptoms of liver damage include nausea, fatigue, lethargy, itching, yellowed skin or eyes, right upper quadrant tenderness, and flulike syndrome. Advise him to stop therapy and call prescriber immediately if he experiences these signs or symptoms.
• Instruct women to inform prescriber of pregnancy or pregnancy plans while taking drug.
• Tell patient to shake oral suspension well before using.
• Tell patient that the most common adverse effects of drug are indigestion, upper abdominal discomfort, heartburn, and nausea. Advise him that taking drug with food may help minimize these effects.

---

## sulindac
Aclin‡, Apo-Sulin†, Clinoril, Novo-Sundac†, Saldac‡

*Pregnancy risk category B; D in 3rd trimester*

**AVAILABLE FORMS**
*Tablets:* 100 mg‡, 150 mg, 200 mg

**INDICATIONS & DOSAGES**
➤ **Osteoarthritis, rheumatoid arthritis, ankylosing spondylitis**
*Adults:* Initially, 150 mg P.O. b.i.d.; increase to 200 mg b.i.d., p.r.n. Maximum dose is 400 mg daily.
➤ **Acute subacromial bursitis or supraspinatus tendinitis, acute gouty arthritis**
*Adults:* 200 mg P.O. b.i.d. for 7 to 14 days. Reduce dosage as symptoms subside. Maximum dose is 400 mg daily.

---

## ACTION

Unknown. Produces anti-inflammatory, analgesic, and antipyretic effects, possibly by inhibiting prostaglandin synthesis.

| Route | Onset | Peak | Duration |
|-------|-------|------|----------|
| P.O. | Unknown | 2-4 hr | Unknown |

## ADVERSE REACTIONS

**CNS:** dizziness, headache, nervousness, psychosis.
**CV:** hypertension, *heart failure,* palpitations, edema.
**EENT:** tinnitus, transient visual disturbances.
**GI:** *epigastric distress,* peptic ulceration, occult blood loss, nausea, constipation, dyspepsia, flatulence, anorexia, GI bleeding.
**GU:** interstitial nephritis.
**Hematologic:** prolonged bleeding time.
**Metabolic:** *hyperkalemia.*
**Skin:** rash, pruritus.
**Other:** drug fever, *anaphylaxis, angioedema,* hypersensitivity reactions.

## INTERACTIONS

**Drug-drug.** *Anticoagulants:* May cause bleeding. Monitor PT and INR closely.
*Aspirin:* May decrease sulindac level and increased risk of GI adverse reactions. Avoid using together.
*Cyclosporine:* May increase nephrotoxicity of cyclosporine. Avoid using together.
*Diflunisal, dimethyl sulfoxide:* May hinder metabolism of sulindac to its metabolite, reducing its effectiveness. Avoid using together.
*Methotrexate:* May increase methotrexate toxicity. Avoid using together.
*Probenecid:* May increase levels of sulindac and its metabolite. Monitor patient for toxicity.
*Sulfonamides, sulfonylureas, other highly protein-bound drugs:* May cause these drugs to be displaced from protein-binding sites, increasing toxicity. Monitor patient closely.
**Drug-herb.** *Dong quai, feverfew, garlic, ginger, horse chestnut, red clover:* May cause bleeding, based on the known effects of components. Discourage use together.

*White willow:* Herb contains components similar to those of aspirin. Discourage use together.
**Drug-lifestyle.** *Alcohol use:* May increase risk of adverse GI reactions. Discourage use together.

## EFFECTS ON LAB TEST RESULTS

● May increase BUN, creatinine, ALT, AST, and potassium levels.

## CONTRAINDICATIONS & CAUTIONS

● Contraindicated in patients hypersensitive to drug and in those for whom aspirin or NSAIDs precipitate acute asthmatic attacks, urticaria, or rhinitis.
● Don't use drug in pregnant women.
● Use cautiously in patients with a history of ulcers and GI bleeding, renal dysfunction, compromised cardiac function, hypertension, or conditions predisposing to fluid retention.

## NURSING CONSIDERATIONS

● Periodically monitor hepatic and renal function and CBC in patient receiving long-term therapy.
● Serious GI toxicity, including peptic ulcers and bleeding, can occur in patient taking NSAIDs, despite lack of symptoms.
● NSAIDs may mask signs and symptoms of infection.

## PATIENT TEACHING

● Tell patient to take drug with food, milk, or antacids.
● Teach patient signs and symptoms of GI bleeding, including blood in vomit, urine, or stool; coffee-ground vomit; and black, tarry stool. Tell him to notify prescriber immediately if any of these occurs.
● *Alert:* Tell patient to notify prescriber immediately if easy bruising or prolonged bleeding occurs.
● Advise patient to avoid hazardous activities that require mental alertness until CNS effects are known.
● Instruct patient to report edema and have blood pressure checked monthly. Drug causes sodium retention but is thought to have less effect on the kidneys than other NSAIDs.
● Advise patient to notify prescriber and have complete eye examination if visual disturbances occur.

---

# valdecoxib
Bextra✦

*Pregnancy risk category C*

## AVAILABLE FORMS
*Tablets:* 10 mg, 20 mg

## INDICATIONS & DOSAGES
➤ **Osteoarthritis, rheumatoid arthritis**
*Adults:* 10 mg P.O. once daily.
➤ **Primary dysmenorrhea**
*Adults:* 20 mg P.O. b.i.d., p.r.n.

## ACTION
Produces anti-inflammatory, analgesic, and antipyretic effects. May inhibit prostaglandin synthesis primarily by inhibiting COX-2. COX-1 doesn't appear to be inhibited at therapeutic levels.

| Route | Onset | Peak | Duration |
|-------|-------|------|----------|
| P.O. | Unknown | 3 hr | Unknown |

## ADVERSE REACTIONS
**CNS:** dizziness, headache, *cerebrovascular disorder.*
**CV:** peripheral edema, *aggravated hypertension, unstable angina, bradycardia, arrhythmia, heart failure, aneurysm.*
**EENT:** sinusitis.
**GI:** abdominal fullness, abdominal pain, diarrhea, dyspepsia, flatulence, nausea.
**GU:** renal impairment.
**Hematologic:** *thrombocytopenia, leukopenia,* anemia.
**Hepatic:** *hepatitis.*
**Metabolic:** hyperglycemia, hypercholesterolemia, hyperkalemia, hyperlipidemia, hyperuricemia, hypocalcemia, hypokalemia, increased or decreased weight.
**Musculoskeletal:** back pain, myalgia.
**Respiratory:** upper respiratory tract infection, *bronchospasm.*
**Skin:** rash.
**Other:** flulike symptoms, accidental injury.

## INTERACTIONS
**Drug-drug.** *ACE inhibitors:* May diminish antihypertensive effect. Monitor blood pressure carefully.
*Aspirin:* May increase risk of GI ulceration. Use together cautiously.

*Dextromethorphan:* May increase dextromethorphan level. Monitor patient carefully.
*Fluconazole, ketoconazole:* May enhance valdecoxib effects. Monitor patient closely.
*Furosemide, thiazide diuretics:* May reduce natriuretic effect. Monitor patient carefully.
*Lithium:* May delay lithium clearance. Monitor lithium level.
*Warfarin:* May increase anticoagulant activity. Monitor INR and PT closely.

## EFFECTS ON LAB TEST RESULTS
● May increase ALT, AST, alkaline phosphatase, BUN, CPK, cholesterol, glucose, potassium, lipid, uric acid, and LDH levels. May decrease calcium and potassium levels.
● May increase platelet and WBC counts and creatinine clearance. May decrease hemoglobin and hematocrit.

## CONTRAINDICATIONS & CAUTIONS
● Contraindicated in patients hypersensitive to this drug and in those with sensitivity to aspirin, sulfonamides, or NSAIDs that results in asthma, urticaria, or allergic reactions.
● Contraindicated in patients with advanced renal or hepatic disease.
● Use with extreme caution in patients with a history of GI bleeding or peptic ulcer disease.
● Use cautiously in elderly and debilitated patients and in patients at increased risk of GI bleeding because of behaviors such as smoking, conditions such as alcoholism, poor general health, or therapies such as corticosteroids, anticoagulants, or long-term NSAIDs.
● Use cautiously in patients with renal impairment, heart failure, hepatic dysfunction, hypertension, and preexisting asthma, and in those taking diuretics or ACE inhibitors. Use cautiously in dehydrated patients and in patients with fluid retention.

## NURSING CONSIDERATIONS
● Monitor patient carefully for signs and symptoms of GI toxicity, such as bleeding or ulceration.

Reactions may be *common*, uncommon, *life-threatening*, or COMMON AND LIFE-THREATENING.

• *Alert:* Drug may cause hypersensitivity reactions, including anaphylaxis, angioedema, and severe skin reactions. Stop therapy at the first sign of skin rash or hypersensitivity.

• Liver function test values may be elevated, and there may be progression to more serious hepatic abnormalities. Notify prescriber if hepatic disease is suspected or if systemic symptoms such as eosinophilia or rash occur.

• Fluid retention and edema may occur.

• Rehydrate dehydrated patients before treatment starts.

• Monitor hemoglobin and hematocrit in patients on long-term therapy; watch for signs and symptoms of anemia.

• *Alert:* Don't confuse Bextra with Arixtra.

## PATIENT TEACHING

• Advise patient to notify his prescriber of signs or symptoms of GI bleeding and ulceration, weight gain, swelling, skin rash, or liver damage (nausea, fatigue, lethargy, yellowed skin or eyes, right upper-quadrant tenderness, flulike symptoms).

• Advise patient to seek emergency attention for trouble breathing, especially if he has a history of aspirin sensitivity.

• Tell patient drug may be taken without regard to meals or antacid administration.

alfentanil hydrochloride
buprenorphine hydrochloride
butorphanol tartrate
codeine phosphate
codeine sulfate
fentanyl citrate
fentanyl transdermal system
fentanyl transmucosal
hydromorphone hydrochloride
meperidine hydrochloride
methadone hydrochloride
morphine hydrochloride
morphine sulfate
morphine tartrate
nalbuphine hydrochloride
oxycodone hydrochloride
oxycodone pectinate
oxymorphone hydrochloride
pentazocine hydrochloride
pentazocine hydrochloride and
    naloxone hydrochloride
pentazocine lactate
propoxyphene hydrochloride
propoxyphene napsylate
remifentanil hydrochloride
tramadol hydrochloride


**COMBINATION PRODUCTS**
222†: aspirin 375 mg, codeine phosphate
8 mg, and caffeine citrate 30 mg.
282 MEP†: aspirin 375 mg, codeine phosphate 15 mg, and caffeine citrate 30 mg.
292†: aspirin 375 mg, codeine phosphate
30 mg, and caffeine citrate 30 mg.
692†: aspirin 375 mg, propoxyphene hydrochloride 65 mg, and caffeine 30 mg.
ACETA WITH CODEINE, EMPRACET-30†,
EMTEC-30†: acetaminophen 300 mg and
codeine phosphate 30 mg.
ANACIN WITH CODEINE†: aspirin 325 mg,
codeine phosphate 8 mg, and caffeine
32 mg.
ANEXSIA 5/500: hydrocodone bitartrate
5 mg and acetaminophen 500 mg.
CAPITAL WITH CODEINE, TYLENOL WITH
CODEINE ELIXIR*: acetaminophen 120 mg
and codeine phosphate 12 mg/5 ml.
DARVOCET A500: 100 mg propoxyphene
napsylate and 500 mg acetaminophen

DARVOCET-N 50: acetaminophen 325 mg
and propoxyphene napsylate 50 mg.
DARVOCET-N 100, PROPACET 100: acetaminophen 650 mg and propoxyphene napsylate 100 mg.
DARVON COMPOUND-65†: aspirin 389 mg,
propoxyphene hydrochloride 65 mg, and
caffeine 32.4 mg.
DARVON-N COMPOUND†: aspirin 375 mg,
propoxyphene napsylate 100 mg, and caffeine 30 mg.
DARVON-N WITH A.S.A.†: aspirin 325 mg
and propoxyphene napsylate 100 mg.
E-LOR, WYGESIC: acetaminophen 650 mg
and propoxyphene hydrochloride 65 mg.
EMPIRIN WITH CODEINE NO. 3, PHENA-
PHEN WITH CODEINE NO. 3: aspirin
325 mg and codeine phosphate 30 mg.
EMPIRIN WITH CODEINE NO. 4, PHENA-
PHEN WITH CODEINE NO. 4: aspirin
325 mg and codeine phosphate 60 mg.
EMPRACET-60†: acetaminophen 300 mg
and codeine phosphate 60 mg.
ENDOCET: acetaminophen 325 mg and
oxycodone 7.5 mg.
ENDOCET: acetaminophen 325 mg and
oxycodone 10 mg
ENDOCET, PERCOCET 7.5/500: oxycodone
7.5 mg and acetaminophen 500 mg.
ENDOCET, PERCOCET 10/650: oxycodone
10 mg and acetaminophen 650 mg.
ENDOCET, OXYCOCET†, PERCOCET 5/325,
ROXICET: oxycodone hydrochloride 5 mg
and acetaminophen 325 mg.
ENDODAN†, OXYCODAN†, PERCODAN†,
ROXIPRIN: aspirin 325 mg and oxycodone
hydrochloride 5 mg.
FIORICET WITH CODEINE CAPSULES: acetaminophen 325 mg, butalbital 50 mg,
caffeine 40 mg, and codeine phosphate
30 mg.
FIORINAL WITH CODEINE CAPSULES: aspirin 325 mg, butalbital 50 mg, caffeine
40 mg, and codeine phosphate 30 mg.
INNOVAR: droperidol 2.5 mg and fentanyl
citrate 0.05 mg/ml.
LORCET 10/650 tablets: hydrocodone
bitartrate 10 mg and acetaminophen
650 mg.

LORCET PLUS TABLETS: acetaminophen
650 mg and hydrocodone bitartrate
7.5 mg.
LORTAB 2.5/500 TABLETS⟁: hydrocodone
bitartrate 2.5 mg and acetaminophen
500 mg.
LORTAB 5/500 TABLETS⟁: hydrocodone
bitartrate 5 mg and acetaminophen
500 mg.
LORTAB 7.5/500 TABLETS⟁: hydrocodone
bitartrate 7.5 mg and acetaminophen
500 mg.
NOVO-GESIC C8†: acetaminophen 300 mg,
codeine phosphate 8 mg, and caffeine
15 mg.
PERCODAN-DEMI TABLETS: aspirin
325 mg, oxycodone hydrochloride
2.25 mg, and oxycodone terephthalate
0.19 mg.
PERCODAN-DEMI†: aspirin 325 mg and
oxycodone hydrochloride 2.5 mg.
PERCODAN, ROXIPRIN TABLETS: aspirin
325 mg, oxycodone hydrochloride 4.5 mg,
and oxycodone terephthalate 0.38 mg.
ROXICET 5/500 CAPLETS, TYLOX CAP-
SULES: oxycodone hydrochloride 5 mg
and acetaminophen 500 mg.
ROXICET ORAL SOLUTION*: acetaminophen 325 mg and oxycodone hydrochloride 5 mg/5 ml.
SUBOXONE (SUBLINGUAL TABLETS):
buprenorphine 2 mg with naloxone
0.5 mg; buprenorphine 8 mg with naloxone 2 mg.
TALACEN: acetaminophen 650 mg and
pentazocine 25 mg.
TALWIN COMPOUND: aspirin 325 mg and
pentazocine 12.5 mg.
TYLENOL WITH CODEINE NO. 1: acetaminophen 300 mg and codeine phosphate
7.5 mg.
TYLENOL WITH CODEINE NO. 2: acetaminophen 300 mg and codeine phosphate
15 mg.
TYLENOL WITH CODEINE NO. 3⟁: acetaminophen 300 mg and codeine phosphate
30 mg.
TYLENOL WITH CODEINE NO. 4: acetaminophen 300 mg and codeine phosphate
60 mg.
ULTRACET⟁: acetaminophen 325 mg and
tramadol hydrochloride 37.5 mg.
VICODIN⟁: hydrocodone bitartrate 5 mg
and acetaminophen 500 mg.

VICODIN ES⟁: hydrocodone bitartrate
7.5 mg and acetaminophen 750 mg.

# alfentanil hydrochloride
Alfenta

*Pregnancy risk category C*
*Controlled substance schedule II*

## AVAILABLE FORMS
*Injection:* 500 mcg/ml

## INDICATIONS & DOSAGES
➤ **Adjunct to general anesthetic**
*Adults:* Initially, 8 to 50 mcg/kg I.V.; then
increments of 3 to 15 mcg/kg I.V. q 5 to
20 minutes.
➤ **As a primary anesthetic**
*Adults:* Initially, 130 to 245 mcg/kg I.V.;
then 0.5 to 1.5 mcg/kg/minute I.V.
➤ **Monitored anesthesia care**
*Adults:* Initially, 3 to 8 mcg/kg I.V.; then
3 to 5 mcg/kg I.V. q 5 to 20 minutes or
0.25 to 1 mcg/kg/minute I.V. Total dose is
3 to 40 mcg/kg I.V.
*Adjust-a-dose:* In debilitated patients,
reduce dosage. In obese patients, base
dosage on lean body weight. In patients
age 65 and older, clearance is reduced by
about 30%, leading to a prolonged half-
life; reduce dosage in these patients.

## I.V. ADMINISTRATION
● Drug is compatible with D₅W, dextrose
5% in lactated Ringer's solution, and normal saline solution. Infusions containing
25 to 80 mcg/ml are used most often.
● Stop infusion at least 10 to 15 minutes
before end of surgery.
● Only individuals specifically trained in
use of I.V. anesthetics should give drug.
● Keep opioid antagonist (naloxone) and
resuscitation equipment available when
giving drug.

## ACTION
Unknown. Binds with opiate receptors in
the CNS, altering both perception of and
emotional response to pain.

| Route | Onset | Peak | Duration |
|---|---|---|---|
| I.V. | 1 min | 1½-2 min | 5-10 min |

**ADVERSE REACTIONS**
**CNS:** anxiety, headache, confusion, dizziness, sedation.
**CV:** *hypotension, hypertension,* BRADYCARDIA, *tachycardia,* ARRHYTHMIAS.
**EENT:** blurred vision.
**GI:** *nausea, vomiting.*
**Musculoskeletal:** skeletal muscle rigidity.
**Respiratory:** *chest wall rigidity, bronchospasm,* RESPIRATORY DEPRESSION, hypercapnia, *respiratory arrest, laryngospasm.*
**Skin:** pruritus, urticaria.

**INTERACTIONS**
**Drug-drug.** *Cimetidine:* May cause CNS toxicity. Monitor patient closely.
*CNS depressants:* May cause additive effects. Use together cautiously.
*Diazepam:* May cause CV depression and decreases blood pressure with high doses of alfentanil. Monitor patient closely.
*Erythromycin:* May increase risk of prolonged respiratory depression. Monitor patient closely.
*Protease inhibitors:* May increase CNS and respiratory depression. Monitor patient.
**Drug-lifestyle.** *Alcohol use:* May cause additive effects. Discourage use together.

**EFFECTS ON LAB TEST RESULTS**
• May increase amylase and lipase levels.

**CONTRAINDICATIONS & CAUTIONS**
• Contraindicated in patients hypersensitive to drug.
• Use cautiously in patients with head injury, pulmonary disease, decreased respiratory reserve, or hepatic or renal impairment.

**NURSING CONSIDERATIONS**
• *Alert:* To give small volumes of alfentanil accurately, use a tuberculin syringe.
• Treat accidental skin contact by rinsing the area with water.
• Periodically monitor postoperative vital signs and bladder function. Because drug decreases both rate and depth of respirations, monitoring arterial oxygen saturation may aid in assessing respiratory depression.
• Hepatobiliary imaging may be compromised.

• *Alert:* Don't confuse alfentanil with Anafranil, fentanyl, or sufentanil; or Alfenta with Sufenta.

**PATIENT TEACHING**
• Explain painkilling effect of drug and preoperative and postoperative care.
• Inform patient that another painkiller will be available to relieve pain after effects of drug have worn off.

---

**buprenorphine hydrochloride**
Buprenex, Temgesic‡

*Pregnancy risk category C*
*Controlled substance schedule V*

**AVAILABLE FORMS**
*Injection:* 0.324 mg (equivalent to 0.3 mg base/ml)

**INDICATIONS & DOSAGES**
➤ **Moderate to severe pain**
*Adults and children age 13 and older:*
0.3 mg I.M. or slow I.V. q 6 hours, p.r.n., or around the clock; repeat dose (up to 0.3 mg), p.r.n., 30 to 60 minutes after first dose.
*Children ages 2 to 12:* 2 to 6 mcg/kg I.M. or I.V. q 4 to 6 hours.
*Elderly patients:* Reduce dose by one-half.
*Adjust-a-dose:* Reduce dose by one-half in high-risk patients, such as debilitated patients.
➤ **Postoperative pain ♦**
*Adults:* 25 to 250 mcg/hr by continuous I.V. infusion. Or, 60 mcg by epidural administration in single doses, up to a mean total dose of 180 mcg over a 48-hour period.
➤ **Adjunct to surgical anesthesia with a local anesthetic ♦**
*Adults:* 0.3 mg by the epidural route.
➤ **Severe, chronic pain in terminally ill patients ♦**
*Adults:* 0.15 to 0.3 mg by the epidural route q 6 hours, up to a mean total daily dose of 0.86 mg (range 0.15 to 7.2 mg).
➤ **Adjunct to surgical anesthesia during circumcision ♦**
*Children 9 months to 9 years old:* 3 mcg/kg I.M., followed by additional 3 mcg/kg doses postoperatively, p.r.n.

---

Reactions may be *common*, uncommon, *life-threatening*, or COMMON AND LIFE-THREATENING.

➤ **To reverse fentanyl-induced anesthesia and provide analgesia after surgery** ◆

*Adults:* 0.3 to 0.8 mg I.M. or I.V. 1 to 4 hours after induction of anesthesia and 30 minutes before surgery ends.

## I.V. ADMINISTRATION

● Give drug by direct I.V. injection, slowly into a vein or through tubing of a free-flowing, compatible I.V. solution over not less than 2 minutes.

● When mixed in a 1:1 volume ratio, drug is compatible with atropine sulfate, diphenhydramine hydrochloride, droperidol, glycopyrrolate, haloperidol lactate, hydroxyzine hydrochloride, promethazine hydrochloride, scopolamine hydrochloride, $D_5W$, 5% dextrose and normal saline solution, sodium chloride, lactated Ringer's solution, and normal saline solution injections.

● Drug is incompatible with diazepam and lorazepam.

## ACTION

Unknown. Binds with opiate receptors in the CNS, altering both perception of and emotional response to pain.

| Route | Onset | Peak | Duration |
|-------|-------|------|----------|
| I.V. | Immediate | 2 min | 6 hr |
| I.M. | 15 min | 1 hr | 6 hr |

## ADVERSE REACTIONS

**CNS:** *dizziness, sedation,* headache, confusion, nervousness, euphoria, *vertigo, increased intracranial pressure,* fatigue, weakness, depression, dreaming, psychosis, slurred speech, paresthesia.

**CV:** hypotension, *bradycardia,* tachycardia, hypertension, Wenckebach block, cyanosis, flushing.

**EENT:** miosis, blurred vision, diplopia, tinnitus, conjunctivitis, visual abnormalities.

**GI:** *nausea,* vomiting, constipation, dry mouth.

**GU:** urine retention.

**Respiratory:** *respiratory depression,* hypoventilation, dyspnea.

**Skin:** pruritus, diaphoresis, injection site reactions.

**Other:** chills, withdrawal syndrome.

## INTERACTIONS

**Drug-drug.** *CNS depressants, MAO inhibitors:* May cause additive effects. Use together cautiously.

*CYP 3A4 inducers (carbamazepine, phenobarbital, phenytoin, rifampin):* May cause increased clearance of buprenorphine. Monitor patient for clinical effects of drug.

*CYP 3A4 inhibitors (erythromycin, indinavir, ketoconazole, ritonavir, saquinavir):* May cause decreased clearance of buprenorphine. Monitor patient for increased adverse effects.

**Drug-lifestyle.** *Alcohol use:* May cause additive effects. Discourage use together.

## EFFECTS ON LAB TEST RESULTS

None reported.

## CONTRAINDICATIONS & CAUTIONS

● Contraindicated in patients hypersensitive to drug.

● Use cautiously in elderly or debilitated patients and in those with head injury, intracranial lesions, and increased intracranial pressure; severe respiratory, liver, or kidney impairment; CNS depression or coma; thyroid irregularities; adrenal insufficiency; and prostatic hypertrophy, urethral stricture, acute alcoholism, delirium tremens, or kyphoscoliosis. Also use cautiously in patients undergoing surgery of the biliary tract.

## NURSING CONSIDERATIONS

● Reassess patient's level of pain 15 and 30 minutes after parenteral administration.

● Buprenorphine 0.3 mg is equal to 10 mg of morphine and 75 mg of meperidine in analgesic potency. It has longer duration of action than morphine or meperidine.

● *Alert:* Naloxone won't completely reverse the respiratory depression caused by buprenorphine overdose; an overdose may necessitate mechanical ventilation. Larger-than-customary doses of naloxone (more than 0.4 mg) and doxapram also may be ordered.

● Treat accidental skin exposure by removing exposed clothing and rinsing skin with water.

● *Alert:* Drug's opioid antagonist properties may cause withdrawal syndrome in opioid-dependent patients.

• If dependence occurs, withdrawal symptoms may appear up to 14 days after drug is stopped.
• *Alert:* Don't confuse Buprenex with Bumex or bupropion.

**PATIENT TEACHING**
• Caution ambulatory patient about getting out of bed or walking.
• When drug is used after surgery, encourage patient to turn, cough, and breathe deeply to prevent breathing problems.

---

## butorphanol tartrate
Stadol, Stadol NS

*Pregnancy risk category C*
*Controlled substance schedule IV*

**AVAILABLE FORMS**
*Injection:* 1 mg/ml, 2 mg/ml
*Nasal spray:* 10 mg/ml

**INDICATIONS & DOSAGES**
➤ **Moderate to severe pain**
*Adults:* 1 to 4 mg I.M. q 3 to 4 hours, p.r.n., or around the clock. Not to exceed 4 mg per dose. Or, 0.5 to 2 mg I.V. q 3 to 4 hours, p.r.n. or around the clock. Or, 1 mg by nasal spray q 3 to 4 hours (1 spray in one nostril); repeat in 60 to 90 minutes if pain relief is inadequate. For severe pain, 2 mg (1 spray in each nostril) q 3 to 4 hours.
*Elderly patients:* 1 mg I.M. or 0.5 mg I.V., allow 6 hours to elapse before repeating dose. For nasal use, 1 mg (1 spray in 1 nostril). May give another 1 mg in 1.5 to 2 hours. Don't repeat this dosing sequence within 6 hours.
*Adjust-a-dose:* For patients with renal or hepatic impairment, increase dosage interval to 6 to 8 hours.
➤ **Labor for patients at full term and in early labor**
*Adults:* 1 or 2 mg I.V. or I.M.; repeat after 4 hours, p.r.n.
➤ **Preoperative anesthesia or preanesthesia**
*Adults:* 2 mg I.M. 60 to 90 minutes before surgery.

➤ **Adjunct to balanced anesthesia**
*Adults:* 2 mg I.V. shortly before induction, or 0.5 to 1 mg I.V. in increments during anesthesia.
*Elderly patients:* One-half usual dose at twice the interval for I.V. use.

**I.V. ADMINISTRATION**
• Compatible solutions include $D_5W$ and normal saline solutions.
• Give by direct injection into a vein or into the tubing of a free-flowing I.V. solution.

**ACTION**
Unknown. Binds with opiate receptors in the CNS, altering both perception of and emotional response to pain.

| Route | Onset | Peak | Duration |
|-------|-------|------|----------|
| I.V. | 1 min | 4-5 min | 2-4 hr |
| I.M. | 10-30 min | 30-60 min | 3-4 hr |
| Nasal | 15 min | 1-2 hr | 2½-5 hr |

**ADVERSE REACTIONS**
**CNS:** confusion, nervousness, lethargy, headache, *somnolence, dizziness, insomnia,* asthenia, anxiety, paresthesia, euphoria, hallucinations, ***increased intracranial pressure.***
**CV:** flushing, palpitations, vasodilation, hypotension.
**EENT:** blurred vision, *nasal congestion,* tinnitus.
**GI:** *nausea, vomiting,* constipation, anorexia, *unpleasant taste.*
**Respiratory:** *respiratory depression.*
**Skin:** rash, hives, clamminess, excessive diaphoresis.
**Other:** sensation of heat.

**INTERACTIONS**
**Drug-drug.** *CNS depressants:* May cause additive effects. Use together cautiously.
**Drug-lifestyle.** *Alcohol use:* May cause additive effects. Discourage use together.

**EFFECTS ON LAB TEST RESULTS**
None reported.

**CONTRAINDICATIONS & CAUTIONS**
• Contraindicated in patients hypersensitive to drug or to preservative, benzethonium chloride, and in those with opioid addiction; may cause withdrawal syndrome.

---

Reactions may be *common,* uncommon, *life-threatening,* or COMMON AND LIFE-THREATENING.

• Use cautiously in patients with head injury, increased intracranial pressure, acute MI, ventricular dysfunction, coronary insufficiency, respiratory disease or depression, and renal or hepatic dysfunction. Also give cautiously to patients who have recently received repeated doses of opioid analgesic.

## NURSING CONSIDERATIONS
• Reassess patient's level of pain 15 and 30 minutes after administration.
• Don't give by S.C. route.
• Respiratory depression apparently doesn't increase with larger dosage.
• Psychological and physical addiction may occur.
• Periodically monitor postoperative vital signs and bladder function. Because drug decreases both rate and depth of respirations, monitoring arterial oxygen saturation may help assess respiratory depression.
• Watch for nasal congestion with nasal spray use.
• **Alert:** Don't confuse Stadol with sotalol.

## PATIENT TEACHING
• Caution ambulatory patient about getting out of bed or walking. Warn outpatient to avoid driving and other hazardous activities that require mental alertness until it is clear how the drug affects the CNS.
• Teach patient how to give and store nasal spray, if applicable.
• Instruct patient to avoid alcohol during therapy.

## codeine phosphate
Paveral†

## codeine sulfate
*Pregnancy risk category C*
*Controlled substance schedule II*

## AVAILABLE FORMS
**codeine phosphate**
*Injection:* 30 mg/ml, 60 mg/ml
*Oral solution:* 15 mg/5 ml, 10 mg/ml†
*Tablets (soluble):* 30 mg, 60 mg
**codeine sulfate**
*Tablets:* 15 mg, 30 mg, 60 mg
*Tablets (soluble):* 15 mg, 30 mg, 60 mg

## INDICATIONS & DOSAGES
➤ **Mild to moderate pain**
*Adults:* 15 to 60 mg P.O. or 15 to 60 mg (phosphate) S.C., I.M., or I.V. q 4 to 6 hours, p.r.n. Maximum daily dose is 360 mg.
*Children older than age 1:* 0.5 mg/kg P.O., S.C., or I.M. q 4 to 6 hours, p.r.n. Don't give I.V. in children.
➤ **Nonproductive cough**
*Adults:* 10 to 20 mg P.O. q 4 to 6 hours. Maximum daily dose is 120 mg.
*Children ages 6 to 12:* 5 to 10 mg P.O. q 4 to 6 hours. Maximum daily dose is 60 mg.
*Children ages 2 to 5:* 2.5 to 5 mg P.O. q 4 to 6 hours. Maximum daily dose is 30 mg.

## I.V. ADMINISTRATION
• Give drug by direct injection into a large vein. Give very slowly.
• Don't give discolored solution.

## ACTION
Unknown. Binds with opiate receptors in the CNS, altering both perception of and emotional response to pain. Drug also suppresses the cough reflex by direct action on the cough center in the medulla.

| Route | Onset | Peak | Duration |
|-------|-------|------|----------|
| P.O. | 30-45 min | 1-2 hr | 4-6 hr |
| I.V. | Immediate | Immediate | 4-6 hr |
| I.M. | 10-30 min | 30-60 min | 4-6 hr |
| S.C. | 10-30 min | Unknown | 4-6 hr |

## ADVERSE REACTIONS
**CNS:** *sedation, clouded sensorium,* euphoria, dizziness, light-headedness, physical dependence.
**CV:** hypotension, **bradycardia,** flushing.
**GI:** nausea, vomiting, *constipation,* dry mouth, ileus.
**GU:** urine retention.
**Respiratory:** *respiratory depression.*
**Skin:** pruritus, *diaphoresis.*

## INTERACTIONS
**Drug-drug.** *CNS depressants, general anesthetics, hypnotics, MAO inhibitors, other opioid analgesics, sedatives, tranquilizers, tricyclic antidepressants:* May cause additive effects. Use together with

extreme caution. Monitor patient response.
**Drug-lifestyle.** *Alcohol use:* May cause additive effects. Discourage use together.

## EFFECTS ON LAB TEST RESULTS
● May increase amylase and lipase levels.

## CONTRAINDICATIONS & CAUTIONS
● Contraindicated in patients hypersensitive to drug.
● I.V. administration contraindicated in children.
● Use with extreme caution in elderly or debilitated patients and in those with head injury, increased intracranial pressure, increased CSF pressure, hepatic or renal disease, hypothyroidism, Addison's disease, acute alcoholism, seizures, severe CNS depression, bronchial asthma, COPD, respiratory depression, and shock.

## NURSING CONSIDERATIONS
● Reassess patient's level of pain at least 15 and 30 minutes after administration.
● *Alert:* Don't mix with other solutions because codeine phosphate is incompatible with many drugs.
● Codeine and aspirin or acetaminophen are commonly prescribed together to provide enhanced pain relief.
● For full analgesic effect, give drug before patient has intense pain.
● Drug is an antitussive and shouldn't be used when cough is a valuable diagnostic sign or is beneficial (as after thoracic surgery).
● Monitor cough type and frequency.
● Monitor respiratory and circulatory status.
● Opiates may cause constipation. Assess bowel function and need for stool softeners or laxatives.
● Codeine may delay gastric emptying, increase biliary tract pressure from contraction of the sphincter of Oddi, and interfere with hepatobiliary imaging studies.
● *Alert:* Don't confuse codeine with Cardene, Lodine, or Cordran.

## PATIENT TEACHING
● Advise patient that GI distress caused by taking drug by mouth can be eased by taking drug with milk or meals.

● Instruct patient to ask for or to take drug before pain is intense.
● Caution ambulatory patient about getting out of bed or walking. Warn outpatient to avoid driving and other hazardous activities that require mental alertness until drug's effects on the CNS are known.
● Advise patient to avoid alcohol during therapy.

# fentanyl citrate
Sublimaze

# fentanyl transdermal system
Duragesic-25, Duragesic-50, Duragesic-75, Duragesic-100

# fentanyl transmucosal
Actiq

*Pregnancy risk category C*
*Controlled substance schedule II*

## AVAILABLE FORMS
*Injection:* 50 mcg/ml
*Transdermal system:* Patches that release 25 mcg, 50 mcg, 75 mcg, or 100 mcg of fentanyl per hour
*Transmucosal:* 200 mcg, 400 mcg, 600 mcg, 800 mcg, 1,200 mcg, 1,600 mcg

## INDICATIONS & DOSAGES
➤ **Adjunct to general anesthetic**
*Adults:* For low-dose therapy, 2 mcg/kg I.V. For moderate-dose therapy, 2 to 20 mcg/kg I.V.; then 25 to 100 mcg I.V., p.r.n. For high-dose therapy, 20 to 50 mcg/kg I.V.; then 25 mcg to one-half initial loading dose I.V., p.r.n.
➤ **Adjunct to regional anesthesia**
*Adults:* 50 to 100 mcg I.M. or slowly I.V. over 1 to 2 minutes, p.r.n.
➤ **Induce and maintain anesthesia**
*Children ages 2 to 12:* 2 to 3 mcg/kg I.V.
➤ **Postoperative pain, restlessness, tachypnea, and emergence delirium**
*Adults:* 50 to 100 mcg I.M. q 1 to 2 hours, p.r.n.
➤ **Preoperative medication**
*Adults:* 50 to 100 mcg I.M. 30 to 60 minutes before surgery.
➤ **To manage chronic pain**
*Adults:* One transdermal system applied to a portion of the upper torso on an area of

skin that isn't irritated and hasn't been ir-radiated. Therapy started with the 25-mcg/hour system; dosage adjusted as needed and tolerated. Each system may be worn for 72 hours, although some patients may need systems to be applied q 48 hours. May increase dose q 3 days after first dose; thereafter, don't increase more often than q 6 days.

➤ **To manage breakthrough cancer pain in patients already receiving and tolerant of opioid therapy**
*Adults:* 200 mcg Actiq initially; may give second dose 15 minutes after completion of the first (30 minutes after first lozenge placed in mouth). Maximum dose is 2 lozenges per breakthrough episode. If several episodes of breakthrough pain requiring 2 lozenges occur, dose may be increased to the next available strength. Once a successful dosage has been reached, patient should limit use to no more than 4 lozenges daily.

**I.V. ADMINISTRATION**
● Only staff trained in administration of I.V. anesthetics and management of their potential adverse effects should give I.V. fentanyl. Inject slowly over 1 to 2 minutes.
● Drug is often used I.V. with droperidol to produce neuroleptanalgesia.
● Keep opioid antagonist (naloxone) and resuscitation equipment available when giving drug I.V.

**ACTION**
Unknown. Binds with opiate receptors in the CNS, altering both perception of and emotional response to pain.

| Route | Onset | Peak | Duration |
|---|---|---|---|
| I.V. | 1-2 min | 3-5 min | 30-60 min |
| I.M. | 7-15 min | 20-30 min | 1-2 hr |
| Trans-dermal | 12-24 hr | 1-3 days | Variable |
| Trans-mucosal | 5-15 min | 20-30 min | Unknown |

**ADVERSE REACTIONS**
**CNS:** *sedation, somnolence, clouded sensorium, euphoria,* dizziness, headache, *confusion, asthenia,* nervousness, hallucinations, anxiety, depression, *seizures.*
**CV:** hypotension, hypertension, *arrhythmias,* chest pain.

**GI:** nausea, vomiting, constipation, ileus, abdominal pain, dry mouth, anorexia, diarrhea, dyspepsia.
**GU:** urine retention.
**Musculoskeletal:** skeletal muscle rigidity (dose-related).
**Respiratory:** *respiratory depression,* hypoventilation, dyspnea, *apnea.*
**Skin:** erythema at application site (transdermal), *pruritus, diaphoresis.*
**Other:** physical dependence.

**INTERACTIONS**
**Drug-drug.** *CNS depressants, general anesthetics, hypnotics, MAO inhibitors, other opioid analgesics, sedatives, tricyclic antidepressants:* May cause additive effects. Use together with extreme caution. Reduce fentanyl dose by one-fourth to one-third; also give above drugs in reduced dosages.
*CYP 3A4 inhibitors (erythromycin, ketoconazole, protease inhibitors such as ritonavir):* May cause increased analgesia, CNS depression, and hypotensive effects. Monitor patient's respiratory status and vital signs.
*CYP 3A4 inducers (carbamazepine, phenytoin, rifampin):* May decrease analgesic effects. Monitor patient for adequate pain relief.
*Diazepam:* May cause CV depression when given with high doses of fentanyl. Monitor patient closely.
*Droperidol:* May cause hypotension and decreases pulmonary arterial pressure. Use together cautiously.
**Drug-lifestyle.** *Alcohol use:* May cause additive effects. Discourage use together.

**EFFECTS ON LAB TEST RESULTS**
● May increase amylase and lipase levels.

**CONTRAINDICATIONS & CAUTIONS**
● Contraindicated in patients intolerant to drug.
● Fentanyl patch is contraindicated in patients hypersensitive to adhesives, for pain management after surgery, mild or intermittent pain that can be managed with nonopioid drugs, and in doses exceeding 25 mcg/hour initially.
● Actiq is contraindicated in children and in management of acute or postoperative pain.

*Rapid onset*   †Canada   ‡Australia   ◇OTC   ◆Off-label use   ⬭Photoguide   *Liquid contains alcohol.

• Don't give transdermal fentanyl to patients younger than age 12 or those younger than age 18 who weigh less than 110 lb (50 kg) or for postoperative pain.
• Use with caution in patients with head injury, increased CSF pressure, COPD, decreased respiratory reserve, potentially compromised respirations, hepatic or renal disease, and cardiac bradyarrhythmias. Also use with caution in elderly or debilitated patients.

## NURSING CONSIDERATIONS
• For better analgesic effect, give drug before patient has intense pain.
• *Alert:* High doses can produce muscle rigidity, which can be reversed with neuromuscular blockers; however, patient must be artificially ventilated.
• Monitor circulatory and respiratory status and urinary function carefully. Drug may cause respiratory depression, hypotension, urine retention, nausea, vomiting, ileus, or altered level of consciousness no matter how it is given.
• Periodically monitor postoperative vital signs and bladder function. Because drug decreases both rate and depth of respirations, monitoring of arterial oxygen saturation ($SaO_2$) may help assess respiratory depression. Immediately report respiratory rate below 12 breaths/minute, decreased respiratory volume, or decreased $SaO_2$.

**Transdermal form**
• Dosage equivalent charts are available to calculate the fentanyl transdermal dose based on the daily morphine intake; for example, for every 90 mg of oral morphine or 15 mg of I.M. morphine per 24 hours, 25 mcg/hour of transdermal fentanyl is needed.
• Make dosage adjustments gradually in patient using the transdermal system. Reaching steady-state level of a new dosage may take up to 6 days; delay dosage adjustment until after at least two applications.
• Monitor patient who develops adverse reactions to the transdermal system for at least 12 hours after removal. Fentanyl level drops gradually and may take as long as 17 hours to decline by 50%.
• Most patients experience good control of pain for 3 days while wearing the transder-

mal system, but a few may need a new application after 48 hours.
• Because the fentanyl level rises for the first 24 hours after application, analgesic effect can't be evaluated on the first day. Be sure patient has adequate supplemental analgesic to prevent breakthrough pain.
• When reducing opiate therapy or switching to a different analgesic, withdraw the transdermal system gradually. Because the fentanyl level drops gradually after removal, give half of the equianalgesic dose of the new analgesic 12 to 18 hours after removal.

**Transmucosal form**
• *Alert:* Actiq is used only to manage breakthrough cancer pain in patients who are already receiving and are tolerant to opioid therapy for their underlying persistent cancer pain.
• Remove foil overwrap of Actiq just before giving.
• The lozenge is placed between the cheek and gum and may occasionally be moved from side to side using the stick. The Actiq lozenge shouldn't be chewed and should be consumed over about 15 minutes. Discard the stick in the trash after use or, if any drug matrix remains on the stick, place under hot running tap water until dissolved or place in child-resistant container provided, and dispose as appropriate for schedule II drugs.
• *Alert:* Don't confuse fentanyl with alfentanil.

## PATIENT TEACHING
• When drug is used for pain control, instruct patient to ask for drug before pain becomes intense.
• When drug is used after surgery, encourage patient to turn, cough, and breathe deeply to prevent lung problems.
• Instruct patient to avoid hazardous activities until CNS effects subside.
• Tell home care patient to avoid drinking alcohol or taking other CNS-type drugs while receiving fentanyl because additive effects can occur.
• Advise patient not to stop drug abruptly.
• Teach patient about proper application of prescribed transdermal patch. Tell patient to clip hair at application site, but not to use a razor, which may irritate skin. Wash area with clear water, if needed, but not

---

Reactions may be *common*, uncommon, *life-threatening*, or COMMON AND LIFE-THREATENING.

with soaps, oils, lotions, alcohol, or other substances that may irritate skin or prevent adhesion. Dry area completely before application.
• Tell patient to remove transdermal system from package just before applying, hold in place for 30 seconds, and be sure the edges of patch stick to skin.
• Teach patient not to alter the transdermal system (e.g., by cutting) in any way before application.
• Teach patient to dispose of the transdermal patch by folding it so the adhesive side adheres to itself, and then flushing it down the toilet.
• Tell patient that, if another patch is needed after 48 to 72 hours, he should apply it to a different skin site.
• Inform patient that heat from fever or environment, such as from heating pads, electric blankets, heat lamps, hot tubs, or water beds, may increase transdermal delivery and cause toxicity requiring dosage adjustment. Instruct patient to notify prescriber if fever occurs or if he'll be spending time in a hot climate.
• *Alert:* Warn patient and patient's family that the amount of fentanyl in one Actiq lozenge can be fatal to a child. Keep well secured and out of children's reach.

## hydromorphone hydrochloride (dihydromorphinone hydrochloride)
Dilaudid, Dilaudid-5, Dilaudid-HP

*Pregnancy risk category C*
*Controlled substance schedule II*

### AVAILABLE FORMS
*Cough syrup:* 1 mg/5 ml
*Injection:* 1 mg/ml, 2 mg/ml, 3 mg/ml, 4 mg/ml, 10 mg/ml
*Liquid:* 5 mg/5 ml
*Suppositories:* 3 mg
*Tablets:* 1 mg, 2 mg, 3 mg, 4 mg, 8 mg

### INDICATIONS & DOSAGES
➤ **Moderate to severe pain**
*Adults:* 2 to 4 mg P.O. q 4 to 6 hours, p.r.n. Or, 1 to 4 mg I.M., S.C., or I.V. (slowly over at least 2 to 5 minutes) q 4 to 6 hours, p.r.n. Or, 3 mg P.R. suppository q 6 to 8 hours, p.r.n.

➤ **Cough**
*Adults and children older than age 12:*
1 mg cough syrup P.O. q 3 to 4 hours, p.r.n.
*Children ages 6 to 12 years:* 0.5 mg cough syrup P.O. q 3 to 4 hours, p.r.n.

### I.V. ADMINISTRATION
• For infusion, drug may be mixed in D₅W, normal saline solution, dextrose 5% in normal saline solution, dextrose 5% in half-normal saline solution, or Ringer's or lactated Ringer's solutions.
• Give by direct injection over no less than 2 minutes.
• Respiratory depression and hypotension can occur. Give slowly, and monitor patient constantly. Keep resuscitation equipment available.

### ACTION
Unknown. Binds with opiate receptors in the CNS, altering both perception of and emotional response to pain. Also suppresses the cough reflex by direct action on the cough center in the medulla.

| Route | Onset | Peak | Duration |
|---|---|---|---|
| P.O. | 30 min | 90-120 min | 4 hr |
| I.V. | 10-15 min | 15-30 min | 2-3 hr |
| I.M. | 15 min | 30-60 min | 4-5 hr |
| S.C. | 15 min | 30-90 min | 4 hr |
| P.R. | Unknown | Unknown | 4 hr |

### ADVERSE REACTIONS
**CNS:** sedation, somnolence, clouded sensorium, dizziness, euphoria, lightheadedness.
**CV:** hypotension, flushing, *bradycardia.*
**EENT:** blurred vision, diplopia, nystagmus.
**GI:** nausea, vomiting, constipation, ileus, dry mouth.
**GU:** urine retention.
**Respiratory:** *respiratory depression, bronchospasm.*
**Skin:** diaphoresis, pruritus.
**Other:** induration with repeated S.C. injections, physical dependence.

### INTERACTIONS
**Drug-drug.** *CNS depressants, general anesthetics, hypnotics, MAO inhibitors, other opioid analgesics, sedatives, tranquilizers, tricyclic antidepressants:* May

cause additive effects. Use together with extreme caution. Reduce hydromorphone dose and monitor patient response.
**Drug-lifestyle.** *Alcohol use:* May cause additive effects. Advise patient to use together cautiously.

**EFFECTS ON LAB TEST RESULTS**
● May increase amylase and lipase levels.

**CONTRAINDICATIONS & CAUTIONS**
● Contraindicated in patients hypersensitive to drug and in those with intracranial lesions that cause increased intracranial pressure; also contraindicated whenever ventilation is depressed, such as in status asthmaticus, COPD, cor pulmonale, emphysema, and kyphoscoliosis.
● Use with extreme caution in elderly or debilitated patients and in those with hepatic or renal disease, hypothyroidism, Addison's disease, prostatic hyperplasia, or urethral stricture.

**NURSING CONSIDERATIONS**
● Reassess patient's level of pain at least 15 and 30 minutes after administration.
● For better analgesic effect, give drug before patient has intense pain.
● Dilaudid-HP, a highly concentrated form (10 mg/ml), may be given in smaller volumes to prevent the discomfort of large-volume I.M. or S.C. injections. Check dosage carefully.
● Rotate injection sites to avoid induration with S.C. injection.
● Monitor respiratory and circulatory status and bowel function.
● Keep opioid antagonist (naloxone) available.
● Drug may delay gastric emptying; increased biliary tract pressure resulting from contraction of the sphincter of Oddi may interfere with hepatobiliary imaging studies.
● Drug may worsen or mask gallbladder pain.
● Drug is a commonly abused opioid.
● *Alert:* Cough syrup may contain tartrazine.
● *Alert:* Don't confuse hydromorphone with morphine or oxymorphone or Dilaudid with Dilantin.

**PATIENT TEACHING**
● Instruct patient to request or take drug before pain becomes intense.
● Tell patient to store suppositories in refrigerator.
● Advise patient to take drug with food if GI upset occurs.
● When drug is used after surgery, encourage patient to turn, cough, and breathe deeply to avoid lung problems.
● Caution ambulatory patient about getting out of bed or walking. Warn outpatient to avoid hazardous activities that require mental alertness until drug's CNS effects are known.
● Advise patient to avoid alcohol during therapy.

---

**meperidine hydrochloride (pethidine hydrochloride)**
Demerol◆

*Pregnancy risk category B; D if used for prolonged periods or in high doses at term*
*Controlled substance schedule II*

**AVAILABLE FORMS**
*Injection:* 10 mg/ml, 25 mg/ml, 50 mg/ml, 75 mg/ml, 100 mg/ml
*Syrup:* 50 mg/5 ml
*Tablets:* 50 mg, 100 mg

**INDICATIONS & DOSAGES**
➤ **Moderate to severe pain**
*Adults:* 50 to 150 mg P.O., I.M., or S.C. q 3 to 4 hours, p.r.n.
*Children:* 1.1 to 1.8 mg/kg P.O., I.M., or S.C. q 3 to 4 hours. Maximum, 100 mg q 4 hours, p.r.n.
➤ **Preoperative analgesia**
*Adults:* 50 to 100 mg I.M. or S.C. 30 to 90 minutes before surgery.
*Children:* 1 to 2.2 mg/kg I.M. or S.C. up to the adult dose 30 to 90 minutes before surgery.
➤ **Adjunct to anesthesia**
*Adults:* Repeated slow I.V. injections of fractional doses (10 mg/ml). Or, continuous I.V. infusion of a more dilute solution (1 mg/ml) titrated to patient's needs.

---

➤ **Obstetric analgesia**
*Adults:* 50 to 100 mg I.M. or S.C. when pain becomes regular; repeated at 1- to 3-hour intervals.

**I.V. ADMINISTRATION**
● Keep opioid antagonist (naloxone) available when giving this drug I.V.
● Give drug slowly by direct I.V. injection.
● Meperidine also may be given by slow continuous I.V. infusion. Drug is compatible with most I.V. solutions, including $D_5W$, normal saline solution, and Ringer's or lactated Ringer's solutions.

**ACTION**
Unknown. Binds with opiate receptors in the CNS, altering both perception of and emotional response to pain.

| Route | Onset | Peak | Duration |
|-------|-------|------|----------|
| P.O. | 15 min | 60-90 min | 2-4 hr |
| I.V. | 1 min | 5-7 min | 2-4 hr |
| I.M. | 10-15 min | 30-50 min | 2-4 hr |
| S.C. | 10-15 min | 30-50 min | 2-4 hr |

**ADVERSE REACTIONS**
**CNS:** physical dependence, *sedation, somnolence, clouded sensorium, euphoria,* paradoxical anxiety, tremor, *dizziness, seizures,* headache, hallucinations, syncope, *light-headedness.*
**CV:** hypotension, *bradycardia,* tachycardia, *cardiac arrest, shock.*
**GI:** constipation, ileus, dry mouth, *nausea, vomiting,* biliary tract spasms.
**GU:** urine retention.
**Musculoskeletal:** muscle twitching.
**Respiratory:** *respiratory depression, respiratory arrest.*
**Skin:** pruritus, urticaria, *diaphoresis.*
**Other:** phlebitis after I.V. delivery, pain at injection site, local tissue irritation, induration.

**INTERACTIONS**
**Drug-drug.** *Aminophylline, barbiturates, heparin, methicillin, morphine sulfate, phenytoin, sodium bicarbonate, sulfonamides:* Incompatible when mixed in same I.V. container. Avoid using together.
*Cimetidine:* May increase respiratory and CNS depression. Monitor patient closely.

*Chlorpromazine:* May cause excessive sedation and hypotension. Avoid using together.
*CNS depressants, general anesthetics, hypnotics, other opioid analgesics, phenothiazines, sedatives, tricyclic antidepressants:* May cause respiratory depression, hypotension, profound sedation, or coma. Use together with extreme caution. Reduce meperidine dosage.
*MAO inhibitors:* May increase CNS excitation or depression that can be severe or fatal. Avoid using together.
*Phenytoin:* May decrease meperidine level. Watch for decreased analgesia.
*Protease inhibitors:* May increase respiratory and CNS depression. Avoid using together.
**Drug-lifestyle.** *Alcohol use:* May cause additive effects. Discourage use together.

**EFFECTS ON LAB TEST RESULTS**
● May increase amylase and lipase levels.

**CONTRAINDICATIONS & CAUTIONS**
● Contraindicated in patients hypersensitive to drug and in those who have received MAO inhibitors within past 14 days.
● Use with caution in elderly or debilitated patients and in those with increased intracranial pressure, head injury, asthma and other respiratory conditions, supraventricular tachycardias, seizures, acute abdominal conditions, hepatic or renal disease, hypothyroidism, Addison's disease, urethral stricture, and prostatic hyperplasia.
● Avoid use in patients with end-stage renal disease.

**NURSING CONSIDERATIONS**
● Active metabolite of meperidine may accumulate in patients with renal dysfunction, causing increased adverse CNS reactions.
● Drug may be used in some patients who are allergic to morphine.
● Reassess patient's level of pain at least 15 and 30 minutes after administration.
● S.C. injection isn't recommended because it's very painful, but it may be suitable for occasional use. Monitor patient for pain at injection site, local tissue irritation, and induration after S.C. injection.

• **Alert:** Oral dose is less than half as effective as parenteral dose. Give I.M., if possible. When changing from parenteral to oral route, increase dosage.

• Syrup has local anesthetic effect. Give with full glass of water.

• Drug and its active metabolite, normeperidine, accumulate in the body. Watch for increased toxic effect, especially in patients with impaired renal function.

• Because drug toxicity frequently appears after several days of treatment, drug isn't recommended for treatment of chronic pain.

• Monitor respirations of neonates exposed to drug during labor. Have resuscitation equipment and naloxone available.

• Monitor respiratory and CV status carefully. Don't give if respirations are below 12 breaths/minute, if respiratory rate or depth is decreased, or if change in pupils is noted.

• Watch for withdrawal symptoms if drug is stopped abruptly after long-term use.

• Monitor bladder function in postoperative patients.

• Monitor bowel function. Patient may need a laxative or stool softener.

• **Alert:** Don't confuse Demerol with Demulen.

**PATIENT TEACHING**

• When drug is used postoperatively, encourage patient to turn, cough, and deep-breathe and to use an incentive spirometer to prevent lung problems.

• Caution ambulatory patient about getting out of bed or walking. Warn outpatient to avoid driving and other potentially hazardous activities that require mental alertness until drug's CNS effects are known.

• Advise patient to avoid alcohol during therapy.

---

## methadone hydrochloride
Dolophine, Methadose,
Physeptone‡

*Pregnancy risk category C*
*Controlled substance schedule II*

**AVAILABLE FORMS**
*Dispersible tablets (for methadone maintenance therapy):* 40 mg

*Injection:* 10 mg/ml
*Oral solution:* 5 mg/5 ml, 10 mg/5 ml, 10 mg/ml (concentrate)
*Tablets:* 5 mg, 10 mg

**INDICATIONS & DOSAGES**
➤ **Severe pain**
*Adults:* 2.5 to 10 mg P.O., I.M., or S.C. q 3 to 4 hours, p.r.n.
➤ **Severe chronic pain**
*Adults:* 5 to 20 mg P.O. q. 6 to 8 hours, p.r.n.
➤ **Opioid withdrawal syndrome**
*Adults:* 15 to 20 mg P.O. daily often suppresses withdrawal symptoms (highly individualized—some patients may require a higher dose). Maintenance dose is 20 to 120 mg P.O. daily. Dosage adjusted, p.r.n.

**ACTION**
Unknown. Binds with opiate receptors in the CNS, altering both perception of and emotional response to pain.

| Route | Onset | Peak | Duration |
|---|---|---|---|
| P.O. | 30-60 min | 90-120 min | 4-6 hr |
| I.M., S.C. | 10-20 min | 1-2 hr | 4-5 hr |

**ADVERSE REACTIONS**
**CNS:** *sedation, somnolence, clouded sensorium,* euphoria, *dizziness,* choreic movements, *seizures,* headache, insomnia, agitation, *light-headedness,* syncope.
**CV:** hypotension, *arrhythmias bradycardia, shock, cardiac arrest,* palpitations, edema.
**EENT:** visual disturbances.
**GI:** *nausea, vomiting,* constipation, ileus, dry mouth, anorexia, biliary tract spasm.
**GU:** urine retention.
**Respiratory:** *respiratory depression, respiratory arrest.*
**Skin:** diaphoresis, pruritus, urticaria.
**Other:** physical dependence, pain at injection site, tissue irritation, induration, decreased libido.

**INTERACTIONS**
**Drug-drug.** *Ammonium chloride, other urine acidifiers, phenytoin:* May reduce methadone effect. Watch for decreased pain control.
*CNS depressants, general anesthetics, hypnotics, MAO inhibitors, sedatives, tranquilizers, tricyclic antidepressants:*

---

Reactions may be *common,* uncommon, *life-threatening,* or COMMON AND LIFE-THREATENING.

May cause respiratory depression, hypotension, profound sedation, or coma. Use together with extreme caution. Monitor patient response.

*Protease inhibitors, cimetidine, fluvoxamine:* May increase respiratory and CNS depression. Monitor patient closely.

*Rifampin:* May cause withdrawal symptoms; reduces level of methadone. Use together cautiously.

**Drug-lifestyle.** *Alcohol use:* May cause additive effects. Discourage use together.

### EFFECTS ON LAB TEST RESULTS
• May increase amylase level.

### CONTRAINDICATIONS & CAUTIONS
• Contraindicated in patients hypersensitive to drug.
• Use with extreme caution in elderly or debilitated patients and in those with acute abdominal conditions, severe hepatic or renal impairment, hypothyroidism, Addison's disease, prostatic hyperplasia, urethral stricture, head injury, increased intracranial pressure, asthma, and other respiratory conditions.

### NURSING CONSIDERATIONS
• Reassess patient's level of pain at least 15 and 30 minutes after parenteral administration and 30 minutes after oral administration.
• When used in opioid withdrawal syndrome, daily doses of more than 120 mg require special state and federal approval.
• Oral liquid form legally required in maintenance programs. Completely dissolve tablets in ½ cup of orange juice or powdered citrus drink.
• For parenteral use, I.M. injection is preferred. Rotate injection sites.
• Monitor patient for pain at injection site, tissue irritation, and induration after S.C. injection.
• Oral dose is one-half as potent as injected dose.
• An around-the-clock regimen is needed to manage severe, chronic pain.
• Patient treated for opioid withdrawal syndrome usually will need an additional analgesic if pain control is needed.
• Monitor patient closely because drug has cumulative effect; marked sedation can occur after repeated doses.

• Monitor circulatory and respiratory status and bladder and bowel function. Patient may need a stool softener or laxative.
• When used as an adjunct in the treatment of opioid addiction (maintenance), withdrawal is usually delayed and mild.
• **Alert:** High doses of methadone may cause or contribute to QT interval prolongation and torsades de point.

### PATIENT TEACHING
• Caution ambulatory patient about getting out of bed or walking. Warn outpatient to avoid hazardous activities that require mental alertness until drug's CNS effects are known.
• Instruct patient to increase fluid and fiber in diet, if not contraindicated, to combat constipation.
• Advise patient to avoid alcohol during therapy.

## morphine hydrochloride
Morphitec†, M.O.S.†, M.O.S.-S.R.†

## morphine sulfate
Anamorph‡, Astramorph PF, Avinza, Duramorph, Epimorph†, Infumorph, Infumorph 500, Kadian, M-Eslon†, Morphine H.P.†, MS Contin, MSIR, MS/L, OMS Concentrate, Oramorph SR, RMS Uniserts, Roxanol, Roxanol 100, Roxanol Rescudose, Roxanol UD, Statex

## morphine tartrate‡

*Pregnancy risk category C*
*Controlled substance schedule II*

### AVAILABLE FORMS
**morphine hydrochloride**
*Oral solution:* 1 mg/ml†, 5 mg/ml†, 10 mg/ml†, 20 mg/ml†, 50 mg/ml†
*Suppositories:* 10 mg†, 20 mg†, 30 mg†
*Syrup:* 1 mg/ml†*, 5 mg/ml†*, 10 mg/ml†*, 20 mg/ml†*, 50 mg/ml†*
*Tablets:* 10 mg†, 20 mg†, 40 mg†, 60 mg†
*Tablets (extended-release):* 30 mg†, 60 mg†
**morphine sulfate**
*Capsules:* 15 mg, 30 mg

*Capsules (extended-release contain immediate and sustained-release morphine beads):* 30 mg, 60 mg, 90 mg, 120 mg
*Capsules (sustained-release):* 20 mg, 50 mg, 100 mg
*Injection (with preservative):* 0.5 mg/ml, 1 mg/ml, 2 mg/ml, 3 mg/ml, 4 mg/ml, 5 mg/ml, 8 mg/ml, 10 mg/ml, 15 mg/ml, 25 mg/ml, 50 mg/ml
*Injection (without preservative):* 0.5 mg/ml, 1 mg/ml, 10 mg/ml, 15 mg/ml, 25 mg/ml
*Oral solution:* 10 mg/2.5 ml (unit dose), 10 mg/5 ml, 20 mg/5 ml, 20 mg/ml (concentrate), 30 mg/1.5 ml, 100 mg/5 ml
*Soluble tablets:* 10 mg, 15 mg, 30 mg
*Suppositories:* 5 mg, 10 mg, 20 mg, 30 mg
*Syrup:* 1 mg/ml, 5 mg/ml
*Tablets:* 15 mg, 30 mg
*Tablets (extended-release):* 15 mg, 30 mg, 60 mg, 100 mg, 200 mg
**morphine tartrate**
*Injection:* 80 mg/ml‡

## INDICATIONS & DOSAGES
➤ **Severe pain**
*Adults:* 5 to 20 mg S.C. or I.M. or 2.5 to 15 mg I.V. q 4 hours, p.r.n. Or, 5 to 30 mg P.O. or 10 to 20 mg P.R. q 4 hours, p.r.n. For continuous I.V. infusion, give loading dose of 15 mg I.V.; then continuous infusion of 0.8 to 10 mg/hour. May also give a 15- or 30-mg extended-release tablet P.O. q 8 to 12 hours. For sustained-release Kadian capsules used as a first opioid, give 20 mg P.O. q 12 hours or 40 mg P.O. once daily; increase conservatively in opioid-naive patients. For epidural injection, give 5 mg by epidural catheter; then, if pain isn't relieved adequately in 1 hour, give supplementary doses of 1 to 2 mg at intervals sufficient to assess efficacy. Maximum total epidural dose shouldn't exceed 10 mg/24 hours. For intrathecal injection, a single dose of 0.2 to 1 mg may provide pain relief for 24 hours (only in the lumbar area). Don't repeat injections.
*Children:* 0.1 to 0.2 mg/kg S.C. or I.M. q 4 hours. Maximum single dose, 15 mg.
➤ **Moderate to severe pain requiring continuous, around-the-clock opioid**
*Adults:* Individualize dosage of Avinza. For patients with no tolerance to opioids, begin with 30 mg Avinza P.O. daily; adjust

dosage by no more than 30 mg q 4 days. When converting from another oral morphine formulation, individualize the dosing schedule according to patient's previous drug dosing schedule.

## I.V. ADMINISTRATION
● For direct injection, dilute 2.5 to 15 mg in 4 or 5 ml of sterile water for injection and give slowly over 4 to 5 minutes.
● For continuous infusion, mix drug with $D_5W$ to yield 0.1 to 1 mg/ml and give by a continuous infusion device.
● In adults with severe, chronic pain, maintenance I.V. infusion is 0.8 to 80 mg/hour; sometimes, higher doses are needed.
● Morphine sulfate is compatible with most common I.V. solutions.

## ACTION
Unknown. Binds with opiate receptors in the CNS, altering both perception of and emotional response to pain.

| Route | Onset | Peak | Duration |
|---|---|---|---|
| P.O. | 1 hr | 1-2 hr | 4-12 hr |
| P.O. (morphine sulfate) | 30 min | Unknown | 24 hr |
| I.V. | 5 min | 20 min | 4-5 hr |
| I.M. | 10-30 min | 30-60 min | 4-5 hr |
| S.C. | 10-30 min | 50-90 min | 4-5 hr |
| P.R. | 20-60 min | 20-60 min | 4-5 hr |
| Epidural | 15-60 min | 15-60 min | 24 hr |
| Intrathecal | 15-60 min | 30-60 min | 24 hr |

## ADVERSE REACTIONS
**CNS:** *sedation, somnolence, clouded sensorium, euphoria,* **seizures,** *dizziness, nightmares,* physical dependence, *lightheadedness,* hallucinations, nervousness, depression, syncope.
**CV:** hypotension, **bradycardia, shock, cardiac arrest,** tachycardia, hypertension.
**GI:** *nausea, vomiting, constipation,* ileus, dry mouth, biliary tract spasms, anorexia.
**GU:** urine retention.
**Hematologic:** *thrombocytopenia.*
**Respiratory:** *respiratory depression, apnea, respiratory arrest.*
**Skin:** pruritus and skin flushing, diaphoresis, edema.
**Other:** decreased libido.

---

Reactions may be *common*, uncommon, *life-threatening*, or COMMON AND LIFE-THREATENING.

## INTERACTIONS

**Drug-drug.** *Cimetidine:* May increase respiratory and CNS depression when given concomitantly with morphine sulfate. Monitor patient closely.

*CNS depressants, general anesthetics, hypnotics, MAO inhibitors, other opioid analgesics, sedatives, tranquilizers, tricyclic antidepressants:* May cause respiratory depression, hypotension, profound sedation, or coma. Use together with extreme caution. Reduce morphine dose and monitor patient response.

**Drug-lifestyle.** *Alcohol use:* May cause additive effects. Advise patient to use together cautiously.

## EFFECTS ON LAB TEST RESULTS

• May increase amylase level.
• May decrease platelet count. Morphine sulfate may decrease hemoglobin and cause abnormal liver function test values.

## CONTRAINDICATIONS & CAUTIONS

• Contraindicated in patients hypersensitive to drug and in those with conditions that would preclude administration of opioids by I.V. route (acute bronchial asthma or upper airway obstruction).
• Contraindicated in patients with GI obstruction.
• Use with extreme caution in elderly or debilitated patients and in those with head injury, increased intracranial pressure, seizures, chronic pulmonary disease, prostatic hyperplasia, severe hepatic or renal disease, acute abdominal conditions, hypothyroidism, Addison's disease, and urethral stricture.
• Use cautiously in patients with circulatory shock, biliary tract disease, CNS depression, toxic psychosis, acute alcoholism, delirium tremens, and seizure disorders.

## NURSING CONSIDERATIONS

• Reassess patient's level of pain at least 15 and 30 minutes after parenteral administration and 30 minutes after oral administration.
• Keep opioid antagonist (naloxone) and resuscitation equipment available.
• Oral solutions of various concentrations and an intensified oral solution (20 mg/ml) are available. Carefully note the strength given.

• ***Alert:*** Don't crush, break, or chew extended-release tablets or sustained release capsules.
• Oral capsules may be carefully opened and the entire bead contents poured into cool, soft foods, such as water, orange juice, applesauce, or pudding; patient should consume mixture immediately.
• S.L. administration may be ordered. Measure oral solution with tuberculin syringe. Give dose a few drops at a time to allow maximal S.L. absorption and minimize swallowing.
• Refrigeration of rectal suppository isn't needed. In some patients, rectal and oral absorption may not be equivalent.
• Preservative-free preparations are available for epidural and intrathecal administration.
• When given epidurally, monitor patient closely for respiratory depression up to 24 hours after the injection. Check respiratory rate and depth every 30 to 60 minutes for 24 hours.
• Watch for pruritus and skin flushing with epidural administration.
• Morphine is drug of choice in relieving MI pain; may cause transient decrease in blood pressure.
• An around-the-clock regimen best manages severe, chronic pain.
• Morphine may worsen or mask gallbladder pain.
• Monitor circulatory, respiratory, bladder, and bowel functions carefully. Drug may cause respiratory depression, hypotension, urine retention, nausea, vomiting, ileus, or altered level of consciousness regardless of the route used. Withhold dose and notify prescriber if respirations are below 12 breaths/minute.
• Constipation is commonly severe with maintenance dose. Ensure that stool softener or other laxative is ordered.
• Give morphine sulfate without regard to food.
• Taper morphine sulfate therapy gradually when stopping therapy.
• Give morphine sulfate whole or open the capsule and sprinkle the beads on a small amount of applesauce immediately before ingestion.
• ***Alert:*** Don't chew, crush, or dissolve morphine sulfate beads due to risk of acute morphine overdose.

---

- Morphine sulfate is not intended for use as a p.r.n. analgesic.
- **Alert:** Don't confuse morphine with hydromorphone or Avinza with Invanz.

## PATIENT TEACHING
- When drug is used after surgery, encourage patient to turn, cough, and deep-breathe and to use incentive spirometer to prevent lung problems.
- Caution ambulatory patient about getting out of bed or walking. Warn outpatient to avoid driving and other potentially hazardous activities that require mental alertness until drug's adverse CNS effects are known.
- Advise patient to avoid alcohol during therapy.
- Tell patient to swallow morphine sulfate whole or to open capsule and sprinkle beads on a small amount of applesauce immediately before ingestion.
- Teach patient that due to the risk of acute overdose, extended release beads can't be crushed, chewed, or dissolved.

---

## nalbuphine hydrochloride
Nubain

*Pregnancy risk category B*

## AVAILABLE FORMS
*Injection:* 10 mg/ml, 20 mg/ml

## INDICATIONS & DOSAGES
➤ **Moderate to severe pain**
*Adults:* For an average-weight (70-kg [154 lb]) person, 10 to 20 mg S.C., I.M., or I.V. q 3 to 6 hours, p.r.n. Maximum, 160 mg daily.
➤ **Adjunct to balanced anesthesia**
*Adults:* 0.3 mg/kg to 3.0 mg/kg I.V. over 10 to 15 minutes; then maintenance doses of 0.25 to 0.50 mg/kg in single I.V. dose, p.r.n.
*Adjust-a-dose:* Decrease dosage in patients with renal or hepatic impairment.

## I.V. ADMINISTRATION
- Inject slowly over at least 2 to 3 minutes into a vein or into an I.V. line containing a compatible, free-flowing I.V. solution, such as $D_5W$, normal saline solution, or lactated Ringer's solution.

- Respiratory depression can be reversed with naloxone. Keep resuscitation equipment available, particularly when giving I.V.

## ACTION
Unknown. Binds with opiate receptors in the CNS, altering both perception of and emotional response to pain.

| Route | Onset | Peak | Duration |
|-------|-------|------|----------|
| I.V. | 2-3 min | 30 min | 3-6 hr |
| I.M. | 15 min | 1 hr | 3-6 hr |
| S.C. | 15 min | Unknown | 3-6 hr |

## ADVERSE REACTIONS
**CNS:** *headache, sedation, dizziness, vertigo,* nervousness, depression, restlessness, crying, euphoria, hostility, unusual dreams, confusion, hallucinations, speech disorders, delusions.
**CV:** hypertension, hypotension, tachycardia, ***bradycardia.***
**EENT:** blurred vision, dry mouth.
**GI:** cramps, dyspepsia, bitter taste, nausea, vomiting, constipation, biliary tract spasms.
**GU:** urinary urgency.
**Respiratory:** *respiratory depression,* dyspnea, asthma, pulmonary edema.
**Skin:** pruritus, burning, urticaria, clamminess, diaphoresis.

## INTERACTIONS
**Drug-drug.** *CNS depressants, general anesthetics, hypnotics, MAO inhibitors, sedatives, tranquilizers, tricyclic antidepressants:* May cause respiratory depression, hypertension, profound sedation, or coma. Use together with extreme caution. Monitor patient response.
*Opioid analgesics:* May decrease analgesic effect. Avoid using together.
**Drug-lifestyle.** *Alcohol use:* May cause additive effects. Discourage use together.

## EFFECTS ON LAB TEST RESULTS
None reported.

## CONTRAINDICATIONS & CAUTIONS
- Contraindicated in patients hypersensitive to drug.
- Use cautiously in patients with history of drug abuse and in those with emotional instability, head injury, increased intracranial pressure, impaired ventilation, MI ac-

---

Reactions may be *common*, uncommon, *life-threatening*, or COMMON AND LIFE-THREATENING.

companied by nausea and vomiting, upcoming biliary surgery, and hepatic or renal disease.
• *Alert:* Certain commercial preparations contain sodium metabisulfite.

## NURSING CONSIDERATIONS
• Reassess patient's level of pain at least 15 and 30 minutes after parenteral administration.
• Drug acts as a opioid antagonist; may cause withdrawal syndrome. For patients who have received opiates long term, give 25% of the usual dose initially. Watch for signs of withdrawal.
• *Alert:* Drug causes respiratory depression, which at 10 mg is equal to respiratory depression produced by 10 mg of morphine.
• Monitor circulatory and respiratory status and bladder and bowel function. Withhold dose and notify prescriber if respirations are shallow or rate is below 12 breaths/minute.
• Constipation is often severe with maintenance therapy. Make sure stool softener or other laxative is ordered.
• Psychological and physical dependence may occur with prolonged use.
• *Alert:* Don't confuse Nubain with Navane.

## PATIENT TEACHING
• Caution ambulatory patient about getting out of bed or walking. Warn outpatient to avoid driving and other hazardous activities that require mental alertness until drug's CNS effects are known.
• Teach patient how to manage troublesome adverse effects such as constipation.

---

## oxycodone hydrochloride
Endocodone, Endonet‡, OxyContin♪, Oxydose, OxyIR, Roxicodone, Roxicodone Intensol, Supeudol†

## oxycodone pectinate
Proladone‡

*Pregnancy risk category B*
*Controlled substance schedule II*

## AVAILABLE FORMS
**oxycodone hydrochloride**
*Capsules:* 5 mg

*Tablets (immediate-release):* 5 mg, 15 mg, 30 mg
*Tablets (controlled-release):* 10 mg, 20 mg, 40 mg, 80 mg
*Oral solution:* 5 mg/5 ml, 20 mg/ml
*Suppository:* 10 mg†, 20 mg†
**oxycodone pectinate**
*Suppositories:* 30 mg‡

## INDICATIONS & DOSAGES
➤ **Moderate to severe pain**
*Adults:* 5 mg P.O. q 6 hours. Or, one suppository P.R. three to four times daily, p.r.n. Patients not currently receiving opiates, who need a continuous, around-the-clock analgesic for an extended period of time, give 10 mg (controlled-release tablets) P.O. q 12 hours. May increase dose q 1 to 2 days as needed. The 80-mg formulation is for opioid-tolerant patients only.

## ACTION
Unknown. Binds with opiate receptors in the CNS, altering both perception of and emotional response to pain.

| Route | Onset | Peak | Duration |
|-------|-------|------|----------|
| P.O. | 10-15 min | 1 hr | 3-6 hr |
| P.R. | Unknown | Unknown | Unknown |

## ADVERSE REACTIONS
**CNS:** sedation, somnolence, clouded sensorium, euphoria, dizziness, lightheadedness, physical dependence.
**CV:** hypotension, ***bradycardia.***
**GI:** *nausea, vomiting,* constipation, ileus.
**GU:** urine retention.
**Respiratory:** ***respiratory depression.***
**Skin:** diaphoresis, pruritus.

## INTERACTIONS
**Drug-drug.** *Anticoagulants:* Oxycodone hydrochloride products containing aspirin may increase anticoagulant effect. Monitor clotting times. Use together cautiously.
*CNS depressants, general anesthetics, hypnotics, MAO inhibitors, other opioid analgesics, sedatives, tranquilizers, tricyclic antidepressants:* May cause additive effects. Use together with extreme caution. Reduce oxycodone dose and monitor patient response.
**Drug-lifestyle.** *Alcohol use:* May cause additive effects. Discourage use together.

---

**EFFECTS ON LAB TEST RESULTS**
● May increase amylase and lipase levels.

**CONTRAINDICATIONS & CAUTIONS**
● Contraindicated in patients hypersensitive to drug.
● Contraindicated in those suspected of having paralytic ileus.
● Use with extreme caution in elderly and debilitated patients and in those with head injury, increased intracranial pressure, seizures, asthma, COPD, prostatic hyperplasia, severe hepatic or renal disease, acute abdominal conditions, urethral stricture, hypothyroidism, Addison's disease, and arrhythmias.

**NURSING CONSIDERATIONS**
● Reassess patient's level of pain at least 15 and 30 minutes after administration.
● For full analgesic effect, give drug before patient has intense pain.
● To minimize GI upset, give drug after meals or with milk.
● Single-drug oxycodone solution or tablets are especially useful for patients who shouldn't take aspirin or acetaminophen.
● Monitor circulatory and respiratory status. Withhold dose and notify prescriber if respirations are shallow or if respiratory rate falls below 12 breaths/minute.
● Monitor patient's bladder and bowel patterns. Patient may need a laxative because drug has a constipating effect.
● Reserve the 80-mg controlled-release tablets for opioid-tolerant patients who are taking daily doses of 160 mg or more.
● Patients taking around-the-clock controlled-release formulations may need to have immediate-release medication available for pain exacerbation or to prevent incident pain.
● For patients who are taking more than 60 mg daily, stop dosing gradually to prevent withdrawal symptoms.
● OxyContin isn't intended for as-needed use or for immediate postoperative pain. Drug is only indicated for postoperative use if patient was receiving it before surgery or if pain is expected to persist for an extended time.
● *Alert:* OxyContin is potentially addictive and abused as much as morphine. Chewing, crushing, snorting, or injecting it can lead to overdose and death.

**PATIENT TEACHING**
● Instruct patient to take drug before pain is intense.
● Tell patient to take drug with milk or after eating.
● Tell patient to swallow extended-release tablets whole.
● Caution ambulatory patient about getting out of bed or walking. Warn outpatient to avoid driving and other hazardous activities that require mental alertness until drug's CNS effects are known.
● Advise patient to avoid alcohol use during therapy.
● Tell patient not to stop drug abruptly.

# oxymorphone hydrochloride
Numorphan

*Pregnancy risk category C; D if used for prolonged periods or high doses at term*
*Controlled substance schedule II*

**AVAILABLE FORMS**
*Injection:* 1 mg/ml, 1.5 mg/ml
*Suppositories:* 5 mg

**INDICATIONS & DOSAGES**
➤ **Moderate to severe pain**
*Adults:* 1 to 1.5 mg I.M. or S.C. q 4 to 6 hours, p.r.n. Or, 0.5 mg I.V. q 4 to 6 hours, p.r.n. Or, 5 mg P.R. q 4 to 6 hours, p.r.n.
➤ **Analgesia during labor**
*Adults:* 0.5 to 1 mg I.M.

**I.V. ADMINISTRATION**
● Give drug by direct I.V. injection.
● If necessary, dilute drug in normal saline solution.

**ACTION**
Unknown. Binds with opiate receptors in the CNS, altering both perception of and emotional response to pain.

| Route | Onset | Peak | Duration |
|-------|-------|------|----------|
| I.V. | 5-10 min | 15-30 min | 3-4 hr |
| I.M. | 10-15 min | 30-90 min | 3-6 hr |
| S.C. | 10-20 min | 60-90 min | 3-6 hr |
| P.R. | 15-30 min | 2 hr | 3-6 hr |

**ADVERSE REACTIONS**
**CNS:** *sedation, somnolence, clouded sensorium, euphoria,* dysphoria, dizziness, **seizures,** physical dependence, lightheadedness, headache, hallucinations, restlessness.
**CV:** *hypotension,* **bradycardia.**
**EENT:** miosis, diplopia, blurred vision.
**GI:** *nausea, vomiting, constipation,* ileus.
**GU:** *urine retention.*
**Respiratory:** *respiratory depression.*
**Skin:** pruritus.

**INTERACTIONS**
**Drug-drug.** *Anticholinergics:* May increase risk of urinary retention or severe constipation, leading to paralytic ileus. Monitor patient for abdominal pain or distention.
*CNS depressants, general anesthetics, MAO inhibitors, phenothiazines, sedative hypnotics, tricyclic antidepressants:* May cause additive effects. Use together with extreme caution.
**Drug-lifestyle.** *Alcohol use:* May cause additive effects. Discourage use together.

**EFFECTS ON LAB TEST RESULTS**
• May increase amylase and lipase levels.

**CONTRAINDICATIONS & CAUTIONS**
• Contraindicated in patients hypersensitive to drug and in those with acute asthma attacks, severe respiratory depression, upper airway obstruction, or paralytic ileus.
• Contraindicated for use in treating pulmonary edema caused by a respiratory irritant.
• Use with extreme caution in elderly or debilitated patients and in those with head injury, increased intracranial pressure, seizures, asthma, COPD, acute abdominal conditions, prostatic hyperplasia, severe hepatic or renal disease, urethral stricture, respiratory depression, hypothyroidism, Addison's disease, and arrhythmias.

**NURSING CONSIDERATIONS**
• Keep opioid antagonist (naloxone) and resuscitation equipment available.
• Use of this drug may worsen gallbladder pain.
• Drug isn't for mild pain. For better effect, give drug before patient has intense pain.

• Monitor CV and respiratory status. Withhold dose and notify prescriber if respirations decrease or rate is below 12 breaths/minute.
• Monitor bladder and bowel function. Patient may need a laxative.
• *Alert:* Don't confuse oxymorphone with oxymetholone or oxycodone, and Numorphan with nalbuphine.

**PATIENT TEACHING**
• Instruct patient to ask for drug before pain is intense.
• When drug is used after surgery, encourage patient to turn, cough, and deep-breathe and to use incentive spirometer to avoid lung problems.
• Caution ambulatory patient about getting out of bed or walking. Warn outpatient to avoid driving and other hazardous activities that require mental alertness until drug's CNS effects are known.
• Instruct patient to store suppositories in refrigerator.
• Advise patient to avoid alcohol during therapy.

---

**pentazocine hydrochloride**
Fortral†‡, Talwin†

**pentazocine hydrochloride and naloxone hydrochloride**
Talwin NX

**pentazocine lactate**
Fortral‡, Talwin

*Pregnancy risk category C*
*Controlled substance schedule IV*

**AVAILABLE FORMS**
**pentazocine hydrochloride**
*Tablets:* 25 mg‡, 50 mg†‡
**pentazocine hydrochloride and naloxone hydrochloride**
*Tablets:* 50 mg pentazocine hydrochloride and 500 mcg naloxone hydrochloride
**pentazocine lactate**
*Injection:* 30 mg/ml

**INDICATIONS & DOSAGES**
➤ **Moderate to severe pain**
*Adults:* 50 to 100 mg P.O. q 3 to 4 hours, p.r.n. Maximum oral dose is 600 mg/day.

Or, 30 mg I.M., I.V., or S.C. q 3 to 4 hours, p.r.n. Maximum parenteral dose is 360 mg/day. Single doses above 30 mg I.V. or 60 mg I.M. or S.C. aren't recommended.

➤ **Labor**
*Adults:* 30 mg I.M. as a single dose or 20 mg I.V. q 2 to 3 hours when contractions become regular for 2 to 3 doses.

## I.V. ADMINISTRATION
● Give drug by direct I.V. injection slowly. Don't mix in syringe with aminophylline, barbiturates, or other alkaline substances.
● Talwin NX, the oral pentazocine available in the United States, contains the opioid antagonist naloxone, which discourages illicit I.V. use.

## ACTION
Unknown. Binds with opiate receptors in the CNS, altering both perception of and emotional response to pain.

| Route | Onset | Peak | Duration |
|-------|-------|------|----------|
| P.O. | 15-30 min | 1-3 hr | 2-3 hr |
| I.V. | 2-3 min | 15-30 min | 2-3 hr |
| I.M., S.C. | 15-20 min | 30-60 min | 2-3 hr |

## ADVERSE REACTIONS
**CNS:** *sedation,* visual disturbances, hallucinations, drowsiness, *dizziness, lightheadedness,* confusion, *euphoria,* headache, psychotomimetic effects.
**CV:** circulatory depression, *shock,* hypertension, hypotension.
**EENT:** dry mouth.
**GI:** *nausea, vomiting,* constipation.
**GU:** urine retention.
**Respiratory:** *respiratory depression,* dyspnea, *apnea.*
**Skin:** induration, nodules, sloughing, sclerosis at injection site; diaphoresis; pruritus.
**Other:** hypersensitivity reactions, *anaphylaxis,* physical and psychological dependence.

## INTERACTIONS
**Drug-drug.** *CNS depressants:* May cause additive effects. Use together cautiously.
*Fluoxetine:* May cause additive effects resulting in serotonin syndrome. Use together cautiously.

*Opioid analgesics:* May decrease analgesic effect. Avoid using together.
**Drug-lifestyle.** *Alcohol use:* May cause additive effects. Discourage use together.
*Smoking:* May increase requirements for pentazocine. Monitor drug's effectiveness.

## EFFECTS ON LAB TEST RESULTS
● May interfere with certain laboratory tests for urinary 17-hydroxycorticosteroids.

## CONTRAINDICATIONS & CAUTIONS
● Contraindicated in patients hypersensitive to drug or its components and in children younger than age 12.
● Use cautiously in patients with hepatic or renal disease, acute MI, head injury, increased intracranial pressure, and respiratory depression.

## NURSING CONSIDERATIONS
● Reassess patient's level of pain at least 15 and 30 minutes after parenteral administration and 30 minutes after oral administration.
● Have naloxone readily available. Respiratory depression can be reversed with naloxone.
● *Alert:* When giving by S.C. or I.M. injection, rotate injection sites to minimize tissue irritation. If possible, avoid giving by S.C. route.
● Drug has opioid antagonist properties. May cause withdrawal syndrome in opioid-dependent patients.
● Psychological and physical dependence may occur with prolonged use.

## PATIENT TEACHING
● Instruct patient to ask for drug before pain is intense.
● Caution ambulatory patient about getting out of bed or walking. Warn outpatient to avoid driving and other hazardous activities that require mental alertness until drug's CNS effects are known.
● Advise patient to avoid alcohol during therapy.
● Instruct patient or family to report skin rash, disorientation, or confusion to prescriber.

---

Reactions may be *common*, uncommon, *life-threatening*, or COMMON AND LIFE-THREATENING.

# propoxyphene hydrochloride (dextropropoxyphene hydrochloride)
Darvon, Darvon Pulvules, 642†

# propoxyphene napsylate (dextropropoxyphene napsylate)
Darvon N, Doloxene‡

*Pregnancy risk category C*
*Controlled substance schedule IV*

## AVAILABLE FORMS
**propoxyphene hydrochloride**
*Capsules:* 65 mg
**propoxyphene napsylate**
*Oral suspension:* 10 mg/ml
*Tablets:* 100 mg

## INDICATIONS & DOSAGES
➤ **Mild to moderate pain**
*Adults:* 65 mg propoxyphene hydrochloride P.O. q 4 hours, p.r.n. Maximum daily dose is 390 mg. Or, 100 mg propoxyphene napsylate P.O. q 4 hours, p.r.n. Maximum daily dose is 600 mg.
**Adjust-a-dose:** For patients with hepatic or renal dysfunction, reduce dosage. Consider increasing dosing interval in elderly patients.

## ACTION
Unknown. Binds with opiate receptors in the CNS, altering both perception of and emotional response to pain.

| Route | Onset | Peak | Duration |
|-------|-------|------|----------|
| P.O. | 15-60 min | 2-2½ hr | 4-6 hr |

## ADVERSE REACTIONS
**CNS:** *dizziness,* headache, *sedation,* euphoria, light-headedness, weakness, hallucinations, psychological and physical dependence.
**GI:** *nausea, vomiting,* constipation, abdominal pain.
**Respiratory:** *respiratory depression.*

## INTERACTIONS
**Drug-drug.** *Carbamazepine:* May increase carbamazepine level. Monitor patient closely.

*CNS depressants:* May cause additive effects. Use together cautiously.
*Tricyclic antidepressants (such as doxepin):* Inhibits antidepressant metabolism. Monitor patient for toxicity.
*Warfarin:* May increase anticoagulant effect. Monitor PT and INR.
**Drug-lifestyle.** *Alcohol use:* May cause additive effects. Discourage use together.
*Smoking:* May increase metabolism of propoxyphene. Monitor patient closely.

## EFFECTS ON LAB TEST RESULTS
● May alter liver function test values.

## CONTRAINDICATIONS & CAUTIONS
● Contraindicated in patients hypersensitive to drug. Contraindicated in patients who are suicidal or addiction-prone.
● Use cautiously in patients with hepatic or renal disease, emotional instability, or history of drug or alcohol abuse.

## NURSING CONSIDERATIONS
● Reassess patient's pain level at least 30 minutes after giving drug.
● Propoxyphene hydrochloride 65 mg equals propoxyphene napsylate 100 mg.
● Drug is considered a mild opioid analgesic, but pain relief is equivalent to that provided by aspirin. Tolerance and physical dependence may occur. Drug is used with aspirin or acetaminophen to maximize analgesia.
● Smokers may need increased dosage because smoking may induce liver enzymes responsible for the metabolism of the drug, thereby decreasing its efficacy.

## PATIENT TEACHING
● Advise patient to take drug with food or milk to minimize GI upset.
● Warn patient not to exceed recommended dosage. Respiratory depression, low blood pressure, profound sedation, coma and death may result if used in excessive doses or with other CNS depressants. Advise patient to avoid alcohol or other CNS-type drugs when taking propoxyphene.
● Caution ambulatory patient about getting out of bed or walking. Warn outpatient to avoid driving and other hazardous activities that require mental alertness until drug's CNS effects are known.

# remifentanil hydrochloride
Ultiva

*Pregnancy risk category C*
*Controlled substance schedule II*

## AVAILABLE FORMS
*Injection (vials):* 1 mg/3 ml, 2 mg/5 ml,
5 mg/10 ml

## INDICATIONS & DOSAGES
➤ **To induce anesthesia through intubation**
*Adults:* 0.5 to 1 mcg/kg/minute with hypnotic or volatile drug; may load with
1 mcg/kg over 30 to 60 seconds if endotracheal intubation is to occur less than
8 minutes after start of drug infusion.
➤ **To maintain anesthesia**
*Adults:* 0.25 to 0.4 mcg/kg/minute, depending on the anesthetic (nitrous oxide, isoflurane, propofol). Increase doses by
25% to 100% and decrease by 25% to
50% q 2 to 5 minutes, p.r.n. If rate exceeds 1 mcg/kg/minute, anesthetic dose
may be increased. May supplement with
1-mcg/kg boluses over 30 to 60 seconds q
2 to 5 minutes, p.r.n.
➤ **To continue as analgesic immediately after surgery**
*Adults:* Initially, 0.1 mcg/kg/minute. Adjust rate by 0.025-mcg/kg/minute increments q 5 minutes, p.r.n. Rates over
0.2 mcg/kg/minute may cause respiratory
depression (under 8 breaths/minute).
➤ **For monitored anesthesia care**
*Adults:* As single I.V. dose, 0.5 to 1 mcg/
kg over 30 to 60 seconds starting 90 seconds before placement of local or regional
anesthetic. As continuous I.V. infusion,
0.1 mcg/kg/minute beginning 5 minutes
before giving local anesthetic; after placement of local anesthetic, titrate rate to
0.05 mcg/kg/minute. Titrate rate by
0.025 mcg/kg/minute q 5 minutes, p.r.n.
Rates over 0.2 mcg/kg/minute may cause
respiratory depression.
*Elderly patients older than age 65:* Decrease first dose by 50%.
**Adjust-a-dose:** For obese patients (more
than 30% over ideal body weight), base
starting dose on ideal body weight.

## I.V. ADMINISTRATION
● Use I.V. bolus administration only during maintenance of general anesthesia. In
nonintubated patients, give single doses
over 30 to 60 seconds.
● To reconstitute solution, add 1 ml of
diluent per mg of drug. Shake well to
dissolve. Reconstituted solution contains
1 mg/ml and should be clear and colorless.
● Further dilute to 25, 50, or 250 mcg/ml
before administration. Drug is stable at
room temperature for 24 hours when in final concentration in $D_5W$, $D_5W$ in normal
saline solution, normal saline solution,
half-normal saline solution, or $D_5W$ in
lactated Ringer's solution. Drug is stable
for 4 hours when mixed in lactated
Ringer's solution.
● Continuous infusion of drug must be
given by infusion device. When the drug
is stopped, clear I.V. tubing to avoid inadvertently giving drug later.
● Hypotension may occur and can be treated by decreasing rate of infusion or giving
I.V. fluids or catecholamine.

## ACTION
Unknown. Binds with mu-opiate receptors
in the CNS, altering both perception of
and emotional response to pain.

| Route | Onset | Peak | Duration |
|---|---|---|---|
| I.V. | Immediate | 1-2 min | 5-10 min |

## ADVERSE REACTIONS
**CNS:** agitation, dizziness, headache,
fever.
**CV: *bradycardia,*** hypertension, *hypotension,* tachycardia.
**EENT:** visual disturbances.
**GI:** *nausea, vomiting.*
**Musculoskeletal:** *muscle rigidity.*
**Respiratory: *apnea, hypoxia, respiratory
depression.***
**Skin:** flushing, pain at injection site, pruritus, sweating.
**Other:** chills, postoperative pain, shivering, warm sensation.

## INTERACTIONS
**Drug-drug.** *Benzodiazepine, hypnotics,
inhaled anesthetics:* Has synergistic effect. Monitor patient closely.

---

**EFFECTS ON LAB TEST RESULTS**
None reported.

**CONTRAINDICATIONS & CAUTIONS**
• Contraindicated in patients hypersensitive to fentanyl analogues. Don't use via epidural or intrathecal routes because of presence of glycine in preparation.
• Use cautiously in breast-feeding women because fentanyl analogues appear in breast milk.

**NURSING CONSIDERATIONS**
• Monitor vital signs and oxygenation continually during drug administration.
• Don't use as a single drug in general anesthesia.
• When giving drug during monitored anesthesia care, decrease dose by 50% if given with 2 mg midazolam. Bolus doses given simultaneously with continuously infusing remifentanil to spontaneously breathing patients aren't recommended.
• Manage respiratory depression in spontaneously breathing patients by decreasing infusion rate by 50% or by temporarily discontinuing infusion.
• Skeletal muscle rigidity may occur. To treat, either stop or decrease the rate of infusion in spontaneously breathing patients.
• Effects of drug use lasting longer than 16 hours in intensive care settings aren't known.
• If bradycardia occurs, consider countering with ephedrine, atropine, or glycopyrrolate.
• Interruption of drug infusion results in rapid reversal (no residual opioid effects within 5 to 10 minutes of infusion discontinuation) of effects; adequate postoperative anesthesia should first be established.
• Drug shouldn't be used outside the monitored anesthesia care setting. Keep opioid antagonist (naloxone) and resuscitation equipment available. Naloxone may be used to manage severe respiratory depression.
• Drug is incompatible with blood products.
• Obtain history from patient regarding previous adverse anesthesia reactions in patient or patient's family.

**PATIENT TEACHING**
• Reassure patient that appropriate monitoring will occur during anesthesia administration.

---

## tramadol hydrochloride
Ultram

*Pregnancy risk category C*

**AVAILABLE FORMS**
*Tablets:* 50 mg

**INDICATIONS & DOSAGES**
➤ **Moderate to moderately severe pain**
*Adults:* Initially, 25 mg P.O. in the morning. Adjust by 25 mg q 3 days to 100 mg/day (25 mg q.i.d.). Thereafter, adjust by 50 mg q 3 days to reach 200 mg/day (50 mg q.i.d.). Thereafter, give 50 to 100 mg P.O. q 4 to 6 hours, p.r.n. Maximum, 400 mg daily.
*Elderly patients:* For patients older than age 75, maximum is 300 mg daily in divided doses.
*Adjust-a-dose:* For renally impaired patients with creatinine clearance below 30 ml/minute, increase dose interval to q 12 hours; maximum is 200 mg daily. For patients with cirrhosis, give 50 mg q 12 hours.

**ACTION**
Unknown. A centrally acting synthetic analgesic compound not chemically related to opiates. Thought to bind to opioid receptors and inhibit reuptake of norepinephrine and serotonin.

| Route | Onset | Peak | Duration |
|-------|---------|------|----------|
| P.O. | Unknown | 2 hr | Unknown |

**ADVERSE REACTIONS**
**CNS:** *dizziness, vertigo, headache, somnolence,* CNS stimulation, asthenia, anxiety, confusion, coordination disturbance, euphoria, nervousness, sleep disorder, *seizures,* malaise.
**CV:** vasodilation.
**EENT:** visual disturbances.
**GI:** *nausea, constipation, vomiting,* dyspepsia, dry mouth, diarrhea, abdominal pain, anorexia, flatulence.

---

**GU:** urine retention, urinary frequency, menopausal symptoms, proteinuria.
**Musculoskeletal:** hypertonia.
**Respiratory:** *respiratory depression.*
**Skin:** pruritus, diaphoresis, rash.

## INTERACTIONS

**Drug-drug.** *Carbamazepine:* May increase tramadol metabolism. Patients receiving long-term carbamazepine therapy at up to 800 mg daily may need up to twice the recommended dose of tramadol.
*CNS depressants:* May cause additive effects. Use together with caution. Dosage of tramadol may need to be reduced.
*Cyclobenzaprine, MAO inhibitors, neuroleptics, other opioids, SSRIs, tricyclic antidepressants:* May increase risk of seizures. Monitor patient closely.
*Quinidine:* May increase level of tramadol. Monitor patient closely.
*SSRIs (paroxetine, sertraline):* May increase risk of serotonin syndrome. Monitor patient for adverse effects.

## EFFECTS ON LAB TEST RESULTS

● May increase liver enzyme level. May decrease creatinine level.
● May decrease hemoglobin.

## CONTRAINDICATIONS & CAUTIONS

● Contraindicated in patients hypersensitive to drug or other opioids, in breast-feeding women, and in those with acute intoxication from alcohol, hypnotics, centrally acting analgesics, opioids, or psychotropic drugs. Serious hypersensitivity reactions can occur, usually after the first dose. Patients with history of anaphylaxis to codeine and other opioids may be at an increased risk.
● Use cautiously in patients at risk for seizures or respiratory depression; in patients with increased intracranial pressure or head injury, acute abdominal conditions, or renal or hepatic impairment; or in patients with physical dependence on opioids.

## NURSING CONSIDERATIONS

● Reassess patient's level of pain at least 30 minutes after administration.
● Monitor CV and respiratory status. Withhold dose and notify prescriber if res-

pirations decrease or rate is below 12 breaths/minute.
● Monitor bowel and bladder function. Anticipate need for laxative.
● For better analgesic effect, give drug before onset of intense pain.
● Monitor patients at risk for seizures. Drug may reduce seizure threshold.
● In the case of an overdose, naloxone may also increase risk of seizures.
● Monitor patient for drug dependence. Drug can produce dependence similar to that of codeine or dextropropoxyphene and thus has potential for abuse.
● Withdrawal symptoms may occur if drug is stopped abruptly. Reduce dosage gradually.
● *Alert:* Don't confuse tramadol with trazodone or trandolapril.

## PATIENT TEACHING

● Tell patient to take drug as prescribed and not to increase dose or dosage interval unless ordered by prescriber.
● Caution ambulatory patient to be careful when rising and walking. Warn outpatient to avoid driving and other potentially hazardous activities that require mental alertness until drug's CNS effects are known.
● Advise patient to check with prescriber before taking OTC drugs because drug interactions can occur.
● Warn patient not to stop the drug abruptly.

---

Reactions may be *common*, uncommon, *life-threatening*, or COMMON AND LIFE-THREATENING.

# 27

## Sedative-hypnotics

**chloral hydrate**
**dexmedetomidine hydrochloride**
**diazepam**
  (See Chapter 30, ANXIOLYTICS.)
**estazolam**
**flurazepam hydrochloride**
**pentobarbital**
**pentobarbital sodium**
**phenobarbital sodium**
  (See Chapter 28, ANTICONVULSANTS.)
**secobarbital sodium**
**temazepam**
**triazolam**
**zaleplon**
**zolpidem tartrate**

### COMBINATION PRODUCTS
TUINAL 100 mg PULVULES: amobarbital sodium 50 mg and secobarbital sodium 50 mg.
TUINAL 200 mg PULVULES: amobarbital sodium 100 mg and secobarbital sodium 100 mg.

---

### chloral hydrate
Aquachloral Supprettes, Novo-Chlorhydrate†

*Pregnancy risk category C*
*Controlled substance schedule IV*

### AVAILABLE FORMS
*Capsules:* 250 mg, 500 mg
*Suppositories:* 324 mg, 500 mg, 648 mg
*Syrup:* 250 mg/5 ml, 500 mg/5 ml

### INDICATIONS & DOSAGES
➤ **Sedation**
*Adults:* 250 mg P.O. or P.R. t.i.d. after meals.
*Children:* 8.3 mg/kg P.O. t.i.d. Maximum dosage is 500 mg t.i.d
➤ **Insomnia**
*Adults:* 500 mg to 1 g P.O. or P.R. 15 to 30 minutes before h.s. Maximum daily dose is 2 g.
*Children:* 50 mg/kg P.O. or P.R. 15 to 30 minutes before h.s. Maximum single dose is 1 g.

➤ **Preoperatively to produce sedation and relieve anxiety**
*Adults:* 500 mg to 1 g P.O. or P.R. 30 minutes before surgery.
➤ **Premedication for EEG**
*Children:* 20 to 25 mg/kg P.O. or P.R. up to 500 mg/single dose. May give divided doses.

### ACTION
Unknown. Sedative effects may be caused by drug's main metabolite, trichloro-ethanol.

| Route | Onset | Peak | Duration |
|-------|-------|------|----------|
| P.O. | 30 min | Unknown | 4-8 hr |
| P.R. | Unknown | Unknown | 4-8 hr |

### ADVERSE REACTIONS
**CNS:** drowsiness, nightmares, dizziness, ataxia, paradoxical excitement, hangover, somnolence, disorientation, delirium, light-headedness, hallucinations, confusion, somnambulism, vertigo, malaise, physical and psychological dependence.
**GI:** *nausea, vomiting, diarrhea,* flatulence.
**Hematologic:** eosinophilia, *leukopenia.*
**Other:** hypersensitivity reactions.

### INTERACTIONS
**Drug-drug.** *CNS depressants, including opioid analgesics:* May cause excessive CNS depression or vasodilation reaction. Use together cautiously.
*Furosemide I.V.:* May cause sweating, flushes, variable blood pressure, nausea, and uneasiness. Use together cautiously or use a different hypnotic drug.
*Oral anticoagulants:* May increase risk of bleeding. Monitor patient closely.
*Phenytoin:* May decrease phenytoin level. Monitor patient closely.
**Drug-lifestyle.** *Alcohol use:* May react synergistically, increasing CNS depression, or, rarely, produce a disulfiram-like reaction. Strongly discourage alcohol use with these drugs.

---

*Rapid onset*　†Canada　‡Australia　◇OTC　♦Off-label use　✏Photoguide　*Liquid contains alcohol.

## EFFECTS ON LAB TEST RESULTS
• May increase eosinophil count. May decrease WBC count.
• May cause false-positive results with urine glucose testing with cupric sulfate, such as Benedict's reagent, and with phentolamine testing.

## CONTRAINDICATIONS & CAUTIONS
• Contraindicated in patients hypersensitive to drug and in those with hepatic or renal impairment.
• Oral administration is contraindicated in patients with gastric disorders.
• Use with extreme caution in patients with severe cardiac disease.
• Use cautiously in patients with mental depression, suicidal tendencies, or history of drug abuse.
• Some products may contain tartrazine; use cautiously in patients with aspirin sensitivity.

## NURSING CONSIDERATIONS
• *Alert:* Note two strengths of oral liquid form. Double-check dose, especially when giving to children. Fatal overdoses have occurred.
• To minimize unpleasant taste and stomach irritation, dilute or give with liquid. Tell patient to take drug after meals.
• Take precautions to prevent hoarding or overdosing by patients who are depressed, suicidal, or drug-dependent or who have history of drug abuse.
• Long-term use isn't recommended; drug loses its effectiveness in promoting sleep after 14 days of continued use. Long-term use may cause drug dependence, and patient may experience withdrawal symptoms if drug is suddenly stopped.
• Monitor BUN level; large doses may raise BUN level.
• Don't give drug for 48 hours before fluorometric test.

## PATIENT TEACHING
• Instruct patient to take capsule with a full glass of water or juice and to swallow capsule whole.
• Tell patient to avoid alcohol during drug therapy.
• Caution patient to avoid performing activities that require mental alertness or physical coordination.

• Advise patient to store drug in dark container and to store suppositories in refrigerator.

---

# dexmedetomidine hydrochloride
Precedex

*Pregnancy risk category C*

---

## AVAILABLE FORMS
*Injection:* 100 mcg/ml in 2-ml vials and 2-ml ampules

## INDICATIONS & DOSAGES
➤ **To sedate initially intubated and mechanically ventilated patients in intensive care unit (ICU)**
*Adults:* Loading infusion of 1 mcg/kg I.V. over 10 minutes; then maintenance infusion of 0.2 to 0.7 mcg/kg/hour for up to 24 hours, titrated to achieve desired level of sedation.

## I.V. ADMINISTRATION
• Dexmedetomidine must be diluted in normal saline solution before administration. To prepare infusion, withdraw 2 ml of drug and add to 48 ml of normal saline injection to total of 50 ml. Shake gently to mix well.
• Don't give through same I.V. catheter with blood or plasma; physical compatibility hasn't been established.
• Infusion is compatible with lactated Ringer's solution, $D_5W$, normal saline solution in water, and 20% mannitol. It's also compatible with thiopental sodium, etomidate, vecuronium bromide, pancuronium bromide, succinylcholine, atracurium besylate, mivacurium chloride, glycopyrrolate bromide, phenylephrine hydrochloride, atropine sulfate, midazolam, morphine sulfate, fentanyl citrate, and plasma substitute.
• *Alert:* Don't give infusion for longer than 24 hours.

## ACTION
Produces sedation by selective stimulation of alpha$_2$-adrenergic receptors in CNS.

| Route | Onset | Peak | Duration |
|-------|---------|---------|----------|
| I.V. | Unknown | Unknown | Unknown |

---

Reactions may be *common*, uncommon, *life-threatening*, or COMMON AND LIFE-THREATENING.

**ADVERSE REACTIONS**
**CNS:** pain.
**CV:** *hypotension, bradycardia, arrhythmias, hypertension,* atrial fibrillation.
**GI:** *nausea,* vomiting, thirst.
**GU:** oliguria.
**Hematologic:** anemia, leukocytosis.
**Respiratory:** *hypoxia,* pleural effusion, *pulmonary edema.*
**Other:** infection, rigors.

**INTERACTIONS**
**Drug-drug.** *Anesthetics, hypnotics, opioids, sedatives:* May enhance effects of dexmedetomidine. May need to reduce dexmedetomidine dose.

**EFFECTS ON LAB TEST RESULTS**
• May increase ALT, AST, and serum glutamic-oxaloacetic transaminase levels.
• May decrease hemoglobin and WBC count.

**CONTRAINDICATIONS & CAUTIONS**
• Contraindicated in patients hypersensitive to dexmedetomidine hydrochloride.
• Use cautiously in patients with advanced heart block or renal or hepatic impairment and in elderly patients.

**NURSING CONSIDERATIONS**
• Only health care professionals skilled in managing patients in the intensive care unit, where cardiac status can be continuously monitored, should give drug.
• *Alert:* Give using controlled infusion device at rate calculated for body weight.
• Determine renal and hepatic function before administration, and consider dosage adjustments in patients with renal or hepatic impairment and in elderly patients.
• Some patients receiving drug can awaken when stimulated. This alone shouldn't be considered evidence of lack of efficacy in absence of other signs and symptoms.
• Drug may be continuously infused in mechanically ventilated patients before, during, and after extubation. It isn't necessary to stop drug before extubation.

**PATIENT TEACHING**
• Tell patient he will be sedated while drug is being given but that he may awaken when stimulated.

• Reassure patient that he will be closely monitored and attended while sedated.

---

# estazolam
ProSom

*Pregnancy risk category X*
*Controlled substance schedule IV*

---

**AVAILABLE FORMS**
*Tablets:* 1 mg, 2 mg

**INDICATIONS & DOSAGES**
➤ **Insomnia**
*Adults:* 1 mg P.O. h.s. Some patients may need 2 mg.
*Elderly patients:* 1 mg P.O. h.s. Use higher doses with extreme care. Frail, elderly, or debilitated patients may take 0.5 mg, but this low dose may be only marginally effective.

**ACTION**
Unknown. Thought to act on the limbic system and thalamus of CNS by binding to specific benzodiazepine receptors.

| Route | Onset | Peak | Duration |
|-------|-------|------|----------|
| P.O. | Unknown | 1-3 hr | Unknown |

**ADVERSE REACTIONS**
**CNS:** fatigue, dizziness, daytime drowsiness, *somnolence, asthenia,* hypokinesia, abnormal thinking.
**GI:** dyspepsia, abdominal pain.
**Musculoskeletal:** back pain, stiffness.
**Respiratory:** cold symptoms, pharyngitis.

**INTERACTIONS**
**Drug-drug.** *Cimetidine, disulfiram, hormonal contraceptives, isoniazid:* May impair metabolism and clearance of benzodiazepines and prolong their plasma half-life. Watch for increased CNS depression.
*CNS depressants, including antihistamines, opiate analgesics, other benzodiazepines:* May increase CNS depression. Avoid using together.
*Digoxin:* May increase digoxin level, resulting in toxicity. Monitor patient closely.
*Fluconazole, itraconazole, ketoconazole, miconazole:* May increase drug level,

CNS depression, and psychomotor impairment. Avoid using together.

*Phenytoin:* May increase phenytoin level, resulting in toxicity. Monitor patient closely.

*Rifampin:* May increase metabolism and clearance and decrease drug half-life of estazolam. Watch for decreased effectiveness.

*Theophylline:* May have antagonistic effect. Watch for decreased effectiveness of estazolam.

**Drug-herb.** *Calendula, hops, kava, lemon balm, passion flower, skullcap, valerian:* May enhance sedative effect of drug. Discourage use together.

**Drug-lifestyle.** *Alcohol use:* May cause additive CNS effects. Discourage use together.

*Smoking:* May increase metabolism and clearance. Advise patient to watch for signs of decreased effectiveness.

### EFFECTS ON LAB TEST RESULTS
• May increase AST level.

### CONTRAINDICATIONS & CAUTIONS
• Contraindicated in pregnant patients and in those hypersensitive to drug.
• Use cautiously in patients with depression, suicidal tendencies, or hepatic, renal, or pulmonary disease.

### NURSING CONSIDERATIONS
• Check liver and renal function and CBC before and periodically during long-term therapy.
• Take precautions to prevent depressed, suicidal, or drug-dependent patients or those with history of drug abuse from hoarding drug.
• Patients who receive prolonged treatment with benzodiazepines may experience withdrawal symptoms if drug is suddenly stopped (possibly after 6 weeks of continuous therapy).
• **Alert:** Don't confuse ProSom with Proscar, Prozac, or Psorcon E.

### PATIENT TEACHING
• Advise patient to notify prescriber about planned, suspected, or known pregnancy during therapy.

• Tell patient not to increase dosage but to inform prescriber if he thinks that drug is no longer effective.
• Caution patient to avoid performing activities that require mental alertness or physical coordination.
• Warn patient that drinking alcohol while taking drug or within 24 hours after taking drug can increase depressant effects.
• Warn patient not to abruptly stop use after taking drug for 1 month or longer.
• Tell breast-feeding patient to avoid using drug.

---

# flurazepam hydrochloride
Apo-Flurazepam†, Dalmane, Novo-Flupam†

*Pregnancy risk category X*
*Controlled substance schedule IV*

### AVAILABLE FORMS
*Capsules:* 15 mg, 30 mg

### INDICATIONS & DOSAGES
➤ **Insomnia**
*Adults:* 15 to 30 mg P.O. h.s. May repeat dose once, p.r.n.
*Elderly patients:* Start with 15-mg dose until response is determined.

### ACTION
Unknown. A benzodiazepine that is thought to act on the limbic system, thalamus, and hypothalamus of CNS to produce hypnotic effects.

| Route | Onset | Peak | Duration |
|-------|-------|------|----------|
| P.O. | Unknown | 30-60 min | Unknown |

### ADVERSE REACTIONS
**CNS:** *daytime sedation, dizziness, drowsiness, disturbed coordination,* lethargy, confusion, physical or psychological dependence, *headache,* light-headedness, nervousness, hallucinations, staggering, ataxia, disorientation, ***coma.***
**GI:** nausea, vomiting, heartburn, diarrhea, abdominal pain.

### INTERACTIONS
**Drug-drug.** *Cimetidine:* May increase sedation. Monitor patient carefully.

---

*CNS depressants, including opioid analgesics:* May cause excessive CNS depression. Use together cautiously.

*Digoxin:* May increase digoxin level, resulting in toxicity. Monitor patient closely.

*Disulfiram, hormonal contraceptives, isoniazid:* May decrease metabolism of benzodiazepines, leading to toxicity. Monitor patient closely.

*Fluconazole, itraconazole, ketoconazole, miconazole:* May increase and prolong drug level, CNS depression, and psychomotor impairment. Avoid using together.

*Phenytoin:* May increase phenytoin level. Watch for toxicity.

*Rifampin:* May enhance metabolism of benzodiazepines. Watch for decreased effectiveness of benzodiazepine.

*Theophylline:* May act as antagonist with flurazepam. Watch for decreased effectiveness of flurazepam.

**Drug-herb.** *Calendula, hops, kava, lemon balm, passion flower, skullcap, valerian:* May enhance sedative effect of drug. Discourage use together.

**Drug-lifestyle.** *Alcohol use:* May cause additive CNS effects. Discourage use together.

*Smoking:* May increase metabolism and clearance and decrease drug half-life. Advise patient to watch for signs of decreased effectiveness.

**EFFECTS ON LAB TEST RESULTS**
● May increase AST, ALT, bilirubin, and alkaline phosphatase levels.

**CONTRAINDICATIONS & CAUTIONS**
● Contraindicated in patients hypersensitive to drug and during pregnancy.
● Use cautiously in patients with impaired hepatic or renal function, chronic pulmonary insufficiency, mental depression, suicidal tendencies, or history of drug abuse.

**NURSING CONSIDERATIONS**
● Check hepatic and renal function and CBC before and periodically during long-term therapy.
● Minor changes in EEG patterns (usually low-voltage, fast activity) may occur during and after flurazepam therapy.
● Assess mental status before starting therapy. Elderly patients are more sensitive to drug's adverse CNS reactions.

● Take precautions to prevent hoarding or self-overdosing by patients who are depressed, suicidal, or drug-dependent or who have history of drug abuse.
● Physical and psychological dependence is possible with long-term use.
● *Alert:* Don't confuse Dalmane with Dialume or Demulen.

**PATIENT TEACHING**
● Inform patient that drug is more effective on second, third, and fourth nights of treatment because drug builds up in the body.
● Warn patient not to abruptly stop after taking drug for 1 month or longer.
● Tell patient to avoid alcohol use while taking drug.
● Caution patient to avoid performing activities that require mental alertness or physical coordination.
● Warn patient that any prolonged use of drug may produce psychological and physical dependence.
● Advise patient to warn prescriber about planned, suspected, or known pregnancy.

# pentobarbital
Nembutal*†

# pentobarbital sodium
Nembutal Sodium*, Nova Rectal†, NovoPentobarb†

*Pregnancy risk category D*
*Controlled substance schedule II;*
*III for suppositories*

**AVAILABLE FORMS**
**pentobarbital**
*Elixir:* 18.2 mg/5 ml
**pentobarbital sodium**
*Capsules:* 50 mg, 100 mg
*Injection:* 50 mg/ml
*Suppositories:* 30 mg, 60 mg, 120 mg, 200 mg

**INDICATIONS & DOSAGES**
➤ **Sedation**
*Adults:* 20 mg P.O. t.i.d. or q.i.d.
*Children:* 2 to 6 mg/kg P.O. daily in three divided doses. Maximum daily dose is 100 mg.

➤ **Insomnia**

*Adults:* 100 to 200 mg P.O. h.s. Or, 150 to 200 mg deep I.M. Or, 100 mg I.V. initially, with further small doses up to total of 500 mg. Or, 120 or 200 mg P.R.
*Children:* 2 to 6 mg/kg or 125 mg/m² I.M. Maximum dose is 100 mg.
*Children ages 12 to 14:* 60 or 120 mg P.R.
*Children ages 5 to 11:* 60 mg P.R.
*Children ages 1 to 4:* 30 or 60 mg P.R.
*Children ages 2 months to 1 year:* 30 mg P.R.

➤ **Preoperative sedation**

*Adults:* 150 to 200 mg I.M.
*Children age 10 and older:* 5 mg/kg P.O. or I.M.
*Children younger than age 10:* 5 mg/kg I.M. or P.R.

## I.V. ADMINISTRATION

● I.V. administration of barbiturates may cause severe respiratory depression, laryngospasm, or hypotension. Keep emergency resuscitation equipment available.
● To minimize deterioration, use I.V. injection solution within 30 minutes after opening container. Don't use cloudy solution.
● Don't mix in syringe or in I.V. solutions or lines with other drugs.
● Reserve I.V. injection for emergency treatment, and give under close supervision. Give slowly at no more than 50 mg/minute.
● Parenteral solution is alkaline. Local tissue reactions and injection site pain may follow I.V. use. Monitor I.V. site for extravasation. Assess patency of I.V. site before and during administration.

## ACTION

Unknown. Probably interferes with transmission of impulses from the thalamus to the cortex of the brain and alters cerebellar function.

| Route | Onset | Peak | Duration |
|-------|-------|------|----------|
| P.O. | 20 min | 30-60 min | 1-4 hr |
| I.V. | Immediate | Immediate | 15 min |
| I.M. | 10-25 min | Unknown | Unknown |
| P.R. | 20 min | Unknown | 1-4 hr |

## ADVERSE REACTIONS

**CNS:** *drowsiness, lethargy, hangover,* paradoxical excitement in elderly patients, somnolence, physical and psychological dependence.
**GI:** nausea, vomiting.
**Hematologic:** worsening porphyria.
**Respiratory:** *respiratory depression.*
**Skin:** rash, urticaria, *Stevens-Johnson syndrome.*
**Other:** *angioedema.*

## INTERACTIONS

**Drug-drug.** *CNS depressants, including opioid analgesics:* May cause excessive CNS and respiratory depression. Use together cautiously.
*Corticosteroids, digitoxin, doxycycline, estrogens and hormonal contraceptives, oral anticoagulants, theophylline, verapamil:* May enhance metabolism of these drugs. Watch for decreased effect.
*Griseofulvin:* May decrease absorption of griseofulvin. Monitor effectiveness of griseofulvin.
*MAO inhibitors, valproic acid:* May inhibit metabolism of barbiturates; may prolong CNS depression. Reduce barbiturate dosage.
*Metoprolol, propranolol:* May reduce effects of these drugs. Consider an increased beta-blocker dose.
*Rifampin:* May decrease barbiturate level. Watch for decreased effect of pentobarbital.
**Drug-herb.** *Kava:* May cause additive effects. Discourage use together.
**Drug-lifestyle.** *Alcohol use:* May impair coordination, increase CNS effects, and cause death. Strongly discourage alcohol use with these drugs.

## EFFECTS ON LAB TEST RESULTS

None reported.

## CONTRAINDICATIONS & CAUTIONS

● Contraindicated in patients hypersensitive to barbiturates and in those with porphyria, bronchopneumonia, or other severe pulmonary insufficiency, and in severe liver or renal dysfunction.
● Use cautiously in elderly or debilitated patients and in patients with acute or chronic pain, mental depression, suicidal tendencies, history of drug abuse, or hepatic impairment.

---

Reactions may be *common,* uncommon, *life-threatening,* or COMMON AND LIFE-THREATENING.

## NURSING CONSIDERATIONS

• Assess mental status before starting therapy and reduce doses in elderly patients; these patients may be more sensitive to drug's adverse CNS effects.

• *Alert:* Give I.M. injection deeply with no more than 5 ml of drug at any one site. Superficial injection may cause pain, sterile abscess, and sloughing.

• To ensure accurate dosage, don't divide suppositories.

• Take precautions to prevent hoarding or overdosing by patients who are depressed, suicidal, or drug-dependent or who have a history of drug abuse.

• Watch for signs of barbiturate toxicity: coma, pupillary constriction, cyanosis, clammy skin, and hypotension. Overdose can be fatal.

• Inspect patient's skin. Skin eruptions may precede potentially fatal reactions to barbiturate therapy. Stop drug when skin reactions occur and call prescriber. In some patients, high temperature, stomatitis, headache, or rhinitis may precede skin reactions.

• Drug has no analgesic effect and may cause restlessness or delirium in patients with pain.

• Long-term use isn't recommended; drug loses its effectiveness in promoting sleep after 14 days of continuous use. Long-term high dosage may cause drug dependence, and patient may experience withdrawal symptoms if drug is suddenly stopped. Withdraw barbiturates gradually.

• EEG patterns show a change in low-voltage fast activity; changes persist after stopping therapy.

• *Alert:* Don't confuse pentobarbital with phenobarbital.

• *Alert:* Nembutal may contain tartrazine.

## PATIENT TEACHING

• Inform patient that morning hangover is common after hypnotic dose, which suppresses REM sleep. Patient may experience increased dreaming after drug is stopped.

• Caution patient to avoid performing activities that require mental alertness or physical coordination.

• Tell patient to avoid alcohol use while taking drug.

• Instruct patient using hormonal contraceptives to consider alternative birth control methods, because drug may decrease contraceptive's effect.

## secobarbital sodium
Seconal Sodium

*Pregnancy risk category D*
*Controlled substance schedule II*

## AVAILABLE FORMS
*Capsules:* 100 mg

## INDICATIONS & DOSAGES
➤ **Preoperative sedation**
*Adults:* 200 to 300 mg P.O. 1 to 2 hours before surgery.
*Children:* 2 to 6 mg/kg P.O. 1 to 2 hours before surgery. Maximum single dose is 100 mg P.O.
➤ **Insomnia**
*Adults:* 100 mg P.O. h.s.
*Adjust-a-dose:* In debilitated, elderly, and renally or hepatically impaired patients, consider reducing dose.

## ACTION
Unknown. Probably interferes with transmission of impulses from the thalamus to the cortex of the brain.

| Route | Onset | Peak | Duration |
|-------|-------|------|----------|
| P.O. | 15 min | 15-30 min | 1-4 hr |

## ADVERSE REACTIONS
**CNS:** *drowsiness, lethargy, hangover,* paradoxical anxiety, somnolence.
**GI:** nausea, vomiting.
**Hematologic:** worsening of porphyria.
**Respiratory:** *respiratory depression.*
**Skin:** rash, urticaria, *Stevens-Johnson syndrome,* tissue reactions.
**Other:** *angioedema,* physical and psychological dependence.

## INTERACTIONS
**Drug-drug.** *Chloramphenicol, MAO inhibitors, valproic acid:* May inhibit metabolism of barbiturates; may cause prolonged CNS depression. Reduce barbiturate dosage.
*CNS depressants, including opioid analgesics:* May cause excessive CNS and res-

piratory depression. Use together cautiously.

*Corticosteroids, digitoxin, doxycycline, estrogens and hormonal contraceptives, oral anticoagulants, theophylline, tricyclic antidepressants, verapamil:* May enhance metabolism of these drugs. Watch for decreased effect.

*Griseofulvin:* May decrease absorption of griseofulvin. Monitor effectiveness of griseofulvin.

*Metoprolol, propranolol:* May reduce the effects of these drugs. Consider increasing beta-blocker dose.

*Rifampin:* May decrease barbiturate level. Watch for decreased effect.

**Drug-lifestyle.** *Alcohol use:* May impair coordination, increase CNS effects, and cause death. Strongly discourage alcohol use with these drugs.

**EFFECTS ON LAB TEST RESULTS**
None reported.

**CONTRAINDICATIONS & CAUTIONS**
● Contraindicated in patients hypersensitive to barbiturates and in those with marked liver or renal impairment, respiratory disease in which dyspnea or obstruction is evident, or porphyria.
● Use cautiously in elderly or debilitated patients and in patients with acute or chronic pain, depression, suicidal tendencies, history of drug abuse, or hepatic or renal impairment.

**NURSING CONSIDERATIONS**
● Assess mental status before starting therapy and reduce doses in elderly patients; these patients may be more sensitive to drug's adverse CNS effects. Also watch for paradoxical excitement in this population.
● Take precautions to prevent hoarding or overdosing by patients who are depressed, suicidal, or drug-dependent or who have history of drug abuse.
● Watch for signs of barbiturate toxicity: coma, pupillary constriction, cyanosis, clammy skin, and hypotension. Overdose can be fatal.
● Inspect patient's skin. Skin eruptions may precede potentially fatal reactions to barbiturate therapy. Stop drug when skin reactions occur and notify prescriber. In

some patients, high temperature, stomatitis, headache, or rhinitis may precede skin reactions.
● Long-term use isn't recommended; drug loses its effect of promoting sleep after 14 days of continued use.
● Drug changes EEG patterns, altering low-voltage fast activity; changes persist for a time after stopping therapy.

**PATIENT TEACHING**
● Tell patient that morning hangover is common after hypnotic dose, which suppresses REM sleep. Patient may experience increased dreaming after drug is stopped.
● Advise patient to avoid alcohol use while taking drug.
● Caution patient to avoid performing activities that require mental alertness or physical coordination.
● Tell patient using hormonal contraceptives to consider a different birth control method.

---

# temazepam
Euhypnos 10‡, Euhypnos 20‡, Nomapam‡, Normison‡, Restoril◆, Temaze‡, Temtabs‡

*Pregnancy risk category X*
*Controlled substance schedule IV*

**AVAILABLE FORMS**
*Capsules:* 7.5 mg, 10 mg‡, 15 mg, 20 mg‡, 30 mg

**INDICATIONS & DOSAGES**
➤ **Insomnia**
*Adults:* 15 or 30 mg P.O. h.s.
*Elderly or debilitated patients:* 15 mg P.O. h.s. until individualized response is determined.

**ACTION**
Unknown. A benzodiazepine that probably acts on the limbic system, thalamus, and hypothalamus of the CNS to produce hypnotic effects.

| Route | Onset | Peak | Duration |
|-------|-------|------|----------|
| P.O. | Unknown | 1-2 hr | Unknown |

## ADVERSE REACTIONS
**CNS:** drowsiness, dizziness, lethargy, disturbed coordination, daytime sedation, confusion, nightmares, vertigo, euphoria, weakness, headache, fatigue, nervousness, anxiety, depression, minor changes in EEG patterns (usually low-voltage fast activity).
**EENT:** blurred vision.
**GI:** diarrhea, nausea, dry mouth.
**Other:** physical and psychological dependence.

## INTERACTIONS
**Drug-drug.** *CNS depressants:* May increase CNS depression. Use together cautiously.
**Drug-herb.** *Calendula, hops, kava, lemon balm, passion flower, skullcap, valerian:* May enhance sedative effect of drug. Discourage use together.
**Drug-lifestyle.** *Alcohol use:* May cause additive CNS effects. Discourage use together.

## EFFECTS ON LAB TEST RESULTS
• May increase liver function test values.

## CONTRAINDICATIONS & CAUTIONS
• Contraindicated in pregnant patients and those hypersensitive to drug or other benzodiazepines.
• Use cautiously in patients with chronic pulmonary insufficiency, impaired hepatic or renal function, severe or latent mental depression, suicidal tendencies, and history of drug abuse.

## NURSING CONSIDERATIONS
• Assess mental status before starting therapy and reduce doses in elderly patients; these patients may be more sensitive to drug's adverse CNS effects.
• Take precautions to prevent hoarding or overdosing by patients who are depressed, suicidal, or drug-dependent or who have history of drug abuse.
• **Alert:** Don't confuse Restoril with Vistaril.

## PATIENT TEACHING
• Tell patient to avoid alcohol during therapy.

• Caution patient to avoid performing activities that require mental alertness or physical coordination.
• Warn patient not to stop drug abruptly if taken for 1 month or longer.
• Tell patient that onset of drug's effects may take as long as 2 to 2¼ hours.

---

# triazolam
Apo-Triazo†, Halcion, Novo-Triolam†

*Pregnancy risk category X*
*Controlled substance schedule IV*

## AVAILABLE FORMS
*Tablets:* 0.125 mg, 0.25 mg

## INDICATIONS & DOSAGES
➤ **Insomnia**
*Adults:* 0.125 to 0.5 mg P.O. h.s.
*Elderly or debilitated patients:* 0.125 mg P.O. h.s.; increased, p.r.n., to 0.25 mg P.O. h.s.

## ACTION
Unknown. A benzodiazepine that probably acts on the limbic system, thalamus, and hypothalamus of the CNS to produce hypnotic effects.

| Route | Onset | Peak | Duration |
|-------|-------|------|----------|
| P.O. | Unknown | 1-2 hr | Unknown |

## ADVERSE REACTIONS
**CNS:** *drowsiness,* dizziness, headache, rebound insomnia, amnesia, lack of coordination, mental confusion, depression, nervousness, ataxia, physical or psychological dependence.
**GI:** nausea, vomiting.

## INTERACTIONS
**Drug-drug.** *Azole antifungals, cimetidine, erythromycin, fluoxetine, fluvoxamine, isoniazid, nefazodone, ranitidine:* May increase triazolam level. Avoid using with azole antifungals or nefazodone. Watch for increased sedation if used with other drugs.
*CNS depressants:* May cause excessive CNS depression. Use together cautiously.

---

*Diltiazem:* May increase CNS depression and prolonged effects of triazolam. Reduce triazolam dose.

*Fluconazole, itraconazole, ketoconazole, miconazole:* May increase and prolong drug level, CNS depression, and psychomotor impairment. Avoid using together.

**Drug-herb.** *Calendula, hops, kava, lemon balm, passion flower, skullcap, valerian:* May enhance sedative effect of drug. Discourage use together.

**Drug-food.** *Grapefruit:* May delay onset and increase drug effects. Discourage use together.

**Drug-lifestyle.** *Alcohol use:* May cause additive CNS effects. Discourage use together.

*Smoking:* May increase metabolism and clearance of drug. Advise patient who smokes to watch for decreased effectiveness of drug.

**EFFECTS ON LAB TEST RESULTS**
● May increase liver function test values.

**CONTRAINDICATIONS & CAUTIONS**
● Contraindicated in pregnant patients and those hypersensitive to benzodiazepines.
● Use cautiously in patients with impaired hepatic or renal function, chronic pulmonary insufficiency, sleep apnea, mental depression, suicidal tendencies, or history of drug abuse.
● Use cautiously in breast-feeding women.

**NURSING CONSIDERATIONS**
● Assess mental status before starting therapy and reduce doses in elderly patients; these patients may be more sensitive to drug's adverse CNS effects.
● Monitor CBC, chemistry, and urinalysis.
● Take precautions to prevent hoarding or overdosing by patients who are depressed, suicidal, or drug-dependent or who have history of drug abuse.
● Minor changes in EEG patterns (usually low-voltage fast activity) may occur during and after therapy.
● *Alert:* Don't confuse Halcion with Haldol or halcinonide.

**PATIENT TEACHING**
● Warn patient not to take more than prescribed amount; overdose can occur at total daily dose of 2 mg (or four times highest recommended amount).
● Tell patient to avoid alcohol use while taking drug.
● Warn patient not to stop drug abruptly after taking for 2 weeks or longer.
● Caution patient to avoid performing activities that require mental alertness or physical coordination.
● Inform patient that drug doesn't tend to cause morning drowsiness.
● Tell patient that rebound insomnia may occur for 1 or 2 nights after stopping therapy.

---

# zaleplon
Sonata

*Pregnancy risk category C*
*Controlled substance schedule IV*

**AVAILABLE FORMS**
*Capsules:* 5 mg, 10 mg

**INDICATIONS & DOSAGES**
➤ **Insomnia**
*Adults:* 10 mg P.O. daily h.s.; may increase to 20 mg, p.r.n. Low-weight adults may respond to 5-mg dose. Limit use to 7 to 10 days. Reevaluate patient if used for more than 2 to 3 weeks.
*Adjust-a-dose:* For elderly or debilitated patients, initially, 5 mg P.O. daily h.s.; doses of more than 10 mg aren't recommended. For patients with mild to moderate hepatic impairment or those also taking cimetidine, 5 mg P.O. daily h.s.

**ACTION**
A hypnotic with chemical structure unrelated to benzodiazepines that interacts with the gamma-aminobutyric acid–benzodiazepine receptor complex in the CNS. Modulation of this complex is thought to be responsible for sedative, anxiolytic, muscle relaxant, and anticonvulsant effects of benzodiazepines.

| Route | Onset | Peak | Duration |
|-------|-------|------|----------|
| P.O. | 1 hr | 1 hr | 3-4 hr |

**ADVERSE REACTIONS**
**CNS:** *headache,* amnesia, dizziness, somnolence, depression, hypertonia, nervous-

ness, depersonalization, hallucinations, vertigo, difficulty concentrating, anxiety, paresthesia, hypesthesia, tremor, asthenia, migraine, malaise, fever.
**CV:** chest pain, peripheral edema.
**EENT:** abnormal vision, conjunctivitis, eye discomfort, ear discomfort, hyperacusis, epistaxis, smell alteration.
**GI:** constipation, dry mouth, anorexia, dyspepsia, nausea, abdominal pain, colitis.
**GU:** dysmenorrhea.
**Musculoskeletal:** arthritis, myalgia, back pain.
**Respiratory:** bronchitis.
**Skin:** pruritus, rash, photosensitivity reactions.

## INTERACTIONS
**Drug-drug.** *Carbamazepine, phenobarbital, phenytoin, rifampin, other CYP 3A4 inducers:* May reduce zaleplon bioavailability and peak level by 80%. Consider using a different hypnotic.
*Cimetidine:* May increase zaleplon bioavailability and peak level by 85%. Use an initial zaleplon dose of 5 mg.
*CNS depressants (imipramine, thioridazine):* May cause additive CNS effects. Use together cautiously.
**Drug-food.** *High-fat foods, heavy meals:* May prolong absorption, delaying peak zaleplon level by about 2 hours; may delay sleep onset. Advise patient to avoid taking with meals.
**Drug-lifestyle.** *Alcohol use:* May increase CNS effects. Discourage use together.

## EFFECTS ON LAB TEST RESULTS
None reported.

## CONTRAINDICATIONS & CAUTIONS
• Contraindicated in patients with severe hepatic impairment.
• Use cautiously in elderly, depressed, or debilitated patients, in breast-feeding women, and in patients with compromised respiratory function.

## NURSING CONSIDERATIONS
• Because drug works rapidly, give immediately before bedtime or after patient has gone to bed and has had difficulty falling asleep.
• Closely monitor patients who have compromised respiratory function caused by

illness or who are elderly or debilitated because they are more sensitive to respiratory depression.
• Start treatment only after carefully evaluating patient because sleep disturbances may be a symptom of an underlying physical or psychiatric disorder.
• Adverse reactions are usually dose-related. Consult prescriber about reducing dose reduction if adverse reactions occur.

## PATIENT TEACHING
• Advise patient that drug works rapidly and should only be taken immediately before bedtime or after he has gone to bed and has had trouble falling asleep.
• Advise patient to take drug only if he will be able to sleep for at least 4 undisturbed hours.
• Caution patient that drowsiness, dizziness, light-headedness, and coordination problems occur most often within 1 hour after taking drug.
• Advise patient to avoid performing activities that require mental alertness until CNS adverse reactions are known.
• Advise patient to avoid alcohol use while taking drug and to notify prescriber before taking other prescription or OTC drugs.
• Tell patient not to take drug after a high-fat or heavy meal.
• Advise patient to report sleep problems that continue despite use of drug.
• Notify patient that dependence can occur and that drug is recommended for short-term use only.
• Warn patient not to abruptly stop drug because of the risk of withdrawal symptoms, including unpleasant feelings, stomach and muscle cramps, vomiting, sweating, shakiness, and seizures.
• Notify patient that insomnia may recur for a few nights after stopping drug, but should resolve on its own.
• Warn patient that drug may cause changes in behavior and thinking, including outgoing or aggressive behavior, loss of personal identity, confusion, strange behavior, agitation, hallucinations, worsening of depression, or suicidal thoughts. Tell patient to notify prescriber immediately if these symptoms occur.

## zolpidem tartrate
Ambien

*Pregnancy risk category B*
*Controlled substance schedule IV*

### AVAILABLE FORMS
*Tablets:* 5 mg, 10 mg

### INDICATIONS & DOSAGES
➤ **Short-term management of insomnia**
*Adults:* 10 mg P.O. immediately before h.s.
*Elderly patients:* 5 mg P.O. immediately before h.s. Maximum daily dose is 10 mg.
***Adjust-a-dose:*** For debilitated patients and those with hepatic insufficiency, 5 mg P.O. immediately before h.s. Maximum daily dose is 10 mg.

### ACTION
Although drug interacts with one of three identified gamma-aminobutyric acid–benzodiazepine receptor complexes, it isn't a benzodiazepine. It exhibits hypnotic activity and minimal muscle relaxant and anticonvulsant properties.

| Route | Onset | Peak | Duration |
|-------|-------|------|----------|
| P.O. | Rapid | 30-120 min | Unknown |

### ADVERSE REACTIONS
**CNS:** daytime drowsiness, lightheadedness, change in dreams, amnesia, dizziness, *headache,* hangover, sleep disorder, nervousness, lethargy, depression.
**CV:** palpitations.
**EENT:** sinusitis, pharyngitis.
**GI:** nausea, vomiting, dry mouth, diarrhea, dyspepsia, constipation, abdominal pain.
**Musculoskeletal:** myalgia, arthralgia.
**Skin:** rash.
**Other:** back or chest pain, flulike syndrome, hypersensitivity reactions.

### INTERACTIONS
**Drug-drug.** *CNS depressants:* May cause excessive CNS depression. Use together cautiously.
*Rifampin:* May decrease effects of zolpidem. Avoid using together, if possible. Consider alternative hypnotic.

**Drug-lifestyle.** *Alcohol use:* May cause excessive CNS depression. Discourage use together.

### EFFECTS ON LAB TEST RESULTS
None reported.

### CONTRAINDICATIONS & CAUTIONS
• No known contraindications.
• Use cautiously in patients with compromised respiratory status.

### NURSING CONSIDERATIONS
• Use hypnotics only for short-term management of insomnia, usually 7 to 10 days.
• Use the smallest effective dose in all patients.
• Take precautions to prevent hoarding or overdosing by patients who are depressed, suicidal, or drug-dependent or who have history of drug abuse.
• *Alert:* Don't confuse Ambien with Amen.

### PATIENT TEACHING
• For rapid sleep onset, instruct patient not to take drug with or immediately after meals.
• Instruct patient to take drug immediately before going to bed; onset of action is rapid.
• Tell patient to avoid alcohol use while taking drug.
• Caution patient to avoid performing activities that require mental alertness or physical coordination during therapy.

---

Reactions may be *common,* uncommon, *life-threatening*, or COMMON AND LIFE-THREATENING.

# 28
# Anticonvulsants

**acetazolamide sodium**
(See Chapter 60, DIURETICS.)
**carbamazepine**
**clonazepam**
**clorazepate dipotassium**
(See Chapter 30, ANXIOLYTICS.)
**diazepam**
(See Chapter 30, ANXIOLYTICS.)
**divalproex sodium**
**fosphenytoin sodium**
**gabapentin**
**lamotrigine**
**levetiracetam**
**magnesium sulfate**
**oxcarbazepine**
**phenobarbital**
**phenobarbital sodium**
**phenytoin**
**phenytoin sodium (extended)**
**phenytoin sodium (prompt)**
**primidone**
**tiagabine hydrochloride**
**topiramate**
**valproate sodium**
**valproic acid**
**zonisamide**

## COMBINATION PRODUCTS
None.

---

## carbamazepine
Apo-Carbamazepine† Atretol,
Carbatrol, Epitol, Novo-
Carbamaz† Tegretol, Tegretol CR†
Tegretol-XR, Teril

*Pregnancy risk category D*

---

### AVAILABLE FORMS
*Capsules (extended-release):* 200 mg,
300 mg
*Oral suspension:* 100 mg/5 ml
*Tablets:* 200 mg
*Tablets (chewable):* 100 mg, 200 mg
*Tablets (extended-release)†:* 100 mg,
200 mg, 400 mg

### INDICATIONS & DOSAGES
➤ **Generalized tonic-clonic and complex partial seizures, mixed seizure patterns**
*Adults and children older than age 12:*
Initially, 200 mg P.O. b.i.d. (tablets), or
100 mg P.O. q.i.d. of suspension with
meals. May be increased weekly by
200 mg P.O. daily in divided doses at 6- to
8-hour intervals, adjusted to minimum
effective level. Maximum, 1 g daily in
children ages 12 to 15, and 1.2 g daily in
patients older than age 15. Usual maintenance dosage is 800 to 1,200 mg/day.
*Children ages 6 to 12:* Initially, 100 mg
P.O. b.i.d. or 50 mg of suspension P.O.
q.i.d. with meals, increased at weekly intervals by up to 100 mg P.O. divided in
three to four doses daily (divided b.i.d. for
extended-release form). Maximum, 1 g
daily. Usual maintenance dosage is 400 to
800 mg/day; or, 20 to 30 mg/kg in divided
doses three to four times daily.
*Children younger than age 6:* 10 to
20 mg/kg in two to three divided doses
(tablets) or four divided doses (suspension). Maximum dose is 35 mg/kg in
24 hours.
➤ **Trigeminal neuralgia**
*Adults:* Initially, 100 mg P.O. b.i.d. or
50 mg of suspension q.i.d. with meals,
increased by 100 mg q 12 hours for tablets or 50 mg of suspension q.i.d. until
pain is relieved. Maximum, 1.2 g daily.
Maintenance dosage is 200 to 400 mg P.O.
b.i.d.
➤ **Restless legs syndrome ◆**
*Adults:* 100 to 300 mg P.O. h.s.
➤ **Non-neuritic pain syndromes
(painful neuromas, phantom limb
pain) ◆**
*Adults:* Initially, 100 mg P.O. b.i.d. Maintenance dose is 600 to 1,400 mg daily.

### ACTION
Unknown. Thought to stabilize neuronal
membranes and limit seizure activity by
either increasing efflux or decreasing influx of sodium ions across cell membranes

---

in the motor cortex during generation of nerve impulses.

| Route | Onset | Peak | Duration |
|-------|-------|------|----------|
| P.O. | Unknown | 1½-12 hr | Unknown |

## ADVERSE REACTIONS

**CNS:** *dizziness, vertigo, drowsiness,* fatigue, *ataxia, worsening of seizures,* confusion, fever, headache, syncope.
**CV:** *heart failure,* hypertension, hypotension, aggravation of coronary artery disease, *arrhythmias, AV block.*
**EENT:** conjunctivitis, dry pharynx, blurred vision, diplopia, nystagmus.
**GI:** dry mouth, *nausea, vomiting,* abdominal pain, diarrhea, anorexia, stomatitis, glossitis.
**GU:** urinary frequency, urine retention, impotence, albuminuria, glycosuria.
**Hematologic:** *aplastic anemia, agranulocytosis,* eosinophilia, leukocytosis, *thrombocytopenia.*
**Hepatic:** *hepatitis.*
**Metabolic:** SIADH, hyponatremia.
**Respiratory:** pulmonary hypersensitivity.
**Skin:** rash, urticaria, *erythema multiforme, Stevens-Johnson syndrome,* excessive diaphoresis.
**Other:** chills.

## INTERACTIONS

**Drug-drug.** *Atracurium, cisatracurium, doxacurium, mivacurium, pancuronium, rocuronium, tubocurarine, vecuronium:* May decrease the effects of nondepolarizing muscle relaxant, causing it to be less effective. May need to increase the dose of the nondepolarizing muscle relaxant.
*Cimetidine, danazol, diltiazem, fluoxetine, fluvoxamine, isoniazid, macrolides, propoxyphene, valproic acid, verapamil:* May increase carbamazepine level. Use together cautiously.
*Clarithromycin, erythromycin, troleandomycin:* May inhibit metabolism of carbamazepine, increasing carbamazepine level and risk of toxicity. Avoid using together.
*Doxycycline, felbamate, haloperidol, hormonal contraceptives, phenytoin, theophylline, tiagabine, topiramate, valproate, warfarin:* May decrease levels of these drugs. Watch for decreased effect.

*Lamotrigine:* May decrease lamotrigine level and increase carbamazepine level. Monitor patient for clinical effects and toxicity.
*Lithium:* May increase CNS toxicity of lithium. Avoid using together.
*MAO inhibitors:* May increase depressant and anticholinergic effects. Avoid using together.
*Phenobarbital, phenytoin, primidone:* May decrease carbamazepine level. Watch for decreased effect.
**Drug-herb.** *Plantains (psyllium seed):* May inhibit GI absorption of drug. Discourage use together.

## EFFECTS ON LAB TEST RESULTS

● May increase BUN level.
● May increase liver function test values and eosinophil count. May decrease thyroid function test values, hemoglobin, hematocrit, and granulocyte, WBC, and platelet counts.
● May interfere with pregnancy test results.

## CONTRAINDICATIONS & CAUTIONS

● Contraindicated in patients hypersensitive to carbamazepine or tricyclic antidepressants and in those with a history of previous bone marrow suppression; also contraindicated in those who have taken an MAO inhibitor within 14 days of therapy.
● Use cautiously in patients with mixed seizure disorders because they may experience an increased risk of seizures. Also, use with caution in patients with hepatic dysfunction.

## NURSING CONSIDERATIONS

● Watch for worsening of seizures, especially in patients with mixed seizure disorders, including atypical absence seizures.
● Obtain baseline determinations of urinalysis, BUN level, liver function, CBC, platelet and reticulocyte counts, and iron level. Monitor these values periodically thereafter.
● Shake oral suspension well before measuring dose.
● Contents of extended-release capsules may be sprinkled over applesauce if patient has difficulty swallowing capsules. Capsules and tablets shouldn't be crushed or chewed, unless labeled as chewable form.

• When giving by nasogastric tube, mix dose with an equal volume of water, normal saline solution, or D$_5$W. Flush tube with 100 ml of diluent after giving dose.
• Never stop drug suddenly when treating seizures. Notify prescriber immediately if adverse reactions occur.
• Adverse reactions may be minimized by gradually increasing dosage.
• Therapeutic carbamazepine level is 4 to 12 mcg/ml. Monitor level and effects closely. Ask patient when last dose was taken to better evaluate drug level.
• When managing seizures, take appropriate precautions.
• *Alert:* Watch for signs of anorexia or subtle appetite changes, which may indicate excessive drug level.
• *Alert:* Don't confuse Tegretol with Toradol or Tegopen.
• *Alert:* Don't confuse Carbatrol with carvedilol.

PATIENT TEACHING
• Instruct patient to take drug with food to minimize GI distress. Tell patient taking suspension form to shake container well before measuring dose.
• Tell patient not to crush or chew extended-release form and not to take broken or chipped tablets.
• Tell patient that Tegretol-XR tablet coating may appear in stool because it isn't absorbed.
• Advise patient to keep tablets in the original container and to keep the container tightly closed and away from moisture. Some formulations may harden when exposed to excessive moisture, so that less is available in the body, decreasing seizure control.
• Inform patient that when drug is used for trigeminal neuralgia, an attempt to decrease dosage or withdraw drug is usually made every 3 months.
• Advise patient to notify prescriber immediately if fever, sore throat, mouth ulcers, or easy bruising or bleeding occurs.
• Tell patient that drug may cause mild to moderate dizziness and drowsiness when first taken. Advise him to avoid hazardous activities until effects disappear, usually within 3 to 4 days.
• Advise patient that periodic eye examinations are recommended.

• Advise woman of risks to fetus if pregnancy occurs while taking carbamazepine.
• Advise woman that breast-feeding isn't recommended during therapy.

# clonazepam
Klonopin⚯

*Pregnancy risk category D*
*Controlled substance schedule IV*

AVAILABLE FORMS
*Tablets:* 0.5 mg, 1 mg, 2 mg

INDICATIONS & DOSAGES
➤ **Lennox-Gastaut syndrome, atypical absence seizures, akinetic and myoclonic seizures**
*Adults:* Initially, no more than 1.5 mg P.O. daily in three divided doses. May be increased by 0.5 to 1 mg q 3 days until seizures are controlled. If given in unequal doses, give largest dose h.s. Maximum recommended daily dose is 20 mg.
*Children up to age 10 or 30 kg (66 lb):* Initially, 0.01 to 0.03 mg/kg P.O. daily (not to exceed 0.05 mg/kg daily) in two or three divided doses. Increase by 0.25 to 0.5 mg q third day to maximum maintenance dose of 0.1 to 0.2 mg/kg daily, p.r.n.
➤ **Panic disorder**
*Adults:* Initially, 0.25 mg P.O. b.i.d.; increase to target dose of 1 mg/day after 3 days. Some patients may benefit from dosages up to maximum of 4 mg/day. To achieve 4 mg/day, increase dosage in increments of 0.125 to 0.25 mg b.i.d. q 3 days, as tolerated, until panic disorder is controlled. Taper drug with decrease of 0.125 mg b.i.d. q 3 days until drug is stopped.
➤ **Acute manic episodes of bipolar disorder ♦**
*Adults:* 0.75 to 16 mg/day P.O.
➤ **Adjunct treatment for schizophrenia ♦**
*Adults:* 0.5 to 2 mg/day P.O.
➤ **Periodic leg movements during sleep ♦**
*Adults:* 0.5 to 2 mg P.O. h.s.
➤ **Parkinsonian (hypokinetic) dysarthria ♦**
*Adults:* 0.25 to 0.5 mg/day P.O.

➤ **Multifocal tic disorders** ◆
*Adults:* 1.5 to 12 mg/day P.O.
➤ **Neuralgias (deafferentation pain syndromes)** ◆
*Adults:* 2 to 4 mg/day P.O.

## ACTION

Unknown. A benzodiazepine that probably acts by facilitating the effects of the inhibitory neurotransmitter gamma-aminobutyric acid.

| Route | Onset | Peak | Duration |
|-------|-------|------|----------|
| P.O. | Unknown | 1-2 hr | Unknown |

## ADVERSE REACTIONS

**CNS:** *drowsiness,* ataxia, behavioral disturbances, slurred speech, tremor, confusion, agitation, depression.
**CV:** palpitations.
**EENT:** nystagmus, abnormal eye movements.
**GI:** sore gums, constipation, gastritis, change in appetite, nausea, vomiting, anorexia, diarrhea.
**GU:** dysuria, enuresis, nocturia, urine retention.
**Hematologic:** *leukopenia, thrombocytopenia,* eosinophilia.
**Respiratory:** *respiratory depression,* chest congestion, shortness of breath.
**Skin:** rash.

## INTERACTIONS

**Drug-drug.** *Carbamazepine, phenobarbital, phenytoin:* Lowers clonazepam levels. Monitor patient closely.
*CNS depressants:* May increase CNS depression. Avoid using together.
*Fluconazole, itraconazole, ketoconazole, miconazole:* May increase and prolong drug levels, CNS depression, and psychomotor impairment. Avoid using together.
**Drug-lifestyle.** *Alcohol use:* May cause additive CNS effects. Discourage use together.
*Smoking:* May increase clearance of clonazepam. Monitor patient for decreased drug effects.

## EFFECTS ON LAB TEST RESULTS

● May increase liver function test values and eosinophil counts. May decrease WBC and platelet counts.

## CONTRAINDICATIONS & CAUTIONS

● Contraindicated in patients hypersensitive to benzodiazepines and in those with significant hepatic disease or acute angle-closure glaucoma.
● Use cautiously in patients with mixed-type seizures because drug may cause generalized tonic-clonic seizures.
● Use cautiously in children and in patients with chronic respiratory disease or open-angle glaucoma.

## NURSING CONSIDERATIONS

● Watch for behavioral disturbances, especially in children.
● Don't stop drug abruptly because this may worsen seizures. Call prescriber at once if adverse reactions develop.
● Assess elderly patient's response closely. Elderly patients are more sensitive to drug's CNS effects.
● Monitor patient for oversedation.
● Monitor CBC and liver function tests.
● Withdrawal symptoms are similar to those of barbiturates.
● To reduce inconvenience of somnolence when drug is used for panic disorder, administration of one dose at bedtime may be desirable.

## PATIENT TEACHING

● Advise patient to avoid driving and other hazardous activities that require mental alertness until drug's CNS effects are known.
● Instruct parent to monitor child's school performance because drug may interfere with attentiveness.
● Warn patient and parents not to stop drug abruptly because seizures may occur.
● Advise patient that drug isn't for use during pregnancy or breast-feeding.

# fosphenytoin sodium
Cerebyx

*Pregnancy risk category D*

## AVAILABLE FORMS

*Injection:* 2 ml (150 mg fosphenytoin sodium equivalent to 100 mg phenytoin sodium), 10 ml (750 mg fosphenytoin sodium equivalent to 500 mg phenytoin sodium)

---

Reactions may be *common,* uncommon, *life-threatening,* or COMMON AND LIFE-THREATENING.

## INDICATIONS & DOSAGES
➤ **Status epilepticus**
*Adults:* 15 to 20 mg phenytoin sodium equivalent (PE)/kg I.V. at 100 to 150 mg PE/minute as loading dose; then 4 to 6 mg PE/kg daily I.V. as maintenance dose.
➤ **To prevent and treat seizures during neurosurgery (nonemergent loading or maintenance dosing)**
*Adults:* Loading dose of 10 to 20 mg PE/kg I.M. or I.V. at infusion rate not exceeding 150 mg PE/minute. Maintenance dose is 4 to 6 mg PE/kg daily I.V. or I.M.
➤ **Short-term substitution for oral phenytoin therapy**
*Adults:* Same total daily dose equivalent as oral phenytoin sodium therapy given as a single daily dose I.M. or I.V. at infusion rate not exceeding 150 mg PE/minute. Some patients may need more frequent dosing.
*Elderly patients:* Phenytoin clearance is decreased slightly in elderly patients; lower or less-frequent dosing may be required.

## I.V. ADMINISTRATION
● Before I.V. infusion, dilute fosphenytoin in D$_5$W or normal saline solution for injection to a level ranging from 1.5 to 25 mg PE/ml. Don't give at a rate exceeding 150 mg PE/minute.
● For status epilepticus, give dose of I.V. fosphenytoin at maximum rate of 150 mg PE/minute. Typical infusion for a 50-kg patient takes 5 to 7 minutes. (An infusion of an identical molar dose of phenytoin can't be accomplished in less than 15 to 20 minutes because of adverse CV effects that accompany direct I.V. administration of phenytoin at rates above 50 mg/minute.) Don't use fosphenytoin I.M. for status epilepticus because therapeutic phenytoin level may not be reached as rapidly as with I.V. administration.
● Patients receiving 20 mg PE/kg at 150 mg PE/minute typically experience discomfort, most often in the groin. To reduce frequency and intensity of discomfort, slow or temporarily stop infusion.
● If rapid phenytoin loading is a primary goal, I.V. administration is preferred.
● Monitor patient's ECG, blood pressure, and respirations continuously during maximal phenytoin level—about 10 to 20 minutes after end of fosphenytoin infusion. Severe CV complications are most common in elderly or gravely ill patients. You may need to reduce the administration rate or stop the drug.

## ACTION
A prodrug of phenytoin, with same anticonvulsant action as phenytoin: it stabilizes neuronal membranes and limits seizure activity by modulating voltage-dependent neuron channels, inhibiting calcium flux across neuronal membranes, and enhancing sodium-potassium ATPase activity.

| Route | Onset | Peak | Duration |
|-------|-------|------|----------|
| I.V. | Unknown | End of infusion | Unknown |
| I.M. | Unknown | 30 min | Unknown |

## ADVERSE REACTIONS
**CNS:** increased or decreased reflexes, speech disorders, asthenia, *intracranial hypertension,* thinking abnormalities, nervousness, hypesthesia, dysarthria, extrapyramidal syndrome, *brain edema,* headache, *dizziness, somnolence, ataxia,* stupor, incoordination, paresthesia, tremor, agitation, vertigo, fever.
**CV:** hypertension, vasodilation, tachycardia, hypotension.
**EENT:** amblyopia, deafness, diplopia, tinnitus, *nystagmus.*
**GI:** constipation, taste perversion, dry mouth, tongue disorder, vomiting.
**Metabolic:** hypokalemia.
**Musculoskeletal:** pelvic pain, back pain, myasthenia.
**Respiratory:** pneumonia.
**Skin:** rash, ecchymoses, *pruritus,* injection site reaction and pain.
**Other:** accidental injury, infection, chills, facial edema.

## INTERACTIONS
**Drug-drug.** *Amiodarone, chloramphenicol, chlordiazepoxide, cimetidine, diazepam, dicumarol, disulfiram, estrogens, ethosuximide, fluoxetine, H$_2$ antagonists, halothane, isoniazid, methylphenidate, phenothiazines, phenylbutazone, salicylates, succinimides, sulfonamides, tolbutamide, trazodone:* May increase

phenytoin level and effect. Use together cautiously.

*Carbamazepine, reserpine:* May decrease phenytoin level. Monitor patient.

*Corticosteroids, coumarin, digitoxin, doxycycline, estrogens, furosemide, oral contraceptives, quinidine, rifampin, theophylline, vitamin D:* May decrease effects of these drugs because of increased hepatic metabolism. Monitor patient closely.

*Lithium:* May increase lithium toxicity. Monitor patient's neurologic status closely. Marked neurologic symptoms have been reported despite normal lithium level.

*Phenobarbital, valproate sodium, valproic acid:* May increase or decrease phenytoin level. May increase or decrease levels of these drugs. Monitor patient.

*Tricyclic antidepressants:* May lower seizure threshold and require adjustments in phenytoin dosage. Use together cautiously.

**Drug-lifestyle.** *Alcohol use:* Acute intoxication may increase phenytoin level and effect. Discourage use together.

*Long-term alcohol use:* May decrease phenytoin level. Monitor patient.

### EFFECTS ON LAB TEST RESULTS
• May increase alkaline phosphatase, GGT, and glucose levels. May decrease potassium, folate, and $T_4$ levels.
• May cause falsely low dexamethasone and metyrapone test results.

### CONTRAINDICATIONS & CAUTIONS
• Contraindicated in patients hypersensitive to drug or its components, phenytoin, or other hydantoins.
• Contraindicated in those with sinus bradycardia, SA block, second- or third-degree AV block, or Adams-Stokes syndrome.
• Use cautiously in patients with porphyria and in those with history of hypersensitivity to similarly structured drugs, such as barbiturates, oxazolidinediones, and succinimide.

### NURSING CONSIDERATIONS
• Most significant drug interactions are those commonly seen with phenytoin.
• *Alert:* Fosphenytoin should always be prescribed and dispensed in phenytoin

sodium equivalent units (PE). Don't make adjustments in the recommended doses when substituting fosphenytoin for phenytoin, and vice versa.
• In status epilepticus, phenytoin may be used instead of fosphenytoin as maintenance, using the appropriate dose.
• Phosphate load provided by fosphenytoin (0.0037 mmol phosphate/mg PE fosphenytoin) must be taken into consideration when treating patients who need phosphate restriction, such as those with severe renal impairment. Monitor laboratory values.
• Stop drug and notify prescriber if patient gets exfoliative, purpuric, or bullous rash or signs and symptoms of lupus erythematosus, Stevens-Johnson syndrome, or toxic epidermal necrolysis. If rash is mild (measleslike or scarlatiniform), you may resume therapy after rash disappears. If rash recurs when therapy is resumed, further fosphenytoin or phenytoin administration is contraindicated. Document that patient is allergic to drug.
• Stop drug in patients with acute hepatotoxicity.
• I.M. administration generates systemic phenytoin levels similar enough to oral phenytoin sodium to allow essentially interchangeable use.
• After administration, phenytoin levels shouldn't be monitored until conversion to phenytoin is essentially complete—about 2 hours after the end of an I.V. infusion or 4 hours after I.M. administration.
• Interpret total phenytoin levels cautiously in patients with renal or hepatic disease or hypoalbuminemia caused by an increased fraction in unbound phenytoin. It may be more useful to monitor unbound phenytoin levels in these patients. When giving drug I.V., monitor patients with renal and hepatic disease because they are at increased risk for more frequent and severe adverse reactions.
• Monitor glucose level closely in diabetic patients; drug may cause hyperglycemia.
• Abrupt withdrawal of drug may precipitate status epilepticus.
• Store drug under refrigeration. Don't store at room temperature longer than 48 hours. Discard vials that develop particulate matter.

• *Alert:* Don't confuse Cerebyx with Cerezyme, Celexa, or Celebrex.

## PATIENT TEACHING
• Warn patient that sensory disturbances may occur with I.V. administration.
• Instruct patient to immediately report adverse reactions, especially rash.
• Warn patient not to stop drug abruptly or adjust dosage without discussing with prescriber.
• Advise woman to discuss drug therapy with prescriber if she's considering pregnancy.
• Advise woman that breast-feeding isn't recommended during therapy.

---

## gabapentin
Neurontin*

*Pregnancy risk category C*

### AVAILABLE FORMS
*Capsules:* 100 mg, 300 mg, 400 mg
*Oral solution:* 250 mg/5 ml
*Tablets:* 600 mg, 800 mg

### INDICATIONS & DOSAGES
➤ **Adjunctive treatment of partial seizures with or without secondary generalization in adults with epilepsy**
*Adults:* Initially, 300 mg P.O. h.s. on day 1; 300 mg P.O. b.i.d. on day 2; then 300 mg P.O. t.i.d. on day 3. Increase dosage as needed and tolerated to 1,800 mg daily in divided doses. Dosages up to 3,600 mg daily have been well tolerated.
➤ **Adjunctive treatment to control partial seizures in children**
*Starting dosage, children ages 3 to 12:* 10 to 15 mg/kg daily P.O. in three divided doses, adjusting over 3 days to reach effective dosage.
*Effective dosage, children ages 5 to 12:* 25 to 35 mg/kg daily P.O. in three divided doses.
*Effective dosage, children ages 3 to 4:* 40 mg/kg daily P.O. in three divided doses.
➤ **Postherpetic neuralgia**
*Adults:* 300 mg P.O. once daily on day 1, 300 mg b.i.d. on day 2, and 300 mg t.i.d. on day 3. Adjust p.r.n. for pain to a maximum daily dose of 1,800 mg in three divided doses.

*Adjust-a-dose:* In patients age 12 and older with creatinine clearance 30 to 59 ml/minute, give 400 to 1,400 mg daily, divided into two doses. For clearance 15 to 29 ml/minute, 200 to 700 mg daily, given in single dose. For clearance less than 15 ml/minute, 100 to 300 mg daily, given in single dose. Reduce daily dose in proportion to creatinine clearance (patients with a clearance of 7.5 ml/minute should receive one-half the daily dose of those with a clearance of 15 ml/minute). Give patients receiving hemodialysis maintenance doses based on estimates of creatinine clearance. Give supplemental dose of 125 to 350 mg after each 4 hours of hemodialysis.

### ACTION
Unknown. Although structurally related to gamma-aminobutyric acid (GABA), drug doesn't interact with GABA receptors and isn't converted metabolically into GABA or a GABA agonist. It doesn't inhibit GABA reuptake and doesn't prevent degradation.

| Route | Onset | Peak | Duration |
|-------|-------|------|----------|
| P.O. | Unknown | Unknown | Unknown |

### ADVERSE REACTIONS
**CNS:** *fatigue, somnolence, dizziness, ataxia,* nystagmus, tremor, nervousness, dysarthria, amnesia, depression, abnormal thinking, twitching, incoordination.
**CV:** peripheral edema, vasodilation.
**EENT:** diplopia, rhinitis, pharyngitis, dry throat, amblyopia.
**GI:** nausea, vomiting, dyspepsia, dry mouth, constipation, increased appetite, dental abnormalities.
**GU:** impotence.
**Hematologic:** *leukopenia.*
**Metabolic:** weight gain.
**Musculoskeletal:** back pain, myalgia, fractures.
**Respiratory:** coughing.
**Skin:** pruritus, abrasion.

### INTERACTIONS
**Drug-drug.** *Antacids:* May decrease absorption of gabapentin. Separate dosage times by at least 2 hours.
*Hydrocodone:* May increase gabapentin level and decrease hydrocodone level.

---

Monitor patient for increased adverse effects or loss of clinical effect.

## EFFECTS ON LAB TEST RESULTS
• May decrease WBC count.
• May cause false-positive results with the Ames-N-Multistix SG dipstick test for urinary protein when used with other antiepileptics.

## CONTRAINDICATIONS & CAUTIONS
• Contraindicated in patients hypersensitive to drug.

## NURSING CONSIDERATIONS
• Give first dose at bedtime to minimize drowsiness, dizziness, fatigue, and ataxia.
• If drug is to be stopped or an alternative drug is substituted, do so gradually over at least 1 week, to minimize risk of precipitating seizures.
• *Alert:* Don't suddenly withdraw other anticonvulsants in patients starting gabapentin therapy.
• Routine monitoring of drug levels isn't necessary. Drug doesn't appear to alter levels of other anticonvulsants.
• *Alert:* Don't confuse Neurontin with Noroxin.

## PATIENT TEACHING
• Advise patient that drug may be taken without regard to meals.
• Instruct patient to take first dose at bedtime to minimize adverse reactions.
• Warn patient to avoid driving and operating heavy machinery until drug's CNS effects are known.
• Advise patient not to stop drug abruptly.
• Advise woman to discuss drug therapy with prescriber if she's considering pregnancy.
• Tell patient to keep oral solution refrigerated.

---

# lamotrigine
Lamictal

*Pregnancy risk category C*

---

## AVAILABLE FORMS
*Tablets:* 25 mg, 100 mg, 150 mg, 200 mg
*Tablets (chewable dispersible):* 2 mg, 5 mg, 25 mg

## INDICATIONS & DOSAGES
➤ **Adjunct treatment of partial seizures caused by epilepsy or generalized seizures of Lennox-Gastout syndrome**
*Adults and children older than age 12:* For patients taking valproic acid with other enzyme-inducing antiepileptics, 25 mg P.O. every other day for 2 weeks; then 25 mg P.O. daily for 2 weeks. Continue to increase, p.r.n., by 25 to 50 mg/day q 1 to 2 weeks until an effective maintenance dosage of 100 to 400 mg daily given in one or two divided doses is reached. When added to valproic acid alone, the usual daily maintenance dose is 100 to 200 mg.

For patients receiving enzyme-inducing antiepileptics but not valproic acid, 50 mg P.O. daily for 2 weeks; then 100 mg P.O. daily in two divided doses for 2 weeks. Increase, p.r.n., by 100 mg daily q 1 to 2 weeks. Usual maintenance dosage is 300 to 500 mg P.O. daily in two divided doses.
*Children ages 2 to 12 years weighing 6.7 to 40 kg (15 to 88 lb.):* For patients taking valproic acid with other enzyme-inducing antiepileptics, 0.15 mg/kg P.O. daily in one or two divided doses (rounded down to nearest whole tablet) for 2 weeks, followed by 0.3 mg/kg daily in one or two divided doses for another 2 weeks. Thereafter, usual maintenance dosage is 1 to 5 mg/kg daily (maximum, 200 mg daily in one to two divided doses).

For patients receiving enzyme-inducing antiepileptics but not valproic acid, 0.6 mg/kg P.O. daily in two divided doses (rounded down to nearest whole tablet) for 2 weeks, followed by 1.2 mg/kg daily in two divided doses for another 2 weeks. Thereafter, usual maintenance dosage is 5 to 15 mg/kg daily (maximum 400 mg/day in two divided doses).
➤ **To convert patients from monotherapy with a hepatic enzyme-inducing anticonvulsant drug to lamotrigine therapy**
*Adults and children age 16 and older:* Add lamotrigine 50 mg P.O. once daily to current drug regimen for 2 weeks, followed by 100 mg P.O. daily in two divided doses for 2 weeks. Then increase daily dosage by 100 mg q 1 to 2 weeks until maintenance dose of 500 mg daily in two divided doses is reached. Then the concomitant

---

hepatic enzyme-inducing anticonvulsant can be gradually withdrawn by 20% decrements weekly for 4 weeks.
*Adjust-a-dose:* For patients with severe renal impairment, use lower maintenance dosage.

## ACTION
Unknown. May inhibit release of glutamate and aspartate (excitatory neurotransmitters) in the brain via an action at voltage-sensitive sodium channels.

| Route | Onset | Peak | Duration |
|-------|-------|------|----------|
| P.O. | Unknown | 1-5 hr | Unknown |

## ADVERSE REACTIONS
**CNS:** *dizziness, headache, ataxia, somnolence,* fever, incoordination, insomnia, tremor, depression, anxiety, *seizures,* irritability, speech disorder, decreased memory, aggravated reaction, concentration disturbance, sleep disorder, emotional lability, vertigo, mind racing, dysarthria, malaise.
**CV:** palpitations.
**EENT:** *diplopia, blurred vision,* vision abnormality, nystagmus, *rhinitis,* pharyngitis.
**GI:** *nausea, vomiting,* diarrhea, dyspepsia, abdominal pain, constipation, anorexia, dry mouth.
**GU:** dysmenorrhea, vaginitis, amenorrhea.
**Musculoskeletal:** muscle spasm, neck pain.
**Respiratory:** cough, dyspnea.
**Skin:** *rash,* **Stevens-Johnson syndrome, toxic epidermal necrolysis,** pruritus, hot flashes, alopecia, acne.
**Other:** flulike syndrome, infection, chills, tooth disorder.

## INTERACTIONS
**Drug-drug.** *Acetaminophen:* May decrease therapeutic effects. Monitor patient.
*Carbamazepine, ethosuximide, oral contraceptives, oxcarbazepine, phenobarbital, phenytoin, primidone:* May decrease steady-state levels of lamotrigine. Monitor patient closely.
*Folate inhibitors, such as co-trimoxazole and methotrexate:* May have additive effect because lamotrigine inhibits dihydrofolate reductase, an enzyme involved in folic acid synthesis. Monitor patient.
*Valproic acid:* May decrease clearance of lamotrigine, which increases the drug's steady-state levels. Also decreases valproic acid levels. Monitor patient for toxicity.
**Drug-lifestyle.** *Sun exposure:* May cause photosensitivity reactions. Advise patient to avoid excessive sun exposure.

## EFFECTS ON LAB TEST RESULTS
None reported.

## CONTRAINDICATIONS & CAUTIONS
● Contraindicated in patients hypersensitive to drug or its components.
● Safety and efficacy of drug in children younger than age 16 (other than those with Lennox-Gastaut syndrome) haven't been established. Don't give drug to children younger than age 16. Children weighing less than 17 kg (37 lb) shouldn't receive drug because therapy can't be initiated using dosing guidelines and currently available tablet strength.
● Use cautiously in patients with renal, hepatic, or cardiac impairment.

## NURSING CONSIDERATIONS
● Drug is also indicated for use in the maintenance of bipolar I disorder. Check manufacturer's package insert for complete dosing instructions.
● Don't stop drug abruptly because this may increase seizure frequency. Instead, taper drug over at least 2 weeks.
● *Alert:* Stop drug at first sign of rash, unless rash is clearly not drug related.
● Reduce lamotrigine dose if drug is added to a multidrug regimen that includes valproic acid.
● Chewable dispersible tablets may be swallowed whole, chewed, or dispersed in water or diluted fruit juice. If tablets are chewed, give a small amount of water or diluted fruit juice to aid in swallowing.
● Evaluate patients for changes in seizure activity. Check adjunct anticonvulsant's levels.
● Encourage enrollment of pregnant patients in national registry before fetal outcome is known.

---

• *Alert:* Don't confuse lamotrigine with lamivudine or Lamictal with Lamisil, Ludiomil, labetalol, or Lomotil.

## PATIENT TEACHING
• Inform patient that drug may cause rash. Combination therapy of valproic acid and lamotrigine may cause a serious rash. Tell patient to report rash or signs or symptoms of hypersensitivity promptly to prescriber because they may warrant drug discontinuation.
• Warn patient not to engage in hazardous activity until drug's CNS effects are known.
• Warn patient that the drug may trigger sensitivity to the sun and to take precautions until tolerance is determined.
• Warn patient not to stop drug abruptly.
• Advise woman to discuss drug therapy with prescriber if she's considering pregnancy.
• Advise woman that breast-feeding isn't recommended during therapy.

---

# levetiracetam
Keppra

*Pregnancy risk category C*

## AVAILABLE FORMS
*Oral solution:* 100 mg/ml
*Tablets:* 250 mg, 500 mg, 750 mg

## INDICATIONS & DOSAGES
➤ **Adjunctive treatment for partial seizures**
*Adults:* Initially, 500 mg b.i.d. Dosage can be increased by 500 mg b.i.d., p.r.n., for seizure control at 2-week intervals to maximum of 1,500 mg b.i.d.
*Adjust-a-dose:* For patients with renal impairment, if creatinine clearance is more than 80 ml/minute, give 500 to 1,500 mg q 12 hours; if clearance is 50 to 80 ml/minute, give 500 to 1,000 mg q 12 hours; if clearance is 30 to 50 ml/minute, give 250 to 750 mg q 12 hours; if clearance is less than 30 ml/minute, give 250 to 500 mg q 12 hours. For dialysis patients, give 500 to 1,000 mg q 24 hours. Give a 250- to 500-mg dose after dialysis.

## ACTION
May act by inhibiting simultaneous neuronal firing that leads to seizure activity.

| Route | Onset | Peak | Duration |
|-------|-------|------|----------|
| P.O. | 1 hr | 1 hr | 12 hr |

## ADVERSE REACTIONS
**CNS:** *asthenia, headache, somnolence,* dizziness, depression, vertigo, paresthesia, nervousness, hostility, emotional lability, ataxia, amnesia, anxiety.
**EENT:** diplopia, pharyngitis, rhinitis, sinusitis.
**GI:** anorexia.
**Hematologic:** *leukopenia, neutropenia.*
**Musculoskeletal:** pain.
**Respiratory:** cough, infection.

## INTERACTIONS
**Drug-drug.** *Antihistamines, benzodiazepines, opioids, other drugs that cause drowsiness, tricyclic antidepressants:* May lead to severe sedation. Avoid using together.
**Drug-lifestyle.** *Alcohol use:* May lead to severe sedation. Discourage use together.

## EFFECTS ON LAB TEST RESULTS
• May alter liver function test results.
• May decrease WBC and neutrophil counts.

## CONTRAINDICATIONS & CAUTIONS
• Contraindicated in patients hypersensitive to drug.
• Leukopenia and neutropenia have been reported with drug use. Use cautiously in immunocompromised patients, such as those with cancer or HIV infection.
• Patients with poor renal function need dosage adjustment.

## NURSING CONSIDERATIONS
• *Alert:* Don't confuse Keppra (levetiracetam) with Kaletra (lopinavir and ritonavir).
• Drug can be taken with or without food.
• Use drug only with other anticonvulsants; it's not recommended for monotherapy.
• Seizures can occur if drug is stopped abruptly. Tapering is recommended.

---

Reactions may be *common,* uncommon, *life-threatening,* or COMMON AND LIFE-THREATENING.

• Monitor patients closely for such adverse reactions as dizziness, which may lead to falls.

## PATIENT TEACHING
• Warn patient to use extra care when sitting or standing to avoid falling.
• Advise patient to call prescriber and not to stop drug suddenly if adverse reactions occur.
• Tell patient to take with other prescribed seizure drugs.
• Inform patient that drug can be taken with or without food.

## magnesium sulfate

*Pregnancy risk category A*

### AVAILABLE FORMS
*Injection:* 4%, 8%, 10%, 12.5%, 25%, 50%
*Injection solution:* 1% in $D_5W$, 2% in $D_5W$

### INDICATIONS & DOSAGES
➤ **To prevent or control seizures in preeclampsia or eclampsia**
*Women:* Initially, 4 g I.V. in 250 ml $D_5W$ or normal saline and 4 to 5 g deep I.M. into each buttock; then 4 to 5 g deep I.M. into alternate buttock q 4 hours, p.r.n. Or, 4 g I.V. loading dose; then 1 to 2 g hourly as I.V. infusion. Total dose shouldn't exceed 30 or 40 g daily.
➤ **Hypomagnesemia**
*Adults:* For mild deficiency, 1 g I.M. q 6 hours for four doses; for severe deficiency, 5 g in 1,000 ml $D_5W$ or normal saline solution infused over 3 hours.
➤ **Seizures, hypertension, and encephalopathy with acute nephritis in children**
*Children:* 0.2 ml/kg of 50% solution I.M. q 4 to 6 hours, p.r.n. For severe symptoms, 100 to 200 mg/kg as a 1% to 3% solution I.V. slowly over 1 hour with 50% of dose given in first 15 to 20 minutes. Adjust dosage according to magnesium level and seizure response.
➤ **To manage paroxysmal atrial tachycardia**
*Adults:* 3 to 4 g I.V. over 30 seconds, with extreme caution.

➤ **To manage life-threatening ventricular arrhythmias, such as sustained ventricular tachycardia or torsades de pointes ◆**
*Adults:* 1 to 6 g I.V. over several minutes; then continuous I.V. infusion of 3 to 20 mg/minute for 5 to 48 hours. Base dosage and duration of therapy on patient response and magnesium level.
➤ **To manage preterm labor ◆**
*Adults:* 4 to 6 g I.V. over 20 minutes, followed by 2 to 4 g/hr I.V. infusion for 12 to 24 hours, as tolerated, after contractions have ceased.

### I.V. ADMINISTRATION
• If necessary, dilute to maximum level of 20%. Infuse no faster than 150 mg/minute (1.5 ml/minute of a 10% solution or 0.75 ml/minute of a 20% solution). Drug is compatible with $D_5W$ and normal saline solution.
• Maximum infusion rate is 150 mg/minute. Too-rapid infusion induces uncomfortable feeling of heat.
• Monitor vital signs every 15 minutes when giving drug I.V.

### ACTION
May decrease acetylcholine released by nerve impulses, but its anticonvulsant mechanism is unknown.

| Route | Onset | Peak | Duration |
|-------|-------|------|----------|
| I.V. | 1-2 min | Rapid | 30 min |
| I.M. | 1 hr | Unknown | 3-4 hr |

### ADVERSE REACTIONS
**CNS:** drowsiness, *depressed reflexes,* flaccid paralysis, hypothermia.
**CV:** *hypotension, flushing, **bradycardia, circulatory collapse,*** depressed cardiac function.
**EENT:** diplopia.
**Metabolic:** hypocalcemia.
**Respiratory:** *respiratory paralysis.*
**Skin:** diaphoresis.

### INTERACTIONS
**Drug-drug.** *Anesthetics, CNS depressants:* May cause additive CNS depression. Use together cautiously.
*Cardiac glycosides:* May worsen arrhythmias. Use together cautiously.

---

*Neuromuscular blockers:* May cause increased neuromuscular blockade. Use together cautiously.

## EFFECTS ON LAB TEST RESULTS
• May increase magnesium level. May decrease calcium level.

## CONTRAINDICATIONS & CAUTIONS
• Parenteral administration contraindicated in patients with heart block or myocardial damage.
• Contraindicated in patients with toxemia of pregnancy during 2 hours preceding delivery.
• Use cautiously in patients with impaired renal function.
• Use cautiously in pregnant women during labor.

## NURSING CONSIDERATIONS
• If used to treat seizures, take appropriate seizure precautions.
• *Alert:* Watch for respiratory depression and signs and symptoms of heart block.
• Keep I.V. calcium gluconate available to reverse magnesium intoxication, but use cautiously in digitalized patients because of danger of arrhythmias.
• Check magnesium level after repeated doses. Disappearance of knee-jerk and patellar reflexes is sign of impending magnesium toxicity.
• Signs of hypermagnesemia begin to appear at levels of 4 mEq/L.
• Effective anticonvulsant level ranges from 2.5 to 7.5 mEq/L.
• Monitor fluid intake and output. Make sure urine output is 100 ml or more in 4-hour period before each dose.
• Observe neonates for signs of magnesium toxicity, including neuromuscular or respiratory depression, when giving I.V. form of drug to toxemic mothers within 24 hours before delivery.
• *Alert:* Don't confuse magnesium sulfate with manganese sulfate.

## PATIENT TEACHING
• Inform patient of short-term need for drug and answer any questions and address concerns.
• Review potential adverse reactions and instruct patient to promptly report any occurrences. Reassure patient that, although adverse reactions can occur, vital signs, reflexes, and drug level will be monitored frequently to ensure safety.

# oxcarbazepine
Trileptal

*Pregnancy risk category C*

## AVAILABLE FORMS
*Oral suspension:* 300 mg/5 ml (60 mg/ml)
*Tablets (film-coated):* 150 mg, 300 mg, 600 mg

## INDICATIONS & DOSAGES
➤ **Adjunctive treatment of partial seizures in patients with epilepsy**
*Adults:* Initially, 300 mg P.O. b.i.d. Increase by a maximum of 600 mg/day (300 mg P.O. b.i.d.) at weekly intervals. Recommended daily dose is 1,200 mg P.O. divided b.i.d.
*Children ages 4 to 16:* Initially, 8 to 10 mg/kg daily P.O. divided b.i.d., not to exceed 600 mg/day. The target maintenance dose depends on patient's weight and should be divided b.i.d. If patient weighs between 20 and 29 kg (44 and 64 lb), then target maintenance dose is 900 mg/day. If between 29 and 39 kg (64 and 86 lb), target maintenance dose is 1,200 mg/day. If more than 39 kg, target maintenance dose is 1,800 mg/day. Target doses should be achieved over 2 weeks.
➤ **To change from multidrug to single-drug treatment of partial seizures in patients with epilepsy**
*Adults:* Initially, 300 mg P.O. b.i.d., with simultaneous reduction in dose of concomitant antiepileptics. Increase oxcarbazepine by a maximum of 600 mg/day at weekly intervals over 2 to 4 weeks. Recommended daily dose is 2,400 mg P.O. divided b.i.d. Withdraw other antiepileptics completely over 3 to 6 weeks.
*Children ages 4 to 16:* Initially, 8 to 10 mg/kg daily P.O. divided b.i.d., with simultaneous reduction in dose of concomitant antiepileptics. Increase oxcarbazepine by a maximum of 10 mg/kg daily at weekly intervals. Withdraw other antiepileptics completely over 3 to 6 weeks.

➤ **To start single-drug treatment of partial seizures in patients with epilepsy**
*Adults:* Initially, 300 mg P.O. b.i.d. Increase dosage by 300 mg/day q third day to a daily dose of 1,200 mg divided b.i.d.
*Children ages 4 to 16:* Initially, 8 to 10 mg/kg daily P.O. divided b.i.d., increasing the dosage by 5 mg/kg daily q third day to the recommended daily dose range shown below.

| Weight (kg) | Dose (mg/day) |
|---|---|
| 20 | 600-900 |
| 25 | 900-1,200 |
| 30 | 900-1,200 |
| 35 | 900-1,500 |
| 40 | 900-1,500 |
| 45 | 1,200-1,500 |
| 50 | 1,200-1,800 |
| 55 | 1,200-1,800 |
| 60 | 1,200-2,100 |
| 65 | 1,200-2,100 |
| 70 | 1,500-2,100 |

*Adjust-a-dose:* In patients with creatinine clearance less than 30 ml/minute, initiate therapy at 150 mg P.O. b.i.d. (one-half usual starting dose), and increase slowly to achieve desired response.

**ACTION**
Unknown. Thought to block voltage-sensitive sodium channels, which ultimately may prevent seizure spread in the brain. Increased potassium conductance and modulation of high-voltage activated calcium channels may also contribute to anticonvulsant effects.

| Route | Onset | Peak | Duration |
|---|---|---|---|
| P.O. | Unknown | Variable | Unknown |

**ADVERSE REACTIONS**
**CNS:** *fatigue,* asthenia, fever, feeling abnormal, *headache, dizziness, somnolence, ataxia, abnormal gait,* insomnia, *tremor,* nervousness, agitation, abnormal coordination, speech disorder, confusion, anxiety, amnesia, *aggravated seizures,* hypesthesia, emotional lability, impaired concentration, *vertigo.*
**CV:** hypotension, edema, chest pain.

**EENT:** *nystagmus, diplopia, abnormal vision,* abnormal accommodation, rhinitis, sinusitis, pharyngitis, epistaxis, ear pain.
**GI:** *nausea, vomiting, abdominal pain,* diarrhea, dyspepsia, constipation, gastritis, anorexia, dry mouth, ***rectal hemorrhage,*** taste perversion, thirst.
**GU:** UTI, urinary frequency, vaginitis.
**Metabolic:** hyponatremia, weight increase.
**Musculoskeletal:** muscular weakness, back pain.
**Respiratory:** *upper respiratory tract infection,* coughing, bronchitis, chest infection.
**Skin:** acne, hot flushes, purpura, rash, bruising, increased sweating.
**Other:** toothache, allergic reaction, lymphadenopathy, infection.

**INTERACTIONS**
**Drug-drug.** *Carbamazepine, valproic acid, verapamil:* May decrease level of active metabolite of oxcarbazepine. Monitor patient and level closely.
*Felodipine:* May decrease felodipine level. Monitor patient closely.
*Hormonal contraceptives:* May decrease levels of ethinyl estradiol and levonorgestrel, rendering hormonal contraceptives less effective. Women of childbearing age should use alternative forms of contraception.
*Phenobarbital:* May decrease level of active metabolite of oxcarbazepine; may increase phenobarbital level. Monitor patient closely.
*Phenytoin:* May decrease level of active metabolite of oxcarbazepine; may increase phenytoin level in adults receiving high doses of oxcarbazepine. Monitor phenytoin level closely when starting therapy in these patients.
**Drug-lifestyle.** *Alcohol use:* May increase CNS depression. Discourage use together.

**EFFECTS ON LAB TEST RESULTS**
● May decrease sodium and thyroxine levels.

**CONTRAINDICATIONS & CAUTIONS**
● Contraindicated in patients hypersensitive to drug or its components.

## NURSING CONSIDERATIONS

• *Alert:* Between 25% and 30% of patients with history of hypersensitivity reaction to carbamazepine may develop hypersensitivities to oxcarbazepine. Question patient about carbamazepine hypersensitivity and stop drug immediately if signs or symptoms of hypersensitivity occur.

• Shake oral suspension well. Suspension can be mixed with water or swallowed directly from syringe.

• Oral suspension and tablets may be interchanged at equal doses.

• *Alert:* Withdraw drug gradually to minimize potential for increased seizure frequency.

• Watch for signs and symptoms of hyponatremia, including nausea, malaise, headache, lethargy, confusion, and decreased sensation.

• Monitor sodium level in patients receiving oxcarbazepine for maintenance treatment, especially patients receiving other therapies that may decrease sodium levels.

• Oxcarbazepine use has been linked to several nervous system–related adverse reactions, including psychomotor slowing, difficulty with concentration, speech or language problems, somnolence, fatigue, and coordination abnormalities, such as ataxia and gait disturbances.

## PATIENT TEACHING

• Drug may be taken with or without food.

• Tell patient to contact prescriber before interrupting or stopping drug.

• Advise patient to report signs and symptoms of low sodium in the blood, such as nausea, malaise, headache, lethargy, and confusion.

• Caution patient to avoid driving and other potentially hazardous activities that require mental alertness until effects of drug are known.

• Instruct woman using oral contraceptives to use alternative form of contraception while taking drug.

• Tell patient to avoid alcohol while taking drug.

• Advise patient to inform prescriber if he has ever experienced hypersensitivity reaction to carbamazepine.

# phenobarbital (phenobarbitone)
Barbita, Solfoton

# phenobarbital sodium
Luminal Sodium

*Pregnancy risk category D*
*Controlled substance schedule IV*

## AVAILABLE FORMS

*Capsules:* 16 mg
*Elixir\*:* 15 mg/5 ml, 20 mg/5 ml
*Injection:* 30 mg/ml, 60 mg/ml, 65 mg/ml, 130 mg/ml
*Tablets:* 15 mg, 16 mg, 30 mg, 60 mg, 90 mg, 100 mg

## INDICATIONS & DOSAGES

➤ **Anticonvulsant, febrile seizures**
*Adults:* 60 to 100 mg P.O. daily. For acute seizures, 200 to 320 mg I.M. or I.V., repeat in 6 hours as necessary.
*Children:* 3 to 6 mg/kg P.O. daily, usually divided q 12 hours. Drug can be given once daily, usually h.s. Or, 10 to 15 mg/kg daily I.V. or I.M.

➤ **Status epilepticus**
*Adults:* 200 to 600 mg I.V.
*Children:* 15 to 20 mg/kg I.V. over 10 to 15 minutes.

➤ **Sedation**
*Adults:* 30 to 120 mg P.O., I.V. or I.M daily in two or three divided doses. Maximum dose is 400 mg/24 hours.
*Children:* 8 to 32 mg P.O.

➤ **Insomnia**
*Adults:* 100 to 200 mg P.O. or 100 to 320 mg I.M. or I.V. h.s.

➤ **Preoperative sedation**
*Adults:* 100 to 200 mg I.M. 60 to 90 minutes before surgery.
*Children:* 1 to 3 mg/kg I.V. or I.M. 60 to 90 minutes before surgery.

## I.V. ADMINISTRATION

• Don't mix parenteral form with acidic solutions; precipitation may result.

• Dilute drug in half-normal or normal saline, $D_5W$, lactated Ringer's, or Ringer's solution.

• I.V. injection is reserved for emergency treatment. Give slowly under close supervision. Monitor respirations closely. Don't give more than 60 mg/minute. Have resuscitation equipment available.

• **Alert:** Inadvertent intra-arterial injection can cause spasm of the artery and severe pain and may even lead to gangrene.

## ACTION

Unknown. A barbiturate that probably depresses monosynaptic and polysynaptic transmission in CNS and increases threshold for seizure activity in motor cortex. As a sedative, drug probably interferes with transmission of impulses from thalamus to cortex of brain.

| Route | Onset | Peak | Duration |
|-------|-------|------|----------|
| P.O. | 1 hr | 8-12 hr | 10-12 hr |
| I.V. | 5 min | 30 min | 4-10 hr |
| I.M. | > 5 min | > 30 min | 4-10 hr |

## ADVERSE REACTIONS

**CNS:** *drowsiness, lethargy, hangover,* paradoxical excitement in elderly patients, somnolence, changes in EEG patterns, physical and psychological dependence.
**CV:** *bradycardia,* hypotension, syncope.
**GI:** nausea, vomiting.
**Hematologic:** exacerbation of porphyria.
**Respiratory:** *respiratory depression, apnea.*
**Skin:** rash, *erythema multiforme, Stevens-Johnson syndrome,* urticaria, pain, swelling, thrombophlebitis, necrosis, nerve injury at injection site.
**Other:** injection site pain, *angioedema.*

## INTERACTIONS

**Drug-drug.** *Chloramphenicol, MAO inhibitors:* May potentiate barbiturate effect. Monitor patient for increased CNS and respiratory depression.
*CNS depressants, including opioid analgesics:* Excessive CNS depression. Monitor patient closely.
*Corticosteroids, digitoxin, doxycycline, estrogens and hormonal contraceptives, oral anticoagulants, tricyclic antidepressants:* May enhance metabolism of these drugs. Watch for decreased effect.
*Diazepam:* May increase effects of both drugs. Use together cautiously.
*Griseofulvin:* May decrease absorption of griseofulvin. Monitor effectiveness of griseofulvin.

*Mephobarbital, primidone:* May cause excessive phenobarbital level. Monitor patient closely.
*Metoprolol, propranolol:* May reduce the effects of these drugs. Consider an increased beta-blocker dose.
*Rifampin:* May decrease barbiturate level. Watch for decreased effect.
*Valproic acid:* May increase phenobarbital level. Watch for toxicity.
**Drug-herb.** *Evening primrose oil:* May increase anticonvulsant dosage requirement. Discourage use together.
**Drug-lifestyle.** *Alcohol use:* May cause impaired coordination, increased CNS effects, and death. Strongly discourage alcohol use with this drug.

## EFFECTS ON LAB TEST RESULTS

• May decrease bilirubin level.
• May cause false-positive phentolamine test result.

## CONTRAINDICATIONS & CAUTIONS

• Contraindicated in patients hypersensitive to barbiturates and in those with history of manifest or latent porphyria; also contraindicated in patients with hepatic or renal dysfunction, respiratory disease with dyspnea or obstruction, or nephritis.
• Use cautiously in patients with acute or chronic pain, depression, suicidal tendencies, history of drug abuse, fever, hyperthyroidism, diabetes mellitus, severe anemia, blood pressure alterations, CV disease, shock, or uremia, and in elderly or debilitated patients.

## NURSING CONSIDERATIONS

• Don't use injectable solution if it contains a precipitate.
• Give I.M. injection deeply into large muscles. Superficial injection may cause pain, sterile abscess, and tissue sloughing.
• Elderly patients are more sensitive to drug's effects; drug may produce paradoxical excitement in this population.
• Up to 30 minutes may be required for maximum effect after I.V. administration; allow time for anticonvulsant effect to develop to avoid overdose.
• **Alert:** Watch for signs of barbiturate toxicity: coma, cyanosis, asthmatic breathing, clammy skin, and hypotension. Overdose can be fatal.

• Therapeutic level is 15 to 40 mcg/ml.
• Don't stop drug abruptly because this may worsen seizures. Call prescriber immediately if adverse reactions develop.
• First withdrawal symptoms occur within 8 to 12 hours and include anxiety, muscle twitching, tremor of hands and fingers, progressive weakness, dizziness, visual distortion, nausea, vomiting, insomnia, and orthostatic hypotension. Convulsions and delirium may occur within 16 hours and last up to 5 days after abruptly stopping drug.
• Some products contain tartrazine; use cautiously in patients with aspirin sensitivity.
• EEG patterns show a change in low-voltage fast activity. Changes persist after therapy ends.
• Drug may decrease bilirubin level in neonates, patients with epilepsy, and those with congenital nonhemolytic, unconjugated hyperbilirubinemia.
• The physiologic effects of drug may impair the absorption of cyanocobalamin Co 57.
• **Alert:** Don't confuse phenobarbital with pentobarbital.

**PATIENT TEACHING**
• Ensure that patient is aware that phenobarbital is available in different milligram strengths and sizes. Advise him to check prescription and refills closely.
• Inform patient that full therapeutic effects aren't seen for 2 to 3 weeks, except when loading dose is used.
• Advise patient to avoid driving and other potentially hazardous activities that require mental alertness until drug's CNS effects are known.
• Warn patient and parents not to stop drug abruptly.
• Tell patient using hormonal contraceptives to consider alternative method because drug may decrease contraceptive effect.

# phenytoin (diphenylhydantoin)
Dilantin 125, Dilantin Infatabs

# phenytoin sodium (prompt)
Dilantin

# phenytoin sodium (extended)
Dilantin Kapseals✔, Phenytek

*Pregnancy risk category D*

**AVAILABLE FORMS**
**phenytoin**
*Oral suspension:* 125 mg/5 ml
*Tablets (chewable):* 50 mg
**phenytoin sodium (extended)**
*Capsules:* 30 mg (27.6-mg base), 100 mg (92-mg base), 200 mg (184 mg base), 300 mg (276 mg base)
**phenytoin sodium (prompt)**
*Capsules:* 100 mg (92-mg base)
*Injection:* 50 mg/ml (46-mg base)

**INDICATIONS & DOSAGES**
➤ **To control tonic-clonic (grand mal) and complex partial (temporal lobe) seizures**
*Adults:* Highly individualized. Initially, 100 mg P.O. t.i.d., increasing by 100 mg P.O. q 2 to 4 weeks until desired response is obtained. Usual range is 300 to 600 mg daily. If patient is stabilized with extended-release capsules, once-daily dosing with 300-mg extended-release capsules is possible as an alternative.
*Children:* 5 mg/kg or 250 mg/m$^2$ P.O. divided b.i.d. or t.i.d. Maximum daily dose is 300 mg.
➤ **For patient requiring a loading dose**
*Adults:* Initially, 1 g P.O. daily divided into three doses and given at 2-hour intervals. Or, 10 to 15 mg/kg I.V. at a rate not exceeding 50 mg/minute. Normal maintenance dosage is started 24 hours after loading dose.
*Children:* 500 to 600 mg in divided doses, followed by maintenance dosage 24 hours after loading dose.
➤ **To prevent and treat seizures occurring during neurosurgery**
*Adults:* 100 to 200 mg I.M. q 4 hours during and after surgery.

---

### ➤ Status epilepticus

*Adults:* Loading dose of 10 to 15 mg/kg I.V. (1 to 1.5 g may be needed) at a rate not exceeding 50 mg/minute; then maintenance dosage of 100 mg P.O. or I.V. q 6 to 8 hours.

*Children:* Loading dose of 15 to 20 mg/kg I.V., at a rate not exceeding 1 to 3 mg/kg/ minute; then highly individualized maintenance dosages.

*Elderly patients:* May need lower dosages.

### I.V. ADMINISTRATION

● Give I.V. bolus slowly (50 mg/minute).
● If giving as an infusion, don't mix drug with $D_5W$ because it will precipitate.
● Clear I.V. tubing first with normal saline solution. Never use cloudy solution.
● May mix with normal saline solution, if needed, and give as an infusion over 30 minutes to 1 hour, when possible.
● Infusion must begin within 1 hour after preparation and should run through an in-line filter.
● *Alert:* Check patency of I.V. catheter before giving. Monitor I.V. site for extravasation because it can cause severe tissue damage.
● If possible, don't give phenytoin by I.V. push into veins on back of hand, to avoid discoloration (purple-glove syndrome). Inject into larger veins or central venous catheter, if available.
● Check vital signs, blood pressure, and ECG during I.V. administration.
● Discard 4 hours after preparation.

### ACTION

Unknown. A hydantoin derivative that probably stabilizes neuronal membranes and limits seizure activity by either increasing efflux or decreasing influx of sodium ions across cell membranes in the motor cortex during generation of nerve impulses.

| Route | Onset | Peak | Duration |
|---|---|---|---|
| P.O. | Unknown | 1½-12 hr | Unknown |
| P.O. (Phenytek) | Unknown | 4-12 hr | Unknown |
| I.V. | Immediate | 1-2 hr | Unknown |
| I.M. | Unknown | Unknown | Unknown |

### ADVERSE REACTIONS

**CNS:** *ataxia, slurred speech,* dizziness, insomnia, nervousness, twitching, headache, *mental confusion, decreased coordination.*
**CV:** periarteritis nodosa.
**EENT:** *nystagmus, diplopia,* blurred vision.
**GI:** *gingival hyperplasia, nausea, vomiting,* constipation.
**Hematologic:** *thrombocytopenia, leukopenia, agranulocytosis, pancytopenia,* macrocythemia, megaloblastic anemia.
**Hepatic:** *toxic hepatitis.*
**Metabolic:** hyperglycemia.
**Musculoskeletal:** osteomalacia.
**Skin:** scarlatiniform or morbilliform rash, bullous or purpuric dermatitis, exfoliative dermatitis, *Stevens-Johnson syndrome,* lupus erythematosus, *toxic epidermal necrolysis,* photosensitivity reactions, discoloration of skin if given by I.V. push in back of hand; hypertrichosis, pain, necrosis, inflammation at injection site.
**Other:** *hirsutism,* lymphadenopathy.

### INTERACTIONS

**Drug-drug.** *Amiodarone, antihistamines, chloramphenicol, cimetidine, cycloserine, diazepam, isoniazid, metronidazole, omeprazole, phenylbutazone, salicylates, sulfamethizole, valproate:* May increase phenytoin activity and toxicity. Monitor patient.

*Atracurium, cisatracurium, doxacurium, mivacurium, pancuronium, rocuronium, tubocurarine, vecuronium:* May decrease the effects of nondepolarizing muscle relaxant, causing it to be less effective. May need to increase the dose of the nondepolarizing muscle relaxant.

*Barbiturates, carbamazepine, dexamethasone, diazoxide, folic acid, rifampin:* May decrease phenytoin activity. Monitor level.

*Carbamazepine, cardiac glycosides, hormonal contraceptives, quinidine, theophylline, valproic acid:* May decrease effects of these drugs. Monitor patient.

*Disulfiram:* May increase toxic effects of phenytoin. Monitor phenytoin level closely and adjust dose as necessary.

**Drug-food.** *Enteral tube feedings:* May interfere with absorption of oral phenytoin. Stop enteral feedings for 2 hours be-

fore and 2 hours after phenytoin administration.
**Drug-lifestyle.** *Long-term alcohol use:*
May decrease phenytoin activity. Inform patient that heavy alcohol use may diminish drug's benefits.

## EFFECTS ON LAB TEST RESULTS
• May increase alkaline phosphatase, GGT, and glucose levels. May decrease urinary 17-hydroxysteroid and 17-ketosteroid levels.
• May increase urine 6-hydroxycortisol excretion. May decrease hemoglobin, hematocrit, and platelet, WBC, RBC, and granulocyte counts.
• May cause falsely reduced protein-bound iodine and free thyroxine levels. May cause decreased dexamethasone suppression and metyrapone test results.

## CONTRAINDICATIONS & CAUTIONS
• Contraindicated in patients hypersensitive to hydantoin and in those with sinus bradycardia, SA block, second- or third-degree AV block, or Adams-Stokes syndrome.
• Use cautiously in patients with hepatic dysfunction, hypotension, myocardial insufficiency, diabetes, or respiratory depression; in elderly or debilitated patients; and in those receiving other hydantoin derivatives.
• Elderly patients tend to metabolize phenytoin slowly and may need reduced dosages.

## NURSING CONSIDERATIONS
• Phenytoin requirements usually increase during pregnancy.
• Use only clear solution for injection. A slight yellow color is acceptable. Don't refrigerate.
• Don't give I.M. unless dosage adjustments are made; drug may precipitate at injection site, cause pain, and be absorbed erratically.
• Divided doses given with or after meals may decrease adverse GI reactions.
• Stop drug if rash appears. If rash is scarlatiniform or morbilliform, resume drug after rash clears. If rash reappears, stop therapy. If rash is exfoliative, purpuric, or bullous, don't resume drug.

• Don't stop drug suddenly because this may worsen seizures. Call prescriber at once if adverse reactions develop.
• Monitor drug level in blood. Therapeutic level is 10 to 20 mcg/ml.
• Allow at least 7 to 10 days to elapse between dosage changes.
• Monitor CBC and calcium level every 6 months, and periodically monitor hepatic function. If megaloblastic anemia is evident, prescriber may order folic acid and vitamin $B_{12}$.
• If using to treat seizures, take appropriate safety precautions.
• Mononucleosis may decrease phenytoin level. Watch for increased seizures.
• Watch for gingival hyperplasia, especially in children.
• *Alert:* Doubling the dose doesn't result in twice initial serum levels but may result in toxic serum levels. Consult pharmacist for specific dosing recommendations.
• If seizure control is established with divided doses, once-a-day dosing may be considered.
• *Alert:* Don't confuse phenytoin with mephenytoin or fosphenytoin or Dilantin with Dilaudid.

## PATIENT TEACHING
• Tell patient to notify prescriber if skin rash develops.
• Advise patient to avoid driving and other potentially hazardous activities that require mental alertness until drug's CNS effects are known.
• Advise patient not to change brands or dosage forms once he's stabilized on therapy.
• Dilantin capsules are the only oral form that can be given once daily. Toxic levels may result if any other brand or form is given once daily. Dilantin tablets and oral suspension should never be taken once daily.
• Tell patient not to use capsules that are discolored.
• Advise patient to avoid alcohol.
• Warn patient and parents not to stop drug abruptly.
• Stress importance of good oral hygiene and regular dental examinations. Surgical removal of excess gum tissue may be needed periodically if dental hygiene is poor.

---

Reactions may be *common,* uncommon, *life-threatening,* or COMMON AND LIFE-THREATENING.

• Caution patient that drug may color urine pink, red, or reddish brown.

# primidone
Apo-Primidone†, Mysoline, PMS Primidone†, Sertan†

*Pregnancy risk category NR*

## AVAILABLE FORMS
*Oral suspension:* 250 mg/5 ml
*Tablets:* 50 mg, 250 mg

## INDICATIONS & DOSAGES
➤ **Tonic-clonic, complex partial, and simple partial seizures**
*Adults and children age 8 and older:* Initially, 100 to 125 mg P.O. h.s. on days 1 to 3; then 100 to 125 mg P.O. b.i.d. on days 4 to 6; then 100 to 125 mg P.O. t.i.d. on days 7 to 9, followed by maintenance dose of 250 mg P.O. t.i.d. Maintenance dose may be increased to 250 mg q.i.d., if needed. Dosage may be increased to maximum of 2 g daily in divided doses.
*Children younger than age 8:* Initially, 50 mg P.O. h.s. for 3 days; then 50 mg P.O. b.i.d. for days 4 to 6; then 100 mg P.O. b.i.d. for days 7 to 9, followed by maintenance dose of 125 to 250 mg P.O. t.i.d. or 10 to 25 mg/kg daily in divided doses.
➤ **Essential tremor** ♦
*Adults:* 750 mg P.O. daily.

## ACTION
Unknown. Some activity may be caused by phenylethylmalonamide and phenobarbital, which are active metabolites.

| Route | Onset | Peak | Duration |
|-------|-------|------|----------|
| P.O. | Unknown | 3-4 hr | Unknown |

## ADVERSE REACTIONS
**CNS:** *drowsiness, ataxia,* emotional disturbances, vertigo, hyperirritability, fatigue, paranoid symptoms.
**EENT:** *diplopia,* nystagmus.
**GI:** anorexia, *nausea, vomiting.*
**GU:** impotence, polyuria.
**Hematologic:** megaloblastic anemia, *thrombocytopenia.*
**Skin:** morbilliform rash.

## INTERACTIONS
**Drug-drug.** *Acetazolamide, succinimide:* May decrease primidone level. Monitor level.
*Carbamazepine:* May increase carbamazepine level and decrease primidone and phenobarbital levels. Watch for toxicity.
*Isoniazid:* May increase primidone level. Monitor level.
*Metoprolol, propranolol:* May reduce effects of these drugs. Consider increasing beta-blocker dose.
*Phenytoin:* May stimulate conversion of primidone to phenobarbital. Watch for increased phenobarbital effect.
**Drug-lifestyle.** *Alcohol use:* May impair coordination, increase CNS effects, and cause death. Strongly discourage alcohol use with this drug.

## EFFECTS ON LAB TEST RESULTS
• May decrease hemoglobin and platelet count. May alter liver function test values.

## CONTRAINDICATIONS & CAUTIONS
• Contraindicated in patients hypersensitive to phenobarbital and in those with porphyria.

## NURSING CONSIDERATIONS
• Shake liquid suspension well.
• Don't withdraw drug suddenly because seizures may worsen. Notify prescriber immediately if adverse reactions develop.
• Therapeutic level of primidone is 5 to 12 mcg/ml. Therapeutic level of phenobarbital is 15 to 40 mcg/ml.
• Monitor CBC and routine blood chemistry every 6 months.
• Brand interchange isn't recommended because of documented bioequivalence problems for primidone products marketed by different manufacturers.
• *Alert:* Don't confuse primidone with prednisone or Prinivil.

## PATIENT TEACHING
• Advise patient to avoid driving and other potentially hazardous activities that require mental alertness until drug's CNS effects are known.
• Warn patient and parents not to stop drug therapy suddenly.

• Tell patient that full therapeutic response may take 2 weeks or longer.
• Advise woman to discuss drug therapy with prescriber if she's considering pregnancy.
• Caution woman that breast-feeding is contraindicated while taking this drug.

---

## tiagabine hydrochloride
Gabitril

*Pregnancy risk category C*

---

### AVAILABLE FORMS
*Tablets:* 4 mg, 12 mg, 16 mg, 20 mg

### INDICATIONS & DOSAGES
➤ **Adjunctive treatment of partial seizures**
*Adults:* Initially, 4 mg P.O. once daily. Total daily dose may be increased by 4 to 8 mg at weekly intervals until clinical response or up to 56 mg/day. Give total daily dose in divided doses b.i.d. to q.i.d.
*Children ages 12 to 18:* Initially, 4 mg P.O. once daily. Total daily dose may be increased by 4 mg at beginning of week 2 and thereafter by 4 to 8 mg/week until clinical response or up to 32 mg/day. Give total daily dose in divided doses b.i.d. to q.i.d.
*Adjust-a-dose:* For patients with hepatic impairment, reduce first and maintenance doses or increase dosing intervals.

### ACTION
Unknown. May act by facilitating the effects of the inhibitory neurotransmitter gamma-aminobutyric acid (GABA). Drug binds to recognition sites associated with the GABA uptake carrier and may thus make more GABA available for binding to receptors on postsynaptic cells.

| Route | Onset | Peak | Duration |
|-------|-------|------|----------|
| P.O. | Rapid | 45 min | 7-9 hr |

### ADVERSE REACTIONS
**CNS:** *dizziness, asthenia, somnolence, nervousness,* tremor, difficulty with concentration and attention, insomnia, ataxia, confusion, speech disorder, difficulty with memory, paresthesia, depression, emo-

tional lability, abnormal gait, hostility, language problems, agitation.
**CV:** vasodilation.
**EENT:** nystagmus, pharyngitis.
**GI:** abdominal pain, *nausea,* diarrhea, vomiting, increased appetite, mouth ulceration.
**Musculoskeletal:** generalized weakness, pain, myasthenia.
**Respiratory:** increased cough.
**Skin:** rash, pruritus.

### INTERACTIONS
**Drug-drug.** *Carbamazepine, phenobarbital, phenytoin:* May increase tiagabine clearance. Monitor patient closely.
*CNS depressants:* May enhance CNS effects. Use together cautiously.
**Drug-lifestyle.** *Alcohol use:* May enhance CNS effects. Discourage use together.

### EFFECTS ON LAB TEST RESULTS
None reported.

### CONTRAINDICATIONS & CAUTIONS
• Contraindicated in patients hypersensitive to drug or its components.
• Use cautiously in breast-feeding women.

### NURSING CONSIDERATIONS
• Never withdraw drug suddenly because seizures may occur more frequently. Withdraw drug gradually unless safety concerns require a more rapid withdrawal.
• *Alert:* Status epilepticus and sudden unexpected death in epilepsy have occurred in patients receiving antiepileptics, including tiagabine.
• *Alert:* Don't confuse tiagabine with tizanidine; both have 4-mg starting doses.
• Patients who aren't receiving at least one enzyme-inducing antiepileptic when starting tiagabine may need lower doses or dosages adjusted more slowly.
• Moderately severe to incapacitating generalized weakness has occurred in patients receiving tiagabine. Weakness resolves after reducing dosages or stopping drug.

### PATIENT TEACHING
• Advise patient to take drug only as prescribed.
• Tell patient to take drug with food.
• Warn patient that drug may cause dizziness, somnolence, and other signs and

---

symptoms of CNS depression. Advise patient to avoid driving and other potentially hazardous activities that require mental alertness until drug's CNS effects are known.
• Tell woman to call prescriber if she becomes pregnant or plans to become pregnant during therapy.
• Instruct woman to notify prescriber if she's planning to breast-feed because drug may appear in breast milk.

---

## topiramate
Topamax

*Pregnancy risk category C*

### AVAILABLE FORMS
*Capsules, sprinkles:* 15 mg, 25 mg, 50 mg
*Tablets:* 25 mg, 100 mg, 200 mg

### INDICATIONS & DOSAGES
➤ **Adjunct treatment for partial onset seizures; Lennox-Gastaut syndrome in children**
*Adults:* Initially, 25 to 50 mg P.O. daily; increase gradually by 25 to 50 mg/week until an effective daily dose is reached. Adjust up to maximum daily dose of 400 mg P.O. in two divided doses.
*Children ages 2 to 16:* 5 to 9 mg/kg P.O. daily in two divided doses. Increase dosage by 1 to 3 mg/kg nightly for 1 week. Then increase at 1- or 2-week intervals by 1 to 3 mg/kg daily in two divided doses to achieve optimal response.
➤ **Adjunct treatment for primary generalized tonic-clonic seizures**
*Adults:* 50 mg P.O. daily in evening for first week; then adjust to maximum daily dose of 400 mg given in two divided doses. Adjustment schedule is as follows: Week 1, give 50 mg P.O. in evening; week 2, give 50 mg P.O. b.i.d. (in morning and evening); week 3, give 50 mg P.O. in morning and 100 mg P.O. in evening; week 4, give 100 mg P.O. b.i.d. (in morning and evening); week 5, give 100 mg P.O. in morning and 150 mg P.O. in evening; week 6, give 150 mg P.O. b.i.d. (in morning and evening); week 7, give 150 mg P.O. in morning and 200 mg P.O. in evening; week 8, give 200 mg P.O. b.i.d. (in morning and evening).

*Children ages 2 to 16:* 5 to 9 mg/kg P.O. daily in two divided doses. Increase dosage by 1 to 3 mg/kg nightly for 1 week. Then increase at 1- or 2-week intervals by 1 to 3 mg/kg daily to achieve optimal response.
*Adjust-a-dose:* For patients with creatinine clearance less than 70 ml/minute, reduce dosage by 50%. For patients on hemodialysis, may need to give supplemental doses to avoid rapid drops in drug level during prolonged dialysis treatment.

### ACTION
Unknown. May block a sodium channel, potentiate the activity of gamma-aminobutyrate, and antagonize the ability of kainate to activate an excitatory amino acid (glutamate) receptor.

| Route | Onset | Peak | Duration |
| --- | --- | --- | --- |
| P.O. | Unknown | 2 hr | Unknown |

### ADVERSE REACTIONS
**CNS:** fever, abnormal coordination, aggressive reaction, agitation, apathy, asthenia, *ataxia, confusion,* depression, depersonalization, *difficulty with memory, dizziness,* emotional lability, euphoria, *generalized tonic-clonic seizures,* hallucination, hyperkinesia, hypertonia, hypoesthesia, hypokinesia, insomnia, mood problems, *nervousness, paresthesia,* personality disorder, *psychomotor slowing,* psychosis, *somnolence, speech disorders,* stupor, *suicide attempts, tremor,* vertigo, malaise, *fatigue,* or difficulty with concentration, attention, or language.
**CV:** chest pain, palpitations, vasodilation, edema.
**EENT:** *abnormal vision,* conjunctivitis, *diplopia,* eye pain, epistaxis, hearing problems, tinnitus, pharyngitis, sinusitis, *nystagmus.*
**GI:** abdominal pain, *anorexia,* constipation, diarrhea, dry mouth, dyspepsia, flatulence, gastroenteritis, gingivitis, *nausea,* vomiting, taste perversion.
**GU:** amenorrhea, dysuria, dysmenorrhea, hematuria, impotence, intermenstrual bleeding, menstrual disorder, menorrhagia, urinary frequency, renal calculi, urinary incontinence, UTI, vaginitis, leukorrhea.
**Hematologic:** anemia, *leukopenia.*

**Metabolic:** increased or *decreased weight.*
**Musculoskeletal:** arthralgia, back or leg pain, muscle weakness, myalgia, rigors.
**Respiratory:** bronchitis, coughing, dyspnea, *upper respiratory tract infection.*
**Skin:** acne, alopecia, increased sweating, pruritus, rash.
**Other:** decreased libido, breast pain, body odor, flulike syndrome, hot flashes, lymphadenopathy.

**INTERACTIONS**
**Drug-drug.** *Carbamazepine:* May decrease topiramate level. Monitor patient.
*Carbonic anhydrase inhibitors (acetazolamide, dichlorphenamide):* May cause renal calculus formation. Avoid using together.
*CNS depressants:* May cause topiramate-induced CNS depression as well as other adverse cognitive and neuropsychiatric events. Use together cautiously.
*Hormonal contraceptives:* May decrease efficacy. Report changes in menstrual patterns. Advise patient to use another contraceptive method.
*Phenytoin:* May decrease topiramate level and increase phenytoin level. Monitor levels.
*Valproic acid:* May decrease valproic acid and topiramate level. Monitor patient.
**Drug-lifestyle.** *Alcohol use:* May cause topiramate-induced CNS depression as well as other adverse cognitive and neuropsychiatric events. Discourage use together.

**EFFECTS ON LAB TEST RESULTS**
● May increase liver enzyme levels.
● May decrease hemoglobin, hematocrit, and WBC count.

**CONTRAINDICATIONS & CAUTIONS**
● Contraindicated in patients hypersensitive to drug or its components.
● Use with caution in breast-feeding or pregnant women and in those with hepatic impairment. Use cautiously in combination with other drugs that predispose patients to heat-related disorders, including other carbonic anhydrase inhibitors and anticholinergics.

**NURSING CONSIDERATIONS**
● If needed, withdraw antiepileptics (including topiramate) gradually to minimize risk of increased seizure activity.
● Monitoring topiramate level isn't necessary.
● Oligohidrosis and hyperthermia have been infrequently reported, mainly in pediatric patients taking topiramate. Monitor patient closely, especially in hot weather.
● Drug is rapidly cleared by dialysis. A prolonged period of dialysis may result in low drug levels and seizures. A supplemental dose may be needed.
● Stop drug if an ocular adverse event occurs, characterized by acute myopia and secondary angle closure glaucoma.
● *Alert:* Don't confuse Topamax with Toprol-XL.

**PATIENT TEACHING**
● Tell patient to drink plenty of fluids during therapy to minimize risk of forming kidney stones.
● Advise patient not to drive or operate hazardous machinery until CNS effects of drug are known. Drug can cause sleepiness, dizziness, confusion, and concentration problems.
● Tell woman that drug may decrease effectiveness of hormonal contraceptives. Advise woman taking hormonal contraceptives to report change in her menstrual patterns.
● Tell patient to avoid crushing or breaking tablets because of bitter taste.
● Inform patient that drug can be taken without regard to food.
● Tell patient that capsules may either be swallowed whole or carefully opened and contents sprinkled on a teaspoonful of soft food. Tell patient to swallow immediately without chewing.
● Tell patient to notify the doctor immediately if he experiences changes in vision.

## valproate sodium
Depacon, Depakene, Epilim‡,
Valpro‡

## valproic acid
Depakene

## divalproex sodium
Depakote✐, Depakote ER,
Depakote Sprinkle✐, Epival†

*Pregnancy risk category D*

## AVAILABLE FORMS
**valproate sodium**
*Injection:* 100 mg/ml
*Syrup:* 250 mg/5 ml
**valproic acid**
*Capsules:* 250 mg
*Syrup:* 200 mg/5 ml‡
*Tablets (crushable):* 100 mg‡
*Tablets (enteric-coated):* 200 mg‡,
500 mg‡
**divalproex sodium**
*Capsules (containing coated particles):*
125 mg
*Tablets (delayed-release):* 125 mg,
250 mg, 500 mg
*Tablets (extended-release):* 250 mg,
500 mg

## INDICATIONS & DOSAGES
➤ **Simple and complex absence sei-
zures, mixed seizure types (including
absence seizures)**
*Adults and children:* Initially, 15 mg/kg
P.O. or I.V. daily; then increase by 5 to
10 mg/kg daily at weekly intervals up to
maximum of 60 mg/kg daily. Don't use
Depakote ER in children younger than 10.
➤ **Complex partial seizures**
*Adults and children age 10 and older:*
10 to 15 mg/kg Depakote or Depakote ER
P.O. or valproate sodium I.V. daily; then
increase by 5 to 10 mg/kg daily at weekly
intervals, up to 60 mg/kg daily.
➤ **Mania**
*Adults:* Initially, 750 mg delayed-release
divalproex sodium daily in divided doses.
Adjust dosage based on patient's response;
maximum dose is 60 mg/kg daily.
➤ **To prevent migraine headache**
*Adults:* Initially, 250 mg delayed-release
divalproex sodium P.O. b.i.d. Some pa-

tients may need up to 1,000 mg/day. Or,
500 mg Depakote ER P.O. daily for 1
week; then 1,000 mg P.O. daily.
*Adjust-a-dose:* For elderly patients, start
at lower dosage. Increase dosage more
slowly and with regular monitoring of fluid and nutritional intake, and watch for dehydration, somnolence, and other adverse
reactions.

## I.V. ADMINISTRATION
● I.V. use is indicated only in patients who
can't take drug orally. Switch patient to
oral form as soon as feasible; effects of
using I.V. dosage for longer than 14 days
are unknown.
● Dilute valproate sodium injection with at
least 50 ml of a compatible diluent. It's
physically compatible and chemically stable in $D_5W$, normal saline, and lactated
Ringer's solution for 24 hours.
● Give drug as a 60-minute I.V. infusion
(but not more than 20 mg/minute) with the
same frequency as oral dosage.
● Monitoring of drug levels and dosage
adjustment may be needed.

## ACTION
Unknown. Probably facilitates the effects
of the inhibitory neurotransmitter gamma-
aminobutyric acid.

| Route | Onset | Peak | Duration |
|-------|-------|------|----------|
| P.O. | Unknown | 15 min-4 hr | Unknown |
| I.V. | Unknown | 1 hr | Unknown |

## ADVERSE REACTIONS
**CNS:** *insomnia, nervousness, somnolence,*
abnormal thinking, amnesia, emotional
upset, depression, *tremor,* ataxia, *headache, dizziness, asthenia,* fever.
**CV:** chest pain, hypertension, hypoten-
sion, tachycardia, edema.
**EENT:** nystagmus, *diplopia, blurred
vision,* rhinitis, pharyngitis, tinnitus.
**GI:** *nausea, vomiting, diarrhea, abdomi-
nal pain, dyspepsia,* constipation, in-
creased appetite, *anorexia,* **pancreatitis.**
**Hematologic:** petechiae, bruising, ***hemor-
rhage, bone marrow suppression.***
**Hepatic:** *hepatotoxicity.*
**Metabolic:** weight gain or loss.
**Musculoskeletal:** back and neck pain.
**Respiratory:** bronchitis, dyspnea.

**Skin:** rash, *alopecia,* pruritus, photosensitivity, *erythema multiforme, Stevens-Johnson syndrome, hypersensitivity reactions,* flu syndrome, infection.

## INTERACTIONS

**Drug-drug.** *Aspirin, chlorpromazine, cimetidine, erythromycin, felbamate:* May cause valproic acid toxicity. Use together cautiously and monitor drug level.

*Benzodiazepines, other CNS depressants:* May cause excessive CNS depression. Avoid using together.

*Carbamazepine:* May cause carbamazepine CNS toxicity; may decrease valproic acid level. Use together cautiously, if at all.

*Lamotrigine:* May increase lamotrigine level; may decrease valproate level. Monitor levels closely.

*Phenobarbital:* May increase phenobarbital level; may increase clearance of valproate. Monitor patient closely.

*Phenytoin:* May increase or decrease phenytoin level; may decrease valproate level. Monitor patient closely.

*Rifampin:* May decrease valproate level. Monitor level.

*Warfarin:* May displace warfarin from binding sites. Monitor PT and INR.

*Zidovudine:* May decrease zidovudine clearance. Avoid using together.

**Drug-lifestyle.** *Alcohol use:* Excessive CNS depression. Discourage use together.

## EFFECTS ON LAB TEST RESULTS

- May increase ALT, AST, and bilirubin levels.
- May increase eosinophil count and bleeding time. May decrease platelet, RBC, and WBC counts.
- May cause false-positive results for urine ketone levels.

## CONTRAINDICATIONS & CAUTIONS

- Contraindicated in patients hypersensitive to drug and in those with hepatic disease or significant hepatic dysfunction, and in patients with a urea cycle disorder (UCD).
- Safety and efficacy of Depakote ER in children younger than age 10 haven't been established.

## NURSING CONSIDERATIONS

- Obtain liver function test results, platelet count, and PT and INR before starting therapy, and monitor these values periodically.
- Don't give syrup to patients who need sodium restriction. Check with prescriber.
- Adverse reactions may not be caused by valproic acid alone because it's usually used with other anticonvulsants.
- When converting adults and children age 10 and older with seizures from Depakote to Depakote ER, make sure the extended-release dose is 8% to 20% higher than the regular dose taken previously. See manufacturer's package insert for more details.
- Divalproex sodium has a lower risk of adverse GI reactions.
- Never withdraw drug suddenly because sudden withdrawal may worsen seizures. Call prescriber at once if adverse reactions develop.
- *Alert:* Serious or fatal hepatotoxicity may follow nonspecific symptoms, such as malaise, fever, and lethargy. If these symptoms occur, notify prescriber at once because drug will need to be stopped in the presence of suspected or apparent substantial hepatic dysfunction.
- Patients at high risk for hepatotoxicity include those with congenital metabolic disorders, mental retardation, or organic brain disease; those taking multiple anticonvulsants; and children younger than age 2.
- Notify prescriber if tremors occur; a dosage reduction may be needed.
- Monitor drug level. Therapeutic level is 50 to 100 mcg/ml.
- Use caution when converting patients from a brand-name drug to a generic drug because breakthrough seizures are possible.
- *Alert:* Sometimes fatal, hyperammonemic encephalopathy, may occur when starting valproate therapy in patients with UCD, a group of uncommon genetic abnormalities (particularly ornithine transcarbamylase deficiency). Evaluate patients with UCD risk factors before starting valproate therapy. Patients who develop symptoms of unexplained hyperammonemic encephalopathy during valproate therapy should stop drug, undergo

prompt appropriate treatment, and be evaluated for underlying UCD.

## PATIENT TEACHING
• Tell patient to take drug with food or milk to reduce adverse GI effects.
• Advise patient not to chew capsules; irritation of mouth and throat may result.
• Tell patient that capsules may be either swallowed whole or carefully opened and contents sprinkled on a teaspoonful of soft food. Tell patient to swallow immediately without chewing.
• Tell patient and parents that syrup shouldn't be mixed with carbonated beverages; mixture may be irritating to mouth and throat.
• Tell patient and parents to keep drug out of children's reach.
• Warn patient and parents not to stop drug therapy abruptly.
• Advise patient to avoid driving and other potentially hazardous activities that require mental alertness until drug's CNS effects are known.
• Instruct patient or parents to call prescriber if malaise, weakness, lethargy, facial swelling, loss of appetite, or vomiting occurs.
• Tell woman to call prescriber if she becomes pregnant or plans to become pregnant during therapy.

## zonisamide
Zonegran

*Pregnancy risk category C*

## AVAILABLE FORMS
*Capsules:* 100 mg

## INDICATIONS & DOSAGES
➤ **Adjunct therapy for partial seizures in adults with epilepsy**
*Adults and children older than age 16:* Initially, 100 mg P.O. as a single daily dose for 2 weeks. Then, dosage may be increased to 200 mg/day for at least 2 weeks. Dosage can be increased to 300 mg and 400 mg P.O. daily, with the dose stable for at least 2 weeks to achieve steady state at each level. Doses can be given once or twice daily except for the

daily dose of 100 mg at start of therapy. Maximum dose is 600 mg/day.

## ACTION
Unknown. May stabilize neuronal membranes and suppress neuronal hypersynchronization, which prevents seizures.

| Route | Onset | Peak | Duration |
|-------|-------|------|----------|
| P.O. | Unknown | 2-6 hr | Unknown |

## ADVERSE REACTIONS
**CNS:** *headache, dizziness,* ataxia, nystagmus, paresthesia, confusion, difficulties in concentration or memory, mental slowing, agitation or irritability, depression, insomnia, anxiety, nervousness, schizophrenic or schizophreniform behavior, *somnolence,* fatigue, asthenia, speech disorders, difficulties in verbal expression, hyperesthesia, incoordination, tremor, *seizures, status epilepticus.*
**EENT:** taste perversion, diplopia, amblyopia, tinnitus, rhinitis, pharyngitis.
**GI:** *anorexia,* nausea, vomiting, diarrhea, dyspepsia, constipation, dry mouth, abdominal pain.
**GU:** kidney stones.
**Hematologic:** ecchymoses.
**Metabolic:** weight loss.
**Respiratory:** cough.
**Skin:** rash, pruritus.
**Other:** flulike syndrome, accidental injury.

## INTERACTIONS
**Drug-drug.** *Drugs that induce or inhibit CYP 3A4:* Alters levels of zonisamide. Clearance of zonisamide is increased by phenytoin, carbamazepine, phenobarbital, and valproate. Monitor patient closely.

## EFFECTS ON LAB TEST RESULTS
• May increase BUN and creatinine levels.

## CONTRAINDICATIONS & CAUTIONS
• Contraindicated in patients hypersensitive to drug or to sulfonamides.
• Contraindicated in those with glomerular filtration rate less than 50 ml/minute.
• Use cautiously in patients with renal and hepatic dysfunction.
• Use cautiously with other drugs that predispose patients to heat-related disorders, including but not limited to carbonic an-

---

hydrase inhibitors and drugs with anticholinergic activity.
- Safety and efficacy in children younger
than age 16 haven't been established.
Children are at an increased risk for oligohidrosis and hyperthermia caused by zonisamide.

## NURSING CONSIDERATIONS
- *Alert:* Rarely, patients receiving sulfonamides have died because of severe reactions such as Stevens-Johnson syndrome,
fulminant hepatic necrosis, aplastic anemia, otherwise unexplained rashes, and
agranulocytosis. If signs and symptoms of
hypersensitivity or other serious reactions
occur, stop drug immediately and notify
prescriber.
- If patient develops acute renal failure or
a significant sustained increase in creatinine or BUN level, stop drug and notify
prescriber.
- Achieving steady-state levels may take
2 weeks.
- Monitor patient for signs and symptoms
of hypersensitivity.
- Don't stop drug abruptly because this
may cause increased seizures or status
epilepticus; reduce dosage or stop drug
gradually.
- Increase fluid intake and urine output to
help prevent kidney stones, especially in
patients with predisposing factors.
- Monitor renal function periodically.

## PATIENT TEACHING
- Tell patient to take drug with or without
food and not to bite or break capsule.
- Advise patient to call prescriber immediately if rash develops or seizures worsen.
- Tell patient to contact prescriber immediately if he develops sudden back or abdominal pain, pain when urinating, bloody
or dark urine, fever, sore throat, mouth
sores or easy bruising, decreased sweating, fever, depression, or speech or language problems.
- Tell patient to drink 6 to 8 glasses of
water a day.
- Caution patient that this drug can cause
drowsiness and not to drive or operate
dangerous machinery until drug's effects
are known.
- Advise patient not to stop taking drug
without prescriber's approval.

- Instruct woman to call prescriber if she
is pregnant or breast-feeding or plans to
become pregnant or breast-feed.
- Advise woman of childbearing potential
to use contraceptives while taking drug.

---

Reactions may be *common*, uncommon, *life-threatening*, or COMMON AND LIFE-THREATENING.

amitriptyline hydrochloride
amitriptyline pamoate
bupropion hydrochloride
citalopram hydrobromide
clomipramine hydrochloride
desipramine hydrochloride
doxepin hydrochloride
escitalopram
fluoxetine hydrochloride
imipramine hydrochloride
imipramine pamoate
mirtazapine
nefazodone hydrochloride
nortriptyline hydrochloride
paroxetine hydrochloride
phenelzine sulfate
sertraline hydrochloride
tranylcypromine sulfate
trazodone hydrochloride
venlafaxine hydrochloride

## COMBINATION PRODUCTS
ETRAFON: perphenazine 2 mg and
amitriptyline hydrochloride 25 mg.
ETRAFON 2-10: perphenazine 2 mg and
amitriptyline hydrochloride 10 mg.
ETRAFON-A: perphenazine 4 mg and
amitriptyline hydrochloride 10 mg.
ETRAFON-FORTE: perphenazine 4 mg and
amitriptyline hydrochloride 25 mg.
LIMBITROL DS: chlordiazepoxide 10 mg
and amitriptyline hydrochloride 25 mg.
TRIAVIL 2-10: perphenazine 2 mg and
amitriptyline hydrochloride 10 mg.
TRIAVIL 4-10: perphenazine 4 mg and
amitriptyline hydrochloride 10 mg.
TRIAVIL 2-25: perphenazine 2 mg and
amitriptyline hydrochloride 25 mg.
TRIAVIL 4-25: perphenazine 4 mg and
amitriptyline hydrochloride 25 mg.

## amitriptyline hydrochloride
Apo-Amitriptyline†, Endep,
Levate†, Novotriptyn†, Tryptanol‡,
Tryptine‡

## amitriptyline pamoate
Elavil Plus†

*Pregnancy risk category C*

## AVAILABLE FORMS
**amitriptyline hydrochloride**
*Injection:* 10 mg/ml
*Tablets:* 10 mg, 25 mg, 50 mg, 75 mg,
100 mg, 150 mg
**amitriptyline pamoate†**
*Syrup:* 10 mg/5 ml*†

## INDICATIONS & DOSAGES
➤ **Depression**
*Adults:* Initially, 50 to 100 mg P.O. h.s.,
increasing to 150 mg daily. Maximum,
300 mg daily, if needed. Maintenance,
50 to 100 mg daily. Or, 20 to 30 mg I.M.
q.i.d.
*Elderly patients and adolescents:* 10 mg
P.O. t.i.d. and 20 mg h.s. daily.

## ACTION
Unknown. A tricyclic antidepressant that
increases the amount of norepinephrine,
serotonin, or both in the CNS by blocking
their reuptake by the presynaptic neurons.

| Route | Onset | Peak | Duration |
|-------|-------|------|----------|
| P.O., I.M. | Unknown | 2-12 hr | Unknown |

## ADVERSE REACTIONS
**CNS:** ataxia, tremor, peripheral neuropathy, anxiety, insomnia, restlessness,
drowsiness, dizziness, weakness, fatigue,
headache, extrapyramidal reactions, *coma,
seizures, CVA,* hallucinations, delusions,
disorientation.
**CV:** *orthostatic hypotension, tachycardia,*
ECG changes, hypertension, edema, *MI,
arrhythmias, heart block.*
**EENT:** blurred vision, tinnitus, mydriasis,
increased intraocular pressure.

---

**GI:** *dry mouth,* nausea, vomiting, anorexia, epigastric pain, diarrhea, constipation, paralytic ileus.
**GU:** urine retention.
**Hematologic:** *agranulocytosis, thrombocytopenia, leukopenia,* eosinophilia.
**Metabolic:** *hypoglycemia,* hyperglycemia.
**Skin:** rash, urticaria, photosensitivity reactions, diaphoresis.
**Other:** hypersensitivity reactions.

## INTERACTIONS
**Drug-drug.** *Barbiturates, CNS depressants:* May enhance CNS depression. Avoid using together.
*Cimetidine, fluoxetine, fluvoxamine, hormonal contraceptives, paroxetine, sertraline:* May increase tricyclic antidepressant level. Watch for increased antidepressant adverse effects.
*Clonidine:* May cause potentially life-threatening elevations in blood pressure. Avoid using together.
*Epinephrine, norepinephrine:* May increase hypertensive effect. Use together cautiously.
*MAO inhibitors:* May cause severe excitation, hyperpyrexia, or seizures, usually with high doses. Avoid using within 14 days of MAO inhibitor therapy.
**Drug-herb.** *Evening primrose:* May cause additive or synergistic effect, resulting in lower seizure threshold and increasing the risk of seizures. Discourage use together.
*St. John's wort, SAM-e, yohimbe:* May cause serotonin syndrome and decrease amitriptyline level. Discourage use together.
**Drug-lifestyle.** *Alcohol use:* May enhance CNS depression. Discourage use together.
*Smoking:* May lower drug level. Watch for lack of effect.
*Sun exposure:* May increase risk of photosensitivity reactions. Advise patient to avoid excessive sunlight exposure.

## EFFECTS ON LAB TEST RESULTS
• May increase or decrease glucose level.
• May increase eosinophil count and liver function test values. May decrease granulocyte, platelet, and WBC counts.

## CONTRAINDICATIONS & CAUTIONS
• Contraindicated in patients hypersensitive to drug and in those who have received an MAO inhibitor within the past 14 days.
• Contraindicated during acute recovery phase of MI.
• Use cautiously in patients with history of seizures, urine retention, angle-closure glaucoma, or increased intraocular pressure; in those with hyperthyroidism, CV disease, diabetes, or impaired liver function; and in those receiving thyroid drugs.
• Use with caution in those receiving electroconvulsive therapy.

## NURSING CONSIDERATIONS
• *Alert:* Parenteral form of drug is for I.M. administration only. Drug shouldn't be given I.V.
• Amitriptyline has strong anticholinergic effects and is one of the most sedating tricyclic antidepressants. Anticholinergic effects have rapid onset even though therapeutic effect is delayed for weeks.
• If signs or symptoms of psychosis occur or increase, expect prescriber to reduce dosage. Record mood changes. Monitor patient for suicidal tendencies and allow only minimum supply of drug.
• Because patients using tricyclic antidepressants may suffer hypertensive episodes during surgery, stop drug gradually several days before surgery.
• Monitor glucose level.
• Watch for nausea, headache, and malaise after abrupt withdrawal of long-term therapy; these symptoms don't indicate addiction.
• Don't withdraw drug abruptly.
• *Alert:* Don't confuse amitriptyline with nortriptyline or aminophylline, or Endep with Depen.

## PATIENT TEACHING
• Whenever possible, advise patient to take full dose at bedtime, but warn him of possible morning orthostatic hypotension.
• Tell patient to avoid alcohol during drug therapy.
• Advise patient to consult prescriber before taking other drugs.
• Warn patient to avoid activities that require alertness and good psychomotor coordination until CNS effects of drug are known. Drowsiness and dizziness usually subside after a few weeks.

---

• Inform patient that dry mouth may be relieved with sugarless hard candy or gum. Saliva substitutes may be useful.
• To prevent photosensitivity reactions, advise patient to use a sunblock, wear protective clothing, and avoid prolonged exposure to strong sunlight.
• Warn patient not to stop drug therapy abruptly.
• Advise patient that it may take as long as 30 days to achieve full therapeutic effect.

## bupropion hydrochloride
Wellbutrin✐, Wellbutrin SR✐, Wellbutrin XL

*Pregnancy risk category B*

### AVAILABLE FORMS
*Tablets (extended-release):* 150 mg, 300 mg
*Tablets (immediate-release):* 75 mg, 100 mg
*Tablets (sustained-release):* 100 mg, 150 mg, 200 mg

### INDICATIONS & DOSAGES
➤ Depression
*Adults:* For immediate-release, initially, 100 mg P.O. b.i.d.; increase after 3 days to 100 mg P.O. t.i.d., if needed. If patient doesn't improve after several weeks of therapy, increase dosage to 150 mg t.i.d. No single dose should exceed 150 mg. Allow at least 6 hours between successive doses. Maximum dosage is 450 mg daily. For sustained-release, initially, 150 mg P.O. q morning; increase to target dose of 150 mg P.O. b.i.d., as tolerated, as early as day 4 of dosing. Allow at least 8 hours between successive doses. Maximum dose is 400 mg daily. For extended-release, initially, 150 mg P.O. q morning; increase to target dosage of 300 mg P.O. daily, as tolerated, as early as day 4 of dosing. Allow at least 24 hours between successive doses. Maximum is 450 mg daily.
*Adjust-a-dose:* In patients with mild to moderate hepatic cirrhosis or renal impairment, reduce frequency and dose. In patients with severe hepatic cirrhosis, don't exceed 75 mg (immediate-release) P.O. daily, 100 mg (sustained-release) P.O. daily, 150 mg (sustained-release) P.O.

every other day, or 150 mg (extended-release) P.O. every other day.

### ACTION
Unknown. Drug doesn't inhibit MAO; it's a weak inhibitor of norepinephrine, dopamine, and serotonin reuptake. Presumed action is through noradrenergic or dopaminergic mechanisms, or both.

| Route | Onset | Peak | Duration |
|---|---|---|---|
| P.O. | Unknown | 2 hr | Unknown |
| P.O. (sustained release) | Unknown | 3 hr | Unknown |
| P.O. (extended release) | Unknown | 5 hr | Unknown |

### ADVERSE REACTIONS
**CNS:** fever, *headache, seizures,* anxiety, confusion, delusions, euphoria, hostility, impaired sleep quality, *insomnia, sedation, tremor,* akinesia, akathisia, *agitation, dizziness,* fatigue, syncope.
**CV:** hypertension, hypotension, palpitations, *tachycardia, **arrhythmias,*** chest pain.
**EENT:** *auditory disturbances,* blurred vision, epistaxis, *pharyngitis,* sinusitis.
**GI:** *nausea, vomiting, anorexia, dry mouth,* taste disturbance, increased appetite, *constipation,* dyspepsia, diarrhea, abdominal pain.
**GU:** impotence, menstrual complaints, urinary frequency, urine retention.
**Metabolic:** *weight loss, weight gain.*
**Musculoskeletal:** arthritis, myalgia, arthralgia, muscle spasm or twitch.
**Respiratory:** upper respiratory complaints, increase in coughing.
**Skin:** pruritus, rash, cutaneous temperature disturbance, *excessive diaphoresis,* urticaria.
**Other:** fever and chills, decreased libido, accidental injury.

### INTERACTIONS
**Drug-drug.** *Carbamazepine:* May decrease bupropion level. Monitor patient.
*Levodopa, phenothiazines, tricyclic antidepressants; recent and rapid withdrawal of benzodiazepines:* May cause adverse reactions, including seizures. Monitor patient closely.

*MAO inhibitors:* May alter seizure threshold. Avoid using together.

*Nicotine replacement agents:* May cause hypertension. Monitor blood pressure.

*Ritonavir:* May increase bupropion level. Monitor closely for adverse reactions.

**Drug-lifestyle.** *Alcohol use:* May alter seizure threshold. Discourage use together.

*Sun exposure:* May increase risk of photosensitivity reactions. Advise patient to avoid excessive sunlight exposure.

**EFFECTS ON LAB TEST RESULTS**
None reported.

**CONTRAINDICATIONS & CAUTIONS**
• Contraindicated in patients hypersensitive to drug, in those who have taken MAO inhibitors within previous 14 days, and in those with seizure disorders or history of bulimia or anorexia nervosa because of a higher risk of seizures. Also contraindicated in patients undergoing abrupt discontinuation of alcohol or sedatives (including benzodiazepines). Don't use with Zyban or other drugs containing bupropion that are used for smoking cessation.

• Use cautiously in patients with recent history of MI, unstable heart disease, or renal or hepatic impairment.

**NURSING CONSIDERATIONS**
• Many patients experience a period of increased restlessness, especially at start of therapy. This may include agitation, insomnia, and anxiety.

• *Alert:* Risk of seizure may be minimized by not exceeding 450 mg/day (immediate-release) and by giving daily dose in three equally divided doses. Increase in doses shouldn't exceed 100 mg/day in a 3-day period. For sustained-release formulation, by not exceeding 400 mg/day and by giving daily dose in two equally divided doses. Increase in doses shouldn't exceed 200 mg/day. For extended-release preparation, by not exceeding 450 mg/day. Patients who experience seizures often have predisposing factors, including history of head trauma, seizures, or CNS tumors, or they may be taking a drug that lowers seizure threshold.

• In switching patients from regular- or sustained-release tablets to extended-release tablets, give the same total daily dose (when possible) as the once-daily dosage provided.

• Closely monitor patient with history of bipolar disorder. Antidepressants can cause manic episodes during the depressed phase of bipolar disorder. This may be less likely to occur with bupropion than with other antidepressants.

• *Alert:* Don't confuse bupropion with buspirone or Wellbutrin with Wellcovorin or Wellferon.

**PATIENT TEACHING**
• Advise patient to take drug as scheduled and to take each day's dose in three divided doses (immediate-release) or two divided doses (sustained-release) to minimize risk of seizures.

• Advise patient to consult prescriber before taking other prescription or OTC drugs.

• Tell patient to avoid alcohol while taking drug because it may contribute to development of seizures.

• Advise patient to avoid hazardous activities that require alertness and good psychomotor coordination until effects of drug are known.

• *Alert:* Advise patient that this drug has the same ingredients as Zyban, used to aid smoking cessation, and that the two shouldn't be used together.

• Tell patient that it may take 4 weeks to reach full therapeutic effect of drug.

• Tell patient to protect drug from light and moisture.

## citalopram hydrobromide
Celexa✍

*Pregnancy risk category C*

**AVAILABLE FORMS**
*Solution:* 10 mg/5 ml
*Tablets:* 10 mg, 20 mg, 40 mg

**INDICATIONS & DOSAGES**
➤ **Depression**
*Adults:* Initially, 20 mg P.O. once daily, increasing to 40 mg daily after no less than

1 week. Maximum recommended dose is 40 mg daily.
*Elderly patients:* 20 mg/day P.O. with adjustment to 40 mg/day only for unresponsive patients.
**Adjust-a-dose:** For patients with hepatic impairment, use 20 mg/day P.O. with adjustment to 40 mg/day only for unresponsive patients.

## ACTION
A selective serotonin reuptake inhibitor whose action is presumed to be linked to potentiation of serotonergic activity in the CNS resulting from inhibition of neuronal reuptake of serotonin.

| Route | Onset | Peak | Duration |
|-------|-------|------|----------|
| P.O. | Unknown | 4 hr | Unknown |

## ADVERSE REACTIONS
**CNS:** tremor, *somnolence, insomnia,* anxiety, agitation, dizziness, paresthesia, migraine, impaired concentration, amnesia, depression, apathy, ***suicide attempt,*** confusion, fatigue, fever.
**CV:** tachycardia, orthostatic hypotension, hypotension.
**EENT:** rhinitis, sinusitis, abnormal accommodation.
**GI:** *dry mouth, nausea,* diarrhea, anorexia, dyspepsia, vomiting, abdominal pain, taste perversion, increased saliva, flatulence, increased appetite.
**GU:** dysmenorrhea, amenorrhea, ejaculation disorder, impotence, anorgasmia, polyuria.
**Metabolic:** decreased or increased weight.
**Musculoskeletal:** arthralgia, myalgia.
**Respiratory:** upper respiratory tract infection, coughing.
**Skin:** rash, pruritus, *increased sweating.*
**Other:** yawning, decreased libido.

## INTERACTIONS
**Drug-drug.** *Carbamazepine:* May increase citalopram clearance. Monitor patient for effects.
*CNS drugs:* May cause additive effects. Use together cautiously.
*Drugs that inhibit cytochrome P-450 isoenzymes 3A4 and 2C19:* May cause decreased clearance of citalopram. Monitor patient for increased adverse effects.

*Imipramine, other tricyclic antidepressants:* May increase level of imipramine metabolite desipramine by about 50%. Use together cautiously.
*Lithium:* May enhance serotonergic effect of citalopram. Use together cautiously, and monitor lithium level.
*MAO inhibitors (phenelzine, selegiline, tranylcypromine):* May cause serotonin syndrome. Avoid using within 14 days of MAO inhibitor therapy.
*Sumatriptan:* May cause weakness, hyperreflexia, and incoordination. Monitor patient closely.
**Drug-lifestyle.** *Alcohol use:* May increase CNS effects. Discourage use together.

## EFFECTS ON LAB TEST RESULTS
None reported.

## CONTRAINDICATIONS & CAUTIONS
• Contraindicated in patients hypersensitive to drug or its inactive components and within 14 days of MAO inhibitor therapy.
• Use cautiously in patients with history of mania, seizures, suicidal ideation, or hepatic or renal impairment.
• Safety and effectiveness of drug haven't been established in children.

## NURSING CONSIDERATIONS
• Although drug hasn't been shown to impair psychomotor performance, any psychoactive drug has the potential to impair judgment, thinking, or motor skills.
• The possibility of a suicide attempt is inherent in depression and may persist until significant remission occurs. Closely supervise high-risk patients at start of drug therapy. Reduce risk of overdose by limiting amount of drug available per refill.
• At least 14 days should elapse between MAO inhibitor therapy and citalopram therapy.
• **Alert:** Don't confuse Celexa with Celebrex or Cerebyx.

## PATIENT TEACHING
• Tell patient that drug may be taken in the morning or evening without regard to meals. If drowsiness occurs, he should take drug in evening.
• Caution patient against use of MAO inhibitors while taking citalopram.

---

*Rapid onset*   †Canada   ‡Australia   ◊OTC   ♦ Off-label use   ✐Photoguide   *Liquid contains alcohol.

• Inform patient that, although improvement may take 1 to 4 weeks, he should continue therapy as prescribed.

• Advise patient not to stop medication abruptly.

• Instruct patient to exercise caution when driving or operating hazardous machinery; drug may impair judgment, thinking, and motor skills.

• Advise patient to consult prescriber before taking other prescription or OTC drugs.

• Advise woman to consult prescriber before breast-feeding.

• Warn patient to avoid alcohol during drug therapy.

• Instruct woman of childbearing potential to use contraceptives during drug therapy and to notify prescriber immediately if pregnancy is suspected.

## clomipramine hydrochloride
Anafranil, Placil‡

*Pregnancy risk category C*

### AVAILABLE FORMS
*Capsules:* 25 mg, 50 mg, 75 mg

### INDICATIONS & DOSAGES
➤ **Obsessive-compulsive disorder**
*Adults:* Initially, 25 mg P.O. daily with meals, gradually increased to 100 mg daily in divided doses during first 2 weeks. Thereafter, increase to maximum dose of 250 mg daily in divided doses with meals, p.r.n. After adjustment, give total daily dose h.s.
*Children and adolescents:* Initially, 25 mg P.O. daily with meals, gradually increased over first 2 weeks to daily maximum of 3 mg/kg or 100 mg P.O. in divided doses, whichever is smaller. Maximum daily dose is 3 mg/kg or 200 mg, whichever is smaller; give h.s. after adjustment. Reassess and adjust dosage periodically.
➤ **To manage panic disorder with or without agoraphobia**
*Adults:* 12.5 to 150 mg P.O. daily (maximum 200 mg).
➤ **Depression, chronic pain ♦**
*Adults:* 100 to 250 mg P.O. daily.

➤ **Cataplexy and associated narcolepsy ♦**
*Adults:* 25 to 200 mg P.O. daily.

### ACTION
Unknown. A tricyclic antidepressant that selectively inhibits reuptake of norepinephrine at the presynaptic neuron.

| Route | Onset | Peak | Duration |
|-------|-------|------|----------|
| P.O. | Unknown | 2-6 hr | Unknown |

### ADVERSE REACTIONS
**CNS:** *somnolence, tremor, dizziness, headache, insomnia, nervousness, myoclonus, fatigue,* EEG changes, **seizures.**
**CV:** *orthostatic hypotension, palpitations,* tachycardia.
**EENT:** *pharyngitis, rhinitis, visual changes.*
**GI:** *dry mouth, constipation, nausea, dyspepsia, increased appetite, diarrhea, anorexia, abdominal pain.*
**GU:** *urinary hesitancy,* urinary tract infection, *dysmenorrhea, ejaculation failure, impotence.*
**Hematologic:** *purpura.*
**Metabolic:** *weight gain.*
**Musculoskeletal:** *myalgia.*
**Skin:** *diaphoresis,* rash, pruritus, dry skin.
**Other:** *altered libido.*

### INTERACTIONS
**Drug-drug.** *Barbiturates:* May decrease tricyclic antidepressant level. Watch for decreased antidepressant effect.
*Cimetidine, fluoxetine, fluvoxamine, paroxetine, sertraline:* May increase tricyclic antidepressant level. Watch for enhanced antidepressant effect.
*Clonidine:* May cause life-threatening blood pressure elevations. Avoid using together.
*CNS depressants:* May enhance CNS depression. Avoid using together.
*Epinephrine, norepinephrine:* May increase hypertensive effect. Use together cautiously.
*MAO inhibitors:* May cause hyperpyretic crisis, seizures, coma, or death. Avoid using within 14 days of MAO inhibitor therapy.
**Drug-herb.** *Evening primrose oil:* May cause additive or synergistic effect, resulting in lower seizure threshold and increas-

ing the risk of seizure. Discourage use together.

*St. John's wort, SAM-e, yohimbe:* May cause serotonin syndrome. Discourage use together.

**Drug-lifestyle.** *Alcohol use:* May enhance CNS depression. Discourage use together.

*Sun exposure:* May increase risk of photosensitivity reactions. Advise patient to avoid excessive sunlight exposure.

**EFFECTS ON LAB TEST RESULTS**
None reported.

**CONTRAINDICATIONS & CAUTIONS**
• Contraindicated in patients hypersensitive to drug or other tricyclic antidepressants, in those who have taken MAO inhibitors within previous 14 days, and in patients in acute recovery period after MI.
• Use cautiously in patients with history of seizure disorders or with brain damage of varying cause; in patients receiving other seizure threshold-lowering drugs; in patients at risk for suicide; in patients with history of urine retention or angle-closure glaucoma, increased intraocular pressure, CV disease, impaired hepatic or renal function, or hyperthyroidism; in patients with tumors of the adrenal medulla; in patients receiving thyroid drug or electroconvulsive therapy; and in those undergoing elective surgery.

**NURSING CONSIDERATIONS**
• Monitor mood and watch for suicidal tendencies. Allow patient to have only minimal amount of drug.
• Don't withdraw drug abruptly.
• Because patients using tricyclic antidepressants may suffer hypertensive episodes during surgery, stop drug gradually several days before surgery.
• Relieve dry mouth with sugarless candy or gum. Saliva substitutes may be needed.
• *Alert:* Don't confuse clomipramine with chlorpromazine or clomiphene, or Anafranil with enalapril, nafarelin, or alfentanil.

**PATIENT TEACHING**
• Warn patient to avoid hazardous activities requiring alertness and good coordination, especially during adjustment. Daytime sedation and dizziness may occur.

• Tell patient to avoid alcohol during drug therapy.
• Warn patient not to stop drug suddenly.
• Advise patient to use sunblock, wear protective clothing, and avoid prolonged exposure to strong sunlight to prevent oversensitivity to the sun.

---

## desipramine hydrochloride
Norpramin, Pertofran‡, Pertofrane†

*Pregnancy risk category NR*

**AVAILABLE FORMS**
*Capsules:* 25 mg, 50 mg
*Tablets:* 10 mg, 25 mg, 50 mg, 75 mg, 100 mg, 150 mg

**INDICATIONS & DOSAGES**
➤ **Depression**
*Adults:* 75 to 150 mg P.O. daily in divided doses; increase to maximum of 300 mg daily. Or, give entire dose h.s.
*Adolescents and elderly patients:* 25 to 100 mg P.O. daily in divided doses; increase gradually to maximum of 150 mg daily, if needed.

**ACTION**
Unknown. A tricyclic antidepressant that increases amount of norepinephrine, serotonin, or both in the CNS by blocking their reuptake by the presynaptic neurons.

| Route | Onset | Peak | Duration |
|---|---|---|---|
| P.O. | Unknown | 4-6 hr | Unknown |

**ADVERSE REACTIONS**
**CNS:** *drowsiness, dizziness,* excitation, tremor, weakness, confusion, anxiety, restlessness, agitation, headache, nervousness, EEG changes, *seizures,* extrapyramidal reactions.
**CV:** orthostatic hypotension, *tachycardia,* ECG changes, hypertension.
**EENT:** *blurred vision,* tinnitus, mydriasis.
**GI:** *dry mouth,* constipation, nausea, vomiting, anorexia, paralytic ileus.
**GU:** urine retention.
**Metabolic:** *hypoglycemia,* hyperglycemia.
**Skin:** rash, urticaria, photosensitivity reactions, diaphoresis.

**Other:** hypersensitivity reactions, *sudden death in children.*

## INTERACTIONS
**Drug-drug.** *Barbiturates, CNS depressants:* May enhance CNS depression. Avoid using together.
*Cimetidine, fluvoxamine, fluoxetine, paroxetine, sertraline:* May increase desipramine level. Monitor patient for adverse reactions.
*Clonidine:* May cause life-threatening blood pressure elevations. Avoid using together.
*Epinephrine, norepinephrine:* May increase hypertensive effect. Use together cautiously.
*MAO inhibitors:* May cause severe excitation, hyperpyrexia, or seizures, usually with high doses. Avoid using within 14 days of MAO inhibitor therapy.
**Drug-herb.** *Evening primrose oil:* May cause additive or synergistic effect, resulting in lower seizure threshold and increasing the risk of seizure. Discourage use together.
*St. John's wort, SAM-e, yohimbe:* May cause serotonin syndrome. Discourage use together.
**Drug-lifestyle.** *Alcohol use:* May enhance CNS depression. Discourage use together.
*Smoking:* May lower desipramine level. Monitor patient for lack of effect.
*Sun exposure:* May increase risk of photosensitivity reactions. Advise patient to avoid excessive sunlight exposure.

## EFFECTS ON LAB TEST RESULTS
• May increase or decrease glucose level.
• May increase liver function test values.

## CONTRAINDICATIONS & CAUTIONS
• Contraindicated in patients hypersensitive to drug, in those who have taken MAO inhibitors within previous 14 days.
• Contraindicated during acute recovery phase after MI.
• Use with extreme caution in patients with CV disease; in those with history of urine retention, glaucoma, seizure disorders, or thyroid disease; and in those taking thyroid drug.
• Avoid use in children.

## NURSING CONSIDERATIONS
• Monitor patient for nausea, headache, and malaise after abrupt withdrawal of long-term therapy; these symptoms don't indicate addiction.
• Don't withdraw drug abruptly.
• Because patients using tricyclic antidepressants may suffer hypertensive episodes during surgery, stop drug gradually several days before surgery.
• If signs or symptoms of psychosis occur or increase, expect prescriber to reduce dosage. Record mood changes. Monitor patient for suicidal tendencies, and allow only a minimum supply of drug.
• Because desipramine produces fewer anticholinergic effects than other tricyclic antidepressants, it's often prescribed for cardiac patients.
• Recommend sugarless hard candy or gum to relieve dry mouth. Saliva substitutes may be needed.
• *Alert:* Norpramin may contain tartrazine.
• *Alert:* Don't confuse desipramine with disopyramide or imipramine.

## PATIENT TEACHING
• Advise patient to take full dose at bedtime, whenever possible.
• Warn patient to avoid hazardous activities that require alertness and good coordination until effects of drug are known. Drowsiness and dizziness usually subside after a few weeks.
• Advise patient to call prescriber if fever and sore throat occur. Blood counts may need to be obtained.
• Tell patient to avoid alcohol during drug therapy because it may antagonize effects of desipramine.
• Tell patient to consult prescriber before taking other prescription or OTC drugs.
• Warn patient not to stop drug suddenly.
• To prevent sensitivity to the sun, advise patient to use sunblock, wear protective clothing, and avoid prolonged exposure to strong sunlight.

---

Reactions may be *common,* uncommon, *life-threatening,* or COMMON AND LIFE-THREATENING.

# doxepin hydrochloride
Deptran‡, Novo-Doxepin†,
Sinequan, Triadapin†

*Pregnancy risk category NR*

## AVAILABLE FORMS
*Capsules:* 10 mg, 25 mg, 50 mg, 75 mg,
100 mg, 150 mg
*Oral concentrate:* 10 mg/ml

## INDICATIONS & DOSAGES
➤ **Depression**
*Adults:* Initially, 30 to 150 mg P.O. daily in
divided doses to maximum of 300 mg daily. Or, entire maintenance dose may be
given once daily with maximum dose of
150 mg.

## ACTION
Unknown. A tricyclic antidepressant that
increases amount of norepinephrine, serotonin, or both in the CNS by blocking
their reuptake by the presynaptic neurons.

| Route | Onset | Peak | Duration |
|-------|-------|------|----------|
| P.O. | Unknown | 2 hr | Unknown |

## ADVERSE REACTIONS
**CNS:** *drowsiness, dizziness,* confusion,
numbness, hallucinations, paresthesia,
ataxia, weakness, headache, *seizures,* ex-
trapyramidal reactions.
**CV:** *orthostatic hypotension, tachycardia,*
ECG changes.
**EENT:** *blurred vision,* tinnitus.
**GI:** *dry mouth, constipation,* nausea, vom-
iting, anorexia.
**GU:** urine retention.
**Metabolic:** *hypoglycemia,* hyperglycemia.
**Skin:** rash, urticaria, photosensitivity re-
actions, *diaphoresis.*
**Other:** hypersensitivity reactions.

## INTERACTIONS
**Drug-drug.** *Barbiturates, CNS depressants:* May enhance CNS depression.
Avoid using together.
*Cimetidine, fluoxetine, fluvoxamine,
paroxetine, sertraline:* May increase doxepin level. Watch for increased adverse reactions.

*Clonidine:* May cause life-threatening
blood pressure elevations. Avoid using together.
*Epinephrine, norepinephrine:* May increase hypertensive effect. Use together
cautiously.
*MAO inhibitors:* May cause severe excitation, hyperpyrexia, or seizures, usually
with high dosage. Avoid using within 14
days of MAO inhibitor therapy.
**Drug-herb.** *Evening primrose oil:* May
cause additive or synergistic effect, resulting in lower seizure threshold and increasing the risk of seizure. Discourage use together.
*St. John's wort, SAM-e, yohimbe:* May
cause serotonin syndrome. Discourage use
together.
**Drug-lifestyle.** *Alcohol use:* May enhance
CNS depression. Discourage use together.
*Sun exposure:* May increase risk of photosensitivity reactions. Advise patient to
avoid excessive sunlight exposure.

## EFFECTS ON LAB TEST RESULTS
● May increase or decrease glucose level.
● May increase liver function test values.

## CONTRAINDICATIONS & CAUTIONS
● Contraindicated in patients hypersensitive to drug and in those with glaucoma or
tendency toward urine retention; also contraindicated in those who have received an
MAO inhibitor within past 14 days and
during acute recovery phase of an MI.

## NURSING CONSIDERATIONS
● Don't withdraw drug abruptly.
● Monitor patient for nausea, headache,
and malaise after abrupt withdrawal of
long-term therapy; these symptoms don't
indicate addiction.
● *Alert:* Because hypertensive episodes
may occur during surgery in patients receiving tricyclic antidepressants, stop drug
gradually several days before surgery.
● If signs or symptoms of psychosis occur
or increase, expect prescriber to reduce
dosage. Record mood changes. Monitor
patient for suicidal tendencies and allow
only a minimum supply of drug.
● Doxepin has strong anticholinergic effects and is one of the most sedating tricyclic antidepressants. Adverse anticholinergic effects can occur rapidly.

• Recommend use of sugarless hard candy or gum to relieve dry mouth.
• *Alert:* Don't confuse doxepin with doxazosin, digoxin, doxapram, or Doxidan; don't confuse Sinequan with saquinavir.

## PATIENT TEACHING
• Tell patient to dilute oral concentrate with 4 ounces (120 ml) of water, milk, or juice (orange, grapefruit, tomato, prune, or pineapple, but not grape); preparation shouldn't be mixed with carbonated beverages.
• Tell patient to take full dose at bedtime whenever he can, but warn him of possible morning dizziness on standing up quickly.
• Advise patient to consult prescriber before taking other prescription or OTC drugs.
• Warn patient to avoid hazardous activities that require alertness and good psychomotor coordination until effects of drug are known. Drowsiness and dizziness usually subside after a few weeks.
• Tell patient to avoid alcohol during drug therapy.
• Tell patient that maximum antidepressant effect may not be evident for 2 to 3 weeks.
• Warn patient not to stop drug suddenly.
• To prevent sensitivity to the sun, advise patient to use sunblock, wear protective clothing, and avoid prolonged exposure to strong sunlight.

---

## escitalopram oxalate
Lexapro◆

*Pregnancy risk category C*

### AVAILABLE FORMS
*Oral solution:* 5 mg/5 ml
*Tablets:* 5 mg, 10 mg, 20 mg

### INDICATIONS & DOSAGES
➤ **Treatment and maintenance therapy for patients with major depressive disorder**
*Adults:* Initially, 10 mg P.O. once daily, increasing to 20 mg if necessary after at least 1 week.
*Adjust-a-dose:* For elderly patients and those with hepatic impairment, 10 mg P.O.

daily, initially and as maintenance dosages.

### ACTIONS
Antidepressant action thought to be linked to potentiation of serotonergic activity in the CNS resulting from inhibition of neuronal reuptake of serotonin. Drug is the S-enantiomer of the racemic compound citalopram and thought to be the active component.

| Route | Onset | Peak | Duration |
|-------|---------|------|----------|
| P.O. | Unknown | 5 hr | Unknown |

### ADVERSE REACTIONS
**CNS:** fever, insomnia, dizziness, somnolence, paresthesia, light-headedness, migraine, tremor, vertigo, abnormal dreams, irritability, impaired concentration, fatigue, lethargy.
**CV:** palpitations, hypertension, flushing, chest pain.
**EENT:** rhinitis, sinusitis, blurred vision, tinnitus, earache.
**GI:** *nausea,* diarrhea, constipation, indigestion, abdominal pain, vomiting, increased or decreased appetite, dry mouth, flatulence, heartburn, cramps, gastroesophageal reflux.
**GU:** ejaculation disorder, impotence, anorgasmia, menstrual cramps, urinary tract infection, urinary frequency.
**Metabolic:** weight gain or loss.
**Musculoskeletal:** arthralgia, myalgia, muscle cramps, pain in arms or legs.
**Respiratory:** bronchitis, cough.
**Skin:** rash, increased sweating.
**Other:** decreased libido, yawning, flulike symptoms.

### INTERACTIONS
**Drug-drug.** *Carbamazepine:* May increase escitalopram clearance. Monitor patient for expected antidepressant effect and adjust dose as needed.
*Cimetidine:* May increase escitalopram level. Monitor patient for increased adverse reactions to escitalopram.
*Citalopram:* May cause additive effects. Avoid using together.
*CNS drugs:* May cause additive effects. Use together cautiously.

---

*Desipramine, other drugs metabolized by CYP 2D6:* May increase levels of these drugs. Use together cautiously.

*Lithium:* May enhance serotonergic effect of escitalopram. Use together cautiously, and monitor lithium level.

*MAO inhibitors:* May cause serious, sometimes fatal, serotonin syndrome. Avoid using within 14 days of MAO inhibitor therapy.

*Sumatriptan:* May increase serotonergic effects, leading to weakness, enhanced reflex response, and incoordination. Use together cautiously.

**Drug-lifestyle.** *Alcohol use:* May increase CNS effects. Discourage use together.

**EFFECTS ON LAB TEST RESULTS**
None reported.

**CONTRAINDICATIONS & CAUTIONS**
• Contraindicated in patients taking MAO inhibitors or within 14 days of MAO inhibitor therapy and in those hypersensitive to escitalopram, citalopram, or any of its inactive ingredients.
• Use cautiously in patients with a history of mania, seizure disorders, suicidal ideation, or renal or hepatic impairment.
• Use cautiously in patients with diseases that produce altered metabolism or hemodynamic responses.
• Use with caution in elderly patients because they may have greater sensitivity to drug.
• Use drug in pregnant patient only if benefits outweigh risks.
• Drug appears in breast milk. Patient should either stop breast-feeding or stop taking drug.

**NURSING CONSIDERATIONS**
• Closely monitor patients at high risk of suicide.
• Evaluate patient for history of drug abuse and observe for signs of misuse or abuse.
• Periodically reassess patient to determine need for maintenance treatment and appropriate dosing.

**PATIENT TEACHING**
• Inform patient that symptoms should improve gradually over several weeks, rather than immediately.

• Tell patient that although improvement may occur within 1 to 4 weeks, he should continue drug should as prescribed.
• Tell patient to use caution while driving or operating hazardous machinery because of drug's potential to impair judgment, thinking, or motor skills.
• Advise patient to consult health care provider before taking other prescription or OTC drugs.
• Tell patient that drug may be taken in the morning or evening without regard to meals.
• Encourage patient to avoid alcohol while taking drug.
• Tell patient to notify health care provider if she's pregnant or breast-feeding.

---

# fluoxetine hydrochloride
Erocap‡, Lovan‡, Prozac🖊, Prozac-20‡, Prozac Weekly, Sarafem🖊, Zactin‡

*Pregnancy risk category C*

**AVAILABLE FORMS**
*Capsules (delayed-release):* 90 mg
*Capsules (pulvules):* 10 mg, 20 mg, 40 mg
*Oral solution:* 20 mg/5 ml
*Tablets:* 10 mg, 20 mg

**INDICATIONS & DOSAGES**
➤ **Depression, obsessive-compulsive disorder (OCD)**
*Adults:* Initially, 20 mg P.O. in the morning; increase dosage based on patient response. Maximum daily dose is 80 mg.
*Children ages 7 to 17 (OCD):* 10 mg P.O. daily. After 2 weeks, increase to 20 mg/day. Dosage is 20 to 60 mg/day.
*Children ages 8 to 18 (depression):* 10 mg P.O. once daily for 1 week; then increase to 20 mg daily.
➤ **Depression in elderly patients**
*Adults age 65 and older:* Initially, 20 mg P.O. daily in the morning. Increase dose based on response. Doses may be given b.i.d., morning and noon. Maximum daily dose is 80 mg. Consider using a lower dosage or less-frequent dosing in these patients, especially those with systemic illness and those who are receiving drugs for other illnesses.

---

➤ **Maintenance therapy for depression in stabilized patients (not for newly diagnosed depression)**
*Adults:* 90 mg Prozac Weekly P.O. once weekly. Start once-weekly dosing 7 days after the last daily dose of Prozac 20 mg.
➤ **Short-term and long-term treatment of bulimia nervosa**
*Adults:* 60 mg P.O. daily in the morning.
➤ **Short-term treatment of panic disorder with or without agoraphobia**
*Adults:* 10 mg P.O. once daily for 1 week, then increase dose as needed to 20 mg daily. Maximum daily dose is 60 mg.
*Adjust-a-dose:* For patients with renal or hepatic impairment, reduce dose or increase dosing interval.
➤ **Anorexia nervosa in weight-restored patients ◆**
*Adults:* 40 mg P.O. daily.
➤ **Depression caused by bipolar disorder ◆**
*Adults:* 20 to 60 mg P.O. daily.
➤ **Cataplexy ◆**
*Adults:* 20 mg P.O. once or twice daily with CNS stimulant therapy.
➤ **Alcohol dependence ◆**
*Adults:* 60 mg P.O. daily.
➤ **Premenstrual dysphoric disorder (PMDD)**
*Sarafem*
*Adults:* 20 mg P.O. daily continuously (every day of the menstrual cycle) or intermittently (daily dose starting 14 days before the anticipated onset of menstruation through the first full day of menses and repeating with each new cycle). Maximum daily dose is 80 mg P.O.
*Adjust-a-dose:* For patients with renal or hepatic impairment and those taking several drugs at the same time, reduce dose or increase dosing interval.

## ACTION
Unknown. Thought to be linked to drug's inhibition of CNS neuronal uptake of serotonin.

| Route | Onset | Peak | Duration |
|-------|-------|------|----------|
| P.O. | Unknown | 6-8 hr | Unknown |

## ADVERSE REACTIONS
**CNS:** *nervousness, somnolence, anxiety, insomnia, headache, drowsiness,* fatigue, *tremor, dizziness, asthenia,* fever.

**CV:** palpitations, hot flashes.
**EENT:** nasal congestion, pharyngitis, sinusitis.
**GI:** *nausea, diarrhea, dry mouth, anorexia,* dyspepsia, constipation, abdominal pain, vomiting, flatulence, increased appetite.
**GU:** sexual dysfunction.
**Metabolic:** weight loss.
**Musculoskeletal:** muscle pain.
**Respiratory:** upper respiratory tract infection, cough, respiratory distress.
**Skin:** rash, pruritus, diaphoresis.
**Other:** flulike syndrome.

## INTERACTIONS
**Drug-drug.** *Benzodiazepines, lithium, tricyclic antidepressants:* May increase CNS effects. Monitor patient closely.
*Beta blockers, carbamazepine, flecainide, vinblastine:* May increase levels of these drugs. Monitor drug levels and monitor patient for adverse reactions.
*Cyproheptadine:* May reverse or decrease fluoxetine effect. Monitor patient closely.
*Dextromethorphan:* May cause unusual side effects, such as visual hallucinations. Advise use of cough suppressant that doesn't contain dextromethorphan while taking fluoxetine.
*Insulin, oral antidiabetics:* May alter glucose level and antidiabetic requirements. Adjust dosage.
*Lithium, tricyclic antidepressants:* May increase adverse CNS effects. Monitor patient closely.
*MAO inhibitors (phenelzine, selegiline, tranylcypromine):* May cause serotonin syndrome. Avoid using with fluoxetine or within a minimum of 5 weeks after stopping fluoxetine.
*Phenytoin:* May increase phenytoin level and risk of toxicity. Monitor phenytoin level and adjust dosage.
*Sumatriptan:* May cause weakness, hyperreflexia, and incoordination. Monitor patient closely.
*Thioridazine:* May increase thioridazine level, increasing risk of serious ventricular arrhythmias and sudden death. Avoid using with fluoxetine or within a minimum of 5 weeks after stopping fluoxetine.
*Tramadol:* May cause serotonin syndrome. Avoid using together.

---

Reactions may be *common*, uncommon, ***life-threatening***, or COMMON AND LIFE-THREATENING.

*Tryptophan:* May increase agitation, restlessness, and GI adverse effects. Use together cautiously.

*Warfarin, other highly protein-bound drugs:* May increase level of fluoxetine or other highly protein-bound drugs. Monitor patient closely.

**Drug-herb.** *St. John's wort:* May increase sedative and hypnotic effects; may cause serotonin syndrome. Discourage use together.

**Drug-lifestyle.** *Alcohol use:* May increase CNS depression. Discourage use together.

**EFFECTS ON LAB TEST RESULTS**
None reported.

**CONTRAINDICATIONS & CAUTIONS**
• Contraindicated in patients hypersensitive to drug and in those taking MAO inhibitors within 14 days of starting therapy. MAO inhibitors shouldn't be started within 5 weeks of stopping fluoxetine therapy. Avoid using thioridazine with fluoxetine or within a minimum of 5 weeks after stopping fluoxetine.
• Use cautiously in patients at high risk for suicide and in those with history of diabetes mellitus, seizures, mania, or hepatic, renal, or CV disease.

**NURSING CONSIDERATIONS**
• Use antihistamines or topical corticosteroids to treat rashes or pruritus.
• Watch for weight change during therapy, particularly in underweight or bulimic patients.
• Record mood changes. Watch for suicidal tendencies.
• *Alert:* Don't confuse fluoxetine with fluvoxamine or fluvastatin.
• *Alert:* Don't confuse Prozac with Proscar, Prilosec, or ProSom.

**PATIENT TEACHING**
• Tell patient to avoid taking drug in the afternoon whenever possible because fluoxetine commonly causes nervousness and insomnia.
• Drug may cause dizziness or drowsiness. Warn patient to avoid driving and other hazardous activities that require alertness and good psychomotor coordination until effects of drug are known.

• Tell patient to consult prescriber before taking other prescription or OTC drugs.
• Advise patient that full therapeutic effect may not be seen for 4 weeks or longer.

---

# imipramine hydrochloride
Apo-Imipramine†, Impril†, Melipramine‡, Norfranil, Novopramine†, Tipramine, Tofranil

# imipramine pamoate
Tofranil-PM

*Pregnancy risk category D*

**AVAILABLE FORMS**
**imipramine hydrochloride**
*Injection:* 12.5 mg/ml
*Tablets:* 10 mg, 25 mg, 50 mg
**imipramine pamoate**
*Capsules:* 75 mg, 100 mg, 125 mg, 150 mg

**INDICATIONS & DOSAGES**
➤ **Depression**
*Adults:* 75 to 100 mg P.O. or (rarely) I.M. daily in divided doses, increased by 25 to 50 mg. Maximum daily dose is 200 mg for outpatients and 300 mg for hospitalized patients. Give entire dose h.s.
*Adolescents and elderly patients:* Initially, 30 to 40 mg daily; maximum shouldn't exceed 100 mg daily.
➤ **Childhood enuresis**
*Children age 5 and older:* 25 mg P.O. 1 hour before bedtime. If patient doesn't improve within 1 week, increase dose to 50 mg if child is younger than age 12; increase dose to 75 mg for children age 12 and older. In either case, maximum daily dose is 2.5 mg/kg.

**ACTION**
Unknown. A tricyclic antidepressant that increases norepinephrine, serotonin, or both in the CNS by blocking their reuptake by the presynaptic neurons.

| Route | Onset | Peak | Duration |
|---|---|---|---|
| P.O. | Unknown | 1-2 hr | Unknown |
| I.M. | Unknown | 30 min | Unknown |

## ADVERSE REACTIONS

**CNS:** *CVA, drowsiness, dizziness,* excitation, tremor, confusion, hallucinations, anxiety, ataxia, paresthesia, nervousness, EEG changes, *seizures,* extrapyramidal reactions.

**CV:** *orthostatic hypotension, tachycardia, ECG changes,* hypertension, *MI, arrhythmias, heart block,* precipitation of heart failure.

**EENT:** *blurred vision,* tinnitus, mydriasis.

**GI:** *dry mouth, constipation,* nausea, vomiting, anorexia, paralytic ileus, abdominal cramps.

**GU:** *urine retention.*

**Metabolic:** *hypoglycemia,* hyperglycemia.

**Skin:** rash, urticaria, photosensitivity reactions, pruritus, diaphoresis.

**Other:** hypersensitivity reactions.

## INTERACTIONS

**Drug-drug.** *Barbiturates, CNS depressants:* May enhance CNS depression. Avoid using together.

*Cimetidine, fluoxetine, paroxetine:* May increase imipramine level. Monitor patient for adverse reactions.

*Clonidine:* May cause potentially life-threatening elevations in blood pressure. Avoid using together.

*Epinephrine, norepinephrine:* May increase hypertensive effect. Use together cautiously.

*MAO inhibitors:* May cause hyperpyretic crisis, severe seizures, and death. Avoid using within 14 days of MAO inhibitor therapy.

**Drug-herb.** *Evening primrose oil:* May cause additive or synergistic effect, resulting in lower seizure threshold and increasing the risk of seizure. Discourage use together.

*St. John's wort, SAM-e, yohimbe:* May cause serotonin syndrome. Discourage use together.

**Drug-lifestyle.** *Alcohol use:* May enhance CNS depression. Discourage use together.

*Smoking:* May lower level of imipramine. Monitor patient for lack of effect.

*Sun exposure:* May increase risk of photosensitivity reactions. Advise patient to avoid excessive sunlight exposure.

## EFFECTS ON LAB TEST RESULTS

• May increase or decrease glucose level.
• May increase liver function test values.

## CONTRAINDICATIONS & CAUTIONS

• Contraindicated in patients hypersensitive to drug and in those receiving MAO inhibitors; also contraindicated during acute recovery phase of MI.
• Use with extreme caution in patients at risk for suicide; in patients with history of urine retention, angle-closure glaucoma, or seizure disorders; in patients with increased intraocular pressure, CV disease, impaired hepatic function, hyperthyroidism, or impaired renal function; and in patients receiving thyroid drugs. Injectable form contains sulfites, which may cause allergic reactions in hypersensitive patients.

## NURSING CONSIDERATIONS

• Monitor patient for nausea, headache, and malaise after abrupt withdrawal of long-term therapy; these symptoms don't indicate addiction.
• Don't withdraw drug abruptly.
• Because of hypertensive episodes during surgery in patients receiving tricyclic antidepressants, stop drug gradually several days before surgery.
• If signs or symptoms of psychosis occur or increase, expect prescriber to reduce dosage. Record mood changes. Monitor patient for suicidal tendencies, and allow only a minimum supply of drug.
• To prevent relapse in children receiving drug for enuresis, withdraw drug gradually.
• Recommend sugarless hard candy or gum to relieve dry mouth. Saliva substitutes may be useful.
• *Alert:* Tofranil and Tofranil PM may contain tartrazine.
• *Alert:* Don't confuse imipramine with desipramine.

## PATIENT TEACHING

• Tell patient to take full dose at bedtime whenever possible, but warn him of possible morning dizziness upon standing up quickly.
• If child is an early night bedwetter, tell parents it may be more effective to divide dose and give the first dose earlier in day.

---

Reactions may be *common,* uncommon, *life-threatening*, or COMMON AND LIFE-THREATENING.

• Tell patient to avoid alcohol while taking this drug.
• Advise patient to consult prescriber before taking other prescription or OTC drugs.
• Warn patient to avoid hazardous activities that require alertness and good coordination until effects of the drug are known. Drowsiness and dizziness usually subside after a few weeks.
• Warn patient not to stop drug suddenly.
• To prevent oversensitivity to the sun, advise patient to use sunblock, wear protective clothing, and avoid prolonged exposure to strong sunlight.

---

## mirtazapine
Remeron, Remeron Soltab

*Pregnancy risk category C*

### AVAILABLE FORMS
*Tablets:* 15 mg, 30 mg, 45 mg
*Tablets (orally disintegrating):* 15 mg, 30 mg, 45 mg

### INDICATIONS & DOSAGES
➤ **Depression**
*Adults:* Initially, 15 mg P.O. h.s. Maintenance dose ranges from 15 to 45 mg daily. Adjust dosage at intervals of at least 1 week.

### ACTION
Thought to be caused by enhancement of central noradrenergic and serotonergic activity.

| Route | Onset | Peak | Duration |
|-------|-------|------|----------|
| P.O. | Unknown | 2 hr | Unknown |

### ADVERSE REACTIONS
**CNS:** *somnolence,* dizziness, asthenia, abnormal dreams, abnormal thinking, tremors, confusion.
**CV:** edema, peripheral edema.
**GI:** nausea, *increased appetite, dry mouth, constipation.*
**GU:** urinary frequency.
**Metabolic:** *weight gain.*
**Musculoskeletal:** back pain, myalgia.
**Respiratory:** dyspnea.
**Other:** flulike syndrome.

### INTERACTIONS
**Drug-drug.** *Diazepam, other CNS depressants:* May cause additive CNS effects. Avoid using together.
*MAO inhibitors:* May cause sometimes-fatal reactions. Avoid using within 14 days of MAO inhibitor therapy.
**Drug-lifestyle.** *Alcohol use:* May cause additive CNS effects. Discourage use together.

### EFFECTS ON LAB TEST RESULTS
• May increase ALT level.

### CONTRAINDICATIONS & CAUTIONS
• Contraindicated in patients hypersensitive to drug and within 14 days of MAO inhibitor therapy.
• Use cautiously in patients with CV or cerebrovascular disease, seizure disorders, suicidal ideations, hepatic or renal impairment, or history of mania or hypomania.
• Use cautiously in patients with conditions that predispose them to hypotension, such as dehydration, hypovolemia, or antihypertensive therapy.

### NURSING CONSIDERATIONS
• Don't use within 14 days of MAO inhibitor therapy.
• Record mood changes. Watch for suicidal tendencies.
• Although agranulocytosis occurs rarely, stop drug and monitor patient closely if he develops a sore throat, fever, stomatitis, or other signs and symptoms of infection with a low WBC count.
• Give drug cautiously to elderly patients; decreased clearance has occurred in this age group.
• Lower dosages tend to be more sedating than higher dosages.

### PATIENT TEACHING
• Caution patient not to perform hazardous activities if he gets too sleepy.
• Tell patient to report signs and symptoms of infection, such as fever, chills, sore throat, mucous membrane irritation, or flulike syndrome.
• Instruct patient not to use alcohol or other CNS depressants while taking drug.
• Stress importance of following prescriber's orders.

• Instruct patient not to take other drugs without prescriber's approval.
• Tell woman of childbearing potential to report suspected pregnancy immediately and to notify prescriber if she is breast-feeding.
• Instruct patient to remove orally disintegrating tablets from blister pack and place immediately on tongue.
• Advise patient not to break or split tablet.

---

# nefazodone hydrochloride
Serzone⬧

*Pregnancy risk category C*

## AVAILABLE FORMS
*Tablets:* 50 mg, 100 mg, 150 mg, 300 mg

## INDICATIONS & DOSAGES
➤ **Depression**
*Adults:* Initially, 200 mg/day P.O. in two divided doses. Dosage may be increased by 100 to 200 mg/day at intervals of at least 1 week, p.r.n. Usual dosage range is 300 to 600 mg/day.
*Elderly patients:* Initially, 100 mg/day P.O. in two divided doses.
*Adjust-a-dose:* For debilitated patients, initially 100 mg/day P.O. in two divided doses.

## ACTION
Unknown. Thought to be linked to drug's inhibition of CNS neuronal uptake of serotonin ($5-HT_2$) and norepinephrine; it also occupies serotonin and alpha$_1$-adrenergic receptors in the CNS.

| Route | Onset | Peak | Duration |
|-------|-------|------|----------|
| P.O. | Unknown | 1 hr | Unknown |

## ADVERSE REACTIONS
**CNS:** fever, *headache, somnolence, dizziness, asthenia, insomnia, lightheadedness, confusion,* memory impairment, paresthesia, vasodilation, abnormal dreams, impaired concentration, ataxia, incoordination, psychomotor retardation, tremor, hypertonia.
**CV:** orthostatic hypotension, hypotension, peripheral edema.
**EENT:** blurred vision, abnormal vision, tinnitus, visual field defect, pharyngitis.

**GI:** *dry mouth, nausea, constipation,* taste perversion, dyspepsia, diarrhea, increased appetite, vomiting.
**GU:** urinary frequency, urinary tract infection, urine retention, vaginitis.
**Musculoskeletal:** neck rigidity, arthralgia.
**Respiratory:** cough.
**Skin:** pruritus, rash.
**Other:** infection, flulike syndrome, chills, breast tenderness, thirst.

## INTERACTIONS
**Drug-drug.** *Alprazolam, triazolam:* May potentiate effects of these drugs. Avoid using together; if use together is unavoidable, greatly reduce doses of alprazolam and triazolam.
*CNS drugs:* May alter CNS activity. Avoid using together.
*Cyclosporine:* May cause cyclosporine toxicity. Monitor cyclosporine level.
*Digoxin:* May increase digoxin level. Use together cautiously and monitor digoxin level.
*Haloperidol:* May increase haloperidol level. Monitor patient for increased adverse reactions.
*HMG-CoA reductase inhibitors:* May increase atorvastatin, lovastatin, and simvastatin levels. Monitor patient for increased adverse effects.
*MAO inhibitors (phenelzine, selegiline, tranylcypromine):* May cause serotonin syndrome. Avoid using within 14 days of MAO inhibitor therapy.
*Other highly protein-bound drugs:* May increase risk and severity of adverse reactions. Monitor patient closely.
**Drug-herb.** *St. John's wort:* May cause additive effects and serotonin syndrome. Discourage use together.
**Drug-lifestyle.** *Alcohol use:* May enhance CNS depression. Discourage use together.

## EFFECTS ON LAB TEST RESULTS
• May decrease hemoglobin and hematocrit.

## CONTRAINDICATIONS & CAUTIONS
• Contraindicated in patients hypersensitive to drug or other phenylpiperazine antidepressants; also contraindicated within 14 days of MAO inhibitor therapy.
• Contraindicated in patients who stopped using nefazodone because of liver injury.

---

• Use cautiously in patients with CV or cerebrovascular disease that could be worsened by hypotension (such as history of MI, angina, or CVA) and conditions that would predispose patients to hypotension (such as dehydration, hypovolemia, and antihypertensive therapy).
• Use cautiously in patients with a history of mania.

**NURSING CONSIDERATIONS**
• *Alert:* Drug may cause hepatic failure. Don't start drug in patients with active liver disease or with elevated baseline transaminase level. Although preexisting hepatic disease doesn't increase the likelihood of developing hepatic failure, baseline abnormalities can complicate patient monitoring. Stop drug if clinical signs and symptoms of hepatic dysfunction appear, such as increased AST or ALT level exceeding three times the upper limit of normal. Don't restart therapy.
• Don't use within 14 days of MAO inhibitor therapy.
• Record mood changes. Monitor patient for suicidal tendencies, and allow only minimum supply of drug.
• *Alert:* Don't confuse Serzone with Seroquel.

**PATIENT TEACHING**
• Warn patient not to engage in hazardous activity until effects of drug are known.
• *Alert:* Instruct men who experience prolonged or inappropriate erections to stop drug immediately and notify prescriber.
• Instruct woman to notify prescriber if she becomes pregnant or is planning pregnancy during therapy, or if she's breast-feeding.
• *Alert:* Teach the patient the signs and symptoms of liver problems, including yellowed skin or eyes, appetite loss, GI complaints, and malaise. Tell the patient to report these adverse events to prescriber immediately.
• Tell patient to notify prescriber if rash, hives, or related allergic reactions occur.
• Instruct patient to avoid alcohol during therapy.
• Tell patient to notify prescriber before taking OTC drugs.
• Inform patient that several weeks of therapy may be needed to obtain full anti-depressant effect. Once improvement occurs, advise him not to stop drug until directed by prescriber.

---

# nortriptyline hydrochloride
Allegron‡, Pamelor*✏

*Pregnancy risk category NR*

**AVAILABLE FORMS**
*Capsules:* 10 mg, 25 mg, 50 mg, 75 mg
*Oral solution:* 10 mg/5 ml*
*Tablets:* 10 mg‡, 25 mg‡

**INDICATIONS & DOSAGES**
➤ **Depression**
*Adults:* 25 mg P.O. t.i.d. or q.i.d., gradually increased to maximum of 150 mg daily. Give entire dose h.s. Monitor level when doses above 100 mg/day are given.
*Adolescents and elderly patients:* 30 to 50 mg daily given once or in divided doses.

**ACTION**
Unknown. A tricyclic antidepressant that increases the amount of norepinephrine, serotonin, or both in the CNS by blocking their reuptake by the presynaptic neurons.

| Route | Onset | Peak | Duration |
|-------|-------|------|----------|
| P.O. | Unknown | 7-8½ hr | Unknown |

**ADVERSE REACTIONS**
**CNS:** *drowsiness, dizziness, seizures,* tremor, weakness, confusion, headache, nervousness, EEG changes, *CVA,* extra-pyramidal syndrome, insomnia, nightmares, hallucinations, paresthesia, ataxia, agitation.
**CV:** ECG changes, *tachycardia,* hypertension, hypotension, *MI, heart block.*
**EENT:** *blurred vision,* tinnitus, mydriasis.
**GI:** dry mouth, *constipation,* nausea, vomiting, anorexia, paralytic ileus.
**GU:** *urine retention.*
**Hematologic:** bone marrow depression, *agranulocytosis,* eosinophilia, *thrombocytopenia.*
**Metabolic:** *hypoglycemia,* hyperglycemia.
**Skin:** rash, urticaria, photosensitivity reactions, diaphoresis.
**Other:** hypersensitivity reactions.

---

## INTERACTIONS
**Drug-drug.** *Barbiturates, CNS depressants:* May enhance CNS depression. Avoid using together.
*Cimetidine, fluoxetine, paroxetine:* May increase nortriptyline level. Watch for adverse reactions.
*Clonidine:* May cause life-threatening blood pressure elevations. Avoid using together.
*Epinephrine, norepinephrine:* May increase hypertensive effect. Use together cautiously.
*MAO inhibitors:* May cause severe excitation, hyperpyrexia, or seizures, usually with high doses. Avoid using within 14 days of MAO inhibitor therapy.
**Drug-herb.** *Evening primrose oil:* May cause additive or synergistic effect, resulting in lower seizure threshold and increasing the risk of seizure. Discourage use together.
*St. John's wort, SAM-e, yohimbe:* May cause serotonin syndrome and reduce drug level. Discourage use together.
**Drug-lifestyle.** *Alcohol use:* May enhance CNS depression. Discourage use together.
*Smoking:* May decrease nortriptyline level. Monitor patient for lack of effect.
*Sun exposure:* May increase risk of photosensitivity reactions. Advise patient to avoid excessive sunlight exposure.

## EFFECTS ON LAB TEST RESULTS
● May increase or decrease glucose level.
● May increase liver function test values and eosinophil count. May decrease WBC, RBC, granulocyte, and platelet counts.

## CONTRAINDICATIONS & CAUTIONS
● Contraindicated in patients hypersensitive to drug and during acute recovery phase of MI; also contraindicated within 14 days of MAO therapy.
● Use with extreme caution in patients with glaucoma, suicidal tendency, history of urine retention or seizures, CV disease, or hyperthyroidism and in those receiving thyroid drugs.

## NURSING CONSIDERATIONS
● Monitor patient for nausea, headache, and malaise after abrupt withdrawal of long-term therapy; these symptoms don't indicate addiction.

● Because patients using tricyclic antidepressants may suffer hypertensive episodes during surgery, stop drug gradually several days before surgery.
● If signs or symptoms of psychosis occur or increase, expect to reduce dosage. Record mood changes. Monitor patient for suicidal tendencies and allow him only a minimum supply of drug.
● *Alert:* Don't confuse nortriptyline with amitriptyline.

## PATIENT TEACHING
● Advise patient to take full dose at bedtime whenever possible, to reduce risk of dizziness upon standing quickly.
● Warn patient to avoid activities that require alertness and good coordination until effects of drug are known. Drowsiness and dizziness usually subside after a few weeks.
● Recommend use of sugarless hard candy or gum to relieve dry mouth. Saliva substitutes may be needed.
● Tell patient to consult prescriber before taking other prescription or OTC drugs.
● Warn patient not to stop drug suddenly.
● To prevent oversensitivity to the sun, advise patient to use sunblock, wear protective clothing, and avoid prolonged exposure to strong sunlight.

---

## paroxetine hydrochloride
Aropax‡, Paxil⊘, Paxil CR

*Pregnancy risk category C*

## AVAILABLE FORMS
*Suspension:* 10 mg/5 ml
*Tablets:* 10 mg, 20 mg, 30 mg, 40 mg
*Tablets (controlled-release):* 12.5 mg, 25 mg, 37.5 mg

## INDICATIONS & DOSAGES
➤ **Depression**
*Adults:* Initially, 20 mg P.O. daily, preferably in morning, as indicated. If patient doesn't improve, dosage may be increased by 10 mg daily at intervals of at least 1 week to maximum of 50 mg daily. If using controlled-release formulation, initially 25 mg P.O. daily. Dose may be increased by 12.5 mg/day at weekly intervals, to maximum of 62.5 mg/day.

*Elderly patients:* Initially, 10 mg P.O. daily, preferably in morning, as indicated. If patient doesn't improve, dose may be increased by 10 mg/day at weekly intervals, to maximum of 40 mg daily. If using controlled-release formulation, start therapy at 12.5 mg P.O. daily. Don't exceed 50 mg/day.

➤ **Obsessive-compulsive disorder (OCD)**
*Adults:* Initially, 20 mg P.O. daily, preferably in morning. Dose may be increased by 10 mg/day at weekly intervals. Recommended daily dose is 40 mg. Maximum daily dose is 60 mg.

➤ **Panic disorder**
*Adults:* Initially, 10 mg P.O. daily. Dose may be increased by 10 mg at no less than weekly intervals, to maximum of 60 mg/day. Or, 12.5 mg P.O. Paxil CR as a single daily dose, usually in the morning, with or without food; may increase dose at intervals of at least 1 week by 12.5 mg/day, up to a maximum of 75 mg/day.
*Adjust a dose:* In elderly or debilitated patients and in those with severe renal or hepatic impairment, the first dose of Paxil CR is 12.5 mg/day; may increase if indicated. Dosage shouldn't exceed 50 mg/day.

➤ **Social anxiety disorder**
*Adults:* Initially, 20 mg P.O. daily, preferably in morning. Dosage range is 20 to 60 mg/day. Adjust dosage to maintain patient on lowest effective dose.

➤ **Generalized anxiety disorder**
*Adults:* 20 mg P.O. daily initially, increasing by 10 mg/day weekly up to 50 mg daily.
*Adjust-a-dose:* For debilitated patients or those with renal or hepatic impairment taking immediate-release formulation, initially, 10 mg P.O. daily, preferably in morning. If patient doesn't respond after full antidepressant effect has occurred, dosage may be increased by 10 mg/day at weekly intervals, to maximum of 40 mg daily. If using controlled-release formulation, start therapy at 12.5 mg/day. Don't exceed 50 mg daily.

➤ **Posttraumatic stress disorder**
*Adults:* Initially, 20 mg P.O. daily. Increase dose by 10 mg/day at intervals of at least 1 week. Maximum daily dose is 50 mg P.O.

✱ *NEW INDICATION:* **Premenstrual dysphoric disorder (PMDD)**
*Adults:* Initially, 12.5 mg P.O Paxil CR as a single daily dose, usually in the morning, with or without food. Dose changes should occur at intervals of at least a week. Maximum dose is 25 mg P.O. daily.

➤ **Premature ejaculation ♦**
*Adults:* 10 to 40 mg P.O. daily. Or, 20 mg P.O. p.r.n. 3 to 4 hours before planned intercourse.

➤ **Diabetic neuropathy ♦**
*Adults:* 40 mg P.O. daily.

## ACTION

Unknown. Thought to be linked to drug's inhibition of CNS neuronal uptake of serotonin.

| Route | Onset | Peak | Duration |
|---|---|---|---|
| P.O. | Unknown | 2-8 hr | Unknown |
| P.O. (controlled-release) | Unknown | 6-10 hr | Unknown |

## ADVERSE REACTIONS

**CNS:** *somnolence, dizziness, insomnia, tremor, nervousness,* anxiety, paresthesia, confusion, *headache,* agitation, *asthenia.*
**CV:** palpitations, vasodilation, orthostatic hypotension.
**EENT:** lump or tightness in throat.
**GI:** *dry mouth, nausea, constipation, diarrhea,* flatulence, vomiting, dyspepsia, dysgeusia, increased or decreased appetite, abdominal pain.
**GU:** *ejaculatory disturbances, sexual dysfunction,* urinary frequency, other urinary disorders.
**Musculoskeletal:** myopathy, myalgia, myasthenia.
**Skin:** rash, pruritus, *diaphoresis.*
**Other:** yawning, *decreased libido.*

## INTERACTIONS

**Drug-drug.** *Cimetidine:* May decrease hepatic metabolism of paroxetine, leading to risk of adverse reactions. Dosage adjustments may be needed.
*Digoxin:* May decrease digoxin level. Use together cautiously.
*MAO inhibitors (phenelzine, selegiline, tranylcypromine):* May cause serotonin syndrome. Avoid using within 14 days of MAO inhibitor therapy.

---

*Rapid onset*   †Canada   ‡Australia   ◇OTC   ♦ Off-label use   ✐Photoguide   *Liquid contains alcohol.

*Phenobarbital, phenytoin:* May alter pharmacokinetics of both drugs. Dosage adjustments may be needed.

*Procyclidine:* May increase procyclidine level. Watch for excessive anticholinergic effects.

*Sumatriptan:* May cause weakness, hyperreflexia, and incoordination. Monitor patient closely.

*Theophylline:* May decrease theophylline clearance. Monitor theophylline level.

*Thioridazine:* May prolong QTc interval and increase risk of serious ventricular arrhythmias, such as torsade de pointes–type arrhythmias, and sudden death. Avoid using together.

*Tramadol:* May cause serotonin syndrome. Monitor patient if used together.

*Tricyclic antidepressants:* May inhibit tricyclic antidepressant metabolism. Dose of tricyclic antidepressant may need to be reduced. Monitor patient closely.

*Tryptophan:* May cause adverse reactions, such as diaphoresis, headache, nausea, and dizziness. Avoid using together.

*Warfarin:* May cause bleeding. Use together cautiously.

**Drug-herb.** *St. John's wort:* May increase sedative-hypnotic effects. Discourage use together.

**Drug-lifestyle.** *Alcohol use:* May alter psychomotor function. Discourage use together.

## EFFECTS ON LAB TEST RESULTS
None reported.

## CONTRAINDICATIONS & CAUTIONS
• Contraindicated in patients hypersensitive to drug, within 14 days of MAO inhibitor therapy, and in those taking thioridazine.
• Contraindicated in children and adolescents under age 18 with major depressive disorder.
• Use cautiously in patients with history of seizure disorders or mania and in those with other severe, systemic illness.
• Use cautiously in patients at risk for volume depletion and monitor them appropriately.

## NURSING CONSIDERATIONS
• Patients taking drug may be at increased risk for developing suicidal behavior, but this hasn't been definitively attributed to use of the drug.
• If signs or symptoms of psychosis occur or increase, expect prescriber to reduce dosage. Record mood changes. Monitor patient for suicidal tendencies, and allow only a minimum supply of drug.
• Monitor patient for complaints of sexual dysfunction. In men, they include anorgasmy, erectile difficulties, delayed ejaculation or orgasm, or impotence; in women, they include anorgasmy or difficulty with orgasm.
• **Alert:** Don't stop drug abruptly. Withdrawal or discontinuation syndrome may occur if drug is stopped abruptly. Symptoms include headache, myalgia, lethargy, and general flulike symptoms. Taper drug slowly over 1 to 2 weeks.
• **Alert:** Don't confuse paroxetine with paclitaxel, or Paxil with Doxil, paclitaxel, Plavix, or Taxol.

## PATIENT TEACHING
• Tell patient that drug may be taken with or without food, usually in morning.
• Tell patient not to break, crush, or chew controlled-release tablets.
• Warn patient to avoid activities that require alertness and good coordination until effects of drug are known.
• Advise woman to contact prescriber if she becomes pregnant or plans to become pregnant during therapy, or if she's currently breast-feeding.
• Tell patient to avoid alcohol and to consult prescriber before taking other prescription or OTC drugs or herbal medicines.
• Instruct patient not to stop taking medication abruptly.

# phenelzine sulfate
Nardil

*Pregnancy risk category C*

## AVAILABLE FORMS
*Tablets:* 15 mg

## INDICATIONS & DOSAGES
➤ **Depression**
*Adults:* 15 mg P.O. t.i.d., increased rapidly to 60 mg daily. Maximum daily dose is

90 mg; dose can usually be reduced to 15 mg daily.

## ACTION
Unknown. An MAO inhibitor that probably promotes accumulation of neurotransmitters by inhibiting their metabolism.

| Route | Onset | Peak | Duration |
| --- | --- | --- | --- |
| P.O. | Unknown | 2-4 hr | 10 days |

## ADVERSE REACTIONS
**CNS:** *dizziness, vertigo, headache,* hyperreflexia, tremor, muscle twitching, *insomnia,* drowsiness, weakness, fatigue.
**CV:** *orthostatic hypotension,* edema.
**GI:** dry mouth, *anorexia,* nausea, *constipation.*
**Metabolic:** weight gain.
**Skin:** diaphoresis.

## INTERACTIONS
**Drug-drug.** *Amphetamines, antihistamines, buspirone, meperidine, methylphenidate, sympathomimetics:* May enhance pressor effects. Avoid using together.
*Antihypertensives containing thiazide diuretics, barbiturates, dextromethorphan, methotrimeprazine, narcotics, other sedatives, spinal anesthetics, tricyclic antidepressants:* May cause unpredictable interaction. Use together cautiously and in reduced dosages.
*Citalopram, fluoxetine, fluvoxamine, nefazodone, paroxetine, sertraline, venlafaxine:* May cause serotonin syndrome. Avoid using within 14 days of MAO inhibitor therapy.
*Dopamine, ephedrine, metaraminol, phenylephrine, pseudoephedrine:* May cause severe headache, hypertension, fever, and hypertensive crisis. Avoid using together.
*Insulin, oral antidiabetics:* May cause hypoglycemia. Use together cautiously and in reduced dosages.
*Levodopa:* May cause hypertensive reaction. Avoid using together.
**Drug-herb.** *Cacao:* May cause potential vasopressor effects. Discourage use together.
*Ephedra:* May cause severe reactions including hypertensive crisis. Discourage use together.
*Ginseng:* May cause headache, tremors, or mania. Discourage use together.
**Drug-food.** *Foods high in caffeine, tryptophan:* May cause hypertensive crisis. Discourage use together; watch for adverse effects.
*Foods with high amine content and tyramine (such as aged, overripe and fermented foods and drinks, broad beans, red wines, chicken or beef liver, caviar, pickled herring, bologna, pepperoni, salami, overripe avocados and various cheeses):* May cause severe hypertension, hypertensive crisis, or hemorrhagic strokes. Warn patient to avoid such foods for at least 1 month after stopping drug therapy.
**Drug-lifestyle.** *Alcohol use:* May cause hypertensive crisis. Discourage use together.

## EFFECTS ON LAB TEST RESULTS
• May increase urinary catecholamine, ALT, and AST levels.

## CONTRAINDICATIONS & CAUTIONS
• Contraindicated in patients hypersensitive to drug and in those with heart failure, pheochromocytoma, hypertension, significant renal impairment, cerebrovascular defect, liver disease, and CV disease. Also contraindicated during therapy with other MAO inhibitors (isocarboxazid, tranylcypromine) or within 10 days of such therapy or within 10 days of elective surgery requiring general anesthesia, cocaine use, or local anesthesia containing sympathomimetic vasoconstrictors.
• Use cautiously with antihypertensives containing thiazide diuretics, with spinal anesthetics, and in patients at risk for suicide, diabetes, or seizure disorders.

## NURSING CONSIDERATIONS
• Obtain baseline blood pressure, heart rate, CBC, and liver function test results before therapy, and continue to monitor them throughout treatment.
• Stop MAO inhibitors 14 days before elective surgery to avoid drug interactions that may occur during anesthesia.
• Monitor patient closely for suicidal tendencies and allow only a minimum supply of drug.

• If patient develops symptoms of over-dose (severe hypotension, palpitations, or frequent headaches), withhold dose and notify prescriber.

• *Alert:* Have phentolamine available to combat severe hypertension.

• Continue precautions 14 days after stopping phenelzine because drug has long-lasting effects.

## PATIENT TEACHING

• Advise patient to consult prescriber before taking other prescription or OTC drugs. Severe adverse effects can occur if MAO inhibitors are taken with OTC cold, hay fever, or diet preparations.

• Warn patient about probability of dizziness upon standing up quickly. Supervise walking. Tell patient to get out of bed slowly, sitting up first for 1 minute.

• Because MAO inhibitors may suppress chest pain, warn patients with angina to engage only in moderate activities and to avoid overexertion.

• Advise patient to avoid anchovies, avocados, bananas, broad beans, canned figs, caviar, cheese, chocolate, dry sausage, liver, meat extract, meat prepared with tenderizers, pickled herring, raisins, sauerkraut, sour cream, soy sauce, yeast extract, yogurt, and any pickled, fermented, or smoked foods. These foods have a high tyramine content, which may interact with the drug and cause a sudden, life-threatening spike in blood pressure (hypertensive crisis). Give patient written MAO inhibitor dietary restrictions, if possible.

• Advise patient to avoid alcohol.

---

## sertraline hydrochloride
Zoloft♦

*Pregnancy risk category C*

---

## AVAILABLE FORMS
*Capsules†:* 25 mg, 50 mg, 100 mg
*Oral concentrate:* 20 mg/ml
*Tablets:* 25 mg, 50 mg, 100 mg

## INDICATIONS & DOSAGES
➤ **Depression**
*Adults:* 50 mg P.O. daily. Adjust dosage as needed and tolerated; dosages range from 50 to 200 mg daily.

➤ **Obsessive-compulsive disorder**
*Adults:* 50 mg P.O. once daily. If patient doesn't improve, increase dosage, up to 200 mg/day.
*Children ages 6 to 17:* Initially, 25 mg P.O. daily in children ages 6 to 12, or 50 mg P.O. daily in children ages 13 to 17. May increase dosage, p.r.n., up to 200 mg/day at intervals of no less than 1 week.
➤ **Panic disorder**
*Adults:* Initially, 25 mg P.O. daily. After 1 week, increase dose to 50 mg P.O. daily. If patient doesn't improve, dose may be increased to maximum of 200 mg/day.
➤ **Posttraumatic stress disorder**
*Adults:* Initially, 25 mg P.O. once daily. Increase dosage to 50 mg P.O. once daily after 1 week. Dosage may be increased at weekly intervals to a maximum of 200 mg daily. Maintain patient on lowest effective dose.
➤ **Premenstrual dysphoric disorder**
*Adults:* Initially, 50 mg daily P.O. either continuously or only during the luteal phase of the menstrual cycle. If patient doesn't respond, dose may be increased 50 mg per menstrual cycle, up to 150 mg daily for dosing throughout the menstrual cycle or 100 mg daily for luteal-phase dosing. If a 100-mg daily dose has been established with luteal-phase dosing, use a 50-mg daily adjustment for 3 days at the beginning of each luteal phase.
✴ *NEW INDICATION:* **Social anxiety disorder**
*Adults:* Initially, 25 mg P.O. once daily. Increase dosage to 50 mg P.O. once daily after 1 week of therapy. Usual dosage range is 50 to 200 mg daily. Adjust to the lowest effective dosage and periodically reassess patient to determine the need for long-term treatment.
➤ **Premature ejaculation ♦**
*Adults:* 25 to 50 mg P.O. daily or p.r.n.
*Adjust-a-dose:* For patients with hepatic disease, use lower or less-frequent doses.

## ACTION
Unknown. Thought to be linked to drug's inhibition of CNS neuronal uptake of serotonin.

| Route | Onset | Peak | Duration |
|-------|---------|--------|----------|
| P.O. | Unknown | 4-8 hr | Unknown |

---

**ADVERSE REACTIONS**
**CNS:** *headache, tremor, dizziness, insomnia, somnolence,* paresthesia, hypesthesia, *fatigue,* nervousness, anxiety, agitation, hypertonia, twitching, confusion.
**CV:** palpitations, chest pain, hot flashes.
**GI:** *dry mouth, nausea, diarrhea, loose stools, dyspepsia,* vomiting, constipation, thirst, flatulence, anorexia, abdominal pain, increased appetite.
**GU:** *male sexual dysfunction.*
**Musculoskeletal:** myalgia.
**Skin:** rash, pruritus, diaphoresis.

**INTERACTIONS**
**Drug-drug.** *Benzodiazepines, tolbutamide:* May decrease clearance of these drugs. Significance unknown; monitor patient for increased drug effects.
*Cimetidine:* May decrease clearance of sertraline. Monitor patient closely.
*Disulfiram:* Oral concentrate contains alcohol, which may react with drug. Avoid using together.
*MAO inhibitors (phenelzine, selegiline, tranylcypromine):* May cause serotonin syndrome. Avoid using within 14 days of MAO inhibitor therapy.
*Pimozide:* May increase pimozide level. Avoid using together.
*Warfarin, other highly protein-bound drugs:* May increase level of sertraline or other highly protein-bound drug. May increase PT or INR may increase by 8%. Monitor patient closely.
**Drug-herb.** *St. John's wort:* May cause additive effects and serotonin syndrome. Discourage use together.

**EFFECTS ON LAB TEST RESULTS**
● May increase ALT and AST levels.

**CONTRAINDICATIONS & CAUTIONS**
● Contraindicated in patients with a hypersensitivity to drug or its components. Contraindicated in patients taking pimozide or MAO inhibitors or within 14 days of MAO inhibitor therapy.
● Use cautiously in patients at risk for suicide and in those with seizure disorders, major affective disorder, or diseases or conditions that affect metabolism or hemodynamic responses.

**NURSING CONSIDERATIONS**
● Give sertraline once daily, either in morning or evening, with or without food.
● Make dosage adjustments at intervals of no less than 1 week.
● Record mood changes. Monitor patient for suicidal tendencies and allow only a minimum supply of drug.
● Don't use the oral concentrate dropper, which is made of rubber, in a patient with latex allergy.

**PATIENT TEACHING**
● Advise patient to use caution when performing hazardous tasks that require alertness.
● Tell patient to avoid alcohol and to consult prescriber before taking OTC drugs.
● Advise patient to mix the oral concentrate with 4 ounces (¼ cup) of water, ginger ale, lemon or lime soda, lemonade, or orange juice only, and to take the dose right away.
● Instruct patient to avoid stopping the medication abruptly.

---

**tranylcypromine sulfate**
Parnate

*Pregnancy risk category C*

---

**AVAILABLE FORMS**
*Tablets:* 10 mg

**INDICATIONS & DOSAGES**
➤ **Depression**
*Adults:* 10 mg P.O. t.i.d. Increase dose by 10 mg P.O. daily at 1- to 3-week intervals to maximum of 60 mg daily, if needed, after 2 weeks of therapy.

**ACTION**
Unknown. An MAO inhibitor that probably promotes accumulation of neurotransmitters by inhibiting their metabolism.

| Route | Onset | Peak | Duration |
|-------|-------|------|----------|
| P.O. | Unknown | 1-3½ hr | 10 days |

**ADVERSE REACTIONS**
**CNS:** *dizziness, headache,* anxiety, agitation, paresthesia, drowsiness, weakness, numbness, tremor, jitters, confusion, *vertigo.*

**CV:** *orthostatic hypotension, tachycardia,* paradoxical hypertension, palpitations, *edema.*
**EENT:** blurred vision, tinnitus.
**GI:** dry mouth, *anorexia,* nausea, diarrhea, constipation, abdominal pain.
**GU:** impotence, urine retention, impaired ejaculation.
**Hematologic:** anemia, *leukopenia, agranulocytosis, thrombocytopenia.*
**Hepatic:** *hepatitis.*
**Metabolic:** SIADH.
**Musculoskeletal:** muscle spasm, myoclonic jerks.
**Skin:** rash.
**Other:** chills.

## INTERACTIONS
**Drug-drug.** *Amphetamines, antihistamines, antihypertensives, diuretics, meperidine, methylphenidate, sympathomimetics:* May enhance pressor effects of these drugs. Avoid using together.
*Antiparkinsonians, barbiturates, dextromethorphan, methotrimeprazine, narcotics, other sedatives, spinal anesthetics, tricyclic antidepressants:* May enhance adverse CNS effects. Avoid using together. If necessary, use with caution and in reduced dosages.
*Buspirone:* May elevate blood pressure. Monitor patient closely.
*Citalopram, fluoxetine, fluvoxamine, nefazodone, paroxetine, sertraline, venlafaxine:* May cause serotonin syndrome. Avoid using within 14 days of MAO inhibitor therapy.
*Dopamine, ephedrine, metaraminol, phenylephrine, pseudoephedrine:* May cause severe headache, hypertension, fever, and hypertensive crisis. Avoid using together.
*Insulin, oral antidiabetics:* May cause hypoglycemia. Use together cautiously and in reduced dosages.
*Levodopa:* May cause hypertensive reaction. Avoid using together.
**Drug-herb.** *Cacao:* May cause potential vasopressor effects. Discourage use together.
*Ephedra:* May cause severe reactions including hypertensive crisis. Discourage use together.
*Ginseng:* May cause headache, tremors, or mania. Monitor patient for effects.

*Licorice:* May cause increase in tranylcypromine activity. Discourage use together.
*Tryptophan:* May cause additive effect leading to serotonin syndrome. Discourage use together.
**Drug-food.** *Foods high in caffeine, tryptophan:* May cause hypertensive crisis. Discourage use together.
*Foods with high amine content and tyramine (such as aged, overripe and fermented foods and drinks, broad beans, red wines, chicken or beef liver, caviar, pickled herring, bologna, pepperoni, salami, overripe avocados and various cheeses):* May cause severe elevation of blood pressure, hypertensive crisis, or hemorrhagic strokes. Warn patient to avoid such foods for at least 1 month after stopping drug therapy.
**Drug-lifestyle.** *Alcohol use:* May enhance CNS effects. Discourage use together.

## EFFECTS ON LAB TEST RESULTS
● May increase urinary catecholamine, ALT, and AST levels.
● May decrease hemoglobin, hematocrit, and WBC, granulocyte, and platelet counts.

## CONTRAINDICATIONS & CAUTIONS
● Contraindicated in patients hypersensitive to drug and in those with pheochromocytoma, cerebrovascular or CV disease, confirmed or suspected cerebrovascular defect, hypertension, heart failure, hepatic disease, significant renal impairment, or history of headache.
● Contraindicated in patients receiving MAO inhibitors or dibenzazepine derivatives within 2 weeks, in those undergoing elective surgery, and debilitated patients.
● Use cautiously in patients with renal disease, diabetes, seizure disorders, Parkinson's disease, or hyperthyroidism, and in those at risk for suicide.

## NURSING CONSIDERATIONS
● Obtain baseline blood pressure, heart rate, CBC, and liver function test results before therapy, and continue to monitor them throughout treatment.
● Dosage usually is reduced to maintenance level as soon as possible.
● Don't withdraw drug abruptly.

---

- Stop MAO inhibitors 14 days before elective surgery, to avoid drug interactions that may occur during anesthesia.
- Monitor patient for suicidal tendencies and allow only a minimum supply of drug.
- If patient develops signs or symptoms of overdose (palpitations, severe hypotension, or frequent headaches), withhold dose and notify prescriber.
- *Alert:* Have phentolamine available to combat severe hypertension.
- Continue precautions for 10 days after stopping drug because it has long-lasting effects.

**PATIENT TEACHING**
- Warn patient to avoid foods high in tyramine, tryptophan, or caffeine. Tranylcypromine is the MAO inhibitor most often reported to cause dangerous, sudden spike in blood pressure after eating tyramine-rich foods, including aged cheese, anchovies, bologna, Chianti wine, beer, avocados, chicken livers, chocolate, bananas, soy sauce, meat tenderizers, salami, broad beans, canned figs, caviar, dry sausage, liver, meat extract, pickled herring, raisins, sauerkraut, sour cream, yeast extract, yogurt, and any pickled, fermented, or smoked foods. Give patient written MAO inhibitor dietary restrictions, if possible.
- Tell patient to avoid alcohol during therapy.
- Advise patient to consult prescriber before taking other prescription or OTC drugs.
- To prevent dizziness caused by standing up too quickly, tell patient to get out of bed slowly, sitting up first for 1 minute.
- Because MAO inhibitors may suppress chest pain, warn patient to perform only moderate activities and to avoid overexertion.
- Warn patient not to stop drug suddenly.

---

**trazodone hydrochloride**
Desyrel◆

*Pregnancy risk category C*

**AVAILABLE FORMS**
*Tablets:* 50 mg, 100 mg, 150 mg, 300 mg

**INDICATIONS & DOSAGES**
➤ **Depression**
*Adults:* Initially, 150 mg P.O. daily in divided doses; then increased by 50 mg daily q 3 to 4 days, p.r.n. Dose ranges from 150 to 400 mg daily. Maximum, 600 mg daily for inpatients and 400 mg daily for outpatients.

**ACTION**
Unknown. Inhibits CNS neuronal uptake of serotonin; not a tricyclic derivative.

| Route | Onset | Peak | Duration |
|-------|-------|------|----------|
| P.O. | Unknown | 1-2 hr | Unknown |

**ADVERSE REACTIONS**
**CNS:** *drowsiness, dizziness,* nervousness, fatigue, confusion, tremor, weakness, hostility, anger, nightmares, vivid dreams, headache, insomnia, syncope.
**CV:** orthostatic hypotension, tachycardia, hypertension, shortness of breath, ECG changes.
**EENT:** blurred vision, tinnitus, nasal congestion.
**GI:** dry mouth, dysgeusia, constipation, nausea, vomiting, anorexia.
**GU:** urine retention; priapism possibly leading to impotence; hematuria.
**Hematologic:** anemia.
**Skin:** rash, urticaria, diaphoresis.
**Other:** decreased libido.

**INTERACTIONS**
**Drug-drug.** *Antihypertensives:* May increase hypotensive effect of trazodone. Antihypertensive dosage may need to be decreased.
*Clonidine, CNS depressants:* May enhance CNS depression. Avoid using together.
*Digoxin, phenytoin:* May increase levels of these drugs. Watch for toxicity.
*MAO inhibitors:* Effects unknown. Use together with extreme caution.
**Drug-herb.** *Ginkgo biloba:* May cause sedation. Discourage use together.
*St. John's wort:* May cause serotonin syndrome. Discourage use together.
**Drug-lifestyle.** *Alcohol use:* May enhance CNS depression. Discourage use together.

**EFFECTS ON LAB TEST RESULTS**
- May increase ALT and AST levels.
- May decrease hemoglobin.

## CONTRAINDICATIONS & CAUTIONS
• Contraindicated in patients hypersensitive to drug.
• Use cautiously in patients with cardiac disease or in the initial recovery phase of MI and in patients at risk for suicide.

## NURSING CONSIDERATIONS
• Give drug after meals or a light snack for optimal absorption and to decrease risk of dizziness.
• Record mood changes. Monitor patient for suicidal tendencies and allow only minimum supply of drug.
• *Alert:* Don't confuse trazodone hydrochloride with tramadol hydrochloride.

## PATIENT TEACHING
• *Alert:* Tell patient to report a persistent, painful erection (priapism) right away because he may need immediate intervention.
• Warn patient to avoid activities that require alertness and good coordination until effects of drug are known. Drowsiness and dizziness usually subside after first few weeks.
• Teach caregivers how to recognize signs and symptoms of suicidal tendency or suicidal thoughts.

---

## venlafaxine hydrochloride
Effexor‡, Effexor♦, Effexor XR♦

*Pregnancy risk category C*

## AVAILABLE FORMS
*Capsules (extended-release):* 37.5 mg, 75 mg, 150 mg
*Tablets:* 25 mg, 37.5 mg, 50 mg, 75 mg, 100 mg

## INDICATIONS & DOSAGES
➤ **Depression**
*Adults:* Initially, 75 mg P.O. daily in two or three divided doses with food. Increase as tolerated and needed by 75 mg/day q 4 days. For moderately depressed outpatients, usual maximum is 225 mg daily; in certain severely depressed patients, dose may be as high as 375 mg daily. For extended-release capsules, 75 mg P.O. daily in a single dose. For some patients, it may be desirable to start at 37.5 mg P.O.

daily for 4 to 7 days before increasing to 75 mg daily. Dosage may be increased by 75 mg/day q 4 days to maximum of 225 mg/day.
➤ **Generalized anxiety disorder**
*Adults:* Initially, 75 mg of Effexor XR P.O. daily in a single dose. For some patients, it may be desirable to start at 37.5 mg P.O. daily for 4 to 7 days before increasing to 75 mg daily. May be increased by 75 mg/day q 4 days to maximum of 225 mg/day.
✳ *NEW INDICATION:* **Social anxiety disorder**
*Adults:* Initially, 75 mg/day extended-release capsule in a single dose. For some patients, it may be desirable to start at 37.5 mg P.O. daily for 4 to 7 days before increasing to 75 mg daily. Increase dosage as needed by 75 mg/day q 4 days. Maximum dosage is 225 mg/day.
*Adjust-a-dose:* For renally impaired patients, reduce daily amount by 25%. For patients undergoing hemodialysis, reduce daily amount by 50% and withhold dose until dialysis is completed. For patients with hepatic impairment, reduce daily amount by 50%.
➤ **To prevent major depressive disorder relapse ◆**
*Adults:* 100 to 200 mg daily P.O. Effexor or 75 to 225 mg daily P.O. Effexor XR.

## ACTION
May increase the amount of norepinephrine, serotonin, or both in the CNS by blocking their reuptake by the presynaptic neurons.

| Route | Onset | Peak | Duration |
|-------|-------|------|----------|
| P.O. | Unknown | 1-2 hr | Unknown |

## ADVERSE REACTIONS
**CNS:** *headache, somnolence, dizziness, nervousness, insomnia,* anxiety, tremor, abnormal dreams, paresthesia, agitation, *asthenia.*
**CV:** hypertension, tachycardia, vasodilation.
**EENT:** blurred vision.
**GI:** *nausea, constipation,* vomiting, *dry mouth, anorexia,* diarrhea, dyspepsia, flatulence.
**GU:** *abnormal ejaculation,* impotence, urinary frequency, impaired urination.
**Metabolic:** weight loss.

---

Reactions may be *common,* uncommon, *life-threatening,* or COMMON AND LIFE-THREATENING.

**Skin:** *diaphoresis,* rash.
**Other:** yawning, chills, infection.

**INTERACTIONS**
**Drug-drug.** *MAO inhibitors (phenelzine, selegiline, tranylcypromine):* May cause serotonin syndrome. Avoid using within 14 days of MAO inhibitor therapy.
**Drug-herb.** *Yohimbe:* May cause additive stimulation. Urge caution.

**EFFECTS ON LAB TEST RESULTS**
None reported.

**CONTRAINDICATIONS & CAUTIONS**
• Contraindicated in patients hypersensitive to drug or within 14 days of MAO inhibitor therapy.
• Use cautiously in patients with renal impairment, diseases or conditions that could affect hemodynamic responses or metabolism, and in those with history of mania or seizures.

**NURSING CONSIDERATIONS**
• Monitor patient for suicidal tendencies. Provide only a minimal supply of drug.
• Carefully monitor blood pressure. Drug therapy may cause sustained, dose-dependent increases in blood pressure. Greatest increases (averaging about 7 mm Hg above baseline) occur in patients taking 375 mg daily.
• Monitor patient's weight, particularly underweight, depressed patients.

**PATIENT TEACHING**
• If medication is to be stopped, inform patient who has received drug for 6 weeks or longer that drug will be gradually stopped by tapering dosage over a 2-week period as instructed by prescriber.
• Warn patient to avoid hazardous activities that require alertness and good coordination until effects of drug are known.
• Tell patient to avoid alcohol and to consult prescriber before taking other prescription or OTC drugs.
• Advise woman to contact prescriber if she becomes pregnant or intends to become pregnant during therapy or if she's breast-feeding.

alprazolam
buspirone hydrochloride
chlordiazepoxide
chlordiazepoxide hydrochloride
clorazepate dipotassium
diazepam
doxepin hydrochloride
(See Chapter 29, ANTIDEPRESSANTS.)
hydroxyzine hydrochloride
hydroxyzine pamoate
lorazepam
midazolam hydrochloride
oxazepam

### COMBINATION PRODUCTS
EQUAGESIC: meprobamate 200 mg and aspirin 325 mg.
LIBRAX: chlordiazepoxide hydrochloride 5 mg and clidinium bromide 2.5 mg.
LIMBITROL DS: chlordiazepoxide 10 mg and amitriptyline hydrochloride 25 mg.

---

### alprazolam
Apo-Alpraz†, Kalma‡, Novo-Alprazol†, Nu-Alpraz†, Xanax♥, Xanax XR

*Pregnancy risk category D*
*Controlled substance schedule IV*

### AVAILABLE FORMS
*Oral solution:* 0.5 mg/5 ml, 1 mg/ml (concentrate)
*Tablets:* 0.25 mg, 0.5 mg, 1 mg, 2 mg
*Tablets (extended-release):* 0.5 mg, 1 mg, 2 mg, 3 mg

### INDICATIONS & DOSAGES
➤ **Anxiety**
*Adults:* Usual first dose, 0.25 to 0.5 mg P.O. t.i.d. Maximum, 4 mg daily in divided doses.
*Elderly patients:* Usual first dose, 0.25 mg P.O. b.i.d. or t.i.d. Maximum, 4 mg daily in divided doses.
➤ **Panic disorders**
*Adults:* 0.5 mg P.O. t.i.d., increased at intervals of 3 to 4 days in increments of no more than 1 mg. Maximum, 10 mg daily

in divided doses. If using extended-release tablets, start with 0.5 to 1 mg P.O. once daily. Increase by no more than 1 mg q 3 to 4 days. Maximum daily dose is 10 mg.
*Adjust-a-dose:* For debilitated patients or those with advanced hepatic disease, usual first dose is 0.25 mg P.O. b.i.d. or t.i.d. Maximum, 4 mg daily in divided doses.

### ACTION
Unknown; a benzodiazepine that probably potentiates the effects of gamma-aminobutyric acid, depresses the CNS, and suppresses the spread of seizure activity.

| Route | Onset | Peak | Duration |
|---|---|---|---|
| P.O. | Unknown | 1-2 hr | Unknown |
| P.O. (extended-release) | Unknown | Unknown | Unknown |

### ADVERSE REACTIONS
**CNS:** *drowsiness, light-headedness, sedation, somnolence, difficulty speaking, impaired coordination, memory impairment, fatigue, depression,* mental impairment, ataxia, paresthesia, dyskinesia, hypoesthesia, lethargy, decreased or increased libido, *confusion, anxiety,* vertigo, malaise, *headache, dizziness,* tremor, *irritability, insomnia,* nervousness, restlessness, agitation, nightmare, syncope, akathisia, mania, **suicide.**
**CV:** hot flushes, palpitation, chest pain, hypotension.
**EENT:** sore throat, allergic rhinitis, blurred vision, nasal congestion
**GI:** *dry mouth, constipation,* nausea, increased or decreased appetite, anorexia, *diarrhea,* vomiting, dyspepsia, abdominal pain.
**GU:** dysmenorrhea, sexual dysfunction, premenstrual syndrome, difficulty urinating
**Metabolic:** increased or decreased weight.
**Musculoskeletal:** arthralgia, myalgia, arm or leg pain, back pain, muscle rigidity, muscle cramps, muscle twitch.

---

Reactions may be *common,* uncommon, *life-threatening,* or COMMON AND LIFE-THREATENING.

**Respiratory:** upper respiratory tract infection, dyspnea, hyperventilation.
**Skin:** pruritus, increased sweating, dermatitis.
**Other:** influenza, injury, emergence of anxiety between doses, dependence.

**INTERACTIONS**
**Drug-drug.** *Anticonvulsants, antidepressants, antihistamines, barbiturates, benzodiazepines, general anesthetics, narcotics, phenothiazines:* May increase CNS depressant effects. Avoid use together.
*Azole antifungals (including fluconazole, itraconazole, ketoconazole, miconazole):* May increase and prolong alprazolam level, CNS depression, and psychomotor impairment. Avoid using together.
*Carbamazepine, propoxyphene:* May decrease alprazolam level. Use together cautiously.
*Cimetidine, fluoxetine, fluvoxamine, hormonal contraceptives, nefazodone:* May increase alprazolam level. Use cautiously together and consider alprazolam dosage reduction.
*Tricyclic antidepressants:* May increase levels of these drugs. Monitor patient closely.
**Drug-herb.** *Kava:* May increase sedation. Discourage use together.
*St. John's wort:* May decrease alprazolam level. Discourage use together.
**Drug-food.** *Grapefruit juice:* May increase alprazolam level. Advise patient to take drug with liquid other than grapefruit juice.
**Drug-lifestyle.** *Alcohol use:* May cause additive CNS effects. Discourage use together.
*Smoking:* May decrease effectiveness of benzodiazepines. Monitor patient closely.

**EFFECTS ON LAB TEST RESULTS**
• May increase ALT and AST levels.

**CONTRAINDICATIONS & CAUTIONS**
• Contraindicated in patients hypersensitive to drug or other benzodiazepines and in those with acute angle-closure glaucoma.
• Use cautiously in patients with hepatic, renal, or pulmonary disease.

**NURSING CONSIDERATIONS**
• Further study is needed to determine the optimum duration of therapy.
• *Alert:* Don't withdraw drug abruptly; withdrawal symptoms, including seizures, may occur. Abuse or addiction is possible.
• Monitor hepatic, renal, and hematopoietic function periodically in patients receiving repeated or prolonged therapy.
• *Alert:* Don't confuse alprazolam with alprostadil.
• *Alert:* Don't confuse Xanax with Zantac or Tenex.

**PATIENT TEACHING**
• Warn patient to avoid hazardous activities that require alertness and good coordination until effects of drug are known.
• Tell patient to avoid alcohol while taking drug.
• Advise patient that smoking may decrease drug's effectiveness.
• Warn patient not to stop drug abruptly because withdrawal symptoms or seizures may occur.
• Tell patient to swallow extended-release tablets whole.

---

**buspirone hydrochloride**
BuSpar♪

*Pregnancy risk category B*

**AVAILABLE FORMS**
*Tablets:* 5 mg, 10 mg, 15 mg, 30 mg

**INDICATIONS & DOSAGES**
➤ **Anxiety disorders, short-term relief of anxiety**
*Adults:* Initially, 10 to 15 mg daily in two or three divided doses. Increase dosage by 5-mg increments at 2- to 4-day intervals. Usual maintenance dosage is 15 to 30 mg daily in divided doses. Don't exceed 60 mg daily.

**ACTION**
Unknown. May inhibit neuronal firing and reduce serotonin turnover in cortical, amygdaloid, and septohippocampal tissue.

| Route | Onset | Peak | Duration |
|---|---|---|---|
| P.O. | Unknown | 40-90 min | Unknown |

## ADVERSE REACTIONS
**CNS:** *dizziness, drowsiness,* nervousness, insomnia, *headache,* light-headedness, fatigue, numbness.
**CV:** tachycardia, nonspecific chest pain.
**EENT:** blurred vision.
**GI:** dry mouth, nausea, diarrhea, abdominal distress.

## INTERACTIONS
**Drug-drug.** *CNS depressants:* May increase CNS depression. Use together cautiously.
*Drugs metabolized by CYP-450 3A4 (erythromycin, itraconazole, nefazodone):* May increase buspirone level. Monitor patient; a decrease in buspirone dosage may be needed.
*MAO inhibitors:* May elevate blood pressure. Avoid using together.
**Drug-food.** *Grapefruit juice:* May increase buspirone level, increasing adverse effects. Give with liquid other than grapefruit juice.
**Drug-lifestyle.** *Alcohol use:* May increase CNS depression. Discourage use together.

## EFFECTS ON LAB TEST RESULTS
None reported.

## CONTRAINDICATIONS & CAUTIONS
● Contraindicated in patients hypersensitive to drug; also contraindicated within 14 days of MAO inhibitor therapy.
● Drug isn't recommended for patients with severe hepatic or renal impairment.

## NURSING CONSIDERATIONS
● Monitor patient closely for adverse CNS reactions. Buspirone is less sedating than other anxiolytics, but CNS effects may be unpredictable.
● *Alert:* Before starting buspirone therapy in a patient already receiving a benzodiazepine, don't stop the benzodiazepine abruptly because a withdrawal reaction may occur.
● Drug has shown no potential for abuse and hasn't been classified as a controlled substance.
● *Alert:* Don't confuse buspirone with bupropion.

## PATIENT TEACHING
● Warn patient to avoid hazardous activities that require alertness and good coordination until effects of drug are known.
● Remind patient that drug effects may not be noticeable for several weeks.
● Warn patient not to abruptly stop a benzodiazepine because of risk of withdrawal symptoms.
● Tell patient to avoid alcohol use during drug therapy.

# chlordiazepoxide
Libritabs

# chlordiazepoxide hydrochloride
Apo-Chlordiazepoxide†, Librium, Novo-Poxide†

*Pregnancy risk category NR*
*Controlled substance schedule IV*

## AVAILABLE FORMS
**chlordiazepoxide**
*Tablets:* 10 mg, 25 mg
**chlordiazepoxide hydrochloride**
*Capsules:* 5 mg, 10 mg, 25 mg
*Powder for injection:* 100-mg ampule

## INDICATIONS & DOSAGES
➤ **Mild to moderate anxiety**
*Adults:* 5 to 10 mg P.O. t.i.d. or q.i.d.
*Children older than age 6:* 5 mg P.O. b.i.d. to q.i.d. Maximum, 10 mg P.O. b.i.d. or t.i.d.
➤ **Severe anxiety**
*Adults:* 20 to 25 mg P.O. t.i.d. or q.i.d.
*Elderly patients:* 5 mg P.O. b.i.d. to q.i.d.
*Adjust-a-dose:* For debilitated patients, 5 mg P.O. b.i.d. to q.i.d.
➤ **Withdrawal symptoms of acute alcoholism**
*Adults:* 50 to 100 mg P.O., I.M., or I.V. Repeat in 2 to 4 hours, p.r.n. Maximum, 300 mg daily.
➤ **Preoperative apprehension and anxiety**
*Adults:* 5 to 10 mg P.O. t.i.d. or q.i.d. on day before surgery; or 50 to 100 mg I.M. 1 hour before surgery.

---

Reactions may be *common,* uncommon, *life-threatening,* or COMMON AND LIFE-THREATENING.

## I.V. ADMINISTRATION

• Parenteral form isn't recommended in children younger than age 12.

• Use 5 ml of normal saline solution or sterile water for injection as diluent for an ampule containing 100 mg of drug. Don't give prepackaged diluent I.V. because air bubbles may form. Give over 1 minute.

• When giving drug I.V., make sure equipment and staff needed for emergency airway management are available. Monitor respirations every 5 to 15 minutes and before each I.V. dose.

## ACTION

Unknown. A benzodiazepine that probably potentiates the effects of gamma-aminobutyric acid, depresses the CNS, and suppresses the spread of seizure activity.

| Route | Onset | Peak | Duration |
|-------|-------|------|----------|
| P.O. | Unknown | ½-4 hr | Unknown |
| I.V. | 1-5 min | Unknown | 15-60 min |
| I.M. | Unknown | Unknown | Unknown |

## ADVERSE REACTIONS

**CNS:** *drowsiness, lethargy,* ataxia, confusion, extrapyramidal reactions, minor changes in EEG patterns.
**CV:** edema.
**GI:** nausea, constipation.
**GU:** menstrual irregularities.
**Hematologic:** *agranulocytosis.*
**Hepatic:** jaundice.
**Skin:** *swelling and pain at injection site,* skin eruptions.
**Other:** altered libido.

## INTERACTIONS

**Drug-drug.** *Cimetidine:* May decrease chlordiazepoxide clearance and increases risk of adverse reactions. Monitor patient carefully.
*CNS depressants:* May increase CNS depression. Use together cautiously.
*Digoxin:* May increase digoxin level and risk of toxicity. Monitor patient and digoxin level closely.
*Disulfiram:* May decrease clearance and increase half-life of chlordiazepoxide. Monitor patient for enhanced effects. Consider dosage adjustment.
*Fluconazole, itraconazole, ketoconazole, miconazole:* May increase and prolong

chlordiazepoxide levels, CNS depression, and psychomotor impairment. Avoid using together.
*Levodopa:* May decrease control of parkinsonian symptoms in patients with Parkinson's disease. Use together cautiously.
**Drug-herb.** *Kava:* May increase sedation. Discourage use together.
**Drug-lifestyle.** *Alcohol use:* May cause additive CNS effects. Discourage use together.
*Smoking:* May decrease effectiveness of benzodiazepines. Monitor patient closely.

## EFFECTS ON LAB TEST RESULTS

• May increase liver function test values. May decrease granulocyte count. May alter urinary 17-ketosteroid (Zimmerman reaction), urine alkaloid (Frings thin-layer chromatography method), and urinary glucose determinations (with Chemstrip uG and Diastix).

## CONTRAINDICATIONS & CAUTIONS

• Contraindicated in patients hypersensitive to drug and in pregnant women, especially in first trimester.
• Use cautiously in patients with mental depression, porphyria, or hepatic or renal disease.

## NURSING CONSIDERATIONS

• *Alert:* Chlordiazepoxide 5-mg and 25-mg unit-dose capsules may look similar in color when viewed through the package. When using unit doses of this or any product, verify contents and read label carefully.
• Long-term effectiveness of drug hasn't been established.
• Injectable form (as hydrochloride) comes in two types of ampules—as diluent and as powdered drug. Read directions carefully.
• Keep powder refrigerated and away from light; mix just before use and discard remainder.
• For I.M. use, add 2 ml of diluent to powder and agitate gently until clear. Use immediately. I.M. form may be absorbed erratically.
• Monitor hepatic, renal, and hematopoietic function periodically in patients receiving repeated or prolonged therapy.
• *Alert:* Use of this drug may lead to abuse and addiction. Don't withdraw drug

abruptly after long-term administration because withdrawal symptoms may occur.
• Drug may cause a false-positive pregnancy test result, depending on method used.

## PATIENT TEACHING
• Warn patient to avoid hazardous activities that require alertness and good coordination until effects of drug are known.
• Tell patient to avoid alcohol while taking drug.
• Notify patient that smoking may decrease drug's effectiveness.
• Warn patient not to abruptly stop the drug because withdrawal symptoms may occur.
• Warn woman to avoid use during pregnancy.

## clorazepate dipotassium
Apo-Clorazepate†, Gen-Xene, Novo-Clopate†, Tranxene, Tranxene-SD

*Pregnancy risk category D*
*Controlled substance schedule IV*

## AVAILABLE FORMS
*Capsules:* 3.75 mg, 7.5 mg, 15 mg
*Tablets:* 3.75 mg, 7.5 mg, 11.25 mg, 15 mg, 22.5 mg

## INDICATIONS & DOSAGES
➤ **Acute alcohol withdrawal**
*Adults:* Day 1, give 30 mg P.O. initially; then 30 to 60 mg P.O. in divided doses. Day 2, give 45 to 90 mg P.O. in divided doses. Day 3, give 22.5 to 45 mg P.O. in divided doses. Day 4, give 15 to 30 mg P.O. in divided doses. Then gradually reduce dosage to 7.5 to 15 mg daily. Maximum dosage is 90 mg daily.
➤ **Anxiety**
*Adults:* 15 to 60 mg P.O. daily.
*Elderly patients:* Initially, 7.5 to 15 mg daily in divided doses or as a single dose h.s.
*Adjust-a-dose:* For debilitated patients, initially, 7.5 to 15 mg daily in divided doses or as a single dose h.s.
➤ **Adjunctive treatment for partial seizure disorder**
*Adults and children older than age 12:* Maximum first dose is 7.5 mg P.O. t.i.d.

Dosage increases shouldn't exceed 7.5 mg weekly. Maximum daily dose is 90 mg.
*Children ages 9 to 12:* Maximum first dose is 7.5 mg P.O. b.i.d. Dosage increases shouldn't exceed 7.5 mg weekly. Maximum daily dose is 60 mg.

## ACTION
Unknown. A benzodiazepine that probably potentiates the effects of gamma-aminobutyric acid, depresses the CNS, and suppresses the spread of seizure activity.

| Route | Onset | Peak | Duration |
|-------|-------|------|----------|
| P.O. | Unknown | 30 min-2 hr | Unknown |

## ADVERSE REACTIONS
**CNS:** *drowsiness, dizziness,* nervousness, confusion, headache, insomnia, depression, irritability, tremor, minor changes in EEG patterns.
**CV:** hypotension.
**EENT:** blurred vision, diplopia.
**GI:** nausea, vomiting, abdominal discomfort, dry mouth.
**GU:** urine retention, incontinence.
**Skin:** rash.

## INTERACTIONS
**Drug-drug.** *Cimetidine:* May decrease clorazepate clearance and increase risk of adverse reactions. Monitor patient carefully.
*CNS depressants:* May increase CNS depression. Use together cautiously.
*Digoxin:* May increase digoxin level and risk of toxicity. Monitor patient and digoxin level closely.
**Drug-herb.** *Kava:* May increase sedation. Discourage use together.
**Drug-lifestyle.** *Alcohol use:* May cause additive CNS effects. Discourage use together.
*Smoking:* May decrease benzodiazepine effectiveness. Urge patient to quit smoking, and monitor patient closely.

## EFFECTS ON LAB TEST RESULTS
• May increase liver function test values.

## CONTRAINDICATIONS & CAUTIONS
• Contraindicated in patients hypersensitive to drug and in those with acute angle-closure glaucoma.

---

Reactions may be *common,* uncommon, *life-threatening,* or COMMON AND LIFE-THREATENING.

- Use cautiously in patients with suicidal tendencies, renal or hepatic impairment, pulmonary disease, or history of drug abuse.
- Don't give drug to pregnant women, especially during first trimester.
- Drug isn't recommended for children younger than age 9.

**NURSING CONSIDERATIONS**
- *Alert:* Monitor hepatic, renal, and hematopoietic function periodically in patients receiving repeated or prolonged therapy.
- *Alert:* Use of this drug may lead to abuse and addiction. Don't withdraw drug abruptly after prolonged use because withdrawal symptoms may occur.
- *Alert:* Don't confuse clorazepate with clofibrate.

**PATIENT TEACHING**
- Warn patient to avoid activities that require alertness and good coordination until effects of drug are known.
- *Alert:* Advise patient taking Tranxene-SD to swallow pill whole and not to crush, break, or chew pill before swallowing it.
- Tell patient to avoid alcohol while taking drug.
- Advise patient that smoking may decrease drug's effectiveness.
- Warn patient not to stop drug abruptly because withdrawal symptoms may occur.
- Warn woman to avoid use during pregnancy.
- Inform patient that sugarless chewing gum or hard candy can relieve dry mouth.

## diazepam
Antenex‡, Apo-Diazepam†, Diastat, Diazemuls†‡, Diazepam Intensol, Ducene‡, Novo-Dipam†, PMS-Diazepam†, Valium♦, Vivol†

*Pregnancy risk category D*
*Controlled substance schedule IV*

**AVAILABLE FORMS**
*Capsules (extended-release):* 15 mg
*Injection:* 5 mg/ml
*Oral solution:* 5 mg/5 ml, 5 mg/ml
*Rectal gel twin packs:* 2.5 mg, 5 mg, 10 mg, 15 mg, 20 mg

*Sterile emulsion for injection:* 5 mg/ml
*Tablets:* 2 mg, 5 mg, 10 mg

**INDICATIONS & DOSAGES**
➤ **Anxiety**
*Adults:* Depending on severity, 2 to 10 mg P.O. b.i.d. to q.i.d. or 15 to 30 mg extended-release capsules P.O. once daily. Or, 2 to 10 mg I.M. or I.V. q 3 to 4 hours, p.r.n.
*Children age 6 months and older:* 1 to 2.5 mg P.O. t.i.d. or q.i.d., increase gradually, as needed and tolerated.
*Elderly patients:* Initially, 2 to 2.5 mg once daily or b.i.d.; increase gradually.
➤ **Acute alcohol withdrawal**
*Adults:* 10 mg P.O. t.i.d. or q.i.d. first 24 hours; reduce to 5 mg P.O. t.i.d. or q.i.d., p.r.n. Or, initially, 10 mg I.M. or I.V. Then, 5 to 10 mg I.M. or I.V. q 3 to 4 hours, p.r.n.
➤ **Before endoscopic procedures**
*Adults:* Adjust I.V. dose to desired sedative response (up to 20 mg). Or, 5 to 10 mg I.M. 30 minutes before procedure.
➤ **Muscle spasm**
*Adults:* 2 to 10 mg P.O. b.i.d. to q.i.d. Or, 15 to 30 mg extended-release capsules once daily. Or, 5 to 10 mg I.M. or I.V. initially; then 5 to 10 mg I.M. or I.V. q 3 to 4 hours, p.r.n. For tetanus, larger doses up to 20 mg q 2 to 8 hours may be needed.
*Children age 5 and older:* 5 to 10 mg I.M. or I.V. q 3 to 4 hours, p.r.n.
*Children ages 1 month to 5 years:* 1 to 2 mg I.M. or I.V. slowly, repeat q 3 to 4 hours, p.r.n.
➤ **Preoperative sedation**
*Adults:* 10 mg I.M. (preferred) or I.V. before surgery.
➤ **Cardioversion**
*Adults:* 5 to 15 mg I.V. within 5 to 10 minutes before procedure.
➤ **Adjunct treatment for seizure disorders**
*Adults:* 2 to 10 mg P.O. b.i.d. to q.i.d.
*Children age 6 months and older:* 1 to 2.5 mg P.O. t.i.d. or q.i.d. initially; increase as needed and as tolerated.
➤ **Status epilepticus, severe recurrent seizures**
*Adults:* 5 to 10 mg I.V. or I.M. initially. Use I.M. route only if I.V. access is unavailable. Repeated q 10 to 15 minutes,

p.r.n., up to maximum dose of 30 mg. Repeat q 2 to 4 hours, if needed.

*Children age 5 and older:* 1 mg I.V. q 2 to 5 minutes up to maximum of 10 mg. Repeat q 2 to 4 hours, if needed.

*Children ages 1 month to 5 years:* 0.2 to 0.5 mg I.V. slowly q 2 to 5 minutes up to maximum of 5 mg. Repeat q 2 to 4 hours, if needed.

➤ **Patients on stable regimens of antiepileptic drugs who need diazepam intermittently to control bouts of increased seizure activity**

*Adults and children age 12 and older:* 0.2 mg/kg P.R. A second dose may be given 4 to 12 hours later.

*Children ages 6 to 11:* 0.3 mg/kg P.R. A second dose may be given 4 to 12 hours later.

*Children ages 2 to 5:* 0.5 mg/kg P.R. A second dose may be given 4 to 12 hours later.

*Adjust-a-dose:* For elderly and debilitated patients, reduce dosage to decrease the likelihood of ataxia and oversedation.

## I.V. ADMINISTRATION

• Keep emergency resuscitation equipment and oxygen at bedside.

• I.V. route is the most reliable parenteral route; I.M. administration isn't recommended because absorption is variable and injection is painful.

• Give I.V. at no more than 5 mg/minute. When injecting, give directly into a large vein. If this is impossible, inject slowly through infusion tubing as near to the insertion site as possible. Watch closely for phlebitis at injection site.

• *Alert:* Monitor respirations every 5 to 15 minutes and before each I.V. dose.

## ACTION

Unknown. A benzodiazepine that probably potentiates the effects of gamma-aminobutyric acid, depresses the CNS, and suppresses the spread of seizure activity.

| Route | Onset | Peak | Duration |
|-------|-------|------|----------|
| P.O. | 30 min | 2 hr | 3-8 hr |
| I.V. | 1-5 min | 1-5 min | 15-60 min |
| I.M. | Unknown | 2 hr | Unknown |
| P.R. | Unknown | 90 min | Unknown |

## ADVERSE REACTIONS

**CNS:** *drowsiness,* dysarthria, slurred speech, tremor, transient amnesia, fatigue, ataxia, headache, insomnia, paradoxical anxiety, hallucinations, minor changes in EEG patterns.

**CV:** hypotension, *CV collapse, bradycardia.*

**EENT:** diplopia, blurred vision, nystagmus.

**GI:** nausea, constipation, diarrhea with rectal form.

**GU:** incontinence, urine retention.

**Hematologic:** *neutropenia.*

**Hepatic:** jaundice.

**Respiratory:** *respiratory depression, apnea.*

**Skin:** rash.

**Other:** altered libido, physical or psychological dependence, *pain, phlebitis at injection site.*

## INTERACTIONS

**Drug-drug.** *Cimetidine, disulfiram, fluoxetine, fluvoxamine, hormonal contraceptives, isoniazid, metoprolol, propoxyphene, propranolol, valproic acid:* May decrease clearance of diazepam and increase risk of adverse effects. Monitor patient for excessive sedation and impaired psychomotor function.

*CNS depressants:* May increase CNS depression. Use together cautiously.

*Digoxin:* May increase digoxin level and risk of toxicity. Monitor patient and digoxin level closely.

*Diltiazem:* May increase CNS depression and prolong effects of diazepam. Reduce dose of diazepam.

*Fluconazole, itraconazole, ketoconazole, miconazole:* May increase and prolong diazepam level, CNS depression, and psychomotor impairment. Avoid using together.

*Phenobarbital:* May increase effects of both drugs. Use together cautiously.

**Drug-herb.** *Kava:* May increase sedation. Discourage use together.

**Drug-lifestyle.** *Alcohol use:* May cause additive CNS effects. Discourage use together.

*Smoking:* May decrease effectiveness of benzodiazepines. Monitor patient closely.

---

Reactions may be *common,* uncommon, *life-threatening,* or COMMON AND LIFE-THREATENING.

**EFFECTS ON LAB TEST RESULTS**
• May increase liver function test values. May decrease neutrophil count.

**CONTRAINDICATIONS & CAUTIONS**
• Contraindicated in patients hypersensitive to drug or soy protein; in patients experiencing shock, coma, or acute alcohol intoxication (parenteral form); in pregnant women, especially in first trimester; and in children younger than age 6 months (oral form).
• Diastat rectal gel is contraindicated in patients with acute angle-closure glaucoma.
• Use cautiously in patients with liver or renal impairment, depression, or chronic open-angle glaucoma. Use cautiously in elderly and debilitated patients.

**NURSING CONSIDERATIONS**
• Use Diastat rectal gel to treat no more than five episodes per month and no more than one episode every 5 days because tolerance may develop.
• Don't mix injectable diazepam with other drugs, and don't store parenteral solution in plastic syringes.
• When using oral concentrate solution, dilute dose just before giving.
• Parenteral emulsion—a stabilized oil-in-water emulsion—should appear milky white and uniform. Avoid mixing with any other drugs or solutions, and avoid infusion sets or containers made from polyvinyl chloride. If dilution is needed, drug may be mixed with I.V. fat emulsion. Use admixture within 6 hours.
• *Alert:* Only caregivers who can distinguish the distinct cluster of seizures or events from the patient's ordinary seizure activity, who have been instructed and can give the treatment competently, who understand which seizures may or may not be treated with Diastat, and who can monitor the clinical response and recognize when immediate professional medical evaluation is needed should give Diastat rectal gel.
• Monitor periodic hepatic, renal, and hematopoietic function studies in patients receiving repeated or prolonged therapy.
• *Alert:* Use of this drug may lead to abuse and addiction. Don't withdraw drug abruptly after long-term use; withdrawal symptoms may occur.

• *Alert:* Don't confuse diazepam with diazoxide.

**PATIENT TEACHING**
• Warn patient to avoid activities that require alertness and good coordination until effects of drug are known.
• Tell patient to avoid alcohol while taking drug.
• Notify patient that smoking may decrease drug's effectiveness.
• Warn patient not to abruptly stop drug because withdrawal symptoms may occur.
• Warn woman to avoid use during pregnancy.
• Instruct patient's caregiver on the proper administration of Diastat rectal gel.

---

# hydroxyzine hydrochloride
Anx, Apo-Hydroxyzine†, Atarax*, Novo-Hydroxyzin†, PMS-Hydroxyzine†, Vistaril

# hydroxyzine pamoate
Vistaril

*Pregnancy risk category NR*

**AVAILABLE FORMS**
**hydroxyzine hydrochloride**
*Capsules:* 10 mg†, 25 mg†, 50 mg†
*Injection:* 25 mg/ml, 50 mg/ml
*Syrup:* 10 mg/5 ml
*Tablets:* 10 mg, 25 mg, 50 mg, 100 mg
**hydroxyzine pamoate**
*Capsules:* 25 mg, 50 mg, 100 mg
*Oral suspension:* 25 mg/5 ml

**INDICATIONS & DOSAGES**
➤ **Anxiety**
*Adults:* 50 to 100 mg P.O. q.i.d.
*Children age 6 and older:* 50 to 100 mg P.O. daily in divided doses.
*Children younger than age 6:* 50 mg P.O. daily in divided doses.
➤ **Preoperative and postoperative adjunctive therapy for sedation**
*Adults:* 25 to 100 mg I.M. q 4 to 6 hours.
*Children:* 1.1 mg/kg I.M. q 4 to 6 hours.
➤ **Pruritus from allergies**
*Adults:* 25 mg P.O. t.i.d. or q.i.d.
*Children age 6 and older:* 50 to 100 mg P.O. daily in divided doses.

---

*Rapid onset*   †Canada   ‡Australia   ◇OTC   ♦Off-label use   ✐Photoguide   *Liquid contains alcohol.

*Children younger than age 6:* 50 mg P.O. daily in divided doses.

➤ **Psychiatric and emotional emergencies, including acute alcoholism**
*Adults:* 50 to 100 mg I.M. q 4 to 6 hours, p.r.n.

➤ **Nausea and vomiting (excluding nausea and vomiting of pregnancy)**
*Adults:* 25 to 100 mg I.M.
*Children:* 1.1 mg/kg I.M.

➤ **Antepartum and postpartum adjunctive therapy**
*Adults:* 25 to 100 mg I.M.

## ACTION

Unknown. A piperazine antihistamine whose action may result from suppression of activity in certain essential regions of the subcortical area of the CNS.

| Route | Onset | Peak | Duration |
|-------|-------|------|----------|
| P.O. | 15-30 min | 2 hr | 4-6 hr |
| I.M. | Unknown | Unknown | 4-6 hr |

## ADVERSE REACTIONS

**CNS:** *drowsiness,* involuntary motor activity.
**GI:** *dry mouth,* constipation.
**Other:** pain at I.M. injection site, hypersensitivity reactions.

## INTERACTIONS

**Drug-drug.** *Anticholinergics:* May cause additive anticholinergic effects. Use together cautiously.
*CNS depressants:* May increase CNS depression. Use together cautiously; dosage adjustments may be needed.
*Epinephrine:* May inhibit and reverse vasopressor effect of epinephrine. Avoid using together.
**Drug-lifestyle.** *Alcohol use:* May increase CNS depression. Discourage use together.

## EFFECTS ON LAB TEST RESULTS

● Falsely increases urinary 17-hydroxycorticosteroid level. May cause false-negative skin allergen tests by attenuating or inhibiting the cutaneous response to histamine.

## CONTRAINDICATIONS & CAUTIONS

● Contraindicated in patients hypersensitive to drug, patients in early pregnancy, and breast-feeding women.

## NURSING CONSIDERATIONS

● Parenteral form (hydroxyzine hydrochloride) is for I.M. use only, preferably by Z-track injection. Never give drug I.V. or S.C.
● Aspirate I.M. injection carefully to prevent inadvertent intravascular injection. Inject deeply into a large muscle.
● If patient takes other CNS drugs, observe for oversedation.
● *Alert:* Don't confuse hydroxyzine with hydroxyurea or hydralazine.

## PATIENT TEACHING

● Warn patient to avoid hazardous activities that require alertness and good coordination until effects of drug are known.
● Tell patient to avoid alcohol while taking drug.
● Advise patient to use sugarless hard candy or gum to relieve dry mouth.
● Warn woman to avoid use during pregnancy and breast-feeding.

# lorazepam

Apo-Lorazepam†, Ativan, Lorazepam Intensol, Novo-Lorazem†, Nu-Loraz† ◇

*Pregnancy risk category D*
*Controlled substance schedule IV*

## AVAILABLE FORMS

*Injection:* 2 mg/ml, 4 mg/ml
*Oral solution (concentrated):* 2 mg/ml
*Tablets:* 0.5 mg, 1 mg, 2 mg
*Tablets (S.L.):* 0.5 mg†, 1 mg†, 2 mg

## INDICATIONS & DOSAGES

➤ **Anxiety**
*Adults:* 2 to 6 mg P.O. daily in divided doses. Maximum, 10 mg daily.
*Elderly patients:* 1 to 2 mg P.O. daily in divided doses. Maximum, 10 mg daily.

➤ **Insomnia from anxiety**
*Adults:* 2 to 4 mg P.O. h.s.

➤ **Preoperative sedation**
*Adults:* 0.05 mg/kg I.M. 2 hours before procedure. Total dose shouldn't exceed 4 mg. Or, 2 mg I.V. total or 0.044 mg/kg I.V., whichever is smaller. Larger doses up to 0.05 mg/kg I.V., to total of 4 mg, may be needed.

➤ **Combined with haloperidol, to manage delirium ♦**
*Adults:* 0.5 go 1 mg I.V. after haloperidol 3 mg I.V. Adjust dosage based on patient's response and tolerance.
➤ **Status epilepticus ♦**
*Adults and children:* 0.05 to 0.1 mg/kg. Repeat dose q 10 to 15 minutes, p.r.n. Or, give adults 4 to 8 mg I.V.
➤ **Nausea and vomiting from emetogenic cancer chemotherapy ♦**
*Adults:* 2.5 mg P.O. the evening before and just after starting chemotherapy. Or, 1.5 mg/m$^2$ (usually up to a maximum dose of 3 mg) I.V. (over 5 minutes) 45 minutes before initiation of chemotherapy.

## I.V. ADMINISTRATION
● Keep emergency resuscitation equipment and oxygen available.
● Dilute with an equal volume of sterile water for injection, normal saline solution for injection, or D$_5$W. Give slowly at no more than 2 mg/minute.
● *Alert:* Monitor respirations every 5 to 15 minutes and before each I.V. dose.

## ACTION
Unknown. A benzodiazepine that probably potentiates the effects of gamma-aminobutyric acid, depresses the CNS, and suppresses the spread of seizure activity.

| Route | Onset | Peak | Duration |
|---|---|---|---|
| P.O. | 1 hr | 2 hr | 12-24 hr |
| I.V. | 5 min | 60-90 min | 6-8 hr |
| I.M. | 15-30 min | 60-90 min | 6-8 hr |

## ADVERSE REACTIONS
**CNS:** *drowsiness,* amnesia, insomnia, agitation, *sedation,* dizziness, weakness, unsteadiness, disorientation, depression, headache.
**CV:** hypotension.
**EENT:** visual disturbances.
**GI:** abdominal discomfort, nausea, change in appetite.

## INTERACTIONS
**Drug-drug.** *CNS depressants:* May increase CNS depression. Use together cautiously.

*Digoxin:* May increase digoxin level and risk of toxicity. Monitor patient and digoxin level closely.
**Drug-herb.** *Kava:* May increase sedation. Discourage use together.
**Drug-lifestyle.** *Alcohol use:* May cause additive CNS effects. Discourage use together.
*Smoking:* May decrease benzodiazepine effectiveness. Monitor patient closely.

## EFFECTS ON LAB TEST RESULTS
● May increase liver function test values.

## CONTRAINDICATIONS & CAUTIONS
● Contraindicated in patients hypersensitive to drug, other benzodiazepines, or the vehicle used in parenteral dosage form; in patients with acute angle-closure glaucoma; and in pregnant women, especially in the first trimester.
● Use cautiously in patients with pulmonary, renal, or hepatic impairment.
● Use cautiously in elderly, acutely ill, or debilitated patients.

## NURSING CONSIDERATIONS
● For I.M. administration, inject deeply into a muscle. Don't dilute.
● Refrigerate parenteral form to prolong shelf life.
● Monitor hepatic, renal, and hematopoietic function periodically in patients receiving repeated or prolonged therapy.
● *Alert:* Use of this drug may lead to abuse and addiction. Don't stop drug abruptly after long-term use because withdrawal symptoms may occur.
● *Alert:* Don't confuse lorazepam with alprazolam.

## PATIENT TEACHING
● When used as a drug before surgery, lorazepam causes substantial preoperative amnesia. Patient teaching requires extra care to ensure adequate recall. Provide written materials or inform a family member, if possible.
● Warn patient to avoid hazardous activities that require alertness or good coordination until effects of drug are known.
● Tell patient to avoid alcohol while taking drug.
● Notify patient that smoking may decrease drug's effectiveness.

● Warn patient not to stop drug abruptly because withdrawal symptoms may occur.
● Warn woman to avoid use during pregnancy.

---

## midazolam hydrochloride
Hypnovel‡, Versed, Versed Syrup

*Pregnancy risk category D*
*Controlled substance schedule IV*

---

### AVAILABLE FORMS
*Injection:* 1 mg/ml, 5 mg/ml
*Syrup:* 2 mg/ml

### INDICATIONS & DOSAGES
➤ **Preoperative sedation (to induce sleepiness or drowsiness and relieve apprehension)**
*Adults:* 0.07 to 0.08 mg/kg I.M. about 1 hour before surgery.
➤ **Conscious sedation before short diagnostic or endoscopic procedures**
*Adults younger than age 60:* Initially, small dose not to exceed 2.5 mg I.V. given slowly; repeat in 2 minutes, if needed, in small increments of first dose over at least 2 minutes to achieve desired effect. Total dose of up to 5 mg may be used. Additional doses to maintain desired level of sedation may be given by slow titration in increments of 25% of dose used to first reach the sedative end point.
*Patients age 60 or older, or debilitated:* 0.5 to 1.5 mg I.V. over at least 2 minutes. Incremental doses shouldn't exceed 1 mg. A total dose of up to 3.5 mg is usually sufficient.
➤ **To induce sleepiness and amnesia and to relieve apprehension before anesthesia or before and during procedures in children**
**P.O.**
*Children ages 6 to 16 and cooperative patients:* 0.25 to 0.5 mg/kg P.O. as a single dose, up to 20 mg.
*Infants and children ages 6 months to 5 years and less-cooperative patients:* 0.25 to 1 mg/kg P.O. as a single dose, up to 20 mg.
**I.V.**
*Children ages 12 to 16:* Initially, no more than 2.5 mg I.V. given slowly; repeat in 2 minutes, if needed, in small increments

of first dose over at least 2 minutes to achieve desired effect. Total dose of up to 10 mg may be used. Additional doses to maintain desired level of sedation may be given by slow titration in increments of 25% of dose used to first reach the sedative end point.
*Children ages 6 to 12:* 0.025 to 0.05 mg/kg I.V. over 2 to 3 minutes. Additional doses may be given in small increments after 2 to 3 minutes. Total dose of up to 0.4 mg/kg, not to exceed 10 mg, may be used.
*Children ages 6 months to 5 years:* 0.05 to 0.1 mg/kg I.V. over 2 to 3 minutes. Additional doses may be given in small increments after 2 to 3 minutes. Total dose of up to 0.6 mg/kg, not to exceed 6 mg, may be used.
**I.M.**
*Children:* 0.1 to 0.15 mg/kg I.M. Use up to 0.5 mg/kg in more anxious patients.
***Adjust-a-dose:*** For obese children, base dose on ideal body weight; high-risk or debilitated children and children receiving other sedatives need lower doses.
➤ **To induce general anesthesia**
*Adults older than age 55:* 0.3 mg/kg I.V. over 20 to 30 seconds if patient hasn't received premedication, or 0.2 mg/kg I.V. over 20 to 30 seconds if patient has received sedative or narcotic premedication. Additional increments of 25% of first dose may be needed to complete induction.
*Adults younger than age 55:* 0.3 to 0.35 mg/kg I.V. over 20 to 30 seconds if patient hasn't received premedication, or 0.25 mg/kg I.V. over 20 to 30 seconds if patient has received sedative or narcotic premedication. Additional increments of 25% of first dose may be needed to complete induction.
***Adjust-a-dose:*** For debilitated patients, initially, 0.2 to 0.25 mg/kg. As little as 0.15 mg/kg may be needed.
➤ **As continuous infusion to sedate intubated patients in critical care unit**
*Adults:* Initially, 0.01 to 0.05 mg/kg may be given I.V. over several minutes, repeated at 10- to 15-minute intervals until adequate sedation is achieved. To maintain sedation, usual initial infusion rate is 0.02 to 0.1 mg/kg/hour. Higher loading dose or infusion rates may be needed in some patients. Use the lowest effective rate.

---

*Children:* Initially, 0.05 to 0.2 mg/kg may be given I.V. over 2 to 3 minutes or longer; then continuous infusion at rate of 0.06 to 0.12 mg/kg/hour. Increase or decrease infusion to maintain desired effect.

*Neonates more than 32 weeks' gestational age:* Initially, 0.06 mg/kg/hour. Adjust rate, p.r.n., using lowest possible rate.

*Neonates less than 32 weeks' gestational age:* Initially, 0.03 mg/kg/hour. Adjust rate, p.r.n., using lowest possible rate.

## I.V. ADMINISTRATION

● When mixing infusion, use 5-mg/ml vial, dilute to 0.5 mg/ml with $D_5W$ or normal saline solution.

● Give slowly over at least 2 minutes, and wait at least 2 minutes when titrating doses to produce therapeutic effect.

## ACTION

Unknown. A benzodiazepine that probably potentiates the effects of gamma-aminobutyric acid, depresses the CNS, and suppresses the spread of seizure activity.

| Route | Onset | Peak | Duration |
|---|---|---|---|
| P.O. | 10-20 min | 45-60 min | 2-6 hr |
| I.V. | 90 sec-5 min | Rapid | 2-6 hr |
| I.M. | 15 min | 15-60 min | 2-6 hr |

## ADVERSE REACTIONS

**CNS:** headache, *oversedation, drowsiness,* amnesia, involuntary movements, nystagmus, paradoxical behavior or excitement.
**CV:** variations in blood pressure and pulse rate.
**GI:** *nausea,* vomiting.
**Respiratory:** *decreased respiratory rate,* APNEA, *hiccups.*
**Other:** *pain at injection site.*

## INTERACTIONS

**Drug-drug.** *CNS depressants:* May cause apnea. Use together cautiously. Prepare to adjust dosage of midazolam if used with opiates or other CNS depressants.
*Diltiazem:* May increase CNS depression and prolonged effects of midazolam. Use lower dose of midazolam.
*Erythromycin:* May alter metabolism of midazolam. Use together cautiously.
*Fluconazole, itraconazole, ketoconazole, miconazole:* May increase and prolong

midazolam level, CNS depression, and psychomotor impairment. Avoid using together.
*Hormonal contraceptives:* May prolong half-life of midazolam. Use together cautiously.
*Rifampin:* May decrease midazolam level. Monitor for midazolam effectiveness.
*Theophylline:* May antagonize sedative effect of midazolam. Use together cautiously.
*Verapamil:* May increase midazolam level. Monitor patient closely.
**Drug-herb.** *St. John's wort:* May decrease midazolam level. Discourage use together.
**Drug-food.** *Grapefruit juice:* May increase bioavailability of oral midazolam. Discourage use together.
**Drug-lifestyle.** *Alcohol use:* May cause additive CNS effects. Discourage use together.

## EFFECTS ON LAB TEST RESULTS
None reported.

## CONTRAINDICATIONS & CAUTIONS

● Contraindicated in patients hypersensitive to drug and in those with acute angle-closure glaucoma, shock, coma, or acute alcohol intoxication.

● Use cautiously in patients with uncompensated acute illness and in elderly or debilitated patients.

## NURSING CONSIDERATIONS

● *Alert:* Before giving drug, have oxygen and resuscitation equipment available in case of severe respiratory depression. Excessive amounts and rapid infusion have been linked to respiratory arrest. Continuously monitor patients who have received midazolam, including children who have received midazolam syrup, to detect potentially life-threatening respiratory depression.

● May be mixed in the same syringe with morphine sulfate, meperidine, atropine, or scopolamine.

● When injecting I.M., give deeply into a large muscle.

● Monitor blood pressure, heart rate and rhythm, respirations, airway integrity, and arterial oxygen saturation during procedure.

---

*Rapid onset*    †Canada    ‡Australia    ◇OTC    ◆ Off-label use    ✐Photoguide    *Liquid contains alcohol.

● *Alert:* Don't confuse Versed with VePesid.

## PATIENT TEACHING
● Because drug's beneficial amnesic effect diminishes patient's recall of events around the time of surgery, provide written information, family member instruction, and follow-up contact to make sure patient has adequate information.
● Warn patient to avoid hazardous activities that require alertness or good coordination until effects of drug are known.
● Tell patient to avoid alcohol while taking drug.
● Tell patient not to take oral form with grapefruit juice.

---

## oxazepam
Alepam‡, Apo-Oxazepam†, Murelax‡, Novoxapam†, Serax, Serepax‡

*Pregnancy risk category D*
*Controlled substance schedule IV*

---

### AVAILABLE FORMS
*Capsules, tablets:* 10 mg, 15 mg, 30 mg

### INDICATIONS & DOSAGES
➤ **Alcohol withdrawal, severe anxiety**
*Adults:* 15 to 30 mg P.O. t.i.d. or q.i.d.
➤ **Mild to moderate anxiety**
*Adults:* 10 to 15 mg P.O. t.i.d. or q.i.d.
*Elderly patients:* Initially, 10 mg t.i.d.; increase to 15 mg t.i.d. to q.i.d.

### ACTION
Unknown. May stimulate gamma-aminobutyric acid receptors in the ascending reticular activating system.

| Route | Onset | Peak | Duration |
|-------|---------|------|----------|
| P.O. | Unknown | 3 hr | Unknown |

### ADVERSE REACTIONS
**CNS:** *drowsiness, lethargy,* dizziness, vertigo, headache, syncope, tremor, slurred speech, changes in EEG patterns.
**CV:** edema.
**GI:** nausea.
**Hepatic:** *hepatic dysfunction.*
**Skin:** rash.
**Other:** altered libido.

## INTERACTIONS
**Drug-drug.** *CNS depressants:* May increase CNS depression. Use together cautiously.
*Digoxin:* May increase digoxin level and risk of toxicity. Monitor patient closely.
**Drug-herb.** *Kava:* May increase sedation. Discourage use together.
**Drug-lifestyle.** *Alcohol use:* May cause additive CNS effects. Discourage use together.

## EFFECTS ON LAB TEST RESULTS
● May increase liver function test values.

## CONTRAINDICATIONS & CAUTIONS
● Contraindicated in patients hypersensitive to drug; in pregnant women, especially in the first trimester; and in those with psychoses.
● Use cautiously in elderly patients and in those with history of drug abuse or in whom a decrease in blood pressure might lead to cardiac problems.

## NURSING CONSIDERATIONS
● Monitor hepatic, renal, and hematopoietic function periodically in patients receiving repeated or prolonged therapy.
● *Alert:* Serax tablets may contain tartrazine.
● *Alert:* Use of this drug may lead to abuse and addiction. Don't stop drug abruptly because withdrawal symptoms may occur.
● *Alert:* Don't confuse oxazepam with oxaprozin.

## PATIENT TEACHING
● Warn patient to avoid hazardous activities that require alertness or good coordination until effects of drug are known.
● Tell patient to avoid alcohol while taking drug.
● Notify patient that smoking may decrease drug's effectiveness.
● Warn patient not to stop drug abruptly because withdrawal symptoms may occur.
● Warn woman to avoid use during pregnancy.

---

Reactions may be *common,* uncommon, *life-threatening,* or COMMON AND LIFE-THREATENING.

aripiprazole
chlorpromazine hydrochloride
clozapine
fluphenazine decanoate
fluphenazine enanthate
fluphenazine hydrochloride
haloperidol
haloperidol decanoate
haloperidol lactate
loxapine hydrochloride
loxapine succinate
mesoridazine besylate
olanzapine
perphenazine
pimozide
prochlorperazine
    (See Chapter 48, ANTIEMETICS.)
quetiapine fumarate
risperidone
thioridazine hydrochloride
thiothixene
thiothixene hydrochloride
trifluoperazine hydrochloride
ziprasidone

### COMBINATION PRODUCTS
ETRAFON: perphenazine 2 mg and
amitriptyline hydrochloride 25 mg.
ETRAFON 2-10: perphenazine 2 mg and
amitriptyline hydrochloride 10 mg.
ETRAFON-A: perphenazine 4 mg and
amitriptyline hydrochloride 10 mg.
ETRAFON-FORTE: perphenazine 4 mg and
amitriptyline hydrochloride 25 mg.
TRIAVIL 2-10: perphenazine 2 mg and
amitriptyline hydrochloride 10 mg.
TRIAVIL 4-10: perphenazine 4 mg and
amitriptyline hydrochloride 10 mg.
TRIAVIL 2-25: perphenazine 2 mg and
amitriptyline hydrochloride 25 mg.
TRIAVIL 4-25: perphenazine 4 mg and
amitriptyline hydrochloride 25 mg.

## aripiprazole
Abilify⚘

*Pregnancy risk category C*

### AVAILABLE FORMS
*Tablets:* 10 mg, 15 mg, 20 mg, 30 mg

### INDICATIONS & DOSAGES
➤ **Schizophrenia**
*Adults:* Initially, 10 to 15 mg P.O. daily;
increase to maximum daily dose of 30 mg
if needed, after at least 2 weeks.
*Adjust-a-dose:* When using with CYP
3A4 inhibitors such as ketoconazole or
CYP 2D6 inhibitors such as quinidine, fluoxetine, or paroxetine, give half the aripiprazole dose. When using with CYP 3A4
inducers such as carbamazepine, double
the aripiprazole dose. Return to original
dosing after the concomitant drugs are
stopped.

### ACTION
Thought to exhibit its antipsychotic effects
through partial agonist activity at D2 and
serotonin 1A receptors and antagonist activity at serotonin 2A receptors.

| Route | Onset | Peak | Duration |
|-------|-------|------|----------|
| P.O. | Unknown | 3-5 hr | Unknown |

### ADVERSE REACTIONS
**CNS:** *headache, anxiety, insomnia, light-
headedness, somnolence, akathisia,*
tremor, asthenia, depression, nervousness,
hostility, **suicidal thoughts,** manic behavior, confusion, abnormal gait, cogwheel
rigidity, **seizures,** fever, tardive dyskinesia,
**neuroleptic malignant syndrome, in-
creased suicide risk.**
**CV:** peripheral edema, chest pain, hypertension, tachycardia, orthostatic hypotension, **bradycardia.**
**EENT:** rhinitis, blurred vision, increased
salivation, conjunctivitis, ear pain.
**GI:** *nausea, vomiting, constipation,*
anorexia, diarrhea, abdominal pain,
esophageal dysmotility.

**GU:** urinary incontinence.
**Hematologic:** ecchymosis, anemia.
**Metabolic:** weight gain, weight loss.
**Musculoskeletal:** neck pain, neck stiffness, muscle cramps.
**Respiratory:** dyspnea, pneumonia, cough.
**Skin:** rash, dry skin, pruritus, sweating, ulcer.
**Other:** flulike syndrome.

### INTERACTIONS

**Drug-drug.** *Antihypertensives:* May enhance antihypertensive effects. Monitor blood pressure.
*Carbamazepine and other CYP 3A4 inducers:* May decrease levels and effectiveness of aripiprazole. Double the usual dose of aripiprazole, and monitor the patient closely.
*Ketoconazole and other CYP 3A4 inhibitors:* May increase risk of serious toxic effects. Start treatment with one-half the usual dose of aripiprazole, and monitor patient closely.
*Potential CYP 2D6 inhibitors (fluoxetine, paroxetine, quinidine):* May increase levels and toxicity of aripiprazole. Give half the usual dose of aripiprazole.
**Drug-food.** *Grapefruit juice:* May increase aripiprazole level. Tell patient not to take drug with grapefruit juice.
**Drug-lifestyle.** *Alcohol use:* May increase CNS effects. Discourage use together.

### EFFECTS ON LAB TEST RESULTS

● May increase creatine phosphokinase level.

### CONTRAINDICATIONS & CAUTIONS

● Contraindicated in patients hypersensitive to aripiprazole.
● Use cautiously in patients with CV disease, cerebrovascular disease, or conditions that could predispose the patient to hypotension, such as dehydration or hypovolemia. Also use cautiously in patients with history of seizures or with conditions that lower the seizure threshold.
● Use cautiously in patients who engage in strenuous exercise, are exposed to extreme heat, take anticholinergic medications, or are susceptible to dehydration.

● Use cautiously in patients at risk for aspiration pneumonia, such as those with Alzheimer's disease.
● Use cautiously in pregnant and breast-feeding patients.

### NURSING CONSIDERATIONS

● *Alert:* Neuroleptic malignant syndrome may occur with aripiprazole use. Monitor patient for hyperpyrexia, muscle rigidity, altered mental status, irregular pulse or blood pressure, tachycardia, diaphoresis, and cardiac dysrhythmias.
● If signs and symptoms of neuroleptic malignant syndrome occur, immediately stop drug and notify prescriber.
● Monitor patient for signs and symptoms of tardive dyskinesia. The elderly, especially elderly women, are at highest risk of developing this adverse effect.
● Treat patient with the smallest dose for the shortest time and periodically reevaluated for continued treatment.
● Give prescriptions only for small quantities of tablets, to reduce risk of overdose.

### PATIENT TEACHING

● Tell patient to use caution while driving or operating hazardous machinery because of psychoactive drugs may impair judgment, thinking, or motor skills.
● Tell patient that drug may be taken without regard to meals.
● Advise patients that grapefruit juice may interact with aripiprazole and to limit or avoid its use.
● Advise patient that gradual improvement in symptoms should occur over several weeks rather than immediately.
● Tell patients to avoid alcohol use while taking drug.
● Advise patients to limit strenuous activity while taking drug, to avoid dehydration.

---

# chlorpromazine hydrochloride
Chlorpromanyl-20†,
Chlorpromanyl-40†, Largactil††,
Novo-Chlorpromazine†, Thorazine

*Pregnancy risk category C*

### AVAILABLE FORMS

*Capsules (extended-release):* 30 mg, 75 mg, 150 mg

---

Reactions may be *common*, uncommon, *life-threatening*, or COMMON AND LIFE-THREATENING.

*Injection:* 25 mg/ml
*Oral concentrate:* 30 mg/ml, 100 mg/ml
*Suppositories:* 25 mg, 100 mg
*Syrup:* 10 mg/5 ml
*Tablets:* 10 mg, 25 mg, 50 mg, 100 mg, 200 mg

## INDICATIONS & DOSAGES
➤ **Psychosis, mania**
*Adults:* For hospitalized patients with acute disease, 25 mg I.M.; may give an additional 25 to 50 mg I.M. in 1 hour if needed. Increase over several days to 400 mg q 4 to 6 hours. Switch to oral therapy as soon as possible. Or, 25 mg P.O. t.i.d. initially; then gradually increase to 400 mg daily in divided doses. For outpatients, 30 to 75 mg daily in two to four divided doses. Increase dosage by 20 to 50 mg twice weekly until symptoms are controlled.
*Children age 6 months and older:*
0.55 mg/kg P.O. q 4 to 6 hours or I.M. q 6 to 8 hours. Or, 1.1 mg/kg P.R. q 6 to 8 hours. Maximum I.M. dose in children younger than age 5 or weighing less than 22.7 kg (50 lb) is 40 mg. Maximum I.M. dose in children ages 5 to 12 or weighing 22.7 to 45.4 kg (50 to 100 lb) is 75 mg.
➤ **Nausea and vomiting**
*Adults:* 10 to 25 mg P.O. q 4 to 6 hours, p.r.n. Or, 50 to 100 mg P.R. q 6 to 8 hours, p.r.n. Or, 25 mg I.M. initially. If no hypotension occurs, 25 to 50 mg I.M. q 3 to 4 hours may be given, p.r.n., until vomiting stops.
*Children age 6 months and older:*
0.55 mg/kg P.O. q 4 to 6 hours or I.M. q 6 to 8 hours. Or, 1.1 mg/kg P.R. q 6 to 8 hours. Maximum I.M. dose in children younger than age 5 or weighing less than 22.7 kg (50 lb) is 40 mg. Maximum I.M. dose in children ages 5 to 12 or weighing 22.7 to 45.4 kg (50 to 100 lb) is 75 mg.
➤ **Acute intermittent porphyria, intractable hiccups**
*Adults:* 25 to 50 mg P.O. t.i.d. or q.i.d. If symptoms persist for 2 to 3 days, 25 to 50 mg I.M. For hiccups, if symptoms still persist, 25 to 50 mg diluted in 500 to 1,000 ml of normal saline solution and infused slowly with patient in supine position.

➤ **Tetanus**
*Adults:* 25 to 50 mg I.V. or I.M. t.i.d. or q.i.d.
*Children age 6 months and older:*
0.55 mg/kg I.M. or I.V. q 6 to 8 hours. Maximum parenteral dosage in children weighing less than 22.7 kg (50 lb) is 40 mg daily; for children weighing 22.7 to 45.4 kg (50 to 100 lb), 75 mg, except in severe cases.
➤ **Surgery**
*Adults:* Preoperatively, 25 to 50 mg P.O. 2 to 3 hours before surgery or 12.5 to 25 mg I.M. 1 to 2 hours before surgery; during surgery, 12.5 mg I.M., repeated in 30 minutes, if needed, or fractional 2-mg doses I.V. at 2-minute intervals to maximum dose of 25 mg; postoperatively, 10 to 25 mg P.O. q 4 to 6 hours or 12.5 to 25 mg I.M., repeated in 1 hour, if needed.
*Children age 6 months and older:* Preoperatively, 0.55 mg/kg P.O. 2 to 3 hours before surgery or I.M. 1 to 2 hours before surgery. During surgery, 0.275 mg/kg I.M., repeated in 30 minutes if needed, or fractional 1-mg doses I.V. at 2-minute intervals to maximum of 0.275 mg/kg. May repeat fractional I.V. regimen in 30 minutes if needed. Postoperatively, 0.55 mg/kg P.O. or I.M. q 4 to 6 hours (oral dose) or 1 hour (I.M. dose), if needed and if hypotension doesn't occur.
*Elderly patients:* Lower dosages are sufficient; dosage increments should be more gradual than in adults.

## I.V. ADMINISTRATION
● Chlorpromazine is compatible with most common I.V. solutions, including D$_5$W, Ringer's injection, lactated Ringer's injection, and normal saline solution for injection.
● For direct injection, drug may be diluted with normal saline solution for injection and given into a large vein or through the tubing of a free-flowing I.V. solution. Don't exceed 1 mg/minute for adults or 0.5 mg/minute for children.
● For intermittent I.V. infusion, dilute with 50 or 100 ml of a compatible solution and infuse over 30 minutes.

---

## ACTION

Unknown. A piperidine phenothiazine that probably blocks postsynaptic dopamine receptors in the brain.

| Route | Onset | Peak | Duration |
|---|---|---|---|
| P.O. | 30-60 min | Unknown | 4-6 hr |
| P.O. (extended) | 30-60 min | Unknown | 10-12 hr |
| I.V., I.M. | Unknown | Unknown | Unknown |
| P.R. | >1 hr | Unknown | 3-4 hr |

## ADVERSE REACTIONS

**CNS:** *extrapyramidal reactions,* drowsiness, *sedation,* **seizures,** *tardive dyskinesia, pseudoparkinsonism,* dizziness, **neuroleptic malignant syndrome.**
**CV:** *orthostatic hypotension,* tachycardia, quinidine-like ECG effects.
**EENT:** ocular changes, blurred vision, nasal congestion.
**GI:** *dry mouth, constipation,* nausea.
**GU:** *urine retention,* menstrual irregularities, inhibited ejaculation, priapism.
**Hematologic:** *leukopenia, agranulocytosis,* eosinophilia, hemolytic anemia, **aplastic anemia, thrombocytopenia.**
**Hepatic:** jaundice.
**Skin:** *mild photosensitivity reactions,* allergic reactions, *pain at I.M. injection site,* sterile abscess, skin pigmentation changes.
**Other:** gynecomastia, lactation, galactorrhea.

## INTERACTIONS

**Drug-drug.** *Antacids:* May inhibit absorption of oral phenothiazines. Separate antacid and phenothiazine doses by at least 2 hours.
*Anticholinergics such as tricyclic antidepressants, antiparkinsonian agents:* May increase anticholinergic activity, aggravated parkinsonian symptoms. Use together cautiously.
*Anticonvulsants:* May lower seizure threshold. Monitor patient closely.
*Barbiturates, lithium:* May decrease phenothiazine effect. Monitor patient.
*Centrally acting antihypertensives:* May decrease antihypertensive effect. Monitor blood pressure.
*CNS depressants:* May increase CNS depression. Use together cautiously.

*Electroconvulsive therapy, insulin:* May cause severe reactions. Monitor patient closely.
*Lithium:* May increase neurologic effects. Monitor patient closely.
*Meperidine:* May cause excessive sedation and hypotension. Don't use together.
*Propranolol:* May increase levels of both propranolol and chlorpromazine. Monitor patient closely.
*Warfarin:* May decrease effect of oral anticoagulants. Monitor PT and INR.
**Drug-herb.** *St. John's wort:* May cause photosensitivity reactions. Advise patient to avoid excessive sunlight exposure.
**Drug-lifestyle.** *Alcohol use:* May increase CNS depression, particularly psychomotor skills. Strongly discourage alcohol use.
*Sun exposure:* May increase risk of photosensitivity reactions. Advise patient to avoid excessive sunlight exposure.

## EFFECTS ON LAB TEST RESULTS

● May increase liver function test values and eosinophil count. May decrease hemoglobin, hematocrit, and WBC, granulocyte, and platelet counts.
● May cause false-positive results for urinary porphyrin, urobilinogen, amylase, and 5-hydroxyindoleacetic acid tests and for urine pregnancy tests that use human chorionic gonadotropin.

## CONTRAINDICATIONS & CAUTIONS

● Contraindicated in patients hypersensitive to drug; in those with CNS depression, bone marrow suppression, or subcortical damage, and in those in coma.
● Use cautiously in elderly or debilitated patients and in patients with hepatic or renal disease, severe CV disease (may suddenly decrease blood pressure), respiratory disorders, hypocalcemia, glaucoma, or prostatic hyperplasia. Also use cautiously in those exposed to extreme heat or cold (including antipyretic therapy) or organophosphate insecticides.
● Use cautiously in acutely ill or dehydrated children.

## NURSING CONSIDERATIONS

● Obtain baseline blood pressure measurements before starting therapy, and monitor regularly. Watch for orthostatic hypotension, especially with parenteral adminis-

tration. Monitor blood pressure before and after I.M. administration; keep patient supine for 1 hour afterward and have him get up slowly.
• Wear gloves when preparing solutions and avoid contact with skin and clothing. Oral liquid and parenteral forms can cause contact dermatitis.
• Slight yellowing of injection or concentrate is common and doesn't affect potency. Discard markedly discolored solutions.
• Protect liquid concentrate from light. Dilute with fruit juice, milk, or semisolid food just before administration.
• Give deep I.M. only in upper outer quadrant of buttocks. Consider giving injection by Z-track method. Massage slowly afterward to prevent sterile abscess. Injection stings. Rotate injection sites.
• Monitor patient for tardive dyskinesia, which may occur after prolonged use. It may not appear until months or years later and may disappear spontaneously or persist for life, despite stopping drug.
• After abrupt withdrawal of long-term therapy, gastritis, nausea, vomiting, dizziness, or tremor may occur.
• *Alert:* Watch for evidence of neuroleptic malignant syndrome (extrapyramidal effects, hyperthermia, autonomic disturbance), which is rare but usually fatal. It may not be related to length of drug use or type of neuroleptic; more than 60% of affected patients are men.
• Monitor therapy with weekly bilirubin tests during first month; with periodic CBCs, liver function tests, and renal function tests; and with ophthalmic tests for long-term use.
• Withhold dose and notify prescriber if jaundice, symptoms of blood dyscrasia (fever, sore throat, infection, cellulitis, weakness), or persistent extrapyramidal reactions (longer than a few hours) develop, or if such reactions occur in children or pregnant women.
• Don't withdraw drug abruptly unless necessitated by severe adverse reactions.
• *Alert:* Don't confuse chlorpromazine with chlorpropamide, a hypoglycemic.
• *Alert:* Don't confuse chlorpromazine with clomipramine.

**PATIENT TEACHING**
• Warn patient to avoid activities that require alertness or good coordination until effects of drug are known. Drowsiness and dizziness usually subside after first few weeks.
• *Alert:* Advise patient not to crush, chew, or break extended release capsule form before swallowing.
• Tell patient to avoid alcohol while taking drug.
• Have patient report signs of urine retention or constipation.
• Tell patient to use sunblock and to wear protective clothing to avoid oversensitivity to the sun. Chlorpromazine is more likely to cause sun sensitivity than any other drug in its class.
• Tell patient to relieve dry mouth with sugarless gum or hard candy.
• Advise patient receiving drug by any method other than by mouth to remain lying down for 1 hour afterward and to rise slowly.

## clozapine
Clozaril

*Pregnancy risk category B*

**AVAILABLE FORMS**
*Tablets:* 25 mg, 100 mg

**INDICATIONS & DOSAGES**
➤ **Schizophrenia in severely ill patients unresponsive to other therapies; to reduce risk of recurrent suicidal behavior in schizophrenia or schizoaffective disorders**
*Adults:* Initially, 12.5 mg P.O. once daily or b.i.d., adjusted upward by 25 to 50 mg daily (if tolerated) to 300 to 450 mg daily by end of 2 weeks. Individual dosage is based on clinical response, patient tolerance, and adverse reactions. Subsequent dosage shouldn't be increased more than once or twice weekly, and shouldn't exceed 50- to 100-mg increments. Many patients respond to dosages of 200 to 600 mg daily, but some may need as much as 900 mg daily. Don't exceed 900 mg daily.

---

## ACTION
Unknown. Binds selectively to dopaminergic receptors (D1 and D2) in the limbic system of the CNS and may interfere with adrenergic, cholinergic, histaminergic, and serotonergic receptors.

| Route | Onset | Peak | Duration |
|-------|---------|-------|----------|
| P.O. | Unknown | 2½ hr | 4-12 hr |

## ADVERSE REACTIONS
**CNS:** *drowsiness, sedation, **seizures**, dizziness,* syncope, *vertigo, headache,* tremor, disturbed sleep or nightmares, restlessness, hypokinesia or akinesia, agitation, rigidity, akathisia, confusion, fatigue, insomnia, hyperkinesia, weakness, lethargy, ataxia, slurred speech, depression, myoclonus, anxiety, fever.
**CV:** *tachycardia,* hypotension, ***cardiomyopathy,*** hypertension, chest pain, ECG changes, orthostatic hypotension, ***myocarditis, pulmonary embolism, cardiac arrest.***
**EENT:** visual disturbances.
**GI:** dry mouth, *constipation,* nausea, vomiting, *excessive salivation,* heartburn, diarrhea.
**GU:** urinary frequency or urgency, urine retention, incontinence, abnormal ejaculation.
**Hematologic:** *leukopenia, agranulocytosis, granulocytopenia,* eosinophilia.
**Metabolic:** weight gain, hyperglycemia.
**Musculoskeletal:** muscle pain or spasm, muscle weakness.
**Respiratory:** *respiratory arrest.*
**Skin:** rash, diaphoresis.

## INTERACTIONS
**Drug-drug.** *Anticholinergics:* May potentiate anticholinergic effects of clozapine. Use together cautiously.
*Antihypertensives:* May potentiate hypotensive effects. Monitor blood pressure.
*Benzodiazepines:* May increase risk of sedation and CV and respiratory arrest. Use together cautiously.
*Bone marrow suppressants:* May increase bone marrow toxicity. Avoid using together.
*Digoxin, other highly protein-bound drugs, warfarin:* May increase levels of these drugs. Monitor patient closely for adverse reactions.
*Fluoroquinolones, fluvoxamine, paroxetine, sertraline:* May increase clozapine level. Use together cautiously, and monitor patient.
*Phenytoin:* May decrease clozapine level and cause breakthrough psychosis. Monitor patient for psychosis and adjust clozapine dosage.
*Psychoactive drugs:* May cause additive effects. Use together cautiously.
**Drug-herb.** *St. John's wort:* May decrease clozapine level. Discourage use together.
**Drug-lifestyle.** *Alcohol use:* May increase CNS depression. Discourage use together.
*Smoking:* May decrease clozapine level. Urge patient to quit smoking. Monitor patient for effectiveness and adjust dosage.

## EFFECTS ON LAB TEST RESULTS
• May increase glucose level.
• May increase eosinophil count. May decrease WBC and granulocyte counts.

## CONTRAINDICATIONS & CAUTIONS
• Contraindicated in patients with uncontrolled epilepsy, history of clozapine-induced agranulocytosis, WBC count below 3,500/mm³, severe CNS depression or coma, and myelosuppressive disorders.
• Contraindicated in patients taking other drugs that suppress bone marrow function.
• Use cautiously in patients with prostatic hyperplasia or angle-closure glaucoma because drug has potent anticholinergic effects.

## NURSING CONSIDERATIONS
• *Alert:* Clozapine carries significant risk of agranulocytosis. If possible, patient should receive at least two trials of drug therapy with a standard antipsychotic before starting clozapine. Baseline WBC and differential counts are needed before therapy. Monitor WBC counts weekly for at least 4 weeks after clozapine therapy ends.
• When giving clozapine, ensure that WBC counts and blood tests are performed weekly and that no more than a 1-week supply of drug is dispensed at a time for first 6 months of therapy. If WBC count stays at 3,000/mm³ or more and absolute neutrophil count stays at 1,500/mm³ or more during first 6 months of continuous therapy, frequency of moni-

toring blood counts may be reduced to every other week.

• If WBC count drops below 3,500/mm³ after therapy begins or if it drops substantially from baseline, monitor patient closely for signs and symptoms of infection. If WBC count is 3,000 to 3,500/mm³ and granulocyte count is above 1,500/mm³, perform WBC and differential count twice weekly. If WBC count drops below 3,000/mm³ and granulocyte count drops below 1,500/mm³, interrupt therapy, notify prescriber, and monitor patient for signs and symptoms of infection. Therapy may be restarted cautiously if WBC count returns to above 3,000/mm³ and granulocyte count returns to above 1,500/mm³. Continue monitoring WBC and differential counts twice weekly until WBC count exceeds 3,500/mm³.

• If WBC count drops below 2,000/mm³ and granulocyte count drops below 1,000/mm³, patient may need protective isolation. If infection develops, prepare cultures according to institutional policy and give antibiotics. Bone marrow aspiration may be needed to assess bone marrow function. Future clozapine therapy is contraindicated in such situations.

• *Alert:* Clozapine causes an increased risk of fatal myocarditis especially during, but not limited to, the first month of therapy. In patients in whom myocarditis is suspected (unexplained fatigue, dyspnea, tachypnea, chest pain, tachycardia, fever, palpitations, and other signs or symptoms of heart failure or ECG abnormalities such as ST-T wave abnormalities or arrhythmias), stop clozapine therapy immediately and don't restart.

• Monitor patient for signs and symptoms of cardiomyopathy.

• Seizures may occur, especially in patients receiving high doses.

• Some patients experience transient fever with temperature higher than 100.4° F (38° C), especially in the first 3 weeks of therapy. Monitor these patients closely.

• After abrupt withdrawal of long-term therapy, abrupt recurrence of psychotic symptoms is possible.

• If clozapine therapy must be stopped, withdraw drug gradually over 1 or 2 weeks. If changes in patient's medical condition (including development of leu-

kopenia) necessitate abrupt discontinuation of drug, monitor patient closely for recurrence of psychotic symptoms.

• If therapy is reinstated in patients withdrawn from drug, follow usual guidelines for dosage increase. Reexposure of patient to drug may increase severity and risk of adverse reactions. If therapy was stopped because WBC counts were below 2,000/mm³ or granulocyte counts were below 1,000/mm³, don't expect drug to be continued.

• *Alert:* Don't confuse clozapine with clonidine, clofazimine, or Klonopin.

### PATIENT TEACHING
• Tell patient about need for weekly blood tests to check for blood cell deficiency. Advise him to report flulike symptoms, fever, sore throat, lethargy, malaise, or other signs of infection.

• Warn patient to avoid hazardous activities that require alertness and good coordination while taking drug.

• Tell patient to check with prescriber before taking alcohol or nonprescription drugs.

• Advise patient that smoking may decrease drug effectiveness.

• Tell patient to rise slowly to avoid dizziness.

• Inform patient that ice chips or sugarless candy or gum may help relieve dry mouth.

---

**fluphenazine decanoate**
Modecate†‡, Modecate Concentrate†, Prolixin Decanoate

**fluphenazine enanthate**
Moditen Enanthate†, Prolixin Enanthate

**fluphenazine hydrochloride**
Anatensol‡*, Apo-Fluphenazine†, Moditen HCl†, Permitil†*, Permitil Concentrate, Prolixin†*, Prolixin Concentrate

*Pregnancy risk category C*

### AVAILABLE FORMS
**fluphenazine decanoate**
*Depot injection:* 25 mg/ml

**fluphenazine enanthate**
*Depot injection:* 25 mg/ml
**fluphenazine hydrochloride**
*Elixir:* 2.5 mg/5 ml*
*I.M. injection:* 2.5 mg/ml
*Oral concentrate:* 5 mg/ml*
*Tablets:* 1 mg, 2.5 mg, 5 mg, 10 mg

## INDICATIONS & DOSAGES
➤ **Psychotic disorders**
*Adults:* Initially, 0.5 to 10 mg fluphenazine hydrochloride P.O. daily in divided doses q 6 to 8 hours; may increase cautiously to 20 mg. Maintenance dose is 1 to 5 mg P.O. daily. I.M. doses are one-third to one-half of oral doses. Usual I.M. dose is 1.25 mg. Give more than 10 mg/day with caution.
Or, 12.5 to 25 mg of long-acting esters (decanoate or enanthate) I.M. or S.C. q 1 to 6 weeks; maintenance dose is 25 to 100 mg, p.r.n.
*Elderly patients:* 1 to 2.5 mg daily.

## ACTION
Unknown. A piperazine phenothiazine that probably blocks postsynaptic dopamine in the brain.

| Route | Onset | Peak | Duration |
|---|---|---|---|
| P.O. | < 1 hr | 30 min | 6-8 hr |
| I.M. (depot) | 24-72 hr | Unknown | 1-6 wk |
| I.M. (hydro-chloride) | < 1 hr | 90-120 min | 6-8 hr |
| S.C. | Unknown | Unknown | Unknown |

## ADVERSE REACTIONS
**CNS:** *extrapyramidal reactions, tardive dyskinesia,* sedation, *pseudoparkinsonism,* EEG changes, drowsiness, *seizures,* dizziness, *neuroleptic malignant syndrome.*
**CV:** orthostatic hypotension, tachycardia, ECG changes.
**EENT:** ocular changes, *blurred vision,* nasal congestion.
**GI:** *dry mouth, constipation,* increased appetite.
**GU:** *urine retention,* dark urine, menstrual irregularities, inhibited ejaculation.
**Hematologic:** *leukopenia, agranulocytosis,* eosinophilia, hemolytic anemia, *aplastic anemia, thrombocytopenia.*
**Hepatic:** cholestatic jaundice.

**Metabolic:** weight gain.
**Skin:** *mild photosensitivity reactions,* allergic reactions.
**Other:** gynecomastia, galactorrhea.

## INTERACTIONS
**Drug-drug.** *Antacids:* May inhibit absorption of oral phenothiazines. Separate antacid and phenothiazine doses by at least 2 hours.
*Anticholinergics:* May increase anticholinergic effects. Use together cautiously.
*Barbiturates, lithium:* May decrease phenothiazine effect and increase neurologic adverse effects. Monitor patient.
*Centrally acting antihypertensives:* May decrease antihypertensive effect. Monitor blood pressure.
*CNS depressants:* May increase CNS depression. Use together cautiously.
**Drug-herb.** *St. John's wort:* May increase risk of photosensitivity reactions. Advise patient to avoid excessive sunlight exposure.
**Drug-lifestyle.** *Alcohol use:* May increase CNS depression, especially that involving psychomotor skills. Strongly discourage alcohol use.
*Sun exposure:* May increase risk of photosensitivity reactions. Advise patient to avoid excessive sunlight exposure.

## EFFECTS ON LAB TEST RESULTS
● May increase liver function test values and eosinophil count. May decrease hemoglobin, hematocrit, and WBC, granulocyte, and platelet counts.
● May cause false-positive results for urinary porphyrin, urobilinogen, amylase, and 5-hydroxyindoleacetic acid tests and for urine pregnancy tests that use human chorionic gonadotropin.

## CONTRAINDICATIONS & CAUTIONS
● Contraindicated in patients hypersensitive to drug and in those with coma, CNS depression, bone marrow suppression or other blood dyscrasia, subcortical damage, or liver damage.
● Use cautiously in elderly or debilitated patients and in those with pheochromocytoma, severe CV disease (may cause sudden drop in blood pressure), peptic ulcer, respiratory disorder, hypocalcemia, seizure disorder (may lower seizure thresh-

old), severe reactions to insulin or electro-convulsive therapy, mitral insufficiency, glaucoma, or prostatic hyperplasia.
• Use cautiously in those exposed to extreme heat or cold (including antipyretic therapy) or phosphorus insecticides. Use parenteral form cautiously in asthmatic patients and in those allergic to sulfites.

**NURSING CONSIDERATIONS**
• Prolixin Concentrate and Permitil Concentrate are 10 times more concentrated than Prolixin elixir (5 mg/ml versus 0.5 mg/ml). Check dosage order carefully.
• Oral liquid and parenteral forms can cause contact dermatitis. Wear gloves when preparing solutions, and avoid contact with skin and clothing.
• Protect drug from light. Slight yellowing of injection or concentrate is common and doesn't affect potency. Discard markedly discolored solutions.
• Dilute liquid concentrate with water, fruit juice, milk, or semisolid food just before administration.
• For long-acting forms (decanoate and enanthate), which are oil preparations, use a dry needle of at least 21G. Allow 24 to 96 hours for onset of action. Note and report adverse reactions in patients taking these drug forms.
• Monitor patient for tardive dyskinesia, which may occur after prolonged use. It may not appear until months or years later and may disappear spontaneously or persist for life, despite ending drug.
• *Alert:* Watch for signs and symptoms of neuroleptic malignant syndrome (extrapyramidal effects, hyperthermia, autonomic disturbance), which is rare but commonly fatal. It may not be related to length of drug use or type of neuroleptic; more than 60% of affected patients are men.
• Monitor therapy with weekly bilirubin tests during first month and with periodic CBCs, liver function tests, renal function tests, and, for long-term use, ophthalmic tests.
• Withhold dose and notify prescriber if signs and symptoms of blood dyscrasia (fever, sore throat, infection, cellulitis, weakness) or extrapyramidal reactions persisting longer than a few hours develop, especially in children and pregnant women.

• Don't withdraw drug abruptly unless serious adverse reactions occur.
• Abrupt withdrawal of long-term therapy may cause gastritis, nausea, vomiting, dizziness, tremor, feeling of warmth or cold, diaphoresis, tachycardia, headache, or insomnia.
• *Alert:* Permitil and Prolixin may contain tartrazine.

**PATIENT TEACHING**
• Warn patient to avoid activities that require alertness and good coordination until effects of drug are known. Drowsiness and dizziness usually subside after first few weeks.
• Warn patient to avoid alcohol while taking drug.
• Tell patient to relieve dry mouth with sugarless gum or hard candy.
• Have patient report signs of urine retention or constipation.
• Advise patient to use sunblock and wear protective clothing to avoid sensitivity to the sun.
• Tell patient that drug may discolor urine.

━━━━━━━━━━━━━━━━━━━━━━

# haloperidol
Apo-Haloperidol† Haldol, Novo-Peridol†, Peridol†, Serenace‡

# haloperidol decanoate
Haldol Decanoate, Haldol LA†

# haloperidol lactate
Haldol, Haldol Concentrate, Haloperidol Intensol

*Pregnancy risk category C*

━━━━━━━━━━━━━━━━━━━━━━

**AVAILABLE FORMS**
**haloperidol**
*Tablets:* 0.5 mg, 1 mg, 2 mg, 5 mg, 10 mg, 20 mg
**haloperidol decanoate**
*Injection:* 50 mg/ml, 100 mg/ml
**haloperidol lactate**
*Injection:* 5 mg/ml
*Oral concentrate:* 2 mg/ml

**INDICATIONS & DOSAGES**
➤ **Psychotic disorders**
*Adults and children older than age 12:*
Dosage varies for each patient. Initially,

0.5 to 5 mg P.O. b.i.d. or t.i.d. Or, 2 to 5 mg I.M. q 4 to 8 hours, although hourly administration may be needed until control is obtained. Maximum, 100 mg P.O. daily.
*Children ages 3 to 12:* 0.05 mg/kg to 0.15 mg/kg P.O. daily. Severely disturbed children may need higher doses.
➤ **Chronic psychosis requiring prolonged therapy**
*Adults:* 50 to 100 mg I.M. decanoate q 4 weeks.
➤ **Nonpsychotic behavior disorders**
*Children ages 3 to 12:* 0.05 mg/kg P.O. daily. Maximum, 6 mg daily.
➤ **Tourette syndrome**
*Adults:* 0.5 to 5 mg P.O. b.i.d., t.i.d., or p.r.n.
*Children ages 3 to 12:* 0.05 to 0.075 mg/kg P.O. daily in two or three divided doses.
*Elderly patients:* 0.5 to 2 mg P.O. b.i.d. or t.i.d.; increase gradually, p.r.n.
*Adjust-a-dose:* For debilitated patients, initially, 0.5 to 2 mg P.O. b.i.d. or t.i.d.; increase gradually, p.r.n.

## ACTION
Unknown. A butyrophenone that probably exerts antipsychotic effects by blocking postsynaptic dopamine receptors in the brain.

| Route | Onset | Peak | Duration |
|---|---|---|---|
| P.O. | Unknown | 3-6 hr | Unknown |
| I.V. | Unknown | Unknown | Unknown |
| I.M. (decanoate) | Unknown | 3-9 days | Unknown |
| I.M. (lactate) | Unknown | 10-20 min | Unknown |

## ADVERSE REACTIONS
**CNS:** *severe extrapyramidal reactions, tardive dyskinesia,* sedation, drowsiness, lethargy, headache, insomnia, confusion, vertigo, *seizures, neuroleptic malignant syndrome.*
**CV:** tachycardia, hypotension, hypertension, ECG changes, *torsades de pointes* with I.V. use.
**EENT:** blurred vision.
**GI:** dry mouth, anorexia, constipation, diarrhea, nausea, vomiting, dyspepsia.
**GU:** urine retention, menstrual irregularities, priapism.
**Hematologic:** *leukopenia,* leukocytosis.

**Hepatic:** jaundice.
**Skin:** rash, other skin reactions, diaphoresis.
**Other:** gynecomastia.

## INTERACTIONS
**Drug-drug.** *Anticholinergics:* May increase anticholinergic effects and glaucoma. Use together cautiously.
*Azole antifungals, buspirone, macrolides:* May increase haloperidol level. Monitor patient for increased adverse reactions; haloperidol dose may need to be adjusted.
*Carbamazepine:* May decrease haloperidol level. Monitor patient.
*CNS depressants:* May increase CNS depression. Use together cautiously.
*Lithium:* May cause lethargy and confusion after high doses. Monitor patient.
*Methyldopa:* May cause dementia. Monitor patient closely.
*Rifampin:* May decrease haloperidol level. Monitor patient for clinical effect.
**Drug-lifestyle.** *Alcohol use:* May increase CNS depression. Discourage use together.

## EFFECTS ON LAB TEST RESULTS
● May increase liver function test values. May increase or decrease WBC count.

## CONTRAINDICATIONS & CAUTIONS
● Contraindicated in patients hypersensitive to drug and in those with parkinsonism, coma, or CNS depression.
● Use cautiously in elderly and debilitated patients; in patients with history of seizures or EEG abnormalities, severe CV disorders, allergies, glaucoma, or urine retention; and in those taking anticonvulsants, anticoagulants, antiparkinsonians, or lithium.

## NURSING CONSIDERATIONS
● Protect drug from light. Slight yellowing of injection or concentrate is common and doesn't affect potency. Discard markedly discolored solutions.
● When switching from tablets to decanoate injection, give 10 to 15 times the oral dose once a month (maximum 100 mg).
● Dilute oral dose with water or a beverage, such as orange juice, apple juice, tomato juice, or cola, immediately before administration.

Reactions may be *common,* uncommon, *life-threatening,* or COMMON AND LIFE-THREATENING.

• *Alert:* Don't give decanoate form I.V.
• Monitor patient for tardive dyskinesia, which may occur after prolonged use. It may not appear until months or years later and may disappear spontaneously or persist for life, despite ending drug.
• *Alert:* Watch for signs and symptoms of neuroleptic malignant syndrome (extrapyramidal effects, hyperthermia, autonomic disturbance), which is rare but commonly fatal. It may not be related to length of drug use or type of neuroleptic; more than 60% of affected patients are men.
• Don't withdraw drug abruptly unless required by severe adverse reactions.
• *Alert:* Haldol may contain tartrazine.
• *Alert:* Don't confuse Haldol with Halcion or Halog.

## PATIENT TEACHING
• Although drug is the least sedating of the antipsychotics, warn patient to avoid activities that require alertness and good coordination until effects of drug are known. Drowsiness and dizziness usually subside after a few weeks.
• Warn patient to avoid alcohol while taking drug.
• Tell patient to relieve dry mouth with sugarless gum or hard candy.

## loxapine hydrochloride
Loxapac†, Loxitane C, Loxitane IM

## loxapine succinate
Loxapac†, Loxitane

*Pregnancy risk category NR*

## AVAILABLE FORMS
**loxapine hydrochloride**
*Injection:* 50 mg/ml
*Oral concentrate:* 25 mg/ml
**loxapine succinate**
*Capsules:* 5 mg, 10 mg, 25 mg, 50 mg
*Tablets:* 5 mg†, 10 mg†, 25 mg†, 50 mg†

## INDICATIONS & DOSAGES
➤ **Psychotic disorders**
*Adults:* 10 mg P.O. b.i.d. to q.i.d., rapidly increasing to 60 to 100 mg P.O. daily for most patients; dosage varies. If patient can't take oral dose, give 12.5 to 50 mg I.M. q 4 to 6 hours or longer; dosage and

interval depend on patient response. Don't exceed 250 mg/day.
*Elderly patients:* Initially, 5 mg P.O. b.i.d. Adjust dosage as needed and as tolerated.

## ACTION
Unknown. A dibenzoxazepine that probably exerts antipsychotic effects by blocking postsynaptic dopamine receptors in the brain.

| Route | Onset | Peak | Duration |
| --- | --- | --- | --- |
| P.O., I.M. | 30 min | 90 min-3 hr | 12 hr |

## ADVERSE REACTIONS
**CNS:** *extrapyramidal reactions, sedation,* drowsiness, *seizures,* numbness, confusion, syncope, *tardive dyskinesia,* pseudoparkinsonism, EEG changes, dizziness, **neuroleptic malignant syndrome.**
**CV:** orthostatic hypotension, tachycardia, ECG changes, hypertension.
**EENT:** *blurred vision,* nasal congestion.
**GI:** *dry mouth, constipation,* nausea, vomiting, paralytic ileus.
**GU:** *urine retention,* menstrual irregularities.
**Hematologic:** *leukopenia, agranulocytosis, thrombocytopenia.*
**Hepatic:** jaundice.
**Metabolic:** weight gain.
**Skin:** allergic reactions, rash, pruritus.
**Other:** gynecomastia, galactorrhea.

## INTERACTIONS
**Drug-drug.** *Anticholinergics:* May increase anticholinergic effect. Use together cautiously.
*CNS depressants:* May increase CNS depression. Use together cautiously.
*Epinephrine:* May inhibit vasopressor effect of epinephrine. Avoid using together.
**Drug-lifestyle.** *Alcohol use:* May increase CNS depression. Discourage use together.

## EFFECTS ON LAB TEST RESULTS
• May increase liver function test values. May decrease WBC, granulocyte, and platelet counts.
• May cause false-positive results for urinary porphyrin, urobilinogen, amylase, and 5-hydroxyindoleacetic acid tests and for urine pregnancy tests that use human chorionic gonadotropin.

**CONTRAINDICATIONS & CAUTIONS**
- Contraindicated in patients hypersensitive to dibenzoxazepines and in those with coma, severe CNS depression, or drug-induced depressed states.
- Use with extreme caution in patients with seizure disorder, CV disorder, glaucoma, or history of urine retention.

**NURSING CONSIDERATIONS**
- Obtain baseline blood pressure measurements before starting therapy and monitor pressure regularly.
- Dilute liquid concentrate with orange or grapefruit juice just before giving it.
- Monitor patient for tardive dyskinesia, which may occur after prolonged use. It may not appear until months or years later and may disappear spontaneously or persist for life, despite ending drug.
- *Alert:* Watch for evidence of neuroleptic malignant syndrome (extrapyramidal effects, hyperthermia, autonomic disturbance), which is rare but commonly fatal. It may not be related to length of drug use or type of neuroleptic; more than 60% of affected patients are men.

**PATIENT TEACHING**
- Warn patient to avoid activities that require alertness and good coordination until effects of drug are known. Drowsiness and dizziness usually subside after first few weeks.
- Advise patient to report bruising, fever, or sore throat immediately.
- Tell patient to avoid alcohol while taking drug.
- Advise patient to get up slowly to avoid dizziness upon standing quickly.
- Tell patient to relieve dry mouth with sugarless gum or hard candy.
- Recommend periodic eye examinations.

## mesoridazine besylate
Serentil*, Serentil Concentrate

*Pregnancy risk category NR*

**AVAILABLE FORMS**
*Injection:* 25 mg/ml
*Oral concentrate:* 25 mg/ml (0.6% alcohol)*
*Tablets:* 10 mg, 25 mg, 50 mg, 100 mg

**INDICATIONS & DOSAGES**
➤ **Schizophrenic patients who don't respond to adequate treatment with other antipsychotic drugs**
*Adults:* Initially, 50 mg P.O. t.i.d. or 25 mg I.M. repeated in 30 to 60 minutes, p.r.n. Maximum, 400 mg P.O. daily or 200 mg I.M. daily.

**ACTION**
Unknown. A piperidine phenothiazine and the major sulfoxide metabolite of thioridazine that probably exerts antipsychotic effects by blocking postsynaptic dopamine receptors in the brain.

| Route | Onset | Peak | Duration |
|---|---|---|---|
| P.O., I.M. | Unknown | Unknown | Unknown |

**ADVERSE REACTIONS**
**CNS:** *extrapyramidal reactions, tardive dyskinesia, sedation,* drowsiness, tremor, rigidity, weakness, EEG changes, dizziness, *neuroleptic malignant syndrome.*
**CV:** *hypotension,* tachycardia, *prolonged QTc interval, torsades de pointes,* ECG changes.
**EENT:** *ocular changes, blurred vision,* retinitis pigmentosa, nasal congestion.
**GI:** *dry mouth, constipation,* nausea, vomiting.
**GU:** *urine retention,* menstrual irregularities, inhibited ejaculation.
**Hematologic:** *leukopenia, agranulocytosis, aplastic anemia,* eosinophilia, *thrombocytopenia.*
**Hepatic:** jaundice.
**Metabolic:** weight gain.
**Skin:** *mild photosensitivity reactions,* allergic reactions, pain at I.M. injection site, sterile abscess, rash.
**Other:** gynecomastia, galactorrhea.

**INTERACTIONS**
**Drug-drug.** *Antacids:* May inhibit absorption of oral phenothiazines. Separate antacid and phenothiazine doses by at least 2 hours.
*Anticholinergics:* May increase anticholinergic effects. Use together cautiously.
*Barbiturates:* May decrease phenothiazine effect. Monitor patient.
*CNS depressants:* May increase CNS depression. Use together cautiously.

Reactions may be *common,* uncommon, *life-threatening,* or **COMMON AND LIFE-THREATENING.**

*Lithium:* May increase neurologic adverse effects. Monitor patient closely.

*Other drugs that prolong QTc interval (disopyramide, procainamide, quinidine):* May increase risk of arrhythmias. Avoid using together.

**Drug-herb.** *St. John's wort:* May cause photosensitivity reactions. Advise patient to avoid excessive sunlight exposure.

**Drug-lifestyle.** *Alcohol use:* May increase CNS depression, particularly psychomotor skills. Strongly discourage alcohol use.

*Sun exposure:* May increase risk of photosensitivity reactions. Advise patient to avoid excessive sunlight exposure.

## EFFECTS ON LAB TEST RESULTS
● May increase liver function test values and eosinophil count. May decrease hemoglobin, hematocrit, and WBC, granulocyte, and platelet counts.
● May cause false-positive results for urinary porphyrin, urobilinogen, amylase, and 5-hydroxyindoleacetic acid tests and for urine pregnancy tests that use human chorionic gonadotropin.

## CONTRAINDICATIONS & CAUTIONS
● Contraindicated in patients hypersensitive to drug and in those with severe CNS depression or coma.
● Contraindicated in patients taking other drugs that prolong the QTc interval and in those with congenital long QT interval syndrome or a history of cardiac arrhythmias.

## NURSING CONSIDERATIONS
● Protect drug from light. Slight yellowing of injection or concentrate is common and doesn't affect potency. Discard markedly discolored solutions.
● Oral liquid and parenteral forms may cause contact dermatitis. Wear gloves when preparing solutions and avoid contact with skin and clothing.
● *Alert:* Before treatment, obtain baseline ECG and measure potassium level. Normalize potassium level before starting treatment. A patient with a QTc interval above 450 msec shouldn't start drug; one with a QTc interval above 500 msec should stop drug.

● Obtain baseline blood pressure measurements before starting therapy and monitor them regularly. Watch for orthostatic hypotension, especially with parenteral administration.
● Give deeply I.M. only in upper outer quadrant of buttocks. Massage slowly afterward to prevent sterile abscess. Injection may sting.
● Monitor patient for tardive dyskinesia, which may occur after prolonged use. It may not appear until months or years later and may disappear spontaneously or persist for life, despite ending drug.
● *Alert:* Watch for evidence of neuroleptic malignant syndrome (extrapyramidal effects, hyperthermia, autonomic disturbance), which is rare but commonly fatal. It may not be related to length of drug use or type of neuroleptic; more than 60% of affected patients are men.
● Monitor therapy with weekly bilirubin tests during first month and with periodic CBCs, liver function tests, renal function tests, and, for long-term use, ophthalmic tests.
● Withhold dose and notify prescriber if jaundice, symptoms of blood dyscrasia (fever, sore throat, infection, cellulitis, weakness), or persistent extrapyramidal reactions (longer than a few hours) develop, especially in children or pregnant women.
● Don't withdraw drug abruptly unless severe adverse reactions occur.
● After abrupt withdrawal of long-term therapy, gastritis, nausea, vomiting, dizziness, tremor, feeling of warmth or cold, diaphoresis, tachycardia, headache, or insomnia may occur.
● *Alert:* Don't confuse Serentil with Serevent or Aventyl.

## PATIENT TEACHING
● Warn patient to avoid activities that require alertness and good coordination until effects of drug are known. Drowsiness and dizziness usually subside after a few weeks.
● Advise patient to report symptoms of dizziness, palpitations, or fainting.
● Tell patient to change positions slowly.
● Warn patient to avoid alcohol while taking drug.

- Have patient report signs of urine retention or constipation.
- Tell patient that drug may discolor urine.
- Instruct patient to relieve dry mouth with sugarless gum or hard candy.
- Advise patient to use sunblock and wear protective clothing to avoid oversensitivity to the sun.

---

## olanzapine
Zyprexa, Zyprexa Zydis

*Pregnancy risk category C*

### AVAILABLE FORMS
*Tablets:* 2.5 mg, 5 mg, 7.5 mg, 10 mg, 15 mg, 20 mg
*Tablets (orally disintegrating):* 5 mg, 10 mg, 15 mg, 20 mg

### INDICATIONS & DOSAGES
➤ **Schizophrenia**
*Adults:* Initially, 5 to 10 mg P.O. once daily. Adjust dose in 5-mg daily increments at intervals of not less than 1 week. Most patients respond to 10 to 15 mg/day. Safety of dosages greater than 20 mg/day hasn't been established.
➤ **Long-term treatment of schizophrenia**
*Adults:* Initially, 5 to 10 mg P.O. daily. Goal is 10 mg P.O. daily within several days of starting therapy. Dosage may be increased weekly by 5 mg daily to a maximum of 20 mg daily. Clinically assess patients whose dosages exceed 10 mg daily.
*Patients age 65 and older:* Start therapy at low end of dosage range. Adjust carefully.
*Adjust-a-dose:* In patients who are debilitated, who are predisposed to hypotensive reactions, who may metabolize olanzapine more slowly than usual (nonsmoking women older than age 65), or who may be more sensitive to olanzapine, start at 5 mg P.O. Increase dose cautiously in these patients.
➤ **Short-term treatment of acute manic episodes linked to bipolar I disorder**
*Adults:* Initially, 10 to 15 mg P.O. daily. Adjust dosage p.r.n. in 5-mg daily increments at intervals of 24 hours or more. Maximum, 20 mg P.O. daily. Duration of treatment is 3 to 4 weeks.

*Adjust-a-dose:* In patients who are debilitated, who are predisposed to hypotensive reactions, who may metabolize olanzapine more slowly than usual (nonsmoking women older than age 65), or who may be more sensitive to olanzapine, start at 5 mg P.O. Increase dose cautiously in these patients.
✴ ***NEW INDICATION:*** **Short-term treatment, with lithium or valproate, of acute manic episodes linked to bipolar I disorder**
*Adults:* 10 mg P.O. once daily. Dosage range is 5 to 20 mg daily. Duration of treatment is 6 weeks.
*Adjust-a-dose:* In patients who are debilitated, who are predisposed to hypotensive reactions, who may metabolize olanzapine more slowly than usual (nonsmoking women older than age 65), or who may be more pharmacodynamically sensitive to olanzapine, start at 5 mg P.O. Increase dose cautiously in these patients.

### ACTION
Unknown. May block dopamine and 5-HT$_2$ receptors.

| Route | Onset | Peak | Duration |
|-------|-------|------|----------|
| P.O. | Unknown | 6 hr | Unknown |

### ADVERSE REACTIONS
**CNS:** *somnolence,* asthenia, abnormal gait, *insomnia, parkinsonism, dizziness,* personality disorder, akathisia, tremor, articulation impairment, ***suicide attempt,*** tardive dyskinesia, ***neuroleptic malignant syndrome,*** fever.
**CV:** orthostatic hypotension, tachycardia, chest pain, hypertension, ecchymosis, peripheral edema
**EENT:** amblyopia, rhinitis, pharyngitis, conjunctivitis.
**GI:** *constipation, dry mouth, dyspepsia,* increased appetite, increased salivation, vomiting, thirst.
**GU:** hematuria, metrorrhagia, urinary incontinence, urinary tract infection, amenorrhea, vaginitis.
**Hematologic:** *leukopenia.*
**Metabolic:** weight gain.
**Musculoskeletal:** joint pain, extremity pain, back pain, neck rigidity, twitching, hypertonia.
**Respiratory:** increased cough, dyspnea.

---

Reactions may be *common,* uncommon, *life-threatening,* or COMMON AND LIFE-THREATENING.

**Skin:** sweating.
**Other:** flulike syndrome, injury.

**INTERACTIONS**
**Drug-drug.** *Antihypertensives:* May potentiate hypotensive effects. Monitor blood pressure closely.
*Carbamazepine, omeprazole, rifampin:* May increase clearance of olanzapine. Monitor patient.
*Ciprofloxacin:* May increase olanzapine level. Monitor patient for increased adverse effects.
*Diazepam:* May increase CNS effects. Monitor patient.
*Dopamine agonists, levodopa:* May cause antagonized activity of these drugs. Monitor patient.
*Fluoxetine:* May increase olanzapine level. Use together cautiously.
*Fluvoxamine:* May increase olanzapine level. Consider lower dose of olanzapine.
**Drug-herb.** *St. John's wort:* May decrease olanzapine level. Discourage use together.
**Drug-lifestyle.** *Alcohol use:* May increase CNS effects. Discourage use together.
*Smoking:* May increase olanzapine clearance. Urge patient to quit smoking.

**EFFECTS ON LAB TEST RESULTS**
• May increase AST, ALT, GGT, CK, triglyceride, and prolactin levels.
• May increase eosinophil count. May decrease WBC count.

**CONTRAINDICATIONS & CAUTIONS**
• Contraindicated in patients hypersensitive to drug.
• Use cautiously in patients with heart disease, cerebrovascular disease, conditions that predispose patient to hypotension, history of seizures or conditions that might lower the seizure threshold, and hepatic impairment. Also use cautiously in elderly patients, those with a history of paralytic ileus, and those at risk for aspiration pneumonia, prostatic hyperplasia, or angle-closure glaucoma.

**NURSING CONSIDERATIONS**
• Monitor patient for abnormal body temperature regulation, especially if he exercises, is exposed to extreme heat, takes anticholinergics, or is dehydrated.

• Obtain baseline and periodic liver function test results.
• Monitor patient for weight gain.
• *Alert:* Watch for evidence of neuroleptic malignant syndrome (hyperpyrexia, muscle rigidity, altered mental status, autonomic instability), which is rare but commonly fatal. Stop drug immediately; monitor and treat patient as needed.
• Monitor patient for tardive dyskinesia, which may occur after prolonged use. It may not appear until months or years later and may disappear spontaneously or persist for life, despite stopping drug.
• *Alert:* Don't confuse olanzapine with olsalazine or Zyprexa with Zyrtec.

**PATIENT TEACHING**
• Warn patient to avoid hazardous tasks until full effects of drug are known.
• Warn patient against exposure to extreme heat; drug may impair body's ability to reduce temperature.
• Inform patient that weight gain may occur.
• Advise patient to avoid alcohol.
• Tell patient to rise slowly to avoid dizziness upon standing up quickly.
• Inform patient that orally disintegrating tablets contain phenylalanine.
• Drug may be taken without regard to food.
• Urge woman to notify prescriber if she becomes pregnant or plans or suspects pregnancy. Tell her not to breast-feed during therapy.

---

**perphenazine**
Apo-Perphenazine†, PMS Perphenazine†, Trilafon, Trilafon Concentrate

*Pregnancy risk category NR*

---

**AVAILABLE FORMS**
*Injection:* 5 mg/ml
*Oral concentrate:* 16 mg/5 ml
*Syrup:* 2 mg/5 ml†
*Tablets:* 2 mg, 4 mg, 8 mg, 16 mg

**INDICATIONS & DOSAGES**
➤ **Psychosis in nonhospitalized patients**
*Adults and children older than age 12:*
Initially, 4 to 8 mg P.O. t.i.d.; reduce as

---

soon as possible to minimum effective dose.

➤ **Psychosis in hospitalized patients**
*Adults and children older than age 12:* Initially, 8 to 16 mg P.O. b.i.d., t.i.d., or q.i.d.; increase to 64 mg daily, p.r.n. Or, 5 to 10 mg I.M. q 6 hours, p.r.n. Maximum dose, 30 mg.

➤ **Severe nausea and vomiting**
*Adults:* 8 to 16 mg P.O. daily in divided doses to maximum of 24 mg. Or, 5 to 10 mg I.M., p.r.n. May be given I.V., diluted to 0.5 mg/ml with saline solution. Dose given I.V. shouldn't exceed 5 mg.

## I.V. ADMINISTRATION

● I.V. administration is intended for use only in recumbent hospitalized patients.
● For fractional I.V. injection, give no more than 1 mg per injection at not less than 1- to 2-minute intervals.
● Drug may also be given by slow I.V. infusion.
● Monitor blood pressure and pulse continuously during I.V. infusion.

## ACTION

Unknown. Probably exerts antipsychotic effects by blocking postsynaptic dopamine receptors in the brain.

| Route | Onset | Peak | Duration |
|-------|-------|------|----------|
| P.O., I.V., I.M. | Unknown | Unknown | Unknown |

## ADVERSE REACTIONS

**CNS:** *extrapyramidal reactions, tardive dyskinesia,* sedation, pseudoparkinsonism, dizziness, *seizures,* drowsiness, *neuroleptic malignant syndrome.*
**CV:** *orthostatic hypotension,* tachycardia, ECG changes.
**EENT:** ocular changes, *blurred vision,* nasal congestion.
**GI:** *dry mouth, constipation,* nausea, vomiting, diarrhea.
**GU:** *urine retention,* dark urine, menstrual irregularities, inhibited ejaculation.
**Hematologic:** *leukopenia, agranulocytosis,* eosinophilia, hemolytic anemia, *thrombocytopenia.*
**Hepatic:** cholestatic jaundice.
**Metabolic:** weight gain.

**Skin:** *mild photosensitivity reactions,* allergic reactions, pain at I.M. injection site, sterile abscess.
**Other:** gynecomastia.

## INTERACTIONS

**Drug-drug.** *Antacids:* May inhibit absorption of oral phenothiazines. Separate antacid and phenothiazine doses by at least 2 hours.
*Barbiturates:* May decrease phenothiazine effect. Monitor patient.
*CNS depressants:* May increase CNS depression. Use together cautiously.
*Fluoxetine, paroxetine, sertraline, tricyclic antidepressants:* May increase phenothiazine level. Monitor patient for increased adverse effects.
*Lithium:* May increase neurologic adverse effects. Monitor patient closely.
**Drug-herb.** *St. John's wort:* May cause photosensitivity reactions. Advise patient to avoid excessive sunlight exposure.
**Drug-lifestyle.** *Alcohol use:* May increase CNS depression, particularly psychomotor skills. Strongly discourage alcohol use.
*Sun exposure:* May increase risk of photosensitivity reactions. Advise patient to avoid excessive sunlight exposure.

## EFFECTS ON LAB TEST RESULTS

● May increase liver function test values and eosinophil count. May decrease hemoglobin, hematocrit, and WBC, granulocyte, and platelet counts.
● May cause false-positive results for urinary porphyrin, urobilinogen, amylase, and 5-hydroxyindoleacetic acid tests and for urine pregnancy tests that use human chorionic gonadotropin.

## CONTRAINDICATIONS & CAUTIONS

● Contraindicated in patients hypersensitive to drug and in those with CNS depression, blood dyscrasia, bone marrow depression, liver damage, or subcortical damage; also contraindicated in those experiencing coma or receiving large doses of CNS depressants.
● Use cautiously in elderly or debilitated patients and in those taking other CNS depressants or anticholinergics.
● Use cautiously in patients with alcohol withdrawal, psychotic depression, suicidal tendency, severe adverse reactions to other

---

Reactions may be *common,* uncommon, *life-threatening,* or **COMMON AND LIFE-THREATENING.**

phenothiazines, renal impairment, CV disease, or respiratory disorders.

## NURSING CONSIDERATIONS
• Obtain baseline blood pressure measurements before starting therapy and monitor pressure regularly. Watch for orthostatic hypotension, especially with parenteral administration. Keep patient supine for 1 hour after giving drug; tell him to change positions slowly.
• Protect drug from light. Slight yellowing of injection or concentrate is common and doesn't affect potency. Discard markedly discolored solutions.
• Prevent contact dermatitis by keeping drug away from skin and clothes. Wear gloves when preparing liquid forms.
• Dilute liquid concentrate with fruit juice, milk, carbonated beverage, or semisolid food just before giving. Don't use colas, black coffee, grape juice, apple juice, or tea because turbidity or precipitation may result.
• Give by deep I.M. injection only in upper outer quadrant of buttocks. Massage slowly afterward to prevent sterile abscess. Injection may sting.
• Monitor patient for tardive dyskinesia, which may occur after prolonged use. It may not appear until months or years later and may disappear spontaneously or persist for life, despite ending drug.
• **Alert:** Watch for evidence of neuroleptic malignant syndrome (extrapyramidal effects, hyperthermia, autonomic disturbance), which is rare but commonly fatal. It may not be related to length of drug use or type of neuroleptic; more than 60% of affected patients are men.
• Monitor therapy with weekly bilirubin tests during first month, periodic blood tests (CBCs and liver function tests), and ophthalmic tests (long-term use).
• Withhold dose and notify prescriber if jaundice, symptoms of blood dyscrasia (fever, sore throat, infection, cellulitis, weakness), or persistent extrapyramidal reactions (longer than a few hours) develop.
• Don't withdraw drug abruptly unless severe adverse reactions occur.
• After abrupt withdrawal of long-term therapy, gastritis, nausea, vomiting, dizziness, tremor, feeling of warmth or cold, diaphoresis, tachycardia, headache, or insomnia may occur.

## PATIENT TEACHING
• Tell patient which beverages to use to dilute oral concentrate.
• Warn patient to avoid activities that require alertness or good coordination until effects of drug are known. Drowsiness and dizziness usually subside after a few weeks.
• Tell patient to avoid alcohol while taking drug.
• Advise patient to report signs of urine retention or constipation.
• Tell patient to use sunblock and wear protective clothing to avoid oversensitivity to the sun.
• Advise patient to relieve dry mouth with sugarless gum or hard candy.

# pimozide
Orap

*Pregnancy risk category C*

## AVAILABLE FORMS
*Tablets:* 2 mg, 4 mg†, 10 mg

## INDICATIONS & DOSAGES
➤ **To suppress motor and phonic tics in patients with Tourette syndrome refractory to first-line therapy**
*Adults and children older than age 12:* Initially, 1 to 2 mg P.O. daily in divided doses; then increased every other day, p.r.n. Maintenance dosage is less than 0.2 mg/kg daily or 10 mg/day, whichever is less. Maximum, 10 mg daily.

## ACTION
Unknown. May block dopamine nonselectively at both presynaptic and postsynaptic receptors on neurons in the CNS.

| Route | Onset | Peak | Duration |
|-------|---------|---------|----------|
| P.O. | Unknown | 4-12 hr | Unknown |

## ADVERSE REACTIONS
**CNS:** *parkinsonian symptoms,* drowsiness, headache, insomnia, other extrapyramidal symptoms, *tardive dyskinesia, sedation, neuroleptic malignant syndrome.*

**CV:** *prolonged QT interval,* hypotension, hypertension, tachycardia.
**EENT:** visual disturbances.
**GI:** *dry mouth, constipation,* excessive salivation.
**GU:** impotence, urinary frequency.
**Musculoskeletal:** muscle rigidity.
**Skin:** rash, diaphoresis.

### INTERACTIONS
**Drug-drug.** *Antiarrhythmics, azole antifungal agents, macrolide antibiotics, phenothiazines, protease inhibitors, tricyclic antidepressants:* May cause ECG abnormalities. Avoid using together.
*CNS depressants:* May increase CNS depression. Use together cautiously.
**Drug-food.** *Grapefruit juice:* May inhibit metabolism of pimozide. Discourage use together.
**Drug-lifestyle.** *Alcohol use:* May increase CNS depression. Discourage use together.

### EFFECTS ON LAB TEST RESULTS
None reported.

### CONTRAINDICATIONS & CAUTIONS
• Contraindicated in patients hypersensitive to drug and in those with severe toxic CNS depression, congenital long QT interval syndrome, coma, or a history of arrhythmias.
• Contraindicated for use with other drugs that cause tics and for treatment of simple tics or tics other than those related to Tourette syndrome.
• Contraindicated with other drugs that prolong the QT interval, such as antiarrhythmics.
• Use cautiously in patients with hepatic or renal dysfunction, glaucoma, prostatic hyperplasia, seizure disorder, or EEG abnormalities.

### NURSING CONSIDERATIONS
• *Alert:* Obtain an ECG before treatment begins and periodically thereafter. Watch for prolonged QT interval.
• Monitor patient for extrapyramidal symptoms such as dystonia, akathisia, hyperreflexia, opisthotonos, and oculogyric crisis.
• Monitor patient for tardive dyskinesia, which may occur after prolonged use. It may not appear until months or years later,

and may disappear spontaneously or persist for life, despite discontinuing drug.
• *Alert:* Watch for evidence of neuroleptic malignant syndrome (extrapyramidal effects, hyperthermia, autonomic disturbance), which is rare but commonly fatal. It may not be related to length of drug use or type of neuroleptic; more than 60% of affected patients are men.
• If patient also takes an anticonvulsant, watch for increased seizure activity. Pimozide may lower the seizure threshold.

### PATIENT TEACHING
• Warn patient not to stop taking drug abruptly and not to exceed prescribed dosage.
• Tell patient to avoid alcohol and grapefruit juice while taking drug.
• Advise patient to use sugarless hard candy, gum, and liquids to relieve dry mouth.

---

## quetiapine fumarate
Seroquel

*Pregnancy risk category C*

### AVAILABLE FORMS
*Tablets:* 25 mg, 100 mg, 200 mg, 300 mg

### INDICATIONS & DOSAGES
➤ **To manage signs and symptoms of psychotic disorders**
*Adults:* Initially, 25 mg P.O. b.i.d., with increases in increments of 25 to 50 mg b.i.d. or t.i.d. on days 2 and 3, as tolerated. Target range is 300 to 400 mg daily divided into two or three doses by day 4. Further dosage adjustments, if indicated, should occur at intervals of not less than 2 days. Dosage can be increased or decreased by 25 to 50 mg b.i.d. Antipsychotic effect generally occurs at 150 to 750 mg/day. Safety of dosages over 800 mg/day hasn't been evaluated.
*Elderly patients:* Give lower dosages, adjust more slowly, and monitor patient carefully in first dosing period.
*Adjust-a-dose:* For debilitated patients and those with hepatic impairment or hypotension, consider lower dosages and slower adjustment.

## ACTION
Unknown. A dibenzothiazepine derivative that may block dopamine D2 receptors and serotonin 5-HT$_2$ receptors in the brain.

| Route | Onset | Peak | Duration |
|-------|-------|------|----------|
| P.O. | Unknown | 1½ hr | Unknown |

## ADVERSE REACTIONS
**CNS:** *dizziness, headache, somnolence,* hypertonia, dysarthria, asthenia, ***neuroleptic malignant syndrome, seizures.***
**CV:** orthostatic hypotension, tachycardia, palpitations, peripheral edema.
**EENT:** ear pain, pharyngitis, rhinitis.
**GI:** dry mouth, dyspepsia, abdominal pain, constipation, anorexia.
**Hematologic:** *leukopenia.*
**Metabolic:** *weight gain.*
**Musculoskeletal:** back pain.
**Respiratory:** increased cough, dyspnea.
**Skin:** rash, diaphoresis.
**Other:** flulike syndrome.

## INTERACTIONS
**Drug-drug.** *Antihypertensives:* May increase effects of antihypertensives. Monitor blood pressure.
*Carbamazepine, glucocorticoids, phenobarbital, phenytoin, rifampin, thioridazine:* May increase quetiapine clearance. Adjust quetiapine dosage, as directed.
*CNS depressants:* May increase CNS effects. Use together cautiously.
*Dopamine agonists, levodopa:* May antagonize the effects of these drugs. Monitor patient.
*Erythromycin, fluconazole, itraconazole, ketoconazole:* May decrease quetiapine clearance. Use together cautiously.
*Lorazepam:* May decrease lorazepam clearance. Monitor patient for increased CNS effects.
**Drug-lifestyle.** *Alcohol use:* May increase CNS effects. Discourage use together.

## EFFECTS ON LAB TEST RESULTS
• May increase liver enzyme, cholesterol, and triglyceride levels. May decrease T$_4$ and thyroid-stimulating hormone levels.
• May decrease WBC count.

## CONTRAINDICATIONS & CAUTIONS
• Contraindicated in patients hypersensitive to drug or its ingredients.
• Use cautiously in patients with CV disease, cerebrovascular disease, conditions that predispose to hypotension, a history of seizures or conditions that lower the seizure threshold, and conditions in which core body temperature may be elevated.
• Use cautiously in patients at risk for aspiration pneumonia.

## NURSING CONSIDERATIONS
• Dispense lowest appropriate quantity of drug to reduce risk of overdose.
• *Alert:* Watch for evidence of neuroleptic malignant syndrome (extrapyramidal effects, hyperthermia, autonomic disturbance), which is rare but commonly fatal. It may not be related to length of drug use or type of neuroleptic; more than 60% of affected patients are men.
• Monitor patient for tardive dyskinesia, which may occur after prolonged use. It may not appear until months or years later and may disappear spontaneously or persist for life, despite ending drug.
• Monitor patient for weight gain.
• Drug use may cause cataract formation. Obtain baseline ophthalmologic examination and reassess every 6 months.
• *Alert:* Don't confuse Seroquel with Serzone.

## PATIENT TEACHING
• Advise patient about risk of dizziness upon standing up quickly. The risk is greatest during the 3- to 5-day period of first dosage adjustment, when resuming treatment, and when increasing dosages.
• Tell patient to avoid becoming overheated or dehydrated.
• Warn patient to avoid activities that require mental alertness until effects of drug are known, especially during first dosage adjustment or dosage increases.
• Remind patient to have an eye examination at start of therapy and every 6 months during therapy to check for cataracts.
• Tell patient to notify prescriber about other prescription or over-the-counter drugs he's taking or plans to take.
• Tell woman to notify prescriber about planned, suspected, or known pregnancy.

---

Advise her not to breast-feed during therapy.
● Advise patient to avoid alcohol while taking drug.
● Tell patient to take drug with or without food.

---

## risperidone
Risperdal✒, Risperdal M-Tab✒

*Pregnancy risk category C*

---

### AVAILABLE FORMS
*Solution:* 1 mg/ml
*Tablets:* 0.25 mg, 0.5 mg, 1 mg, 2 mg, 3 mg, 4 mg
*Orally disintegrating tablets:* 0.5 mg, 1 mg, 2 mg

### INDICATIONS & DOSAGES
➤ **Short-term (6 to 8 weeks) treatment of schizophrenia**
*Adults:* Initially, 1 mg P.O. b.i.d. Increase by 1 mg b.i.d. on days 2 and 3 of treatment to a target dose of 3 mg b.i.d. Or, 1 mg P.O. on day 1, increase to 2 mg once daily on day 2, and 4 mg once daily on day 3. Wait at least 1 week before adjusting dosage further. Adjust doses by 1 to 2 mg. Maximum, 8 mg/day.
➤ **To delay relapse in long-term (1 to 2 years) treatment of schizophrenia**
*Adults:* Initially, 1 mg P.O. on day 1, increase to 2 mg once daily on day 2, and 4 mg once daily on day 3. Dosage range is 2 to 8 mg daily.
*Adjust-a-dose:* In elderly or debilitated patients, hypotensive patients, or those with severe renal or hepatic impairment, start with 0.5 mg P.O. b.i.d. Increase dosage by 0.5 mg b.i.d. Increase in dosages above 1.5 mg b.i.d. should occur at intervals of at least 1 week. Subsequent switches to once-daily dosing may be made after patient is on a twice-daily regimen for 2 to 3 days at the target dose.

### ACTION
Blocks dopamine and 5-HT$_2$ receptors in the brain.

| Route | Onset | Peak | Duration |
|-------|-------|------|----------|
| P.O. | Unknown | 1 hr | Unknown |

### ADVERSE REACTIONS
**CNS:** fever, somnolence, *extrapyramidal reactions,* **suicide attempt,** headache, insomnia, agitation, anxiety, **stroke or transient ischemic attack (TIA) in elderly patients with dementia,** tardive dyskinesia, aggressiveness, **neuroleptic malignant syndrome.**
**CV:** tachycardia, chest pain, orthostatic hypotension, *prolonged QT interval.*
**EENT:** *rhinitis,* sinusitis, pharyngitis, abnormal vision.
**GI:** *constipation, nausea, vomiting, dyspepsia.*
**GU:** diminished sexual desire, erectile dysfunction, ejaculatory dysfunction, orgastic dysfunction.
**Metabolic:** weight gain.
**Musculoskeletal:** arthralgia, back pain.
**Respiratory:** coughing, upper respiratory tract infection.
**Skin:** rash, dry skin, photosensitivity reactions.

### INTERACTIONS
**Drug-drug.** *Antihypertensives:* May enhance hypotensive effects. Monitor blood pressure.
*Carbamazepine:* May increase risperidone clearance and decreases effectiveness. Monitor patient closely.
*Clozapine:* May decrease risperidone clearance, increasing toxicity. Monitor patient closely.
*CNS depressants:* Causes additive CNS depression. Use together cautiously.
*Dopamine agonists, levodopa:* May antagonize effects of these drugs. Use together cautiously and monitor patient.
**Drug-lifestyle.** *Alcohol use:* Causes additive CNS depression. Discourage use together.
*Sun exposure:* May increase risk of photosensitivity reactions. Advise patient to avoid excessive sunlight exposure.

### EFFECTS ON LAB TEST RESULTS
● May increase prolactin level.

### CONTRAINDICATIONS & CAUTIONS
● Contraindicated in patients hypersensitive to drug and in breast-feeding women.
● Use cautiously in patients with prolonged QT interval, CV disease, cerebrovascular disease, dehydration, hypo-

---

volemia, history of seizures, or conditions that could affect metabolism or hemodynamic responses.
• Use cautiously in patients exposed to extreme heat.
• Use caution in patients at risk for aspiration pneumonia.

**NURSING CONSIDERATIONS**
• *Alert:* Obtain baseline blood pressure measurements before starting therapy, and monitor pressure regularly. Watch for orthostatic hypotension, especially during first dosage adjustment.
• Cerebrovascular adverse events (stroke, TIA), including fatalities, may occur in elderly patients with dementia. Risperidone isn't safe or effective in these patients.
• Phenylalanine contents of orally disintegrating tablets are as follows: 0.5-mg tablet contains 0.14 mg phenylalanine; 1-mg tablet contains 0.28 mg phenylalanine; 2-mg tablet contains 0.56 mg phenylalanine.
• Monitor patient for tardive dyskinesia, which may occur after prolonged use. It may not appear until months or years later and may disappear spontaneously or persist for life, despite ending drug.
• Monitor patient for weight gain.
• Dosages above 6 mg/day may be no more effective than lower doses and may cause more extrapyramidal reactions. Safety of dosages above 16 mg/day hasn't been evaluated.
• *Alert:* Watch for evidence of neuroleptic malignant syndrome (extrapyramidal effects, hyperthermia, autonomic disturbance), which is rare but commonly fatal. It may not be related to length of drug use or type of neuroleptic; more than 60% of patients are men.
• *Alert:* Don't confuse risperidone with reserpine.

**PATIENT TEACHING**
• Warn patient to avoid activities that require alertness until effects of drug are known.
• Warn patient to rise slowly, avoid hot showers, and use extra caution during first few days of therapy to avoid fainting.
• Advise patient to use caution in hot weather to prevent heatstroke.

• Tell patient to take drug with or without food.
• Instruct patient to release the orally disintegrating tablets from their blister pack just before taking them.
• Advise patient to open the pack and dissolve orally disintegrating tablet on tongue; tell him not to split or chew tablet.
• Tell patient to use sunblock and wear protective clothing outdoors.
• Advise woman to notify prescriber if she is or plans to become pregnant during therapy.

**thioridazine hydrochloride**
Aldazine‡, Apo-Thioridazine†, Mellaril*, Mellaril Concentrate, Novo-Ridazine†, PMS Thioridazine†

*Pregnancy risk category C*

**AVAILABLE FORMS**
*Oral concentrate:* 30 mg/ml, 100 mg/ml (3% to 4.2% alcohol)
*Oral suspension:* 25 mg/5 ml, 100 mg/5 ml
*Tablets:* 10 mg, 15 mg, 25 mg, 50 mg, 100 mg, 150 mg, 200 mg

**INDICATIONS & DOSAGES**
➤ **Schizophrenia in patients who don't respond to treatment with other antipsychotic drugs**
*Adults:* Initially, 50 to 100 mg P.O. t.i.d., increased gradually to 800 mg daily in divided doses, if needed. Dosage varies.
*Children:* Initially, 0.5 mg/kg daily in divided doses. Increase gradually to optimum therapeutic effect; maximum dose is 3 mg/kg daily.

**ACTION**
Unknown. A piperidine phenothiazine that probably blocks postsynaptic dopamine receptors in the brain.

| Route | Onset | Peak | Duration |
|-------|-------|------|----------|
| P.O. | Unknown | Unknown | Unknown |

**ADVERSE REACTIONS**
**CNS:** *tardive dyskinesia, sedation,* EEG changes, dizziness, ***neuroleptic malignant syndrome.***

**CV:** *orthostatic hypotension,* tachycardia, *prolonged QTc interval, torsades de pointes,* ECG changes.
**EENT:** *ocular changes, blurred vision,* retinitis pigmentosa.
**GI:** *dry mouth, constipation,* increased appetite.
**GU:** *urine retention,* dark urine, menstrual irregularities, inhibited ejaculation.
**Hematologic:** *transient leukopenia, agranulocytosis,* hyperprolactinemia.
**Hepatic:** cholestatic jaundice.
**Metabolic:** weight gain.
**Skin:** *mild photosensitivity reactions,* allergic reactions.
**Other:** gynecomastia, galactorrhea.

## INTERACTIONS
**Drug-drug.** *Antacids:* May inhibit absorption of oral phenothiazines. Separate antacid and phenothiazine doses by at least 2 hours.
*Barbiturates:* May decrease phenothiazine effect. Monitor patient.
*Centrally acting antihypertensives:* May decrease antihypertensive effect. Monitor blood pressure.
*Fluoxetine, fluvoxamine, pindolol, propranolol; other drugs that inhibit cytochrome P-450 2D6 enzyme; drugs that prolong QTc interval (disopyramide, procainamide, quinidine):* May inhibit metabolism of thioridazine; may cause arrhythmias resulting from QTc interval prolongation. Avoid using together.
*Lithium:* May decrease phenothiazine effect and increase neurologic adverse effects. Monitor patient closely.
*Other CNS depressants:* May increase CNS depression. Use together cautiously.
**Drug-herb.** *St. John's wort:* May cause photosensitivity reactions. Advise patient to avoid excessive sunlight exposure.
**Drug-lifestyle.** *Alcohol use:* May increase CNS depression, particularly psychomotor skills. Strongly discourage alcohol use.
*Sun exposure:* May increase risk of photosensitivity reactions. Advise patient to avoid excessive sunlight exposure.

## EFFECTS ON LAB TEST RESULTS
● May increase liver enzyme levels.
● May decrease granulocyte and WBC counts.

● May cause false-positive results for urinary porphyrin, urobilinogen, amylase, and 5-hydroxyindoleacetic acid tests and for urine pregnancy tests that use human chorionic gonadotropin.

## CONTRAINDICATIONS & CAUTIONS
● Contraindicated in patients hypersensitive to drug and in those with CNS depression, coma, or severe hypertensive or hypotensive cardiac disease.
● Contraindicated with fluvoxamine, propranolol, pindolol, fluoxetine, drugs that inhibit the cytochrome P-450 2D6 enzyme, and drugs that prolong the QTc interval.
● Contraindicated in patients with reduced levels of cytochrome P-450 2D6 enzyme, patients with congenital long QT interval syndrome, or patients with a history of cardiac arrhythmias.
● Use cautiously in elderly or debilitated patients and in patients with hepatic disease, CV disease, respiratory disorders, hypocalcemia, seizure disorders, or severe reactions to insulin or electroconvulsive therapy.
● Use cautiously in those exposed to extreme heat or cold (including antipyretic therapy) or organophosphate insecticides.

## NURSING CONSIDERATIONS
● *Alert:* Before starting treatment, obtain baseline ECG and potassium level. Patients with a QTc interval greater than 450 msec shouldn't receive Mellaril. Patients with a QTc interval greater than 500 msec should stop drug.
● *Alert:* Drug isn't used in first treatment of schizophrenia.
● *Alert:* Different liquid formulations have different concentrations. Check dosage carefully.
● Prevent contact dermatitis by keeping drug away from skin and clothes. Wear gloves when preparing liquid forms.
● Dilute liquid concentrate with water or fruit juice just before giving.
● Shake suspension well before using.
● Monitor patient for tardive dyskinesia, which may occur after prolonged use. It may not appear until months or years later and may disappear spontaneously or persist for life, despite ending drug.

---

Reactions may be *common,* uncommon, *life-threatening,* or COMMON AND LIFE-THREATENING.

- *Alert:* Watch for evidence of neuroleptic malignant syndrome (extrapyramidal effects, hyperthermia, autonomic disturbance), which is rare but commonly fatal. It may not be related to length of drug use or type of neuroleptic; more than 60% of patients are men.
- Monitor therapy with weekly bilirubin tests during first month, periodic blood tests (CBCs and liver function tests), and ophthalmic tests (long-term use).
- Withhold dose and notify prescriber if jaundice, blood dyscrasia (fever, sore throat, infection, cellulitis, weakness), or persistent extrapyramidal reactions develop, especially in children or pregnant women.
- Don't stop drug abruptly unless required by severe adverse reactions.
- After abrupt withdrawal of long-term therapy, gastritis, nausea, vomiting, dizziness, tremor, feeling of warmth or cold, diaphoresis, tachycardia, headache, or insomnia may occur.
- *Alert:* Don't confuse thioridazine with Thorazine or Mellaril with Elavil.

**PATIENT TEACHING**
- Tell patient to shake suspension before use.
- Warn patient to avoid activities that require alertness until effects of drug are known.
- Tell patient to watch for dizziness when standing quickly. Advise patient to change positions slowly.
- Instruct patient to report symptoms of dizziness, palpitations, or fainting to prescriber.
- Tell patient to avoid alcohol use.
- Have patient report signs of urine retention, constipation, or blurred vision.
- Tell patient that drug may discolor the urine.
- Advise patient to relieve dry mouth with sugarless gum or hard candy.
- Instruct patient to use sunblock and to wear protective clothing outdoors.

# thiothixene
Navane

# thiothixene hydrochloride
Navane*

*Pregnancy risk category C*

**AVAILABLE FORMS**
**thiothixene**
*Capsules:* 1 mg, 2 mg, 5 mg, 10 mg, 20 mg
**thiothixene hydrochloride**
*Injection:* 2 mg/ml, 5 mg/ml
*Oral concentrate:* 5 mg/ml*

**INDICATIONS & DOSAGES**
➤ **Mild to moderate psychosis**
*Adults:* Initially, 2 mg P.O. t.i.d. Increased gradually to 15 mg daily, p.r.n.
➤ **Severe psychosis**
*Adults:* Initially, 5 mg P.O. b.i.d. Increase gradually to 20 to 30 mg daily, p.r.n. Maximum dose is 60 mg daily. Or, 4 mg I.M. b.i.d. to q.i.d. Maximum, 30 mg I.M. daily. Switch to oral form as soon as possible.

**ACTION**
Unknown. A thioxanthene that probably blocks dopamine receptors in the brain.

| Route | Onset | Peak | Duration |
|---|---|---|---|
| P.O., I.M. | Unknown | Unknown | Unknown |

**ADVERSE REACTIONS**
**CNS:** *extrapyramidal reactions, drowsiness,* restlessness, agitation, insomnia, *tardive dyskinesia,* sedation, EEG changes, pseudoparkinsonism, dizziness, *neuroleptic malignant syndrome.*
**CV:** *hypotension,* tachycardia, ECG changes.
**EENT:** ocular changes, *blurred vision,* nasal congestion.
**GI:** *dry mouth, constipation.*
**GU:** *urine retention,* menstrual irregularities, inhibited ejaculation.
**Hematologic:** *transient leukopenia,* leukocytosis, *agranulocytosis.*
**Hepatic:** jaundice.
**Metabolic:** weight gain.

**Skin:** *mild photosensitivity reactions,* allergic reactions, pain at I.M. injection site, sterile abscess, exfoliative dermatitis.
**Other:** gynecomastia.

## INTERACTIONS
**Drug-drug.** *CNS depressants:* May increase CNS depression. Use together cautiously.
**Drug-lifestyle.** *Alcohol use:* May increase CNS depression. Discourage use together. *Sun exposure:* May increase risk of photosensitivity reactions. Advise patient to avoid excessive sunlight exposure.

## EFFECTS ON LAB TEST RESULTS
• May increase liver enzyme levels.
• May decrease WBC and granulocyte counts.
• May cause false-positive results for urinary porphyrin, urobilinogen, amylase, and 5-hydroxyindoleacetic acid tests and for urine pregnancy tests that use human chorionic gonadotropin.

## CONTRAINDICATIONS & CAUTIONS
• Contraindicated in patients hypersensitive to drug and in those with CNS depression, circulatory collapse, coma, or blood dyscrasia.
• Use with extreme caution in patients with history of seizure disorder and in those undergoing alcohol withdrawal.
• Use cautiously in elderly or debilitated patients and in those with CV disease (may cause sudden drop in blood pressure), hepatic disease, heat exposure, glaucoma, or prostatic hyperplasia.

## NURSING CONSIDERATIONS
• Prevent contact dermatitis by keeping drug off skin and clothes. Wear gloves when preparing liquid forms.
• Dilute liquid concentrate with fruit juice, milk, or semisolid food just before giving.
• Slight yellowing of injection or concentrate is common and doesn't affect potency. Discard markedly discolored solutions.
• Give I.M. only in upper outer quadrant of buttocks or midlateral thigh. Massage slowly afterward to prevent sterile abscess. Injection may sting.
• Monitor patient for tardive dyskinesia, which may occur after prolonged use; it may not appear until months or years later,

and may disappear spontaneously or persist for life, despite stopping drug.
• *Alert:* Watch for evidence of neuroleptic malignant syndrome (extrapyramidal effects, hyperthermia, autonomic disturbance), which is rare but commonly fatal. It may not be related to length of drug use or type of neuroleptic; more than 60% of patients are men.
• Monitor therapy with weekly bilirubin tests during first month; with periodic CBCs, liver function tests, and renal function tests; and with ophthalmic tests for long-term use.
• Watch for orthostatic hypotension, especially with parenteral administration. Keep patient supine for 1 hour after drug administration, and tell him to change positions slowly.
• Withhold dose and notify prescriber if jaundice, blood dyscrasia (fever, sore throat, infection, cellulitis, weakness), or persistent extrapyramidal reactions develop, especially in pregnant women.
• Don't withdraw drug abruptly unless severe adverse reactions occur.
• After abrupt withdrawal of long-term therapy, gastritis, nausea, vomiting, dizziness, tremor, feeling of warmth or cold, diaphoresis, tachycardia, headache, or insomnia may occur.
• *Alert:* Don't confuse Navane with Nubain or Norvasc.

## PATIENT TEACHING
• Warn patient to avoid activities that require alertness until effects of drug are known.
• Tell patient to watch for dizziness upon standing quickly. Advise him to change positions slowly.
• Instruct patient to dilute liquid appropriately.
• Tell patient to avoid alcohol use during therapy.
• Have patient report signs of urine retention, constipation, or blurred vision.
• Instruct patient to use sunblock and to wear protective clothing outdoors.

---

# trifluoperazine hydrochloride
Apo-Trifluoperazine†, Novo-
Trifluzine†, PMS Trifluoperazine†,
Stelazine, Stelazine Concentrate

*Pregnancy risk category NR*

## AVAILABLE FORMS
*Injection:* 2 mg/ml
*Oral concentrate:* 10 mg/ml
*Tablets (regular and film-coated):* 1 mg,
2 mg, 5 mg, 10 mg

## INDICATIONS & DOSAGES
➤ **Anxiety states**
*Adults:* 1 to 2 mg P.O. b.i.d. Maximum,
6 mg daily. Don't give drug for longer
than 12 weeks for this indication.
➤ **Schizophrenia, other psychotic
disorders**
*Adults:* 2 to 5 mg P.O. b.i.d., gradually increased until therapeutic response occurs.
Or, 1 to 2 mg deeply I.M. q 4 to 6 hours,
p.r.n. Most patients respond to 15 to
20 mg P.O. daily, although some may need
40 mg/day or more. More than 6 mg I.M.
in 24 hours is rarely needed.
*Children ages 6 to 12:* 1 mg P.O. daily or
b.i.d.; may increase gradually to 15 mg
daily, if needed.

## ACTION
Unknown. A piperazine phenothiazine
that probably blocks dopamine receptors
in the brain.

| Route | Onset | Peak | Duration |
|---|---|---|---|
| P.O., I.M. | Unknown | Unknown | Unknown |

## ADVERSE REACTIONS
**CNS:** *extrapyramidal reactions, tardive
dyskinesia,* pseudoparkinsonism, dizzi-
ness, drowsiness, insomnia, fatigue, head-
ache, **neuroleptic malignant syndrome.**
**CV:** *orthostatic hypotension,* tachycardia,
ECG changes.
**EENT:** ocular changes, *blurred vision.*
**GI:** *dry mouth, constipation,* nausea.
**GU:** *urine retention,* menstrual irregulari-
ties, inhibited ejaculation.
**Hematologic:** *transient leukopenia,
agranulocytosis.*
**Hepatic:** cholestatic jaundice.
**Metabolic:** weight gain.

**Skin:** *photosensitivity reactions,* allergic
reactions, pain at I.M. injection site, sterile
abscess, rash.
**Other:** gynecomastia.

## INTERACTIONS
**Drug-drug.** *Antacids:* May inhibit absorption of oral phenothiazines. Separate
antacid and phenothiazine doses by at
least 2 hours.
*Barbiturates, lithium:* May decrease phenothiazine effect. Monitor patient.
*Centrally acting antihypertensives:* May
decrease antihypertensive effect. Monitor
blood pressure.
*CNS depressants:* May increase CNS depression. Use together cautiously.
*Propranolol:* May increase propranolol
and trifluoperazine levels. Monitor patient.
*Warfarin:* May decrease effect of oral anticoagulants. Monitor PT and INR.
**Drug-herb.** *St. John's wort:* May cause
photosensitivity reactions. Advise patient
to avoid excessive sunlight exposure.
**Drug-lifestyle.** *Alcohol use:* May increase
CNS depression, particularly psychomotor
skills. Strongly discourage alcohol use.
*Sun exposure:* May increase risk of photosensitivity reactions. Advise patient to
avoid excessive sunlight exposure.

## EFFECTS ON LAB TEST RESULTS
• May increase liver enzyme levels.
• May decrease WBC and granulocyte
counts.
• May cause false-positive results for urinary porphyrin, urobilinogen, amylase,
and 5-hydroxyindoleacetic acid tests and
for urine pregnancy tests that use human
chorionic gonadotropin.

## CONTRAINDICATIONS & CAUTIONS
• Contraindicated in patients hypersensitive to phenothiazines and in those with
CNS depression, coma, bone marrow suppression, or liver damage.
• Use cautiously in elderly or debilitated
patients and in patients with CV disease
(may decrease blood pressure), seizure
disorder, glaucoma, or prostatic hyperplasia; also, use cautiously in those exposed
to extreme heat.
• Reserve use in children for those who
are hospitalized or under close supervision.

## NURSING CONSIDERATIONS
● Wear gloves when preparing liquid forms.
● Dilute liquid concentrate with 60 ml of tomato or fruit juice, carbonated beverage, coffee, tea, milk, water, or semisolid food just before giving.
● Protect drug from light. Slight yellowing of injection or concentrate is common and doesn't affect potency. Discard markedly discolored solutions.
● Give deeply I.M. only in upper outer quadrant of buttocks. Massage slowly afterward to prevent sterile abscess. Injection may sting.
● Watch for orthostatic hypotension, especially with parenteral administration. Keep patient supine for 1 hour after giving drug, and tell him to change positions slowly.
● Monitor patient for tardive dyskinesia, which may occur after prolonged use. It may not appear until months or years later and may disappear spontaneously or persist for life, despite ending drug.
● *Alert:* Watch for evidence of neuroleptic malignant syndrome (extrapyramidal effects, hyperthermia, autonomic disturbance), which is rare but commonly fatal. It may not be related to length of drug use or type of neuroleptic; more than 60% of patients are men.
● Monitor therapy with weekly bilirubin tests during first month, periodic blood tests (CBCs and liver function tests), and ophthalmic tests (long-term use).
● Withhold dose and notify prescriber if jaundice, signs and symptoms of blood dyscrasia (fever, sore throat, infection, cellulitis, weakness), or persistent extrapyramidal reactions (longer than a few hours) develop, especially in children or pregnant women.
● Don't withdraw drug abruptly unless severe adverse reactions occur.
● After abrupt withdrawal of long-term therapy, gastritis, nausea, vomiting, dizziness, tremor, feeling of warmth or cold, diaphoresis, tachycardia, headache, insomnia, anorexia, muscle rigidity, altered mental status, or evidence of autonomic instability may occur.
● *Alert:* Don't confuse trifluoperazine with triflupromazine.

## PATIENT TEACHING
● Warn patient to avoid activities that require alertness until effects of drug are known.
● Tell patient to avoid alcohol while taking drug.
● Instruct patient to properly dilute liquid.
● Tell patient to report signs of urine retention or constipation.
● Tell patient to use sunblock and to wear protective clothing outdoors.
● Advise patient to relieve dry mouth with sugarless gum or hard candy.

## ziprasidone
Geodon

*Pregnancy risk category C*

### AVAILABLE FORMS
*Capsules:* 20 mg, 40 mg, 60 mg, 80 mg
*I.M. injection:* 20 mg/ml single-dose vials (after reconstitution)

### INDICATIONS & DOSAGES
➤ **Symptomatic treatment of schizophrenia**
*Adults:* Initially, 20 mg b.i.d. with food. Dosages are highly individualized. Adjust dosage, if necessary, no more frequently than q 2 days; to allow for lowest possible doses, the interval should be several weeks to assess symptom response. Effective dosage range is usually 20 to 80 mg b.i.d. Maximum dosage is 100 mg b.i.d.
➤ **Rapid control of acute agitation in schizophrenic patients**
*Adults:* 10 to 20 mg I.M. p.r.n., up to a maximum dosage of 40 mg daily. Doses of 10 mg may be given q 2 hours; doses of 20 mg may be given q 4 hours.

### ACTION
May inhibit dopamine and serotonin-2 receptors, causing reduction in schizophrenia symptoms.

| Route | Onset | Peak | Duration |
|-------|-------|------|----------|
| P.O. | 1-3 days | 6-8 hr | 12 hr |
| I.M. | Unknown | 1 hr | Unknown |

### ADVERSE REACTIONS
**CNS:** *somnolence,* akathisia, dizziness, extrapyramidal symptoms, hypertonia, as-

---

thenia; dystonia (P.O.); *headache, dizziness,* anxiety, **suicide attempt,** insomnia, agitation, cogwheel rigidity, paresthesia, personality disorder, psychosis, speech disorder (I.M.).
**CV:** orthostatic hypotension, *QT interval prolongation;* tachycardia (P.O.); hypertension, **bradycardia,** vasodilation (I.M.).
**EENT:** rhinitis; abnormal vision (P.O.).
**GI:** *nausea,* constipation, dyspepsia, diarrhea, dry mouth, anorexia; abdominal pain, rectal hemorrhage, vomiting, dyspepsia, tooth disorder (I.M.).
**GU:** dysmenorrhea, priapism (I.M.).
**Musculoskeletal:** myalgia (P.O.); back pain (I.M.)
**Respiratory:** cough (P.O.).
**Skin:** rash (P.O.); injection site pain, furunculosis, sweating (I.M.).
**Other:** flulike syndrome (I.M.).

## INTERACTIONS
**Drug-drug.** *Antihypertensives:* may enhance hypotensive effects. Monitor blood pressure.
*Carbamazepine:* May decrease ziprasidone level. May need to increase ziprasidone dose to achieve desired effect.
*Drugs that decrease potassium or magnesium, such as diuretics:* May increase risk of arrhythmias. Monitor potassium and magnesium levels if using these drugs together.
*Drugs that prolong QT interval, such as dofetilide, moxifloxacin, pimozide, quinidine, sotalol, sparfloxacin, thioridazine:* May increase risk of arrhythmias. Avoid using together.
*Itraconazole, ketoconazole:* May increase ziprasidone level. May need to reduce ziprasidone dose to achieve desired effect.

## EFFECTS ON LAB TEST RESULTS
None reported.

## CONTRAINDICATIONS & CAUTIONS
● Contraindicated in patients hypersensitive to drug and in those with recent MI or uncompensated heart failure.
● Contraindicated in those with history of prolonged QT interval or congenital long QT interval syndrome and in those taking other drugs that prolong QT interval, such as dofetilide, sotalol, quinidine, other class Ia and III antiarrhythmics, mesoridazine,

thioridazine, chlorpromazine, droperidol, pimozide, sparfloxacin, gatifloxacin, moxifloxacin, halofantrine, mefloquine, pentamidine, arsenic trioxide, levomethadyl acetate, dolasetron mesylate, probucol, and tacrolimus.
**P.O.**
● Contraindicated in patients with a history of QT interval prolongation or congenital QT syndrome and in those taking other drugs that prolong QT interval.
● Use cautiously in patients with history of seizures, bradycardia, hypokalemia, or hypomagnesemia; in those with acute diarrhea; and in those with conditions that may lower the seizure threshold (such as Alzheimer's dementia).
● Use cautiously in patients at risk for aspiration pneumonia.
**I.M.**
● Contraindicated in schizophrenic patients already taking P.O. ziprasidone.
● Use cautiously in elderly patients and in those with hepatic or renal impairment.

## NURSING CONSIDERATIONS
**P.O.**
● Stop drug in patients with a QTc interval more than 500 msec.
● Dizziness, palpitations, or syncope may be symptoms of a life-threatening arrhythmia such as torsades de pointes. Further CV evaluation and monitoring are needed in patients who experience these symptoms.
● Don't give to patients experiencing electrolyte disturbances, such as hypokalemia or hypomagnesemia, because these increase the risk of developing an arrhythmia.
● Patient taking an antipsychotic is at risk for developing neuroleptic malignant syndrome or tardive dyskinesia. Hyperpyrexia, muscle rigidity, altered mental status, and autonomic instability are signs and symptoms of neuroleptic malignant syndrome, which can be fatal. Assess abnormal involuntary movement before starting therapy, at dosage changes, and periodically thereafter, to monitor patient for tardive dyskinesia.
● Monitor patient for abnormal body temperature regulation, especially if patient is exercising strenuously, exposed to extreme

heat, receiving concomitant anticholinergics, or being subject to dehydration.
● Symptoms may not improve for 4 to 6
weeks.
● Always give drug with food for optimal
effect.
● Don't use drug in breast-feeding patients.

**I.M.**
● To prepare I.M. ziprasidone, add 1.2 ml
of sterile water for injection to the vial and
shake vigorously until all the drug is dissolved.
● Don't mix injection with other medicinal
products or solvents other than sterile
water for injection.
● Inspect parenteral drug products visually
for particulate matter and discoloration
before administration, whenever solution
and container permit.
● The effects of giving I.M. ziprasidone
for more than 3 consecutive days haven't
been studied. If long-term therapy of
ziprasidone is indicated, switch to P.O. as
soon as possible.
● Store injection at controlled room temperature, 15° to 30° C (59° to 86° F) in
dry form, and protect from light. After reconstituting the drug, it may be stored
away from light for up to 24 hours at 15°
to 30° C (59° to 86° F) or up to 7 days refrigerated, 2° to 8° C (36° to 46° F).

**PATIENT TEACHING**
● Tell patient to take drug with food.
● Tell patient to immediately report to prescriber signs or symptoms of dizziness,
fainting, irregular heartbeat, or relevant
heart problems.
● Advise patient to report any recent
episodes of diarrhea, abnormal movements, sudden fever, muscle rigidity, or
change in mental status.
● Advise patient that symptoms may not
improve for 4 to 6 weeks.

**dexmethylphenidate
  hydrochloride**
**dextroamphetamine sulfate**
**doxapram hydrochloride**
**methylphenidate hydrochloride**
**modafinil**
**pemoline**
**phentermine hydrochloride**

### COMBINATION PRODUCTS
ADDERALL 5 MG, ADDERALL XR 5 MG:
amphetamine aspartate 1.25 mg, amphetamine sulfate 1.25 mg, dextroamphetamine
saccharate 1.25 mg, dextroamphetamine
sulfate 1.25 mg, total amphetamine base
equivalence 3.13 mg.
ADDERALL 10 MG, ADDERALL XR 10 MG:
amphetamine aspartate 2.5 mg, amphetamine sulfate 2.5 mg, dextroamphetamine
saccharate 2.5 mg, dextroamphetamine
sulfate 2.5 mg, total amphetamine base
equivalence 6.3 mg.
ADDERALL 15 MG, ADDERALL XR 15 MG:
amphetamine aspartate 3.75 mg, amphetamine sulfate 3.75 mg, dextroamphetamine
sulfate 3.75 mg, total amphetamine base
equivalence 9.4 mg.
ADDERALL 20 MG, ADDERALL XR 20 MG:
amphetamine aspartate 5 mg, amphetamine sulfate 5 mg, dextroamphetamine
saccharate 5 mg, dextroamphetamine sulfate 5 mg, total amphetamine base equivalence 12.5 mg.
ADDERALL 30 MG, ADDERALL XR 30 MG:
amphetamine aspartate 7.5 mg, amphetamine sulfate 7.5 mg, dextroamphetamine
saccharate 7.5 mg, dextroamphetamine
sulfate 7.5 mg, total amphetamine base
equivalence 18.8 mg.
ADDERALL XR 7.5 MG: dextroamphetamine saccharate 1.875 mg, amphetamine
aspartate monohydrate 1.875 mg, dextroamphetamine sulfate USP 1.875 mg, amphetamine sulfate USP 1.875 mg.
ADDERALL XR 12.5 MG: dextroamphetamine saccharate 3.125 mg, amphetamine
aspartate monohydrate 3.125 mg, dextroamphetamine sulfate USP 3.125 mg,
amphetamine sulfate USP 3.125 mg. Total
amphetamine equivalence 12.5 mg.

ADDERALL XR 25 mg: dextroamphetamine saccharate 6.25 mg, amphetamine
aspartate monohydrate 6.25 mg, dextroamphetamine sulfate USP 6.25 mg, amphetamine sulfate USP 6.25 mg. Total amphetamine equivalence 15.6 mg.

## dexmethylphenidate hydrochloride
Focalin

*Pregnancy risk category C*
*Controlled substance schedule II*

### AVAILABLE FORMS
*Tablets:* 2.5 mg, 5 mg, 10 mg

### INDICATIONS & DOSAGES
➤ **Attention deficit hyperactivity disorder (ADHD)**
*Children ages 6 to 17:* For patients who
aren't currently taking methylphenidate,
initially, 2.5 mg P.O. b.i.d., given at least
4 hours apart. Make weekly increases of
2.5 to 5 mg daily, up to a maximum of
20 mg daily in divided doses.
  For patients who are currently taking
methylphenidate, initially, give half the
current methylphenidate dosage, up to a
maximum of 20 mg P.O. daily in divided
doses.

### ACTION
Blocks presynaptic reuptake of norepinephrine and dopamine and increases their
release, leading to an increased concentration in the synapse.

| Route | Onset | Peak | Duration |
|-------|-------|------|----------|
| P.O. | Unknown | 1-1½ hr | Unknown |

### ADVERSE REACTIONS
**CNS:** fever, insomnia, nervousness.
**CV:** tachycardia.
**GI:** anorexia, *abdominal pain,* nausea.
**Musculoskeletal:** twitching (motor or vo-
cal tics).
**Other:** hypersensitivity reactions.

## INTERACTIONS

**Drug-drug.** *Anticoagulants, phenobarbital, phenytoin, primidone, SSRIs, tricyclic antidepressants:* May inhibit metabolism of these drugs. May need to decrease dosage of these drugs; monitor drug levels.

*Antihypertensives:* May decrease effectiveness of these drugs. Use together cautiously; monitor blood pressure.

*Clonidine, other centrally acting alpha agonists:* May cause serious adverse effects. Use together cautiously.

*MAO inhibitors:* May cause risk of hypertensive crisis. Avoid using within 14 days of MAO inhibitor therapy.

## EFFECTS ON LAB TEST RESULTS

None reported.

## CONTRAINDICATIONS & CAUTIONS

● Contraindicated in patients hypersensitive to methylphenidate or other components.

● Contraindicated in patients with severe anxiety, tension, or agitation, glaucoma, and in those who have motor tics or a family history or diagnosis of Tourette syndrome.

● Contraindicated within 14 days of MAO inhibitor therapy.

● Use cautiously in patients with a history of drug abuse or alcoholism.

● Use cautiously in patients with psychosis, seizures, hypertension, hyperthyroidism, heart failure, or recent MI.

● Use in pregnant women only if the benefits outweigh the risks; drug may delay skeletal ossification, suppress weight gain, and impair organ development in the fetus.

● It's unknown if drug appears in breast milk. Use cautiously in breast-feeding women.

## NURSING CONSIDERATIONS

● Diagnosis of ADHD must be based on complete history and evaluation of the child by psychological and educational experts.

● Refer patient for psychological, educational, and social support during treatment.

● Periodically reevaluate the long-term usefulness of the drug.

● Stop treatment or reduce dosage if symptoms worsen or adverse reactions occur.

● Long-term stimulant use may temporarily suppress growth. Monitor children for growth and weight gain. Stop treatment if growth slows or if weight gain is lower than expected.

● Monitor blood pressure and pulse routinely.

● Monitor patient for signs of drug dependence or abuse.

● Stop treatment if seizures occur.

## PATIENT TEACHING

● Stress the importance of taking the correct dose of drug at the same time every day. Report accidental overdose immediately.

● Advise parents to monitor child for medication abuse or sharing.

● Advise parents to monitor child's height and weight and to tell the prescriber if they suspect growth is slowing.

● Advise patient to report blurred vision to the prescriber.

---

# dextroamphetamine sulfate
Dexedrine*, Dexedrine Spansule

*Pregnancy risk category C*
*Controlled substance schedule II*

---

## AVAILABLE FORMS

*Capsules (extended-release):* 5 mg, 10 mg, 15 mg
*Tablets:* 5 mg, 10 mg

## INDICATIONS & DOSAGES

➤ **Narcolepsy**

*Adults:* 5 to 60 mg P.O. daily in divided doses.

*Children ages 6 to 12:* 5 mg P.O. daily. Increase by 5 mg at weekly intervals p.r.n.

*Children age 12 and older:* 10 mg P.O. daily. Increase by 10 mg at weekly intervals, p.r.n. Give first dose on awakening; additional doses (one or two) given at intervals of 4 to 6 hours.

➤ **Attention deficit hyperactivity disorder (ADHD)**

*Children age 6 and older:* 5 mg P.O. once daily or b.i.d. Increase by 5 mg at weekly intervals, p.r.n. It is rarely necessary to exceed 40 mg/day.

---

*Children ages 3 to 5:* 2.5 mg P.O. daily. Increase by 2.5 mg at weekly intervals, p.r.n.
➤ **Short-term adjunct in exogenous obesity** ◆
*Adults and children age 12 and older:* 5 to 30 mg P.O. daily 30 to 60 minutes before meals in divided doses of 5 to 10 mg. Or, one 10- or 15-mg extended-release capsule daily as a single dose in the morning.

## ACTION
Unknown. Probably promotes nerve impulse transmission by releasing stored dopamine and norepinephrine from nerve terminals in the brain. Main sites of activity appear to be the cerebral cortex and the reticular activating system.

| Route | Onset | Peak | Duration |
|---|---|---|---|
| P.O. | 30-60 min | 2 hr | 4 hr |
| P.O. (extended) | 60 min | 2 hr | 8 hr |

## ADVERSE REACTIONS
**CNS:** *restlessness,* tremor, *insomnia,* dizziness, headache, chills, overstimulation, dysphoria, euphoria, *nervousness.*
**CV:** *tachycardia, palpitations,* hypertension, *arrhythmias.*
**GI:** dry mouth, taste perversion, diarrhea, constipation, anorexia, other GI disturbances.
**GU:** impotence.
**Metabolic:** weight loss.
**Skin:** urticaria.
**Other:** increased libido.

## INTERACTIONS
**Drug-drug.** *Acetazolamide, alkalizing drugs, antacids, sodium bicarbonate:* May increase renal reabsorption. Monitor patient for enhanced amphetamine effects.
*Acidifying drugs, ammonium chloride, ascorbic acid:* May decrease level and increase renal clearance of dextroamphetamine. Monitor patient for decreased amphetamine effects.
*Adrenergic blockers:* May inhibit adrenergic blocking effects. Avoid using together.
*Chlorpromazine:* May inhibit central stimulant effects of amphetamines. May use to treat amphetamine poisoning.
*Insulin, oral antidiabetics:* May decrease antidiabetic requirements. Monitor glucose level.

*MAO inhibitors:* May cause severe hypertension or hypertensive crisis. Avoid using within 14 days of MAO inhibitor therapy.
*Meperidine:* May potentiate analgesic effect. Use together cautiously.
*Methenamine:* May increase urinary excretion of amphetamines and reduce efficacy. Monitor drug effects.
*Norepinephrine:* May enhance adrenergic effect of norepinephrine. Monitor patient.
*Phenobarbital, phenytoin:* May delay absorption of these drugs. Monitor patient closely.
**Drug-food.** *Caffeine:* May increase amphetamine and related amine effects. Urge caution.

## EFFECTS ON LAB TEST RESULTS
• May increase corticosteroid level.

## CONTRAINDICATIONS & CAUTIONS
• Contraindicated in patients hypersensitive to or with idiosyncratic reactions to sympathomimetic amines, and in those with hyperthyroidism, moderate to severe hypertension, symptomatic CV disease, glaucoma, advanced arteriosclerosis, or history of drug abuse.
• Contraindicated within 14 days of MAO inhibitor therapy.
• Contraindicated as first-line treatment for obesity. Use as an anorexigenic is prohibited in some states.
• Use cautiously in agitated patients and patients with motor tics, phonic tics, or Tourette syndrome.

## NURSING CONSIDERATIONS
• Drug shouldn't be used to prevent fatigue.
• In children with ADHD, dextroamphetamine has a paradoxical calming effect.
• Patients with obesity should follow a weight-reduction program.
• Drug has a high abuse potential and may cause dependence.
• Certain formulations may contain tartrazine.
• *Alert:* Overdose may cause seizures.
• If tolerance to anorexigenic effect develops, stop drug and notify prescriber.
• *Alert:* Don't confuse Dexedrine with dextran or Excedrin.

## PATIENT TEACHING
• Tell patient to take drug 30 to 60 minutes before meals if used for weight reduction and at least 6 hours before bedtime to avoid sleep interference.
• Warn patient to avoid activities that require alertness or good coordination until CNS effects of drug are known.
• Tell patient he may get tired as drug effects wear off.
• Ask patient to report signs and symptoms of excessive stimulation.
• Advise patient to consume caffeine-containing products cautiously.
• Warn patient with seizure disorder that drug may decrease seizure threshold. Instruct him to notify prescriber if seizure occurs.

---

## doxapram hydrochloride
Dopram

*Pregnancy risk category B*

### AVAILABLE FORMS
*Injection:* 20 mg/ml (benzyl alcohol 0.9%)

### INDICATIONS & DOSAGES
➤ **Postanesthesia respiratory stimulation**
*Adults:* 0.5 to 1 mg/kg as a single I.V. injection (not to exceed 1.5 mg/kg) or as multiple injections q 5 minutes, total not to exceed 2 mg/kg. Or, 250 mg in 250 ml of normal saline solution or $D_5W$ infused at initial rate of 5 mg/minute I.V. until satisfactory response is achieved. Maintain at 1 to 3 mg/minute. Don't exceed total dose for infusion of 4 mg/kg.
➤ **Drug-induced CNS depression**
*Adults:* For injection, priming dosage of 2 mg/kg I.V., repeated in 5 minutes and again q 1 to 2 hours until patient awakens (and if relapse occurs). Maximum daily dosage is 3 g.
   For infusion, priming dosage of 2 mg/kg I.V., repeated in 5 minutes and again in 1 to 2 hours, if needed. If response occurs, give I.V. infusion (1 mg/ml) at 1 to 3 mg/minute until patient awakens. Don't infuse for longer than 2 hours or give more than 3 g/day. May resume I.V. infusion after

rest period of 30 minutes to 2 hours, if needed.
➤ **Chronic pulmonary disease related to acute hypercapnia**
*Adults:* 1 to 2 mg/minute by I.V. infusion using 2 mg/ml solution. Maximum, 3 mg/minute for up to 2 hours.

### I.V. ADMINISTRATION
• Doxapram is incompatible with strongly alkaline drugs, such as thiopental sodium, aminophylline, and sodium bicarbonate. Drug is compatible with $D_5W$, dextrose 10% in water, and normal saline solution.
• Give slowly; rapid infusion may cause hemolysis.
• Watch for irritation and infiltration; extravasation can cause tissue damage and necrosis.

### ACTION
Not clearly defined. Directly stimulates the central respiratory centers in the medulla and may indirectly act on carotid, aortic, or other peripheral chemoreceptors.

| Route | Onset | Peak | Duration |
|-------|-------|------|----------|
| I.V. | 20-40 sec | 1-2 min | 5-12 min |

### ADVERSE REACTIONS
**CNS:** *seizures,* headache, dizziness, apprehension, disorientation, hyperactivity, bilateral Babinski's signs, paresthesia.
**CV:** *chest pain and tightness, variations in heart rate, hypertension, arrhythmias,* T-wave depression on ECG, flushing.
**EENT:** sneezing, *laryngospasm.*
**GI:** nausea, vomiting, diarrhea.
**GU:** urine retention, bladder stimulation with incontinence, albuminuria.
**Musculoskeletal:** muscle spasms.
**Respiratory:** cough, *bronchospasm,* dyspnea, rebound hypoventilation, hiccups.
**Skin:** pruritus, diaphoresis.

### INTERACTIONS
**Drug-drug.** *General anesthetics:* May cause self-limiting arrhythmias. Avoid using doxapram within 10 minutes of an anesthetic that sensitizes the myocardium to catecholamines.
*MAO inhibitors, sympathomimetics:* May potentiate adverse CV effects. Use together cautiously.

---

Reactions may be *common,* uncommon, *life-threatening,* or COMMON AND LIFE-THREATENING.

## EFFECTS ON LAB TEST RESULTS
● May increase BUN level.
● May decrease hemoglobin, hematocrit, and erythrocyte, WBC, and RBC counts.

## CONTRAINDICATIONS & CAUTIONS
● Contraindicated in patients with seizure disorders; head injury; CV disorders; frank, uncompensated heart failure; severe hypertension; CVA; respiratory failure or incompetence secondary to neuromuscular disorders, muscle paresis, flail chest, obstructed airway, pulmonary embolism, pneumothorax, restrictive respiratory disease, acute bronchial asthma, or extreme dyspnea; or hypoxia not related to hypercapnia.
● Use cautiously in patients with bronchial asthma, severe tachycardia or arrhythmias, cerebral edema, increased intracranial pressure, hyperthyroidism, pheochromocytoma, or metabolic disorders.

## NURSING CONSIDERATIONS
● Drug is used only in surgical or emergency department situations.
● Separate end of anesthetic treatment and start of doxapram by at least 10 minutes.
● *Alert:* Establish an adequate airway before giving drug. Prevent patient from aspirating vomitus by placing him on his side.
● Monitor blood pressure, heart rate, deep tendon reflexes, and arterial blood gases before giving drug and every 30 minutes afterward.
● Monitor patient for evidence of overdose, such as hypertension, tachycardia, arrhythmias, skeletal muscle hyperactivity, and dyspnea. Hold drug and notify prescriber if patient needs mechanical ventilation or shows signs of increased arterial carbon dioxide or oxygen tension.
● *Alert:* Don't confuse doxapram with doxorubicin, doxepin, doxacurium, or doxazosin.

## PATIENT TEACHING
● Inform family and patient about need for drug.
● Answer patient's questions and address his concerns.

# methylphenidate hydrochloride
Concerta♦, Metadate CD, Metadate ER, Methylin, Methylin ER, Ritalin♦, Ritalin LA, Ritalin-SR♦

*Pregnancy risk category NR (C for Concerta, Metadate CD, Ritalin LA)*
*Controlled substance schedule II*

## AVAILABLE FORMS
*Tablets (Ritalin, Methylin):* 5 mg, 10 mg, 20 mg
*Oral solution (Methylin):* 5 mg/5 ml, 10 mg/5 ml
**Extended-release**
*Capsules (Metadate CD):* 20 mg
*Capsules (Ritalin LA):* 20 mg, 30 mg, 40 mg
*Tablets (Concerta):* 18 mg, 27, mg, 36 mg, 54 mg
*Tablets (Metadate ER, Methylin ER):* 10 mg, 20 mg
**Sustained-release**
*Tablets (Ritalin-SR):* 20 mg

## INDICATIONS & DOSAGES
➤ **Attention deficit hyperactivity disorder (ADHD)**
*Children age 6 and older:* Initially, 5 mg P.O. b.i.d. immediate-release form before breakfast and lunch, increasing by 5 to 10 mg at weekly intervals, p.r.n., until an optimum daily dosage of 2 mg/kg is reached, not to exceed 60 mg/day. To use Ritalin-SR, Metadate ER, and Methylin ER tablets in place of immediate-release methylphenidate tablets, calculate methylphenidate dosage in 8-hour intervals.
*Concerta*
*Children age 6 and older not currently taking methylphenidate or patients taking stimulants other than methylphenidate:* 18 mg P.O. (extended-release) once daily q morning. Adjust dosage by 18 mg at weekly intervals to a maximum of 54 mg/ day q morning.
*Children age 6 and older currently taking methylphenidate:* If previous methylphenidate dosage was 5 mg b.i.d. or t.i.d. or 20 mg sustained-release, give 18 mg P.O. q morning. If previous methylphenidate dosage was 10 mg b.i.d. or t.i.d. or 40 mg

sustained-release, give 36 mg P.O. q
morning. If previous methylphenidate
dosage was 15 mg b.i.d. or t.i.d. or 60 mg
sustained-release, give 54 mg P.O. q morning. Maximum daily dosage is 54 mg.
*Metadate CD*
*Children age 6 and older:* Initially, 20 mg
P.O. daily before breakfast, increasing by
20 mg at weekly intervals to a maximum
of 60 mg/day.
*Ritalin LA*
*Children age 6 and older:* 20 mg P.O. once
daily. Increase by 10 mg at weekly intervals to a maximum of 60 mg daily. If previous methylphenidate dosage was 10 mg
b.i.d. or 20 mg sustained-release, give
20 mg P.O. once daily. If previous methylphenidate dosage was 15 mg b.i.d., give
30 mg P.O. once daily. If previous methylphenidate dosage was 20 mg b.i.d. or
40 mg sustained-release, give 40 mg P.O.
once daily. If previous methylphenidate
dosage was 30 mg b.i.d. or 60 mg
sustained-release, give 60 mg P.O. once
daily.
➤ **Narcolepsy**
*Adults:* 10 mg P.O. b.i.d. or t.i.d.
immediate-release, 30 to 45 minutes
before meals. Dosage varies; average is
40 to 60 mg/day. To use Ritalin-SR, Metadate ER, or Methylin ER tablets in place
of immediate-release methylphenidate
tablets, calculate the dose of methylphenidate in 8-hour intervals.

## ACTION
Releases nerve terminal stores of norepinephrine, promoting nerve impulse transmission. At high doses, effects are mediated by dopamine.

| Route | Onset | Peak | Duration |
|---|---|---|---|
| P.O.<br>(Methylin,<br>Ritalin) | Unknown | 2 hr | Unknown |
| P.O.<br>(Methylin ER,<br>Ritalin-SR) | Unknown | 5 hr | 8 hr |
| P.O.<br>(Metadate<br>CD) | Unknown | 1½ hr and<br>4½ hr | Unknown |
| P.O.<br>(Ritalin LA) | Unknown | 1-3 hr and<br>4-7 hr | Unknown |
| P.O.<br>(Concerta) | Unknown | 6-8 hr | Unknown |

## ADVERSE REACTIONS
**CNS:** *nervousness, insomnia,* tics, dizziness, *headache,* akathisia, dyskinesia,
*seizures,* drowsiness.
**CV:** *palpitations, tachycardia,* hypertension, *arrhythmias.*
**EENT:** pharyngitis, sinusitis.
**GI:** nausea, abdominal pain, anorexia,
vomiting.
**Hematologic:** *thrombocytopenia, thrombocytopenic purpura, leukopenia,* anemia.
**Metabolic:** weight loss.
**Respiratory:** cough, upper respiratory
tract infection.
**Skin:** rash, urticaria, *exfoliative dermatitis, erythema multiforme.*

## INTERACTIONS
**Drug-drug.** *Centrally acting alpha-2 agonists, clonidine:* May cause serious adverse events. Avoid using together.
*Centrally acting antihypertensives:* May
decrease antihypertensive effect. Monitor
blood pressure.
*MAO inhibitors:* May cause severe hypertension or hypertensive crisis. Avoid using
within 14 days of MAO inhibitor therapy.
*Tricyclic antidepressants:* May increase
levels of these drugs. Monitor patient for
adverse reactions.
**Drug-food.** *Caffeine:* May increase amphetamine and related amine effects. Discourage use together.

## EFFECTS ON LAB TEST RESULTS
• May decrease hemoglobin, hematocrit,
and platelet and WBC counts.

## CONTRAINDICATIONS & CAUTIONS
• Contraindicated in patients hypersensitive to drug and in those with glaucoma,
motor tics, family history or diagnosis of
Tourette syndrome, or history of marked
anxiety, tension, or agitation.
• Because it doesn't dissolve, Concerta is
contraindicated in patients with severe GI
narrowing (such as small bowel inflammatory disease, short-gut syndrome caused
by adhesions or decreased transit time,
history of peritonitis, cystic fibrosis,
chronic intestinal pseudo-obstruction, or
Meckel's diverticulum).

• Ritalin, Ritalin-SR, and Ritalin LA are contraindicated within 14 days of MAO inhibitor therapy.
• Use cautiously in patients with a history of seizures, EEG abnormalities, or hypertension, and in patients whose underlying medical conditions might be compromised by increases in blood pressure or heart rate, such as those with preexisting hypertension, heart failure, recent MI, or hyperthyroidism.
• Use cautiously in patients who are emotionally unstable or who have a history of drug dependence or alcoholism.

**NURSING CONSIDERATIONS**
• Like amphetamines, drug has a paradoxical calming effect in hyperactive children.
• Don't use drug to prevent fatigue or to treat severe depression.
• Drug may trigger Tourette syndrome in children. Monitor patient, especially at start of therapy.
• Observe patient for signs of excessive stimulation. Monitor blood pressure.
• Monitor results of periodic CBC, differential, and platelet counts with long-term use.
• Monitor height and weight in children on long-term therapy. Drug may delay growth spurt, but children will attain normal height when drug is stopped.
• Monitor patient for tolerance or psychological dependence.
• *Alert:* Don't confuse Ritalin with Rifadin.

**PATIENT TEACHING**
• Tell patient or caregiver to give last daily dose at least 6 hours before bedtime to prevent insomnia and after meals to reduce appetite-suppressant effects.
• Warn patient against chewing sustained-release tablets.
• Metadate CD may be swallowed whole, or the contents of the capsule may be sprinkled onto a small amount of applesauce and taken immediately.
• Caution patient to avoid activities that require alertness or good psychomotor coordination until CNS effects of drug are known.
• Warn patient with seizure disorder that drug may decrease seizure threshold. Urge him to notify prescriber if seizure occurs.

• Advise patient to avoid beverages containing caffeine while taking drug.

## modafinil
Provigil

*Pregnancy risk category C*
*Controlled substance schedule IV*

**AVAILABLE FORMS**
*Tablets:* 100 mg, 200 mg

**INDICATIONS & DOSAGES**
➤ **To improve wakefulness in patients with excessive daytime sleepiness caused by narcolepsy, obstructive sleep apnea–hypoapnea syndrome, and shift-work sleep disorder**
*Adults:* 200 mg P.O. daily, as single dose in the morning. Patients with shift-work sleep disorder should take dose about 1 hour before the start of their shift.
*Adjust-a-dose:* In patients with severe hepatic impairment, give 100 mg P.O. daily, as single dose in the morning.

**ACTION**
Unknown. Similar to action of sympathomimetics, including amphetamines, but drug is structurally distinct from amphetamines and doesn't alter release of dopamine or norepinephrine to produce CNS stimulation.

| Route | Onset | Peak | Duration |
|-------|-------|------|----------|
| P.O. | Unknown | 2-4 hr | Unknown |

**ADVERSE REACTIONS**
**CNS:** *headache, nervousness, dizziness,* fever, depression, anxiety, cataplexy, *insomnia,* paresthesia, dyskinesia, hypertonia, confusion, syncope, amnesia, emotional lability, ataxia, tremor.
**CV:** hypotension, hypertension, vasodilation, *arrhythmias,* chest pain.
**EENT:** *rhinitis,* pharyngitis, epistaxis, amblyopia, abnormal vision.
**GI:** *nausea,* diarrhea, dry mouth, anorexia, vomiting, mouth ulcer, gingivitis, thirst.
**GU:** abnormal urine, urine retention, abnormal ejaculation, albuminuria.
**Hematologic:** eosinophilia.
**Metabolic:** hyperglycemia.

**Musculoskeletal:** joint disorder, neck pain, neck rigidity.
**Respiratory:** lung disorder, dyspnea, asthma.
**Skin:** dry skin.
**Other:** herpes simplex, chills.

## INTERACTIONS

**Drug-drug.** *Carbamazepine, phenobarbital, rifampin, and other inducers of CYP 3A4:* May alter modafinil level. Monitor patient closely.
*Cyclosporine, theophylline:* May reduce levels of these drugs. Use together cautiously.
*Diazepam, phenytoin, propranolol, and other drugs metabolized by CYP 2C19:* May inhibit CYP 2C19 and lead to higher levels of drugs metabolized by this enzyme. Use together cautiously; adjust dosage as needed.
*Hormonal contraceptives:* May reduce contraceptive effectiveness. Advise patient to use alternative or additional method of contraception during modafinil therapy and for 1 month after drug is stopped.
*Itraconazole, ketoconazole, other inhibitors of CYP 3A4:* May alter modafinil level. Monitor patient closely.
*Methylphenidate:* May cause 1-hour delay in absorption of modafinil when given together. Separate dosage times.
*Phenytoin, warfarin:* May inhibit CYP 2C9 and increase phenytoin and warfarin levels. Monitor patient closely for toxicity.
*Tricyclic antidepressants (such as clomipramine, desipramine):* May increase tricyclic antidepressant level. Reduce dosage of these drugs.

## EFFECTS ON LAB TEST RESULTS
● May increase glucose, GGT, and AST levels.
● May increase eosinophil count.

## CONTRAINDICATIONS & CAUTIONS
● Contraindicated in patients hypersensitive to drug and in those with a history of left ventricular hypertrophy or ischemic ECG changes, chest pain, arrhythmias, or other evidence of mitral valve prolapse linked to CNS stimulant use.
● Use cautiously in patients with recent MI or unstable angina and in those with history of psychosis.

● Use cautiously and give reduced dosage to patients with severe hepatic impairment, with or without cirrhosis.
● Use cautiously in patients taking MAO inhibitors.
● Safety and efficacy in patients with severe renal impairment haven't been determined.

## NURSING CONSIDERATIONS
● Monitor hypertensive patients closely.
● Although single daily 400-mg doses have been well tolerated, the larger dose is no more beneficial than the 200-mg dose.
● Food has no effect on overall bioavailability but may delay absorption of drug by 1 hour.

## PATIENT TEACHING
● Advise woman to notify prescriber about planned, suspected, or known pregnancy, or if she's breast-feeding.
● Caution patient that use of hormonal contraceptives (including depot or implantable contraceptives) together with modafinil tablets may reduce contraceptive effectiveness. Recommend an alternative method of contraception during modafinil therapy and for 1 month after drug is stopped.
● Instruct patient to confer with prescriber before taking prescription or OTC drugs to avoid drug interactions.
● Tell patient to avoid alcohol while taking drug.
● Tell patient to notify prescriber if rash, hives, or related allergic reaction develops.
● Warn patient to avoid activities that require alertness or good coordination until CNS effects of drug are known.

# pemoline
Cylert, Cylert Chewable, PemADD, PemADD CT

*Pregnancy risk category B*
*Controlled substance schedule IV*

## AVAILABLE FORMS
*Tablets:* 18.75 mg, 37.5 mg, 75 mg
*Tablets (chewable and containing povidone):* 37.5 mg

---

## INDICATIONS & DOSAGES
➤ **Attention deficit hyperactivity disorder**
*Children age 6 and older:* Initially, 37.5 mg P.O. in the morning, with daily dosage raised by 18.75 mg weekly, p.r.n. Usual effective dosage is 56.25 to 75 mg daily; maximum is 112.5 mg daily.

## ACTION
Unknown. Probably promotes nerve impulse transmission by releasing stored norepinephrine from nerve terminals in the brain. Main sites of activity appear to be the cerebral cortex and the reticular activating system.

| Route | Onset | Peak | Duration |
|-------|-------|------|----------|
| P.O. | Unknown | 2-4 hr | Unknown |

## ADVERSE REACTIONS
**CNS:** *insomnia,* dyskinetic movements, irritability, fatigue, mild depression, dizziness, headache, drowsiness, hallucinations, **seizures,** *Tourette syndrome,* abnormal oculomotor function.
**CV:** tachycardia.
**GI:** anorexia, abdominal pain, nausea.
**GU:** prostatic enlargement.
**Hematologic:** *aplastic anemia.*
**Hepatic:** *acute hepatic failure, hepatitis,* jaundice.
**Skin:** rash.

## INTERACTIONS
**Drug-drug.** *CNS stimulants:* May increase CNS effects. Monitor patient closely.
*Insulin, oral antidiabetics:* May decrease antidiabetic requirements. Monitor glucose level.

## EFFECTS ON LAB TEST RESULTS
• May increase liver enzyme and prostate-specific antigen levels.
• May decrease hemoglobin and hematocrit.

## CONTRAINDICATIONS & CAUTIONS
• Contraindicated in patients hypersensitive to drug, in those with idiosyncratic reactions to drug, and in those with hepatic dysfunction.
• Use cautiously in patients with renal impairment.

## NURSING CONSIDERATIONS
• Obtain liver function tests before starting, and periodically during therapy; however, tests may not predict onset of acute hepatic failure. Start treatment only in patients without hepatic disease and with normal baseline liver function test results.
• Closely monitor patients on long-term therapy for possible blood or hepatic function abnormalities and for growth suppression.
• **Alert:** Stop drug if patient experiences significant hepatic dysfunction during therapy.
• Drug is structurally dissimilar to amphetamines or methylphenidate, but it may produce similar adverse reactions. Drug has greater risk of abuse and dependence than previously thought.
• Drug may trigger Tourette syndrome in children. Monitor patient, especially at start of therapy.
• **Alert:** Don't confuse pemoline with Pelamine or pimozide.

## PATIENT TEACHING
• Tell patient to take drug at least 6 hours before bedtime to avoid sleep interference.
• Tell patient to avoid activities that require alertness or good coordination until CNS effects of drug are known.
• Warn patient with seizure disorder that drug may decrease seizure threshold. Urge him to notify prescriber if seizure occurs.

---

# phentermine hydrochloride
Adipex-P, Duromine‡, Ionamin, Pro-Fast HS, Pro-Fast SA, Pro-Fast SR

*Pregnancy risk category NR*
*Controlled substance schedule IV*

## AVAILABLE FORMS
*Capsules:* 18.75 mg, 30 mg, 37.5 mg
*Capsules (resin complex, sustained-release):* 15 mg, 30 mg
*Tablets:* 8 mg, 37.5 mg

## INDICATIONS & DOSAGES
➤ **Short-term adjunct in exogenous obesity**
*Adults:* 8 mg P.O. t.i.d. 30 minutes before meals. Or, 15 to 37.5 mg or 15 to 30 mg

---

(as resin complex) P.O. daily as a single dose in the morning. Take Pro-Fast HS and Pro-Fast SR 2 hours after breakfast. Take Adipex-P before breakfast or 1 to 2 hours after breakfast.

## ACTION

Unknown. Drug probably promotes nerve impulse transmission by releasing stored norepinephrine from nerve terminals in the brain. Main sites of activity appear to be the cerebral cortex and the reticular activating system.

| Route | Onset | Peak | Duration |
|-------|-------|------|----------|
| P.O. | Unknown | Unknown | 12-14 hr |

## ADVERSE REACTIONS

**CNS:** overstimulation, headache, euphoria, dysphoria, dizziness, *insomnia.*
**CV:** *palpitations, tachycardia,* increased blood pressure.
**GI:** dry mouth, dysgeusia, constipation, diarrhea, unpleasant taste, other GI disturbances.
**GU:** impotence.
**Skin:** urticaria.
**Other:** altered libido.

## INTERACTIONS

**Drug-drug.** *Acetazolamide, antacids, sodium bicarbonate:* May increase renal reabsorption. Monitor patient for enhanced effects.
*Ammonium chloride, ascorbic acid:* May decrease level and increase renal excretion of phentermine. Monitor patient for decreased phentermine effects.
*Insulin, oral antidiabetics:* May alter antidiabetic requirements. Monitor glucose level.
*MAO inhibitors:* May cause severe hypertension or hypertensive crisis. Avoid using within 14 days of MAO inhibitor therapy.
**Drug-food.** *Caffeine:* May increase CNS stimulation. Discourage use together.

## EFFECTS ON LAB TEST RESULTS

None reported.

## CONTRAINDICATIONS & CAUTIONS

● Contraindicated in patients hypersensitive to sympathomimetic amines, in those with idiosyncratic reactions to them, in agitated patients, and in those with hyperthyroidism, moderate-to-severe hypertension, advanced arteriosclerosis, symptomatic CV disease, or glaucoma.
● Contraindicated within 14 days of MAO inhibitor therapy.
● Use cautiously in patients with mild hypertension.

## NURSING CONSIDERATIONS

● Use drug with a weight-reduction program.
● Monitor patient for tolerance or dependence.
● *Alert:* Don't confuse phentermine with phentolamine.

## PATIENT TEACHING

● Tell patient to take drug at least 10 hours before bedtime to avoid sleep interference.
● Advise patient to avoid products that contain caffeine. Tell him to report evidence of excessive stimulation.
● Warn patient that fatigue may result as drug effects wear off, and that he'll need more rest.
● Warn patient that drug may lose its effectiveness over time.

# 33

## Antiparkinsonians

**amantadine hydrochloride**
(See Chapter 15, ANTIVIRALS.)
**benztropine mesylate**
**bromocriptine mesylate**
**entacapone**
**levodopa**
**levodopa-carbidopa**
**levodopa-carbidopa-entacapone**
**pergolide mesylate**
**pramipexole dihydrochloride**
**ropinirole hydrochloride**
**selegiline hydrochloride**
**tolcapone**
**trihexyphenidyl hydrochloride**

### COMBINATION PRODUCTS
MADOPAR‡: levodopa 200 mg and benser-azide 50 mg.
MADOPAR HBS‡: levodopa 100 mg and benserazide 25 mg.
MADOPAR Q‡: levodopa 50 mg and benserazide 12.5 mg.
SINEMET 10-100: carbidopa 10 mg and levodopa 100 mg.
SINEMET 25-100: carbidopa 25 mg and levodopa 100 mg.
SINEMET 25-250: carbidopa 25 mg and levodopa 250 mg.
SINEMET CR: carbidopa 50 mg and lev-odopa 200 mg, in extended-release tablets; carbidopa 25 mg and levodopa 100 mg in extended-release tablets.

---

### benztropine mesylate
Apo-Benztropine†, Cogentin, PMS Benztropine†

*Pregnancy risk category NR*

#### AVAILABLE FORMS
*Injection:* 1 mg/ml in 2-ml ampules
*Tablets:* 0.5 mg, 1 mg, 2 mg

#### INDICATIONS & DOSAGES
➤ **Drug-induced extrapyramidal dis-orders (except tardive dyskinesia)**
*Adults:* 1 to 4 mg P.O. or I.M. once or twice daily.

➤ **Acute dystonic reaction**
*Adults:* 1 to 2 mg I.V. or I.M.; then 1 to 2 mg P.O. b.i.d. to prevent recurrence.
➤ **Parkinsonism**
*Adults:* 0.5 to 6 mg P.O. or I.M. daily. First dosage is 0.5 mg to 1 mg, increased by 0.5 mg q 5 to 6 days. Adjust dosage to meet individual requirements. Maximum, 6 mg daily.

#### I.V. ADMINISTRATION
● The I.V. route is seldom used because no clinically significant difference exists be-tween it and the I.M. route.

#### ACTION
Unknown. May block central cholinergic receptors, helping to balance cholinergic activity in the basal ganglia.

| Route | Onset | Peak | Duration |
|-------|-------|------|----------|
| P.O. | 1-2 hr | Unknown | 24 hr |
| I.M., I.V. | 15 min | Unknown | 24 hr |

#### ADVERSE REACTIONS
**CNS:** confusion, memory impairment, nervousness, depression, disorientation, hallucinations, toxic psychosis.
**CV:** tachycardia.
**EENT:** dilated pupils, blurred vision.
**GI:** *dry mouth, constipation,* nausea, vom-iting, paralytic ileus.
**GU:** urine retention, dysuria.
**Skin:** decreased sweating.

#### INTERACTIONS
**Drug-drug.** *Amantadine, phenothiazines, tricyclic antidepressants:* May cause addi-tive anticholinergic adverse reactions, such as confusion and hallucinations. Re-duce dosage before giving.

#### EFFECTS ON LAB TEST RESULTS
None reported.

#### CONTRAINDICATIONS & CAUTIONS
● Contraindicated in patients hypersensi-tive to drug or its components, in those

---

with angle-closure glaucoma, and in children younger than age 3.
• Use cautiously in hot weather, in patients with mental disorders, and in children age 3 and older. Also, use cautiously in patients with prostatic hyperplasia, arrhythmias, and seizure disorders.

## NURSING CONSIDERATIONS
• Monitor vital signs carefully. Watch closely for adverse reactions, especially in elderly or debilitated patients. Call prescriber promptly if adverse reactions occur.
• Some adverse reactions are dose related and may be caused by atropine-like toxicity.
• Drug produces atropine-like adverse reactions and may aggravate tardive dyskinesia.
• Watch for intermittent constipation and abdominal distention and pain, which may indicate onset of paralytic ileus.
• *Alert:* Never stop drug abruptly. Reduce dosage gradually.
• *Alert:* Don't confuse benztropine with bromocriptine.

## PATIENT TEACHING
• Warn patient to avoid activities that require alertness until CNS effects of drug are known.
• If patient takes a single daily dose, tell him to do so at bedtime.
• Advise patient to report signs and symptoms of urinary hesitancy or urine retention.
• Tell patient to relieve dry mouth with cool drinks, ice chips, sugarless gum, or hard candy.
• Advise patient to limit hot weather activities because drug-induced lack of sweating may cause overheating.

---

# bromocriptine mesylate
Parlodel

*Pregnancy risk category B*

## AVAILABLE FORMS
*Capsules:* 5 mg
*Tablets:* 2.5 mg

## INDICATIONS & DOSAGES
➤ **Parkinson's disease**
*Adults:* 1.25 mg P.O. b.i.d. with meals. Increase dosage by 2.5 mg/day q 14 to 28 days, up to 100 mg daily.
➤ **Amenorrhea and galactorrhea from hyperprolactinemia; female infertility; macroprolactinoma**
*Adults:* 1.25 to 2.5 mg P.O. daily, increased by 2.5 mg daily at 3- to 7-day intervals until desired effect occurs. Therapeutic daily dosage is 2.5 to 15 mg. Safety and efficacy of dosages exceeding 100 mg daily haven't been established.
➤ **Acromegaly**
*Adults:* 1.25 to 2.5 mg P.O. with h.s. snack for 3 days. Another 1.25 to 2.5 mg may be added q 3 to 7 days until patient experiences therapeutic benefit. Maximum, 100 mg daily.

## ACTION
Inhibits secretion of prolactin and acts as a dopamine-receptor agonist by activating postsynaptic dopamine receptors.

| Route | Onset | Peak | Duration |
|-------|-------|------|----------|
| P.O. | 2 hr | 8 hr | 24 hr |

## ADVERSE REACTIONS
**CNS:** *CVA, dizziness, headache, fatigue,* mania, light-headedness, drowsiness, delusions, nervousness, insomnia, depression, *seizures.*
**CV:** *hypotension, acute MI.*
**EENT:** nasal congestion, blurred vision.
**GI:** *nausea,* vomiting, *abdominal cramps, constipation,* diarrhea, anorexia.
**GU:** urine retention, urinary frequency.
**Skin:** coolness and pallor of fingers and toes.

## INTERACTIONS
**Drug-drug.** *Amitriptyline, haloperidol, imipramine, loxapine, MAO inhibitors, methyldopa, metoclopramide, phenothiazines, reserpine:* May interfere with bromocriptine's effects. Bromocriptine dosage may need to be increased.
*Antihypertensives:* May increase hypotensive effects. Adjust dosage of antihypertensive.

---

*Erythromycin:* May increase bromocriptine levels and risk of adverse reactions. Use together cautiously.
*Estrogens, hormonal contraceptives, progestins:* May interfere with effects of bromocriptine. Avoid using together.
*Levodopa:* May have additive effects. Adjust dosage of levodopa, if needed.
**Drug-lifestyle.** *Alcohol use:* May cause disulfiram-like reaction. Discourage use together.

### EFFECTS ON LAB TEST RESULTS
● May increase BUN, alkaline phosphatase, uric acid, AST, ALT, and CK levels.

### CONTRAINDICATIONS & CAUTIONS
● Contraindicated in patients hypersensitive to ergot derivatives and in those with uncontrolled hypertension, toxemia of pregnancy, severe ischemic heart disease, or peripheral vascular disease.
● Use cautiously in patients with impaired renal or hepatic function and in those with a history of MI with residual arrhythmias.

### NURSING CONSIDERATIONS
● For Parkinson's disease, bromocriptine usually is given with either levodopa or levodopa-carbidopa. The levodopa-carbidopa dose may need to be reduced.
● Adverse reactions may be minimized if drug is given in the evening with food.
● *Alert:* Monitor patient for adverse reactions, which occur in 68% of patients, particularly at start of therapy. Most reactions are mild to moderate; nausea is most common. Minimize adverse reactions by gradually adjusting dosages to effective levels. Adverse reactions are more common when drug is used for Parkinson's disease.
● Baseline and periodic evaluations of cardiac, hepatic, renal, and hematopoietic function are recommended during prolonged therapy.
● Drug may lead to early postpartum conception. After menses resumes, test for pregnancy every 4 weeks or as soon as a period is missed.
● *Alert:* Don't confuse bromocriptine with benztropine or brimonidine, or Parlodel with pindolol.

### PATIENT TEACHING
● Instruct patient to take drug with meals.
● Advise patient to use contraceptive methods during treatment other than oral contraceptives or subdermal implants.
● Instruct patient to avoid dizziness and fainting by rising slowly to an upright position and avoiding sudden position changes.
● Inform patient that it may take 8 weeks or longer for menses to resume and excess production of milk to slow down.
● Advise patient to avoid alcohol while taking drug.

# entacapone
Comtan

*Pregnancy risk category C*

### AVAILABLE FORMS
*Tablets:* 200 mg

### INDICATIONS & DOSAGES
➤ **Adjunct to levodopa-carbidopa for treatment of idiopathic Parkinson's disease in patients with signs and symptoms of end-of-dose wearing off**
*Adults:* 200 mg P.O. with each dose of levodopa-carbidopa to maximum of eight times daily. Maximum, 1,600 mg daily. May need to reduce daily levodopa dose or extend the interval between doses to optimize patient's response.

### ACTION
A reversible catechol-*O*-methyltransferase (COMT) inhibitor that is given with levodopa-carbidopa. Giving together is believed to cause higher levels of levodopa and optimal control of parkinsonian symptoms.

| Route | Onset | Peak | Duration |
|-------|-------|------|----------|
| P.O. | 1 hr | 1 hr | 6 hr |

### ADVERSE REACTIONS
**CNS:** *dyskinesia, hyperkinesia,* hypokinesia, dizziness, anxiety, somnolence, agitation, fatigue, asthenia, hallucinations.
**GI:** *nausea, diarrhea,* abdominal pain, constipation, vomiting, dry mouth, dyspepsia, flatulence, gastritis, taste perversion.

**GU:** *urine discoloration.*
**Hematologic:** purpura.
**Musculoskeletal:** back pain.
**Respiratory:** dyspnea.
**Skin:** sweating.
**Other:** bacterial infection.

## INTERACTIONS

**Drug-drug.** *Ampicillin, chloramphenicol, cholestyramine, erythromycin, probenecid:* May block biliary excretion, resulting in higher levels of entacapone. Use together cautiously.

*CNS depressants:* May cause additive effect. Use together cautiously.

*Drugs metabolized by COMT (dobutamine, dopamine, epinephrine, isoetharine, isoproterenol, norepinephrine):* May cause higher levels of these drugs, resulting in increased heart rate, changes in blood pressure, or arrhythmias. Use together cautiously.

*Nonselective MAO inhibitors (such as phenelzine, tranylcypromine):* May inhibit normal catecholamine metabolism. Avoid using together.

**Drug-lifestyle.** *Alcohol use:* May cause additive CNS effects. Discourage use together.

## EFFECTS ON LAB TEST RESULTS

None reported.

## CONTRAINDICATIONS & CAUTIONS

• Contraindicated in patients hypersensitive to drug.
• Use cautiously in patients with hepatic impairment, biliary obstruction, or orthostatic hypotension.

## NURSING CONSIDERATIONS

• Use drug only with levodopa-carbidopa; no antiparkinsonian effects occur when drug is given as monotherapy.
• Levodopa-carbidopa dosage requirements are usually lower when drug is given with entacapone; lower levodopa-carbidopa dose or increase dosing interval to avoid adverse effects.
• Drug may cause or worsen dyskinesia, even if levodopa dose is lowered.
• Hallucinations may occur or worsen during therapy with this drug.
• Monitor blood pressure closely, and watch for orthostatic hypotension.

• Diarrhea most often begins within 4 to 12 weeks of starting therapy but may begin as early as 1 week or as late as many months after starting treatment.
• Drug may discolor urine.
• Rarely, rhabdomyolysis has occurred with drug use.
• Rapid withdrawal or abrupt reduction in dose could lead to signs and symptoms of Parkinson's disease; it may also lead to hyperpyrexia and confusion, a group of symptoms resembling neuroleptic malignant syndrome. Stop drug gradually, and monitor patient closely. Adjust other dopaminergic treatments, as needed.
• Drug can be given with immediate or sustained-release levodopa-carbidopa and can be taken with or without food.

## PATIENT TEACHING

• Instruct patient not to crush or break tablet and to take it at same time as levodopa-carbidopa.
• Warn patient to avoid hazardous activities until CNS effects of drug are known.
• Advise patient to avoid alcohol during treatment.
• Instruct patient to use caution when standing after a prolonged period of sitting or lying down because dizziness may occur. This effect is more common during initial therapy.
• Warn patient that hallucinations, increased difficulty with voluntary movements, nausea, and diarrhea could occur.
• Inform patient that drug may turn urine brownish orange.
• Advise patient to notify prescriber about planned, suspected, or known pregnancy, and to notify prescriber if she's breast-feeding.

# levodopa
Larodopa

*Pregnancy risk category NR*

## AVAILABLE FORMS

*Capsules:* 100 mg, 250 mg, 500 mg
*Tablets:* 100 mg, 250 mg, 500 mg

## INDICATIONS & DOSAGES

➤ **Idiopathic parkinsonism, postencephalitic parkinsonism, and sympto-**

matic parkinsonism after carbon monoxide or manganese intoxication or with cerebral arteriosclerosis

*Adults and children older than age 12:* Initially, 0.5 to 1 g P.O. daily, divided in two or more doses with food; increased by no more than 0.75 g daily q 3 to 7 days until maximum response is achieved. Don't exceed 8 g daily. Dosage adjusted to patient requirements, tolerance, and response. Higher dosage needs close supervision.

## ACTION

Unknown. May be decarboxylated to dopamine, countering the depletion of striatal dopamine in extrapyramidal centers; this depletion is thought to produce parkinsonism.

| Route | Onset | Peak | Duration |
|-------|---------|--------|----------|
| P.O. | Unknown | 1-3 hr | 5 hr |

## ADVERSE REACTIONS

**CNS:** *aggressive behavior; involuntary grimacing; head movements; myoclonic body jerks;* **seizures;** *ataxia; tremor; muscle twitching; bradykinetic episodes; psychiatric disturbances; mood changes; nervousness; anxiety; disturbing dreams; euphoria; malaise; fatigue; severe depression;* **suicidal tendencies;** *dementia; delirium; hallucinations; choreiform, dystonic, and dyskinetic movements.*

**CV:** *orthostatic hypotension,* phlebitis, cardiac irregularities.

**EENT:** blepharospasm, blurred vision, diplopia, mydriasis or miosis, activation of latent Horner's syndrome, oculogyric crises.

**GI:** dry mouth, bitter taste, *nausea, vomiting, anorexia,* constipation, flatulence, diarrhea, abdominal pain, excessive salivation.

**GU:** urinary frequency, urine retention, incontinence, darkened urine, priapism.

**Hematologic:** *leukopenia,* hemolytic anemia, *agranulocytosis.*

**Hepatic:** *hepatotoxicity.*

**Metabolic:** weight loss.

**Respiratory:** hiccups, hyperventilation.

**Skin:** dark perspiration.

## INTERACTIONS

**Drug-drug.** *Antacids:* May increase absorption of levodopa. Give antacids 1 hour after levodopa.

*Furazolidone, MAO inhibitors, phenelzine, procarbazine, tranylcypromine:* May cause severe hypertension. Avoid using together.

*Inhaled anesthetics, sympathomimetics:* May increase risk of arrhythmias. Monitor patient closely.

*Iron salts:* May reduce bioavailability of levodopa. Separate dosage times.

*Metoclopramide:* May accelerate gastric emptying of levodopa. Give metoclopramide 1 hour after levodopa.

*Papaverine, phenothiazines, other antipsychotics, phenytoin, rauwolfia alkaloids:* May decrease levodopa effect. Avoid using together.

*Pyridoxine (vitamin $B_6$):* May decrease the effectiveness of levodopa. Avoid using pyridoxine with levodopa. Pyridoxine has little to no effect on the combination drug levodopa and carbidopa.

**Drug-herb.** *Kava:* May increase parkinsonian symptoms. Discourage kava use altogether.

**Drug-food.** *Foods high in protein:* May decrease levodopa absorption. Discourage use together.

**Drug-lifestyle.** *Cocaine use:* May increase risk of arrhythmias. Inform patient of this interaction.

## EFFECTS ON LAB TEST RESULTS

● May increase BUN, ALT, AST, alkaline phosphatase, LDH, and bilirubin levels; may cause transient elevations in protein-bound iodine levels.

● May decrease hemoglobin, hematocrit, and WBC and granulocyte counts.

● May falsely elevate levels of colorimetric test for uric acid and urinary catecholamine, and may falsely decrease urinary vanillylmandelic acid levels. May cause false-positive Coombs' test result during extended therapy. May cause copper-reduction method to show false-positive results for urine glucose; glucose oxidase method has shown false-negative results. May interfere with tests for urine ketones. Levodopa may interfere with urine screening tests for phenylketonuria.

---

**CONTRAINDICATIONS & CAUTIONS**
• Contraindicated in patients hypersensitive to drug and in those with acute angle-closure glaucoma, melanoma, or undiagnosed skin lesions; also contraindicated within 14 days of MAO inhibitor therapy.
• Use cautiously in patients with severe CV, renal, hepatic, and pulmonary disorders; peptic ulcer; psychiatric illness; MI with residual arrhythmias; bronchial asthma; emphysema; and endocrine disease.

**NURSING CONSIDERATIONS**
• Capsules may contain tartrazine.
• Patients who need surgery should continue levodopa therapy as long as oral intake is permitted, usually until 6 to 24 hours before surgery. Resume therapy as soon as patient can take drug orally.
• *Alert:* Because of risk of precipitating a symptom complex resembling neuroleptic malignant syndrome, observe patient closely if levodopa dosage is reduced abruptly or stopped.
• Levodopa-carbidopa typically decreases amount of levodopa needed by 75%, reducing risk of adverse reactions.
• Monitor vital signs, especially while adjusting dosage. Report changes.
• *Alert:* Watch for muscle twitching and blepharospasm, which may be early signs of drug overdose; report immediately.
• *Alert:* Hallucinations may require reduction or withdrawal of drug.
• An accurate measure for urine glucose can be obtained if paper strip is partially immersed in the urine sample. Urine migrates up the strip, as with an ascending chromatographic system. Read only the top of the strip.
• Test patients receiving long-term therapy regularly for diabetes and acromegaly; also periodically monitor renal, hepatic, and hematopoietic function.

**PATIENT TEACHING**
• Tell patient to take drug with food to minimize GI upset. However, high-protein meals can impair absorption and reduce effectiveness.
• If patient has trouble swallowing pills, tell him or caregiver to crush tablets and mix with applesauce or pureed fruit.

• Warn patient or caregiver not to increase dosage unless ordered. Daily dosage shouldn't exceed 8 g.
• Tell patient to protect drug from heat, light, and moisture. If preparation darkens, it has lost potency; discard.
• Warn patient about possible dizziness upon standing quickly, especially at start of therapy. Tell him to change positions slowly and dangle legs before rising. Elastic stockings may control these adverse reactions.
• Advise patient and caregivers that multivitamin preparations, fortified cereals, and certain OTC drugs may contain pyridoxine (vitamin $B_6$), which can block the effects of levodopa by enhancing its peripheral metabolism.

# levodopa-carbidopa
Sinemet✓, Sinemet CR✓

*Pregnancy risk category C*

**AVAILABLE FORMS**
*Tablets:* 100 mg levodopa with 10 mg carbidopa (Sinemet 10-100), 100 mg levodopa with 25 mg carbidopa (Sinemet 25-100), 250 mg levodopa with 25 mg carbidopa (Sinemet 25-250)
*Tablets (extended-release):* 200 mg levodopa with 50 mg carbidopa (Sinemet CR); 100 mg levodopa with 25 mg carbidopa

**INDICATIONS & DOSAGES**
➤ **Idiopathic Parkinson's disease, postencephalitic parkinsonism, and symptomatic parkinsonism resulting from carbon monoxide or manganese intoxication**
*Adults:* 1 tablet of 100 mg levodopa with 25 mg carbidopa P.O. t.i.d.; then increased by 1 tablet daily or every other day, p.r.n., to maximum daily dosage of 8 tablets. May use 250 mg levodopa with 25 mg carbidopa or 100 mg levodopa with 10 mg carbidopa tablets, as directed, to obtain maximum response. Optimum daily dose must be determined by careful adjustment for each patient.
   Patients given conventional tablets may receive extended-release tablets; dosage is calculated on current levodopa intake.

Extended-release tablets should provide 10% more levodopa daily, increased p.r.n. and as tolerated to 30% more levodopa daily. Give in divided doses at intervals of 4 to 8 hours.

## ACTION
Levodopa, a dopamine precursor, relieves parkinsonian symptoms by being converted to dopamine in the brain. Carbidopa inhibits the decarboxylation of peripheral levodopa, which allows more intact levodopa to travel to the brain.

| Route | Onset | Peak | Duration |
|---|---|---|---|
| P.O. | Unknown | 40-150 min | Unknown |

## ADVERSE REACTIONS
**CNS:** *choreiform, dystonic, dyskinetic movements; involuntary grimacing, head movements, myoclonic body jerks, ataxia,* tremor, muscle twitching; bradykinetic episodes; psychiatric disturbances, anxiety, disturbing dreams, euphoria, malaise, fatigue; severe depression, *suicidal tendencies,* dementia, delirium, hallucinations, confusion, insomnia, agitation.
**CV:** *orthostatic hypotension,* cardiac irregularities, phlebitis.
**EENT:** blepharospasm, blurred vision, diplopia, mydriasis or miosis, oculogyric crises, excessive salivation.
**GI:** *dry mouth,* bitter taste, *nausea, vomiting,* anorexia, constipation, flatulence, diarrhea, abdominal pain.
**GU:** urinary frequency, urine retention, urinary incontinence, darkened urine, priapism.
**Hematologic:** hemolytic anemia, *thrombocytopenia, leukopenia, agranulocytosis.*
**Hepatic:** *hepatotoxicity.*
**Metabolic:** weight loss.
**Respiratory:** hiccups, hyperventilation.
**Skin:** dark perspiration.

## INTERACTIONS
**Drug-drug.** *Antihypertensives:* May cause additive hypotensive effects. Use together cautiously.
*Iron salts:* May reduce bioavailability of levodopa and carbidopa. Give iron 1 hour before or 2 hours after Sinemet.
*MAO inhibitors:* May cause risk of severe hypertension. Avoid using together.

*Papaverine, phenytoin:* May antagonize antiparkinsonian actions. Avoid using together.
*Phenothiazines, other antipsychotics:* May antagonize antiparkinsonian actions. Use together cautiously.
*Kava:* May decrease action of drug. Discourage kava use altogether.
*Octacosanol:* May worsen dyskinesias. Discourage use together.
**Drug-food.** *Foods high in protein:* May decrease levodopa absorption. Don't give levodopa with high-protein foods.

## EFFECTS ON LAB TEST RESULTS
• May increase uric acid, ALT, AST, alkaline phosphatase, LDH, and bilirubin levels.
• May decrease hemoglobin, hematocrit, and WBC, granulocyte, and platelet counts.
• May falsely increase urinary catecholamine level and serum and urinary uric acid levels in colorimetric tests. May falsely decrease urinary vanillylmandelic acid level. May cause false-positive results in urine ketone tests using sodium nitroprusside reagent and in urinary glucose tests using cupric sulfate reagent. May cause false-negative results in tests using glucose oxidase. May alter results of urine screening tests for phenylketonuria.

## CONTRAINDICATIONS & CAUTIONS
• Contraindicated in patients hypersensitive to drug and in those with angle-closure glaucoma, melanoma, or undiagnosed skin lesions.
• Contraindicated within 14 days of MAO inhibitor therapy.
• Use cautiously in patients with severe CV, renal, hepatic, endocrine, or pulmonary disorders; history of peptic ulcer; psychiatric illness; MI with residual arrhythmias; bronchial asthma; emphysema; and well-controlled, chronic open-angle glaucoma.

## NURSING CONSIDERATIONS
• If patient takes levodopa, stop drug at least 8 hours before starting levodopa-carbidopa.
• Levodopa-carbidopa typically decreases amount of levodopa needed by 75%, reducing risk of adverse reactions.

- Therapeutic and adverse reactions occur more rapidly with levodopa-carbidopa than with levodopa alone. Observe patient and monitor vital signs, especially while adjusting dosage. Report significant changes.
- *Alert:* Because of risk of precipitating a symptom complex resembling neuroleptic malignant syndrome, observe patient closely if levodopa dosage is reduced abruptly or stopped.
- Hallucinations may require reduction or withdrawal of drug.
- *Alert:* Muscle twitching and blepharospasm may be early signs of drug overdose; report immediately.
- Test patients receiving long-term therapy regularly for diabetes and acromegaly, and periodically for hepatic, renal, and hematopoietic function.

**PATIENT TEACHING**
- Tell patient to take drug with food to minimize GI upset; however, high-protein meals can impair absorption and reduce effectiveness.
- Tell patient not to chew or crush extended-release form.
- Warn patient and caregivers not to increase dosage without prescriber's orders.
- Caution patient about possible dizziness when standing up quickly, especially at start of therapy. Tell him to change positions slowly and dangle his legs before getting out of bed. Elastic stockings may control these adverse reactions in some patients.
- Instruct patient to report adverse reactions and therapeutic effects.
- Inform patient that pyridoxine (vitamin $B_6$) doesn't reverse beneficial effects of levodopa-carbidopa. Multivitamins can be taken without reversing levodopa's effects.

✳ *NEW DRUG*
_____

# levodopa, carbidopa, entacapone
Stalevo⊘

*Pregnancy risk category C*

**AVAILABLE FORMS**
*Tablets (film-coated):* 50 mg levodopa, 12.5 mg carbidopa, 200 mg entacapone;

100 mg levodopa, 25 mg carbidopa, 200 mg entacapone; 150 mg levodopa, 37.5 mg carbidopa, 200 mg entacapone

**INDICATIONS & DOSAGES**
➤ **Idiopathic Parkinson's disease to replace (with equivalent strengths) levodopa-carbidopa and entacapone given individually or to replace immediate-release levodopa-carbidopa for a patient with end-of-dose "wearing off" taking a total daily levodopa dose of 600 mg or less and no dyskinesia—**
*Adults:* 1 tablet P.O.; determine dose and interval by therapeutic response. Maximum, 8 tablets daily.

**ACTION**
Levodopa, a dopamine precursor, relieves parkinsonian symptoms by converting to dopamine in the brain. Carbidopa inhibits the decarboxylation of peripheral levodopa, which allows more intact levodopa to travel to the brain. Entacapone is a reversible catecholamine-*O*-methyltransferase (COMT) inhibitor that increases levodopa level.

| Route | Onset | Peak | Duration |
|-------|-------|------|----------|
| P.O. | Unknown | 1½ hr | Unknown |

**ADVERSE REACTIONS**
**levodopa-carbidopa**
**CNS:** agitation, asthenia, confusion, delusions, dementia, depression, dizziness, dyskinesia, hallucinations, headache, increased libido, insomnia, *neuroleptic malignant syndrome,* nightmares, paranoid ideation, paresthesias, psychosis, somnolence, syncope.
**CV:** cardiac irregularities, chest pain, hypertension, hypotension, orthostatic hypotension, palpitations, phlebitis.
**GI:** anorexia, constipation, dark saliva, diarrhea, dry mouth, duodenal ulcer, dyspepsia, GI bleeding, nausea, taste alterations, vomiting.
**GU:** dark urine, urinary frequency, UTI.
**Hematologic:** *agranulocytosis,* anemia, *leukopenia, thrombocytopenia.*
**Musculoskeletal:** back pain, muscle cramps, shoulder pain.
**Respiratory:** dyspnea, upper respiratory infection.

**Skin:** alopecia, bullous lesions, dark sweat, Henoch-Schönlein purpura, increased sweating, pruritus, rash, urticaria.
**Other:** *angioedema.*

**entacapone**
**CNS:** agitation, anxiety, asthenia, dizziness, *dyskinesia,* fatigue, *hyperkinesia,* hypokinesia, somnolence.
**GI:** abdominal pain, constipation, *diarrhea,* dry mouth, dyspepsia, flatulence, gastritis, *nausea,* taste perversion, vomiting.
**GU:** *urine discoloration.*
**Musculoskeletal:** back pain.
**Respiratory:** dyspnea.
**Skin:** increased sweating, purpura.
**Other:** bacterial infection.

## INTERACTIONS
**Drug-drug.** *Ampicillin, chloramphenicol, cholestyramine, erythromycin, probenecid, rifampicin:* May interfere with entacapone excretion. Use together cautiously.
*Antihypertensives:* May cause orthostatic hypotension. Adjust antihypertensive dosage as needed.
*CNS depressants:* Additive effects. Use together cautiously.
*Dopamine D2 receptor antagonists, such as butyrophenones, iron salts, isoniazid, metoclopramide, papaverine, phenothiazines, phenytoin, and risperidone:* May decrease levodopa-carbidopa-entacapone effects. Monitor patient for effectiveness.
*Drugs metabolized by COMT, such as alpha-methyldopa, apomorphine, bitolterol, dobutamine, dopamine, epinephrine, isoproterenol, isoetharine, and norepinephrine:* May increase heart rate, arrhythmias, and excessive blood pressure changes. Use together cautiously.
*Metoclopramide:* May increase availability of levodopa-carbidopa by increasing gastric emptying. Monitor patient for adverse effects.
*Nonselective MAO inhibitor:* May disrupt catecholamine metabolism. Avoid using together.
*Selegiline:* May cause severe hypotension. Use together cautiously, and monitor blood pressure.
*Tricyclic antidepressants:* May increase risk of hypertension and dyskinesia. Monitor patient closely.

## EFFECTS ON LAB TEST RESULTS
● May increase alkaline phosphatase, AST, ALT, LDH, glucose, BUN, and bilirubin levels.
● May decrease hemoglobin, hematocrit, and platelet and WBC counts.
● May cause false-positive reaction for urinary ketone bodies on a test tape. May cause false-negative result for glucosuria with glucose-oxidase testing methods.

## CONTRAINDICATIONS & CAUTIONS
● Contraindicated in patients hypersensitive to drug or its ingredients.
● Contraindicated in patients with angle-closure glaucoma, suspicious undiagnosed skin lesions, or a history of melanoma.
● Contraindicated within 2 weeks of MAO inhibitor therapy.
● Use cautiously in patients with past or current psychosis and in patients with severe cardiovascular or pulmonary disease, bronchial asthma, biliary obstruction, or renal, hepatic, or endocrine disease.
● Use cautiously in patients with chronic open-angle glaucoma or a history of MI and residual atrial, nodal, or ventricular arrhythmias.

## NURSING CONSIDERATIONS
● Certain CNS effects, such as dyskinesia, may occur at lower dosages and sooner with levodopa-carbidopa-entacapone than with levodopa alone. Dyskinesia may require a reduced dosage.
● During the first adjustment period, monitor a patient with CV disease carefully and in a facility equipped to provide intensive cardiac care.
● Neuroleptic malignant syndrome may develop when levodopa-carbidopa is reduced or stopped, especially in patients taking antipsychotic drugs. Watch patient carefully for fever, hyperthermia, muscle rigidity, involuntary movements, altered consciousness, mental status changes, and autonomic dysfunction.
● During extended therapy, periodically monitor hepatic, hematopoietic, CV, and renal function.
● Diarrhea is common; it usually develops 4 to 12 weeks after treatment starts but may appear as early as the first week or as late as many months after treatment starts.

- Monitor patient for hallucinations, depression, and suicidal tendencies.

## PATIENT TEACHING
- Advise patient to take drug exactly as prescribed.
- Tell patient to report a "wearing-off" effect, which may occur at the end of the dosing interval.
- Tell patient that urine, sweat, and saliva may turn dark (red, brown, or black) during treatment.
- Advise patient to notify the prescriber if problems making voluntary movements increase.
- Tell patient that diarrhea is common with this treatment.
- Inform patient that hallucinations may occur.
- Urge patient to immediately report depression or suicidal thoughts.
- Explain that he may become dizzy if he rises quickly. Urge patient to use caution when rising.
- Tell patient that a high-protein diet, excessive acidity, and iron salts may reduce the drug's effectiveness.
- Urge patient to avoid hazardous activities until the CNS effects of the drug are known.
- Advise patient to notify prescriber if she becomes pregnant.

---

## pergolide mesylate
Permax

*Pregnancy risk category B*

### AVAILABLE FORMS
*Tablets:* 0.05 mg, 0.25 mg, 1 mg

### INDICATIONS & DOSAGES
➤ **Adjunctive treatment with levodopa-carbidopa to manage signs and symptoms of Parkinson's disease**
*Adults:* Initially, 0.05 mg P.O. daily for first 2 days; then increase by 0.1 to 0.15 mg q third day over 12 days. Increase subsequent dosage by 0.25 mg q third day, if needed, until optimum response is achieved. Maximum dose is 5 mg daily. Drug is usually given in divided doses t.i.d. Gradual reduction in levodopa-

carbidopa dosage may be needed during dosage adjustment.

### ACTION
Dopamine agonist that directly stimulates dopamine receptors in the nigrostriatal system.

| Route | Onset | Peak | Duration |
|-------|-------|------|----------|
| P.O. | Unknown | Unknown | Unknown |

### ADVERSE REACTIONS
**CNS:** headache, chills, asthenia, *dyskinesia, dizziness, hallucinations, dystonia, confusion, somnolence,* insomnia, anxiety, depression, tremor, abnormal dreams, personality disorder, psychosis, abnormal gait, akathisia, extrapyramidal syndrome, incoordination, akinesia, hypertonia, neuralgia, speech disorder, syncope, twitching, paresthesia.
**CV:** *orthostatic hypotension,* vasodilation, palpitations, hypotension, hypertension, *arrhythmias, MI.*
**EENT:** *rhinitis,* epistaxis, abnormal vision, diplopia, eye disorder.
**GI:** dry mouth, taste perversion, abdominal pain, *nausea, constipation,* diarrhea, dyspepsia, anorexia, vomiting.
**GU:** urinary frequency, UTI, hematuria.
**Metabolic:** weight gain.
**Musculoskeletal:** arthralgia; bursitis; myalgia; chest, neck, and back pain.
**Respiratory:** dyspnea.
**Skin:** rash, diaphoresis.
**Other:** flu syndrome; infection; facial, peripheral, and generalized edema.

### INTERACTIONS
**Drug-drug.** *Dopamine antagonists:* May antagonize effects of pergolide. Avoid using together.

### EFFECTS ON LAB TEST RESULTS
None reported.

### CONTRAINDICATIONS & CAUTIONS
- Contraindicated in patients hypersensitive to drug or to ergot alkaloids.
- Use cautiously in patients prone to arrhythmias.
- Use cautiously in patients with a history of pleuritis, pleural effusion, pleural fibrosis, pericarditis, pericardial effusion, car-

---

diac valvulopathy, or retroperitoneal fibrosis.

### NURSING CONSIDERATIONS
● *Alert:* Monitor blood pressure. Symptomatic orthostatic or sustained hypotension may occur, especially at start of therapy.
● *Alert:* Don't confuse Permax with Permitil.

### PATIENT TEACHING
● Inform patient about possible adverse reactions, especially hallucinating, being confused, and suddenly falling asleep performing activities of daily living.
● Warn patient to avoid activities that could result in injury from fainting or dizziness upon standing up quickly.
● Advise patient to take drug with food.

---

## pramipexole dihydrochloride
Mirapex

*Pregnancy risk category C*

---

### AVAILABLE FORMS
*Tablets:* 0.125 mg, 0.25 mg, 0.5 mg, 1 mg, 1.5 mg

### INDICATIONS & DOSAGES
➤ **Signs and symptoms of idiopathic Parkinson's disease**
*Adults:* Initially, 0.375 mg P.O. daily in three divided doses. Titrate doses slowly (not more often than q 5 to 7 days) over several weeks until desired therapeutic effect is achieved. Maintenance dosage is 1.5 to 4.5 mg daily in three divided doses.
*Adjust-a-dose:* For patients with creatinine clearance over 60 ml/minute, first dosage is 0.125 mg P.O. t.i.d., up to 1.5 mg t.i.d. For those with clearance 35 to 59 ml/minute, first dosage is 1.25 mg P.O. b.i.d., up to 1.5 mg b.i.d. For those with clearance 15 to 34 ml/minute, first dosage is 0.125 mg P.O. daily, up to 1.5 mg daily.

### ACTION
Unknown. Non–ergot-derivative dopamine receptor agonist that is thought to stimulate dopamine (D2) receptors in striatum.

| Route | Onset | Peak | Duration |
|-------|-------|------|----------|
| P.O. | Rapid | 2 hr | 8-12 hr |

### ADVERSE REACTIONS
**CNS:** drowsiness, akathisia, amnesia, *asthenia, confusion,* delusions, *dizziness, dream abnormalities, dyskinesia,* dystonia, *extrapyramidal syndrome,* gait abnormalities, *hallucinations,* hypoesthesia, hypertonia, *insomnia,* myoclonus, paranoid reaction, malaise, *somnolence,* sleep disorders, thought abnormalities, fever.
**CV:** chest pain, peripheral edema, *orthostatic hypotension.*
**EENT:** accommodation abnormalities, diplopia, rhinitis, vision abnormalities.
**GI:** dry mouth, anorexia, *constipation,* dysphagia, *nausea.*
**GU:** impotence, urinary frequency, UTI, urinary incontinence.
**Metabolic:** weight loss.
**Musculoskeletal:** arthritis, bursitis, myasthenia, twitching.
**Respiratory:** dyspnea, pneumonia.
**Skin:** skin disorders.
**Other:** decreased libido, *accidental injury,* general edema.

### INTERACTIONS
**Drug-drug.** *Cimetidine, diltiazem, quinidine, quinine, ranitidine, triamterene, verapamil:* May decrease pramipexole clearance. Adjust dosage as needed.
*Dopamine antagonists:* May reduce pramipexole effectiveness. Monitor patient closely.

### EFFECTS ON LAB TEST RESULTS
None reported.

### CONTRAINDICATIONS & CAUTIONS
● Contraindicated in patients hypersensitive to drug or its components.
● It's unknown if drug appears in breast milk. Use cautiously in breast-feeding women.

### NURSING CONSIDERATIONS
● If drug must be stopped, withdraw over 1 week.
● Drug may cause orthostatic hypotension, especially during dosage increases. Monitor patient carefully.
● Adjust dosage gradually to achieve maximum therapeutic effect, balanced against the main adverse effects of dyskinesia, hallucinations, somnolence, and dry mouth.

---

534 Central nervous system drugs

## PATIENT TEACHING

• Instruct patient not to rise rapidly after sitting or lying down because of risk of dizziness.
• Caution patient to avoid hazardous activities until CNS response to drug is known.
• Tell patient to use caution before taking drug with other CNS depressants.
• Tell patient (especially elderly patient) that hallucinations may occur.
• Advise patient to take drug with food if nausea develops.
• Tell woman to notify prescriber if she is breast-feeding or intends to do so.
• Advise patient that it may take 4 weeks for effects of drug to be noticed because of slow adjustment schedule.

---

## ropinirole hydrochloride
Requip

*Pregnancy risk category C*

---

### AVAILABLE FORMS
*Tablets:* 0.25 mg, 0.5 mg, 1 mg, 2 mg, 3 mg, 4 mg, 5 mg

### INDICATIONS & DOSAGES
➤ **Idiopathic Parkinson's disease**
*Adults:* Initially, 0.25 mg P.O., t.i.d. Increase dose by 0.25 mg t.i.d. at weekly intervals for 4 weeks. After week 4, dosage may be increased by 1.5 mg daily divided t.i.d. at weekly intervals, up to 9 mg daily divided t.i.d.; then dosage may be increased by up to 3 mg daily divided t.i.d.; at weekly intervals, up to 24 mg daily divided t.i.d.
*Elderly patients:* Adjust dosages individually, according to patient response; clearance is reduced in these patients.

### ACTION
Unknown. Non–ergot-derivative dopamine receptor agonist that is thought to stimulate dopamine (D2) receptors in striatum.

| Route | Onset | Peak | Duration |
|-------|---------|--------|----------|
| P.O. | Unknown | 1-2 hr | 6 hr |

### ADVERSE REACTIONS
**Early Parkinson's disease (without levodopa)**
**CNS:** hallucinations, *dizziness,* aggravated Parkinson's disease, *somnolence,* headache, confusion, hyperkinesia, hypoesthesia, vertigo, amnesia, impaired concentration, *syncope, fatigue,* malaise, asthenia.
**CV:** orthostatic hypotension, orthostatic symptoms, hypertension, edema, chest pain, extrasystoles, atrial fibrillation, palpitations, tachycardia, flushing.
**EENT:** pharyngitis, abnormal vision, eye abnormality, xerophthalmia, rhinitis, sinusitis.
**GI:** dry mouth, *nausea, vomiting, dyspepsia,* flatulence, abdominal pain, anorexia, constipation.
**GU:** UTI, impotence.
**Respiratory:** bronchitis, dyspnea, yawning.
**Other:** *viral infection,* pain, increased sweating, peripheral ischemia.
**Advanced Parkinson's disease (with levodopa)**
**CNS:** *dizziness,* aggravated parkinsonism, *somnolence, headache,* insomnia, *hallucinations,* abnormal dreaming, confusion, tremor, anxiety, nervousness, amnesia, paresis, paresthesia, syncope.
**CV:** hypotension.
**EENT:** diplopia.
**GI:** *nausea,* abdominal pain, dry mouth, vomiting, constipation, diarrhea, dysphagia, flatulence, increased saliva.
**GU:** UTI, pyuria, urinary incontinence.
**Hematologic:** anemia.
**Metabolic:** weight decrease, suppressed prolactin.
**Musculoskeletal:** arthralgia, arthritis, *dyskinesia,* hypokinesia.
**Respiratory:** upper respiratory tract infection, dyspnea.
**Skin:** increased sweating.
**Other:** injury, *falls,* viral infection, pain.

### INTERACTIONS
**Drug-drug.** *Cimetidine, ciprofloxacin, fluvoxamine, inhibitors or substrates of cytochrome P450 1A2, ritonavir:* May alter ropinirole clearance. Adjust ropinirole dose if other drugs are started or stopped during treatment.
*CNS depressants:* May increase CNS effects. Use together cautiously.

---

Reactions may be *common,* uncommon, *life-threatening,* or COMMON AND LIFE-THREATENING.

*Dopamine antagonists (neuroleptics) or metoclopramide:* May decrease ropinirole effects. Avoid using together.

*Estrogens:* May decrease ropinirole clearance. Adjust ropinirole dosage if estrogen therapy is started or stopped during treatment.

**Drug-lifestyle.** *Alcohol use:* May increase sedative effect. Advise patient to use cautiously.

*Smoking:* May increase ropinirole clearance. Discourage use together.

## EFFECTS ON LAB TEST RESULTS
● May increase BUN and alkaline phosphatase levels.
● May decrease hemoglobin.
● May cause positive result for amphetamine on urine drug screen.

## CONTRAINDICATIONS & CAUTIONS
● Contraindicated in patients hypersensitive to drug.
● Use cautiously in patients with severe hepatic or renal impairment.

## NURSING CONSIDERATIONS
● *Alert:* Monitor patient carefully for orthostatic hypotension, especially during dosage increases.
● Drug may potentiate the dopaminergic adverse effects of levodopa and may cause or worsen dyskinesia. Dosage may be decreased.
● Although not reported with ropinirole, other adverse reactions reported with dopaminergic therapy include hyperpyrexia, fibrotic complications, and confusion, which may occur with rapid dosage reduction or withdrawal of medication.
● Patient may have syncope, with or without bradycardia. Monitor patient carefully, especially for 4 weeks after start of therapy and with dosage increases.
● Withdraw drug gradually over 7 days.

## PATIENT TEACHING
● Advise patient to take drug with food if nausea occurs.
● Inform patient (especially elderly patient) that hallucinations can occur.
● Instruct patient not to rise rapidly after sitting or lying down because of risk of dizziness, which may occur more frequently early in therapy or when dosage increases.
● Sleepiness can occur early in therapy. Warn patient to minimize hazardous activities until CNS effects of drug are known.
● Advise patient to avoid alcohol.
● Tell woman to notify prescriber about planned, suspected, or known pregnancy; also tell her to inform prescriber if she's breast-feeding.

---

## selegiline hydrochloride (L-deprenyl hydrochloride)
Carbex, Eldepryl

*Pregnancy risk category C*

## AVAILABLE FORMS
*Capsules:* 5 mg
*Tablets:* 5 mg

## INDICATIONS & DOSAGES
➤ **Adjunctive treatment with levodopa-carbidopa in managing signs and symptoms of Parkinson's disease**
*Adults:* 10 mg P.O. daily, 5 mg at breakfast and 5 mg at lunch. After 2 or 3 days, gradual decrease of levodopa-carbidopa dosage may be needed.

## ACTION
Unknown. May selectively inhibit MAO type B (found mostly in the brain) and dopamine metabolism. At higher than recommended doses, it's a nonselective inhibitor of MAO, including MAO type A (found in the GI tract). May also directly increase dopaminergic activity by decreasing the reuptake of dopamine into nerve cells.

| Route | Onset | Peak | Duration |
|-------|-------|------|----------|
| P.O. | Unknown | 30-120 min | Unknown |

## ADVERSE REACTIONS
**CNS:** *dizziness,* increased tremor, chorea, loss of balance, restlessness, increased bradykinesia, facial grimacing, stiff neck, dyskinesia, involuntary movements, twitching, increased apraxia, behavioral changes, fatigue, headache, confusion, hallucinations, vivid dreams, anxiety, insomnia, lethargy, malaise, syncope.

**CV:** orthostatic hypotension, hypertension, hypotension, ***arrhythmias,*** palpitations, new or increased angina, tachycardia, peripheral edema.
**EENT:** blepharospasm.
**GI:** dry mouth, *nausea,* vomiting, constipation, abdominal pain, anorexia or poor appetite, dysphagia, diarrhea, heartburn.
**GU:** slow urination, transient nocturia, prostatic hyperplasia, urinary hesitancy, urinary frequency, urine retention, sexual dysfunction.
**Metabolic:** weight loss.
**Skin:** rash, hair loss, diaphoresis.

## INTERACTIONS
**Drug-drug.** *Sympathomimetics:* May cause increased pressor response, particularly in patients who have taken an overdose of selegiline. Use together cautiously.
*MAO inhibitors:* May cause hypertensive crisis. Avoid using together.
*Meperidine:* May cause stupor, muscle rigidity, severe agitation, and fever. Avoid using together.
*Tricyclic antidepressants:* May cause mental status change. Avoid using together.
*Citalopram, fluoxetine, fluvoxamine, nefazodone, paroxetine, sertraline, venlafaxine:* May cause serotonin syndrome (CNS irritability, shivering, and altered consciousness). Separate dosages by at least 2 weeks.
**Drug-herb.** *Cacao:* May cause vasopressor effects. Discourage use together.
*Ginseng:* May cause headache, tremors, or mania. Discourage use together.
**Drug-food.** *Foods high in tyramine:* May cause hypertensive crisis. Monitor blood pressure.

## EFFECTS ON LAB TEST RESULTS
• May cause positive result for amphetamine on urine drug screen.

## CONTRAINDICATIONS & CAUTIONS
• Contraindicated in patients hypersensitive to drug and in those receiving meperidine.

## NURSING CONSIDERATIONS
• *Alert:* Some patients experience increased adverse reactions to levodopa when it's used with selegiline and need a 10% to 30% reduction of levodopa-carbidopa dosage.
• *Alert:* Don't confuse selegiline with Stelazine or Eldepryl with enalapril.
• *Alert:* Severe adverse reactions may occur if used with antidepressants.

## PATIENT TEACHING
• Warn patient to move cautiously at start of therapy because he may become dizzy.
• Advise patient not to take more than 10 mg daily. A larger amount may increase adverse reactions.

# tolcapone
Tasmar

*Pregnancy risk category C*

## AVAILABLE FORMS
*Tablets:* 100 mg, 200 mg

## INDICATIONS & DOSAGES
➤ **Adjunct to levodopa and carbidopa for treating signs and symptoms of idiopathic Parkinson's disease in patients who have symptom fluctuation or haven't responded to other adjunctive treatment**
*Adults:* Initially, 100 mg P.O. t.i.d. with levodopa-carbidopa. Recommended daily dosage is 100 mg P.O. t.i.d. Reducing levodopa dosage by 20% to 30% may be needed to minimize risk of dyskinesias. Maximum, 600 mg daily. Stop drug if patient shows no benefit within 3 weeks.

## ACTION
Unknown. May reversibly inhibit catechol-*O*-methyltransferase when given with levodopa-carbidopa, increasing levodopa bioavailability. This causes a more constant dopaminergic stimulation in the brain.

| Route | Onset | Peak | Duration |
|-------|-------|------|----------|
| P.O. | Unknown | 2 hr | Unknown |

## ADVERSE REACTIONS
**CNS:** fever, *dyskinesia, sleep disorder, dystonia, excessive dreaming, somnolence,* dizziness, *confusion, headache, hallucinations,* hyperkinesia, hypertonia, fatigue, falling, syncope, balance loss,

depression, tremor, speech disorder, paresthesia, agitation, irritability, mental deficiency, hyperactivity, hypokinesia.
**CV:** *orthostatic complaints,* chest pain, chest discomfort, palpitations, hypotension.
**EENT:** pharyngitis, tinnitus, sinus congestion.
**GI:** *nausea, anorexia, diarrhea,* flatulence, *vomiting,* constipation, abdominal pain, dyspepsia, dry mouth.
**GU:** UTI, urine discoloration, hematuria, micturition disorder, urinary incontinence, impotence.
**Hematologic:** bleeding.
**Hepatic:** *hepatotoxicity.*
**Musculoskeletal:** *muscle cramps,* stiffness, arthritis, neck pain.
**Respiratory:** bronchitis, dyspnea, upper respiratory tract infection.
**Skin:** increased sweating, rash.
**Other:** influenza.

## INTERACTIONS
**Drug-drug.** *CNS depressants:* May cause additive effects. Monitor patient closely.
*Desipramine, SSRIs, tricyclic antidepressants:* May increase risk of adverse effects. Use together cautiously.
*Nonselective MAO inhibitors (phenelzine, tranylcypromine):* May cause hypertensive crisis. Avoid using together.
*Warfarin:* May cause increased warfarin levels. Monitor INR, and adjust warfarin dosage, as needed.

## EFFECTS ON LAB TEST RESULTS
● May increase liver function test values.

## CONTRAINDICATIONS & CAUTIONS
● Contraindicated in patients hypersensitive to drug or its components and in those with hepatic disease, elevated ALT or AST levels, or history of drug-related confusion and nontraumatic rhabdomyolysis or hyperpyrexia. Also contraindicated in those who were withdrawn from tolcapone because of drug-induced hepatocellular injury.
● Use cautiously in patients with severe renal impairment and in breast-feeding women.

## NURSING CONSIDERATIONS
● Because of risk of liver toxicity, stop treatment if patient shows no benefit within 3 weeks.
● Because of fatal hepatic failure risk, drug should only be used in patients taking levodopa-carbidopa who don't respond to or who aren't appropriate candidates for other adjunctive therapies.
● *Alert:* Make sure patient provides written informed consent before using drug.
● Monitor liver function test results before starting drug, every 2 weeks for first year of therapy, every 4 weeks for next 6 months, and every 8 weeks thereafter. Stop drug if results are abnormal or if patient appears jaundiced.
● Because drug is highly protein-bound, it isn't significantly removed during dialysis.
● Monitor patient for orthostatic hypotension and syncope.
● Give first dose of the day with first daily dose of levodopa-carbidopa.

## PATIENT TEACHING
● Advise patient to take drug exactly as prescribed.
● Teach patient to immediately report the signs and symptoms of liver injury (yellow eyes or skin, fatigue, loss of appetite, persistent nausea, itching, dark urine, or right upper abdominal tenderness).
● Warn patient about risk of dizziness upon standing up quickly; tell him to stand up cautiously.
● Advise patient to avoid hazardous activities until CNS effects of drug are known.
● Tell patient that nausea may occur early in therapy.
● Inform patient that diarrhea is common, sometimes occurring 2 to 12 weeks after therapy begins, and usually resolves when therapy stops.
● Advise patient about risk of increased problems making voluntary movements or impaired muscle tone.
● Inform patient that hallucinations may occur.
● Tell woman to notify prescriber about planned, suspected, or known pregnancy.
● Inform patient that drug may be taken without regard to meals.

# trihexyphenidyl hydrochloride
Apo-Trihex†, Trihexy-2, Trihexy-5

*Pregnancy risk category NR*

## AVAILABLE FORMS
*Capsules (sustained-release):* 5 mg
*Tablets:* 2 mg, 5 mg

## INDICATIONS & DOSAGES
➤ **All forms of parkinsonism, including drug-induced parkinsonism; adjunct to levodopa in managing signs and symptoms of parkinsonism**
*Adults:* 1 mg P.O. on day 1, 2 mg on day 2; then increased in 2-mg increments q 3 to 5 days up to total of 6 to 10 mg daily. Usually given t.i.d. with meals; sometimes given q.i.d. (last dose h.s.) or switched to extended-release form b.i.d.

Patients with postencephalitic parkinsonism may need total daily dose of 12 to 15 mg.

## ACTION
Unknown. Drug blocks central cholinergic receptors, helping to balance cholinergic activity in the basal ganglia.

| Route | Onset | Peak | Duration |
|-------|-------|------|----------|
| P.O. | 1 hr | 1-1½ hr | 6-12 hr |

## ADVERSE REACTIONS
**CNS:** nervousness, dizziness, headache, hallucinations, drowsiness, weakness.
**CV:** tachycardia.
**EENT:** blurred vision, mydriasis, increased intraocular pressure.
**GI:** *dry mouth,* constipation, *nausea,* vomiting.
**GU:** urinary hesitancy, urine retention.

## INTERACTIONS
**Drug-drug.** *Amantadine, other anticholinergics:* May cause additive anticholinergic adverse reactions, such as confusion and hallucinations. Reduce dose of trihexyphenidyl before giving.
*Levodopa:* May decrease total bioavailability of levodopa. May require lower doses of both drugs.
**Drug-lifestyle.** *Alcohol use:* May increase sedative effects. Discourage use together.

## EFFECTS ON LAB TEST RESULTS
None reported.

## CONTRAINDICATIONS & CAUTIONS
● Contraindicated in patients hypersensitive to drug.
● Use cautiously in patients with glaucoma, cardiac disorders, hepatic disorders, renal disorders, obstructive GI or GU disorders, and prostatic hyperplasia.

## NURSING CONSIDERATIONS
● Dosage may need to be gradually increased in patients who develop tolerance to drug.
● Monitor patient. Adverse reactions are dose related and transient.
● *Alert:* Don't confuse Artane with Anturane or Altace.

## PATIENT TEACHING
● Tell patient that drug may cause nausea if taken before meals.
● Tell patient to avoid activities that require alertness, until CNS effects of drug are known.
● Advise patient to report signs and symptoms of urinary hesitancy or urine retention.
● Tell patient to relieve dry mouth with cool drinks, ice chips, or sugarless gum or hard candy.
● Advise patient to avoid alcohol while taking drug.
● Advise patient to avoid OTC sleep aids or cold medicines because of possibility of increased anticholinergic effects.

# 34

## Miscellaneous central nervous system drugs

almotriptan malate
atomoxetine hydrochloride
bupropion hydrochloride
donepezil hydrochloride
droperidol
eletriptan hydrobromide
fluvoxamine maleate
frovatriptan succinate
galantamine hydrobromide
lithium carbonate
lithium citrate
memantine hydrochloride
naratriptan hydrochloride
propofol
rivastigmine tartrate
rizatriptan benzoate
sibutramine hydrochloride
    monohydrate
sumatriptan succinate
tacrine hydrochloride
zolmitriptan

**COMBINATION PRODUCTS**
None.

---

## almotriptan malate
Axert

*Pregnancy risk category C*

**AVAILABLE FORMS**
*Tablets:* 6.25 mg, 12.5 mg

**INDICATIONS & DOSAGES**
➤ **Acute migraine with or without aura**
*Adults:* 6.25-mg or 12.5-mg tablet P.O.,
with one additional dose after 2 hours if
headache is unresolved or recurs. Maximum, two doses within 24 hours.
*Adjust-a-dose:* For patients with hepatic
or renal impairment, initially 6.25 mg,
with maximum daily dosage of 12.5 mg.

**ACTION**
Not fully understood. Believed to relieve
migraine through selective vasoconstriction of certain cranial blood vessels, inhibition of neuropeptide release, and re-

duced pain transmission down trigeminal
pathway.

| Route | Onset | Peak | Duration |
|-------|-------|------|----------|
| P.O. | 1-3 hr | 1-3 hr | 3-4 hr |

**ADVERSE REACTIONS**
**CNS:** paresthesia, headache, dizziness,
somnolence.
**CV:** *coronary artery vasospasm, transient
myocardial ischemia, MI, ventricular
tachycardia, ventricular fibrillation.*
**GI:** nausea, dry mouth.

**INTERACTIONS**
**Drug-drug.** *MAO inhibitors, verapamil:*
May increase almotriptan level. No dose
adjustment is necessary.
*CYP3A4 inhibitors such as ketoconazole:*
May increase almotriptan level. Monitor
patient for potential adverse reaction. May
need to reduce dosage.
*Ergot-containing drugs, serotonin
5-HT$_{1B/1D}$ agonists:* May cause additive
effects. Avoid using within 24 hours of
almotriptan.
*SSRIs:* May cause additive serotonin effects, resulting in weakness, hyperreflexia,
or incoordination. Monitor patient closely
if given together.

**EFFECTS ON LAB TEST RESULTS**
None reported.

**CONTRAINDICATIONS & CAUTIONS**
● Contraindicated in patients hypersensitive to drug.
● Contraindicated in those with angina
pectoris, history of MI, silent ischemia,
coronary artery vasospasm, Prinzmetal's
variant angina, or other CV disease; uncontrolled hypertension; and hemiplegic
or basilar migraine.
● Don't give within 24 hours after treatment with other 5-HT$_{1B/1D}$ agonists or ergotamine drugs.
● Use cautiously in patients with renal or
hepatic impairment and in those with
cataracts because of the potential for
corneal opacities.

• Use cautiously in patients with risk factors for coronary artery disease (CAD), such as obesity, diabetes, and family history of CAD.

**NURSING CONSIDERATIONS**
• Patients with poor renal or hepatic function should receive a reduced dosage.
• Repeat dose after 2 hours, if needed and don't give more than two doses within 24 hours.
• *Alert:* Don't confuse Axert (almotriptan) with Antivert (meclizine).

**PATIENT TEACHING**
• Tell patient that drug can be taken with or without food.
• Advise patient to take drug only when he's having a migraine; explain that drug isn't taken on a regular schedule.
• Advise patient to use only one repeat dose within 24 hours, no sooner than 2 hours after first dose.
• Advise patient that other commonly prescribed migraine medications can interact with almotriptan.
• Advise patient to report chest or throat tightness, pain, or heaviness.
• Teach patient to avoid possible migraine triggers such as cheese, chocolate, citrus fruits, caffeine, and alcohol.

---

## atomoxetine hydrochloride
Strattera✒

*Pregnancy risk category C*

---

**AVAILABLE FORMS**
*Capsules:* 10 mg, 18 mg, 25 mg, 40 mg, 60 mg

**INDICATIONS & DOSAGES**
➤ **Attention-deficit hyperactivity disorder (ADHD)**
*Adults, children, and adolescents weighing more than 70 kg (154 lb):* Initially, 40 mg P.O. daily; increase after at least 3 days to a total of 80 mg/day P.O., as a single dose in the morning or two evenly divided doses in the morning and late afternoon or early evening. After 2 to 4 weeks, total dosage may be increased to a maximum of 100 mg, if needed.

*Children weighing 70 kg or less:* Initially, 0.5 mg/kg P.O. daily; increase after a minimum of 3 days to a target total daily dose of 1.2 mg/kg P.O. as a single dose in the morning or two evenly divided doses in the morning and late afternoon or early evening. Don't exceed 1.4 mg/kg or 100 mg daily, whichever is less.
*Adjust-a-dose:* In patients with moderate hepatic impairment, reduce to 50% of the normal dose; in those with severe hepatic impairment, reduce to 25% of the normal dose. Poor metabolizers of CYP2D6 may require a reduced dose.

In children weighing less than 70 kg, adjust dosage to 0.5 mg/kg daily and increase to 1.2 mg/kg daily if symptoms don't improve after 4 weeks and if first dose is tolerated. In children and adults weighing more than 70 kg, start at 40 mg daily and increase to 80 mg daily if symptoms don't improve after 4 weeks and if first dose is tolerated.

**ACTION**
Unknown. Thought to be related to selective inhibition of the presynaptic norepinephrine transporter.

| Route | Onset | Peak | Duration |
|-------|-------|------|----------|
| P.O. | Rapid | 1-2 hr | Unknown |

**ADVERSE REACTIONS**
**CNS:** dizziness, *headache,* somnolence, crying, irritability, mood swings, pyrexia, fatigue, *insomnia,* sedation, depression, tremor, early morning awakening, paresthesia, abnormal dreams, sleep disorder.
**CV:** orthostatic hypotension, tachycardia, hypertension, palpitations, hot flashes.
**EENT:** ear infection, rhinorrhea, sore throat, nasal congestion, nasopharyngitis, sinus congestion, mydriasis, sinusitis.
**GI:** *abdominal pain, constipation,* dyspepsia, *nausea, vomiting, decreased appetite,* gastroenteritis, *dry mouth,* flatulence.
**GU:** urinary retention, urinary hesitation, ejaculatory problems, difficulty in micturition, dysmenorrhea, erectile disturbance, impotence, delayed menses, menstrual disorder, prostatitis.
**Metabolic:** weight loss.
**Musculoskeletal:** arthralgia, myalgia.

---

Reactions may be *common,* uncommon, **life-threatening**, or COMMON AND LIFE-THREATENING.

**Respiratory:** *cough,* upper respiratory tract infection.
**Skin:** *dermatitis, pruritus, increased sweating.*
**Other:** influenza, decreased libido, rigors.

## INTERACTIONS
**Drug-drug.** *Albuterol:* May increase CV effects. Use together cautiously.
*MAO inhibitors:* May cause hyperthermia, rigidity, myoclonus, autonomic instability with possible rapid fluctuations of vital signs, and mental status changes. Avoid use within 2 weeks of MAO inhibitor therapy.
*Pressor agents:* May increase blood pressure. Use together cautiously.
*Strong CYP 2D6 inhibitors (paroxetine, fluoxetine, quinidine):* May increase atomoxetine level. Reduce first dose.

## EFFECTS ON LAB TEST RESULTS
None reported.

## CONTRAINDICATIONS & CAUTIONS
• Contraindicated in patients hypersensitive to atomoxetine or to components of drug, in those who have used an MAO inhibitor within the past 2 weeks, and in those with angle-closure glaucoma.
• Use cautiously in patients with hypertension, tachycardia, or CV or cerebrovascular disease, and in pregnant or breast-feeding patients.
• Safety and efficacy haven't been established in patients younger than age 6.

## NURSING CONSIDERATIONS
• Use drug as part of a total treatment program for ADHD, including psychological, educational, and social intervention.
• Effectiveness of treatment lasting longer than 10 weeks hasn't been evaluated. Patients taking drug for extended periods must be reevaluated periodically to determine drug's usefulness.
• Monitor growth during treatment. If growth or weight gain is unsatisfactory, consider interrupting therapy.
• Monitor blood pressure and pulse at baseline, after each dose increase and periodically during treatment.
• Monitor for urinary hesitancy or retention and sexual dysfunction.

• Patient can stop taking drug without tapering off.

## PATIENT TEACHING
• Tell pregnant women, women planning to become pregnant, and breast-feeding women to consult prescriber before taking atomoxetine.
• Tell patient to use caution when operating a vehicle or machinery until the effects of atomoxetine are known.

# bupropion hydrochloride
Zyban⧸

*Pregnancy risk category B*

## AVAILABLE FORMS
*Tablets (sustained-release):* 100 mg, 150 mg, 200 mg

## INDICATIONS & DOSAGES
➤ **Aid to smoking cessation treatment**
*Adults:* 150 mg P.O. daily for 3 days; increased to maximum of 300 mg P.O. daily in two divided doses at least 8 hours apart.

## ACTION
Unknown. Relatively weak inhibitor of the neuronal uptake of norepinephrine, serotonin, and dopamine. Drug doesn't inhibit MAO.

| Route | Onset | Peak | Duration |
|-------|-------|------|----------|
| P.O. | Unknown | 3 hr | Unknown |

## ADVERSE REACTIONS
**CNS:** agitation, asthenia, depression, *dizziness,* fever, headache, *insomnia,* irritability, somnolence, tremor, thinking or dream abnormalities, disturbed concentration, anxiety, nervousness.
**CV: *complete AV block,*** hypertension, hypotension, *tachycardia,* palpitations, hot flashes.
**EENT:** amblyopia, epistaxis, *pharyngitis,* sinusitis, tinnitus, *rhinitis, blurred vision.*
**GI:** *anorexia,* dyspepsia, increased appetite, abdominal pain, *nausea, constipation,* diarrhea, flatulence, *vomiting, dry mouth,* taste perversion, mouth ulcer.
**GU:** urinary frequency.
**Musculoskeletal:** arthralgia, leg cramps and twitching, myalgia, neck pain.

**Respiratory:** bronchitis, increased cough, dyspnea.
**Skin:** dry skin, pruritus, rash, urticaria, *excessive sweating.*
**Other:** allergic reactions, injury.

## INTERACTIONS
**Drug-drug.** *Antidepressants, antipsychotics, systemic corticosteroids, theophylline:* May lower seizure threshold. Use together cautiously.
*Carbamazepine, phenobarbital, phenytoin:* May enhance metabolism of bupropion and decrease its effect. Monitor patient closely.
*Cimetidine:* May inhibit metabolism of bupropion and lead to increased levels. Monitor patient closely.
*Levodopa:* May increase risk of adverse reactions. If used together, give small first doses of bupropion and increase dosage gradually.
*MAO inhibitors (phenelzine):* May increase toxicity. Avoid using within 2 weeks of MAO inhibitor therapy.
*Nicotine-replacement agents:* May cause hypertension. Monitor blood pressure.
*Other drugs containing bupropion (Wellbutrin, Wellbutrin SR):* Contains same active ingredient as bupropion. Avoid using together.
*Ritonavir:* May increase bupropion level. Monitor patient closely for adverse reactions.
**Drug-lifestyle.** *Alcohol use:* May increase risk of seizures. Discourage use together.
*Sun exposure:* Photosensitivity reactions may occur. Advise patient to avoid excessive sunlight exposure.

## EFFECTS ON LAB TEST RESULTS
None reported.

## CONTRAINDICATIONS & CAUTIONS
• Contraindicated in patients allergic to drug or its components, in those with seizure disorders or a current or prior diagnosis of bulimia or anorexia nervosa, and in those being treated with other drugs containing bupropion (such as Wellbutrin and Wellbutrin SR).
• Contraindicated within 2 weeks of MAO inhibitor therapy.
• Use cautiously in patients with recent MI or unstable heart disease.
• Use cautiously in patients with history of seizures, head trauma, or other predisposition to seizures, and in those being treated with drugs that lower seizure threshold.

## NURSING CONSIDERATIONS
• *Alert:* Excessive use of alcohol, abrupt withdrawal from alcohol or other sedatives, and addiction to cocaine, opiates, or stimulants during therapy may increase risk of seizures. Seizure risk is also increased in those using OTC stimulants, in anorectics, and in diabetic patients using oral antidiabetics or insulin.
• *Alert:* Different trade names for separate indications using bupropion exist. Be certain the patient isn't already taking Wellbutrin.
• To reduce seizure risk, don't exceed 300 mg daily. Give 150 mg twice daily so that no single dosage exceeds 150 mg.
• Therapy should stop if patient hasn't made progress toward abstinence by week 7 of therapy.
• Patient can stop taking drug without tapering off.
• Therapy should begin while patient is still smoking; about 1 week is needed to achieve steady-state drug levels.
• *Alert:* Don't confuse bupropion with buspirone.

## PATIENT TEACHING
• Stress importance of combining drug therapy with behavioral interventions, counseling, and support services.
• Advise patient to take doses at least 8 hours apart. If insomnia occurs, tell him not to take dose at bedtime.
• Tell patient not to chew, divide, or crush tablets.
• Tell patient that it may take 1 week for effects of drug to appear, and that he should set a target date for smoking cessation during the second week of therapy.
• Tell patient that treatment usually lasts 7 to 12 weeks.
• Inform patient that tablets may have a characteristic odor.
• Advise patient to avoid alcohol while taking drug.
• Tell patient to avoid hazardous activities that require mental alertness until drug's CNS effects are known.

• Warn patient not to use drug with nicotine patches unless directed by prescriber because this could increase blood pressure.

• Inform patient that risk of seizures increases if he has a seizure or eating disorder, exceeds the recommended dosage, or takes other drugs that either contain bupropion or lower seizure threshold.

• Advise patient to read accompanying patient information before starting drug.

• Advise patient to notify prescriber about planned, suspected, or known pregnancy.

## donepezil hydrochloride
Aricept

*Pregnancy risk category C*

### AVAILABLE FORMS
*Tablets:* 5 mg, 10 mg

### INDICATIONS & DOSAGES
➤ **Mild to moderate Alzheimer's dementia**
*Adults:* Initially, 5 mg P.O. daily h.s. After 4 to 6 weeks, increase to 10 mg daily.

### ACTION
Thought to increase acetylcholine concentration by inhibiting the cholinesterase enzyme, which causes hydrolysis of acetylcholine. May improve cognitive function in patients with Alzheimer's disease.

| Route | Onset | Peak | Duration |
|-------|-------|------|----------|
| P.O. | Unknown | 3-4 hr | Unknown |

### ADVERSE REACTIONS
**CNS:** *headache, insomnia,* dizziness, fatigue, depression, abnormal dreams, somnolence, *seizures,* tremor, irritability, paresthesia, aggression, vertigo, ataxia, restlessness, abnormal crying, nervousness, aphasia, syncope, pain.
**CV:** chest pain, hypertension, vasodilation, atrial fibrillation, hot flashes, hypotension.
**EENT:** cataract, blurred vision, eye irritation, sore throat.
**GI:** *nausea, diarrhea,* vomiting, anorexia, fecal incontinence, GI bleeding, bloating, epigastric pain.
**GU:** urinary frequency.

**Metabolic:** weight loss, dehydration.
**Musculoskeletal:** muscle cramps, arthritis, bone fracture.
**Respiratory:** dyspnea, bronchitis.
**Skin:** pruritus, urticaria, diaphoresis, ecchymoses.
**Other:** toothache, influenza, increased libido.

### INTERACTIONS
**Drug-drug.** *Anticholinergics:* May decrease donepezil effects. Avoid using together.
*Anticholinesterases, cholinomimetics:* May cause synergistic effect. Monitor patient closely.
*Bethanechol, succinylcholine:* May have additive effects. Monitor patient closely.
*Carbamazepine, dexamethasone, phenobarbital, phenytoin, rifampin:* May increase rate of donepezil elimination. Monitor patient.

### EFFECTS ON LAB TEST RESULTS
None reported.

### CONTRAINDICATIONS & CAUTIONS
• Contraindicated in patients hypersensitive to drug or piperidine derivatives and in breast-feeding patients.
• Use cautiously in pregnant patients and in those who take NSAIDs or have CV disease, asthma, obstructive pulmonary disease, urinary outflow impairment, or history of ulcer disease.

### NURSING CONSIDERATIONS
• Monitor patient for evidence of active or occult GI bleeding.
• *Alert:* Don't confuse Aricept with Ascriptin.

### PATIENT TEACHING
• Stress that drug doesn't alter underlying degenerative disease but can temporarily stabilize or relieve symptoms. Effectiveness depends on taking drug at regular intervals.
• Tell caregiver to give drug just before patient's bedtime.
• Advise patient and caregiver to immediately report significant adverse effects or changes in overall health status and to inform health care team that patient is taking drug before he receives anesthesia.

● Tell patient to avoid OTC cold or sleep remedies because of risk of increased anticholinergic effects.

## droperidol
Inapsine

*Pregnancy risk category C*

### AVAILABLE FORMS
*Injection:* 2.5 mg/ml in 1-, 2-, and 5-ml ampules, and 2-, 5-, and 10-ml vials

### INDICATIONS & DOSAGES
➤ **To prevent nausea and vomiting caused by surgical or diagnostic procedures**
*Adults and children older than age 12:* Maximum first dose, 2.5 mg I.M. or slow I.V. Give additional 1.25 mg cautiously, if needed. Give additional doses only if benefit outweighs risk.
*Children ages 2 to 12:* Maximum first dose, 0.1 mg/kg, considering patient's age and other factors. Give additional doses cautiously and only if benefit outweighs risk.
***Adjust-a-dose:*** In elderly or debilitated patients and those who have received other CNS depressant drugs, give reduced dosage.

### I.V. ADMINISTRATION
● Give I.V. doses slowly.
● For high-risk patients, dilute calculated dose in $D_5W$ or lactated Ringer's injection and give as a slow I.V. infusion.

### ACTION
Unknown. Tranquilizes, sedates, and provides antiemetic effects without affecting reflex alertness; also causes mild alpha blockade.

| Route | Onset | Peak | Duration |
|---|---|---|---|
| I.V., I.M. | 3-10 min | 30 min | 2-4 hr |

### ADVERSE REACTIONS
**CNS:** *drowsiness,* restlessness, hyperactivity, anxiety, extrapyramidal symptoms, dizziness, hallucinations, dysphoria, *neuroleptic malignant syndrome.*
**CV:** hypotension, tachycardia.

**Respiratory:** *laryngospasm, bronchospasm.*
**Other:** chills, shivering.

### INTERACTIONS
**Drug-drug.** *CNS depressants:* May cause additive CNS effects. Adjust dosage, as needed.
*Cyclobenzaprine:* May have additive effects on prolonging QT interval. Monitor patient closely.
*Fentanyl citrate:* May cause hypertension and respiratory depression. Use together cautiously.

### EFFECTS ON LAB TEST RESULTS
None reported.

### CONTRAINDICATIONS & CAUTIONS
● Contraindicated in patients hypersensitive to drug.
● Contraindicated in patients with prolonged QT interval, including patients with congenital long QT interval syndrome.
● Use cautiously in those at risk for prolonged QT interval syndrome (those with heart failure, bradycardia, cardiac hypertrophy, hypokalemia, or hypomagnesemia and those taking drugs that prolong QT interval or worsen hypokalemia or hypomagnesemia).
● Use cautiously in patients with hepatic or renal dysfunction and in breast-feeding patients.
● Use with caution in patients with suspected or diagnosed pheochromocytoma because severe hypertension and tachycardia can occur.

### NURSING CONSIDERATIONS
● When used for induction of general anesthesia, give drug with an analgesic.
● If used in procedures such as bronchoscopy, appropriate topical anesthesia is still needed.
● **Alert:** Keep fluids and other measures to manage hypotension readily available.
● Monitor patient for signs and symptoms of neuroleptic malignant syndrome (fever, altered consciousness, extrapyramidal symptoms, tachycardia).
● **Alert:** Don't confuse droperidol with dronabinol.

---

Reactions may be *common,* uncommon, *life-threatening*, or COMMON AND LIFE-THREATENING.

## PATIENT TEACHING
• Warn patient to rise slowly to minimize dizziness.
• Advise patient to avoid alcohol for 24 hours after receiving droperidol.

✳ NEW DRUG

# eletriptan hydrobromide
Relpax✔

*Pregnancy risk category C*

## AVAILABLE FORMS
*Tablets:* 20 mg, 40 mg

## INDICATIONS & DOSAGES
➤ **Acute migraine with or without aura**
*Adults:* 20 to 40 mg P.O. at first migraine symptom. If headache recurs, dose may be repeated at least 2 hours later to a maximum of 80 mg daily.

## ACTION
Binds to $5-HT_1$ receptors and may constrict intracranial blood vessels and inhibit proinflammatory neuropeptide release.

| Route | Onset | Peak | Duration |
|---|---|---|---|
| P.O. | ½ hr | 1½-2 hr | Unknown |

## ADVERSE REACTIONS
**CNS:** *asthenia,* dizziness, headache, hypertonia, hypesthesia, pain, paresthesia, somnolence, vertigo.
**CV:** chest tightness, pain, and pressure; flushing; palpitations.
**EENT:** pharyngitis.
**GI:** abdominal pain, discomfort, or cramps; dry mouth; dyspepsia; dysphagia; nausea.
**Musculoskeletal:** back pain.
**Skin:** increased sweating.
**Other:** chills.

## INTERACTIONS
**Drug-drug.** *CYP 3A4 inhibitors (such as clarithromycin, itraconazole, ketoconazole, nefazodone, nelfinavir, ritonavir, troleandomycin):* May decrease eletriptan metabolism. Avoid use within 72 hours of these drugs.
*Ergotamine-containing or ergot-type drugs (such as dihydroergotamine or methysergide), other $5-HT_1$ agonists:* May

prolong vasospastic reactions. Avoid use within 24 hours of these drugs.

## EFFECTS ON LAB TEST RESULTS
None known.

## CONTRAINDICATIONS & CAUTIONS
• Contraindicated in patients hypersensitive to drug or its components and in those with severe hepatic impairment; ischemic heart disease, such as angina pectoris, a history of MI, or silent ischemia; coronary artery vasospasm, including Prinzmetal's variant angina; and other significant CV conditions.
• Contraindicated in patients with cerebrovascular syndromes, such as CVA or transient ischemic attack; peripheral vascular disease, including ischemic bowel disease; uncontrolled hypertension; or hemiplegic or basilar migraine.
• Contraindicated within 24 hours of another $5-HT_1$ agonist, drug containing ergotamine, or ergot-type drug.
• Contraindicated in patients with risk factors for coronary artery disease (hypertension, hypercholesterolemia, smoking, obesity, diabetes, strong family history of coronary artery disease), in postmenopausal women, and in men older than age 40, unless there's no underlying CV disease. In these patients, give the first dose under medical supervision.
• Safety of treating more than three migraine headaches in 30 days hasn't been established.

## NURSING CONSIDERATIONS
• Drug isn't intended for migraine prevention.
• Use drug only when patient has a clear diagnosis of migraine. If the first use produces no response, reconsider the migraine diagnosis.
• *Alert:* Serious cardiac events including acute MI, arrhythmias, and death occur rarely within a few hours after use of $5-HT_1$ agonists.
• Ophthalmologic effects may occur with long-term use.
• Older patients may develop higher blood pressure than younger patients after taking drug.

## PATIENT TEACHING
• Instruct patient to take dose at the first sign of a migraine headache. If the headache comes back after the first dose, he may take a second dose after 2 hours. Caution patient not to take more than 80 mg in 24 hours.
• Warn patient to avoid driving and operating machinery if he feels dizzy or fatigued after taking the drug.
• Tell patient to immediately report pain, tightness, heaviness, or pressure in the chest, throat, neck, or jaw.

---

# fluvoxamine maleate
Luvox

*Pregnancy risk category C*

---

## AVAILABLE FORMS
*Tablets:* 25 mg, 50 mg, 100 mg

## INDICATIONS & DOSAGES
➤ **Obsessive-compulsive disorder (OCD)**
*Adults:* Initially, 50 mg P.O. daily h.s.; increase by 50 mg q 4 to 7 days. Maximum, 300 mg daily. Give total daily amounts above 100 mg in two divided doses.
*Children ages 8 to 17:* Initially, 25 mg P.O. daily h.s.; increase by 25 mg q 4 to 7 days. Maximum, 200 mg daily for children ages 8 to 11 and 300 mg daily for children ages 11 to 17. Give total daily amounts over 50 mg in two divided doses.
*Adjust-a-dose:* In elderly patients and those with hepatic impairment, give lower first dose and adjust dose more slowly.

## ACTION
Unknown. Selectively inhibits the presynaptic neuronal uptake of serotonin, which may improve OCD.

| Route | Onset | Peak | Duration |
|-------|---------|--------|----------|
| P.O. | Unknown | 3-8 hr | Unknown |

## ADVERSE REACTIONS
**CNS:** *headache, asthenia, somnolence, insomnia, nervousness, dizziness,* tremor, anxiety, hypertonia, *agitation,* depression, CNS stimulation.
**CV:** palpitations, vasodilation.
**EENT:** amblyopia.

**GI:** *nausea, diarrhea, constipation, dyspepsia,* anorexia, *vomiting,* flatulence, dysphagia, *dry mouth,* taste perversion.
**GU:** abnormal ejaculation, urinary frequency, impotence, anorgasmia, urine retention.
**Respiratory:** upper respiratory tract infection, dyspnea, yawning.
**Skin:** sweating.
**Other:** tooth disorder, flulike syndrome, chills, decreased libido.

## INTERACTIONS
**Drug-drug.** *Benzodiazepines, theophylline, warfarin:* May reduce clearance of these drugs. Use together cautiously (except for diazepam, which shouldn't be used with fluvoxamine). Adjust dosage as needed.
*Carbamazepine, clozapine, methadone, metoprolol, propranolol, theophylline, tricyclic antidepressants:* May increase levels of these drugs. Use together cautiously, and monitor patient closely for adverse reactions. Dosage adjustments may be needed.
*Diltiazem:* May cause bradycardia. Monitor heart rate.
*Lithium, tryptophan:* May enhance effects of fluvoxamine. Use together cautiously.
*Pimodize, thioridazine:* May increase risk of prolonged QTc interval. Avoid using together.
*Sumatriptan:* May cause weakness, hyperreflexia, and incoordination. Monitor patient closely.
*MAO inhibitors (phenelzine, selegiline, tranylcypromine):* May cause serotonin syndrome (CNS irritability, shivering, and altered consciousness). Avoid using within 2 weeks of MAO inhibitor therapy.
**Drug-lifestyle.** *Alcohol use:* May increase CNS effects. Discourage use together.
*Smoking:* May decrease drug's effectiveness. Urge patient to stop smoking.

## EFFECTS ON LAB TEST RESULTS
None reported.

## CONTRAINDICATIONS & CAUTIONS
• Contraindicated in patients hypersensitive to drug or to other phenyl piperazine antidepressants, in those receiving pimozide or thioridazine therapy, and within 2 weeks of MAO inhibitor therapy.

---

Reactions may be *common,* uncommon, *life-threatening*, or COMMON AND LIFE-THREATENING.

• Use cautiously in patients with hepatic dysfunction, other conditions that may affect hemodynamic responses or metabolism, or history of mania or seizures.

**NURSING CONSIDERATIONS**
• Record mood changes. Monitor patient for suicidal tendencies.
• **Alert:** Don't confuse Luvox with Lasix, or fluvoxamine with fluoxetine.
• Abruptly stopping drug may cause withdrawal syndrome, with symptoms including headache, muscle ache, and flulike symptoms.

**PATIENT TEACHING**
• Warn patient to avoid hazardous activities until CNS effects of drug are known.
• Tell woman to notify prescriber about planned, suspected, or known pregnancy.
• Tell patient who develops a rash, hives, or a related allergic reaction to notify prescriber.
• Inform patient that several weeks of therapy may be needed to obtain full therapeutic effect. Once improvement occurs, advise patient not to stop drug until directed by prescriber.
• Advise patient to check with prescriber before taking OTC drugs; drug interactions can occur.
• Tell patient drug can be taken with or without food.

## frovatriptan succinate
Frova*✓*

*Pregnancy risk category C*

**AVAILABLE FORMS**
*Tablets:* 2.5 mg

**INDICATIONS & DOSAGES**
➤ **Acute treatment of migraine attacks with or without aura**
*Adults:* 2.5 mg P.O. taken at the first sign of migraine attack. If the headache recurs, a second tablet may be taken at least 2 hours after the first dose. The total daily dose shouldn't exceed 7.5 mg.

**ACTION**
May inhibit excessive dilation of extracerebral and intracranial arteries during migraine headaches.

| Route | Onset | Peak | Duration |
|-------|-------|------|----------|
| P.O. | Unknown | 2-4 hr | Unknown |

**ADVERSE REACTIONS**
**CNS:** dizziness, headache, fatigue, paresthesia, insomnia, anxiety, somnolence, dysesthesia, hypoesthesia, hot or cold sensation, pain.
**CV:** flushing, palpitations, chest pain, *coronary artery vasospasm, transient myocardial ischemia, MI, ventricular tachycardia, ventricular fibrillation.*
**EENT:** abnormal vision, tinnitus, sinusitis, rhinitis.
**GI:** dry mouth, dyspepsia, vomiting, abdominal pain, diarrhea, nausea.
**Musculoskeletal:** skeletal pain.
**Skin:** increased sweating.

**INTERACTIONS**
**Drug-drug.** *5-HT$_1$ agonists:* May cause additive effects. Separate doses by 24 hours.
*Ergotamine-containing or ergot-type medications (such as dihydroergotamine or methysergide):* May cause prolonged vasospastic reactions. Separate doses by 24 hours.
*SSRIs (such as citalopram, fluoxetine, fluvoxamine, paroxetine, sertraline):* May cause weakness, hyperreflexia, and incoordination. Monitor patient closely.

**EFFECTS ON LAB TEST RESULTS**
None reported.

**CONTRAINDICATIONS & CAUTIONS**
• Contraindicated in patients hypersensitive to drug or to any of its components.
• Contraindicated in patients with history or symptoms of ischemic heart disease or coronary artery vasospasm, including Prinzmetal's variant angina; in those with cerebrovascular or peripheral vascular disease, including ischemic bowel disease; in those with uncontrolled hypertension; and in those with hemiplegic or basilar migraine.

• Contraindicated within 24 hours of another 5-HT$_1$ agonist, drug containing ergotamine, or ergot-type drug.

• Contraindicated in patients with coronary artery disease (CAD) risk factors (such as hypertension, hypercholesterolemia, smoking, obesity, strong family history of CAD, postmenopausal women, men older than age 40), unless patient has no underlying CV disease. If drug is used in such a patient, give first dose under medical supervision. Consider obtaining an ECG after the first dose. Intermittent, long-term users of 5-HT$_1$ agonists or those with risk factors should undergo periodic cardiac evaluation while using frovatriptan.

• It's unknown whether drug appears in breast milk. Use cautiously in breast-feeding patients.

## NURSING CONSIDERATIONS

• **Alert:** Serious cardiac events, including acute MI, life-threatening cardiac arrhythmias, and death have been reported within a few hours of administration of 5-HT$_1$ agonists.

• Use drug only when patient has a clear diagnosis of migraine. If a patient has no response for the first migraine attack treated with frovatriptan, reconsider the diagnosis of migraine.

• The safety of treating an average of more than four migraine headaches in a 30-day period hasn't been established.

## PATIENT TEACHING

• Instruct patient to take dose at first sign of migraine headache. If headache comes back after first dose, he may take a second dose after 2 hours. Tell patient not to take more than 3 tablets in 24-hours.

• Caution patient to take extra care or avoid driving and operating machinery if dizziness or fatigue develops after taking drug.

• Stress importance of immediately reporting pain, tightness, heaviness, or pressure in chest, throat, neck, or jaw, or rash or itching after taking drug.

• Instruct the patient not to take drug within 24 hours of taking another serotonin-receptor agonist or ergot-type drug.

# galantamine hydrobromide
Reminyl

*Pregnancy risk category B*

## AVAILABLE FORMS
*Oral solution:* 4 mg/ml
*Tablets:* 4 mg, 8 mg, 12 mg

## INDICATIONS AND DOSAGES
➤ **Mild to moderate Alzheimer's dementia**
*Adults:* Initially, 4 mg b.i.d., preferably with morning and evening meals. If dose is well tolerated after minimum of 4 weeks of therapy, increase dosage to 8 mg b.i.d. A further increase to 12 mg b.i.d. may be attempted, but only after at least 4 weeks of therapy at the previous dosage. Dosage range is 16 to 24 mg daily in two divided doses.
*Adjust-a-dose:* For patients with Child-Pugh score of 7 to 9, dosage usually shouldn't exceed 16 mg daily. Drug isn't recommended for patients with Child-Pugh score of 10 to 15.

For patients with moderate renal impairment, dosage usually shouldn't exceed 16 mg daily. For patients with creatinine clearance less than 9 ml/minute, drug isn't recommended.

## ACTION
Exact mechanism of action is unknown. A competitive and reversible inhibitor of acetylcholinesterase, which is believed to enhance cholinergic function by increasing the level of acetylcholine in the brain.

| Route | Onset | Peak | Duration |
|-------|-------|------|----------|
| P.O. | Unknown | 1 hr | Unknown |

## ADVERSE REACTIONS
**CNS:** depression, dizziness, headache, tremor, insomnia, somnolence, fatigue, syncope.
**CV:** *bradycardia.*
**EENT:** rhinitis.
**GI:** *nausea, vomiting,* anorexia, *diarrhea,* abdominal pain, dyspepsia, anorexia.
**GU:** UTI, hematuria.
**Hematologic:** anemia.
**Metabolic:** weight loss.

---

Reactions may be *common*, uncommon, *life-threatening*, or COMMON AND LIFE-THREATENING.

## INTERACTIONS

**Drug-drug.** *Amitriptyline, fluoxetine, fluvoxamine, quinidine:* May decrease galantamine clearance. Monitor patient closely.

*Anticholinergics:* May antagonize anticholinergic activity. Monitor patient.

*Cholinergics (such as bethanechol, succinylcholine):* May have synergistic effect. Monitor patient closely. May need to avoid use before procedures using general anesthesia with succinylcholine-type neuromuscular blockers.

*Cimetidine, clarithromycin, erythromycin, ketoconazole, paroxetine:* May increase galantamine bioavailability. Monitor patient closely.

## EFFECTS ON LAB TEST RESULTS
None reported.

## CONTRAINDICATIONS & CAUTIONS
• Contraindicated in patients hypersensitive to drug or its components.
• Use cautiously in patients with supraventricular cardiac conduction disorders and in those taking other drugs that significantly slow heart rate.
• Use cautiously during or before procedures involving anesthesia using succinylcholine-type or similar neuromuscular blockers.
• Use cautiously in patients with history of peptic ulcer disease and in those taking NSAIDs. Because of the potential for cholinomimetic effects, use cautiously in patients with bladder outflow obstruction, seizures, asthma, or COPD.
• Safety and efficacy in children haven't been established.

## NURSING CONSIDERATIONS
• Bradycardia and heart block may occur in patients with and without underlying cardiac conduction abnormalities. Consider all patients at risk for adverse effects on cardiac conduction.
• Give drug with food and antiemetics and ensure adequate fluid intake to decrease the risk of nausea and vomiting.
• Use proper technique when dispensing the oral solution with the pipette. Dispense measured amount in a nonalcoholic beverage and give right away.

• If drug is stopped for several days or longer, restart at the lowest dose and gradually increase, at 4-week or longer intervals, to the previous dosage level.
• Because of the risk of increased gastric acid secretion, monitor patients closely for symptoms of active or occult GI bleeding, especially those with an increased risk of developing ulcers.

## PATIENT TEACHING
• Advise caregiver to give drug with morning and evening meals.
• Inform patient that nausea and vomiting are common adverse effects.
• Teach caregiver the proper technique when measuring the oral solution with the pipette. Place measured amount in a nonalcoholic beverage and have patient drink right away.
• Urge patient or caregiver to report slow heartbeat immediately.
• Advise patient and caregiver that although drug may improve cognitive function, it doesn't alter the underlying disease process.

---

## lithium carbonate
Carbolith†, Duralith†, Eskalith, Eskalith CR, Lithane, Lithicarb‡, Lithizine†, Lithobid, Lithonate, Lithotabs, Quilonum SR‡

## lithium citrate
Cibalith-S*

*Pregnancy risk category D*

---

## AVAILABLE FORMS
**lithium carbonate**
*Capsules:* 150 mg, 300 mg, 600 mg
*Tablets:* 250 mg‡, 300 mg (300 mg equals 8.12 mEq lithium)
*Tablets (controlled-release):* 300 mg, 450 mg
**lithium citrate**
*Syrup (sugarless):* 8 mEq lithium/5 ml
Lithium citrate liquid 5 ml contains 8 mEq lithium, equal to 300 mg lithium carbonate.

## INDICATIONS & DOSAGES
➤ **To prevent or control mania**
*Adults:* 300 to 600 mg P.O. up to q.i.d. Or, 900-mg controlled-release tablets P.O. q 12 hours. Increase dosage based on blood levels to achieve optimal dosage. Recommended therapeutic lithium levels are 1.0 to 1.5 mEq/L for acute mania and 0.6 to 1.2 mEq/L for maintenance therapy.

## ACTION
Unknown. Probably alters chemical transmitters in the CNS, possibly by interfering with ionic pump mechanisms in brain cells, and may compete with or replace sodium ions.

| Route | Onset | Peak | Duration |
|-------|-------|------|----------|
| P.O. | Unknown | 30 min-3 hr | Unknown |

## ADVERSE REACTIONS
**CNS:** tremors, drowsiness, headache, confusion, restlessness, dizziness, psychomotor retardation, *lethargy, coma,* blackouts, *epileptiform seizures,* EEG changes, worsened organic mental syndrome, impaired speech, ataxia, incoordination, *fatigue.*
**CV:** reversible ECG changes, *arrhythmias,* hypotension, *bradycardia.*
**EENT:** tinnitus, blurred vision.
**GI:** dry mouth, metallic taste, nausea, *vomiting, anorexia, diarrhea, thirst,* abdominal pain, flatulence, indigestion.
**GU:** *polyuria,* glycosuria, decreased creatinine clearance, albuminuria, *renal toxicity* with long-term use.
**Hematologic:** *leukocytosis with leukocyte count of 14,000 to 18,000/mm³.*
**Metabolic:** transient hyperglycemia; goiter; hypothyroidism, hyponatremia.
**Musculoskeletal:** *muscle weakness.*
**Skin:** pruritus, rash, diminished or absent sensation, drying and thinning of hair, psoriasis, acne, alopecia.
**Other:** ankle and wrist edema.

## INTERACTIONS
**Drug-drug.** *ACE inhibitors:* May increase lithium level. Monitor lithium level; adjust lithium dosage, as needed.
*Aminophylline, sodium bicarbonate, urine alkalinizers:* May increase lithium excretion. Avoid excessive salt, and monitor lithium levels.

*Calcium channel blockers (verapamil):* May decrease lithium levels and may increase risk of neurotoxicity. Use together cautiously.
*Carbamazepine, fluoxetine, methyldopa, NSAIDs, probenecid:* May increase effect of lithium. Monitor patient for lithium toxicity.
*Neuromuscular blockers:* May cause prolonged paralysis or weakness. Monitor patient closely.
*Thiazide diuretics:* May increase reabsorption of lithium by kidneys, with possible toxic effect. Use with caution, and monitor lithium and electrolyte levels (especially sodium).
**Drug-food.** *Caffeine:* May decrease lithium level and drug effect. Advise patient who ingests large amounts of caffeine to tell prescriber before stopping caffeine. Adjust lithium dosage, as needed.

## EFFECTS ON LAB TEST RESULTS
• May increase glucose and creatinine levels. May decrease sodium, $T_3$, $T_4$, and protein-bound iodine levels.
• May increase $^{131}I$ uptake and WBC and neutrophil counts.

## CONTRAINDICATIONS & CAUTIONS
• Contraindicated if therapy can't be closely monitored.
• Avoid using in pregnant patient unless benefits outweigh risks.
• Use with caution in patients receiving neuromuscular blockers and diuretics; in elderly or debilitated patients; and in patients with thyroid disease, seizure disorder, infection, renal or CV disease, severe debilitation or dehydration, or sodium depletion.

## NURSING CONSIDERATIONS
• Lithane may contain tartrazine.
• *Alert:* Determination of lithium level is crucial to safe use of drug. Don't use drug in patients who can't have regular tests. Monitor lithium level 8 to 12 hours after first dose, the morning before second dose is given, two or three times weekly for the first month, then weekly to monthly during maintenance therapy.
• When level of lithium is below 1.5 mEq/L, adverse reactions are usually mild.

• Monitor baseline ECG, thyroid studies, renal studies, and electrolyte levels.
• Check fluid intake and output, especially when surgery is scheduled.
• Weigh patient daily; check for edema or sudden weight gain.
• Adjust fluid and salt ingestion to compensate if excessive loss occurs from protracted diaphoresis or diarrhea. Under normal conditions, patient fluid intake should be 2½ to 3 L daily and he should follow a balanced diet with adequate salt intake.
• Check urine specific gravity and report level below 1.005, which may indicate diabetes insipidus.
• Drug alters glucose tolerance in diabetics. Monitor glucose level closely.
• Perform outpatient follow-up of thyroid and renal functions every 6 to 12 months. Palpate thyroid to check for enlargement.
• *Alert:* Don't confuse Lithobid with Levbid, Lithonate with Lithostat, or Lithotabs with Lithobid or Lithostat.

## PATIENT TEACHING
• Tell patient to take drug with plenty of water and after meals to minimize GI upset.
• Explain that lithium has a narrow therapeutic margin of safety. A level that's even slightly high can be dangerous.
• Warn patient and caregivers to expect transient nausea, large amounts of urine, thirst, and discomfort during first few days of therapy and to watch for evidence of toxicity (diarrhea, vomiting, tremor, drowsiness, muscle weakness, incoordination).
• Instruct patient to withhold one dose and call prescriber if signs and symptoms of toxicity appear, but not to stop drug abruptly.
• Warn patient to avoid hazardous activities that require alertness and good psychomotor coordination until CNS effects of drug are known.
• Tell patient not to switch brands of lithium or take other prescription or OTC drugs without prescriber's guidance.
• Tell patient to wear or carry medical identification at all times.

✳ *NEW DRUG*

# memantine hydrochloride
Namenda

*Pregnancy risk category B*

## AVAILABLE FORMS
*Tablets:* 5 mg, 10 mg

## INDICATIONS & DOSAGES
➤ **Moderate to severe dementia of the Alzheimer's type**
*Adults:* Initially, 5 mg P.O. once daily. Increase by 5 mg/day q week until target dose is reached. Maximum, 10 mg P.O. b.i.d. Doses greater than 5 mg should be divided b.i.d.
*Adjust-a-dose:* Reduce dosage in patients with moderate renal impairment.

## ACTION
Antagonizes N-methyl-D-aspartate (NMDA) receptors, the persistent activation of which seems to increase Alzheimer's symptoms.

| Route | Onset | Peak | Duration |
|-------|-------|------|----------|
| P.O. | Unknown | 3-7 hr | Unknown |

## ADVERSE REACTIONS
**CNS:** aggressiveness, agitation, anxiety, ataxia, confusion, *CVA,* depression, dizziness, fatigue, hallucinations, headache, hypokinesia, insomnia, pain, somnolence, syncope, transient ischemic attack, vertigo.
**CV:** edema, *heart failure,* hypertension.
**EENT:** cataracts, conjunctivitis.
**GI:** anorexia, constipation, diarrhea, nausea, vomiting.
**GU:** incontinence, urinary frequency, UTI.
**Hematologic:** anemia.
**Metabolic:** weight loss.
**Musculoskeletal:** arthralgia, back pain.
**Respiratory:** bronchitis, coughing, dyspnea, flulike symptoms, pneumonia, upper respiratory tract infection.
**Skin:** rash.
**Other:** abnormal gait, falls, injury.

## INTERACTIONS
**Drug-drug.** *Cimetidine, hydrochlorothiazide, quinidine, ranitidine, triamterene:* May alter levels of both drugs. Monitor patient.

*NMDA antagonists (amantadine, dextromethorphan, ketamine):* Combined use not studied. Use together cautiously.
*Urine alkalinizers (carbonic anhydrase inhibitors, sodium bicarbonate):* May decrease memantine clearance. Monitor patient for adverse effects.
**Drug-herb.** *Herbs that alkalinize urine:* May increase drug level and adverse effects. Use together cautiously.
**Drug-food.** *Foods that alkalinize urine:* May increase drug level and adverse effects. Use together cautiously.
**Drug-lifestyle.** *Alcohol use:* May alter drug adherence, decrease its effectiveness, or increase adverse effects. Discourage use together.
*Nicotine:* May alter levels of drug and nicotine. Discourage use together.

**EFFECTS ON LAB TEST RESULTS**
● May increase alkaline phosphatase level.
● May decrease hemoglobin and hematocrit.

**CONTRAINDICATIONS & CAUTIONS**
● Contraindicated in patients allergic to drug or its components.
● Not recommended for patients with severe renal impairment.
● Use cautiously in patients with seizures, hepatic impairment, or moderate renal impairment.
● Use cautiously in patients who may have an increased urine pH (from drugs, diet, renal tubular acidosis, or severe UTI, for example).

**NURSING CONSIDERATIONS**
● Memantine isn't indicated for mild Alzheimer's disease or other types of dementia.
● The effects of memantine on a fetus haven't been adequately studied. Give memantine to pregnant patient only if benefit justifies use.
● Use cautiously in breast-feeding patients; it's unknown if drug appears in breast milk.
● In elderly patients, even those with a normal creatinine level, use of this drug may impair renal function. Estimate creatinine clearance; reduce dosage in patients with moderate renal impairment. Don't

give drug to patients with severe renal impairment.

**PATIENT TEACHING**
● Explain that memantine doesn't cure Alzheimer's disease but may improve the symptoms.
● Tell patient to report adverse effects.
● Urge patient to avoid alcohol during treatment.
● To avoid possible interactions, advise patient not to take herbal or OTC products without consulting prescriber.

## naratriptan hydrochloride
Amerge, Naramig‡

*Pregnancy risk category C*

**AVAILABLE FORMS**
*Tablets:* 1 mg, 2.5 mg

**INDICATIONS & DOSAGES**
➤ **Acute migraine attacks with or without aura**
*Adults:* 1 or 2.5 mg P.O. as a single dosage. If headache returns or responds only partially, dose may be repeated after 4 hours. Maximum, 5 mg in 24 hours.
*Adjust-a-dose:* For patients with mild to moderate renal or hepatic impairment, reduce dosage. Maximum, 2.5 mg in 24 hours.

**ACTION**
May selectively activate serotonin receptors in intracranial blood vessels, resulting in vasoconstriction and migraine headache relief. Or the inhibition of neuropeptide release may reduce pain transmission in the trigeminal pathways.

| Route | Onset | Peak | Duration |
|-------|-------|------|----------|
| P.O. | Unknown | 2-3 hr | Unknown |

**ADVERSE REACTIONS**
**CNS:** paresthesia, dizziness, drowsiness, malaise, fatigue, vertigo, syncope.
**CV:** palpitations, increased blood pressure, *tachyarrhythmias, abnormal ECG changes, coronary artery vasospasm, transient myocardial ischemia, MI, ventricular tachycardia, ventricular fibrillation.*

---

Reactions may be *common,* uncommon, *life-threatening,* or COMMON AND LIFE-THREATENING.

**EENT:** ear, nose, and throat infections; photophobia.
**GI:** nausea, hyposalivation, vomiting.
**Other:** sensations of warmth, cold, pressure, tightness, or heaviness.

## INTERACTIONS
**Drug-drug.** *Ergot-containing or ergot-type drugs (dihydroergotamine, methysergide), other 5-HT$_1$ agonists:* May prolong vasospastic reactions. Avoid using within 24 hours of naratriptan.
*Hormonal contraceptives:* May slightly increase naratriptan level. Monitor patient.
*SSRIs (fluoxetine, fluvoxamine, paroxetine, sertraline):* May cause weakness, hyperreflexia, and incoordination. Monitor patient.
**Drug-herb.** *St. John's wort:* May increase serotonergic effect. Discourage use together.
**Drug-lifestyle.** *Smoking:* May increase naratriptan clearance. Discourage use together.

## EFFECTS ON LAB TEST RESULTS
None reported.

## CONTRAINDICATIONS & CAUTIONS
● Contraindicated in patients hypersensitive to drug or its components, in those with prior or current cardiac ischemia, in those with cerebrovascular or peripheral vascular syndromes, and in those with uncontrolled hypertension.
● Contraindicated in elderly patients, patients with creatinine clearance below 15 ml/minute, patients with Child-Pugh grade C, and patients who have used ergot-containing, ergot-type, or other 5-HT$_1$ agonists within 24 hours.
● Use cautiously in patients with risk factors for coronary artery disease, such as hypertension, hypercholesterolemia, obesity, diabetes, or strong family history of coronary artery disease.
● Use cautiously in postmenopausal women, in men older than age 40, and in patients who smoke, unless patient is free from cardiac disease. If patient has cardiac risk factors but satisfactory CV evaluation results, monitor him closely after first dose.
● Use cautiously in patients with renal or hepatic impairment.

## NURSING CONSIDERATIONS
● Assess cardiac status in patients who develop risk factors for coronary artery disease.
● *Alert:* Drug can cause coronary artery vasospasm and increased risk of cerebrovascular events.
● Drug isn't intended to prevent migraines or manage hemiplegic or basilar migraine.
● Safety and effectiveness of treating cluster headaches or more than four headaches in a 30-day period haven't been established.
● Use drug only when patient has a clear diagnosis of migraine.

## PATIENT TEACHING
● Instruct patient to take drug only as prescribed and to read the accompanying patient instruction leaflet before using drug.
● Tell patient that drug is intended to relieve, not prevent, migraines.
● Instruct patient to take dose soon after headache starts. If no response occurs with first tablet, tell patient to seek medical approval before taking second tablet. Tell patient that if more relief is needed after first tablet (if a partial response occurs or headache returns), and prescriber has approved a second dose, he may take a second tablet (but not sooner than 4 hours after first tablet). Tell him not to exceed two tablets within 24 hours.
● Advise patient to increase fluid intake.
● Advise patient not to use drug if she suspects or knows that she's pregnant.
● Tell patient to alert prescriber about bothersome adverse effects.

# propofol
Diprivan

*Pregnancy risk category B*

## AVAILABLE FORMS
*Injection:* 10 mg/ml in 20-ml ampules; 50-ml prefilled syringes; 50-ml and 100-ml infusion vials

## INDICATIONS & DOSAGES
➤ **To induce anesthesia**
*Adults younger than age 55 classified as American Society of Anesthesiologists (ASA) Physical Status (PS) category I or*

*II:* 2 to 2.5 mg/kg. Give in 40-mg boluses q 10 seconds until desired response is achieved.

*Children ages 3 to 16 classified as ASA I or II:* 2.5 to 3.5 mg/kg over 20 to 30 seconds.

**Adjust-a-dose:** In geriatric, debilitated, hypovolemic, or ASA PS III or IV patients, give half the usual induction dose, in 20-mg boluses, q 10 seconds. For cardiac anesthesia, give 20 mg (0.5 to 1.5 mg/kg) q 10 seconds until desired response is achieved. For neurosurgical patients, give 20 mg (1 to 2 mg/kg) q 10 seconds until desired response is achieved.

➤ **To maintain anesthesia**
*Healthy adults younger than age 55:* 0.1 to 0.2 mg/kg/minute (6 to 12 mg/kg/hour). Or, give in 20- to 50-mg intermittent boluses, p.r.n.
*Healthy children ages 2 months to 16 years:* 125 to 300 mcg/kg/minute (7.5 to 18 mg/kg/hour).

**Adjust-a-dose:** In geriatric, debilitated, hypovolemic, or ASA PS III or IV patients, give half the usual maintenance dose (0.05 to 0.1 mg/kg/minute or 3 to 6 mg/kg/hour). For cardiac anesthesia with secondary opioid, 100 to 150 mcg/kg/minute; low dose with primary opioid, 50 to 100 mcg/kg/minute. For neurosurgical patients, 100 to 200 mcg/kg/minute (6 to 12 mg/kg/hour).

➤ **Monitored anesthesia care**
*Healthy adults younger than age 55:* Initially, 100 to 150 mcg/kg/minute (6 to 9 mg/kg/hour) for 3 to 5 minutes or a slow injection of 0.5 mg/kg over 3 to 5 minutes. For maintenance dose, give infusion of 25 to 75 mcg/kg/minute (1.5 to 4.5 mg/kg/hour), or incremental 10- or 20-mg boluses.

**Adjust-a-dose:** In geriatric, debilitated, or ASA PS III or IV patients, give 80% of usual adult maintenance dose. Don't use rapid bolus.

➤ **To sedate intubated intensive care unit (ICU) patients**
*Adults:* Initially, 5 mcg/kg/minute (0.3 mg/kg/hour) for 5 minutes. Increments of 5 to 10 mcg/kg/minute (0.3 to 0.6 mg/kg/hour) over 5 to 10 minutes may be used until desired sedation is achieved. Maintenance rate, 5 to 50 mcg/kg/minute (0.3 to 3 mg/kg/hour).

**I.V. ADMINISTRATION**
● Maintain strict aseptic technique when handling the solution. Drug can support the growth of microorganisms; don't use if solution might be contaminated.
● Allow an adequate time interval (3 to 5 minutes) between dosage adjustments to assess effects.
● Protect drug from light. Shake well. Dilute only with D₅W. Don't dilute to less than 2 g/ml. Don't infuse through a filter with a pore size smaller than 5 microns. Give via larger veins in arms to decrease injection site pain.
● Don't mix drug with other therapeutic drugs before infusion.
● Don't give drug in same I.V. line as blood or plasma. Discard tubing and unused portions of drug after 12 hours.
● Don't use if phases of emulsion show evidence of separation.

**ACTION**
Unknown. Rapid-acting I.V. sedative-hypnotic.

| Route | Onset | Peak | Duration |
|---|---|---|---|
| I.V. | < 40 sec | Unknown | 10-15 min |

**ADVERSE REACTIONS**
**CNS:** movement.
**CV: *bradycardia,*** hypotension, hypertension, decreased cardiac output.
**Metabolic:** hyperlipemia.
**Respiratory:** APNEA, respiratory acidosis.
**Skin:** rash.
**Other:** *burning or stinging at injection site.*

**INTERACTIONS**
**Drug-drug.** *Inhaled anesthetics (such as enflurane, halothane, isoflurane), opioids (alfentanil, fentanyl, meperidine, morphine), sedatives (such as barbiturates, benzodiazepines, chloral hydrate, droperidol):* May increase anesthetic and sedative effects and further decrease blood pressure and cardiac output. Monitor patient closely.
**Drug-herb.** *St. John's wort:* May prolong anesthetic effects. Advise patient to stop using herb 5 days before surgery.

**EFFECTS ON LAB TEST RESULTS**
● May increase lipid levels.

## CONTRAINDICATIONS & CAUTIONS

• Contraindicated in patients hypersensitive to drug or its components (including egg lecithin, soybean oil, and glycerol) and in those unable to undergo general anesthesia or sedation.
• Use cautiously in patients who are hemodynamically unstable or who have seizures, disorders of lipid metabolism, or increased intracranial pressure.
• Contraindicated in pregnant women because it may cause fetal depression.
• Because drug appears in breast milk, avoid using in breast-feeding patients.

## NURSING CONSIDERATIONS

• Urine may turn green if drug is used for prolonged sedation in ICU.
• Titrate drug daily to maintain minimum effective level.
• For general anesthesia or monitored anesthesia care sedation, trained staff not involved in the surgical or diagnostic procedure should give drug. For ICU sedation, persons skilled in managing critically ill patients and trained in cardiopulmonary resuscitation and airway management should give drug.
• Continuously monitor vital signs.
• Monitor patient at risk for hyperlipidemia for elevated triglyceride levels.
• Drug contains 0.1 g of fat (1.1 kcal)/ml. Reduce other lipid products if given together.
• Drug contains ethylenediamine-tetraacetic acid, a strong metal chelator. Consider supplemental zinc during prolonged therapy.
• When giving drug in the ICU, assess patient's CNS function daily to determine minimum dose needed.
• Stop drug gradually to prevent abrupt awakening and increased agitation.
• **Alert:** Don't confuse Diprivan with Diprivefrin.

## PATIENT TEACHING

• Advise patient that performance of activities requiring mental alertness may be impaired for some time after drug use.

# rivastigmine tartrate
Exelon

*Pregnancy risk category B*

## AVAILABLE FORMS

*Capsules:* 1.5 mg, 3 mg, 4.5 mg, 6 mg

## INDICATIONS & DOSAGES

➤ **Symptomatic treatment of patients with mild to moderate Alzheimer's disease**
*Adults:* Initially, 1.5 mg P.O. b.i.d. with food. If tolerated, may increase to 3 mg b.i.d. after 2 weeks. Following 2 weeks at this dose, may increase to 4.5 mg b.i.d. and 6 mg b.i.d., as tolerated. Effective dosage range is 6 to 12 mg daily; maximum, 12 mg daily.

## ACTION

Thought to increase acetylcholine concentration by reversibly inhibiting the cholinesterase enzyme, which causes hydrolysis of acetylcholine. This may result in some memory improvement.

| Route | Onset | Peak | Duration |
|-------|-------|------|----------|
| P.O. | Unknown | 1 hr | 12 hr |

## ADVERSE REACTIONS

**CNS:** syncope, fatigue, asthenia, malaise, *dizziness, headache,* somnolence, tremor, insomnia, confusion, depression, anxiety, hallucinations, aggressive reaction, vertigo, agitation, nervousness, delusion, paranoid reaction.
**CV:** hypertension, chest pain, peripheral edema.
**EENT:** rhinitis, pharyngitis.
**GI:** *nausea, vomiting, diarrhea, anorexia, abdominal pain,* dyspepsia, constipation, flatulence, eructation.
**GU:** UTI, urinary incontinence.
**Metabolic:** weight loss.
**Musculoskeletal:** back pain, arthralgia, bone fracture.
**Respiratory:** upper respiratory tract infection, cough, bronchitis.
**Skin:** increased sweating, rash.
**Other:** *accidental trauma,* flulike symptoms, pain.

## INTERACTIONS
**Drug-drug.** *Bethanechol, succinylcholine, other neuromuscular blocking drugs or cholinergic antagonists:* May have synergistic effect. Monitor patient closely.
**Drug-lifestyle.** *Smoking:* May increase rivastigmine clearance. Discourage use together.

## EFFECTS ON LAB TEST RESULTS
None reported.

## CONTRAINDICATIONS & CAUTIONS
• Contraindicated in patients hypersensitive to drug, other carbamate derivatives, or other components of the drug.

## NURSING CONSIDERATIONS
• Expect significant GI adverse effects (such as nausea, vomiting, anorexia, and weight loss). These effects are less common during maintenance doses.
• Monitor patient for evidence of active or occult GI bleeding.
• Dramatic memory improvement is unlikely. As disease progresses, the benefits of rivastigmine may decline.
• Monitor patient for severe nausea, vomiting, and diarrhea, which may lead to dehydration and weight loss.
• Carefully monitor patient with a history of GI bleeding, NSAID use, arrhythmias, seizures, or pulmonary conditions for adverse effects.

## PATIENT TEACHING
• Tell caregiver to give rivastigmine with food in the morning and evening.
• Advise patient that memory improvement may be subtle and that drug more likely slows memory loss.
• Tell patient to report nausea, vomiting, or diarrhea.
• Tell patient to consult prescriber before using OTC medications.

---

## rizatriptan benzoate
Maxalt, Maxalt-MLT

*Pregnancy risk category C*

## AVAILABLE FORMS
*Tablets:* 5 mg, 10 mg

*Tablets (orally disintegrating):* 5 mg, 10 mg

## INDICATIONS & DOSAGES
➤ **Acute migraine headaches with or without aura**
*Adults:* Initially, 5 or 10 mg P.O. If first dose is ineffective, another dose can be given at least 2 hours after first. Maximum, 30 mg in a 24-hour period. For patients receiving propranolol, 5 mg P.O. up to maximum of 15 mg in 24 hours.

## ACTION
May act as an agonist at serotonin receptors on extracerebral intracranial blood vessels, which constricts the affected vessels, inhibits neuropeptide release, and reduces pain transmission in the trigeminal pathways.

| Route | Onset | Peak | Duration |
|-------|-------|------|----------|
| P.O. | Unknown | 60-90 min | Unknown |

## ADVERSE REACTIONS
**CNS:** dizziness, headache, somnolence, paresthesia, asthenia, fatigue, decreased mental acuity, euphoria, tremor, pain.
**CV:** chest pain, pressure, or heaviness, palpitations, flushing, *coronary artery vasospasm, transient myocardial ischemia, MI, ventricular tachycardia, ventricular fibrillation.*
**EENT:** neck, throat, and jaw pain.
**GI:** dry mouth, nausea, diarrhea, vomiting.
**Respiratory:** dyspnea.
**Other:** hot flashes, warm or cold feelings.

## INTERACTIONS
**Drug-drug.** *Ergot-containing or ergot-type drugs (dihydroergotamine, methysergide), other 5-HT₁ agonists:* May prolong vasospastic reactions. Avoid using within 24 hours of rizatriptan.
*MAO inhibitors:* May increase rizatriptan level. Avoid using within 2 weeks of MAO inhibitor therapy.
*Propranolol:* May increase rizatriptan level. Reduce rizatriptan dose to 5 mg.
*SSRIs (fluoxetine, fluvoxamine, paroxetine, sertraline):* May cause weakness, hyperreflexia, and incoordination. Monitor patient.

---

## EFFECTS ON LAB TEST RESULTS
None reported.

## CONTRAINDICATIONS & CAUTIONS
• Contraindicated in patients hypersensitive to drug or its components and in those with a history or symptoms of ischemic heart disease, coronary artery vasospasm (Prinzmetal's variant angina), or other significant underlying CV disease.
• Contraindicated in patients with uncontrolled hypertension; within 24 hours of another 5-HT$_1$ agonist, drug containing ergotamine, or ergot-type drug, such as dihydroergotamine or methysergide; or within 2 weeks of MAO inhibitor therapy.
• Contraindicated in patients with hemiplegic or basilar migraine.
• Use cautiously in patients with risk factors for coronary artery disease (hypertension, hypercholesterolemia, smoking, obesity, diabetes, strong family history of coronary artery disease, postmenopausal women, or men older than age 40), unless patient is free from cardiac disease. Monitor patient closely after first dose.
• Use cautiously in patients with hepatic or renal impairment.
• Safety of treating more than four headaches in a 30-day period hasn't been established.
• Safety and effectiveness in children is unknown.

## NURSING CONSIDERATIONS
• Assess CV status in patients who develop risk factors for coronary artery disease during treatment.
• Use drug only when patient has a clear diagnosis of migraine.
• Don't use drug to prevent migraines or to treat hemiplegic or basilar migraine or cluster headaches.
• The orally disintegrating tablets contain phenylalanine.

## PATIENT TEACHING
• Inform patient that drug doesn't prevent migraine headache.
• For Maxalt-MLT, tell patient to remove blister pack from pouch and remove drug from blister pack immediately before use. Tablet shouldn't be popped out of blister pack; tell patient to carefully peel away package with dry hands, place tablet on tongue, and allow tablet to dissolve. Tablet is then swallowed with saliva. No water is needed or recommended. Tell patient that orally dissolving tablet doesn't relieve headache more quickly.
• Advise patient that, if headache returns after first dose, he may take a second dose at least 2 hours after the first dose. Warn against taking more than 30 mg in a 24-hour period.
• Inform patient that drug may cause sleepiness and dizziness, and warn him to avoid hazardous activities until effects are known.
• Tell patient that food may delay onset of drug action.
• Advise patient to notify prescriber about suspected or known pregnancy.
• Instruct patient not to breast-feed during therapy because effects on the infant are unknown.

---

# sibutramine hydrochloride monohydrate
Meridia

*Pregnancy risk category C*
*Controlled substance schedule IV*

## AVAILABLE FORMS
*Capsules:* 5 mg, 10 mg, 15 mg

## INDICATIONS & DOSAGES
➤ **To manage obesity**
*Adults:* 10 mg P.O. given once daily with or without food. May increase to 15 mg P.O. daily after 4 weeks if weight loss is inadequate. Patients who don't tolerate 10 mg daily may receive 5 mg P.O. daily. Don't exceed 15 mg daily.

## ACTION
Inhibits reuptake of norepinephrine, and to a lesser extent, serotonin and dopamine.

| Route | Onset | Peak | Duration |
|-------|-------|------|----------|
| P.O. | Unknown | 3-4 hr | Unknown |

## ADVERSE REACTIONS
**CNS:** *headache, insomnia,* dizziness, nervousness, anxiety, depression, paresthesia, somnolence, CNS stimulation, emotional lability, asthenia, migraine.

**CV:** tachycardia, vasodilation, hypertension, palpitations, chest pain.
**EENT:** *rhinitis, pharyngitis,* sinusitis, ear disorder, ear pain.
**GI:** *anorexia, constipation,* increased appetite, nausea, dyspepsia, gastritis, vomiting, *dry mouth,* taste perversion, abdominal pain, rectal disorder.
**GU:** dysmenorrhea, UTI, vaginal candidiasis, metrorrhagia.
**Musculoskeletal:** arthralgia, myalgia, tenosynovitis, joint disorder, neck or back pain.
**Respiratory:** increased cough, laryngitis.
**Skin:** rash, sweating, acne.
**Other:** herpes simplex, flulike syndrome, accidental injury, allergic reaction, generalized edema.

**INTERACTIONS**
**Drug-drug.** *CNS depressants:* May enhance CNS depression. Use together cautiously.
*Dextromethorphan, dihydroergotamine, fentanyl, fluoxetine, fluvoxamine, lithium, MAO inhibitors, meperidine, paroxetine, pentazocine, sertraline, sumatriptan, tryptophan, venlafaxine:* May cause hyperthermia, tachycardia, and loss of consciousness. Avoid using together.
*Ephedrine, pseudoephedrine:* May increase blood pressure or heart rate. Use together cautiously.
**Drug-lifestyle.** *Alcohol use:* May enhance CNS depression. Discourage use together.

**EFFECTS ON LAB TEST RESULTS**
• May increase ALT, AST, GGT, LDH, alkaline phosphatase, and bilirubin levels.

**CONTRAINDICATIONS & CAUTIONS**
• Contraindicated in patients hypersensitive to drug or its active ingredients, in those taking MAO inhibitors or other centrally acting appetite suppressants, and in those with anorexia nervosa.
• Contraindicated in patients with severe renal or hepatic dysfunction, history of hypertension, coronary artery disease, heart failure, arrhythmias, or CVA.
• Contraindicated in elderly patients.
• Use cautiously in patients with history of seizures or angle-closure glaucoma.

**NURSING CONSIDERATIONS**
• Drug is recommended for obese patients with a body mass index of 30 kg/m² or more (27 kg/m² or more if patient has other risk factors, such as hypertension, diabetes, or dyslipidemia).
• Rule out organic causes of obesity before starting therapy.
• Measure blood pressure and pulse before starting therapy, with dosage changes, and at regular intervals during therapy.
• Avoid using within 2 weeks of MAO inhibitor therapy.

**PATIENT TEACHING**
• Advise patient to report rash, hives, or other allergic reactions immediately.
• Instruct patient to notify prescriber before taking other prescription or OTC drugs.
• Advise patient to have blood pressure and pulse monitored at regular intervals. Stress importance of regular follow-up visits with health care provider.
• Advise patient to follow a reduced-calorie diet.
• Tell patient that weight loss can cause gallstones. Teach signs and symptoms, and tell patient to notify prescriber promptly if they occur.

---

sumatriptan succinate
Imitrex❧

*Pregnancy risk category C*

**AVAILABLE FORMS**
*Injection:* 6 mg/0.5 ml (12 mg/ml) in 0.5-ml prefilled syringes and vials
*Nasal solution:* 5 mg/0.1 ml, 20 mg/0.1 ml
*Tablets:* 25 mg, 50 mg, 100 mg (base)†

**INDICATIONS & DOSAGES**
➤ **Acute migraine attacks (with or without aura)**
*Adults:* For injection, 6 mg S.C. Maximum dose is two 6-mg injections in 24 hours, separated by at least 1 hour.
   For tablets, 25 to 100 mg P.O., initially. If desired response isn't achieved in 2 hours, may give second dose of 25 to 100 mg. Additional doses may be used in at least 2-hour intervals. Maximum daily dose, 200 mg.

---

Reactions may be *common*, uncommon, *life-threatening*, or COMMON AND LIFE-THREATENING.

For nasal spray, give 5 mg, 10 mg, or 20 mg once in one nostril; may repeat once after 2 hours, for maximum daily dose of 40 mg. A 10-mg dose may be achieved by giving a 5-mg dose in each nostril.

➤ **Cluster headache**
*Adults:* 6 mg S.C. Maximum recommended dose is two 6-mg injections in 24 hours, separated by at least 1 hour.
*Adjust-a-dose:* In patients with hepatic impairment, the maximum single oral dose shouldn't exceed 50 mg.

## ACTION

May act as an agonist at serotonin receptors on extracerebral intracranial blood vessels, which constricts the affected vessels, inhibits neuropeptide release, and reduces pain transmission in the trigeminal pathways.

| Route | Onset | Peak | Duration |
|-------|-------|------|----------|
| P.O. | 30 min | 90 min | Unknown |
| S.C. | 10 min | 12 min | Unknown |
| Intranasal | Rapid | 1-2 hr | Unknown |

## ADVERSE REACTIONS

**CNS:** *dizziness, vertigo,* drowsiness, headache, anxiety, malaise, fatigue.
**CV:** *atrial fibrillation, ventricular fibrillation, ventricular tachycardia, coronary artery vasospasm, transient myocardial ischemia, MI,* pressure or tightness in chest.
**EENT:** discomfort of throat, nasal cavity or sinus, mouth, jaw, or tongue; altered vision.
**GI:** abdominal discomfort, dysphagia, diarrhea; nausea, vomiting, unusual or bad taste (nasal spray).
**Musculoskeletal:** myalgia, muscle cramps, neck pain.
**Respiratory:** upper respiratory inflammation and dyspnea (P.O.).
**Skin:** diaphoresis; flushing, *tingling, injection site reaction* (S.C.).
**Other:** *warm or hot sensation; burning sensation;* heaviness, pressure or tightness; tight feeling in head; cold sensation, numbness.

## INTERACTIONS

**Drug-drug.** *Ergot and ergot derivatives; other 5HT₁ agonists:* May prolong vasospastic effects. Don't use within 24 hours of sumatriptan therapy.
*MAO inhibitors:* May reduce sumatriptan clearance. Avoid using within 2 weeks of MAO inhibitor therapy. Use injection cautiously in patients and decrease sumatriptan dose.
*SSRIs:* May cause weakness, hyperreflexia, and incoordination. Monitor patient closely if concomitant therapy is clinically warranted.
**Drug-herb.** *Horehound:* May enhance serotonergic effects. Discourage use together.

## EFFECTS ON LAB TEST RESULTS

None reported.

## CONTRAINDICATIONS & CAUTIONS

• Contraindicated in patients with hypersensitivity to drug or its components; those with history, symptoms, or signs of ischemic cardiac, cerebrovascular (such as stroke or transient ischemic attack), or peripheral vascular syndromes (such as ischemic bowel disease); significant underlying CV diseases, including angina pectoris, MI, and silent myocardial ischemia; uncontrolled hypertension; or severe hepatic impairment.
• Contraindicated within 24 hours of another 5-HT agonist or drug containing ergotamine and within 2 weeks of MAO inhibitor therapy.

## NURSING CONSIDERATIONS

• Use cautiously in patient who is or intends to become pregnant.
• Use cautiously in patients who may have unrecognized coronary artery disease (CAD), such as postmenopausal women, men older than age 40, or patients with such risk factors as hypertension, hypercholesterolemia, obesity, diabetes, smoking, or family history of CAD.
• **Alert:** When giving drug to patient at risk for unrecognized CAD, consider giving first dose in presence of other medical personnel. Serious adverse cardiac effects can follow administration of drug, but such events are rare.
• After S.C. injection, most patients experience relief in 1 to 2 hours.

• Redness or pain at injection site should subside within 1 hour after injection.
• *Alert:* Don't confuse sumatriptan with somatropin.

## PATIENT TEACHING
• Inform patient that drug is intended only to treat migraine attacks, not to prevent them or reduce their occurrence.
• If patient is pregnant or intends to become pregnant, tell her not to use drug but to discuss with prescriber the risks and benefits of using drug during pregnancy.
• Tell patient that drug may be taken any time during a migraine attack, as soon as signs or symptoms appear.
• Review information about drug's injectable form, which is available in a spring-loaded injector system for easier patient use. Make sure patient understands how to load the injector, give the injection, and dispose of used syringes.
• *Alert:* Tell patient to tell prescriber immediately about persistent or severe chest pain. Warn him to stop using drug and to call prescriber if he develops pain or tightness in the throat, wheezing, heart throbbing, rash, lumps, hives, or swollen eyelids, face, or lips.

---

## tacrine hydrochloride
Cognex

*Pregnancy risk category C*

## AVAILABLE FORMS
*Capsules:* 10 mg, 20 mg, 30 mg, 40 mg

## INDICATIONS & DOSAGES
➤ **Mild to moderate Alzheimer's dementia**
*Adults:* Initially, 10 mg P.O. q.i.d. After 4 weeks, if patient tolerates treatment and has no increase in transaminase levels, increase dosage to 20 mg q.i.d. After an additional 4 weeks, increase to 30 mg q.i.d. If still tolerated, increase dosage to 40 mg q.i.d. after another 4 weeks.

## ACTION
Reversibly inhibits the enzyme cholinesterase in the CNS, preventing or blocking the breakdown of acetylcholine and thereby temporarily improving cognitive function in patients with Alzheimer's disease.

| Route | Onset | Peak | Duration |
|-------|-------|------|----------|
| P.O. | Unknown | 30 min-3 hr | Unknown |

## ADVERSE REACTIONS
**CNS:** agitation, ataxia, insomnia, abnormal thinking, somnolence, depression, anxiety, *headache,* fatigue, *dizziness,* confusion.
**CV:** chest pain.
**EENT:** rhinitis.
**GI:** *nausea, vomiting, diarrhea,* dyspepsia, loose stools, changes in stool color, anorexia, abdominal pain, flatulence, constipation.
**Metabolic:** weight loss.
**Musculoskeletal:** myalgia.
**Respiratory:** upper respiratory tract infection, cough.
**Skin:** rash, jaundice, facial flushing.

## INTERACTIONS
**Drug-drug.** *Anticholinergics:* May lessen the effects of tacrine. Avoid using together.
*Cholinergics such as bethanechol, anticholinesterases:* May have additive effects. Monitor patient for toxicity.
*Cimetidine, ciprofloxacin, fluvoxamine, ritonavir:* May increase tacrine level. Monitor for adverse effects.
*Succinylcholine:* May enhance neuromuscular blockade and prolong duration of action. Monitor patient closely.
*Theophylline:* May increase theophylline level and prolong theophylline half-life. Carefully monitor theophylline level and adjust dosage.
**Drug-food.** *Any food:* May delay drug absorption. Give drug 1 hour before meals.
**Drug-lifestyle.** *Smoking:* May decrease drug levels. Ask patient about nicotine use, and monitor him closely.

## EFFECTS ON LAB TEST RESULTS
• May increase ALT and AST levels.

## CONTRAINDICATIONS & CAUTIONS
• Contraindicated in patients hypersensitive to drug or to acridine derivatives.
• Contraindicated in patients for whom tacrine-related jaundice has previously been confirmed, with a total bilirubin level of more than 3 mg/dl.

---

Reactions may be *common,* uncommon, *life-threatening,* or COMMON AND LIFE-THREATENING.

• Use cautiously in patients with sick sinus syndrome or bradycardia, in patients at risk for peptic ulcers (including those taking NSAIDs or those with history of peptic ulcer), and in those with a history of hepatic disease.

• Use cautiously in patients with renal disease, asthma, prostatic hyperplasia, or other urine outflow impairment.

## NURSING CONSIDERATIONS

• Monitor ALT level weekly during first 18 weeks of therapy. If ALT is modestly elevated (twice the upper limit of normal range) after first 18 weeks, continue weekly monitoring. If no problems are detected, ALT tests may be decreased to once every 3 months. On each occasion that dosage is increased, resume weekly monitoring for at least 6 weeks.

• If drug is stopped for 4 weeks or longer, full dosage adjustment and monitoring schedule must be restarted.

## PATIENT TEACHING

• Stress that drug doesn't alter the underlying degenerative disease but can stabilize or alleviate symptoms. Effect of therapy depends on regular drug administration.

• *Alert:* Remind caregiver that dosage adjustment is an integral part of safe drug use. Abrupt discontinuation or a large reduction in daily dosage (80 mg daily or more) may cause behavioral disturbances and a decline in cognitive function.

• Tell caregiver to give drug between meals whenever possible. If GI upset becomes a problem, drug may be taken with meals, although doing so may reduce plasma levels by 30% to 40%.

• Advise patient and caregiver to immediately report significant adverse reactions or changes in status.

## zolmitriptan
Zomig, Zomig ZMT

*Pregnancy risk category C*

## AVAILABLE FORMS

*Nasal spray:* 5 mg
*Tablets (immediate-release):* 2.5 mg, 5 mg
*Tablets (oral disintegrating):* 2.5 mg, 5 mg

## INDICATIONS & DOSAGES

➤ **Acute migraine headaches**

*Adults:* Initially, 2.5 mg or less P.O., increased to 5 mg per dose, p.r.n. Or, disintegrating tablets: initially, 2.5 mg P.O. Don't break tablets in half. Or, 1 spray (5 mg) into nostril. If headache returns after first dose, a second dose may be given after 2 hours. Maximum dosage is 10 mg in 24-hour period.

*Adjust-a-dose:* In patients with hepatic disease, use doses less than 2.5 mg. Don't use orally disintegrating tablets because they shouldn't be broken in half or nasal spray because 5 mg is the lowest deliverable dose.

## ACTION

May act as an agonist at serotonin receptors on extracerebral intracranial blood vessels, which constricts the affected vessels, inhibits neuropeptide release, and reduces pain transmission in the trigeminal pathways.

| Route | Onset | Peak | Duration |
|-------|-------|------|----------|
| P.O. | Unknown | 2 hr | 3 hr |
| Nasal | 5 min | 3 hr | Unknown |

## ADVERSE REACTIONS

**CNS:** somnolence, vertigo, *dizziness,* hypesthesia, paresthesia, asthenia, pain.
**CV:** palpitations, *coronary artery vasospasm, transient myocardial ischemia, MI, ventricular tachycardia, ventricular fibrillation;* pain, tightness, pressure, or heaviness in chest.
**EENT:** *pain, tightness, or pressure in the neck, throat, or jaw.*
**GI:** dry mouth, dyspepsia, dysphagia, nausea.
**Musculoskeletal:** myalgia, myasthenia.
**Skin:** sweating.
**Other:** warm or cold sensations.

## INTERACTIONS

**Drug-drug.** *Cimetidine:* May double half-life of zolmitriptan. Monitor patient closely.
*Ergot-containing drugs, 5HT₁ agonists:* May cause additive effects. Avoid using within 24 hours of almotriptan.
*Hormonal contraceptives, propranolol:* May increase zolmitriptan level. Monitor patient closely.

*MAO inhibitors:* May increase zolmitriptan level. Avoid using within 2 weeks of MAO inhibitor therapy.

*SSRIs:* May cause additive serotonin effects, resulting in weakness, hyperreflexia, or incoordination. Monitor patient closely if given together.

**EFFECTS ON LAB TEST RESULTS**
● May increase glucose levels.

**CONTRAINDICATIONS & CAUTIONS**
● Contraindicated in patients hypersensitive to drug or its components, pregnant or breast-feeding patients, and those with uncontrolled hypertension, hemiplegic or basilar migraine, ischemic heart disease (angina pectoris, history of MI or documented silent ischemia); symptoms of ischemic heart disease, coronary artery vasospasm, including Prinzmetal's variant angina, or other significant heart disease.
● Contraindicated within 24 hours of other 5-HT₁ agonists or drugs containing ergot or within 2 weeks of stopping MAO inhibitor therapy.
● Use cautiously in patients with liver disease.
● Use cautiously in patients who may be at risk for coronary artery disease (such as postmenopausal women or men older than age 40) or those with risk factors such as hypertension, hypercholesterolemia, obesity, diabetes, smoking, or family history.

**NURSING CONSIDERATIONS**
● Drug isn't intended for preventing migraines or treating hemiplegic or basilar migraines.
● Safety of drug hasn't been established for cluster headaches.

**PATIENT TEACHING**
● Tell patient that drug is intended to relieve, not prevent, signs and symptoms of migraine.
● Advise patient to take drug as prescribed and not to take a second dose unless instructed by prescriber. Tell patient if a second dose is indicated and permitted, he should take it 2 hours after first dose.
● Instruct patient to release the orally disintegrating tablets from the blister pack just before taking; tablet should dissolve on tongue.

● Advise patient not to break the orally disintegrating tablets in half.
● Advise patient to immediately report pain or tightness in the chest or throat, heart throbbing, rash, skin lumps, or swelling of the face, lips, or eyelids.
● Tell patient not to take drug if she suspects, plans to become, or knows that she's pregnant.

---

Reactions may be *common,* uncommon, *life-threatening,* or COMMON AND LIFE-THREATENING.

# 35
## Cholinergics (parasympathomimetics)

bethanechol chloride
cevimeline hydrochloride
neostigmine bromide
neostigmine methylsulfate
physostigmine salicylate
pilocarpine hydrochloride
pyridostigmine bromide

**COMBINATION PRODUCTS**
None.

---

## bethanechol chloride
Duvoid, Myotonachol, Urabeth,
Urocarb‡

*Pregnancy risk category C*

---

**AVAILABLE FORMS**
*Injection:* 5 mg/ml
*Tablets:* 5 mg, 10 mg, 25 mg, 50 mg

**INDICATIONS & DOSAGES**
➤ **Acute postoperative and postpartum nonobstructive (functional) urine retention, neurogenic atony of urinary bladder with urine retention**
*Adults:* 10 to 50 mg P.O. t.i.d. to q.i.d. Or, 2.5 to 5 mg S.C. Never give I.M. or I.V.

Test dosage is 2.5 mg S.C., repeated at 15- to 30-minute intervals to total of four doses to determine the minimal effective dose; then, minimal effective dose used q 6 to 8 hours. All doses must be adjusted individually.

**ACTION**
Directly stimulates primarily muscarinic cholinergic receptors, mimicking the action of acetylcholine, increasing tone and peristalsis in the GI tract, and increasing contraction of the detrusor muscle of the urinary bladder.

| Route | Onset | Peak | Duration |
|-------|-------|------|----------|
| P.O. | 30-90 min | 1 hr | 6 hr |
| S.C. | 5-15 min | 15-30 min | 2 hr |

**ADVERSE REACTIONS**
**CNS:** headache, malaise.
**CV:** *bradycardia,* profound hypotension with reflexive tachycardia, flushing.
**EENT:** lacrimation, miosis.
**GI:** *abdominal cramps, diarrhea,* excessive salivation, nausea, belching, borborygmus.
**GU:** urinary urgency.
**Respiratory:** *bronchoconstriction,* increased bronchial secretions.
**Skin:** diaphoresis.

**INTERACTIONS**
**Drug-drug.** *Anticholinergics, atropine, procainamide, quinidine:* May reverse cholinergic effects. Observe patient for lack of drug effect.
*Cholinesterase inhibitors, cholinergic agonists:* May cause additive effects or increase toxicity. Avoid using together.
*Ganglionic blockers:* May cause critical drop in blood pressure, usually preceded by severe abdominal pain. Avoid using together.

**EFFECTS ON LAB TEST RESULTS**
• May increase liver enzyme, amylase, and lipase levels.

**CONTRAINDICATIONS & CAUTIONS**
• Contraindicated in patients hypersensitive to drug or its components and in those with uncertain strength or integrity of bladder wall, mechanical obstruction of GI or urinary tract, hyperthyroidism, peptic ulceration, latent or active bronchial asthma, obstructive pulmonary disease, pronounced bradycardia or hypotension, vasomotor instability, cardiac or coronary artery disease, atrioventricular conduction defects, hypertension, seizure disorder, Parkinson's disease, spastic GI disturbances, acute inflammatory lesions of the GI tract, peritonitis, or marked vagotonia.
• Contraindicated for I.M. or I.V. use and when increased muscular activity of the GI or urinary tract is harmful.
• Use cautiously in pregnant patient.

## NURSING CONSIDERATIONS
● Give drug on empty stomach, as it may cause nausea and vomiting.
● Adverse effects are rare with P.O. dosing.
● *Alert:* Never give I.M. or I.V. because of possible circulatory collapse, hypotension, severe abdominal cramping, bloody diarrhea, shock, or cardiac arrest.
● Monitor vital signs frequently, especially respirations. Always have atropine injection available, and be prepared to give 0.6 mg S.C. or by slow I.V. push. Provide respiratory support, if needed.
● Watch for toxicity, especially with S.C. administration.
● Watch closely for adverse reactions that may indicate drug toxicity.
● Oral drug absorption is poor and variable, requiring larger oral doses. Oral and S.C. doses aren't interchangeable.

## PATIENT TEACHING
● Tell patient to take oral form on an empty stomach and at regular intervals.
● Inform patient that drug is usually effective 30 to 90 minutes after oral use and 5 to 15 minutes after S.C. administration.

---

# cevimeline hydrochloride
Evoxac

*Pregnancy risk category C*

## AVAILABLE FORMS
*Capsules:* 30 mg

## INDICATIONS & DOSAGES
➤ **Dry mouth in patients with Sjögren's syndrome**
*Adults:* 30 mg P.O. t.i.d.

## ACTION
Stimulates the muscarinic receptors of the saliva-producing glands.

| Route | Onset | Peak | Duration |
|-------|-------|------|----------|
| P.O. | Unknown | 1½-2 hr | Unknown |

## ADVERSE REACTIONS
**CNS:** anxiety, depression, fever, dizziness, fatigue, *headache,* hypoesthesia, insomnia, migraine, pain, tremor, vertigo.
**CV:** chest pain, palpitations, peripheral edema.
**EENT:** abnormal vision, conjunctivitis, earache, epistaxis, eye infection, eye pain, otitis media, pharyngitis, *rhinitis, sinusitis,* xerophthalmia, eye abnormality.
**GI:** abdominal pain, anorexia, constipation, *diarrhea,* dry mouth, eructation, excessive salivation, flatulence, gastroesophageal reflux, *nausea,* salivary gland enlargement and pain, salivary calculi, ulcerative stomatitis, vomiting, dyspepsia, increased amylase.
**GU:** cystitis, candidiasis, urinary tract infection, vaginitis.
**Hematologic:** anemia.
**Musculoskeletal:** arthralgia, back pain, hypertonia, hyporeflexia, leg cramps, myalgia, rigors, skeletal pain, tooth disorder, toothache.
**Respiratory:** *upper respiratory tract infection,* bronchitis, pneumonia, coughing, hiccups.
**Skin:** rash, pruritus, skin disorder, erythematous rash, *excessive sweating.*
**Other:** fungal infections, flulike symptoms, injury, hot flushes, postoperative pain, allergic reaction, infection, abscess.

## INTERACTIONS
**Drug-drug.** *Antimuscarinics:* May cause antagonistic effects. Monitor patient for effectiveness.
*Beta blockers:* May cause conduction disturbances. Use together cautiously.
*Drugs that inhibit CYP:* May inhibit metabolism of cevimeline. Monitor patient closely.
*Parasympathomimetics:* May have additive effects. Use together cautiously.

## EFFECTS ON LAB TEST RESULTS
● May increase amylase level.
● May decrease hemoglobin.

## CONTRAINDICATIONS & CAUTIONS
● Contraindicated in patients hypersensitive to drug and in those for whom miosis is undesirable (as in those who have acute iritis or angle-closure glaucoma).
● Contraindicated in patients with uncontrolled asthma.
● Use cautiously in patients with significant CV disease, controlled asthma,

---

chronic bronchitis, or COPD and in those with a history of kidney stones or gallstones.

## NURSING CONSIDERATIONS
• Monitor patients with a history of asthma, COPD, or chronic bronchitis for an increase in signs or symptoms, such as wheezing, increased sputum production, or cough.
• Monitor patients with a history of cardiac disease for changes in heart rate or increased frequency, severity, or duration of angina.
• Monitor elderly patients closely because they have an increased risk of impaired renal, hepatic, and cardiac function.

## PATIENT TEACHING
• Advise patient not to interrupt or stop treatment without consulting prescriber.
• Tell patient that sweating is a common adverse effect. Urge adequate fluid intake to prevent dehydration.
• Inform patient that drug may cause visual disturbances that can impair driving ability, especially at night.

---

## neostigmine bromide
Prostigmin

## neostigmine methylsulfate
Prostigmin

*Pregnancy risk category C*

## AVAILABLE FORMS
**neostigmine bromide**
*Tablets:* 15 mg
**neostigmine methylsulfate**
*Injection:* 0.25 mg/ml, 0.5 mg/ml, 1 mg/ml

## INDICATIONS & DOSAGES
➤ **To control myasthenia gravis symptoms**
*Adults:* Initially, 15 mg P.O. t.i.d.; increase gradually, p.r.n. Range is 15 to 375 mg/day. Average dosage is 150 mg/day with intervals individualized. Or, 0.5 mg S.C. or I.M.; base subsequent parenteral doses on patient's response.

*Children:* 2 mg/kg/day P.O. divided q 3 to 4 hours, or 0.01 to 0.04 mg/kg/dose I.M. or S.C. q 2 to 3 hours, p.r.n.
➤ **To prevent and treat postoperative distention and urinary retention**
*Adults:* For prevention, 0.25 mg I.M. or S.C. as soon as possible after surgery; then q 4 to 6 hours for 2 to 3 days. For treatment, 0.5 mg I.M. or S.C. If urination hasn't occurred in 1 hour, catheterize. Continue 0.5 mg injections q 3 hours for at least 5 doses.
➤ **Antidote for nondepolarizing neuromuscular blockers**
*Adults:* 0.5 to 2 mg I.V. slowly. Repeat, p.r.n., to total of 5 mg. Before antidote dose, give 0.6 to 1.2 mg atropine sulfate I.V. if patient is bradycardic.

## I.V. ADMINISTRATION
• Give at a slow, controlled rate, not exceeding 1 mg/minute in adults.
• If patient's muscle weakness is severe, prescriber will determine whether severity is caused by drug-induced toxicity or worsening of myasthenia gravis. Test dose of edrophonium I.V. will aggravate drug-induced weakness but will temporarily relieve disease-induced weakness.

## ACTION
Competitively inhibits acetylcholinesterase, thus blocking the destruction of acetylcholine that has been released from the parasympathetic and somatic efferent nerves. Acetylcholine accumulates, promoting increased stimulation of the receptors.

| Route | Onset | Peak | Duration |
|---|---|---|---|
| P.O. | 45-75 min | 1-2 hr | 2-4 hr |
| I.V. | 4-8 min | 1-2 hr | 2-4 hr |
| I.M., S.C. | 20-30 min | 1-2 hr | 2-4 hr |

## ADVERSE REACTIONS
**CNS:** dizziness, headache, muscle weakness, loss of consciousness, drowsiness, syncope, *seizures.*
**CV:** *bradycardia,* hypotension, tachycardia, *AV block,* flushing, *cardiac arrest.*
**EENT:** blurred vision, lacrimation, miosis.

**GI:** *nausea, vomiting, diarrhea, abdominal cramps,* excessive salivation, flatulence, increased peristalsis.
**GU:** urinary frequency.
**Musculoskeletal:** *muscle cramps,* muscle fasciculations, arthralgia.
**Respiratory:** *bronchospasm,* dyspnea, *respiratory depression, respiratory arrest,* increased secretions, *laryngospasm, paralysis of respiratory muscles, central respiratory paralysis.*
**Skin:** rash, urticaria, diaphoresis.
**Other:** hypersensitivity reactions, *anaphylaxis.*

**INTERACTIONS**
**Drug-drug.** *Aminoglycosides, anticholinergics, atropine, corticosteroids, local and general anesthetics, magnesium sulfate, procainamide, quinidine:* May reverse cholinergic effects; watch for lack of drug effect. Stop all other cholinergics before giving this drug.
*Succinylcholine:* May worsen blockade produced by succinylcholine when used to reverse the effects of nondepolarizing neuromuscular blockers in surgical patients. Monitor patient.

**EFFECTS ON LAB TEST RESULTS**
None reported.

**CONTRAINDICATIONS & CAUTIONS**
● Contraindicated in patients hypersensitive to cholinergics or bromides and in those with peritonitis or mechanical obstruction of the intestinal or urinary tract.
● Use cautiously in patients with bronchial asthma, bradycardia, seizure disorders, recent coronary occlusion, vagotonia, hyperthyroidism, arrhythmias, and peptic ulcer.

**NURSING CONSIDERATIONS**
● Dosage for the treatment of myasthenia gravis must be highly individualized, depending on response and tolerance of adverse effects. Therapy may be needed day and night.
● In myasthenia gravis, schedule doses before periods of fatigue. For example, if patient has difficulty swallowing, schedule dose 30 minutes before each meal.
● *Alert:* Monitor vital signs frequently, especially respirations. Keep atropine injec-

tion available, and be prepared to provide respiratory support, as needed.
● *Alert:* Don't confuse neostigmine with etomidate (Amidate) vials, which may look alike.
● Monitor and document patient's response after each dose. Optimum dosage is difficult to judge. Watch closely for improvement in strength, vision, and ptosis, 45 to 60 minutes after each dose.
● When drug is used to prevent abdominal distention and GI distress, insertion of a rectal tube may help passage of gas.
● When drug is given for postoperative abdominal distention and bladder atony, rule out mechanical obstruction before doses are given. If no response within 1 hour after first dose, catheterize patient.
● Patients sometimes develop resistance to neostigmine.
● If appropriate, obtain order for hospitalized patient to have bedside supply of tablets. Many patients with long-standing disease insist on self-administration.

**PATIENT TEACHING**
● Tell patient to take drug with food or milk to reduce adverse GI reactions.
● When giving drug for myasthenia gravis, explain that it will relieve ptosis, double vision, chewing and swallowing problems, and trunk and limb weakness. Stress the importance of taking drug exactly as prescribed, including nighttime doses. Explain that patient may need to take drug for life.
● Teach patient how to observe and record variations in muscle strength.
● Advise patient to wear or carry medical identification of myasthenia gravis condition.

---

**physostigmine salicylate (eserine salicylate)**
Antilirium

*Pregnancy risk category C*

**AVAILABLE FORMS**
*Injection:* 1 mg/ml

## INDICATIONS & DOSAGES

➤ **To reverse CNS toxicity from clinical or toxic dosages of drugs capable of producing anticholinergic syndrome**
*Adults:* 0.5 to 2 mg I.M. or I.V. or 1 mg/minute I.V. repeated q 20 minutes p.r.n. until patient responds or adverse cholinergic effects occur. Additional dosages of 1 to 4 mg I.M. or I.V. q 30 to 60 minutes may be given if life-threatening problems such as coma, seizures, and arrhythmias recur.
*Children:* Reserved for life-threatening situations. Give 0.02 mg/kg I.M. or slow I.V., repeated q 5 to 10 minutes until response occurs. Maximum dose is 2 mg.

## I.V. ADMINISTRATION

● Give I.V. at controlled rate; use direct injection at no more than 1 mg/minute in adults or 0.5 mg/minute in children.
● Monitor vital signs frequently, especially respirations. Position patient to ease breathing. Keep atropine injection available, and be prepared to give 0.5 mg S.C. or by slow I.V. push. Provide respiratory support, as needed. Best given in presence of prescriber.

## ACTION

Reversibly inhibits acetylcholinesterase, thus blocking the destruction of acetylcholine that has been released from the parasympathetic and somatic efferent nerves. Acetylcholine accumulates, promoting increased stimulation of the receptor.

| Route | Onset | Peak | Duration |
|-------|-------|------|----------|
| I.V. | 3-5 min | 5 min | 30 min-5 hr |
| I.M. | 3-5 min | 20-30 min | 30 min-5 hr |

## ADVERSE REACTIONS

**CNS:** *seizures,* muscle weakness, *restlessness, excitability.*
**CV:** *bradycardia,* hypotension, palpitation, irregular pulse.
**EENT:** miosis, lacrimation.
**GI:** nausea, vomiting, epigastric pain, *diarrhea, excessive salivation.*
**GU:** urinary urgency.
**Respiratory:** *bronchospasm, bronchial constriction,* dyspnea, *respiratory paralysis.*
**Skin:** diaphoresis.

## INTERACTIONS

**Drug-drug.** *Anticholinergics, atropine, local and general anesthetics, procainamide, quinidine:* May reverse cholinergic effects. Observe patient for lack of drug effect.
*Ganglionic blockers:* May decrease blood pressure. Avoid using together.
*Neuromuscular blockers (succinylcholine):* May increase neuromuscular blockade, respiratory depression. Use together cautiously.
**Drug-herb.** *Jaborandi tree, pill-bearing spurge:* May have additive effect. Ask patient about use of herbal remedies, and recommend caution.

## EFFECTS ON LAB TEST RESULTS

None reported.

## CONTRAINDICATIONS & CAUTIONS

● Contraindicated in patients with mechanical obstruction of the intestine or urogenital tract; in patients with asthma, gangrene, diabetes, CV disease, or vagotonia; and in patients receiving choline esters or depolarizing neuromuscular blockers.
● Use cautiously in pregnant patients and patients with epilepsy, parkinsonian syndrome, or bradycardia.

## NURSING CONSIDERATIONS

● Use only clear solution. Darkening may indicate loss of potency.
● *Alert:* Watch closely for adverse reactions, particularly CNS disturbances. Raise side rails of bed if patient becomes restless or hallucinates. Adverse reactions may indicate drug toxicity.
● Effectiveness is typically immediate and dramatic but may be transient. Patient may need repeated doses.

## PATIENT TEACHING

● Inform patient of need for drug, explain its use and adverse reactions, and answer any questions or concerns.
● Tell patient to report adverse reactions promptly.
● Instruct patient to report discomfort at I.V. site.

# pilocarpine hydrochloride
Salagen

*Pregnancy risk category C*

## AVAILABLE FORMS
*Tablets:* 5 mg

## INDICATIONS & DOSAGES
➤ **Xerostomia from salivary gland hypofunction caused by radiotherapy for cancer of head and neck**
*Adults:* 5 mg P.O. t.i.d.; may increase to 10 mg P.O. t.i.d., p.r.n.
➤ **Dry mouth in patients with Sjögren's syndrome**
*Adults:* 5 mg P.O. q.i.d.

## ACTION
A cholinergic parasympathomimetic that increases secretion of salivary glands, eliminating dryness.

| Route | Onset | Peak | Duration |
|-------|-------|------|----------|
| P.O. | 20 min | 1 hr | 3-5 hr |

## ADVERSE REACTIONS
**CNS:** *dizziness, headache,* tremor, *asthenia.*
**CV:** hypertension, tachycardia, *flushing,* edema.
**EENT:** *rhinitis,* lacrimation, amblyopia, pharyngitis, voice alteration, conjunctivitis, epistaxis, *sinusitis, abnormal vision.*
**GI:** *nausea,* dyspepsia, diarrhea, abdominal pain, vomiting, dysphagia, taste perversion.
**GU:** *urinary frequency.*
**Musculoskeletal:** myalgia.
**Skin:** rash, pruritus, *sweating.*
**Other:** *chills.*

## INTERACTIONS
**Drug-drug.** *Beta blockers:* May increase risk of conduction disturbances. Use together cautiously.
*Drugs with anticholinergic effects:* May antagonize anticholinergic effects. Use together cautiously.
*Drugs with parasympathomimetic effects:* May result in additive pharmacologic effects. Monitor patient closely.

**Drug-food.** *High-fat meals:* May reduce drug absorption. Discourage patient from eating high-fat meals.

## EFFECTS ON LAB TEST RESULTS
None reported.

## CONTRAINDICATIONS & CAUTIONS
● Contraindicated in patients hypersensitive to pilocarpine, in breast-feeding patients, in those with uncontrolled asthma, and in those for whom miosis is undesirable, as in acute iritis or angle-closure glaucoma.
● Use cautiously in patients with CV disease, controlled asthma, chronic bronchitis, COPD, cholelithiasis, biliary tract disease, nephrolithiasis, or cognitive or psychiatric disturbances.
● Safety and efficacy of drug in children haven't been established.

## NURSING CONSIDERATIONS
● Examine patient's fundus carefully before beginning therapy because retinal detachment may occur in patients with retinal disease.
● Monitor patient for signs and symptoms of toxicity: headache, visual disturbance, lacrimation, sweating, respiratory distress, GI spasm, nausea, vomiting, diarrhea, AV block, tachycardia, bradycardia, hypotension, hypertension, shock, mental confusion, arrhythmia, and tremors. Immediately notify prescriber of suspected toxicity.

## PATIENT TEACHING
● Warn patient that driving ability may be impaired, especially at night, by drug-induced visual disturbances.
● Advise patient to drink plenty of fluids to prevent dehydration.
● Tell elderly patient with Sjögren's syndrome that he may be especially prone to urinary frequency, diarrhea, and dizziness.
● Advise patient not to take drug with a high-fat meal.

---

Reactions may be *common,* uncommon, *life-threatening,* or COMMON AND LIFE-THREATENING.

# pyridostigmine bromide
Mestinon*, Mestinon-SR†,
Mestinon Timespans, Regonol

*Pregnancy risk category C*

## AVAILABLE FORMS
*Injection:* 5 mg/ml in 2-ml ampules or
5-ml vials
*Syrup:* 60 mg/5 ml
*Tablets:* 30 mg (for military use only),
60 mg
*Tablets (extended-release):* 180 mg

## INDICATIONS & DOSAGES
➤ **Antidote for nondepolarizing neuro-
muscular blockers**
*Adults:* 10 to 20 mg I.V., preceded by at-
ropine sulfate 0.6 to 1.2 mg I.V.
➤ **Myasthenia gravis**
*Adults:* 60 to 120 mg P.O. q 3 or 4 hours.
Usual dosage is 600 mg daily but dosages
up to 1,500 mg daily may be needed. For
I.M. or I.V. use, give 1/30th of oral dose.
Dosage must be adjusted for each patient,
based on response and tolerance. Or,
180 to 540 mg extended-release tablets
P.O. b.i.d., with at least 6 hours between
doses.
*Children:* 7 mg/kg or 200 mg/m² daily in
five or six divided doses.
➤ **To increase survival after exposure to
the nerve agent soman**
*Adults in military:* 30 mg P.O. q 8 hours
starting at least several hours before soman exposure.
**Adjust-a-dose:** Smaller doses may be required in patients with renal disease. Adjust dosage to achieve desired effect.

## I.V. ADMINISTRATION
● *Alert:* Give I.V. injection no faster than
1 mg/minute. Rapid I.V. infusion may
cause bradycardia and seizures. Monitor
vital signs frequently, especially respirations. Position patient to ease breathing.
Keep atropine injection available, and be
prepared to give it immediately; provide
respiratory support, as needed.
● If patient's muscle weakness is severe,
prescriber will determine whether symptom is caused by drug-induced toxicity or
worsening of myasthenia gravis. Test
dose of edrophonium I.V. will aggravate

drug-induced weakness but will temporarily relieve disease-induced weakness.

## ACTION
Competitively inhibits acetylcholinesterase, thus blocking the destruction of
acetylcholine that was released from the
parasympathetic and somatic efferent
nerves. Acetylcholine accumulates, promoting increased stimulation of the receptors.

| Route | Onset | Peak | Duration |
|---|---|---|---|
| P.O. | 20-30 min | 1-2 hr | 3-6 hr |
| P.O. (extended) | 30-60 min | 1-2 hr | 6-12 hr |
| I.V. | 2-5 min | Unknown | 2-4 hr |
| I.M. | 15 min | Unknown | 2-4 hr |

## ADVERSE REACTIONS
**CNS:** headache with high doses, weakness, syncope.
**CV:** *bradycardia,* hypotension, *cardiac
arrest,* thrombophlebitis.
**EENT:** miosis.
**GI:** abdominal cramps, *nausea, vomiting,*
diarrhea, excessive salivation, increased
peristalsis.
**Musculoskeletal:** muscle cramps, muscle
fasciculations.
**Respiratory:** *bronchospasm, bronchoconstriction,* increased bronchial secretions.
**Skin:** rash, diaphoresis.

## INTERACTIONS
**Drug-drug.** *Aminoglycosides:* May prolong or enhance muscle weakness. Use together cautiously.
*Anticholinergics, atropine, corticoste-
roids, general or local anesthetics, magnesium, procainamide, quinidine:* May antagonize cholinergic effects. Observe
patient for lack of drug effect.
*Ganglionic blockers:* May increase risk of
hypotension. Monitor patient closely.

## EFFECTS ON LAB TEST RESULTS
None reported.

## CONTRAINDICATIONS & CAUTIONS
● Contraindicated in patients hypersensitive to anticholinesterases or bromides and
in those with mechanical obstruction of
the intestinal or urinary tract.

• Use cautiously in patients with bronchial asthma, bradycardia, arrhythmias, epilepsy, recent coronary occlusion, vagotonia, hyperthyroidism, or peptic ulcer.
• Use cautiously in pregnant women.

## NURSING CONSIDERATIONS
• *Alert:* If taken immediately before or during soman exposure, drug may be ineffective against soman and may worsen soman's effects.
• Stop all other cholinergics before giving this drug.
• Don't crush extended-release tablets.
• When using sweet syrup for patients who have trouble swallowing, give over ice chips if patient can't tolerate flavor.
• Monitor and document patient's response after each dose. Optimum dosage is difficult to judge.
• *Alert:* In the United States, Regonol contains benzyl ethanol preservative, which may cause toxicity in neonates if given in high doses. The Canadian formulation of this drug doesn't contain benzyl ethanol.
• If appropriate, obtain order for hospitalized patient to have bedside supply of tablets. Many patients with long-standing disease insist on self-administration.
• *Alert:* Don't confuse Mestinon with Mesantoin or Metatensin.

## PATIENT TEACHING
• When giving drug for myasthenia gravis, stress importance of taking it exactly as prescribed, on time, in evenly spaced doses. If using extended-release tablets, explain that patient must take tablets at same time each day, at least 6 hours apart.
• Advise patient not to crush or chew extended-release tablets.
• Explain that patient may have to take drug for life.
• Advise patient to wear or carry medical identification that identifies his myasthenia gravis.
• Stress importance to military personnel of taking nerve agent antidotes atropine and pralidoxime rather than pyridostigmine bromide at first sign of nerve agent poisoning.

---

Reactions may be *common*, uncommon, *life-threatening*, or COMMON AND LIFE-THREATENING.

# 36
## Anticholinergics

**atropine sulfate**
   (See Chapter 19, ANTIARRHYTHMICS.)
**dicyclomine hydrochloride**
**glycopyrrolate**
**hyoscyamine**
**hyoscyamine sulfate**
**scopolamine**
**scopolamine butylbromide**
**scopolamine hydrobromide**

### COMBINATION PRODUCTS
ARCO-LASE TABLETS: amylase 30 mg, protease 6 mg, lipase 25 mg, cellulase 2 mg.
BARBIDONNA No. 2 TABLETS: atropine sulfate 0.025 mg, scopolamine hydrobromide 0.0074 mg, hyoscyamine hydrobromide or sulfate 0.1286 mg, and phenobarbital 32 mg.
BARBIDONNA TABLETS: atropine sulfate 0.025 mg, scopolamine hydrobromide 0.0074 mg, hyoscyamine hydrobromide or sulfate 0.1286 mg, and phenobarbital 16 mg.
DONNATAL CAPSULES AND TABLETS: atropine sulfate 0.0194 mg, scopolamine hydrobromide 0.0065 mg, hyoscyamine hydrobromide or sulfate 0.1037 mg, and phenobarbital 16.2 mg.
DONNATAL ELIXIR*: atropine sulfate 0.0194 mg/5 ml, scopolamine hydrobromide 0.0065 mg/5 ml, ethanol 23%, hyoscyamine hydrobromide or sulfate 0.1037 mg/5 ml, and phenobarbital 16 mg/5 ml.
DONNATAL EXTENTABS: atropine sulfate 0.0582 mg, scopolamine hydrobromide 0.0195 mg, hyoscyamine sulfate 0.3111 mg, and phenobarbital 48.6 mg.
PROSED TABLETS: methenamine 81.6 mg, phenyl salicylate 36.2 mg, methylene blue 10.8 mg, benzoic acid 9 mg, atropine sulfate 0.06 mg, hyoscyamine sulfate 0.06 mg.
URIMAX TABLETS: methenamine 81.6 mg, sodium biphosphate 40.8 mg, phenyl salicylate 36.2 mg, methylene blue 10.8 mg, hyoscyamine sulfate 0.12 mg.
URISED TABLETS: methenamine 40.8 mg, phenyl salicylate 18.1 mg, methylene blue 5.4 mg, benzoic acid 4.5 mg, atropine sulfate 0.03 mg, hyoscyamine sulfate 0.03 mg.

---

### dicyclomine hydrochloride
Antispas, A-Spas, Bentyl, Bentylol†, Byclomine, Dibent, Di-Spaz, Formulex†, Lominet†, Merbentyl‡, Or-Tyl, Spasmoban†

*Pregnancy risk category B*

---

#### AVAILABLE FORMS
*Capsules:* 10 mg, 20 mg
*Injection:* 10 mg/ml
*Syrup:* 5 mg/5 ml‡, 10 mg/5 ml
*Tablets:* 10 mg‡, 20 mg

#### INDICATIONS & DOSAGES
➤ **Irritable bowel syndrome, other functional GI disorders**
*Adults:* Initially, 20 mg P.O. q.i.d., increased to 40 mg q.i.d. Or, 20 mg I.M. q.i.d.

#### ACTION
Inhibits action of acetylcholine on postganglionic, parasympathetic muscarinic receptors, decreasing GI motility. Also, possesses local anesthetic properties that may be partly responsible for spasmolysis.

| Route | Onset | Peak | Duration |
|-------|-------|------|----------|
| P.O., I.M. | Unknown | 1-1½ hr | Unknown |

#### ADVERSE REACTIONS
**CNS:** *headache; dizziness;* fever; insomnia; light-headedness; drowsiness; nervousness, confusion, and excitement in elderly patients.
**CV:** *palpitations,* tachycardia.
**EENT:** blurred vision, increased intraocular pressure, mydriasis, photophobia.
**GI:** nausea, vomiting, *constipation, dry mouth, thirst,* abdominal distention, heartburn, paralytic ileus.
**GU:** *urinary hesitancy, urine retention,* impotence.

---

*Rapid onset*   †Canada   ‡Australia   ◇OTC   ♦ Off-label use   ✐Photoguide   *Liquid contains alcohol.

**Skin:** urticaria, decreased sweating or inability to sweat, local irritation.
**Other:** allergic reactions.

**INTERACTIONS**
**Drug-drug.** *Amantadine, antihistamines, antiparkinsonians, disopyramide, glutethimide, meperidine, phenothiazines, procainamide, quinidine, tricyclic antidepressants:* May have additive adverse effects. Avoid using together.

**EFFECTS ON LAB TEST RESULTS**
None reported.

**CONTRAINDICATIONS & CAUTIONS**
• Contraindicated in patients hypersensitive to anticholinergics and in those with obstructive uropathy, obstructive disease of the GI tract, reflux esophagitis, severe ulcerative colitis, toxic megacolon, myasthenia gravis, unstable CV status in acute hemorrhage, tachycardia secondary to cardiac insufficiency or thyrotoxicosis, or glaucoma.
• Contraindicated in breast-feeding patients and in children younger than age 6 months.
• Use cautiously in patients with autonomic neuropathy, hyperthyroidism, coronary artery disease, arrhythmias, heart failure, hypertension, hiatal hernia, hepatic or renal disease, prostatic hyperplasia, known or suspected GI infection, and ulcerative colitis.
• Use cautiously in patients in hot or humid environments; drug can cause heat stroke.

**NURSING CONSIDERATIONS**
• Give drug 30 to 60 minutes before meals and at bedtime. Bedtime dose can be larger; give at least 2 hours after last meal of day.
• *Alert:* Don't give S.C. or I.V.
• Adjust dosage based on patient's needs and response. Dosages up to 40 mg P.O. q.i.d. have been used in adults, but safety and efficacy for longer than 2 weeks haven't been established.
• Dicyclomine is a synthetic tertiary derivative that may have atropine-like adverse reactions.

• *Alert:* Overdose may cause curarelike effects, such as respiratory paralysis. Keep emergency equipment available.
• Monitor patient's vital signs and urine output carefully.
• *Alert:* The dicyclomine labeling may be misleading. The ampule label reads 10 mg/ml but doesn't indicate that the ampule contains 2 ml of solution (20 mg of drug).
• *Alert:* Don't confuse dicyclomine with dyclonine or doxycycline; don't confuse Bentyl with Aventyl or Benadryl.

**PATIENT TEACHING**
• Tell patient when to take drug, and stress importance of doing so on time and at evenly spaced intervals.
• Advise patient to avoid driving and other hazardous activities if drowsiness, dizziness, or blurred vision occurs; to drink plenty of fluids to help prevent constipation; and to report rash or other skin eruption.

# glycopyrrolate
Robinul, Robinul Forte

*Pregnancy risk category B*

**AVAILABLE FORMS**
*Injection:* 0.2 mg/ml
*Tablets:* 1 mg, 2 mg

**INDICATIONS & DOSAGES**
➤ **Blockade of adverse cholinergic effects caused by anticholinesterases used to reverse neuromuscular blockade**
*Adults and children:* 0.2 mg I.V. for each 1 mg of neostigmine or 5 mg of pyridostigmine. May be given I.V. without dilution or may be added to dextrose injection and given by infusion.
➤ **Preoperatively to diminish secretions and block cardiac vagal reflexes**
*Adults and children age 2 and older:* 0.0044 mg/kg I.M. 30 to 60 minutes before anesthesia.
*Children younger than age 2:* 0.0088 mg/kg I.M. 30 to 60 minutes before anesthesia.

➤ **Adjunctive therapy in peptic ulcerations and other GI disorders**
*Adults:* 1 to 2 mg P.O. t.i.d. or 0.1 to 0.2 mg I.M. or I.V. t.i.d. or q.i.d. Dosage must be individualized. Maximum oral dosage, 8 mg daily.

## I.V. ADMINISTRATION
● Give by direct injection without dilution, or inject into tubing of a free-flowing I.V. solution.
● Don't mix with I.V. solutions that contain sodium bicarbonate or alkaline solutions with a pH of 6 or higher. Alkaline drugs, such as barbiturates, chloramphenicol, dexamethasone, diazepam, dimenhydrinate, methylprednisolone, and pentazocine, are incompatible.

## ACTION
Inhibits cholinergic (muscarinic) actions of acetylcholine on autonomic effectors innervated by postganglionic cholinergic nerves.

| Route | Onset | Peak | Duration |
|---|---|---|---|
| P.O. | Unknown | Unknown | 8-12 hr |
| I.V. | 1 min | Unknown | 2-7 hr |
| I.M., S.C. | 15-30 min | 30-45 min | 2-7 hr |

## ADVERSE REACTIONS
**CNS:** fever, weakness, nervousness, insomnia, drowsiness, dizziness, headache, confusion, excitement.
**CV:** palpitations, tachycardia.
**EENT:** *dilated pupils, blurred vision,* photophobia, increased intraocular pressure.
**GI:** *constipation, dry mouth,* nausea, loss of taste, abdominal distention, vomiting, epigastric distress.
**GU:** urinary hesitancy, urine retention, impotence.
**Skin:** urticaria, decreased sweating or anhidrosis.
**Other:** allergic reactions, *anaphylaxis.*

## INTERACTIONS
**Drug-drug.** *Amantadine, antihistamines, antiparkinsonians, disopyramide, glutethimide, meperidine, phenothiazines, procainamide, quinidine, tricyclic antidepressants:* May have additive adverse effects. Avoid using together.
*Potassium chloride:* May slow transit time and increase risk of potassium-induced GI lesions. Avoid wax-based potassium products.

## EFFECTS ON LAB TEST RESULTS
None reported.

## CONTRAINDICATIONS & CAUTIONS
● Contraindicated in patients hypersensitive to drug, in neonates, and in those with glaucoma, obstructive uropathy, obstructive disease of the GI tract, myasthenia gravis, paralytic ileus, intestinal atony, unstable CV status in acute hemorrhage, tachycardia secondary to cardiac insufficiency or thyrotoxicosis, severe ulcerative colitis, toxic megacolon, or known or suspected GI infection.
● Use cautiously in patients with autonomic neuropathy, hyperthyroidism, coronary artery disease, arrhythmias, heart failure, hypertension, hiatal hernia, hepatic or renal disease, ulcerative colitis, and known or suspected GI infection.
● Use cautiously in patients in hot or humid environments; drug can cause heat stroke.

## NURSING CONSIDERATIONS
● Give oral form 30 to 60 minutes before meals.
● *Alert:* Check all dosages carefully; slight overdose can lead to toxicity.
● *Alert:* Overdose may cause curarelike effects, such as respiratory paralysis. Keep emergency equipment available.
● Monitor vital signs carefully. Watch closely for adverse reactions, especially in geriatric or debilitated patients. Call prescriber promptly if reactions occur.
● Elderly patients may be more susceptible to adverse effects and typically receive smaller doses.

## PATIENT TEACHING
● Tell patient to take oral drug 30 to 60 minutes before meals.
● Tell patient not to crush or chew extended release products.
● Warn patient to avoid activities that require alertness until drug's CNS effects are known.
● Advise patient to report signs and symptoms of urinary hesitancy or urine retention.

# hyoscyamine
Cystospaz

## hyoscyamine sulfate
Anaspaz, Cystospaz,
Cystospaz-M, Gastrosed,
Levbid, Levsin*, Levsin Drops*,
Levsin SL, Levsinex Timecaps,
Neoquess, NuLev

*Pregnancy risk category C*

## AVAILABLE FORMS
**hyoscyamine**
*Tablets:* 0.15 mg
**hyoscyamine sulfate**
*Capsules (extended-release):* 0.375 mg
*Elixir:* 0.125 mg/5 ml
*Injection:* 0.5 mg/ml
*Oral solution:* 0.125 mg/ml
*Tablets:* 0.125 mg, 0.13 mg, 0.15 mg

## INDICATIONS & DOSAGES
➤ **GI tract disorders caused by spasm;
to diminish secretions and block cardiac
vagal reflexes preoperatively; as adjunctive therapy for peptic ulcers, cystitis,
renal colic; as drying agent to relieve
symptoms of allergic rhinitis**
*Adults and children age 12 and older:*
0.125 to 0.25 mg P.O. or S.L. t.i.d. or q.i.d.
before meals and h.s. Or, 0.375 to 0.75 mg
extended-release form P.O. q 8 to 12 hours.
Or, 0.25 to 0.5 mg or 1 or 2 ml I.M., I.V.,
or S.C. b.i.d. to q.i.d. Oral drug is substituted when symptoms are controlled.
Maximum, 1.5 mg daily.
*Children younger than age 12:* Dosage individualized according to weight. Usual
dose is ½ to 1 tablet P.O. q 4 hours or
p.r.n. Don't exceed 6 tablets or 0.75 mg in
24 hours.

## I.V. ADMINISTRATION
● I.V. form used when P.O. or S.L. route
isn't feasible or rapid effect is needed.

## ACTION
Competitively blocks the action of acetylcholine at muscarinic receptors, which decreases GI motility and inhibits gastric
acid secretion.

| Route | Onset | Peak | Duration |
|---|---|---|---|
| P.O. | 20-30 min | ½-1 hr | 4-12 hr |
| P.O. (extended) | 20-30 min | 40-90 min | 12 hr |
| I.V. | 2-3 min | 15-30 min | 4 hr |
| I.M., S.C. | Unknown | 15-30 min | 4-12 hr |
| S.L. | 5-20 min | ½-1 hr | 4 hr |

## ADVERSE REACTIONS
**CNS:** fever , headache, insomnia, drowsiness, dizziness, *confusion or excitement in
elderly patients,* nervousness, weakness.
**CV:** *palpitations,* tachycardia.
**EENT:** *blurred vision,* mydriasis, increased intraocular pressure, cycloplegia,
photophobia.
**GI:** *dry mouth,* dysphagia, *constipation,*
heartburn, loss of taste, nausea, vomiting,
*paralytic ileus.*
**GU:** *urinary hesitancy, urine retention,*
impotence.
**Skin:** urticaria, decreased or lack of
sweating.
**Other:** hypersensitivity reactions.

## INTERACTIONS
**Drug-drug.** *Amantadine, antihistamines,
antiparkinsonians, disopyramide, glutethimide, MAO inhibitors, meperidine, phenothiazines, procainamide, quinidine, tricyclic antidepressants:* May have additive
adverse effects. Avoid using together.
*Antacids:* May decrease absorption of oral
anticholinergics. Separate doses by 2 or
3 hours.
*Ketoconazole:* May interfere with ketoconazole absorption. Separate doses by
2 or 3 hours.

## EFFECTS ON LAB TEST RESULTS
None reported.

## CONTRAINDICATIONS & CAUTIONS
● Contraindicated in patients hypersensitive to anticholinergics and in those with
glaucoma, obstructive uropathy, obstructive disease of the GI tract, severe ulcerative colitis, myasthenia gravis, paralytic
ileus, intestinal atony, unstable CV status
in acute hemorrhage, tachycardia secondary to cardiac insufficiency of thyrotoxicosis, or toxic megacolon.
● Use cautiously in patients with autonomic neuropathy, hyperthyroidism, coronary

artery disease, arrhythmias, heart failure, hypertension, hiatal hernia with reflux esophagitis, hepatic or renal disease, known or suspected GI infection, and ulcerative colitis.
• Use cautiously in patients in hot or humid environments; drug can cause heat stroke.

## NURSING CONSIDERATIONS
• Give drug 30 minutes to 1 hour before meals and at bedtime. Bedtime dose can be larger; give at least 2 hours after last meal of day.
• *Alert:* Overdose may cause curarelike effects, such as respiratory paralysis. Keep emergency equipment available.
• Monitor patient's vital signs and urine output carefully.
• Injection contains sodium metabisulfite, which may cause allergic reaction in certain people.

## PATIENT TEACHING
• Urge patient to take drug as prescribed.
• Caution patient not to crush or chew extended-release tablets.
• Advise patient to avoid driving and other hazardous activities if drowsiness, dizziness, or blurred vision occurs; to drink plenty of fluids to help prevent constipation; and to report rash or other skin eruption.

---

## scopolamine (hyoscine)
Transderm-Scop

## scopolamine butylbromide (hyoscine butylbromide)
Buscopan†

## scopolamine hydrobromide (hyoscine hydrobromide)
Scopolamine Hydrobromide Injection

*Pregnancy risk category C*

---

## AVAILABLE FORMS
**scopolamine**
*Transdermal patch:* 1.5 mg/2.5 cm$^2$ (1 mg/72 hours)
**scopolamine butylbromide**
*Capsules:* 0.25 mg

*Suppositories:* 10 mg†
*Tablets:* 10 mg†
**scopolamine hydrobromide**
*Injection:* 0.3 mg, 0.4 mg, 0.5 mg, 0.6 mg, and 1 mg/ml in 1-ml vials and ampules; 0.86 mg/ml in 0.5-ml ampules

## INDICATIONS & DOSAGES
➤ **Spastic states**
*Adults:* 10 to 20 mg P.O. t.i.d. or q.i.d. or 10 mg P.R. t.i.d. or q.i.d. Adjust dosage, p.r.n. Or, 10 to 20 mg butylbromide S.C., I.M., or I.V., t.i.d. or q.i.d.
➤ **Delirium, preanesthetic sedation, and obstetric amnesia with analgesics**
*Adults:* 0.3 to 0.65 mg I.M., S.C., or I.V. Dilute solution with sterile water for injection before giving I.V.
*Children:* 0.006 mg/kg I.M., S.C., or I.V. Maximum dose, 0.3 mg. Dilute solution with sterile water for injection before giving I.V.
➤ **Prevention of nausea and vomiting from motion sickness**
*Adults:* One Transderm-Scop, formulated to deliver 1 mg scopolamine over 3 days, applied to the skin behind the ear at least 4 hours before antiemetic is needed. Or, 300 to 600 mcg hydrobromide S.C., I.M., or I.V.
*Children:* 6 mcg/kg or 200 mcg/m$^2$ hydrobromide S.C., I.M., or I.V.

## I.V. ADMINISTRATION
• Intermittent and continuous infusions aren't recommended. For direct injection, dilute with sterile water and inject diluted drug at ordered rate through patent I.V. line.
• Protect I.V. solutions from freezing and light, and store at room temperature.

## ACTION
Inhibits muscarinic actions of acetylcholine on autonomic effectors innervated by postganglionic cholinergic neurons. May affect neural pathways originating in the inner ear to inhibit nausea and vomiting.

| Route | Onset | Peak | Duration |
|---|---|---|---|
| P.O., I.M. | 1 hr | 1-2 hr | 4-6 hr |
| I.V. | 10 min | 50-80 min | 2 hr |
| Transdermal | 4 hr | Unknown | 72 hr |
| P.R., S.C. | Unknown | Unknown | Unknown |

## ADVERSE REACTIONS

**CNS:** disorientation, restlessness, irritability, dizziness, drowsiness, headache, confusion, hallucinations, delirium, impaired memory.

**CV:** palpitations, tachycardia, *paradoxical bradycardia,* flushing.

**EENT:** dilated pupils, blurred vision, photophobia, increased intraocular pressure, difficulty swallowing.

**GI:** *constipation, dry mouth, nausea, vomiting, epigastric distress.*

**GU:** urinary hesitancy, urine retention.

**Respiratory:** bronchial plugging, depressed respirations.

**Skin:** rash, dryness, contact dermatitis with transdermal patch.

## INTERACTIONS

**Drug-drug.** *Amantadine, antihistamines, antiparkinsonians, disopyramide, glutethimide, meperidine, phenothiazines, procainamide, quinidine, tricyclic antidepressants:* May increase risk of adverse CNS reactions. Avoid using together.

*Antacids:* May decrease oral absorption of anticholinergics. Separate doses by 2 or 3 hours.

*CNS depressants:* May increase risk of CNS depression. Monitor patient closely.

*Digoxin:* May increase digoxin level. Monitor patient for digoxin toxicity.

*Ketoconazole:* May interfere with ketoconazole absorption. Separate doses by 2 or 3 hours.

**Drug-herb.** *Jaborandi tree:* May decrease drug effects. Discourage use together.

*Pill-bearing spurge:* May decrease drug effects. Inform patient of this interaction.

*Squaw vine:* May decrease metabolic breakdown. Discourage use together.

**Drug-lifestyle.** *Alcohol use:* May increase risk of CNS depression. Discourage use together.

## EFFECTS ON LAB TEST RESULTS

None reported.

## CONTRAINDICATIONS & CAUTIONS

● Contraindicated in patients with angle-closure glaucoma, obstructive uropathy, obstructive disease of the GI tract, asthma, chronic pulmonary disease, myasthenia gravis, paralytic ileus, intestinal atony, unstable CV status in acute hemorrhage, tachycardia from cardiac insufficiency, or toxic megacolon.

● Use cautiously in patients with autonomic neuropathy, hyperthyroidism, coronary artery disease, arrhythmias, heart failure, hypertension, hiatal hernia with reflux esophagitis, hepatic or renal disease, known or suspected GI infection, or ulcerative colitis.

● Use cautiously in children younger than age 6.

● Use cautiously in patients in hot or humid environments; drug can cause heat stroke.

## NURSING CONSIDERATIONS

● Raise side rails as a precaution because some patients become temporarily excited or disoriented and some develop amnesia or become drowsy. Reorient patient, as needed.

● Tolerance may develop when therapy is prolonged.

● Atropine-like toxicity may cause dose-related adverse reactions. Individual tolerance varies greatly.

● *Alert:* Overdose may cause curarelike effects, such as respiratory paralysis. Keep emergency equipment available.

## PATIENT TEACHING

● Advise patient to apply patch the night before a planned trip. Transdermal method releases a controlled therapeutic amount of scopolamine. Transderm-Scop is effective if applied 2 or 3 hours before experiencing motion but is more effective if applied 12 hours before.

● Instruct patient to wash and dry hands thoroughly before and after applying the transdermal patch (on dry skin behind the ear) and before touching the eye, because pupil may dilate. Tell patient to discard patch after removing it and to wash application site thoroughly.

● Tell patient that if patch becomes displaced, he should remove it and apply another patch on a fresh skin site behind the ear.

● Alert patient to possible withdrawal signs or symptoms (nausea, vomiting,

headache, dizziness) when transdermal
system is used for longer than 72 hours.
● Advise patient that eyes may be more
sensitive to light while wearing patch.
● Warn patient to avoid activities that require alertness until CNS effects of drug
are known.
● Instruct patient to ask pharmacist for
brochure that comes with the transdermal
product.
● Urge patient to report urinary hesitancy
or urine retention.

**dobutamine hydrochloride
dopamine hydrochloride
norepinephrine bitartrate
phenylephrine hydrochloride
pseudoephedrine hydrochloride
pseudoephedrine sulfate**

### COMBINATION PRODUCTS
CHILDREN'S ADVIL COLD: pseudoephedrine 15 mg and ibuprofen 100 mg per 5 ml.
ENTEX PSE: pseudoephedrine 120 mg and guaifenesin 600 mg.
SEMPREX-D: acrivastine 8 mg and pseudoephedrine hydrochloride 60 mg.

---

## dobutamine hydrochloride
Dobutrex

*Pregnancy risk category B*

---

### AVAILABLE FORMS
*Injection:* 12.5 mg/ml in 20-ml vials (parenteral)

### INDICATIONS & DOSAGES
➤ **Increased cardiac output in short-term treatment of cardiac decompensation caused by depressed contractility, such as during refractory heart failure; adjunctive therapy in cardiac surgery**
*Adults:* 0.5 to 1 mcg/kg/minute I.V. infusion, titrating to optimal dosage of 2 to 20 mcg/kg/minute. Rarely, rates up to 40 mcg/kg/minute may be needed.

### I.V. ADMINISTRATION
● Dilute concentrate before giving injection. Compatible solutions include D₅W, half-normal or normal saline solution for injection, and lactated Ringer's injection. Contents of 1 vial (250 mg) diluted with 1,000 ml of solution yields 250 mcg/ml. Diluting with 500 ml yields 500 mcg/ml. Diluting with 250 ml yields 1,000 mcg/ml. Don't exceed maximum of 5 mg/ml.

● Oxidation of drug may slightly discolor admixtures containing dobutamine. This doesn't indicate a significant loss of potency provided drug is used within 24 hours of reconstitution.
● Don't give through same I.V. line with other drugs. Drug is incompatible with heparin, hydrocortisone sodium succinate, cefazolin, cefamandole, neutral cephalothin, penicillin, sodium bicarbonate, and ethacrynate sodium.
● Give through a central venous catheter or large peripheral vein. Titrate infusion according to prescriber's orders and patient's condition. Use an infusion pump. Infusions for up to 72 hours produce no more adverse effects than shorter infusions.
● Watch for irritation and infiltration; extravasation can cause tissue damage and necrosis. Change I.V. sites regularly to avoid phlebitis.
● I.V. solutions remain stable for 24 hours.

### ACTION
Directly stimulates beta₁ receptors of heart to increase myocardial contractility and stroke volume. At therapeutic dosages, drug decreases peripheral vascular resistance (afterload), reduces ventricular filling pressure (preload), and may facilitate AV node conduction. Net result is increased cardiac output.

| Route | Onset | Peak | Duration |
|---|---|---|---|
| I.V. | 1-2 min | 10 min | < 5 min after infusion ends |

### ADVERSE REACTIONS
**CNS:** headache.
**CV:** *increased heart rate, hypertension,* PVCs, angina, phlebitis, nonspecific chest pain, palpitations, hypotension.
**GI:** nausea, vomiting.
**Respiratory:** shortness of breath, *asthma attacks.*
**Other:** hypersensitivity reactions, *anaphylaxis.*

---

Reactions may be *common,* uncommon, *life-threatening,* or COMMON AND LIFE-THREATENING.

## INTERACTIONS

**Drug-drug.** *Beta blockers:* May antagonize dobutamine effects. Avoid using together.

*General anesthetics:* May have greater risk of ventricular arrhythmias. Monitor ECG closely.

*Guanethidine, oxytocic drugs:* May increase pressor response, possibly resulting in severe hypertension. Monitor blood pressure closely.

*Tricyclic antidepressants:* May potentiate the pressor response and cause arrhythmias. Use together cautiously.

**Drug-herb.** *Rue:* May increase inotropic potential. Discourage use together.

## EFFECTS ON LAB TEST RESULTS

• May decrease potassium levels.

## CONTRAINDICATIONS & CAUTIONS

• Contraindicated in patients hypersensitive to drug or its components and in those with idiopathic hypertrophic subaortic stenosis.

• Use cautiously in patients with history of hypertension. Drug may cause exaggerated pressor response. Also, use cautiously in patients with history of sulfite sensitivity.

## NURSING CONSIDERATIONS

• Before starting therapy with dobutamine, correct hypovolemia with plasma volume expanders.

• Give a cardiac glycoside before dobutamine. Because drug increases AV node conduction, patients with atrial fibrillation may develop a rapid ventricular rate.

• Continuously monitor ECG, blood pressure, pulmonary artery wedge pressure, cardiac output, and urine output.

• Monitor electrolyte levels. Drug may lower potassium levels.

• *Alert:* Don't confuse dobutamine with dopamine.

## PATIENT TEACHING

• Tell patient to report adverse reactions promptly, especially labored breathing and drug-induced headache.

• Instruct patient to report discomfort at I.V. insertion site.

# dopamine hydrochloride
Intropin, Revimine†

*Pregnancy risk category C*

## AVAILABLE FORMS

*Injection:* 40 mg/ml, 80 mg/ml, 160 mg/ml parenteral concentrate for injection for I.V. infusion; 0.8 mg/ml (200 or 400 mg) in $D_5W$; 1.6 mg/ml (400 or 800 mg) in $D_5W$; 3.2 mg/ml (800 mg) in $D_5W$ parenteral injection for I.V. infusion

## INDICATIONS & DOSAGES

➤ **To treat shock and correct hemodynamic imbalances, to improve perfusion to vital organs, to increase cardiac output, to correct hypotension**
*Adults:* Initially, 1 to 5 mcg/kg/minute by I.V. infusion. Titrate dosage to desired hemodynamic or renal response. Infusion may be increased by 1 to 4 mcg/kg/minute at 10- to 30-minute intervals.

## I.V. ADMINISTRATION

• Dilute with $D_5W$, normal saline solution, or a combination of $D_5W$ and normal saline solution. Mix just before use.

• Don't mix other drugs in I.V. container with dopamine. Don't give alkaline drugs, oxidizing drugs, or iron salts through I.V. line containing dopamine.

• Use a continuous infusion pump to regulate flow rate. Dosages of 0.5 to 2 mcg/kg/minute predominantly stimulate dopamine receptors and produce vasodilation of the renal vasculature. Dosages of 2 to 10 mcg/kg/minute stimulate beta receptors for a positive inotropic effect. Higher dosages also stimulate alpha receptors, constricting blood vessels and increasing blood pressure. Most patients are satisfactorily maintained on dosages of less than 20 mcg/kg/minute.

• Use a central line or large vein, as in the antecubital fossa, to minimize risk of extravasation. Watch infusion site carefully for signs of extravasation; if it occurs, stop infusion immediately and call prescriber. Extravasation may require treatment by infiltrating the area with 5 to 10 mg phentolamine in 10 to 15 ml normal saline solution.

• Discard after 24 hours (dopamine solutions deteriorate after 24 hours), or earlier if solution is discolored.

## ACTION
Stimulates dopaminergic and alpha and beta receptors of the sympathetic nervous system. Action is dose-related; large doses cause mainly alpha stimulation.

| Route | Onset | Peak | Duration |
|-------|-------|------|----------|
| I.V. | 5 min | Unknown | < 10 min after infusion ends |

## ADVERSE REACTIONS
**CNS:** headache.
**CV:** ectopic beats, tachycardia, angina, palpitations, *hypotension.*
**GI:** nausea, vomiting.
**Metabolic:** azotemia, hyperglycemia.
**Respiratory:** dyspnea, asthmatic episodes.
**Skin:** necrosis and tissue sloughing with extravasation, piloerection.
**Other:** *anaphylactic reactions.*

## INTERACTIONS
**Drug-drug.** *Alpha-adrenergic blockers, beta blockers:* May antagonize dopamine effects. Monitor patient closely.
*Ergot alkaloids:* May cause extremely high blood pressure. Avoid using together.
*Inhaled anesthetics:* May increase risk of arrhythmias or hypertension. Monitor patient closely.
*Oxytocics:* May cause severe, persistent hypertension. Use together cautiously.
*Phenytoin:* May cause seizures, severe hypotension, and bradycardia. Monitor patient carefully.
*MAO inhibitors (phenelzine, tranylcypromine):* May cause severe headache, hypertension, fever and hypertensive crisis. Avoid using together.
*Tricyclic antidepressants:* May decrease pressor response. Monitor patient closely.

## EFFECTS ON LAB TEST RESULTS
• May increase glucose, urine urea, and catecholamine levels.

## CONTRAINDICATIONS & CAUTIONS
• Contraindicated in patients with uncorrected tachyarrhythmias, pheochromocytoma, or ventricular fibrillation.
• Use cautiously in patients with occlusive vascular disease, cold injuries, diabetic endarteritis, and arterial embolism; in pregnant patients; in those with a history of sulfite sensitivity; and in those taking MAO inhibitors.

## NURSING CONSIDERATIONS
• Drug isn't a substitute for blood or fluid volume deficit. If deficit exists, replace fluid before giving vasopressors.
• During infusion, frequently monitor ECG, blood pressure, cardiac output, central venous pressure, pulmonary artery wedge pressure, pulse rate, urine output, and color and temperature of limbs.
• If diastolic pressure rises disproportionately (a marked decrease in pulse pressure) in a patient receiving dopamine, decrease infusion rate, and watch carefully for further evidence of predominant vasoconstrictor activity, unless such an effect is desired.
• Observe patient closely for adverse reactions; dosage may need to be adjusted or drug stopped.
• Check urine output often. If urine flow decreases without hypotension, notify prescriber because dosage may need to be reduced.
• *Alert:* After drug is stopped, watch closely for sudden drop in blood pressure. Taper dosage slowly to evaluate stability of blood pressure.
• Acidosis decreases effectiveness of dopamine.
• *Alert:* Don't confuse dopamine with dobutamine.

## PATIENT TEACHING
• Tell patient to report adverse reactions promptly.
• Instruct patient to report discomfort at I.V. insertion site.

---

## norepinephrine bitartrate (levarterenol bitartrate, noradrenaline acid tartrate)
Levophed

*Pregnancy risk category C*

### AVAILABLE FORMS
*Injection:* 1 mg/ml

### INDICATIONS & DOSAGES
➤ **To restore blood pressure in acute hypotensive states**
*Adults:* Initially, 8 to 12 mcg/minute by I.V. infusion; then titrated to maintain normal blood pressure. Average maintenance dose is 2 to 4 mcg/minute.
*Children:* 2 mcg/m$^2$/minute by I.V. infusion; adjust dosage based on patient response.
➤ **Severe hypotension during cardiac arrest**
*Children:* First I.V. infusion rate is 0.1 mcg/kg/minute. Titrate infusion rate based on patient response.

### I.V. ADMINISTRATION
• Avoid mixing with alkaline solutions, oxidizing drugs, or iron salts.
• Use a central venous catheter or large vein, as in the antecubital fossa, to minimize risk of extravasation. Give in D$_5$W in normal saline solution for injection; normal saline solution for injection alone isn't recommended. Use continuous infusion pump to regulate infusion flow rate and a piggyback setup so I.V. line stays open if norepinephrine is stopped.
• Check site frequently for signs of extravasation. If they appear, stop infusion immediately and call prescriber. Infiltrate area with 5 to 10 mg phentolamine in 10 to 15 ml of normal saline solution to counteract effect of extravasation. Also, check for blanching along course of infused vein, which may progress to superficial sloughing.
• Protect drug from light. Discard discolored solutions or solutions that contain a precipitate. Norepinephrine solutions deteriorate after 24 hours.
• If prolonged I.V. therapy is needed, change injection site frequently.

### ACTION
Stimulates alpha and beta$_1$ receptors in the sympathetic nervous system, causing vasoconstriction and cardiac stimulation.

| Route | Onset | Peak | Duration |
|---|---|---|---|
| I.V. | Immediate | Immediate | 1-2 min after infusion ends |

### ADVERSE REACTIONS
**CNS:** *headache,* anxiety, weakness, dizziness, tremor, restlessness, insomnia.
**CV:** *bradycardia, severe hypertension, arrhythmias.*
**Respiratory:** respiratory difficulties, *asthma attacks.*
**Skin:** irritation with extravasation, necrosis and gangrene secondary to extravasation.
**Other:** *anaphylaxis.*

### INTERACTIONS
**Drug-drug.** *Alpha-adrenergic blockers:* May antagonize drug effects. Avoid using together.
*Antihistamines, ergot alkaloids, guanethidine, MAO inhibitors, methyldopa, oxytocics:* When given with sympathomimetics, may cause severe hypertension (hypertensive crisis). Avoid using together.
*Inhaled anesthetics:* May increase risk of arrhythmias. Monitor ECG.
*Tricyclic antidepressants:* May potentiate the pressor response and cause arrhythmias. Use together cautiously.

### EFFECTS ON LAB TEST RESULTS
None reported.

### CONTRAINDICATIONS & CAUTIONS
• Contraindicated in patients with mesenteric or peripheral vascular thrombosis, profound hypoxia, hypercarbia, or hypotension resulting from blood volume deficit.
• Contraindicated during cyclopropane and halothane anesthesia.
• Use with extreme caution in patients receiving MAO inhibitors or triptyline- or imipramine-type antidepressants.
• Use cautiously in patients with sulfite sensitivity.

**NURSING CONSIDERATIONS**
• Drug isn't a substitute for blood or fluid replacement therapy. If patient has volume deficit, replace fluids before giving vasopressors.
• *Alert:* Never leave patient unattended during infusion. Check blood pressure every 2 minutes until stabilized; then check every 5 minutes. In previously hypertensive patients, blood pressure should increase no more than 40 mm Hg below baseline systolic pressure.
• During infusion, frequently monitor ECG, cardiac output, central venous pressure, pulmonary artery wedge pressure, pulse rate, urine output, and color and temperature of limbs. Titrate infusion rate based on findings and prescriber guidelines.
• Keep emergency drugs on hand to reverse effects of norepinephrine: atropine for reflex bradycardia, phentolamine to decrease vasopressor effects, and propranolol for arrhythmias.
• Notify prescriber immediately of decreased urine output.
• When stopping drug, gradually slow infusion rate. Continue monitoring vital signs, watching for possible severe drop in blood pressure.
• *Alert:* Don't confuse norepinephrine with epinephrine.

**PATIENT TEACHING**
• Tell patient to report adverse reactions promptly.
• Advise patient to report discomfort at I.V. insertion site.

---

**phenylephrine hydrochloride**
Neo-Synephrine

*Pregnancy risk category C*

**AVAILABLE FORMS**
*Injection:* 10 mg/ml

**INDICATIONS & DOSAGES**
➤ **Hypotensive emergencies during spinal anesthesia**
*Adults:* Initially, 0.2 mg I.V.; subsequent doses shouldn't exceed the preceding dose by more than 0.2 mg. Maximum single dosage is 0.5 mg.

➤ **To maintain blood pressure during spinal or inhaled anesthesia**
*Adults:* 2 to 3 mg S.C. or I.M. 3 to 4 minutes before anesthesia.
*Children:* 0.044 mg to 0.088 mg/kg S.C. or I.M.
➤ **To prolong spinal anesthesia**
*Adults:* 2 to 5 mg added to anesthetic solution.
➤ **Vasoconstrictor for regional anesthesia**
*Adults:* 1 mg phenylephrine added to each 20 ml local anesthetic.
➤ **Mild to moderate hypotension**
*Adults:* 2 to 5 mg S.C. or I.M.; repeated in 1 or 2 hours as needed and tolerated. First dose shouldn't exceed 5 mg. Or, 0.1 to 0.5 mg slow I.V., not to be repeated more often than 10 to 15 minutes.
*Children:* 0.1 mg/kg I.M. or S.C.; repeated in 1 or 2 hours as needed and tolerated.
➤ **Severe hypotension and shock (including drug-induced)**
*Adults:* 10 mg in 250 to 500 ml of $D_5W$ or normal saline solution for injection. I.V. infusion started at 100 to 180 mcg/minute; then decreased to maintenance infusion of 40 to 60 mcg/minute when blood pressure stabilizes.
➤ **Paroxysmal supraventricular tachycardia**
*Adults:* Initially, 0.5 mg rapid I.V., increased in increments of 0.1 to 0.2 mg Use cautiously; maximum single dose is 1 mg.

**I.V. ADMINISTRATION**
• For direct injection, dilute 10 mg (1 ml) with 9 ml sterile water for injection to provide 1 mg/ml. Infusions are usually prepared by adding 10 mg of drug to 500 ml of $D_5W$ or normal saline solution for injection. The first I.V. infusion rate is usually 100 to 180 mcg/minute; maintenance rate is usually 40 to 60 mcg/minute.
• Use a central venous catheter or large vein, as in the antecubital fossa, to minimize risk of extravasation. Use a continuous infusion pump to regulate infusion flow rate.
• To treat extravasation, infiltrate site promptly with 10 to 15 ml of normal saline solution for injection containing 5 to 10 mg phentolamine. Use a fine needle.
• During infusion, frequently monitor ECG, blood pressure, cardiac output, cen-

---

tral venous pressure, pulmonary artery wedge pressure, pulse rate, urine output, and color and temperature of limbs. Titrate infusion rate according to findings and prescriber guidelines. Maintain blood pressure slightly below patient's normal level. In previously normotensive patients, maintain systolic blood pressure at 80 to 100 mm Hg; in previously hypertensive patients, maintain systolic blood pressure at 30 to 40 mm Hg below usual level.
• Avoid abrupt withdrawal after prolonged I.V. infusions.

## ACTION
Stimulates alpha receptors in the sympathetic nervous system, causing vasoconstriction.

| Route | Onset | Peak | Duration |
|-------|-------|------|----------|
| I.V. | Immediate | Unknown | 15-20 min |
| I.M. | 10-15 min | Unknown | 30-120 min |
| S.C. | 10-15 min | Unknown | 50-60 min |

## ADVERSE REACTIONS
**CNS:** *headache,* excitability, restlessness, anxiety, nervousness, dizziness, weakness.
**CV:** *bradycardia, arrhythmias,* hypertension.
**Respiratory:** *asthmatic episodes.*
**Skin:** tissue sloughing with extravasation.
**Other:** tachyphylaxis and decreased organ perfusion with continued use, *anaphylaxis.*

## INTERACTIONS
**Drug-drug.** *Alpha-adrenergic blockers, phenothiazines:* May decrease vasopressor response. Monitor patient closely.
*Beta blockers:* May block cardiostimulatory effects. Monitor patient closely.
*Halogenated hydrocarbon anesthetics, sympathomimetics:* May cause serious arrhythmias. Use together with extreme caution.
*Guanethidine, oxytocics:* May increase pressor response. Monitor patient.
*MAO inhibitors (phenelzine, tranylcypromine):* May cause severe headache, hypertension, fever and hypertensive crisis. Avoid using together.
*Tricyclic antidepressants:* May potentiate the pressor response and cause arrhythmias. Use together cautiously.

## EFFECTS ON LAB TEST RESULTS
None reported.

## CONTRAINDICATIONS & CAUTIONS
• Contraindicated in patients hypersensitive to drug and in those with severe hypertension or ventricular tachycardia.
• Use with extreme caution in elderly patients and in patients with heart disease, hyperthyroidism, severe atherosclerosis, bradycardia, partial heart block, myocardial disease, or sulfite sensitivity.

## NURSING CONSIDERATIONS
• Drug causes little or no CNS stimulation.
• Drug may lower intraocular pressure in normal eyes or in open-angle glaucoma. It also may cause false-normal tonometry readings.
• Drug is incompatible with butacaine sulfate, alkalis, ferric salts, and oxidizing drugs.
• Drug used in eyedrops and OTC cold preparations for decongestant effects.

## PATIENT TEACHING
• Tell patient to report adverse reactions promptly.
• Instruct patient to report discomfort at I.V. insertion site.

# pseudoephedrine hydrochloride
Cenafed ◇  Decofed ◇, Dimetapp, Genaphed ◇, PediaCare Infants' Decongestant Drops ◇, Sudafed ◇, Triaminic

# pseudoephedrine sulfate
Drixoral Non-Drowsy Formula ◇

*Pregnancy risk category C*

## AVAILABLE FORMS
**pseudoephedrine hydrochloride**
*Capsules:* 60 mg ◇
*Capsules (extended-release):* 120 mg
*Oral solution:* 7.5 mg/0.8 ml ◇, 15 mg/ 5 ml ◇, 30 mg/5 ml ◇
*Syrup:* 30 mg/5 ml
*Tablets:* 30 mg ◇, 60 mg ◇
*Tablets (chewable):* 15 mg ◇

---

*Tablets (extended-release):* 120 mg ◇,
240 mg ◇
**pseudoephedrine sulfate**
*Tablets (extended-release):* 120 mg
(60 mg immediate-release, 60 mg
delayed-release) ◇

## INDICATIONS & DOSAGES
➤ **To decongest nose and eustachian tube**
*Adults and children age 12 and over:*
60 mg P.O. q 4 to 6 hours; or 120 mg P.O.
extended-release tablet q 12 hours; or
240 mg P.O. extended-release tablet once
daily. Maximum dosage is 240 mg daily.
*Children ages 6 to 12:* 30 mg P.O. q 4 to
6 hours. Maximum dosage is 120 mg
daily.
*Children ages 2 to 5:* 15 mg P.O. q 4 to
6 hours. Maximum dosage is 60 mg daily,
or 4 mg/kg or 125 mg/m$^2$ P.O. divided
q.i.d.
*Children ages 1 to 2:* 7 drops or 0.2 ml/kg
P.O. q 4 to 6 hours, up to four doses daily.
*Children ages 3 to 12 months:* 3 drops/kg
P.O. q 4 to 6 hours, up to four doses daily.

## ACTION
Stimulates alpha receptors in the respiratory tract, constricting blood vessels,
shrinking swollen nasal mucous membranes, increasing airway patency, and reducing tissue hyperemia, edema, and nasal
congestion.

| Route | Onset | Peak | Duration |
|-------|-------|------|----------|
| P.O. | 30 min | 30-60 min | 4-12 hr |

## ADVERSE REACTIONS
**CNS:** *anxiety,* transient stimulation,
tremor, dizziness, headache, insomnia,
*nervousness.*
**CV:** **arrhythmias,** *palpitations,* tachycardia, **CV collapse.**
**GI:** anorexia, nausea, vomiting, dry
mouth.
**GU:** difficulty urinating.
**Respiratory:** respiratory difficulties.
**Skin:** pallor.

## INTERACTIONS
**Drug-drug.** *Antihypertensives:* May inhibit hypotensive effect. Monitor blood
pressure closely.

*MAO inhibitors (phenelzine, tranylcypromine):* May cause severe headache, hypertension, fever, and hypertensive crisis.
Avoid using together.
*Methyldopa:* May increase pressor response. Monitor patient closely.

## EFFECTS ON LAB TEST RESULTS
None reported.

## CONTRAINDICATIONS & CAUTIONS
● Contraindicated in patients with severe
hypertension or severe coronary artery
disease, in those receiving MAO inhibitors, and in breast-feeding women.
Extended-release forms are contraindicated in children younger than age 12.
● Use cautiously in patients with hypertension, cardiac disease, diabetes, glaucoma,
hyperthyroidism, and prostatic hyperplasia.

## NURSING CONSIDERATIONS
● Elderly patients are more sensitive to
drug's effects. Extended-release tablets
shouldn't be given to elderly patients until
safety with short-acting preparations has
been established.

## PATIENT TEACHING
● Tell patient not to crush or break
extended-release forms.
● Warn against using OTC products containing other sympathomimetics.
● Instruct patient not to take drug within
2 hours of bedtime because it can cause
insomnia.
● Tell patient to stop drug and notify prescriber if he becomes unusually restless.

---

Reactions may be *common,* uncommon, *life-threatening*, or COMMON AND LIFE-THREATENING.

**baclofen**
**carisoprodol**
**cyclobenzaprine hydrochloride**
**dantrolene sodium**
**methocarbamol**
**tizanidine hydrochloride**

## COMBINATION PRODUCTS

NORGESIC: orphenadrine citrate 25 mg, aspirin 385 mg, and caffeine 30 mg.
NORGESIC FORTE: orphenadrine citrate 50 mg, aspirin 770 mg, and caffeine 60 mg.
ROBAXISAL: methocarbamol 400 mg and aspirin 325 mg.
SOMA COMPOUND: carisoprodol 200 mg and aspirin 325 mg.
SOMA COMPOUND WITH CODEINE: carisoprodol 200 mg, aspirin 325 mg, and codeine phosphate 16 mg.

---

## baclofen
Clofen‡, Lioresal, Lioresal Intrathecal

*Pregnancy risk category C*

## AVAILABLE FORMS
*Intrathecal injection:* 500 mcg/ml, 2,000 mcg/ml
*Tablets:* 10 mg, 20 mg, 25 mg‡

## INDICATIONS & DOSAGES
➤ **Spasticity in multiple sclerosis; spinal cord injury**
*Adults:* Initially, 5 mg P.O. t.i.d. for 3 days; then 10 mg t.i.d. for 3 days, 15 mg t.i.d. for 3 days, 20 mg t.i.d. for 3 days. Increase daily dosage based on response, to maximum of 80 mg.
*Adjust-a-dose:* For patients with psychiatric or brain disorders and in the elderly, increase dose gradually.
➤ **To manage severe spasticity in patients who don't respond to or can't tolerate oral baclofen therapy**
*Adults:* For screening phase, after test dose to check responsiveness, give drug via implantable infusion pump. Give test dosage of 1 ml of 50-mcg/ml dilution into intra-

thecal space by barbotage over 1 minute or longer. Significantly decreased severity or frequency of muscle spasm or reduced muscle tone should appear within 4 to 8 hours. If response is inadequate, give second test dosage of 75 mcg/1.5 ml 24 hours after the first. If response is still inadequate, give final test dosage of 100 mcg/2 ml after 24 hours. Patients unresponsive to the 100-mcg dose shouldn't be considered candidates for implantable pump.

For maintenance therapy, adjust first dose based on screening dose that elicited an adequate response. Double this effective dose and give over 24 hours. However, if screening dose efficacy was maintained for 12 hours or longer, don't double the dose. After the first 24 hours, increase dose slowly as needed and tolerated by 10% to 30% daily. During prolonged maintenance therapy, increase daily dose by 10% to 40% if needed; if patient experiences adverse effects, decrease dosage by 10% to 20%. Maintenance dosages range from 12 mcg to 2,000 mcg daily, but experience with dosages over 1,000 mcg daily is limited. Most patients need 300 to 800 mcg daily.
*Adjust-a-dose:* For patients with impaired renal function, decrease oral and intrathecal doses.

## ACTION
Hyperpolarizes fibers to reduce impulse transmission. Appears to reduce transmission of impulses from the spinal cord to skeletal muscle, thus decreasing the frequency and amplitude of muscle spasms in patients with spinal cord lesions.

| Route | Onset | Peak | Duration |
|-------|-------|------|----------|
| P.O. | Unknown | 2-3 hr | Unknown |
| Intrathecal | 30 min–1 hr | 4 hr | 4-8 hr |

## ADVERSE REACTIONS
**CNS:** *drowsiness, **high fever,** dizziness,* headache, *weakness, fatigue,* **paresthesias,** hypotonia, *confusion,* insomnia, dysarthria, ***seizures with intrathecal use.***
**CV:** hypotension, hypertension.

**EENT:** blurred vision, nasal congestion, slurred speech.
**GI:** *nausea,* constipation, *vomiting.*
**GU:** urinary frequency.
**Metabolic:** hyperglycemia, weight gain.
**Musculoskeletal:** muscle rigidity or spasticity, *rhabdomyolysis,* muscle weakness.
**Respiratory:** dyspnea.
**Skin:** rash, pruritus, excessive sweating.
**Other:** *multiple organ-system failure.*

## INTERACTIONS
**Drug-drug.** *CNS depressants:* May increase CNS depression. Avoid using together.
**Drug-lifestyle.** *Alcohol use:* May increase CNS depression. Discourage use together.

## EFFECTS ON LAB TEST RESULTS
• May increase AST, alkaline phosphatase, CPK, and glucose levels.

## CONTRAINDICATIONS & CAUTIONS
• Contraindicated in patients hypersensitive to drug.
• Use cautiously in patients with impaired renal function or seizure disorder or when spasticity is used to maintain motor function.

## NURSING CONSIDERATIONS
• Give oral form with meals or with milk to prevent GI distress.
• *Alert:* Don't use oral drug to treat muscle spasm caused by rheumatic disorders, cerebral palsy, Parkinson's disease, or CVA because drug's efficacy for these indications hasn't been established. Don't give intrathecal injection by I.V., I.M., S.C., or epidural route.
• Watch for sensitivity reactions, such as fever, skin eruptions, and respiratory distress.
• Expect an increased risk of seizures in patients with seizure disorder.
• The amount of relief determines whether dosage (and drowsiness) can be reduced.
• Don't withdraw drug abruptly after long-term use unless severe adverse reactions demand it; doing so may precipitate seizures, hallucinations or rebound spasticity.
• Experience with long-term intrathecal use suggests that about 5% of patients may develop tolerance to drug. In some

cases, it may be treated by hospitalizing patient and slowly withdrawing drug over a 2-week period.
• *Alert:* Don't confuse baclofen with Bactroban.

## PATIENT TEACHING
• Instruct patient to take oral form with meals or milk.
• Tell patient to avoid activities that require alertness until CNS effects of drug are known. Drowsiness usually is transient.
• Tell patient to avoid alcohol and OTC antihistamines while taking drug.
• Advise patient to follow prescriber's orders regarding rest and physical therapy.

# carisoprodol
Soma◆, Vanadom

*Pregnancy risk category C*

## AVAILABLE FORMS
*Tablets:* 350 mg

## INDICATIONS & DOSAGES
➤ **Adjunctive treatment for acute, painful musculoskeletal conditions**
*Adults:* 350 mg P.O. t.i.d. and h.s.

## ACTION
Unknown. Appears to modify central perception of pain without modifying pain reflexes. Muscle relaxant effects may be related to sedative properties.

| Route | Onset | Peak | Duration |
|-------|-------|------|----------|
| P.O. | ½ hr | 4 hr | 4-6 hr |

## ADVERSE REACTIONS
**CNS:** fever, *drowsiness, dizziness,* vertigo, ataxia, tremor, agitation, irritability, headache, depressive reactions, insomnia, syncope.
**CV:** *orthostatic hypotension,* tachycardia, facial flushing.
**GI:** nausea, vomiting, epigastric distress.
**Hematologic:** eosinophilia.
**Respiratory:** *asthmatic episodes,* hiccups.
**Skin:** rash, *erythema multiforme,* pruritus.
**Other:** *angioedema, anaphylaxis.*

---

Reactions may be *common,* uncommon, *life-threatening,* or COMMON AND LIFE-THREATENING.

## INTERACTIONS

**Drug-drug.** *CNS depressants:* May increase CNS depression. Avoid using together.
**Drug-lifestyle.** *Alcohol use:* May increase CNS depression. Discourage use together.

## EFFECTS ON LAB TEST RESULTS
• May increase eosinophil count.

## CONTRAINDICATIONS & CAUTIONS
• Contraindicated in patients hypersensitive to related compounds (such as meprobamate or tybamate) and in those with intermittent porphyria.
• Use cautiously in patients with impaired hepatic or renal function.
• Safety and efficacy in children younger than age 12 haven't been established.

## NURSING CONSIDERATIONS
• *Alert:* Watch for idiosyncratic reactions after first to fourth doses (weakness, ataxia, visual and speech difficulties, fever, skin eruptions, and mental changes) and for severe reactions, including bronchospasm, hypotension, and anaphylactic shock. After unusual reactions, withhold dose and notify prescriber immediately.
• Record amount of relief to help prescriber determine whether dosage can be reduced.
• Don't stop drug abruptly, which may cause mild withdrawal effects such as insomnia, headache, nausea, and abdominal cramps.
• Drug may be habit forming.

## PATIENT TEACHING
• Warn patient to avoid activities that require alertness until CNS effects of drug are known. Drowsiness is transient.
• Advise patient to avoid combining drug with alcohol or other CNS depressants.
• Tell patient to ask prescriber before using OTC cold or hay fever remedies.
• Instruct patient to follow prescriber's orders regarding rest and physical therapy.
• Advise patient to avoid sudden changes in posture if dizziness occurs.
• Tell patient to take drug with food or milk if GI upset occurs.

# cyclobenzaprine hydrochloride
Flexeril

*Pregnancy risk category B*

## AVAILABLE FORMS
*Tablets:* 5 mg, 10 mg

## INDICATIONS & DOSAGES
➤ **Adjunct to rest and physical therapy to relieve muscle spasm from acute, painful musculoskeletal conditions**
*Adults:* 5 mg P.O. t.i.d. Based on response, dose may be increased to 10 mg t.i.d. Use for periods longer than 2 or 3 weeks isn't recommended.
*Adjust-a-dose:* In elderly patients and in those with mild hepatic impairment, start with 5 mg and adjust slowly upward. Drug isn't recommended in patients with moderate-to-severe impairment.

## ACTION
Unknown. Relieves skeletal muscle spasm of local origin without disrupting muscle function.

| Route | Onset | Peak | Duration |
|-------|-------|------|----------|
| P.O. | 1 hr | 3-8 hr | 12-24 hr |

## ADVERSE REACTIONS
**CNS:** *drowsiness,* headache, insomnia, fatigue, asthenia, nervousness, confusion, paresthesia, *dizziness,* depression, **seizures,** dysarthria, ataxia, syncope.
**CV:** tachycardia, **arrhythmias,** palpitations, hypotension, vasodilation.
**EENT:** visual disturbances, blurred vision.
**GI:** dyspepsia, abnormal taste, constipation, *dry mouth,* nausea.
**GU:** urine retention, urinary frequency.
**Skin:** rash, urticaria, pruritus.

## INTERACTIONS
**Drug-drug.** *Anticholinergics:* May have additive anticholinergic effects. Avoid using together.
*CNS depressants:* May increase CNS depression. Avoid using together.
*MAO inhibitors:* May cause hyperpyretic crisis, seizures, and death when MAO inhibitors are used with tricyclic antidepres-

sants; may also occur with cyclobenzaprine. Avoid using within 2 weeks of MAO inhibitor therapy.
**Drug-lifestyle.** *Alcohol use:* May increase CNS depression. Discourage use together.

## EFFECTS ON LAB TEST RESULTS
None reported.

## CONTRAINDICATIONS & CAUTIONS
• Contraindicated in patients hypersensitive to drug and in those with hyperthyroidism, heart block, arrhythmias, conduction disturbances, or heart failure; also contraindicated in those who have received MAO inhibitors within 14 days and those who are in the acute recovery phase of an MI.
• Use cautiously in elderly or debilitated patients, and those with a history of urine retention, acute angle-closure glaucoma, or increased intraocular pressure.
• Safety and efficacy in children younger than age 15 haven't been established.

## NURSING CONSIDERATIONS
• Cyclobenzaprine may cause toxic reactions similar to tricyclic antidepressants. Observe precautions as when giving tricyclic antidepressants.
• Monitor patient for nausea, headache, and malaise, which may occur if drug is stopped abruptly after long-term use.
• *Alert:* Notify prescriber immediately of signs and symptoms of overdose, including cardiac toxicity.
• *Alert:* Don't confuse Flexeril with Floxin or Flaxedil.

## PATIENT TEACHING
• Advise patient to report urinary hesitancy or urine retention. If constipation is a problem, suggest that patient increase fluid intake and use a stool softener.
• Warn patient to avoid activities that require alertness until CNS effects of drug are known.
• Warn patient not to combine with alcohol or other CNS depressants, including OTC cold or allergy remedies.
• Instruct patient not to attempt splitting the generic 10-mg tablets because of a high potential for dosing inconsistencies.

---

# dantrolene sodium
Dantrium, Dantrium Intravenous

*Pregnancy risk category C*

## AVAILABLE FORMS
*Capsules:* 25 mg, 50 mg, 100 mg
*Injection:* 20 mg/vial

## INDICATIONS & DOSAGES
➤ **Spasticity and sequelae from severe chronic disorders, such as multiple sclerosis, cerebral palsy, spinal cord injury, CVA**
*Adults:* 25 mg P.O. daily. Increase gradually by 25-mg, up to 100 mg b.i.d. to q.i.d. Maximum, 400 mg daily. Maintain each dosage level for 4 to 7 days to determine response.
*Children:* Initially, 0.5 mg/kg P.O. q.d. for 7 days, then 0.5 mg/kg t.i.d. for 7 days, then 1 mg/kg t.i.d. for 7 days, then 2 mg/kg, t.i.d. for 7 days. Maximum, 100 mg q.i.d.
➤ **To manage malignant hyperthermic crisis**
*Adults and children:* Initially, 1 mg/kg I.V. push. Repeat, p.r.n., up to cumulative dose of 10 mg/kg.
➤ **To prevent or attenuate malignant hyperthermic crisis in susceptible patients who need surgery**
*Adults:* 4 to 8 mg/kg P.O. daily in three or four divided doses for 1 or 2 days before procedure. Give final dose 3 or 4 hours before procedure.
➤ **To prevent recurrence of malignant hyperthermic crisis**
*Adults:* 4 to 8 mg/kg P.O. daily in four divided doses for up to 3 days after hyperthermic crisis.

## I.V. ADMINISTRATION
• Give as soon as malignant hyperthermia reaction is recognized.
• Reconstitute drug by adding 60 ml of sterile water for injection and shaking vial until clear. Don't use a diluent that contains a bacteriostatic drug.
• Protect contents from light, and use within 6 hours.

## ACTION
Acts directly on skeletal muscle to decrease excitation and contraction coupling

---

and reduce muscle strength by interfering with intracellular calcium movement.

| Route | Onset | Peak | Duration |
|-------|-------|------|----------|
| P.O. | Unknown | 5 hr | Unknown |
| I.V. | Unknown | Unknown | 3 hr after infusion ends |

## ADVERSE REACTIONS
**CNS:** *drowsiness, dizziness,* headache, light-headedness, *malaise, fatigue,* confusion, nervousness, insomnia, *seizures,* fever, depression.
**CV:** tachycardia, blood pressure changes, phlebitis, thrombophlebitis.
**EENT:** excessive lacrimation, speech disturbance, diplopia, visual disturbances.
**GI:** anorexia, constipation, cramping, dysphagia, metallic taste, severe diarrhea, GI bleeding, vomiting.
**GU:** urinary frequency, hematuria, incontinence, nocturia, dysuria, crystalluria, difficult erection, urine retention.
**Hepatic:** *hepatitis.*
**Musculoskeletal:** myalgia, back pain, *muscle weakness.*
**Respiratory:** pleural effusion with pericarditis, pulmonary edema.
**Skin:** eczematous eruption, pruritus, urticaria, abnormal hair growth, diaphoresis.
**Other:** chills.

## INTERACTIONS
**Drug-drug.** *Clofibrate, warfarin:* May decrease plasma protein binding of dantrolene. Use together cautiously.
*CNS depressants:* May increase CNS depression. Avoid using together.
*Estrogens:* May increase risk of hepatotoxicity. Use together cautiously.
*I.V. verapamil and other calcium channel blockers:* May result in CV collapse. Stop verapamil before giving I.V. dantrolene.
*Vecuronium:* May increase neuromuscular blockade effect. Use together cautiously.
**Drug-lifestyle.** *Alcohol use:* May increase CNS depression. Discourage use together.
*Sun exposure:* May cause photosensitivity reactions. Advise patient to avoid excessive sunlight exposure.

## EFFECTS ON LAB TEST RESULTS
● May increase BUN, ALT, AST, and bilirubin levels.

## CONTRAINDICATIONS & CAUTIONS
● Contraindicated for spasms in rheumatic disorders and when spasticity is used to maintain motor function.
● Contraindicated in breast-feeding patients and patients with upper motor neuron disorders or active hepatic disease.
● Use cautiously in women, patients older than age 35, and patients with hepatic disease or severely impaired cardiac or pulmonary function.

## NURSING CONSIDERATIONS
● Because of risk of liver damage with long-term use, stop therapy within 45 days if benefits don't occur.
● Obtain liver function test results at start of therapy.
● Prepare oral suspension for single dose by dissolving capsule contents in juice or other liquid. For multiple doses, use acid vehicle, and refrigerate. Use within several days.
● *Alert:* Watch for hepatitis (fever and jaundice), severe diarrhea, severe weakness, and sensitivity reactions (fever or skin eruptions). Withhold dose and notify prescriber.
● The amount of relief obtained determines whether dosage (and drowsiness) can be reduced.
● *Alert:* Don't confuse Dantrium with Daraprim.

## PATIENT TEACHING
● Instruct patient to take drug with meals or milk in four divided doses.
● Tell patient to eat cautiously to avoid choking. Some patients may have trouble swallowing during therapy.
● Warn patient to avoid driving and other hazardous activities until CNS effects of drug are known.
● Advise patient to avoid combining drug with alcohol and other CNS depressants.
● Advise patient to notify prescriber if skin or eyes turn yellow, skin itches, or fever develops.
● Tell patient to avoid photosensitivity reactions by using sunblock and wearing protective clothing, to report abdominal discomfort or GI problems immediately, and to follow prescriber's orders regarding rest and physical therapy.

---

# methocarbamol
Carbacot, Robaxin, Robaxin-750, Skelex

*Pregnancy risk category C*

## AVAILABLE FORMS
*Injection:* 100 mg/ml
*Tablets:* 500 mg, 750 mg

## INDICATIONS & DOSAGES
➤ **Adjunctive treatment in acute, painful musculoskeletal conditions**
*Adults:* 1.5 g P.O. q.i.d. for 2 to 3 days, then 1 g P.O. q.i.d. Or, no more than 500 mg or 5 ml I.M. into each gluteal region, repeated q 8 hours, p.r.n. Or, 1 to 3 g or 10 to 30 ml daily I.V. directly into vein at 3 ml/minute. Or, 10 ml may be added to no more than 250 ml of $D_5W$ or normal saline solution. Maximum I.V. or I.M. dosage is 3 g daily for no longer than 3 days.
➤ **Supportive therapy in tetanus management**
*Adults:* 1 to 2 g by direct I.V. or 1 to 3 g as infusion q 6 hours until nasogastric tube can be inserted; then give oral doses through nasogastric tube. Maximum total daily oral dose is 24 g.
*Children:* 15 mg/kg I.V. q 6 hours p.r.n.

## I.V. ADMINISTRATION
● Dilute 10 ml of drug in no more than 250 ml of solution. Use $D_5W$ or normal saline solution for injection. Infuse slowly; maximum rate is 300 mg (3 ml)/minute.
● Drug irritates veins and, if injected rapidly, may cause phlebitis or fainting and aggravate seizures. Make sure patient stays supine during infusion and for 10 to 15 minutes after infusion. Watch for irritation and infiltration; extravasation can cause tissue damage and necrosis.

## ACTION
Unknown. Probably modifies central perception of pain through sedative effects without modifying pain reflexes.

| Route | Onset | Peak | Duration |
|-------|-------|------|----------|
| P.O. | 30 min | 2 hr | Unknown |
| I.V. | Immediate | Immediate | Unknown |
| I.M. | Unknown | Unknown | Unknown |

## ADVERSE REACTIONS
**CNS:** *drowsiness, dizziness,* headache, fever, *light-headedness,* syncope, mild muscular incoordination with I.M. or I.V. use, *seizures with I.V. use,* vertigo.
**CV:** hypotension, *bradycardia with I.M. or I.V. use,* thrombophlebitis, flushing.
**EENT:** blurred vision, conjunctivitis, nystagmus, diplopia.
**GI:** nausea, GI upset, metallic taste.
**GU:** hematuria with I.V. use, discoloration of urine.
**Skin:** urticaria, pruritus, rash.
**Other:** extravasation with I.V. use, *anaphylactic reactions with I.M. or I.V. use.*

## INTERACTIONS
**Drug-drug.** *CNS depressants:* May increase CNS depression. Avoid using together.
**Drug-lifestyle.** *Alcohol use:* May increase CNS depression. Discourage use together.

## EFFECTS ON LAB TEST RESULTS
● May cause false-positive results for urine 5-hydroxyindoleacetic acid using Udenfriend method and for vanillylmandelic acid using Gitlow screening test (though not when using Sunderman method).

## CONTRAINDICATIONS & CAUTIONS
● Contraindicated in patients hypersensitive to drug.
● Injectable form contraindicated in those with impaired renal function or seizure disorder.

## NURSING CONSIDERATIONS
● For nasogastric tube administration, prepare liquid by crushing tablets into water or saline solution.
● In tetanus management, methocarbamol is used with tetanus antitoxin, penicillin, tracheotomy, and aggressive supportive care. Long course of I.V. methocarbamol therapy is needed.
● Give I.M. deeply, only into upper outer quadrant of buttocks, with maximum of 5 ml in each buttock.
● Don't give by S.C. route.
● Watch for orthostatic hypotension, especially with parenteral use. Keep patient in a supine position for 15 minutes after-

---

ward, have patient rise slowly, and supervise ambulation.
• Watch for sensitivity reactions, such as fever and skin eruptions.
• Keep epinephrine, antihistamines, and corticosteroids available.
• *Alert:* Don't confuse methocarbamol with mephobarbital.

## PATIENT TEACHING
• Instruct patient to take drug with food or milk at evenly spaced intervals.
• Tell patient that a metallic taste may develop and that urine may turn green, black, or brown.
• Advise patient to follow prescriber's orders regarding physical activity.
• Warn patient to avoid activities that require alertness until CNS effects of drug are known.
• Advise patient not to combine drug with alcohol or other CNS depressants.

---

## tizanidine hydrochloride
Zanaflex

*Pregnancy risk category C*

## AVAILABLE FORMS
*Capsules:* 2 mg, 4 mg, 6 mg
*Tablets:* 2 mg, 4 mg

## INDICATIONS & DOSAGES
➤ **Acute and intermittent management of increased muscle tone with spasticity**
*Adults:* Initially, 4 mg P.O. q 6 to 8 hours, p.r.n., to maximum of three doses in 24 hours. Dosage can be increased gradually in 2- to 4-mg increments. Maximum, 36 mg daily.
*Adjust-a-dose:* For patients with renal failure, reduce dosage. If higher dosages are needed, increase individual doses rather than frequency.

## ACTION
Unknown. Acts as an alpha$_2$ agonist. May reduce spasticity by increasing presynaptic inhibition of motor neurons at the level of the spinal cord.

| Route | Onset | Peak | Duration |
|-------|-------|------|----------|
| P.O. | Unknown | 1-2 hr | 3-6 hr |

## ADVERSE REACTIONS
**CNS:** *somnolence, sedation, asthenia, dizziness,* speech disorder, dyskinesia, nervousness, hallucinations.
**CV:** *hypotension.*
**EENT:** amblyopia, pharyngitis, rhinitis.
**GI:** *dry mouth,* constipation, vomiting.
**GU:** *urinary tract infection,* urinary frequency.
**Hepatic:** hepatic injury.
**Other:** infection, flulike syndrome.

## INTERACTIONS
**Drug-drug.** *Antihypertensives, other alpha agonists such as clonidine:* May cause hypotension; monitor patient closely. Avoid using together.
*Baclofen, benzodiazepines, other CNS depressants:* May have additive CNS depressant effects. Avoid using together.
*Hormonal contraceptives:* May decrease tizanidine clearance. Dosage of tizanidine may be reduced.
**Drug-lifestyle.** *Alcohol use:* May increase CNS depression. Discourage use together.

## EFFECTS ON LAB TEST RESULTS
• May increase AST and ALT levels.

## CONTRAINDICATIONS & CAUTIONS
• Contraindicated in patients hypersensitive to drug and in pregnant or breast-feeding women.
• Use cautiously in patients who are taking antihypertensives, in those with renal and hepatic impairment, and in elderly patients.
• Safety and effectiveness in children haven't been established.

## NURSING CONSIDERATIONS
• *Alert:* Don't confuse tizanidine with tiagabine; both have 4-mg starting doses.
• Obtain liver function test results before treatment; during treatment at 1, 3, and 6 months; and then periodically thereafter.

## PATIENT TEACHING
• Caution patient to avoid alcohol and activities that require alertness. Drug may cause drowsiness.
• Inform patient that dizziness upon standing quickly can be minimized by rising slowly and avoiding sudden position changes.

---

**atracurium besylate**
**cisatracurium besylate**
**doxacurium chloride**
**mivacurium chloride**
**pancuronium bromide**
**rocuronium bromide**
**succinylcholine chloride**
**tubocurarine chloride**
**vecuronium bromide**

**COMBINATION PRODUCTS**
None.

---

## atracurium besylate
Tracrium

*Pregnancy risk category C*

---

**AVAILABLE FORMS**
*Injection:* 10 mg/ml

**INDICATIONS & DOSAGES**
➤ **Adjunct to general anesthesia to facilitate endotracheal intubation and relax skeletal muscles during surgery or mechanical ventilation**
*Adults and children older than age 2:* 0.4 to 0.5 mg/kg by I.V. bolus. Give maintenance dosage of 0.08 to 0.1 mg/kg within 20 to 45 minutes during prolonged surgery. Give maintenance doses q 12 to 25 minutes in patients receiving balanced anesthesia. For prolonged procedures, use a constant infusion of 5 to 9 mcg/kg/minute.
*Children ages 1 month to 2 years:* First dose, 0.3 to 0.4 mg/kg I.V. for children under halothane anesthesia. Frequent maintenance doses may be needed.

**I.V. ADMINISTRATION**
• Use drug only under direct supervision by medical staff skilled in using neuromuscular blockers and maintaining patent airway. Keep available emergency respiratory support (endotracheal equipment, ventilator, oxygen, atropine, edrophonium, neostigmine, and epinephrine).

• Give sedatives or general anesthetics before neuromuscular blockers, which don't obtund consciousness or alter pain threshold.
• Drug usually is given by rapid I.V. bolus injection but may be given by intermittent infusion or continuous infusion. At concentrations of 0.2 mg/ml to 0.5 mg/ml, atracurium is compatible for 24 hours in $D_5W$, normal saline solution for injection, or dextrose 5% in normal saline solution for injection.
• Don't use lactated Ringer's solution. In lactated Ringer's injection, atracurium is stable for 8 hours at 0.5 mg/ml, but, because of increased degradation in this solution, it isn't recommended.
• Don't mix with alkaline solutions such as barbiturates, because precipitates may form.
• Stable if undiluted for 6 weeks.
• Store in refrigerator. Don't freeze. Once removed, use within 14 days.

**ACTION**
A nondepolarizing drug that keeps acetylcholine from binding to receptors on motor end plate, thus blocking neuromuscular transmission.

| Route | Onset | Peak | Duration |
|-------|-------|------|----------|
| I.V. | 2 min | 3-5 min | 35-70 min |

**ADVERSE REACTIONS**
**CV:** *bradycardia,* hypotension, tachycardia.
**Respiratory:** *prolonged, dose-related apnea;* wheezing; increased bronchial secretions; dyspnea; *bronchospasm; laryngospasm.*
**Skin:** *skin flushing,* erythema, pruritus, urticaria, rash.
**Other:** *anaphylaxis.*

**INTERACTIONS**
**Drug-drug.** *Amikacin, gentamicin, neomycin, streptomycin, tobramycin:* May increase the effects of nondepolarizing muscle relaxant including prolonged respiratory depression. Use together cau-

---

tiously. May reduce nondepolarizing muscle relaxant dose.
*Carbamazepine, phenytoin, theophylline:* May reverse, or cause resistance to, neuromuscular blockade. May need to increase atracurium dose.
*Clindamycin, general anesthetics (enflurane, halothane, isoflurane), kanamycin, polymyxin antibiotics (colistin, polymyxin B sulfate), procainamide, quinidine, quinine, thiazide and loop diuretics, trimethaphan, verapamil:* May enhance neuromuscular blockade, increasing skeletal muscle relaxation and prolonging effect of atracurium. Use together cautiously during and after surgery.
*Corticosteroids:* May cause prolonged weakness. Monitor patient closely.
*Edrophonium, neostigmine, pyridostigmine:* May inhibit drug and reverse neuromuscular block. Monitor patient closely.
*Lithium, magnesium salts, opioid analgesics:* May enhance neuromuscular blockade, increasing skeletal muscle relaxation and possibly causing respiratory paralysis. Reduce atracurium dosage.
*Succinylcholine:* May cause quicker onset of atracurium; may increase depth of neuromuscular blockade. Monitor patient.

**EFFECTS ON LAB TEST RESULTS**
None reported.

**CONTRAINDICATIONS & CAUTIONS**
● Contraindicated in patients hypersensitive to drug.
● Use cautiously in elderly or debilitated patients and in those with CV disease; severe electrolyte disorder; bronchogenic carcinoma; hepatic, renal, or pulmonary impairment; neuromuscular disease; or myasthenia gravis.

**NURSING CONSIDERATIONS**
● Dosage depends on anesthetic used, individual needs, and response. Recommended dosages are only representative.
● Give analgesics for pain. Patient may have pain but not be able to express it.
● Don't give drug by I.M. injection.
● Once spontaneous recovery starts, be prepared to reverse atracurium-induced neuromuscular blockade with an anticholinesterase (such as neostigmine or edrophonium). Usually given together

with an anticholinergic such as atropine. Complete reversal of neuromuscular blockade is usually achieved within 8 to 10 minutes after using an anticholinesterase.
● Monitor respirations and vital signs closely until patient has fully recovered from neuromuscular blockade, as indicated by tests of muscle strength (hand grip, head lift, and ability to cough).
● A nerve stimulator and train-of-four monitoring are recommended to confirm antagonism of neuromuscular blockade and recovery of muscle strength. Make sure spontaneous recovery is evident before attempting reversal with neostigmine.
● Prior use of succinylcholine doesn't prolong duration of action, but quickens onset and may deepen neuromuscular blockade.
● *Alert:* Careful dosage calculation is essential. Always verify dosage with another health care professional.

**PATIENT TEACHING**
● Explain all events and procedures to patient because he can still hear.

---

## cisatracurium besylate
Nimbex

*Pregnancy risk category B*

**AVAILABLE FORMS**
*Injection:* 2 mg/ml, 10 mg/ml

**INDICATIONS & DOSAGES**
➤ **Adjunct to general anesthesia to facilitate endotracheal intubation and relax skeletal muscles during surgery**
*Adults:* First dose of 0.15 mg/kg I.V., then maintenance dosages of 0.03 mg/kg I.V. q 40 to 50 minutes, p.r.n. Or, first dose of 0.2 mg/kg I.V., then maintenance dosages of 0.03 mg/kg I.V. q 50 to 60 minutes, p.r.n. Or, after first dose, a maintenance infusion may be given at 3 mcg/kg/minute, reduced to 1 to 2 mcg/kg/minute, p.r.n.
*Children ages 2 to 12:* 0.1 mg/kg I.V. over 5 to 10 seconds. After first dose, a maintenance infusion may be given at 3 mcg/kg/minute, reduced to 1 to 2 mcg/kg/minute, p.r.n.

➤ **To maintain neuromuscular blockade during mechanical ventilation in
intensive care unit (ICU)**
*Adults:* Principles for infusion in operating room apply to use in ICU. After first
dose, give 3 mcg/kg/minute by I.V. infusion. Range, 0.5 to 5 mcg/kg/minute.
**Adjust-a-dose:** In patients with neuromuscular disease such as myasthenia
gravis or Eaton-Lambert syndrome, don't
exceed 0.02 mg/kg. Patients with burns
may need increased amount.

## I.V. ADMINISTRATION
● Use only under direct supervision by
medical staff skilled in using neuromuscular blockers and maintaining airway patency. Don't use unless resources for intubation, mechanical ventilation, and oxygen
therapy are within reach.
● The 20-ml vial is intended for use only
in ICU. Drug isn't compatible with propofol injection or ketorolac injection for
Y-site use. Drug is acidic and may not be
compatible with an alkaline solution of
more than 8.5 pH (such as barbiturate solutions for Y-site use). Drug shouldn't be
diluted in lactated Ringer's injection because of chemical instability.
● Drug is colorless to slightly yellow or
green-yellow. Inspect vials for particulates
and discoloration before use. Unclear solutions or those with visible particulates
shouldn't be used.
● Drug has no known effect on consciousness, pain threshold, or cerebration. To
avoid patient distress, don't induce neuromuscular block before unconsciousness.

## ACTION
Nondepolarizing drug that binds to
cholinergic receptors on the motor end
plate, antagonizing acetylcholine and
blocking neuromuscular transmission.

| Route | Onset | Peak | Duration |
|-------|-------|------|----------|
| I.V. | 1-2 min | 2-5 min | 25-44 min |

## ADVERSE REACTIONS
**CV:** *bradycardia,* hypotension, flushing.
**Respiratory:** *bronchospasm, prolonged
apnea.*
**Skin:** rash.

## INTERACTIONS
**Drug-drug.** *Aminoglycosides, bacitracin,
clindamycin, colistimethate sodium, colistin, lithium, local anesthetics, magnesium salts, polymyxins, procainamide,
quinidine, quinine, tetracyclines:* May enhance neuromuscular blocking action of
cisatracurium. Use together cautiously.
*Carbamazepine, phenytoin:* May decrease
the effects of cisatracurium. May need to
increase cisatracurium dose.
*Enflurane or isoflurane given with nitrous
oxide or oxygen:* May prolong cisatracurium duration of action. Patient may need
less frequent maintenance dosing, lower
maintenance doses, or reduced infusion
rate of cisatracurium.
*Succinylcholine:* May shorten time to onset of maximum neuromuscular block.
Monitor patient.

## EFFECTS ON LAB TEST RESULTS
None reported.

## CONTRAINDICATIONS & CAUTIONS
● Contraindicated in patients hypersensitive to drug, other bis-benzylisoquolini-
um drugs, or benzyl alcohol (found in
10-ml vial).
● Use cautiously in pregnant or breast-
feeding women.

## NURSING CONSIDERATIONS
● Drug isn't recommended for rapid-
sequence endotracheal intubation because
of its intermediate onset.
● Dosage requirements vary widely
among patients.
● Monitor neuromuscular function with
nerve stimulator during drug administration. If stimulation doesn't elicit a response, stop infusion until response returns.
● To avoid inaccurate dosing, perform
neuromuscular monitoring on a nonparetic
arm or leg in patients with hemiparesis or
paraparesis.
● In patients with neuromuscular disease
(myasthenia gravis or myasthenic syndrome [Eaton-Lambert syndrome]), prolonged neuromuscular block is possible.
A peripheral nerve stimulator and a dosage of no more than 0.02 mg/kg is recommended to assess the level of neuromuscu-

lar block and to monitor dosage requirements.
• Monitor acid-base balance and electrolyte levels. Abnormalities may potentiate or antagonize the action of cisatracurium.
• Monitor patient for malignant hyperthermia.
• Give analgesics, if appropriate. Patient can feel pain but can't indicate its presence.
• *Alert:* Careful dosage calculation is essential. Always verify dosage with another health care professional.

**PATIENT TEACHING**
• Explain purpose of drug.
• Assure patient that monitoring will be continuous.
• Explain all procedures and events because patient can still hear.

---

## doxacurium chloride
Nuromax

*Pregnancy risk category C*

**AVAILABLE FORMS**
*Injection:* 1 mg/ml

**INDICATIONS & DOSAGES**
➤ **Adjunct to general anesthesia to relax skeletal muscles during surgery**
*Adults:* 0.05 mg/kg rapid I.V. produces adequate conditions for endotracheal intubation in 5 minutes in about 90% of patients when used as part of a thiopental-narcotic induction technique. Lower doses may need longer delay before intubation is possible. Neuromuscular blockade at this dose lasts for an average of 100 minutes.
*Children older than age 2:* A first dose of 0.03 mg/kg I.V. given during halothane anesthesia produces effective blockade in 7 minutes with duration of 30 minutes. Under the same conditions, 0.05 mg/kg produces blockade in 4 minutes with duration of 45 minutes.
➤ **To maintain neuromuscular blockade during long procedures**
*Adults:* After first dose of 0.05 mg/kg I.V., maintenance doses of 0.005 to 0.01 mg/kg will prolong neuromuscular blockade for an average of 30 to 45 minutes.

*Adjust-a-dose:* Patients with renal or hepatic insufficiency may need dosage adjustment. In obese patients 30% or more above their ideal weight, adjust dosage to ideal body weight to avoid prolonged neuromuscular blockade. In patients with severe burns and in some patients with severe liver disease, higher first doses may be needed. Doses of 0.8 mg/kg will produce intubating conditions more rapidly, within 4 minutes, with neuromuscular blockade for 160 minutes or longer. Consequently, reserve these higher doses for long procedures. Administration during steady-state anesthesia with enflurane, halothane, or isoflurane may allow 33% reduction of dose.

**I.V. ADMINISTRATION**
• Use drug only under direct supervision by medical staff skilled in using neuromuscular blockers and maintaining patent airway. Don't use unless an antagonist and resources for mechanical ventilation, oxygen therapy, and intubation are within reach.
• Drug has no known effect on consciousness, pain threshold, or cerebration. To avoid patient distress, don't induce neuromuscular block before unconsciousness.
• Prepare drug for I.V. use with $D_5W$, normal saline solution for injection, dextrose 5% in normal saline solution for injection, lactated Ringer's injection, or dextrose 5% in lactated Ringer's injection.
• When diluted as directed, drug is compatible with alfentanil, fentanyl, and sufentanil.
• Give drug immediately after reconstitution. Diluted solutions are stable for 24 hours at room temperature, but, because reconstitution dilutes the preservative, risk of contamination increases. Discard unused solutions after 8 hours.

**ACTION**
Nondepolarizing neuromuscular blocker that competes with acetylcholine for receptor sites at the motor end plate. Because this action may be antagonized by anticholinesterases, doxacurium is considered a competitive antagonist.

| Route | Onset | Peak | Duration |
|-------|-------|------|----------|
| I.V. | Variable | Variable | Variable |

**ADVERSE REACTIONS**
**Musculoskeletal:** prolonged muscle weakness.
**Respiratory:** dyspnea, *respiratory depression, respiratory insufficiency or apnea.*

**INTERACTIONS**
**Drug-drug.** *Alkaline solutions:* Physically incompatible; precipitate may form. Don't give through same I.V. line.
*Aminoglycosides (amikacin, gentamicin, neomycin, streptomycin, tobramycin):* May increase the effects of nondepolarizing muscle relaxant, including prolonged respiratory depression. Use together only when necessary. Dose of nodepolarizing muscle relaxant may need to be reduced.
*Bacitracin, clindamycin, colistimethate sodium, colistin, lincomycin, polymyxin B sulfate, tetracyclines:* May enhance neuromuscular blockade, increasing skeletal muscle relaxation and prolonging effect of doxacurium. Use together cautiously.
*Beta blockers, lithium, local anesthetics, magnesium salts, procainamide, quinidine, quinine:* May enhance neuromuscular blockade. Monitor patient for excessive weakness.
*Carbamazepine, phenytoin:* May decrease the effects of doxacurium. May need to increase doxacurium dose.
*Inhalation anesthetics:* May enhance or prolong action of nondepolarizing neuromuscular blockers. Monitor patient.

**EFFECTS ON LAB TEST RESULTS**
• May increase glucose and urine urea levels.

**CONTRAINDICATIONS & CAUTIONS**
• Contraindicated in patients hypersensitive to drug; also contraindicated in neonates because drug contains benzyl alcohol, which has been linked to neonatal deaths.
• Use cautiously, possibly at reduced dosage, in elderly or debilitated patients; in patients with metastatic cancer, severe electrolyte disturbances, renal or hepatic impairment, or neuromuscular diseases; and in those for whom potentiation or difficulty in reversing neuromuscular blockade is anticipated. Patients with myasthenia gravis or myasthenic syndrome

(Eaton-Lambert syndrome) are particularly sensitive to the effects of nondepolarizing relaxants. Shorter-acting drugs are recommended in such patients.
• Because of lack of data supporting drug's safety, drug isn't recommended for patients who need prolonged mechanical ventilation in the intensive care unit. Also not recommended before or after use of nondepolarizing neuromuscular blockers or during cesarean section.

**NURSING CONSIDERATIONS**
• Dosage is highly individualized. All times of onset and duration are averages; considerable individual variation is normal.
• Drug isn't metabolized; it's excreted in urine and bile. Patients with renal or hepatic insufficiency may need dosage adjustment.
• A nerve stimulator and train-of-four monitoring are recommended to document antagonism of neuromuscular blockade and recovery of muscle strength. Make sure there is some evidence of spontaneous recovery before attempting pharmacologic reversal with neostigmine.
• Because drug has minimal vagolytic action, monitor patient for bradycardia, which may occur during anesthesia.
• Monitor respirations until patient recovers fully from neuromuscular blockade, as indicated by tests of muscle strength (hand grip, head lift, and ability to cough).
• Acid-base and electrolyte balance may influence the actions of nondepolarizing neuromuscular blockers. Alkalosis may counteract paralysis; acidosis may enhance it.
• *Alert:* Careful dosage calculation is essential. Always verify dosage with another health care professional.
• *Alert:* Don't confuse doxacurium with doxapram or doxorubicin.

**PATIENT TEACHING**
• Explain drug's purpose.
• Assure patient that monitoring will be continuous.
• Explain all procedures and events because patient can still hear.

# mivacurium chloride
Mivacron

*Pregnancy risk category C*

## AVAILABLE FORMS
*Infusion:* 0.5 mg/ml in 50 ml of $D_5W$
*Injection:* 2 mg/ml in 5-ml and 10-ml vials

## INDICATIONS & DOSAGES
➤ **Adjunct to general anesthesia to facilitate endotracheal intubation and relax skeletal muscles during surgery or mechanical ventilation**
*Adults:* Dosage is highly individualized. Usually, 0.15 mg/kg by I.V. push over 5 to 15 seconds provides adequate muscle relaxation in 2½ to 3 minutes for endotracheal intubation. Supplemental dosages of 0.1 mg/kg I.V. q 15 minutes are usually sufficient to maintain muscle relaxation. Or, maintain neuromuscular blockade with a continuous infusion of 4 mcg/kg/minute begun simultaneously with the first dose. Or, 9 to 10 mcg/kg/minute started after evidence of spontaneous recovery caused by the first dose. When used with isoflurane or enflurane anesthesia, dosage is usually reduced up to 40%.
*Children ages 2 to 12:* 0.2 mg/kg by I.V. push given over 5 to 15 seconds. Neuromuscular blockade is usually evident in less than 2 minutes. Maintenance doses are usually needed more frequently in children.

Or, neuromuscular blockade can be maintained with a continuous I.V. infusion titrated to effect. Most children respond to 5 to 31 mcg/kg/minute (average, 14 mcg/kg/minute).
*Adjust-a-dose:* In obese patients 30% or more above their ideal weight, adjust dosage to ideal body weight to avoid prolonged neuromuscular blockade.

## I.V. ADMINISTRATION
● Use only under direct supervision by medical staff skilled in using neuromuscular blockers and maintaining patent airway. Don't use unless an antagonist and resources for mechanical ventilation, oxygen therapy, and intubation are within reach.
● Drug has no known effect on consciousness, pain threshold, or cerebration. To avoid patient distress, don't induce neuromuscular block before unconsciousness.
● Prepare drug for I.V. use with $D_5W$, normal saline solution for injection, dextrose 5% in normal saline solution for injection, lactated Ringer's injection, or dextrose 5% in lactated Ringer's injection. Diluted solutions are stable for 24 hours at room temperature.
● For drug available as premixed infusion in $D_5W$, remove the protective outer wrap, and then check container for minor leaks by squeezing the bag before giving. Don't add other drugs to the container, and don't use the container in series connections.
● When diluted as directed, mivacurium is compatible with alfentanil, fentanyl, sufentanil, droperidol, and midazolam.
● Alkaline solutions, such as barbiturate solutions, are physically incompatible; precipitate may form. Don't give through same I.V. line.

## ACTION
Nondepolarizing drug that competes with acetylcholine for receptor sites at the motor end plate, blocking neuromuscular transmission. Because this action may be antagonized by anticholinesterases, mivacurium is considered a competitive antagonist. Drug is a mixture of three stereoisomers, each with neuromuscular blocking activity.

| Route | Onset | Peak | Duration |
|-------|-------|------|----------|
| I.V. | 1-2 min | 2-5 min | 20-35 min |

## ADVERSE REACTIONS
**CNS:** dizziness.
**CV:** *flushing,* tachycardia, **bradycardia, arrhythmias,** hypotension, phlebitis.
**Musculoskeletal:** prolonged muscle weakness, muscle spasms.
**Respiratory:** **bronchospasm,** wheezing, *respiratory insufficiency or apnea.*
**Skin:** rash, urticaria, erythema.

## INTERACTIONS
**Drug-drug.** *Aminoglycosides (amikacin, gentamicin, neomycin, streptomycin, tobramycin):* May increase nondepolarizing muscle relaxant effects, including prolonged respiratory depression. Use togeth-

er only when necessary. May reduce non-depolarizing muscle relaxant dose.

*Bacitracin, clindamycin, colistimethate sodium, colistin, lincomycin, polymyxin B sulfate, tetracyclines:* May enhance neuromuscular blockade, increasing skeletal muscle relaxation and prolonging effect of mivacurium. Use together cautiously.

*Beta blockers, lithium, local anesthetics, magnesium salts, procainamide, quinidine, quinine:* May enhance neuromuscular blockade. Monitor patient for excessive weakness.

*Carbamazepine, phenytoin:* May decrease effects of mivacurium. May need to increase mivacurium dose.

*Inhaled anesthetics (enflurane, isoflurane):* May enhance or prolong action of nondepolarizing neuromuscular blockers. Monitor patient for excessive weakness.

**EFFECTS ON LAB TEST RESULTS**
None reported.

**CONTRAINDICATIONS & CAUTIONS**
• Contraindicated in patients hypersensitive to drug, other bis-benzylisoquinolinium drugs, or benzyl alcohol.
• Use cautiously (possibly at reduced dosage) in debilitated patients; in those with metastatic cancer, severe electrolyte disturbances, or neuromuscular diseases; and in those for whom potentiation or difficulty in reversing neuromuscular blockade is anticipated. Patients with myasthenia gravis or myasthenic syndrome (Eaton-Lambert syndrome) are particularly sensitive to effects of nondepolarizing relaxants. Test dosage of 0.015 to 0.02 mg/kg may be used to assess patient's sensitivity to drug.
• **Alert:** Use cautiously, if at all, in patients who are homozygous for the atypical plasma pseudocholinesterase gene. Drug is metabolized to inactive compound by plasma pseudocholinesterase.

**NURSING CONSIDERATIONS**
• Certain patients may be adversely affected by histamine release (such as asthmatic patients). To avoid hypotension, use lower first dose or give drug over longer period (60 seconds).
• Give a test dose to assess patient's sensitivity to drug. Patients with severe burns

can develop resistance to nondepolarizing neuromuscular blockers; however, they also may have reduced plasma pseudocholinesterase activity.
• Like other neuromuscular blockers, dosage requirements for children are higher on a milligram per kilogram basis than those for adults. Onset and recovery of neuromuscular blockade occur more rapidly in children.
• A nerve stimulator and train-of-four monitoring are recommended to document antagonism of neuromuscular blockade and recovery of muscle strength. Make sure there is some evidence of spontaneous recovery before attempting pharmacologic reversal with neostigmine or edrophonium.
• Monitor respirations closely until patient recovers fully from neuromuscular blockade, as indicated by tests of muscle strength (hand grip, head lift, and ability to cough).
• Experimental evidence suggests that acid-base and electrolyte balances may influence the actions of nondepolarizing neuromuscular blockers. Alkalosis may counteract the paralysis; acidosis may enhance it.
• Duration of drug effect is increased about 150% in patients with end-stage renal disease and 300% in patients with hepatic dysfunction.
• **Alert:** Careful dosage calculation is essential. Always verify dosage with another health care professional.
• **Alert:** Don't confuse Mivacron with Mevacor.

**PATIENT TEACHING**
• Explain purpose of drug.
• Assure patient that monitoring will be continuous.
• Explain all procedures and events because patient can still hear.

## pancuronium bromide

*Pregnancy risk category C*

**AVAILABLE FORMS**
*Injection:* 1 mg/ml, 2 mg/ml

## INDICATIONS & DOSAGES
➤ **Adjunct to anesthesia to relax skeletal muscle, facilitate intubation, assist with mechanical ventilation**
*Adults and children age 1 month and older:* Initially, 0.04 to 0.1 mg/kg I.V.; then 0.01 mg/kg q 30 to 60 minutes.
*Neonates:* Individualized.

## I.V. ADMINISTRATION
● Keep emergency respiratory support equipment (endotracheal equipment, ventilator, oxygen, atropine, edrophonium, epinephrine, and neostigmine) immediately available.
● Drug has no known effect on consciousness, pain threshold, or cerebration. To avoid patient distress, don't induce neuromuscular block before unconsciousness.
● Don't mix with alkaline solutions (such as barbiturates) because precipitate will form; use only fresh solutions.
● Store in refrigerator. Don't store in plastic containers or syringes, although plastic syringes may be used for administration.

## ACTION
Nondepolarizing drug that prevents acetylcholine from binding to receptors on the motor end plate, thus blocking neuromuscular transmission.

| Route | Onset | Peak | Duration |
|-------|-------|------|----------|
| I.V. | 30-45 sec | 3-4½ min | 35-65 min |

## ADVERSE REACTIONS
**CV:** tachycardia, increased blood pressure.
**EENT:** excessive salivation.
**Musculoskeletal:** residual muscle weakness.
**Respiratory:** *prolonged respiratory insufficiency or apnea.*
**Skin:** transient rashes.
**Other:** *allergic or idiosyncratic hypersensitivity reactions.*

## INTERACTIONS
**Drug-drug.** *Aminoglycosides (amikacin, gentamicin, neomycin, streptomycin, tobramycin):* May increase the effects of nondepolarizing muscle relaxant including prolonged respiratory depression. Use together only when necessary. Dose of nondepolarizing muscle relaxant may need to be reduced.

*Azathioprine:* May reverse neuromuscular blockade induced by pancuronium. Monitor patient.
*Beta blockers, clindamycin, general anesthetics (such as enflurane, halothane, isoflurane), lincomycin, magnesium sulfate, polymyxin antibiotics (colistin, polymyxin B sulfate), quinidine, quinine:* May enhance neuromuscular blockade, increasing skeletal muscle relaxation and prolonging effect of pancuronium. Use together cautiously during and after surgery.
*Carbamazepine, phenytoin:* May decrease effects of pancuronium. May need to increase pancuronium dose.
*Lithium, opioid analgesics:* May enhance neuromuscular blockade, increasing skeletal muscle relaxation and possibly causing respiratory paralysis. Use with extreme caution, and reduce dose of pancuronium.
*Succinylcholine:* May increase intensity and duration of neuromuscular blockade. Allow effects of succinylcholine to subside before giving pancuronium.

## EFFECTS ON LAB TEST RESULTS
None reported.

## CONTRAINDICATIONS & CAUTIONS
● Contraindicated in patients hypersensitive to bromides, those with tachycardia, and those for whom even a minor increase in heart rate is undesirable.
● Use cautiously in elderly or debilitated patients; in patients with renal, hepatic, or pulmonary impairment; and in those with respiratory depression, myasthenia gravis, myasthenic syndrome related to lung cancer, dehydration, thyroid disorders, CV disease, collagen diseases, porphyria, electrolyte disturbances, hyperthermia, and toxemic states. Also, use large doses cautiously in patients undergoing cesarean section.

## NURSING CONSIDERATIONS
● Dosage depends on anesthetic used, individual needs, and response. Dosages are representative and must be adjusted.
● Only staff skilled in airway management should use drug.
● Allow succinylcholine effects to subside before giving pancuronium.
● Monitor baseline electrolyte determinations (electrolyte imbalance can potentiate

neuromuscular effects) and vital signs, especially respirations and heart rate.
• Measure fluid intake and output; renal dysfunction may prolong duration of action because 25% of drug is excreted unchanged in the urine.
• A nerve stimulator and train-of-four monitoring are recommended to confirm antagonism of neuromuscular blockade and recovery of muscle strength. Make sure there is some evidence of spontaneous recovery before attempting pharmacologic reversal with neostigmine.
• Monitor respirations closely until patient recovers fully from neuromuscular blockade, as indicated by tests of muscle strength (hand grip, head lift, and ability to cough).
• Once spontaneous recovery starts, pancuronium-induced neuromuscular blockade may be reversed with an anticholinesterase (such as neostigmine or edrophonium), which is usually given with an anticholinergic (such as atropine).
• Drug doesn't cause histamine release or hypotension, but it may raise heart rate and blood pressure.
• Give analgesics for pain.
• *Alert:* Careful dosage calculation is essential. Always verify dosage with another health care professional.
• *Alert:* Don't confuse pancuronium with pipecuronium or Pavulon with Peptavlon.

**PATIENT TEACHING**
• Explain all events and procedures to patient because he can still hear.

---

## rocuronium bromide
Zemuron

*Pregnancy risk category C*

**AVAILABLE FORMS**
*Injection:* 10 mg/ml

**INDICATIONS & DOSAGES**
➤ **Adjunct to general anesthesia to facilitate endotracheal intubation and relax skeletal muscles during surgery or mechanical ventilation**
*Adults:* Initially, 0.6 mg/kg I.V. bolus. In most patients, tracheal intubation may be performed within 2 minutes; muscle

paralysis should last about 31 minutes. A maintenance dosage of 0.1 mg/kg should provide an additional 12 minutes of muscle relaxation; 0.15 mg/kg will add 17 minutes; or 0.2 mg/kg will add 24 minutes to the duration of effect.
*Children ages 3 months to 12 years receiving halothane anesthesia:* Initially, 0.6 mg/kg I.V. bolus. In most patients, tracheal intubation may be performed within 1 minute; muscle paralysis should last about 41 minutes in children ages 3 to 12 months and 27 minutes in children ages 13 months to 12 years. A maintenance dose of 0.075 to 0.125 mg/kg should provide an additional 7 to 10 minutes of muscle relaxation.

**I.V. ADMINISTRATION**
• Keep airway clear. Keep available emergency respiratory support (endotracheal equipment, ventilator, oxygen, atropine, edrophonium, epinephrine, and neostigmine).
• Drug has no known effect on consciousness, pain threshold, or cerebration. To avoid patient distress, don't induce neuromuscular block before unconsciousness.
• Give by rapid I.V. injection or by continuous I.V. infusion. Infusion rates are highly individualized. Compatible solutions include $D_5W$, normal saline solution for injection, dextrose 5% in normal saline solution for injection, sterile water for injection, and lactated Ringer's injection.
• Store vials at room temperature for up to 30 days. Use diluted infusion solutions within 24 hours.

**ACTION**
Nondepolarizing drug that prevents acetylcholine from binding to receptors on the motor end plate, thus blocking neuromuscular transmission.

| Route | Onset | Peak | Duration |
|-------|-------|------|----------|
| I.V.  | 1 min | 2 min | 20-60 min |

**ADVERSE REACTIONS**
**CV:** tachycardia, abnormal ECG, transient hypotension, hypertension, edema.
**GI:** nausea, vomiting.
**Respiratory:** asthma, hiccups, *respiratory insufficiency, apnea.*
**Skin:** rash, pruritus.

---

Reactions may be *common*, uncommon, *life-threatening*, or COMMON AND LIFE-THREATENING.

## INTERACTIONS

**Drug-drug.** *Aminoglycosides (amikacin, gentamicin, neomycin, streptomycin, tobramycin):* May increase the effects of nondepolarizing muscle relaxant including prolonged respiratory depression. Use together only when necessary. May need to reduce nondepolarizing muscle relaxant dose.

*Anticonvulsants, beta blockers, clindamycin, general anesthetics (enflurane, halothane, isoflurane), magnesium salts, opiate analgesics, polymyxin antibiotics (colistin, polymyxin B sulfate), quinidine, quinine, succinylcholine, tetracyclines:* May enhance neuromuscular blockade, increasing skeletal muscle relaxation and potentiating effect. Use together cautiously during and after surgery.

*Carbamazepine, phenytoin:* May decrease effect of rocuronium. May need to increase rocuronium dose.

## EFFECTS ON LAB TEST RESULTS
None reported.

## CONTRAINDICATIONS & CAUTIONS
• Contraindicated in patients hypersensitive to drug or to bromides.
• Use cautiously in patients with hepatic disease, severe obesity, bronchogenic carcinoma, electrolyte disturbances, neuromuscular disease, and an altered circulation time caused by CV disease, old age, or edema.
• Drug isn't recommended for use during rapid sequence induction for cesarean section.

## NURSING CONSIDERATIONS
• Dosage depends on anesthetic used, individual needs, and response. Recommended dosages are representative and must be adjusted.
• Only staff skilled in airway management should use drug.
• Rocuronium provides conditions for intubation within 3 minutes.
• A nerve stimulator and train-of-four monitoring are recommended to confirm antagonism of neuromuscular blockade and recovery of muscle strength. Make sure there is some evidence of spontaneous recovery before attempting pharmacologic reversal with neostigmine

• Prior use of succinylcholine may enhance neuromuscular blocking effect and duration of action.
• Monitor patients with liver disease because they may need higher doses to achieve adequate muscle relaxation. However, such patients have prolonged drug effects.
• Monitor respirations closely until patient recovers fully from neuromuscular blockade, as indicated by tests of muscle strength (hand grip, head lift, and ability to cough).
• Rocuronium is well tolerated in patients with renal failure.
• Give analgesics for pain.
• *Alert:* Careful drug calculation is essential. Always verify dosage with another health care professional.

## PATIENT TEACHING
• Explain all events and procedures to patient because he can still hear.

---

## succinylcholine chloride (suxamethonium chloride)
Anectine, Anectine Flo-Pack, Quelicin, Scoline‡, Sucostrin

*Pregnancy risk category C*

## AVAILABLE FORMS
*Injection:* 20 mg/ml, 50 mg/ml, 100 mg/ml, 100-mg vial, 500-mg vial, 1-g vial

## INDICATIONS & DOSAGES
➤ **Adjunct to anesthesia to relax skeletal muscles for surgery and orthopedic manipulations; to facilitate intubation and assist with mechanical ventilation; to lessen muscle contractions in pharmacologically or electrically induced seizures**
*Adults:* 0.6 mg/kg I.V. given over 10 to 30 seconds. For longer response, give continuous infusion at 0.5 to 10 mg/minute, or give 0.04 to 0.07 mg/kg intermittently, p.r.n., to maintain relaxation. Or, 2.5 to 4 mg/kg I.M. Maximum I.M. dose is 150 mg.
*Children:* 1 to 2 mg/kg I.V. or 3 to 4 mg/kg I.M. Maximum I.M. dose is 150 mg.

---

## I.V. ADMINISTRATION

● Drug has no known effect on consciousness, pain threshold, or cerebration. To avoid patient distress, don't induce neuromuscular block before unconsciousness.

● Give test dose (5 to 10 mg I.V.) after patient has been anesthetized. Normal response (no respiratory depression or transient depression for up to 5 minutes) indicates patient can metabolize drug and it may be given. Don't give if patient develops respiratory paralysis sufficient to permit endotracheal intubation. (Recovery should occur within 30 to 60 minutes.)

● Store injectable form in refrigerator. Store powder form at room temperature in tightly closed container. Use immediately after reconstitution. Don't mix with alkaline solutions (thiopental sodium, sodium bicarbonate, or barbiturates).

## ACTION

Binds with a high affinity to cholinergic receptors, prolonging depolarization of the motor end plate and ultimately producing muscle paralysis.

| Route | Onset | Peak | Duration |
|-------|-------|------|----------|
| I.V. | 30-60 sec | 1-2 min | 4-10 min |
| I.M. | 2-3 min | Unknown | 10-30 min |

## ADVERSE REACTIONS

**CV:** *bradycardia,* tachycardia, hypertension, hypotension, *arrhythmias,* flushing, *cardiac arrest.*
**EENT:** increased intraocular pressure.
**GI:** excessive salivation.
**Metabolic:** hyperkalemia.
**Musculoskeletal:** muscle fasciculation, *postoperative muscle pain,* jaw rigidity.
**Respiratory:** *prolonged respiratory depression, apnea, bronchoconstriction.*
**Skin:** rash.
**Other:** *malignant hyperthermia, allergic or idiosyncratic hypersensitivity reactions, anaphylaxis.*

## INTERACTIONS

**Drug-drug.** *Aminoglycosides, anticholinesterases (such as echothiophate, edrophonium, neostigmine, physostigmine, pyridostigmine), general anesthetics (such as enflurane, halothane, isoflurane), glucocorticoids, hormonal contraceptives, polymyxin antibiotics (colistin, polymyxin B sulfate):* May enhance neuromuscular blockade, increasing skeletal muscle relaxation and potentiating effect. Use together cautiously during and after surgery.
*Cardiac glycosides:* May cause arrhythmias. Use together cautiously.
*Cyclophosphamide, lithium, MAO inhibitors:* May prolong apnea. Use together cautiously.
*Opioid analgesics:* May enhance neuromuscular blockade, increasing skeletal muscle relaxation and possibly causing respiratory paralysis. Use together with extreme caution.
*Parenteral magnesium sulfate:* May enhance neuromuscular blockade, may increase skeletal muscle relaxation, and may cause respiratory paralysis. Use together cautiously, preferably at reduced doses.
**Drug-herb.** *Melatonin:* May potentiate blocking properties of succinylcholine. Ask patient about herbal remedy use, and recommend caution.

## EFFECTS ON LAB TEST RESULTS

● May increase myoglobin and potassium levels.

## CONTRAINDICATIONS & CAUTIONS

● Contraindicated in patients hypersensitive to drug and in those with abnormally low plasma pseudocholinesterase, angle-closure glaucoma, personal or family history of malignant hyperthermia, myopathies with elevated CK, acute major burns, multiple trauma, skeletal muscle denervation, upper motor neuron injury, or penetrating eye injuries.

● Use cautiously in elderly or debilitated patients; in patients receiving quinidine or cardiac glycoside therapy; in patients with hepatic, renal, or pulmonary impairment; in those with respiratory depression, severe burns or trauma, electrolyte imbalances, hyperkalemia, paraplegia, spinal CNS injury, CVA, degenerative or dystrophic neuromuscular disease, myasthenia gravis, myasthenic syndrome related to lung cancer, dehydration, thyroid disorders, collagen diseases, porphyria, fractures, muscle spasms, eye surgery, and pheochromocytoma. Also, use large doses cautiously in patients undergoing cesarean section.

## NURSING CONSIDERATIONS

● Dosage depends on anesthetic used, individual needs, and response. Recommended dosages are representative.

● Children may be less sensitive to succinylcholine than adults.

● Succinylcholine is the drug of choice for short procedures (less than 3 minutes) and for orthopedic manipulations; use cautiously with fractures or dislocations.

● Only staff skilled in airway management should use drug.

● When giving drug by I.M. route, inject deeply, preferably high into deltoid muscle.

● Monitor baseline electrolyte determinations and vital signs. Check respirations every 5 to 10 minutes during infusion.

● Monitor respirations closely until patient recovers fully from neuromuscular blockade, as indicated by tests of muscle strength (hand grip, head lift, and ability to cough).

● *Alert:* Don't use reversing drugs. Unlike nondepolarizing drugs, neostigmine or edrophonium may worsen neuromuscular blockade.

● Repeated or continuous infusions of succinylcholine aren't advisable; they may cause reduced response or prolonged muscle relaxation and apnea.

● Give analgesics for pain.

● Keep airway clear. Have emergency respiratory support equipment (endotracheal equipment, ventilator, oxygen, atropine, and epinephrine) immediately available.

● *Alert:* Careful dosage calculation is essential. Always verify dosage with another health care professional.

## PATIENT TEACHING

● Explain all events and procedures to patient because he can still hear.

● Reassure patient that postoperative stiffness is normal and will soon subside.

---

## tubocurarine chloride

*Pregnancy risk category C*

## AVAILABLE FORMS

*Injection:* 3 mg (20 units)/ml

## INDICATIONS & DOSAGES

➤ **Adjunct to anesthesia to relax skeletal muscles; to facilitate intubation and orthopedic manipulations; adjunct during pharmacologically or electrically induced convulsive therapy**

*Adults:* 1.1 units/kg or 0.165 mg/kg I.V. slowly over 60 to 90 seconds. Average dose is initially 40 to 60 units I.V. May give 20 to 30 units in 3 to 5 minutes. For longer procedures, give 20 units, p.r.n.

➤ **To assist with mechanical ventilation**

*Adults and children:* Initially, 0.0165 mg/kg I.V. (average, 1 mg or 7 units); then adjust subsequent doses to patient response.

➤ **To lessen muscle contractions in pharmacologically or electrically induced seizures**

*Adults and children:* 1.1 units/kg or 0.165 mg/kg over 60 to 90 seconds. As a precaution, make first dose 20 units (3 mg) less than calculated dose.

➤ **Diagnosis of myasthenia gravis**

*Adults:* 4 to 33 mcg/kg as a single I.V. dose.

## I.V. ADMINISTRATION

● Keep airway clear. Have available emergency respiratory support (endotracheal equipment, ventilator, oxygen, atropine, edrophonium, epinephrine, and neostigmine).

● Drug has no known effect on consciousness, pain threshold, or cerebration. To avoid patient distress, don't induce neuromuscular block before unconsciousness.

● Allow succinylcholine effects to subside before giving tubocurarine.

● Don't mix with barbiturates or other alkaline solutions because a precipitate will form. Use only fresh solutions, and discard if discolored.

● Give I.V. over 60 to 90 seconds.

## ACTION

Nondepolarizing neuromuscular blocker that prevents acetylcholine from binding to receptors on the motor end plate, thus blocking neuromuscular transmission.

| Route | Onset | Peak | Duration |
|-------|-------|------|----------|
| I.V. | 1 min | 2-5 min | 25-90 min |

---

## ADVERSE REACTIONS
**CV:** hypotension, *arrhythmias, cardiac arrest, bradycardia.*
**GI:** increased salivation.
**Musculoskeletal:** profound and prolonged muscle relaxation, residual muscle weakness.
**Respiratory:** *respiratory depression or apnea, bronchospasm.*
**Other:** hypersensitivity reactions.

## INTERACTIONS
**Drug-drug.** *Aminoglycosides (amikacin, gentamicin, neomycin, streptomycin, tobramycin):* May increase the effects of nondepolarizing muscle relaxant including prolonged respiratory depression. Use together only when necessary. May need to reduce nondepolarizing muscle relaxant dose.
*Amphotericin B, ethacrynic acid, furosemide, methotrimeprazine, opioid analgesics, propranolol, thiazide diuretics, verapamil:* May enhance neuromuscular blockade, increasing skeletal muscle relaxation and possibly causing respiratory paralysis. Use together with extreme caution during and after surgery.
*Carbamazepine, phenytoin:* May decrease effects of tubocurarine. May need to increase tubocurarine dose.
*Clindamycin, general anesthetics (enflurane, halothane, isoflurane), lincomycin, magnesium salts, polymyxin antibiotics (colistin, polymyxin B sulfate):* May enhance neuromuscular blockade, increasing skeletal muscle relaxation and potentiating effect. Use together cautiously during and after surgery.
*Quinidine, quinine:* May prolong neuromuscular blockade. Use together cautiously. Monitor patient closely.

## EFFECTS ON LAB TEST RESULTS
None reported.

## CONTRAINDICATIONS & CAUTIONS
● Contraindicated in patients hypersensitive to drug and in those for whom histamine release is a hazard (such as patients with asthma).
● Use cautiously in elderly or debilitated patients and in those with hepatic or pulmonary impairment, hypothermia, respiratory depression, myasthenia gravis, myasthenic syndrome related to lung cancer, sulfite sensitivity, dehydration, thyroid disorders, collagen diseases, porphyria, electrolyte disturbances, fractures, and muscle spasms.
● Use large doses cautiously in patients undergoing cesarean section.

## NURSING CONSIDERATIONS
● Dosage depends on anesthetic used, individual needs, and response. Recommended dosages are representative and must be adjusted.
● Only staff skilled in airway management should use drug.
● Assess baseline electrolyte determinations because electrolyte imbalance can potentiate neuromuscular blocking effects.
● Check vital signs every 15 minutes. Notify prescriber at once of changes.
● Measure fluid intake and output; renal dysfunction prolongs duration of action because much of drug is excreted unchanged in urine.
● A nerve stimulator and train-of-four monitoring are recommended to confirm antagonism of neuromuscular blockade and recovery of muscle strength. Make sure there is some evidence of spontaneous recovery before attempting pharmacologic reversal with neostigmine.
● Large doses produce a factor that interferes with detection of urinary catecholamines by fluorometric measures in patients with tetanus.
● Monitor respirations closely until patient recovers fully from neuromuscular blockade, as indicated by tests of muscle strength (hand grip, head lift, and ability to cough).
● Give analgesics for pain.
● Premedication with an antihistamine will reduce the risk of histamine-related hypotension.
● *Alert:* Careful dosage calculation is essential. Always verify dosage with another health care professional.

## PATIENT TEACHING
● Explain all events and procedures to patient because he can still hear.

# vecuronium bromide
Norcuron

*Pregnancy risk category C*

## AVAILABLE FORMS
*Injection:* 10-mg vial, 20-mg vial

## INDICATIONS & DOSAGES
➤ **Adjunct to general anesthesia to facilitate endotracheal intubation and relax skeletal muscles during surgery or mechanical ventilation**
*Adults and children older than age 9:* Initially, 0.08 to 0.1 mg/kg I.V. bolus. Give maintenance doses of 0.01 to 0.015 mg/kg within 25 to 40 minutes of first dose during prolonged surgical procedures. Maintenance doses may be given q 12 to 15 minutes in patients receiving balanced anesthesia.
*Children ages 1 to 9:* May need a slightly higher first dose and may need supplementation slightly more often than adults. Or, drug may be given by continuous I.V. infusion of 1 mcg/kg/minute initially; then 0.8 to 1.2 mcg/kg/minute.
*Children ages 7 weeks to 1 year:* Doses comparable to those used in adults are appropriate, but less frequent use of maintenance doses may be needed.

## I.V. ADMINISTRATION
● Keep airway clear. Have available emergency respiratory support (endotracheal equipment, ventilator, oxygen, atropine, edrophonium, epinephrine, and neostigmine).
● Drug has no known effect on consciousness, pain threshold, or cerebration. To avoid patient distress, don't induce neuromuscular block before unconsciousness.
● Allow succinylcholine effects to subside before giving tubocurarine.
● Don't mix with barbiturates or other alkaline solutions because a precipitate will form. Use only fresh solutions, and discard if discolored.
● Give I.V. over 60 to 90 seconds.

## ACTION
Nondepolarizing drug that prevents acetylcholine from binding to receptors on the motor end plate, thus blocking neuromuscular transmission.

| Route | Onset | Peak | Duration |
|-------|-------|------|----------|
| I.V. | 1 min | 3-5 min | 15-25 min |

## ADVERSE REACTIONS
**Musculoskeletal:** skeletal muscle weakness.
**Respiratory:** *prolonged respiratory insufficiency or apnea.*

## INTERACTIONS
**Drug-drug.** *Aminoglycoside (amikacin, gentamicin, neomycin, streptomycin, tobramycin):* May increase the effects of nondepolarizing muscle relaxant including prolonged respiratory depression. Use together only when necessary. May need to reduce nondepolarizing muscle relaxant dose.
*Bacitracin, beta blockers, clindamycin, general anesthetics (enflurane, halothane, isoflurane), magnesium salts, other skeletal muscle relaxants, polymyxin antibiotics (colistin, polymyxin B sulfate), quinidine, quinine, succinylcholine, tetracyclines:* May enhance neuromuscular blockade, increasing skeletal muscle relaxation and potentiating effect. Use together cautiously during and after surgery.
*Carbamazepine, phenytoin:* May decrease effects of vecuronium. May need to increase vecuronium dose.
*Opioid analgesics:* May enhance neuromuscular blockade, increasing skeletal muscle relaxation and possibly causing respiratory paralysis. Use together with extreme caution, and reduce vecuronium dose.

## EFFECTS ON LAB TEST RESULTS
None reported.

## CONTRAINDICATIONS & CAUTIONS
● Contraindicated in patients hypersensitive to drug or to bromides.
● Use cautiously in elderly patients; in patients with altered circulation caused by CV disease or edema; and in those with hepatic disease, severe obesity, bronchogenic carcinoma, electrolyte disturbances, and neuromuscular disease.
● Not recommended for use in infants younger than 7 weeks old.

## NURSING CONSIDERATIONS

• Dosage depends on anesthetic used, individual needs, and response. Recommended dosages are representative and must be adjusted.

• Only staff skilled in airway management should use drug.

• A nerve stimulator and train-of-four monitoring are recommended to confirm antagonism of neuromuscular blockade and recovery of muscle strength. Make sure there is some evidence of spontaneous recovery before attempting pharmacologic reversal with neostigmine.

• Monitor respirations closely until patient recovers fully from neuromuscular blockade, as indicated by tests of muscle strength (hand grip, head lift, and ability to cough).

• Prior use of succinylcholine may enhance the neuromuscular blocking effect and duration of action.

• Vecuronium is well tolerated in patients with renal failure.

• Give analgesics for pain.

• *Alert:* Careful dosage calculation is essential. Always verify dosage with another health care professional.

## PATIENT TEACHING

• Explain all events and procedures to patient because he can still hear.

# 40

## Antihistamines

cetirizine hydrochloride
chlorpheniramine maleate
clemastine fumarate
desloratadine
diphenhydramine hydrochloride
fexofenadine hydrochloride
loratadine
promethazine hydrochloride
promethazine theoclate

### COMBINATION PRODUCTS

ALLEGRA-D: fexofenadine hydrochloride 60 mg and pseudoephedrine sulfate 120 mg.

ALLEREST MAXIMUM STRENGTH TABLETS ◊: pseudoephedrine hydrochloride 30 mg and chlorpheniramine maleate 2 mg.

CHLOR-TRIMETON ALLERGY 4-HOUR DECONGESTANT ◊: chlorpheniramine maleate 4 mg and pseudoephedrine sulfate 60 mg.

CHLOR-TRIMETON 12 HOUR RELIEF TABLETS ◊: chlorpheniramine maleate 8 mg and pseudoephedrine sulfate 120 mg.

CLARITIN-D: loratadine 5 mg and pseudoephedrine sulfate 120 mg; loratadine 10 mg and pseudoephedrine sulfate 240 mg.

CONTAC SEVERE COLD & FLU CAPLETS ◊: acetaminophen 500 mg, dextromethorphan hydrobromide 15 mg, pseudoephedrine hydrochloride 30 mg, and chlorpheniramine maleate 2 mg.

CORICIDIN D COLD, FLU, & SINUS ◊: chlorpheniramine maleate 2 mg, acetaminophen 325 mg, and pseudoephedrine sulfate 30 mg.

CORICIDIN D TABLETS ◊: chlorpheniramine maleate 2 mg and acetaminophen 325 mg.

DECONAMINE: pseudoephedrine hydrochloride 60 mg and chlorpheniramine maleate 4 mg.

FEDAHIST: pseudoephedrine hydrochloride 60 mg and chlorpheniramine maleate 4 mg.

NOVAFED A: pseudoephedrine hydrochloride 120 mg and chlorpheniramine maleate 8 mg.

NOVAHISTINE ELIXIR ◊ *: phenylephrine 5 mg, chlorpheniramine maleate 2 mg.

P-V-TUSSIN SYRUP*: chlorpheniramine maleate 2 mg/5 ml, phenindamine tartrate 5 mg/5 ml, phenylephrine hydrochloride 5 mg/5 ml, and pyrilamine maleate 6 mg/5 ml.

SUDAFED PLUS ◊: pseudoephedrine hydrochloride 60 mg and chlorpheniramine maleate 4 mg.

TRIAMINIC COLD & ALLERGY ◊: pseudoephedrine hydrochloride 15 mg and chlorpheniramine maleate 1 mg.

TRIAMINIC COLD & COUGH ◊: pseudoephedrine hydrochloride 15 mg, dextromethorphan hydrobromide 5 mg, and chlorpheniramine maleate 1 mg.

TRIAMINIC COLD & NIGHTTIME COUGH ◊: pseudoephedrine hydrochloride 15 mg, dextromethorphan hydrobromide 7.5 mg, and chlorpheniramine maleate 1 mg.

ZYRTEC-D 12 HOUR EXTENDED-RELEASE TABLETS: cetirizine hydrochloride 5 mg and pseudoephedrine hydrochloride 120 mg.

---

## cetirizine hydrochloride
Zyrtec⬥

*Pregnancy risk category B*

### AVAILABLE FORMS
*Oral solution:* 5 mg/5 ml
*Tablets:* 5 mg, 10 mg

### INDICATIONS & DOSAGES
➤ **Seasonal allergic rhinitis**
*Adults and children age 6 and older:* 5 to 10 mg P.O. once daily.
*Children ages 2 to 5:* 2.5 mg P.O. once daily. Maximum daily dosage is 5 mg.
➤ **Perennial allergic rhinitis, chronic urticaria**
*Adults and children age 6 and older:* 5 to 10 mg P.O. once daily.

*Children age 6 months to 5 years:* 2.5 mg
P.O. once daily; in children ages 1 to 5, increase to maximum of 5 mg daily in two
divided doses.
**Adjust-a-dose:** In adults and children age
6 and older on hemodialysis, those with
hepatic impairment, and those with creatinine clearance less than 31 ml/minute,
give 5 mg P.O. daily. Don't use in children
younger than age 6 with renal or hepatic
impairment.

**ACTION**
A long-acting nonsedating antihistamine
that selectively inhibits peripheral $H_1$ receptors.

| Route | Onset | Peak | Duration |
|-------|-------|------|----------|
| P.O. | 20-60 min | 30-90 min | 24 hr |

**ADVERSE REACTIONS**
**CNS:** *somnolence,* fatigue, dizziness,
headache.
**EENT:** pharyngitis.
**GI:** dry mouth, nausea, vomiting, abdomi-
nal distress.

**INTERACTIONS**
**Drug-drug.** *CNS depressants:* May cause
additive effect. Avoid using together.
*Theophylline:* May decrease cetirizine
clearance. Monitor patient closely.
**Drug-lifestyle.** *Alcohol use:* May cause
additive effect. Discourage use together.

**EFFECTS ON LAB TEST RESULTS**
• May prevent, reduce, or mask positive
result in diagnostic skin test.

**CONTRAINDICATIONS & CAUTIONS**
• Contraindicated in patients hypersensitive to drug or to hydroxyzine or in breast-
feeding women.
• Use cautiously in patients with renal or
liver impairment.

**NURSING CONSIDERATIONS**
• Stop drug 4 days before patient undergoes diagnostic skin tests. Drug can prevent, reduce, or mask positive skin test response.
• **Alert:** Don't confuse Zyrtec with
Zyprexa or Zantac.

**PATIENT TEACHING**
• Warn patient not to perform hazardous
activities until CNS effects of drug are
known. Somnolence is a common adverse
reaction.
• Advise patient not to use alcohol or other CNS depressants while taking drug.
• Tell patient that coffee or tea may reduce
drowsiness.
• Inform patient that sugarless gum, hard
candy, or ice chips may relieve dry mouth.

---

# chlorpheniramine maleate
Aller-Chlor, Allergy, Chlo-Amine,
Chlor-Trimeton Allergy 4 hour,
Chlor-Trimeton Allergy 8 hour,
Chlor-Trimeton Allergy 12 hour,
Chlor-Tripolon†

*Pregnancy risk category B*

**AVAILABLE FORMS**
*Capsules (sustained-release):* 8 mg,
12 mg
*Syrup* ◊ : 2 mg/5 ml*
*Tablets* ◊ : 4 mg
*Tablets (chewable)* ◊ : 2 mg
*Tablets (timed-release)* ◊ : 8 mg, 12 mg
**Aller-Chlor**
*Capsules (sustained-release)* (Chlor-
Tripolon)† ◊ : 8 mg, 12 mg
*Syrup* (Aller-Chlor) ◊ : 2 mg/5 ml*
*Tablets* (Aller-Chlor) ◊ : 4 mg
*Tablets* (Allergy) ◊ : 4 mg
*Tablets (chewable)* (Chlo-Amine) ◊ : 2 mg
*Tablets* (Chlor-Trimeton Allergy 4
hour) ◊ : 4 mg
*Tablets* (Chlor-Trimeton Allergy 8
hour) ◊ : 8 mg
*Tablets* (Chlor-Trimeton Allergy 12
hour) ◊ : 12 mg

**INDICATIONS & DOSAGES**
➤ **Rhinitis, allergy symptoms**
*Adults and children older than age 12:*
4 mg P.O. q 4 to 6 hours, not to exceed
24 mg daily. Or, 8 to 12 mg timed-release
P.O. q 8 to 12 hours, not to exceed 24 mg
daily.
*Children ages 6 to 12:* 2 mg P.O. q 4 to
6 hours, not to exceed 12 mg daily. Or,
8 mg timed-release P.O. h.s.
*Children ages 2 to 5:* 1 mg P.O. q 4 to
6 hours, not to exceed 4 mg daily.

---

Reactions may be *common,* uncommon, *life-threatening,* or COMMON AND LIFE-THREATENING.

*Children younger than age 2:* 0.35 mg/kg daily in divided doses q 4 to 6 hours.

### ACTION
Competes with histamine for H₁-receptor sites on effector cells. It prevents, but doesn't reverse, histamine-mediated responses.

| Route | Onset | Peak | Duration |
|-------|-------|------|----------|
| P.O. | 15-60 min | 2-6 hr | 24 hr |

### ADVERSE REACTIONS
**CNS:** *stimulation,* sedation, *drowsiness,* excitability in children.
**CV:** hypotension, palpitations, weak pulse.
**GI:** epigastric distress, *dry mouth.*
**GU:** urine retention.
**Respiratory:** thick bronchial secretions.
**Skin:** rash, urticaria, pallor.

### INTERACTIONS
**Drug-drug.** *CNS depressants:* May increase sedation. Use together cautiously.
*MAO inhibitors:* May increase anticholinergic effects. Avoid using together.
**Drug-lifestyle.** *Alcohol use:* May increase CNS depression. Discourage use together.

### EFFECTS ON LAB TEST RESULTS
• May prevent, reduce, or mask positive result in diagnostic skin test.

### CONTRAINDICATIONS & CAUTIONS
• Contraindicated in patients having acute asthmatic attacks and in those with angle-closure glaucoma, symptomatic prostatic hyperplasia, pyloroduodenal obstruction, or bladder neck obstruction.
• Contraindicated in breast-feeding women and in patients taking MAO inhibitors.
• Use cautiously in elderly patients and in those with increased intraocular pressure, hyperthyroidism, CV or renal disease, hypertension, bronchial asthma, urine retention, prostatic hyperplasia, and stenosing peptic ulcerations.

### NURSING CONSIDERATIONS
• Stop drug 4 days before performing diagnostic skin tests. Antihistamines can prevent, reduce, or mask positive skin test response.

### PATIENT TEACHING
• Warn patient to avoid alcohol and hazardous activities that require alertness until CNS effects of drug are known.
• Tell patient that coffee or tea may reduce drowsiness.
• Inform patient that sugarless gum, hard candy, or ice chips may relieve dry mouth.
• Instruct patient to notify prescriber if tolerance develops because a different antihistamine may need to be prescribed.
• Tell parent that drug (including timed- and sustained-release products) shouldn't be used in children younger than age 12 unless directed by prescriber.

## clemastine fumarate
Tavist Allergy ◇

*Pregnancy risk category B*

### AVAILABLE FORMS
*Syrup:* 0.5 mg/5 ml
*Tablets:* 1.34 mg ◇ (equivalent to 1 mg clemastine), 2.68 mg

### INDICATIONS & DOSAGES
➤ **Rhinitis, allergy symptoms**
*Adults and children age 12 and older:* 1.34 mg P.O. b.i.d.; not to exceed 8.04 mg/day for syrup and 2.68 mg/day for tablets.
*Children age 6 to 11:* 0.67 mg syrup P.O. b.i.d.; not to exceed 4.02 mg/day.
➤ **Allergic skin manifestation of urticaria and angioedema**
*Adults and children age 12 and older:* 2.68 mg P.O. b.i.d; not to exceed 8.04 mg daily.
*Children age 6 to 11:* 1.34 mg syrup P.O. b.i.d.; not to exceed 4.02 mg/day.

### ACTION
Competes with histamine for H₁-receptor sites on effector cells. It prevents, but doesn't reverse, histamine-mediated responses.

| Route | Onset | Peak | Duration |
|-------|-------|------|----------|
| P.O. | 15-60 min | 5-7 hr | 12 hr |

### ADVERSE REACTIONS
**CNS:** *sedation, drowsiness,* **seizures,** nervousness, tremor, confusion, restlessness,

vertigo, headache, *sleepiness, dizziness, incoordination,* fatigue.
**CV:** hypotension, palpitations, tachycardia.
**GI:** *epigastric distress,* anorexia, diarrhea, nausea, vomiting, constipation, *dry mouth.*
**GU:** urine retention, urinary frequency.
**Hematologic:** hemolytic anemia, ***thrombocytopenia, agranulocytosis.***
**Respiratory:** *thick bronchial secretions.*
**Skin:** rash, urticaria, photosensitivity, diaphoresis.
**Other:** *anaphylactic shock.*

## INTERACTIONS
**Drug-drug.** *CNS depressants:* May increase sedation. Use together cautiously.
*MAO inhibitors:* May increase anticholinergic effects. Avoid using together.
**Drug-lifestyle.** *Alcohol use:* May increase CNS depression. Discourage use together.
*Sun exposure:* May cause photosensitivity reactions. Advise patient to avoid extensive sunlight exposure.

## EFFECTS ON LAB TEST RESULTS
● May decrease hemoglobin and platelet and granulocyte counts.
● May prevent, reduce, or mask positive result in diagnostic skin test.

## CONTRAINDICATIONS & CAUTIONS
● Contraindicated in patients hypersensitive to drug or other antihistamines of similar chemical structure, in those taking MAO inhibitors, and in those with acute asthma, angle-closure glaucoma, stenosing peptic ulcer, symptomatic prostatic hyperplasia, bladder neck obstruction, or pyloroduodenal obstruction.
● Contraindicated in neonates, premature infants, and breast-feeding women.
● Use cautiously in elderly patients or in those with increased intraocular pressure, hyperthyroidism, CV disease, hypertension, bronchial asthma, and prostatic hyperplasia.
● Use in children younger than age 12 only as directed by prescriber.

## NURSING CONSIDERATIONS
● Stop drug 4 days before patient undergoes diagnostic skin tests. Antihistamines can prevent, reduce, or mask positive skin test result.

● Monitor blood counts during long-term therapy; observe for signs of blood dyscrasias.

## PATIENT TEACHING
● Warn patient to avoid alcohol and hazardous activities that require alertness until CNS effects of drug are known.
● Tell patient that coffee or tea may reduce drowsiness. Urge caution if palpitations develop.
● Inform patient that sugarless gum, hard candy, or ice chips may relieve dry mouth.
● Warn patient of possible photosensitivity reactions. Advise use of a sunblock.
● Tell patient to notify prescriber if tolerance develops because a different antihistamine may need to be prescribed.

---

# desloratadine
Clarinex❤, Clarinex Reditabs

*Pregnancy risk category C*

## AVAILABLE FORMS
*Tablets:* 5 mg
*Tablets (orally disintegrating):* 5 mg

## INDICATIONS & DOSAGES
➤ **Symptomatic relief from seasonal and perennial allergic rhinitis; symptomatic relief from pruritus; to reduce number and size of hives in patients with chronic idiopathic urticaria**
*Adults and children age 12 and older:* 5 mg P.O. once daily.
*Adjust-a-dose:* In patients with hepatic or renal impairment, start dosage at 5 mg P.O. every other day.

## ACTION
Long-acting tricyclic antihistamine with selective $H_1$-receptor histamine antagonist activity. It inhibits histamine release from human mast cells in vitro. Drug doesn't cross the blood-brain barrier.

| Route | Onset | Peak | Duration |
|---|---|---|---|
| P.O. | Unknown | 3 hr | Unknown |
| P.O. (orally disinte-grating) | Unknown | 2½-4 hr | Unknown |

## ADVERSE REACTIONS
**CNS:** somnolence, fatigue, dizziness.
**EENT:** pharyngitis, dry throat.
**GI:** nausea, dry mouth.
**Musculoskeletal:** myalgia.
**Other:** flulike symptoms.

## INTERACTIONS
None reported.

## EFFECTS ON LAB TEST RESULTS
• May increase liver enzyme and bilirubin levels.
• May prevent, reduce, or mask positive result in diagnostic skin test.

## CONTRAINDICATIONS & CAUTIONS
• Contraindicated in patients hypersensitive to drug, to any of its components, or to loratadine.
• Use cautiously in elderly patients because of the greater likelihood of decreased hepatic, renal, or cardiac function, and concomitant disease or other drug therapy.
• Contraindicated in breast-feeding women.
• Safety and effectiveness haven't been established in children younger than age 12.

## NURSING CONSIDERATIONS
• Store tablets from 36° to 86° F (2° to 30° C); store orally disintegrating tablets from 59° to 86° F (15° to 30° C).

## PATIENT TEACHING
• Advise patient not to exceed recommended dosage. Higher doses don't increase effectiveness and may cause somnolence.
• Tell patient that drug can be taken without regard to meals.
• Instruct patient to remove orally disintegrating tablets from blister pack and place on tongue immediately to dissolve.
• Orally disintegrating tablets may be taken with or without water.
• Tell patient to report adverse effects.

# diphenhydramine hydrochloride
Allerdryl† ◇ , AllerMax Allergy and Cough Formula, AllerMax Caplets ◇ , Aller-med ◇ , Banophen ◇ , Banophen Caplets ◇ , Benadryl ◇ , Benadryl Allergy, Benylin Cough ◇ , Bydramine Cough ◇ , Compoz ◇ , Diphen Cough ◇ , Diphenadryl ◇ , Diphenhist ◇ , Diphenhist Captabs ◇ , Dormarex 2 ◇ , Genahist ◇ , Hydramine ◇ , Hydramine Cough ◇ , Hyrexin-50, Nervine Nighttime Sleep-Aid ◇ , Nordryl Cough ◇ , Sleep-eze 3 ◇ , Sominex ◇ , Tusstat ◇ , Twilite Caplets ◇ , Uni-Bent Cough ◇

*Pregnancy risk category B*

## AVAILABLE FORMS
*Capsules:* 25 mg ◇ , 50 mg ◇
*Elixir:* 12.5 mg/5 ml* ◇
*Injection:* 10 mg/ml, 50 mg/ml
*Liquid:* 6.25 mg/5 ml
*Syrup:* 12.5 mg/5 ml* ◇
*Tablets:* 25 mg ◇ , 50 mg ◇
*Tablets (chewable):* 12.5 mg ◇

## INDICATIONS & DOSAGES
➤ **Rhinitis, allergy symptoms, motion sickness, Parkinson's disease**
*Adults and children age 12 and older:*
25 to 50 mg P.O. t.i.d. or q.i.d. Maximum, 300 mg P.O. daily. Or, 10 to 50 mg deep I.M. or I.V. Maximum by I.M. or I.V. route, 400 mg daily.
*Children younger than age 12:* 5 mg/kg/ day P.O., deep I.M., or I.V., in divided doses q.i.d. Maximum, 300 mg daily.
➤ **Sedation**
*Adults:* 25 to 50 mg P.O. or deep I.M., p.r.n.
➤ **Nighttime sleep aid**
*Adults:* 25 to 50 mg P.O. h.s.
➤ **Nonproductive cough**
*Adults and children age 12 and older:*
25 mg P.O. q 4 to 6 hours. Don't exceed 150 mg daily.
*Children ages 6 to 11:* 12.5 mg P.O. q 4 to 6 hours. Don't exceed 75 mg daily.
*Children ages 2 to 5:* 6.25 mg P.O. q 4 to 6 hours. Don't exceed 25 mg daily.

## I.V. ADMINISTRATION
• Make sure I.V. site is patent. Drug given perivascularly causes tissue irritation.
• I.V. use shouldn't exceed 25 mg/minute.

## ACTION
Competes with histamine for $H_1$-receptor sites on effector cells. Prevents, but doesn't reverse, histamine-mediated responses, particularly the effects of histamine on the smooth muscle of the bronchial tubes, GI tract, uterus, and blood vessels. Structurally related to local anesthetics, diphenhydramine provides local anesthesia by preventing initiation and transmission of nerve impulses. Also suppresses cough reflex by a direct effect on the medulla.

| Route | Onset | Peak | Duration |
|-------|-------|------|----------|
| P.O. | 15 min | 1-4 hr | 6-8 hr |
| I.V. | Immediate | 1-4 hr | 6-8 hr |
| I.M. | Unknown | 1-4 hr | 6-8 hr |

## ADVERSE REACTIONS
**CNS:** *drowsiness,* confusion, insomnia, headache, vertigo, *sedation, sleepiness, dizziness, incoordination,* fatigue, restlessness, tremor, nervousness, ***seizures.***
**CV:** palpitations, hypotension, tachycardia.
**EENT:** diplopia, blurred vision, nasal congestion, tinnitus.
**GI:** *nausea,* vomiting, diarrhea, *dry mouth,* constipation, *epigastric distress,* anorexia.
**GU:** dysuria, urine retention, urinary frequency.
**Hematologic:** hemolytic anemia, ***thrombocytopenia, agranulocytosis.***
**Respiratory:** *thickening of bronchial secretions.*
**Skin:** urticaria, photosensitivity, rash.
**Other:** ***anaphylactic shock.***

## INTERACTIONS
**Drug-drug.** *CNS depressants:* May increase sedation. Use together cautiously.
*MAO inhibitors:* May increase anticholinergic effects. Avoid using together.
*Other diphenhydramine-containing products (including topical therapy):* May increase risk of adverse reactions. Avoid using together.

**Drug-lifestyle.** *Alcohol use:* May increase CNS depression. Discourage use together.
*Sun exposure:* May cause photosensitivity reactions. Advise patient to avoid extensive sunlight exposure.

## EFFECTS ON LAB TEST RESULTS
• May decrease hemoglobin and platelet and granulocyte counts.
• May prevent, reduce, or mask positive result in diagnostic skin test.

## CONTRAINDICATIONS & CAUTIONS
• Contraindicated in patients hypersensitive to drug, in newborns, in premature neonates, in breast-feeding women, and in patients with angle-closure glaucoma, stenosing peptic ulcer, symptomatic prostatic hyperplasia, bladder neck obstruction, or pyloroduodenal obstruction; also contraindicated during acute asthmatic attacks.
• Avoid use in patients taking MAO inhibitors.
• Use with caution in patients with prostatic hyperplasia, asthma, COPD, increased intraocular pressure, hyperthyroidism, CV disease, and hypertension.
• Children younger than age 12 should use drug only as directed by prescriber.

## NURSING CONSIDERATIONS
• Stop drug 4 days before patient undergoes diagnostic skin tests because antihistamines can prevent, reduce, or mask positive skin test response.
• Alternate injection sites to prevent irritation. Give I.M. injection deeply into large muscle.
• *Alert:* Don't confuse diphenhydramine with dimenhydrinate; don't confuse Benadryl with Bentyl, Benylin, or benazepril.

## PATIENT TEACHING
• Warn patient not to take this drug with any other diphenhydramine-containing products (including topical therapy) because of increased adverse reactions.
• Instruct patient to take drug 30 minutes before travel to prevent motion sickness.
• Tell patient to take diphenhydramine with food or milk to reduce GI distress.
• Warn patient to avoid alcohol and hazardous activities that require alertness until CNS effects of drug are known.

---

Reactions may be *common,* uncommon, *life-threatening*, or COMMON AND LIFE-THREATENING.

• Tell patient that coffee or tea may reduce drowsiness. Urge caution if palpitations develop.
• Inform patient that sugarless gum, hard candy, or ice chips may relieve dry mouth.
• Tell patient to notify prescriber if tolerance develops because a different antihistamine may need to be prescribed.
• Diphenhydramine is contained in many OTC sleep and cold products. Advise patient to consult prescriber before using these products.
• Warn patient of possible photosensitivity reactions. Advise use of a sunblock.

## fexofenadine hydrochloride
Allegra✐, Telfast‡

*Pregnancy risk category C*

### AVAILABLE FORMS
*Capsules:* 60 mg
*Tablets:* 30 mg, 60 mg, 120 mg‡, 180 mg

### INDICATIONS & DOSAGES
➤ **Seasonal allergic rhinitis**
*Adults and children age 12 and older:* 60 mg P.O. b.i.d. or 180 mg P.O. once daily.
*Children ages 6 to 11:* 30 mg P.O. b.i.d.
➤ **Chronic idiopathic urticaria**
*Adults and children age 12 and older:* 6 mg P.O. b.i.d.
*Children ages 6 to 11:* 30 mg P.O. b.i.d.
*Adjust-a-dose:* For patients with impaired renal function or a need for dialysis, adults should receive 60 mg daily and children should receive 30 mg daily.

### ACTION
A long-acting nonsedating antihistamine that selectively inhibits peripheral $H_1$ receptors.

| Route | Onset | Peak | Duration |
|-------|-------|------|----------|
| P.O. | Unknown | 3 hr | 14 hr |

### ADVERSE REACTIONS
**CNS:** fatigue, drowsiness, headache.
**GI:** nausea, dyspepsia.
**GU:** dysmenorrhea.
**Other:** viral infection.

### INTERACTIONS
**Drug-drug.** *Aluminum or magnesium antacids:* May decrease fexofenadine concentrations. Separate administration times.
*Erythromycin, ketoconazole:* May increase fexofenadine plasma concentrations. Monitor patient for side effects.
**Drug-food.** *Apple juice, grapefruit juice, orange juice:* May decrease effects of fexofenadine. Patients should take drug with liquid other than these juices.
**Drug-lifestyle.** *Alcohol use:* May increase CNS depression. Discourage use together.

### EFFECTS ON LAB TEST RESULTS
• May prevent, reduce, or mask positive result in diagnostic skin test.

### CONTRAINDICATIONS & CAUTIONS
• Contraindicated in patients hypersensitive to drug or its components.
• Use cautiously in patients with impaired renal function.

### NURSING CONSIDERATIONS
• Stop drug 4 days before patient undergoes diagnostic skin tests because drug can prevent, reduce, or mask positive skin test response.
• No data exist to demonstrate whether drug appears in breast milk; use caution when giving drug to breast-feeding woman. Advise woman taking drug to avoid breast-feeding.

### PATIENT TEACHING
• Instruct patient not to exceed prescribed dosage and to take drug only when needed.
• Warn patient to avoid alcohol and hazardous activities that require alertness until CNS effects of drug are known. Explain that drug may cause drowsiness.
• Avoid taking antacids within 2 hours of fexofenadine.
• Inform patient that sugarless gum, hard candy, or ice chips may relieve dry mouth.

---

# loratadine
Alavert ◇, Claratyne‡, Clarinase‡,
Claritin ◇, Claritin Reditabs ◇,
Claritin Syrup ◇, Tavist ND
Allergy ◇

*Pregnancy risk category B*

## AVAILABLE FORMS
*Syrup:* 1 mg/ml ◇
*Tablets:* 10 mg ◇
*Tablets (rapidly disintegrating):* 10 mg ◇

## INDICATIONS & DOSAGES
➤ **Hay fever or other upper respiratory allergies; chronic idiopathic urticaria**
*Adults and children age 6 and older:*
10 mg P.O. daily.
*Children ages 2 to 5 years:* 5 mg P.O. daily.
***Adjust-a-dose:*** In adults and children age 6 and older with liver failure or creatinine clearance less than 30 ml/minute, adjust dose to 10 mg every other day. In children ages 2 to 5 years with liver failure or renal insufficiency, adjust dose to 5 mg every other day.

## ACTION
Blocks effects of histamine at $H_1$-receptor sites. Loratadine is a nonsedating antihistamine; its chemical structure prevents entry into the CNS.

| Route | Onset | Peak | Duration |
|-------|-------|------|----------|
| P.O. | 1-3 hr | 8-10 hr | 24 hr |

## ADVERSE REACTIONS
**CNS:** *headache,* drowsiness, fatigue, insomnia, nervousness.
**GI:** dry mouth.

## INTERACTIONS
**Drug-drug.** *Cimetidine, ketoconazole, macrolide antibiotics (clarithromycin, erythromycin, troleandomycin):* May increase plasma loratadine levels. Monitor patient closely.
**Drug-lifestyle.** *Alcohol use:* May increase CNS depression. Discourage use together.

## EFFECTS ON LAB TEST RESULTS
● May prevent, reduce, or mask positive result in diagnostic skin test.

## CONTRAINDICATIONS & CAUTIONS
● Contraindicated in patients hypersensitive to drug.
● Use cautiously in patients with liver or renal impairment and in breast-feeding patients.

## NURSING CONSIDERATIONS
● Stop drug 4 days before patient undergoes diagnostic skin tests because drug can prevent, reduce, or mask positive skin test response.

## PATIENT TEACHING
● Make sure patient understands to take drug once daily. If symptoms persist or worsen, tell him to contact prescriber.
● Advise patient taking Claritin Reditabs to place tablet on the tongue where it disintegrates within a few seconds. It can be swallowed with or without water.
● Warn patient to avoid alcohol and hazardous activities that require alertness until CNS effects of drug are known.
● Tell patient that dry mouth can be relieved with sugarless gum, hard candy, or ice chips.

# promethazine hydrochloride
Anergan 50, Phenadoz,
Phenergan*✔

# promethazine theoclate‡
Avomine‡

*Pregnancy risk category C*

## AVAILABLE FORMS
**promethazine hydrochloride**
*Injection:* 25 mg/ml, 50 mg/ml
*Suppositories:* 12.5 mg, 25 mg, 50 mg
*Syrup:* 6.25 mg/5 ml*
*Tablets:* 12.5 mg, 25 mg, 50 mg
**promethazine theoclate‡**
*Tablets:* 25 mg‡

## INDICATIONS & DOSAGES
➤ **Motion sickness**
*Adults:* 25 mg P.O. or P.R. b.i.d. with the first dose taken 30 minutes to 1 hour before departure.
*Children older than age 2:* 12.5 to 25 mg P.O. or P.R. b.i.d. 30 minutes to 1 hour before departure.

➤ **Nausea and vomiting**
*Adults:* 12.5 to 25 mg P.O., I.M., or P.R. q 4 to 6 hours, p.r.n.
*Children older than age 2:* 12.5 to 25 mg P.O. or P.R. q 4 to 6 hours, p.r.n. Or, 6.25 to 12.5 mg I.M. q 4 to 6 hours, p.r.n.
➤ **Rhinitis, allergy symptoms**
*Adults:* 12.5 mg P.O. or P.R. q.i.d.; or 25 mg P.O. or P.R. h.s.
*Children older than age 2:* 6.25 to 12.5 mg P.O. or P.R. t.i.d., or 25 mg P.O. or P.R. h.s.
➤ **Nighttime sedation**
*Adults:* 25 to 50 mg P.O., P.R., I.V., or I.M. h.s.
*Children older than age 2:* 12.5 to 25 mg P.O., I.M., or P.R. h.s.
➤ **Adjunct to analgesics for routine preoperative or postoperative sedation**
*Adults:* 25 to 50 mg I.M. or I.V., or 25 to 50 mg P.O. or P.R.
*Children older than age 2:* 0.5 to 1.1 mg/ kg P.O., P.R., or I.M.

## I.V. ADMINISTRATION
• Discard injection if solution is discolored or contains a precipitate.
• Give injection through a free-flowing I.V. line.
• Don't give at a concentration above 25 mg/ml or a rate above 25 mg/minute.

## ACTION
Phenothiazine derivative that competes with histamine for $H_1$-receptor sites on effector cells. Prevents, but doesn't reverse, histamine-mediated responses. At high doses, it also has local anesthetic effects.

| Route | Onset | Peak | Duration |
|---|---|---|---|
| P.O. | 15-60 min | Unknown | < 12 hr |
| I.V. | 3-5 min | Unknown | < 12 hr |
| I.M., P.R. | 20 min | Unknown | < 12 hr |

## ADVERSE REACTIONS
**CNS:** *sedation,* confusion, sleepiness, dizziness, disorientation, extrapyramidal symptoms, *drowsiness.*
**CV:** hypotension, hypertension.
**EENT:** blurred vision.
**GI:** nausea, vomiting, *dry mouth.*
**GU:** urine retention.
**Hematologic:** *leukopenia, agranulocytosis, thrombocytopenia.*

**Metabolic:** hyperglycemia.
**Skin:** photosensitivity, rash.

## INTERACTIONS
**Drug-drug.** *Anticholinergics, phenothiazines, tricyclic antidepressants:* May increase anticholinergic effects. Avoid using together.
*CNS depressants:* May increase sedation. Use together cautiously.
*Epinephrine:* May block or reverse effects of epinephrine. Use other pressor drugs instead.
*Levodopa:* May decrease antiparkinsonian action of levodopa. Avoid using together.
*Lithium:* May reduce GI absorption or enhance renal elimination of lithium. Avoid using together.
*MAO inhibitors:* May increase extrapyramidal effects. Avoid using together.
**Drug-herb.** *Yohimbe:* May increase risk of yohimbe toxicity. Ask patient about use of herbal remedies, and recommend caution.
**Drug-lifestyle.** *Alcohol use:* May increase sedation. Discourage use together.
*Sun exposure:* May cause photosensitivity reactions. Advise patient to avoid extensive sunlight exposure.

## EFFECTS ON LAB TEST RESULTS
• May increase hemoglobin. May decrease WBC, platelet, and granulocyte counts.
• May prevent, reduce, or mask positive result in diagnostic skin test. May cause false-positive or false-negative pregnancy test result. May interfere with blood grouping in the ABO system.

## CONTRAINDICATIONS & CAUTIONS
• Contraindicated in patients hypersensitive to drug and in those who have experienced adverse reactions to phenothiazines. Also contraindicated in newborns, premature neonates, breast-feeding women, and acutely ill or dehydrated children.
• Use cautiously in patients with asthma or pulmonary, hepatic, or CV disease, and in those with intestinal obstruction, prostatic hyperplasia, bladder-neck obstruction, angle-closure glaucoma, seizure disorders, coma, CNS depression, and stenosis or peptic ulcerations.

## NURSING CONSIDERATIONS
• Monitor patient for neuroleptic malignant syndrome: altered mental status, autonomic instability, muscle rigidity, and hyperpyrexia.
• Stop drug 4 days before patient undergoes diagnostic skin tests because antihistamines can prevent, reduce, or mask positive skin test response.
• Pronounced sedative effect limits use in many ambulatory patients.
• Promethazine is used as an adjunct to analgesics (usually to increase sedation); it has no analgesic activity.
• Reduce GI distress by giving drug with food or milk.
• Inject deep I.M. into large muscle mass. Rotate injection sites.
• *Alert:* Don't give by S.C. route.
• Drug may be mixed with meperidine in same syringe.
• In patients scheduled for a myelogram, stop drug 48 hours before procedure. Don't resume drug until 24 hours after procedure because of the risk of seizures.
• *Alert:* Don't confuse promethazine with promazine.

## PATIENT TEACHING
• Tell patient to take oral form with food or milk.
• When treating motion sickness, tell patient to take first dose 30 to 60 minutes before travel. On succeeding days of travel, patient should take dose upon arising and with evening meal.
• Warn patient to avoid alcohol and hazardous activities that require alertness until CNS effects of drug are known.
• Inform patient that sugarless gum, hard candy, or ice chips may relieve dry mouth.
• Warn patient about possible photosensitivity reactions. Advise use of a sunblock.

---

Reactions may be *common*, uncommon, *life-threatening*, or COMMON AND LIFE-THREATENING.

albuterol sulfate
aminophylline
atropine sulfate
(See Chapter 19, ANTIARRHYTHMICS.)
ephedrine sulfate
epinephrine
epinephrine bitartrate
epinephrine hydrochloride
formoterol fumarate inhalation
powder
ipratropium bromide
isoproterenol
isoproterenol hydrochloride
isoproterenol sulfate
levalbuterol hydrochloride
metaproterenol sulfate
pirbuterol acetate
salmeterol xinafoate
terbutaline sulfate
theophylline

### COMBINATION PRODUCTS
**Inhalants**
ADVAIR: salmeterol xinafoate 50 mcg and fluticasone propionate 100 mcg, salmeterol xinafoate 50 mcg and fluticasone propionate 250 mcg, salmeterol xinafoate 50 mcg and fluticasone propionate 500 mcg.
COMBIVENT: ipratropium bromide 18 mcg and albuterol sulfate 103 mcg.
**Oral bronchodilators**
BRONCHIAL CAPSULES: theophylline 150 mg and guaifenesin 90 mg.
DILOR-G TABLETS: dyphylline 200 mg and guaifenesin 200 mg.
DYFLEX-G TABLETS: dyphylline 200 mg and guaifenesin 200 mg.
DYLINE-GG TABLETS: dyphylline 200 mg and guaifenesin 200 mg.
GLYCERYL-T CAPSULES: theophylline 150 mg and guaifenesin 90 mg.
MARAX*: theophylline 130 mg, ephedrine sulfate 25 mg, and hydroxyzine hydrochloride 10 mg.
MUDRANE GG-2 TABLETS: theophylline 111 mg and guaifenesin 100 mg.
QUIBRON CAPSULES: theophylline 150 mg and guaifenesin 90 mg.

SLO-PHYLLIN GG SYRUP: theophylline 150 mg and guaifenesin 90 mg.
SYNOPHYLATE-GG SYRUP*: guaifenesin 33.3 mg/5 ml and theophylline sodium glycinate 100 mg/5 ml.
**Decongestants**
ELIXOPHYLLIN KI ELIXIR: theophylline 80 mg and potassium iodide 130 mg.
MARAX-DF SYRUP: theophylline 97.5 mg, ephedrine sulfate 18.75 mg, hydroxyzine hydrochloride 7.5 mg.

---

## albuterol sulfate (salbutamol sulfate)
AccuNeb, Airomir‡, Proventil, Proventil HFA, Proventil Repetabs, Ventolin, Ventolin HFA, Ventolin Obstetric Injection‡, Ventolin Rotacaps‡, Volmax

*Pregnancy risk category C*

### AVAILABLE FORMS
*Capsules for inhalation:* 200 mcg‡
*Injection:* 1 mg/ml‡
*Solution for inhalation:* 0.083%, 0.5%, 0.63 mg/ml, 1.25 mg/3 ml
*Syrup:* 2 mg/5 ml
*Tablets:* 2 mg, 4 mg
*Tablets (extended-release):* 4 mg, 8 mg

### INDICATIONS & DOSAGES
➤ **To prevent or treat bronchospasm in patients with reversible obstructive airway disease**
*Capsules for inhalation*
*Adults and children age 4 and older:* 200 mcg inhaled q 4 to 6 hours using a Rotahaler inhalation device. Some patients may need 400 mcg q 4 to 6 hours.
*Solution for inhalation*
*Adults and children age 12 and older:* 2.5 mg t.i.d. or q.i.d. by nebulizer. To prepare solution, use 0.5 ml of 0.5% solution diluted with 2.5 ml of normal saline solution. Or, use 3 ml of 0.083% solution.
*Children ages 2 to 12:* Initially, 0.1 to 0.15 mg/kg by nebulizer, with subsequent

dosing titrated to response. Don't exceed 2.5 mg t.i.d. or q.i.d. by nebulization.

*Syrup*
*Adults and children age 14 and older:* 2 to 4 mg (1 to 2 tsp) P.O. t.i.d. or q.i.d. Maximum, 8 mg q.i.d.
*Children ages 6 to 14:* 2 mg (1 tsp) P.O. t.i.d. or q.i.d. Maximum, 24 mg daily in divided doses.
*Children ages 2 to 6:* Initially, 0.1 mg/kg P.O. t.i.d. Starting dosage shouldn't exceed 2 mg (1 tsp) t.i.d. Maximum, 4 mg (2 tsp) t.i.d.

*Oral tablets*
*Adults and children age 12 and older:* 2 to 4 mg P.O. t.i.d. or q.i.d. Maximum, 8 mg q.i.d.
*Children ages 6 to 12:* 2 mg P.O. t.i.d. or q.i.d. Maximum, 6 mg q.i.d.

*Extended-release tablets*
*Adults and children age 12 and older:* 4 to 8 mg P.O. q 12 hours. Maximum, 16 mg b.i.d.
*Children ages 6 to 12:* 4 mg P.O. q 12 hours. Maximum, 12 mg b.i.d.

*Adjust-a-dose:* For elderly patients and those sensitive to beta stimulators, 2 mg P.O. t.i.d. or q.i.d. as oral tablets or syrup. Maximum, 8 mg t.i.d. or q.i.d.

➤ **To prevent exercise-induced bronchospasm**
*Adults and children age 4 and older:* 200-mcg capsule for inhalation inhaled using a Rotahaler inhalation device 15 minutes before exercise.

**I.V. ADMINISTRATION‡**
• Where available, I.V. form may be used to prevent premature labor. To prepare infusion, use saline solution, $D_5W$ for injection, or saline solution and dextrose for injection.
• Don't give drug undiluted.
• Don't mix with other drugs.
• Discard unused diluted solution after 24 hours.

**ACTION**
Relaxes bronchial, uterine, and vascular smooth muscle by stimulating $beta_2$ receptors.

| Route | Onset | Peak | Duration |
|---|---|---|---|
| P.O. | 15-30 min | 2-3 hr | 6-12 hr |
| P.O. (extended) | Unknown | Unknown | 12 hr |
| I.V. | Variable | Unknown | 4-6 hr |
| Inhalation | 5-15 min | 30-120 min | 2-6 hr |

**ADVERSE REACTIONS**
**CNS:** *tremor, nervousness,* dizziness, insomnia, *headache, hyperactivity,* weakness, CNS stimulation, malaise.
**CV:** *tachycardia, palpitations,* hypertension.
**EENT:** dry and irritated nose and throat with inhaled form, nasal congestion, epistaxis, hoarseness.
**GI:** heartburn, *nausea, vomiting,* anorexia, bad taste, increased appetite.
**Metabolic:** hypokalemia.
**Musculoskeletal:** muscle cramps.
**Respiratory:** *bronchospasm,* cough, wheezing, dyspnea, bronchitis, increased sputum.
**Other:** hypersensitivity reactions.

**INTERACTIONS**
**Drug-drug.** *CNS stimulants:* May increase CNS stimulation. Avoid using together.
*Digoxin:* May decrease digoxin level. Monitor digoxin level closely.
*MAO inhibitors, tricyclic antidepressants:* May increase adverse CV effects. Monitor patient closely.
*Propranolol, other beta blockers:* May cause mutual antagonism. Monitor patient carefully.

**EFFECTS ON LAB TEST RESULTS**
• May decrease potassium level.

**CONTRAINDICATIONS & CAUTIONS**
• Contraindicated in patients hypersensitive to drug or its ingredients.
• Use cautiously in patients with CV disorders (including coronary insufficiency and hypertension), hyperthyroidism, or diabetes mellitus and in those who are unusually responsive to adrenergics.
• Give extended-release tablets cautiously to patients with GI narrowing.

---

Reactions may be *common,* uncommon, *life-threatening,* or COMMON AND LIFE-THREATENING.

## NURSING CONSIDERATIONS

- Albuterol may decrease sensitivity of spirometry used for diagnosis of asthma.
- When switching from regular-release to extended-release tablets, remember that a regular-release 2-mg tablet every 6 hours is equivalent to an extended-release 4-mg tablet every 12 hours.
- Syrup may be taken by children as young as age 2; it contains no alcohol or sugar.
- Rarely, erythema multiforme or Stevens-Johnson syndrome has been linked to use of syrup in children.
- Ventolin HFA is a newer version of the Ventolin metered-dose inhaler (MDI) for asthma and other obstructive lung diseases. Ventolin HFA uses the propellant hydrofluoroalkane as an alternative to chlorofluorocarbons to propel the medication.
- **Alert:** Patient may use tablets and aerosol together. Monitor these patients closely for signs and symptoms of toxicity.
- **Alert:** Don't confuse albuterol with atenolol or Albutein or Flomax with Volmax.

## PATIENT TEACHING

- Warn patient about possibility of paradoxical bronchospasm. Tell him to stop drug immediately if it occurs.
- Teach patient to perform oral inhalation correctly. Give the following instructions for using the MDI:
  – Shake the inhaler.
  – Clear nasal passages and throat.
  – Breathe out, expelling as much air from lungs as possible.
  – Place mouthpiece well into mouth, seal lips around mouthpiece, and inhale deeply as you release a dose from inhaler. Or, you may hold inhaler about 1 inch (two finger widths) from your open mouth; inhale while dose is released.
  – Hold breath for several seconds, remove mouthpiece, and exhale slowly.
- If prescriber orders more than 1 inhalation, tell patient to wait at least 2 minutes before repeating procedure.
- Tell patient that use of an AeroChamber may improve drug delivery to lungs.
- If patient is also using a corticosteroid inhaler, instruct him to use the bronchodilator first and then wait about 5 minutes before using the corticosteroid. This allows the bronchodilator to open the air passages for maximum effectiveness of the corticosteroid.

- Tell patient to remove canister and wash inhaler with warm, soapy water at least once a week.
- Advise patient not to chew or crush extended-release tablets and not to mix them with food.

---

# aminophylline (theophylline ethylenediamine)
Aminophylline, Phyllocontin, Phyllocontin-350, Truphylline

*Pregnancy risk category C*

---

## AVAILABLE FORMS
*Injection:* 250 mg/10 ml, 500 mg/20 ml, 100 mg/100 ml in half-normal saline solution, 200 mg/100 ml in half-normal saline solution
*Oral liquid:* 105 mg/5 ml
*Rectal suppositories:* 250 mg, 500 mg
*Tablets:* 100 mg, 200 mg
*Tablets (extended-release):* 350 mg†

## INDICATIONS & DOSAGES
➤ **Symptomatic relief of bronchospasm (aminophylline doses)**
*Patients not currently receiving theophylline products who need rapid relief from symptoms:* Loading dosage is 6 mg/kg (equivalent to 4.7 mg/kg anhydrous theophylline) I.V. at 25 mg/minute or less; then maintenance infusion.
*Nonsmoking adults and adolescents older than age 16:* 0.7 mg/kg/hour I.V. for 12 hours; then 0.5 mg/kg/hour.
*Children ages 9 to 16:* 1 mg/kg/hour I.V. for 12 hours; then 0.8 mg/kg/hour.
*Children ages 6 months to 9 years:* 1.2 mg/kg/hour for 12 hours; then 1 mg/kg/hour.
*Adjust-a-dose:* For otherwise healthy adult smokers, 1 mg/kg/hour I.V. for 12 hours; then 0.8 mg/kg/hour. For elderly patients and those with cor pulmonale, 0.6 mg/kg/hour I.V. for 12 hours; then 0.3 mg/kg/hour. For adults with heart failure or liver disease, 0.5 mg/kg/hour I.V. for 12 hours; then 0.1 to 0.2 mg/kg/hour.

---

*Rapid onset*   †Canada   ‡Australia   ◊OTC   ♦Off-label use   *♦*Photoguide   *Liquid contains alcohol.

*Patients currently receiving theophylline products:* First, determine time, amount, route of administration, and dosage form of patient's last theophylline dose. Aminophylline infusions of 0.63 mg/kg (0.5 mg/kg anhydrous theophylline) will increase theophylline level by 1 mcg/ml. Some prescribers recommend a dose of 3.1 mg/kg (2.5 mg/kg anhydrous theophylline) if no obvious signs or symptoms of theophylline toxicity develop.

➤ **Chronic bronchial asthma**
*Adults and children:* Dosage is highly individualized. The P.R. route and the P.O. route use the same dosage. Doses reflect anhydrous theophylline equivalents: 100 mg aminophylline hydrous = 78.9 mg theophylline anhydrous (tablets, suppositories, and parenteral injection); 100 mg aminophylline hydrous = 85.7 mg theophylline anhydrous.

Usual first P.O. dosage is 16 mg/kg or 400 mg (whichever is less) daily in three or four divided doses q 6 to 8 hours if using rapidly absorbed dosage forms. Dosage may be increased, if tolerated, in increments of 25% q 2 to 3 days. Or, if using extended-release preparations, 12 mg/kg or 400 mg (whichever is less) P.O. daily in two to three divided doses q 8 to 12 hours. Dosage may be increased, if tolerated, by 2 to 3 mg/kg daily q 3 days.

Regardless of dosage form, the following are recommended maximum doses: For adults and children age 16 and older, 13 mg/kg daily or 900 mg/day, whichever is less; children ages 12 to 16, give 18 mg/kg daily; children ages 9 to 12, give 20 mg/kg daily; and children ages 1 to 8, give 24 mg/kg daily.

When recommended maximum dosage is reached, adjust dosages based on measurement of peak theophylline level. Target theophylline levels are generally between 10 and 20 mcg/ml.

### I.V. ADMINISTRATION
● I.V. drug use can cause burning; dilute with compatible I.V. solution, and inject at no more than 25 mg/minute.
● Drug is compatible with most I.V. solutions except invert sugar, fructose, and fat emulsions.

### ACTION
Inhibits phosphodiesterase, the enzyme that degrades cAMP, resulting in relaxation of smooth muscle of the bronchial airways and pulmonary blood vessels.

| Route | Onset | Peak | Duration |
|---|---|---|---|
| P.O. (extended) | Variable | Variable | Variable |
| P.O. (solution) | 15-60 min | 1-7 hr | Variable |
| I.V. | 15 min | Immediate | Variable |
| P.R. | Unknown | Unknown | Unknown |

### ADVERSE REACTIONS
**CNS:** fever, *nervousness, restlessness,* headache, *insomnia,* **seizures,** muscle twitching, irritability, *dizziness,* confusion, psychosis.
**CV:** *palpitations, sinus tachycardia,* extrasystoles, flushing, marked hypotension, ***arrhythmias.***
**GI:** *nausea, vomiting,* diarrhea, epigastric pain, hematemesis, irritation with rectal suppositories, anorexia.
**Metabolic:** hyperglycemia.
**Respiratory:** tachypnea, ***respiratory arrest.***
**Skin:** urticaria.
**Other:** hypersensitivity reactions.

### INTERACTIONS
**Drug-drug.** *Adenosine:* May decrease antiarrhythmic effectiveness. Higher adenosine doses may be needed.
*Alkali-sensitive drugs:* May reduce activity. Don't add to I.V. fluids containing aminophylline.
*Barbiturates, nicotine, phenytoin, rifampin:* May enhance metabolism and decrease theophylline level. Monitor patient for decreased aminophylline effect.
*Calcium channel blockers, cimetidine, disulfiram, influenza virus vaccine, interferon, macrolide antibiotics (such as erythromycin), methotrexate, hormonal contraceptives, quinolone antibiotics (ciprofloxacin):* May decrease hepatic clearance of theophylline; may elevate theophylline level. Monitor patient for signs and symptoms of toxicity. Monitor theophylline level.
*Carbamazepine, isoniazid, loop diuretics:* May increase or decrease theophylline level. Monitor theophylline level closely.

*Carteolol, pindolol, propranolol, timolol:* May act antagonistically, reducing the effects of one or both drugs. Monitor patient closely.

*Ephedrine, other sympathomimetics:* May exhibit synergistic toxicity with these drugs, predisposing patient to arrhythmias. Monitor patient closely.

*Lithium:* May increase lithium excretion. Monitor lithium level.

**Drug-herb.** *Cayenne:* May increase risk of theophylline toxicity. Advise patient to use together cautiously.

*Ipriflavone:* May increase risk of theophylline toxicity. Urge caution.

*St. John's wort:* May lower theophylline level. Monitor theophylline level and discourage use together.

**Drug-lifestyle.** *Smoking:* May increase elimination of theophylline, increasing dosing requirements. Monitor theophylline response and level.

**EFFECTS ON LAB TEST RESULTS**
● May increase glucose and free fatty acid levels.
● May alter results of the assay for uric acid. May falsely elevate theophylline level when used with furosemide, phenylbutazone, probenecid, theobromine, caffeine, tea, chocolate, cola beverages, or acetaminophen.

**CONTRAINDICATIONS & CAUTIONS**
● Contraindicated in patients hypersensitive to xanthine compounds (caffeine, theobromine) and ethylenediamine and in those with active peptic ulcer disease and seizure disorders (unless they receive adequate anticonvulsant therapy). Rectal suppositories are contraindicated in patients who have an irritation or infection of the rectum or lower colon.
● Use cautiously in neonates, infants, young children, and elderly patients; also, use cautiously in patients with heart failure, other cardiac or circulatory impairment, COPD, cor pulmonale, renal or hepatic disease, hyperthyroidism, diabetes mellitus, glaucoma, peptic ulcer, severe hypoxemia, or hypertension.

**NURSING CONSIDERATIONS**
● Relieve GI symptoms by giving oral drug with full glass of water at meals,

although food in stomach delays absorption. No evidence exists that antacids reduce adverse GI reactions. Enteric-coated tablets may delay or impair absorption.
● *Alert:* Before giving loading dose, make sure patient hasn't had recent theophylline therapy.
● Suppositories are slowly and erratically absorbed. Give rectal suppository if patient can't take drug orally. Schedule dose after bowel evacuation, if possible; drug may be retained better if given before a meal. Have patient remain recumbent 15 to 20 minutes after insertion.
● Monitor vital signs; measure and record fluid intake and output. Expect improved quality of pulse and respirations.
● Aminophylline is a soluble salt of theophylline. Dosage is adjusted by monitoring response, tolerance, pulmonary function, and theophylline levels. Drug levels should range from 10 to 20 mcg/ml; toxicity may occur with levels above 20 mcg/ml.
● *Alert:* Evidence of toxicity includes tachycardia, anorexia, nausea, vomiting, diarrhea, restlessness, irritability, and headache. Check theophylline level, and adjust dosage as directed.
● Patients who develop urticaria may tolerate other theophylline preparations. Urticaria may be caused by the ethylenediamine salt.
● *Alert:* Don't confuse aminophylline with amitriptyline or ampicillin.

**PATIENT TEACHING**
● Provide dosage schedule and instructions for home use of prescribed form. Some patients may need an around-the-clock dosage schedule.
● Warn elderly patient that dizziness is common at start of therapy.
● Warn patient to check with prescriber before combining aminophylline with other drugs. Prescription or OTC remedies may contain ephedrine and theophylline salts; excessive CNS stimulation may result.
● Caution patient not to switch brands without first checking with prescriber.
● If patient smokes, tell him to notify prescriber if he quits.

---

*Rapid onset*   †Canada   ‡Australia   ◇OTC   ◆Off-label use   ✐Photoguide   *Liquid contains alcohol.

# ephedrine sulfate
Pretz-D ◊

*Pregnancy risk category C*

## AVAILABLE FORMS
*Capsules:* 25 mg, 50 mg
*Injection:* 25 mg/ml, 30 mg/ml‡, 50 mg/ml
*Nasal spray:* 0.25%◊

## INDICATIONS & DOSAGES
➤ **To correct hypotension**
*Adults:* 25 mg one to four times daily P.O.
Or, 25 to 50 mg I.M. or S.C. Or, 10 to
25 mg I.V., p.r.n., to maximum of 150 mg/
24 hours.
*Children:* 3 mg/kg or 25 to 100 mg/m²
S.C. or I.V. daily, in four to six divided
doses.
➤ **Bronchodilation, nasal decongestion**
*Adults and children older than age 12:*
12.5 to 50 mg P.O. q 3 to 4 hours, p.r.n.,
not to exceed 150 mg in 24 hours. As a
nasal decongestant, 2 to 3 sprays in each
nostril q 4 hours.
*Children age 2 to 12:* 2 to 3 mg/kg or
100 mg/m² P.O. daily in four to six divided doses. Or, for children ages 6 to 12,
6.25 to 12.5 mg P.O. q 4 hours, not to
exceed 75 mg in 24 hours. As a nasal decongestant, 1 to 2 sprays in each nostril q
4 hours.

## I.V. ADMINISTRATION
● Compatible with most common I.V. solutions.
● Give 10 to 25 mg by I.V. injection slowly; repeat in 5 to 10 minutes, if needed.

## ACTION
Relaxes bronchial smooth muscle by stimulating beta₂ receptors; also, stimulates
alpha and beta receptors and is a direct-
and indirect-acting sympathomimetic.

| Route | Onset | Peak | Duration |
| --- | --- | --- | --- |
| P.O. | 15-60 min | Unknown | 3-5 hr |
| I.V. | 5 min | Unknown | 60 min |
| I.M., S.C. | 10-20 min | Unknown | 30-60 min |

## ADVERSE REACTIONS
**CNS:** *insomnia, nervousness,* dizziness,
headache, muscle weakness, euphoria,
confusion, delirium, tremor, ***cerebral he-
morrhage.***
**CV:** *palpitations,* tachycardia, hyperten-
sion, precordial pain, ***arrhythmias.***
**EENT:** dry nose and throat.
**GI:** nausea, vomiting, anorexia.
**GU:** urine retention, painful urination
caused by visceral sphincter spasm.
**Skin:** diaphoresis.

## INTERACTIONS
**Drug-drug.** *Acetazolamide:* May increase
ephedrine level. Monitor patient for tox-
icity.
*Alpha-adrenergic blockers:* May reduce vasopressor response. Monitor patient closely.
*Antihypertensives:* May decrease effects.
Monitor blood pressure.
*Beta blockers:* May block the effects of
ephedrine. Monitor patient closely.
*Cardiac glycosides, general anesthetics
(halogenated hydrocarbons):* May in-
crease risk of ventricular arrhythmias.
Monitor ECG closely.
*Guanethidine:* May decrease pressor ef-
fects of ephedrine. Monitor patient closely.
*MAO inhibitors (phenelzine, tranylcypro-
mine):* May cause severe headache, hyper-
tension, fever, and hypertensive crisis.
Avoid use together.
*Methyldopa, reserpine:* May inhibit
ephedrine effects. Use together cautiously.
*Oxytocics:* May cause severe hypotension.
Don't use together.
*Tricyclic antidepressants:* May decrease
pressor response. Monitor patient closely.

## EFFECTS ON LAB TEST RESULTS
None reported.

## CONTRAINDICATIONS & CAUTIONS
● Contraindicated in patients hypersensitive to ephedrine and other sympathomimetics and in those with porphyria,
severe coronary artery disease, arrhythmias, angle-closure glaucoma, psychoneurosis, angina pectoris, substantial organic heart disease, or CV disease.
● Contraindicated in those receiving MAO
inhibitors or general anesthesia with cyclopropane or halothane.
● Use with caution in elderly patients and
in those with hypertension, hyperthyroidism, nervous or excitable states, diabetes,
or prostatic hyperplasia.

## NURSING CONSIDERATIONS

• *Alert:* Hypoxia, hypercapnia, and acidosis must be identified and corrected before or during ephedrine therapy because they may reduce effectiveness or increase adverse reactions.

• Drug isn't a substitute for blood or fluid volume replenishment. Volume deficit must be corrected before giving vasopressors.

• To prevent insomnia, avoid giving drug within 2 hours of bedtime.

• Effectiveness decreases after 2 to 3 weeks as tolerance develops. Prescriber may increase dosage. Drug isn't addictive.

• Use ephedrine in children younger than age 12 only under direction of prescriber.

• Rebound congestion and tachyphylaxis may occur with topical decongestant formulations.

• *Alert:* Don't confuse ephedrine with epinephrine.

## PATIENT TEACHING

• Tell patient taking oral form of drug at home to take last dose of day at least 2 hours before bedtime.

• Warn patient not to take OTC drugs or herbs that contain ephedrine without consulting prescriber.

---

## epinephrine (adrenaline)
Bronkaid Mist ◊ , Bronkaid
Mistometer† , Primatene Mist ◊

## epinephrine bitartrate
AsthmaHaler Mist ◊ , Bronkaid
Mist ◊ , Primatene Mist*

## epinephrine hydrochloride
Adrenalin Chloride,
AsthmaNefrin ◊ , EpiPen, EpiPen
Jr., MicroNefrin ◊ , Nephron ◊ ,
Sus-Phrine, Vaponefrin

*Pregnancy risk category C*

---

## AVAILABLE FORMS
*Aerosol inhaler:* 160 mcg ◊ , 200 mcg ◊ ,
220 mcg ◊ , 250 mcg/metered spray ◊
*Injection:* 0.01 mg/ml (1:100,000),
0.1 mg/ml (1:10,000), 0.5 mg/ml

(1:2,000), 1 mg/ml (1:1,000) parenteral;
5 mg/ml (1:200) parenteral suspension
*Nebulizer inhaler:* 1% (1:100)† ◊ ,
1.25%† ◊ , 2.25%† ◊

## INDICATIONS & DOSAGES
➤ **Bronchospasm, hypersensitivity reactions, anaphylaxis**
*Adults:* 0.1 to 0.5 ml of 1:1,000 solution S.C. or I.M. Repeat q 10 to 15 minutes, p.r.n. Or, 0.1 to 0.25 ml of 1:1,000 solution I.V. slowly over 5 to 10 minutes (1 to 2.5 ml of a commercially available 1:10,000 injection or of a 1:10,000 dilution prepared by diluting 1 ml of a commercially available 1:1,000 injection with 10 ml of water for injection or normal saline solution for injection). May repeat q 5 to 15 minutes, p.r.n., or follow with a continuous I.V. infusion, starting at 1 mcg/minute and increasing to 4 mcg/minute, p.r.n.
*Children:* 0.01 ml/kg (10 mcg) of 1:1,000 solution S.C.; repeat q 20 minutes to 4 hours, p.r.n. Maximum single dose shouldn't exceed 0.5 mg. Or, 0.004 to 0.005 ml/kg of 1:200 Sus-Phrine S.C.; repeat q 8 to 12 hours, p.r.n. Maximum single dose shouldn't exceed 0.75 mg.
➤ **Hemostasis**
*Adults:* 1:50,000 to 1:1,000, sprayed or applied topically.
➤ **Acute asthma attacks**
*Adults and children age 4 and older:*
160 to 250 mcg metered aerosol, which is equivalent to 1 inhalation, repeated once if needed after at least 1 minute; subsequent doses shouldn't be given for at least 3 hours. Or, 1% (1:100) solution of epinephrine or 2.25% solution of racepinephrine used with a hand-bulb nebulizer as 1 to 3 deep inhalations, repeated q 3 hours, p.r.n.
➤ **To prolong local anesthetic effect**
*Adults and children:* With local anesthetics, may be used in concentrations of 1:500,000 to 1:50,000. The most commonly used concentration is 1:200,000.
➤ **To restore cardiac rhythm in cardiac arrest**
*Adults:* Usual adult dosage is 0.5 to 1 mg I.V. Doses may be repeated q 3 to 5 minutes, if needed. Higher dose epinephrine may be used if 1-mg doses fail: 3 to 5 mg (about 0.1 mg/kg) doses of epinephrine repeated q 3 to 5 minutes.

---

*Children:* Usual dose is 0.01 mg/kg (0.1 ml/kg of 1:10,000 injection) I.V. First endotracheal dose is 0.1 mg/kg (0.1 ml/kg of a 1:1,000 injection) diluted in 1 to 2 ml of half-normal or normal saline solution. Subsequent I.V. or intratracheal doses range from 0.1 to 0.2 mg/kg (0.1 to 0.2 ml/kg of a 1:1,000 injection). I.V. or intratracheal doses may be repeated q 3 to 5 minutes, if needed.

## I.V. ADMINISTRATION
● Don't mix with alkaline solutions. Use $D_5W$, normal saline solution for injection, lactated Ringer's injection, or combinations of dextrose in saline solution. Mix just before use.
● Monitor blood pressure, heart rate, and ECG when therapy starts and frequently thereafter.

## ACTION
Relaxes bronchial smooth muscle by stimulating $beta_2$ receptors; also stimulates alpha and beta receptors in the sympathetic nervous system.

| Route | Onset | Peak | Duration |
|---|---|---|---|
| I.V. | Immediate | 5 min | Short |
| I.M. | Variable | Unknown | 1-4 hr |
| S.C. | 5-15 min | 30 min | 1-4 hr |
| Inhalation | 1-5 min | Unknown | 1-3 hr |

## ADVERSE REACTIONS
**CNS:** *nervousness, tremor,* vertigo, pain, *headache,* disorientation, agitation, *drowsiness,* fear, dizziness, weakness, **cerebral hemorrhage, CVA.**
**CV:** *palpitations,* widened pulse pressure, hypertension, tachycardia, **ventricular fibrillation, shock,** anginal pain, altered ECG, including a decreased T-wave amplitude.
**GI:** *nausea, vomiting.*
**Respiratory:** dyspnea.
**Skin:** urticaria, hemorrhage at injection site, pallor.
**Other:** tissue necrosis.

## INTERACTIONS
**Drug-drug.** *Alpha blockers:* May cause hypotension from unopposed beta-adrenergic effects. Avoid using together.
*Antihistamines, thyroid hormones:* When given with sympathomimetics, may cause severe adverse cardiac effects. Avoid using together.
*Cardiac glycosides, general anesthetics (halogenated hydrocarbons):* May increase risk of ventricular arrhythmias. Monitor ECG closely.
*Doxapram, mazindol, methylphenidate:* May enhance CNS stimulation or pressor effects. Monitor patient closely.
*Ergot alkaloids:* May decrease vasoconstrictor activity. Monitor patient closely.
*Guanadrel, guanethidine:* May enhance pressor effects of epinephrine. Monitor patient closely.
*Levodopa:* May enhance risk of arrhythmias. Monitor ECG closely.
*MAO inhibitors:* May increase risk of hypertensive crisis. Monitor blood pressure closely.
*Carteolol, nadolol, penbutolol, pindolol, propranolol, timolol:* May cause a hypertensive episode followed by bradycardia. Stop the beta blocker 3 days before anticipated epinephrine use. Monitor patient closely.
*Tricyclic antidepressants:* May potentiate the pressor response and cause arrhythmias. Use with caution.

## EFFECTS ON LAB TEST RESULTS
● May increase BUN, glucose, and lactic acid levels.

## CONTRAINDICATIONS & CAUTIONS
● Contraindicated in patients with angle-closure glaucoma, shock (other than anaphylactic shock), organic brain damage, cardiac dilation, arrhythmias, coronary insufficiency, or cerebral arteriosclerosis.
● Contraindicated in patients receiving general anesthesia with halogenated hydrocarbons or cyclopropane and in patients in labor (may delay second stage).
● Some commercial products contain sulfites and are contraindicated in patients with sulfite allergies, except when epinephrine is being used to treat serious allergic reactions or other emergency situations. With local anesthetics, epinephrine is contraindicated for use in fingers, toes, ears, nose, or genitalia.
● Use with caution in patients with long-standing bronchial asthma or emphysema who have developed degenerative heart disease.

• Use cautiously in elderly patients and in those with hyperthyroidism, CV disease, hypertension, psychoneurosis, and diabetes.

**NURSING CONSIDERATIONS**
• Drug increases rigidity and tremor in patients with Parkinson's disease.
• Epinephrine therapy interferes with tests for urinary catecholamines.
• One mg equals 1 ml of 1:1,000 solution or 10 ml of 1:10,000 solution.
• Epinephrine is drug of choice in emergency treatment of acute anaphylactic reactions.
• Discard epinephrine solution after 24 hours, or if it's discolored or contains precipitate. Keep solution in light-resistant container, and don't remove before use.
• *Alert:* Avoid I.M. use of parenteral suspension into buttocks. Gas gangrene may occur because epinephrine reduces oxygen tension of the tissues, encouraging the growth of contaminating organisms.
• Massage site after I.M. injection to counteract possible vasoconstriction. Repeated local injection can cause necrosis caused by vasoconstriction at injection site.
• Observe patient closely for adverse reactions. Notify prescriber if adverse reactions develop; dosage adjustment or drug discontinuation may be necessary.
• If blood pressure increases sharply, rapid-acting vasodilators such as nitrates or alpha blockers can be given to counteract the marked pressor effect of large doses of epinephrine.
• Epinephrine is rapidly destroyed by oxidizing products, such as iodine, chromates, nitrites, oxygen, and salts of easily reducible metals (such as iron).
• *Alert:* Don't confuse epinephrine with ephedrine or norepinephrine.
• When treating reactions caused by other drugs given I.M. or S.C., to minimize further absorption epinephrine may be injected into the site where the other drug was given.

**PATIENT TEACHING**
• Teach patient to perform oral inhalation correctly. Give the following instructions for using an MDI:
– Shake canister.
– Clear nasal passages and throat.

– Breathe out, expelling as much air from lungs as possible.
– Place mouthpiece well into mouth, and inhale deeply as you release dose from inhaler. Or, hold inhaler about 1 inch (two finger widths) from open mouth, and inhale while releasing dose.
– Hold breath for several seconds, remove mouthpiece, and exhale slowly.
• If more than one inhalation is prescribed, advise patient to wait at least 2 minutes before repeating procedure.
• Tell patient that use of an AeroChamber may improve drug delivery to lungs.
• If patient is also using a corticosteroid inhaler, instruct him to use the bronchodilator first and then to wait about 5 minutes before using the corticosteroid. This allows the bronchodilator to open the air passages for maximum effectiveness.
• Instruct patient to remove canister and wash inhaler with warm, soapy water at least once weekly.
• If patient has acute hypersensitivity reactions (such as to bee stings), you may need to teach him to self-inject epinephrine.

---

## formoterol fumarate inhalation powder
Foradil Aerolizer

*Pregnancy risk category C*

---

**AVAILABLE FORMS**
*Capsules for inhalation:* 12 mcg

**INDICATIONS & DOSAGES**
➤ **Maintenance treatment and prevention of bronchospasm in patients with reversible obstructive airway disease or nocturnal asthma, who usually require treatment with short-acting inhaled beta$_2$ agonists**
*Adults and children age 5 and older:* One 12-mcg capsule by inhalation via Aerolizer inhaler q 12 hours. Total daily dosage shouldn't exceed 1 capsule b.i.d. (24 mcg/day). If symptoms are present between doses, use a short-acting beta$_2$ agonist for immediate relief.
➤ **To prevent exercise-induced bronchospasm**
*Adults and children age 12 and older:* One 12-mcg capsule by inhalation via Aeroliz-

er inhaler at least 15 minutes before exercise, p.r.n. Don't give additional doses within 12 hours of first dose.

## ACTION
Long-acting selective beta$_2$ agonist that causes bronchodilation. It ultimately increases cAMP, leading to relaxation of bronchial smooth muscle and inhibition of mediator release from mast cells.

| Route | Onset | Peak | Duration |
|-------|-------|------|----------|
| Inhalation | 15 min | 1-3 hr | 12 hr |

## ADVERSE REACTIONS
**CNS:** tremor, dizziness, insomnia, nervousness, headache, fatigue, malaise.
**CV:** chest pain, angina, hypertension, hypotension, tachycardia, *arrhythmias,* palpitations.
**EENT:** dry mouth, tonsillitis, dysphonia.
**GI:** nausea.
**Metabolic:** hypokalemia, hyperglycemia, metabolic acidosis.
**Musculoskeletal:** muscle cramps.
**Respiratory:** bronchitis, chest infection, dyspnea.
**Skin:** rash.
**Other:** viral infection.

## INTERACTIONS
**Drug-drug.** *Adrenergics:* May potentiate sympathetic effects of formoterol. Use together cautiously.
*Beta blockers:* May antagonize effects of beta agonists, causing bronchospasm in asthmatic patients. Avoid use except when benefit outweighs risks. Use cardioselective beta blockers with caution to minimize risk of bronchospasm.
*Diuretics, steroids, xanthine derivatives:* May increase hypokalemic effect of formoterol. Use together cautiously.
*MAO inhibitors, tricyclic antidepressants, other drugs that prolong QT interval:* May increase risk of ventricular arrhythmias. Use together cautiously.
*Non–potassium-sparing diuretics (such as loop or thiazide diuretics):* May worsen ECG changes or hypokalemia. Use together cautiously, and monitor patient for toxicity.

## EFFECTS ON LAB TEST RESULTS
• May increase glucose level. May decrease potassium level.

## CONTRAINDICATIONS & CAUTIONS
• Contraindicated in patients hypersensitive to drug or its components.
• Use cautiously in patients with CV disease, particularly coronary insufficiency, cardiac arrhythmias, and hypertension, and in those who are unusually responsive to sympathomimetic amines.
• Use cautiously in patients with preexisting diabetes mellitus because instances of hyperglycemia and ketoacidosis have occurred rarely with the use of beta agonists.
• Use cautiously in patients with seizure disorders or thyrotoxicosis.

## NURSING CONSIDERATIONS
• Drug isn't indicated for patients who can control asthma symptoms with just occasional use of inhaled, short-acting beta$_2$ agonists or for treatment of acute bronchospasm requiring immediate reversal with short-acting beta$_2$ agonists.
• Drug may be used along with short-acting beta$_2$ agonists, inhaled corticosteroids, and theophylline therapy for asthma management.
• Patients using drug twice daily shouldn't take additional doses to prevent exercise-induced bronchospasm.
• Don't use as a substitute for short-acting beta$_2$ agonists for immediate relief of bronchospasm, or as a substitute for inhaled or oral corticosteroids.
• Don't begin use in patients with rapidly deteriorating or significantly worsening asthma.
• If usual dose doesn't control symptoms of bronchoconstriction, and patient's short-acting beta$_2$ agonist becomes less effective, reevaluate patient and treatment regimen.
• For patients formerly using regularly scheduled short-acting beta$_2$ agonists, decrease use of the short-acting drug to an as-needed basis when starting long-acting formoterol.
• As with all beta$_2$ agonists, formoterol may produce life-threatening paradoxical bronchospasm. If bronchospasm occurs, stop formoterol immediately and use an alternative drug.

• *Alert:* If patient develops tachycardia, hypertension, or other CV adverse effects occur, drug may need to be stopped.

• Watch for immediate hypersensitivity reactions, such as anaphylaxis, urticaria, angioedema, rash, and bronchospasm.

• Give Foradil capsules only by oral inhalation and only with the Aerolizer inhaler. They aren't for oral ingestion. Patient shouldn't exhale into the device. Capsules should remain in the unopened blister until administration time and only be removed immediately before use.

• Don't use Foradil Aerolizer with a spacer device.

• Pierce capsules only once. In rare instances, the gelatin capsule may break into small pieces and get delivered to the mouth or throat upon inhalation. The Aerolizer contains a screen that should catch any broken pieces before they leave the device. To minimize the possibility of shattering the capsule, strictly follow storage and use instructions.

• No overall differences in safety or efficacy have been observed in elderly patients, but increased sensitivity is possible.

• It's unknown if drug appears in breast milk. Use cautiously in breast-feeding women.

• *Alert:* Don't confuse Foradil (formoterol fumarate) with Toradol (ketorolac).

**PATIENT TEACHING**

• Tell patient not to increase the dosage or frequency of use without medical advice.

• Warn patient not to stop or reduce other medication taken for asthma.

• Advise patient that drug isn't to be used for acute asthmatic episodes. Prescriber should give a short-acting beta₂ agonist for this use.

• Advise patient to report worsening symptoms, treatment that becomes less effective, or increased use of short-acting beta₂ agonists.

• Tell patient to report nausea, vomiting, shakiness, headache, fast or irregular heartbeat, or sleeplessness.

• Warn patient not to exceed the recommended daily dosage.

• Tell patient being treated for exercise-induced bronchospasm to take drug at least 15 minutes before exercise and not to take additional doses for 12 hours.

• Warn patient of possible side effects, which may include palpitations, chest pain, rapid heart rate, tremor, and nervousness.

• Tell patient not to use the Foradil Aerolizer with a spacer device or to exhale or blow into the Aerolizer inhaler.

• Advise patient to avoid washing the Aerolizer and to always keep it dry. Each refill contains a new device to replace the old one.

• Tell patient to avoid exposing capsules to moisture and to handle them only with dry hands.

• Advise patient to notify prescriber if she becomes pregnant or is breast-feeding.

# ipratropium bromide
Atrovent

*Pregnancy risk category B*

**AVAILABLE FORMS**
*Inhaler:* Each metered dose supplies 18 mcg.
*Nasal spray:* 0.03% (each metered dose supplies 21 mcg), 0.06% (each metered dose supplies 42 mcg)
*Solution (for inhalation):* 0.02% (500 mcg/vial)
*Solution (for nebulizer):* 0.025% (250 mcg/ml)‡

**INDICATIONS & DOSAGES**
➤ **Bronchospasm in chronic bronchitis and emphysema**
*Adults:* Usually, 2 inhalations (36 mcg) q.i.d.; patient may take additional inhalations p.r.n. but shouldn't exceed 12 inhalations in 24 hours or 500 mcg q 6 to 8 hours via oral nebulizer.
➤ **Rhinorrhea caused by allergic and nonallergic perennial rhinitis**
*Adults and children age 6 and older:* Two 0.03% nasal sprays (42 mcg) per nostril b.i.d. or t.i.d.
➤ **Rhinorrhea caused by the common cold**
*Adults and children age 12 and older:* Two 0.06% nasal sprays (84 mcg) per nostril t.i.d. or q.i.d.
*Children ages 5 to 11:* Two 0.06% nasal sprays (84 mcg) per nostril t.i.d.

✳ *NEW INDICATION:* **Rhinorrhea caused by seasonal allergic rhinitis**
*Adults and children age 5 and older:* Two 0.06% nasal sprays (84 mcg) per nostril q.i.d.

## ACTION
Inhibits vagally mediated reflexes by antagonizing acetylcholine at muscarinic receptors on bronchial smooth muscle.

| Route | Onset | Peak | Duration |
|---|---|---|---|
| Inhalation | 5-15 min | 1-2 hr | 3-6 hr |

## ADVERSE REACTIONS
**CNS:** dizziness, pain, headache, nervousness.
**CV:** palpitations, hypertension, chest pain.
**EENT:** blurred vision, rhinitis, pharyngitis, sinusitis, epistaxis.
**GI:** nausea, GI distress, dry mouth.
**Musculoskeletal:** back pain.
**Respiratory:** *upper respiratory tract infection, bronchitis,* cough, dyspnea, ***bronchospasm,*** increased sputum.
**Skin:** rash.
**Other:** flulike symptoms, hypersensitivity reactions.

## INTERACTIONS
**Drug-drug.** *Anticholinergics:* May increase anticholinergic effects. Avoid using together.
**Drug-herb.** *Jaborandi tree:* May decrease effect of ipratropium when used together. Advise patient to use together cautiously.
*Pill-bearing spurge:* Choline, a chemical component of the herb, may decrease effect of ipratropium. Advise patient to use together cautiously.

## EFFECTS ON LAB TEST RESULTS
None reported.

## CONTRAINDICATIONS & CAUTIONS
● Contraindicated in patients hypersensitive to drug, atropine, or its derivatives and in those hypersensitive to soy lecithin or related food products, such as soybeans and peanuts.
● Use cautiously in patients with angle-closure glaucoma, prostatic hyperplasia, or bladder-neck obstruction.

● Safety and efficacy of nebulization or inhaler in children younger than age 12 haven't been established.

## NURSING CONSIDERATIONS
● If patient uses a face mask for a nebulizer, take care to prevent leakage around the mask because eye pain or temporary blurring of vision may occur.
● Safety and efficacy of use beyond 4 days in patients with a common cold haven't been established.
● *Alert:* Patient with a severe peanut allergy could have an anaphylactic reaction after using Atrovent inhalation aerosol (MDI). Get a thorough allergy history from patient before giving any drug.
● *Alert:* Don't confuse Atrovent with Alupent.

## PATIENT TEACHING
● Warn patient that drug isn't effective for treating acute episodes of bronchospasm when rapid response is needed.
● Teach patient to perform oral inhalation correctly. Give the following instructions for using an MDI:
– Shake canister.
– Clear nasal passages and throat.
– Breathe out, expelling as much air from lungs as possible.
– Place mouthpiece well into mouth, and inhale deeply as you release dose from inhaler. (Patient may want to close eyes.)
– Hold breath for several seconds, remove mouthpiece, and exhale slowly.
● Inform patient that use of AeroChamber with MDI may improve drug delivery to lungs.
● Warn patient to avoid accidentally spraying drug into eyes. Temporary blurring of vision may result.
● If more than 1 inhalation is ordered, tell patient to wait at least 2 minutes before repeating procedure.
● Instruct patient to remove canister and wash inhaler in warm, soapy water at least once weekly.
● If patient also uses a corticosteroid inhaler, tell him to use ipratropium first, and then wait about 5 minutes before using the corticosteroid. This method allows the bronchodilator to open air passages for maximum effectiveness of the corticosteroid.

# isoproterenol hydrochloride
Isuprel

*Pregnancy risk category C*

## AVAILABLE FORMS
*Injection:* 20 mcg/ml, 200 mcg/ml

## INDICATIONS & DOSAGES
➤ **Bronchospasm during anesthesia**
*Adults:* Dilute 1 ml of a 1:5,000 solution with 10 ml of normal saline or $D_5W$. Give 0.01 to 0.02 mg I.V. and repeat as necessary. Or, give 1:50,000 solution undiluted using same dose.
➤ **Heart block, ventricular arrhythmias**
*Adults:* Initially, 0.02 to 0.06 mg I.V.; then 0.01 to 0.2 mg I.V. or 5 mcg/minute I.V. Or, initially, 0.2 mg I.M.; then 0.02 to 1 mg I.M., p.r.n.
*Children:* Initial I.V. infusion of 0.1 mcg/kg/minute. Adjust dosage based on patient's response. Usual dosage range is 0.1 to 1 mcg/kg/minute.
➤ **Shock**
*Adults and children:* 0.5 to 5 mcg/minute isoproterenol hydrochloride by continuous I.V. infusion. Usual concentration is 1 mg or 5 ml in 500 ml $D_5W$. Titrate infusion rate according to heart rate, central venous pressure, blood pressure, and urine flow.
➤ **Postoperative cardiac patients with bradycardia ♦**
*Children:* I.V. infusion of 0.029 mcg/kg/minute.
➤ **As an aid in diagnosing the cause of mitral regurgitation ♦**
*Adults:* 4 mcg/minute I.V. infusion.
➤ **As an aid in diagnosing coronary artery disease or lesions ♦**
*Adults:* 1 to 3 mcg/minute I.V. infusion.

## I.V. ADMINISTRATION
● Give by direct injection or I.V. infusion. For infusion, drug may be diluted with most common I.V. solutions, but don't use with sodium bicarbonate injection; drug decomposes rapidly in alkaline solutions.
● When giving I.V. to treat shock, closely monitor blood pressure, central venous pressure, ECG, arterial blood gas measurements, and urine output. Carefully titrate infusion rate according to these measurements. Use a continuous infusion pump to regulate flow rate.

## ACTION
Relaxes bronchial smooth muscle by stimulating $beta_2$ receptors. As a cardiac stimulant, acts on $beta_1$ receptors in the heart.

| Route | Onset | Peak | Duration |
|-------|-------|------|----------|
| I.V. | Immediate | Unknown | < 60 min |

## ADVERSE REACTIONS
**CNS:** headache, mild tremor, weakness, dizziness, nervousness, insomnia, anxiety.
**CV:** *palpitations, tachycardia, angina, arrhythmias, cardiac arrest, rapid rise and fall in blood pressure.*
**GI:** nausea, vomiting.
**Metabolic:** hyperglycemia.
**Skin:** diaphoresis.
**Other:** swelling of parotid glands with prolonged use.

## INTERACTIONS
**Drug-drug.** *Epinephrine, other sympathomimetics:* May increase risk of arrhythmias. Use together cautiously. If used together, give at least 4 hours apart.
*Halogenated general anesthetics or cyclopropane:* May increase risk of arrhythmias. Avoid using together.
*Propranolol, other beta blockers:* May block bronchodilating effect of isoproterenol. Monitor patient carefully.

## EFFECTS ON LAB TEST RESULTS
● May increase glucose level.

## CONTRAINDICATIONS & CAUTIONS
● Contraindicated in patients with tachycardia or AV block caused by digoxin intoxication, arrhythmias (other than those that may respond to treatment with isoproterenol), angina pectoris, or angle-closure glaucoma.
● Contraindicated when used with general anesthetics with halogenated drugs or cyclopropane.
● Use cautiously in elderly patients and in those with renal or CV disease, coronary insufficiency, diabetes, hyperthyroidism, or history of sensitivity to sympathomimetic amines.

## NURSING CONSIDERATIONS
• Drug isn't a substitute for blood or fluid volume deficit. Correct volume deficit before giving vasopressors.
• Don't use solution if it's discolored or contains precipitate.
• *Alert:* Notify prescriber if heart rate exceeds 110 beats/minute with I.V. infusion. Doses sufficient to increase the heart rate to more than 130 beats/minute may induce ventricular arrhythmias.
• Isoproterenol may cause a slight increase in systolic blood pressure and a slight-to-marked decrease in diastolic blood pressure.
• Monitor patient for adverse reactions.
• *Alert:* Don't confuse Isuprel with Isordil.

## PATIENT TEACHING
• Tell patient to report chest pain, fluttering in chest or other adverse reactions.
• Remind patient to report pain at the I.V. injection site.

---

# levalbuterol hydrochloride
Xopenex

*Pregnancy risk category C*

## AVAILABLE FORMS
*Solution for inhalation:* 0.31 mg, 0.63 mg, or 1.25 mg in 3-ml vials

## INDICATIONS & DOSAGES
➤ **To prevent or treat bronchospasm in patients with reversible obstructive airway disease**
*Adults and adolescents age 12 and older:* 0.63 mg given t.i.d. q 6 to 8 hours, by oral inhalation via a nebulizer. Patients with more severe asthma who don't respond adequately to 0.63 mg t.i.d. may benefit from 1.25 mg t.i.d.
*Children ages 6 to 11:* 0.31 mg inhaled t.i.d. by nebulizer. Routine dosing shouldn't exceed 0.63 mg t.i.d.

## ACTION
Relaxes bronchial smooth muscle by stimulating beta$_2$ receptors; also, inhibits release of mediators from mast cells in the airway.

| Route | Onset | Peak | Duration |
|---|---|---|---|
| Inhalation | 10-17 min | 1½ hr | 5-8 hr |

## ADVERSE REACTIONS
**CNS:** dizziness, migraine, nervousness, pain, tremor, anxiety.
**CV:** tachycardia.
**EENT:** *rhinitis,* sinusitis, turbinate edema.
**GI:** dyspepsia.
**Musculoskeletal:** leg cramps.
**Respiratory:** increased cough.
**Other:** flulike syndrome, accidental injury, *viral infection.*

## INTERACTIONS
**Drug-drug.** *Beta blockers:* May block pulmonary effect of the drug and cause severe bronchospasm. Avoid using together, if possible. If use together is necessary, consider a cardioselective beta blocker, but give with caution.
*Digoxin:* May decrease digoxin level up to 22%. Monitor digoxin level.
*Loop or thiazide diuretics:* May cause ECG changes and hypokalemia. Use together cautiously.
*MAO inhibitors, tricyclic antidepressants:* May potentiate action of levalbuterol on the vascular system. Avoid using within 2 weeks of MAO inhibitor or tricyclic antidepressant therapy.
*Other short-acting sympathomimetic aerosol bronchodilators, epinephrine:* May increase adrenergic adverse effects. Use together cautiously.

## EFFECTS ON LAB TEST RESULTS
None reported.

## CONTRAINDICATIONS & CAUTIONS
• Contraindicated in patients hypersensitive to drug or to racemic albuterol.
• Use cautiously in patients with CV disorders, especially coronary insufficiency, hypertension, and arrhythmias.
• Use cautiously in patients with seizure disorders, hyperthyroidism, or diabetes mellitus and in those who are unusually responsive to sympathomimetic amines.

## NURSING CONSIDERATIONS
• *Alert:* Like other inhaled beta agonists, levalbuterol can produce paradoxical bronchospasm, which may be life-threatening.

---

Reactions may be *common*, uncommon, *life-threatening*, or COMMON AND LIFE-THREATENING.

If this occurs, stop drug immediately and start alternative therapy.

• *Alert:* Like all other beta agonists, levalbuterol can produce significant CV effects in some patients. Although such effects are uncommon at recommended doses, stop drug as directed if they occur.

• Drug may worsen diabetes mellitus and ketoacidosis.

• Potassium level may be transiently decreased, but potassium supplementation is usually unnecessary.

• The compatibility, efficacy, and safety of levalbuterol mixed with other drugs in a nebulizer haven't been established.

PATIENT TEACHING

• Warn patient that he may experience worsened breathing. Tell him to stop drug and contact prescriber immediately if this occurs.

• Tell patient not to increase dosage without consulting prescriber.

• Urge patient to seek medical attention immediately if levalbuterol becomes less effective, if signs and symptoms become worse, or if he's using levalbuterol more frequently than usual.

• Tell patient that the effects of levalbuterol may last up to 8 hours.

• Tell patient not to double the next dose if he misses a dose. Tell him to take doses at least 6 hours apart.

• Advise patient to use other inhalations and antiasthmatics only as directed while taking levalbuterol.

• Inform patient that common adverse reactions include palpitations, rapid heart rate, headache, dizziness, tremor, and nervousness.

• Encourage patient to contact prescriber if she becomes pregnant or is breast-feeding.

• Tell patient to keep unopened vials in foil pouch. Once the foil pouch is opened, vials must be used within 2 weeks. Inform patient that vials removed from the pouch, if not used immediately, should be protected from light and excessive heat and used within 1 week.

• Teach patient to use drug correctly by oral inhalation via a nebulizer.

• Instruct patient to breathe as calmly, deeply, and evenly as possible until no more mist is formed in the nebulizer reservoir (5 to 15 minutes).

---

## metaprotenerol sulfate
Alupent, Arm-a-Med
Metaproterenol, Dey-Lute
Metaproterenol

*Pregnancy risk category C*

---

AVAILABLE FORMS
*Aerosol inhaler:* 0.65 mg/metered spray
*Nebulizer inhaler:* 0.4%, 0.6%, 5% solution
*Syrup:* 10 mg/5 ml
*Tablets:* 10 mg, 20 mg

INDICATIONS & DOSAGES
➤ **Acute episodes of bronchial asthma**
*Adults and children age 12 and older:* 2 or 3 inhalations q 3 to 4 hours. Don't exceed 12 inhalations daily.
➤ **Bronchial asthma and reversible bronchospasm**
*Adults:* 20 mg P.O. q 6 to 8 hours.
*Children older than age 9, or weighing more than 27 kg (60 lb):* 20 mg P.O. q 6 to 8 hours.
*Children ages 6 to 9, or weighing less than 27 kg:* 10 mg P.O. q 6 to 8 hours.
*Children younger than age 6:* 1.3 to 2.6 mg/kg/day P.O. in divided doses of syrup.
*IPPB or nebulizer*
*Adults and children age 12 and older:* 0.2 to 0.3 ml of 5% solution diluted in about 2.5 ml of half-normal or normal saline solution. Or, 2.5 ml of a commercially available 0.4% or 0.6% solution q 4 hours, p.r.n.
*Children ages 6 to 12:* 0.1 to 0.2 ml of a 5% solution diluted in normal saline solution to final volume of 3 ml q 4 hours, p.r.n.

ACTION
Relaxes bronchial smooth muscle by stimulating beta$_2$ receptors.

| Route | Onset | Peak | Duration |
|-------|-------|------|----------|
| P.O. | 15 min | 1 hr | 4 hr |
| Inhalation | 1 min | 1 hr | 1½ hr |
| Nebulizer | 5-30 min | 1 hr | 1½ hr |

---

## ADVERSE REACTIONS
**CNS:** *nervousness, weakness,* drowsiness, *tremor,* vertigo, headache, dizziness, insomnia.
**CV:** *tachycardia,* hypertension, palpitations, **cardiac arrest with excessive use.**
**EENT:** dry and irritated throat.
**GI:** *vomiting, nausea,* heartburn, dry mouth.
**Respiratory:** ***paradoxical bronchiolar constriction with excessive use,*** cough.
**Skin:** rash.
**Other:** hypersensitivity reactions.

## INTERACTIONS
**Drug-drug.** *Epinephrine, other sympathomimetics:* May increase risk of arrhythmias. Use together cautiously.
*MAO inhibitors, tricyclic antidepressants:* May potentiate the effect of metaproterenol on the vascular system. Use together cautiously.
*Propranolol, other beta blockers:* May block bronchodilating effect of metaproterenol. Monitor patient carefully.

## EFFECTS ON LAB TEST RESULTS
None reported.

## CONTRAINDICATIONS & CAUTIONS
• Contraindicated in patients hypersensitive to drug or its ingredients and in those with tachycardia, arrhythmias linked to tachycardia, peripheral or mesenteric vascular thrombosis, profound hypoxia or hypercapnia.
• Contraindicated in those receiving general anesthesia with cyclopropane or halogenated hydrocarbon anesthetics.
• Use cautiously in patients receiving cardiac glycosides and in patients with hypertension, hyperthyroidism, heart disease, diabetes, or cirrhosis.

## NURSING CONSIDERATIONS
• Patients may use tablets and aerosol together. Watch closely for toxicity.
• Drug may reduce the sensitivity of spirometry in the diagnosis of asthma.
• Inhalant solution can be given by IPPB with drug diluted in normal saline solution or with a hand nebulizer at full strength.
• **Alert:** Don't confuse metaproterenol with metoprolol or metipranolol; don't confuse Alupent with Atrovent.

## PATIENT TEACHING
• Teach patient to perform oral inhalation correctly. Give the following instructions for using an MDI:
– Shake canister.
– Clear nasal passages and throat.
– Breathe out, expelling as much air from lungs as possible.
– Place mouthpiece well into mouth, and inhale deeply as you release dose from inhaler. Or, hold inhaler about 1 inch (two finger widths) from open mouth; inhale while dose is released.
– Hold breath for several seconds, remove mouthpiece, and exhale slowly. Allow 2 minutes between inhalations.
• Inform patient that use of AeroChamber with MDI may improve drug delivery to lungs.
• Advise patient to store drug in light-resistant container.
• Tell patient who is also using a corticosteroid inhaler to use bronchodilator first, and then wait about 5 minutes before using the corticosteroid. This method allows bronchodilator to open air passages for maximum effectiveness of the corticosteroid.
• Tell patient to remove canister and wash inhaler in warm, soapy water at least once weekly.
• Warn patient to stop drug immediately and notify prescriber if paradoxical bronchospasm occurs.
• Warn patient to notify prescriber if he has no response to drug.

---

# pirbuterol acetate
Maxair, Maxair Autohaler

*Pregnancy risk category C*

---

## AVAILABLE FORMS
*Inhaler:* 0.2 mg/metered dose

## INDICATIONS & DOSAGES
➤ **To prevent and reverse bronchospasm; asthma**
*Adults and children age 12 and older:* 1 or 2 inhalations (0.2 to 0.4 mg), repeated q 4 to 6 hours. Don't exceed 12 inhalations daily.

---

## ACTION
Relaxes bronchial smooth muscle by stimulating beta$_2$ receptors.

| Route | Onset | Peak | Duration |
|---|---|---|---|
| Inhalation | 5 min | 30-60 min | 5 hr |

## ADVERSE REACTIONS
**CNS:** tremor, nervousness, dizziness, insomnia, headache, vertigo.
**CV:** tachycardia, palpitations, chest tightness.
**EENT:** dry or irritated throat.
**GI:** nausea, vomiting, diarrhea, dry mouth.
**Respiratory:** cough.

## INTERACTIONS
**Drug-drug.** *Beta blockers, propranolol:*
May decrease bronchodilating effects. Avoid using together.
*MAO inhibitors, tricyclic antidepressants:*
May potentiate action of beta agonist on vascular system. Use together cautiously.

## EFFECTS ON LAB TEST RESULTS
None reported.

## CONTRAINDICATIONS & CAUTIONS
• Contraindicated in patients hypersensitive to drug.
• Use cautiously in patients unusually responsive to sympathomimetic amines and patients with CV disorders, hyperthyroidism, diabetes, and seizure disorders.

## NURSING CONSIDERATIONS
• Monitor patient for increased pulse or blood pressure during therapy.
• Stop drug immediately and notify prescriber if paradoxical bronchospasm occurs.
• The likelihood of paradoxical bronchospasm is increased with the first use of a new canister or vial.
• Notify prescriber of decreasing effectiveness of the drug.

## PATIENT TEACHING
• Teach patient to perform oral inhalation correctly. Give the following instructions for using an MDI:
– Shake canister.
– Clear nasal passages and throat.

– Breathe out, expelling as much air from lungs as possible.
– Place mouthpiece well into mouth, and inhale deeply as you release dose from inhaler.
– Hold breath for several seconds, remove mouthpiece, and exhale slowly.
• If more than one inhalation is ordered, tell patient to wait at least 2 minutes before repeating procedure.
• Give the following instructions for using Autohaler:
– Remove mouthpiece cover by pulling down lip on back cover. Inspect mouthpiece for foreign objects. Locate "Up" arrows and air vents.
– Hold Autohaler upright so that arrows point up; raise lever until it snaps into place.
– Hold Autohaler around the middle, and shake gently several times.
– Continue to hold upright, and be careful not to block air vents at bottom. Exhale normally before use.
– Seal lips around mouthpiece. Inhale deeply through mouthpiece with steady, moderate force to trigger release of the drug. You'll hear a click and feel a soft puff when drug is released. Continue to take a full, deep breath.
– Take Autohaler away from mouth when done inhaling. Hold breath for 10 seconds; then exhale slowly.
– Continue to hold Autohaler upright while lowering lever. Lower lever after each puff. If additional puffs are ordered, wait 1 minute before repeating process to obtain the next puff.
• Have patient clean inhaler per manufacturer's instructions.
• If patient also uses a corticosteroid inhaler, tell him to use the bronchodilator first, and then wait about 5 minutes before using the corticosteroid. This allows the bronchodilator to open air passages for maximum effectiveness of the corticosteroid.
• Instruct patient to call prescriber if bronchospasm increases after using drug.
• Advise patient to seek medical attention if a previously effective dosage doesn't control symptoms; this change may signal worsening of disease.

## salmeterol xinafoate
Serevent Diskus

*Pregnancy risk category C*

### AVAILABLE FORMS
*Inhalation powder:* 50 mcg/blister

### INDICATIONS & DOSAGES
➤ **Long-term maintenance of asthma; to prevent bronchospasm in patients with nocturnal asthma or reversible obstructive airway disease who need regular treatment with short-acting beta agonists**
*Adults and children age 4 and older:* 1 inhalation (50 mcg) q 12 hours, morning and evening.
➤ **To prevent exercise-induced bronchospasm**
*Adults and children age 4 and older:* 1 inhalation (50 mcg) at least 30 minutes before exercise. Additional doses shouldn't be taken for at least 12 hours.
➤ **COPD or emphysema**
*Adults:* 1 inhalation (50 mcg) b.i.d. in the morning and evening, about 12 hours apart.

### ACTION
Not clearly defined. Selectively activates beta$_2$ receptors, which results in bronchodilation; also, blocks the release of allergic mediators from mast cells lining the respiratory tract.

| Route | Onset | Peak | Duration |
|-------|-------|------|----------|
| Inhalation | 10-20 min | 3 hr | 12 hr |

### ADVERSE REACTIONS
**CNS:** headache, sinus headache, tremor, nervousness, giddiness, dizziness.
**CV:** tachycardia, palpitations, *ventricular arrhythmias.*
**EENT:** *nasopharyngitis,* pharyngitis, nasal cavity or sinus disorder.
**GI:** nausea, vomiting, diarrhea, heartburn.
**Musculoskeletal:** joint and back pain, myalgia.
**Respiratory:** cough, lower respiratory tract infection, *upper respiratory tract infection,* **bronchospasm.**
**Other:** hypersensitivity reactions.

### INTERACTIONS
**Drug-drug.** *Beta agonists, other methylxanthines, theophylline:* May cause adverse cardiac effects with excessive use. Monitor patient.
*MAO inhibitors:* May cause risk of severe adverse CV effects. Avoid use within 14 days of MAO inhibitor therapy.
*Tricyclic antidepressants:* May cause risk of moderate to severe adverse CV effects. Use together with caution.

### EFFECTS ON LAB TEST RESULTS
None reported.

### CONTRAINDICATIONS & CAUTIONS
● Contraindicated in patients hypersensitive to drug or its ingredients.
● Use cautiously in patients unusually responsive to sympathomimetics and those with coronary insufficiency, arrhythmias, hypertension, other CV disorders, thyrotoxicosis, or seizure disorders.

### NURSING CONSIDERATIONS
● Drug isn't indicated for acute bronchospasm.
● *Alert:* Monitor patient for rash and urticaria, which may signal a hypersensitivity reaction.
● *Alert:* Don't confuse Serevent with Serentil.

### PATIENT TEACHING
● Remind patient to take drug at about 12-hour intervals for optimum effect and to take drug even when feeling better.
● If patient is taking drug to prevent exercise-induced bronchospasm, tell him to take it 30 to 60 minutes before exercise.
● *Alert:* Tell patient that although drug is a beta agonist, it shouldn't be used to treat acute bronchospasm. He must be given a short-acting beta agonist, such as albuterol, to treat worsening symptoms.
● *Alert:* Rare serious asthma episodes or asthma-related deaths have occurred in patients using salmeterol, with African Americans at greatest risk.
● Tell patient to contact prescriber if the short-acting agonist no longer provides sufficient relief or if he needs more than 4 inhalations daily. This may be a sign that the asthma symptoms are worsening. Tell

him not to increase the dosage of salmeterol.

• If patient takes an inhaled corticosteroid, he should continue to use it regularly. Warn patient not to take other drugs without prescriber's consent.

• If patient takes the inhalation powder (Diskus device), instruct him not to exhale into the device. He should activate and use it only in a level, horizontal position.

• Tell patient not to use Diskus with a spacer.

• Instruct patient never to wash the mouthpiece or any part of the Diskus; it must be kept dry.

---

## terbutaline sulfate
Brethine, Bricanyl

*Pregnancy risk category B*

### AVAILABLE FORMS
*Injection:* 1 mg/ml
*Tablets:* 2.5 mg, 5 mg

### INDICATIONS & DOSAGES
➤ **Bronchospasm in patients with reversible obstructive airway disease**
*Injection*
*Adults and children age 12 and older:* 0.25 mg S.C. May be repeated in 15 to 30 minutes, p.r.n. Maximum, 0.5 mg in 4 hours.
*Tablets*
*Adults and adolescents older than age 15:* 2.5 to 5 mg P.O. q 6 hours t.i.d. during waking hours. Maximum, 15 mg daily.
*Children ages 12 to 15:* 2.5 mg P.O. q 6 hours t.i.d. during waking hours. Maximum, 7.5 mg daily.

### ACTION
Relaxes bronchial smooth muscle by stimulating beta$_2$ receptors.

| Route | Onset | Peak | Duration |
|-------|-------|------|----------|
| P.O. | 30 min | 2-3 hr | 4-8 hr |
| S.C. | 15 min | 30 min | 1½-4 hr |

### ADVERSE REACTIONS
**CNS:** *nervousness, tremor, drowsiness, dizziness, headache,* weakness.

**CV:** *palpitations,* tachycardia, ***arrhythmias,*** flushing.
**GI:** *vomiting, nausea,* heartburn.
**Metabolic:** hypokalemia.
**Respiratory:** ***paradoxical bronchospasm with prolonged use,*** dyspnea.
**Skin:** diaphoresis.

### INTERACTIONS
**Drug-drug.** *Cardiac glycosides, cyclopropane, halogenated inhaled anesthetics, levodopa:* May increase risk of arrhythmias. Monitor patient closely, and avoid using together with levodopa.
*CNS stimulants:* May increase CNS stimulation. Avoid using together.
*MAO inhibitors:* When given with sympathomimetics, may cause severe hypertension (hypertensive crisis). Avoid using together.
*Propranolol, other beta blockers:* May block bronchodilating effects of terbutaline. Avoid using together.

### EFFECTS ON LAB TEST RESULTS
• May decrease potassium levels.

### CONTRAINDICATIONS & CAUTIONS
• Contraindicated in patients hypersensitive to drug or sympathomimetic amines.
• Use cautiously in patient with CV disorders, hyperthyroidism, diabetes, or seizure disorders.

### NURSING CONSIDERATIONS
• Give S.C. injections in lateral deltoid area.
• Protect injection from light. Don't use if discolored.
• Terbutaline may reduce the sensitivity of spirometry for the diagnosis of bronchospasm.
• *Alert:* Don't confuse terbutaline with tolbutamide or terbinafine.

### PATIENT TEACHING
• Make sure patient and caregivers understand why patient needs drug.

---

## theophylline

*Immediate-release liquids*
Accurbron*, Aerolate, Aquaphyllin, Asmalix*, Bronkodyl*, Elixomin*, Elixophyllin*, Lanophyllin*, Slo-Phyllin, Theoclear-80, Theolair Liquid, Theostat 80*

*Immediate-release tablets and capsules*
Bronkodyl, Elixophyllin, Nuelin‡, Quibron T Dividose, Slo-Phyllin

*Timed-release tablets*
Quibron-T/SR, Respbid, Sustaire, Theochron, Theolair-SR, Theo-Sav, Theo-Time, T-Phyl, Uniphyl

*Timed-release capsules*
Aerolate, Elixophyllin, Nuelin-SR‡, Slo-bid Gyrocaps, Slo-Phyllin, Theobid Duracaps, Theochron, Theoclear L.A., Theospan-SR, Theo-24, Theovent Long-Acting

*Pregnancy risk category C*

**AVAILABLE FORMS**
*Capsules:* 100 mg, 200 mg
*Capsules (extended-release):* 50 mg, 60 mg, 65 mg, 75 mg, 100 mg, 125 mg, 130 mg, 200 mg, 250 mg, 260 mg, 300 mg
*$D_5W$ injection:* 200 mg in 50 ml or 100 ml; 400 mg in 100 ml, 250 ml, 500 ml, or 1,000 ml; 800 mg in 500 ml or 1,000 ml
*Elixir:* 27 mg/5 ml*, 50 mg/5 ml*
*Oral solution:* 27 mg/5 ml, 50 mg/5 ml
*Syrup:* 27 mg/5 ml, 50 mg/5 ml
*Tablets:* 100 mg, 125 mg, 200 mg, 250 mg, 300 mg
*Tablets (chewable):* 100 mg
*Tablets (extended-release):* 100 mg, 200 mg, 250 mg, 300 mg, 400 mg, 500 mg, 600 mg

**INDICATIONS & DOSAGES**
Extended-release preparations shouldn't be used to treat acute bronchospasm.

➤ **Oral theophylline for acute broncho-spasm in patients not currently receiving theophylline**
*Adult nonsmokers and children older than age 16:* 5 mg/kg P.O., then 3 mg/kg q 6 hours for two doses. Maintenance dosage is 3 mg/kg q 8 hours.
*Children ages 9 to 16:* 5 mg/kg P.O.; then 3 mg/kg q 4 hours for three dosages. Maintenance dosage is 3 mg/kg q 6 hours.
*Children ages 6 months to 9 years:* 5 mg/ kg P.O.; then 4 mg/kg q 4 hours for three dosages. Maintenance dosage is 4 mg/kg q 6 hours.
*Adjust-a-dose:* For otherwise healthy adult smokers, 5 mg/kg P.O.; then 3 mg/kg q 4 hours for three dosages. Maintenance dosage is 3 mg/kg q 6 hours.
    For older adults and patients with cor pulmonale, 5 mg/kg P.O.; then 2 mg/kg q 6 hours for two dosages. Maintenance dosage is 2 mg/kg q 8 hours.
    For adults with heart failure or liver disease, 5 mg/kg P.O.; then 2 mg/kg q 8 hours for two dosages. Maintenance dosage is 1 to 2 mg/kg q 12 hours.
➤ **Parenteral theophylline for patients not currently receiving theophylline**
*Loading dosage:* 4.7 mg/kg I.V. slowly; then maintenance infusion.
*Adult nonsmokers and children older than age 16:* 0.55 mg/kg/hour I.V. for 12 hours; then 0.39 mg/kg/hour.
*Children ages 9 to 16:* 0.79 mg/kg/hour I.V. for 12 hours; then 0.63 mg/kg/hour.
*Children ages 6 months to 9 years:* 0.95 mg/kg/hour I.V. for 12 hours; then 0.79 mg/kg/hour.
*Adjust-a-dose:* For otherwise healthy adult smokers, 0.79 mg/kg/hour I.V. for 12 hours; then 0.63 mg/kg/hour.
    For older adults and patients with cor pulmonale, 0.47 mg/kg/hour I.V. for 12 hours; then 0.24 mg/kg/hour.
    For adults with heart failure or liver disease, 0.39 mg/kg/hour I.V. for 12 hours; then 0.08 to 0.16 mg/kg/hour.
➤ **Oral and parenteral theophylline for acute bronchospasm in patients cur-rently receiving theophylline**
*Adults and children:* Ideally, dose is based on current theophylline level. Each 0.5 mg/kg I.V. or P.O. loading dose will increase drug level by 1 mcg/ml. In emer-gencies, some prescribers recommend a

2.5-mg/kg P.O. dose of rapidly absorbed form if patient develops no obvious signs or symptoms of theophylline toxicity.

➤ **Chronic bronchospasm**

*Adults and children:* Initially, 16 mg/kg or 400 mg P.O. daily, whichever is less, given in three or four divided doses at 6- to 8-hour intervals. Or, 12 mg/kg or 400 mg P.O. daily, whichever is less, in an extended-release preparation given in two or three divided doses at 8- or 12-hour intervals. Dosage may be increased, as tolerated, at 2- to 3-day intervals to the following maximums: adults and children older than age 16, 13 mg/kg or 900 mg P.O. daily, whichever is less; children ages 12 to 16, 18 mg/kg P.O. daily; children ages 9 to 12, 20 mg/kg P.O. daily; children younger than age 9, 24 mg/kg P.O. daily.

**I.V. ADMINISTRATION**
● Use commercially available infusion solution, or mix in $D_5W$ solution.
● Use infusion pump for continuous infusion.

**ACTION**
Inhibits phosphodiesterase, the enzyme that degrades cAMP, resulting in relaxation of smooth muscle of the bronchial airways and pulmonary blood vessels.

| Route | Onset | Peak | Duration |
|---|---|---|---|
| P.O. | 15-60 min | 1-2 hr | Unknown |
| P.O. (extended) | 15-60 min | 4-7 hr | Unknown |
| I.V. | 15 min | 15-30 min | Unknown |

**ADVERSE REACTIONS**
**CNS:** *restlessness, dizziness,* headache, *insomnia,* irritability, ***seizures,*** muscle twitching.
**CV:** *palpitations, sinus tachycardia,* extrasystoles, flushing, marked hypotension, ***arrhythmias.***
**GI:** *nausea, vomiting,* diarrhea, epigastric pain.
**Metabolic:** urinary catecholamines.
**Respiratory:** tachypnea, ***respiratory arrest.***

**INTERACTIONS**
**Drug-drug.** *Adenosine:* May decrease antiarrhythmic effectiveness. Higher doses of adenosine may be needed.

*Allopurinol, calcium channel blockers, cimetidine, disulfiram, influenza virus vaccine, interferon, macrolide antibiotics (such as erythromycin), methotrexate, hormonal contraceptives, quinolone antibiotics (such as ciprofloxacin):* May decrease hepatic clearance of theophylline; may increase theophylline level. Monitor patient for toxicity.
*Barbiturates, nicotine, phenytoin, rifampin:* May enhance metabolism and decrease theophylline level. Monitor patient for decreased effect.
*Carbamazepine, isoniazid, loop diuretics:* May increase or decrease theophylline level. Monitor theophylline level.
*Carteolol, pindolol, propranolol, timolol:* May act antagonistically, reducing the effects of one or both drugs; may reduce elimination of theophylline. Monitor theophylline level and patient closely.
*Ephedrine, other sympathomimetics:* May exhibit synergistic toxicity with these drugs, predisposing patient to arrhythmias. Monitor patient closely.
*Lithium:* May increase lithium excretion. Monitor patient closely.
**Drug-herb.** *Cacao tree:* May inhibit theophylline metabolism. Discourage use together.
*Cayenne:* May increase risk of theophylline toxicity. Advise patient to use together cautiously.
*Ephedra:* May increase risk of adverse reactions. Discourage use together.
*Guarana:* May cause additive CNS and CV effects. Discourage use together.
*Ipriflavone:* May increase risk of theophylline toxicity. Advise patient to use together cautiously.
*St. John's wort:* May decrease theophylline level. Discourage use together.
**Drug-food.** *Any food:* May cause accelerated release of theophylline from extended-release products. Tell patient to take Theo-24 on an empty stomach.
*Caffeine:* May decrease hepatic clearance of theophylline; may increase theophylline level. Monitor patient for toxicity.
**Drug-lifestyle.** *Smoking:* May increase elimination of theophylline, increasing dosage requirements. Monitor theophylline response and level.

**EFFECTS ON LAB TEST RESULTS**
• May increase free fatty acid levels.

**CONTRAINDICATIONS & CAUTIONS**
• Contraindicated in patients hypersensitive to xanthine compounds (caffeine, theobromine) and in those with active peptic ulcer or poorly controlled seizure disorders.
• Use cautiously in young children, infants, neonates, elderly patients, and those with COPD, cardiac failure, cor pulmonale, renal or hepatic disease, peptic ulceration, hyperthyroidism, diabetes mellitus, glaucoma, severe hypoxemia, hypertension, compromised cardiac or circulatory function, angina, acute MI, or sulfite sensitivity.

**NURSING CONSIDERATIONS**
• *Alert:* Don't confuse extended-release forms with regular-release forms.
• Dosage may need to be increased in cigarette smokers and in habitual marijuana smokers because smoking causes drug to be metabolized faster.
• Give drug around-the-clock, using extended-release product at bedtime.
• Depending on assay used, theophylline levels may be falsely elevated in the presence of furosemide, phenylbutazone, probenecid, theobromine, caffeine, tea, chocolate, cola beverages, and acetaminophen.
• Monitor vital signs; measure and record fluid intake and output. Expect improved quality of pulse and respirations.
• People metabolize xanthines at different rates; dosage is determined by monitoring response, tolerance, pulmonary function, and theophylline level. Theophylline levels range from 10 to 20 mcg/ml; toxicity may occur at levels above 20 mcg/ml.
• *Alert:* Evidence of toxicity includes tachycardia, anorexia, nausea, vomiting, diarrhea, restlessness, irritability, and headache. The presence of any of these signs in patients taking theophylline warrants checking theophylline level and adjusting dosage, as indicated.
• *Alert:* Don't confuse Theolair with Thyrolar.

**PATIENT TEACHING**
• Supply instructions for home care and dosage schedule.
• Warn patient not to dissolve, crush, or chew extended-release products. Small children unable to swallow these can ingest (without chewing) the contents of capsules sprinkled over soft food.
• Tell patient to relieve GI symptoms by taking oral drug with full glass of water after meals, although food in stomach delays absorption.
• Warn patient to take drug regularly, only as directed. Patients tend to want to take extra "breathing pills."
• Inform elderly patient that dizziness is common at start of therapy.
• Urge patient to tell prescriber about any other medications used. OTC drugs or herbal remedies may contain ephedrine or theophylline salts; excessive CNS stimulation may result.
• If patient smokes, have him inform prescriber if he quits. A dosage reduction may be necessary to prevent toxicity.

# 42
# Expectorants and antitussives

**benzonatate**
**codeine phosphate**
(See Chapter 26, OPIOID ANALGESICS.)
**codeine sulfate**
(See Chapter 26, OPIOID ANALGESICS.)
**dextromethorphan hydrobromide**
**diphenhydramine hydrochloride**
(See Chapter 40, ANTIHISTAMINES.)
**guaifenesin**
**hydromorphone hydrochloride**
(See Chapter 26, OPIOID ANALGESICS.)

## COMBINATION PRODUCTS
Preparations are available in the following combinations:
• Expectorants with decongestants, antihistamines, or both
• Antitussives with decongestants, antihistamines, or both
• Expectorants and antitussives
• Expectorants and antitussives with decongestants, antihistamines, or both

---

## benzonatate
Tessalon, Tessalon Perles

*Pregnancy risk category C*

### AVAILABLE FORMS
*Capsules:* 100 mg, 200 mg

### INDICATIONS & DOSAGES
➤ **Symptomatic relief of cough**
*Adults and children older than age 10:*
100 to 200 mg P.O. t.i.d.; up to 600 mg daily may be needed.

### ACTION
Chemical relative of tetracaine that suppresses the cough reflex by direct action on the cough center in the medulla and through an anesthetic action on stretch receptors of vagal afferent fibers in the respiratory passages, lungs, and pleura.

| Route | Onset | Peak | Duration |
|-------|-------|------|----------|
| P.O. | 15-20 min | Unknown | 3-8 hr |

### ADVERSE REACTIONS
**CNS:** dizziness, headache, sedation.
**EENT:** nasal congestion, burning sensation in eyes.
**GI:** nausea, constipation, GI upset.
**Other:** chills, hypersensitivity reactions.

### INTERACTIONS
None significant.

### EFFECTS ON LAB TEST RESULTS
None reported.

### CONTRAINDICATIONS & CAUTIONS
• Contraindicated in patients hypersensitive to drug or related compounds.
• Use cautiously in patients hypersensitive to PABA anesthetics (procaine, tetracaine) because cross-sensitivity reactions may occur.

### NURSING CONSIDERATIONS
• Don't use benzonatate when cough is a valuable diagnostic sign or is beneficial (as after thoracic surgery).
• Monitor cough type and frequency.
• Use with percussion and chest vibration.

### PATIENT TEACHING
• Warn patient not to chew capsules or dissolve in mouth. Produces either local anesthesia that may result in aspiration or CNS stimulation that may cause restlessness, tremor, and seizures.
• Instruct patient to report adverse reactions.
• Instruct patient to protect drug from light and moisture.
• *Alert:* Make sure patient understands that persistent cough may indicate a serious condition and that he should contact his prescriber if cough lasts longer than 1 week, recurs frequently, or is accompanied by high fever, rash, or severe headache.

---

# dextromethorphan hydrobromide

Balminil DM◇ Benylin DM◇, Broncho-Grippol-DM†, Buckley's DM, Children's Hold◇, Delsym, Hold◇, Koffex DM†, Pertussin CS◇, Pertussin ES◇, Robitussin Pediatric◇, St. Joseph Cough Suppressant for Children◇, Trocal◇, Vicks Formula 44e Pediatric◇

*More commonly available in combination products, such as* Anti-Tuss DM Expectorant◇, Benylin Expectorant◇, Cheracol D Cough◇, Glycotuss-dM◇, Guiamid D.M. Liquid◇, Guiatuss-DM◇, Halotussin-DM◇, Kolephrin GG/DM◇, Mytussin DM◇, Naldecon Senior DX◇, Pertussin CS◇, Rhinosyn-DMX Expectorant◇, Robitussin-DM◇, Scot-Tussin DM Cough Chasers◇, Tolu-Sed DM◇, Tuss-DM◇, Unproco◇, Vicks Pediatric 44E◇

*Pregnancy risk category C*

## AVAILABLE FORMS
*Liquid (extended-release):* 30 mg/5 ml◇
*Lozenges:* 5 mg◇, 7.5 mg◇, 15 mg◇
*Solution:* 3.5 mg/5 ml, 5 mg/5 ml*◇, 7.5 mg/5 ml◇, 10 mg/5 ml*◇, 15 mg/5 ml*◇, 15 mg/15 ml*◇, 12.5 mg/5 ml

## INDICATIONS & DOSAGES
➤ **Nonproductive cough**
*Adults and children age 12 and older:* 10 to 20 mg P.O. q 4 hours, or 30 mg q 6 to 8 hours. Or, 60 mg extended-release liquid b.i.d. Maximum, 120 mg daily.
*Children ages 6 to 11:* 5 to 10 mg P.O. q 4 hours, or 15 mg q 6 to 8 hours. Or, 30 mg extended-release liquid b.i.d. Maximum, 60 mg daily.
*Children ages 2 to 5:* 2.5 to 5 mg P.O. q 4 hours, or 7.5 mg q 6 to 8 hours. Or, 15 mg extended-release liquid b.i.d. Maximum, 30 mg daily.
*Children younger than age 2:* Individualize dosages.

## ACTION
Antitussive that suppresses the cough reflex by direct action on the cough center in the medulla.

| Route | Onset | Peak | Duration |
|-------|-------|------|----------|
| P.O. | < 30 min | Unknown | 3-6 hr |

## ADVERSE REACTIONS
**CNS:** drowsiness, dizziness.
**GI:** nausea, vomiting, stomach pain.

## INTERACTIONS
**Drug-drug.** *MAO inhibitors:* May cause risk of hypotension, coma, hyperpyrexia, and death. Avoid using together.
*Selegiline:* May cause risk of confusion, coma, hyperpyrexia. Avoid using together.
**Drug-herb.** *Parsley:* May promote or produce serotonin syndrome. Discourage use together.

## EFFECTS ON LAB TEST RESULTS
None reported.

## CONTRAINDICATIONS & CAUTIONS
● Contraindicated in patients currently taking MAO inhibitors or within 2 weeks of discontinuing MAO inhibitors.
● Use cautiously in atopic children, sedated or debilitated patients, and patients confined to the supine position. Also, use cautiously in patients sensitive to aspirin or tartrazine dyes.

## NURSING CONSIDERATIONS
● Don't use dextromethorphan when cough is a valuable diagnostic sign or is beneficial (as after thoracic surgery).
● Dextromethorphan 15 to 30 mg is equivalent to 8 to 15 mg codeine as an antitussive.
● Drug produces no analgesia or addiction and little or no CNS depression.
● Use drug with chest percussion and vibration.
● Monitor cough type and frequency.

## PATIENT TEACHING
● Instruct patient to take drug exactly as prescribed.
● Tell patient to report adverse reactions.
● *Alert:* Make sure patient understands that persistent cough may indicate a serious condition and that he should contact his

prescriber if cough lasts longer than 1 week, recurs frequently, or is accompanied by high fever, rash, or severe headache.

---

## guaifenesin (glyceryl guaiacolate)
Anti-Tuss*◇, Balminil Expectorant†, Breonesin◇, Gee-Gee◇, GG-CEN*◇, Glyate*◇, Glycotuss◇, Glytuss◇, Guiatuss*◇, Halotussin, Hytuss◇, Hytuss 2X◇, Mucinex◇, Naldecon Senior EX◇, Resyl†◇, Robitussin*◇, Scot-Tussin Expectorant◇, Uni-tussin*◇

*Pregnancy risk category C*

### AVAILABLE FORMS
*Capsules:* 200 mg◇
*Solution:* 100 mg/5 ml*◇, 200 mg/5 ml
*Tablets:* 100 mg◇, 200 mg◇
*Tablets (extended-release):* 600 mg◇, 1,200 mg◇

### INDICATIONS & DOSAGES
➤ **Expectorant**
*Adults and children age 12 and older:* 200 to 400 mg P.O. q 4 hours, or 600 to 1,200 mg extended-release capsules or tablets q 12 hours. Maximum, 2,400 mg daily.
*Children ages 6 to 11:* 100 to 200 mg P.O. q 4 hours. Maximum, 1,200 mg daily.
*Children ages 2 to 5:* 50 to 100 mg P.O. q 4 hours. Maximum, 600 mg daily.

### ACTION
Increases production of respiratory tract fluids to help liquefy and reduce the viscosity of tenacious secretions.

| Route | Onset | Peak | Duration |
|-------|-------|------|----------|
| P.O. | Unknown | Unknown | Unknown |

### ADVERSE REACTIONS
**CNS:** dizziness, headache.
**GI:** vomiting, nausea.
**Skin:** rash.

### INTERACTIONS
None significant.

### EFFECTS ON LAB TEST RESULTS
None reported.

### CONTRAINDICATIONS & CAUTIONS
● Contraindicated in patients hypersensitive to drug.

### NURSING CONSIDERATIONS
● Drug is used to liquefy thick, tenacious sputum. Evidence suggests that guaifenesin is effective as an expectorant, but no evidence exists to support its role as an antitussive.
● Monitor cough type and frequency.
● *Alert:* Don't confuse guaifenesin with guanfacine.

### PATIENT TEACHING
● *Alert:* Make sure patient understands that persistent cough may indicate a serious condition and that he should contact his prescriber if cough lasts longer than 1 week, recurs frequently, or is accompanied by high fever, rash, or severe headache.
● Inform patient that drug shouldn't be used for chronic or persistent cough, such as with smoking, asthma, chronic bronchitis, or emphysema.
● Advise patient to take each dose with one glass of water; increasing fluid intake may prove beneficial.
● Encourage deep-breathing exercises.

# 43

# Miscellaneous respiratory tract drugs

acetylcysteine
beclomethasone dipropionate
beractant
budesonide
calfactant
cromolyn sodium
dornase alfa
flunisolide
fluticasone propionate
fluticasone propionate and
    salmeterol inhalation powder
montelukast sodium
omalizumab
palivizumab
triamcinolone acetonide
zafirlukast

---

## acetylcysteine
Mucomyst, Mucosil-10, Mucosil-20

*Pregnancy risk category B*

### AVAILABLE FORMS
*Solution:* 10%, 20%

### INDICATIONS & DOSAGES
➤ **Adjunct therapy for abnormal viscid or inspissated mucous secretions in patients with pneumonia, bronchitis, bronchiectasis, primary amyloidosis of the lung, tuberculosis, cystic fibrosis, emphysema, atelectasis, pulmonary complications of thoracic surgery, or CV surgery**
*Adults and children:* 1 to 2 ml 10% or 20% solution by direct instillation into trachea as often as q hour. Or, 1 to 10 ml of 20% solution or 2 to 20 ml of 10% solution by nebulization q 2 to 6 hours, p.r.n.
➤ **Acetaminophen toxicity**
*Adults and children:* Initially, 140 mg/kg P.O., then 70 mg/kg P.O. q 4 hours for 17 doses (total).

### ACTION
Mucolytic that reduces the viscosity of pulmonary secretions by splitting disulfide [bond]s between mucoprotein molecular [   ]. Also, restores liver stores of

glutathione to treat acetaminophen toxicity.

| Route | Onset | Peak | Duration |
|-------|-------|------|----------|
| P.O., inhalation | Unknown | Unknown | Unknown |

### ADVERSE REACTIONS
**CNS:** fever, drowsiness.
**CV:** tachycardia, hypotension, hypertension, chest tightness.
**EENT:** *rhinorrhea.*
**GI:** *stomatitis, nausea, vomiting.*
**Respiratory:** *bronchospasm.*
**Skin:** rash, clamminess, urticaria.
**Other:** *angioedema,* chills.

### INTERACTIONS
**Drug-drug.** *Activated charcoal:* May limit acetylcysteine's effectiveness. Avoid using activated charcoal before or with acetylcysteine.

### EFFECTS ON LAB TEST RESULTS
None reported.

### CONTRAINDICATIONS & CAUTIONS
• Contraindicated in patients hypersensitive to drug.
• Use cautiously in elderly or debilitated patients with severe respiratory insufficiency.

### NURSING CONSIDERATIONS
• Use plastic, glass, stainless steel, or another nonreactive metal when giving by nebulization. Hand-bulb nebulizers aren't recommended because output is too small and particle size too large.
• Drug is physically or chemically incompatible with tetracyclines, erythromycin lactobionate, amphotericin B, and ampicillin sodium. If given by aerosol inhalation, nebulize these drugs separately. Iodized oil, trypsin, and hydrogen peroxide are physically incompatible with acetylcysteine; don't add to nebulizer.
• Drug smells strongly of sulfur. Mixing oral form with juice or cola improves its palatability.

• If drug is to be delivered through naso-gastric tube, you may dilute it with water.
• Monitor cough type and frequency.
• *Alert:* Monitor patient for bronchospasm, especially if he has asthma.
• Use fresh dilutions used within 1 hour. Store undiluted solutions that have been opened in the refrigerator for up to 96 hours.
• *Alert:* Acetylcysteine is given to treat ac-etaminophen overdose within 24 hours after ingestion. Start treatment immediately as prescribed; don't wait for results of ac-etaminophen level.
• Ingestion of acetaminophen in amounts exceeding 150 mg/kg may cause liver tox-icity. Obtain plasma or serum acetamino-phen level 4 hours after ingestion to deter-mine the risk of liver toxicity.
• When used orally to treat acetaminophen overdose, dilute oral doses with cola, fruit juice, or water before giving. Dilute the 20% solution to 5% (add 3 ml of diluent to each ml of acetylcysteine). If patient vomits within 1 hour of receiving loading or maintenance dose, repeat dose. Use di-luted solution within 1 hour.
• When acetaminophen level returns to below toxic level according to nomogram, acetylcysteine therapy may be stopped.
• *Alert:* Don't confuse acetylcysteine with acetylcholine.

## PATIENT TEACHING
• Warn patient that drug may have a foul taste or smell that some patients find dis-tressing.
• For maximum effect, instruct patient to clear his airway by coughing before aerosol administration.

---

## beclomethasone dipropionate
Qvar

*Pregnancy risk category C*

## AVAILABLE FORMS
*Oral inhalation aerosol:* 40 mcg/metered spray, 80 mcg/metered spray

## INDICATIONS & DOSAGES
➤ Chronic asthma
*Adults and children age 12 and older:* Starting dose, 40 to 80 mcg b.i.d. when

used with bronchodilators alone, or 40 to 160 mcg b.i.d. when used with inhaled corticosteroids. Maximum, 320 mcg b.i.d. *Children ages 5 to 12:* 40 mcg b.i.d., up to 80 mcg b.i.d. when used with bronchodila-tors alone or with inhaled corticosteroids.

## ACTION
Unknown. May decrease inflammation by decreasing the number and activity of in-flammatory cells, inhibiting bronchocon-strictor mechanisms producing direct smooth-muscle relaxation, and decreasing airway hyperresponsiveness.

| Route | Onset | Peak | Duration |
|---|---|---|---|
| Inhalation | 1-4 wk | Unknown | Unknown |

## ADVERSE REACTIONS
**EENT:** *hoarseness,* fungal infection of throat, *throat irritation.*
**GI:** dry mouth, *fungal infection of mouth.*
**Metabolic:** suppression of hypothalamic-pituitary-adrenal function, adrenal insuffi-ciency.
**Respiratory:** *bronchospasm,* wheezing, cough.
**Other:** *angioedema,* hypersensitivity re-actions, facial edema.

## INTERACTIONS
None significant.

## EFFECTS ON LAB TEST RESULTS
None reported.

## CONTRAINDICATIONS & CAUTIONS
• Contraindicated in patients hypersensi-tive to drug or its ingredients and in those with status asthmaticus, nonasthmatic bronchial diseases, or asthma controlled by bronchodilators or other noncorticos-teroids alone.
• Use with extreme caution, if at all, in pa-tients with tuberculosis, fungal or bacterial infections, ocular herpes simplex, or sys-temic viral infections.
• Use cautiously in patients receiving sys-temic corticosteroid therapy.

## NURSING CONSIDERATIONS
• Check mucous membranes frequently for signs and symptoms of fungal infec-tion.

• During times of stress (trauma, surgery, or infection), systemic corticosteroids may be needed to prevent adrenal insufficiency in previously corticosteroid-dependent patients.
• Periodic measurement of growth and development may be needed during high-dose or prolonged therapy in children.
• *Alert:* Taper oral corticosteroid therapy slowly. Acute adrenal insufficiency and death have occurred in patients with asthma who changed abruptly from oral corticosteroids to beclomethasone.

## PATIENT TEACHING
• Tell patient to prime the inhaler before first use, or after 10 days of not using it, by depressing cannister twice into the air.
• Inform patient that drug doesn't relieve acute asthma attacks.
• Tell patient who needs a bronchodilator to use it several minutes before beclomethasone.
• Instruct patient to carry or wear medical identification indicating his need for supplemental systemic corticosteroids during stress.
• Advise patient to allow 1 minute to elapse between inhalations of drug and to hold his breath for a few seconds to enhance drug action.
• Tell patient it may take up to 4 weeks to feel the full benefit of the drug.
• Tell patient to keep inhaler clean by wiping it weekly with a dry tissue or cloth; don't get it wet.
• Advise patient to prevent oral fungal infections by gargling or rinsing his mouth with water after each use. Caution him not to swallow the water.
• Tell patient to report evidence of corticosteroid withdrawal, including fatigue, weakness, arthralgia, orthostatic hypotension, and dyspnea.
• Instruct patient to store drug at 77° F (25° C). Advise patient to ensure delivery of proper dose by gently warming canister to room temperature before using.

# beractant (natural lung surfactant)
Survanta

*Pregnancy risk category NR*

**AVAILABLE FORMS**
*Suspension for intratracheal instillation:* 25 mg/ml

**INDICATIONS & DOSAGES**
➤ **To prevent respiratory distress syndrome (RDS), also known as hyaline membrane disease, in premature neonates weighing 1,250 g (2 lb, 12 ounces) or less at birth or having symptoms consistent with surfactant deficiency**
*Neonates:* 4 ml/kg intratracheally. Divide each dose into four quarter-doses and give each quarter-dose with infant in a different position to ensure even distribution of drug; between quarter-doses, use a hand-held resuscitation bag at 60 breaths/minute and sufficient oxygen to prevent cyanosis. Give drug as soon as possible, preferably within 15 minutes of birth. Repeat in 6 hours if respiratory distress continues. Give no more than four doses in 48 hours.
➤ **Rescue treatment of RDS in premature infants**
*Neonates:* 4 ml/kg intratracheally; before giving, increase ventilator rate to 60 breaths/minute with an inspiratory time of 0.5 second and a fraction of inspired oxygen of 1. Divide each dose into four quarter-doses and give each quarter-dose with infant in a different position to ensure even distribution of drug; between quarter-doses, continue mechanical ventilation for at least 30 seconds or until stable. Give dose as soon as RDS is confirmed by X-ray, preferably within 8 hours of birth. Repeat in 6 hours if respiratory distress continues. Give no more than four doses in 48 hours.

**ACTION**
Lowers alveolar surface tension during respiration and stabilizes alveoli against collapse. This extract of bovine lung contains neutral lipids, fatty acids, surfactant-related proteins, and phospholipids that mimics naturally occurring surfactant;

palmitic acid, tripalmitin, and colfosceril palmitate are added to standardize the solution's composition.

| Route | Onset | Peak | Duration |
|-------|-------|------|----------|
| Intra-tracheal | 30-120 min | Unknown | 2-3 days |

## ADVERSE REACTIONS

**CV:** TRANSIENT BRADYCARDIA, vasoconstriction, hypotension.
**Hematologic:** decreased oxygen saturation, hypocapnia, hypercapnia.
**Respiratory:** *endotracheal tube reflux or blockage, apnea.*
**Skin:** pallor.

## INTERACTIONS
None significant.

## EFFECTS ON LAB TEST RESULTS
None reported.

## CONTRAINDICATIONS & CAUTIONS
No known contraindications.

## NURSING CONSIDERATIONS
● Give beractant only by staff experienced in caring for clinically unstable premature neonates, including neonatal intubation and airway management.
● Accurate weight determination is essential for proper measurement of dosage.
● Continuously monitor neonate before, during, and after beractant administration. The endotracheal tube may be suctioned before giving drug; allow neonate to stabilize before proceeding with administration.
● Refrigerate at 36° to 46° F (2° to 8° C). Warm before use by allowing drug to stand at room temperature for at least 20 minutes or by holding in hand for at least 8 minutes. Don't use artificial warming methods. Unopened vials that have been warmed to room temperature may be returned to the refrigerator within 24 hours; however, warm and return drug to the refrigerator only once. Vials are for single use only; discard unused drug.
● Beractant doesn't need sonication or reconstitution before use. Inspect contents before giving; make sure color is off-white to light brown and that contents are uni-

form. If settling occurs, swirl vial gently; don't shake. Some foaming is normal.
● Use a large-bore needle (20G or larger) to draw up drug; don't use a filter. Give drug using a #5 French end-hole catheter. Premeasure and shorten catheter before use. Fill catheter with beractant and discard excess drug so that only total dose to be given remains in the syringe. Insert catheter into neonate's endotracheal tube; make sure catheter tip protrudes just beyond end of tube above neonate's carina. Don't instill drug into a mainstream bronchus.
● Even distribution of drug is important. For example, give each dose in four quarter-doses, with each quarter-dose being given over 2 to 3 seconds and with the patient positioned differently after each use. Between giving quarter-doses, remove the catheter and ventilate the patient. Give the first quarter-dose with the patient's head and body inclined slightly downward, and the head turned to the right. Give the second quarter-dose with the head turned to the left. Then, incline the head and body slightly upward with the head turned to the right to give the third quarter-dose. Turn the head to the left for the fourth quarter-dose.
● Immediately after giving, moist breath sounds and crackles can occur. Don't suction the neonate for 1 hour unless he has other signs or symptoms of airway obstruction.
● Continuous monitoring of ECG and transcutaneous oxygen saturation are essential; frequent arterial blood pressure monitoring and frequent arterial blood gas sampling are highly desirable.
● Transient bradycardia and oxygen desaturation are common after dosing.
● *Alert:* Beractant can rapidly affect oxygenation and lung compliance. Peak ventilator inspiratory pressures may need to be adjusted if chest expansion improves substantially after drug administration. Notify prescriber and adjust immediately as directed because lung overdistention and fatal pulmonary air leakage may result.
● Audiovisual materials that describe dosage and usage procedures are available from the manufacturer.
● *Alert:* Don't confuse Survanta with Sufenta.

## PATIENT TEACHING
• Inform parents of neonate's need for drug, and explain drug action and use.
• Encourage parents to ask questions, and address their concerns.

---

## budesonide
Pulmicort Respules, Pulmicort Turbuhaler

*Pregnancy risk category B*

### AVAILABLE FORMS
*Dry powder inhaler:* 200 mcg/dose
*Suspension:* 0.25 mg, 0.5 mg

### INDICATIONS & DOSAGES
➤ **As a preventative in maintenance treatment of asthma**
In all patients, use lowest effective dose after stabilization of asthma.
*Adults previously on bronchodilators alone:* Initially, inhaled dose of 200 to 400 mcg b.i.d. to maximum of 400 mcg b.i.d.
*Adults previously on inhaled corticosteroids:* Initially, inhaled dose of 200 to 400 mcg b.i.d. to maximum of 800 mcg b.i.d.
*Adults previously on oral corticosteroids:* Initially, inhaled dose of 400 to 800 mcg b.i.d. to maximum of 800 mcg b.i.d.
*Children older than age 6 previously on bronchodilators alone or inhaled corticosteroids:* Initially, inhaled dose of 200 mcg b.i.d. to maximum of 400 mcg b.i.d.
*Children older than age 6 previously on oral corticosteroids:* Highest recommended dose is 400 mcg b.i.d.
*Children ages 1 to 8:* 0.25 mg Respules via jet nebulizer with compressor once daily. Increase to 0.5 mg daily or 0.25 mg b.i.d. in child not receiving systemic or inhaled corticosteroids or 1 mg daily or 0.5 mg b.i.d. if child is receiving oral corticosteroids.

### ACTION
Anti-inflammatory corticosteroid that exhibits potent glucocorticoid activity and weak mineralocorticoid activity. The exact ~~nism~~ of the corticosteroids isn't ~~they have a wide range of in-~~ ~~against such cell types~~

as mast cells and macrophages and mediators (such as leukotrienes) involved in allergic and nonallergic inflammation.

| Route | Onset | Peak | Duration |
|-------|-------|------|----------|
| Inhalation | 24 hr | 1-2 wk | Unknown |

### ADVERSE REACTIONS
**CNS:** *headache,* fever, asthenia, pain, insomnia, syncope, hypertonia.
**EENT:** *sinusitis, pharyngitis,* rhinitis, voice alteration.
**GI:** oral candidiasis, dyspepsia, gastroenteritis, nausea, dry mouth, taste perversion, vomiting, abdominal pain.
**Metabolic:** weight gain.
**Musculoskeletal:** back pain, fractures, myalgia.
**Respiratory:** *respiratory tract infections,* increased cough, **bronchospasm.**
**Skin:** ecchymoses.
**Other:** flulike symptoms, hypersensitivity reactions.

### INTERACTIONS
**Drug-drug.** *Ketoconazole:* May inhibit metabolism and increase level of budesonide. Monitor patient.

### EFFECTS ON LAB TEST RESULTS
None reported.

### CONTRAINDICATIONS & CAUTIONS
• Contraindicated in patients hypersensitive to drug and in those with status asthmaticus or other acute asthma episodes.
• Use cautiously, if at all, in patients with active or quiescent tuberculosis of the respiratory tract, ocular herpes simplex, or untreated systemic fungal, bacterial, viral, or parasitic infections.

### NURSING CONSIDERATIONS
• When transferring from systemic corticosteroid to budesonide, use caution and gradually decrease corticosteroid dose to prevent adrenal insufficiency.
• Drug doesn't remove the need for systemic corticosteroid therapy in some situations.
• If bronchospasm occurs after using budesonide, stop therapy and treat with a bronchodilator.
• Improved lung function has been observed within 24 hours of starting budes-

onide treatment, although maximum benefit may not be achieved for 1 to 2 weeks or
longer.
● Watch for *Candida* infections of the
mouth or pharynx.
● *Alert:* Corticosteroids may increase risk
of developing serious or fatal infections in
patients exposed to viral illnesses, such as
chickenpox or measles.
● In rare cases, inhaled corticosteroids
have been linked to increased intraocular
pressure and cataract development. Stop
drug if local irritation occurs.

**PATIENT TEACHING**
● Tell patient that budesonide inhaler isn't
a bronchodilator and isn't intended to treat
acute episodes of asthma.
● Instruct patient to use the inhaler at regular intervals as follows because effectiveness depends on twice-daily use on a regular basis:
– Tell patient to keep Pulmicort Turbuhaler
upright (mouthpiece on top) during loading, to provide the correct dose.
– Instruct patient to prime Turbuhaler
when using it for the first time. To prime,
hold unit upright and turn brown grip fully
to the right, then fully to the left until it
clicks. Repeat priming.
– Tell patient to load first dose by holding
unit upright and turning brown grip to the
right and then to the left until it clicks.
– Tell patient to turn his head away from
the inhaler and breathe out.
– During inhalation, Turbuhaler must be in
the upright or horizontal position.
– Tell patient not to shake inhaler.
– Instruct patient to place mouthpiece between lips and to inhale forcefully and
deeply.
– Tell patient that he may not taste the
drug or sense it entering his lungs, but this
doesn't mean it isn't effective.
– Tell patient not to exhale through the
Turbuhaler. If more than one dose is required, repeat steps.
– Advise patient to rinse his mouth with
water and then spit out the water after
each dose to decrease the risk of developing oral candidiasis.
– When 20 doses remain in the Turbuhaler,
a red mark appears in the indicator win-
dow. When red mark reaches the bottom,
the unit's empty.

– Tell patient not to use Turbuhaler with a
spacer device and not to chew or bite the
mouthpiece.
– Replace mouthpiece cover after use and
always keep it clean and dry.
● Tell patient that improvement in asthma
control may be seen within 24 hours, although the maximum benefit may not appear for 1 to 2 weeks. If signs or symptoms worsen during this time, patient
should contact prescriber.
● Advise patient to avoid exposure to
chickenpox or measles and to contact prescriber if exposure occurs.
● Instruct patient to carry or wear medical
identification indicating need for supplementary corticosteroids during periods of
stress or an asthma attack.
● Tell patient to read and follow the patient information leaflet contained in the
package.

# calfactant
Infasurf

*Pregnancy risk category NR*

**AVAILABLE FORMS**
*Intratracheal suspension:* 35 mg phospholipids and 0.65 mg proteins/ml; 6-ml vial

**INDICATIONS & DOSAGES**
➤ **To prevent respiratory distress syndrome (RDS) in premature infants under 29 weeks' gestational age at high
risk for RDS; to treat infants younger
than 72 hours of age who develop RDS
(confirmed by clinical and radiologic
findings) and who need endotracheal
intubation**
*Newborns:* 3 ml/kg of body weight at
birth intratracheally, given in two aliquots
of 1.5 ml/kg each, q 12 hours for total of
three doses.

**ACTION**
Nonpyrogenic lung surfactant that modifies alveolar surface tension, thereby stabilizing the alveoli.

| Route | Onset | Peak | Duration |
|---|---|---|---|
| Intra-tracheal | 24-48 hr | Unknown | Unknown |

**ADVERSE REACTIONS**
**CV:** BRADYCARDIA.
**Respiratory:** AIRWAY OBSTRUCTION, APNEA, *hypoventilation, cyanosis.*
**Other:** *reflux of drug into endotracheal tube,* dislodgment of endotracheal tube.

**INTERACTIONS**
None significant.

**EFFECTS ON LAB TEST RESULTS**
None reported.

**CONTRAINDICATIONS & CAUTIONS**
None known.

**NURSING CONSIDERATIONS**
● Give drug under supervision of medical staff experienced in the acute care of newborn infants with respiratory failure who need intubation.
● Store drug at 36° to 46° F (2° to 8° C). It isn't necessary to warm drug before use.
● Unopened, unused vials that have warmed to room temperature can be re-refrigerated within 24 hours for future use. Avoid repeated warming to room temperature.
● Suspension settles during storage. Gentle swirling or agitation of the vial is commonly needed for redispersion. Don't shake vial. Visible flecks in the suspension and foaming at the surface are normal.
● *Alert:* Drug is intended only for intratracheal use; to prevent RDS, give to infant as soon as possible after birth, preferably within 30 minutes.
● Withdraw dose into a syringe from single-use vial using a 20G or larger needle; avoid excessive foaming.
● Give through a side-port adapter into the endotracheal tube. Make sure two medical staff are present during dosing. Give dose in two aliquots of 1.5 ml/kg each. Place infant on one side after first aliquot and other side after second aliquot. Give while ventilation is continued over 20 to 30 breaths for each aliquot, with small bursts timed only during the inspiratory cycles. Evaluate respiratory status and reposition infant between each aliquot.
● Monitor patient for reflux of drug into ~~~al tube, cyanosis, bradycardia, ~~~tion during the dosing ~~~ur, stop drug and

take appropriate measures to stabilize infant. After infant is stable, resume dosing with appropriate monitoring.
● After giving drug, carefully monitor infant so that oxygen therapy and ventilatory support can be modified in response to improvements in oxygenation and lung compliance.
● Enter each single-use vial only once; discard unused material.

**PATIENT TEACHING**
● Explain to parents the function of drug in preventing and treating RDS.
● Notify parents that, although infant may improve rapidly after treatment, he may continue to need intubation and mechanical ventilation.
● Notify parents of possible adverse effects of drug, including bradycardia, reflux into endotracheal tube, airway obstruction, cyanosis, dislodgment of endotracheal tube, and hypoventilation.
● Reassure parents that infant will be carefully monitored.

---

## cromolyn sodium (sodium cromoglycate)
Crolom, Gastrocrom, Intal Inhaler, Intal Nebulizer Solution, Nasalcrom, Rynacrom†

*Pregnancy risk category B*

**AVAILABLE FORMS**
*Aerosol:* 800 mcg/metered spray
*Nasal solution:* 5.2 mg/metered spray (40 mg/ml)
*Ophthalmic solution:* 4%
*Oral concentrate:* 20 mg/ml
*Solution (for nebulization):* 20 mg/2 ml

**INDICATIONS & DOSAGES**
➤ **Mild to moderate persistent asthma**
*Adults and children age 5 and older:*
2 metered sprays using inhaler q.i.d. at regular intervals. Or, 20 mg via nebulization q.i.d. at regular intervals.
➤ **To prevent and treat seasonal and perennial allergic rhinitis**
*Adults and children older than age 2:*
1 spray in each nostril t.i.d. or q.i.d. Maximum, six times daily.

*~~~ contains alcohol.*

~n, *life-threatening*, or COMMON AND LIFE-THREATENING.

➤ **To prevent exercise-induced bron-chospasm**
*Adults and children age 5 and older:*
2 metered sprays inhaled no longer than
1 hour before anticipated exercise.
➤ **Conjunctivitis**
*Adults and children age 4 and older:* 1 or
2 drops in each eye four to six times daily
at regular intervals.
➤ **Systemic mastocytosis**
*Adults and children older than age 12:*
200 mg P.O. q.i.d. before meals and h.s.
*Children ages 2 to 12:* 100 mg P.O. q.i.d.
30 minutes before meals and h.s.

**ACTION**
Inhibits the degranulation of sensitized
mast cells that occurs after exposure to
specific antigens. Also, inhibits release of
histamine and slow-reacting substance of
anaphylaxis.

| Route | Onset | Peak | Duration |
|---|---|---|---|
| P.O., ophthalmic, inhalation, intranasal | Unknown | Unknown | Unknown |

**ADVERSE REACTIONS**
**CNS:** dizziness, headache.
**EENT:** *irritated throat and trachea,*
lacrimation, nasal congestion, pharyngeal
irritation, *sneezing,* nasal burning and irritation, epistaxis, ocular burning and stinging.
**GI:** nausea, esophagitis, abdominal pain,
*bad taste,* diarrhea.
**GU:** dysuria, urinary frequency.
**Musculoskeletal:** joint swelling and pain.
**Respiratory:** *bronchospasm* after inhalation of dry powder, *cough,* wheezing,
*eosinophilic pneumonia.*
**Skin:** rash, urticaria.
**Other:** swollen parotid gland, *angioedema.*

**INTERACTIONS**
None significant.

**EFFECTS ON LAB TEST RESULTS**
None reported.

**CONTRAINDICATIONS & CAUTIONS**
• Contraindicated in patients hypersensitive to drug and in those experiencing

acute asthma attacks and status asthmaticus.
• Use with caution in children. Use of cromolyn oral inhalation solution isn't recommended in children younger than age
2. Cromolyn powder or aerosol for oral inhalation isn't recommended for children
younger than age 5. Cromolyn ophthalmic
solution isn't recommended for children
younger than age 4. Cromolyn nasal solution isn't recommended for children
younger than age 6.
• Use inhalation form cautiously in patients with coronary artery disease or a
history of arrhythmias.

**NURSING CONSIDERATIONS**
• Use drug (except for ophthalmic solution) only when acute episode of asthma
has been controlled, airway is cleared, and
patient can breathe independently.
• *Alert:* For full-term neonates and infants,
use oral cromolyn sodium only for severe,
incapacitating disease when benefits clearly outweigh risks.
• Dissolve powder in capsules for oral
dose in hot water, and further dilute with
cold water before ingestion. Don't mix
with fruit juice, milk, or food.
• Stop drug if eosinophilic pneumonia develops, as evidenced by eosinophilia and
infiltrates on chest X-ray.
• Watch for recurrence of asthma signs and
symptoms when dosage is decreased, especially when corticosteroids are also used.

**PATIENT TEACHING**
• Teach patient how to use prescribed
form of drug.
• Advise patient that full effects of drug
may not be noted for 4 weeks.
• Tell patient that esophagitis may be relieved by antacids or a glass of milk.
• Warn patient that nasal solution may
cause stinging or sneezing.

## dornase alfa
Pulmozyme

*Pregnancy risk category B*

**AVAILABLE FORMS**
*Inhalation solution:* 2.5-mg ampule
(1 mg/ml)

## INDICATIONS & DOSAGES
➤ **To improve pulmonary function and decrease the frequency of moderate to severe respiratory tract infections in patients with cystic fibrosis**
*Adults and children age 5 and older:*
1 ampule or 2.5 mg inhaled once daily. Treatment usually takes 10 to 15 minutes. Use drug only with an approved nebulizer.

## ACTION
Hydrolyzes DNA in sputum of cystic fibrosis patients, causing decreased viscosity and elasticity of pulmonary secretions.

| Route | Onset | Peak | Duration |
|---|---|---|---|
| Inhalation | 3-7 days | 9 days | Unknown |

## ADVERSE REACTIONS
**CV:** *chest pain.*
**EENT:** *pharyngitis, voice alteration,* laryngitis, conjunctivitis.
**Skin:** *rash,* urticaria.

## INTERACTIONS
None significant.

## EFFECTS ON LAB TEST RESULTS
None reported.

## CONTRAINDICATIONS & CAUTIONS
● Contraindicated in patients hypersensitive to drug or to products derived from Chinese hamster ovary cells.
● Safety and efficacy haven't been established for use longer than 12 months, for children younger than age 5, and for children with forced vital capacity below 40% of normal value.

## NURSING CONSIDERATIONS
● Drug is used with other standard therapies for cystic fibrosis.
● Patients older than age 21 and those with a forced vital capacity over 85% may benefit from twice-daily use.
● **Alert:** Give only with the Hudson T Updraft II disposable jet nebulizer, the Marquest Acorn II disposable jet nebulizer along with Pulmo-Aide compressor, or the LC Jet+ reusable nebulizer or the PARI BABY along with the PARI PRONEB or the Durable sidestream MOBILAIRE or Porta Neb

● Discard cloudy or discolored solution.
● Don't mix with other drugs in the nebulizer. Mixing could lead to a physical or chemical reaction that may inactivate dornase alfa.
● Refrigerate drug in its protective foil pouch to protect it from strong light.
● Once opened, the entire ampule must be used or discarded.

## PATIENT TEACHING
● Teach patient how to use drug at home.
● Remind patient to breathe only through his mouth when using the nebulizer. If this is difficult, suggest that he use a nose clip.
● Tell patient that if he begins coughing during treatment, he should turn off nebulizer without spilling drug. To resume, he should turn on nebulizer and continue breathing through the mouthpiece until the nebulizer cup is empty or mist is no longer produced.

# flunisolide
AeroBid, AeroBid-M, Bronalide†, Nasalide, Nasarel

*Pregnancy risk category C*

## AVAILABLE FORMS
*Nasal solution:* 25 mcg/metered spray
*Oral inhalant:* 250 mcg/metered spray (at least 100 metered inhalations/container)

## INDICATIONS & DOSAGES
➤ **Chronic asthma**
*Adults and adolescents older than age 15:*
2 inhalations (500 mcg) b.i.d. Maximum, 8 inhalations (2,000 mcg) daily.
*Children ages 6 to 15:* 2 inhalations (500 mcg) b.i.d. Higher dosages haven't been studied. Maximum, 1,000 mcg daily.
➤ **Seasonal or perennial rhinitis**
*Adults and adolescents older than age 14:*
2 sprays (50 mcg) in each nostril b.i.d. May be increased to t.i.d. if necessary. Maximum dose is 8 sprays in each nostril daily (400 mcg).
*Children ages 6 to 14:* 1 spray (25 mcg) in each nostril t.i.d. or 2 sprays (50 mcg) in each nostril b.i.d. Maximum dose is 4 sprays in each nostril daily (200 mcg).

† *life-threatening*, or COMMON AND LIFE-THREATENING.

## ACTION

Unknown. May decrease inflammation through inhibitory activities against such cell types as mast cells or macrophages, and mediators such as leukotrienes. In nasal passages it has anti-inflammatory and vasoconstricting effects.

| Route | Onset | Peak | Duration |
|---|---|---|---|
| Inhalation (nasal) | < 3 wk | Unknown | Unknown |
| Inhalation (oral) | 1-4 wk | Unknown | Unknown |

## ADVERSE REACTIONS

**CNS:** fever, dizziness, irritability, nervousness, *headache.*
**CV:** palpitations, chest pain, edema.
**EENT:** throat irritation, hoarseness, nasopharyngeal fungal infections, *sore throat, nasal congestion,* nasal irritation, nasal burning or stinging.
**GI:** *nausea, vomiting,* dry mouth, *unpleasant taste, diarrhea, upset stomach,* abdominal pain, decreased appetite.
**Respiratory:** *upper respiratory tract infection, cold symptoms.*
**Skin:** rash, pruritus.
**Other:** *influenza.*

## INTERACTIONS

None significant.

## EFFECTS ON LAB TEST RESULTS

None reported.

## CONTRAINDICATIONS & CAUTIONS

• Contraindicated in patients hypersensitive to drug and in those with status asthmaticus or respiratory tract infections.
• Drug isn't recommended in patients with nonasthmatic bronchial diseases or with asthma controlled by bronchodilators or other noncorticosteroids alone.

## NURSING CONSIDERATIONS

• A spacer device may help to ensure proper dosage administration and decrease oral adverse effects.
• Store drug between 59° and 86° F (15° and 30° C).
• Stop nasal spray after 3 weeks if symptoms don't improve.

• **Alert:** Withdraw drug slowly in patients who have received long-term oral corticosteroid therapy.
• After withdrawing systemic corticosteroids, patient may need supplemental systemic corticosteroids if stress (trauma, surgery, or infection) causes adrenal insufficiency.
• **Alert:** Don't confuse flunisolide with fluocinonide.

## PATIENT TEACHING
### Oral inhalant

• Warn patient that flunisolide doesn't relieve acute asthma attacks.
• Advise patient to ensure delivery of proper dose by gently warming the canister to room temperature before using. Some patients carry the canister in a pocket to keep it warm.
• Tell patient who also is using a bronchodilator to use it several minutes before beginning flunisolide treatment.
• Instruct patient to allow 1 minute to elapse before repeating inhalations and to hold his breath for a few seconds to enhance drug action.
• Teach patient to keep inhaler clean and unobstructed. He should wash it with warm water and dry it thoroughly after use.
• Teach patient to check mucous membranes frequently for signs and symptoms of fungal infection.
• Advise patient to prevent oral fungal infections by gargling or rinsing mouth with water after each inhaler use. Caution him not to swallow the water.
• Warn patient to avoid exposure to chicken pox or measles. If exposed, contact prescriber immediately.
• Advise parents of a child receiving long-term therapy that the child should have periodic growth measurements and be checked for evidence of hypothalamic-pituitary-adrenal axis suppression.
### Nasal spray
• Tell patient to prime the nasal inhaler (5 to 6 sprays) before first use and after long periods of no use.
• Advise patient to clear nasal passageways before use.
• Patient should follow manufacturer's instructions for use and cleaning. Discard open containers after 3 months.

• Advise patient that therapeutic results may take several weeks.

---

## fluticasone propionate
Flonase, Flovent, Flovent Diskus, Flovent Rotadisk

*Pregnancy risk category C*

---

### AVAILABLE FORMS
*Nasal spray:* 50 mcg/metered spray
*Oral inhalation aerosol:* 44 mcg, 110 mcg, 220 mcg
*Oral inhalation powder:* 50 mcg, 100 mcg, 250 mcg

### INDICATIONS & DOSAGES
➤ **As preventative in maintenance treatment of patients requiring oral corticosteroid for chronic asthma**
*Flovent*
*Adults and children age 12 and older:* In those previously taking bronchodilators alone, initially, inhaled dose of 88 mcg b.i.d. to maximum of 440 mcg b.i.d.
*Patients previously taking inhaled corticosteroids:* Initially, inhaled dose of 88 to 220 mcg b.i.d. to maximum of 440 mcg b.i.d.
*Patients previously taking oral corticosteroids:* Inhaled dose of 880 mcg b.i.d.
*Flovent Rotadisk and Diskus*
*Adults and children ages 12 and older:* In patients previously taking bronchodilators alone, initially, inhaled dose of 100 mcg b.i.d. to maximum of 500 mcg b.i.d.
*Patients previously taking inhaled corticosteroids:* Initially, inhaled dose of 100 to 250 mcg b.i.d. to maximum of 500 mcg b.i.d.
*Patients previously taking oral corticosteroids:* Inhaled dose of 1,000 mcg b.i.d.
*Children ages 4 to 11:* For patients previously on bronchodilators alone or on inhaled corticosteroids, initially, inhaled dose of 50 mcg b.i.d. to maximum of 100 mcg b.i.d.
*Flonase*
➤ **Nasal symptoms of seasonal and perennial allergic and nonallergic rhinitis**

*Adults:* Initially, 2 sprays (100 mcg) in each nostril ... 1 spray b.i.d. Once ... decrease to

1 spray in each nostril daily. Or, for seasonal allergic rhinitis, 2 sprays in each nostril once daily, as needed, for symptom control.
*Adolescents and children age 4 and older:* Initially, 1 spray (50 mcg) in each nostril daily. If not responding, increase to 2 sprays in each nostril daily. Once symptoms are controlled, decrease to 1 spray in each nostril daily. Maximum dose is 2 sprays in each nostril daily.

### ACTION
Synthetic glucocorticoid with potent anti-inflammatory activity. Inflammation is an important cause of asthma. Glucocorticoids inhibit many cell types and mediator production or secretion involved in the asthmatic response and produce anti-inflammatory and vasoconstrictor effects in nasal passages.

| Route | Onset | Peak | Duration |
|---|---|---|---|
| Inhalation (nasal) | 12 hr | Several days | 1-2 wk |
| Inhalation (oral) | 24 hr | Several days | 1-2 wk |

### ADVERSE REACTIONS
**CNS:** fever, *headache,* dizziness, migraine, nervousness.
**EENT:** *pharyngitis,* acute nasopharyngitis, nasal congestion, sinusitis, dysphonia, rhinitis, otitis media, tonsillitis, nasal discharge, earache, laryngitis, epistaxis, sneezing, hoarseness, conjunctivitis, eye irritation.
**GI:** mouth irritation, *oral candidiasis,* diarrhea, abdominal pain, viral gastroenteritis, colitis, abdominal discomfort, nausea, vomiting.
**GU:** dysmenorrhea, candidiasis of vagina, pelvic inflammatory disease, vaginitis, vulvovaginitis, irregular menstrual cycle.
**Metabolic:** cushingoid features, growth retardation in children, weight gain.
**Musculoskeletal:** joint pain, aches and pains, disorder or symptoms of neck sprain or strain, muscular soreness.
**Respiratory:** *upper respiratory tract infection,* bronchitis, chest congestion, dyspnea, irritation from inhalant, cough.
**Skin:** dermatitis, urticaria.
**Other:** influenza, dental problems.

---

*life-threatening,* or COMMON AND LIFE-THREATENING.

## INTERACTIONS

**Drug-drug.** *Ketoconazole and other cytochrome P-450 3A4 inhibitors:* May increase mean fluticasone level. Use together cautiously.

## EFFECTS ON LAB TEST RESULTS
None reported.

## CONTRAINDICATIONS & CAUTIONS
• Contraindicated in patients hypersensitive to ingredients in these preparations.
• Contraindicated as primary treatment of patients with status asthmaticus or other acute episodes of asthma requiring more intensive measures.
• Use cautiously in breast-feeding patients.

## NURSING CONSIDERATIONS
• Because of risk of systemic absorption of inhaled corticosteroids, observe patient carefully for evidence of systemic corticosteroid effects.
• Some patients on high doses of fluticasone may have an abnormal response to the 6-hour cosyntropin stimulation test.
• Monitor patient, especially postoperatively or during periods of stress, for evidence of inadequate adrenal response.
• During withdrawal from oral corticosteroids, some patients may experience signs and symptoms of systemically active corticosteroid withdrawal, such as joint or muscle pain, lassitude, and depression, despite maintenance or even improvement of respiratory function.
• For patients starting therapy who are currently receiving oral corticosteroid therapy, reduce dose of prednisone to no more than 2.5 mg/day on a weekly basis, beginning after at least 1 week of therapy with fluticasone.
• *Alert:* As with other inhaled asthma drugs, bronchospasm may occur with an immediate increase in wheezing after dosing. If bronchospasm occurs after dosing with fluticasone inhalation aerosol, treat immediately with a fast-acting inhaled bronchodilator.

## PATIENT TEACHING
• Tell patient that drug isn't indicated for the relief of acute bronchospasm.

• For proper use of drug and to attain maximum improvement, tell patient to carefully follow the accompanying patient instructions.
• Advise patient to use drug at regular intervals, as directed.
• Instruct patient to contact prescriber if nasal spray doesn't improve condition after 4 days of treatment.
• Instruct patient to immediately contact prescriber if asthma episodes unresponsive to bronchodilators occur during treatment with fluticasone. During such episodes, patient may need therapy with oral corticosteroids.
• Warn patient to avoid exposure to chickenpox or measles and, if exposed, to consult prescriber immediately.
• Tell patient to carry or wear medical identification indicating that he may need supplementary corticosteroids during stress or a severe asthma attack.
• During periods of stress or a severe asthma attack, instruct patient who has been withdrawn from systemic corticosteroids to resume oral corticosteroids (in prescribed doses) immediately and to contact prescriber for further instruction. Instruct him to rinse his mouth and spit water out after inhalation.
• Advise patient to avoid spraying inhalation aerosol into eyes.
• Instruct patient to shake canister well before using inhalation aerosol.
• Advise patient to store fluticasone powder in a dry place.

**Flonase nasal spray**
• Tell patient to prime the nasal inhaler before first use or after 1 week or longer of non-use.
• Have patient clear nasal passages before use.
• Advise patient to follow manufacturer's recommendations for use and cleaning.
• Advise patient to use at regular intervals for full benefit.
• Tell patient to contact provider if signs or symptoms don't improve within 4 days or if signs or symptoms worsen.

---

# fluticasone propionate and salmeterol inhalation powder
Advair Diskus 100/50, Advair Diskus 250/50, Advair Diskus 500/50

*Pregnancy risk category C*

## AVAILABLE FORMS
*Inhalation powder:* 100 mcg fluticasone/50 mcg salmeterol, 250 mcg fluticasone/50 mcg salmeterol, 500 mcg fluticasone/50 mcg salmeterol

## INDICATIONS & DOSAGES
➤ **Long-term maintenance therapy for asthma**
*Adults and children older than age 12:*
1 inhalation b.i.d., at least 12 hours apart.
*Adults and children older than age 12 not currently taking an inhaled corticosteroid:*
1 inhalation of Advair Diskus 100/50 b.i.d.
*Adults and children older than age 12 currently taking beclomethasone dipropionate:* If beclomethasone dipropionate daily dose is 420 mcg or less, start with 1 inhalation of Advair Diskus 100/50 b.i.d. If beclomethasone dipropionate daily dose is 462 to 840 mcg, start with 1 inhalation of Advair Diskus 250/50 b.i.d.
*Adults and children older than age 12 currently taking budesonide:* If budesonide daily dose is 400 mcg or less, start with 1 inhalation of Advair Diskus 100/50 b.i.d. If budesonide daily dose is 800 to 1,200 mcg, start with 1 inhalation of Advair Diskus 250/50 b.i.d. If budesonide daily dose is 1,600 mcg, start with 1 inhalation of Advair Diskus 500/50 b.i.d.
*Adults and children older than age 12 currently taking flunisolide:* If flunisolide daily dose is 1,000 mcg or less, start with 1 inhalation of Advair Diskus 100/50 b.i.d. If flunisolide daily dose is 1,250 to 2,000 mcg, start with 1 inhalation of Advair Diskus 250/50 b.i.d.
*Adults and children older than age 12 currently taking fluticasone propionate inhalation aerosol:* If fluticasone propionate inhalation aerosol daily dose is 176 mcg or less, start with 1 inhalation of Advair Diskus 100/50 b.i.d. If fluticasone propionate inhalation aerosol daily dose is 440 mcg, start with 1 inhalation of Advair

Diskus 250/50 b.i.d. If fluticasone propionate inhalation aerosol daily dose is 660 to 880 mcg, start with 1 inhalation of Advair Diskus 500/50 b.i.d.
*Adults and children older than age 12 currently taking fluticasone propionate inhalation powder:* If fluticasone propionate inhalation powder daily dose is 200 mcg or less, start with 1 inhalation of Advair Diskus 100/50 b.i.d. If fluticasone propionate inhalation powder daily dose is 500 mcg, start with 1 inhalation of Advair Diskus 250/50 b.i.d. If fluticasone propionate inhalation powder daily dose is 1,000 mcg, start with 1 inhalation of Advair Diskus 500/50 b.i.d.
*Adults and children older than age 12 currently taking triamcinolone acetonide:* If triamcinolone acetonide daily dose is 1,000 mcg or less, start with 1 inhalation of Advair Diskus 100/50 b.i.d. If triamcinolone acetonide daily dose is 1,100 to 1,600 mcg, start with 1 inhalation of Advair Diskus 250/50 b.i.d.

For patients already using an inhaled corticosteroid, maximum inhalation of Advair Diskus is 500/50 b.i.d.
**❋ NEW INDICATION: Maintenance therapy for airflow obstruction in patients with COPD from chronic bronchitis**
*Adults:* 1 inhalation of Advair Diskus 250/50 only, b.i.d., about 12 hours apart.

## ACTION
Fluticasone is a synthetic corticosteroid with potent anti-inflammatory activity, although precise mechanisms of action in asthma are unknown.

Salmeterol xinafoate, a long-acting beta agonist, relaxes bronchial smooth muscle and inhibits release of mediators of immediate hypersensitivity from cells.

| Route | Onset | Peak | Duration |
|---|---|---|---|
| Inhalation (fluticasone) | Unknown | 1-2 hr | Unknown |
| Inhalation (salmeterol) | Unknown | 5 min | Unknown |

## ADVERSE REACTIONS
**CNS:** sleep disorders, tremors, hypnagogic effects, compressed nerve syndromes, *headache.*
**CV:** palpitations, pain.

**EENT:** *pharyngitis,* sinusitis, hoarseness or dysphonia, oral candidiasis, dental discomfort and pain, rhinorrhea, rhinitis, sneezing, nasal irritation, blood in nasal mucosa, keratitis, conjunctivitis, eye redness, viral eye infections, congestion.
**GI:** nausea, vomiting, abdominal pain and discomfort, diarrhea, gastroenteritis, oral discomfort and pain, constipation, oral ulcerations, oral erythema and rashes, appendicitis, unusual taste.
**Musculoskeletal:** muscle pain, arthralgia, articular rheumatism, muscle stiffness, tightness, rigidity, bone and cartilage disorders.
**Respiratory:** *upper respiratory tract infection,* lower respiratory tract infections, bronchitis, cough, pneumonia.
**Skin:** infection, urticaria, skin flakiness, disorders of sweat and sebum, sweating.
**Other:** viral or bacterial infections, chest symptoms, fluid retention, allergic reactions.

**INTERACTIONS**
**Drug-drug.** *Beta blockers:* Blocked pulmonary effect of salmeterol may produce severe bronchospasm in patients with asthma. Avoid using together. If necessary, use a cardioselective beta blocker cautiously.
*Ketoconazole, other inhibitors of cytochrome P-450:* May increase fluticasone level and adverse effects. Use together cautiously.
*Loop diuretics, thiazide diuretics:* Potassium-wasting diuretics may cause or worsen ECG changes or hypokalemia. Use together cautiously.
*MAO inhibitors, tricyclic antidepressants:* May potentiate the action of salmeterol on the vascular system. Separate doses by 2 weeks.

**EFFECTS ON LAB TEST RESULTS**
● May increase liver enzyme level.

**CONTRAINDICATIONS & CAUTIONS**
● Contraindicated in patients hypersensitive to drug or its components.
● Contraindicated as primary treatment of status asthmaticus or other acute asthmatic episodes.
● Use cautiously, if at all, in patients with active or quiescent respiratory tuberculo-

sis infection; untreated systemic fungal, bacterial, viral, or parasitic infection; or ocular herpes simplex.
● Use cautiously in patients with CV disorders, seizure disorders or thyrotoxicosis; in patients unusually responsive to sympathomimetic amines; and in patients with hepatic impairment.

**NURSING CONSIDERATIONS**
● Patient shouldn't be switched from systemic corticosteroids to Advair Diskus because of hypothalamic-pituitary-adrenal axis suppression. Death from adrenal insufficiency can occur. Several months are required for recovery of hypothalamic-pituitary-adrenal function after withdrawal of systemic corticosteroids.
● Don't start therapy during rapidly deteriorating or potentially life-threatening episodes of asthma. Serious acute respiratory events, including fatality, can occur.
● Monitor patient for urticaria, angioedema, rash, bronchospasm, or other signs of hypersensitivity.
● Don't use Advair Diskus to stop an asthma attack. Patients using Advair Diskus should carry an inhaled, short-acting beta$_2$ agonist (such as albuterol) for acute symptoms.
● If Advair Diskus causes paradoxical bronchospasm, treat immediately with a short-acting inhaled bronchodilator (such as albuterol), and notify prescriber.
● Monitor patient for increased use of inhaled short-acting beta$_2$-agonist. The dose of Advair Diskus may need to be increased.
● Closely monitor children for growth suppression.

**PATIENT TEACHING**
● Instruct patient on proper use of Diskus device to provide effective treatment.
● Tell patient to avoid exhaling into the Diskus and to activate and use the Diskus in a level, horizontal position and not to use Advair Diskus with a spacer device.
● Instruct patient to keep the Diskus in a dry place, away from direct heat or sunlight, to avoid washing the mouthpiece or other parts of the device. Patient should discard device 1 month after removal from the moisture-protective overwrap pouch or after every blister has been used, whichev-

er comes first. He shouldn't attempt to take device apart.
• Instruct patient to rinse mouth after inhalation to prevent oral candidiasis.
• Inform patient that improvement may occur within 30 minutes after an Advair dose, but the full benefit may not occur for 1 week or more.
• Advise patient not to exceed recommended prescribing dose.
• Instruct patient not to relieve acute symptoms with Advair Diskus. Treat acute symptoms with an inhaled short-acting beta₂-agonist.
• Instruct patient to report decreasing effects or use of increasing doses of their short-acting inhaled beta₂-agonist.
• Tell patient to report palpitations, chest pain, rapid heart rate, tremor, or nervousness.
• Instruct patient to call immediately if exposed to chickenpox or measles.

---

## montelukast sodium
Singulair✷

*Pregnancy risk category B*

### AVAILABLE FORMS
*Oral granules:* 4-mg packet
*Tablets (chewable):* 4 mg, 5 mg
*Tablets (film-coated):* 10 mg

### INDICATIONS & DOSAGES
➤ **Asthma, seasonal allergic rhinitis**
*Adults and children age 15 and older:*
10 mg P.O. once daily in evening.
*Children ages 6 to 14:* 5 mg (chewable tablet) P.O. once daily in evening.
*Children ages 2 to 5:* 4 mg chewable tablet or 1 packet of oral granules P.O. once daily in the evening.
*Children ages 12 to 23 months (asthma only):* 1 packet of oral granules P.O. once daily in the evening.

### ACTION
A selective, competitive leukotriene-receptor antagonist that inhibits airway cysteinyl leukotriene (CysLT₁) receptors. Binds with high affinity and selectivity to the CysLT₁ receptor and inhibits physiologic action of the cysteinyl leukotriene LTD₄. This receptor inhibition reduces

early- and late-phase bronchoconstriction from antigen challenge.

| Route | Onset | Peak | Duration |
|---|---|---|---|
| P.O. (chewable, granules) | Unknown | 2-2½ hr | ≥ 24 hr |
| P.O. (film-coated) | Unknown | 3-4 hr | ≥ 24 hr |

### ADVERSE REACTIONS
**CNS:** fever, *headache*, dizziness, fatigue, asthenia.
**EENT:** nasal congestion, dental pain.
**GI:** dyspepsia, infectious gastroenteritis, abdominal pain.
**GU:** pyuria.
**Respiratory:** cough.
**Skin:** rash.
**Other:** trauma, influenza.

### INTERACTIONS
**Drug-drug.** *Phenobarbital, rifampin:* May decrease bioavailability of montelukast because of hepatic metabolism induction. Monitor for effectiveness.

### EFFECTS ON LAB TEST RESULTS
• May increase ALT and AST levels.

### CONTRAINDICATIONS & CAUTIONS
• Contraindicated in patients hypersensitive to drug or its ingredients.
• Use cautiously and with appropriate monitoring in patients whose dosages of systemic corticosteroids are reduced.

### NURSING CONSIDERATIONS
• Assess patient's underlying condition, and monitor patient for effectiveness.
• *Alert:* Don't abruptly substitute drug for inhaled or oral corticosteroids. Dose of inhaled corticosteroids may be reduced gradually.
• Drug isn't indicated for use in patients with acute asthmatic attacks, status asthmaticus, or as monotherapy for management of exercise-induced bronchospasm. Continue appropriate rescue drug for acute worsening.
• Give oral granules either directly in the mouth or mixed with a teaspoonful of cold or room-temperature applesauce, carrots, rice, or ice cream. Don't open packet until ready to use. After opening packet, give full dose within 15 minutes. If mixed with

---

food, don't store excess for future use; discard any unused portion.
● Don't dissolve oral granules in liquid; let the patient take a drink after receiving the granules.
● Oral granules may be given without regard to meals.

**PATIENT TEACHING**
● Teach patient how to mix granules with applesauce, carrots, rice, or ice cream.
● Tell patient to discard any unused portion.
● Advise patient to take drug daily, even if asymptomatic, and to contact his prescriber if asthma isn't well controlled.
● Warn patient not to reduce or stop taking other prescribed antasthmatics without prescriber's approval.
● Advise patient to seek medical attention if short-acting inhaled bronchodilators are needed more often than usual during drug therapy.
● Warn patient that drug isn't beneficial in acute asthma attacks or in exercise-induced bronchospasm, and advise him to keep appropriate rescue drugs available.
● Advise patient with known aspirin sensitivity to continue to avoid using aspirin and NSAIDs during drug therapy.
● Advise patient with phenylketonuria that chewable tablet contains phenylalanine.

✳ *NEW DRUG*

## omalizumab
Xolair

*Pregnancy risk category B*

**AVAILABLE FORMS**
*Powder for injection:* 150 mg in 5-ml vial

**INDICATIONS & DOSAGES**
➤ **Moderate to severe persistent asthma in patients with positive skin test or in vitro reactivity to a perennial aeroallergen and whose symptoms aren't adequately controlled by inhaled corticosteroids**
*Adults and adolescents age 12 and older:* 150 to 375 mg S.C. q 2 or 4 weeks. Dose and frequency vary with pretreatment IgE level (IU/ml) and patient. Divide doses

larger than 150 mg among more than one injection site.

**ACTION**
Inhibits binding of IgE to the high-affinity receptor (FceRI) on the surface of mast cells and basophils, which limits release of allergic response mediators; also reduces number of FceRI receptors on basophils in atopic patients.

| Route | Onset | Peak | Duration |
|-------|-------|------|----------|
| S.C. | Unknown | 7-8 days | Unknown |

**ADVERSE REACTIONS**
**CNS:** dizziness, fatigue, *headache,* pain.
**EENT:** earache, *pharyngitis, sinusitis.*
**Musculoskeletal:** arm pain, arthralgia, fracture, leg pain.
**Respiratory:** *upper respiratory tract infection.*
**Skin:** dermatitis, *injection site reaction,* pruritus.
**Other:** *viral infections.*

**INTERACTIONS**
None reported.

**EFFECTS ON LAB TEST RESULTS**
● May increase IgE level.

**CONTRAINDICATIONS & CAUTIONS**
● Contraindicated in patients severely hypersensitive to omalizumab.
● Safety and effectiveness haven't been established in children younger than age 12.

**NURSING CONSIDERATIONS**
● *Alert:* Don't use this drug to treat acute bronchospasm or status asthmaticus.
● Don't abruptly stop systemic or inhaled corticosteroid when omalizumab therapy starts; taper the dose gradually and under supervision.
● Because the solution is slightly viscous, it may take 5 to 10 seconds to give.
● Injection site reactions may occur, such as bruising, redness, warmth, burning, stinging, itching, hives, pain, induration, and inflammation. Most occur within 1 hour after the injection, last fewer than 8 days, and decrease in frequency with subsequent injections.
● *Alert:* Observe patient after the injection, and keep drugs available to respond to

anaphylactic reactions. If the patient has a severe hypersensitivity reaction, stop treatment.

• Drug increases IgE level, so it can't be used to determine appropriate dosage during therapy or for 1 year after therapy ends.

## PATIENT TEACHING
• Tell patients not to stop or reduce the dosage of any other asthma drugs unless directed by the prescriber.
• Explain that patient may not notice an immediate improvement in asthma after omalizumab therapy starts.

## palivizumab
Synagis

*Pregnancy risk category C*

## AVAILABLE FORMS
*Injection:* 50-mg vial, 100-mg vial

## INDICATIONS & DOSAGES
➤ **To prevent serious lower respiratory tract disease caused by respiratory syncytial virus (RSV) in children at high risk**
*Children:* 15 mg/kg I.M. monthly throughout RSV season (November to April in the northern hemisphere). Give first dose before start of RSV season.

## ACTION
Exhibits neutralizing and fusion-inhibitory activity against RSV, which inhibits RSV replication.

| Route | Onset | Peak | Duration |
|-------|-------|------|----------|
| I.M. | Unknown | Unknown | Unknown |

## ADVERSE REACTIONS
**CNS:** nervousness, pain.
**EENT:** *otitis media, rhinitis,* pharyngitis, sinusitis, conjunctivitis.
**GI:** diarrhea, vomiting, gastroenteritis, oral candidiasis.
**Hematologic:** anemia.
**Respiratory:** *upper respiratory tract infection,* cough, wheeze, bronchiolitis, ̶  pneumonia, bronchitis, asthma,
̶   ̶matitis, eczema, se-

**Other:** hernia, *failure to thrive,* injection site reaction, viral infection, flu syndrome.

## INTERACTIONS
None significant.

## EFFECTS ON LAB TEST RESULTS
• May increase ALT and AST levels.
• May decrease hemoglobin.

## CONTRAINDICATIONS & CAUTIONS
• Contraindicated in children hypersensitive to drug or its components.
• Use cautiously in patients with thrombocytopenia or other coagulation disorders.

## NURSING CONSIDERATIONS
• Patients should receive monthly doses throughout RSV season, even if RSV infection develops. In the northern hemisphere, RSV season typically lasts from November to April.
• To reconstitute, slowly add 1 ml of sterile water for injection into a 100-mg vial or 0.6 ml of sterile water for injection into a 50-mg vial. Gently swirl the vial for 30 seconds to avoid foaming. Don't shake vial. Let reconstituted solution stand at room temperature for 20 minutes until the solution clears. Give within 6 hours of reconstitution.
• Give drug into anterolateral aspect of thigh. Don't use gluteal muscle routinely as an injection site because of risk of damage to sciatic nerve. Give injection volumes over 1 ml as a divided dose.
• *Alert:* Rarely, patient may have an anaphylactoid reaction after using this drug. If anaphylaxis or severe allergic reaction occurs, give epinephrine (1:1,000), and provide supportive care as needed. If reaction is mild, use caution when giving again; if severe, stop therapy.

## PATIENT TEACHING
• Explain to parent or caregiver that drug is used to prevent RSV and not to treat it.
• Advise parent that monthly injections are recommended throughout RSV season (November to April in the northern hemisphere).
• Tell parent to immediately report adverse reactions or any unusual bruising, bleeding, or weakness.

̶reatening, or COMMON AND LIFE-THREATENING.

Liquid contains alcohol.

# triamcinolone acetonide
Azmacort, Nasacort, Nasacort AQ

*Pregnancy risk category C*

## AVAILABLE FORMS
*Inhalation aerosol:* 100 mcg/metered spray, 55 mcg/metered spray
*Nasal spray:* 55 mcg/metered spray, 50 mcg/metered spray

## INDICATIONS & DOSAGES
➤ **Persistent asthma**
*Adults and children older than age 12:* 2 inhalations t.i.d. to q.i.d. Maximum, 16 inhalations daily. In some patients, maintenance can be achieved when total daily dose is given b.i.d.
*Children ages 6 to 12:* 1 to 2 inhalations t.i.d. to q.i.d. Maximum, 12 inhalations daily.
➤ **Nasal treatment of symptoms of seasonal and perennial allergic rhinitis**
*Adults and children older than age 12:* 2 sprays Nasacort in each nostril daily, up to 4 sprays per nostril daily. Or, 2 sprays Nasacort AQ in each nostril daily; may decrease to 1 spray per nostril daily.
*Children ages 6 to 12:* Initially, 1 spray Nasacort AQ in each nostril daily. If no response occurs, increase to 2 sprays in each nostril daily. Or, 2 sprays Nasacort per nostril daily.

## ACTION
Unknown. May decrease inflammation through inhibitory activities against such cell types as mast cells and macrophages and against mediators such as leukotrienes.

| Route | Onset | Peak | Duration |
|---|---|---|---|
| Inhalation (nasal) | 12-24 hr | Several days | 1-2 wk |
| Inhalation (oral) | 1-4 wk | Unknown | Unknown |

## ADVERSE REACTIONS
**EENT:** dry or irritated nose or throat, hoarseness, *pharyngitis.*
**GI:** oral candidiasis, dry or irritated tongue or mouth.
**Metabolic:** hypothalamic-pituitary-adrenal function suppression, adrenal insufficiency.

**Respiratory:** cough, wheezing.
**Other:** facial edema.

## INTERACTIONS
None significant.

## EFFECTS ON LAB TEST RESULTS
None reported.

## CONTRAINDICATIONS & CAUTIONS
• Contraindicated in patients hypersensitive to drug or its ingredients and in those with status asthmaticus.
• Use with extreme caution, if at all, in patients with tuberculosis of the respiratory tract, ocular herpes simplex, or untreated fungal, bacterial, or systemic viral infections.
• It's unknown if drug appears in breast milk. Because of risk of severe adverse effects, don't use in breast-feeding women.

## NURSING CONSIDERATIONS
• Unlike other corticosteroids, drug has a spacer built into the drug-delivery device.
• Use cautiously in patients receiving systemic corticosteroids.
• Most adverse reactions to corticosteroids are dose- or duration-dependent.
• Patients who have recently been switched from systemic corticosteroids to oral inhaled corticosteroids may need to resume systemic corticosteroid therapy during periods of stress or severe asthma attacks.
• Taper oral therapy slowly.
• Store drug between 59° and 86° F (15° and 30° C).
• For nasal spray, if symptoms don't improve after 2 to 3 weeks, reevaluate the patient.
• *Alert:* Don't confuse triamcinolone with Triaminicin.

## PATIENT TEACHING
**Inhalation aerosol**
• Inform patient that inhaled corticosteroids don't relieve emergency asthma attacks.
• Advise patient to warm canister to room temperature before using. Some patients carry canister in a pocket to keep it warm.
• If patient needs a bronchodilator, tell him to use it several minutes before triamcinolone. Tell patient to allow 1 minute to elapse before repeat inhalations and to

hold his breath for a few seconds to enhance drug action.
● Teach patient to check mucous membranes frequently for evidence of fungal infection. Advise patient to avoid exposure to chickenpox or measles and to contact provider if exposure occurs.
● Tell patient to prevent oral fungal infections by gargling or rinsing mouth with water after each use of the inhaler. Remind him not to swallow the water.
● Tell patient to keep inhaler clean and unobstructed and to wash it with warm water and dry it thoroughly after use.
● Instruct patient to contact prescriber if response to therapy decreases; dosage may need adjustment. Tell him not to exceed recommended dosage on his own.
● Instruct patient to wear or carry medical identification indicating his need for supplemental systemic glucocorticoids during periods of stress.

**Nasal spray**
● Advise patient to use at regular intervals for full therapeutic effect.
● Advise patient to clear nasal passages before use.
● Have patient follow manufacturer's recommendations for use and cleaning.

---

### zafirlukast
Accolate

*Pregnancy risk category B*

---

### AVAILABLE FORMS
*Tablets:* 10 mg, 20 mg

### INDICATIONS & DOSAGES
➤ **Prevention and long-term treatment of asthma**
*Adults and children age 12 and older:* 20 mg P.O. b.i.d. taken 1 hour before or 2 hours after meals.
*Children ages 5 to 11:* 10 mg P.O. b.i.d. taken 1 hour before or 2 hours after meals.

### ACTION
Selectively competes for leukotriene receptor sites, blocking inflammatory ac-

### ADVERSE REACTIONS
**CNS:** *headache,* asthenia, dizziness, pain.
**GI:** nausea, diarrhea, abdominal pain, vomiting, dyspepsia, gastritis.
**Musculoskeletal:** myalgia, back pain.
**Other:** infection, accidental injury, fever.

### INTERACTIONS
**Drug-drug.** *Aspirin:* May increase zafirlukast level. Monitor for adverse effects.
*Erythromycin, theophylline:* May decrease zafirlukast level. Monitor for decreased effectiveness.
*Warfarin:* May increase PT. Monitor PT and INR, and adjust anticoagulant dosage.
**Drug-food.** *Food:* May reduce rate and extent of zafirlukast absorption. Give 1 hour before or 2 hours after a meal.

### EFFECTS ON LAB TEST RESULTS
● May increase liver enzyme level.

### CONTRAINDICATIONS & CAUTIONS
● Contraindicated in patients hypersensitive to drug.
● Drug isn't indicated for reversing bronchospasm in acute asthma attacks.
● Give cautiously to geriatric patients and those with hepatic impairment.
● Give drug to pregnant patients only if clearly needed. Don't give to breast-feeding women.

### NURSING CONSIDERATIONS
● *Alert:* Reducing oral corticosteroid dose has been followed in rare cases by eosinophilia, vasculitic rash, worsening pulmonary symptoms, cardiac complications, or neuropathy, sometimes presenting as Churg-Strauss syndrome.

### PATIENT TEACHING
● Tell patient that drug is used for long-term treatment of asthma and to keep taking it even if symptoms resolve.
● Advise patient to continue taking other antiasthma drugs, as prescribed.
● Instruct patient to take drug 1 hour before or 2 hours after meals.

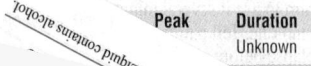

| | Peak | Duration |
|---|---|---|
| | | Unknown |

**aluminum hydroxide**
**calcium carbonate**
**magaldrate**
**magnesium hydroxide**
   (See Chapter 47, LAXATIVES.)
**magnesium oxide**
**simethicone**
**sodium bicarbonate**
   (See Chapter 62, ACIDIFIERS AND
   ALKALINIZERS.)

## COMBINATION PRODUCTS

ALKA-SELTZER GOLD ◊: sodium bicarbonate 958 mg, citric acid 832 mg, and potassium bicarbonate 312 mg.
ALKA-SELTZER ORIGINAL ◊: aspirin 325 mg, citric acid 1,000 mg, and phenylalanine 9 mg and sodium bicarbonate 1,700 mg.
ALUDROX ◊: aluminum hydroxide 307 mg and magnesium hydroxide 103 mg per 5 ml.
DI-GEL, ADVANCED: magnesium hydroxide 128 mg and calcium carbonate 280 mg, and simethicone 20 mg.
EXTRA STRENGTH ALKA-SELTZER ◊: aspirin 500 mg and citric acid 1,000 mg.
GAVISCON TABLETS ◊: aluminum hydroxide 80 mg and magnesium trisilicate 20 mg.
GELUSIL-II ◊: aluminum hydroxide 400 mg, magnesium hydroxide 400 mg, and simethicone 30 mg.
MAALOX PLUS EXTRA STRENGTH: aluminum hydroxide 350 mg, magnesium hydroxide 350 mg, and simethicone 30 mg.
MAALOX PLUS ◊: aluminum hydroxide 200 mg, magnesium hydroxide 200 mg, and simethicone 25 mg.
MAALOX THERAPEUTIC CONCENTRATE SUSPENSION: aluminum hydroxide 600 mg and magnesium hydroxide 300 mg/5 ml.
MYLANTA LIQUID: aluminum hydroxide 200 mg, magnesium hydroxide 200 mg, and simethicone 20 mg/5 ml.
MYLANTA TABLETS ◊: aluminum hydroxide 200 mg, magnesium hydroxide 200 mg, and simethicone 20 mg.

PEPCID COMPLETE: calcium carbonate 800 mg, magnesium hydroxide 165 mg, and famotidine 10 mg.
RIOPAN PLUS CHEWABLE TABLETS ◊: magaldrate 480 mg and simethicone 20 mg.
RIOPAN PLUS DOUBLE STRENGTH CHEWABLE TABLETS: magaldrate 1,080 mg and simethicone 20 mg.
RIOPAN PLUS DOUBLE STRENGTH SUSPENSION: magaldrate 1,080 mg and simethicone 40 mg/5 ml.
RIOPAN PLUS SUSPENSION ◊: magaldrate 540 mg and simethicone 40 mg/5 ml.
TITRALAC PLUS ◊: calcium carbonate 420 mg and simethicone 21 mg.
UNIVOL† ◊: aluminum hydroxide and magnesium carbonate co-dried gel 300 mg and magnesium hydroxide 100 mg.

---

## aluminum hydroxide
AlternaGEL ◊, Aluminum Hydroxide Gel ◊, Aluminum Hydroxide Gel Concentrated ◊, Alu-Tab ◊, Amphojel ◊, Dialume ◊

*Pregnancy risk category C*

## AVAILABLE FORMS
*Capsules:* 400 mg ◊, 500 mg ◊
*Oral suspension:* 450 mg/5 ml ◊, 675 mg/5 ml ◊
*Tablets:* 300 mg ◊, 500 mg ◊, 600 mg ◊

## INDICATIONS & DOSAGES
➤ **Antacid**
*Adults:* 500 to 1,500 mg P.O. 1 hour after meals and h.s. Or, 300-mg tablet or 600-mg tablet, chewed before swallowing, taken with milk or water five to six times daily after meals and h.s.

## ACTION
Antacid that reduces total acid load in the GI tract, elevates gastric pH to reduce pepsin activity, strengthens the gastric mu-

cosal barrier, and increases esophageal sphincter tone.

| Route | Onset | Peak | Duration |
|-------|-------|------|----------|
| P.O. | Variable | Unknown | 20-180 min |

### ADVERSE REACTIONS
**CNS:** *encephalopathy.*
**GI:** *constipation, **intestinal obstruction.***
**Metabolic:** hypophosphatemia.
**Musculoskeletal:** osteomalacia.

### INTERACTIONS
**Drug-drug.** *Allopurinol, antibiotics (tetracyclines), corticosteroids, diflunisal, digoxin, ethambutol, $H_2$-receptor antagonists, iron salts, isoniazid, penicillamine, phenothiazines, thyroid hormones, ticlopidine:* May decrease pharmacologic effect of these drugs because of possible impaired absorption. Separate doses by 1 to 2 hours.
*Ciprofloxacin, gatifloxacin, levofloxacin, lomefloxacin, moxifloxacin, norfloxacin, ofloxacin:* May decrease effects of quinolone. Give antacid at least 6 hours before or 2 hours after the quinolone.
*Enteric-coated drugs:* May be released prematurely in stomach. Separate doses by at least 1 hour.

### EFFECTS ON LAB TEST RESULTS
● May increase gastrin level. May decrease phosphate level.

### CONTRAINDICATIONS & CAUTIONS
● No known contraindications.
● Use cautiously in patients with chronic renal disease.

### NURSING CONSIDERATIONS
● When giving through nasogastric tube, make sure tube is placed correctly and is patent; after instilling drug, flush tube with water to ensure passage to stomach and to clear tube.
● *Alert:* Monitor long-term, high-dose use in patient on restricted sodium intake. Each tablet, capsule, or 5 ml of suspension may contain 2 or 3 mg of sodium. Refer to manufacturer's label for specific sodium content.
● Record amount and consistency of stools. Manage constipation with laxa-

tives or stool softeners; alternate with magnesium-containing antacids (if patient doesn't have renal disease).
● Monitor phosphate level.
● Watch for evidence of hypophosphatemia (anorexia, malaise, and muscle weakness) with prolonged use; also can lead to resorption of calcium and bone demineralization.
● Aluminum hydroxide therapy may interfere with imaging techniques using sodium pertechnetate Tc99m, and thus impair evaluation of Meckel's diverticulum. It also may interfere with reticuloendothelial imaging of liver, spleen, or bone marrow using technetium Tc99m sulfur colloid. It may antagonize effect of pentagastrin during gastric acid secretion tests.
● Because drug contains aluminum, it's used in patients with renal failure to help control hyperphosphatemia by binding with phosphate in the GI tract.

### PATIENT TEACHING
● Instruct patient to shake suspension well and to follow with a small amount of milk or water to facilitate passage.
● Advise patient not to take aluminum hydroxide indiscriminately or to switch antacids without prescriber's advice.
● Urge patient to notify prescriber about signs and symptoms of GI bleeding, such as tarry stools or coffee-ground vomitus.
● Instruct pregnant patient to seek medical advice before taking drug.

---

## calcium carbonate
Alka-Mints◊, Amitone◊, Calci-Chew, Cal-Supp‡, Caltrate, Chooz◊, Dicarbosil◊, Maalox Antacid Caplets◊, Oscal, Rolaids Calcium Rich◊, Tums◊, Tums E-X◊, Tums Ultra◊

*Pregnancy risk category C*

### AVAILABLE FORMS
Calcium carbonate contains 40% calcium; 20 mEq calcium per gram.
*Chewing gum:* 500 mg/piece
*Lozenges:* 600 mg◊
*Oral suspension:* 1,250 mg/5 ml

*Tablets:* 500 mg◊, 600 mg◊, 650 mg◊, 1,000 mg◊, 1,250 mg◊
*Tablets (chewable):* 350 mg◊, 420 mg◊, 500 mg◊, 750 mg, 850 mg, 1,000 mg, 1,250 mg‡

## INDICATIONS & DOSAGES
➤ **Antacid, calcium supplement**
*Adults:* 350 mg to 1.5 g P.O. or 2 pieces of chewing gum 1 hour after meals and h.s., p.r.n.

## ACTION
Reduces total acid load in the GI tract, elevates gastric pH to reduce pepsin activity, strengthens the gastric mucosal barrier, and increases esophageal sphincter tone.

| Route | Onset | Peak | Duration |
|---|---|---|---|
| P.O. | 20 min | Unknown | 20-180 min |

## ADVERSE REACTIONS
**CNS:** headache, irritability, weakness.
**GI:** rebound hyperacidity, *nausea,* constipation, flatulence.

## INTERACTIONS
**Drug-drug.** *Antibiotics (tetracyclines), hydantoins, iron salts, isoniazid, salicylates:* May decrease pharmacologic effect of these drugs because of impaired absorption. Separate doses by 2 hours.
*Ciprofloxacin, gatifloxacin, levofloxacin, lomefloxacin, moxifloxacin, norfloxacin, ofloxacin:* May decrease effects of quinolone. Give antacid at least 6 hours before or 2 hours after the quinolone.
*Enteric-coated drugs:* May be released prematurely in stomach. Separate doses by at least 1 hour.
**Drug-food.** *Milk, other foods high in vitamin D:* May cause milk-alkali syndrome (headache, confusion, distaste for food, nausea, vomiting, hypercalcemia, hypercalciuria). Discourage use together.

## EFFECTS ON LAB TEST RESULTS
● May decrease phosphate level.

## CONTRAINDICATIONS & CAUTIONS
● Contraindicated in patients with ventricular fibrillation or hypercalcemia.

● Use cautiously, if at all, if patient takes a cardiac glycoside or has sarcoidosis or renal or cardiac disease.

## NURSING CONSIDERATIONS
● Record amount and consistency of stools. Manage constipation with laxatives or stool softeners.
● Monitor calcium level, especially in patients with mild renal impairment.
● Watch for evidence of hypercalcemia (nausea, vomiting, headache, confusion, and anorexia).

## PATIENT TEACHING
● Advise patient not to take calcium carbonate indiscriminately or to switch antacids without prescriber's advice.
● Tell patient who takes chewable tablets to chew thoroughly before swallowing and to follow with a glass of water.
● Tell patient who uses suspension form to shake well and take with a small amount of water to facilitate passage.
● Urge patient to notify prescriber about signs and symptoms of GI bleeding, such as tarry stools, or coffee-ground vomitus.

---

# magaldrate (aluminum-magnesium complex)
Isopan, Lowsium◊, Lowsium Plus, Riopan, Riopan Plus

*Pregnancy risk category C*

## AVAILABLE FORMS
*Oral suspension:* 540 mg/5 ml◊

## INDICATIONS & DOSAGES
➤ **Antacid**
*Adults:* 540 to 1,080 mg (5 to 10 ml) of suspension P.O. with water between meals and h.s.

## ACTION
Antacid that reduces total acid load in the GI tract, elevates gastric pH to reduce pepsin activity, strengthens the gastric mucosal barrier, and increases esophageal sphincter tone.

| Route | Onset | Peak | Duration |
|---|---|---|---|
| P.O. | 20 min | Unknown | 20-180 min |

**ADVERSE REACTIONS**
**GI:** mild constipation, diarrhea.
**GU:** increased urine pH.
**Metabolic:** hypokalemia.

**INTERACTIONS**
**Drug-drug.** *Allopurinol, antibiotics (including quinolones, tetracyclines), diflunisal, digoxin, iron salts, isoniazid, penicillamine, phenothiazines, quinidine, salicylates, ticlopidine:* May decrease effects of these drugs because of impaired absorption. Separate doses by 1 to 2 hours.
*Enteric-coated drugs:* May be released prematurely in stomach. Separate doses by at least 1 hour.

**EFFECTS ON LAB TEST RESULTS**
• May increase gastrin level. May decrease potassium level.

**CONTRAINDICATIONS & CAUTIONS**
• Contraindicated in patients with severe renal disease.
• Use cautiously in patients with mild renal impairment.

**NURSING CONSIDERATIONS**
• When giving drug through nasogastric tube, make sure tube is placed properly and is patent. After instilling drug, flush tube with water to ensure passage to stomach and to clear tube.
• Monitor magnesium level in patients with mild renal impairment. Symptomatic hypermagnesemia usually occurs only in severe renal failure.
• Drug may antagonize effect of pentagastrin during gastric acid secretion tests.
• *Alert:* Drug isn't typically used in patients with renal failure to help control hypophosphatemia because it contains magnesium, which may accumulate in the body.
• Drug has a low sodium content and is good for patients on sodium restriction.

**PATIENT TEACHING**
• Instruct patient to shake suspension well and to follow dose with water.
• Advise patient not to take magaldrate indiscriminately or to switch antacids without prescriber's advice.

• Urge patient to notify prescriber about signs and symptoms of GI bleeding, such as tarry stools, or coffee-ground vomitus.

---

# magnesium oxide
Mag-Ox 400 ◊  Maox ◊ , Uro-Mag ◊

*Pregnancy risk category B*

**AVAILABLE FORMS**
*Capsules:* 140 mg ◊
*Tablets:* 400 mg ◊ , 420 mg ◊ , 500 mg

**INDICATIONS & DOSAGES**
➤ **Antacid**
*Adults:* 140 mg P.O. with water or milk after meals and h.s.
➤ **Laxative**
*Adults:* 4 g P.O. with water or milk, usually h.s.
➤ **Oral replacement therapy in mild hypomagnesemia**
*Adults:* 400 to 840 mg P.O. daily. Monitor magnesium level.

**ACTION**
Reduces total acid load in the GI tract, elevates gastric pH, strengthens the gastric mucosal barrier, and increases esophageal sphincter tone.

| Route | Onset | Peak | Duration |
|-------|-------|------|----------|
| P.O. | 20 min | Unknown | 20-180 min |

**ADVERSE REACTIONS**
**GI:** *diarrhea,* nausea, abdominal pain.
**Metabolic:** hypermagnesemia.

**INTERACTIONS**
**Drug-drug.** *Allopurinol, antibiotics, digoxin, iron salts, penicillamine, phenothiazines:* May decrease effects of these drugs because of impaired absorption. Separate doses by 1 to 2 hours.
*Enteric-coated drugs:* May be released prematurely in stomach. Separate doses by at least 1 hour.

**EFFECTS ON LAB TEST RESULTS**
• May increase magnesium level.

---

## CONTRAINDICATIONS & CAUTIONS
• Contraindicated in patients with severe renal disease.
• Use cautiously in patients with mild renal impairment.

## NURSING CONSIDERATIONS
• When using drug as a laxative, don't give within 1 to 2 hours of other oral drugs.
• *Alert:* Monitor magnesium level. With prolonged use and renal impairment, watch for evidence of hypermagnesemia (hypotension, nausea, vomiting, depressed reflexes, respiratory depression, and coma).
• If diarrhea occurs, be prepared to suggest alternative preparation.

## PATIENT TEACHING
• Advise patient not to take magnesium oxide indiscriminately or to switch antacids without prescriber's advice.
• Urge patient to report signs of GI bleeding, such as tarry stools, or coffee-ground vomitus.

---

## simethicone
Flatulex◊, Gas Relief◊, Gas-X◊, Gas-X Extra Strength◊, Mylanta Gas◊, Mylanta Anti-Gas Extra Strength◊, Mylicon◊, Ovol†, Ovol-40†, Ovol-80†, Phazyme◊, Phazyme 95◊, Phazyme-125 Maximum Strength◊, Ultra-strength Phazyme-180

*Pregnancy risk category C*

## AVAILABLE FORMS
*Capsules:* 125 mg, 180 mg
*Drops:* 40 mg/0.6 ml ◊
*Tablets:* 40 mg◊, 55 mg†◊, 60 mg◊, 80 mg◊, 95 mg◊, 125 mg◊

## INDICATIONS & DOSAGES
➤ **Flatulence, functional gastric bloating**
*Adults and children older than age 12:* 40 to 125 mg P.O. after each meal and h.s., up to 500 mg daily. For drops, 40 to 80 mg P.O. after each meal and h.s., up to 500 mg daily.

*Children ages 2 to 12:* 40 mg after meals and h.s., up to 240 mg daily.
*Children younger than age 2:* 20 mg after meals and h.s., up to 240 mg daily.

## ACTION
By its defoaming action, drug disperses or prevents formation of mucus-surrounded gas pockets in the GI tract.

| Route | Onset | Peak | Duration |
|-------|-------|------|----------|
| P.O. | Immediate | Immediate | Unknown |

## ADVERSE REACTIONS
**GI:** belching, flatus.

## INTERACTIONS
None significant.

## EFFECTS ON LAB TEST RESULTS
None reported.

## CONTRAINDICATIONS & CAUTIONS
• Contraindicated in patients hypersensitive to drug.
• Drug isn't recommended for treating infant colic because information on safety in children is limited.

## NURSING CONSIDERATIONS
• Drug doesn't prevent formation of gas.
• *Alert:* Don't confuse simethicone with cimetidine.

## PATIENT TEACHING
• Tell patient to chew tablet before swallowing.
• Advise patient that changing positions often and walking will help pass flatus.

---

# 45

# Digestive enzymes and gallstone solubilizers

**pancreatin**
**pancrelipase**
**ursodiol**

## COMBINATION PRODUCTS
None.

---

## pancreatin
Creon, Digepepsin, Hi-Vegi-Lip
Tablets ◊ , 4X Pancreatin 600
mg ◊ , 8X Pancreatin 900 mg ◊ ,
Pancrezyme 4X Tablets ◊

*Pregnancy risk category C*

---

## AVAILABLE FORMS
**Hi-Vegi-Lip Tablets** ◊
*Tablets (enteric-coated):* 2,400 mg pancreatin, 4,800 units lipase, 60,000 units protease, and 60,000 units amylase ◊
**4X Pancreatin** ◊
*Tablets (enteric-coated):* 600 mg pancreatin, 12,000 units lipase, 60,000 units protease, and 60,000 units amylase ◊
**8X Pancreatin** ◊
*Tablets (enteric-coated):* 900 mg pancreatin, 22,500 units lipase, 180,000 units protease, and 180,000 units amylase ◊
**Creon**
*Capsules (enteric-coated microspheres):* 300 mg pancreatin, 8,000 units lipase, 13,000 units protease, and 30,000 units amylase
**Digepepsin**
*Tablets (enteric-coated):* 300 mg pancreatin

## INDICATIONS & DOSAGES
➤ **Exocrine pancreatic secretion insufficiency; digestive aid in diseases related to deficiency of pancreatic enzymes, such as cystic fibrosis**
*Adults and children:* Dosage varies with condition being treated. Usual initial dose is 8,000 to 24,000 units of lipase activity P.O. before or with each meal or snack. Total daily dose also may be given in divided doses at 1- to 2-hour intervals throughout day.

## ACTION
Replaces endogenous exocrine pancreatic enzymes and aids digestion of starches, fats, and proteins.

| Route | Onset | Peak | Duration |
|-------|-------|------|----------|
| P.O. | Unknown | Unknown | 1-2 hr |

## ADVERSE REACTIONS
**GI:** nausea, diarrhea with high doses.
**Skin:** perianal irritation.
**Other:** allergic reactions.

## INTERACTIONS
**Drug-drug.** *Antacids:* May negate pancreatin's beneficial effect. Avoid using together.
*Iron:* May reduce oral iron supplement level. Separate doses.

## EFFECTS ON LAB TEST RESULTS
● May increase uric acid level.

## CONTRAINDICATIONS & CAUTIONS
● Contraindicated in patients hypersensitive to drug, pork protein, or pork enzymes and in those with acute pancreatitis or acute worsening of chronic pancreatitis.
● Use with caution in pregnant or breastfeeding women.

## NURSING CONSIDERATIONS
● Minimal USP standards dictate that each milligram of bovine or porcine pancreatin contains lipase 2 units, protease 25 units, and amylase 25 units.
● To avoid indigestion, monitor patient's diet to ensure proper balance of fat, protein, and starch. Dosage varies according to degree of maldigestion and malabsorption, amount of fat in diet, and enzyme activity of individual preparations.
● Fewer bowel movements and improved stool consistency indicate effective therapy.
● Drug isn't effective in GI disorders unrelated to pancreatic enzyme deficiency.
● Enteric coating on some products may reduce available enzyme in upper portion of jejunum.

## PATIENT TEACHING

• Instruct patient to take before or with meals and snacks.

• Tell patient not to crush or chew enteric-coated forms. Capsules containing enteric-coated microspheres may be opened and sprinkled on a small quantity of cool, soft food. Stress importance of swallowing immediately, without chewing, and following with a glass of water or juice.

• Warn patient not to inhale powder form or powder from capsules; it may irritate skin or mucous membranes.

• Tell patient to store in airtight container at room temperature.

• Instruct patient not to change brands without consulting prescriber.

## pancrelipase

Cotazym Capsules, Cotazym S Capsules, Creon 5, Creon 10, Creon 20, Kutrase, Ku-Zyme, Ku-Zyme HP, Lipram 4500, Lipram-CR5, Lipram-CR10, Lipram-CR20, Lipram-PN10, Lipram-PN16, Lipram-PN20, Lipram-UL12, Lipram-UL18, Lipram-UL20, Pancrease, Pancrease MT4, Pancrease MT10, Pancrease MT 16, Pancrease MT 20, Pancrecarb MS4, Pancrecarb MS8, Panokase, Plaretase 8000, Ultrase MT12, Ultrase, Ultrase MT18, Ultrase MT20, Viokase, Viokase 8, Viokase 16, Viokase Powder, Viokase Tablets

*Pregnancy risk category C*

## AVAILABLE FORMS
**Creon 5, Lipram-CR5**
*Capsules (enteric-coated microspheres):*
5,000 units lipase, 18,750 units protease, and 16,600 units amylase
**Creon 10, Lipram-CR10**
*Capsules (enteric-coated microspheres):*
10,000 units lipase, 37,500 units protease, and 33,200 units amylase
**Creon 20, Lipram-CR20**
*Capsules (enteric-coated microspheres):*
20,000 units lipase, 75,000 units protease, and 66,400 units amylase

**Ku-Zyme**
*Capsules:* 1,200 units lipase; 15,000 units protease; 15,000 units amylase
**Ku-Zyme HP, PanoKase, Plaretase 8000, Viokase 8**
*Capsules or tablets:* 8,000 units lipase, 30,000 units protease, and 30,000 units amylase
**Lipram-PN10, Pancrease MT10**
*Capsules (enteric-coated contents):*
10,000 units lipase, 30,000 units protease, and 30,000 units amylase
**Lipram-PN16, Pancrease MT16**
*Capsules (enteric-coated contents):*
16,000 units lipase, 48,000 units protease, and 48,000 units amylase
**Lipram-PN20, Pancrease MT20**
*Capsules (enteric-coated contents):*
20,000 units lipase, 44,000 units protease, and 56,000 units amylase
**Lipram-UL12, Ultrase MT12**
*Capsules (enteric-coated contents):*
12,000 units lipase, 39,000 units protease, and 39,000 units amylase
**Lipram-UL18, Ultrase MT18**
*Capsules (enteric-coated contents):*
18,000 units lipase, 58,500 units protease, and 58,500 units amylase
**Lipram-UL20, Ultrase MT20**
*Capsules (enteric-coated contents):*
20,000 units lipase, 65,000 units protease, and 65,000 units amylase
**Pancrease, Lipram 4,500, Ultrase**
*Capsules (enteric-coated microspheres):*
4,500 units lipase, 25,000 units protease, and 20,000 units amylase
**Pancrease MT4**
*Capsules (enteric-coated microtablets):*
4,000 units lipase, 12,000 units protease, and 12,000 units amylase
**Pancrecarb MS4**
*Capsules (enteric-coated microspheres):*
4,000 units lipase; 25,000 units protease; 25,000 units amylase
**Pancrecarb MS8**
*Capsules (enteric-coated microspheres):*
8,000 units lipase; 45,000 units protease; 40,000 units amylase
**Viokase**
*Powder:* 16,800 units lipase, 70,000 units protease, and 70,000 units amylase per 0.7 g powder
**Viokase 16**
*Tablets:* 16,000 units lipase, 6,000 units protease, and 6,000 units amylase

## INDICATIONS & DOSAGES
➤ **Exocrine pancreatic secretion insufficiency; cystic fibrosis in adults and children; steatorrhea and other disorders of fat metabolism caused by insufficient pancreatic enzymes**
*Adults and children older than age 12:*
Dosage adjusted to patient's response. Usual first dosage, 4,000 to 48,000 units of lipase with each meal.
*Children ages 7 to 12:* 4,000 to 12,000 units of lipase activity with each meal or snack. More can be taken, if needed.
*Children ages 1 to 6:* 4,000 to 8,000 units of lipase with each meal and 4,000 units of lipase with each snack.
*Children ages 6 months to 11 months:* 2,000 units of lipase with each meal.

## ACTION
Replaces endogenous exocrine pancreatic enzymes and aids digestion of starches, fats, and proteins.

| Route | Onset | Peak | Duration |
|-------|-------|------|----------|
| P.O. | Variable | Variable | Variable |

## ADVERSE REACTIONS
**GI:** *nausea,* cramping, diarrhea with high doses.

## INTERACTIONS
**Drug-drug.** *Antacids:* May destroy enteric coating and enhance degradation of pancrelipase. Avoid using together.
*Oral iron:* May decrease iron response. Monitor patient for decreased effectiveness.

## EFFECTS ON LAB TEST RESULTS
• May increase uric acid level.

## CONTRAINDICATIONS & CAUTIONS
• Contraindicated in patients with severe hypersensitivity to pork and in those with acute pancreatitis or acute worsening of chronic pancreatic diseases.

## NURSING CONSIDERATIONS
• *Alert:* Use drug only for confirmed exocrine pancreatic insufficiency. It isn't effective in GI disorders unrelated to enzyme deficiency.
• Lipase activity is greater than with other pancreatic enzymes.

• For infants, mix powder with applesauce and give with meals. Avoid contact with or inhalation of powder because it may be highly irritating. Older children may take capsules with food.
• Monitor patient's stools. Adequate replacement decreases number of bowel movements and improves stool consistency.
• Minimal USP standards dictate that each milligram of pancrelipase contains 24 units lipase, 100 units protease, and 100 units amylase.
• Dosage varies with degree of maldigestion and malabsorption, amount of fat in diet, and enzyme activity of individual preparations.
• Enteric coating on some products may reduce available enzyme in upper portion of jejunum.

## PATIENT TEACHING
• Instruct patient to take before or with meals and snacks.
• Advise patient not to crush or chew enteric-coated forms. Capsules containing enteric-coated microspheres may be opened and sprinkled on a small quantity of cool, soft food. Stress importance of swallowing immediately, without chewing, and following with glass of water or juice.
• Warn patient not to inhale powder form or powder from capsules; it may irritate skin or mucous membranes.
• Tell patient to store in airtight container at room temperature.
• Instruct patient not to change brands without consulting prescriber.

# ursodiol
Actigall, Urso

*Pregnancy risk category B*

## AVAILABLE FORMS
*Capsules:* 300 mg
*Tablets:* 250 mg

## INDICATIONS & DOSAGES
➤ **Dissolution of gallstones less than 20 mm in diameter when surgery is prohibited**
*Adults:* 8 to 10 mg/kg P.O. daily in two or three divided doses.

➤ **To prevent gallstone formation in obese patients experiencing rapid weight loss**
*Adults:* 300 mg P.O. b.i.d.

## ACTION
Unknown. Drug is a naturally occurring bile acid that probably suppresses hepatic synthesis and secretion of cholesterol as well as intestinal cholesterol absorption. With long-term use, ursodiol can solubilize cholesterol from gallstones.

| Route | Onset | Peak | Duration |
|-------|-------|------|----------|
| P.O. | Unknown | 1-3 hr | Unknown |

## ADVERSE REACTIONS
**CNS:** *headache,* fatigue, anxiety, depression, *dizziness,* sleep disorders.
**EENT:** rhinitis.
**GI:** *nausea, vomiting, dyspepsia,* metallic taste, *abdominal pain,* biliary pain, cholecystitis, *diarrhea, constipation,* stomatitis, flatulence.
**GU:** *urinary tract infection.*
**Musculoskeletal:** arthralgia, myalgia, *back pain.*
**Respiratory:** cough.
**Skin:** pruritus, rash, dry skin, urticaria, hair thinning, diaphoresis.

## INTERACTIONS
**Drug-drug.** *Aluminum-containing antacids, cholestyramine, colestipol:* May bind ursodiol, preventing its absorption. Avoid using together.
*Clofibrate, estrogens, hormonal contraceptives:* May increase hepatic cholesterol secretion; may counteract effects of ursodiol. Avoid using together.

## EFFECTS ON LAB TEST RESULTS
None reported.

## CONTRAINDICATIONS & CAUTIONS
● Contraindicated in patients hypersensitive to ursodiol or other bile acids and in those with chronic hepatic disease, unremitting acute cholecystitis, cholangitis, biliary obstruction, gallstone-induced pancreatitis, or biliary fistula.

## NURSING CONSIDERATIONS
● Drug won't dissolve calcified cholesterol stones, radiolucent bile pigment stones, or radiopaque stones.
● *Alert:* Monitor liver function test results, including AST and ALT, at the start of therapy and after 1 month, 3 months, and then every 6 months during therapy. Abnormal test results may indicate worsening of the disease. There is a theoretical risk that a hepatotoxic metabolite of ursodiol may form in some patients.
● Therapy usually is long-term, with ultrasound images of the gallbladder taken every 6 months. If stones don't partially dissolve within 12 months, eventual success is unlikely. Safety of use for longer than 24 months hasn't been established.

## PATIENT TEACHING
● Advise patient about alternative therapies, including watchful waiting (no intervention) and cholecystectomy, because the relapse rate may be as high as 50% after 5 years.
● Tell patient to report adverse effects.
● Advise patient that dissolution of gallstones requires months of treatment.

bismuth subsalicylate
calcium polycarbophil
(See Chapter 47, LAXATIVES.)
diphenoxylate hydrochloride and
atropine sulfate
loperamide
octreotide acetate
opium tincture
opium tincture, camphorated

## COMBINATION PRODUCTS
IMODIUM ADVANCED: loperamide 2 mg
and simethicone 125 mg chewable tablets.
KAODENE NON-NARCOTIC ◊: 3.9 g kaolin
and 194.4 mg pectin in 30-ml bismuth
subsalicylate liquid.
KAPECTOLIN: 90 g kaolin and 2 g pectin in
30-ml suspension.
K-C SUSPENSION ◊: 5.2 g kaolin, 260 mg
pectin, 260 mg bismuth subsalicylate in
30-ml suspension.

---

## bismuth subsalicylate
Bismatrol ◊, Bismatrol Extra
Strength ◊, Children's
Kaopectate ◊, Extra Strength
Kaopectate ◊, Kaopectate ◊,
Pepto-Bismol ◊, Pepto-Bismol
Maximum Strength Liquid ◊, Pink
Bismuth ◊

*Pregnancy risk category NR*

---

## AVAILABLE FORMS
*Caplets:* 262 mg
*Oral suspension:* 262 mg/15 ml ◊,
524 mg/15 ml ◊, 130 mg/15 ml
*Tablets (chewable):* 262 mg ◊
*Liquid:* 87 mg/5 ml ◊, 87.3 mg/5 ml ◊,
175 mg /5 ml ◊

## INDICATIONS & DOSAGES
➤ **Mild, nonspecific diarrhea**
*Adults and children older than age 12:*
30 ml or 2 tablets P.O. q 30 minutes to
1 hour, up to maximum of eight doses and
for no longer than 2 days.
*Children ages 9 to 12:* 15 ml or 1 tablet
P.O. q 30 minutes to 1 hour, up to maxi-

mum of eight doses and for no longer than
2 days.
*Children ages 6 to 9:* 10 ml or ⅔ tablet P.O.
q 30 minutes to 1 hour, up to maximum of
eight doses and for no longer than 2 days.
*Children ages 3 to 6:* 5 ml or ⅓ tablet P.O.
q 30 minutes to 1 hour, up to maximum of
eight doses and for no longer than 2 days.
➤ **Traveler's diarrhea**
*Adults:* 2 tablets P.O. q.i.d., before meals
and h.s. for up to 3 weeks when traveling
in high-risk areas during instances of
high-risk.

## ACTION
Bismuth subsalicylate may have antisecre-
tory, antimicrobial, and anti-inflammatory
effects.

| Route | Onset | Peak | Duration |
|-------|-------|------|----------|
| P.O. | 1 hr | Unknown | Unknown |

## ADVERSE REACTIONS
**GI:** temporary darkening of tongue and
stools.
**Other:** salicylism with high doses.

## INTERACTIONS
**Drug-drug.** *Aspirin, other salicylates:*
May cause salicylate toxicity. Monitor patient.
*Oral anticoagulants, oral antidiabetics:*
May increase effects of these drugs after
high doses of bismuth subsalicylate. Monitor patient closely.
*Tetracycline:* May decrease tetracycline
absorption. Separate doses by at least 2
hours.

## EFFECTS ON LAB TEST RESULTS
None reported.

## CONTRAINDICATIONS & CAUTIONS
● Contraindicated in patients hypersensi-
tive to salicylates.
● Use cautiously in patients taking aspirin.
Stop therapy if tinnitus occurs.
● Use cautiously in children and in pa-
tients with bleeding disorders or salicylate
sensitivity.

---

## NURSING CONSIDERATIONS

• Avoid use before GI radiologic procedures because bismuth is radiopaque and
may interfere with X-rays.

## PATIENT TEACHING

• Advise patient that bismuth subsalicylate
contains salicylate. Each tablet has
102 mg salicylate. Regular-strength liquid
has 130 mg/15 ml. Extra-strength liquid
has 230 mg/15 ml.
• Instruct patient to shake liquid before
measuring dose and to chew tablets well
before swallowing.
• Tell patient to call prescriber if diarrhea
lasts longer than 2 days or is accompanied
by high fever.
• Advise patient to drink plenty of clear
fluids to help prevent dehydration, which
may accompany diarrhea.
• Urge patient to consult with prescriber
before giving bismuth subsalicylate to
children or teenagers during or after recovery from the flu or chickenpox.
• Inform patient that all forms of Pepto-
Bismol are effective against traveler's diarrhea. Tablets and caplets may be more
convenient to carry.

---

## diphenoxylate hydrochloride and atropine sulfate
Logen, Lomanate, Lomotil*, Lonox

*Pregnancy risk category C*
*Controlled substance schedule V*

---

## AVAILABLE FORMS

*Liquid:* 2.5 mg/5 ml (with atropine sulfate
0.025 mg/5 ml)*
*Tablets:* 2.5 mg (with atropine sulfate
0.025 mg)

## INDICATIONS & DOSAGES

➤ **Acute, nonspecific diarrhea**
*Adults and children older than age 12:*
Initially, 5 mg P.O. q.i.d.; then adjusted,
p.r.n. Maximum dosage 20 mg/day.
*Children ages 2 to 12:* 0.3 to 0.4 mg/kg
liquid form P.O. daily in four divided doses. For maintenance, reduce first dose
p.r.n., up to 75%. Maximum dosage
20 mg/day.

## ACTION

Unknown. Probably increases smooth
muscle tone in GI tract, inhibits motility
and propulsion, and diminishes secretions.

| Route | Onset | Peak | Duration |
|-------|-------|------|----------|
| P.O. | 45-60 min | 3 hr | 3-4 hr |

## ADVERSE REACTIONS

**CNS:** *sedation, dizziness,* headache,
drowsiness, lethargy, restlessness, depression, euphoria, malaise, confusion, numbness in limbs.
**CV:** tachycardia.
**EENT:** blurred vision.
**GI:** *dry mouth,* nausea, vomiting, abdominal discomfort or distention, *paralytic
ileus,* anorexia, fluid retention in bowel or
megacolon, *pancreatitis,* swollen gums.
**GU:** urine retention.
**Respiratory:** *respiratory depression.*
**Skin:** pruritus, rash, dry skin.
**Other:** *angioedema, anaphylaxis,* possible physical dependence with long-term
use.

## INTERACTIONS

**Drug-drug.** *Barbiturates, CNS depres-
sants, opioids, tranquilizers:* May enhance
CNS depression. Monitor patient closely.
*MAO inhibitors:* May cause hypertensive
crisis. Avoid using together.
**Drug-lifestyle.** *Alcohol use:* May enhance
CNS depression. Discourage use together.

## EFFECTS ON LAB TEST RESULTS

None reported.

## CONTRAINDICATIONS & CAUTIONS

• Contraindicated in patients hypersensitive to diphenoxylate or atropine, in those
with obstructive jaundice, and in children
younger than age 2.
• Contraindicated in those with acute
diarrhea resulting from poison (until toxic
material is eliminated from GI tract), from
organisms that penetrate intestinal mucosa, or from antibiotic-induced pseudomembranous enterocolitis.
• Use cautiously in children age 2 and older; in patients with hepatic disease, opioid
dependence, or acute ulcerative colitis;
and in pregnant patients.

---

## NURSING CONSIDERATIONS

- *Alert:* Monitor fluid and electrolyte balance. Correct fluid and electrolyte disturbances before starting drug. Dehydration, especially in young children, may increase risk of delayed toxicity. Fluid retention in bowel or megacolon may occur with drug use and may mask depletion of extracellular fluid and electrolytes, especially in young children treated for acute gastroenteritis.
- Stop therapy immediately and notify prescriber if abdominal distention or other signs or symptoms of toxic megacolon develop.
- Don't use to treat antibiotic-induced diarrhea.
- Drug is unlikely to be effective if no response occurs within 48 hours.
- Risk of physical dependence increases with high dosage and long-term use. Atropine sulfate helps discourage abuse.
- Monitor for signs of overdose, which may include restlessness, flushing, hyperthermia, and tachycardia, initially, followed by lethargy, coma, pinpoint pupils, hypotonicity, and respiratory depression.
- *Alert:* Don't confuse Lomotil with Lamictal.

## PATIENT TEACHING

- Tell patient not to exceed recommended dosage.
- Warn patient not to use drug to treat acute diarrhea for longer than 2 days and to seek medical attention if diarrhea continues.
- Advise patient to avoid hazardous activities, such as driving, until CNS effects of drug are known.

---

# loperamide
Imodium, Imodium A-D ◊,
Kaopectate II Caplets ◊, Maalox
Anti-Diarrheal Caplets ◊, Pepto
Diarrhea Control ◊

*Pregnancy risk category B*

---

## AVAILABLE FORMS
*Caplets:* 2 mg ◊
*Capsules:* 2 mg
*Oral liquid:* 1 mg/5 ml ◊

## INDICATIONS & DOSAGES
➤ **Acute, nonspecific diarrhea**
*Adults and children older than age 12:*
Initially, 4 mg P.O.; then 2 mg after each unformed stool. Maximum, 8 mg daily, unless directed.
*Children ages 8 to 12:* 2 mg P.O. t.i.d. on first day. Subsequent dosages of 5 ml or 0.1 mg/kg of body weight may be given after each unformed stool. Maximum, 6 mg daily.
*Children ages 6 to 8:* 2 mg P.O. b.i.d. on first day. If diarrhea persists, contact prescriber. Maximum, 4 mg daily.
*Children ages 2 to 5:* 1 mg P.O. t.i.d. on first day. If diarrhea persists, contact prescriber.
➤ **Chronic diarrhea**
*Adults:* Initially, 4 mg P.O.; then 2 mg after each unformed stool until diarrhea subsides. Dosage adjusted to individual response.

## ACTION
Inhibits peristaltic activity, prolonging transit of intestinal contents.

| Route | Onset | Peak | Duration |
|-------|-------|------|----------|
| P.O. | Unknown | 2½-5 hr | 24 hr |

## ADVERSE REACTIONS
**CNS:** drowsiness, fatigue, dizziness.
**GI:** dry mouth; abdominal pain, distention, or discomfort; *constipation;* nausea; vomiting.
**Skin:** rash, hypersensitivity reactions.

## INTERACTIONS
None significant.

## EFFECTS ON LAB TEST RESULTS
None reported.

## CONTRAINDICATIONS & CAUTIONS
- Contraindicated in patients hypersensitive to drug and in those in whom constipation must be avoided.
- Contraindicated in patients with bloody diarrhea or diarrhea with fever greater than 101° F (38° C), in breast-feeding women, and in children younger than age 2.
- Use cautiously in patients with hepatic disease.

---
Reactions may be *common*, uncommon, *life-threatening*, or COMMON AND LIFE-THREATENING.

## NURSING CONSIDERATIONS

• If clinical symptoms don't improve within 48 hours, stop therapy and consider other alternatives.

• Drug produces antidiarrheal action similar to that of diphenoxylate but without as many adverse CNS effects.

• *Alert:* Monitor children closely for CNS effects; children may be more sensitive to these effects than adults.

• *Alert:* Don't confuse Imodium with Ionamin.

## PATIENT TEACHING

• Advise patient not to exceed recommended dosage.

• Tell patient with acute diarrhea to stop drug and seek medical attention if no improvement occurs within 48 hours. In chronic diarrhea, tell patient to notify prescriber and to stop drug if no improvement occurs after taking 16 mg daily for at least 10 days.

• Advise patient with acute colitis to stop drug immediately and notify prescriber about abdominal distention.

• Warn patient to avoid activities that require mental alertness until CNS effects of drug are known.

• Tell patient to report nausea, abdominal pain, or abdominal discomfort.

• Advise patient to relieve dry mouth with ice chips or sugarless gum.

• Advise breast-feeding patients to avoid use.

---

## octreotide acetate
Sandostatin, Sandostatin LAR

*Pregnancy risk category B*

### AVAILABLE FORMS

*Injection ampules:* 0.05 mg/ml, 0.1 mg/ml, 0.2 mg/ml, 0.5 mg/ml, 1.0 mg/ml
*Injection (long-acting):* 10 mg, 20 mg, 30 mg
*Injection (multidose vials):* 0.2 mg/ml, 1 mg/ml

### INDICATIONS & DOSAGES

➤ **Flushing and diarrhea from carcinoid tumors**
*Adults:* 0.1 to 0.6 mg daily S.C. in two to four divided doses for first 2 weeks of therapy. Usual daily dosage is 0.3 mg. Subsequent dosage based on individual response.

➤ **Watery diarrhea from vasoactive intestinal polypeptide-secreting tumors (VIPomas)**
*Adults:* 0.2 to 0.3 mg daily S.C. in two to four divided doses for first 2 weeks of therapy. Subsequent dosage based on individual response; usually shouldn't exceed 0.45 mg daily.

➤ **Acromegaly**
*Adults:* Initially, 50 mcg S.C. t.i.d., then adjusted based on somatomedin C levels q 2 weeks. If Sandostatin LAR is used, give 20 mg I.M. (intragluteally) at 4-week intervals.

➤ **GI fistula** ♦
*Adults:* 50 to 200 mcg S.C. q 8 hours.

➤ **Variceal bleeding** ♦
*Adults:* 25 to 50 mcg/hour via continuous I.V. infusion, over 18 hours to 5 days.

➤ **AIDS-related diarrhea** ♦
*Adults:* 100 to 500 mcg S.C. t.i.d.

➤ **Short bowel syndrome** ♦
*Adults:* I.V. infusion of 25 mcg/hour or 50 mcg S.C. b.i.d.

➤ **Diarrhea caused by chemotherapy or radiation therapy** ♦
*Adults:* 50 to 100 mcg S.C. t.i.d. for 1 to 3 days.

➤ **Pancreatic fistula** ♦
*Adults:* 50 to 200 mcg q 8 hours.

➤ **Irritable bowel syndrome** ♦
*Adults:* Initially, 100 mcg S.C. as single dose; maximum, 125 mcg S.C. b.i.d.

### ACTION

Mimics action of naturally occurring somatostatin.

| Route | Onset | Peak | Duration |
|-------|-------|------|----------|
| S.C. | 30 min | 30 min | < 12 hr |

### ADVERSE REACTIONS

**CNS:** dizziness, light-headedness, fatigue, headache.
**CV:** *bradycardia,* edema, conduction abnormalities, *arrhythmias.*
**EENT:** blurred vision.
**GI:** *nausea, diarrhea, abdominal pain or discomfort, loose stools,* vomiting, fat malabsorption, *gallbladder abnormalities,* flatulence, constipation, *pancreatitis.*
**GU:** pollakiuria, urinary tract infection.

---

**Metabolic:** hyperglycemia; *hypoglycemia;* hypothyroidism; suppressed secretion of growth hormone and of the gastroenterohepatic peptides gastrin, vasoactive intestinal polypeptide, insulin, glucagon, secretin, motilin, and pancreatic polypeptide.
**Musculoskeletal:** backache, joint pain.
**Skin:** flushing, wheal, erythema or pain at injection site, alopecia.
**Other:** pain or burning at S.C. injection site, cold symptoms, flulike symptoms.

**INTERACTIONS**
**Drug-drug.** *Cyclosporine:* May decrease cyclosporine level. Monitor patient closely.

**EFFECTS ON LAB TEST RESULTS**
● May decrease vitamin $B_{12}$ level. May increase or decrease glucose level.
● May alter liver function test result.

**CONTRAINDICATIONS & CAUTIONS**
● Contraindicated in patients hypersensitive to drug or its components.

**NURSING CONSIDERATIONS**
● Monitor baseline thyroid function tests.
● Monitor IGF-I (somatomedin C) levels every 2 weeks. Dosage adjustments are based on this level.
● Periodically monitor laboratory tests such as thyroid function, glucose, urine 5-hydroxyindoleacetic acid, plasma serotonin, and plasma substance P (for carcinoid tumors).
● Monitor patient regularly for gallbladder disease. Octreotide therapy may be related to the development of cholelithiasis because of its effect on gallbladder motility or fat absorption.
● Monitor patient closely for signs and symptoms of glucose imbalance. Patients with type 1 diabetes mellitus and patients receiving oral antidiabetics or oral diazoxide may need dosage adjustments during therapy. Monitor glucose level.
● Octreotide therapy may alter fluid and electrolyte balance and may cause need for adjustment of other drugs used to control symptoms of the disease, such as beta blockers.

● Half-life may be altered in patients with end-stage renal failure who are receiving dialysis.
● **Alert:** Don't confuse Sandostatin with Sandimmune or Sandoglobulin.

**PATIENT TEACHING**
● Urge patient to report signs and symptoms of abdominal discomfort immediately.
● Stress importance of the need for periodic laboratory testing during octreotide therapy.

---

**opium tincture\***

**opium tincture, camphorated\* (paregoric)**

*Pregnancy risk category B (D for high doses or long-term use)*
*Controlled substance schedule II (opium tincture); III (camphorated)*

**AVAILABLE FORMS**
**opium tincture**
*Oral solution:* Equivalent to morphine 10 mg/ml\*
**opium tincture, camphorated**
*Oral solution:* Each 5 ml contains morphine 2 mg, anise oil 0.2 ml, benzoic acid 20 mg, camphor 20 mg, glycerin 0.2 ml, and alcohol\*

**INDICATIONS & DOSAGES**
➤ **Acute, nonspecific diarrhea**
*Opium tincture*
*Adults:* 0.6 ml P.O. q.i.d. Maximum, 6 ml daily.
*Opium tincture, camphorated*
*Adults:* 5 to 10 ml P.O. once daily, b.i.d., t.i.d., or q.i.d. until diarrhea subsides.
*Children:* 0.25 to 0.5 ml/kg P.O. once daily, b.i.d., t.i.d., or q.i.d. until diarrhea subsides.

**ACTION**
Increases smooth muscle tone in GI tract, inhibits motility and propulsion, and diminishes secretions.

| Route | Onset | Peak | Duration |
|-------|-------|------|----------|
| P.O. | Unknown | Unknown | Unknown |

**ADVERSE REACTIONS**
**CNS:** dizziness, light-headedness.
**GI:** nausea, vomiting.
**Other:** physical dependence after long-term use.

**INTERACTIONS**
None significant.

**EFFECTS ON LAB TEST RESULTS**
• May increase amylase and lipase levels.

**CONTRAINDICATIONS & CAUTIONS**
• Contraindicated in patients with acute diarrhea caused by poisoning until toxic material is removed from GI tract. Also contraindicated in patients with diarrhea caused by organisms that penetrate intestinal mucosa.
• Use cautiously in patients with asthma, prostatic hyperplasia, hepatic disease, and history of opioid dependence.

**NURSING CONSIDERATIONS**
• *Alert:* Opium tincture has 25 times more opium content than camphorated opium tincture. Camphorated opium tincture is more dilute, and teaspoon doses are easier to measure than dropper quantities of opium tincture.
• *Alert:* For overdose, use the opioid antagonist, naloxone, to reverse respiratory depression.
• Mix with sufficient water to ensure passage to stomach.
• Opium tincture and camphorated opium tincture may prevent delivery of Tc99m disofenin to small intestine during hepatobiliary imaging tests; delay test until 24 hours after last dose.
• A milky fluid forms when camphorated opium tincture is added to water.
• Store in tightly capped, light-resistant container.
• *Alert:* Don't confuse opium tincture with camphorated opium tincture.

**PATIENT TEACHING**
• Advise patient against long-term use of drug, because risk of physical dependence increases with long-term use.
• Warn patient to avoid activities that require mental alertness until CNS effects of drug are known.

• Instruct patient to measure dose carefully to avoid overdose.
• Tell patient to notify prescriber if diarrhea persists.

bisacodyl
calcium polycarbophil
docusate calcium
docusate sodium
glycerin
lactulose
magnesium citrate
magnesium hydroxide
magnesium sulfate
methylcellulose
polyethylene glycol and
  electrolyte solution
psyllium
senna
sodium phosphate monohydrate,
  sodium phosphate dibasic
  anhydrous

## COMBINATION PRODUCTS

DIALOSE PLUS‡ ◊ : docusate sodium
100 mg and danthron 30 mg.
DOXIDAN ◊ : docusate sodium 100 mg and
casanthranol 30 mg.
HALEY'S M-O ◊ : mineral oil 3.75 ml and
magnesium hydroxide 900 mg per 15 ml.
PERDIEM ◊ : psyllium 3.25 g and senna
0.74g/6 mg tsp.
PERI-COLACE CAPSULES†: docusate sodium 100 mg and casanthranol 30 mg.
PERI-COLACE SYRUP†: docusate sodium
60 mg and casanthranol 30 mg/15 ml.
SENOKOT-S ◊ : docusate sodium 50 mg
and 8.6 mg sennosides.

## bisacodyl
Bisacolax‡ ◊ , Bisalax‡, Bisco-
Lax ◊ , Correctol, Dulcolax ◊ ,
Durolax‡, Feen-a-Mint, Fleet
Bisacodyl ◊ , Fleet Bisacodyl
Enema ◊ , Fleet Laxatives ◊ ,
Laxit† ◊

*Pregnancy risk category B*

## AVAILABLE FORMS
*Enema:* 0.33 mg/ml ◊ , 10 mg/5 ml
(microenema)‡

*Powder for rectal solution (bisacodyl tan-
nex):* 1.5 mg bisacodyl and 2.5 g tannic
acid
*Suppositories:* 5 mg ◊ , 10 mg ◊
*Tablets (enteric-coated):* 5 mg ◊

## INDICATIONS & DOSAGES
➤ **Chronic constipation; preparation
for childbirth, surgery, or rectal or
bowel examination**
*Adults and children age 12 and older:*
10 to 15 mg P.O. in evening or before
breakfast. Up to 30 mg P.O., p.r.n. Or,
10 mg P.R. for evacuation before examination or surgery.
*Children ages 6 to 11:* 5 mg P.O. or P.R.
h.s. or before breakfast. Oral dose isn't recommended if child can't swallow tablet
whole.

## ACTION
Unknown. Stimulant laxative that increases peristalsis, probably by direct effect on
smooth muscle of the intestine. Thought to
either irritate the musculature or stimulate
the colonic intramural plexus. Drug also
promotes fluid accumulation in colon and
small intestine.

| Route | Onset | Peak | Duration |
|-------|-------|------|----------|
| P.O. | 6-12 hr | Variable | Variable |
| P.R. | 15-60 min | Variable | Variable |

## ADVERSE REACTIONS
**CNS:** muscle weakness with excessive
use, dizziness, faintness.
**GI:** *nausea, vomiting, abdominal cramps,*
diarrhea with high doses, *burning sensation in rectum* with suppositories, laxative
dependence with long-term or excessive
use, protein-losing enteropathy with excessive use.
**Metabolic:** alkalosis, hypokalemia, fluid
and electrolyte imbalance.
**Musculoskeletal:** tetany.

## INTERACTIONS
**Drug-drug.** *Antacids:* May cause gastric
irritation or dyspepsia from premature dis-

solution of enteric coating. Separate doses by at least 1 or 2 hours.

**Drug-food.** *Milk:* May cause gastric irritation or dyspepsia from premature dissolution of enteric coating. Don't use within 1 or 2 hours of drinking milk.

**EFFECTS ON LAB TEST RESULTS**
• May increase phosphate and sodium levels. May decrease calcium, magnesium, and potassium levels.

**CONTRAINDICATIONS & CAUTIONS**
• Contraindicated in patients hypersensitive to drug or its components and in those with rectal bleeding, gastroenteritis, intestinal obstruction, abdominal pain, nausea, vomiting, or other symptoms of appendicitis or acute surgical abdomen.

**NURSING CONSIDERATIONS**
• Give drug at times that don't interfere with scheduled activities or sleep. Soft, formed stools are usually produced 15 to 60 minutes after rectal use.
• Before giving for constipation, determine whether patient has adequate fluid intake, exercise, and diet.
• Tablets and suppositories are used together to clean the colon before and after surgery and before barium enema.
• Insert suppository as high as possible into the rectum, and try to position suppository against the rectal wall. Avoid embedding within fecal material because doing so may delay onset of action.
• Bisco-Lax may contain tartrazine.

**PATIENT TEACHING**
• Advise patient to swallow enteric-coated tablet whole to avoid GI irritation. Instruct him not to take within 1 hour of milk or antacid.
• Tell patient that drug is for short-term (1 week) treatment only (stimulant laxatives are commonly abused). Discourage excessive use.
• Advise patient to report adverse effects to prescriber.
• Teach patient about dietary sources of bulk, including bran and other cereals, fresh fruit, and vegetables.

• Tell patient to take drug with a full glass of water or juice.

---

# calcium polycarbophil
Equalactin◇, Fiberall◇, FiberCon◇, Fiber-Lax◇, Mitrola◇, Phillips' Fibercaps

*Pregnancy risk category A*

**AVAILABLE FORMS**
*Tablets:* 500 mg◇, 625 mg◇
*Tablets (chewable):* 500 mg◇

**INDICATIONS & DOSAGES**
➤ **Constipation**
*Adults and children older than age 12:* 1 g P.O. q.i.d., p.r.n. Maximum, 4 g in 24-hour period.
*Children ages 7 to 12:* 500 mg P.O. once daily to t.i.d., p.r.n. Maximum, 2 g in 24-hour period.
➤ **Diarrhea from irritable bowel syndrome; acute, nonspecific diarrhea**
*Adults and children older than age 12:* 1 g P.O. q.i.d., p.r.n. Maximum, 4 g in 24-hour period.
*Children ages 7 to 12:* 500 mg P.O. t.i.d., p.r.n. Maximum, 2 g in 24-hour period.

**ACTION**
Bulk-forming laxative that absorbs water and expands to increase bulk and moisture content of stools. The increased bulk encourages peristalsis and bowel movement. As an antidiarrheal, drug absorbs free fecal water, thereby producing formed stools.

| Route | Onset | Peak | Duration |
|-------|-------|------|----------|
| P.O. | 12-24 hr | 3 days | Variable |

**ADVERSE REACTIONS**
**GI:** abdominal fullness and increased flatus, *intestinal obstruction.*
**Other:** laxative dependence with long-term or excessive use.

**INTERACTIONS**
**Drug-drug.** *Tetracyclines:* May impair tetracycline absorption. Avoid using together.

---

**EFFECTS ON LAB TEST RESULTS**
None reported.

**CONTRAINDICATIONS & CAUTIONS**
● Contraindicated in patients with signs or symptoms of GI obstruction or those with swallowing difficulty.

**NURSING CONSIDERATIONS**
● Before giving drug for constipation, determine whether patient has adequate fluid intake, exercise, and diet.
● In children younger than age 6, use must be directed by prescriber.
● *Alert:* Rectal bleeding or failure to respond to therapy may indicate need for surgery.

**PATIENT TEACHING**
● Full benefit of drug may take 1 to 3 days.
● Advise patient to chew Equalactin or Mitrolan tablets thoroughly before swallowing and to drink an 8-ounce glass of water with each dose. When drug is used as an antidiarrheal, tell patient not to drink the glass of water.
● Advise patient to seek medical attention if he experiences vomiting, chest pain, or difficulty breathing or swallowing after taking medication.
● Teach patient about dietary sources of bulk, including bran and other cereals, fresh fruit, and vegetables.
● For severe diarrhea, advise patient to repeat dose every 30 minutes, but not to exceed maximum daily dose. Tell patient not to use for longer than 2 days, unless directed by a prescriber.

---

**docusate calcium (dioctyl calcium sulfosuccinate)**
DC Softgels ◇ , Surfak ◇

**docusate sodium (dioctyl sodium sulfosuccinate)**
Colace ◇ , Coloxyl‡, Coloxyl Enema Concentrate‡, Diocto ◇ , Dioeze ◇ , Diosuccin ◇ , Di-Sosul ◇ , D.O.S. ◇ , D-S-S ◇ , Duosol ◇ , Ex-Lax Stool Softener Caplets, Modane Soft ◇ , Phillips'

Liqui-Gels, Pro-Sof ◇ , Regulax SS ◇ , Regulex† ◇

*Pregnancy risk category C*

**AVAILABLE FORMS**
**docusate calcium**
*Capsules:* 50 mg ◇ , 240 mg ◇
**docusate sodium**
*Capsules:* 50 mg ◇ , 100 mg ◇ , 240 mg ◇ , 250 mg ◇
*Enema concentrate:* 18 g/100 ml (must be diluted)‡
*Oral liquid:* 150 mg/15 ml ◇
*Oral solution:* 10 mg/ml ◇ , 50 mg/ml ◇
*Syrup:* 20 mg/5 ml, 50 mg/15 ml ◇ , 60 mg/15 ml ◇
*Tablets:* 50 mg ◇ , 100 mg ◇

**INDICATIONS & DOSAGES**
➤ **Stool softener**
*Adults and children older than age 12:* 50 to 500 mg docusate calcium or sodium P.O. daily until bowel movements are normal. Or, give enema. Dilute 1:24 with sterile water before use, and give 100 to 150 ml retention enema, 300 to 500 ml evacuation enema, or 0.5 to 1.5 L flushing enema P.R.
*Children ages 6 to 12:* 40 to 120 mg docusate sodium P.O. daily.
*Children ages 3 to 6:* 20 to 60 mg docusate sodium P.O. daily.
*Children younger than age 3:* 10 to 40 mg docusate sodium P.O. daily.
   Higher dosages are used for initial therapy. Dosages are adjusted to individual response.

**ACTION**
Stool softener that reduces surface tension of interfacing liquid contents of the bowel. This detergent activity promotes incorporation of additional liquid into stools, thus forming a softer mass.

| Route | Onset | Peak | Duration |
|-------|-------|------|----------|
| P.O. | 1-3 days | Unknown | Unknown |
| P.R. | Unknown | Unknown | Unknown |

**ADVERSE REACTIONS**
**GI:** bitter taste, mild abdominal cramping, diarrhea.
**Other:** laxative dependence with long-term or excessive use.

## INTERACTIONS
**Drug-drug.** *Mineral oil:* May increase mineral oil absorption and cause toxicity and lipid pneumonia. Separate doses.

## EFFECTS ON LAB TEST RESULTS
None reported.

## CONTRAINDICATIONS & CAUTIONS
● Contraindicated in patients hypersensitive to drug and in those with intestinal obstruction or signs and symptoms of appendicitis, fecal impaction, or acute surgical abdomen, such as undiagnosed abdominal pain or vomiting.

## NURSING CONSIDERATIONS
● Drug isn't used to treat existing constipation but prevents constipation from developing.
● Before giving drug, determine whether patient has adequate fluid intake, exercise, and diet.
● Give liquid (not syrups) in milk, fruit juice, or infant formula to mask bitter taste.
● Drug is laxative of choice for patients who shouldn't strain during defecation, including patients recovering from MI or rectal surgery, those with rectal or anal disease that makes passage of firm stools difficult, and those with postpartum constipation.
● Store drug at 59° to 86° F (15° to 30° C), and protect liquid from light.

## PATIENT TEACHING
● Teach patient about dietary sources of bulk, including bran and other cereals, fresh fruit, and vegetables.
● Instruct patient to use drug only occasionally and not for longer than 1 week without prescriber's knowledge.
● Tell patient to stop drug and notify prescriber if severe cramping occurs.
● Notify patient that it may take from 1 to 3 days to soften stools.

# glycerin
Fleet Babylax ◊ , Sani-Supp ◊

*Pregnancy risk category NR*

## AVAILABLE FORMS
*Enema (pediatric):* 4 ml/applicator ◊
*Suppositories:* Adult, children, and infant sizes ◊

## INDICATIONS & DOSAGES
➤ **Constipation**
*Adults and children age 6 and older:* 2 to 3 g as rectal suppository; or 5 to 15 ml as enema.
*Children ages 2 to 6:* 1 to 1.7 g as rectal suppository; or 2 to 5 ml as enema.

## ACTION
Hyperosmolar laxative that draws water from the tissues into the feces, thus stimulating evacuation.

| Route | Onset | Peak | Duration |
|-------|-------|------|----------|
| P.R. | 15-30 min | Unknown | Unknown |

## ADVERSE REACTIONS
**GI:** *cramping pain,* rectal discomfort, hyperemia of rectal mucosa.

## INTERACTIONS
None significant.

## EFFECTS ON LAB TEST RESULTS
None reported.

## CONTRAINDICATIONS & CAUTIONS
● Contraindicated in patients hypersensitive to drug and in those with intestinal obstruction or signs and symptoms of appendicitis, fecal impaction, or acute surgical abdomen, such as undiagnosed abdominal pain or vomiting.

## NURSING CONSIDERATIONS
● Drug is used mainly to reestablish proper toilet habits in laxative-dependent patients.

## PATIENT TEACHING
● Tell patient that drug must be retained for at least 15 minutes and that it usually acts within 1 hour. Entire suppository need not melt to be effective.
● Warn patient about adverse GI reactions.

---

# lactulose
Cephulac, Cholac, Chronulac,
Constilac, Constulose, Duphalac,
Enulose, Kristalose, Lactulax†

*Pregnancy risk category B*

## AVAILABLE FORMS
*Packets:* 10 g, 20 g
*Syrup:* 10 g/15 ml

## INDICATIONS & DOSAGES
➤ **Constipation**
*Adults:* 10 to 20 g or 15 to 30 ml P.O. daily, increased to 60 ml/day, if needed.
➤ **To prevent and treat hepatic encephalopathy, including hepatic precoma and coma in patients with severe hepatic disease**
*Adults:* Initially, 20 to 30 g or 30 to 45 ml P.O. t.i.d. or q.i.d., until two or three soft stools are produced daily. Usual dose is 60 to 100 g daily in divided doses. Or, 200 g or 300 ml diluted with 700 ml of water or normal saline solution and given as retention enema P.R. q 4 to 6 hours, p.r.n.

## ACTION
Produces an osmotic effect in colon; resulting distention promotes peristalsis. Also decreases ammonia, probably as a result of bacterial degradation, which lowers the pH of colon contents.

| Route | Onset | Peak | Duration |
|---|---|---|---|
| P.O. | 24-48 hr | Variable | Variable |
| P.R. | Unknown | Unknown | Unknown |

## ADVERSE REACTIONS
**GI:** *abdominal cramps, belching, diarrhea, gaseous distention, flatulence,* nausea, vomiting.

## INTERACTIONS
**Drug-drug.** *Antacids, antibiotics, oral neomycin:* May decrease lactulose effectiveness. Avoid using together.

## EFFECTS ON LAB TEST RESULTS
None reported.

## CONTRAINDICATIONS & CAUTIONS
• Contraindicated in patients on a low-galactose diet.
• Use cautiously in patients with diabetes mellitus.

## NURSING CONSIDERATIONS
• To minimize sweet taste, dilute with water or fruit juice or give with food.
• Prepare enema (not commercially available) by adding 200 g (300 ml) to 700 ml of water or normal saline solution. The diluted solution is given as retention enema for 30 to 60 minutes. Use a rectal balloon.
• If enema isn't retained for at least 30 minutes, be prepared to repeat dose.
• Monitor sodium level for hypernatremia, especially when giving in higher doses to treat hepatic encephalopathy.
• Monitor mental status and potassium levels when giving to patients with hepatic encephalopathy.
• Be prepared to replace fluid loss.
• *Alert:* Don't confuse lactulose with lactose.

## PATIENT TEACHING
• Show home care patient how to mix and use drug.
• Inform patient about adverse reactions and tell him to notify prescriber if reactions become bothersome or if diarrhea occurs.
• Instruct patient not to take other laxatives during lactulose therapy.

# magnesium citrate (citrate of magnesia)
Citroma◊, Citro-Mag†

# magnesium hydroxide (milk of magnesia)
Milk of Magnesia◊, Milk of Magnesia-Concentrated◊, Phillips' Milk of Magnesia◊

# magnesium sulfate (epsom salts)◊

*Pregnancy risk category B*

## AVAILABLE FORMS
**magnesium citrate**
*Oral solution:* about 168 mEq magnesium/240 ml◊

**magnesium hydroxide**
*Chewable tablets:* 300 mg, 600 mg
*Oral suspension:* 400 mg/5 ml, 800 mg/5 ml
**magnesium sulfate**
*Granules:* about 40 mEq magnesium/5 g ◊

## INDICATIONS & DOSAGES
➤ **Constipation, to evacuate bowel before surgery**
*Adults and children age 12 and older:*
11 to 25 g magnesium citrate P.O. daily as a single or divided dose. Or, 2.4 to 4.8 g or 30 to 60 ml magnesium hydroxide P.O. (2 to 4 tablespoons at bedtime or upon arising, followed by 8 ounces of liquid) daily as a single dose or divided. Or, 10 to 30 g magnesium sulfate P.O. daily as a single or divided dose.
*Children ages 6 to 11:* 5.5 to 12.5 g magnesium citrate P.O. daily as a single or divided dose. Or, 1.2 to 2.4 g or 15 to 30 ml magnesium hydroxide P.O. (1 to 2 tablespoons, followed by 8 ounces of liquid) daily as a single or divided dose. Or, 5 to 10 g magnesium sulfate P.O. daily as a single or divided dose. Don't use dosage cup.
*Children ages 2 to 5:* 2.7 to 6.25 g magnesium citrate P.O. daily as a single or divided dose. Or, 0.4 to 1.2 g or 5 to 15 ml magnesium hydroxide P.O. (1 to 3 tsp, followed by 8 ounces of liquid) *and older:* 1 to ... directed. Don't use dosage cup.

## ACTION
Saline laxative that produces an osmotic effect in the small intestine by drawing water into the intestinal lumen.

| Route | Onset | Peak | Duration |
|-------|-------|------|----------|
| P.O. | 30 min-3 hr | Variable | Variable |

## ADVERSE REACTIONS
**GI:** abdominal cramping, nausea, diarrhea.
**Metabolic:** fluid and electrolyte disturbances with daily use.

**Other:** laxative dependence with long-term or excessive use.

## INTERACTIONS
**Drug-drug.** *Oral drugs:* May impair absorption. Separate doses.

## EFFECTS ON LAB TEST RESULTS
● May alter fluid and electrolyte levels with prolonged use.

## CONTRAINDICATIONS & CAUTIONS
● Contraindicated in pregnant patients about to deliver and in patients with myocardial damage, heart block, fecal impaction, rectal fissures, intestinal obstruction or perforation, renal disease, or signs and symptoms of appendicitis or acute surgical abdomen, such as abdominal pain, nausea, or vomiting.
● Use cautiously in patients with rectal bleeding.

## NURSING CONSIDERATIONS
● Give drug at times that don't interfere with scheduled activities or sleep. Drug produces watery stools in 3 to 6 hours.
● Before giving drug for constipation, determine whether patient has adequate fluid intake, exercise, and diet.
● Chill magnesium citrate before use to improve its palatability.
● Shake suspension well; give with a large amount of water if used as laxative.
After instilling drug, flush tube with water to ensure passage to stomach and maintain tube patency.
● **Alert:** Monitor electrolyte levels during prolonged use. Magnesium may accumulate if patient has renal insufficiency.
● Drug is recommended for short-term use only.
● Magnesium sulfate is more potent than other saline laxatives.

## PATIENT TEACHING
● Teach patient how to use drug as ...
● Teach patient about ... bulk, including that frequent or prolonged ... as a laxative may cause dependence.

## methylcellulose
Citrucel◇, Citrucel Orange
Flavor◇, Citrucel Sugar-Free
Orange Flavor◇

*Pregnancy risk category NR*

### AVAILABLE FORMS
*Powder:* 2g◇

### INDICATIONS & DOSAGES
➤ **Chronic constipation**
*Adults and children older than age 12:*
1 packet in 8 ounces cold water up to t.i.d.
*Children ages 6 to 12:* ½ packet in 8
ounces cold water up to t.i.d.

### ACTION
Bulk-forming laxative that absorbs water
and expands to increase bulk and moisture
content of stools. The increased bulk encourages peristalsis and bowel movement.

| Route | Onset | Peak | Duration |
|-------|-------|------|----------|
| P.O. | 12-24 hr | < 3 days | Variable |

### ADVERSE REACTIONS
**GI:** *nausea,* vomiting, diarrhea with excessive use; esophageal, gastric, small intestinal, or colonic strictures when drug is
chewed or taken in dry form; *abdominal
cramps,* especially in severe constipation.
**Other:** laxative dependence with long-
term or excessive use.

### INTERACTIONS
None significant.

### EFFECTS ON LAB TEST RESULTS
None reported.

### CONTRAINDICATIONS & CAUTIONS
• Contraindicated in patients with intestinal obstruction, intestinal ulceration, disabling adhesions, difficulty swallowing, or
signs and symptoms of appendicitis or
acute surgical abdomen, such as abdominal pain, nausea, and vomiting.

### NURSING CONSIDERATIONS
• Determine whether patient has adequate
fluid intake, exercise, and diet. Elimination, de-

• Drug is especially useful in debilitated
patients and in those with postpartum constipation, irritable bowel syndrome, diverticulitis, and colostomies. It's also used to
treat laxative abuse and to empty colon
before barium enema examinations.
• Drug isn't absorbed systemically and is
nontoxic.
• *Alert:* Don't confuse Citrucel with Citracal.

### PATIENT TEACHING
• Tell patient to take drug with at least
8 ounces (240 ml) of liquid to mask grittiness.
• Teach patient about dietary sources of
bulk, including bran and other cereals,
fresh fruit, and vegetables.
• Tell patient to increase fluid intake.

## polyethylene glycol and electrolyte solution
Co-Lav, CoLyte, Glycoprep‡,
Go-Evac, GoLYTELY, Miralax,
NuLytely, OCL

*Pregnancy risk category C*

### AVAILABLE FORMS
*Powder for oral solution:* PEG 3350
(240 g), sodium sulfate (22.72 g), NaCl
(5.84 g), potassium chloride (2.98 g),
sodium bicarbonate (6.72 g) per 4 L
(CoLyte); PEG 3350 (60 g), NaCl
(745 mg), potassium chloride (0.745 g),
sodium sulfate decahydrate
PEG 3350 (236 g), sodium sul-
(22.74 g), sodium bicarbonate
NaCl (5.86 g), potassium chlo-
per 4 L (GoLYTELY); PEG 3350 (420 g),
sodium sulfate (5.685 g), sodium bicarbonate (1.685 g), NaCl (1.465 g), potassium chloride (0.743 g)/L (Go-Evac); PEG
3350 (420 g), sodium bicarbonate
(5.72 g), NaCl (11.2 g), potassium chloride (1.48 g) per 4 L (NuLYTELY); PEG
3350 (6 g), sodium sulfate decahydrate
(1.29 g), NaCl (146 mg), potassium chloride (75 mg), sodium bicarbonate

(168 mg), polysorbate-80 (30 mg) per 100 ml (OCL)

## INDICATIONS & DOSAGES
➤ **Bowel preparation before GI examination**
*Adults:* 240 ml P.O. q 10 minutes until 4 L are consumed or until watery stool is clear. Typically, give 4 hours before examination, allowing 3 hours for drinking and 1 hour for bowel evacuation.

## ACTION
PEG 3350, a nonabsorbable solution, acts as an osmotic product. Sodium sulfate greatly reduces sodium absorption. The electrolyte level causes virtually no net absorption or secretion of ions.

| Route | Onset | Peak | Duration |
|-------|-------|------|----------|
| P.O. | 1 hr | Variable | Variable |

## ADVERSE REACTIONS
**EENT:** rhinorrhea.
**GI:** *nausea, bloating, cramps, vomiting, abdominal fullness.*
**Skin:** urticaria, dermatitis, allergic reaction, anal irritation.

## INTERACTIONS
**Drug-drug.** *Oral drugs:* May decrease absorption if given within 1 hour of starting therapy. Give at least 2 to 3 hours before starting therapy.

## EFFECTS ON LAB TEST RESULTS
None reported.

## CONTRAINDICATIONS & CAUTIO...
• Contraindicated in patients w... struction or perforation... toxic colitis, or... solution, but use

...flavoring or additional ...the solution or give chilled ...ngesting large amounts of chilled solution.
• Give solution early in the morning... tient is scheduled for a mid-...ng ex-

amination. Oral solution induces diarrhea (onset 30 to 60 minutes) that rapidly cleans the bowel, usually within 4 hours.
• When using to prepare for barium enema, give solution the evening before the examination to avoid interfering with barium coating of the colonic mucosa.
• If given to semiconscious patient or to patient with impaired gag reflex, take care to prevent aspiration.
• No major shifts in fluid or electrolyte balance have been reported.
• Patient preparation for barium enema may be less satisfactory with this solution because it may interfere with the barium coating of the colonic mucosa using the double-contrast technique.

## PATIENT TEACHING
• Tell patient to fast for 3 to 4 hours before taking the solution, and thereafter to drink only clear fluids until examination is complete.
• Warn patient about adverse reactions.

---

## psyllium
Fiberall ◇, Genfiber ◇, Hydrocil Instant ◇, Konsyl ◇, Konsyl-D ◇, Metamucil ◇, Metamucil Effervescent Sugar Free ◇, Metamucil Sugar Free ◇, ...odane Bulk ◇, Mylanta N...ral Fiber Supplement ◇, Perdiem Fiber ◇, Prodiem Plain ◇, P...uloid ◇, Natural ◇, Syllact ◇

...category B

...LE FORMS
...escent powder: 3.4 g/packet ◇,
*Granules:* 2.5 g/tsp ◇,
*Powder:* 3.3 g/tsp ◇, 4.03 g/tsp ◇,
tsp ◇, 4.94 g/tsp ◇, 3.4 g/tsp ◇, 3.5 g/
3.4 g/tablespoon, 6 g/tsp, 3.4 g/packet, packet
3.5 g/scoopful, 6 g/
*Wafers:* 3.4 g/wafer ◇

## INDICATIONS & DOS...
➤ **Constipation**...
*Adults:* ...quid once daily, b.i.d., or t.i.d., ...ollowed by second glass of liquid. Or,

1 packet dissolved in water once daily, b.i.d., or t.i.d. Up to 30 g daily.
*Children older than age 6:* ½ rounded tsp P.O. in a full glass of liquid 1 to 3 times daily.

## ACTION
Bulk-forming laxative that absorbs water and expands to increase bulk and moisture content of stool, thus encouraging peristalsis and bowel movement.

| Route | Onset | Peak | Duration |
|---|---|---|---|
| P.O. | 12-24 hr | 3 days | Variable |

## ADVERSE REACTIONS
**GI:** nausea, vomiting, diarrhea with excessive use; esophageal, gastric, small intestine, and rectal obstruction when drug is taken in dry form; abdominal cramps, especially in severe constipation.

## INTERACTIONS
None significant.

## EFFECTS ON LAB TEST RESULTS
None reported.

## CONTRAINDICATIONS & CAUTIONS
● Contraindicated in patients hypersensitive to drug and in those with intestinal obstruction, intestinal ulceration, disabling adhesions, difficulty swallowing, or signs or symptoms of appendicitis, such as abdominal pain, nausea, or vomiting.

## NURSING CONSIDERATIONS
● Before giving drug for constipation, determine whether patient has adequate fluid intake, exercise, and diet.
● Mix with at least 8 ounces (240 ml) of cold, pleasant-tasting liquid such as orange juice to mask grittiness, and stir only a few seconds. Have patient drink mixture immediately so it doesn't congeal. Follow with additional glass of liquid.
● For dosages in children younger than age 6, consult prescriber.
● Drug may reduce appetite if taken before meals.
● Drug isn't absorbed systemically and is nontoxic; it's especially useful in debilitated patients and in those with postpartum constipation, irritable bowel syndrome, and diverticular disease. It's also used to treat

chronic laxative abuse and with other laxatives to empty colon before barium enema examinations.
● Patients with phenylketonuria should avoid psyllium products, which contain phenylalanine (Nutrasweet).

## PATIENT TEACHING
● Teach patient how to properly mix drug. Tell him to take drug with plenty of water (at least 8 ounces). Advise patient that inhaling powder may cause allergic reactions.
● Advise patient to seek medical attention if he experiences vomiting, chest pain, or difficulty breathing or swallowing after taking medication.
● Tell patient that laxative effect usually occurs in 12 to 24 hours, but may be delayed 3 days.
● Advise diabetic patient to check label and use a brand of psyllium that doesn't contain sugar.
● Teach patient about dietary sources of bulk, including bran and other cereals, fresh fruit, and vegetables.

---

## senna
Black-Draught◇*, Fletcher's Castoria◇, Senexon◇, Senna-Gen◇, Senokot◇, SenokotXTRA◇, X-Prep Liquid*◇

*Pregnancy risk category C*

## AVAILABLE FORMS
Liquid◇: as sennosides (active
Suppositories◇: 8.8 mg
Syrup◇: 8.8 mg
Tablets◇: 6 mg, 8.6 mg,
25 mg

## INDICATIONS & DOSAGES
➤ **Acute constipation, preparation for bowel examination**
*Black-Draught*
*Adults:* 2 tablets, or ¼ to ½ level tsp of granules mixed with water.

### Other preparations
*Adults and children age 12 and older:*
Usual dose is 2 tablets, 1 tsp of granules
dissolved in water, 1 suppository, or 10 to
15 ml syrup h.s. Maximum dose varies
with preparation used.
*Children ages 6 to 12:* ½ to 1 tablet, ½ tsp
of granules dissolved in water, ½ suppository h.s., or 1 to 1½ tsp syrup. Maximum
dose is 2 tablets b.i.d., 1 tsp of granules
b.i.d., or 1½ tsp of syrup b.i.d.
*Children ages 2 to 6:* ½ tablet, or ¼ tsp of
granules dissolved in water, or ½ to ¾ tsp
of syrup. Maximum dose is 1 tablet b.i.d.,
½ tsp of granules b.i.d., or ¾ tsp of syrup
b.i.d.

### ACTION
Unknown. Stimulant laxative that increases peristalsis, probably by direct effect on
smooth muscle of the intestine. It's
thought to either irritate the musculature
or stimulate the colonic intramural plexus.
Drug also promotes fluid accumulation in
colon and small intestine.

| Route | Onset | Peak | Duration |
|-------|-------|------|----------|
| P.O. | 6-10 hr | Variable | Variable |
| P.R. | 30-120 min | Unknown | Unknown |

### ADVERSE REACTIONS
**GI:** *nausea,* vomiting, diarrhea, loss of
normal bowel function with excessive use,
*abdominal cramps* especially in severe
constipation, malabsorption of nutrients,
cathartic colon with long-term misuse,
possible constipation after catharsis, yellow or yellow-green cast to feces, diarrhea
in breast-feeding infants of mothers taking
senna, darkened pigmentation of rectal
mucosa with long-term use, protein-losing
enteropathy.
**GU:** red-pink discoloration in alkaline
urine, yellow-brown discoloration in
acidic urine.
**Metabolic:** electrolyte imbalance such as
hypokalemia.
**Other:** laxative dependence with long-
term or excessive use.

### INTERACTIONS
None significant.

### EFFECTS ON LAB TEST RESULTS
• May alter fluid and electrolyte levels,
with prolonged use.

### CONTRAINDICATIONS & CAUTIONS
• Contraindicated in patients with ulcerative bowel lesions, fecal impaction, intestinal obstruction, intestinal perforation, or
signs and symptoms of appendicitis or
acute surgical abdomen, such as nausea,
vomiting, and abdominal pain.

### NURSING CONSIDERATIONS
• Before giving drug for constipation, determine whether patient has adequate fluid
intake, exercise, and diet.
• In phenolsulfonphthalein excretion test,
senna may turn urine pink to red, red to vi-
olet, or red to brown.
• Limit diet to clear liquids after X-Prep
Liquid is taken.
• Avoid exposing product to excessive
heat or light.
• Drug is for short-term use.
• Senna is one of the most effective laxatives for counteracting constipation caused
by narcotic analgesics.

### PATIENT TEACHING
• Teach patient about dietary sources of
bulk, including bran and other cereals,
fresh fruit, and vegetables.
• Tell patient to report persistent or severe
reactions.

## sodium phosphates
Fleet Phospho-soda ◇

*Pregnancy risk category* NR

### AVAILABLE FORMS
*Enema:* 160 mg/ml sodium phosphate and
60 mg/ml sodium biphosphate ◇
*Liquid:* 2.4 g/5 ml sodium phosphate and
900 mg sodium biphosphate/5 ml ◇

### INDICATIONS & DOSAGES
➤ **Constipation**
*Adults:* 20 to 30 ml solution ⌐⌐ 135 ml
120 ml cold water. ⌐ ⌐ ⌐ mixed with
P.R. as ⌐⌐⌐ to 15 ml solution mixed with
120 ml cold water P.O. Or, 67.5 ml P.R. as
enema.

## ACTION
Saline laxative that produces an osmotic effect in the small intestine by drawing water into the intestinal lumen.

| Route | Onset | Peak | Duration |
|-------|-------|------|----------|
| P.O. | 30-180 min | Variable | Variable |
| P.R. | 5-10 min | With effect | With effect |

## ADVERSE REACTIONS
**GI:** *abdominal cramping.*
**Metabolic:** fluid and electrolyte disturbances, such as hypernatremia and hyperphosphatemia, with daily use.
**Other:** laxative dependence with long-term or excessive use.

## INTERACTIONS
None significant.

## EFFECTS ON LAB TEST RESULTS
● May increase sodium and phosphate levels. May decrease electrolyte level with prolonged use.

## CONTRAINDICATIONS & CAUTIONS
● Contraindicated in patients on sodium-restricted diets and in patients with intestinal obstruction, intestinal perforation, edema, heart failure, megacolon, impaired renal function, or signs and symptoms of appendicitis or acute surgical abdomen, such as abdominal pain, nausea, or vomiting.
● Use cautiously in patients with large hemorrhoids or anal excoriations.

## NURSING CONSIDERATIONS
● Before giving drug for constipation, determine whether patient has adequate fluid intake, exercise, and diet.
● *Alert:* Up to 10% of sodium content of drug may be absorbed.
● *Alert:* Severe electrolyte imbalances may occur if recommended dosage is exceeded.

## PATIENT TEACHING
● Teach patient about dietary sources of fiber, including bran and other cereals, and stress importance of ~~vegetables.~~
● Warn patient ~~~~
for short-term therapy.

---

## sodium phosphate monohydrate and sodium phosphate dibasic anhydrous
Visicol

*Pregnancy risk category C*

## AVAILABLE FORMS
*Tablets:* 1.5 g sodium phosphate (1.102 g sodium phosphate monohydrate and 0.398 g sodium phosphate dibasic anhydrous)

## INDICATIONS & DOSAGES
➤ **To cleanse the bowel before colonoscopy**
*Adults:* 40 tablets taken in the following manner. The evening before the procedure, 3 tablets P.O. with at least 8 ounces of clear liquid q 15 minutes, for a total of 20 tablets. The last dose will be only 2 tablets. The day of the procedure, 3 tablets P.O. with at least 8 ounces of clear liquid q 15 minutes, for a total of 20 tablets, starting 3 to 5 hours before the procedure. The last dose will be only 2 tablets.

## ACTION
Induces diarrhea that rapidly and effectively evacuates the colon by causing large amounts of water to be drawn into the colon, promoting evacuation.

| Route | Onset | Peak | Duration |
|-------|-------|------|----------|
| P.O. | Rapid | Varies | 1-3 hr |

## ADVERSE REACTIONS
**CNS:** headache, dizziness.
**GI:** nausea, vomiting, abdominal bloating, abdominal pain.

## INTERACTIONS
**Drug-drug.** *Any drugs:* Reduces absorption of these drugs. Separate doses.

## EFFECTS ON LAB TEST RESULTS
● May increase phosphorus level (typically normalizes 48 to 72 hours after giving drug). May decrease potassium and calcium levels.

## CONTRAINDICATIONS & CAUTIONS
● Contraindicated in patients hypersensitive to sodium phosphate or any of its in-

gredients. Avoid giving drug to patients with heart failure, ascites, unstable angina, gastric retention, ileus, acute intestinal obstruction, pseudo-obstruction, severe chronic constipation, bowel perforation, acute colitis, toxic megacolon, or hypomotility syndrome (hypothyroidism, scleroderma).

• Use cautiously in patients with a history of electrolyte abnormalities, current electrolyte abnormalities, or impaired renal function. Also use cautiously in patients who take drugs that can induce electrolyte abnormalities or prolong the QT interval.

• Use cautiously in elderly patients because they may be more sensitive to drug effects.

## NURSING CONSIDERATIONS

• Correct electrolyte imbalances before giving drug.

• As with other sodium phosphate cathartic preparations, this drug may induce colonic mucosal ulceration.

• Monitor patient for signs of dehydration.

• Don't repeat administration within 7 days.

• No enema or laxative is needed in addition to drug. Patients shouldn't take any additional purgatives, particularly those that contain sodium phosphate.

• *Alert:* Administration of other sodium phosphate products has caused death from significant fluid shifts, electrolyte abnormalities, and cardiac arrhythmias. Patients with electrolyte disturbances have an increased risk of prolonged QT interval. Use drug cautiously in patients who are taking other drugs known to prolong the QT interval.

## PATIENT TEACHING

• Urge patient to drink at least 8 ounces of clear liquid with each dose. Inadequate fluid intake may lead to excessive fluid loss and hypovolemia.

• Tell patient to drink only clear liquids for at least 12 hours before starting the purgative regimen.

• Caution patient against taking an additional enema or laxative, particularly one that contains sodium phosphate.

• Tell patient that undigested or partially digested Visicol tablets and other drugs may appear in the stool.

---

aprepitant
chlorpromazine hydrochloride
   (See Chapter 31, ANTIPSYCHOTICS.)
dimenhydrinate
dolasetron mesylate
dronabinol
granisetron hydrochloride
meclizine hydrochloride
metoclopramide hydrochloride
ondansetron hydrochloride
palonosetron
perphenazine
   (See Chapter 31, ANTIPSYCHOTICS.)
prochlorperazine
prochlorperazine edisylate
prochlorperazine maleate
promethazine hydrochloride
   (See Chapter 40, ANTIHISTAMINES.)
scopolamine
   (See Chapter 36, ANTICHOLINERGICS.)
trimethobenzamide hydrochloride

**COMBINATION PRODUCTS**
None.

✳ *NEW DRUG*

## aprepitant
Emend

*Pregnancy risk category B*

**AVAILABLE FORMS**
*Capsules:* 80 mg, 125 mg

**INDICATIONS & DOSAGES**
➤ **To prevent nausea and vomiting
after highly emetogenic chemotherapy
(including cisplatin); given with a
5-HT$_3$ antagonist and a corticosteroid**
*Adults:* On day 1 of chemotherapy,
125 mg P.O. 1 hour before treatment; then
80 mg P.O. q morning on days 2 and 3 of
chemotherapy.

**ACTION**
Selectively antagonizes substance P and
neurokinin-1 receptors in the brain; appears to be synergistic with 5-HT$_3$ antagonists and corticosteroids.

| Route | Onset | Peak | Duration |
|-------|-------|------|----------|
| P.O. | Unknown | 4 hr | Unknown |

**ADVERSE REACTIONS**
**CNS:** *asthenia,* dizziness, *fatigue,* fever,
headache, insomnia.
**EENT:** mucous membrane disorder, tinni-
tus.
**GI:** abdominal pain, *anorexia, constipa-
tion, diarrhea,* epigastric pain, gastritis,
heartburn, *nausea,* vomiting.
**Hematologic:** *neutropenia.*
**Respiratory:** hiccups.
**Other:** dehydration.

**INTERACTIONS**
**Drug-drug.** *Alprazolam, midazolam, triazolam:* May increase levels of these drugs.
Watch for CNS effects, such as increased
sedation. Decrease benzodiazepine dose
by 50%.
*Carbamazepine, phenytoin, rifampin,
other CYP3A4 inducers:* May decrease
aprepitant level. Watch for decreased antiemetic effect.
*Clarithromycin, diltiazem, erythromycin,
itraconazole, ketoconazole, nefazodone,
nelfinavir, ritonavir, troleandomycin, and
other CYP3A4 inhibitors:* May increase
aprepitant level and risk of toxicity. Use
together cautiously.
*Dexamethasone, methylprednisolone:*
May increase levels of these drugs and
risk of toxicity. Decrease oral corticosteroid dose by 50%; decrease I.V. methylprednisolone dose by 25%.
*Diltiazem:* May increase diltiazem level.
Monitor heart rate and blood pressure.
Avoid using together.
*Docetaxel, etoposide, ifosfamide, imatinib,
irinotecan, paclitaxel, vinorelbine, vinblastine, vincristine:* May increase levels
and risk of toxicity of these drugs. Use together cautiously.
*Hormonal contraceptives:* May decrease
contraceptive effectiveness. Tell women to

use additional birth control method during therapy.

*Paroxetine:* May decrease paroxetine and aprepitant effects. Monitor patient for effectiveness.

*Phenytoin:* May decrease phenytoin level. Monitor level carefully, and increase phenytoin dose as needed during therapy. Avoid using together.

*Pimozide:* May increase pimozide level. Avoid using together.

*Tolbutamide:* May decrease tolbutamide effects. Monitor glucose level.

*Warfarin:* May decrease warfarin effectiveness. Monitor INR carefully for 2 weeks after each aprepitant treatment.

**Drug-herb.** *St. John's wort:* May decrease antiemetic effects by inducing CYP 3A4. Discourage use together.

**Drug-food.** *Grapefruit juice:* May increase aprepitant level and risk of toxicity. Discourage use together.

### EFFECTS ON LAB TEST RESULTS
● May increase creatinine, AST, ALT, alkaline phosphatase, BUN, glucose, and urine protein levels. May decrease sodium level.
● May increase RBC and WBC counts. May decrease neutrophil count.

### CONTRAINDICATIONS & CAUTIONS
● Contraindicated in patients hypersensitive to aprepitant or its components.
● Use cautiously in patients receiving chemotherapy drugs metabolized mainly via CYP 3A4 and in those with severe hepatic disease.
● Give drug to pregnant women only when benefit clearly outweighs risk.
● It's unknown if drug appears in breast milk. Don't give to breast-feeding women.
● Safety and efficacy haven't been established in children.

### NURSING CONSIDERATIONS
● Avoid giving drug for more than 3 days per chemotherapy cycle.
● *Alert:* Before giving drug, screen patient carefully for possible drug or herb interactions.
● Don't give drug for existing nausea or vomiting.
● Expect to give drug with other antiemetics to treat breakthrough emesis.

● Monitor CBC, liver function test results, and creatinine level periodically during therapy.

### PATIENT TEACHING
● Tell patient that aprepitant is given with other antiemetics and shouldn't be taken alone to prevent chemotherapy-induced nausea and vomiting.
● If nausea or vomiting occurs, instruct patient to take breakthrough antiemetics rather than taking more aprepitant.
● Urge patient to report use of any other prescription, nonprescription, or herbal medicines.
● Caution patient against taking drug with grapefruit juice.
● Advise woman who takes a hormonal contraceptive to use an additional form of birth control during aprepitant therapy.
● Tell patient who takes warfarin that PT and INR will be monitored closely for 2 weeks after aprepitant therapy starts.

## dimenhydrinate
Andrumin‡, Apo-Dimenhydrinate†, Calm-X ◇, Children's Dramamine ◇ *, Dramamine ◇ *, Dramamine Liquid ◇ *, Driminate, Dymenate, Gravol†, Gravol L/A†, Hydrate, PMS-Dimenhydrinate†, Triptone Caplets ◇

*Pregnancy risk category B*

### AVAILABLE FORMS
*Elixir:* 15 mg/5 ml†
*Injection:* 50 mg/ml
*Syrup:* 12.5 mg/4 ml* ◇, 15.62 mg/5 ml
*Tablets:* 50 mg ◇
*Tablets (chewable):* 50 mg ◇

### INDICATIONS & DOSAGES
➤ **To prevent and treat motion sickness**
*Adults and children age 12 and older:* 50 to 100 mg P.O. q 4 to 6 hours; 50 mg I.M., p.r.n.; or 50 mg I.V. diluted in 10 ml normal saline solution for injection, injected over 2 minutes. Maximum, 400 mg daily. For prevention, take 30 minutes before motion exposure.
*Children ages 6 to 11:* 25 to 50 mg P.O. q 6 to 8 hours, not to exceed 150 mg in 24 hours. Or, 1.25 mg/kg or 37.5 mg/m$^2$

I.M. or P.O. q.i.d. Maximum, 300 mg
daily.
*Children ages 2 to 5:* 12.5 to 25 mg P.O. q
6 to 8 hours, not to exceed 75 mg in
24 hours. Or, 1.25 mg/kg or 37.5 mg/m$^2$
I.M. or P.O. q.i.d. Maximum, 300 mg
daily.

## I.V. ADMINISTRATION
● Dilute each milliliter (50 mg) of drug
with 10 ml of sterile water for injection,
$D_5W$, or normal saline solution for injection.
● Give by direct injection over at least 2
minutes.

## ACTION
Unknown. May affect neural pathways
originating in the labyrinth to inhibit nausea and vomiting.

| Route | Onset | Peak | Duration |
|-------|-------|------|----------|
| P.O. | 15-30 min | Unknown | 3-6 hr |
| I.V. | Immediate | Unknown | 3-6 hr |
| I.M. | 20-30 min | Unknown | 3-6 hr |

## ADVERSE REACTIONS
**CNS:** *drowsiness,* headache, dizziness,
confusion, nervousness, vertigo, tingling
and weakness of hands, lassitude, excitation, insomnia.
**CV:** palpitations, hypotension, tachycardia.
**EENT:** blurred vision, dry respiratory
passages, diplopia, nasal congestion.
**GI:** dry mouth, nausea, vomiting, diarrhea, epigastric distress, constipation,
anorexia.
**GU:** urine retention.
**Respiratory:** wheezing, thickened
bronchial secretions.
**Skin:** photosensitivity, urticaria, rash.
**Other:** *anaphylaxis,* tightness of chest.

## INTERACTIONS
**Drug-drug.** *CNS depressants:* May cause
additive CNS depression. Avoid using together.
*Ototoxic drugs:* Dimenhydrinate may
mask symptoms of ototoxicity. Use together cautiously.
*Tricyclic antidepressants, other anti-
cholinergics:* May increase anticholinergic
activity. Monitor patient.

**Drug-lifestyle.** *Alcohol use:* May cause
additive CNS depression. Discourage use
together.

## EFFECTS ON LAB TEST RESULTS
● May prevent, reduce, or mask diagnostic
skin test response. May alter xanthine test
results.

## CONTRAINDICATIONS & CAUTIONS
● Contraindicated in patients hypersensitive to drug or its components.
● Use cautiously in elderly patients, patients receiving ototoxic drugs, and patients with seizures, acute angle-closure
glaucoma, or enlarged prostate gland.

## NURSING CONSIDERATIONS
● Elderly patients may be more susceptible
to adverse CNS effects.
● Undiluted solution irritates veins and
may cause sclerosis.
● Drug may alter or confuse test results for
xanthines (caffeine, aminophylline) because of its 8-chlorotheophylline content.
● Stop drug 4 days before diagnostic skin
tests to prevent falsifying test response.
● Dramamine may contain tartrazine.
● *Alert:* Drug may mask symptoms of ototoxicity, brain tumor, or intestinal obstruction.
● *Alert:* Don't confuse dimenhydrinate
with diphenhydramine.

## PATIENT TEACHING
● Advise patient to avoid activities that require alertness until CNS effects of drug
are known.
● Instruct patient to report adverse reactions promptly.

## dolasetron mesylate
Anzemet

*Pregnancy risk category B*

## AVAILABLE FORMS
*Injection:* 20 mg/ml as 12.5 mg/0.625 ml
ampule or 100 mg/5 ml vials
*Tablets:* 50 mg, 100 mg

# Nursing2005 Drug Handbook
## Photoguide to tablets and capsules

This photoguide presents nearly 400 tablets and capsules, representing the most commonly prescribed generic and trade name drugs. These drugs, organized alphabetically by generic name, are shown in actual size and color with cross-references to drug information. Each product is labeled with its trade name and its strength.

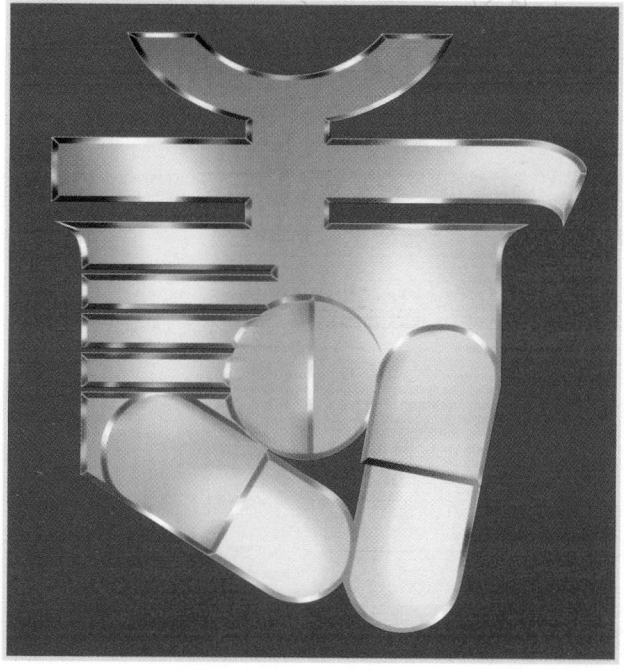

Adapted from Facts and Comparisons, St. Louis, Missouri.
For the list of companies permitting use of these photographs,
see pages 1343-1344.

## ACETAMINOPHEN WITH CODEINE

### Tylenol with Codeine No. 3
(page 383)

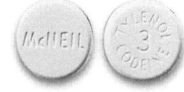

300/30 mg

## ACYCLOVIR

### Zovirax
(page 150)

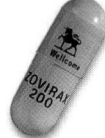 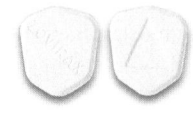 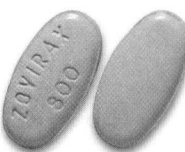

200 mg          400 mg          800 mg

## ALENDRONATE SODIUM

### Fosamax
(page 841)

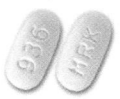  

10 mg          40 mg          70 mg

## ALFUZOSIN HYDROCHLORIDE

### UroXatral
(page 1267)

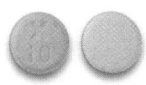

10 mg

## ALOSETRON HYDROCHLORIDE

### Lotronex
(page 715)

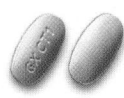

1 mg

## ALPRAZOLAM

### Xanax
(page 472)

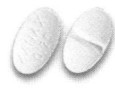 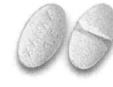 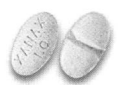

0.25 mg          0.5 mg          1 mg

## AMIODARONE

**Cordarone**
(page 233)

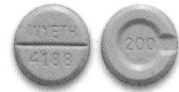

200 mg

## AMLODIPINE BESYLATE

**Norvasc**
(page 256)

 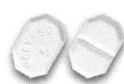

2.5 mg          5 mg

## AMOXICILLIN AND CLAVULANATE POTASSIUM

**Augmentin**
(page 75)

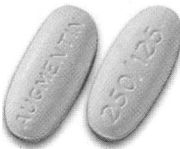 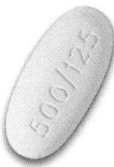 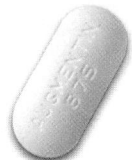

250 mg          500 mg          875 mg

**Augmentin Chewable**
(page 75)

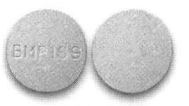 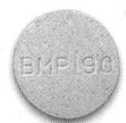

125 mg          250 mg

## AMOXICILLIN TRIHYDRATE

**Amoxil**
(page 77)

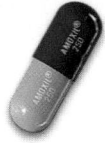 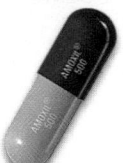

250 mg          500 mg

## ANASTROZOLE

**Arimidex**
(page 973)

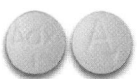

1 mg

## ARIPIPRAZOLE

**Abilify**
(page 485)

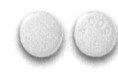

15 mg

## ATAZANAVIR SULFATE

**Reyataz**
(page 156)

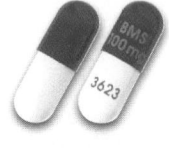 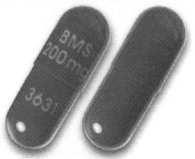

100 mg       200 mg

## ATENOLOL

**Tenormin**
(page 272)

 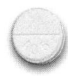 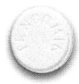

25 mg     50 mg     100 mg

## ATOMOXETINE HYDROCHLORIDE

**Strattera**
(page 540)

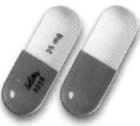 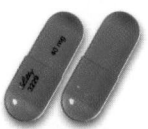

25 mg      40 mg

## ATORVASTATIN CALCIUM

**Lipitor**
(page 322)

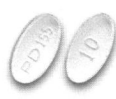 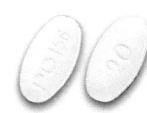

10 mg      20 mg

## AZITHROMYCIN

**Zithromax**
(page 201)

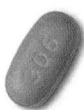

250 mg

## BENAZEPRIL HYDROCHLORIDE

### Lotensin
(page 274)

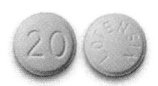 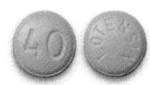

20 mg 40 mg

## BUMETANIDE

### Bumex
(page 854)

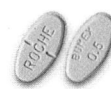 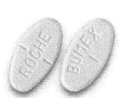 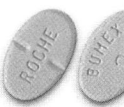

0.5 mg 1 mg 2 mg

## BUPROPION HYDROCHLORIDE

### Wellbutrin
(page 447)

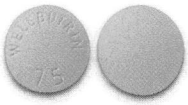 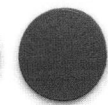 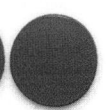

75 mg 100 mg

### Wellbutrin SR
(page 447)

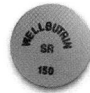 

150 mg

### Zyban
(page 541)

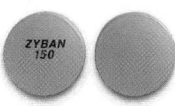

150 mg

## BUSPIRONE HYDROCHLORIDE

### BuSpar
(page 473)

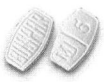 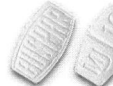

5 mg 10 mg

## CAPTOPRIL

**Capoten**
(page 278)

12.5 mg

25 mg

## CARISOPRODOL

**Soma**
(page 586)

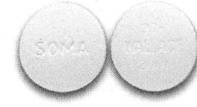
350 mg

## CARVEDILOL

**Coreg**
(page 281)

3.125 mg

6.25 mg

12.5 mg

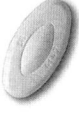
25 mg

## CEFADROXIL

**Duricef**
(page 97)

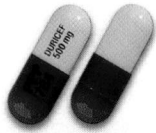
500 mg

1000 mg

## CEFPROZIL

**Cefzil**
(page 111)

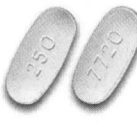
250 mg

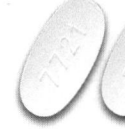
500 mg

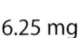

**CEFUROXIME AXETIL**

**Ceftin**
(page 116)

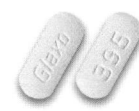 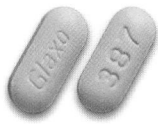 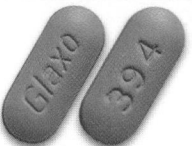

125 mg         250 mg         500 mg

**CELECOXIB**

**Celebrex**
(page 359)

 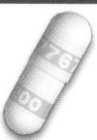

100 mg         200 mg

**CETIRIZINE HYDROCHLORIDE**

**Zyrtec**
(page 607)

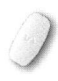 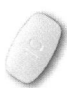

5 mg         10 mg

**CILOSTAZOL**

**Pletal**
(page 342)

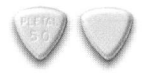 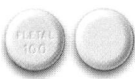

50 mg         100 mg

**CIMETIDINE**

**Tagamet**
(page 701)

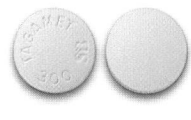 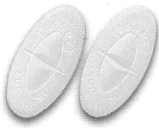 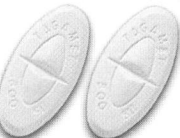

300 mg         400 mg         800 mg

**CIPROFLOXACIN**

**Cipro**
(page 135)

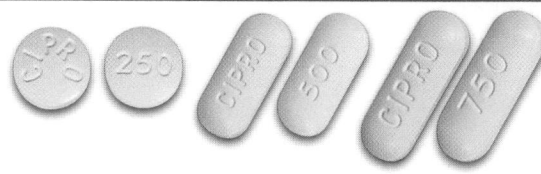

250 mg         500 mg         750 mg

## CITALOPRAM HYDROBROMIDE

**Celexa**
(page 448)

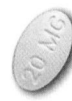 

20 mg            40 mg

## CLARITHROMYCIN

**Biaxin**
(page 203)

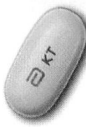 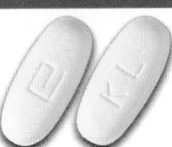

250 mg        500 mg

**Biaxin XL**
(page 203)

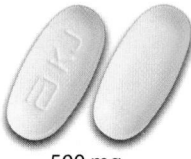

500 mg

## CLONAZEPAM

**Klonopin**
(page 421)

0.5 mg            1 mg            2 mg

## CO-TRIMOXAZOLE

**Bactrim DS**
(page 130)

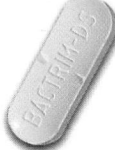

160/800 mg

## DESLORATADINE

**Clarinex**
(page 610)

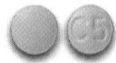

5 mg

### DIAZEPAM

**Valium**
(page 477)

2 mg          5 mg          10 mg

### DIGOXIN

**Lanoxin**
(page 227)

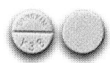 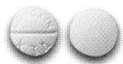

0.125 mg          0.25 mg

### DILTIAZEM HYDROCHLORIDE

**Cardizem**
(page 257)

 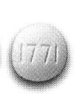 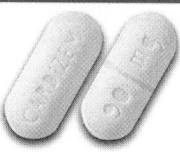

30 mg          90 mg

**Cardizem CD**
(page 257)

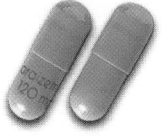 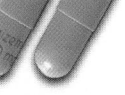 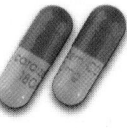 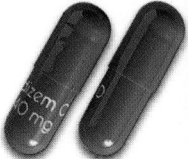

120 mg          180 mg          240 mg

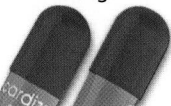 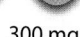 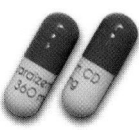

300 mg          360 mg

**Cardizem LA**
(page 257)

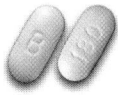 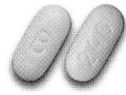 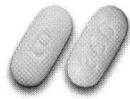

180 mg          240 mg          360 mg

## DILTIAZEM HYDROCHLORIDE

### Cardizem SR
(page 257)

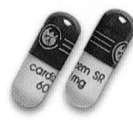 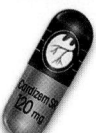

60 mg      120 mg

## DIVALPROEX SODIUM

### Depakote
(page 441)

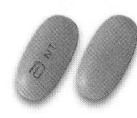 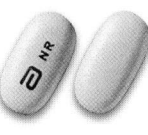 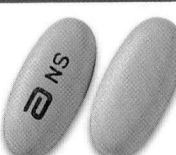

125 mg      250 mg      500 mg

### Depakote Sprinkle
(page 441)

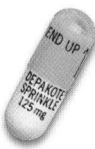

125 mg

## DOXAZOSIN MESYLATE

### Cardura
(page 286)

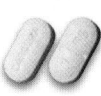 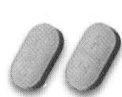 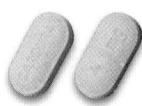

1 mg      2 mg      4 mg

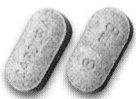

8 mg

## ELETRIPTAN HYDROBROMIDE

### Relpax
(page 545)

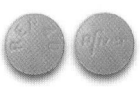

40 mg

## ENALAPRIL MALEATE

**Vasotec**
(page 287)

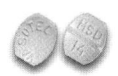 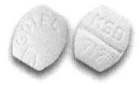 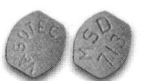

2.5 mg      5 mg      10 mg

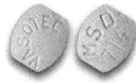

20 mg

## ERYTHROMYCIN BASE

**E-Mycin**
(page 205)

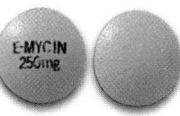 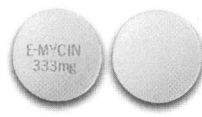

250 mg      333 mg

**Eryc**
(page 205)

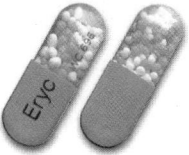

250 mg

**Ery-Tab**
(page 205)

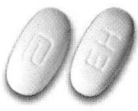

333 mg

## ESCITALOPRAM OXALATE

**Lexapro**
(page 454)

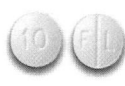 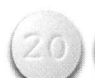 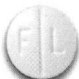

10 mg      20 mg

## ESTRADIOL

**Estrace**
(page 758)

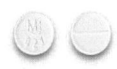

0.5 mg       1 mg       2 mg

## ESTROGENS, CONJUGATED

**Premarin**
(page 763)

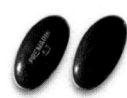 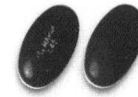 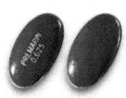

0.3 mg       0.45 mg       0.625 mg

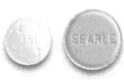 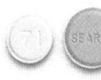

0.9 mg       1.25 mg       2.5 mg

## ETHINYL ESTRADIOL AND ETHYNODIOL DIACETATE

**Demulen**
(page 769)

1 mg/35 mcg       1 mg/50 mcg

## ETHINYL ESTRADIOL AND NORETHINDRONE

**Ovcon-35**
(page 770)

0.4 mg/35 mcg

## EZETIMIBE

**Zetia**
(page 325)

10 mg

## FAMOTIDINE

**Pepcid**
(page 704)

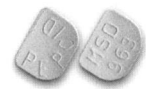 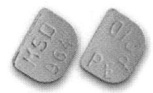

20 mg          40 mg

## FEXOFENADINE HYDROCHLORIDE

**Allegra**
(page 613)

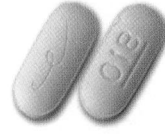

180 mg

## FLUCONAZOLE

**Diflucan**
(page 37)

50 mg          100 mg          150 mg

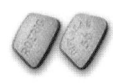                              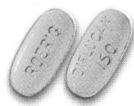

200 mg

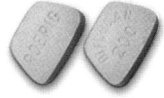

## FLUOXETINE HYDROCHLORIDE

**Prozac**
(page 455)

10 mg          20 mg          90 mg

**Sarafem**
(page 455)

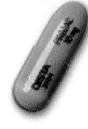 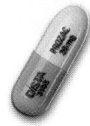

10 mg          20 mg

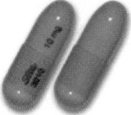 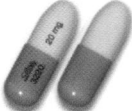

## FLUVASTATIN SODIUM

**Lescol**
(page 328)

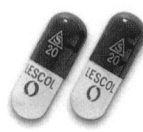 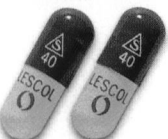

20 mg      40 mg

## FOSINOPRIL SODIUM

**Monopril**
(page 292)

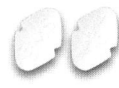 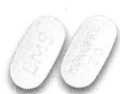 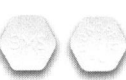

10 mg      20 mg      40 mg

## FROVATRIPTAN

**Frova**
(page 547)

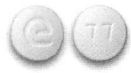

2.5 mg

## FUROSEMIDE

**Lasix**
(page 857)

 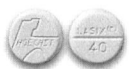 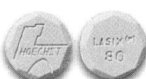

20 mg      40 mg      80 mg

## GABAPENTIN

**Neurontin**
(page 425)

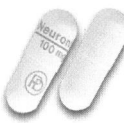 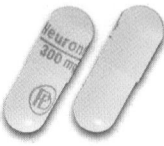 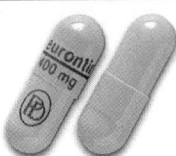

100 mg      300 mg      400 mg

## GEMFIBROZIL

**Lopid**
(page 329)

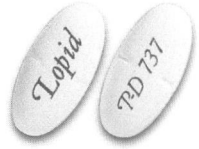

600 mg

## GLIPIZIDE

**Glucotrol**
(page 793)

5 mg          10 mg

**Glucotrol XL**
(page 793)

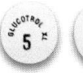  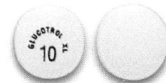

2.5 mg        5 mg        10 mg

## GLYBURIDE

**DiaBeta**
(page 797)

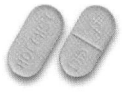  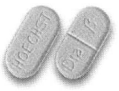 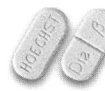

1.25 mg       2.5 mg       5 mg

**Micronase**
(page 797)

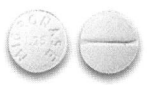  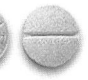 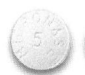 

1.25 mg       2.5 mg       5 mg

## HYDROCHLOROTHIAZIDE

**HydroDIURIL**
(page 859)

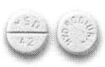 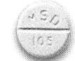 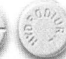

25 mg          50 mg

## HYDROCODONE BITARTRATE AND ACETAMINOPHEN

**Lortab**
(page 383)

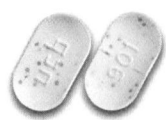 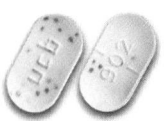 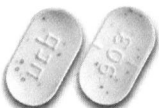

2.5 mg/500 mg     5 mg/500 mg     7.5 mg/500 mg

**Vicodin**
(page 383)

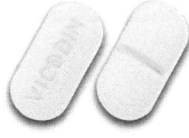

5 mg/500 mg

**Vicodin ES**
(page 383)

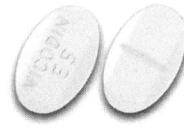

7.5 mg/750 mg

## IBUPROFEN

**Motrin**
(page 364)

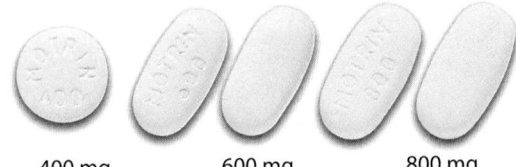

400 mg     600 mg     800 mg

## IMATINIB MESYLATE

**Gleevec**
(page 1007)

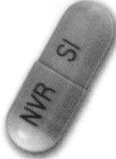

100 mg

## INDINAVIR SULFATE

**Crixivan**
(page 174)

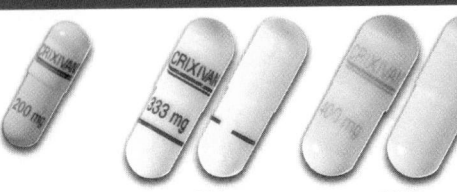

200 mg     333 mg     400 mg

## LAMIVUDINE AND ZIDOVUDINE

**Combivir**
(page 178)

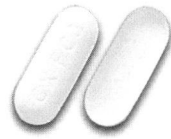

150 mg/300 mg

## LANSOPRAZOLE

**Prevacid**
(page 705)

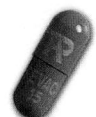 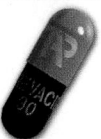

15 mg                30 mg

## LEVODOPA AND CARBIDOPA

**Sinemet**
(page 528)

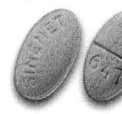 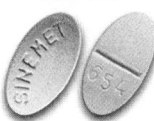

10 mg/100 mg     25 mg/250 mg

**Sinemet CR**
(page 528)

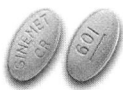

25 mg/100 mg

## LEVODOPA, CARBIDOPA, AND ENTACAPONE

**Stalevo**
(page 530)

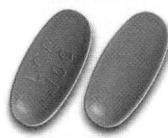 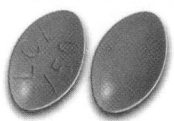

100 mg            150 mg

## LEVOFLOXACIN

**Levaquin**
(page 141)

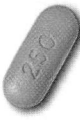 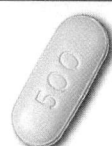

250 mg            500 mg

**LEVOTHYROXINE SODIUM**

### Levoxyl
(page 821)

25 mcg

50 mcg

75 mcg

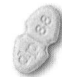

88 mcg

100 mcg

112 mcg

125 mcg

137 mcg

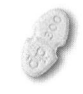

150 mcg

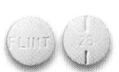

175 mcg

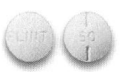

200 mcg

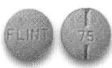

300 mcg

### Synthroid
(page 821)

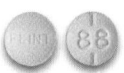

0.025 mg

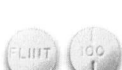

0.05 mg

0.075 mg

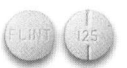

0.088 mg

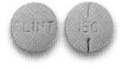

0.1 mg

0.112 mg

0.125 mg

0.15 mg

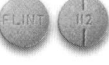

0.175 mg

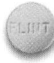

0.2 mg

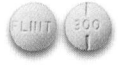

0.3 mg

## LISINOPRIL

**Prinivil**
(page 297)

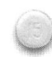  

| 2.5 mg | 5 mg | 10 mg |

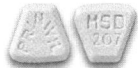 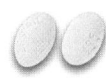  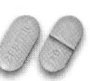  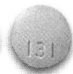

| 20 mg | 40 mg |

**Zestril**
(page 297)

| 2.5 mg | 5 mg | 10 mg |

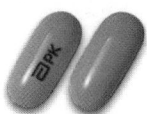

| 20 mg | 40 mg |

## LOPINAVIR AND RITONAVIR

**Kaletra**
(page 179)

133.3 mg/33.3 mg

## LOSARTAN POTASSIUM

**Cozaar**
(page 298)

| 25 mg | 50 mg |

## LOVASTATIN

### Mevacor
(page 330)

  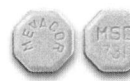  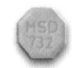

|       |       |       |
|-------|-------|-------|
| 10 mg | 20 mg | 40 mg |

## MEDROXYPROGESTERONE ACETATE

### Provera
(page 776)

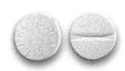  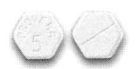  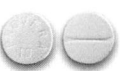

|        |      |       |
|--------|------|-------|
| 2.5 mg | 5 mg | 10 mg |

## MEPERIDINE HYDROCHLORIDE

### Demerol
(page 392)

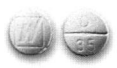  

|       |        |
|-------|--------|
| 50 mg | 100 mg |

## METFORMIN HYDROCHLORIDE

### Glucophage
(page 810)

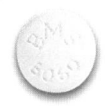  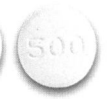  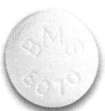  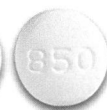

|        |        |
|--------|--------|
| 500 mg | 850 mg |

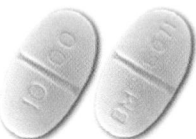

1000 mg

### Glucophage XR
(page 810)

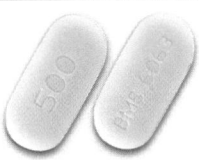

500 mg

## METHYLPHENIDATE HYDROCHLORIDE

**Concerta**
(page 517)

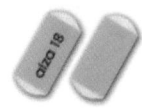 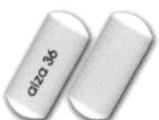 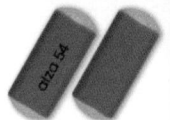

| 18 mg | 36 mg | 54 mg |

**Ritalin**
(page 517)

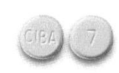 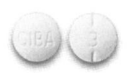 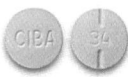

| 5 mg | 10 mg | 20 mg |

**Ritalin-SR**
(page 517)

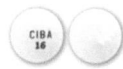

20 mg

## METHYLPREDNISOLONE

**Medrol**
(page 733)

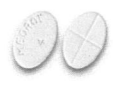 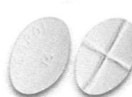

| 4 mg | 16 mg |

## METOPROLOL SUCCINATE

**Toprol-XL**
(page 302)

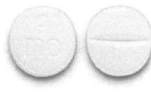 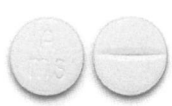 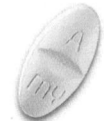

| 50 mg | 100 mg | 200 mg |

## MONTELUKAST SODIUM

**Singulair**
(page 656)

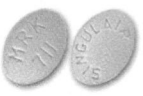  

| 4 mg | 5 mg | 10 mg |

**NABUMETONE**

**Relafen**
(page 373)

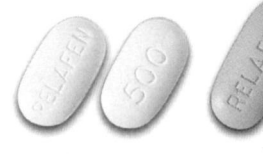

500 mg          750 mg

**NAPROXEN**

**Naprosyn**
(page 374)

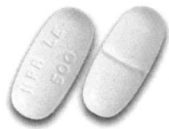

500 mg

**NEFAZODONE HYDROCHLORIDE**

**Serzone**
(page 460)

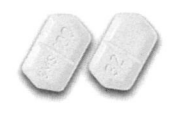       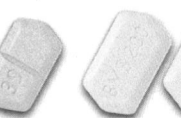

100 mg          150 mg          200 mg

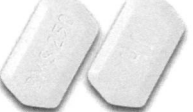

250 mg

**NIFEDIPINE**

**Procardia**
(page 263)

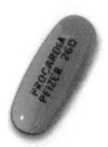       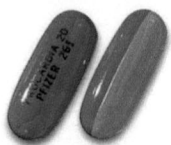

10 mg          20 mg

**Procardia XL**
(page 263)

              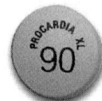

30 mg          60 mg          90 mg

## NITROFURANTOIN MACROCRYSTALS

**Macrobid**
(page 221)

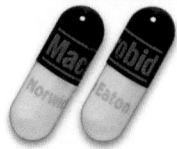

100 mg

## NITROGLYCERIN

**Nitrostat**
(page 264)

0.4 mg

## NORTRIPTYLINE HYDROCHLORIDE

**Pamelor**
(page 461)

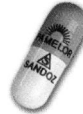        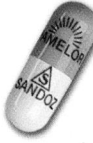        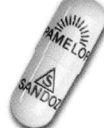

10 mg                25 mg                50 mg

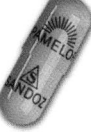

75 mg

## OFLOXACIN

**Floxin**
(page 146)

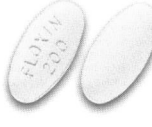        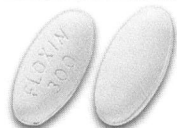        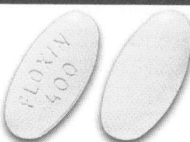

200 mg            300 mg            400 mg

## OLMESARTAN MEDOXOMIL

**Benicar**
(page 307)

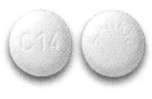        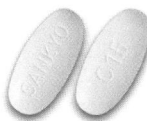

20 mg                40 mg

## OMEPRAZOLE

**Prilosec**
(page 708)

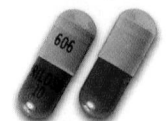 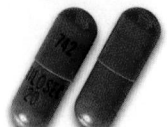 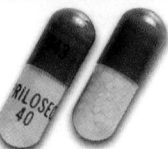

10 mg          20 mg          40 mg

## OXYCODONE HYDROCHLORIDE

**OxyContin**
(page 399)

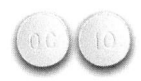 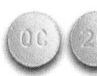 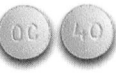

10 mg          20 mg          40 mg

80 mg

## PAROXETINE HYDROCHLORIDE

**Paxil**
(page 462)

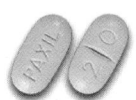 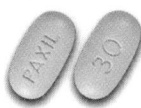

20 mg          30 mg

## PENTOXIFYLLINE

**Trental**
(page 348)

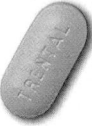

400 mg

## PHENYTOIN SODIUM

**Dilantin Kapseals**
(page 434)

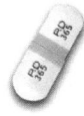 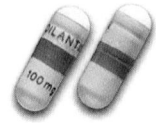

30 mg          100 mg

## POTASSIUM CHLORIDE

**K-Dur 20**
(page 876)

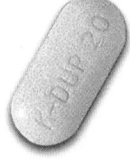

20 mEq

## PRAVASTATIN SODIUM

**Pravachol**
(page 332)

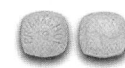 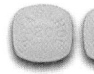 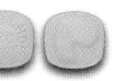 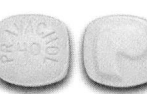

10 mg          20 mg          40 mg

## PREDNISONE

**Deltasone**
(page 738)

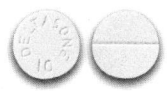 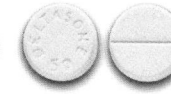

10 mg          50 mg

## PROCHLORPERAZINE

**Compazine**
(page 698)

 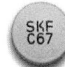

5 mg          10 mg

## PROMETHAZINE HYDROCHLORIDE

**Phenergan**
(page 614)

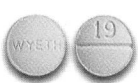 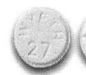 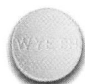 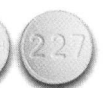

12.5 mg          25 mg          50 mg

## PROPRANOLOL HYDROCHLORIDE

### Inderal
(page 266)

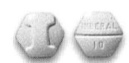

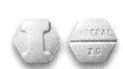

10 mg          20 mg          40 mg

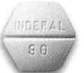

60 mg          80 mg

### Inderal LA
(page 266)

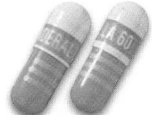

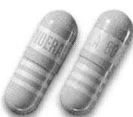

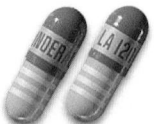

60 mg          80 mg          120 mg

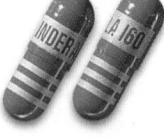

160 mg

## QUINAPRIL HYDROCHLORIDE

### Accupril
(page 312)

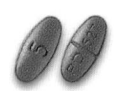

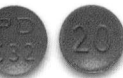

5 mg          10 mg          20 mg

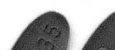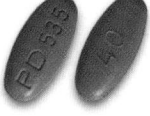

40 mg

## RALOXIFENE HYDROCHLORIDE

### Evista
(page 1287)

60 mg

## RANITIDINE HYDROCHLORIDE

**Zantac**
(page 712)

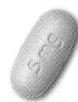 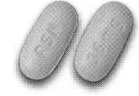

150 mg          300 mg

## RISEDRONATE SODIUM

**Actonel**
(page 846)

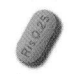 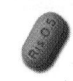

5 mg          35 mg

## RISPERIDONE

**Risperdal**
(page 504)

          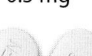          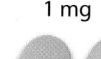

0.25 mg          0.5 mg          1 mg

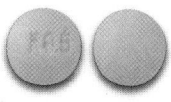

2 mg          3 mg          4 mg

**Risperdal M-Tab**
(page 504)

0.5 mg

## ROFECOXIB

**Vioxx**
(page 377)

                    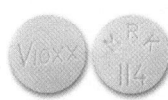

12.5 mg          25 mg          50 mg

## ROSIGLITAZONE MALEATE

**Avandia**
(page 817)

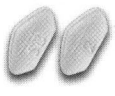          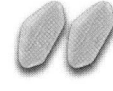          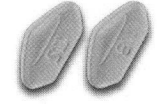

2 mg          4 mg          8 mg

## ROSUVASTATIN CALCIUM

### Crestor
(page 333)

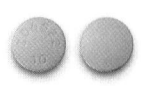 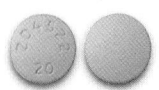

10 mg        20 mg

## SERTRALINE HYDROCHLORIDE

### Zoloft
(page 466)

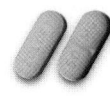 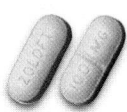

50 mg        100 mg

## SILDENAFIL CITRATE

### Viagra
(page 1289)

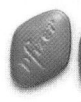 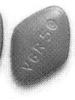 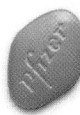 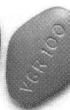

50 mg        100 mg

## SIMVASTATIN

### Zocor
(page 335)

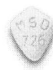  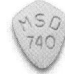

5 mg        10 mg        20 mg

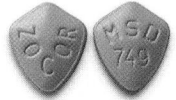

40 mg

## SUCRALFATE

### Carafate
(page 713)

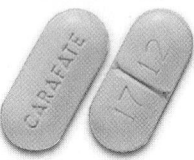

1 g

## SUMATRIPTAN SUCCINATE

**Imitrex**
(page 558)

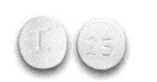 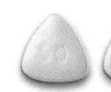 

25 mg          50 mg

## TAMOXIFEN CITRATE

**Nolvadex**
(page 982)

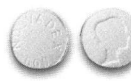  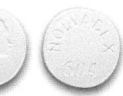

10 mg          20 mg

## TEMAZEPAM

**Restoril**
(page 414)

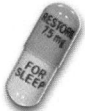 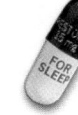 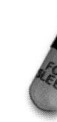

7.5 mg          15 mg          30 mg

## TENOFOVIR DISOPROXIL FUMARATE

**Viread**
(page 192)

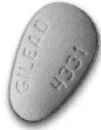

300 mg

## TERAZOSIN HYDROCHLORIDE

**Hytrin**
(page 317)

   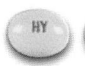    

1 mg          2 mg          5 mg

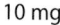

10 mg

## TICLOPIDINE HYDROCHLORIDE

**Ticlid**
(page 349)

250 mg

## TOLTERODINE TARTRATE

**Detrol**
(page 1245)

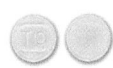        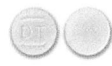

1 mg                       2 mg

## TRAMADOL HYDROCHLORIDE AND ACETAMINOPHEN

**Ultracet**
(page 383)

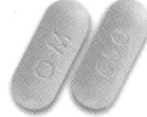

37.5 mg/325 mg

## TRAZODONE HYDROCHLORIDE

**Desyrel**
(page 469)

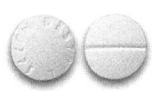        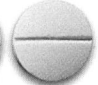

50 mg                      100 mg

## VALDECOXIB

**Bextra**
(page 380)

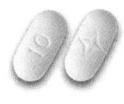        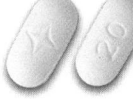

10 mg                      20 mg

## VARDENAFIL HYDROCHLORIDE

**Levitra**
(page 1297)

    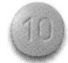    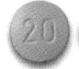

5 mg                 10 mg                 20 mg

## VENLAFAXINE HYDROCHLORIDE

### Effexor
(page 470)

25 mg     37.5 mg     50 mg

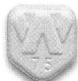 

75 mg     100 mg

### Effexor XR
(page 470)

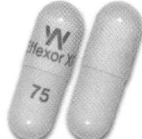 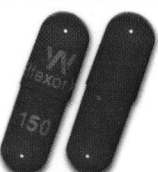

75 mg     150 mg

## VERAPAMIL HYDROCHLORIDE

### Calan
(page 268)

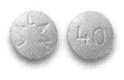 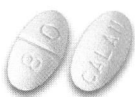 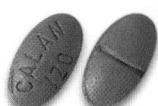

40 mg     80 mg     120 mg

### Isoptin SR
(page 268)

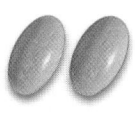 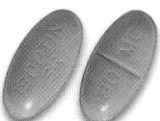 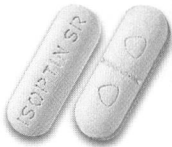

120 mg     180 mg     240 mg

### Verelan
(page 268)

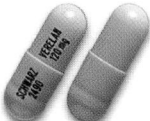 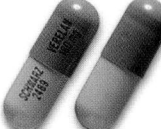 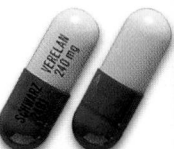

120 mg     180 mg     240 mg

## WARFARIN SODIUM

### Coumadin
(page 904)

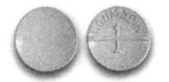 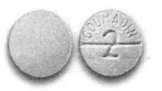 

1 mg  2 mg  2.5 mg

 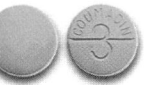 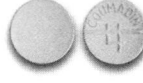 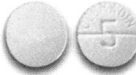

3 mg  4 mg  5 mg

    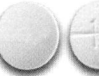

6 mg  7.5 mg  10 mg

## ZIDOVUDINE

### Retrovir
(page 198)

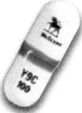 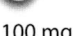 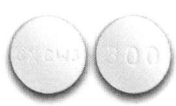

100 mg  300 mg

## ZOLPIDEM TARTRATE

### Ambien
(page 418)

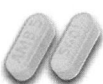 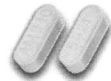

5 mg  10 mg

## INDICATIONS & DOSAGES

➤ **To prevent nausea and vomiting from cancer chemotherapy**

*Adults:* 100 mg P.O. given as a single dose 1 hour before chemotherapy. Or, 1.8 mg/kg or a fixed dose of 100 mg as a single I.V. dose given 30 minutes before chemotherapy.

*Children ages 2 to 16:* 1.8 mg/kg P.O. given 1 hour before chemotherapy. Or, 1.8 mg/kg as a single I.V. dose given 30 minutes before chemotherapy. Injectable formulation can be mixed with apple juice and given P.O. Maximum dose is 100 mg.

➤ **To prevent postoperative nausea and vomiting**

*Adults:* 100 mg P.O. within 2 hours before surgery. Or, 12.5 mg as a single I.V. dose about 15 minutes before cessation of anesthesia or as soon as nausea or vomiting presents.

*Children ages 2 to 16:* 1.2 mg/kg P.O. given within 2 hours before surgery, to maximum of 100 mg. Or, 0.35 mg/kg, up to 12.5 mg given as a single I.V. dose about 15 minutes before cessation of anesthesia or as soon as nausea or vomiting presents. Injectable formulation can be mixed with apple juice and given P.O.

➤ **Postoperative nausea and vomiting**

*Adults:* 12.5 mg as a single I.V. dose as soon as nausea or vomiting occurs.

*Children ages 2 to 16:* 0.35 mg/kg, to maximum dosage of 12.5 mg, given as a single I.V. dose as soon as nausea or vomiting occurs.

## I.V. ADMINISTRATION

● Drug can be injected as rapidly as 100 mg over 30 seconds or diluted in 50 ml compatible solution and infused over 15 minutes.

## ACTION

Selective serotonin 5-HT$_3$ receptor antagonist that blocks the action of serotonin. Blocking the activity of the serotonin receptors prevents serotonin from stimulating the vomiting reflex.

| Route | Onset | Peak | Duration |
|-------|-------|------|----------|
| P.O. | Rapid | 1 hr | 8 hr |
| I.V. | Rapid | 36 min | 7 hr |

## ADVERSE REACTIONS

**CNS:** fever, *headache,* dizziness, drowsiness, fatigue.
**CV:** *arrhythmias,* ECG changes, edema, hypotension, hypertension, tachycardia.
**GI:** *diarrhea,* dyspepsia, abdominal pain, constipation, anorexia.
**GU:** polyuria, hematuria, urine retention.
**Skin:** pruritus, rash.
**Other:** chills, pain at injection site.

## INTERACTIONS

**Drug-drug.** *Drugs that prolong ECG intervals, such as antiarrhythmics:* May increase risk of arrhythmia. Monitor patient closely.
*Drugs that inhibit CYP enzymes, such as cimetidine:* May increase hydrodolasetron level. Monitor patient for adverse effects.
*Drugs that induce CYP enzymes, such as rifampin:* May decrease hydrodolasetron level. Monitor patient for decreased efficacy of antiemetic.

## EFFECTS ON LAB TEST RESULTS

● May increase PTT, ALT, and AST levels.

## CONTRAINDICATIONS & CAUTIONS

● Contraindicated in patients hypersensitive to drug.
● *Alert:* Give with caution in patients who have or may develop prolonged cardiac conduction intervals, such as those with electrolyte abnormalities, history of arrhythmia, and cumulative high-dose anthracycline therapy.
● Drug isn't recommended for use in children younger than age 2. Use cautiously in breast-feeding women.

## NURSING CONSIDERATIONS

● Injection for oral use is stable in apple or apple-grape juice for 2 hours at room temperature.
● *Alert:* Don't confuse Anzemet with Aldomet or Avandamet.

## PATIENT TEACHING

● Tell patient about possible adverse effects.
● Instruct patient not to mix injection in juice for oral use until just before dosing.
● Tell patient to report nausea or vomiting.

# dronabinol (delta-9-tetrahydrocannabinol)
Marinol

*Pregnancy risk category C*
*Controlled substance schedule III*

## AVAILABLE FORMS
*Capsules:* 2.5 mg, 5 mg, 10 mg

## INDICATIONS & DOSAGES
➤ **Nausea and vomiting from cancer chemotherapy**
*Adults:* 5 mg/m$^2$ P.O. 1 to 3 hours before chemotherapy session. Then same dose q 2 to 4 hours after chemotherapy, for total of four to six doses daily. If needed, increase dosage in 2.5-mg/m$^2$ increments to maximum of 15 mg/m$^2$ per dose.
➤ **Anorexia and weight loss in patients with AIDS**
*Adults:* 2.5 mg P.O. b.i.d. before lunch and dinner. If patient can't tolerate it, decrease to 2.5 mg P.O. given as a single dose daily in evening or h.s. May gradually increase to maximum of 20 mg daily given in divided doses.

## ACTION
Unknown. A derivative of marijuana.

| Route | Onset | Peak | Duration |
|-------|-------|------|----------|
| P.O. | 30-60 min | 2-4 hr | 4-6 hr |

## ADVERSE REACTIONS
**CNS:** *dizziness, drowsiness, euphoria, ataxia,* depersonalization, hallucinations, somnolence, headache, muddled thinking, asthenia, amnesia, confusion, *paranoia.*
**CV:** tachycardia, orthostatic hypotension, palpitations, vasodilation.
**EENT:** visual disturbances.
**GI:** *dry mouth, nausea, vomiting, abdominal pain,* diarrhea.

## INTERACTIONS
**Drug-drug.** *CNS depressants, psychomimetic substances, sedatives:* May cause additive CNS depression. Avoid using together.
**Drug-lifestyle.** *Alcohol use:* May cause additive CNS depression. Discourage use together.

## EFFECTS ON LAB TEST RESULTS
None reported.

## CONTRAINDICATIONS & CAUTIONS
● Contraindicated in patients hypersensitive to sesame oil or cannabinoids.
● Use cautiously in elderly, pregnant, or breast-feeding patients and in those with heart disease, psychiatric illness, or history of drug abuse.

## NURSING CONSIDERATIONS
● Expect drug to be prescribed only for patients who haven't responded satisfactorily to other antiemetics.
● *Alert:* Dronabinol is the principal active substance in *Cannabis sativa* (marijuana). This substance can produce both physiological and psychological dependence and has a high risk of abuse.
● CNS effects are intensified at higher dosages.
● Drug effects may persist for days after treatment ends.
● *Alert:* Don't confuse dronabinol with droperidol.

## PATIENT TEACHING
● Tell patient that drug may induce unusual changes in mood or other adverse behavioral effects.
● Advise patient against performing activities that require alertness until CNS effects of drug are known.
● Warn caregivers to supervise patient during and immediately after treatment.
● Advise patient to take drug 1 to 3 hours before chemotherapy use.

# granisetron hydrochloride
Kytril

*Pregnancy risk category B*

## AVAILABLE FORMS
*Injection:* 1 mg/ml
*Oral solution:* 1 mg/5 ml
*Tablets:* 1 mg

## INDICATIONS & DOSAGES
➤ **To prevent nausea and vomiting from emetogenic cancer chemotherapy**
*Adults and children age 2 and older:* 10 mcg/kg I.V. undiluted and given by

direct injection over 30 seconds, or diluted and infused over 5 minutes. Begin administration within 30 minutes before use of chemotherapy. Or, for adults, 1 mg P.O. up to 1 hour before chemotherapy and repeated 12 hours later. Or, for adults, 2 mg P.O. daily given up to 1 hour before chemotherapy.

➤ **To prevent nausea and vomiting from radiation, including total body irradiation and fractionated abdominal radiation**
*Adults:* 2 mg P.O. once daily within 1 hour of radiation.

➤ **Postoperative nausea and vomiting**
*Adults:* 1 mg I.V. undiluted and given over 30 seconds. For prevention, give before anesthesia induction or immediately before reversal.

**I.V. ADMINISTRATION**
• Dilute drug with normal saline solution for injection or $D_5W$ to a volume of 20 to 50 ml. Infuse over 5 minutes, beginning within 30 minutes before chemotherapy, and only on days chemotherapy is given. Diluted solutions are stable for 24 hours at room temperature.
• For direct I.V. injection, the drug is given undiluted over 30 seconds.

**ACTION**
Selective antagonist of a specific type of serotonin receptor ($5\text{-}HT_3$) located in the CNS in the chemoreceptor trigger zone and in the peripheral nervous system on nerve terminals of the vagus nerve. Drug's blocking action may occur at both sites.

| Route | Onset | Peak | Duration |
|---|---|---|---|
| P.O., I.V. | Unknown | Unknown | Unknown |

**ADVERSE REACTIONS**
**CNS:** *headache, asthenia, fever,* somnolence, dizziness, anxiety, agitation, CNS stimulation, insomnia.
**CV:** hypertension, hypotension, ***bradycardia.***
**GI:** diarrhea, *constipation,* abdominal pain, *nausea, vomiting,* decreased appetite, taste disorder, flatulence, dyspepsia.
**GU:** UTI, oliguria.
**Hematologic:** *leukopenia, anemia, thrombocytopenia, leukocytosis.*

**Respiratory:** cough, increased sputum.
**Skin:** alopecia rash dermatitis.
**Other:** *hypersensitivity reactions (anaphylaxis, urticaria, dyspnea, hypotension), pain,* infection.

**INTERACTIONS**
**Drug-herb.** *Horehound:* May enhance serotoninergic effects. Discourage use together.

**EFFECTS ON LAB TEST RESULTS**
• May increase ALT and AST levels. May alter fluid and electrolyte levels with prolonged use.
• May decrease hemoglobin and WBC and platelet counts.

**CONTRAINDICATIONS & CAUTIONS**
• Contraindicated in patients hypersensitive to drug.

**NURSING CONSIDERATIONS**
• Drug regimen is given only on days when chemotherapy is given. Treatment at other times hasn't been found useful.
• *Alert:* Don't mix with other drugs; data regarding compatibility are limited.

**PATIENT TEACHING**
• Stress importance of taking second dose of oral drug 12 hours after the first for maximum effectiveness.
• Tell patient to report adverse reactions immediately.

---

# meclizine hydrochloride (meclozine hydrochloride)
Antivert, Antivert/25 ◊, Antivert/50, Bonamine†, Bonine ◊, Dramamine Less Drowsy Formula

*Pregnancy risk category B*

**AVAILABLE FORMS**
*Capsules:* 25 mg, 30 mg ◊
*Tablets:* 12.5 mg, 25 mg ◊, 50 mg
*Tablets (chewable):* 25 mg ◊

**INDICATIONS & DOSAGES**
➤ **Vertigo**
*Adults:* 25 to 100 mg P.O. daily in divided doses. Dosage varies with response.

---

➤ **Motion sickness**
*Adults and children age 12 and older:*
25 to 50 mg P.O. 1 hour before travel; then daily for duration of trip.

**ACTION**
Unknown. May affect neural pathways originating in the labyrinth to inhibit nausea and vomiting.

| Route | Onset | Peak | Duration |
|-------|-------|------|----------|
| P.O. | 1 hr | Unknown | 8-24 hr |

**ADVERSE REACTIONS**
**CNS:** *drowsiness,* restlessness, excitation, nervousness, auditory and visual hallucinations.
**CV:** hypotension, palpitations, tachycardia.
**EENT:** blurred vision, diplopia, tinnitus, dry nose and throat.
**GI:** dry mouth, constipation, anorexia, nausea, vomiting, diarrhea.
**GU:** urine retention, urinary frequency.
**Skin:** urticaria, rash.

**INTERACTIONS**
**Drug-drug.** *CNS depressants:* May increase drowsiness. Use together cautiously.

**EFFECTS ON LAB TEST RESULTS**
● May prevent, reduce, or mask diagnostic skin test response.

**CONTRAINDICATIONS & CAUTIONS**
● Contraindicated in patients hypersensitive to drug.
● Use cautiously in patients with asthma, glaucoma, or prostatic hyperplasia.

**NURSING CONSIDERATIONS**
● Stop drug 4 days before diagnostic skin tests to avoid interference with test response.
● Drug may mask signs and symptoms of ototoxicity, brain tumor, or intestinal obstruction.
● **Alert:** Don't confuse Antivert (meclizine) with Axert (almotriptan).

**PATIENT TEACHING**
● Advise patient to avoid hazardous activities that require alertness until CNS effects of drug are known.

● Urge patient to report persistent or serious adverse reactions promptly.

---

# metoclopramide hydrochloride
Apo-Metoclop†, Clopra, Maxeran†, Maxolon‡, Octamide PFS, Pramin‡, Reglan

*Pregnancy risk category B*

**AVAILABLE FORMS**
*Injection:* 5 mg/ml
*Syrup:* 5 mg/5 ml, 10 mg/ml
*Tablets:* 5 mg, 10 mg

**INDICATIONS & DOSAGES**
➤ **To prevent or reduce nausea and vomiting from emetogenic cancer chemotherapy**
*Adults:* 1 to 2 mg/kg I.V. 30 minutes before chemotherapy; repeat q 2 hours for two doses, then q 3 hours for three doses.
➤ **To prevent or reduce postoperative nausea and vomiting**
*Adults:* 10 to 20 mg I.M. near end of surgical procedure; repeat q 4 to 6 hours, p.r.n.
➤ **To facilitate small-bowel intubation, to aid in radiologic examinations**
*Adults and children age 14 and older:*
10 mg or 2 ml I.V. as a single dose over 1 to 2 minutes.
*Children ages 6 to 14:* 2.5 to 5 mg or 0.5 to 1 ml I.V.
*Children younger than age 6:* 0.1 mg/kg I.V.
➤ **Delayed gastric emptying secondary to diabetic gastroparesis**
*Adults:* 10 mg P.O. for mild symptoms. Slow I.V. infusion over 1 to 2 minutes for severe symptoms 30 minutes before meals and h.s. for up to 10 days; then P.O. dose may be started and continued for 2 to 8 weeks.
➤ **Gastroesophageal reflux disease**
*Adults:* 10 to 15 mg P.O. q.i.d., p.r.n., 30 minutes before meals and h.s.
*Adjust-a-dose:* For patients with creatinine clearance below 40 ml/minute, decrease dosage by half.
➤ **Emesis during pregnancy ♦**
*Adults:* 5 to 10 mg P.O. or 5 to 20 mg I.V. or I.M. t.i.d.

---

Reactions may be *common,* uncommon, *life-threatening,* or **COMMON AND LIFE-THREATENING.**

# Antiemetics  695

## I.V. ADMINISTRATION
• Give lower doses (10 mg or less) by direct injection over 1 to 2 minutes. Dilute doses larger than 10 mg in 50 ml of compatible diluent, and infuse over at least 15 minutes. No need to protect from light if infusion mixture is given within 24 hours. If protected from light and refrigerated, it's stable for 48 hours.
• Drug is compatible with D₅W, normal saline solution for injection, dextrose 5% in half-normal saline solution, Ringer's injection, and lactated Ringer's injection. Normal saline solution is the preferred diluent because drug is most stable in this solution.
• Closely monitor blood pressure.

## ACTION
Stimulates motility of upper GI tract, increases lower esophageal sphincter tone, and blocks dopamine receptors at the chemoreceptor trigger zone.

| Route | Onset | Peak | Duration |
|-------|-------|------|----------|
| P.O. | 30-60 min | 1-2 hr | 1-2 hr |
| I.V. | 1-3 min | Unknown | 1-2 hr |
| I.M. | 10-15 min | Unknown | 1-2 hr |

## ADVERSE REACTIONS
**CNS:** *restlessness, anxiety, drowsiness, fatigue, lassitude,* fever, depression, akathisia, insomnia, confusion, **suicide ideation, seizures, neuroleptic malignant syndrome,** hallucinations, headache, dizziness, extrapyramidal symptoms, tardive dyskinesia, *dystonic reactions.*
**CV:** transient hypertension, hypotension, **supraventricular tachycardia, bradycardia.**
**GI:** nausea, bowel disorders, diarrhea.
**GU:** urinary frequency, incontinence.
**Hematologic:** **neutropenia, agranulocytosis.**
**Skin:** rash, urticaria.
**Other:** prolactin secretion, loss of libido.

## INTERACTIONS
**Drug-drug.** *Anticholinergics, opioid analgesics:* May antagonize GI motility effects of metoclopramide. Use together cautiously.
*CNS depressants:* May cause additive CNS effects. Avoid using together.

*Levodopa:* Levodopa and metoclopramide have opposite effects on dopamine receptors. Avoid using together.
*MAO inhibitors:* May increase release of catecholamines in patients with hypertension. Use together cautiously.
*Phenothiazines:* May increase risk of extrapyramidal effects. Monitor patient closely.
**Drug-lifestyle.** *Alcohol use:* May cause additive CNS effects. Discourage use together.

## EFFECTS ON LAB TEST RESULTS
• May increase aldosterone and prolactin levels.
• May decrease neutrophil and granulocyte counts.

## CONTRAINDICATIONS & CAUTIONS
• Contraindicated in patients hypersensitive to drug and in those with pheochromocytoma or seizure disorders.
• Contraindicated in patients for whom stimulation of GI motility might be dangerous (those with hemorrhage, obstruction, or perforation).
• Use cautiously in patients with history of depression, Parkinson's disease, or hypertension.

## NURSING CONSIDERATIONS
• Monitor bowel sounds.
• Safety and effectiveness of drug haven't been established for therapy lasting longer than 12 weeks.
• When oral solution is used (10 mg/ml) dilute in pudding, applesauce, juice, or water just before using.
• *Alert:* Use diphenhydramine 25 mg I.V., to counteract extrapyramidal adverse effects from high metoclopramide doses.

## PATIENT TEACHING
• Tell patient to avoid activities that require alertness for 2 hours after doses.
• Urge patient to report persistent or serious adverse reactions promptly.
• Advise patient to avoid alcohol ingestion during therapy.

*Rapid onset  †Canada  ‡Australia  ◊OTC  ♦ Off-label use  ♪Photoguide  *Liquid contains alcohol.*

# ondansetron hydrochloride
Zofran, Zofran ODT

*Pregnancy risk category B*

## AVAILABLE FORMS
*Injection:* 2 mg/ml
*Oral solution:* 4 mg/5 ml
*Premixed injection:* 32 mg/50 ml
*Tablets:* 4 mg, 8 mg, 24 mg
*Tablets (disintegrating):* 4 mg, 8 mg

## INDICATIONS & DOSAGES
➤ **To prevent nausea and vomiting from emetogenic chemotherapy**
*Adults and children age 12 and older:*
8 mg P.O. 30 minutes before chemotherapy. Then, 8 mg P.O. 8 hours after first dose. Then, 8 mg q 12 hours for 1 to 2 days. Or, a single dose of 32 mg by I.V. infusion over 15 minutes beginning 30 minutes before chemotherapy. Or, three divided doses of 0.15 mg/kg I.V. Give first dose 30 minutes before chemotherapy and subsequent doses 4 and 8 hours after first dose. Infuse drug over 15 minutes.
*Children ages 4 to 11:* 4 mg P.O. 30 minutes before chemotherapy. Then, 4 mg P.O. 4 and 8 hours after first dose. Then, 4 mg q 8 hours for 1 to 2 days. Or, three doses of 0.15 mg/kg I.V. Give first dose 30 minutes before chemotherapy; use subsequent doses 4 and 8 hours after first dose. Infuse drug over 15 minutes.
➤ **To prevent postoperative nausea and vomiting**
*Adults:* 4 mg I.V. undiluted over 2 to 5 minutes. Or, 16 mg P.O. 1 hour before induction of anesthesia.
*Children weighing more than 40 kg (88 lb):* 4 mg I.V. as a single dose.
*Children weighing 40 kg or less:* 0.1 mg/kg I.V. as a single dose.
➤ **To prevent nausea and vomiting from radiotherapy in patients receiving total body irradiation, single high-dose fraction to abdomen, or daily fractions to abdomen**
*Adults:* 8 mg P.O. t.i.d.
*Adjust-a-dose:* For patients with severe hepatic impairment, total daily dose shouldn't exceed 8 mg.

## I.V. ADMINISTRATION
● Dilute drug in 50 ml of $D_5W$ injection or normal saline solution for injection before using.
● Drug is stable for up to 48 hours after dilution in $D_5W$, 5% dextrose in half-normal saline solution for injection, 5% dextrose in normal saline solution, and 3% sodium chloride solution for injection.
● *Alert:* Give as I.V. infusion over 15 minutes.

## ACTION
Selective antagonist of a specific type of serotonin receptor ($5\text{-}HT_3$) located in the CNS at the chemoreceptor trigger zone and in the peripheral nervous system on nerve terminals of the vagus nerve. Drug's blocking action may occur at both sites.

| Route | Onset | Peak | Duration |
|---|---|---|---|
| P.O., I.V. | Unknown | Unknown | Unknown |

## ADVERSE REACTIONS
**CNS:** *headache, malaise, fatigue, dizziness,* fever, *sedation,* extrapyramidal syndrome.
**CV:** chest pain, ***arrhythmias.***
**GI:** *diarrhea, constipation,* abdominal pain, xerostomia, decreased appetite.
**GU:** urine retention, gynecologic disorders.
**Musculoskeletal:** *pain.*
**Respiratory:** hypoxia.
**Skin:** rash, pruritus.
**Other:** chills, injection site reaction.

## INTERACTIONS
**Drug-drug.** *Drugs that alter hepatic drug-metabolizing enzymes, such as cimetidine, phenobarbital, rifampin:* May change pharmacokinetics of ondansetron. No need to adjust dosage.
**Drug-herb.** *Horehound:* May enhance serotoninergic effects. Discourage use together.

## EFFECTS ON LAB TEST RESULTS
● May increase ALT and AST levels.

## CONTRAINDICATIONS & CAUTIONS
● Contraindicated in patients hypersensitive to drug.
● Use cautiously in patients with hepatic impairment.

---

## NURSING CONSIDERATIONS
● *Alert:* Don't confuse Zofran with Zosyn, Zantac, or Zoloft.
● Monitor liver function test results. Don't exceed 8 mg in patients with hepatic impairment.

## PATIENT TEACHING
● Instruct patient to immediately report difficulty breathing after drug administration.
● Tell patient receiving drug I.V. to report discomfort at insertion site.
● Instruct patient, when using disintegrating tablets, to open blister just before use by peeling backing off. Don't push through foil blister. Using with a liquid isn't necessary.

---

**✳ NEW DRUG**

# palonosetron hydrochloride
Aloxi

*Pregnancy risk category B*

---

## AVAILABLE FORMS
*Injection:* 0.25 mg in 5-ml, single-use vial

## INDICATIONS & DOSAGES
➤ **To prevent acute and delayed nausea and vomiting from moderately or highly emetogenic chemotherapy**
*Adults:* 0.25 mg given I.V. over 30 seconds, 30 minutes before chemotherapy starts. Drug is given once per cycle, no more than q 7 days.

## I.V. ADMINISTRATION
● Flush with normal saline solution before and after injection.
● Give by rapid I.V. injection over 30 seconds. Drug may be given through a peripheral or central I.V. line.

## ACTION
Antagonizes 5-HT$_3$ receptors in the GI tract and brain, which inhibits emesis caused by cytotoxic chemotherapy.

| Route | Onset | Peak | Duration |
|-------|-------|------|----------|
| I.V. | 30 min | Unknown | 5 days |

## ADVERSE REACTIONS
**CNS:** anxiety, dizziness, headache, weakness.
**CV:** *bradycardia,* hypotension, *nonsustained ventricular tachycardia.*
**GI:** constipation, diarrhea.
**Metabolic:** *hyperkalemia.*

## INTERACTIONS
**Drug-drug.** *Antiarrhythmics or other drugs that may prolong the QTc interval, diuretics that may induce electrolyte abnormalities, high-dose anthracycline:* May increase risk of prolonged QTc interval. Use together cautiously.

## EFFECTS ON LAB TEST RESULTS
● May increase potassium level.

## CONTRAINDICATIONS & CAUTIONS
● Contraindicated in patents hypersensitive to palonosetron or its ingredients.
● Use cautiously in patients hypersensitive to other 5-HT$_3$ antagonists. Use cautiously in patients taking drugs that affect cardiac conduction and those with cardiac conduction abnormalities, hypokalemia, or hypomagnesemia.
● Safety and efficacy haven't been established in children.

## NURSING CONSIDERATIONS
● Before giving this drug, check patient's potassium level.
● Give drug 30 minutes before chemotherapy on the first day of each cycle.
● Consider adding corticosteroids to the antiemetic regimen, particularly for patients receiving highly emetogenic chemotherapy.
● Make sure patient has additional antiemetics to take for breakthrough nausea or vomiting.
● If patient has cardiac conduction abnormalities, check the ECG before giving drug.
● No differences in safety and efficacy have been noted in elderly versus younger patients; no dosage changes are needed.

## PATIENT TEACHING
● Advise patient to take a different antiemetic for breakthrough nausea or vomiting.

---

• Instruct patient to take the breakthrough antiemetic at the first sign of nausea rather than waiting until symptoms are severe.

• Urge patient with a history of cardiac conduction abnormalities to report any changes in medication regimen (such as adding or stopping an antiarrhythmic).

## prochlorperazine
Compazine⊘, PMS
Prochlorperazine†, Stemetil†

## prochlorperazine edisylate
Compazine, Compazine Syrup

## prochlorperazine maleate
Compazine, Compazine Spansule,
PMS Prochlorperazine†, Stemetil†

*Pregnancy risk category C*

### AVAILABLE FORMS
**prochlorperazine**
*Injection:* 5 mg/ml
*Suppositories:* 2.5 mg, 5 mg, 25 mg
*Tablets:* 5 mg, 10 mg
**prochlorperazine edisylate**
*Injection:* 5 mg/ml
*Syrup:* 5 mg/5 ml
**prochlorperazine maleate**
*Capsules (extended-release):* 10 mg,
15 mg, 30 mg
*Tablets:* 5 mg, 10 mg, 25 mg

### INDICATIONS & DOSAGES
➤ **To control preoperative nausea**
*Adults:* 5 to 10 mg I.M. 1 to 2 hours before induction of anesthesia; repeat once in 30 minutes, if needed. Or, 5 to 10 mg I.V. 15 to 30 minutes before induction of anesthesia; repeat once, if needed.
➤ **Severe nausea and vomiting**
*Adults:* 5 to 10 mg P.O., t.i.d. or q.i.d.;
15 mg sustained-release form P.O. on rising; 10 mg sustained-release form P.O. q 12 hours; 25 mg P.R., b.i.d.; or 5 to 10 mg I.M., repeated q 3 to 4 hours, p.r.n. Maximum I.M. dose is 40 mg daily. Or, 2.5 to 10 mg I.V. at no more than 5 mg/minute.
*Children weighing 18 to 39 kg (39 to 86 lb):* 2.5 mg P.O. or P.R., t.i.d.; or 5 mg P.O. or P.R., b.i.d. Maximum, 15 mg daily.

Or, 0.132 mg/kg by deep I.M. injection. Control is usually achieved with one dose.
*Children weighing 14 to 17 kg (30 to 38 lb):* 2.5 mg P.O. or P.R., b.i.d. or t.i.d. Maximum, 10 mg daily. Or, 0.132 mg/kg by deep I.M. injection. Control is usually achieved with one dose.
*Children weighing 9 to 13 kg (20 to 29 lb):* 2.5 mg P.O. or P.R. once daily or b.i.d. Maximum, 7.5 mg daily. Or, 0.132 mg/kg by deep I.M. injection. Control is usually achieved with one dose.
➤ **To manage symptoms of psychotic disorders**
*Adults and children age 12 and older:* 5 to 10 mg P.O., t.i.d. or q.i.d.
*Children ages 2 to 12:* 2.5 mg P.O. or P.R., b.i.d. or t.i.d. Don't exceed 10 mg on day 1. Increase dosage gradually to maximum, if needed. In children ages 2 to 5, maximum is 20 mg daily. In children ages 6 to 12, maximum is 25 mg daily.
➤ **To manage symptoms of severe psychosis**
*Adults and children age 12 and older:*
10 to 20 mg I.M., repeated in 1 to 4 hours, if needed. Rarely, patients may receive 10 to 20 mg q 4 to 6 hours. Start oral therapy after symptoms are controlled.
*Children ages 2 to 12:* 0.13 mg/kg I.M.
➤ **Nonpsychotic anxiety**
*Adults:* 5 to 10 mg P.O., t.i.d. or q.i.d. Or, 15 mg extended-release capsule once daily. Or, 10 mg extended-release capsule q 12 hours. Don't exceed 20 mg daily, and don't give for longer than 12 weeks.

### I.V. ADMINISTRATION
• Add 20 mg prochlorperazine per liter D₅W and normal saline solution 15 to 30 minutes before induction. Infusion rate shouldn't exceed 5 mg/minute. Maximum parenteral dose is 40 mg daily. Infuse slowly, never as a bolus.
• Watch for orthostatic hypotension, especially when giving drug I.V.

### ACTION
Acts on the chemoreceptor trigger zone to inhibit nausea and vomiting; in larger doses, it partially depresses vomiting center.

| Route | Onset | Peak | Duration |
|---|---|---|---|
| P.O. | 30-40 min | Unknown | 3-12 hr |
| P.O. (extended) | 30-40 min | Unknown | 10-12 hr |
| I.V. | Unknown | Unknown | Unknown |
| I.M. | 10-20 min | Unknown | 3-4 hr |
| P.R. | 1 hr | Unknown | 3-4 hr |

## ADVERSE REACTIONS
**CNS:** *extrapyramidal reactions,* sedation, pseudoparkinsonism, EEG changes, dizziness.
**CV:** *orthostatic hypotension,* tachycardia, ECG changes.
**EENT:** *ocular changes,* blurred vision.
**GI:** *dry mouth, constipation,* increased appetite.
**GU:** *urine retention,* dark urine, menstrual irregularities, inhibited ejaculation.
**Hematologic:** *transient leukopenia, agranulocytosis.*
**Hepatic:** cholestatic jaundice.
**Metabolic:** weight gain.
**Skin:** *mild photosensitivity,* allergic reactions, exfoliative dermatitis.
**Other:** gynecomastia, hyperprolactinemia.

## INTERACTIONS
**Drug-drug.** *Antacids:* May inhibit absorption of oral phenothiazines. Separate antacid and phenothiazine doses by at least 2 hours.
*Anticholinergics, including antidepressants and antiparkinsonians:* May increase anticholinergic activity and may aggravate parkinsonian symptoms. Use together cautiously.
*Barbiturates:* May decrease phenothiazine effect. Monitor patient for decreased antiemetic effect.
**Drug-herb.** *Dong quai, St. John's wort:* May increase risk of photosensitivity. Advise patient to avoid excessive sun exposure.
*Kava:* May increase risk of dystonic reactions. Discourage use together.
**Drug-lifestyle.** *Alcohol use:* May increase CNS depression, particularly psychomotor skills. Strongly discourage use together.

## EFFECTS ON LAB TEST RESULTS
• May decrease WBC and granulocyte counts.

• May cause false-positive results for urinary porphyrins, urobilinogen, amylase, and 5-hydroxyindoleacetic acid, and false-positive urine pregnancy results in tests using human chorionic gonadotropin. May cause abnormal liver function test results.

## CONTRAINDICATIONS & CAUTIONS
• Contraindicated in patients hypersensitive to phenothiazines and in those with CNS depression, including coma. Also contraindicated during pediatric surgery, when using spinal or epidural anesthetic or adrenergic blockers, and in children younger than age 2.
• Use cautiously in patients with impaired CV function, glaucoma, seizure disorders, and Parkinson's disease; in those who have been exposed to extreme heat; and in children with acute illness.

## NURSING CONSIDERATIONS
• Dilute oral solution with tomato juice, fruit juice, milk, coffee, carbonated beverage, tea, water, or soup. Or, mix with pudding.
• For I.M. use, inject deeply into upper outer quadrant of gluteal region.
• Don't give by S.C. route or mix in syringe with another drug.
• To prevent contact dermatitis, avoid getting concentrate or injection solution on hands or clothing.
• Monitor CBC and liver function studies during long-term therapy.
• *Alert:* Use drug only when vomiting can't be controlled by other measures or when only a few doses are needed. If more than four doses are needed in 24 hours, notify prescriber.
• Store in light-resistant container. Slight yellowing doesn't affect potency; discard extremely discolored solutions.

## PATIENT TEACHING
• Teach patient what to use to dilute oral solution.
• Advise patient to wear protective clothing when exposed to sunlight.
• Tell patient to call prescriber if more than four doses are needed within 24 hours.

# trimethobenzamide hydrochloride
Arrestin, Tebamide, T-Gen, Ticon, Tigan, Triban, Trimazide

*Pregnancy risk category C*

## AVAILABLE FORMS
*Capsules:* 250 mg, 300 mg
*Injection:* 100 mg/ml
*Suppositories:* 100 mg, 200 mg

## INDICATIONS & DOSAGES
➤ **Nausea and vomiting**
*Adults:* 250 to 300 mg P.O. t.i.d. or q.i.d.; or 200 mg I.M. or P.R., t.i.d. or q.i.d.
*Children weighing 13 to 40 kg (29 to 88 lb):* 100 to 200 mg P.O. or P.R., t.i.d. or q.i.d.
*Children weighing less than 13 kg:* 100 mg P.R., t.i.d. or q.i.d.

## ACTION
Unknown. Probably acts on the chemoreceptor trigger zone to inhibit nausea and vomiting.

| Route | Onset | Peak | Duration |
|-------|-------|------|----------|
| P.O. | 10-20 min | Unknown | 3-4 hr |
| I.M. | 15-35 min | Unknown | 2-3 hr |
| P.R. | Unknown | Unknown | Unknown |

## ADVERSE REACTIONS
**CNS:** *drowsiness,* dizziness with large doses, headache, disorientation, depression, parkinsonian-like symptoms, *coma, seizures.*
**CV:** hypotension.
**EENT:** blurred vision.
**GI:** diarrhea.
**Hepatic:** jaundice.
**Musculoskeletal:** muscle cramps.
**Other:** hypersensitivity reactions.

## INTERACTIONS
**Drug-drug.** *CNS depressants:* May cause additive CNS depression. Avoid using together.
**Drug-lifestyle.** *Alcohol use:* May cause additive CNS depression. Discourage use together.

## EFFECTS ON LAB TEST RESULTS
None reported.

## CONTRAINDICATIONS & CAUTIONS
• Contraindicated in patients hypersensitive to drug. Suppositories contraindicated in patients hypersensitive to benzocaine hydrochloride or similar local anesthetic.
• Use cautiously in children because drug may be linked to Reye's syndrome.

## NURSING CONSIDERATIONS
• For I.M. use, inject deeply into upper outer quadrant of gluteal region to reduce pain and local irritation.
• Drug may mask signs and symptoms of toxic drug overdose, intestinal obstruction, brain tumor, or other conditions.
• Drug may cause pain, stinging, burning, redness, or swelling at I.M. injection site. Withhold drug if skin hypersensitivity reaction occurs.
• *Alert:* Don't confuse Tigan with Ticar.

## PATIENT TEACHING
• Tell patient to refrigerate suppositories.
• Advise patient of possible drowsiness and dizziness; caution against performing hazardous activities requiring alertness until CNS effects of drug are known.

---

Reactions may be *common,* uncommon, *life-threatening,* or COMMON AND LIFE-THREATENING.

# 49

# Antiulcer drugs

cimetidine
cimetidine hydrochloride
esomeprazole magnesium
famotidine
lansoprazole
misoprostol
omeprazole
omeprazole magnesium
pantoprazole sodium
rabeprazole sodium
ranitidine hydrochloride
sucralfate

## COMBINATION PRODUCTS

ARTHROTEC: 50 mg diclofenac sodium and 200 mcg misoprostol; 75 mg diclofenac sodium and 200 mcg misoprostol.
PEPCID COMPLETE ◊ : 800 mg calcium carbonate, 165 mg magnesium hydroxide, and 10 mg famotidine.
PREVPAK: 4 capsules of amoxicillin 500 mg, 2 capsules of delayed-release lansoprazole 30 mg, and 2 tablets of film-coated clarithromycin 500 mg (in a daily administration pack).

---

## cimetidine
Tagamet✐, Tagamet HB ◊

## cimetidine hydrochloride
Tagamet

*Pregnancy risk category B*

---

## AVAILABLE FORMS
*Injection:* 300 mg/2 ml, 300 mg in 50 ml normal saline solution, 300 mg/2 ml ADD-Vantage vial
*Oral liquid:* 300 mg/5 ml*
*Tablets:* 100 mg ◊ , 200 mg, 300 mg, 400 mg, 800 mg

## INDICATIONS & DOSAGES
➤ **To prevent upper GI bleeding in critically ill patients**
*Adults:* 50 mg/hour by continuous I.V. infusion for up to 7 days; 25 mg/hour to patients with creatinine clearance below 30 ml/minute.

➤ **Short-term treatment of duodenal ulcer; maintenance therapy**
*Adults and children age 16 and older:*
800 mg P.O. h.s. Or, 400 mg P.O. b.i.d. or 300 mg q.i.d. (with meals and h.s.). Or, 200 mg t.i.d. with a 400-mg h.s. dose. Treatment lasts 4 to 6 weeks unless endoscopy shows healing. For maintenance therapy, 400 mg h.s. For parenteral therapy, 300 mg diluted to 20 ml total volume with normal saline solution or other compatible I.V. solution by I.V. push over at least 5 minutes q 6 to 8 hours; or 300 mg diluted in 50 ml $D_5W$ or other compatible I.V. solution by I.V. infusion over 15 to 20 minutes q 6 to 8 hours; or 300 mg I.M. q 6 to 8 hours (no dilution needed). To increase dosage, give 300-mg doses more frequently to maximum of 2,400 mg daily, p.r.n. Or, 900 mg/day (37.5 mg/hour) I.V. diluted in 100 to 1,000 ml of compatible solution by continuous I.V. infusion.

➤ **Active benign gastric ulceration**
*Adults:* 800 mg P.O. h.s. or 300 mg P.O. q.i.d. (with meals and h.s.) for up to 8 weeks.

➤ **Pathologic hypersecretory conditions, such as Zollinger-Ellison syndrome, systemic mastocytosis, and multiple endocrine adenomas**
*Adults and children age 16 and older:*
300 mg P.O. q.i.d. with meals and h.s.; adjusted to patient needs. Maximum oral amount, 2,400 mg daily.

For parenteral therapy, 300 mg diluted to 20 ml with normal saline solution or other compatible I.V. solution by I.V. push over at least 5 minutes q 6 to 8 hours; or 300 mg diluted in 50 ml $D_5W$ or other compatible I.V. solution by I.V. infusion over 15 to 20 minutes q 6 to 8 hours. Increase parenteral dosage by giving 300-mg doses more frequently to maximum of 2,400 mg daily, p.r.n.

➤ **Gastroesophageal reflux disease**
*Adults:* 800 mg P.O. b.i.d. or 400 mg q.i.d. before meals and h.s. for up to 12 weeks.
*Adjust-a-dose:* In patients with renal impairment, decrease dosage to 300 mg P.O. or I.V. q 12 hours, increasing dosing fre-

quency to q 8 hours with caution. A renally impaired patient who also has liver dysfunction may require even further dose reduction.

➤ **Heartburn**
*Adults:* 200 mg Tagamet HB P.O. with water as symptoms occur, or as directed, up to b.i.d. Maximum, 400 mg daily. Drug shouldn't be taken daily for longer than 2 weeks.

## I.V. ADMINISTRATION
● *Alert:* Dilute I.V. solutions with normal saline solution, $D_5W$, dextrose 10% in water (and combinations of these), lactated Ringer's solution, or 5% sodium bicarbonate injection. Don't dilute with sterile water for injection. Cimetidine is also commonly added to total parenteral nutrition solutions with or without fat emulsion.
● Give direct injection over 5 minutes. Rapid I.V. injection may result in arrhythmias and hypotension.
● Infuse drug over at least 30 minutes to minimize risk of adverse cardiac effects. Use infusion pump if cimetidine is given as continuous I.V. infusion in a total volume of 250 ml over 24 hours or less.

## ACTION
Competitively inhibits action of histamine on the $H_2$ at receptor sites of parietal cells, decreasing gastric acid secretion.

| Route | Onset | Peak | Duration |
|-------|-------|------|----------|
| P.O. | Unknown | 45-90 min | 4-5 hr |
| I.V. | Unknown | Immediate | Unknown |
| I.M. | Unknown | Unknown | Unknown |

## ADVERSE REACTIONS
**CNS:** confusion, dizziness, headache, peripheral neuropathy, somnolence, hallucinations.
**GI:** mild and transient diarrhea.
**GU:** impotence.
**Musculoskeletal:** muscle pain, arthralgia.
**Other:** mild gynecomastia if used longer than 1 month, hypersensitivity reactions.

## INTERACTIONS
**Drug-drug.** *Antacids:* May interfere with cimetidine absorption. Separate doses by at least 1 hour, if possible.
*Fosphenytoin, phenytoin, some benzodiazepines, theophylline, warfarin:* May in-

hibit hepatic microsomal enzyme metabolism of these drugs. Monitor drug level.
*Digoxin, fluconazole, indomethacin, iron salts, ketoconazole, tetracycline:* May decrease drug absorption. Separate doses by at least 2 hours.
*I.V. lidocaine:* May decrease clearance of lidocaine, increasing the risk of toxicity. Consider using a different $H_2$ antagonist if possible. Monitor lidocaine level closely.
*Metoprolol, propranolol, timolol:* May increase the effects of beta-blocker. Consider another $H_2$ agonist or decrease the dose of beta-blocker.
*Procainamide:* May increase procainamide level. Avoid this combination if possible. Monitor procainamide level closely and adjust the dose as necessary.
**Drug-herb.** *Guarana:* May increase caffeine level or prolong caffeine half-life. Monitor patient.
*Pennyroyal:* May change rate at which toxic metabolites of pennyroyal form. Monitor patient.
*Yerba maté:* May decrease clearance of yerba maté methylxanthines and cause toxicity. Discourage use together.
**Drug-lifestyle.** *Alcohol use:* May increase blood alcohol level. Discourage use together.
*Smoking:* May decrease the ability of cimetidine to inhibit nocturnal gastric secretion. Urge patient to quit smoking.

## EFFECTS ON LAB TEST RESULTS
● May increase creatinine, AST, and ALT levels.
● May antagonize pentagastrin's effect during gastric acid secretion tests; it may cause false-negative results in skin tests using allergen extracts. FD&C blue dye number 2 used in Tagamet tablets may impair interpretation of Hemoccult and Gastroccult test results on gastric content aspirate.

## CONTRAINDICATIONS & CAUTIONS
● Contraindicated in patients hypersensitive to drug.
● Use cautiously in elderly or debilitated patients because they may be more susceptible to cimetidine-induced confusion.

---

Reactions may be *common*, uncommon, *life-threatening*, or COMMON AND LIFE-THREATENING.

## NURSING CONSIDERATIONS
• Assess patient for abdominal pain. Note blood in emesis, stool, or gastric aspirate.
• Identify tablet strength when obtaining a drug history.
• Schedule cimetidine dose at end of hemodialysis treatment because hemodialysis reduces blood levels of cimetidine. Adjust dosage for patients with renal impairment.
• Wait at least 15 minutes after giving Tagamet tablet before drawing sample for Hemoccult or Gastroccult test, and follow test manufacturer's instructions closely.
• I.M. injection may be given undiluted.
• Treatment of gastric ulcer isn't as effective as treatment of duodenal ulcer.
• Up to 10 g overdose can occur without adverse reactions.
• **Alert:** Don't confuse cimetidine with simethicone.

## PATIENT TEACHING
• Remind patient taking cimetidine once daily to take it at bedtime and to take multiple daily doses with meals.
• Instruct patient taking Tagamet HB not to exceed recommended dosage and not to take daily for longer than 14 days.
• Warn patient receiving drug I.M. that injection may be painful.
• Urge patient to avoid cigarette smoking because it may increase gastric acid secretion and worsen disease.
• Advise patient to report abdominal pain and blood in stools or emesis.

## esomeprazole magnesium
Nexium

*Pregnancy risk category B*

### AVAILABLE FORMS
*Capsules (delayed-release):* 20 mg, 40 mg

### INDICATIONS & DOSAGES
➤ **Gastroesophageal reflux disease (GERD), healing erosive esophagitis**
*Adults:* 20 or 40 mg P.O. daily for 4 to 8 weeks.
➤ **Maintenance of healing erosive esophagitis**
*Adults:* 20 mg P.O. daily. Don't use for longer than 6 months.

➤ **Symptomatic GERD**
*Adults:* 20 mg P.O. daily for 4 weeks. If symptoms are unresolved, may continue treatment for 4 more weeks.
➤ *Helicobacter pylori* **eradication**
*Adults:* Use the following drugs together to reduce duodenal ulcer recurrence: esomeprazole magnesium 40 mg P.O. daily for 10 days, amoxicillin 1,000 mg P.O. b.i.d. for 10 days, clarithromycin 500 mg P.O. b.i.d. for 10 days.
*Adjust-a-dose:* For patients with mild to moderate hepatic failure, no dosage adjustment is needed. For patients with severe hepatic failure, maximum daily dose is 20 mg.

### ACTION
Proton pump inhibitor that reduces gastric acid secretion and decreases gastric acidity.

| Route | Onset | Peak | Duration |
|-------|-------|------|----------|
| P.O. | Unknown | 1½ hr | 13-17 hr |

### ADVERSE REACTIONS
**CNS:** headache.
**GI:** dry mouth, diarrhea, abdominal pain, nausea, flatulence, vomiting, constipation.

### INTERACTIONS
**Drug-drug.** *Amoxicillin, clarithromycin:* May increase levels of esomeprazole. Monitor patient for toxicity.
*Diazepam:* May decrease clearance of diazepam. Monitor patient for diazepam toxicity.
*Drugs metabolized by cytochrome P-450 2C19:* May alter clearance of esomeprazole, especially in elderly patients or patients with hepatic insufficiency. Monitor patient for toxicity.
**Drug-food.** *Any food:* May reduce drug levels. Advise patient to take drug 1 hour before food.

### EFFECTS ON LAB TEST RESULTS
None reported.

### CONTRAINDICATIONS & CAUTIONS
• Contraindicated in patients hypersensitive to drug or components of esomeprazole or omeprazole.

---

• Use cautiously in patients with hepatic insufficiency and in pregnant or breast-feeding patients.

## NURSING CONSIDERATIONS
• Give drug at least 1 hour before meals. If patient has difficulty swallowing the capsule, contents of the capsule can be emptied and mixed with 1 tablespoon of applesauce and swallowed (without chewing the enteric-coated pellets).
• Antacids can be used while taking drug, unless otherwise directed by prescriber.
• Monitor patient for rash or signs and symptoms of hypersensitivity. Monitor GI symptoms for improvement or worsening. Monitor liver function tests, especially in patients with preexisting hepatic disease.
• Long-term therapy has resulted in atrophic gastritis with omeprazole, of which esomeprazole is the s-isomer.
• It's unknown if drug appears in breast milk. Because omeprazole, a similar drug, does appear in breast milk, use cautiously in breast-feeding women.

## PATIENT TEACHING
• Instruct patient to take drug exactly as prescribed.
• Tell patient to take drug at least 1 hour before a meal.
• Advise patient that antacids can be used while taking drug unless otherwise directed by prescriber.
• Warn patient not to chew or crush drug pellets because this makes the drug ineffective.
• If patient has difficulty swallowing capsule, tell him to mix contents of capsule with 1 tablespoon of soft applesauce and swallow immediately.
• Advise patient to store capsules at room temperature in a tight container.
• Tell patient to inform prescriber of worsening signs and symptoms or pain.
• Instruct patient to alert prescriber if rash or other signs and symptoms of allergy occur.

# famotidine
Mylanta-AR◊ , Pepcid✐ , Pepcid AC◊ , Pepcid RPD, Pepcidine‡

*Pregnancy risk category B*

## AVAILABLE FORMS
*Gelcaps:* 10 mg◊
*Injection:* 10 mg/ml
*Powder for oral suspension:* 40 mg/5 ml after reconstitution
*Premixed injection:* 20 mg/50 ml in normal saline solution
*Tablets:* 10 mg◊ , 20 mg◊ , 40 mg
*Tablets (chewable):* 10 mg◊

## INDICATIONS & DOSAGES
➤ **Short-term treatment for duodenal ulcer**
*Adults:* For acute therapy, 40 mg P.O. once daily h.s. or 20 mg P.O. b.i.d. Healing usually occurs within 4 weeks. For maintenance therapy, 20 mg P.O. once daily h.s.
➤ **Short-term treatment for benign gastric ulcer**
*Adults:* 40 mg P.O. daily h.s. for 8 weeks.
*Children ages 1 to 16:* 0.5 mg/kg/day P.O. at h.s. or divided b.i.d. up to 40 mg daily.
➤ **Pathologic hypersecretory conditions (such as Zollinger-Ellison syndrome)**
*Adults:* 20 mg P.O. q 6 hours, up to 160 mg q 6 hours.
➤ **Hospitalized patients who can't take oral drug or who have intractable ulcers or hypersecretory conditions**
*Adults:* 20 mg I.V. q 12 hours.
➤ **Gastroesophageal reflux disease (GERD)**
*Adults:* 20 mg P.O. b.i.d. for up to 6 weeks. For esophagitis caused by GERD, 20 to 40 mg b.i.d. for up to 12 weeks.
*Children ages 1 to 16:* 1 mg/kg/day P.O. divided twice daily up to 40 mg b.i.d.
➤ **To prevent or treat heartburn**
*Adults:* 10 mg Pepcid AC P.O. 1 hour before meals to prevent symptoms, or 10 mg Pepcid AC P.O. with water when symptoms occur. Maximum daily dose is 20 mg. Drug shouldn't be taken daily for longer than 2 weeks.
*Adjust-a-dose:* For patients with creatinine clearance below 50 ml/minute, give half the dose, or increase dosing interval to q 36 to 48 hours.

## I.V. ADMINISTRATION
● To prepare I.V. injection, dilute 2 ml (20 mg) famotidine with compatible I.V. solution to a total volume of either 5 or 10 ml, and inject over at least 2 minutes. Compatible solutions include sterile water for injection, normal saline solution for injection, $D_5W$ or dextrose 10% in water for injection, 5% sodium bicarbonate injection, and lactated Ringer's injection. Famotidine also can be added to total parenteral nutrition solutions.
● To give drug by intermittent I.V. infusion, dilute 20 mg (2 ml) famotidine in 100 ml compatible solution; the premixed solution is 50 ml and doesn't need further dilution. Infuse over 15 to 30 minutes. After dilution, solution is stable for 48 hours refrigerated.
● Store I.V. injection in refrigerator at 36° to 46° F (2° to 8° C).

## ACTION
Competitively inhibits action of histamine on the H2 at receptor sites of parietal cells, decreasing gastric acid secretion.

| Route | Onset | Peak | Duration |
|-------|-------|------|----------|
| P.O. | 1 hr | 1-3 hr | 12 hr |
| I.V. | 1 hr | 1-4 hr | 12 hr |

## ADVERSE REACTIONS
**CNS:** *headache,* fever, dizziness, vertigo, malaise, paresthesia.
**CV:** palpitations, flushing.
**EENT:** tinnitus, orbital edema.
**GI:** diarrhea, constipation, anorexia, taste perversion, dry mouth.
**Musculoskeletal:** bone and muscle pain.
**Skin:** acne, dry skin.
**Other:** transient irritation at I.V. site.

## INTERACTIONS
None significant.

## EFFECTS ON LAB TEST RESULTS
● May increase BUN, creatinine, and liver enzyme levels.
● May cause false-negative results in skin tests using allergen extracts.

## CONTRAINDICATIONS & CAUTIONS
● Contraindicated in patients hypersensitive to drug.

## NURSING CONSIDERATIONS
● Assess for abdominal pain. Note blood in emesis, stool, or gastric aspirate.
● Oral suspension must be reconstituted and shaken before use.
● Store reconstituted suspension below 86° F (30° C). Discard after 30 days.
● Drug may antagonize pentagastrin during gastric acid secretion tests.

## PATIENT TEACHING
● Instruct patient in proper use of OTC product (Pepcid AC), if appropriate.
● Tell patient to take prescription drug with a snack, if desired.
● Remind patient that prescription drug is most effective if taken at bedtime. Tell patient taking 20 mg twice daily to take one dose at bedtime.
● Advise patient not to take prescription drug for longer than 8 weeks, unless ordered by prescriber, and to limit use of OTC drug to no longer than 2 weeks.
● With prescriber's knowledge, allow patient to take antacids together, especially at beginning of therapy when pain is severe.
● Urge patient to avoid cigarette smoking because it may increase gastric acid secretion and worsen disease.
● Advise patient to report abdominal pain or blood in stools or vomit.

# lansoprazole
Prevacid✐, Prevacid SoluTab

*Pregnancy risk category B*

## AVAILABLE FORMS
*Capsules (delayed-release):* 15 mg, 30 mg
*Oral suspension (delayed-release):* 15 mg/packet, 30 mg/packet
*Orally disintegrating tablet (delayed-release):* 15 mg, 30 mg

## INDICATIONS & DOSAGES
➤ **Short-term treatment of active duodenal ulcer**
*Adults:* 15 mg P.O. daily before eating for 4 weeks.
➤ **Maintenance of healed duodenal ulcers**
*Adults:* 15 mg P.O. daily.

---

*Rapid onset*    †Canada    ‡Australia    ◊ OTC    ◆ Off-label use    ✐Photoguide    *Liquid contains alcohol.

➤ **Short-term treatment of active benign gastric ulcer**
*Adults:* 30 mg P.O. once daily for up to 8 weeks.
➤ **Short-term treatment of erosive esophagitis**
*Adults:* 30 mg P.O. daily before eating for up to 8 weeks. If healing doesn't occur, 8 more weeks of therapy may be given. Maintenance dosage for healing is 15 mg P.O. daily.
➤ **Maintenance of healing of erosive esophagitis**
*Adults:* 15 mg P.O. once daily.
➤ **Long-term treatment of pathologic hypersecretory conditions, including Zollinger-Ellison syndrome**
*Adults:* Initially, 60 mg P.O. once daily. Increase dosage, p.r.n. Give daily amounts above 120 mg in evenly divided doses.
➤ **Helicobacter pylori eradication to reduce risk of duodenal ulcer recurrence**
*Adults:* For patients receiving dual therapy, 30 mg P.O. lansoprazole with 1 g P.O. amoxicillin, each given t.i.d. for 14 days. For patients receiving triple therapy, 30 mg P.O. lansoprazole with 1 g P.O. amoxicillin and 500 mg P.O. clarithromycin, all given b.i.d. for 10 to 14 days.
➤ **Short-term treatment of symptomatic gastroesophageal reflux disease (GERD)**
*Adults:* 15 mg P.O. once daily for up to 8 weeks.
➤ **Short-term treatment of symptomatic GERD; short-term treatment of erosive esophagitis**
*Children ages 1 to 11, weighing more than 30 kg:* 30 mg P.O. once daily for up to 12 weeks.
*Children ages 1 to 11, weighing 30 kg (66 lb) or less:* 15 mg P.O. once daily for up to 12 weeks.
➤ **NSAID-related ulcer in patients who take NSAIDs**
*Adults:* 30 mg P.O. daily for 8 weeks.
➤ **To reduce risk of NSAID-related ulcer in patients with history of gastric ulcer who need NSAIDs**
*Adults:* 15 mg P.O. daily for up to 12 weeks.

**ACTION**
Inhibits activity of proton pump and binds to hydrogen-potassium adenosine triphosphatase, located at secretory surface of gastric parietal cells, to block secretion of gastric acid.

| Route | Onset | Peak | Duration |
|-------|-------|------|----------|
| P.O. | 1-3 hr | Unknown | Unknown |

**ADVERSE REACTIONS**
**GI:** diarrhea, nausea, abdominal pain.

**INTERACTIONS**
**Drug-drug.** *Ampicillin esters, digoxin, iron salts, ketoconazole:* May inhibit absorption of these drugs. Monitor patient closely.
*Sucralfate:* May cause delayed lansoprazole absorption. Give lansoprazole at least 30 minutes before sucralfate.
*Theophylline:* May mildly increase theophylline clearance. Dosage adjustment of theophylline may be needed when lansoprazole is started or stopped. Use together cautiously.
**Drug-herb.** *Male fern:* May cause alkaline environment, in which herb is inactivated. Discourage use together.
*St. John's wort:* May increase risk of sun sensitivity. Advise patient to avoid excessive sunlight exposure.
**Drug-food.** *Food:* May decrease rate and extent of GI absorption. Advise patient to take before meals.

**EFFECTS ON LAB TEST RESULTS**
None reported.

**CONTRAINDICATIONS & CAUTIONS**
• Contraindicated in patients hypersensitive to drug.

**NURSING CONSIDERATIONS**
• Patients with severe liver disease may need dosage adjustment, but don't adjust dosage for elderly patients or those with renal insufficiency.
• The contents of capsule can be mixed with 40 ml of apple juice in a syringe and given within 3 to 5 minutes via a nasogastric tube. Flush with additional apple juice to give entire dose and maintain patency of the tube.
• Orally disintegrating tablets contain 2.5 mg phenylalanine/15-mg tablet and 5.1 mg phenylalanine/30-mg tablet.

---

Reactions may be *common*, uncommon, *life-threatening*, or COMMON AND LIFE-THREATENING.

• A symptomatic response to lansoprazole therapy doesn't preclude presence of gastric malignancy.

• Because it's unknown if lansoprazole appears in breast milk, breast-feeding women should either stop breast-feeding or stop drug.

**PATIENT TEACHING**
• For best effect, instruct patient to take drug no more than 30 minutes before eating.

• Tell patient he may mix the capsule's contents with a small amount (about 2 ounces) of apple, cranberry, grape, orange, pineapple, prune, tomato, or vegetable juice. The patient must drink the mixture within 30 minutes. To ensure complete delivery of the dose, the patient should rinse the glass with two or more volumes of juice and swallow the contents immediately.

• Contents of capsule can be mixed with 1 tablespoon of applesauce, Ensure pudding, cottage cheese, yogurt, or strained pears and swallowed immediately. The granules shouldn't be chewed or crushed.

• For the oral suspension, empty packet contents into 30 ml of water. Stir well and drink immediately. Don't crush or chew the granules. Don't use with other liquids or food. If any material remains after drinking, add more water, stir, and drink immediately.

• Inform patient not to crush or chew any formulations of lansoprazole.

• Tell patient taking orally disintegrating tablets to allow tablet to dissolve on tongue until all particles can be swallowed.

---

**misoprostol**
Cytotec

*Pregnancy risk category X*

---

**AVAILABLE FORMS**
*Tablets:* 100 mcg, 200 mcg

**INDICATIONS & DOSAGES**
➤ To prevent NSAID-induced gastric ulcer in elderly or debilitated patients at high risk for complications from gastric ulcer and in patients with history of NSAID-induced ulcer
*Adults:* 200 mcg P.O. q.i.d. with food; if not tolerated, decrease to 100 mcg P.O. q.i.d. Give dosage for duration of NSAID therapy. Give last dose h.s.

**ACTION**
A synthetic prostaglandin $E_1$ analogue that replaces gastric prostaglandins depleted by NSAID therapy. Also decreases basal and stimulated gastric acid secretion and may increase gastric mucus and bicarbonate production.

| Route | Onset | Peak | Duration |
|-------|-------|------|----------|
| P.O. | 30 min | 60-90 min | 3 hr |

**ADVERSE REACTIONS**
**CNS:** headache.
**GI:** *diarrhea, abdominal pain,* nausea, flatulence, dyspepsia, vomiting, constipation.
**GU:** hypermenorrhea, dysmenorrhea, spotting, cramps, menstrual disorders, postmenopausal vaginal bleeding.

**INTERACTIONS**
**Drug-food.** *Any food:* May decrease absorption rate of drug. However, manufacturer recommends that patient take drug with food.

**EFFECTS ON LAB TEST RESULTS**
None reported.

**CONTRAINDICATIONS & CAUTIONS**
• Contraindicated in those allergic to prostaglandins. Drug shouldn't be taken by pregnant women to reduce the risk of NSAID-induced ulcers.
• Use with caution in patients with inflammatory bowel disease.

**NURSING CONSIDERATIONS**
• *Alert:* Take special precautions to prevent use of drug during pregnancy. Uterine rupture is linked to certain risk factors, including later-trimester pregnancies, higher doses of the drug, prior cesarean delivery or uterine surgery, or five or more previous pregnancies. Make sure patient understands dangers of drug to herself and the fetus and that she receives both oral and written warnings about these dangers.

---

*Rapid onset* †Canada ‡Australia ◇OTC ♦ Off-label use ⊘Photoguide *Liquid contains alcohol.

Also, make sure she can comply with effective contraception and that the result of a serum pregnancy test performed within 2 weeks of starting therapy is negative. Patient shouldn't breast-feed during therapy.
• Drug causes modest decrease in basal pepsin secretion.
• *Alert:* Don't confuse misoprostol (Cytotec) with mifepristone (Mifeprex).

**PATIENT TEACHING**
• Instruct patient not to share misoprostol.
• Remind pregnant patient that drug may cause miscarriage, often with potentially life-threatening bleeding.
• Advise woman not to begin therapy until second or third day of next normal menstrual period.
• Advise patient to take drug as prescribed for duration of NSAID therapy.
• Tell patient that diarrhea usually occurs early in the course of therapy and is usually self-limiting. Taking drug with food helps minimize the diarrhea.

---

**omeprazole**
Losec†‡, Prilosec✒

**omeprazole magnesium**
Prilosec OTC◇

*Pregnancy risk category C*

**AVAILABLE FORMS**
*Capsules (delayed-release):* 10 mg, 20 mg, 40 mg
*Tablets (delayed-release):* 20 mg ◇

**INDICATIONS & DOSAGES**
➤ **Symptomatic gastroesophageal reflux disease (GERD) without esophageal lesions**
*Adults:* 20 mg P.O. daily for 4 weeks for patients who respond poorly to customary medical treatment, usually including an adequate course of H₂-receptor antagonists.
➤ **Erosive esophagitis and accompanying symptoms caused by GERD**
*Adults:* 20 mg P.O. daily for 4 to 8 weeks.
➤ **Maintenance of healing erosive esophagitis**
*Adults:* 20 mg P.O. daily.

➤ **Pathologic hypersecretory conditions (such as Zollinger-Ellison syndrome)**
*Adults:* Initially, 60 mg P.O. daily; adjust dosage based on patient response. If daily dose exceeds 80 mg, give in divided doses. Doses up to 120 mg t.i.d. have been given. Continue therapy as long as clinically indicated.
➤ **Duodenal ulcer (short-term treatment)**
*Adults:* 20 mg P.O. daily for 4 to 8 weeks.
➤ **Helicobacter pylori infection and duodenal ulcer disease, to eradicate H. pylori with clarithromycin (dual therapy)**
*Adults:* 40 mg P.O. q morning with clarithromycin 500 mg P.O. t.i.d. for 14 days. For patients with an ulcer at start of therapy, give another 14 days of omeprazole 20 mg P.O. once daily.
➤ **H. pylori infection and duodenal ulcer disease, to eradicate H. pylori with clarithromycin and amoxicillin (triple therapy)**
*Adults:* 20 mg P.O. with clarithromycin 500 mg P.O. and amoxicillin 1,000 mg P.O., each given b.i.d. for 10 days. For patients with an ulcer at start of therapy, give another 18 days of omeprazole 20 mg P.O. once daily.
➤ **Short-term treatment of active benign gastric ulcer**
*Adults:* 40 mg P.O. once daily for 4 to 8 weeks.
✻ *NEW INDICATION:* **Frequent heartburn (2 or more days a week)**
*Adults:* 20 mg P.O. Prilosec OTC once daily before breakfast for 14 days. May repeat the 14-day course q 4 months.

**ACTION**
Inhibits activity of acid (proton) pump and binds to hydrogen-potassium adenosine triphosphatase at secretory surface of gastric parietal cells to block formation of gastric acid.

| Route | Onset | Peak | Duration |
|-------|-------|------|----------|
| P.O. | 1 hr | 2 hr | < 3 days |

**ADVERSE REACTIONS**
**CNS:** headache, dizziness, asthenia.
**GI:** diarrhea, abdominal pain, nausea, vomiting, constipation, flatulence.
**Musculoskeletal:** back pain.

---

Reactions may be *common,* uncommon, *life-threatening,* or COMMON AND LIFE-THREATENING.

**Respiratory:** cough, upper respiratory tract infection.
**Skin:** rash.

**INTERACTIONS**
**Drug-drug.** *Ampicillin esters, iron derivatives, ketoconazole:* May exhibit poor bioavailability in patients taking omeprazole because these drugs need a low gastric pH for optimal absorption. Avoid using together.
*Diazepam, fosphenytoin, phenytoin, warfarin:* May decrease hepatic clearance, possibly leading to increased serum levels. Monitor drug levels.
**Drug-herb.** *Male fern.* May cause alkaline environment in which herb is inactivated. Discourage use together.
*Pennyroyal:* May change rate at which toxic metabolites of pennyroyal form. Ask patient about the use of herbal remedies, and discourage use together.
*St. John's wort:* May increase risk of sun sensitivity. Advise patient to avoid excessive sunlight exposure.

**EFFECTS ON LAB TEST RESULTS**
None reported.

**CONTRAINDICATIONS & CAUTIONS**
• Contraindicated in patients hypersensitive to drug or its components.

**NURSING CONSIDERATIONS**
• Dosage adjustments may be necessary in Asian patients and patients with hepatic impairment.
• Omeprazole increases its own bioavailability with repeated doses. Drug is labile in gastric acid; less drug is lost to hydrolysis because drug increases gastric pH.
• *Alert:* Don't confuse Prilosec with Prozac, Prilocaine, or Prinivil.
• Gastrin level rises in most patients during the first 2 weeks of therapy.

**PATIENT TEACHING**
• Tell patient to swallow tablets or capsules whole and not to open, crush, or chew them.
• Instruct patient to take drug 30 minutes before meals.
• Caution patient to avoid hazardous activities if he gets dizzy.

• Advise patient that Prilosec OTC isn't intended to treat infrequent heartburn (one episode of heartburn a week or less), or for those who want immediate relief of heartburn.
• Inform patient that Prilosec OTC may take 1 to 4 days for full effect, although some patients may get complete relief of symptoms within 24 hours.

# pantoprazole sodium
Protonix, Protonix I.V.

*Pregnancy risk category B*

**AVAILABLE FORMS**
*Injection:* 40 mg per vial
*Tablet (delayed-release):* 20 mg, 40 mg

**INDICATIONS & DOSAGES**
➤ **Erosive esophagitis with gastroesophageal reflux disease (GERD)**
*Adults:* 40 mg P.O. once daily for up to 8 weeks. For patients who haven't healed after 8 weeks of treatment, another 8-week course may be considered.
➤ **Short-term treatment of GERD in patients who can't take delayed-release tablets orally**
*Adults:* 40 mg I.V. daily for 7 to 10 days.
➤ **Short-term treatment of GERD linked to history of erosive esophagitis**
*Adults:* 40 mg I.V. once daily for 7 to 10 days. Switch to P.O. form as soon as patient can take P.O. medications.
➤ **Long-term maintenance of healing erosive esophagitis and reduction in relapse rates of daytime and nighttime heartburn symptoms in patients with GERD**
*Adults:* 40 mg PO once daily.
➤ **Short-term treatment of pathological hypersecretion conditions caused by Zollinger-Ellison syndrome or other neoplastic conditions**
*Adults:* Individualize dosage. Usual dose is 80 mg I.V. q 12 hours for no more than 6 days. For those needing a higher dose, 80 mg q 8 hours is expected to maintain acid output below 10 mEq/hour. Maximum daily dose is 240 mg/day.

➤ **Long-term treatment of pathological hypersecretory conditions, including with Zollinger-Ellison syndrome**
*Adults:* Individualize dosage. Usual starting dose is 40 mg P.O. b.i.d. Adjust dose to a maximum of 240 mg/day.

Stop treatment with I.V. pantoprazole when P.O. pantoprazole is warranted.

**I.V. ADMINISTRATION**
● Reconstitute each vial with 10 ml of normal saline solution.
● Compatible diluents for infusion include normal saline solution, $D_5W$, or lactated Ringer's solution for injection.
● For patients with GERD, further dilute with 100 ml of diluent to yield 0.4 mg/ml.
● For patients with hypersecretion conditions, combine 2 reconstituted vials and further dilute with 80 ml of diluent to a total volume of 100 ml, to yield 0.8 mg/ml.
● Infuse diluted solutions I.V. using inline filter provider by manufacturer, over 15 minutes at a rate no greater than 3 mg/minute (7 ml/minute) for GERD and 6 mg/minute (7 ml/minute) for pathological hypersecretory conditions.
● Don't give another infusion simultaneously through the same line.
● The reconstituted solution may be stored for up to 2 hours at room temperature, and the diluted solutions may be stored for up to 12 hours at room temperature.

**ACTION**
Inhibits proton pump activity by binding to hydrogen-potassium adenosine triphosphatase, located at secretory surface of gastric parietal cells, to suppress gastric acid secretion.

| Route | Onset | Peak | Duration |
|-------|-------|------|----------|
| P.O. | Unknown | 2½ hr | > 24 hr |
| I.V. | 15-30 min | Unknown | 24 hr |

**ADVERSE REACTIONS**
**CNS:** headache, insomnia, asthenia, migraine, anxiety, dizziness.
**CV:** chest pain.
**EENT:** pharyngitis, rhinitis, sinusitis.
**GI:** diarrhea, flatulence, abdominal pain, eructation, constipation, dyspepsia, gastroenteritis, GI disorder, nausea, vomiting, rectal disorder.

**GU:** urinary frequency, urinary tract infection.
**Metabolic:** hyperglycemia, hyperlipemia.
**Musculoskeletal:** back pain, neck pain, arthralgia, hypertonia.
**Respiratory:** bronchitis, increased cough, dyspnea, upper respiratory tract infection.
**Skin:** rash.
**Other:** flu syndrome, infection, pain.

**INTERACTIONS**
**Drug-drug.** *Ampicillin esters, iron salts, ketoconazole:* May decrease absorption of these drugs. Monitor patient closely and separate doses.
**Drug-herb.** *St. John's wort:* May increase risk of sunburn. Advise patient to avoid excessive sunlight exposure.
**Drug-lifestyle.** *Sunlight:* May increase risk of sunburn. Advise patient to avoid excessive sunlight exposure.

**EFFECTS ON LAB TEST RESULTS**
● May increase glucose and lipid levels.
● May increase liver function test result values.

**CONTRAINDICATIONS & CAUTIONS**
● Contraindicated in patients hypersensitive to any component of the formulation.
● Safety and efficacy of using the I.V. formulation to start therapy for GERD are unknown.

**NURSING CONSIDERATIONS**
● Stop treatment with I.V. pantoprazole when P.O. form is warranted.
● *Alert:* Don't confuse Protonix with Prilosec, Prozac, or Prevacid.
● Drug can be given without regard to meals.
● Symptomatic response to therapy doesn't preclude the presence of gastric malignancy.

**PATIENT TEACHING**
● Instruct patient to take exactly as prescribed and at about the same time every day.
● Advise patient that drug can be taken without regard to meals.
● Tell patient to swallow tablet whole and not to crush, split, or chew it.
● Tell patient that antacids don't affect pantoprazole absorption.

---

Reactions may be *common,* uncommon, *life-threatening*, or COMMON AND LIFE-THREATENING.

## rabeprazole sodium
Aciphex

*Pregnancy risk category B*

### AVAILABLE FORMS
*Tablets (delayed-release):* 20 mg

### INDICATIONS & DOSAGES
➤ **Healing of erosive or ulcerative gastroesophageal reflux disease (GERD)**
*Adults:* 20 mg P.O. daily for 4 to 8 weeks. Additional 8-week course may be considered, if needed.
➤ **Maintenance of healing of erosive or ulcerative GERD**
*Adults:* 20 mg P.O. daily.
➤ **Healing of duodenal ulcers**
*Adults:* 20 mg P.O. daily after morning meal for up to 4 weeks.
➤ **Pathologic hypersecretory conditions, including Zollinger-Ellison syndrome**
*Adults:* 60 mg P.O. daily; may be increased, p.r.n., to 100 mg P.O. daily or 60 mg P.O. b.i.d.
➤ **Symptomatic GERD, including daytime and nighttime heartburn**
*Adults:* 20 mg P.O. daily for 4 weeks. Additional 4-week course may be considered, if necessary.
➤ *Helicobacter pylori* **eradication, to reduce the risk of duodenal ulcer recurrence**
*Adults:* 20 mg P.O. b.i.d., combined with amoxicillin 1,000 mg P.O. b.i.d. and clarithromycin 500 mg P.O. b.i.d., for total of 7 days.

### ACTION
Blocks proton pump activity by inhibiting gastric hydrogen-potassium adenosine triphosphatase at secretory surface of gastric parietal cells, thereby blocking gastric acid secretion.

| Route | Onset | Peak | Duration |
|-------|-------|------|----------|
| P.O. | < 1 hr | 2-5 hr | > 24 hr |

### ADVERSE REACTIONS
**CNS:** headache.

### INTERACTIONS
**Drug-drug.** *Clarithromycin:* May increase rabeprazole level. Monitor patient closely.
*Cyclosporine:* May inhibit cyclosporine metabolism. Use together cautiously.
*Digoxin, ketoconazole, other gastric pH-dependent drugs:* May decrease or increase drug absorption at increased pH values. Monitor patient closely.
*Warfarin:* May inhibit warfarin metabolism. Monitor PT and INR.

### EFFECTS ON LAB TEST RESULTS
None reported.

### CONTRAINDICATIONS & CAUTIONS
● Contraindicated in patients hypersensitive to drug, other benzimidazoles (lansoprazole, omeprazole), or components of these formulations.
● In *H. pylori* eradication, clarithromycin is contraindicated in pregnant patients, patients hypersensitive to macrolides, and those taking pimozide; amoxicillin is contraindicated in patients hypersensitive to penicillin.
● Use cautiously in patients with severe hepatic impairment.

### NURSING CONSIDERATIONS
● Consider additional courses of therapy if duodenal ulcer or GERD isn't healed after first course of therapy.
● If *H. pylori* eradication is unsuccessful, do susceptibility testing. If patient is resistant to clarithromycin or susceptibility testing isn't possible, expect to start therapy using a different antimicrobial.
● *Alert:* Amoxicillin may trigger anaphylaxis in patients with a history of penicillin hypersensitivity.
● Symptomatic response to therapy doesn't preclude presence of gastric malignancy.
● *Alert:* Patients treated for *H. pylori* eradication have developed pseudomembranous colitis with nearly all antibacterial agents, including clarithromycin and amoxicillin. Monitor patient closely.

### PATIENT TEACHING
● Explain importance of taking drug exactly as prescribed.

● Advise patient to swallow delayed-release tablets whole and not to crush, chew, or split it.
● Inform patient that drug may be taken without regard to meals.

---

# ranitidine hydrochloride
Apo-Ranitidine†, Zantac*✏,
Zantac-C†, Zantac 75◊, Zantac
150, Zantac EFFERdose Tablets,
Zantac 150 GELdose, Zantac 300,
Zantac 300 GELdose

*Pregnancy risk category B*

---

## AVAILABLE FORMS
*Granules (effervescent):* 150 mg
*Infusion:* 0.5 mg/ml in 100-ml containers
*Injection:* 25 mg/ml
*Syrup:* 15 mg/ml*
*Tablets:* 75 mg◊, 150 mg, 300 mg
*Tablets (dispersible):* 150 mg‡
*Tablets (effervescent):* 150 mg

## INDICATIONS & DOSAGES
➤ **Duodenal and gastric ulcer (short-term treatment); pathologic hypersecretory conditions, such as Zollinger-Ellison syndrome**
*Adults:* 150 mg P.O. b.i.d. or 300 mg daily h.s. Or, 50 mg I.V. or I.M. q 6 to 8 hours. Patients with Zollinger-Ellison syndrome may need doses up to 6 g P.O. daily.
*Children ages 1 month to 16 years:* 2 to 4 mg/kg daily, divided b.i.d. up to 300 mg/day.
➤ **Maintenance therapy for duodenal or gastric ulcer**
*Adults:* 150 mg P.O. h.s.
➤ **Gastroesophageal reflux disease**
*Adults:* 150 mg P.O. b.i.d.
*Children ages 1 month to 16 years:* 5 to 10 mg/kg daily given as two divided doses P.O.
➤ **Erosive esophagitis**
*Adults:* 150 mg P.O. q.i.d. Maintenance dosage is 150 mg P.O. b.i.d.
*Children ages 1 month to 16 years:* 5 to 10 mg/kg daily given as two divided doses P.O.
➤ **Heartburn**
*Adults and children age 12 and older:* 75 mg of Zantac 75 P.O. as symptoms oc-

cur, up to 150 mg daily, not to exceed 2 weeks of continuous treatment.
*Adjust-a-dose:* For patients with creatinine clearance below 50 ml/minute, 150 mg P.O. q 24 hours or 50 mg I.V. q 18 to 24 hours.

## I.V. ADMINISTRATION
● To prepare I.V. injection, dilute 2 ml (50 mg) ranitidine with compatible I.V. solution to a total volume of 20 ml, and inject over at least 5 minutes. Compatible solutions include sterile water for injection, normal saline solution for injection, $D_5W$ or lactated Ringer's injection.
● To give drug by intermittent I.V. infusion, dilute 50 mg (2 ml) ranitidine in 100 ml compatible solution and infuse at a rate of 5 to 7 ml/minute. The premixed solution is 50 ml and doesn't need further dilution. Infuse over 15 to 20 minutes. After dilution, solution is stable for 48 hours at room temperature.
● Store I.V. injection at 39° to 86° F (4° to 30° C). Store premixed containers at 36° to 77° F (2° to 25° C)

## ACTION
Competitively inhibits action of histamine on the $H_2$ at receptor sites of parietal cells, decreasing gastric acid secretion.

| Route | Onset | Peak | Duration |
|-------|-------|------|----------|
| P.O. | 1 hr | 1-3 hr | 13 hr |
| I.V. | Unknown | Unknown | Unknown |

## ADVERSE REACTIONS
**CNS:** vertigo, malaise, headache.
**EENT:** blurred vision.
**Hepatic:** jaundice.
**Other:** burning and itching at injection site, *anaphylaxis, angioedema.*

## INTERACTIONS
**Drug-drug.** *Antacids:* May interfere with ranitidine absorption. Stagger doses, if possible.
*Diazepam:* May decrease absorption of diazepam. Monitor patient closely.
*Glipizide:* May increase hypoglycemic effect. Adjust glipizide dosage, as directed.
*Procainamide:* May decrease renal clearance of procainamide. Monitor patient closely for toxicity.

---

Reactions may be *common*, uncommon, *life-threatening*, or COMMON AND LIFE-THREATENING.

*Warfarin:* May interfere with warfarin clearance. Monitor patient closely.

## EFFECTS ON LAB TEST RESULTS
• May increase creatinine and ALT levels.
• May cause false-positive results in urine protein tests using Multistix.

## CONTRAINDICATIONS & CAUTIONS
• Contraindicated in patients hypersensitive to drug and those with acute porphyria.
• Use cautiously in patients with hepatic dysfunction. Adjust dosage in patients with impaired renal function.

## NURSING CONSIDERATIONS
• Assess patient for abdominal pain. Note presence of blood in emesis, stool, or gastric aspirate.
• Ranitidine may be added to total parenteral nutrition solutions.
• *Alert:* Don't confuse ranitidine with rimantadine; don't confuse Zantac with Xanax or Zyrtec.

## PATIENT TEACHING
• Instruct patient on proper use of OTC preparation, as indicated.
• Remind patient to take once-daily prescription drug at bedtime for best results.
• Instruct patient to take without regard to meals because absorption isn't affected by food.
• Tell patient taking EFFERdose to dissolve drug in 6 to 8 ounces of water before taking.
• Urge patient to avoid cigarette smoking because this may increase gastric acid secretion and worsen disease.
• Advise patient to report abdominal pain and blood in stool or emesis.
• Warn patients with phenylketonuria that EFFERdose granules and tablets contain aspartame.

---

## sucralfate
Carafate⚕

*Pregnancy risk category B*

## AVAILABLE FORMS
*Suspension:* 1 g/10 ml
*Tablets:* 1 g

## INDICATIONS & DOSAGES
➤ **Short-term (up to 8 weeks) treatment of duodenal ulcer**
*Adults:* 1 g P.O. q.i.d. 1 hour before meals and h.s.
➤ **Maintenance therapy for duodenal ulcer**
*Adults:* 1 g P.O. b.i.d.

## ACTION
Unknown. Probably adheres to and protects surface of ulcer by forming a barrier.

| Route | Onset | Peak | Duration |
|-------|-------|------|----------|
| P.O. | Unknown | Unknown | 6 hr |

## ADVERSE REACTIONS
**CNS:** dizziness, sleepiness, headache, vertigo.
**GI:** *constipation,* nausea, gastric discomfort, diarrhea, bezoar formation, vomiting, flatulence, dry mouth, indigestion.
**Musculoskeletal:** back pain.
**Skin:** rash, pruritus.

## INTERACTIONS
**Drug-drug.** *Antacids:* May decrease binding of drug to gastroduodenal mucosa, impairing effectiveness. Separate doses by 30 minutes.
*Cimetidine, digoxin, fosphenytoin, ketoconazole, phenytoin, quinidine, ranitidine, tetracycline, theophylline:* May decrease absorption. Separate doses by at least 2 hours.
*Ciprofloxacin, lomefloxacin, moxifloxacin, norfloxacin, ofloxacin:* May decrease absorption of the quinolone reducing antiinfective response. If use together can't be avoided, give at least 6 hours apart.

## EFFECTS ON LAB TEST RESULTS
None reported.

## CONTRAINDICATIONS & CAUTIONS
• Use cautiously in patients with chronic renal failure.

## NURSING CONSIDERATIONS
• Reconstitute drug before instillation through a nasogastric tube. Flush tube with water to ensure passage into stomach.
• Drug is minimally absorbed and causes few adverse reactions.

---

• Monitor patient for severe, persistent constipation.
• Sucralfate is as effective as cimetidine in healing duodenal ulcer.
• Drug contains aluminum but isn't classified as an antacid. Monitor patient with renal insufficiency for aluminum toxicity.

## PATIENT TEACHING
• Tell patient to take sucralfate on an empty stomach, 1 hour before each meal and at bedtime.
• Instruct patient to continue prescribed regimen to ensure complete healing. Pain and other ulcer signs and symptoms may subside within first few weeks of therapy.
• Urge patient to avoid cigarette smoking because it may increase gastric acid secretion and worsen disease.
• Antacids may be used while taking sucralfate, but separate antacid and sucralfate doses by 30 minutes.

# 50

## Miscellaneous gastrointestinal tract drugs

alosetron hydrochloride
balsalazide disodium
budesonide
mesalamine
olsalazine sodium
sulfasalazine
tegaserod maleate

**COMBINATION PRODUCTS**
None.

---

## alosetron hydrochloride
Lotronex◆

*Pregnancy risk category B*

**AVAILABLE FORMS**
*Tablets:* 1 mg

**INDICATIONS & DOSAGES**
➤ **Severe diarrhea-predominant irritable bowel syndrome (IBS) in women who have had chronic IBS symptoms for 6 months or longer, who have no anatomic or biochemical GI tract abnormalities, and who don't respond to conventional therapy**
*Adults:* 1 mg P.O. once daily with or without food. May increase dosage to 1 mg b.i.d., if necessary, after 4 weeks. If adequate control isn't reached after 4 weeks on twice-daily therapy, stop drug.

**ACTION**
Selectively inhibits 5-HT$_3$ receptors on enteric neurons in the GI tract. By inhibiting activation of these cation channels, neuronal depolarization is blocked, resulting in less visceral pain, colonic transit, and GI secretions, which usually contribute to the symptoms of IBS.

| Route | Onset | Peak | Duration |
|-------|-------|------|----------|
| P.O. | Unknown | 1 hr | Variable |

**ADVERSE REACTIONS**
**CNS:** headache.
**GI:** CONSTIPATION, nausea, GI discomfort and pain, abdominal discomfort and pain,

abdominal distention, hemorrhoids, regurgitation, reflux, *ileus perforation, ischemic colitis, small bowel mesenteric ischemia, impaction, obstruction.*
**Skin:** rash.

**INTERACTIONS**
**Drug-drug.** *Hydralazine, isoniazid, and procainamide:* May cause slower metabolism of these drugs because of *N*-acetyltransferase inhibition. Monitor patient for toxicity.

**EFFECTS ON LAB TEST RESULTS**
• May increase ALT level.

**CONTRAINDICATIONS & CAUTIONS**
• Contraindicated in patients hypersensitive to alosetron or any of its components, and in those with a history of or current chronic or severe constipation, sequelae from constipation, intestinal obstruction, stricture, toxic megacolon, GI perforation, GI adhesions, ischemic colitis, impaired intestinal circulation, thrombophlebitis, or hypercoagulable state.
• Contraindicated in patients with a history of or current Crohn's disease, ulcerative colitis, or diverticulitis, and in those who are unable to understand or comply with the Patient-Physician Agreement.
• Alosetron shouldn't be used in patient whose predominant symptom is constipation.
• Use cautiously in patients who are pregnant, breast-feeding, or planning to become pregnant.
• Use in patients younger than age 18 hasn't been studied.

**NURSING CONSIDERATIONS**
• Diarrhea-predominant IBS is considered severe if one or more of the following accompanies the diarrhea:
– frequent and severe abdominal pain or discomfort
– frequent bowel urgency or fecal incontinence
– disability or restriction of daily activities

---

*Rapid onset* †Canada ‡Australia ◇OTC ◆Off-label use ✐Photoguide *Liquid contains alcohol.

● *Alert:* Patients taking drug have developed ischemic colitis and serious complications of constipation, resulting in death. If patient develops ischemic colitis (acute colitis, rectal bleeding, or sudden worsening of abdominal pain) while taking drug, stop therapy.
● If patient taking drug develops constipation, stop drug until symptoms subside.
● Drug is approved for use only in women with IBS. This drug isn't indicated for use in men.
● Elderly people may be at greater risk for complications of constipation.

**PATIENT TEACHING**
● Tell patient she must sign a Patient-Physician Agreement before starting therapy.
● Urge patient to read the Medication Guide before starting alosetron and each time she refills the prescription.
● Tell patient that this drug won't cure but may alleviate some IBS symptoms.
● Inform patient that most women notice their symptoms improving after about 1 week of therapy, but some may take up to 4 weeks to get relief from abdominal pain, discomfort, and diarrhea. Let patient know that symptoms usually return within 1 week after stopping the drug.
● Advise patient that drug may be taken with or without food.
● If constipation or signs of ischemic colitis occur (rectal bleeding, bloody diarrhea, or worsened abdominal pain or cramping), tell patient to stop the drug and consult prescriber immediately. Therapy can be resumed after the situation is discussed with prescriber and constipation resolves.
● Inform patient not to share alosetron with other people having similar symptoms. This drug hasn't been shown to be safe or effective for men.
● Tell patient to notify the prescriber immediately if she becomes pregnant.

---

**balsalazide disodium**
Colazal

*Pregnancy risk category B*

---

**AVAILABLE FORMS**
*Capsules:* 750 mg

**INDICATIONS & DOSAGES**
➤ **Ulcerative colitis**
*Adults:* 2.25 g P.O. (three 750-mg capsules) t.i.d., for a total of 6.75 g/day, for 8 weeks.

**ACTION**
Unknown; probably topical. Drug converted first to mesalamine, then to 5-aminosalicylic acid; may decrease inflammation by blocking production of arachidonic acid metabolites in the colon.

| Route | Onset | Peak | Duration |
|-------|-------|------|----------|
| P.O. | Unknown | 1-2 hr | Unknown |

**ADVERSE REACTIONS**
**CNS:** fever, dizziness, fatigue, headache, insomnia.
**EENT:** pharyngitis, rhinitis, sinusitis.
**GI:** abdominal pain, anorexia, constipation, cramps, diarrhea, dyspepsia, flatulence, frequent stools, nausea, rectal bleeding, vomiting, dry mouth.
**GU:** urinary tract infection.
**Musculoskeletal:** arthralgia, back pain, myalgia.
**Respiratory:** cough, respiratory infection.
**Other:** flulike syndrome, pain.

**INTERACTIONS**
**Drug-drug.** *Oral antibiotics:* May interfere with release of mesalamine in the colon. Monitor patient for effect.

**EFFECTS ON LAB TEST RESULTS**
● May increase AST, ALT, LDH, or bilirubin levels.

**CONTRAINDICATIONS & CAUTIONS**
● Contraindicated in patients hypersensitive to salicylates or to any component of balsalazide disodium or balsalazide metabolites.
● Use cautiously in patients with history of renal disease or renal dysfunction.
● It isn't known if balsalazide appears in breast milk; use caution when giving drug to a breast-feeding patient.
● Safety and effectiveness of use of drug for longer than 12 weeks are unknown.
● Safety and effectiveness in children haven't been established.

---

Reactions may be *common*, uncommon, *life-threatening*, or COMMON AND LIFE-THREATENING.

## NURSING CONSIDERATIONS
• Hepatotoxicity, including elevated liver function test values, jaundice, cirrhosis, liver necrosis, and liver failure, has occurred with other products containing or metabolized to mesalamine. Although no signs of hepatotoxicity have been reported with balsalazide disodium, monitor patient closely for evidence of hepatic dysfunction.
• Patients with pyloric stenosis may have prolonged retention of drug.

## PATIENT TEACHING
• Advise patient not to take drug if he's allergic to aspirin.
• Instruct patient to swallow capsules whole.
• Advise patient to report adverse reactions promptly.

# budesonide
Entocort EC

*Pregnancy risk category B*

## AVAILABLE FORMS
*Capsules:* 3 mg

## INDICATIONS AND DOSAGES
➤ **Mild to moderate active Crohn's disease involving the ileum, ascending colon, or both**
*Adults:* 9 mg P.O. once daily in morning for up to 8 weeks. For recurrent episodes of active Crohn's disease, a repeat 8-week course may be given. Treatment can be tapered to 6 mg P.O. daily for 2 weeks before complete cessation.
*Adjust-a-dose:* Dosage may need to be reduced in patients with moderate to severe liver disease, if they have increased signs or symptoms of hypercorticism.

## ACTION
Significant glucocorticoid effects caused by drug's high affinity for glucocorticoid receptors, which leads to improvement of Crohn's disease.

| Route | Onset | Peak | Duration |
|-------|-------|------|----------|
| P.O. | Unknown | 30 min-10 hr | Unknown |

## ADVERSE REACTIONS
**CNS:** *headache,* dizziness, asthenia, hyperkinesia, paresthesia, tremor, vertigo, fatigue, malaise, agitation, confusion, insomnia, nervousness, somnolence.
**CV:** chest pain, hypertension, palpitations, tachycardia, flushing.
**EENT:** facial edema, ear infection, eye abnormality, abnormal vision.
**GI:** *nausea,* dyspepsia, abdominal pain, flatulence, vomiting, anal disorder, aggravated Crohn's disease, enteritis, epigastric pain, fistula, glossitis, hemorrhoids, intestinal obstruction, tongue edema, tooth disorder, increased appetite.
**GU:** dysuria, micturition frequency, nocturia, intermenstrual bleeding, menstrual disorder, hematuria, pyuria.
**Hematologic:** leukocytosis, anemia.
**Metabolic:** *hypercorticism,* dependent edema, hypokalemia, increased weight.
**Musculoskeletal:** back pain, aggravated arthritis, cramps, myalgia.
**Respiratory:** *respiratory tract infection,* bronchitis, dyspnea.
**Skin:** *acne,* alopecia, dermatitis, eczema, skin disorder, increased sweating.
**Other:** flulike disorder, sleep disorder, candidiasis, pain.

## INTERACTIONS
**Drug-drug.** *CYP inhibitors (erythromycin, indinavir, itraconazole, ketoconazole, ritonavir, saquinavir):* May increase effects of budesonide. If use together is unavoidable, reduce budesonide dosage.
**Drug-food.** *Grapefruit juice:* May increase drug effects. Discourage use together.

## EFFECTS ON LAB TEST RESULTS
• May increase alkaline phosphatase and C-reactive protein levels. May decrease potassium level.
• May increase erythrocyte sedimentation rate and WBC count. May decrease hemoglobin.

## CONTRAINDICATIONS & CAUTIONS
• Contraindicated in patients hypersensitive to budesonide.
• Use cautiously in patients with tuberculosis, hypertension, diabetes mellitus, osteoporosis, peptic ulcer disease, glaucoma, or cataracts; those with a family history of

---

diabetes or glaucoma; and those with any other condition in which glucocorticosteroids may have unwanted effects.
● Glucocorticoids appear in breast milk, and infants may have adverse reactions. Use cautiously in breast-feeding women only if benefits outweigh risks.

## NURSING CONSIDERATIONS
● Reduced liver function affects elimination of this drug; systemic availability of drug may increase in patients with liver cirrhosis.
● Patients undergoing surgery or other stressful situations may need systemic glucocorticoid supplementation in addition to budesonide therapy.
● Carefully monitor patients transferred from systemic glucocorticoid therapy to budesonide for signs and symptoms of corticosteroid withdrawal. Watch for immunosuppression, especially in patients who haven't had diseases such as chickenpox or measles; these can be fatal in patients who are immunosuppressed or receiving glucocorticoids.
● Replacement of systemic glucocorticoids with this drug may unmask allergies, such as eczema and rhinitis, which were previously controlled by systemic drug.
● Long-term use of drug may cause hypercorticism and adrenal suppression.

## PATIENT TEACHING
● Tell patient to swallow capsules whole and not to chew or break them.
● Advise patient to avoid grapefruit juice while taking drug.
● Tell patient to notify prescriber immediately if he is exposed to or develops chickenpox or measles.

## mesalamine
Asacol, Canasa, Mesasal, Pentasa, Rowasa, Salofalk

*Pregnancy risk category B*

## AVAILABLE FORMS
*Capsules (controlled-release):* 250 mg
*Rectal suspension:* 4 g/60 ml
*Suppositories:* 500 mg
*Tablets (delayed-release):* 400 mg

## INDICATIONS & DOSAGES
➤ **Active mild to moderate distal ulcerative colitis, proctitis, or proctosigmoiditis**
*Adults:* 800 mg P.O. (tablets) t.i.d. for total dose of 2.4 g/day for 6 weeks; or 1 g P.O. (capsules) q.i.d. for total dose of 4 g up to 8 weeks; or 500 mg P.R. (suppository) retained in the rectum for 1 to 3 hours or longer, b.i.d., increased to t.i.d. after 2 weeks; or 4 g as retention enema once daily (preferably h.s.). Patient should retain rectal dosage form overnight (for about 8 hours). Usual course of therapy for rectal form is 3 to 6 weeks.

## ACTION
Unknown. An active metabolite of sulfasalazine; probably acts topically by inhibiting prostaglandin production in the colon.

| Route | Onset | Peak | Duration |
|---|---|---|---|
| P.O., P.R. | Unknown | 3-12 hr | Unknown |

## ADVERSE REACTIONS
**CNS:** *headache,* dizziness, fever, fatigue, malaise, asthenia.
**CV:** chest pain.
**EENT:** *pharyngitis.*
**GI:** abdominal pain, cramps, discomfort, flatulence, diarrhea, rectal pain, bloating, nausea, *pancolitis,* vomiting, constipation, eructation.
**GU:** interstitial nephritis, nephropathy, *nephrotoxicity.*
**Musculoskeletal:** arthralgia, myalgia, back pain, hypertonia.
**Respiratory:** wheezing.
**Skin:** itching, rash, urticaria, hair loss.
**Other:** chills, acne.

## INTERACTIONS
**Drug-drug.** *Lactulose:* May impair release of delayed or extended-release products. Monitor patient closely.
*Omeprazole:* May increase absorption of mesalamine. Monitor patient closely.

## EFFECTS ON LAB TEST RESULTS
● May increase BUN, creatinine, AST, ALT, alkaline phosphatase, LDH, amylase, and lipase levels.

---

Reactions may be *common,* uncommon, *life-threatening*, or COMMON AND LIFE-THREATENING.

## CONTRAINDICATIONS & CAUTIONS

• Contraindicated in patients allergic to mesalamine, any salicylates, or any component of the preparation; also contraindicated in children.
• Use cautiously in elderly, pregnant, and breast-feeding patients and in those with renal impairment. Problems haven't been documented, but nephrotoxic potential from absorbed mesalamine exists.

## NURSING CONSIDERATIONS

• Shake suspension well before each use and remove sheath before inserting into rectum.
• Intact or partially intact tablets may be seen in the stool. Notify prescriber if this occurs repeatedly.
• Monitor periodic renal function studies in patients on long-term therapy.
• Because the mesalamine rectal suspension contains potassium metabisulfite, it may cause hypersensitivity reactions in patients sensitive to sulfites.
• **Alert:** Don't confuse Asacol with Os-Cal.

## PATIENT TEACHING

• Instruct patient to carefully follow instructions supplied with drug and to swallow tablets whole without crushing or chewing.
• Advise patient to stop drug if fever or rash occurs. Patient intolerant of sulfasalazine may also be hypersensitive to mesalamine.
• Tell patient to remove foil wrapper from suppositories before inserting into rectum.
• Teach patient about proper use of retention enema.
• Tell patient that enema solution may stain bedsheets and clothing. Patient should use protective underpads and linens.

## olsalazine sodium
Dipentum

*Pregnancy risk category C*

## AVAILABLE FORMS
*Capsules:* 250 mg

## INDICATIONS & DOSAGES
➤ **Maintenance of remission of ulcerative colitis in patients intolerant of sulfasalazine**
*Adults:* 500 mg P.O. b.i.d. with meals.

## ACTION
Unknown. After oral administration, converts to 5-aminosalicylic acid (5-ASA or mesalamine) in the colon, where it has local anti-inflammatory effect.

| Route | Onset | Peak | Duration |
|-------|-------|------|----------|
| P.O. | Unknown | 1 hr | Unknown |

## ADVERSE REACTIONS
**CNS:** headache, depression, vertigo, dizziness, fatigue.
**GI:** *diarrhea,* nausea, *abdominal pain,* dyspepsia, bloating, anorexia.
**Musculoskeletal:** arthralgia.
**Skin:** rash, itching.

## INTERACTIONS
**Drug-drug.** *Anticoagulants, coumarin derivatives:* May prolong PT or INR. Monitor bleeding studies.
**Drug-food.** *Any food:* May decrease GI irritation. Advise patient to take drug with food.

## EFFECTS ON LAB TEST RESULTS
None reported.

## CONTRAINDICATIONS & CAUTIONS
• Contraindicated in patients hypersensitive to salicylates.
• Use cautiously in patients with renal disease. Although problems haven't been reported, possibility of renal tubular damage from absorbed drug or its metabolites must be considered.

## NURSING CONSIDERATIONS
• Regularly monitor BUN and creatinine levels and urinalysis in patients with renal disease.
• Some patients have reported diarrhea during therapy. Although diarrhea appears to be dose-related, it's difficult to distinguish from worsening of disease symptoms.
• Similar drugs have caused worsening of disease.

● *Alert:* Don't confuse olsalazine with olanzapine.

**PATIENT TEACHING**
● Teach patient to take drug in evenly divided doses and with food to minimize adverse GI reactions.
● Instruct patient to report persistent or severe adverse reactions promptly.

---

## sulfasalazine
## (salazosulfapyridine, sulphasalazine)
Azulfidine, Azulfidine EN-tabs, PMS-Sulfasalazine E.C.†, Salazopyrin†‡, Salazopyrin EN-Tabs†‡

*Pregnancy risk category B*

---

**AVAILABLE FORMS**
*Tablets:* 500 mg with or without enteric coating

**INDICATIONS & DOSAGES**
➤ **Mild to moderate ulcerative colitis, adjunctive therapy in severe ulcerative colitis, Crohn's disease**
*Adults:* Initially, 3 to 4 g P.O. daily in evenly divided doses; usual maintenance dose is 2 g P.O. daily in divided doses q 6 hours. Dosage may be started with 1 to 2 g, with gradual increase in dosage to minimize adverse effects.
*Children older than age 2:* Initially, 40 to 60 mg/kg P.O. daily, divided into three to six doses; then 30 mg/kg daily in four doses. Dosage may be started at lower dose if GI intolerance occurs.
➤ **Rheumatoid arthritis in patients who have responded inadequately to salicylates or NSAIDs**
*Adults:* 2 g P.O. daily in evenly divided doses. Dosage may be started at 0.5 to 1 g daily to reduce possible GI intolerance.
➤ **Polyarticular-course juvenile rheumatoid arthritis in patients who have responded inadequately to salicylates or other NSAIDS**
*Children age 6 and older:* 30 to 50 mg/kg P.O. daily in two divided doses. Maximum dose is 2 g daily. To reduce possible GI intolerance, start with one-quarter to one-third of planned maintenance dose and in-

crease weekly until reaching maintenance dose at 1 month.

**ACTION**
Unknown.

| Route | Onset | Peak | Duration |
|-------|-------|------|----------|
| P.O. | Unknown | 3-12 hr | Unknown |

**ADVERSE REACTIONS**
**CNS:** headache, depression, *seizures,* hallucinations.
**GI:** *nausea, vomiting, diarrhea,* abdominal pain, anorexia, stomatitis.
**GU:** *toxic nephrosis with oliguria and anuria,* crystalluria, hematuria, oligospermia, infertility.
**Hematologic:** *agranulocytosis,* aplastic anemia, megaloblastic anemia, *thrombocytopenia, leukopenia,* hemolytic anemia.
**Hepatic:** jaundice, *hepatotoxicity.*
**Skin:** *erythema multiforme, Stevens-Johnson syndrome, generalized skin eruption,* epidermal necrolysis, exfoliative dermatitis, photosensitivity reaction, urticaria, pruritus.
**Other:** hypersensitivity reactions, *serum sickness, drug fever, anaphylaxis.*

**INTERACTIONS**
**Drug-drug.** *Antibiotics:* May alter action of sulfasalazine by altering internal flora. Monitor patient closely.
*Digoxin:* May reduce absorption of digoxin. Monitor patient closely.
*Folic acid:* May decrease absorption. Monitor patient.
*Hormonal contraceptives:* May decrease contraceptive effectiveness and increased risk of breakthrough bleeding. Suggest nonhormonal form of contraception.
*Iron:* May decrease blood levels of sulfasalazine caused by iron chelation. Monitor patient closely.
*Oral anticoagulants:* May increase anticoagulant effect. Watch for bleeding.
*Oral antidiabetics:* May increase hypoglycemic effect. Monitor glucose levels.

**EFFECTS ON LAB TEST RESULTS**
● May increase AST and ALT levels.
● May decrease hemoglobin and granulocyte, platelet, and WBC counts.

---

## CONTRAINDICATIONS & CAUTIONS

• Contraindicated in patients hypersensitive to drug or its metabolites, in those with porphyria or intestinal and urinary obstruction, and in children younger than age 2.

• Use cautiously and in reduced doses in patients with impaired hepatic or renal function, severe allergy, bronchial asthma, or G6PD deficiency.

## NURSING CONSIDERATIONS

• Although therapeutic response in rheumatoid arthritis has been noted as soon as 4 weeks after starting therapy, it may take 12 weeks of therapy before some patients show benefit.

• May cause urine discoloration.

• Give drug with food to decrease GI irritation.

• *Alert:* Stop drug immediately and notify prescriber if patient shows signs and symptoms of hypersensitivity.

• *Alert:* Don't confuse sulfasalazine with sulfisoxazole, salsalate, or sulfadiazine.

## PATIENT TEACHING

• Instruct patient to take drug after eating and to space doses evenly.

• Advise patient to drink plenty of water.

• Tell patient to take tablets whole.

• Warn patient to avoid ultraviolet light.

• Advise patient that drug may produce an orange-yellow discoloration of skin and urine, and may cause contact lenses to turn yellow.

• Instruct patient to notify prescriber immediately if discoloration of skin or urine occurs.

• Tell patient to make sure fluid intake is adequate and to swallow tablets intact without crushing or chewing.

---

## tegaserod maleate
Zelnorm

*Pregnancy risk category B*

## AVAILABLE FORMS

*Tablets:* 2 mg, 6 mg

## INDICATIONS & DOSAGES

➤ **Short-term treatment of women with irritable bowel syndrome, when the primary bowel symptom is constipation**

*Women:* 6 mg P.O. b.i.d. before meals for 4 to 6 weeks. May add another 4- to 6-week course for patients who respond to therapy at 4 to 6 weeks.

## ACTION

Binds with high affinity to 5-HT$_4$ receptors and acts as an agonist. The activation of 5-HT$_4$ receptors in the GI tract stimulates the peristaltic reflex and intestinal secretion and inhibits visceral sensitivity.

| Route | Onset | Peak | Duration |
|-------|-------|------|----------|
| P.O. | Unknown | 1 hr | Unknown |

## ADVERSE REACTIONS

**CNS:** *headache,* dizziness, migraine.
**GI:** *abdominal pain,* diarrhea, nausea, flatulence.
**Musculoskeletal:** back pain, leg pain, arthropathy.
**Other:** accidental injury.

## INTERACTIONS

**Drug-drug.** *Digoxin:* May reduce peak plasma level and exposure of digoxin by 15%. No need to adjust digoxin dose.
**Drug-food.** *Food:* May reduce bioavailability of tegaserod. Advise patient to take drug on an empty stomach.

## EFFECTS ON LAB TEST RESULTS

None reported.

## CONTRAINDICATIONS & CAUTIONS

• Contraindicated in patients hypersensitive to drug or its components and in those with severe renal impairment, moderate or severe hepatic impairment, a history of bowel obstruction, symptomatic gallbladder disease, suspected sphincter of Oddi dysfunction or abdominal adhesions, or frequently or currently occurring diarrhea.

• Use cautiously in patient who now has or often has diarrhea.

## NURSING CONSIDERATIONS

• Stop drug if patient has new or sudden worsening of abdominal pain.

• Patients have developed diarrhea during therapy. Diarrhea usually occurs in the first week of treatment and resolves as therapy continues.

---

*Rapid onset*   †Canada   ‡Australia   ◊OTC   ♦Off-label use   ⌗Photoguide   *Liquid contains alcohol.

## PATIENT TEACHING

- Tell patient to take drug on an empty stomach, before a meal.
- Inform patient that diarrhea might develop during therapy.
- Tell patient to consult her prescriber if she gets severe diarrhea or diarrhea accompanied by severe cramping, abdominal pain, or dizziness.
- Advise patient not to start therapy if she now has or often has diarrhea.
- Warn patient not to use drug during pregnancy or breast-feeding.

# 51

## Corticosteroids

betamethasone
betamethasone acetate and
    betamethasone sodium
    phosphate
betamethasone sodium
    phosphate
cortisone acetate
dexamethasone
dexamethasone acetate
dexamethasone sodium
    phosphate
fludrocortisone acetate
hydrocortisone
hydrocortisone acetate
hydrocortisone cypionate
hydrocortisone sodium
    phosphate
hydrocortisone sodium succinate
methylprednisolone
methylprednisolone acetate
methylprednisolone sodium
    succinate
prednisolone
prednisolone acetate
prednisolone sodium phosphate
prednisolone tebutate
prednisone
triamcinolone
triamcinolone acetonide
triamcinolone diacetate
triamcinolone hexacetonide

### COMBINATION PRODUCTS

DECADRON PHOSPHATE WITH
XYLOCAINE: dexamethasone phosphate
4 mg and lidocaine hydrochloride 10 mg
per ml.

---

### betamethasone
Celestone*

### betamethasone acetate and
### betamethasone sodium
### phosphate
Celestone Chronodose‡,
Celestone Soluspan

### betamethasone sodium
### phosphate
Celestone Phosphate

*Pregnancy risk category C*

### AVAILABLE FORMS
**betamethasone**
*Syrup:* 600 mcg/5 ml*
*Tablets:* 600 mcg
*Tablets (effervescent):* 500 mcg†
**betamethasone acetate and betametha-
sone sodium phosphate**
*Injection (suspension):* betamethasone
acetate 3 mg and betamethasone sodium
phosphate (equivalent to 3-mg base) per
ml
**betamethasone sodium phosphate**
*Injection:* 4 mg (equivalent to 3-mg base)
per ml in 5-ml vials

### INDICATIONS & DOSAGES
➤ **Conditions with severe inflammation,
conditions requiring immunosuppression**
*Adults:* 0.6 to 7.2 mg P.O. daily. Or, 0.5 to
9 mg I.M. or into joint or soft tissue daily.
Betamethasone sodium phosphate-acetate
suspension 6 to 12 mg injected into large
joints or 1.5 to 6 mg injected into smaller
joints. Both injections may be given q 1 to
2 weeks, p.r.n.
*Children:* 0.0175 to 0.25 mg/kg daily or
0.5 to 7.5 mg/m² daily; given in three or
four divided doses. Not recommended for
long-term use; especially likely to inhibit
growth.

### ACTION
Not completely defined. Decreases inflammation, mainly by stabilizing leukocyte
lysosomal membranes; suppresses immune response; stimulates bone marrow;
and influences protein, fat, and carbohydrate metabolism.

| Route | Onset | Peak | Duration |
|-------|-------|------|----------|
| P.O. | Rapid | Unknown | 3-25 days |
| I.M. | Rapid | 1-3 hr | 7-14 days |

---

## ADVERSE REACTIONS

**CNS:** *euphoria, insomnia,* psychotic behavior, ***pseudotumor cerebri,*** vertigo, headache, paresthesia, *seizures.*
**CV:** ***heart failure,*** hypertension, edema, ***arrhythmias,*** thrombophlebitis, ***thromboembolism.***
**EENT:** cataracts, glaucoma.
**GI:** *peptic ulceration,* GI irritation, increased appetite, ***pancreatitis,*** nausea, vomiting.
**GU:** menstrual irregularities.
**Metabolic:** hypokalemia, hyperglycemia, carbohydrate intolerance, hypercholesterolemia, hypocalcemia.
**Musculoskeletal:** muscle weakness, osteoporosis; growth suppression in children.
**Skin:** hirsutism, delayed wound healing, acne, various skin eruptions.
**Other:** susceptibility to infections; *acute adrenal insufficiency* after increased stress or abrupt withdrawal after long-term use, cushingoid state.
**After abrupt withdrawal:** rebound inflammation, fatigue, weakness, arthralgia, fever, dizziness, lethargy, depression, fainting, orthostatic hypotension, dyspnea, anorexia, *hypoglycemia. After prolonged use, sudden withdrawal may be fatal.*

## INTERACTIONS

**Drug-drug.** *Antidiabetics, including insulin:* May increase glucose level. May need dosage adjustment of antidiabetic therapy.
*Aspirin, indomethacin, other NSAIDs:* May increase risk of GI distress and bleeding. Use together cautiously.
*Barbiturates, carbamazepine, fosphenytoin, phenytoin, rifampin:* May decrease corticosteroid effect. Corticosteroid dosage may need to be increased.
*Cardiac glycosides:* May increase risk of arrhythmia resulting from hypokalemia. Monitor potassium level.
*Cyclosporine:* May increase toxicity. Monitor patient closely.
*Oral anticoagulants:* May alter dosage requirements. Monitor PT and INR closely.
*Potassium-depleting drugs such as thiazide diuretics:* May enhance potassium-wasting effects of betamethasone. Monitor potassium level.

*Salicylates:* May reduce salicylate level. Monitor patient for lack of salicylate effectiveness.
*Skin-test antigens:* May decrease response. Postpone skin testing until therapy is completed.
*Toxoids, vaccines:* May decrease antibody response and increase risk of neurologic complications. Avoid using together.
**Drug-herb.** *Echinacea:* May increase immune-stimulating effects. Discourage use together.
*Ginseng:* May increase immune-modulating response. Discourage use together.
**Drug-lifestyle.** *Alcohol use:* May increase risk of gastric irritation and GI ulceration. Discourage use together.

## EFFECTS ON LAB TEST RESULTS

● May increase glucose and cholesterol levels. May decrease potassium and calcium levels.
● May suppress reactions to skin tests. May cause false-negative results in nitroblue tetrazolium test for systemic bacterial infections. May cause decreased $^{131}I$ uptake and protein-bound iodine level in thyroid function tests.

## CONTRAINDICATIONS & CAUTIONS

● Contraindicated in patients hypersensitive to drug or its ingredients, in those with systemic fungal infections, and in those receiving immunosuppressive doses together with live virus vaccines.
● Use with caution and only in life-threatening situations if patient has recent MI or active peptic ulcer.
● Use cautiously in patients with renal disease, hypertension, osteoporosis, diabetes mellitus, hypothyroidism, cirrhosis, diverticulitis, nonspecific ulcerative colitis, recent intestinal anastomoses, thromboembolic disorders, active hepatitis, lactation, seizures, myasthenia gravis, heart failure, tuberculosis, ocular herpes simplex, emotional instability, or psychotic tendencies.
● Because some formulations contain sulfite preservatives, also use cautiously in patients hypersensitive to sulfites.

## NURSING CONSIDERATIONS

● Check for sensitivity to other corticosteroids.

---

Reactions may be *common,* uncommon, *life-threatening,* or COMMON AND LIFE-THREATENING.

• Betamethasone sodium phosphate and betamethasone acetate suspension combination product shouldn't be given by I.V. route.

• *Alert:* Don't use drug for alternate-day therapy.

• *Alert:* Avoid using wrong salt formulation of drug; salt formulations aren't interchangeable.

• Obtain baseline weight before starting therapy, and weigh patient daily; report sudden weight gain to prescriber.

• For better results and less toxicity, give once-daily dose in morning.

• Most adverse reactions to corticosteroids are dose- or duration-dependent.

• To reduce GI irritation, give drug with milk or food.

• To prevent muscle atrophy, give I.M. injection deeply. Rotate injection sites.

• Always adjust drug to lowest effective dose.

• Monitor patient for cushingoid symptoms, including moon face, buffalo hump, central obesity, thinning hair, hypertension, and increased susceptibility to infection.

• Monitor glucose and potassium levels regularly. Diabetic patient may need adjustments in insulin dosage.

• Watch for depression or mood changes, especially in patient receiving long-term therapy.

• A calorie- or sodium-restricted diet with protein supplementation may be needed for patient receiving long-term therapy.

• Elderly patients may be more susceptible to osteoporosis with long-term use.

• Adrenal suppression may last up to 1 year after drug is stopped.

• Gradually reduce drug dosage after long-term therapy.

• Observe patient for evidence of infection, especially after corticosteroid withdrawal.

**PATIENT TEACHING**

• Tell patient not to stop drug abruptly or without prescriber's consent.

• Instruct patient to take drug with food or milk; tell patient using effervescent tablets to dissolve them in water immediately before ingestion.

• Teach patient about drug's effects. Warn patient on long-term therapy about cushingoid effects (moon face, buffalo hump) and to notify prescriber about sudden weight gain or swelling.

• Instruct patient to report signs and symptoms of corticosteroid withdrawal, including fatigue, weakness, joint pain, dizziness upon standing, and shortness of breath.

• Tell patient to contact prescriber if signs and symptoms worsen or drug is no longer effective. Tell him not to increase dosage without prescriber's consent.

• Advise elderly patient receiving long-term therapy to consider exercise or physical therapy. Tell him to ask prescriber about vitamin D or calcium supplement.

• Advise patient receiving prolonged therapy to have periodic eye examinations.

• Tell patient to report slow healing of wounds.

• Instruct patient to carry or wear medical identification indicating his need for supplemental glucocorticoids during stress. This card should contain prescriber's name and drug name and dosage.

• Advise patient to avoid exposure to infections (such as chickenpox or measles) and to notify prescriber if exposure occurs.

• Tell patient to report signs and symptoms of infection (fever, sore throat, painful urination, muscle pain) or injuries during therapy and within 12 months after therapy stops.

---

## cortisone acetate
Cortate‡, Cortone Acetate

*Pregnancy risk category C*

**AVAILABLE FORMS**
*Injection (suspension):* 50 mg/ml
*Tablets:* 5 mg, 10 mg, 25 mg

**INDICATIONS & DOSAGES**
➤ **Adrenal insufficiency, allergy, inflammation**
*Adults:* 25 to 300 mg P.O. or 20 to 300 mg I.M. daily. Dosages are highly individualized, depending on severity of disease.

**ACTION**
Not completely defined. Decreases inflammation, mainly by stabilizing leukocyte

lysosomal membranes; suppresses immune response; stimulates bone marrow; and influences protein, fat, and carbohydrate metabolism.

| Route | Onset | Peak | Duration |
|---|---|---|---|
| P.O., I.M. | Variable | Variable | Variable |

## ADVERSE REACTIONS

**CNS:** *euphoria, insomnia,* psychotic behavior, *pseudotumor cerebri,* vertigo, headache, paresthesia, *seizures.*
**CV:** *heart failure,* hypertension, edema, *arrhythmias,* thrombophlebitis, *thromboembolism.*
**EENT:** cataracts, glaucoma.
**GI:** *peptic ulceration,* GI irritation, increased appetite, *pancreatitis,* nausea, vomiting.
**GU:** menstrual irregularities, increased urine glucose levels.
**Metabolic:** hypokalemia, hyperglycemia, carbohydrate intolerance, hypercholesterolemia, hypocalcemia.
**Musculoskeletal:** growth suppression in children, muscle weakness, osteoporosis.
**Skin:** hirsutism, delayed wound healing, acne, various skin eruptions; atrophy at I.M. injection site.
**Other:** susceptibility to infections; *acute adrenal insufficiency* after increased stress or abrupt withdrawal after long-term therapy, cushingoid state.
**After abrupt withdrawal:** rebound inflammation, fatigue, weakness, arthralgia, fever, dizziness, lethargy, depression, fainting, orthostatic hypotension, dyspnea, anorexia, *hypoglycemia. After prolonged use, sudden withdrawal may be fatal.*

## INTERACTIONS

**Drug-drug.** *Antidiabetics, including insulin:* May decrease response. May need dosage adjustment.
*Aspirin, indomethacin, other NSAIDs:* May increase risk of GI distress and bleeding. Use together cautiously.
*Barbiturates, fosphenytoin, phenytoin, rifampin:* May decrease corticosteroid effect. Increase corticosteroid dosage.
*Cyclosporine:* May increase toxicity. Monitor patient closely.
*Live attenuated virus vaccines, other toxoids and vaccines:* May decrease antibody response and may increase risk of neurologic complications. Avoid using together.
*Oral anticoagulants:* May alter dosage requirements. Monitor PT and INR closely.
*Potassium-depleting drugs such as thiazide diuretics:* May enhance potassium-wasting effects of cortisone. Monitor potassium level.
*Salicylates:* May decrease salicylate level. Watch for lack of salicylate effectiveness.
*Skin-test antigens:* May decrease response. Postpone skin testing until therapy is completed.
**Drug-herb.** *Echinacea:* May increase immune-stimulating effects. Discourage use together.
*Ginseng:* May increase immune-modulating response. Discourage use together.
**Drug-lifestyle.** *Alcohol use:* May increase risk of gastric irritation and GI ulceration. Discourage use together.

## EFFECTS ON LAB TEST RESULTS

• May increase glucose and cholesterol levels. May decrease potassium, calcium, $T_3$, and $T_4$ levels.
• May suppress reactions to skin tests. May cause false-negative results in nitroblue tetrazolium test for systemic bacterial infections. May cause decreased $^{131}I$ uptake and protein-bound iodine level in thyroid function tests.

## CONTRAINDICATIONS & CAUTIONS

• Contraindicated in patients hypersensitive to drug or its ingredients, in those with systemic fungal infections, and in those receiving immunosuppressive doses with live virus vaccines.
• Use with caution in patients with recent MI.
• Use cautiously in patients with GI ulcer, renal disease, hypertension, osteoporosis, diabetes mellitus, hypothyroidism, cirrhosis, diverticulitis, nonspecific ulcerative colitis, recent intestinal anastomoses, thromboembolic disorders, seizures, myasthenia gravis, heart failure, tuberculosis, active hepatitis, lactation, ocular herpes simplex, emotional instability, or psychotic tendencies.

## NURSING CONSIDERATIONS
- Check for sensitivity to other corticosteroids.
- Most adverse reactions to corticosteroids are dose- or duration-dependent.
- To reduce GI irritation, give with milk or food. Patient may need adjunctive medication to prevent GI irritation.
- For better results and less toxicity, give a once-daily dose in morning.
- The I.M. route has slow onset of action and shouldn't be used for acute conditions that need rapid effect. This route may be used on a twice-daily schedule matching diurnal variation. Rotate injection sites to prevent muscle atrophy. The I.M. route is usually reserved for patients unable to take the P.O. form.
- Mixing or diluting parenteral suspension may alter absorption rate and decrease drug effectiveness.
- *Alert:* Drug isn't for I.V. use.
- Drug should always be adjusted to lowest effective dose.
- Monitor electrolyte and glucose levels. Diabetic patient may need adjustment in insulin dosage.
- Monitor patient for fluid and electrolyte imbalances. Patient may need low-sodium diet and potassium supplements.
- Monitor patient for cushingoid effects, including moon face, buffalo hump, central obesity, thinning hair, hypertension, and increased susceptibility to infection.
- Elderly patients may be more susceptible to osteoporosis with long-term use.
- Gradually reduce dosage after long-term therapy.
- Watch for evidence of infection, especially after corticosteroid withdrawal.

## PATIENT TEACHING
- Tell patient not to stop drug abruptly or without prescriber's consent.
- Instruct patient to take drug with milk or food.
- Advise patient receiving long-term therapy to consider exercise or physical therapy. Also, tell him to ask prescriber about vitamin D or calcium supplement.
- Tell patient to report slow healing of wounds.
- Warn patient on long-term therapy about cushingoid effects (moon face, buffalo hump) and the need to notify prescriber about sudden weight gain or swelling.
- Instruct patient to carry or wear medical identification indicating his need for supplemental glucocorticoids during stress. This card should contain prescriber's name, and drug name and dosage.
- Instruct patient to avoid exposure to infections (such as measles and chickenpox) and to notify prescriber if such exposure occurs.

---

## dexamethasone
Decadron*, Dexone, Hexadrol

## dexamethasone acetate
Cortastat LA, Dalalone D.P., Decaject LA, Dexasone LA, Dexone LA, Solurex LA

## dexamethasone sodium phosphate
Cortastat, Dalalone, Decadron Phosphate, Decaject, Dexasone, Hexadrol Phosphate, Solurex

*Pregnancy risk category C*

---

## AVAILABLE FORMS
**dexamethasone**
*Elixir:* 0.5 mg/5 ml*
*Oral solution:* 0.5 mg/5 ml, 1 mg/ml
*Tablets:* 0.25 mg, 0.5 mg, 0.75 mg, 1 mg, 1.5 mg, 2 mg, 4 mg, 6 mg
**dexamethasone acetate**
*Injection:* 8 mg/ml, 16 mg/ml
**dexamethasone sodium phosphate**
*Injection:* 4 mg/ml, 10 mg/ml, 20 mg/ml, 24 mg/ml

## INDICATIONS & DOSAGES
➤ **Cerebral edema**
*Adults:* Initially, 10 mg phosphate I.V.; then 4 to 6 mg I.M. q 6 hours until symptoms subside (usually 2 to 4 days); then tapered over 5 to 7 days.
➤ **Inflammatory conditions, allergic reactions, neoplasias**
*Adults:* 0.75 to 9 mg/day P.O. or 0.5 to 9 mg/day phosphate I.M. Or, 8 to 16 mg acetate I.M. into joint or soft tissue q 1 to 3 weeks. Or, 0.8 to 1.6 mg acetate into lesions q 1 to 3 weeks.

---

➤**Shock**
*Adults:* 20 mg phosphate as single first dose; then 3 mg/kg/24 hours via continuous I.V. infusion. Or, 1 to 6 mg/kg phosphate I.V. as single dose. Or, 40 mg phosphate I.V. q 2 to 6 hours, p.r.n., continued only until patient is stabilized (usually not longer than 48 to 72 hours).

➤**Dexamethasone suppression test for Cushing's syndrome**
*Adults:* After determining baseline 24-hour urine levels of 17-hydroxycorticosteroids, 0.5 mg P.O. q 6 hours for 48 hours. Repeat 24-hour urine collection to determine 17-hydroxycorticosteroid excretion during second 24 hours of dexamethasone administration. Or, 1 mg P.O. as single dose at 11:00 p.m. with determination of plasma cortisol at 8 a.m. the next morning.

➤**Adrenocortical insufficiency**
*Children:* 0.024 to 0.34 mg/kg or 0.66 to 10 mg/m$^2$ P.O. daily, in four divided doses.

## I.V. ADMINISTRATION
• For direct injection, inject undiluted over at least 1 minute.
• For intermittent or continuous infusion, dilute solution according to manufacturer's instructions, and give over prescribed duration. If used for continuous infusion, change solution every 24 hours.

## ACTION
Not clearly defined. Decreases inflammation, mainly by stabilizing leukocyte lysosomal membranes; suppresses immune response; stimulates bone marrow; and influences protein, fat, and carbohydrate metabolism.

| Route | Onset | Peak | Duration |
|---|---|---|---|
| P.O. | 1-2 hr | 1-2 hr | 2½ days |
| I.V. | 1 hr | 1 hr | Variable |
| I.M. | 1 hr | 1 hr | 6 days |
| I.M. (acetate) | 1 hr | 8 hr | Unknown |

## ADVERSE REACTIONS
**CNS:** *euphoria, insomnia,* psychotic behavior, *pseudotumor cerebri,* vertigo, headache, paresthesia, *seizures.*
**CV:** *heart failure,* hypertension, edema, *arrhythmias,* thrombophlebitis, *thromboembolism.*
**EENT:** cataracts, glaucoma.

**GI:** *peptic ulceration,* GI irritation, increased appetite, *pancreatitis,* nausea, vomiting.
**GU:** menstrual irregularities, increased urine glucose and calcium levels.
**Metabolic:** hypokalemia, hyperglycemia, carbohydrate intolerance, hypercholesterolemia, hypocalcemia.
**Musculoskeletal:** growth suppression in children, muscle weakness, osteoporosis.
**Skin:** hirsutism, delayed wound healing, acne, various skin eruptions, atrophy at I.M. injection site.
**Other:** cushingoid state, susceptibility to infections, *acute adrenal insufficiency* after increased stress or abrupt withdrawal after long-term therapy.
**After abrupt withdrawal:** rebound inflammation, fatigue, weakness, arthralgia, fever, dizziness, lethargy, depression, fainting, orthostatic hypotension, dyspnea, anorexia, *hypoglycemia. After prolonged use, sudden withdrawal may be fatal.*

## INTERACTIONS
**Drug-drug.** *Aminoglutethimide:* May cause loss of dexamethasone-induced adrenal suppression. Use together cautiously.
*Antidiabetics, including insulin:* May decrease response. May need dosage adjustment.
*Aspirin, indomethacin, other NSAIDs:* May increase risk of GI distress and bleeding. Use together cautiously.
*Barbiturates, carbamazepine, phenytoin, rifampin:* May decrease corticosteroid effect. Increase corticosteroid dosage.
*Cardiac glycosides:* May increase risk of arrhythmia resulting from hypokalemia. May need dosage adjustment.
*Cyclosporine:* May increase toxicity. Monitor patient closely.
*Ephedrine:* May cause decreased half-life and increased clearance of dexamethasone.
*Oral anticoagulants:* May alter dosage requirements. Monitor PT and INR closely.
*Potassium-depleting drugs such as thiazide diuretics:* May enhance potassium-wasting effects of dexamethasone. Monitor potassium level.

---

Reactions may be *common,* uncommon, *life-threatening,* or COMMON AND LIFE-THREATENING.

*Salicylates:* May decrease salicylate level. Monitor patient for lack of salicylate effectiveness.

*Skin-test antigens:* May decrease response. Postpone skin testing until therapy is completed.

*Toxoids, vaccines:* May decrease antibody response and increases risk of neurologic complications. Avoid using together.

**Drug-herb.** *Echinacea:* May increase immune-stimulating effects. Discourage use together.

*Ginseng:* May increase immune-modulating response. Discourage use together.

**Drug-lifestyle.** *Alcohol use:* May increase risk of gastric irritation and GI ulceration. Discourage use together.

### EFFECTS ON LAB TEST RESULTS
• May increase glucose and cholesterol levels. May decrease potassium, calcium, $T_3$, and $T_4$ levels.
• May cause decreased $^{131}I$ uptake and protein-bound iodine levels in thyroid function tests. May cause false-negative results in nitroblue tetrazolium test for systemic bacterial infections. May alter reactions to skin tests.

### CONTRAINDICATIONS & CAUTIONS
• Contraindicated in patients hypersensitive to drug or its ingredients, in those with systemic fungal infections, and in those receiving immunosuppressive doses together with live virus vaccines.
• Use with caution in patient with recent MI.
• Use cautiously in patients with GI ulcer, renal disease, hypertension, osteoporosis, diabetes mellitus, hypothyroidism, cirrhosis, diverticulitis, nonspecific ulcerative colitis, recent intestinal anastomoses, thromboembolic disorders, seizures, myasthenia gravis, heart failure, tuberculosis, active hepatitis, lactation, ocular herpes simplex, emotional instability, or psychotic tendencies.
• Because some formulations contain sulfite preservatives, also use cautiously in patients sensitive to sulfites.

### NURSING CONSIDERATIONS
• Determine whether patient is sensitive to other corticosteroids.

• Most adverse reactions to corticosteroids are dose- or duration-dependent.
• For better results and less toxicity, give once-daily dose in morning.
• Give oral dose with food when possible. Patient may need medication to prevent GI irritation.
• Give I.M. injection deeply into gluteal muscle. Rotate injection sites to prevent muscle atrophy. Avoid S.C. injection because atrophy and sterile abscesses may occur.
• Always adjust to lowest effective dose.
• Monitor patient's weight, blood pressure, and electrolyte levels.
• Monitor patient for cushingoid effects, including moon face, buffalo hump, central obesity, thinning hair, hypertension, and increased susceptibility to infection.
• Watch for depression or psychotic episodes, especially in high-dose therapy.
• Diabetic patient may need increased insulin; monitor glucose levels.
• Drug may mask or worsen infections, including latent amebiasis.
• Elderly patients may be more susceptible to osteoporosis with long-term use.
• Inspect patient's skin for petechiae.
• Gradually reduce dosage after long-term therapy.
• **Alert:** Don't confuse dexamethasone with desoximetasone.

### PATIENT TEACHING
• Tell patient not to stop drug abruptly or without prescriber's consent.
• Instruct patient to take drug with food or milk.
• Teach patient signs and symptoms of early adrenal insufficiency: fatigue, muscle weakness, joint pain, fever, anorexia, nausea, shortness of breath, dizziness, and fainting.
• Instruct patient to carry or wear medical identification indicating his need for supplemental systemic glucocorticoids during stress, especially when dosage is decreased. This card should contain prescriber's name, and name and dosage of drug.
• Warn patient on long-term therapy about cushingoid effects (moon face, buffalo hump) and the need to notify prescriber about sudden weight gain or swelling.
• Warn patient about easy bruising.

• Advise patient receiving long-term therapy to consider exercise or physical therapy. Tell him to ask prescriber about vitamin D or calcium supplement.
• Instruct patient receiving long-term therapy to have periodic eye examinations.
• Advise patient to avoid exposure to infections (such as measles and chickenpox) and to notify prescriber if such exposure occurs.

---

## fluorocortisone acetate
### Florinef Acetate

*Pregnancy risk category C*

### AVAILABLE FORMS
*Tablets:* 0.1 mg

### INDICATIONS & DOSAGES
➤ **Salt-losing adrenogenital syndrome**
*Adults:* 0.1 to 0.2 mg P.O. daily.
➤ **Addison's disease (adrenocortical insufficiency)**
*Adults:* 0.1 mg P.O. daily. Usual dosage range is 0.1 mg three times weekly to 0.2 mg daily. Decrease dosage to 0.05 mg daily if transient hypertension develops as a result of drug therapy.

### ACTION
Increases sodium reabsorption and potassium and hydrogen secretion at the distal convoluted tubules of nephrons.

| Route | Onset | Peak | Duration |
|-------|-------|------|----------|
| P.O. | Variable | 2 hr | 1-2 days |

### ADVERSE REACTIONS
**CV:** hypertension, cardiac hypertrophy, edema, *heart failure.*
**Hematologic:** bruising.
**Metabolic:** *sodium and water retention,* hypokalemia.
**Skin:** diaphoresis, urticaria, allergic rash.

### INTERACTIONS
**Drug-drug.** *Barbiturates, carbamazepine, fosphenytoin, phenytoin, rifampin:* May increase clearance of fluorocortisone acetate. Monitor patient for possible diminished effect of corticosteroid. Corticosteroid dosage may need to be increased.

*Potassium-depleting drugs such as amphotericin B, thiazide diuretics:* May enhance potassium-wasting effects of fluorocortisone. Monitor potassium level.
**Drug-food.** *Sodium-containing drugs or foods:* May increase blood pressure. Sodium intake may need adjustment.

### EFFECTS ON LAB TEST RESULTS
• May decrease potassium level.

### CONTRAINDICATIONS & CAUTIONS
• Contraindicated in patients hypersensitive to drug and in those with systemic fungal infections.
• Use cautiously in patients with hypothyroidism, recent MI, cirrhosis, ocular herpes simplex, emotional instability, psychotic tendencies, diverticulitis, fresh intestinal anastomoses, active or latent peptic ulcer, renal insufficiency, hypertension, osteoporosis, myasthenia gravis, active hepatitis, lactation, or nonspecific ulcerative colitis.

### NURSING CONSIDERATIONS
• Drug is used with cortisone or hydrocortisone in adrenal insufficiency.
• Perform glucose tolerance tests only if needed because addisonian patients tend to develop severe hypoglycemia within 3 hours of the test.
• *Alert:* Monitor patient's blood pressure and electrolyte levels. If hypertension occurs, notify prescriber and expect dosage to be decreased by 50%.
• Weigh patient daily; notify prescriber about sudden weight gain.
• Unless contraindicated, give low-sodium diet that is high in potassium and protein. Potassium supplements may be needed.
• Drug may cause adverse effects similar to those of glucocorticoids.

### PATIENT TEACHING
• Tell patient to notify prescriber if low blood pressure, weakness, cramping, or palpitations worsen, or if changes in mental status occur.
• Warn patient that mild swelling is common.

---

## hydrocortisone
Aquacort†, Cortef, Cortenema, Hydrocortone

## hydrocortisone acetate
Anucort-HC, Anusol-HC, Cortifoam, Proctocort

## hydrocortisone cypionate
Cortef

## hydrocortisone sodium phosphate

## hydrocortisone sodium succinate
A-Hydrocort, Solu-Cortef

*Pregnancy risk category C*

---

## AVAILABLE FORMS
**hydrocortisone**
*Enema:* 100 mg/60 ml
*Tablets:* 5 mg, 10 mg, 20 mg
**hydrocortisone acetate**
*Injection:* 25 mg/ml\*, 50 mg/ml\* suspension
*Rectal aerosol foam:* 10% aerosol foam (provides 90 mg/application)
*Rectal suppository:* 25 mg, 30 mg
**hydrocortisone cypionate**
*Oral suspension:* 2 mg/ml
**hydrocortisone sodium phosphate**
*Injection:* 50 mg/ml solution
**hydrocortisone sodium succinate**
*Injection:* 100-mg vial\*, 250-mg vial\*, 500-mg vial\*, 1,000-mg vial\*

## INDICATIONS & DOSAGES
➤ **Severe inflammation, adrenal insufficiency**
*Adults:* 5 to 30 mg P.O. b.i.d., t.i.d., or q.i.d. (as much as 80 mg q.i.d. may be given in acute situations). Or, initially, 100 to 500 mg succinate I.M. or I.V.; then 50 to 100 mg I.M., as indicated. Or, 15 to 240 mg phosphate I.M., S.C., or I.V. daily in divided doses q 12 hours. Or, 5 to 75 mg acetate into joints or soft tissue repeated at 3 to 5 days for bursae and 1 to 4 weeks for joints. Dosage varies with size of joint. Local anesthetics commonly are injected with dose.

➤ **Shock**
*Adults:* Initially, 50 mg/kg succinate I.V., repeated in 4 hours. Repeat dosage q 24 hours, p.r.n. Or, 100 to 500 mg to 2 g q 2 to 6 hours, continued until patient is stabilized (usually not longer than 48 to 72 hours).
*Children:* Phosphate (I.M.) or succinate (I.M. or I.V.) 0.16 to 1 mg/kg or 6 to 30 mg/m² given once or twice daily.
➤ **Adjunct treatment for ulcerative colitis and proctitis**
*Adults:* 1 enema (100 mg) P.R. nightly for 21 days. Or, 1 applicatorful (90-mg foam) P.R. daily or b.i.d. for 14 to 21 days. Or, 25 mg rectal suppository b.i.d. for 2 weeks. For severe proctitis, 25 mg P.R. t.i.d. or 50 mg b.i.d.

## I.V. ADMINISTRATION
• Don't use acetate or suspension form for I.V. route.
• Hydrocortisone sodium phosphate may be added directly to $D_5W$ or normal saline solution for I.V. use.
• Reconstitute hydrocortisone sodium succinate with bacteriostatic water or bacteriostatic saline solution before adding to I.V. solutions. For direct injection, inject over 30 seconds to 10 minutes. For infusion, dilute with $D_5W$, normal saline solution, or dextrose 5% in normal saline solution to 1 mg/ml or less.

## ACTION
Not clearly defined. Decreases inflammation, mainly by stabilizing leukocyte lysosomal membranes; suppresses immune response; stimulates bone marrow; and influences protein, fat, and carbohydrate metabolism.

| Route | Onset | Peak | Duration |
|---|---|---|---|
| P.O., I.V., I.M., P.R. | Variable | Variable | Variable |

## ADVERSE REACTIONS
**CNS:** *euphoria, insomnia,* psychotic behavior, ***pseudotumor cerebri,*** vertigo, headache, paresthesia, ***seizures.***
**CV:** ***heart failure,*** hypertension, edema, ***arrhythmias,*** thrombophlebitis, ***thromboembolism.***
**EENT:** cataracts, glaucoma.

---

*Rapid onset*   †Canada   ‡Australia   ◇OTC   ◆Off-label use   🖉Photoguide   \*Liquid contains alcohol.

**GI:** *peptic ulceration,* GI irritation, increased appetite, *pancreatitis,* nausea, vomiting.

**GU:** menstrual irregularities, increased urine calcium levels.

**Hematologic:** easy bruising.

**Metabolic:** hypokalemia, hyperglycemia, carbohydrate intolerance, hypercholesterolemia, hypocalcemia.

**Musculoskeletal:** growth suppression in children, muscle weakness, osteoporosis.

**Skin:** hirsutism, delayed wound healing, acne, skin eruptions.

**Other:** cushingoid state, susceptibility to infections, *acute adrenal insufficiency after increased stress or abrupt withdrawal after long-term therapy.*

**After abrupt withdrawal:** rebound inflammation, fatigue, weakness, arthralgia, fever, dizziness, lethargy, depression, fainting, orthostatic hypotension, dyspnea, anorexia, *hypoglycemia. After prolonged use, sudden withdrawal may be fatal.*

**INTERACTIONS**

**Drug-drug.** *Aspirin, indomethacin, other NSAIDs:* May increase risk of GI distress and bleeding. Use together cautiously.

*Barbiturates, carbamazepine, fosphenytoin, phenytoin, rifampin:* May decrease corticosteroid effect. Increase corticosteroid dosage.

*Cyclosporine:* May increase toxicity. Monitor patient closely.

*Live attenuated virus vaccines, other toxoids and vaccines:* May decrease antibody response and increase risk of neurologic complications. Avoid using together.

*Oral anticoagulants:* May alter dosage requirements. Monitor PT and INR closely.

*Potassium-depleting drugs such as thiazide diuretics:* May enhance potassium-wasting effects of hydrocortisone. Monitor potassium level.

*Skin-test antigens:* May decrease response. Postpone skin testing until after therapy.

**Drug-herb.** *Echinacea:* May increase immune-stimulating effects. Discourage use together.

*Ginseng:* May increase immune-modulating response. Discourage use together.

**EFFECTS ON LAB TEST RESULTS**

● May increase glucose and cholesterol levels. May decrease $T_3$, $T_4$, potassium, and calcium levels.

● May cause decreased $^{131}I$ uptake and protein-bound iodine levels in thyroid function tests. May cause false-negative results in nitroblue tetrazolium test for systemic bacterial infections. May alter reactions to skin tests.

**CONTRAINDICATIONS & CAUTIONS**

● Contraindicated in patients hypersensitive to drug or its ingredients, in those with systemic fungal infections, in those receiving immunosuppressive doses together with live virus vaccines, and in premature infants (succinate).

● Use with caution in patient with recent MI.

● Use cautiously in patients with GI ulcer, renal disease, hypertension, osteoporosis, diabetes mellitus, hypothyroidism, cirrhosis, diverticulitis, nonspecific ulcerative colitis, active hepatitis, lactation, recent intestinal anastomoses, thromboembolic disorders, seizures, myasthenia gravis, heart failure, tuberculosis, ocular herpes simplex, emotional instability, and psychotic tendencies.

**NURSING CONSIDERATIONS**

● Determine whether patient is sensitive to other corticosteroids.

● Most adverse reactions to corticosteroids are dose- or duration-dependent.

● For better results and less toxicity, give a once-daily dose in morning.

● Give oral dose with food when possible. Patient may need medication to prevent GI irritation.

● *Alert:* Salt formulations aren't interchangeable.

● Give I.M. injection deeply into gluteal muscle. Rotate injection sites to prevent muscle atrophy. Avoid S.C. injection because atrophy and sterile abscesses may occur.

● Injectable forms aren't used for alternate-day therapy.

● *Alert:* Only hydrocortisone sodium phosphate and sodium succinate can be given I.V.

● Enema may produce same systemic effects as other forms of hydrocortisone. If

---

enema therapy must exceed 21 days, stop gradually by reducing use to every other night for 2 to 3 weeks.
● High-dose therapy usually isn't continued beyond 48 hours.
● Always adjust to lowest effective dose.
● Monitor patient's weight, blood pressure, and electrolyte level.
● Monitor patient for cushingoid effects, including moon face, buffalo hump, central obesity, thinning hair, hypertension, and increased susceptibility to infection.
● Unless contraindicated, give a low-sodium diet that is high in potassium and protein. Give potassium supplements.
● Drug may mask or worsen infections, including latent amebiasis.
● Stress (fever, trauma, surgery, and emotional problems) may increase adrenal insufficiency. Increase dosage.
● Watch for depression or psychotic episodes, especially during high-dose therapy.
● Inspect patient's skin for petechiae.
● Diabetic patient may need increased insulin; monitor glucose level.
● Periodic measurement of growth and development may be needed during high-dose or prolonged therapy in children.
● Elderly patients may be more susceptible to osteoporosis with prolonged use.
● Gradually reduce dosage after long-term therapy.
● *Alert:* Don't confuse Solu-Cortef with Solu-Medrol (methylprednisolone sodium succinate), or hydrocortisone with hydroxychloroquine.

**PATIENT TEACHING**
● Tell patient not to stop drug abruptly or without prescriber's consent.
● Instruct patient to take oral form of drug with milk or food.
● Warn patient on long-term therapy about cushingoid effects (moon face, buffalo hump) and the need to notify prescriber about sudden weight gain or swelling.
● Teach patient signs and symptoms of early adrenal insufficiency: fatigue, muscle weakness, joint pain, fever, anorexia, nausea, shortness of breath, dizziness, and fainting.
● Instruct patient to carry or wear medical identification indicating his need for supplemental systemic glucocorticoids during stress. This card should contain pre-

scriber's name and name and dosage of drug.
● Warn patient about easy bruising.
● Urge patient receiving long-term therapy to consider exercise or physical therapy. Also, tell him to ask prescriber about vitamin D or calcium supplement.
● Advise patient receiving long-term therapy to have periodic eye examinations.
● Caution patient to avoid exposure to infections (such as chickenpox or measles) and to notify prescriber if such exposure occurs.

---

# methylprednisolone
Medrol✍

# methylprednisolone acetate
depMedalone 40, depMedalone 80, Depo-Medrol, Depopred-40, Depopred-80

# methylprednisolone sodium succinate
A-Methapred, Solu-Medrol

*Pregnancy risk category C*

---

**AVAILABLE FORMS**
**methylprednisolone**
*Tablets:* 2 mg, 4 mg, 8 mg, 16 mg, 24 mg, 32 mg
**methylprednisolone acetate**
*Injection (suspension):* 20 mg/ml, 40 mg/ml, 80 mg/ml
**methylprednisolone sodium succinate**
*Injection:* 40-mg vial, 125-mg vial, 500-mg vial, 1,000-mg vial, 2,000-mg vial

**INDICATIONS & DOSAGES**
➤ **Severe inflammation or immunosuppression**
*Adults:* 2 to 60 mg base P.O. usually in four divided doses, 10 to 80 mg acetate I.M. daily, or 10 to 250 mg succinate I.M. or I.V. up to six times daily. Or, 4 to 40 mg acetate into smaller joints or 20 to 80 mg acetate into larger joints. Intralesional use is usually 20 to 60 mg acetate. Intralesional and intra-articular injections may be repeated q 1 to 5 weeks.
*Children:* 0.03 to 0.2 mg/kg or 1 to 6.25 mg/m$^2$ succinate I.M. once daily or b.i.d.

➤ **Shock**
*Adults:* 100 to 250 mg succinate I.V. at 2-
to 6-hour intervals. Or, 30 mg/kg I.V. initially, repeated q 4 to 6 hours, p.r.n. Give
over 3 to 15 minutes. Continue therapy for
2 to 3 days or until patient is stable.

## I.V. ADMINISTRATION
• Use only methylprednisolone sodium
succinate for I.V. route; never use acetate
form. Reconstitute according to manufacturer's directions using supplied diluent, or
use bacteriostatic water for injection with
benzyl alcohol.
• For direct injection, inject diluted drug
into vein or free-flowing compatible I.V.
solution over at least 1 minute.
• For shock, give massive doses over at
least 10 minutes to prevent arrhythmias
and circulatory collapse.
• For intermittent or continuous infusion,
dilute solution according to manufacturer's instructions, and give over prescribed
duration. If used for continuous infusion,
change solution every 24 hours.
• Compatible solutions include $D_5W$, normal saline solution, and dextrose 5% in
normal saline solution.

## ACTION
Not clearly defined. Decreases inflammation, mainly by stabilizing leukocyte lysosomal membranes; suppresses immune response; stimulates bone marrow; and
influences protein, fat, and carbohydrate
metabolism.

| Route | Onset | Peak | Duration |
|---|---|---|---|
| P.O. | Rapid | 2-3 hr | 30-36 hr |
| I.V. | Rapid | Immediate | 1 wk |
| I.M. | 6-48 hr | 4-8 days | 4-8 days |
| Intra-articular | Rapid | 7 days | 1-5 wk |

## ADVERSE REACTIONS
**CNS:** *euphoria, insomnia,* psychotic behavior, *pseudotumor cerebri,* vertigo,
headache, paresthesia, *seizures.*
**CV:** *heart failure,* hypertension, edema,
*arrhythmias,* thrombophlebitis, *thromboembolism, cardiac arrest, circulatory
collapse* after rapid use of large I.V. doses.
**EENT:** cataracts, glaucoma.

**GI:** *peptic ulceration,* GI irritation, increased appetite, *pancreatitis,* nausea,
vomiting.
**GU:** menstrual irregularities, increased
urine calcium levels.
**Metabolic:** hypokalemia, hyperglycemia,
carbohydrate intolerance, hypercholesterolemia, hypocalcemia.
**Musculoskeletal:** growth suppression in
children, muscle weakness, osteoporosis.
**Skin:** hirsutism, delayed wound healing,
acne, various skin eruptions.
**Other:** cushingoid state, susceptibility to
infections, *acute adrenal insufficiency after increased stress or abrupt withdrawal
after long-term therapy.*
**After abrupt withdrawal:** rebound inflammation, fatigue, weakness, arthralgia,
fever, dizziness, lethargy, depression,
fainting, orthostatic hypotension, dyspnea,
anorexia, *hypoglycemia. After prolonged
use, sudden withdrawal may be fatal.*

## INTERACTIONS
**Drug-drug.** *Aspirin, indomethacin, other
NSAIDs:* May increase risk of GI distress
and bleeding. Use together cautiously.
*Barbiturates, carbamazepine, phenytoin,
rifampin:* May decrease corticosteroid ef-
fect. Increase corticosteroid dosage.
*Cyclosporine:* May increase toxicity.
Monitor patient closely.
*Ketoconazole and macrolide antibiotics:*
May decrease methylprednisolone clear-
ance. Decreased dose may be required.
*Oral anticoagulants:* May alter dosage re-
quirements. Monitor PT and INR closely.
*Potassium-depleting drugs such as thi-
azide diuretics:* May enhance potassium-
wasting effects of methylprednisolone.
Monitor potassium level.
*Salicylates:* May decrease salicylate levels. Monitor patient for lack of salicylate
effectiveness.
*Skin-test antigens:* May decrease response.
Postpone skin testing until after therapy.
*Toxoids, vaccines:* May decrease antibody
response and may increase risk of neurologic complications. Avoid using together.
**Drug-herb.** *Echinacea:* May increase
immune-stimulating effects. Discourage
use together.
*Ginseng:* May increase immune-
modulating response. Discourage use
together.

---

Reactions may be *common,* uncommon, *life-threatening,* or COMMON AND LIFE-THREATENING.

## EFFECTS ON LAB TEST RESULTS
• May increase glucose and cholesterol levels. May decrease $T_3$, $T_4$, potassium, and calcium levels.
• May cause decreased [131]I uptake and protein-bound iodine levels in thyroid function tests. May cause false-negative results in nitroblue tetrazolium test for systemic bacterial infections. May alter reactions to skin tests.

## CONTRAINDICATIONS & CAUTIONS
• Contraindicated in patients hypersensitive to drug or its ingredients, in those with systemic fungal infections, in premature infants (acetate and succinate), and in patients receiving immunosuppressive doses together with live virus vaccines.
• Use cautiously in patients with GI ulceration or renal disease, hypertension, osteoporosis, diabetes mellitus, hypothyroidism, cirrhosis, diverticulitis, nonspecific ulcerative colitis, recent intestinal anastomoses, thromboembolic disorders, seizures, active hepatitis, lactation, myasthenia gravis, heart failure, tuberculosis, ocular herpes simplex, emotional instability, and psychotic tendencies.

## NURSING CONSIDERATIONS
• Determine whether patient is sensitive to other corticosteroids.
• Medrol may contain tartrazine.
• Drug may be used for alternate-day therapy.
• Most adverse reactions to corticosteroids are dose- or duration-dependent.
• For better results and less toxicity, give a once-daily dose in the morning.
• Give oral dose with food when possible. Critically ill patients may need to take drug together with antacid or $H_2$-receptor antagonist.
• *Alert:* Salt formulations aren't interchangeable.
• *Alert:* Don't give Solu-Medrol intrathecally because severe adverse reactions may occur.
• Give I.M. injection deeply into gluteal muscle. Avoid S.C. injection because atrophy and sterile abscesses may occur.
• Dermal atrophy may occur with large doses of acetate salt. Use several small injections rather than a single large dose, and rotate injection sites.

• Don't use acetate if immediate onset of action is needed.
• Discard reconstituted solution after 48 hours.
• Always adjust to lowest effective dose.
• Monitor patient's weight, blood pressure, electrolyte level, and sleep patterns. Euphoria may initially interfere with sleep, but patients typically adjust to therapy in 1 to 3 weeks.
• Monitor patient for cushingoid effects, including moon face, buffalo hump, central obesity, thinning hair, hypertension, and increased susceptibility to infection.
• Drug may mask or worsen infections, including latent amebiasis.
• Watch for depression or psychotic episodes, especially in high-dose therapy.
• Diabetic patient may need increased insulin; monitor glucose level.
• Watch for an enhanced response to drug in patients with hypothyroidism or cirrhosis.
• Watch for allergic reaction to tartrazine in patients with sensitivity to aspirin.
• Unless contraindicated, give low-sodium diet that's high in potassium and protein. Give potassium supplements, as needed.
• Elderly patients may be more susceptible to osteoporosis with prolonged use.
• Gradually reduce dosage after long-term therapy.
• *Alert:* Don't confuse Solu-Medrol with Solu-Cortef (hydrocortisone sodium succinate) or methylprednisolone with medroxyprogesterone.

## PATIENT TEACHING
• Tell patient not to stop drug abruptly or without prescriber's consent.
• Instruct patient to take oral form of drug with milk or food.
• Teach patient signs and symptoms of early adrenal insufficiency: fatigue, muscle weakness, joint pain, fever, anorexia, nausea, shortness of breath, dizziness, and fainting.
• Instruct patient to carry or wear medical identification indicating his need for supplemental systemic glucocorticoids during stress. This card should contain prescriber's name, name of drug, and dosage taken.
• Warn patient on long-term therapy about cushingoid effects (moon face, buffalo

hump) and the need to notify prescriber about sudden weight gain or swelling.
• Advise patient receiving long-term therapy to consider exercise or physical therapy. Also, tell patient to ask prescriber about vitamin D or calcium supplement.
• Instruct patient to avoid exposure to infections (such as chickenpox or measles) and to contact prescriber if such exposure occurs.

---

## prednisolone
Delta-Cortef, Panafcortelone‡, Prelone

## prednisolone acetate
Key-Pred 25, Key-Pred 50, Predalone 50, Predcor-50

## prednisolone sodium phosphate
Hydeltrasol, Key-Pred-SP, Orapred, Pediapred, Predsol Retention Enema‡, Predsol Suppositories‡, Prelone

## prednisolone tebutate
Prednisol TBA, Nor-Pred T.B.A., Predate TBA, Predcor-TBA

*Pregnancy risk category C*

---

### AVAILABLE FORMS
**prednisolone**
*Syrup:* 5 mg/5 ml, 15 mg/5 ml\*
*Tablets:* 1 mg‡, 5 mg, 25 mg‡
**prednisolone acetate**
*Injection (suspension):* 25 mg/ml, 50 mg/ml
**prednisolone sodium phosphate**
*Injection:* 20 mg/ml
*Oral solution:* 5 mg/5 ml, 20 mg/5 ml
*Retention enema:* 20 mg/100 ml‡
*Suppositories:* 5 mg‡
**prednisolone tebutate**
*Injection (suspension):* 20 mg/ml

### INDICATIONS & DOSAGES
➤ **Severe inflammation, immunosuppression**
*prednisolone*
*Adults:* 2.5 to 15 mg P.O. b.i.d., t.i.d., or q.i.d.

*Children:* Initially, 0.14 to 2 mg/kg/day P.O. or 4 to 60 mg/m$^2$/day in four divided doses.
*prednisolone acetate*
*Adults:* 2 to 30 mg I.M. q 12 hours.
*Children:* 0.04 to 0.25 mg/kg or 1.5 to 7.5 mg/m$^2$ I.M. once daily or b.i.d.
*prednisolone sodium phosphate*
*Adults:* 4 to 60 mg I.M., I.V., or P.O. daily
*Children:* Initially, 0.14 to 2 mg/kg/day or 4 to 60 mg/m$^2$/day in three or four divided doses I.M., I.V., or P.O.
*prednisolone tebutate*
*Adults:* 4 to 40 mg into joints and lesions, p.r.n.
➤ **Uncontrolled asthma in those taking inhaled corticosteroids and long-acting bronchodilators**
*Children:* 1 to 2 mg/kg/day prednisolone sodium phosphate P.O. in single or divided doses. Continue short course, or "burst," therapy until a child achieves a peak expiratory flow rate of 80% of his or her personal best, or until symptoms resolve. This usually requires 3 to 10 days of treatment but can take longer. Tapering the dose after improvement doesn't necessarily prevent relapse.
➤ **Acute exacerbations of multiple sclerosis**
*Adults and children:* 200 mg/day prednisolone sodium phosphate P.O. as single or divided dose for 7 days; then 80 mg every other day for 1 month.
➤ **Nephrotic syndrome**
*Children:* 60 mg/m$^2$/day prednisolone sodium phosphate P.O. in three divided doses for 4 weeks, followed by 4 weeks of single-dose alternate-day therapy at 40 mg/m$^2$/day.
➤ **Proctitis‡**
*Adults:* 1 suppository b.i.d., preferably in the morning and h.s.
➤ **Ulcerative colitis‡**
*Adults:* 1 retention enema h.s. for 2 to 4 weeks. Patient should retain contents of enema overnight.

### I.V. ADMINISTRATION
• Use only prednisolone sodium phosphate.
• For direct injection, inject undiluted over at least 1 minute.
• For intermittent or continuous infusion, dilute solution according to manufactur-

---

er's instructions, and give over prescribed duration.

• Use $D_5W$ or normal saline solution as diluent for I.V. infusion.

## ACTION

Not clearly defined. Decreases inflammation, mainly by stabilizing leukocyte lysosomal membranes; suppresses immune response; stimulates bone marrow; and influences protein, fat, and carbohydrate metabolism.

| Route | Peak | Onset | Duration |
|---|---|---|---|
| P.O. | Rapid | 1-2 hr | 3-36 hr |
| I.V. | Rapid | 1 hr | Unknown |
| I.M. | Rapid | 1 hr | 4 wk |
| P.R. | Unknown | Unknown | Unknown |
| Intra-articular | 1-2 days | Unknown | < 4 wk |

## ADVERSE REACTIONS

**CNS:** *euphoria, insomnia,* psychotic behavior, *pseudotumor cerebri,* vertigo, headache, paresthesia, *seizures.*
**CV:** *heart failure,* hypertension, edema, *arrhythmias,* thrombophlebitis, *thromboembolism.*
**EENT:** cataracts, glaucoma.
**GI:** *peptic ulceration,* GI irritation, increased appetite, *pancreatitis,* nausea, vomiting.
**GU:** menstrual irregularities, increased urine calcium levels.
**Metabolic:** hypokalemia, hyperglycemia, carbohydrate intolerance, hypercholesterolemia, hypocalcemia.
**Musculoskeletal:** growth suppression in children, muscle weakness, osteoporosis.
**Skin:** hirsutism, delayed wound healing, acne, various skin eruptions.
**Other:** susceptibility to infections, cushingoid state, *acute adrenal insufficiency* after increased stress or abrupt withdrawal after long-term therapy.
**After abrupt withdrawal:** rebound inflammation, fatigue, weakness, arthralgia, fever, dizziness, lethargy, depression, fainting, orthostatic hypotension, dyspnea, anorexia, *hypoglycemia. After prolonged use, sudden withdrawal may be fatal.*

## INTERACTIONS

**Drug-drug.** *Aspirin, indomethacin, other NSAIDs:* May increase risk of GI distress and bleeding. Use together cautiously.
*Barbiturates, carbamazepine, fosphenytoin, phenytoin, rifampin:* May decrease corticosteroid effect. Increase corticosteroid dosage.
*Cyclosporine:* May increase toxicity. Monitor patient closely.
*Oral anticoagulants:* May alter dosage requirements. Monitor PT and INR closely.
*Potassium-depleting drugs such as thiazide diuretics:* May enhance potassium-wasting effects of prednisolone. Monitor potassium level.
*Salicylates:* May decrease salicylate level. Monitor patient for lack of salicylate effectiveness.
*Skin-test antigens:* May decrease response. Postpone skin testing until therapy is completed.
*Toxoids, vaccines:* May decrease antibody response and may increase risk of neurologic complications. Avoid using together.
**Drug-herb.** *Echinacea:* May increase immune-stimulating effects. Discourage use together.
*Ginseng:* May increase immune-modulating response. Discourage use together.

## EFFECTS ON LAB TEST RESULTS

• May increase glucose and cholesterol levels. May decrease $T_3$, $T_4$, potassium, and calcium levels.
• May cause decreased [131]I uptake and protein-bound iodine levels in thyroid function tests. May cause false-negative results in nitroblue tetrazolium test for systemic bacterial infections. May alter reactions to skin tests.

## CONTRAINDICATIONS & CAUTIONS

• Contraindicated in patients hypersensitive to drug or its ingredients, in those with systemic fungal infections, and in those receiving immunosuppressive doses together with live virus vaccines.
• Use with caution in patients with recent MI.
• Use cautiously in patients with GI ulcer, renal disease, hypertension, osteoporosis, diabetes mellitus, hypothyroidism, cirrhosis, active hepatitis, lactation, diverticuli-

---

tis, nonspecific ulcerative colitis, recent intestinal anastomoses, thromboembolic disorders, seizures, myasthenia gravis, heart failure, tuberculosis, ocular herpes simplex, emotional instability, and psychotic tendencies.

## NURSING CONSIDERATIONS
● Determine whether patient is sensitive to other corticosteroids.
● Always adjust to lowest effective dose.
● Prednisolone salts (sodium phosphate and tebutate) are less often used parenterally than other corticosteroids that have more potent anti-inflammatory action.
● Drug may be used for alternate-day therapy.
● Most adverse reactions to corticosteroids are dose- or duration-dependent.
● Give oral dose with food, when possible, to reduce GI irritation. Patient may need medication to prevent GI irritation.
● Give I.M. injection deeply into gluteal muscle. Rotate injection sites to prevent muscle atrophy. Avoid S.C. injection because atrophy and sterile abscesses may occur.
● *Alert:* Prednisolone acetate and tebutate aren't for I.V. use.
● Monitor patient's weight, blood pressure, and electrolyte level.
● Monitor patient for cushingoid effects, including moon face, buffalo hump, central obesity, thinning hair, hypertension, and increased susceptibility to infection.
● Watch for depression or psychotic episodes, especially during high-dose therapy.
● Diabetic patient may need increased insulin; monitor glucose level.
● Unless contraindicated, give low-sodium diet that's high in potassium and protein. Give potassium supplements as needed.
● Drug may mask or worsen infections, including latent amebiasis.
● Elderly patients may be more susceptible to osteoporosis with long-term use.
● Gradually reduce dosage after long-term therapy.
● *Alert:* Don't confuse prednisolone with prednisone.

## PATIENT TEACHING
● Tell patient not to stop drug abruptly or without prescriber's consent.

● Instruct patient to take oral form of drug with food or milk.
● Teach patient signs and symptoms of early adrenal insufficiency: fatigue, muscle weakness, joint pain, fever, anorexia, nausea, shortness of breath, dizziness, and fainting.
● Instruct patient to carry or wear medical identification indicating his need for supplemental systemic glucocorticoids during stress. It should include prescriber's name, and name and dosage of drug.
● Warn patient on long-term therapy about cushingoid effects (moon face, buffalo hump) and the need to notify prescriber about sudden weight gain or swelling.
● Tell patient to report slow healing.
● Advise patient receiving long-term therapy to consider exercise or physical therapy. Also, tell him to ask prescriber about vitamin D or calcium supplement.
● Instruct patient to avoid exposure to infections and to notify prescriber if exposure occurs.
● Tell patient to avoid immunizations while taking drug.
● Tell patient to store Orapred in the refrigerator between 36° to 46° F.

# prednisone
Apo-Prednisone†, Deltasone⬦, Liquid Pred*, Meticorten, Orasone, Panafcort‡, Panasol-S, Prednicen-M, Prednisone Intensol*, Sterapred, Winpred†

*Pregnancy risk category C*

## AVAILABLE FORMS
*Oral solution:* 5 mg/5 ml*, 5 mg/ml (concentrate)*
*Syrup:* 5 mg/5 ml*
*Tablet:* 1 mg, 2.5 mg, 5 mg, 10 mg, 20 mg, 50 mg
*Tablet (film-coated):* 5 mg

## INDICATIONS & DOSAGES
➤ **Severe inflammation, immunosuppression**
*Adults:* 5 to 60 mg P.O. daily in single dose or as two to four divided doses. Maintenance dose given once daily or every other day. Dosage must be individualized.

---

Reactions may be *common,* uncommon, *life-threatening,* or COMMON AND LIFE-THREATENING.

*Children:* 0.14 to 2 mg/kg or 4 to 60 mg/m² daily P.O. in four divided doses.
➤ **Acute exacerbations of multiple sclerosis**
*Adults:* 200 mg P.O. daily for 7 days; then 80 mg P.O. every other day for 1 month.

## ACTION

Not clearly defined. Decreases inflammation, mainly by stabilizing leukocyte lysosomal membranes; suppresses immune response; stimulates bone marrow; and influences protein, fat, and carbohydrate metabolism.

| Route | Onset | Peak | Duration |
|-------|-------|------|----------|
| P.O. | Variable | Variable | Variable |

## ADVERSE REACTIONS

**CNS:** *euphoria, insomnia,* psychotic behavior, ***pseudotumor cerebri,*** vertigo, headache, paresthesia, ***seizures.***
**CV:** ***heart failure,*** hypertension, edema, ***arrhythmias,*** thrombophlebitis, ***thromboembolism.***
**EENT:** cataracts, glaucoma.
**GI:** *peptic ulceration,* GI irritation, increased appetite, ***pancreatitis,*** nausea, vomiting.
**GU:** menstrual irregularities, increased urine calcium level.
**Metabolic:** hypokalemia, hyperglycemia, carbohydrate intolerance, hypercholesterolemia, hypocalcemia.
**Musculoskeletal:** growth suppression in children, muscle weakness, osteoporosis.
**Skin:** hirsutism, delayed wound healing, acne, various skin eruptions.
**Other:** cushingoid state, susceptibility to infections, *acute adrenal insufficiency* after increased stress or abrupt withdrawal after long-term therapy.
**After abrupt withdrawal:** rebound inflammation, fatigue, weakness, arthralgia, fever, dizziness, lethargy, depression, fainting, orthostatic hypotension, dyspnea, anorexia, *hypoglycemia. After prolonged use, sudden withdrawal may be fatal.*

## INTERACTIONS

**Drug-drug.** *Aspirin, indomethacin, other NSAIDs:* May increase risk of GI distress and bleeding. Use together cautiously.
*Barbiturates, carbamazepine, fosphenytoin, phenytoin, rifampin:* May decrease

corticosteroid effect. Increase corticosteroid dosage.
*Cyclosporine:* May increase toxicity. Monitor patient closely.
*Oral anticoagulants:* May alter dosage requirements. Monitor PT and INR closely.
*Potassium-depleting drugs such as thiazide diuretics:* May enhance potassium-wasting effects of prednisone. Monitor potassium level.
*Salicylates:* May decrease salicylate level. Monitor patient for lack of salicylate effectiveness.
*Skin-test antigens:* May decrease response. Postpone skin testing until therapy is completed.
*Toxoids, vaccines:* May decrease antibody response and may increase risk of neurologic complications. Avoid using together.
**Drug-herb.** *Echinacea:* May increase immune-stimulating effects. Discourage use together.
*Ginseng:* May increase immune-modulating response. Discourage use together.

## EFFECTS ON LAB TEST RESULTS

● May increase glucose and cholesterol levels. May decrease $T_3$, $T_4$, potassium, and calcium levels.
● May decrease $^{131}$I uptake and protein-bound iodine values in thyroid function tests. May cause false-negative results in nitroblue tetrazolium test for systemic bacterial infections. May alter reactions to skin tests.

## CONTRAINDICATIONS & CAUTIONS

● Contraindicated in patients hypersensitive to drug or its ingredients, in those with systemic fungal infections, and in those receiving immunosuppressive doses together with live virus vaccines.
● Use cautiously in patients with recent MI, GI ulcer, renal disease, hypertension, osteoporosis, diabetes mellitus, hypothyroidism, cirrhosis, active hepatitis, lactation, diverticulitis, nonspecific ulcerative colitis, recent intestinal anastomoses, thromboembolic disorders, seizures, myasthenia gravis, heart failure, tuberculosis, ocular herpes simplex, emotional instability, and psychotic tendencies.

## NURSING CONSIDERATIONS

- Determine whether patient is sensitive to other corticosteroids.
- Drug may be used for alternate-day therapy.
- Always adjust to lowest effective dose.
- Most adverse reactions to corticosteroids are dose- or duration-dependent.
- For better results and less toxicity, give a once-daily dose in the morning.
- Unless contraindicated, give oral dose with food when possible to reduce GI irritation. Patient may need medication to prevent GI irritation.
- The oral solution may be diluted in juice or other flavored diluent or semi-solid food (such as applesauce) before using.
- Monitor patient's blood pressure, sleep patterns, and potassium level.
- Weigh patient daily; report sudden weight gain to prescriber.
- Monitor patient for cushingoid effects, including moon face, buffalo hump, central obesity, thinning hair, hypertension, and increased susceptibility to infection.
- Watch for depression or psychotic episodes, especially during high-dose therapy.
- Diabetic patient may need increased insulin; monitor glucose level.
- Elderly patients may be more susceptible to osteoporosis with long-term use.
- Drug may mask or worsen infections, including latent amebiasis.
- Unless contraindicated, give low-sodium diet that's high in potassium and protein. Give potassium supplements, as needed.
- Gradually reduce dosage after long-term therapy.
- *Alert:* Don't confuse prednisone with prednisolone, primidone, or prednimustine.

## PATIENT TEACHING

- Tell patient not to stop drug abruptly or without prescriber's consent.
- Instruct patient to take drug with food or milk.
- Teach patient signs and symptoms of early adrenal insufficiency: fatigue, muscle weakness, joint pain, fever, anorexia, nausea, shortness of breath, dizziness, and fainting.
- Instruct patient to carry or wear medical identification indicating his need for supplemental systemic glucocorticoids during stress. It should include prescriber's name and name and dosage of drug.
- Warn patient on long-term therapy about cushingoid effects (moon face, buffalo hump) and the need to notify prescriber about sudden weight gain or swelling.
- Advise patient receiving long-term therapy to consider exercise or physical therapy. Also, tell patient to ask prescriber about vitamin D or calcium supplement.
- Tell patient to report slow healing.
- Advise patient receiving long-term therapy to have periodic eye examinations.
- Instruct patient to avoid exposure to infections and to contact prescriber if exposure occurs.

# triamcinolone
Aristocort, Atolone, Kenacort

# triamcinolone acetonide
Azmacort, Kenaject-40, Kenalog-10, Kenalog-40, Tac-3, Tac-40, Triam-A, Triamonide 40, Tri-Kort, Trilog

# triamcinolone diacetate
Amcort, Aristocort Forte, Aristocort Intralesional, Clinacort, Kenacort, Triam Forte, Trilone, Tristoject

# triamcinolone hexacetonide
Aristospan Intra-Articular, Aristospan Intralesional

*Pregnancy risk category C*

## AVAILABLE FORMS

**triamcinolone**
*Tablets:* 4 mg, 8 mg
**triamcinolone acetonide**
*Injection (suspension):* 3 mg/ml, 10 mg/ml, 40 mg/ml
*Metered spray:* 100 mcg/spray
**triamcinolone diacetate**
*Injection (suspension):* 25 mg/ml, 40 mg/ml
*Oral syrup:* 4 mg/5 ml
**triamcinolone hexacetonide**
*Injection (suspension):* 5 mg/ml (intralesional); 20 mg/ml (intra-articular)

---

Reactions may be *common*, uncommon, *life-threatening*, or COMMON AND LIFE-THREATENING.

## INDICATIONS & DOSAGES
➤ **Severe inflammation, immunosuppression**

*Adults:* 4 to 48 mg P.O. daily in single dose or divided doses. Or, 40 to 80 mg I.M. acetonide at 4-week intervals. Or, 1 mg acetonide into lesions. Or, initially, 2.5 to 15 mg acetonide into joints (depending on joint size) or soft tissue; then, may increase to 40 mg for larger areas. A local anesthetic is commonly injected with triamcinolone into the joint. For triamcinolone hexacetonide, up to 0.5 mg (of 5 mg/ml suspension) intralesional or sublesional injection per square inch of affected skin. Additional injections based on patient's response. Or, 2 to 20 mg (using the 20 mg/ml suspension) via intra-articular injection. Dose may be repeated q 3 to 4 weeks.

➤ **Adrenocortical insufficiency**

*Children:* 0.117 to 1.66 mg/kg/day or 3.3 to 50 mg/m$^2$/day P.O. in four divided doses.

➤ **Asthma**

*Adults and children age 12 and older:* 2 inhalations t.i.d. or q.i.d. Maximum, 16 inhalations daily.

*Children ages 6 to 12:* 1 to 2 inhalations t.i.d. or q.i.d. Maximum, 12 inhalations daily.

## ACTION

Not clearly defined. Decreases inflammation, mainly by stabilizing leukocyte lysosomal membranes; suppresses immune response; stimulates bone marrow; and influences protein, fat, and carbohydrate metabolism.

| Route | Onset | Peak | Duration |
|---|---|---|---|
| P.O., I.M., inhalation, intra-articular, intralesional | Variable | Variable | Variable |

## ADVERSE REACTIONS

**CNS:** *euphoria, insomnia,* psychotic behavior, *pseudotumor cerebri,* vertigo, headache, paresthesia, *seizures.*

**CV:** *heart failure,* hypertension, edema, *arrhythmias,* thrombophlebitis, *thromboembolism.*

**EENT:** cataracts, glaucoma.

**GI:** *peptic ulceration,* GI irritation, increased appetite, *pancreatitis,* nausea, vomiting.

**GU:** menstrual irregularities, increased urine calcium level.

**Metabolic:** hypokalemia, hyperglycemia, and carbohydrate intolerance; hypercholesterolemia; hypokalemia; hypocalcemia.

**Musculoskeletal:** growth suppression in children, muscle weakness, osteoporosis.

**Skin:** hirsutism, delayed wound healing, acne, various skin eruptions.

**Other:** cushingoid state, susceptibility to infections, *acute adrenal insufficiency* after increased stress or abrupt withdrawal after long-term therapy.

**After abrupt withdrawal:** rebound inflammation, fatigue, weakness, arthralgia, fever, dizziness, lethargy, depression, fainting, orthostatic hypotension, dyspnea, anorexia, *hypoglycemia. After prolonged use, sudden withdrawal may be fatal.*

## INTERACTIONS

**Drug-drug.** *Aspirin, indomethacin, other NSAIDs:* May increase risk of GI distress and bleeding. Use together cautiously.

*Barbiturates, carbamazepine, fosphenytoin, phenytoin, rifampin:* May decrease corticosteroid effect. Increase corticosteroid dosage.

*Cyclosporine:* May increase toxicity. Monitor patient closely.

*Oral anticoagulants:* May alter dosage requirements. Monitor PT and INR closely.

*Potassium-depleting drugs such as thiazide diuretics:* May enhance potassium-wasting effects of triamcinolone. Monitor potassium level.

*Salicylates:* May decrease salicylate level. Monitor patient for lack of salicylate effectiveness.

*Skin-test antigens:* May decrease response. Postpone skin testing until after therapy.

*Toxoids, vaccines:* May decrease antibody response and increase risk of neurologic complications. Avoid using together.

**Drug-herb.** *Echinacea:* May increase immune-stimulating effects. Discourage use together.

*Ginseng:* May increase immune-modulating response. Discourage use together.

**EFFECTS ON LAB TEST RESULTS**
• May increase glucose and cholesterol levels. May decrease potassium and calcium levels.
• May cause decreased $^{131}$I uptake and protein-bound iodine values in thyroid function tests. May cause false-negative results in nitroblue tetrazolium test for systemic bacterial infections. May alter reactions to skin tests.

**CONTRAINDICATIONS & CAUTIONS**
• Contraindicated in patients hypersensitive to drug or its ingredients, in those with systemic fungal infections, and in those receiving immunosuppressive doses together with live virus vaccines.
• Use cautiously in patients with recent MI, GI ulcer, renal disease, hypertension, osteoporosis, diabetes mellitus, hypothyroidism, cirrhosis, diverticulitis, nonspecific ulcerative colitis, recent intestinal anastomoses, thromboembolic disorders, seizures, myasthenia gravis, active hepatitis, lactation, heart failure, tuberculosis, ocular herpes simplex, emotional instability, or psychotic tendencies.

**NURSING CONSIDERATIONS**
• Determine whether patient is sensitive to other corticosteroids.
• Kenacort may contain tartrazine.
• Drug isn't used for alternate-day therapy.
• Always adjust to lowest effective dose.
• Most adverse reactions to corticosteroids are dose- or duration-dependent.
• For better results and less toxicity, give a once-daily oral dose in the morning with food.
• *Alert:* Parenteral form isn't for I.V. use.
• *Alert:* Salt formulations aren't interchangeable.
• Don't use 40 mg/ml strength for intradermal or intralesional use.
• Don't use 10 mg/ml strength for I.M. use.
• Don't use diluents that contain preservatives; flocculation may occur.
• Give I.M. injection deeply into gluteal muscle. Rotate injection sites to prevent muscle atrophy.
• Monitor patient's weight, blood pressure, and electrolyte level.
• Monitor patient for cushingoid effects, including moon face, buffalo hump, central obesity, thinning hair, hypertension, and increased susceptibility to infection.
• Watch for allergic reaction to tartrazine in patients with sensitivity to aspirin.
• Watch for depression or psychotic episodes, especially during high-dose therapy.
• Diabetic patient may need increased insulin dosage; monitor glucose level.
• Drug may mask or worsen infections, including latent amebiasis.
• Elderly patients may be more susceptible to osteoporosis with long-term use.
• Unless contraindicated, give low-sodium diet that's high in potassium and protein. Give potassium supplements, as needed.
• Gradually reduce dosage after long-term therapy. Drug may affect patient's sleep.
• *Alert:* Don't confuse triamcinolone with Triaminicin or Triaminicol.

**PATIENT TEACHING**
• Tell patient not to stop drug abruptly or without prescriber's consent.
• Instruct patient to take drug with food or milk.
• Teach patient signs and symptoms of early adrenal insufficiency: fatigue, muscle weakness, joint pain, fever, anorexia, nausea, shortness of breath, dizziness, and fainting.
• Instruct patient to carry or wear medical identification indicating his need for supplemental systemic glucocorticoids during stress. It should include prescriber's name and drug's name and dosage.
• Warn patient on long-term therapy about cushingoid effects (moon face, buffalo hump) and the need to notify prescriber about sudden weight gain and swelling.
• Tell patient to report slow healing.
• Advise patient receiving long-term therapy to consider exercise or physical therapy. Also, tell patient to ask prescriber about vitamin D or calcium supplement.
• Instruct patient to avoid exposure to infections and to notify prescriber if exposure occurs.

# 52

## Androgens and anabolic steroids

**fluoxymesterone**
**methyltestosterone**
**nandrolone decanoate**
**testosterone**
**testosterone cypionate**
**testosterone enanthate**
**testosterone propionate**
**testosterone transdermal system**

### COMBINATION PRODUCTS
DEPO-TESTADIOL, DEPOTESTOGEN, DUO-CYP: testosterone cypionate 50 mg/ml and estradiol cypionate 2 mg/ml in cottonseed oil
ESTRATEST: esterified estrogens 1.25 mg and methyltestosterone 2.5 mg
ESTRATEST H.S.: esterified estrogens 0.625 mg and methyltestosterone 1.25 mg
VALERTEST NO. 1: testosterone enanthate 90 mg/ml and estradiol valerate 4 mg/ml in sesame oil

---

## fluoxymesterone
Halotestin

*Pregnancy risk category X*
*Controlled substance schedule III*

### AVAILABLE FORMS
*Tablets:* 2 mg, 5 mg, 10 mg

### INDICATIONS & DOSAGES
➤ **Hypogonadism from testicular deficiency**
*Adults:* 5 to 20 mg P.O. daily.
➤ **Delayed puberty in boys**
*Adolescents:* Highly individualized; usually 2.5 to 10 mg daily for 4 to 6 months.
➤ **Palliation of breast cancer in women**
*Adults:* 10 to 40 mg P.O. daily in divided doses. Individualize and use lowest effective dose.

### ACTION
Stimulates target tissues to develop normally in androgen-deficient men. May have some antiestrogen properties, making it useful in treating certain estrogen-dependent breast cancers.

| Route | Onset | Peak | Duration |
|-------|-------|------|----------|
| P.O. | Unknown | Unknown | 9 hr |

### ADVERSE REACTIONS
**CNS:** headache, anxiety, depression, paresthesia, sleep apnea.
**CV:** edema.
**GI:** nausea.
**Hematologic:** polycythemia, *suppression of clotting factors.*
**Hepatic:** reversible jaundice.
**Metabolic:** hypercalcemia, hypernatremia, hyperkalemia, hyperphosphatemia.
**Skin:** hypersensitivity reactions.
**Other:** *hypoestrogenic effects in women,* excessive hormonal effects in men, androgenic effects in women, altered libido.

### INTERACTIONS
**Drug-drug.** *Hepatotoxic drugs:* May increase risk of hepatotoxicity. Monitor liver function closely.
*Insulin, oral antidiabetics:* May alter dosage requirements. Monitor glucose levels in diabetic patients.
*Oral anticoagulants:* May increase sensitivity to oral anticoagulants; may alter dosage requirements. Monitor INR.

### EFFECTS ON LAB TEST RESULTS
● May increase liver enzyme, lipid, sodium, potassium, phosphate, and calcium levels. May decrease thyroxine-binding globulin and total $T_4$ levels.
● May increase RBC count and resin uptake of $T_3$ and $T_4$.
● May cause abnormal glucose tolerance test results.

### CONTRAINDICATIONS & CAUTIONS
● Contraindicated in patients hypersensitive to drug; in men with breast cancer or known or suspected prostate cancer; in patients with cardiac, hepatic, or renal decompensation; and in pregnant or breast-feeding women.
● Use cautiously in prepubertal boys or patients with benign prostatic hyperplasia or aspirin sensitivity.

---

## NURSING CONSIDERATIONS
• *Alert:* Don't use in women of childbearing age until pregnancy is ruled out.
• Monitor INR in patients taking oral anticoagulants because dosage may need adjustment.
• Unless contraindicated, use with high-calorie, high-protein diet. Give small, frequent feedings.
• Watch for evidence of jaundice, and periodically evaluate hepatic function. If liver function test results are abnormal, notify prescriber because therapy should be stopped.
• Edema can be controlled with sodium restriction or diuretics. Monitor weight routinely.
• Monitor male patients for evidence of excessive hormonal effects. If patient is prepubertal, watch for premature epiphyseal closure, acne, priapism, growth of body and facial hair, and phallic enlargement. If postpubertal, watch for testicular atrophy, oligospermia, decreased ejaculatory volume, impotence, gynecomastia, epididymitis.
• Evaluate semen routinely every 3 to 4 months, especially in adolescent boys.
• *Alert:* Hypercalcemia symptoms may be difficult to distinguish from those caused by the condition being treated, unless anticipated and thought of as a symptom cluster. Hypercalcemia is particularly likely to occur in immobilized patients or in women with metastatic breast cancer, and may indicate bone metastases.
• *Alert:* Don't give drug to enhance patient's athletic performance or physique.
• Watch for signs and symptoms of hypoglycemia in diabetic patients. Check glucose levels. Dosage of antidiabetic may need adjustment.
• When given for breast cancer, subjective effects may not occur for about 1 month; objective effects on clinical symptoms may take 3 months.
• Hypoestrogenic effects in women include flushing, diaphoresis, vaginal bleeding, nervousness, emotional lability, menstrual irregularities, and vaginitis, including itching, dryness, and burning.
• Halotestin may contain tartrazine.

## PATIENT TEACHING
• If GI upset occurs, tell patient to take drug with food or meals.
• Make sure patient understands importance of using an effective nonhormonal contraceptive during therapy.
• Advise woman to wear cotton underwear and to wash after intercourse to decrease risk of vaginitis.
• Tell woman to report menstrual irregularities and to stop drug until she can be examined.
• Instruct patient to stop drug immediately and notify prescriber if she suspects that she's pregnant.
• Explain to patient taking drug for palliation of breast cancer that virilization usually occurs. Give emotional support. Tell patient to immediately report androgenic effects (acne, swelling, weight gain, increased hair growth, hoarseness, clitoral enlargement, deepening voice, decreased breast size, changes in libido, male-pattern baldness, and oily skin or hair).
• Tell patient that stopping drug prevents further androgenic changes but probably won't reverse existing effects.
• Warn patient with diabetes to be alert for signs and symptoms of hypoglycemia and to notify prescriber if these occur.
• Tell patient to report sudden weight gain.

## methyltestosterone
Android, Metandren†, Methitest, Testred, Virilon

*Pregnancy risk category X*
*Controlled substance schedule III*

## AVAILABLE FORMS
*Capsules:* 10 mg
*Tablets:* 10 mg, 25 mg
*Tablets (buccal):* 10 mg

## INDICATIONS & DOSAGES
➤ **Breast cancer in women 1 to 5 years postmenopausal**
*Women:* 50 to 200 mg P.O. daily; or 25 to 100 mg buccally daily.
➤ **Male hypogonadism**
*Men:* 10 to 50 mg P.O. daily; or 5 to 25 mg buccally daily.

➤ **Postpubertal cryptorchidism**
*Men:* 30 mg P.O. daily; or 15 mg buccally daily.

**ACTION**
Stimulates target tissues to develop normally in androgen-deficient men. May have some antiestrogen properties, making it useful in treating certain estrogen-dependent breast cancers. Action in postpartum breast engorgement isn't known because testosterone doesn't suppress lactation.

| Route | Onset | Peak | Duration |
|-------|-------|------|----------|
| P.O. | Unknown | 2 hr | Unknown |
| Buccal | Unknown | 1 hr | Unknown |

**ADVERSE REACTIONS**
**CNS:** headache, anxiety, depression, paresthesia.
**CV:** edema.
**GI:** irritation of oral mucosa with buccal administration, nausea.
**Hematologic:** *suppression of clotting factors,* polycythemia.
**Hepatic:** reversible jaundice, *cholestatic hepatitis.*
**Metabolic:** hypernatremia, hyperkalemia, hyperphosphatemia, hypercholesterolemia, hypercalcemia.
**Musculoskeletal:** muscle cramps or spasms.
**Skin:** hypersensitivity reactions.
**Other:** androgenic effects in women, altered libido, *hypoestrogenic effects in women,* excessive hormonal effects in men.

**INTERACTIONS**
**Drug-drug.** *Hepatotoxic drugs:* May increase risk of hepatotoxicity. Monitor liver function closely.
*Imipramine:* May cause dramatic paranoid response. Monitor patient closely.
*Insulin, oral antidiabetics:* May decrease glucose level; may alter dosage requirements. Monitor glucose level in diabetic patients.
*Oral anticoagulants:* May increase sensitivity to oral anticoagulants; may alter dosage requirements. Monitor PT and INR.

**EFFECTS ON LAB TEST RESULTS**
● May increase sodium, potassium, phosphate, liver enzyme, lipid, and calcium levels. May decrease thyroxine-binding globulin and total $T_4$ levels.
● May increase RBC count and resin uptake of $T_3$ and $T_4$.

**CONTRAINDICATIONS & CAUTIONS**
● Contraindicated in pregnant or breast-feeding women and in men with breast or prostate cancer.
● Contraindicated in patients with cardiac, hepatic, or renal disease.
● Use cautiously in elderly patients; patients with cardiac, renal, or hepatic disease; or healthy males with delayed puberty.

**NURSING CONSIDERATIONS**
● Don't give to women of childbearing age until pregnancy is ruled out.
● In children, obtain X-rays of wrist bones before therapy begins to establish bone maturation level. During treatment, bones may mature more rapidly than they grow in length. Periodically review X-rays to monitor bone maturation.
● Drug is typically used only for intermittent therapy. Because of potential hepatotoxicity, watch closely for jaundice.
● Promptly report evidence of virilization in women, such as deepening of the voice, hirsutism, acne, or baldness.
● Watch for hypoestrogenic effects in women (flushing, diaphoresis, vaginal bleeding, nervousness, emotional lability, menstrual irregularities, and vaginitis, including itching, dryness, and burning).
● Watch for excessive hormonal effects in men. If patient is prepubertal, watch for premature epiphyseal closure, acne, priapism, growth of body and facial hair, and phallic enlargement. If he's postpubertal, watch for testicular atrophy, oligospermia, decreased ejaculatory volume, impotence, gynecomastia, and epididymitis.
● Unless contraindicated, use with high-calorie, high-protein diet. Give small, frequent meals.
● Periodically check hemoglobin, hematocrit, cholesterol, and calcium levels and cardiac and liver function test results.
● Check weight regularly. Control edema with sodium restriction or diuretics.

● *Alert:* Therapeutic response in breast cancer usually occurs within 3 months. Drug should be stopped if signs of disease progression appear.
● Report signs of hypercalcemia. In metastatic breast cancer, hypercalcemia may indicate progression of bone metastases.
● Evaluate semen routinely every 3 to 4 months, especially in adolescent boys.
● *Alert:* Don't use to enhance athletic performance or physique.
● *Alert:* Testosterone and methyltestosterone aren't interchangeable. Don't confuse methyltestosterone with medroxyprogesterone.

### PATIENT TEACHING
● Make sure patient understands importance of using effective contraception during therapy.
● Tell woman to report menstrual irregularities and to stop drug pending examination.
● Instruct patient to stop drug immediately and notify prescriber if pregnancy is suspected.
● Buccal tablets are twice as potent as oral tablets. Place in upper or lower buccal pouch between cheek and gum; tablet needs 30 to 60 minutes to dissolve. Tell patient not to eat, drink, chew, or smoke while buccal tablet is in place and not to swallow tablet.
● Instruct patient to change buccal tablet absorption site with each dose to minimize risk of irritation. Advise patient to rinse mouth after using buccal tablet.
● Tell woman to immediately report evidence of virilization, such as acne, swelling, weight gain, excessive hairiness, hoarseness, clitoral enlargement, decreased breast size, deepening of voice, changes in libido, male-pattern baldness, and oily skin or hair.
● Teach patient signs and symptoms of low blood sugar (hypoglycemia) and method for checking glucose level; drug enhances hypoglycemia. Instruct patient to report signs or symptoms of hypoglycemia immediately.
● Advise woman to wear cotton underwear and to wash after intercourse to decrease risk of vaginitis.

# nandrolone decanoate
Deca-Durabolin

*Pregnancy risk category X*
*Controlled substance schedule III*

### AVAILABLE FORMS
*Injection (in oil):* 50 mg/ml, 100 mg/ml, 200 mg/ml

### INDICATIONS & DOSAGES
➤ **Severe debility or disease states, refractory anemias**
*Adults and children older than age 13:* 50 to 100 mg I.M. at 1- to 4-week intervals for women; 50 to 200 mg I.M. at 1- to 4-week intervals for men. Therapy should be intermittent and should be stopped if no improvement in 6 months.
*Children ages 2 to 13:* 25 to 50 mg I.M. q 3 to 4 weeks.

### ACTION
An anabolic steroid that promotes tissue-building processes, reverses catabolism, and stimulates erythropoiesis.

| Route | Onset | Peak | Duration |
|-------|-------|------|----------|
| I.M. | Unknown | 3-6 days | Unknown |

### ADVERSE REACTIONS
**CNS:** excitation, insomnia, habituation, depression.
**CV:** edema.
**GI:** nausea, vomiting, diarrhea.
**GU:** bladder irritability.
**Hematologic:** *suppression of clotting factors.*
**Hepatic:** reversible jaundice, *peliosis hepatis, liver cell tumors.*
**Metabolic:** hypernatremia, hyperkalemia, hypercalcemia, hyperphosphatemia, hypercholesterolemia.
**Skin:** pain, induration at injection site, acne.
**Other:** *hypoestrogenic effects in women,* excessive hormonal effects in men, androgenic effects in women.

### INTERACTIONS
**Drug-drug.** *Hepatotoxic drugs:* May increase risk of hepatotoxicity. Monitor liver function closely.

---

Reactions may be *common,* uncommon, *life-threatening,* or COMMON AND LIFE-THREATENING.

*Insulin, oral antidiabetics:* May alter dosage requirements. Monitor glucose level in diabetic patients.

*Oral anticoagulants:* May alter dosage requirements. Monitor PT and INR.

**EFFECTS ON LAB TEST RESULTS**
● May increase creatinine, lipid, sodium, potassium, calcium, phosphate, cholesterol, and liver enzyme levels.
● May increase $T_3$ uptake. May decrease protein-bound iodine, thyroxine-binding capacity, and radioactive iodine uptake.
● May cause abnormal results of fasting glucose, glucose tolerance, and metyrapone tests.

**CONTRAINDICATIONS & CAUTIONS**
● Contraindicated in patients hypersensitive to anabolic steroids, in patients with nephrosis or the nephrotic phase of nephritis, in men with breast cancer or known or suspected prostate cancer, in women with breast cancer and hypercalcemia, in pregnant or breast-feeding women, and in those who want to enhance their physical appearance or athletic performance.
● Use cautiously in patients with diabetes; cardiac, renal, or hepatic disease; epilepsy; or migraine or other conditions that may be aggravated by fluid retention.

**NURSING CONSIDERATIONS**
● Don't give to women of childbearing age until pregnancy is ruled out.
● Make sure patient understands importance of using an effective nonhormonal contraceptive during therapy.
● Instruct patient to stop drug immediately and notify prescriber if she suspects pregnancy.
● In children, obtain X-rays of wrist bones before therapy begins to establish bone maturation level. During treatment, bones may mature more rapidly than they grow in length. Periodically review X-ray results to monitor bone maturation.
● Inject I.M. drug deeply, preferably into upper outer quadrant of gluteal muscle in adults. Rotate injection sites to prevent muscle atrophy.
● Unless contraindicated, use with high-calorie, high-protein diet. Give small, frequent feedings.

● Watch for signs of virilization, which may be irreversible even if drug is stopped. Androgenic effects in women include acne, edema, weight gain, hirsutism, hoarseness, clitoral enlargement, decreased breast size, changes in libido, male-pattern baldness, and oily skin or hair.
● Watch for hypoestrogenic effects in women, such as flushing, diaphoresis, vaginal bleeding, nervousness, emotional lability, menstrual irregularities, and vaginitis, including itching, dryness, and burning.
● Watch for excessive hormonal effects in male patients. If patient is prepubertal, watch for premature epiphyseal closure, acne, priapism, growth of body and facial hair, and phallic enlargement. If postpubertal, watch for testicular atrophy, oligospermia, decreased ejaculatory volume, impotence, gynecomastia, and epididymitis.
● Closely observe boys younger than age 7 for precocious development of male sexual characteristics.
● Evaluate semen routinely every 3 to 4 months, especially in adolescent boys.
● *Alert:* Periodically evaluate hepatic function. Watch for jaundice; dosage adjustment may reverse condition. If liver function test results are abnormal, therapy should be stopped.
● Check weight regularly. Edema usually can be controlled with sodium restriction or diuretics.
● Watch for evidence of hypoglycemia in diabetic patients. Check glucose levels and adjust dosage of antidiabetic.
● Check quantitative urine and serum calcium levels. Hypercalcemia is most likely to occur in patients with breast cancer.
● When used to promote erythropoiesis in patient with refractory anemia, make sure he has adequate daily iron intake.
● Anabolic steroids may alter results of laboratory studies performed during therapy and for 2 to 3 weeks after therapy ends.

**PATIENT TEACHING**
● Make sure patient understands importance of using an effective nonhormonal contraceptive during therapy.

• Review signs and symptoms of virilization with woman, and instruct her to notify prescriber immediately if they occur.
• Advise woman to wear cotton underwear and to wash after intercourse to decrease risk of vaginitis.
• Warn diabetic patient to be alert for hypoglycemia, and tell him to notify prescriber if it occurs.
• Tell patient to report sudden weight gain to prescriber.
• Tell woman to report menstrual irregularities and to stop drug when these occur, pending examination.

---

## testosterone
Testopel Pellets

## testosterone cypionate
Depo-Testosterone

## testosterone enanthate
Delatestryl

## testosterone propionate
Malogen†

*Pregnancy risk category X*
*Controlled substance schedule III*

---

### AVAILABLE FORMS
**testosterone**
*Pellets (S.C. implant):* 75 mg
**testosterone cypionate**
*Injection (in oil):* 100 mg/ml, 200 mg/ml
**testosterone enanthate**
*Injection (in oil):* 200 mg/ml
**testosterone propionate**
*Injection (in oil):* 100 mg/ml

### INDICATIONS & DOSAGES
➤ **Male hypogonadism**
*Men:* 10 to 25 mg propionate I.M. two to three times weekly; or 50 to 400 mg cypionate or enanthate I.M. q 2 to 4 weeks. Or, 150 to 450 mg (2 to 6 pellets) implanted S.C. q 3 to 6 months.
➤ **Metastatic breast cancer in women 1 to 5 years after menopause**
*Women:* 50 to 100 mg propionate I.M. three times weekly; or 200 to 400 mg cypionate or enanthate I.M. q 2 to 4 weeks.

### ACTION
Stimulates target tissues to develop normally in androgen-deficient men. Testosterone may have some antiestrogen properties, making it useful in treating certain estrogen-dependent breast cancers. Its action in postpartum breast engorgement isn't known because testosterone doesn't suppress lactation.

| Route | Onset | Peak | Duration |
|-------|-------|------|----------|
| I.M. | Unknown | 10-100 min | Unknown |
| S.C. | Unknown | Unknown | 3-6 mo |

### ADVERSE REACTIONS
**CNS:** headache, anxiety, depression, paresthesia, sleep apnea.
**CV:** edema.
**GI:** nausea.
**GU:** amenorrhea.
**Hematologic:** polycythemia, *suppression of clotting factors.*
**Hepatic:** reversible jaundice, *cholestatic hepatitis.*
**Metabolic:** hypernatremia, hyperkalemia, hypercalcemia, hyperphosphatemia, hypercholesterolemia.
**Skin:** pain, induration at injection site, local edema, acne.
**Other:** androgenic effects in women, gynecomastia, hypersensitivity reactions, hypoestrogenic effects in women, excessive hormonal effects in men.

### INTERACTIONS
**Drug-drug.** *Hepatotoxic drugs:* May increase risk of hepatotoxicity. Monitor liver function closely.
*Insulin, oral antidiabetics:* May decrease glucose level; may alter dosage requirements. Monitor glucose level in diabetic patients.
*Oral anticoagulants:* May increase sensitivity; may alter dosage requirements. Monitor PT and INR.

### EFFECTS ON LAB TEST RESULTS
• May increase sodium, potassium, phosphate, cholesterol, liver enzyme, calcium, and creatinine levels. May decrease thyroxine-binding globulin and total $T_4$ levels.
• May increase resin uptake of $T_3$ and $T_4$ and RBC count.

---

## CONTRAINDICATIONS & CAUTIONS
● Contraindicated in patients hypersensitive to drug and in those with hypercalcemia or cardiac, hepatic, or renal decompensation.
● Contraindicated in men with breast or prostate cancer and in pregnant or breast-feeding women.
● Use cautiously in elderly patients.

## NURSING CONSIDERATIONS
● Don't give to women of childbearing age until pregnancy is ruled out.
● Store I.M. preparations at room temperature. If crystals appear, warm and shake bottle to disperse them.
● Cypionate and enanthate are long-acting solutions.
● Inject deep into upper outer quadrant of gluteal muscle. Rotate injection sites; report soreness at site.
● Unless contraindicated, give with diet high in calories and protein. Provide small, frequent meals to help avoid nausea.
● Monitor patient's liver function test results.
● Testosterone may cause abnormal glucose tolerance test results.
● In patients with metastatic breast cancer, hypercalcemia usually indicates progression of bone metastases. Report signs and symptoms of hypercalcemia.
● Report evidence of virilization in women. Androgenic effects include acne, edema, weight gain, hirsutism, hoarseness, clitoral enlargement, decreased breast size, changes in libido, male-pattern baldness, and oily skin or hair.
● Watch for hypoestrogenic effects in women (flushing; diaphoresis; vaginitis, including itching, drying, and burning; vaginal bleeding; menstrual irregularities).
● Watch for excessive hormonal effects in male patients. If patient is prepubertal, watch for premature epiphyseal closure, acne, priapism, growth of body and facial hair, and phallic enlargement. If postpubertal, watch for testicular atrophy, oligospermia, decreased ejaculatory volume, impotence, gynecomastia, epididymitis.
● Monitor patient's weight and blood pressure routinely.

● Monitor prepubertal boys by X-ray for rate of bone maturation.
● *Alert:* Therapeutic response in breast cancer is usually apparent within 3 months. Therapy should be stopped if disease progresses.
● Androgens may alter results of laboratory studies during therapy and for 2 to 3 weeks after therapy ends.
● *Alert:* Don't confuse testosterone with testolactone.
● *Alert:* Testosterone salts aren't interchangeable.

## PATIENT TEACHING
● Make sure patient understands importance of using an effective nonhormonal contraceptive during therapy.
● Instruct patient to stop drug immediately and notify prescriber if pregnancy is suspected.
● Review signs and symptoms of virilization with woman, and instruct her to notify prescriber if they occur.
● Advise woman to wear cotton underwear and to wash after intercourse to decrease risk of vaginitis.
● Instruct man to notify prescriber about priapism, reduced ejaculatory volume, or gynecomastia.
● Warn diabetic patient to be alert for hypoglycemia and to notify prescriber if it occurs.
● Instruct boys using testosterone for delayed puberty to have X-rays of hand and wrist obtained every 6 months during treatment.
● Tell patient to report sudden weight gain.
● Warn patient that drug shouldn't be used to enhance athletic performance.

## testosterone transdermal system
Androderm, Androgel, Testoderm, Testoderm TTS, Testoderm w/Adhesive

*Pregnancy risk category X*
*Controlled substance schedule III*

## AVAILABLE FORMS
*1% gel:* 25 mg, 50 mg per unit dose
*Transdermal system:* 2.5 mg/day, 4 mg/day, 5 mg/day, 6 mg/day

---

## INDICATIONS & DOSAGES
➤ **Primary or hypogonadotropic hypogonadism in men**
*Androderm*
*Men:* One or two patches applied to back, abdomen, arm, or thigh h.s. for total dose of 5 mg/day.
*AndroGel*
*Men:* First, 50 mg applied q morning to shoulders, upper arms, or abdomen. Check testosterone level after about 2 weeks. If response is inadequate, may increase dose to 75 mg daily. Subsequently, adjust to 100 mg, if needed.
*Testoderm*
*Men:* One 6-mg/day patch applied to scrotal area daily; or 4 mg/day if scrotal area is small. Patch is worn for 22 to 24 hours daily.
*Testoderm TTS*
*Men:* One 5-mg/day patch applied to arm, back, or upper buttock.

## ACTION
Releases testosterone, which stimulates target tissues to develop normally in androgen-deficient men.

| Route | Onset | Peak | Duration |
|-------|-------|------|----------|
| Trans-dermal | Unknown | 2-4 hr | 2 hr after removal |

## ADVERSE REACTIONS
**CNS:** *CVA,* asthenia, depression, headache.
**GI:** GI bleeding.
**GU:** prostatitis, prostate abnormalities, UTI.
**Hepatic:** reversible jaundice, *cholestatic hepatitis.*
**Metabolic:** hypernatremia, hyperkalemia, hypercalcemia, hyperphosphatemia, hypercholesterolemia.
**Skin:** acne irritation, *pruritus, blister under system,* allergic contact dermatitis, burning.
**Other:** gynecomastia, breast tenderness, flulike syndrome.

## INTERACTIONS
**Drug-drug.** *Insulin:* May alter insulin dosage requirements. Monitor glucose level.

*Oral anticoagulants:* May alter anticoagulant dosage requirements. Monitor PT and INR.

## EFFECTS ON LAB TEST RESULTS
• May increase sodium, potassium, phosphate, cholesterol, liver enzyme, calcium, and creatinine levels.
• May increase RBC count.

## CONTRAINDICATIONS & CAUTIONS
• Contraindicated in patients hypersensitive to drug, in women, in men with known or suspected breast or prostate cancer, and in patients with CV, renal, or hepatic disease.
• Use cautiously in elderly men.

## NURSING CONSIDERATIONS
• Apply Androderm system to clean, dry skin on back, abdomen, upper arms, or thigh. Apply Testoderm TTS to arm, back, or upper buttock. Rotate application site every 7 days.
• Wear gloves when handling transdermal patches. Fold used patches with adhesive sides together, and discard so they can't be handled.
• Periodically assess liver function test results, lipid profiles, hemoglobin level, hematocrit (with long-term use), and levels of prostatic acid phosphatase and prostate-specific antigen.
• Monitor for excessive hormonal effects in male patients.
• **Alert:** Don't confuse Testoderm with Estraderm.
• **Alert:** Testoderm and Androderm are not interchangeable.

## PATIENT TEACHING
• Teach patient how to apply transdermal system. Warn him that adequate serum level won't be attained if Testoderm patch isn't applied to genital skin. Scrotal area may be dry-shaved for best contact. Application sites should be rotated, with 7 days between applications to same site. Avoid bony prominences.
• Don't interchange patch brands.
• Tell patient not to apply Androderm or Testoderm TTS to scrotum.
• Tell patient that if the patch falls off, it may be reapplied. If patch falls off and can't be reapplied, and it has been worn at

---

least 12 hours, a new patch may be applied at the next application time.
• Advise patient to wear underwear briefs to prevent patch from falling off.
• Instruct patient that system must be changed every 24 hours.
• Tell patient to apply gel to clean, dry, intact skin of the shoulders, upper arms, or abdomen only. Don't apply to scrotum.
• Tell patient to wash his hands thoroughly with soap and water after applying gel.
• Advise patient for best results to wait to swim or shower for at least 5 hours after applying gel. Showering or swimming 1 hour after gel application, if done infrequently, should have minimal effects on drug absorption.
• Warn diabetic patient that testosterone may decrease glucose level and to be alert for hypoglycemia.
• Tell patient that topical testosterone has caused virilization in women partners, who should report acne or changes in body hair distribution.
• Advise patient to report persistent erections, nausea, vomiting, changes in skin color, ankle swelling, or sudden weight gain to prescriber.
• Tell patient that Androderm doesn't have to be removed during sexual intercourse or while showering.

# 53

# Estrogens and progestins

17 beta-estradiol and
   norgestimate
drospirenone and ethinyl
   estradiol
esterified estrogens
estradiol
estradiol cypionate
estradiol hemihydrate
estradiol valerate
estradiol and norethindrone
   acetate transdermal system
estrogens, conjugated
estropipate
ethinyl estradiol
ethinyl estradiol and desogestrel
ethinyl estradiol and ethynodiol
   diacetate
ethinyl estradiol and
   levonorgestrel
ethinyl estradiol and
   norethindrone
ethinyl estradiol and
   norethindrone acetate
ethinyl estradiol and
   norgestimate
ethinyl estradiol and norgestrel
ethinyl estradiol, norethindrone
   acetate, and ferrous fumarate
etonogestrel and ethinyl estradiol
   ring
medroxyprogesterone acetate
medroxyprogesterone acetate
   and estradiol cypionate
mestranol and norethindrone
norelgestromin and ethinyl
   estradiol transdermal system
norethindrone
norethindrone acetate
progesterone

## COMBINATION PRODUCTS

ACTIVELLA: estradiol 1 mg and norethindrone acetate 0.5 mg.
ESTRATEST: esterified estrogens 1.25 mg and methyltestosterone 2.5 mg.
ESTRATEST H.S.: esterified estrogens 0.625 mg and methyltestosterone 1.25 mg.
FEMHRT: ethinyl estradiol 5 mcg and norethindrone acetate 1 mg.

PREMPHASE: conjugated estrogens 0.625 mg and conjugated estrogens 0.625 mg with medroxyprogesterone acetate 5 mg.
PREMPRO 0.45 MG/1.5 MG: 0.45 mg conjugated estrogens and 1.5 mg medroxyprogesterone acetate.
PREMPRO 0.625 MG /2.5 MG: 0.625 mg conjugated estrogens and 2.5 mg medroxyprogesterone acetate.
PREMPRO 0.625 MG /5 MG: 0.625 mg conjugated estrogens and 5 mg medroxyprogesterone acetate.
PREVEN EMERGENCY: ethinyl estradiol 50 mcg and levonorgestrel 0.25 mg.

## 17 beta-estradiol and norgestimate
Ortho-Prefest

*Pregnancy risk category X*

### AVAILABLE FORMS
*Tablets:* Blister card of 15 pink and 15 white tablets, for a total of 30 tablets
Pink tablets—1 mg estradiol
White tablets—1 mg estradiol and 0.09 mg norgestimate

### INDICATIONS & DOSAGES
➤ **Moderate to severe vasomotor symptoms caused by menopause; vulvar and vaginal atrophy; to prevent osteoporosis in women with an intact uterus**
*Women:* 1 mg estradiol (pink tablet) P.O. daily for 3 days; then 1 mg estradiol/ 0.09 mg norgestimate (white tablet) P.O. daily for 3 days. Repeat continuously until blister card is finished.

### ACTION
Circulating estrogens modulate the pituitary secretion of luteinizing hormone and follicle-stimulating hormone through a negative feedback mechanism. Estrogen replacement therapy lowers high levels of these hormones in postmenopausal women. Norgestimate binds to androgen and progesterone receptors. Progestins

counter the estrogenic effects by decreasing the number of estradiol receptors and suppressing synthesis of endometrial tissue.

| Route | Onset | Peak | Duration |
|-------|-------|------|----------|
| P.O. | Unknown | 7 hr (estradiol) 2 hr (norgestimate) | Unknown |

## ADVERSE REACTIONS
**CNS:** depression, dizziness, fatigue, pain, *headache.*
**CV:** *venous thromboembolism, MI, pulmonary embolism,* thrombophlebitis, edema.
**EENT:** steepening of corneal curvature, intolerance to contact lenses, pharyngitis, sinusitis.
**GI:** flatulence, nausea, *abdominal pain,* gallbladder disease.
**GU:** dysmenorrhea, vaginal bleeding, vaginitis.
**Metabolic:** weight changes, reduced carbohydrate tolerance, aggravation of porphyria.
**Musculoskeletal:** arthralgia, myalgia, *back pain.*
**Respiratory:** cough, *upper respiratory tract infection.*
**Skin:** chloasma, melasma, hirsutism, *erythema multiforme,* erythema nodosum, hemorrhagic eruption, loss of scalp hair.
**Other:** changes in libido, *flulike symptoms,* viral infection, tooth disorder, breast pain, galactorrhea.

## INTERACTIONS
**Drug-herb.** *Black cohosh:* May increase adverse effects of estrogens. Discourage use together.
*Saw palmetto:* May have antiestrogenic effects. Discourage use together.
*St. John's wort:* May decrease effects of estrogens. Discourage use together.
**Drug-lifestyle.** *Smoking:* May increase risk of CV effects. Advise patient to avoid smoking.

## EFFECTS ON LAB TEST RESULTS
● May increase thyroid-binding globulin; factor II, VII antigen, VIII antigen, VIII coagulant activity, IX, X, XII, VII-X complex, II-VII-X complex; beta-thromboglobulin; HDL; triglyceride; corticosteroid; sex steroid; angiotensin and renin substrate; alpha$_1$-antitrypsin; ceruloplasmin; fibrinogen; and plasminogen antigen levels. May decrease folate, LDL, anti-factor Xa, and antithrombin III levels.
● May increase PT, PTT, platelet aggregation time, and platelet count. May decrease T$_3$ resin uptake and glucose tolerance.
● May decrease metyrapone test results.

## CONTRAINDICATIONS & CAUTIONS
● Contraindicated in patients hypersensitive to any of its components, in postmenopausal women, in women who are or may be pregnant, and in patients with breast cancer, estrogen-dependent neoplasia, undiagnosed abnormal genital bleeding, and active or previous thrombophlebitis or thromboembolic disorders.

## NURSING CONSIDERATIONS
● Give Ortho-Prefest cautiously to women who have had a hysterectomy, to overweight women, to women with abnormal lipid profiles, and to women with impaired liver function.
● Reassess patient at 6-month intervals to determine whether treatment for symptoms is still necessary.
● Use of estrogens is linked to development of endometrial hyperplasia. Giving progestin with estrogen significantly reduces this risk.
● Users of estrogen replacement have an increased risk of venous thromboembolism.
● Hormone replacement therapy may increase the risk of breast cancer in postmenopausal women.
● Estrogens can lead to severe hypercalcemia in patients with breast cancer and bone metastases. If this occurs, stop the drug and take appropriate measures to reduce calcium level.
● Monitor glucose level closely in patients with diabetes.

## PATIENT TEACHING
● Inform patient about the risks of estrogen therapy, such as breast cancer, uterine cancer, abnormal blood clotting, and gallbladder disease.

• Tell patient to immediately report undiagnosed, persistent, or recurring abnormal vaginal bleeding.
• Instruct patient to perform monthly breast self-examinations and to obtain yearly mammograms after age 50.
• Tell patient to report warning signals of blood clots, including pain in the calves or chest, sudden shortness of breath, coughing of blood, severe headaches, vomiting, dizziness, faintness, changes in vision or speech, and weakness or numbness in arms or legs.
• Urge patient to report evidence of liver problems, such as yellowing of skin or eyes, or upper right quadrant pain.
• Instruct patient to report abdominal pain, swelling, or tenderness, which may suggest gallbladder problems.
• Encourage patient to stop smoking or reduce number of cigarettes smoked because of the risk of CV complications.
• Tell patient to store Ortho-Prefest at room temperature away from excessive heat and moisture. Product will remain stable for 18 months.

# drospirenone and ethinyl estradiol
Yasmin

*Pregnancy risk category X*

## AVAILABLE FORMS
*Tablets:* 3 mg drospirenone and 0.03 mg ethinyl estradiol as 21 yellow tablets and 7 white (inert) tablets

## INDICATIONS & DOSAGES
➤ **Contraception**
*Women:* 1 yellow tablet P.O. daily for 21 days beginning on day 1 of menstrual cycle or the first Sunday after the onset of menstruation. Then take 1 white inert tablet P.O. daily on days 22 through 28. Begin the next and all subsequent 28-day regimens on the same day of the week that the first regimen began, following the same schedule. Restart taking yellow tablets on the next day after taking the last white tablet.

## ACTION
Reduces the chance for conception by inhibiting ovulation, inhibiting progression of sperm, and reducing chance of implantation.

| Route | Onset | Peak | Duration |
|---|---|---|---|
| P.O. | Unknown | 1-3 hr | Unknown |

## ADVERSE REACTIONS
**CNS:** asthenia, *cerebral hemorrhage, cerebral thrombosis,* depression, dizziness, emotional lability, headache, migraine, nervousness.
**CV:** *arterial thromboembolism,* hypertension, *mesenteric thrombosis, MI,* thrombophlebitis.
**EENT:** cataracts, steepening of corneal curvature, intolerance to contact lenses, pharyngitis, retinal thrombosis, sinusitis.
**GI:** abdominal pain, abdominal cramping, bloating, changes in appetite, colitis, diarrhea, gastroenteritis, nausea, vomiting, gallbladder disease.
**GU:** amenorrhea, breakthrough bleeding, change in cervical erosion and secretion, change in menstrual flow, cystitis, cystitis-like syndrome, dysmenorrhea, *hemolytic-uremic syndrome,* impaired renal function, leukorrhea, menstrual disorder, premenstrual syndrome, spotting, temporary infertility after discontinuing treatment, UTI, vaginal candidiasis, vaginitis.
**Hepatic:** *Budd-Chiari syndrome,* cholestatic jaundice, *hepatic adenomas,* benign liver tumors.
**Metabolic:** reduced tolerance to carbohydrates, porphyria, weight change.
**Musculoskeletal:** back pain.
**Respiratory:** bronchitis, *pulmonary embolism,* upper respiratory tract infection.
**Skin:** acne, *erythema multiforme,* erythema nodosum, hemorrhagic eruption, hirsutism, loss of scalp hair, melasma, pruritus, rash.
**Other:** changes in libido.

## INTERACTIONS
**Drug-drug.** *ACE inhibitors, aldosterone antagonists, angiotensin II receptor antagonists, NSAIDs, potassium-sparing diuretics:* May increase risk of hyperkalemia. Monitor potassium level.
*Acetaminophen:* May increase level of contraceptive and decrease effectiveness

of acetaminophen. Monitor patient for adverse effects. Adjust acetaminophen dose as needed.

*Ampicillin, griseofulvin, tetracycline:* May decrease contraceptive effect. Encourage use of additional method of birth control while taking the antibiotic.

*Ascorbic acid, atorvastatin:* May increase level of contraceptive. Monitor patient for adverse effects.

*Carbamazepine, phenobarbital, phenytoin:* May increase metabolism of ethinyl estradiol and decrease contraceptive effectiveness. Encourage use of alternative method of birth control.

*Clofibrate, morphine, salicylic acid, temazepam:* May decrease levels and increase clearance of these drugs. Monitor patient for effectiveness.

*Cyclosporine, prednisolone, theophylline:* May increase levels of these drugs. Monitor patient for adverse effects and toxicity.

*Phenylbutazone, rifampin:* May decrease contraceptive effectiveness and increase menstrual irregularities. Advise patient to use alternative method of birth control.

**Drug-herb.** *St. John's wort:* May decrease contraceptive effectiveness and may increase breakthrough bleeding. Encourage use of additional method of birth control or discourage use together.

**Drug-lifestyle.** *Smoking:* May increase risk of CV adverse effects. Advise patient to avoid smoking.

## EFFECTS ON LAB TEST RESULTS

• May increase thyroid-binding globulin, total thyroid hormone, total circulating sex steroid, prothrombin, corticoid, folate, triglyceride, and factor VII, VIII, IX, and X levels. May decrease antithrombin III level.

• May increase norepinephrine-induced platelet aggregability. May decrease free $T_3$ resin uptake and glucose tolerance.

## CONTRAINDICATIONS & CAUTIONS

• Contraindicated in women with hepatic dysfunction, tumor, or disease; renal or adrenal insufficiency; thrombophlebitis, thromboembolic disorders, or history of deep vein thrombosis or thromboembolic disorders; cerebrovascular or coronary artery disease; known or suspected breast cancer, endometrial cancer, or other estrogen-dependent neoplasia; abnormal genital bleeding; or cholestatic jaundice of pregnancy or jaundice with other contraceptive pill use. Also contraindicated in women who are pregnant or suspect they may be pregnant and in women older than age 35 who smoke 15 or more cigarettes daily.

• Use cautiously in patients with risk factors for CV disease, such as hypertension, hyperlipidemias, obesity, and diabetes. Also use cautiously in patients with conditions aggravated by fluid retention.

## NURSING CONSIDERATIONS

• The use of contraceptives causes increased risk of MI, thromboembolism, stroke, hepatic neoplasia, gallbladder disease, and hypertension. Risk increases in patients with hypertension, diabetes, hyperlipidemia, and obesity.

• Smoking increases the risk of serious CV adverse effects. The risk increases with age (especially age older than 35 years) and in patients who smoke 15 or more cigarettes daily.

• The relationship between the use of hormonal contraceptives and breast and cervical cancers is unclear. Encourage women to schedule a complete gynecologic examination at least yearly and to perform breast self-examinations monthly.

• In patients scheduled to have elective surgery that may increase the risk of thromboembolism, stop contraceptive use from at least 4 weeks before until 2 weeks after surgery. Also stop use during and after prolonged immobilization.

• Because of increased risk of thromboembolism in the postpartum period, don't start contraceptive earlier than 4 to 6 weeks after delivery.

• Stop use and evaluate patient if loss of vision, proptosis, diplopia, papilledema, or retinal vascular lesions occur. Recommend that contact lens wearers be evaluated by an ophthalmologist if visual changes or lens intolerance occurs.

• If patient misses two consecutive periods, she should obtain a negative pregnancy test result before continuing contraceptive.

• Immediately stop use if pregnancy is confirmed.

• Closely monitor patient with diabetes. Glucose intolerance may occur.
• Closely monitor patient with hypertension or a history of depression. Stop drug if these events occur.
• In patient taking medications that may increase potassium, check potassium level during the first treatment cycle.
• Stop drug and evaluate patient if persistent, severe headaches occur or if migraines occur or are worsened.
• Evaluate patient for malignancy or pregnancy if she experiences breakthrough bleeding or spotting.
• Closely monitor patient with hyperlipidemias.
• Stop use if jaundice occurs.

**PATIENT TEACHING**
• Advise patient to use additional method of birth control during the first 7 days of the first cycle of hormonal contraceptive.
• Inform patient that pills don't protect against sexually transmitted diseases, such as HIV.
• Advise patient of the dangers of smoking while taking hormonal contraceptives. Suggest smokers choose a different form of birth control.
• Tell patient to schedule gynecologic examinations yearly and perform breast self-examination monthly.
• Inform patient that spotting, light bleeding, or stomach upset may occur during the first 1 to 3 packs of pills. Tell her to continue taking the pills and to notify her health care provider if these symptoms persist.
• Tell patient to take the pill at the same time each day.
• Tell patient to immediately report sharp chest pain; coughing of blood or sudden shortness of breath; calf pain; crushing chest pain or chest heaviness; sudden severe headache or vomiting, dizziness or fainting, visual or speech disturbances, weakness or numbness in an arm or leg; vision loss; breast lumps; severe stomach pain or tenderness; difficulty sleeping; lack of energy, fatigue, or change in mood; jaundice with fever, fatigue, loss of appetite, dark urine, or light-colored bowel movements.
• Tell patient to notify health care provider if she wears contact lenses and notices a

change in vision or has trouble wearing the lenses.
• Tell patient that the risk of pregnancy increases with each active yellow tablet she forgets to take. Inform patient what to do if she misses pills.
• Tell patient to use an additional method of birth control and notify health care provider if she isn't sure what to do about missed pills.
• Small amounts of hormonal contraceptives are excreted in breast milk. Yellow skin and eyes (jaundice) and breast enlargement may occur in breast-feeding infants.

## esterified estrogens
Estratab, Menest, Neo-Estrone†

*Pregnancy risk category X*

**AVAILABLE FORMS**
*Tablets:* 0.3 mg, 0.625 mg, 1.25 mg, 2.5 mg
*Tablets (film-coated):* 0.3 mg, 0.625 mg, 1.25 mg, 2.5 mg

**INDICATIONS & DOSAGES**
➤ **Inoperable prostate cancer**
*Men:* 1.25 to 2.5 mg P.O. t.i.d.
➤ **Breast cancer**
*Men and postmenopausal women:* 10 mg P.O. t.i.d. for 3 or more months.
➤ **Female hypogonadism**
*Women:* 2.5 to 7.5 mg daily in divided doses in cycles of 20 days on, 10 days off.
➤ **Castration, primary ovarian failure**
*Women:* 1.25 mg daily in cycles of 3 weeks on, 1 week off. Adjust for symptoms. Can be given continuously.
➤ **Vasomotor menopausal symptoms**
*Women:* 1.25 mg P.O. daily in cycles of 3 weeks on, 1 week off. Dosage may be increased to 2.5 to 3.75 mg P.O. daily if needed.
➤ **Atrophic vaginitis, atrophic urethritis**
*Women:* 0.3 to 1.25 mg or more P.O. daily in cycles of 3 weeks on, 1 week off.

**ACTION**
Increases synthesis of DNA, RNA, and protein in responsive tissues. Also, reduces release of follicle-stimulating and

luteinizing hormones from the pituitary gland.

| Route | Onset | Peak | Duration |
|-------|-------|------|----------|
| P.O. | Unknown | Unknown | Unknown |

## ADVERSE REACTIONS
**CNS:** headache, dizziness, chorea, depression, *CVA, seizures.*
**CV:** thrombophlebitis, *thromboembolism,* hypertension, *edema, pulmonary embolism, MI.*
**EENT:** worsening myopia or astigmatism, intolerance of contact lenses.
**GI:** *nausea,* vomiting, abdominal cramps, bloating, anorexia, increased appetite, *pancreatitis,* increased risk of gallbladder disease.
**GU:** breakthrough bleeding, altered menstrual flow, dysmenorrhea, amenorrhea, *increased risk of endometrial cancer,* cervical erosion, altered cervical secretions, enlargement of uterine fibromas, vaginal candidiasis, testicular atrophy, impotence.
**Hepatic:** cholestatic jaundice, *hepatic adenoma.*
**Metabolic:** hypercalcemia, weight changes.
**Skin:** melasma, rash, hirsutism or hair loss, erythema nodosum, dermatitis.
**Other:** *breast tenderness, enlargement, or secretion; gynecomastia; increased risk of breast cancer.*

## INTERACTIONS
**Drug-drug.** *Carbamazepine, fosphenytoin, phenobarbital, phenytoin, rifampin:* May decrease effectiveness of estrogen therapy. Monitor patient closely.
*Corticosteroids:* May enhance effects. Monitor patient closely.
*Cyclosporine:* May increase risk of toxicity. Use together with caution, and monitor cyclosporine level frequently.
*Dantrolene, hepatotoxic drugs:* May increase risk of hepatotoxicity. Monitor liver function closely.
*Oral anticoagulants:* May decrease anticoagulant effects. Dosage adjustments may be needed. Monitor PT and INR.
*Tamoxifen:* May interfere with tamoxifen effectiveness. Avoid using together.

**Drug-herb.** *Black cohosh:* May increase adverse effects of estrogens. Discourage use together.
*Saw palmetto:* May have antiestrogenic effects. Discourage use together.
*St. John's wort:* May decrease effects of estrogens. Discourage use together.
**Drug-food.** *Caffeine:* May increase caffeine level. Advise caution.
**Drug-lifestyle.** *Smoking:* May increase risk of CV effects. If smoking continues, may need alternative form of therapy.

## EFFECTS ON LAB TEST RESULTS
• May increase calcium and clotting factor VII, VIII, IX, and X levels.
• May increase PT and norepinephrine-induced platelet aggregation. May reduce metyrapone test results.

## CONTRAINDICATIONS & CAUTIONS
• Contraindicated in pregnant patients, in patients hypersensitive to drug, and in patients with breast cancer (except metastatic disease), estrogen-dependent neoplasia, active thrombophlebitis, thromboembolic disorders, undiagnosed abnormal genital bleeding, or history of thromboembolic disease.
• Use cautiously in patients with history of hypertension, mental depression, cardiac or renal dysfunction, liver impairment, bone disease, migraine, seizures, or diabetes mellitus.

## NURSING CONSIDERATIONS
• When used for vasomotor symptoms in menstruating women, cyclic administration is started on day 5 of bleeding.
• Make sure patient has thorough physical examination before starting estrogen therapy. Patients receiving long-term therapy should have annual examinations. Periodically monitor body weight, blood pressure, lipid levels, and hepatic function.
• Notify pathologist about patient's estrogen therapy when sending specimens to laboratory for evaluation.
• Because of risk of thromboembolism, stop therapy at least 1 month before procedures that cause prolonged immobilization or increased risk of thromboembolism, such as knee or hip surgery.

---

*Rapid onset*   †Canada   ‡Australia   ◇OTC   ◆ Off-label use   ✐Photoguide   *Liquid contains alcohol.

• Glucose tolerance may be impaired. Monitor glucose level closely in patients with diabetes.

• **Alert:** Don't confuse Estratab with Estratest.

## PATIENT TEACHING

• Tell patient to read package insert describing estrogen's adverse effects; also, give patient verbal explanation.

• Emphasize importance of regular physical examinations. Postmenopausal women who use estrogen replacement for longer than 5 years to treat menopausal symptoms may be at increased risk for endometrial cancer. This risk is reduced by using cyclic rather than continuous therapy and the lowest possible estrogen dose. Adding progestins to the regimen decreases risk of endometrial hyperplasia; however, it isn't known whether progestins affect risk of endometrial cancer.

• **Alert:** Warn patient to immediately report abdominal pain; pain, numbness, or stiffness in legs or buttocks; pressure or pain in chest or shortness of breath; severe headaches; visual disturbances such as blind spots, flashing lights, or blurriness; vaginal bleeding or discharge; breast lumps; swelling of hands or feet; yellow skin or sclera; dark urine; or light-colored stools.

• Tell diabetic patient to report elevated glucose level so that antidiabetic dosage can be adjusted.

• Explain to patient on cyclic therapy for postmenopausal symptoms that she may experience withdrawal bleeding during week off drug. Tell her to report unusual vaginal bleeding.

• Teach woman to perform routine breast self-examination.

• Advise woman of childbearing age to consult prescriber before taking drug and to advise prescriber immediately if she becomes pregnant.

• Teach patient methods to decrease risk of blood clots.

• Encourage patient to stop smoking or reduce number of cigarettes smoked because of the risk of CV complications.

# estradiol (oestradiol)
Alora, Climara, Esclim, Estrace✐, Estrace Vaginal Cream, Estraderm, Estring Vaginal Ring, FemPatch, Femring, Gynodiol, Vivelle, Vivelle-Dot

# estradiol cypionate
depGynogen, Depo-Estradiol Cypionate, Depogen

# estradiol hemihydrate
Vagifem

# estradiol valerate (oestradiol valerate)
Delestrogen, Estra-L 40, Gynogen L.A., Primogyn Depot‡, Valergen

*Pregnancy risk category X*

## AVAILABLE FORMS
**estradiol**
*Tablets (micronized):* 0.5 mg, 1 mg, 1.5 mg, 2 mg
*Transdermal:* 0.025 mg/24 hours, 0.0375 mg/24 hours, 0.05 mg/24 hours, 0.075 mg/24 hours, 0.1 mg/24 hours
*Vaginal cream (in nonliquefying base):* 0.1 mg/g
*Vaginal ring:* 0.0075 mg/24 hours; 0.05 mg/24 hours; 0.1 mg/24 hours
**estradiol cypionate**
*Injection (in oil):* 5 mg/ml
**estradiol hemihydrate**
*Vaginal tablets:* 25 mcg
**estradiol valerate**
*Injection (in oil):* 10 mg/ml, 20 mg/ml, 40 mg/ml

## INDICATIONS & DOSAGES
➤ **Vasomotor menopausal symptoms, female hypogonadism, female castration, primary ovarian failure**
*Women:* 0.5 to 2 mg P.O. estradiol daily in cycles of 21 days on and 7 days off or cycles of 5 days on and 2 days off. Or, for vasomotor symptoms, 1 to 5 mg cypionate I.M. once q 3 to 4 weeks; for female hypogonadism, 1.5 to 2 mg cypionate I.M. once q month.
*Transdermal patch*
Esclim 0.025 mg/24 hours, Estraderm 0.05 mg/24 hours, Vivelle 0.0375 mg/

24 hours, Vivelle 0.05 mg/24 hours twice weekly, Climara 0.05 mg/24 hours, or FemPatch 0.025 mg/24 hours once weekly. Apply to clean, dry area of the trunk. Adjust dose if necessary after the first 2 or 3 weeks of therapy, then q 3 to 6 months p.r.n. Rotate application sites weekly, with an interval of at least 1 week between particular sites used. Adjust dosage p.r.n.

➤ **Postmenopausal urogenital symptoms**

*Women:* One ring inserted into the upper third of the vagina. Ring is kept in place for 3 months.

➤ **Atrophic vaginitis, kraurosis vulvae**

*Women:* 0.05 mg/24 hours Estraderm applied twice weekly in a cyclic regimen. Or, 0.05 mg/24 hours Climara applied weekly in a cyclic regimen. Or, 2 to 4 g intravaginal applications of cream daily for 1 to 2 weeks. When vaginal mucosa is restored, maintenance dose is 1 g one to three times weekly in a cyclic regimen. If using Vagifem for atrophic vaginitis, give 1 tablet vaginally once daily for 2 weeks. Maintenance dose is 1 tablet inserted vaginally twice weekly. Or, 10 to 20 mg valerate I.M. q 4 weeks, p.r.n. Or, 1 to 5 mg estradiol cypionate I.M. once q 3 to 4 weeks.

➤ **Palliative treatment of advanced, inoperable breast cancer**

*Men and postmenopausal women:* 10 mg P.O. estradiol t.i.d. for 3 months.

➤ **Palliative treatment of advanced, inoperable prostate cancer**

*Men:* 30 mg valerate I.M. q 1 to 2 weeks, or 1 to 2 mg P.O. estradiol t.i.d.

➤ **To prevent postmenopausal osteoporosis**

*Women:* Place a 6.5-cm² (0.025 mg/day) Climara patch once weekly on clean, dry skin of lower abdomen or upper quadrant of buttock; press firmly in place for about 10 seconds; ensure complete contact, especially around edges. Or, 0.025-mg/day Vivelle, Vivelle-Dot, or Alora system applied to a clean, dry area of the trunk twice weekly.

## ACTION

Increases synthesis of DNA, RNA, and protein in responsive tissues. Also reduces release of follicle-stimulating and luteinizing hormones from the pituitary gland.

| Route | Onset | Peak | Duration |
|---|---|---|---|
| P.O., I.M., intravaginal | Unknown | Unknown | Unknown |
| Transdermal (Esclim) | Unknown | 27-30 hr | Unknown |

## ADVERSE REACTIONS

**CNS:** *increased risk of CVA,* headache, dizziness, chorea, depression, *seizures;* insomnia (Vagifem).

**CV:** thrombophlebitis, *thromboembolism,* hypertension, *edema, pulmonary embolism, MI.*

**EENT:** worsening myopia or astigmatism, intolerance of contact lenses; sinusitis (Vagifem).

**GI:** *nausea,* vomiting, abdominal cramps, bloating, increased appetite, *pancreatitis,* anorexia, gallbladder disease, dyspepsia (Vagifem).

**GU:** breakthrough bleeding, altered menstrual flow, dysmenorrhea, amenorrhea, *increased risk of endometrial cancer,* cervical erosion, altered cervical secretions, enlargement of uterine fibromas, vaginal candidiasis in women; testicular atrophy, impotence in men; genital pruritus, hematuria, vaginal discomfort, vaginitis (Vagifem).

**Hepatic:** cholestatic jaundice, *hepatic adenoma.*

**Metabolic:** weight changes.

**Respiratory:** upper respiratory tract infection, allergy, bronchitis (Vagifem).

**Skin:** melasma, urticaria, erythema nodosum, dermatitis, hair loss.

**Other:** gynecomastia; *increased risk of breast cancer;* hot flashes, pain (Vagifem), *breast tenderness, enlargement, or secretion.*

## INTERACTIONS

**Drug-drug.** *Carbamazepine, fosphenytoin, phenobarbital, phenytoin, rifampin:* May decrease effectiveness of estrogen therapy. Monitor patient closely.

*Corticosteroids:* May enhance effects of corticosteroids. Monitor patient closely.

*Cyclosporine:* May increase risk of toxicity. Use together with caution and monitor cyclosporine level frequently.

*Dantrolene, other hepatotoxic drugs:* May increase risk of hepatotoxicity. Monitor liver function closely.

*Oral anticoagulants:* May decrease anticoagulant effect. Dosage adjustments may be needed. Monitor PT and INR.

*Tamoxifen:* May interfere with tamoxifen effectiveness. Avoid using together.

**Drug-herb.** *Black cohosh:* May increase estrogen adverse effects. Discourage use together.

*Saw palmetto:* May have antiestrogenic effects. Discourage use together.

*St. John's wort:* May decrease effects of estrogens. Discourage use together.

**Drug-food.** *Caffeine:* May increase caffeine level. Advise patient to avoid or minimize use of caffeine.

*Grapefruit juice:* May elevate estrogen level. Tell patient to take drug with liquid other than grapefruit juice.

**Drug-lifestyle.** *Smoking:* May increase risk of adverse CV effects. If smoking continues, may need alternative therapy.

### EFFECTS ON LAB TEST RESULTS
● May increase clotting factor VII, VIII, IX, and X, total $T_4$, thyroid-binding globulin, and triglyceride levels.
● May increase PT and norepinephrine-induced platelet aggregation.
● May decrease metyrapone test results.

### CONTRAINDICATIONS & CAUTIONS
● Contraindicated in pregnant patients and patients with thrombophlebitis or thromboembolic disorders, estrogen-dependent neoplasia, breast or reproductive organ cancer (except for palliative treatment), undiagnosed abnormal genital bleeding, or history of thrombophlebitis or thromboembolic disorders linked to previous estrogen use (except for palliative treatment of breast and prostate cancer).
● Use cautiously in patients with cerebrovascular or coronary artery disease, asthma, bone disease, migraine, seizures, or cardiac, hepatic, or renal dysfunction. Also, use cautiously in women with strong family history of breast cancer or who have breast nodules, fibrocystic breasts, or abnormal mammograms.

### NURSING CONSIDERATIONS
● Ensure that patient has physical examination before starting therapy. Patients receiving long-term therapy should have yearly examinations. Monitor lipid levels, blood pressure, body weight, and hepatic function.
● Ask patient about allergies, especially to foods and plants. Estradiol is available as an aqueous solution or as a solution in peanut oil; estradiol cypionate, as a solution in cottonseed oil; estradiol valerate, as a solution in castor oil or sesame oil.
● To give I.M. injection, make sure drug is well dispersed by rolling vial between palms. Inject deeply into large muscle. Rotate injection sites to prevent muscle atrophy. Never give drug I.V.
● Apply transdermal patch to clean, dry, hairless, intact skin on abdomen or buttock. Don't apply it to breasts, waistline, or other areas where clothing can loosen patch. When applying, ensure thorough contact between patch and skin, especially around edges, and hold in place for about 10 seconds. Apply patch immediately after opening and removing protective cover. Rotate application sites.
● In women also taking oral estrogen, treatment with the Estraderm transdermal patch can begin 1 week after withdrawal of oral therapy, or sooner if menopausal symptoms appear before the end of the week.
● Transdermal systems are sometimes used on a continuous basis (not cyclic). Other alternatives are 1 to 5 mg (cypionate) I.M. q 3 to 4 weeks; or 10 to 20 mg (valerate) I.M. q 4 weeks, p.r.n.
● Instruct patients using Vagifem who have severely atrophic vaginal mucosa to exercise care when inserting the applicator. After gynecologic surgery, tell patient to use any vaginal applicator with caution and only if clearly indicated.
● The prescriber should assess the patient's need to continue Vagifem therapy. Make attempts to stop or taper at 3- to 6-month intervals.
● Because of risk of thromboembolism, stop therapy at least 1 month before high-risk procedures or those that cause prolonged immobilization, such as knee or hip surgery.

---

• Glucose tolerance may be impaired. Monitor glucose level closely in patients with diabetes.
• Notify pathologist about estrogen therapy when sending specimens to laboratory for evaluation.
• Estrace may contain tartrazine.

**PATIENT TEACHING**
• Tell patient to read package insert describing estrogen's adverse effects and give verbal explanation.
• Emphasize importance of regular physical examinations. Postmenopausal women who use estrogen replacement for longer than 5 years may be at increased risk for endometrial cancer. Risk is reduced by using cyclic rather than continuous therapy and the lowest possible dosages of estrogen. Adding progestins to the regimen decreases risk of endometrial hyperplasia; however, it isn't known whether progestins affect risk of endometrial cancer. No increased risk of breast cancer has been reported.
• Teach patient how to use cream. Patient should wash vaginal area with soap and water before applying and insert cream high into the vagina (about two-thirds the length of the applicator). Patient should take drug at bedtime, or lie flat for 30 minutes after instillation to minimize drug loss.
• Tell patient to use transdermal system correctly, to rotate sites, to avoid breasts and waistline, and to reapply patch if it falls off.
• Tell patient to insert Vagifem by the applicator as far into vagina as it can comfortably go, without using force.
• **Alert:** Warn patient to immediately report abdominal pain; pressure or pain in chest, shortness of breath, severe headaches, visual disturbances, vaginal bleeding or discharge, breast lumps, swelling of hands or feet, yellow skin or sclera, dark urine, light-colored stools, and pain, numbness, or stiffness in legs or buttocks.
• Explain to patient on cyclic therapy for postmenopausal symptoms that withdrawal bleeding may occur during week off drug. Tell her to report unusual vaginal bleeding.

• Tell diabetic patient to report elevated glucose level so that antidiabetic dosage can be adjusted.
• Teach woman how to perform routine breast self-examination.
• Teach patient methods to decrease risk of blood clots.
• Advise woman not to become pregnant during estrogen therapy.
• Advise woman of childbearing age to consult prescriber before taking drug and to advise prescriber immediately if she becomes pregnant.
• Encourage patient to stop or reduce smoking because of the risk of CV complications.

## estradiol and norethindrone acetate transdermal system
CombiPatch

*Pregnancy risk category X*

**AVAILABLE FORMS**
*Transdermal:* 9-cm$^2$ system releasing 0.05 mg estradiol and 0.14 mg norethindrone acetate per day; 16-cm$^2$ system releasing 0.05 mg estradiol and 0.25 mg norethindrone acetate per day

**INDICATIONS & DOSAGES**
➤ **Moderate to severe vasomotor symptoms from menopause; vulvar and vaginal atrophy; hypoestrogenemia from hypogonadism, castration, or primary ovarian failure in women with intact uterus**
*Continuous combined regimen*
*Women:* 9-cm$^2$ patch worn continuously on lower abdomen. Remove old system removed and apply new system twice weekly during a 28-day cycle. May increase to 16-cm$^2$ patch.
*Continuous sequential regimen*
*Women:* Patch can be applied as a sequential regimen with an estradiol transdermal system (such as Alora, Esclim, Estraderm, Vivelle). A 0.05-mg estradiol transdermal patch is worn for first 14 days of a 28-day cycle; replace system twice weekly. For rest of 28-day cycle, patient should wear 9-cm$^2$ patch system on lower abdomen. May increase to 16-cm$^2$ patch, p.r.n.

## ACTION

A matrix transdermal system in which estradiol and norethindrone are released continuously. Estrogen replacement therapy can reduce frequency of menopausal symptoms and release of follicle-stimulating and luteinizing hormones from the pituitary gland in postmenopausal women.

| Route | Onset | Peak | Duration |
|---|---|---|---|
| Transdermal | 12-24 hr | Unknown | 3-4 days |

## ADVERSE REACTIONS

**CNS:** *asthenia, **increased risk of CVA,*** depression, insomnia, nervousness, dizziness, *headache.*
**CV:** ***thromboembolism,*** thrombophlebitis, hypertension, *edema,* ***pulmonary embolism, MI.***
**EENT:** pharyngitis, *rhinitis, sinusitis.*
**GI:** *abdominal pain, diarrhea,* dyspepsia, flatulence, *nausea,* constipation.
**GU:** *dysmenorrhea, leukorrhea, menstrual disorder,* suspicious Papanicolaou smears, *vaginitis,* menorrhagia, vaginal hemorrhage.
**Musculoskeletal:** arthralgia, *back pain.*
**Respiratory:** *respiratory disorder,* bronchitis.
**Skin:** application site reactions, acne.
**Other:** *accidental injury, flulike syndrome, pain, breast pain,* tooth disorder, peripheral edema, breast enlargement, infection.

## INTERACTIONS

**Drug-drug.** *Carbamazepine, fosphenytoin, phenobarbital, phenytoin, rifampin:* May decrease estrogen therapy effectiveness. Monitor patient closely.
*Corticosteroids:* May enhance effects of corticosteroids. Monitor patient closely.
*Cyclosporine:* May increase risk of toxicity. Use together with caution, and monitor cyclosporine level frequently.
*Dantrolene, hepatotoxic drugs:* May increase risk of hepatotoxicity. Monitor liver function closely.
*Oral anticoagulants:* May decrease effect of anticoagulant. May need to adjust dose. Monitor PT and INR.
*Tamoxifen:* May interfere with tamoxifen effectiveness. Avoid using together.

**Drug-herb.** *Black cohosh:* May increase adverse effects of estrogens. Discourage use together.
*Saw palmetto:* May cause antiestrogenic effects. Discourage use together.
*St. John's wort:* May decrease effects of estrogens. Discourage use together.
**Drug-food.** *Caffeine:* May increase caffeine level. Advise patient to avoid caffeine.
*Grapefruit juice:* May elevate estrogen level. Advise patient to take with liquid other than grapefruit juice.
**Drug-lifestyle.** *Smoking:* May increase risk of adverse CV effects. If smoking continues, may need alternative therapy.

## EFFECTS ON LAB TEST RESULTS

● May increase $T_3$ and $T_4$ levels. May decrease total cholesterol, HDL cholesterol, LDL cholesterol, and triglyceride levels.
● May increase platelet count and fibrinogen activity. May decrease $T_3$ resin uptake. May alter INR, activated PTT, and platelet aggregation times.
● May reduce metyrapone test values. May alter glucose tolerance test results.

## CONTRAINDICATIONS & CAUTIONS

● Contraindicated in women hypersensitive to estrogen, progestin, or any component of the patch; in pregnant patients; and in patients with known or suspected breast cancer, known or suspected estrogen-dependent neoplasia, undiagnosed abnormal genital bleeding, active thrombophlebitis, thromboembolic disorders, or CVA.
● Use cautiously in breast-feeding patients and in patients with impaired liver function, asthma, epilepsy, migraine, or cardiac or renal dysfunction.

## NURSING CONSIDERATIONS

● Women not receiving continuous estrogen or combined estrogen and progestin therapy may start therapy at any time.
● Women receiving continuous hormone replacement therapy should complete the current cycle before starting therapy. Women commonly have withdrawal bleeding at completion of cycle; first day of withdrawal bleeding is appropriate time to start therapy.

---

• Store norethindrone patches in refrigerator before dispensing. Patient may then store patches at room temperature for up to 3 months.

• Reevaluate therapy at 3- to 6-month intervals.

• A combined estrogen and progestin regimen is indicated for a woman with an intact uterus. Progestins taken with estrogen significantly reduce, but don't eliminate, risk of endometrial cancer linked to use of estrogen alone.

• Blood pressure increases have been linked to estrogen use. Monitor patient's blood pressure regularly.

• Treatment of postmenopausal symptoms usually starts during menopausal stage when vasomotor symptoms occur.

• Apply patch system to a smooth (fold-free), clean, dry, nonirritated area of skin on lower abdomen, avoiding the waistline. Rotate application sites, with an interval of at least 1 week between applications to same site.

• Don't apply patch on or near breasts.

• Avoid applying to areas that may get prolonged sun exposure.

• Reapply patch, if needed, to another area of lower abdomen. If patch fails to adhere, replace with a new one.

• Monitor glucose level closely in patients with diabetes.

• **Alert:** Don't interchange CombiPatch with other estrogen patches. Verify therapy before application.

## PATIENT TEACHING
• Teach patient how to apply patch properly. She should wear only one patch at any time during the dosing intervals. Apply patch immediately after opening protective cover.

• Tell patient an oil-based cream or lotion may help remove adhesive from the skin once patch has been removed and the area allowed to dry for 15 minutes.

• Advise patient not to use patch if she's pregnant or plans to become pregnant.

• Urge woman of childbearing age to consult prescriber before applying patch and to advise prescriber immediately if she becomes pregnant.

• Instruct patient that the continuous combined regimen may lead to irregular bleeding, particularly in the first 6 months, but

that it usually decreases with time, and often stops completely.

• Tell patient that, for the continuous sequential regimen, monthly withdrawal bleeding is common.

• Advise patient to alert prescriber and remove patch at first sign of clotting disorders (thrombophlebitis, cerebrovascular disorders, and pulmonary embolism).

• Instruct patient to stop using patch and call prescriber about any loss of vision, sudden onset of protrusion of the eyeball (proptosis), double vision, or migraine.

• Encourage patient to stop or reduce smoking because of the risk of CV complications.

• Advise patient not to store patches where extreme temperatures can occur.

---

# estrogens, conjugated (estrogenic substances, conjugated; oestrogens, conjugated)
C.E.S.†, Cenestin, Premarin✐, Premarin Intravenous

*Pregnancy risk category X*

## AVAILABLE FORMS
*Injection:* 25 mg/5 ml
*Tablets:* 0.3 mg, 0.45 mg, 0.625 mg, 0.9 mg, 1.25 mg, 2.5 mg
*Vaginal cream:* 0.625 mg/g

## INDICATIONS & DOSAGES
➤ **Abnormal uterine bleeding (hormonal imbalance)**
*Adults:* 25 mg I.V. or I.M. Repeat dose in 6 to 12 hours, if necessary.
➤ **Vulvar or vaginal atrophy**
*Adults:* 0.5 to 2 g cream intravaginally once daily in cycles of 3 weeks on, 1 week off.
➤ **Castration and primary ovarian failure**
*Adults:* Initially, 1.25 mg P.O. daily in cycles of 3 weeks on, 1 week off. Adjust dose p.r.n.
➤ **Female hypogonadism**
*Adults:* 0.3 to 0.625 mg P.O. daily, given cyclically 3 weeks on, 1 week off.

➤ **Moderate to severe vasomotor symptoms with or without moderate to severe symptoms of vulvar and vaginal atrophy associated with menopause**
*Adults:* 0.3 mg P.O. daily, or cyclically 25 days on, 5 days off.

➤ **To prevent osteoporosis**
*Adults:* 0.3 to 0.625 mg P.O. daily, or cyclically, 25 days on, 5 days off.

➤ **Palliative treatment of inoperable prostatic cancer**
*Adults:* 1.25 to 2.5 mg P.O. t.i.d.

➤ **Palliative treatment of breast cancer**
*Adults:* 10 mg P.O. t.i.d. for 3 months or more.

## I.V. ADMINISTRATION

● Refrigerate before reconstituting. Reconstitute only with diluent provided. Agitate gently after adding diluent. Drug is compatible with normal saline, dextrose, or invert sugar solutions. I.V. solution isn't compatible with protein hydrolysate, ascorbic acid, or solutions with an acid pH.

● Use reconstituted solution within a few hours. Don't use parenteral preparations if darkening or precipitation is noted.

● When giving drug by direct I.V. injection, give slowly to avoid flushing reaction.

## ACTION

Increases synthesis of DNA, RNA, and protein in responsive tissues. Also reduces release of follicle-stimulating and luteinizing hormones from the pituitary gland.

| Route | Onset | Peak | Duration |
|---|---|---|---|
| P.O., I.V., I.M., intra-vaginal | Unknown | Unknown | Unknown |

## ADVERSE REACTIONS

**CNS:** headache, dizziness, chorea, depression, *increased risk of CVA, seizures.*
**CV:** flushing with rapid I.V. administration; thrombophlebitis; *thromboembolism;* hypertension; *edema; pulmonary embolism, MI.*
**EENT:** worsening myopia or astigmatism, intolerance of contact lenses.
**GI:** *nausea,* vomiting, abdominal cramps, bloating, anorexia, increased appetite, *pancreatitis,* gallbladder disease.

**GU:** breakthrough bleeding, altered menstrual flow, dysmenorrhea, amenorrhea, *increased risk of endometrial cancer,* cervical erosion, altered cervical secretions, enlargement of uterine fibromas, vaginal candidiasis, testicular atrophy, impotence.
**Hepatic:** cholestatic jaundice, *hepatic adenoma.*
**Metabolic:** weight changes.
**Skin:** melasma, urticaria, hirsutism or hair loss, erythema nodosum, dermatitis.
**Other:** *breast tenderness, enlargement, or secretion; gynecomastia; increased risk of breast cancer.*

## INTERACTIONS

**Drug-drug.** *Carbamazepine, fosphenytoin, phenobarbital, phenytoin, rifampin:* May decrease effectiveness of estrogen therapy. Monitor patient closely.
*Corticosteroids:* May enhance corticosteroid effects. Monitor patient closely.
*Cyclosporine:* May increase risk of toxicity. Use together with caution, and monitor cyclosporine level frequently.
*Dantrolene, other hepatotoxic drugs:* May increase risk of hepatotoxicity. Monitor liver function closely.
*Oral anticoagulants:* May decrease anticoagulant effects. May need to adjust dosage. Monitor PT and INR.
*Tamoxifen:* May interfere with tamoxifen effectiveness. Avoid using together.
**Drug-herb.** *Black cohosh:* May increase adverse effects of estrogens. Discourage use together.
*Red clover:* May interfere with hormonal therapies. Discourage use together.
*Saw palmetto:* May have antiestrogenic effects. Discourage use together.
*St. John's wort:* May decrease effects of estrogens. Discourage use together.
**Drug-food.** *Caffeine:* May increase caffeine level. Advise caution.
**Drug-lifestyle.** *Smoking:* May increase risk of adverse CV effects. If smoking continues, may need alternative therapy.

## EFFECTS ON LAB TEST RESULTS

● May increase clotting factor VII, VIII, IX, and X, total $T_4$, thyroid-binding globulin, phospholipid, and triglyceride levels.
● May increase PT and norepinephrine-induced platelet aggregation.
● May decrease metyrapone test results.

Reactions may be *common,* uncommon, *life-threatening,* or COMMON AND LIFE-THREATENING.

## CONTRAINDICATIONS & CAUTIONS

• Contraindicated in pregnant patients and in patients with thrombophlebitis, thromboembolic disorders, estrogen-dependent neoplasia, breast or reproductive cancer (except for palliative treatment), or undiagnosed abnormal genital bleeding.

• Use cautiously in patients with cerebrovascular or coronary artery disease, asthma, bone disease, migraine, seizures, or cardiac, hepatic, or renal dysfunction. Also, use cautiously in women with family history (mother, grandmother, sister) of breast or genital tract cancer or who have breast nodules, fibrocystic breasts, or abnormal mammogram findings.

## NURSING CONSIDERATIONS

• Make sure patient has thorough physical examination before starting estrogen therapy. Patients receiving long-term therapy should have annual examinations. Periodically monitor lipid levels, blood pressure, body weight, and hepatic function.

• Rapid treatment of dysfunctional uterine bleeding or reduction of surgical bleeding usually demands delivery by I.V. or I.M. route.

• *Alert:* Estrogens and progestins shouldn't be used to prevent CV disease. The Women's Health Initiative (WHI) study reported increased risks of MI, stroke, invasive breast cancer, pulmonary emboli, and deep vein thrombosis in postmenopausal women during 5 years of combination therapy. Because of these risks, estrogens and progestins should be prescribed at the lowest effective doses and for the shortest duration consistent with treatment goals and risks for the individual woman.

• *Alert:* Postmenopausal women who use estrogen replacement for longer than 5 years to treat menopausal symptoms may be at increased risk for endometrial cancer. This risk is reduced by using cyclic rather than continuous therapy and lowest possible estrogen dosage. Adding progestins to the regimen decreases risk of endometrial hyperplasia; however, it isn't known whether progestins affect risk of endometrial cancer.

• When giving by I.M. injection, inject deeply into large muscle. Rotate injection sites to prevent muscle atrophy.

• Notify pathologist about estrogen therapy when sending specimens to laboratory for evaluation.

• Because of thromboembolism risk, stop therapy at least 1 month before procedures that prolong immobilization or raise the risk of thromboembolism, such as knee or hip surgery.

• Glucose tolerance may be impaired. Monitor glucose level closely in patients with diabetes.

• *Alert:* Don't confuse Premarin with Primaxin.

## PATIENT TEACHING

• Tell patient to read package insert describing estrogen's adverse effects and explain effects verbally.

• Emphasize importance of regular physical examinations.

• Teach patient how to use vaginal cream. Patient should wash the vaginal area with soap and water before applying and insert cream high into the vagina (about two-thirds the length of the applicator). Tell her to use drug at bedtime or to lie flat for 30 minutes after instillation to minimize drug loss.

• Explain to patient that cyclic therapy for postmenopausal symptoms may cause withdrawal bleeding during week off drug. Tell her to report unusual vaginal bleeding.

• *Alert:* Warn patient to immediately report abdominal pain; pain, numbness, or stiffness in legs or buttocks; pressure or pain in chest; shortness of breath; severe headaches; visual disturbances, such as blind spots, flashing lights, or blurriness; vaginal bleeding or discharge; breast lumps; swelling of hands or feet; yellow skin or sclera; dark urine; and light-colored stools.

• Tell diabetic patient to report elevated glucose level so that antidiabetic dosage can be adjusted.

• Teach woman how to perform routine breast self-examination.

• Advise patient not to become pregnant during estrogen therapy.

• Advise woman of childbearing age to consult prescriber before taking drug and to advise prescriber immediately if she becomes pregnant.

---

• Encourage patient to stop smoking or reduce number of cigarettes smoked because of the risk of CV complications.

---

# estropipate (piperazine estrone sulfate)
Ogen, Ortho-Est

*Pregnancy risk category X*

---

## AVAILABLE FORMS
*Tablets:* 0.75 mg, 1.5 mg, 3 mg, 6 mg
*Vaginal cream:* 1.5 mg/g

## INDICATIONS & DOSAGES
➤ **Vulvar and vaginal atrophy**
*Women:* 0.75 to 6 mg P.O. daily, 3 weeks on and 1 week off; or 2 to 4 g vaginal cream daily. Typically, drug is given on a cyclic, short-term basis. Can be given continuously.
➤ **Primary ovarian failure, female castration, female hypogonadism**
*Women:* 1.5 to 9 mg P.O. daily for first 3 weeks; then a rest period of 8 to 10 days. If bleeding doesn't occur by end of rest period, cycle is repeated. Can be given continuously.
➤ **Vasomotor menopausal symptoms**
*Women:* 0.75 to 6 mg P.O. daily in cyclic method, 3 weeks on and 1 week off. Can be given continuously.
➤ **To prevent osteoporosis**
*Women:* 0.75 mg P.O. daily for 25 days of a 31-day cycle.

## ACTION
Increases synthesis of DNA, RNA, and proteins in responsive tissues. Also reduces release of follicle-stimulating and luteinizing hormones from the pituitary gland.

| Route | Onset | Peak | Duration |
|---|---|---|---|
| P.O., intravaginal | Unknown | Unknown | Unknown |

## ADVERSE REACTIONS
**CNS:** depression, headache, dizziness, migraine, *seizures, increased risk of CVA.*
**CV:** *edema;* thrombophlebitis, *increased risk of pulmonary embolism and MI, thromboembolism.*
**GI:** nausea, vomiting, gallbladder disease, abdominal cramps, bloating.
**GU:** increased size of uterine fibromas, *increased risk of endometrial cancer,* vaginal candidiasis, cystitis-like syndrome, dysmenorrhea, amenorrhea, breakthrough bleeding, condition resembling premenstrual syndrome.
**Hepatic:** cholestatic jaundice, *hepatic adenoma.*
**Metabolic:** weight changes.
**Skin:** hemorrhagic eruption, erythema nodosum, *erythema multiforme,* hirsutism or hair loss, melasma.
**Other:** breast engorgement or enlargement; *possible increased risk of breast cancer.*

## INTERACTIONS
**Drug-drug.** *Carbamazepine, fosphenytoin, phenobarbital, phenytoin, rifampin:* May decrease effectiveness of estrogen therapy. Monitor patient closely.
*Corticosteroids:* May enhance effects of corticosteroids. Monitor patient closely.
*Cyclosporine:* May increase risk of toxicity. Use together with caution and frequently monitor cyclosporine level.
*Dantrolene, other hepatotoxic drugs:* May increase risk of hepatotoxicity. Monitor liver function closely.
*Oral anticoagulants:* May decrease effect of anticoagulant. Dosage adjustments may be needed. Monitor PT and INR.
*Tamoxifen:* May interfere with tamoxifen effectiveness. Avoid using together.
**Drug-herb.** *Black cohosh:* May increase adverse effects of estrogens. Discourage use together.
*Red clover:* May interfere with hormonal therapies. Discourage use together.
*Saw palmetto:* May have antiestrogenic effects. Discourage use together.
*St. John's wort:* May decrease effects of estrogens. Discourage use together.
**Drug-food.** *Caffeine:* May increase caffeine level. Advise caution.
**Drug-lifestyle.** *Smoking:* May increase risk of adverse CV effects. If smoking continues, may need alternative therapy.

## EFFECTS ON LAB TEST RESULTS
• May increase clotting factor VII, VIII, IX, and X, total $T_4$, thyroid-binding globulin, phospholipid, and triglyceride levels.

---

Reactions may be *common*, uncommon, *life-threatening*, or COMMON AND LIFE-THREATENING.

• May increase PT and norepinephrine-induced platelet aggregation.
• May reduce metyrapone test results.

## CONTRAINDICATIONS & CAUTIONS
• Contraindicated in pregnant patients and those with active thrombophlebitis, thromboembolic disorders, estrogen-dependent neoplasia, undiagnosed genital bleeding, and breast, reproductive organ, or genital cancer.
• Use cautiously in patients with cerebrovascular or coronary artery disease, asthma, mental depression, bone disease, migraine, seizures, or cardiac, hepatic, or renal dysfunction. Also, use cautiously in women with family history (mother, grandmother, sister) of breast or genital tract cancer or who have breast nodules, fibrocystic breasts, or abnormal mammogram findings.

## NURSING CONSIDERATIONS
• Make sure patient has thorough physical examination before starting estrogen therapy. Patients receiving long-term therapy should have examinations yearly. Periodically monitor lipid levels, blood pressure, body weight, and hepatic function.
• *Alert:* Estrogens and progestins shouldn't be used to prevent CV disease. The Women's Health Initiative (WHI) study reported increased risks of MI, stroke, invasive breast cancer, pulmonary emboli, and deep vein thrombosis in postmenopausal women during 5 years of combination therapy. Because of these risks, estrogens and progestins should be prescribed at the lowest effective doses and for the shortest duration consistent with treatment goals and risks for the individual woman.
• When used to treat hypogonadism, duration of therapy needed to produce withdrawal bleeding depends on patient's endometrial response to drug. If satisfactory withdrawal bleeding doesn't occur, an oral progestin is added to the regimen. Explain to patient that, despite return of withdrawal bleeding, pregnancy can't occur because she doesn't ovulate.
• Estropipate/estrone equivalents are:
0.75 mg estropipate = 0.625 mg estrone
1.5 mg estropipate = 1.25 mg estrone
3 mg estropipate = 2.5 mg estrone
6 mg estropipate = 5 mg estrone.

• May give with meals to minimize GI upset.
• Because of risk of thromboembolism, stop therapy at least 1 month before procedures that prolong immobilization or raise the risk of thromboembolism, such as knee or hip surgery.
• Glucose tolerance may be impaired. Monitor glucose level closely in patients with diabetes.

## PATIENT TEACHING
• Tell patient to read package insert describing estrogen's adverse effects; also explain effects verbally.
• Teach patient how to use vaginal cream. Patient should wash the vaginal area with soap and water and then insert vaginal cream high into the vagina (about two-thirds the length of the applicator). Tell her to use drug at bedtime or to lie flat for 30 minutes after application to minimize drug loss.
• Tell diabetic patient to report elevated glucose level to prescriber.
• Stress importance of regular physical examinations. Postmenopausal women who use estrogen replacement for longer than 5 years may have increased risk of endometrial cancer. Using cyclic therapy and lowest possible estrogen dosage reduces risk. Adding progestins to regimen decreases risk of endometrial hyperplasia; however, it isn't known whether progestins affect risk of endometrial cancer.
• *Alert:* Warn patient to immediately report abdominal pain; pain, stiffness, or numbness in legs or buttocks; pressure or pain in chest; shortness of breath; severe headaches; visual disturbances, such as blind spots or flashing lights; vaginal bleeding or discharge; breast lumps; swelling of hands or feet; yellow skin or sclera; dark urine; and light-colored stools.
• Teach woman how to perform routine breast self-examination.
• Advise patient not to become pregnant while on estrogen therapy.
• Encourage patient to stop or reduce smoking because of the risk of CV complications.
• Advise woman of childbearing age to consult prescriber before taking drug and

to tell prescriber immediately if she becomes pregnant.

---

# ethinyl estradiol (ethinyloestradiol)
Estinyl

*Pregnancy risk category X*

---

## AVAILABLE FORMS
*Tablets:* 0.02 mg, 0.05 mg, 0.5 mg

## INDICATIONS & DOSAGES
➤ **Palliative treatment of metastatic breast cancer (at least 5 years after menopause)**
*Women:* 1 mg P.O. t.i.d. for at least 3 months.
➤ **Female hypogonadism**
*Women:* 0.05 mg P.O. once daily to t.i.d. 2 weeks per month; then 2 weeks of progesterone therapy. Continued for 3 to 6 monthly dosing cycles; then 2 months off. Can be given continuously.
➤ **Vasomotor menopausal symptoms**
*Women:* 0.02 to 0.05 mg P.O. daily for cycles of 3 weeks on and 1 week off. Can be given continuously.
➤ **Palliative treatment of metastatic inoperable prostate cancer**
*Men:* 0.15 to 2 mg P.O. daily.

## ACTION
Increases synthesis of DNA, RNA, and protein in responsive tissues. Also reduces release of follicle-stimulating and luteinizing hormones from the pituitary gland.

| Route | Onset | Peak | Duration |
|-------|-------|------|----------|
| P.O. | Unknown | Unknown | Unknown |

## ADVERSE REACTIONS
**CNS:** *increased risk of CVA,* headache, dizziness, chorea, depression, *seizures.*
**CV:** thrombophlebitis, *thromboembolism,* hypertension, *edema, pulmonary embolism, MI.*
**EENT:** worsening myopia or astigmatism, intolerance to contact lenses.
**GI:** *nausea,* vomiting, gallbladder, abdominal cramps, bloating, anorexia, increased appetite.

**GU:** breakthrough bleeding, altered menstrual flow, dysmenorrhea, amenorrhea, cervical erosion, *increased risk of endometrial cancer,* altered cervical secretions, enlargement of uterine fibromas, vaginal candidiasis; testicular atrophy, impotence in men.
**Hepatic:** cholestatic jaundice, *hepatic adenoma.*
**Metabolic:** weight changes.
**Skin:** melasma, urticaria, acne, seborrhea, oily skin, hirsutism or hair loss, erythema nodosum, dermatitis.
**Other:** *breast tenderness, enlargement, or secretion; increased risk of breast cancer;* gynecomastia.

## INTERACTIONS
**Drug-drug.** *Carbamazepine, fosphenytoin, phenobarbital, phenytoin, rifampin:* May decrease effectiveness of estrogen therapy. Monitor patient closely.
*Corticosteroids:* May enhance effects of corticosteroids. Monitor patient closely.
*Cyclosporine:* May increase risk of toxicity. Use together cautiously, and monitor cyclosporine level frequently.
*Dantrolene, other hepatotoxic drugs:* May increase risk of hepatotoxicity. Monitor liver function closely.
*Oral anticoagulants:* May decrease effects of anticoagulant. Dosage adjustments may be needed. Monitor PT and INR.
*Tamoxifen:* May interfere with tamoxifen effectiveness. Avoid using together.
**Drug-herb.** *Black cohosh:* May increase adverse effects of estrogens. Discourage use together.
*Saw palmetto:* May have antiestrogenic effects. Discourage use together.
*St. John's wort:* May decrease effects of estrogens. Discourage use together.
**Drug-food.** *Caffeine:* May increase caffeine level. Advise patient to avoid caffeine.
*Grapefruit juice:* May elevate estrogen level. Advise patient to take with liquid other than grapefruit juice.
**Drug-lifestyle.** *Smoking:* May increase risk of adverse CV effects. If smoking continues, may need alternative therapy.

---

Reactions may be **common**, uncommon, *life-threatening*, or COMMON AND LIFE-THREATENING.

## EFFECTS ON LAB TEST RESULTS
• May increase clotting factor VII, VIII, IX, and X, total $T_4$, thyroid-binding globulin, phospholipid, and triglyceride levels.
• May increase PT and norepinephrine-induced platelet aggregation. May decrease antithrombin III activity.
• May reduce metyrapone test results.

## CONTRAINDICATIONS & CAUTIONS
• Contraindicated in pregnant patients and in those with thrombophlebitis, thromboembolic disorders, estrogen-dependent neoplasia, breast or reproductive organ cancer (except for palliative treatment), or undiagnosed abnormal genital bleeding.
• Use cautiously in patients with cerebrovascular or coronary artery disease, asthma, depression, bone disease, or cardiac, hepatic, or renal dysfunction.
• Use cautiously in women with family history (mother, grandmother, sister) of breast or genital tract cancer or who have breast nodules, fibrocystic breasts, or abnormal mammogram findings.

## NURSING CONSIDERATIONS
• Make sure patient has thorough physical examination before starting estrogen therapy. Patients receiving long-term therapy should have yearly examinations. Periodically monitor lipid levels, blood pressure, body weight, and hepatic function.
• Because of risk of thromboembolism, stop therapy at least 1 month before procedures that prolong immobilization or raise the risk of thromboembolism, such as knee or hip surgery.
• Notify pathologist about estrogen therapy when sending specimens to laboratory for evaluation.
• Glucose tolerance may be impaired. Monitor glucose level closely in patients with diabetes.
• Drug may contain tartrazine.

## PATIENT TEACHING
• Tell patient to read package insert describing estrogen's adverse effects; also, give verbal explanation.
• Emphasize importance of regular physical examinations. Postmenopausal women who use estrogen replacement for longer than 5 years to treat menopausal symptoms may be at increased risk for endometrial cancer. This risk is reduced by using cyclic rather than continuous therapy and the lowest possible dosages of estrogen. Adding progestins to the regimen decreases risk of endometrial hyperplasia; however, it isn't known whether progestins affect risk of endometrial cancer.
• Explain to patient that cyclic therapy for postmenopausal symptoms may cause withdrawal bleeding during week off drug. Tell her to report unusual vaginal bleeding.
• *Alert:* Warn patient to immediately report abdominal pain; pain, numbness, or stiffness in legs or buttocks; pressure or pain in chest; shortness of breath; severe headaches; visual disturbances such as blind spots, flashing lights, or blurriness; vaginal bleeding or discharge; breast lumps; swelling of hands or feet; yellow skin or sclera; dark urine; or light-colored stools.
• Tell diabetic patient to report elevated glucose level; antidiabetic dosage may be adjusted.
• Teach woman how to perform routine breast self-examination.
• Teach patient methods to decrease risk of thromboembolism.
• Encourage patient to stop or reduce smoking because of the risk of CV complications.

## ethinyl estradiol and desogestrel
*monophasic:* Apri, Desogen, Ortho-Cept

*biphasic:* Kariva, Mircette

*triphasic:* Cyclessa

## ethinyl estradiol and ethynodiol diacetate
*monophasic:* Demulen 1/35◆, Demulen 1/50◆, Zovia 1/35E, Zovia 1/50E

## ethinyl estradiol and levonorgestrel
*monophasic:* Alesse-21, Alesse-28, Aviane, Lessina, Levlen,

---

Levlite, Levora-21, Levora-28, Nordette-21, Nordette-28, Portia

*biphasic:* Preven Emergency Contraceptive Kit

*triphasic:* Enpresse, Tri-Levlen, Triphasil, Trivora-28

## ethinyl estradiol and norethindrone
*monophasic:* Brevicon, Genora 0.5/35, Genora 1/35, Junel 21-1/20, Junel 21-1.5/30, ModiCon, N.E.E. 1/35, Necon 1/35-21, Necon 1/35-28, Necon 0.5/35-21, Necon 0.5/35-28, Nelova 0.5/35E, Nelova 1/35E, Norethin 1/35E, Norinyl 1 + 35, Ortho-Novum 1/35, Ovcon-35◔, Ovcon-50

*biphasic:* Necon 10/11-21, Necon 10/11-28, Ortho-Novum 10/11

*triphasic:* Necon 7/7/7, Nortel 7/7/7, Ortho-Novum 7/7/7, Tri-Norinyl

## ethinyl estradiol and norethindrone acetate
*monophasic:* Junel 21-1/20, Junel 21-1.5/30, Loestrin 1/20, Loestrin 1.5/30

*triphasic:* Estrostep 21

## ethinyl estradiol and norgestimate
*monophasic:* MonoNessa, Ortho-Cyclen, Sprintec

*triphasic:* Ortho Tri-Cyclen, Ortho Tri-Cyclen Lo, Tri-Sprintec

## ethinyl estradiol and norgestrel
*monophasic:* Cryselle, Lo/Ovral, Lo-Ogestrel, Ogestrel, Ovral

## ethinyl estradiol, norethindrone acetate, and ferrous fumarate
*monophasic:* Loestrin Fe 1/20, Loestrin Fe 1.5/30, Microgesin Fe 1/20, Microgesin Fe 1.5/30

*triphasic:* Estrostep Fe

## mestranol and norethindrone
*monophasic:* Genora 1/50, Necon 1/50-21, Necon 1/50-28, Nelova 1/50M, Norethin 1/50M, Norinyl 1+50, Ortho-Novum 1/50

*Pregnancy risk category X*

**AVAILABLE FORMS**
**monophasic hormonal contraceptives**
*ethinyl estradiol and desogestrel*
*Tablets:* ethinyl estradiol 30 mcg and des-ogestrel 0.15 mg (Apri, Desogen, Ortho-Cept)
*ethinyl estradiol and ethynodiol diacetate*
*Tablets:* ethinyl estradiol 35 mcg and ethynodiol diacetate 1 mg (Demulen 1/35, Zovia 1/35E); ethinyl estradiol 50 mcg and ethynodiol diacetate 1 mg (Demulen 1/50, Zovia 1/50E)
*ethinyl estradiol and levonorgestrel*
*Tablets:* ethinyl estradiol 20 mcg and lev-onorgestrel 0.1 mg (Alesse-21, Alesse-28, Aviane, Lessina); ethinyl estradiol 30 mcg and levonorgestrel 0.15 mg (Levlen, Lev-lite, Levora, Nordette-21, Nordette-28, Portia)
*ethinyl estradiol and norethindrone*
*Tablets:* ethinyl estradiol 35 mcg and norethindrone 0.4 mg (Ovcon-35); ethinyl estradiol 35 mcg and norethindrone 0.5 mg (Brevicon, Genora 0.5/35, Modi-Con, Necon 0.5/35-21, Necon 0.5/35-28, Nelova 0.5/35E); ethinyl estradiol 35 mcg and norethindrone 1 mg (Genora 1/35, N.E.E. 1/35, Necon 1/35-21, Necon 1/35-28, Nelova 1/35E, Norethin 1/35E, Norinyl 1+35, Ortho-Novum 1/35); ethinyl estradiol 50 mcg and norethin-drone 1 mg (Ovcon-50)
*ethinyl estradiol and norethindrone ac-etate*
*Tablets:* ethinyl estradiol 20 mcg and norethindrone acetate 1 mg (Loestrin 1/20); ethinyl estradiol 30 mcg and norethindrone acetate 1.5 mg (Loestrin 1.5/30)
*ethinyl estradiol and norgestimate*
*Tablets:* ethinyl estradiol 35 mcg and norgestimate 0.25 mg (MonoNessa, Ortho-Cyclen, Sprintec)
*ethinyl estradiol and norgestrel*
*Tablets:* ethinyl estradiol 30 mcg and norgestrel 0.3 mg (Cryselle, Lo/Ovral,

Lo-Ogestrel); ethinyl estradiol 50 mcg and norgestrel 0.5 mg (Ogestrel, Ovral)

*ethinyl estradiol, norethindrone acetate, and ferrous fumarate*
*Tablets:* ethinyl estradiol 20 mcg, norethindrone acetate 1 mg, and ferrous fumarate 75 mg (Loestrin Fe 1/20, Microgesin Fe 1/20); ethinyl estradiol 30 mcg, norethindrone acetate 1.5 mg, and ferrous fumarate 75 mg (Loestrin Fe 1.5/30, Microgesin Fe 1.5/30)

*mestranol and norethindrone*
*Tablets:* mestranol 50 mcg and norethindrone 1 mg (Genora 1/50, Nelova 1/50M, Norethin 1/50M, Norinyl 1/50, Ortho-Novum 1/50)

**biphasic hormonal contraceptives**
*ethinyl estradiol and desogestrel*
*Tablets:* ethinyl estradiol 20 mcg and desogestrel 0.15 mg (21 days), then inert tablets (2 days), then ethinyl estradiol 10 mcg (5 days) (Kariva, Mircette)

*ethinyl estradiol and levonorgestrel*
*Tablets:* ethinyl estradiol 50 mcg and levonorgestrel 0.25 mg (Preven Emergency Contraceptive Kit)

*ethinyl estradiol and norethindrone*
*Tablets:* ethinyl estradiol 35 mcg and norethindrone 0.5 mg (10 days); ethinyl estradiol 35 mcg and norethindrone 1 mg (11 days) (Necon 10/11-21, Necon 10/11-28, Ortho-Novum 10/11)

**triphasic hormonal contraceptives**
*ethinyl estradiol and desogestrel*
*Tablets:* 0.1 mg desogestrel with 25 mcg ethinyl estradiol (7 tablets); 0.125 mg desogestrel with 25 mcg ethinyl estradiol (7 tablets); 0.15 mg desogestrel with 25 mcg ethinyl estradiol (7 tablets) (Cyclessa)

*ethinyl estradiol and levonorgestrel*
*Tablets:* ethinyl estradiol 30 mcg and levonorgestrel 0.05 mg (6 days); ethinyl estradiol 40 mcg and levonorgestrel 0.075 mg (5 days); ethinyl estradiol 30 mcg and levonorgestrel 0.125 mg (10 days) (Enpresse, Tri-Levlen, Triphasil, Trivora-28)

*ethinyl estradiol and norethindrone*
*Tablets:* ethinyl estradiol 35 mcg and norethindrone 0.5 mg (7 days); ethinyl estradiol 35 mcg and norethindrone 1 mg (9 days); ethinyl estradiol 35 mcg and norethindrone 0.5 mg (5 days) (Tri-Norinyl); ethinyl estradiol 35 mcg and norethindrone 0.5 mg (7 days); ethinyl estradiol 35 mcg and norethindrone 0.75 mg (7 days); ethinyl estradiol 35 mcg and norethindrone 1 mg (7 days) (Necon 7/7/7, Nortel 7/7/7, Ortho-Novum 7/7/7).

*ethinyl estradiol and norethindrone acetate*
*Tablets:* ethinyl estradiol 20 mcg and norethindrone acetate 1 mg (5 days); ethinyl estradiol 30 mcg and norethindrone acetate 1 mg (7 days); ethinyl estradiol 35 mcg and norethindrone acetate 1 mg (9 days) (Estrostep 21)

*ethinyl estradiol, norethindrone acetate, and ferrous fumarate*
*Tablets:* ethinyl estradiol 20 mcg and norethindrone acetate 1 mg (5 days); ethinyl estradiol 30 mcg and norethindrone acetate 1 mg (7 days); ethinyl estradiol 35 mcg and norethindrone acetate 1 mg (9 days); and 75-mg ferrous fumarate tablets (7 days) (Estrostep Fe)

*ethinyl estradiol and norgestimate*
*Tablets:* ethinyl estradiol 25 mcg and norgestimate 0.18 mg (7 days); ethinyl estradiol 25 mcg and norgestimate 0.215 mg (7 days); ethinyl estradiol 25 mcg and norgestimate 0.25 mg (7 days) (Ortho Tri-Cyclen Lo); ethinyl estradiol 35 mcg and norgestimate 0.18 mg (7 days); ethinyl estradiol 35 mcg and norgestimate 0.215 mg (7 days); ethinyl estradiol 35 mcg and norgestimate 0.25 mg (7 days) (Ortho Tri-Cyclen, Tri-Sprintec)

## INDICATIONS & DOSAGES
➤**Contraception**
*Monophasic hormonal contraceptives*
*Women:* 1 tablet P.O. daily beginning on the first day of menstrual cycle or the first Sunday after menstrual cycle begins. With 20- and 21-tablet package, new dosing cycle begins 7 days after last tablet taken. With 28-tablet package, dosage is 1 tablet daily without interruption; extra tablets taken on days 22 to 28 are placebos or contain iron.
*Biphasic hormonal contraceptives*
*Women:* 1 color tablet P.O. daily for 10 days; then next color tablet for 11 days. With 21-tablet packages, new dosing cycle begins 7 days after last tablet taken. With 28-tablet packages, dosage is 1 tablet daily without interruption.

*Triphasic hormonal contraceptives*
*Women:* 1 tablet P.O. daily in the sequence specified by the brand. With 21-tablet packages, new dosing cycle begins 7 days after last tablet taken. With 28-tablet packages, dosage is 1 tablet daily without interruption.

➤ **To prevent pregnancy after intercourse**
*Women:* For Preven Emergency Contraceptive Kit, 2 tablets P.O. within 72 hours of unprotected intercourse; take second dose 12 hours after the first dose.

➤ **Moderate acne vulgaris in women age 15 and older, who have no known contraindications to hormonal contraceptive therapy, who desire oral contraception for at least 6 months, who have achieved menarche, and who are unresponsive to topical anti-acne medications**
*Women age 15 and older:* 1 tablet Estrostep or Ortho Tri-Cyclen. P.O. daily (21 tablets contain active ingredients and 7 are inert).

## ACTION
Hormonal contraceptives inhibit ovulation through a negative feedback mechanism directed at the hypothalamus. These contraceptives also may prevent transport of the ovum through the fallopian tubes.

Estrogen suppresses secretion of follicle-stimulating hormone, blocking follicular development and ovulation.

Progestin suppresses secretion of luteinizing hormone so that ovulation can't occur even if the follicle develops. Progestin thickens cervical mucus, which interferes with sperm migration and causes endometrial changes that prevent implantation of the fertilized ovum.

| Route | Onset | Peak | Duration |
|-------|-------|------|----------|
| P.O. | Unknown | 30 min-4 hr | Unknown |

## ADVERSE REACTIONS
**CNS:** *headache, dizziness,* depression, lethargy, migraine, ***CVA.***
**CV:** ***thromboembolism,*** hypertension, edema, ***pulmonary embolism.***
**EENT:** worsening myopia or astigmatism, intolerance of contact lenses, exophthalmos, diplopia.
**GI:** *nausea,* vomiting, abdominal cramps, bloating, anorexia, changes in appetite, gallbladder disease, ***pancreatitis.***
**GU:** *breakthrough bleeding, spotting,* granulomatous colitis, dysmenorrhea, amenorrhea, cervical erosion or abnormal secretions, enlargement of uterine fibromas, vaginal candidiasis.
**Hepatic:** cholestatic jaundice, ***liver tumors.***
**Metabolic:** weight gain.
**Skin:** rash, acne, ***erythema multiforme.***
**Other:** breast tenderness, enlargement, or secretion.

## INTERACTIONS
**Drug-drug.** *Beta blockers:* May increase beta blocker level. Dosage adjustments may be necessary.
*Carbamazepine, fosphenytoin, phenobarbital, phenytoin, rifampin:* May decrease effectiveness of estrogen therapy. Use cautiously.
*Corticosteroids:* May enhance effects of corticosteroids. Monitor patient closely.
*Griseofulvin, penicillins, sulfonamides, tetracyclines:* May decrease effectiveness of hormonal contraceptives. Avoid using together, if possible.
*Insulin, sulfonylureas:* Glucose intolerance may decrease effects of antidiabetics. Monitor effects.
*Oral anticoagulants:* May decrease anticoagulant effect. Dosage adjustments may be needed. Monitor PT and INR.
*Tamoxifen:* May interfere with tamoxifen effectiveness. Avoid using together.
**Drug-herb.** *Black cohosh:* May increase adverse effects of estrogens. Discourage use together.
*Red clover:* May interfere with hormonal therapies. Discourage use together.
*Saw palmetto:* May have antiestrogenic effects. Discourage use together.
*St. John's wort:* May decrease efficacy of the hormonal contraceptive because of increased hepatic metabolism. Discourage use together or advise patient to use an additional method of contraception.
**Drug-food.** *Caffeine:* May increase caffeine level. Advise caution.
*Grapefruit juice:* May elevate estrogen level. Advise patient to take with liquid other than grapefruit juice.

---

Reactions may be *common*, uncommon, ***life-threatening***, or **COMMON AND LIFE-THREATENING.**

**Drug-lifestyle.** *Smoking:* May increase risk of adverse CV effects. If smoking continues, may need alternative therapy.

## EFFECTS ON LAB TEST RESULTS
● May increase fibrinogen, triglyceride, total $T_4$, thyroid-binding globulin, plasminogen, phospholipid, and clotting factor II, VII, VIII, IX, X, and XII levels.
● May increase PT and norepinephrine-induced platelet aggregation.
● May reduce metyrapone test results. May cause false-positive result in nitro-blue tetrazolium test.

## CONTRAINDICATIONS & CAUTIONS
● Contraindicated in patients with thromboembolic disorders, cerebrovascular or coronary artery disease, diplopia or ocular lesions arising from ophthalmic vascular disease, classic migraine, MI, known or suspected breast cancer, known or suspected estrogen-dependent neoplasia, benign or malignant liver tumors, active liver disease or history of cholestatic jaundice with pregnancy or previous use of hormonal contraceptives, and undiagnosed abnormal vaginal bleeding. Also, contraindicated in women who are or may be pregnant and in breast-feeding women.
● Use cautiously in patients with hyperlipidemia, hypertension, migraines, seizure disorders, asthma, or cardiac, renal, or hepatic insufficiency.

## NURSING CONSIDERATIONS
● Use estrogen-containing hormonal contraceptives with caution in patients who smoke.
● Triphasic hormonal contraceptives may cause fewer adverse reactions, such as breakthrough bleeding and spotting.
● The Centers for Disease Control and Prevention reports that use of hormonal contraceptives may decrease ovarian and endometrial cancers. Also, hormonal contraceptives don't appear to increase woman's risk of breast cancer. However, the FDA reports that hormonal contraceptives may be linked to an increase in cervical cancer.
● Monitor lipid levels, blood pressure, body weight, and hepatic function.

● **Alert:** Many hormonal contraceptives share similar names. Make sure to check the hormone strength for verification.
● Estrogens and progestins may alter glucose tolerance, thus changing dosage requirements for antidiabetics. Monitor glucose level.
● Stop hormonal contraceptives for a few weeks before adrenal function tests.
● Stop hormonal contraceptive and notify prescriber if patient develops granulomatous colitis.
● Stop drug at least 1 week before surgery to decrease risk of thromboembolism. Tell patient to use an alternative method of birth control.

## PATIENT TEACHING
● Tell patient to take tablets at same time each day; nighttime dosing may reduce nausea and headaches.
● Advise patient to use an additional method of birth control, such as condoms or a diaphragm with spermicide, for the first week of the first cycle.
● Tell patient that missing doses in midcycle greatly increases likelihood of pregnancy.
● Tell patient that missing a dose may cause spotting or light bleeding.
● Tell patient that hormonal contraceptives don't protect against HIV or other sexually transmitted diseases.
● If 1 tablet is missed, tell patient to take it as soon as she remembers or to take 2 tablets the next day and continue regular schedule. If patient misses 2 consecutive days, instruct her to take 2 tablets daily for 2 days and then resume normal schedule. Also, advise her to use an additional method of birth control for 7 days after two missed doses. If she misses three or more doses, tell her to discard remaining tablets in monthly package and to substitute another contraceptive method. If next menstrual period doesn't begin on schedule, warn patient to rule out pregnancy before starting new dosing cycle. If menstrual period begins, have patient start new dosing cycle 7 days after last tablet was taken.
● Warn patient of common initial adverse effects such as headache, nausea, dizziness, breast tenderness, spotting, and

breakthrough bleeding. These effects should diminish after 3 to 6 months.
● Instruct patient to weigh herself at least twice a week and to report any sudden weight gain or swelling to prescriber.
● Warn patient to avoid exposure to ultraviolet light or prolonged exposure to sunlight.
● *Alert:* Warn patient to immediately report abdominal pain; numbness, stiffness, or pain in legs or buttocks; pressure or pain in chest; shortness of breath; severe headache; visual disturbances such as blind spots, blurriness, or flashing lights; undiagnosed vaginal bleeding or discharge; two consecutive missed menstrual periods; lumps in the breast; swelling of hands or feet; or severe pain in the abdomen (tumor rupture in liver).
● Advise patient of increased risks created by simultaneous use of cigarettes and hormonal contraceptives.
● If one menstrual period is missed and tablets have been taken on schedule, tell patient to continue taking them. If two consecutive menstrual periods are missed, tell patient to stop drug and have pregnancy test. Progestins may cause birth defects if taken early in pregnancy.
● Advise patient not to take same drug for longer than 12 months without consulting prescriber. Stress importance of Pap tests and annual gynecologic examinations.
● Advise patient to check with prescriber about how soon pregnancy may be attempted after hormonal therapy is stopped. Many prescribers recommend that women not become pregnant within 2 months after stopping drug.
● Warn patient of possible delay in achieving pregnancy when drug is stopped.
● Teach woman how to perform routine breast self-examination.
● Teach patient methods to decrease risk of thromboembolism.
● Advise patient taking hormonal contraceptives to use additional form of birth control during concurrent treatment with certain antibiotics.
● Advise patient that hormonal contraceptives may change the fit of contact lenses.

## etonogestrel and ethinyl estradiol vaginal ring
NuvaRing

*Pregnancy risk category X*

**AVAILABLE FORMS**
*Vaginal ring:* Delivers 0.12 mg etonogestrel and 0.015 mg ethinyl estradiol daily

**INDICATIONS & DOSAGES**
➤ **Contraception**
*Women:* Insert one ring into the vagina and leave in place for 3 weeks. Insert new ring 1 week after the previous ring is removed.

**ACTION**
Suppresses gonadotropins, which inhibits ovulation, increases the viscosity of cervical mucus (decreasing the ability of sperm to enter the uterus), and alters the endometrial lining (reducing potential for implantation).

| Route | Onset | Peak | Duration |
|-------|-------|------|----------|
| Vaginal | Immediate | Unknown | Unknown |

**ADVERSE REACTIONS**
**CNS:** *headache,* emotional lability, ***cerebral thrombosis.***
**CV:** hypertension, ***thromboembolic events,*** coagulation abnormalities.
**EENT:** *sinusitis.*
**GI:** *nausea.*
**GU:** *vaginitis, leukorrhea,* device-related events (such as foreign body sensation, coital difficulties, device expulsion), vaginal discomfort.
**Hepatic:** *hepatic adenomas,* benign liver tumors.
**Metabolic:** weight gain.
**Respiratory:** *upper respiratory tract infection.*

**INTERACTIONS**
**Drug-drug.** *Acetaminophen:* May decrease acetaminophen level and increase ethinyl estradiol level. Monitor patient for effects.
*Ampicillin, barbiturates, carbamazepine, felbamate, griseofulvin, oxcarbazepine, phenylbutazone, phenytoin, rifampin,*

*tetracyclines, topiramate:* May decrease contraceptive efficacy and increase risk of pregnancy, breakthrough bleeding, or both. Tell patient to use an additional form of contraception while taking these drugs.

*Ascorbic acid, atorvastatin, itraconazole:* May increase ethinyl estradiol level. Monitor patient for adverse effects.

*Clofibric acid, morphine, salicylic acid, temazepam:* May increase clearance of these drugs. Monitor patient for effectiveness.

*Cyclosporine, prednisolone, theophylline:* May increase levels of these drugs. Monitor levels if appropriate and adjust dosage.

*HIV protease inhibitors:* May affect efficacy of contraception. Refer to the specific protease inhibitor drug literature. May need to use a back-up method of contraception.

**Drug-herb.** *St. John's wort:* May reduce contraceptive effectiveness and increase the risk of breakthrough bleeding and pregnancy. Discourage use together.

**Drug-lifestyle.** *Smoking:* May increase risk of serious CV adverse effects, especially in those older than age 35 who smoke 15 or more cigarettes daily. Urge patient to avoid smoking.

### EFFECTS ON LAB TEST RESULTS
● May increase levels of prothrombin; factors VII, VIII, IX, and X; thyroid-binding globulin (leading to increased circulating total thyroid hormone levels); other binding proteins; sex hormone–binding globulins; and triglycerides. May decrease antithrombin III and folate levels.
● May increase norepinephrine-induced platelet aggregability. May decrease $T_3$ resin uptake.

### CONTRAINDICATIONS & CAUTIONS
● Contraindicated in patients hypersensitive to any component of drug, patients who are or may be pregnant, patients older than age 35 who smoke 15 or more cigarettes daily, and patients with thrombophlebitis, thromboembolic disorder, history of deep vein thrombophlebitis, cerebral vascular or coronary artery disease (current or previous), valvular heart disease with complications, severe hypertension, diabetes with vascular complications, headache with focal neurologic

symptoms, major surgery with prolonged immobilization, known or suspected cancer of the endometrium or breast, estrogen-dependent neoplasia, abnormal undiagnosed genital bleeding, jaundice related to pregnancy or previous use of hormonal contraceptive, active liver disease, or benign or malignant hepatic tumors.
● Use cautiously in patients with hypertension, hyperlipidemias, obesity, or diabetes. Also use cautiously in patients with conditions that could be aggravated by fluid retention, and in patients with a history of depression.

### NURSING CONSIDERATIONS
● *Alert:* Drug may increase the risk of MI, thromboembolism, CVA, hepatic neoplasia, and gallbladder disease.
● Cigarette smoking increases the risk of serious adverse cardiac effects. The risk increases with age and in patients who smoke 15 or more cigarettes daily.
● Stop drug at least 4 weeks before and for 2 weeks after procedures that may increase the risk of thromboembolism, and during and after prolonged immobilization.
● Stop drug and notify prescriber if patient develops unexplained partial or complete loss of vision, proptosis, diplopia, papilledema, retinal vascular lesions, migraines, depression or jaundice.
● Monitor blood pressure closely if patient has hypertension or renal disease.
● Ring should remain in place continuously for a full 3 weeks to maintain efficacy. It is then removed for 1 week. During this time, withdrawal bleeding occurs (usually starting 2 or 3 days after removal). A new ring should be inserted 1 week after removal of the previous one, regardless of whether the patient is still menstruating.
● Rule out pregnancy if patient hasn't adhered to the prescribed regimen and a period is missed, if prescribed regimen is adhered to and two periods are missed, or if the patient has retained the ring for longer than 4 weeks.

### PATIENT TEACHING
● Emphasize the importance of having regular annual physical examinations to check for adverse effects or developing contraindications.

---

*Rapid onset*    †Canada    ‡Australia    ◇OTC    ◆Off-label use    ✐Photoguide    *Liquid contains alcohol.

• Tell patient that drug doesn't protect against HIV and other sexually transmitted diseases.

• Advise patient not to smoke while using contraceptive.

• Tell patient not to use a diaphragm if a back-up method of birth control is needed.

• Tell patient who wears contact lenses to contact an ophthalmologist if vision or lens tolerance changes.

• Advise patient to follow the manufacturer's instructions for use if switching from a different form of hormonal contraceptive.

• Tell patient to insert ring into the vagina (using fingers) and keep it in place continuously for 3 weeks to maintain efficacy. Save the foil package for later disposal. It is then removed for 1 full week. Explain that, during this time, withdrawal bleeding occurs (usually starting 2 or 3 days after removal). Tell patient to insert a new ring 1 week after removing the previous one, regardless of menstrual bleeding. Tell patient to reseal the ring in the package after removing it from the vagina.

• Advise patient that, if the ring is removed or expelled (such as while removing a tampon, straining, or moving bowels), it should be washed with cool to lukewarm (not hot) water and reinserted immediately. Stress that contraceptive efficacy may be compromised if the ring stays out for longer than 3 hours and to use a back-up method of contraception until the newly reinserted ring is used continuously for 7 days.

---

## medroxyprogesterone acetate
Amen, Cycrin, Depo-Provera†, Provera◆

*Pregnancy risk category X*

---

### AVAILABLE FORMS
*Tablets:* 2.5 mg, 5 mg, 10 mg
*Injection (suspension):* 150 mg/ml, 400 mg/ml

### INDICATIONS & DOSAGES
➤ **Abnormal uterine bleeding caused by hormonal imbalance**
*Women:* 5 to 10 mg P.O. daily for 5 to 10 days beginning on day 16 of menstrual cycle. If patient also has received estrogen, give 10 mg P.O. daily for 10 days beginning on day 16 or 21 of cycle.
➤ **Secondary amenorrhea**
*Women:* 5 to 10 mg P.O. daily for 5 to 10 days. Start at any time during menstrual cycle (usually during latter half of cycle).
➤ **Endometrial or renal cancer**
*Adults:* 400 to 1,000 mg I.M. weekly. Dosage may be decreased to 400 mg/month when disease has stabilized.
➤ **Contraception**
*Women:* 150 mg I.M. once q 3 months.

### ACTION
Suppresses ovulation, possibly by inhibiting pituitary gonadotropin secretion, thus preventing follicular maturation and causing endometrial thinning.

| Route | Onset | Peak | Duration |
|---|---|---|---|
| P.O., I.M. | Unknown | Unknown | Unknown |

### ADVERSE REACTIONS
**CNS:** depression, *CVA,* pain.
**CV:** thrombophlebitis, *pulmonary embolism,* edema, *thromboembolism.*
**EENT:** exophthalmos, diplopia.
**GI:** *bloating, abdominal pain.*
**GU:** *breakthrough bleeding,* dysmenorrhea, *amenorrhea,* cervical erosion, abnormal secretions.
**Hepatic:** cholestatic jaundice.
**Metabolic:** weight changes.
**Skin:** rash, induration, sterile abscesses, acne, pruritus, melasma, alopecia, hirsutism.
**Other:** breast tenderness, enlargement, or secretion.

### INTERACTIONS
**Drug-drug.** *Aminoglutethimide, carbamazepine, fosphenytoin, phenobarbital, phenytoin, rifampin:* May decrease progestin effects. Monitor patient for diminished therapeutic response. Tell patient to use a nonhormonal contraceptive during therapy with these drugs.
**Drug-food.** *Caffeine:* May increase caffeine level. Advise caution.
**Drug-lifestyle.** *Smoking:* May increase risk of adverse CV effects. If smoking continues, may need alternative therapy.

---

Reactions may be *common*, uncommon, *life-threatening*, or COMMON AND LIFE-THREATENING.

## EFFECTS ON LAB TEST RESULTS
• May increase liver function test values. May cause abnormal thyroid function test results.
• May reduce metyrapone test results.

## CONTRAINDICATIONS & CAUTIONS
• Contraindicated in patients hypersensitive to drug and in those with active thromboembolic disorders or history of thromboembolic disorders, cerebrovascular disease, apoplexy, breast cancer, undiagnosed abnormal vaginal bleeding, missed abortion, or hepatic dysfunction; also contraindicated during pregnancy. Tablets are contraindicated in patients with liver dysfunction or known or suspected malignant disease of genital organs.
• Use cautiously in patients with diabetes mellitus, seizures, migraine, cardiac or renal disease, asthma, and depression.

## NURSING CONSIDERATIONS
• Drug shouldn't be used as test for pregnancy; it may cause birth defects and masculinization of female fetus.
• I.M. injection may be painful. Monitor sites for evidence of sterile abscess. Rotate injection sites to prevent muscle atrophy.
• Monitor patient for pain and swelling, warmth, or redness in calves; sudden, severe headaches; visual disturbances; numbness in extremities; signs of depression; signs of liver dysfunction (abdominal pain, dark urine, jaundice).

## PATIENT TEACHING
• According to FDA regulations, patient must read package insert explaining possible adverse effects of progestins before receiving first dose. Also, give patient verbal explanation.
• Advise patient to take medication with food if GI upset occurs.
• *Alert:* Tell patient to report unusual symptoms immediately and to stop drug and notify prescriber about visual disturbances or migraine.
• Teach woman how to perform routine breast self-examination.
• Advise patient to immediately report to prescriber any breast abnormalities, vaginal bleeding, swelling, yellowed skin or eyes, dark urine, clay-colored stools,

shortness of breath, chest pain, or pregnancy.
• Advise patient that injection must be given every 3 months to maintain adequate contraceptive effects.
• Tell patient to immediately report to prescriber a suspected pregnancy.

---

# medroxyprogesterone acetate and estradiol cypionate
Lunelle

*Pregnancy risk category X*

## AVAILABLE FORMS
*Injection:* 25 mg medroxyprogesterone acetate and 5 mg estradiol cypionate per 0.5 ml

## INDICATIONS & DOSAGES
➤ **Contraception**
*Women older than age 16 who have achieved menarche:* 0.5 ml I.M. into deltoid, gluteus maximus, or anterior thigh. Give first injection within first 5 days of onset of a normal menstrual period, within 5 days of a complete first trimester abortion, or at least 4 weeks postpartum if not breast-feeding (at least 6 weeks postpartum if breast-feeding). Give second and subsequent injections monthly (28 to 30 days, not to exceed 33 days) after previous injection.

## ACTION
Medroxyprogesterone acetate and estradiol cypionate inhibit gonadotropin secretion, which prevents follicular maturation and ovulation. Other possible mechanisms of action include thinning of the endometrium and thickening of reduced volume of cervical mucus.

| Route | Onset | Peak | Duration |
|-------|-------|------|----------|
| I.M. | 1 day | 7-10 days | 28-30 days |

## ADVERSE REACTIONS
**CNS:** emotional lability, depression, headache, nervousness, dizziness, asthenia.
**CV:** *thromboembolism,* edema.
**EENT:** intolerance to contact lenses.
**GI:** abdominal pain, nausea, enlarged abdomen, gallbladder disease.

**GU:** amenorrhea, dysmenorrhea, menorrhagia, metrorrhagia, vaginal candidiasis, vulvovaginal disorder.
**Hepatic:** *tumors,* cholestatic jaundice.
**Metabolic:** weight gain.
**Skin:** acne, alopecia.
**Other:** breast tenderness or pain, decreased libido, hypersensitivity reactions.

## INTERACTIONS
**Drug-drug.** *Acetaminophen:* May decrease acetaminophen level. Monitor patient.
*Aminoglutethimide:* May decrease medroxyprogesterone acetate level. Recommend additional birth control.
*Antibiotics (ampicillin, griseofulvin, tetracycline):* May decrease contraceptive effectiveness. Recommend additional birth control.
*Anticonvulsants (carbamazepine, phenobarbital, phenytoin):* May increase metabolism of some synthetic estrogens and progestins, which could reduce contraceptive effectiveness. Recommend additional birth control.
*Clofibric acid, morphine, salicylic acid, temazepam:* May increase clearance of these drugs. Monitor levels, or recommend alternative therapy.
*Cyclosporine, prednisolone, theophylline:* May increase levels of these drugs. Monitor levels, and adjust as needed.
*Phenylbutazone:* May decrease contraceptive effectiveness and increase menstrual irregularities. Recommend additional birth control.
*Rifampin:* May increase metabolism of some synthetic estrogens and progestins, decreasing contraceptive effectiveness and increasing irregular bleeding. Recommend additional birth control.
**Drug-herb.** *St. John's wort:* May induce hepatic enzymes (cytochrome P-450) and transporter proteins. May reduce the effectiveness of contraceptives and may cause breakthrough bleeding. Discourage use together or advise using a second method of contraception.
**Drug-lifestyle.** *Smoking:* May increase risk of thromboembolic disorders. Discourage smoking.

## EFFECTS ON LAB TEST RESULTS
● May increase levels of total circulating sex steroid, corticoid, triglyceride, plasma and urinary steroid, gonadotropin, sulfobromophthalein, folate, prothrombin, and factor VII, VIII, IX, and X. May decrease antithrombin III level.
● May increase liver function test values, norepinephrine-induced platelet aggregability, thyroid-binding globulin, and total thyroid hormone. May decrease free $T_3$ resin uptake, glucose tolerance, and sex hormone-binding globulin concentration.

## CONTRAINDICATIONS & CAUTIONS
● Contraindicated in patients who are or may be pregnant and in those with thrombophlebitis or thromboembolic disorders, a history of deep vein thrombophlebitis or thromboembolic disorders, and cerebral vascular or coronary artery disease.
● Contraindicated in those with undiagnosed abnormal genital bleeding; liver dysfunction or disease, such as history of hepatic adenoma or cancer; history of cholestatic jaundice of pregnancy or jaundice with prior hormonal contraceptive use, including severe pruritus of pregnancy.
● Contraindicated in patients with cancer of the endometrium, breast, or other known or suspected estrogen-dependent neoplasia.
● Contraindicated in patients hypersensitive to drug components, in women older than age 35 who smoke 15 or more cigarettes daily, and those with severe hypertension, diabetes with vascular involvement, headaches with focal neurologic symptoms, or valvular heart disease with complications.
● Use cautiously in patients with hypertension, hyperlipidemia, obesity, diabetes, and liver dysfunction.
● Use cautiously in patients who smoke and in those with a history of depression.

## NURSING CONSIDERATIONS
● The use of hormonal contraceptives is linked to increased risk of MI, CVA, hepatic neoplasia, and gallbladder disease.
● Monthly injection is effective for contraception during the first cycle of use when given as recommended.

---

• If more than 33 days have elapsed since last injection, consider pregnancy and don't give another injection until pregnancy is ruled out.

• Shortening the injection interval could lead to a change in menstrual pattern.

• Don't use bleeding episodes to guide the injection schedule.

• Shake the aqueous suspension vigorously just before use to ensure a uniform suspension.

• Provide yearly physical examinations. Monitor breast examination closely in women with breast nodules or family history of breast cancer.

• When switching patients from other methods of birth control, give drug in a manner that ensures continuous contraceptive coverage based on the mechanism of action from both methods. For example, patients switching from hormonal contraceptives should have their first injection within 7 days after taking their last active pill.

• Stop use at least 4 weeks before and for 2 weeks after elective surgery that may be linked to increased risk of thromboembolism.

• Don't use during periods of prolonged immobilization or within 4 weeks after childbirth.

• Store injection at 59° to 86° F (15° to 30° C).

• Effects of drug in breast-feeding women are unknown, but estrogen use by breast-feeding women may decrease quality and quantity of milk.

• Small amounts of combined hormonal contraceptives have been identified in milk with no deleterious effects to the child. However, breast-feeding women shouldn't begin a combined hormonal contraceptive until 6 weeks postpartum.

**PATIENT TEACHING**

• **Alert:** Teach patient that this product is intended to prevent pregnancy and won't protect against sexually transmitted diseases.

• Advise patient that injection must be given every 28 to 30 days. If more than 33 days have passed since an injection, pregnancy must be ruled out before another injection can be given.

• Tell patient that menstrual bleeding patterns may be disrupted while she is receiving drug. Advise patient to report excessive or prolonged bleeding.

• Tell patient that weight gain may occur while she is taking drug.

• Advise patient who wears contact lenses to have an eye examination if visual changes or changes in lens tolerance develop while she is taking drug.

• Inform patient that monthly injection is effective for contraception during the first cycle of use when given as recommended.

# norelgestromin and ethinyl estradiol transdermal system
Ortho Evra

*Pregnancy risk category X*

**AVAILABLE FORMS**
*Transdermal patch:* norelgestromin 6 mg and ethinyl estradiol 0.75 mg per patch, delivering 150 mcg norelgestromin and 20 mcg ethinyl estradiol daily.

**INDICATIONS & DOSAGES**
➤ **Contraception**
*Women:* Apply 1 patch weekly for 3 weeks. Apply each new patch on the same day of the week. Week 4 is patch free. On the day after week 4 ends, apply a new patch to start a new 4-week cycle. The patch-free interval between cycles should never be longer than 7 days.

**ACTION**
Combination hormonal contraceptives act by suppressing gonadotropins. The primary mechanism of this action is ovulation inhibition. However, changes in cervical mucus increase the difficulty of sperm entry into the uterus, and changes in the endometrium decrease the likelihood of implantation.

| Route | Onset | Peak | Duration |
|-------|-------|------|----------|
| Transdermal | Rapid | 2 days | Unknown |

**ADVERSE REACTIONS**
**CNS:** *headache,* emotional lability.
**CV:** ***thromboembolic events, MI,*** hypertension, ***cerebral hemorrhage.***
**EENT:** contact lens intolerance.

**GI:** *nausea, abdominal pain,* vomiting, gallbladder disease.
**GU:** *menstrual cramps,* changes in menstrual flow, vaginal candidiasis.
**Hepatic:** *hepatic adenomas,* benign liver tumors.
**Metabolic:** weight changes.
**Respiratory:** *upper respiratory tract infection.*
**Skin:** *application site reaction.*
**Other:** *breast tenderness, enlargement, or secretion.*

## INTERACTIONS
**Drug-drug.** *Acetaminophen, clofibric acid, morphine, salicylic acid, temazepam:* May decrease levels or increase clearance of these drugs. Monitor patient for lack of effect.
*Ampicillin, barbiturates, carbamazepine, felbamate, griseofulvin, oxcarbazepine, phenylbutazone, phenytoin, rifampin, topiramate:* May reduce contraceptive effectiveness, resulting in unintended pregnancy or breakthrough bleeding. Encourage back-up method of contraception if used together.
*Ascorbic acid, atorvastatin, itraconazole, ketoconazole:* May increase hormone levels. Use together cautiously.
*Cyclosporine, prednisolone, theophylline:* May increase levels of these drugs. Monitor patient for adverse reactions.
*HIV protease inhibitors:* May affect contraceptive effectiveness and safety. Use together cautiously.
**Drug-herb.** *St. John's wort:* May reduce effectiveness of contraceptive and cause breakthrough bleeding. Discourage use together.
**Drug-lifestyle.** *Smoking:* May increase risk of CV adverse effects of hormonal contraceptive use, related to age and smoking 15 or more cigarettes daily. Urge patient not to smoke.

## EFFECTS ON LAB TEST RESULTS
● May increase circulating total thyroid hormone, triglyceride, other binding protein, sex hormone binding globulin, total circulating endogenous sex steroid, corticoid, and factor VII, VIII, IX, and X levels. May decrease antithrombin III and folate levels.

● May increase prothrombin. May decrease free $T_3$ resin uptake and glucose tolerance.

## CONTRAINDICATIONS & CAUTIONS
● Contraindicated in patients hypersensitive to any component of this drug and in those with past history of deep vein thrombosis or related disorder, current or past history of cerebrovascular or coronary artery disease, past or current known or suspected breast cancer, endometrial cancer or other known or suspected estrogen-dependent neoplasia, or hepatic adenoma or cancer, and in those who are or may be pregnant.
● Contraindicated in patients with thrombophlebitis, thromboembolic disorders, valvular heart disease with complications, severe hypertension, diabetes with vascular involvement, headaches with focal neurologic symptoms, major surgery with prolonged immobilization, undiagnosed abnormal genital bleeding, cholestatic jaundice of pregnancy or jaundice with previous hormonal contraceptive use, or acute or chronic hepatocellular disease with abnormal liver function.
● Use cautiously in patients with CV disease risk factors, with conditions that might be aggravated by fluid retention, or with a history of depression.

## NURSING CONSIDERATIONS
● **Alert:** Patients taking combination hormonal contraceptives may be at increased risk for thrombophlebitis, venous thrombosis with or without embolism, pulmonary embolism, MI, cerebral hemorrhage, cerebral thrombosis, hypertension, gallbladder disease, hepatic adenomas, benign liver tumors, mesenteric thrombosis, and retinal thrombosis.
● Increased risk of MI occurs primarily in smokers and women with hypertension, hypercholesterolemia, morbid obesity, and diabetes.
● Encourage women with a history of hypertension or renal disease to use a different method of contraception. If Ortho Evra is used, monitor blood pressure closely and stop use if hypertension occurs.
● Drug may be less effective in women weighing 198 lb (90 kg) or more.

---

Reactions may be *common*, uncommon, ***life-threatening***, or COMMON AND LIFE-THREATENING.

- Cigarette smoking increases the risk of serious adverse cardiac effects. The risk increases with age and in those who smoke 15 or more cigarettes daily.
- The risk of thromboembolic disease increases if therapy is used postpartum or postabortion.
- Rule out pregnancy if withdrawal bleeding fails to occur for two consecutive cycles.
- If skin becomes irritated, the patch may be removed and a new patch applied at a different site.
- Stop drug and notify prescriber at least 4 weeks before and for 2 weeks after an elective surgery that increases the risk of thromboembolism, and during and after prolonged immobilization.
- Stop drug and notify prescriber if patient has headaches, vision loss, proptosis, diplopia, papilledema, retinal vascular lesions, jaundice, or depression.

**PATIENT TEACHING**
- Emphasize the importance of having regular annual physical examinations to check for adverse effects or developing contraindications.
- Tell patient that drug doesn't protect against HIV and other sexually transmitted diseases.
- Advise patient to immediately apply a new patch once the used patch is removed, on the same day of the week every 7 days for 3 weeks. Week 4 is patch free. Bleeding is expected to occur during this time.
- Tell patient to apply each patch to a clean, dry area of the skin on the buttocks, abdomen, upper outer arm, or upper torso. Tell patient not to apply to the breasts or to skin that is red, irritated, or cut.
- Tell patient to carefully fold the used patch in half so that it sticks to itself, before discarding.
- Tell patient to immediately stop use if pregnancy is confirmed.
- Tell patient who wears contact lenses to report visual changes or changes in lens tolerance.
- Advise patient not to smoke while using the patch.
- Stress that if patient isn't sure what to do about mistakes with patch use, she should use a back-up method of birth control and contact her health care provider.

# norethindrone
Camila, Errin, Micronor, Nora-BE, Nor-QD

# norethindrone acetate
Aygestin

*Pregnancy risk category X*

**AVAILABLE FORMS**
**norethindrone**
*Tablets:* 0.35 mg
**norethindrone acetate**
*Tablets:* 5 mg

**INDICATIONS & DOSAGES**
➤ **Amenorrhea, abnormal uterine bleeding**
*Women:* 2.5 to 10 mg norethindrone acetate P.O. daily on days 5 to 25 of menstrual cycle.
➤ **Endometriosis**
*Women:* 5 mg norethindrone acetate P.O. daily for 14 days; then increased by 2.5 mg daily q 2 weeks, up to 15 mg daily.
➤ **Contraception**
*Women:* Initially, 0.35 mg norethindrone P.O. on first day of menstruation; then 0.35 mg daily.

**ACTION**
Suppresses ovulation, possibly by inhibiting pituitary gonadotropin secretion, and forms thick cervical mucus.

| Route | Onset | Peak | Duration |
|-------|-------|------|----------|
| P.O. | Unknown | Unknown | Unknown |

**ADVERSE REACTIONS**
**CNS:** depression, *CVA.*
**CV:** thrombophlebitis, *pulmonary embolism,* edema, *thromboembolism.*
**EENT:** exophthalmos, diplopia.
**GI:** *bloating, abdominal pain or cramping.*
**GU:** *breakthrough bleeding,* dysmenorrhea, *amenorrhea,* cervical erosion, abnormal secretions.
**Hepatic:** cholestatic jaundice.
**Metabolic:** weight changes.
**Skin:** melasma, rash, acne, pruritus.
**Other:** breast tenderness, enlargement, or secretion.

## INTERACTIONS

**Drug-drug.** *Barbiturates, carbamazepine, fosphenytoin, phenytoin, rifampin:* May decrease progestin effects. Monitor patient for diminished therapeutic response.

**Drug-food.** *Caffeine:* May increase caffeine level. Advise caution.

**Drug-lifestyle.** *Smoking:* May increase risk of adverse CV effects. If smoking continues, may need alternative therapy.

## EFFECTS ON LAB TEST RESULTS
● May increase liver function test values.
● May decrease metyrapone test results.

## CONTRAINDICATIONS & CAUTIONS
● Contraindicated in pregnant patients, patients hypersensitive to drug, and patients with breast cancer, undiagnosed abnormal vaginal bleeding, severe hepatic disease, missed abortion, or current or previous thromboembolic disorders.
● Use cautiously in patients with diabetes mellitus, seizures, migraines, cardiac or renal disease, asthma, and depression.

## NURSING CONSIDERATIONS
● If switching from combined oral contraceptives to progestin-only pills (POPs), take the first POP the day after the last active combined pill.
● If switching from POPs to combined pills, take the first active combined pill on the first day of menstruation, even if the POP pack is not finished.
● Norethindrone acetate is twice as potent as norethindrone. Norethindrone acetate shouldn't be used for contraception.
● Preliminary estrogen treatment is usually needed in those with menstrual disorders.
● Watch patient closely for signs of edema.
● Monitor blood pressure.
● *Alert:* Don't confuse Micronor with Micro K or Micronase.

## PATIENT TEACHING
● According to FDA regulations, patient must read package insert explaining possible adverse effects of progestins before receiving first dose. Also, give patient verbal explanation.
● Tell patient to take drug at the same time every day when used as a contraceptive. If she is more than 3 hours late taking the pill or if she has missed a pill, she should take the pill as soon as she remembers, then continue the normal schedule. Also tell her to use a backup method of contraception for the next 48 hours.
● *Alert:* Tell patient to report unusual symptoms immediately and to stop drug and notify prescriber about visual disturbances or migraine.
● Teach woman how to perform routine breast self-examination.
● Tell patient to report suspected pregnancy to prescriber.
● Encourage patient to stop or reduce smoking because of the risk of CV complications.

# progesterone

*Pregnancy risk category X*

## AVAILABLE FORMS
*Injection (in oil):* 50 mg/ml

## INDICATIONS & DOSAGES
➤ **Amenorrhea**
*Women:* 5 to 10 mg I.M. daily for 6 to 10 days, usually beginning 8 to 10 days before anticipated start of menstruation. Or as a single 100- to 150-mg I.M. dose.
➤ **Dysfunctional uterine bleeding**
*Women:* 5 to 10 mg I.M. daily for six doses.

## ACTION
Suppresses ovulation, possibly by inhibiting pituitary gonadotropin secretion, and forms thick cervical mucus.

| Route | Onset | Peak | Duration |
|-------|-------|------|----------|
| I.M. | Unknown | Unknown | Unknown |

## ADVERSE REACTIONS
**CNS:** depression, *CVA.*
**CV:** thrombophlebitis, *thromboembolism, pulmonary embolism, edema,* hypertension.
**GU:** *breakthrough bleeding,* dysmenorrhea, *amenorrhea,* cervical erosion, abnormal secretions.
**Hepatic:** cholestatic jaundice.
**Skin:** melasma, rash, acne, pruritus, *pain at injection site.*

---

**Other:** breast tenderness, enlargement, or secretion.

## INTERACTIONS
**Drug-drug.** *Barbiturates, carbamazepine, fosphenytoin, phenytoin, rifampin:* May decrease progestin effects. Monitor patient for diminished therapeutic response.
**Drug-herb.** *Red clover:* May interfere with hormonal therapies. Discourage use together.

## EFFECTS ON LAB TEST RESULTS
● May decrease pregnanediol excretion.
● May increase liver function test values. May reduce metyrapone test results. May cause abnormal thyroid function test results.

## CONTRAINDICATIONS & CAUTIONS
● Contraindicated in pregnant patients, patients hypersensitive to drug, and patients with breast cancer, undiagnosed abnormal vaginal bleeding, severe hepatic disease, missed abortion, or current or previous thromboembolic disorders. Because of possible allergic reaction, drug shouldn't be given to patients allergic to peanuts or sesame.
● Use cautiously in patients with diabetes mellitus, seizures, migraine, cardiac or renal disease, asthma, or depression.

## NURSING CONSIDERATIONS
● Preliminary estrogen treatment is usually needed in those with menstrual disorders.
● **Alert:** Ask patient about food allergies (peanuts, sesame).
● Give oil solutions (peanut oil or sesame oil) via deep I.M. injection. Check sites frequently for irritation. Rotate injection sites.
● Advise woman of childbearing age to consult prescriber before taking drug and to advise prescriber immediately if she becomes pregnant.

## PATIENT TEACHING
● According to FDA regulations, patient must read the package insert explaining possible adverse effects of progestins before receiving her first dose. Also give patient verbal explanation.
● **Alert:** Tell patient to report unusual symptoms immediately and to stop drug

and notify prescriber about visual disturbances or migraine.
● **Alert:** Tell patient to report increased depression immediately; drug may need to be stopped.
● Teach woman how to perform routine breast self-examination.
● Tell patient to report suspected pregnancy to prescriber immediately.
● Encourage patient to stop smoking or reduce number of cigarettes because of the risk of CV complications.

**cetrorelix acetate**
**histrelin acetate**
**menotropins**

### COMBINATION PRODUCTS
None.

---

### cetrorelix acetate
Cetrotide

*Pregnancy risk category X*

### AVAILABLE FORMS
*Powder for injection:* 0.25 mg, 3 mg

### INDICATIONS & DOSAGES
➤ **To inhibit premature luteinizing hormone (LH) surges in women undergoing controlled ovarian stimulation**
*Women:* 3 mg S.C. once during early to middle follicular phase, given when estradiol level indicates an appropriate stimulation response, usually on stimulation day 7 (range, days 5 to 9). If human chorionic gonadotropin (hCG) hasn't been given within 4 days after injection, give cetrorelix 0.25 mg S.C. once daily until the day of hCG administration. Or, give 0.25-mg S.C. multiple-dose regimen on stimulation day 5 (morning or evening) or day 6 (morning) and continue once daily until the day of hCG administration.

### ACTION
Competes with natural gonadotropin-releasing hormone (GnRH) for binding to membrane receptors on pituitary cells, which controls the release of LH and follicle-stimulating hormone (FSH).

| Route | Onset | Peak | Duration |
|-------|-------|------|----------|
| S.C. | 1-2 hr | 1-2 hr | > 4 days |

### ADVERSE REACTIONS
**CNS:** headache.
**GI:** nausea.
**GU:** ovarian hyperstimulation syndrome.

### INTERACTIONS
None reported.

### EFFECTS ON LAB TEST RESULTS
● May increase ALT, AST, GGT, and alkaline phosphatase levels.

### CONTRAINDICATIONS & CAUTIONS
● Contraindicated in patients hypersensitive to cetrorelix acetate, extrinsic peptide hormones, mannitol, GnRH, or any other GnRH analogues.
● Contraindicated in pregnant and breast-feeding women.

### NURSING CONSIDERATIONS
● Rule out pregnancy before starting treatment.
● Prescriber should be experienced in fertility treatment.
● Adjust dose according to patient response.
● When ultrasound shows enough follicles of adequate size, give hCG to induce ovulation and maturation of oocytes.
● To reduce the risk of ovarian hyperstimulation syndrome, don't give hCG if ovaries show an excessive response to treatment.

### PATIENT TEACHING
● Instruct patient to store 3-mg form at room temperature (77° F [25° C]) and to store 0.25-mg form in refrigerator (36° to 46° F [2° to 8° C]). Tell patient to keep this product away from children.
● Tell patient to report any adverse effects that become bothersome.
● Teach patient the importance of following the regimen exactly as prescribed, to achieve optimal results.
● Instruct patient on the proper administration technique, as follows: Wash hands thoroughly with soap and water. Flip off the plastic cover of the vial and wipe the top with an alcohol swab. Attach the needle with the yellow mark to the prefilled syringe. Push the needle through the rubber stopper of the vial and slowly inject

the liquid into the vial. Leave the syringe in place and gently swirl the vial until the solution is clear and without residue. Don't shake. Draw liquid from the vial into the syringe. If necessary, invert the vial and pull the needle back as far as needed to withdraw the entire contents of the vial. Detach the needle with the yellow mark from the syringe and replace it with the needle with the gray mark. Invert the syringe and push the plunger until all air bubbles are gone.

• Tell patient to choose an injection site on the lower abdomen, around the navel. If she receives a multiple-dose (0.25-mg) regimen, tell her to choose a different site each day to minimize local irritation. Instruct her to clean the site with an alcohol swab and gently pinch a skinfold surrounding injection site. Instruct her to insert the needle completely into the skin at about a 45-degree angle and, once the needle has been inserted completely, to release her grasp of the skin. Tell her to gently pull back the plunger of the syringe to check for correct positioning of the needle. If no blood appears, tell her to inject the entire solution by slowly pushing the plunger. She should then withdraw the needle and gently press an alcohol swab onto the injection site.

• If blood appears when the patient pulls back on the plunger, tell her to withdraw the needle and gently press an alcohol swab onto the injection site. Explain that she'll need to discard the syringe and the drug vial and to repeat the procedure using a new pack.

• Urge patient to use a syringe and needle only once and then to dispose of them properly, in a medical waste container, if available.

## histrelin acetate
Supprelin

*Pregnancy risk category X*

### AVAILABLE FORMS
*Injection:* 120 mcg/0.6 ml, 300 mcg/0.6 ml, 600 mcg/0.6 ml

### INDICATIONS & DOSAGES
➤ **Centrally mediated (idiopathic or neurogenic) precocious puberty**
*Children (girls ages 2 to 8; boys ages 2 to 9½):* 10 mcg/kg S.C. daily.

### ACTION
Mimics effects of, but is more potent than, gonadotropin-releasing hormone (GnRH). Long-term use desensitizes responsiveness of pituitary gonadotropin, decreasing sex hormone production by testes or ovaries.

| Route | Onset | Peak | Duration |
|-------|-------|------|----------|
| S.C. | Unknown | Unknown | Unknown |

### ADVERSE REACTIONS
**CNS:** malaise, *mood changes, nervousness, dizziness, depression, headache, insomnia, anxiety,* paresthesia, cognitive changes, syncope, somnolence, lethargy, impaired consciousness, tremor, hyperkinesia, *seizures,* hot flashes, conduct disorder, *fever,* fatigue.
**CV:** *vasodilation,* edema, palpitations, pallor, tachycardia, hypertension.
**EENT:** epistaxis, ear congestion, abnormal pupillary function, otalgia, visual disturbances, hearing loss, polyopia, photophobia, rhinorrhea, sinusitis, nasal infections.
**GI:** *abdominal pain, nausea, vomiting, diarrhea, flatulence, decreased appetite, dyspepsia,* cramps, constipation, thirst, gastritis, GI distress.
**GU:** *menstrual changes, vaginal dryness, leukorrhea, hypermenorrhea, vaginal bleeding, vaginitis, dysmenorrhea,* tenderness of female genitalia, polyuria, incontinence, dysuria, hematuria, nocturia, glycosuria.
**Hematologic:** anemia, purpura.
**Metabolic:** hyperlipidemia, *weight gain.*
**Musculoskeletal:** *arthralgia, muscle stiffness, muscle cramps.*
**Respiratory:** *upper respiratory tract infection, respiratory congestion, cough,* asthma, breathing disorder, bronchitis, hyperventilation.
**Skin:** *redness, swelling, acne, rash, diaphoresis,* urticaria, pruritus, alopecia.
**Other:** *libido changes, breast pain or edema,* breast discharge, decreased breast size, *body pains,* chills, ***acute hypersensi-***

*tivity reactions, anaphylaxis, angioede-ma.*

**INTERACTIONS**
None significant.

**EFFECTS ON LAB TEST RESULTS**
• May increase lipid levels.
• May decrease hemoglobin.

**CONTRAINDICATIONS & CAUTIONS**
• Contraindicated in patients hypersensitive to drug or its ingredients and in pregnant or breast-feeding women.

**NURSING CONSIDERATIONS**
• Drug is indicated only for patients who will comply with daily schedule. Noncompliance or inadequate dosing may result in inadequate control of pubertal process, possibly allowing recurrence of symptoms, including onset of menses, breast development, or testicular growth; long-term consequences may involve decreased adult height.
• Perform a complete physical and endocrinologic evaluation before therapy starts; reexamine several indices at 3 months and every 6 to 12 months thereafter. Such evaluations should include height and weight, hand and wrist X-rays for bone-age determination, sex steroid (estradiol or testosterone) levels, and GnRH stimulation test. Monitor these tests periodically to determine effectiveness of therapy.
• Further tests to rule out other causes of precocious puberty include beta hCG levels (to detect chorionic gonadotropin–secreting tumor); pelvic, adrenal, or testicular ultrasound (to detect corticosteroid-secreting tumor); and computed tomography scan of the head (to detect undiagnosed intracranial tumors). Work-up also sets baseline of gonad size for serial monitoring.
• Refrigerate drug (36° to 46° F [2° to 8° C]) and protect from light in its original container. Use vials only once because drug doesn't contain preservatives. Allow drug to reach room temperature before use.
• Give by S.C. route and rotate injection sites to minimize local reactions.

• Decreases in follicle-stimulating hormone, luteinizing hormone, and sex corticosteroid levels occur within 3 months.
• Reevaluate patient if prepubertal sex steroid levels or GnRH test responses aren't achieved within 3 months of therapy.
• Safety and efficacy of drug haven't been established in children younger than age 2.

**PATIENT TEACHING**
• Before therapy, make sure patient and caregiver understand importance of adhering to daily schedules. Tell parents to give drug at same time each day to aid compliance and ensure adequate dosing.
• Drug is dispensed as a 30-day kit that contains a patient information leaflet. Make sure caregiver reads and understands leaflet.
• Inform patient that because drug is a peptide, it's destroyed in GI tract and so must be given parenterally.
• Explain importance of rotating injection sites daily. Sites should include upper arms, thighs, and abdomen.
• Warn patient of potential risks and adverse effects of therapy. During first month of treatment, girls commonly experience a slight menstrual flow, which probably is related to decreasing estrogen levels brought on by treatment. As estrogen levels decrease, menstruation begins because estrogens support the endometrium.
• Advise patient to seek medical attention immediately if signs of hypersensitivity reaction occur: sudden rash, difficulty breathing or swallowing, or rapid heartbeat. Also tell patient to notify prescriber about severe or persistent swelling, redness, or irritation at injection site.

---

# menotropins
**Pergonal, Repronex**

*Pregnancy risk category X*

**AVAILABLE FORMS**
*Injection:* 75 IU of luteinizing hormone (LH) and 75 IU of follicle-stimulating hormone (FSH) activity per ampule;

---

150 IU of LH and 150 IU of FSH activity per ampule.

## INDICATIONS & DOSAGES
➤ **Anovulation**
*Women:* 75 IU each of FSH and LH I.M. daily for 7 to 12 days; then 5,000 to 10,000 units of hCG I.M. 1 day after last dose of menotropins. Don't exceed 12 days of menotropins. Repeat for one to three menstrual cycles, until ovulation occurs.

➤ **Infertility with ovulation**
*Women:* 75 IU each of FSH and LH I.M. daily for 7 to 12 days; then 10,000 units hCG I.M. 1 day after last dose of menotropins. Repeated for two menstrual cycles. Then 150 IU each of FSH and LH daily for 7 to 12 days, followed by 10,000 units hCG I.M. 1 day after last dose of menotropins. Repeat for two menstrual cycles.

➤ **Infertility in men**
*Men:* Initially, 5,000 units hCG three times a week for 4 to 6 months; then 75 IU each of FSH and LH I.M. three times a week (given with 2,000 units hCG twice a week) for at least 4 months. If spermatogenesis doesn't improve, increase to 150 IU each of FSH and LH three times a week (no change in hCG dose).

## ACTION
In women who haven't had primary ovarian failure, drug mimics FSH in inducing follicular growth and LH in aiding follicular maturation. In men, drug induces spermatogenesis.

| Route | Onset | Peak | Duration |
|-------|-------|------|----------|
| I.M. | 9-12 days | Unknown | Unknown |

## ADVERSE REACTIONS
**CNS:** headache, malaise, fever, dizziness, *CVA.*
**CV:** tachycardia, venous thrombophlebitis, *arterial occlusion, pulmonary embolism.*
**GI:** nausea, vomiting, diarrhea, abdominal cramps, bloating.
**GU:** *ovarian enlargement with pain and abdominal distention,* multiple births, ovarian hyperstimulation syndrome, ovarian cysts, ectopic pregnancy.

**Musculoskeletal:** aches, joint pains.
**Respiratory:** atelectasis, *adult respiratory distress syndrome, pulmonary infarction,* dyspnea, tachypnea.
**Skin:** rash.
**Other:** *gynecomastia,* hypersensitivity reactions, *anaphylaxis,* chills.

## INTERACTIONS
None significant.

## EFFECTS ON LAB TEST RESULTS
• May increase or decrease AST and ALT levels in men.

## CONTRAINDICATIONS & CAUTIONS
• Contraindicated in patients hypersensitive to drug and in those with primary ovarian failure, uncontrolled thyroid or adrenal dysfunction, pituitary tumor, abnormal uterine bleeding, uterine fibromas, ovarian cysts or enlargement, or any cause of infertility other than anovulation.
• Contraindicated in pregnant women and in men with normal pituitary function, primary testicular failure, or infertility disorders other than hypogonadotropic hypogonadism.

## NURSING CONSIDERATIONS
• Prescriber should be experienced in fertility treatment.
• Monitor patient closely to ensure adequate ovarian stimulation without hyperstimulation.
• Watch for ovarian hyperstimulation syndrome, which may progress rapidly to a serious medical event characterized by dramatic increase in vascular permeability, which causes rapid accumulation of fluid in the peritoneal cavity, thorax, and pericardium. Evidence includes hypovolemia, hemoconcentration, electrolyte imbalance, ascites, hemoperitoneum, pleural effusion, hydrothorax, and thromboembolitic events. Condition is common and severe if patient becomes pregnant.
• Refrigerate powder or store at room temperature.
• Reconstitute with 1 to 2 ml of sterile normal saline solution for injection. Use immediately.
• Rotate injection sites.

**PATIENT TEACHING**
• Tell patient about possibility of multiple births. (It occurs about 20% of the time.)
• In women being treated for infertility, encourage daily intercourse from day before hCG is given until ovulation occurs.
• Instruct patient to immediately report severe abdominal pain, bloating, swelling of hands or feet, nausea, vomiting, diarrhea, substantial weight gain, or shortness of breath.

# 55

## Antidiabetics and glucagon

acarbose
chlorpropamide
glimepiride
glipizide
glipizide and metformin
   hydrochloride
glucagon
glyburide
glyburide and metformin
   hydrochloride
insulins
insulin aspart (rDNA origin)
   injection
insulin glargine (rDNA origin)
   injection
metformin hydrochloride
miglitol
nateglinide
pioglitazone hydrochloride
repaglinide
rosiglitazone maleate
rosiglitazone maleate and
   metformin hydrochloride

### COMBINATION PRODUCTS

AVANDAMET: 1 mg rosiglitazone and
500 mg metformin, 2 mg rosiglitazone
and 500 mg metformin, 4 mg rosiglitazone and 500 mg metformin
GLUCOVANCE: 1.25 mg glyburide and
250 mg metformin, 2.5 mg glyburide and
500 mg metformin, 5 mg glyburide and
500 mg metformin
METAGLIP: 2.5 mg glipizide and 250 mg
metformin, 2.5 mg glipizide and 500 mg
metformin, 5 mg glipizide and 500 mg
metformin

---

## acarbose
Prandase†, Precose

*Pregnancy risk category B*

### AVAILABLE FORMS
*Tablets:* 25 mg, 50 mg, 100 mg

### INDICATIONS & DOSAGES
➤ **Adjunct to diet to lower glucose level
in patients with type 2 (non–insulin-
dependent) diabetes mellitus whose hyperglycemia can't be managed by diet
alone or by diet and a sulfonylurea;
adjunct to insulin or metformin therapy
in patients with type 2 (non–insulin-
dependent) diabetes mellitus whose hyperglycemia can't be managed by diet,
exercise, and insulin or metformin alone**
*Adults:* Individualized. Initially, 25 mg
P.O. t.i.d. with first bite of each main meal.
Adjust dosage q 4 to 8 weeks, based on
1-hour postprandial glucose level and tolerance. Maintenance dosage is 50 to
100 mg P.O. t.i.d.
*Adjust-a-dose:* For patients weighing less
than 60 kg (132 lb), don't exceed 50 mg
P.O. t.i.d. For patients weighing more than
60 kg, don't exceed 100 mg P.O. t.i.d.

### ACTION
An alpha-glucosidase inhibitor that delays
digestion of carbohydrates, resulting in a
smaller increase in glucose level after
meals.

| Route | Onset | Peak | Duration |
|-------|-------|------|----------|
| P.O. | Unknown | 1 hr | 2-4 hr |

### ADVERSE REACTIONS
**GI:** *abdominal pain, diarrhea, flatulence.*
**Metabolic:** hypocalcemia.

### INTERACTIONS
**Drug-drug.** *Calcium channel blockers,
corticosteroids, estrogens, fosphenytoin,
hormonal contraceptives, isoniazid,
nicotinic acid, phenothiazine, phenytoin,
sympathomimetics, thiazides and other
diuretics, thyroid products:* May cause hyperglycemia when used together or hypoglycemia when withdrawn. Monitor glucose level.
*Digestive enzyme preparations containing
carbohydrate-splitting enzymes (such as
amylase, pancreatin), intestinal adsor-
bents (such as activated charcoal):* May
reduce effect of acarbose. Avoid using together.
*Digoxin:* May reduce digoxin concentration. Monitor digoxin level.

## EFFECTS ON LAB TEST RESULTS
• May increase ALT and AST levels. May decrease calcium and vitamin B$_6$ levels.
• May decrease hematocrit and hemoglobin.

## CONTRAINDICATIONS & CAUTIONS
• Contraindicated in patients hypersensitive to drug and in those with diabetic ketoacidosis, cirrhosis, inflammatory bowel disease, colonic ulceration, renal impairment, partial intestinal obstruction, predisposition to intestinal obstruction, chronic intestinal disease with marked disorder of digestion or absorption, or conditions that may deteriorate because of increased intestinal gas formation.
• Contraindicated in pregnant or breast-feeding patients and those with creatinine level greater than 2 mg/dl.
• Use cautiously in patients receiving a sulfonylurea or insulin.
• Safety and efficacy of drug haven't been established in children.

## NURSING CONSIDERATIONS
• Closely monitor patients receiving a sulfonylurea or insulin; acarbose may increase risk of hypoglycemia. If hypoglycemia occurs, treat patient with oral glucose (dextrose). Severe hypoglycemia may require I.V. glucose infusion or glucagon administration. Because dosage adjustments may be needed to prevent further hypoglycemia, report hypoglycemia and treatment required to prescriber.
• Insulin therapy may be needed during increased stress (infection, fever, surgery, or trauma). Monitor patient closely for hyperglycemia.
• Monitor patient's 1-hour postprandial glucose level to determine therapeutic effectiveness of acarbose and to identify appropriate dose. Report hyperglycemia to prescriber. Thereafter, measure glycosylated hemoglobin every 3 months.
• Monitor transaminase level every 3 months in first year of therapy and periodically thereafter in patients receiving more than 50 mg three times a day. Report abnormalities; dosage adjustment or drug withdrawal may be needed.

## PATIENT TEACHING
• Tell patient to take drug daily with first bite of each of three main meals.
• Explain that therapy relieves symptoms but doesn't cure disease.
• Stress importance of adhering to therapeutic regimen, specific diet, weight reduction, exercise, and hygiene programs. Show patient how to monitor glucose level and to recognize and treat hyperglycemia.
• Teach patient taking a sulfonylurea how to recognize hypoglycemia. Advise treating symptoms with a form of dextrose rather than with a product containing table sugar.
• Urge patient to wear or carry medical identification at all times.
• Advise patient that adverse reactions usually occur in the first few weeks of therapy and diminish over time.

---

# chlorpropamide
Apo-Chlorpropamide†, Diabinese

*Pregnancy risk category C*

---

## AVAILABLE FORMS
*Tablets:* 100 mg, 250 mg

## INDICATIONS & DOSAGES
➤ **Adjunct to diet to lower glucose level in patients with type 2 (non–insulin-dependent) diabetes mellitus**
*Adults:* Initially, 250 mg P.O. daily with breakfast. Increase first dose after 5 to 7 days because of extended duration of action; then increase q 3 to 5 days by 50 to 125 mg, if needed, to maximum of 750 mg daily. Some patients with mild diabetes respond well to 100 mg daily or less.
*Adjust-a-dose:* In patients older than age 65, initially, 100 to 125 mg P.O. daily; then increase as with adult dose. In patients with renal or hepatic impairment, use lower first doses, and increase dosage as tolerated.
➤ **To change from insulin to oral therapy**
*Adults:* If insulin dosage is 40 units or less daily, stop insulin and start oral therapy as above. If insulin dosage is more than 40 units daily, start oral therapy as above with insulin reduced by 50%. Further reduce insulin dosage, according to response.

---

## ACTION

Unknown. A sulfonylurea that probably stimulates insulin release from pancreatic beta cells, reduces glucose output by the liver, increases peripheral sensitivity to insulin, and has an antidiuretic effect in patients with diabetes insipidus.

| Route | Onset | Peak | Duration |
|-------|-------|------|----------|
| P.O. | 1 hr | 2-4 hr | 24-60 hr |

## ADVERSE REACTIONS

**CNS:** paresthesia, fatigue, dizziness, vertigo, malaise, headache.
**CV:** *increased risk of cardiovascular death.*
**EENT:** tinnitus.
**GI:** nausea, heartburn, epigastric distress.
**GU:** tea-colored urine.
**Hematologic:** *leukopenia, thrombocytopenia, aplastic anemia, agranulocytosis,* hemolytic anemia.
**Hepatic:** cholestatic jaundice.
**Metabolic:** *prolonged hypoglycemia,* dilutional hyponatremia.
**Skin:** rash, pruritus, erythema, urticaria.
**Other:** *disulfiram-like reactions,* hypersensitivity reactions.

## INTERACTIONS

**Drug-drug.** *Anabolic steroids, chloramphenicol, clofibrate, guanethidine, MAO inhibitors, salicylates, sulfonamides:* May increase hypoglycemic activity. Monitor glucose level.
*Beta blockers:* May prolong hypoglycemic effect and masks symptoms of hypoglycemia. Use together cautiously.
*Corticosteroids, glucagon, phenytoin, rifampin, thiazide diuretics:* May decrease hypoglycemic response. Monitor glucose level.
*Oral anticoagulants:* May increase hypoglycemic activity or enhances anticoagulant effect. Monitor glucose level, PT, and INR.
**Drug-herb.** *Bitter melon (karela), burdock, dandelion, eucalyptus, ginkgo biloba, marshmallow:* May increase hypoglycemic effects. Discourage use together.
**Drug-lifestyle.** *Alcohol use:* May alter glycemic control, most commonly causing hypoglycemia. May also cause a disulfiram-like reaction. Discourage use together.

## EFFECTS ON LAB TEST RESULTS
• May increase BUN, creatinine, alkaline phosphatase, bilirubin, AST, LDH, and cholesterol levels. May decrease glucose and sodium levels.
• May decrease hemoglobin and WBC, platelet, and granulocyte counts.

## CONTRAINDICATIONS & CAUTIONS
• Contraindicated in pregnant women, breast-feeding women, patients hypersensitive to drug, and those with type 2 diabetes complicated by ketosis, acidosis, diabetic coma, major surgery, severe infections, or severe trauma.
• Contraindicated for treating type 1 (insulin-dependent) diabetes or diabetes that can be adequately controlled by diet.
• Use cautiously in patients with porphyria or impaired hepatic or renal function, or in debilitated, malnourished, or elderly patients.
• Use cautiously in patients allergic to sulfonamides.

## NURSING CONSIDERATIONS
• Elderly patients may be more sensitive to therapeutic and adverse effects.
• Drug may accumulate in patients with renal insufficiency. Watch for and report signs of impending renal insufficiency, such as dysuria, anuria, and hematuria.
• *Alert:* Adverse effects of drug, especially hypoglycemia, may be more frequent, prolonged, or severe than with some other sulfonylureas because of drug's long duration of action. If hypoglycemia occurs, monitor patient closely for minimum of 3 to 5 days.
• Patients switching from another oral antidiabetic don't usually need a transition period.
• Patients may need hospitalization during transition from insulin to an oral antidiabetic. Monitor patient's glucose level at least three times daily before meals.
• *Alert:* Don't confuse chlorpropamide with chlorpromazine.

## PATIENT TEACHING
• Instruct patient about nature of disease and importance of following therapeutic regimen, adhering to specific diet, losing weight, getting exercise, following personal hygiene programs, and avoiding infec-

tion. Explain how and when to monitor glucose level, and teach recognition of and intervention for both low and high glucose levels. .

● Make sure patient understands that therapy relieves symptoms but doesn't cure the disease. He should also understand potential risks and advantages of taking drug and of other treatment methods.

● Advise woman planning pregnancy to consult prescriber before becoming pregnant. Insulin may be needed during pregnancy and breast-feeding.

● Tell patient not to change drug dosage without prescriber's consent and to report abnormal blood or urine glucose test results.

● Teach patient to carry candy or other simple sugars to treat mild low glucose episodes. Patient experiencing severe episode may need hospital treatment.

● Advise patient not to take other drugs, including OTC drugs, without first checking with prescriber.

● *Alert:* Advise patient to avoid alcohol consumption. Signs and symptoms of chlorpropamide-alcohol flush are facial flushing, light-headedness, headache, and occasional breathlessness. Even very small amounts of alcohol can produce this reaction.

● Advise patient to wear or carry medical identification at all times.

● *Alert:* Tell patient to report rash, skin eruptions, and other signs and symptoms of hypersensitivity to prescriber immediately.

---

## glimepiride
Amaryl

*Pregnancy risk category C*

---

### AVAILABLE FORMS
*Tablets:* 1 mg, 2 mg, 4 mg

### INDICATIONS & DOSAGES
➤ **Adjunct to diet and exercise to lower glucose level in patients with type 2 (non–insulin-dependent) diabetes mellitus whose hyperglycemia can't be managed by diet and exercise alone**
*Adults:* Initially, 1 or 2 mg P.O. once daily with first main meal of day; usual mainte-

nance dose is 1 to 4 mg P.O. once daily. After reaching 2 mg, dosage is increased in increments not exceeding 2 mg q 1 to 2 weeks, based on patient's glucose level response. Maximum dose is 8 mg/day.
➤ **Adjunct to diet and exercise in conjunction with insulin or metformin therapy in patients with type 2 diabetes mellitus whose hyperglycemia can't be managed with the maximum dosage of glimepiride alone**
*Adults:* 8 mg P.O. once daily with first main meal of day; used with low-dose insulin or metformin. Increase insulin or metformin dosage weekly, p.r.n., based on patient's glucose level response.
***Adjust-a-dose:*** For renally or hepatically impaired patients, initially, 1 mg P.O. once daily with first main meal of day; then adjust to appropriate dosage, p.r.n.

### ACTION
Unknown. Lowers glucose level, possibly by stimulating release of insulin from functioning pancreatic beta cells. Drug also can lead to increased sensitivity of peripheral tissues to insulin.

| Route | Onset | Peak | Duration |
|-------|-------|--------|----------|
| P.O. | 1 hr | 2-3 hr | > 24 hr |

### ADVERSE REACTIONS
**CNS:** dizziness, asthenia, headache.
**EENT:** changes in accommodation.
**GI:** nausea.
**Hematologic:** *leukopenia,* hemolytic anemia, *agranulocytosis, thrombocytopenia, aplastic anemia, pancytopenia.*
**Hepatic:** cholestatic jaundice.
**Metabolic:** *hypoglycemia,* dilutional hyponatremia.
**Skin:** pruritus, erythema, urticaria, morbilliform or maculopapular eruptions, photosensitivity reactions.

### INTERACTIONS
**Drug-drug.** *Beta blockers:* May mask symptoms of hypoglycemia. Monitor glucose level.
*Drugs that tend to produce hyperglycemia (such as corticosteroids, estrogens, fosphenytoin, hormonal contraceptives, isoniazid, nicotinic acid, other diuretics, phenothiazines, phenytoin, sympathomimetic*

---

*thiazides, thyroid products):* May lead to loss of glucose control. Adjust dosage.
*Insulin:* May increase risk of hypoglycemia. Avoid using together.
*NSAIDs, other drugs that are highly protein-bound (such as beta blockers, chloramphenicol, coumarin, MAO inhibitors, probenecid, salicylates, sulfonamides):* May increase hypoglycemic action of sulfonylureas such as glimepiride. Monitor glucose level carefully.
**Drug-herb.** *Burdock, dandelion, eucalyptus, marshmallow:* May increase hypoglycemic effects. Discourage use together.
**Drug-lifestyle.** *Alcohol use:* May alter glycemic control, most commonly causing hypoglycemia. May also cause disulfiram-like reaction. Discourage use together.

### EFFECTS ON LAB TEST RESULTS
● May increase BUN, creatinine, alkaline phosphatase, and AST levels. May decrease glucose and sodium levels.
● May decrease hemoglobin and WBC, RBC, platelet, and granulocyte counts.

### CONTRAINDICATIONS & CAUTIONS
● Contraindicated in patients hypersensitive to drug and in those with diabetic ketoacidosis, which should be treated with insulin.
● Contraindicated in pregnant or elderly patients and as sole therapy for type 1 diabetes.
● Contraindicated in breast-feeding patients because it may cause hypoglycemia in breast-fed infants.
● Use cautiously in debilitated or malnourished patients and in those with adrenal, pituitary, hepatic, or renal insufficiency; these patients are more susceptible to the hypoglycemic action of glucose-lowering drugs.
● Use cautiously in patients allergic to sulfonamides.
● Safety and effectiveness of drug in children haven't been established.

### NURSING CONSIDERATIONS
● Glimepiride and insulin may be used together in patients who lose glucose control after first responding to therapy.
● Monitor fasting glucose level periodically to determine therapeutic response. Also monitor glycosylated hemoglobin, usually

every 3 to 6 months, to precisely assess long-term glycemic control.
● Use of oral hypoglycemics may carry higher risk of CV mortality than use of diet alone or of diet and insulin therapy.
● When changing patient from other sulfonylureas to glimepiride, a transition period isn't needed.
● *Alert:* Don't confuse glimepiride with glyburide or glipizide.

### PATIENT TEACHING
● Tell patient to take drug with first meal of the day.
● Make sure patient understands that therapy relieves symptoms but doesn't cure the disease. He should also understand potential risks and advantages of taking drug and of other treatment methods.
● Stress importance of adhering to diet, weight reduction, exercise, and personal hygiene programs. Explain to patient and family how and when to monitor glucose level, and teach recognition of and intervention for signs and symptoms of high and low glucose levels.
● Advise patient to wear or carry medical identification at all times.
● Advise woman to consult prescriber before planning pregnancy. Insulin may be needed during pregnancy and breast-feeding.
● Advise patient to consult prescriber before taking any OTC products.
● Teach patient to carry candy or other simple sugars to treat mild episodes of low glucose level. Patient experiencing severe episode may need hospital treatment.
● Advise patient to avoid alcohol, which lowers glucose level.

## glipizide
Glucotrol⌀, Glucotrol XL⌀, Minidiab‡

*Pregnancy risk category C*

### AVAILABLE FORMS
*Tablets (extended-release):* 2.5 mg, 5 mg, 10 mg
*Tablets (immediate-release):* 5 mg, 10 mg

## INDICATIONS & DOSAGES
➤ **Adjunct to diet to lower glucose level in patients with type 2 (non–insulin-dependent) diabetes mellitus**
*Immediate-release tablets*
*Elderly patients:* For patients older than age 65, first dose is 2.5 mg P.O. daily.
*Adults:* Initially, 5 mg P.O. daily 30 minutes before breakfast. Maximum once-daily dose is 15 mg. Divide doses of more than 15 mg. Maximum total daily dose is 40 mg.
*Extended-release tablets*
*Adults:* Initially, 5 mg P.O. with breakfast daily. Increase by 5 mg q 3 months, depending on level of glycemic control. Maximum daily dose is 20 mg.
*Adjust-a-dose:* For patients with liver disease, first dose is 2.5 mg P.O. daily.
➤ **To replace insulin therapy**
*Adults:* If insulin dosage is more than 20 units daily, start patient at usual dosage in addition to 50% of insulin. If insulin dosage is less than or equal to 20 units daily, insulin may be stopped when glipizide starts.

## ACTION
Unknown. A sulfonylurea that probably stimulates insulin release from pancreatic beta cells, reduces glucose output by the liver, and increases peripheral sensitivity to insulin.

| Route | Onset | Peak | Duration |
|---|---|---|---|
| P.O. (immediate-release) | 15-30 min | 1-3 hr | 24 hr |
| P.O. (extended-release) | 2-3 hr | 6-12 hr | 24 hr |

## ADVERSE REACTIONS
**CNS:** dizziness, drowsiness, headache.
**GI:** nausea, constipation, diarrhea.
**Hematologic:** *leukopenia,* hemolytic anemia, *agranulocytosis, thrombocytopenia, aplastic anemia.*
**Hepatic:** cholestatic jaundice.
**Metabolic:** *hypoglycemia.*
**Skin:** rash, pruritus, photosensitivity.

## INTERACTIONS
**Drug-drug.** *Amantadine, anabolic steroids, antifungal antibiotics (miconazole, fluconazole), chloramphenicol, clofi-brate, guanethidine, MAO inhibitors, probenecid, salicylates, sulfonamides:* May increase hypoglycemic activity. Monitor glucose level.
*Beta blockers:* May prolong hypoglycemic effect and mask symptoms of hypoglycemia. Use together cautiously.
*Corticosteroids, glucagon, phenytoin, rifampin, thiazide diuretics:* May decrease hypoglycemic response. Monitor glucose level.
*Oral anticoagulants:* May increase hypoglycemic activity or enhanced anticoagulant effect. Monitor glucose level, PT, and INR.
**Drug-herb.** *Burdock, dandelion, eucalyptus, marshmallow:* May increase hypoglycemic effects. Discourage use together.
**Drug-lifestyle.** *Alcohol use:* May alter glycemic control, most commonly causing hypoglycemia. May cause disulfiram-like reaction. Discourage use together.

## EFFECTS ON LAB TEST RESULTS
● May increase BUN, creatinine, alkaline phosphatase, AST, and cholesterol levels. May decrease glucose level.
● May decrease hemoglobin and WBC, platelet, and granulocyte counts.

## CONTRAINDICATIONS & CAUTIONS
● Contraindicated in patients hypersensitive to drug and in those with diabetic ketoacidosis with or without coma.
● Contraindicated in pregnant or breast-feeding women and as sole therapy in type 1 diabetes.
● Use cautiously in patients with renal or hepatic disease, in those allergic to sulfonamides, and in debilitated, malnourished, or elderly patients.

## NURSING CONSIDERATIONS
● Give immediate-release tablet about 30 minutes before meals.
● Some patients may attain effective control on a once-daily regimen, whereas others respond better with divided dosing.
● Patient may switch from immediate-release dose to extended-release tablets at the nearest equivalent total daily dose.
● Glipizide is a second-generation sulfonylurea. The frequency of adverse reactions appears to be lower than with first-generation drugs such as chlorpropamide.

• During periods of increased stress, patient may need insulin therapy. Monitor patient closely for hyperglycemia in these situations.

• Patient switching from insulin therapy to an oral antidiabetic should check glucose level at least three times a day before meals. Patient may need hospitalization during transition.

• **Alert:** Don't confuse glipizide with glyburide or glimepiride.

## PATIENT TEACHING
• Instruct patient about disease and importance of following therapeutic regimen, adhering to diet, losing weight, getting exercise, following personal hygiene programs, and avoiding infection. Explain how and when to monitor glucose level, and teach recognition of episodes of low and high glucose levels.

• Tell patient to carry candy or other simple sugars to treat mild low glucose episodes. Patient experiencing severe episode may need hospital treatment.

• Instruct patient not to change drug dosage without prescriber's consent and to report abnormal blood or urine glucose test results.

• Tell patient not to take other drugs, including OTC drugs, without first checking with prescriber.

• Advise patient to wear or carry medical identification at all times.

• Advise woman planning pregnancy to first consult prescriber. Insulin may be needed during pregnancy and breast-feeding.

• Advise patient to avoid alcohol, which lowers glucose level.

---

## glipizide and metformin hydrochloride
Metaglip

*Pregnancy risk category C*

## AVAILABLE FORMS
*Tablets:* 2.5 mg glipizide and 250 mg metformin hydrochloride; 2.5 mg glipizide and 500 mg metformin; 5 mg glipizide and 500 mg metformin

## INDICATIONS & DOSAGES
➤ **First-line therapy, adjunct to diet and exercise, to improve glycemic control in patients with type 2 diabetes**
*Adults:* Initially, 2.5 mg/250 mg P.O. once daily with a meal. In patients whose fasting glucose is 280 to 320 mg/dl, start with 2.5 mg/500 mg P.O. b.i.d. Dosage may be increased in increments of one tablet per day q 2 weeks, up to a maximum of 10 mg/1,000 mg or 10 mg/2,000 mg daily in divided doses.
➤ **Second-line therapy in patients with type 2 diabetes for whom diet, exercise, and initial treatment with a sulfonylurea or metformin don't provide adequate glycemic control**
*Adults:* Initially, 2.5 mg/500 mg or 5 mg/500 mg P.O. b.i.d. with the morning and evening meals. Increase in increments of no more than 5 mg/500 mg, up to the minimum effective dose needed to adequately control glucose or to a maximum daily dose of 20 mg/2,000 mg.

## ACTION
Appears to lower glucose level by stimulating the pancreas to release insulin. Metformin decreases hepatic glucose production and intestinal absorption of glucose and improves insulin sensitivity.

| Route | Onset | Peak | Duration |
|---|---|---|---|
| P.O. (glipizide) | 15-30 min | 1-3 hr | Unknown |
| P.O. (metformin) | Unknown | Unknown | Unknown |

## ADVERSE REACTIONS
**CNS:** *headache*, dizziness.
**CV:** hypertension.
**GI:** nausea, *diarrhea*, vomiting, abdominal pain.
**GU:** UTI.
**Metabolic:** hypoglycemia, *lactic acidosis*.
**Musculoskeletal:** pain.
**Respiratory:** *upper respiratory tract infection*.

## INTERACTIONS
**Drug-drug.** *Azoles, beta blockers, chloramphenicol, coumarins, MAO inhibitors, NSAIDs, probenecid, salicylates, sulfonamides:* May increase the effect of sulfonylureas. Monitor closely for hypogly-

cemia. May increase loss of glucose control when these drugs are withdrawn.

*Calcium channel blockers, corticosteroids, estrogens, highly protein-bound drugs, isoniazid, hormonal contraceptives, nicotinic acid, phenytoin, phenothiazines, sympathomimetics, thyroid products, thiazides and other diuretics:* May increase risk of hyperglycemia and loss of glucose control. May increase risk of hypoglycemia when these drugs are withdrawn. Monitor glucose level.

*Cationic drugs (amiloride, digoxin, morphine, procainamide, quinidine, quinine, ranitidine, triamterene, trimethoprim, vancomycin):* May increase metformin level. Monitor patient carefully.

*Furosemide:* May increase metformin level and decreases furosemide level. Monitor patient closely.

*Iodinated contrast material used in radiologic studies:* May increase risk of acute renal failure. Stop the drug for 48 hours before and after such tests.

*Nifedipine:* May increase metformin level. Metformin dose may need to be decreased.

**Drug-herb.** *Juniper berries, ginseng, garlic, fenugreek, coriander, dandelion root, celery:* May increase risk of hypoglycemia. Discourage use together.

**Drug-lifestyle.** *Alcohol use:* May increase risk of hypoglycemia and lactic acidosis. Discourage use together.

### EFFECTS ON LAB TEST RESULTS
• May decrease glucose and vitamin $B_{12}$ levels.

### CONTRAINDICATIONS & CAUTIONS
• Contraindicated in patients hypersensitive to any components of the drug and in those with renal disease, creatinine level at least 1.5 mg/dl in men and at least 1.4 mg/dl in women, abnormal creatinine clearance, heart failure, shock, acute MI, septicemia, or acute or chronic metabolic acidosis, including diabetic ketoacidosis.
• Contraindicated after surgical procedures, in pregnant or breast-feeding patients, and in patients age 80 or older unless renal function is normal..
• Use cautiously in elderly patients and in patients with hepatic dysfunction, malnourished or debilitated patients, and

those with adrenal or pituitary insufficiency. Don't give elderly patients the maximum dose.
• Use cautiously in patients with abnormal vitamin $B_{12}$ level or hypoglycemia and in those who consume alcohol.

### NURSING CONSIDERATIONS
• Temporarily stop drug in patients undergoing radiologic studies involving iodinated contrast materials or any surgical procedure.
• To reduce the risk of lactic acidosis, use the minimum effective dose and monitor renal function regularly during treatment.
• Stop drug in patients with any condition linked to hypoxemia, dehydration, or sepsis.
• Evaluate patient for ketoacidosis or lactic acidosis if laboratory abnormalities or vague, poorly defined illness occurs. Stop drug immediately if acidosis occurs.
• Periodically monitor fasting glucose level and glycosylated hemoglobin.
• Monitor CBC and renal function annually.
• Drug shouldn't be used in pregnant patients unless the benefits outweigh the risks. If the drug is used, stop therapy at least 1 month before delivery.

### PATIENT TEACHING
• Tell patient to take once daily with breakfast or twice daily with breakfast and dinner.
• Tell patient to immediately report signs of lactic acidosis—unexplained hyperventilation, myalgia, malaise, unusual drowsiness, suddenly developing a slow or irregular heartbeat, or feeling cold, dizzy, or light-headed.
• Tell patient that GI symptoms are common during initial therapy but should resolve. Tell patient to report persistent or new onset of GI symptoms.
• Advise patient to avoid alcohol intake.
• Teach patient about diabetes and the warning signs of hypoglycemia and hyperglycemia, along with how to self-monitor glucose level. Also teach patient the importance of good hygiene to help avoid infections and of adhering to diet, exercise, and medication schedule.
• Instruct patient to wear or carry medical identification.

---

Reactions may be *common,* uncommon, *life-threatening,* or COMMON AND LIFE-THREATENING.

# glucagon
GlucaGen Diagnostic Kit,
Glucagon Diagnostic Kit,
Glucagon Emergency Kit

*Pregnancy risk category B*

## AVAILABLE FORMS
*Powder for injection:* 1-mg (1-unit) vial

## INDICATIONS & DOSAGES
➤ **Hypoglycemia**
*Adults and children weighing more than
20 kg (44 lb):* 1 mg (1 unit) I.V., I.M., S.C.
*Children weighing 20 kg or less:* 0.5 mg
(0.5 units) or 20 to 30 mcg/kg I.V., I.M.,
S.C.; maximum dose 1 mg. May repeat in
15 minutes, if needed. I.V. glucose must
be given if patient fails to respond.
➤ **Diagnostic aid for radiologic examination**
*Adults:* 0.25 to 2 mg I.V. or I.M. before radiologic examination.

## I.V. ADMINISTRATION
• Reconstitute drug in 1-unit vial with
1 ml of diluent. Use only diluent supplied
by manufacturer when preparing doses of
2 mg or less. For larger doses, dilute with
sterile water for injection.
• Unstable hypoglycemic diabetic patients
may not respond to glucagon; give dextrose I.V. instead.

## ACTION
Raises glucose level by promoting catalytic depolymerization of hepatic glycogen to
glucose. Relaxes the smooth muscle of the
stomach, duodenum, small bowel, and
colon.

| Route | Onset | Peak | Duration |
|---|---|---|---|
| I.V. (hyper-glycemia) | Immediate | 30 min | 60-90 min |
| I.V. (gastric relaxation) | 1 min | 30 min | 9-25 min |
| I.M., S.C. | 4-10 min | Unknown | 12-32 min |

## ADVERSE REACTIONS
**GI:** nausea, vomiting.
**Respiratory:** *bronchospasm, respiratory
distress.*
**Other:** hypersensitivity reactions.

## INTERACTIONS
**Drug-drug.** *Anticoagulants:* May enhance
anticoagulant effect. Monitor prothrombin
activity, and watch for signs of bleeding.

## EFFECTS ON LAB TEST RESULTS
• May decrease potassium level.

## CONTRAINDICATIONS & CAUTIONS
• Contraindicated in patients hypersensitive to drug and in those with pheochromocytoma.
• Use cautiously in patients with history
of insulinoma or pheochromocytoma.

## NURSING CONSIDERATIONS
• Use drug only in emergency situations.
• Monitor glucose level before, during,
and after administration.
• *Alert:* Arouse patient from coma as
quickly as possible and give additional
carbohydrates orally to prevent secondary
hypoglycemic reactions.
• *Alert:* Don't confuse glucagon with
Glaucon.

## PATIENT TEACHING
• Instruct patient and caregivers how to
give glucagon and recognize a low glucose episode.
• Explain importance of calling prescriber
at once in emergencies.

# glyburide (glibenclamide)
DiaBeta✐, Euglucon†, Glynase
PresTab, Micronase✐

*Pregnancy risk category B*

## AVAILABLE FORMS
*Tablets:* 1.25 mg, 2.5 mg, 5 mg
*Tablets (micronized):* 1.5 mg, 3 mg,
4.5 mg, 6 mg

## INDICATIONS & DOSAGES
➤ **Adjunct to diet to lower glucose level
in patients with type 2 (non–insulin-
dependent) diabetes mellitus**
*Nonmicronized*
*Adults:* Initially, 2.5 to 5 mg P.O. once
daily with breakfast or first main meal.
Usual daily maintenance dosage is 1.25 to
20 mg, as single dose or divided doses.
Maximum daily dose is 20 mg P.O.

*Micronized*
*Adults:* Initially, 1.5 to 3 mg daily with breakfast or first main meal. Usual daily maintenance dosage is 0.75 to 12 mg. Dosages exceeding 6 mg daily may have better response with b.i.d. dosing. Maximum dose is 12 mg P.O. daily.
*Adjust-a-dose:* For patients who are more sensitive to antidiabetics and for those with adrenal or pituitary insufficiency, start with 1.25 mg daily. When using micronized tablets, patients who are more sensitive to antidiabetics should start with 0.75 mg daily.
➤ **To replace insulin therapy**
*Adults:* If insulin dosage is less than 40 units/day, patient may be switched directly to glyburide when insulin is stopped. If insulin dosage is 40 or more units/day, initially, 5-mg regular tablets or 3-mg micronized formulation can be given P.O. once daily in addition to 50% of insulin dosage.

## ACTION
Unknown. A sulfonylurea that probably stimulates insulin release from pancreatic beta cells, reduces glucose output by the liver, and increases peripheral sensitivity to insulin.

| Route | Onset | Peak | Duration |
|---|---|---|---|
| P.O. (micronized) | 1 hr | 1 hr | 12-24 hr |
| P.O. (non-micronized) | 2-4 hr | 2-4 hr | 16-24 hr |

## ADVERSE REACTIONS
**EENT:** changes in accommodation or blurred vision.
**GI:** nausea, epigastric fullness, heartburn.
**Hematologic:** *leukopenia,* hemolytic anemia, *agranulocytosis, thrombocytopenia, aplastic anemia.*
**Hepatic:** cholestatic jaundice, *hepatitis.*
**Metabolic:** *hypoglycemia.*
**Musculoskeletal:** arthralgia, myalgia.
**Skin:** rash, pruritus, other allergic reactions.
**Other:** *angioedema.*

## INTERACTIONS
**Drug-drug.** *Anabolic steroids, chloramphenicol, clofibrate, guanethidine, MAO inhibitors, probenecid, phenylbutazone,*

*salicylates, sulfonamides:* May increase hypoglycemic activity. Monitor glucose level.
*Beta blockers:* May prolong hypoglycemic effect and mask symptoms of hypoglycemia. Use together cautiously.
*Carbamazepine, corticosteroids, glucagon, rifampin, thiazide diuretics:* May decrease hypoglycemic response. Monitor glucose level.
*Oral anticoagulants:* May increase hypoglycemic activity or enhance anticoagulant effect. Monitor glucose level, PT, and INR.
**Drug-herb.** *Burdock, dandelion, eucalyptus, marshmallow:* May increase hypoglycemic effect. Discourage use together.
**Drug-lifestyle.** *Alcohol use:* May alter glycemic control, most commonly causing hypoglycemia. May cause disulfiram-like reaction. Discourage use together.

## EFFECTS ON LAB TEST RESULTS
● May increase BUN, alkaline phosphatase, bilirubin, AST, ALT, and cholesterol levels. May decrease glucose level.
● May decrease hemoglobin and WBC, platelet, and granulocyte counts.

## CONTRAINDICATIONS & CAUTIONS
● Contraindicated in patients hypersensitive to drug and in those with diabetic ketoacidosis with or without coma.
● Contraindicated as sole therapy for type 1 diabetes and in pregnant or breast-feeding women.
● Use cautiously in patients with hepatic or renal impairment; in debilitated, malnourished, or elderly patients; and in patients allergic to sulfonamides.

## NURSING CONSIDERATIONS
● *Alert:* Micronized glyburide (Glynase PresTab) contains drug in a smaller particle size and isn't bioequivalent to regular glyburide tablets. Patients who have been taking Micronase or DiaBeta need dosage readjustment.
● Although most patients may take drug once daily, those taking more than 10 mg daily may achieve better results with twice-daily dosage.
● Glyburide is a second-generation sulfonylurea. Adverse effects are less common with second-generation drugs than

---

Reactions may be *common,* uncommon, *life-threatening,* or COMMON AND LIFE-THREATENING.

with first-generation drugs such as chlor-propamide.
- During periods of increased stress, such as infection, fever, surgery, or trauma, patient may need insulin therapy. Monitor patient closely for hyperglycemia in these situations.
- Patient switching from insulin therapy to an oral antidiabetic should check glucose level at least three times a day before meals. Patient may need hospitalization during transition.
- *Alert:* Don't confuse glyburide with glimepiride or glipizide.
- DiaBeta may contain tartrazine.

## PATIENT TEACHING
- Instruct patient about nature of disease and importance of following therapeutic regimen, adhering to specific diet, losing weight, getting exercise, following personal hygiene programs, and avoiding infection. Explain how and when to monitor glucose level, and teach recognition of and intervention for low and high glucose episodes.
- Tell patient not to change drug dosage without prescriber's consent and to report abnormal blood or urine glucose test results.
- Teach patient to carry candy or other simple sugars to treat mild low glucose episodes. Patient experiencing severe episode may need hospital treatment.
- Advise patient not to take other drugs, including OTC drugs, without first checking with prescriber.
- Advise patient to wear or carry medical identification at all times.
- *Alert:* Instruct patient to report episodes of low glucose to prescriber immediately; severe low glucose is sometimes fatal in patients receiving as little as 2.5 to 5 mg glyburide daily.
- Advise patient to avoid alcohol, which may lower glucose level.

# glyburide and metformin hydrochloride
Glucovance

*Pregnancy risk category B*

## AVAILABLE FORMS
*Tablets:* 1.25 mg glyburide/250 mg metformin hydrochloride, 2.5 mg glyburide/500 mg metformin hydrochloride, 5 mg glyburide/500 mg metformin hydrochloride

## INDICATIONS & DOSAGES
➤ **Adjunct to diet and exercise to improve glycemic control in patients with type 2 (non–insulin-dependent) diabetes whose hyperglycemia can't be controlled with diet and exercise alone**
*Adults:* Initially, 1.25 mg glyburide/250 mg metformin hydrochloride P.O. once daily or b.i.d. with meals. In patients with $HbA_{1c}$ greater than 9% or a fasting glucose level greater than 200 mg/dl, start with 1.25 mg glyburide/250 mg metformin hydrochloride b.i.d. with morning and evening meals. May increase daily dose by 1.25 mg glyburide/250 mg metformin hydrochloride q 2 weeks, up to the minimum effective dose needed to achieve adequate control of glucose level. Maximum daily dose is 20 mg glyburide/2,000 mg metformin.
➤ **Second-line therapy in patients with type 2 diabetes when diet, exercise, and first-line treatment with a sulfonylurea or metformin don't adequately control glucose level**
*Adults:* Initially, 2.5 mg glyburide/500 mg metformin hydrochloride or 5 mg glyburide/500 mg metformin hydrochloride b.i.d. with meals. Increase by no more than 5 mg glyburide/500 mg metformin hydrochloride, up to the minimum effective dose needed to achieve adequate glucose level control. Maximum daily dose is 20 mg glyburide/2,000 mg metformin hydrochloride.
*Adjust-a-dose:* In elderly patients, first and maintenance dosing is conservative because of the potential for decreased renal function in these patients. Any dosage adjustment requires careful assessment of renal function. In elderly, debilitated, or

malnourished patients, don't give the maximum dosage to avoid the risk of hypoglycemia.

## ACTION
Unknown. Glyburide may lower glucose level by stimulating the release of insulin from the pancreas. Metformin decreases hepatic glucose production and intestinal absorption of glucose and improves insulin sensitivity.

| Route | Onset | Peak | Duration |
| --- | --- | --- | --- |
| P.O. (glyburide) | 1 hr | 4 hr | 16-24 hr |
| P.O. (metformin) | Unknown | Unknown | Unknown |

## ADVERSE REACTIONS
**CNS:** headache, dizziness.
**GI:** *diarrhea,* nausea, vomiting, abdominal pain.
**Metabolic:** *hypoglycemia, lactic acidosis.*
**Respiratory:** *upper respiratory tract infection.*

## INTERACTIONS
**Drug-drug.** *Beta blockers, chloramphenicol, ciprofloxacin, coumarin, highly protein-bound drugs, MAO inhibitors, miconazole, NSAIDs, probenecid, salicylates, sulfonamides:* May increase hypoglycemic activity of glyburide. Monitor glucose level.
*Calcium channel blockers, corticosteroids, estrogens, hormonal contraceptives, isoniazid, nicotinic acid, phenothiazines, phenytoin, sympathomimetics, thiazides and other diuretics, thyroid agents:* May cause hyperglycemia. Monitor glucose level.
*Cationic drugs (such as amiloride, cimetidine, digoxin, morphine, procainamide, quinidine, quinine, ranitidine, triamterene, trimethoprim, vancomycin):* May increase metformin level. Monitor glucose level.
*Furosemide:* May increase metformin level and decrease furosemide level. Monitor patient closely.
*Nifedipine:* May increase metformin level. Metformin dosage may need to be decreased.
**Drug-lifestyle.** *Alcohol use:* May alter glycemic control, most commonly causing hypoglycemia. May cause disulfiram-like reaction with glyburide component. Discourage use together.

## EFFECTS ON LAB TEST RESULTS
● May increase lactate level. May decrease glucose and vitamin $B_{12}$ levels.

## CONTRAINDICATIONS & CAUTIONS
● Contraindicated in patients hypersensitive to glyburide or metformin and in those with renal disease, renal dysfunction, or metabolic acidosis (including diabetic ketoacidosis).
● Contraindicated in breast-feeding women and patients with heart failure requiring pharmacologic treatment.
● Use cautiously in elderly, hepatically impaired, debilitated, or malnourished patients and in those with adrenal or pituitary insufficiency because of increased risk of hypoglycemia.

## NURSING CONSIDERATIONS
● In elderly patients, monitor renal function regularly.
● For patients requiring additional glycemic control, a thiazolidinedione may be added to Glucovance therapy.
● Assess glucose level before and regularly after therapy. Monitor glycosylated hemoglobin to assess long-term therapy.
● *Alert:* Obtain baseline renal function studies and don't start drug if creatinine level is 1.5 mg/dl or greater (in men) or 1.4 mg/dl or greater (in women). Monitor renal function at least once yearly while patient is on long-term therapy and more often if renal dysfunction is anticipated. If renal impairment is detected, stop drug.
● Temporarily stop drug in patients undergoing radiologic studies involving intravascular administration of iodinated contrast materials because these products may acutely alter renal function.
● For patients previously treated with glyburide or metformin, the starting dose of drug shouldn't exceed daily dose of the glyburide (or equivalent dose of another sulfonylurea) and metformin already being taken.
● Monitor patient closely during times of increased stress, such as infection, fever, surgery, or trauma; insulin therapy may be needed. Temporarily suspend drug for any surgical procedure that requires restricted

intake of food and fluids, and don't restart until patient's oral intake has resumed.

• Lactic acidosis is a rare but serious (50% fatal) metabolic complication caused by metformin accumulation. Lactic acidosis occurs primarily in diabetic patients with significant renal insufficiency; multiple medical or surgical problems; and multiple drug regimens. The risk of lactic acidosis increases with the degree of renal impairment and patient age.

• Early symptoms of lactic acidosis may include malaise, myalgias, respiratory distress, increasing somnolence, and nonspecific abdominal distress.

• GI symptoms that occur after patient is stabilized on drug are unlikely to be drug-related and could be caused by lactic acidosis or other serious disease.

• Suspect lactic acidosis in any diabetic patient with metabolic acidosis lacking evidence of ketoacidosis.

• Monitor patient's hematologic status for megaloblastic anemia. Patients with inadequate vitamin $B_{12}$ or calcium intake or absorption seem predisposed to developing subnormal vitamin $B_{12}$ levels when taking metformin. These patients should have vitamin $B_{12}$ level determinations every 2 to 3 years.

• Stop drug if CV collapse, acute heart failure, acute MI, or other conditions characterized by hypoxemia occur, because these conditions may be linked to lactic acidosis and may cause prerenal azotemia.

• Watch for ketoacidosis or lactic acidosis in patient who develops laboratory abnormalities or clinical illness, by evaluating laboratory values, including electrolyte, ketone, glucose, pH, lactate, pyruvate, and metformin levels. Stop drug if there is evidence of acidosis.

• Obtain a baseline creatinine level that indicates normal renal function before starting therapy. Don't start therapy in patients age 80 or older, unless creatinine clearance level demonstrates that renal function is normal.

• Drug shouldn't usually be increased to maximum dose.

**PATIENT TEACHING**
• Tell patient to take once-daily dose with breakfast and twice-daily dose with breakfast and dinner.

• Teach patient about diabetes and importance of following therapeutic regimen; adhering to diet, weight reduction, regular exercise and hygiene programs; and avoiding infection. Explain how and when to self-monitor glucose level and how to differentiate between symptoms of low and high glucose levels.

• Instruct patient to stop drug and tell prescriber of unexplained hyperventilation, muscle pain, malaise, unusual sleepiness, or other symptoms of early lactic acidosis.

• Tell patient that GI symptoms are common with initial drug therapy. He should report promptly GI symptoms occurring after prolonged therapy, as they may be related to lactic acidosis or other serious disease.

• Advise patient not to drink too much alcohol.

• Advise patient not to take any other drugs, including OTC drugs, without checking with prescriber.

• Instruct patient to carry medical identification.

## insulins

### insulin (regular)
Actrapid‡, Actrapid Penfill‡, Humulin R ◇, Humulin R Regular U-500 (concentrated), Hypurin Neutral‡, Iletin II Regular ◇, Novolin R ◇, Novolin R PenFill ◇, Novolin R Prefilled ◇, Velosulin BR ◇

### insulin (lispro)
Humalog

### insulin lispro protamine and insulin lispro
Humalog Mix25‡, Humalog Mix 50/50, Humalog Mix 75/25

### insulin zinc suspension (lente)
Humulin L ◇, Lente Iletin II ◇

### extended zinc insulin suspension (ultralente)
Humulin-U Ultralente ◇

## isophane insulin suspension (NPH)

Humulin N◇, Humulin NPH‡, Hypurin Isophane‡, Novolin N◇, Novolin N PenFill◇, Novolin N Prefilled◇, NPH Iletin II◇, Protaphane‡, Protaphane Prefill‡

## isophane insulin suspension and insulin injection (70% isophane insulin and 30% insulin injection)

Humulin 70/30◇, Novolin 70/30◇, Novolin 70/30 PenFill◇, Novolin 70/30 Prefilled◇, Mixtard 30/70‡, Mixtard 30/70 Penfill‡

## isophane insulin suspension and insulin injection (50% isophane insulin and 50% insulin injection)

Humulin 50/50◇, Mixtard 50/50‡, Mixtard Penfill 50/50‡

## isophane insulin suspension and insulin injection (80% isophane insulin and 20% insulin injection)

Mixtard 80/20‡, Mixtard Penfill 80/20‡

*Pregnancy risk category B*

---

**AVAILABLE FORMS**
**Available without a prescription**
*insulin (regular)*
*Injection (pork):* 100 units/ml (Iletin II Regular)
*Injection (human):* 100 units/ml (Humulin R, Novolin R, Novolin R PenFill, Novolin R Prefilled, Velosulin BR)
*isophane insulin suspension (NPH)*
*Injection (pork):* 100 units/ml (NPH Iletin II)
*Injection (human):* 100 units/ml (Humulin N, Novolin N, Novolin N PenFill, Novolin N Prefilled)
*insulin zinc suspension (lente)*
*Injection (pork):* 100 units/ml (Lente Iletin II)
*Injection (human):* 100 units/ml (Humulin L, Novolin L)

*extended zinc insulin suspension (ultra-lente)*
*Injection (human):* 100 units/ml (Humulin U Ultralente)
*isophane insulin suspension and insulin injection combinations*
*Injection (human):* 100 units/ml (Humulin 70/30, Novolin 70/30, Novolin 70/30 PenFill, Novolin 70/30 Prefilled, Humulin 50/50)
**Available by prescription only**
*insulin (regular)*
*Injection (human):* 100 units/ml (Actrapid‡, Actrapid Penfill‡), 500 units/ml (Humulin R Regular U-500 [concentrated])
*Injection (bovine):* 100 units/ml (Hypurin Neutral‡)
*insulin (lispro)*
*Injection (human):* 100 units/ml (Humalog)
*insulin lispro protamine and insulin lispro*
*Injection (human):* 100 units/ml (Humalog Mix25‡, Humalog Mix 50/50, Humalog Mix 75/25)
*isophane insulin suspension (NPH)*
*Injection (human):* 100 units/ml (Humulin NPH‡, Protaphane‡, Protaphane Prefill‡)
*Injection (bovine):* 100 units/ml (Hypurin Isophane‡)
*isophane insulin suspension and insulin injection combinations*
*Injection (human):* 100 units/ml (Mixtard 30/70‡, Mixtard 30/70 Penfill‡, Mixtard 50/50‡, Mixtard Penfill 50/50‡, Mixtard 80/20‡, Mixtard Penfill 80/20‡)

**INDICATIONS & DOSAGES**
➤ **Moderate to severe diabetic ketoacidosis or hyperosmolar hyperglycemia (regular insulin)**
*Adults older than age 20:* Give loading dose of 0.15 units/kg I.V. direct injection, followed by 0.1 unit/kg/hour as a continuous infusion. Decrease rate of insulin infusion to 0.05 to 0.1 unit/kg/hour when glucose level reaches 250 to 300 mg/dl. Start infusion of $D_5W$ in half-normal saline solution separately from the insulin infusion when glucose level is 150 to 200 mg/dl in patients with diabetic ketoacidosis or 250 to 300 mg/dl in those with hyperosmolar hyperglycemia. Give dose of insulin S.C. 1 to 2 hours before stopping insulin

---

infusion (intermediate-acting insulin is recommended).

*Adults and children age 20 or younger:*
Loading dose isn't recommended. Begin therapy at 0.1 unit/kg/hour I.V. infusion. Once condition improves, decrease rate of insulin infusion to 0.05 unit/kg/hour. Start infusion of $D_5W$ in half-normal saline solution separately from the insulin infusion when glucose level is 250 mg/dl.

➤**Mild diabetic ketoacidosis (regular insulin)**
*Adults older than age 20:* Give loading dose of 0.4 to 0.6 unit/kg divided in two equal parts, with half the dose given by direct I.V. injection and half given I.M. or S.C. Subsequent doses can be based on 0.1 unit/kg/hour I.M. or S.C.

➤**Newly diagnosed diabetes mellitus (regular insulin)**
*Adults older than age 20:* Individualize therapy. Initially, 0.5 to 1 unit/kg/day S.C. as part of a regimen with short-acting and long-acting insulin therapy.
*Adults and children age 20 or younger:*
Individualize therapy. Initially, 0.1 to 0.25 unit/kg S.C. q 6 to 8 hours for 24 hours then adjust accordingly.

➤**Control of hyperglycemia with Humalog and longer-acting insulin in patients with type 1 diabetes mellitus**
*Adults:* Dosage varies among patients and must be determined by prescriber familiar with patient's metabolic needs, eating habits, and other lifestyle variables. Inject S.C. within 15 minutes before or after a meal.

➤**Control of hyperglycemia with Humalog and sulfonylureas in patients with type 2 diabetes mellitus**
*Adults and children older than age 3:*
Dosage varies among patients and must be determined by prescriber familiar with patient's metabolic needs, eating habits, and other lifestyle variables. Inject S.C. within 15 minutes before or after a meal.

➤**Hyperkalemia ♦**
*Adults:* 50 ml of dextrose 50% given over 5 minutes, followed by 5 to 10 units of regular insulin by I.V. push.

**I.V. ADMINISTRATION**
● Give only regular insulin I.V. Inject directly into vein or into a port close to I.V. access site. Intermittent infusion isn't re-

commended. If given by continuous infusion, infuse drug diluted in normal saline solution at prescribed rate.

● **Alert:** Regular insulin is used in patients with circulatory collapse, diabetic ketoacidosis, or hyperkalemia. Don't use Humulin R (concentrated) U-500 I.V. Don't use intermediate or long-acting insulins for coma or other emergency requiring rapid drug action. Also, ketosis-prone type 1, severely ill, and newly diagnosed diabetic patients with very high glucose level may need hospitalization and I.V. treatment with regular fast-acting insulin.

**ACTION**
Increases glucose transport across muscle and fat cell membranes to reduce glucose level. Promotes conversion of glucose to its storage form, glycogen; triggers amino acid uptake and conversion to protein in muscle cells and inhibits protein degradation; stimulates triglyceride formation and inhibits release of free fatty acids from adipose tissue; and stimulates lipoprotein lipase activity, which converts circulating lipoproteins to fatty acids.

| Route | Onset | Peak | Duration |
| --- | --- | --- | --- |
| I.V. (regular) | Immediate | Unknown | Unknown |
| S.C. (rapid) | ¼-1½ hr | 2-3 hr | 5-7 hr |
| S.C. (intermediate) | 1-2½ hr | 4-15 hr | 24 hr |
| S.C. (long-acting) | 4-8 hr | 10-30 hr | 36 hr |

**ADVERSE REACTIONS**
**Metabolic:** *hypoglycemia,* hyperglycemia, hypomagnesemia, hypokalemia.
**Skin:** rash, urticaria, pruritus, swelling, redness, stinging, warmth at injection site.
**Other:** *lipoatrophy, lipohypertrophy,* hypersensitivity reactions, **anaphylaxis.**

**INTERACTIONS**
**Drug-drug.** *ACE inhibitors, anabolic steroids, antidiabetic agents, beta blockers, calcium, chloroquine, clofibrate, clonidine, disopyramide, fluoxetine, guanethidine, lithium, MAO inhibitors, mebendazole, octreotide, pentamidine,*

---

*Rapid onset    †Canada    ‡Australia    ◇OTC    ♦Off-label use    ✒Photoguide    *Liquid contains alcohol.*

*propoxyphene, pyridoxine, salicylates, sulfinpyrazone, sulfonamides, tetracyclines:* May enhance hypoglycemic effects of insulin. Monitor glucose level.

*Acetazolamide, adrenocorticosteroids, AIDS antivirals, albuterol, asparaginase, calcitonin, cyclophosphamide, danazol, diazoxide, diltiazem, diuretics, dobutamine, epinephrine, estrogen-containing hormonal contraceptives, estrogens, ethacrynic acid, isoniazid, lithium, morphine, niacin, nicotine, phenothiazines, phenytoin, somatropin, terbutaline, thyroid hormones:* May diminish insulin response. Monitor glucose level.

*Carteolol, nadolol, pindolol, propranolol, timolol:* May mask symptoms of hypoglycemia as a result of beta blockade (such as tachycardia). Use with extreme caution in patients with diabetes.

*Rosiglitazone:* May cause fluid retention that may lead to or worsen heart failure. Monitor patient closely.

**Drug-herb.** *Basil, bay, bee pollen, burdock, ginseng, glucomannan, horehound, marshmallow, myrrh, sage:* May affect glycemic control. Monitor glucose level carefully and discourage use together.

**Drug-food.** *Unregulated diet:* May cause hyperglycemia or hypoglycemia. Monitor diet.

**Drug-lifestyle.** *Alcohol use:* May cause hypoglycemic effect. Discourage use together.

*Marijuana use:* May increase glucose level. Tell patient to avoid marijuana.

*Smoking:* May increase glucose level and decrease response to insulin administration. Monitor glucose level.

**EFFECTS ON LAB TEST RESULTS**
● May decrease glucose, magnesium, and potassium levels.

**CONTRAINDICATIONS & CAUTIONS**
● Contraindicated in patients with history of systemic allergic reaction to pork when porcine-derived products are used or hypersensitivity to any component of preparation.
● Contraindicated during episodes of hypoglycemia.

**NURSING CONSIDERATIONS**
● Insulin is drug of choice to treat diabetes during pregnancy. Insulin requirements increase in pregnant diabetic women and then decline immediately postpartum. Monitor patient closely.
● Dosage is always expressed in USP units. Use only the syringes calibrated for the particular concentration of insulin given.
● Some patients may develop insulin resistance and need large insulin doses to control symptoms of diabetes. U-500 insulin is available as Humulin R (concentrated) U-500 for such patients. Give pharmacy sufficient notice when requesting refill prescription. Never store U-500 insulin in same area with other insulin preparations because of danger of severe overdose if given accidentally to other patients.
● To mix insulin suspension, swirl vial gently or rotate between palms or between palm and thigh. Don't shake vigorously— this causes bubbling and air in syringe.
● Lente, semilente, and ultralente insulins may be mixed in any proportion. Regular insulin may be mixed with NPH or lente insulins in any proportion. When mixing regular insulin with intermediate or long-acting insulin, always draw up regular insulin into syringe first.
● Switching from separate injections to a prepared mixture may alter patient response. When NPH or lente is mixed with regular insulin in the same syringe, give immediately to avoid loss of potency.
● Lispro insulin may be mixed with Humulin N or Humulin U; give within 15 minutes before a meal to prevent a hypoglycemic reaction.
● Don't use insulin that changes color or becomes clumped or granular in appearance.
● Check expiration date on vial before using contents.
● Usual administration route is S.C. For proper S.C. administration, pinch a fold of skin with fingers at least 3 inches (7.6 cm) apart, and insert needle at a 45- to 90-degree angle.
● Press but don't rub site after injection. Rotate injection sites to avoid overuse of one area. Diabetic patients may achieve

---

Reactions may be *common*, uncommon, ***life-threatening***, or COMMON AND LIFE-THREATENING.

better control if injection site is rotated within same anatomic region.
- Monitor patient for hyperglycemia (rebound, or Somogyi effect).
- Store insulin in cool area. Refrigeration is desirable but not essential, except with Humulin R (concentrated) U-500.

**PATIENT TEACHING**
- Make sure patient knows that drug relieves symptoms but doesn't cure disease.
- Instruct patient about nature of disease and importance of following therapeutic regimen, adhering to specific diet, losing weight, getting exercise, following personal hygiene program, and avoiding infection. Emphasize importance of timing injections with eating and of not skipping meals.
- Stress that accuracy of measurement is important, especially with concentrated regular insulin. Aids, such as magnifying sleeve or dose magnifier, may improve accuracy. Show patient and caregivers how to measure and give insulin.
- Advise patient not to change order in which insulins are mixed or model or brand of insulin, syringe, or needle. Be sure patient knows when mixing two insulins, always draw the regular into the syringe first.
- Teach patient that glucose level and urine ketone tests provide essential guides to dosage and success of therapy. It's important for patient to recognize symptoms of high and low glucose levels. Insulin-induced low glucose level is hazardous and may cause brain damage if prolonged; most adverse effects are temporary. Instruct patient on insulin peak times and their importance.
- Instruct patient on proper use of equipment for monitoring glucose level.
- Advise patient not to smoke within 30 minutes after insulin injection because smoking decreases amount of insulin absorbed by S.C. route.
- Advise patient to avoid vigorous exercise immediately after insulin injection, especially of the area where injection was given, because it increases absorption and risk of high glucose episodes.
- Inform patient that marijuana use may increase insulin requirements.

- Teach patient to avoid alcohol use because it lowers glucose level.
- Advise patient to wear or carry medical identification at all times, to carry ample insulin and syringes on trips, to keep carbohydrates (lump of sugar or candy) on hand for emergencies, and to note time zone changes for dosage schedule when traveling.
- Advise woman planning pregnancy to first consult prescriber.
- Advise patient to store insulin at 36° to 46° F (2° to 8° C). Don't freeze or expose vials to excessive heat or sunlight.

---

# insulin aspart (rDNA origin) injection
NovoLog

# insulin aspart (rDNA origin) protamine suspension and insulin aspart (rDNA origin) injection
NovoLog 70/30

*Pregnancy risk category C*

---

**AVAILABLE FORMS**
*PenFill cartridges:* 3 ml
*Prefilled syringes:* 3 ml
*Vial:* 10 ml, containing 100 units of insulin aspart per ml (U-100)

**INDICATIONS & DOSAGES**
➤ **Control of hyperglycemia in patients with diabetes mellitus**
*NovoLog*
*Adults and children age 6 and older:*
Dosage is highly individualized. Typical daily insulin requirement is 0.5 to 1 unit/kg/day, divided in a meal-related treatment regimen. About 50% to 70% of dose is provided with NovoLog and the remainder by an intermediate- or long-acting insulin. Give 5 to 10 minutes before start of meal by S.C. injection in the abdominal wall, thigh, or upper arm. External insulin infusion pumps: initially, based on the total daily insulin dose of the previous regimen. Usually 50% of the total dose is given as meal-related boluses, and the remainder as basal infusion. Adjust dose p.r.n.

➤ **Control of hyperglycemia in patients with diabetes mellitus**
*NovoLog 70/30*
*Adults:* Dosage is individualized based on the needs of the patient. Doses are usually given twice daily within 15 minutes of meals.

## ACTION

The primary action of NovoLog is the regulation of glucose metabolism. It has the same glucose-lowering effect as regular human insulin, but its effect is more rapid and of shorter duration.

| Route | Onset | Peak | Duration |
|---|---|---|---|
| S.C. | 15 min | 1-3 hr | 3-5 hr |
| S.C. (70/30) | Rapid | 1-4 hr | ≤ 24 hr |

## ADVERSE REACTIONS

**Metabolic:** *hypoglycemia,* hypokalemia.
**Skin:** injection site reactions, lipodystrophy, pruritus, rash.
**Other:** *allergic reactions.*

## INTERACTIONS

**Drug-drug.** *ACE inhibitors, disopyramide, fibrates, fluoxetine, MAO inhibitors, oral antidiabetics, propoxyphene, salicylates, somatostatin analogue (octreotide), sulfonamide antibiotics:* May enhance the glucose-lowering effect of insulin and potentiate hypoglycemia. Monitor glucose level, and watch for signs and symptoms of hypoglycemia. May need insulin dose adjustment.
*Beta blockers, clonidine:* May increase or decrease the glucose-lowering effect of insulin and cause hypoglycemia or hyperglycemia. May reduce or mask symptoms of hypoglycemia. Monitor glucose level.
*Corticosteroids, danazol, diuretics, estrogens, progestins (as in hormonal contraceptives), isoniazid, niacin, phenothiazine derivatives, somatropin, sympathomimetics (epinephrine, salbutamol, terbutaline), and thyroid hormones:* May decrease the glucose-lowering effect of insulin and cause hyperglycemia. Monitor glucose level. May require insulin dose adjustment.
*Crystalline zinc preparations:* May be incompatible with NovoLog. Don't mix together.

*Guanethidine, reserpine:* May reduce or mask symptoms of hypoglycemia. Monitor glucose level.
*Lithium salts, pentamidine:* May increase or decrease glucose-lowering effect of insulin and may cause hypoglycemia or hyperglycemia. Pentamidine may cause hypoglycemia, sometimes followed by hyperglycemia. Monitor glucose level.
**Drug-herb.** *Burdock, dandelion, eucalyptus, marshmallow:* May increase hypoglycemic effects. Discourage use together.
**Drug-lifestyle.** *Alcohol use:* May increase or decrease glucose-lowering effect of insulin, causing hypoglycemia or hyperglycemia. Advise patient to monitor glucose level.
*Exercise:* May alter the need for insulin, requiring dose adjustment. Advise patient to report changes in physical activity.
*Marijuana use:* May increase glucose level. Tell patient to avoid marijuana use.
*Smoking:* May increase glucose level and decrease response to insulin. Monitor glucose level.

## EFFECTS ON LAB TEST RESULTS

• May decrease glucose and potassium levels.

## CONTRAINDICATIONS & CAUTIONS

• Contraindicated during episodes of hypoglycemia and in patients hypersensitive to NovoLog or one of its components.
• Use cautiously in patients susceptible to hypoglycemia and hypokalemia, such as those who have autonomic neuropathy or are fasting, using potassium-lowering drugs, or using drugs sensitive to potassium level.

## NURSING CONSIDERATIONS

• Give NovoLog 5 to 10 minutes before the start of a meal. Give NovoLog 70/30 up to 15 minutes before the start of a meal. Because of its rapid onset of action and short duration of action, patients also may need longer-acting insulins to prevent pre-meal hyperglycemia.
• Let insulin warm to room temperature before administering to minimize discomfort. Then give by S.C. injection into the abdominal wall, thigh, or upper arm. Rotate sites to minimize lipodystrophies.

---

Reactions may be *common,* uncommon, *life-threatening,* or COMMON AND LIFE-THREATENING.

• The time course of NovoLog action may vary among people or at different times in the same person and depends on the site of injection, blood supply, temperature, and physical activity.

• Adjustments in the dose of NovoLog or of any insulin may be needed with changes in physical activity or meal routine. Insulin requirements also may be altered during emotional disturbances, illness, or other stresses.

• When giving and mixing NovoLog with NPH human insulin, draw up NovoLog into syringe first and give immediately after dose is drawn up.

• Adjust dose regularly, according to patient's glucose measurements. Monitor glucose level regularly.

• Store drug between 36° and 46° F (2° and 8° C). Don't freeze. Don't expose vials to excessive heat or sunlight. Open vials of NovoLog 70/30 and open vials and cartridges of NovoLog are stable at room temperature for 28 days. Punctured cartridges of NovoLog 70/30 may be stored at room temperature up to 14 days; don't refrigerate punctured NovoLog 70/30 cartridges.

• *Alert:* Don't confuse NovoLog 70/30 with Novolin 70/30.

• Periodically monitor glycosylated hemoglobin.

• Assess patient for rash (including pruritus) over whole body, shortness of breath, wheezing, hypotension, rapid pulse, or sweating, which may signify a generalized allergy to insulin. Severe cases, including anaphylactic reactions, may be life threatening.

• Patients with renal dysfunction and hepatic impairment may need close glucose monitoring and dose adjustments of NovoLog.

• Observe injection sites for reactions such as redness, swelling, itching, or burning. These reactions should resolve within a few days to a few weeks.

• *Alert:* Don't give I.V.

• Assess patient for evidence of hypoglycemia (sweating, shaking, trembling, confusion, headache, irritability, hunger, rapid pulse, nausea) and hyperglycemia (drowsiness, fruity breath odor, frequent urination, thirst). Notify prescriber if any of these warning signs occur.

• Symptoms of hypoglycemia may occur in patients with diabetes, regardless of glucose value.

• Patients with long duration of diabetes, diabetic nerve disease, or intensified diabetes control may experience different or less-pronounced early warning symptoms of hypoglycemia. Severe hypoglycemia may occur without warning.

• Inspect insulin vials before use. NovoLog is a clear, colorless solution. It should never contain particulate matter or appear cloudy, viscous, or discolored. NovoLog 70/30 should appear uniformly white and cloudy and should never contain particulate matter or be discolored.

**For external pump use with NovoLog**

• Monitor patient with an external insulin pump for erythematous, pruritic, or thickened skin at injection site.

• *Alert:* Pump or infusion set malfunctions or insulin degradation can lead to hyperglycemia and ketosis in a short time because there is an S.C. depot of fast-acting insulin.

• Don't dilute or mix insulin aspart with any other insulin, when using an external insulin pump.

• Teach patient how to properly use the external insulin pump.

• Insulin aspart is recommended for use with Disetronic H-TRON plus V100 with Disetronic 3.15 plastic cartridges and Classic or Tender infusion sets, Polyfin or Sof-set infusion sets, and MiniMed Models 505, 506, and 507 with MiniMed 3-ml syringes.

• Replace infusion sets, insulin aspart in the reservoir, and choose a new infusion site every 48 hours or less to avoid insulin degradation and infusion set malfunction.

• Discard insulin exposed to temperatures higher than 98.6° F (37° C). The temperature of the insulin may exceed ambient temperature when the pump housing, cover, tubing, or sport case is exposed to sunlight or radiant heat.

**PATIENT TEACHING**

• Tell patient not to stop insulin therapy without medical approval.

• Advise patient of the warning signs of low glucose (shaking, sweating, moodiness, irritability, confusion, or agitation).

Tell patient to carry sugar (candy, sugar packets) to counteract low glucose.
• Teach patient proper insulin injection technique and importance of timing dose to meals and adhering to meal plans.
• Tell patient to report swelling, redness, and itching at injection site, and instruct patient on the importance of rotating injection sites to avoid lipodystrophies.
• Instruct patient to use the same brand of insulin, especially if mixing insulin. Changing brands of insulin may necessitate dosage changes.
• Tell patient not to dilute or mix insulin aspart with any other insulin when using an external insulin pump.
• Instruct patient to monitor glucose regularly.
• Advise patient to avoid vigorous exercise immediately after insulin injection, especially of the area where injection was given; it causes increased absorption and increased risk of high glucose.
• Advise patient to store insulin at 36° to 46° F (2° to 8° C), and avoid freezing or excessive heat or sunlight.
• Advise woman to notify prescriber about planned, suspected, or known pregnancy.
• Urge patient to wear or carry medical identification at all times.
• Instruct patient about the importance of diet and exercise. Explain long-term complications of diabetes and the importance of yearly eye and foot examinations.

## insulin glargine (rDNA origin) injection
Lantus

*Pregnancy risk category C*

### AVAILABLE FORMS
*Vial:* 10 ml, containing 100 units of insulin aspart per ml (U-100)

### INDICATIONS & DOSAGES
➤ **To manage type 1 (insulin-dependent) diabetes mellitus in patients who need basal (long-acting) insulin to control hyperglycemia**
*Adults and children age 6 and older:* Individualize dosage, and give S.C. once daily at the same time each day.

➤ **To manage type 2 (non–insulin-dependent) diabetes mellitus in patients who need basal (long-acting) insulin to control hyperglycemia**
*Adults:* Individualize dosage, and give S.C. once daily at the same time each day.

### ACTION
Insulin glargine lowers glucose level by stimulating peripheral glucose uptake, especially by skeletal muscle and fat, and by inhibiting hepatic glucose production.

| Route | Onset | Peak | Duration |
|-------|-------|------|----------|
| S.C. | 1 hr | None | 24 hr |

### ADVERSE REACTIONS
**Metabolic:** *hypoglycemia.*
**Skin:** lipodystrophy, pruritus, rash.
**Other:** allergic reactions, pain at injection site.

### INTERACTIONS
**Drug-drug.** *ACE inhibitors, disopyramide, fibrates, fluoxetine, MAO inhibitors, octreotide, oral antidiabetics, propoxyphene, salicylates, sulfonamide antibiotics:* May cause hypoglycemia and increase insulin effect. Monitor glucose level. May need to adjust dosage of insulin glargine.
*Beta blockers, clonidine:* May mask signs of hypoglycemia and may either increase or reduce insulin's glucose-lowering effect. Avoid using together, if possible. If used together, monitor glucose level carefully.
*Corticosteroids, danazol, diuretics, estrogens, isoniazid, phenothiazines (such as prochlorperazine, promethazine hydrochloride), progestins (such as hormonal contraceptives), somatropin, sympathomimetics (such as albuterol, epinephrine, terbutaline), thyroid hormones:* May reduce the glucose-lowering effect of insulin. Monitor glucose level. May need to adjust dosage of insulin glargine.
*Guanethidine, reserpine:* May mask the signs of hypoglycemia. Avoid using together, if possible. Monitor glucose level carefully.
*Lithium:* May either increase or decrease the glucose-lowering effect of insulin. Monitor glucose level. May require dosage adjustments of insulin glargine.

*Pentamidine:* May cause hypoglycemia, which may be followed by hyperglycemia. Avoid using together, if possible.

**Drug-herb.** *Burdock, dandelion, eucalyptus, marshmallow:* May increase hypoglycemic effects. Discourage use together.

*Licorice root:* May increase dosage requirements of insulin. Discourage use together.

**Drug-lifestyle.** *Alcohol use, emotional stress:* May increase or decrease the glucose-lowering effect of insulin. Advise patient to self-monitor glucose level.

**EFFECTS ON LAB TEST RESULTS**
● May decrease glucose level.

**CONTRAINDICATIONS & CAUTIONS**
● Contraindicated in patients hypersensitive to insulin glargine or its excipients.
● Contraindicated during episodes of hypoglycemia.
● Use cautiously in patients with renal or hepatic impairment.

**NURSING CONSIDERATIONS**
● *Alert:* Drug isn't intended for I.V. use. It's only for S.C. use. Prolonged duration of activity depends on injection into S.C. space.
● Because of prolonged duration, this isn't the insulin of choice for diabetic ketoacidosis.
● Desired glucose level, as well as the doses and timing of antidiabetic medication, must be determined individually, as with any insulin. Glucose monitoring is recommended for all patients with diabetes.
● The rate of absorption, onset, and duration of action may be affected by exercise and other variables, such as illness and emotional stress.
● *Alert:* Insulin glargine must not be diluted or mixed with any other insulin or solution.
● As with any insulin therapy, lipodystrophy may occur at the site of injection and may delay insulin absorption. Continuously rotate injection sites within a given area to reduce lipodystrophy.
● Hypoglycemia is the most common adverse effect of insulin. Early symptoms may be different or less pronounced in patients with long duration of diabetes, diabetic nerve disease, or intensified diabetes

control. Monitor glucose level closely in these patients because severe hypoglycemia may result before the patient develops symptoms.
● *Alert:* Don't confuse Lente with Lantus.

**PATIENT TEACHING**
● Teach proper glucose monitoring, injection techniques, and diabetes management.
● Tell patient to take dose once daily at the same time each day.
● *Alert:* Educate diabetic patients about signs and symptoms of low glucose, such as fatigue, weakness, confusion, headache, pallor, and profuse sweating.
● Urge patient to wear or carry medical identification at all times.
● Advise patient to treat mild episodes of low glucose with oral glucose tablets. Encourage patient to always carry glucose tablets in case of a low glucose episode.
● Educate patients on the importance of maintaining a diabetic diet, and explain that adjustments in drug dosage, meal patterns, and exercise may be needed to regulate glucose.
● *Alert:* Advise patient not to dilute or mix any other insulin or solution with insulin glargine. If the solution is cloudy, urge patient to discard the vial. Use solution only if it is clear and colorless.
● *Alert:* Make any change of insulin cautiously and only under medical supervision. Changes in insulin type, strength, manufacturer, type (such as regular, NPH, or insulin analogues), species (animal, human), or method of manufacturer (rDNA versus animal source insulin) may require a change in dosage. Oral antidiabetic treatment taken at the same time may need to be adjusted.
● Tell patient to consult prescriber before using OTC medications.
● Inform patient to avoid alcohol, which lowers glucose level.
● Advise patient to avoid vigorous exercise immediately after insulin injection, especially of the area where injection was given; it causes increased absorption and increased risk of high glucose.
● Advise woman planning pregnancy to first consult prescriber.
● Advise patient to store unopened insulin vials in the refrigerator. Opened vials may

be stored at 86° F or less and away from direct heat. Discard opened vials after 28 days whether refrigerated or not. Don't freeze.

# metformin hydrochloride
Glucophage⚕, Glucophage XR⚕

*Pregnancy risk category B*

## AVAILABLE FORMS
*Tablets:* 500 mg, 850 mg, 1,000 mg
*Tablets (extended-release):* 500 mg, 750 mg

## INDICATIONS & DOSAGES
➤ **Adjunct to diet to lower glucose level in patients with type 2 (non–insulin-dependent) diabetes mellitus**
*Adults:* Initially, 500 mg P.O. b.i.d. given with morning and evening meals, or 850 mg P.O. once daily given with morning meal. When 500-mg form is used, increase dosage by 500 mg weekly to maximum dose of 2,500 mg P.O. daily in divided doses, p.r.n. When 850-mg form is used, increase dosage by 850 mg every other week to maximum dose of 2,550 mg P.O. daily in divided doses, p.r.n. If using extended-release formulation, start therapy at 500 mg P.O. once daily with the evening meal. May increase dose weekly in increments of 500 mg/day, up to a maximum dose of 2,000 mg once daily. If higher doses are required, consider using the regular release formulation up to its maximum dose.
*Children ages 10 to 16:* 500 mg P.O. b.i.d. using the regular release formulation only. Increase dosage in increments of 500 mg weekly up to a maximum of 2,000 mg daily in divided doses.
*Adjust-a-dose:* For debilitated and elderly patients, dosing should be conservative because of potential decrease in renal function.

## ACTION
Decreases hepatic glucose production and intestinal absorption of glucose and improves insulin sensitivity (increases peripheral glucose uptake and use).

| Route | Onset | Peak | Duration |
|---|---|---|---|
| P.O. (conventional) | Unknown | 2-4 hr | Unknown |
| P.O. (extended release) | Unknown | 4-8 hr | Unknown |

## ADVERSE REACTIONS
**GI:** diarrhea, nausea, vomiting, abdominal bloating, flatulence, anorexia, taste perversion.
**Hematologic:** megaloblastic anemia.
**Metabolic:** *lactic acidosis.*

## INTERACTIONS
**Drug-drug.** *Calcium channel blockers, corticosteroids, estrogens, fosphenytoin, hormonal contraceptives, isoniazid, nicotinic acid, phenothiazines, phenytoin, sympathomimetics, thiazide and other diuretics, thyroid drugs:* May produce hyperglycemia. Monitor patient's glycemic control. Metformin dosage may need to be increased.
*Cationic drugs (such as amiloride, cimetidine, digoxin, morphine, procainamide, quinidine, quinine, ranitidine, triamterene, trimethoprim, vancomycin):* Have potential to compete for common renal tubular transport systems, which may increase metformin level. Monitor glucose level.
*Nifedipine:* May increase metformin level. Monitor patient closely. Metformin dosage may need to be decreased.
*Radiologic contrast dye:* May cause acute renal failure. Withhold metformin for 24 hours before procedure.
**Drug-herb.** *Guar gum:* May decrease hypoglycemic effect. Discourage use together.
**Drug-lifestyle.** *Alcohol use:* May increase drug effects. Discourage use together.

## EFFECTS ON LAB TEST RESULTS
● May decrease hemoglobin and vitamin $B_{12}$ level.

## CONTRAINDICATIONS & CAUTIONS
● Contraindicated in patients hypersensitive to drug and in those with renal disease, hepatic disease, or metabolic acidosis.
● Contraindicated in patients with heart failure requiring pharmacologic interven-

tion, conditions predisposing to renal dysfunction, CV collapse, MI, hypoxia, and septicemia. Temporarily withhold from patients having X-rays involving injection of iodinated contrast materials.
• Use caution when giving drug to elderly, debilitated, or malnourished patients and to those with adrenal or pituitary insufficiency because of increased risk of hypoglycemia.

## NURSING CONSIDERATIONS
• Before therapy begins and at least annually thereafter, assess patient's renal function. If renal impairment is detected, expect prescriber to switch patient to a different antidiabetic. This is particularly important in elderly patients.
• Give with meals; give once-daily dosage with breakfast and twice-daily dosage with breakfast and dinner. Maximum doses may be better tolerated if total dose is divided into t.i.d. dosing and given with meals.
• When switching patients from standard oral hypoglycemics (except chlorpropamide) to metformin, no transition period is usually needed. When switching patients from chlorpropamide to metformin, take care during the first 2 weeks of metformin therapy because the prolonged retention of chlorpropamide increases the risk of hypoglycemia during this time.
• Monitor patient's glucose level regularly to evaluate effectiveness of therapy. Notify prescriber if glucose level increase despite therapy.
• If patient hasn't responded to 4 weeks of therapy with maximum dosage, prescriber may add an oral sulfonylurea while keeping metformin at maximum dosage. If patient still doesn't respond after several months of therapy with both drugs at maximum dosage, prescriber may stop both and start insulin therapy.
• Monitor patient closely during times of increased stress, such as infection, fever, surgery, or trauma. Insulin therapy may be needed in these situations.
• Risk of drug-induced lactic acidosis is very low. Reported cases have occurred primarily in diabetic patients with significant renal insufficiency; in those with other medical or surgical problems; and in those with other drug regimens. Risk in-

creases with degree of renal impairment and patient age.
• *Alert:* Stop drug immediately and notify prescriber if patient develops a condition related to hypoxemia or dehydration because of risk of lactic acidosis.
• Expect drug therapy to be temporarily suspended for surgical procedures (except minor procedures that don't restrict intake of food and fluids) and for patients undergoing radiologic studies involving use of contrast media containing iodine. Therapy shouldn't be restarted until patient's oral intake has resumed and renal function has been deemed normal by prescriber.
• Monitor patient's hematologic status for evidence of megaloblastic anemia. Patients with inadequate vitamin $B_{12}$ or calcium intake or absorption appear to be predisposed to developing subnormal vitamin $B_{12}$ level. These patients should have routine vitamin $B_{12}$ level determinations every 2 to 3 years.
• *Alert:* Don't confuse Glucophage with Glucovance.

## PATIENT TEACHING
• Instruct patient about nature of diabetes and importance of following therapeutic regimen, adhering to specific diet, losing weight, getting exercise, following personal hygiene programs, and avoiding infection. Explain how and when to monitor glucose level. Teach evidence of low and high glucose levels. Explain emergency measures.
• *Alert:* Instruct patient to stop drug and immediately notify prescriber about unexplained hyperventilation, muscle pain, malaise, unusual sleepiness, or other nonspecific symptoms of early lactic acidosis.
• Warn patient not to consume excessive alcohol while taking drug.
• Tell patient not to change drug dosage without prescriber's consent. Encourage patient to report abnormal glucose level test results.
• Advise patient not to take other drugs, including OTC drugs, without first checking with prescriber.
• Instruct patient to wear or carry medical identification at all times.

# miglitol
Glyset

*Pregnancy risk category B*

## AVAILABLE FORMS
*Tablets:* 25 mg, 50 mg, 100 mg

## INDICATIONS & DOSAGES
➤ **Adjunct to diet to improve glycemic control in patients with type 2 (non–insulin-dependent) diabetes mellitus whose hyperglycemia can't be managed with diet alone; with a sulfonylurea when diet plus either miglitol or sulfonylurea doesn't adequately control glucose level**
*Adults:* 25 mg P.O. t.i.d. with first bite of each main meal; may start with 25 mg P.O. daily and increase gradually to t.i.d. to minimize GI upset; dosage may be increased after 4 to 8 weeks to 50 mg P.O. t.i.d. Dosage may then be further increased after 3 months, based on glycosylated hemoglobin level, to maximum of 100 mg P.O. t.i.d.

## ACTION
Lowers glucose level by inhibiting the alpha-glucosidases in the small intestine, which convert carbohydrates to glucose. Inhibiting these enzymes delays the digestion of carbohydrates after a meal, resulting in a smaller increase in postprandial glucose level.

| Route | Onset | Peak | Duration |
|-------|-------|------|----------|
| P.O. | Unknown | 2-3 hr | Unknown |

## ADVERSE REACTIONS
**GI:** *abdominal pain, diarrhea, flatulence.*
**Skin:** rash.

## INTERACTIONS
**Drug-drug.** *Digoxin, propranolol, ranitidine:* May decrease bioavailability of these drugs. Watch for loss of efficacy of these drugs and adjust dosage.
*Intestinal absorbents (such as charcoal), digestive enzyme preparations (such as amylase, pancreatin):* May reduce effectiveness of miglitol. Discourage use together.

## EFFECTS ON LAB TEST RESULTS
● May decrease iron level.

## CONTRAINDICATIONS & CAUTIONS
● Contraindicated in patients hypersensitive to drug or its components and in those with diabetic ketoacidosis, inflammatory bowel disease, colonic ulceration, partial intestinal obstruction, chronic intestinal diseases with marked disorders of digestion or absorption, or conditions that may deteriorate because of increased gas formation in the intestine.
● Contraindicated in those predisposed to intestinal obstruction and in those with creatinine level greater than 2 mg/dl.
● Use cautiously in patients also receiving insulin or oral sulfonylureas because drug may increase hypoglycemic potential of insulin or sulfonylureas.

## NURSING CONSIDERATIONS
● In patients also taking insulin or oral sulfonylureas, dosages of these drugs may be needed. Monitor patient for increased frequency of hypoglycemia.
● Management of type 2 diabetes should include diet control, exercise program, and regular testing of urine and glucose level.
● Monitor glucose level regularly, especially during situations of increased stress, such as infection, fever, surgery, or trauma.
● Besides checking glucose level regularly, monitor glycosylated hemoglobin level every 3 months to evaluate long-term glycemic control.
● Treat mild to moderate hypoglycemia with a form of dextrose, such as glucose tablets or gel. Severe hypoglycemia may necessitate I.V. glucose or glucagon.
● Give drug with the first bite of each main meal.
● Monitor patient for adverse GI effects.

## PATIENT TEACHING
● Stress importance of adhering to diet, weight reduction, and exercise instructions. Urge patient to have glucose level and glycosylated hemoglobin tested regularly.
● Inform patient that drug treatment relieves symptoms but doesn't cure diabetes.
● Teach patient how to recognize high and low glucose levels.

---

• Instruct patient to have a source of glucose readily available to treat low glucose when miglitol is taken with a sulfonylurea or with insulin.
• Advise patient to seek medical advice promptly during periods of stress, such as fever, trauma, infection, or surgery, because dosage may have to be adjusted.
• Instruct patient to take drug three times daily with first bite of each main meal.
• Show patient how and when to monitor glucose level.
• Advise patient that sucrose (table sugar, cane sugar) or fruit juices shouldn't be used to treat low glucose reactions with miglitol. Oral glucose (dextrose) or glucagon is necessary to increase glucose.
• Advise patient that adverse GI effects are most common during first few weeks of therapy and should improve over time.
• Urge patient to wear or carry medical identification at all times.

---

## nateglinide
Starlix

*Pregnancy risk category C*

### AVAILABLE FORMS
*Tablets:* 60 mg, 120 mg

### INDICATIONS & DOSAGES
➤ **As monotherapy, or with metformin, to lower glucose level in patients with type 2 (non–insulin-dependent) diabetes whose hyperglycemia isn't adequately controlled by diet and exercise and who haven't had long-term treatment with other antidiabetics**
*Adults:* 120 mg P.O. t.i.d. taken 1 to 30 minutes before meals. Patients near goal HbA$_{1c}$ when treatment is started may receive 60 mg P.O. t.i.d.

### ACTION
Lowers glucose level by stimulating insulin secretion from pancreatic beta cells.

| Route | Onset | Peak | Duration |
|-------|-------|------|----------|
| P.O. | 20 min | 1 hr | 4 hr |

### ADVERSE REACTIONS
**CNS:** dizziness.
**GI:** diarrhea.

**Metabolic:** *hypoglycemia.*
**Musculoskeletal:** back pain, arthropathy.
**Respiratory:** *upper respiratory tract infection,* bronchitis, coughing.
**Other:** flulike symptoms, accidental trauma.

### INTERACTIONS
**Drug-drug.** *Corticosteroids, sympathomimetics, thiazides, thyroid products:* May reduce hypoglycemic action of nateglinide. Monitor glucose level closely.
*MAO inhibitors, nonselective beta blockers, NSAIDs, salicylates:* May increase hypoglycemic action of nateglinide. Monitor glucose level closely.

### EFFECTS ON LAB TEST RESULTS
• May decrease glucose level.

### CONTRAINDICATIONS & CAUTIONS
• Contraindicated in patients hypersensitive to drug, in those with type 1 diabetes or diabetic ketoacidosis, and in breast-feeding patients.
• Use cautiously in patients with moderate to severe liver dysfunction or adrenal or pituitary insufficiency, and in elderly and malnourished patients.

### NURSING CONSIDERATIONS
• Don't use with or as a substitute for glyburide or other oral antidiabetics; may use with metformin.
• Give drug 1 to 30 minutes before a meal. If patient misses a meal, skip the scheduled dose.
• Monitor glucose level regularly to evaluate drug's efficacy.
• Observe patient for signs and symptoms of hypoglycemia (sweating, rapid pulse, trembling, confusion, headache, irritability, and nausea). To minimize risk of hypoglycemia, make sure that patient has a meal immediately after dose. If hypoglycemia occurs and patient remains conscious, give him an oral form of glucose. If he is unconscious, treat with I.V. glucose.
• Risk of hypoglycemia increases with strenuous exercise, alcohol ingestion, or insufficient caloric intake.
• Symptoms of hypoglycemia may be masked in patients with autonomic neu-

ropathy and in those who use beta blockers.

● Insulin therapy may be needed for glycemic control in patients with fever, infection, or trauma and in those undergoing surgery.

● Monitor glucose level closely when other drugs are started or stopped, to evaluate for possible drug interactions.

● Periodically monitor $HbA_{1c}$ level.

● Drug's effectiveness may decrease over time.

● No special dosage adjustments are usually necessary in elderly patients, but some elderly patients may have greater sensitivity to glucose-lowering effect.

**PATIENT TEACHING**

● Tell patient to take drug 1 to 30 minutes before a meal.

● Advise patient to skip the scheduled dose if he skips a meal, to reduce risk of low glucose level.

● Instruct patient on risk of low glucose level, its signs and symptoms (sweating, rapid pulse, trembling, confusion, headache, irritability, and nausea), and ways to treat these symptoms by eating or drinking something containing sugar.

● Teach patient how to monitor and log glucose levels to evaluate diabetes control.

● Advise patient to notify prescriber for persistent low or high glucose level.

● Instruct patient to adhere to prescribed diet and exercise regimen.

● Explain possible long-term complications of diabetes and importance of regular preventive therapy.

● Encourage patient to wear a medical identification bracelet.

---

# pioglitazone hydrochloride
Actos

*Pregnancy risk category C*

**AVAILABLE FORMS**
*Tablets:* 15 mg, 30 mg, 45 mg

**INDICATIONS & DOSAGES**
➤ **Adjunct to diet and exercise to improve glycemic control in patients with type 2 (non–insulin-dependent) diabetes mellitus; or when diet, exercise, and a sulfonylurea, metformin, or insulin fail to yield adequate glycemic control**
*Adults:* Initially, 15 or 30 mg P.O. once daily. For patients who respond inadequately to first dosage, it may be increased incrementally; maximum dosage is 45 mg/day. If used in combination therapy, maximum dosage shouldn't exceed 30 mg/day.

**ACTION**
Lowers glucose level by decreasing insulin resistance and hepatic glucose production. Improves sensitivity of insulin in muscle and adipose tissue.

| Route | Onset | Peak | Duration |
|-------|---------|----------|----------|
| P.O. | Unknown | ≤ 2 hr | Unknown |

**ADVERSE REACTIONS**
**CNS:** headache.
**CV:** *edema,* **heart failure.**
**EENT:** sinusitis, pharyngitis.
**Hematologic:** anemia.
**Metabolic:** *hypoglycemia with combination therapy,* aggravated diabetes mellitus, weight gain.
**Musculoskeletal:** myalgia.
**Respiratory:** upper respiratory tract infection.
**Other:** tooth disorder.

**INTERACTIONS**
**Drug-drug.** *Ketoconazole:* May inhibit pioglitazone metabolism. Monitor glucose level more frequently.
*Hormonal contraceptives:* May decrease level of hormonal contraceptives, reducing contraceptive effectiveness. Advise patient taking drug and hormonal contraceptives to consider additional birth control measures.
**Drug-herb.** *Burdock, dandelion, eucalyptus, marshmallow:* May increase hypoglycemic effects. Discourage use together.
**Drug-lifestyle.** *Alcohol use:* May alter glycemic control; hypoglycemia. Discourage use together.

**EFFECTS ON LAB TEST RESULTS**
● May decrease glucose and triglyceride levels. May increase ALT, HDL, LDL, and total cholesterol levels.
● May decrease hemoglobin.

---

Reactions may be *common,* uncommon, *life-threatening*, or COMMON AND LIFE-THREATENING.

**CONTRAINDICATIONS & CAUTIONS**

- Contraindicated in patients hypersensitive to drug or its components and in those with type 1 (insulin-dependent) diabetes mellitus, clinical evidence of active liver disease, ALT level greater than 2½ times the upper limit of normal, or New York Heart Association (NYHA) Class III or IV heart failure.
- Contraindicated in patients with diabetic ketoacidosis and in those who experienced jaundice while taking troglitazone.
- Use cautiously in patients with edema or heart failure.

**NURSING CONSIDERATIONS**

- ***Alert:*** Measure liver enzyme levels at start of therapy, every 2 months for first year of therapy, and periodically thereafter. Obtain liver function test results in patients who develop signs and symptoms of liver dysfunction, such as nausea, vomiting, abdominal pain, fatigue, anorexia, or dark urine. Stop drug if patient develops jaundice or if liver function test results show ALT level greater than 3 times the upper limit of normal.
- Pioglitazone hydrochloride alone or with insulin can cause fluid retention that may lead to or worsen heart failure. Observe patients for these signs or symptoms of heart failure. Stop drug if cardiac status deteriorates. This drug isn't recommended for NYHA Class III or IV cardiac status patients.
- Because ovulation may resume in premenopausal, anovulatory women with insulin resistance, recommend use of additional contraceptive measures.
- Use drug in pregnant patients only if the benefit justifies risk to fetus. Insulin is the preferred antidiabetic for use during pregnancy.
- Monitor patients with heart failure for increased edema.
- Hemoglobin and hematocrit may drop, usually during first 4 to 12 weeks of therapy.
- Management of type 2 diabetes should include diet control. Because caloric restrictions, weight loss, and exercise help improve insulin sensitivity and help make drug therapy effective, these measures are essential for proper diabetes management.
- Watch for hypoglycemia, especially in patients receiving combination therapy. Dosage adjustments of these drugs may be needed.
- Monitor glucose level regularly, especially during situations of increased stress, such as infection, fever, surgery, and trauma.
- Check glucose level and glycosylated hemoglobin periodically to evaluate therapeutic response to drug.
- Safety and efficacy of drug in children haven't been evaluated.
- ***Alert:*** Don't confuse pioglitazone with rosiglitazone.

**PATIENT TEACHING**

- Instruct patient to adhere to dietary instructions and to have glucose level and glycosylated hemoglobin tested regularly.
- Teach patient taking pioglitazone with insulin or oral antidiabetics the signs and symptoms of low glucose.
- Advise patient to notify prescriber during periods of stress, such as fever, trauma, infection, or surgery, because dosage may have to be changed.
- Instruct patient how and when to monitor glucose level.
- Notify patient that blood tests of liver function will be performed before therapy starts, every 2 months for the first year, and periodically thereafter.
- Tell patient to report unexplained nausea, vomiting, abdominal pain, fatigue, anorexia, or dark urine immediately because they may indicate liver problems.
- Warn patient to contact his health care provider if he has signs or symptoms of heart failure (unusually rapid increase in weight or swelling, shortness of breath).
- Advise anovulatory, premenopausal women with insulin resistance that therapy may cause resumption of ovulation; recommend using contraceptive measures.

## repaglinide
Prandin

*Pregnancy risk category C*

**AVAILABLE FORMS**

*Tablets:* 0.5 mg, 1 mg, 2 mg

## INDICATIONS & DOSAGES

➤ **Adjunct to diet and exercise to lower the glucose in patients with type 2 diabetes mellitus whose hyperglycemia can't be controlled satisfactorily by diet and exercise alone; adjunct to diet, exercise and metformin; adjunct to diet, exercise, and pioglitazone hydrochloride or rosiglitazone maleate**

*Adults:* For patients not previously treated or whose $HbA_{1c}$ is below 8%, starting dose is 0.5 mg P.O. taken about 15 minutes before each meal; time may vary from immediately before to as long as 30 minutes before meal. For patients previously treated with glucose-lowering drugs and whose $HbA_{1c}$ is 8% or more, first dose is 1 to 2 mg P.O. with each meal. Recommended dosage range is 0.5 to 4 mg with meals b.i.d., t.i.d., or q.i.d. Maximum daily dose is 16 mg.

Determine dosage by glucose response. May double dosage up to 4 mg with each meal until satisfactory glucose response is achieved. At least 1 week should elapse between dosage adjustments to assess response to each dose.

Metformin may be added if repaglinide monotherapy is inadequate; no repaglinide dosage adjustment is necessary.

*Adjust a dose:* In patients with severe renal impairment, starting dose is 0.5 mg P.O. with meals.

## ACTION

Stimulates insulin release from beta cells in the pancreas by closing ATP-dependent potassium channels in beta cell membranes, which causes calcium channels to open. Increased calcium influx induces insulin secretion; the overall effect is to lower glucose level.

| Route | Onset | Peak | Duration |
|-------|-------|------|----------|
| P.O. | 30 min | 1 hr | Unknown |

## ADVERSE REACTIONS

**CNS:** *headache,* paresthesia.
**CV:** angina.
**EENT:** rhinitis, sinusitis.
**GI:** constipation, diarrhea, dyspepsia, nausea, vomiting.
**GU:** UTI.
**Metabolic:** HYPOGLYCEMIA, hyperglycemia.

**Musculoskeletal:** arthralgia, back pain.
**Respiratory:** bronchitis, *upper respiratory tract infection.*
**Other:** tooth disorder.

## INTERACTIONS

**Drug-drug.** *Barbiturates, carbamazepine, rifampin:* May increase repaglinide metabolism. Monitor glucose level.
*Beta blockers, chloramphenicol, coumarins, MAO inhibitors, NSAIDs, other drugs that are highly protein-bound, probenecid, salicylates, sulfonamides:* May increase hypoglycemic action of repaglinide. Monitor glucose level.
*Calcium channel blockers, corticosteroids, estrogens, fosphenytoin, hormonal contraceptives, isoniazid, nicotinic acid, phenothiazines, phenytoin, sympathomimetics, thiazides and other diuretics, thyroid products:* May produce hyperglycemia, resulting in a loss of glycemic control. Monitor glucose level.
*Erythromycin, inhibitors of CYP, ketoconazole, miconazole:* May inhibit repaglinide metabolism. Monitor glucose level.
**Drug-herb.** *Burdock, dandelion, eucalyptus, marshmallow:* May increase hypoglycemic effects. Discourage use together.
**Drug-food.** *Grapefruit juice:* May inhibit metabolism of repaglinide. Discourage use together.
**Drug-lifestyle.** *Alcohol use:* May alter glycemic control, most commonly causing hypoglycemia. Discourage use together.

## EFFECTS ON LAB TEST RESULTS

● May increase or decrease glucose level.

## CONTRAINDICATIONS & CAUTIONS

● Contraindicated in patients hypersensitive to drug or its inactive ingredients and in those with type 1 (insulin-dependent) diabetes mellitus or diabetic ketoacidosis.
● Use cautiously in patients with hepatic insufficiency in whom reduced metabolism could cause hypoglycemia and elevated blood level of repaglinide.
● Use cautiously in elderly, debilitated, or malnourished patients and in those with adrenal or pituitary insufficiency because these patients are more susceptible to hypoglycemic effect of glucose-lowering drugs.

---

Reactions may be *common,* uncommon, *life-threatening,* or COMMON AND LIFE-THREATENING.

## NURSING CONSIDERATIONS

● Increase dosage carefully in patients with impaired renal function or renal failure requiring dialysis.

● Adjust dosage by glucose level response. May double dosage up to 4 mg with each meal until satisfactory glucose level is achieved. At least 1 week should elapse between dosage adjustments to assess response.

● Metformin may be added if repaglinide monotherapy is inadequate.

● Administration of oral antidiabetics may cause increased CV mortality compared with diet alone or diet plus insulin treatment. This association may also apply to repaglinide.

● Loss of glycemic control can occur during stress, such as fever, trauma, infection, or surgery. Stop drug and give insulin.

● Hypoglycemia may be difficult to recognize in elderly patients and in patients taking beta blockers.

● When switching to another oral hypoglycemic, begin new drug on day after last dose of repaglinide.

## PATIENT TEACHING

● Stress importance of diet and exercise with drug therapy.

● Discuss symptoms of low glucose level with patient and family.

● Tell patient to monitor glucose level periodically to determine minimum effective dose.

● Encourage patient to keep regular appointments and have his HbA$_{1c}$ level checked every 3 months to determine long-term glucose control.

● Tell patient to give drug before meals, usually 15 minutes before start of meal; however, time can vary from immediately preceding meal to up to 30 minutes before meal.

● Tell patient that, if a meal is skipped or added, he should skip dose or add an extra dose of drug for that meal, respectively.

● Instruct patient to monitor glucose level carefully and tell him what to do when he's ill, undergoing surgery, or under added stress.

● Advise woman planning pregnancy to first consult prescriber. Insulin may be needed during pregnancy and breast-feeding.

● Teach patient to carry candy or other simple sugars to treat mild low glucose episodes. Patient experiencing severe episode may need hospital treatment.

● Advise patient to avoid alcohol, which lowers glucose level.

## rosiglitazone maleate
Avandia⚘

*Pregnancy risk category C*

## AVAILABLE FORMS
*Tablets:* 2 mg, 4 mg, 8 mg

## INDICATIONS & DOSAGES
➤ **Adjunct to diet and exercise (as monotherapy) to improve glycemic control in patients with type 2 diabetes mellitus, or (as combination therapy) with sulfonylurea or metformin, or insulin when diet, exercise, and a single agent don't result in adequate glycemic control**

*Adults:* Initially, 4 mg P.O. daily in the morning or in divided doses b.i.d. in the morning and evening. Dosage may be increased to 8 mg P.O. daily or in divided doses b.i.d. if fasting glucose level doesn't improve after 12 weeks of treatment.

*Adjust-a-dose:* For patients stabilized on insulin, continue the insulin dose when rosiglitazone therapy starts. Don't give doses of rosiglitazone greater than 4 mg daily with insulin. Decrease insulin dose by 10% to 25% if patient reports hypoglycemia or if fasting glucose level falls to below 100 mg/dl. Individualize further adjustments based on glucose-lowering response.

## ACTION
Lowers glucose level by improving insulin sensitivity.

| Route | Onset | Peak | Duration |
|-------|-------|------|----------|
| P.O. | Unknown | 1 hr | Unknown |

## ADVERSE REACTIONS
**CNS:** headache, fatigue.
**CV:** edema.
**EENT:** sinusitis.
**GI:** diarrhea.
**Hematologic:** anemia.

**Metabolic:** hyperglycemia.
**Musculoskeletal:** back pain.
**Respiratory:** upper respiratory tract infection.
**Other:** accidental injury.

**INTERACTIONS**
None significant.

**EFFECTS ON LAB TEST RESULTS**
• May increase glucose, HDL, LDL, total cholesterol, and ALT levels.
• May decrease hemoglobin and hematocrit.

**CONTRAINDICATIONS & CAUTIONS**
• Contraindicated in patients hypersensitive to drug or its components and in those with New York Heart Association Class III or IV cardiac status unless expected benefits outweigh risks.
• Contraindicated in patients with active liver disease, increased baseline liver enzyme levels (ALT level greater than 2½ times upper limit of normal), type 1 (insulin-dependent) diabetes, or diabetic ketoacidosis and in those who experienced jaundice while taking troglitazone.
• Because metformin is contraindicated in patients with renal impairment, combination therapy with rosiglitazone is also contraindicated in patients with renal impairment. Rosiglitazone can be used as monotherapy in patients with renal impairment.
• Use cautiously in patients with edema or heart failure.

**NURSING CONSIDERATIONS**
• Before starting drug therapy, treat patient for other causes of poor glycemic control, such as infection.
• *Alert:* Check liver enzyme levels before therapy starts. Don't use drug in patients with increased baseline liver enzyme levels. In patients with normal baseline liver enzyme levels, monitor these levels every 2 months for first 12 months and periodically thereafter. If ALT level is elevated during treatment, recheck levels as soon as possible. Stop drug if levels remain elevated.
• Rosiglitazone alone or in combination with insulin can cause fluid retention that may lead to or worsen heart failure. Ob-

serve patients for these signs or symptoms of heart failure. Stop drug if any deterioration in cardiac status occurs. This drug is not recommended for NYHA Class III or IV cardiac status patients.
• Because ovulation may resume in premenopausal, anovulatory women with insulin resistance, recommend use of contraceptives.
• Management of type 2 diabetes should include diet control. Because caloric restriction, weight loss, and exercise help improve insulin sensitivity and improve effectiveness of drug therapy, these measures are essential to proper diabetes treatment.
• Check glucose level and glycosylated hemoglobin periodically to monitor therapeutic response to drug.
• Monitor patient with heart failure for increased edema.
• Hemoglobin and hematocrit may drop during therapy, usually during first 4 to 8 weeks. Increases in total cholesterol, low-density lipoprotein, and high-density lipoprotein levels and decreases in free fatty acid level also may occur.
• For patients inadequately controlled with a maximum dose of a sulfonylurea or metformin, add rosiglitazone to, rather than substitute it for, a sulfonylurea or metformin.
• *Alert:* Don't confuse rosiglitazone with pioglitazone.

**PATIENT TEACHING**
• Advise patient that drug can be taken with or without food.
• Notify patient that blood will be tested to check liver function before therapy starts, every 2 months for first 12 months, and then periodically thereafter.
• Tell patient to immediately notify prescriber about unexplained signs and symptoms, such as nausea, vomiting, abdominal pain, fatigue, anorexia, or dark urine; these may indicate liver problems.
• Warn patient to contact his health care provider if they have signs or symptoms of heart failure (unusually rapid increase in weight or swelling, shortness of breath).
• Recommend use of contraceptives to premenopausal, anovulatory women with insulin resistance because ovulation may resume with therapy.

---

Reactions may be *common*, uncommon, *life-threatening*, or COMMON AND LIFE-THREATENING.

• Advise patient that management of diabetes should include diet control. Because caloric restriction, weight loss, and exercise help improve insulin sensitivity and improve effectiveness of drug therapy, these measures are essential to proper diabetes treatment.

• Instruct patient to monitor glucose level carefully and tell him what to do when he's ill, undergoing surgery, or under added stress.

## rosiglitazone maleate and metformin hydrochloride
Avandamet

*Pregnancy risk category C*

### AVAILABLE FORMS

*Tablets:* 1 mg rosiglitazone maleate and 500 mg metformin hydrochloride, 2 mg rosiglitazone maleate and 500 mg metformin hydrochloride, 4 mg rosiglitazone maleate and 500 mg metformin hydrochloride

### INDICATIONS & DOSAGES

➤ **Adjunct to diet and exercise in patients with type 2 diabetes mellitus already treated with rosiglitazone and metformin or in patients who are inadequately controlled on metformin or rosiglitazone alone**

*Adults:* Dosage is based on patient's current doses of rosiglitazone or metformin (or both), individualized on the basis of efficacy and tolerability, and given in two divided doses with meals.

For patients inadequately controlled on metformin alone, give 2 mg rosiglitazone P.O. b.i.d., plus the dose of metformin already being taken (500 mg or 1,000 mg P.O. b.i.d.). Dosage increases may occur after 8 to 12 weeks.

For patients inadequately controlled on rosiglitazone alone, give 500 mg metformin P.O. b.i.d., plus the dose of rosiglitazone already being taken (2 mg or 4 mg P.O. b.i.d.). Dosage increases may occur after 1 to 2 weeks.

The total daily dose of Avandamet may be increased in increments of 4 mg rosiglitazone or 500 mg metformin, or both, up to the maximum daily dose of 8 mg/2,000 mg in two divided doses.

*Adjust-a-dose:* In elderly patients, initial and maintenance doses should be conservative because kidney function may be reduced in this population. Don't give elderly, malnourished, and debilitated patients the maximum dose.

### ACTION

Drug contains two antidiabetic agents with different mechanisms of action to lower glucose level. Rosiglitazone is an insulin-sensitizing agent that enhances peripheral glucose use. It's a highly selective and potent agonist of receptors found in key target tissues for insulin action such as adipose tissue, skeletal muscle, and the liver. Metformin hydrochloride decreases hepatic glucose production and intestinal absorption of glucose and increases insulin sensitivity (peripheral glucose uptake and use).

| Route | Onset | Peak | Duration |
|---|---|---|---|
| P.O. (rosiglitazone) | Unknown | 1 hr | Unknown |
| P.O. (metformin) | Unknown | 2-4 hr | Unknown |

### ADVERSE REACTIONS

**CNS:** headache, fatigue.
**CV:** edema.
**EENT:** sinusitis.
**GI:** *diarrhea.*
**Hematologic:** anemia.
**Metabolic:** hyperglycemia, hypoglycemia.
**Musculoskeletal:** back pain, arthralgia.
**Respiratory:** *upper respiratory tract infection.*
**Other:** accidental injury, viral infection.

### INTERACTIONS

**Drug-drug.** *Cationic drugs (amiloride, digoxin, morphine, procainamide, quinidine, quinine, ranitidine, triamterene, trimethoprim, vancomycin):* May decrease metformin excretion. Monitor glucose level; may need to adjust cationic drugs or metformin.
*Furosemide:* May increase metformin level and decrease furosemide level. Monitor patient closely.
*Nifedipine:* May increase absorption of metformin. Monitor patient closely.

---

*Thiazides, corticosteroids, phenothiazines, thyroid products, estrogens, hormonal contraceptives, phenytoin, nicotinic acid, sympathomimetics, calcium channel blocking drugs, isoniazid:* May affect glycemic control. Monitor glucose level; may need to adjust dosage.

**Drug-herb.** *Guar gum:* May decrease hypoglycemic effect. Monitor glucose level.

**Drug-lifestyle.** *Alcohol use:* May increase effect of metformin on lactate metabolism and increase risk of lactic acidosis. Discourage use together.

## EFFECTS ON LAB TEST RESULTS
• May increase ALT level. May decrease vitamin $B_{12}$ level.
• May decrease hemoglobin and hematocrit.

## CONTRAINDICATIONS & CAUTIONS
• Contraindicated in patients hypersensitive to rosiglitazone or metformin and in those with renal disease or renal dysfunction (abnormal creatinine clearance, or creatinine level 1.5 mg/dl or greater in men or 1.4 mg/dl or greater in women); heart failure requiring drug therapy; type 1 diabetes; acute or chronic metabolic acidosis, including diabetic ketoacidosis, with or without coma; clinical evidence of active liver disease or increased transaminase level (ALT more than 2.5 times the upper limit of normal).
• Contraindicated in pregnant and breastfeeding patients.
• Contraindicated if combined with insulin.
• Use cautiously in patients with edema or at high risk for heart failure.

## NURSING CONSIDERATIONS
• Because aging often causes reduced renal function, use drug with caution in elderly patients. Make dose selection carefully and monitor renal function regularly. Don't give elderly patients the maximum daily dose. Don't start treatment in patients older than age 80 unless renal function is normal.
• In patients undergoing radiologic studies involving iodinated contrast materials, stop drug before or during the procedure, and withhold for 48 hours after the procedure. Resume treatment only after renal function has been reevaluated and documented to be normal.
• Stop drug temporarily in patients having surgery. Don't restart until oral intake has resumed and renal function is normal.
• Monitor transaminase level at baseline, every 2 months for the first 12 months, and periodically thereafter. If ALT level increases to more than 3 times the upper limit of normal, recheck liver enzymes as soon as possible. If ALT remains more than 3 times the upper limit of normal, stop drug.
• Monitor CBC and vitamin $B_{12}$ level.
• Monitor for signs and symptoms of heart failure and hepatic dysfunction. Stop drug use if jaundice occurs.
• Monitor renal function at baseline and at least annually during therapy.
• Monitor glycosylated hemoglobin every 3 months.
• Stop drug if shock, acute heart failure, acute MI, or other conditions linked to hypoxemia occur.

## PATIENT TEACHING
• Stress the importance of dietary instructions, weight loss, and a regular exercise program.
• Tell patient to immediately report unexplained hyperventilation, myalgia, malaise, or unusual somnolence.
• Instruct patients to report a rapid increase in weight, swelling, shortness of breath, or other symptoms of heart failure.
• Tell patient to report unexplained nausea, vomiting, abdominal pain, fatigue, anorexia, or dark urine.
• Explain that it may take 1 to 2 weeks for drug to take effect and up to 2 to 3 months for the full effect to occur.
• Stress the importance of avoiding excessive alcohol intake.
• Discuss the possible need for contraception with premenopausal women as ovulation may resume.
• Advise patient to take the medication in divided doses with meals to reduce GI side effects.

levothyroxine sodium
liothyronine sodium
liotrix
thyroid, desiccated

**COMBINATION PRODUCTS**
None.

---

## levothyroxine sodium
## ($T_4$, L-thyroxine sodium)
Eltroxin†, Levo-T, Levotect†,
Levothroid, Levoxine, Levoxyl✐,
Novothyrox, Oroxine‡, Synthroid✐,
Thyro-Tabs, Unithroid

*Pregnancy risk category A*

**AVAILABLE FORMS**
*Injection:* 200-mcg vial, 500-mcg vial
*Tablets:* 25 mcg, 50 mcg, 75 mcg, 88 mcg,
100 mcg, 112 mcg, 125 mcg, 137 mcg,
150 mcg, 175 mcg, 200 mcg, 300 mcg

**INDICATIONS & DOSAGES**
➤ **Myxedema coma**
*Adults:* 300 to 500 mcg I.V., followed by
parenteral maintenance dose of 75 to
100 mcg I.V. daily. Switch patient to oral
maintenance as soon as possible.
➤ **Thyroid hormone replacement**
*Adults:* Initially, 25 to 50 mcg P.O. daily;
increase by 25 mcg P.O. q 4 to 8 weeks
until desired response occurs. Maintenance dosage is 75 to 200 mcg P.O. daily.
*Children older than age 12:* More than
150 mcg or 2 to 3 mcg/kg P.O. daily.
*Children ages 6 to 12:* 100 to 150 mcg or
4 to 5 mcg/kg P.O. daily.
*Children ages 1 to 5:* 75 to 100 mcg or
5 to 6 mcg/kg P.O. daily.
*Children ages 6 months to 1 year:* 50 to
75 mcg or 6 to 8 mcg/kg P.O. daily.
*Children younger than age 6 months:*
25 to 50 mcg or 8 to 10 mcg/kg P.O. daily.
*Patients older than age 65:* 12.5 to 50 mcg
P.O. daily; increase by 12.5 to 25 mcg q
6 to 8 weeks, depending on response.

**I.V. ADMINISTRATION**
• Prepare I.V. dose immediately before injection. Dilute Synthroid powder for injection with 5 ml of normal saline solution
for injection to 200- or 500-mcg vial;
don't use other diluents. Resulting solutions contain 40 or 100 mcg/ml, respectively. Don't mix with other I.V. infusion
solutions. Inject into vein over 1 to 2 minutes.
• First I.V. dose is about half the previously established oral dose of Synthroid
tablets.
• Monitor blood pressure and heart rate
closely. High initial I.V. dosage is usually
well tolerated by patients in myxedema
coma. Normal $T_4$ level should occur within 24 hours, followed by a threefold increase in $T_3$ in 3 days.

**ACTION**
Not completely defined. Stimulates metabolism of all body tissues by accelerating rate of cellular oxidation.

| Route | Onset | Peak | Duration |
|-------|-------|------|----------|
| P.O. | 24 hr | Unknown | Unknown |
| I.V. | Unknown | Unknown | Unknown |

**ADVERSE REACTIONS**
**CNS:** *nervousness, insomnia, tremor,*
headache, fever.
**CV:** *tachycardia, palpitations,* **arrhyth-
mias,** *angina pectoris,* **cardiac arrest.**
**GI:** diarrhea, vomiting.
**GU:** menstrual irregularities.
**Metabolic:** weight loss.
**Musculoskeletal:** decreased bone density.
**Skin:** allergic skin reactions, diaphoresis.
**Other:** heat intolerance.

**INTERACTIONS**
**Drug-drug.** *Beta blockers:* May reduce
beta blocker effects. Monitor patient.
*Cholestyramine, colestipol:* May impair
levothyroxine absorption. Separate doses
by 4 to 5 hours.
*Digoxin:* May decrease glycoside effects.
Monitor patient for clinical effect.

---

*Estrogens:* May decrease free levothyroxines. Monitor patient for decreased effectiveness of thyroid hormone.

*Fosphenytoin, phenytoin:* May release free thyroid. Monitor patient for tachycardia.

*Insulin, oral antidiabetics:* May alter glucose level. Monitor glucose level. Dosage adjustments may be needed.

*Oral anticoagulants:* May alter PT. Monitor PT and INR. Dosage adjustments may be needed.

*Sympathomimetics such as epinephrine:* May increase risk of coronary insufficiency. Monitor patient closely.

*Theophylline:* May decrease theophylline clearance in hypothyroidism; clearance may return to normal when euthyroid state is achieved. Monitor theophylline level.

**Drug-herb.** *Horseradish:* May cause abnormal thyroid function. Discourage use in patients undergoing thyroid function tests.

*Lemon balm:* May have antithyroid effects; may inhibit thyroid-stimulating hormone. Discourage use together.

### EFFECTS ON LAB TEST RESULTS
• May decrease thyroid function test result values.

### CONTRAINDICATIONS & CAUTIONS
• Contraindicated in patients hypersensitive to drug and in those with acute MI uncomplicated by hypothyroidism, untreated thyrotoxicosis, or uncorrected adrenal insufficiency.
• Use cautiously in elderly patients and in those with angina pectoris, hypertension, other CV disorders, renal insufficiency, or ischemia.
• Use cautiously in patients with diabetes mellitus, diabetes insipidus, or myxedema and during rapid replacement in those with arteriosclerosis. Patients with diabetes mellitus may need increased antidiabetic doses when starting thyroid hormone replacement.

### NURSING CONSIDERATIONS
• *Alert:* Drug may be given I.V. or I.M. when P.O. ingestion is precluded for long periods. However, dosage adjustment is needed.

• Watch for angina, coronary occlusion, or CVA in patients with arteriosclerosis who are receiving rapid replacement.
• In patients with coronary artery disease who must receive thyroid hormone, observe carefully for possible coronary insufficiency.
• Thyroid hormone replacement requirements are about 25% lower in patients older than age 60 than in young adults.
• Patients with adult hypothyroidism are unusually sensitive to thyroid hormone. Start at lowest dosage and adjust to higher dosages according to patient's symptoms and laboratory data until euthyroid state is reached.
• When changing from levothyroxine to liothyronine, stop levothyroxine and begin liothyronine. Increase dosage in small increments after residual effects of levothyroxine have disappeared. When changing from liothyronine to levothyroxine, levothyroxine is started several days before withdrawing liothyronine to avoid relapse. Drugs aren't interchangeable.
• Long-term therapy causes bone loss in premenopausal and postmenopausal women. Consider a basal bone density measurement and monitor closely for osteoporosis.
• Thyroid hormones alter thyroid function test results.
• Patients taking levothyroxine who need to have [131]I uptake studies performed must stop drug 4 weeks before test.
• Patients taking anticoagulants may need their dosage modified; they require careful monitoring of coagulation status.
• Results of liothyronine, protein-bound iodine, and radioactive [131]I uptake studies may be altered.
• *Alert:* Don't confuse levothyroxine with liothyronine or liotrix.
• Synthroid may contain tartrazine.

### PATIENT TEACHING
• Teach patient the importance of compliance. Tell him to take thyroid hormones at same time each day, preferably ½ to 1 hour before breakfast, to maintain constant hormone levels and help prevent insomnia.
• Make sure patient understands that replacement therapy is usually for a lifetime.

---

Reactions may be *common*, uncommon, *life-threatening*, or COMMON AND LIFE-THREATENING.

The drug should never be stopped unless directed by prescriber.

• Warn patient (especially elderly patient) to notify prescriber at once about chest pain, palpitations, sweating, nervousness, shortness of breath, or other signals of overdose or aggravated CV disease.

• Tell caregiver of infant or child who can't swallow tablets to crush tablet and suspend in small amount of formula (except soy formula which may decrease the absorption), breast milk, or water and give by spoon or dropper. Crushed tablet can be sprinkled over food, avoiding foods containing large amounts of soybean, fiber, or iron.

• Advise patient who has achieved stable response not to change brands.

• Tell patient to report unusual bleeding and bruising.

• Advise patient not to take OTC or other prescription medications without first consulting prescriber.

---

## liothyronine sodium (T₃)
Cytomel, Tertroxin‡, Triostat

*Pregnancy risk category A*

### AVAILABLE FORMS
*Injection:* 10 mcg/ml
*Tablets:* 5 mcg, 20 mcg‡, 25 mcg, 50 mcg

### INDICATIONS & DOSAGES
➤ **Congenital hypothyroidism**
*Children:* 5 mcg P.O. daily; increase by 5 mcg q 3 to 4 days until desired response is achieved.
➤ **Myxedema**
*Adults:* Initially, 2.5 to 5 mcg P.O. daily; increase by 5 to 10 mcg q 1 to 2 weeks until daily dose reaches 25 mcg. Then, increase by 12.5 to 25 mcg daily q 1 to 2 weeks. Maintenance dosage is 50 to 100 mcg daily.
➤ **Myxedema coma, premyxedema coma**
*Adults:* Initially, 10 to 20 mcg I.V. for patients with CV disease; 25 to 50 mcg I.V. for patients who don't have CV disease. Adjust dosage based on patient's condition and response. Switch patient to oral therapy as soon as possible.

➤ **Simple (nontoxic) goiter**
*Adults:* Initially, 5 mcg P.O. daily; may increase by 5 to 10 mcg daily q 1 to 2 weeks, until daily dose reaches 25 mcg. Then, increase by 12.5 to 25 mcg daily q 1 to 2 weeks. Usual maintenance dosage is 75 mcg daily.
➤ **Thyroid hormone replacement**
*Adults:* Initially, 25 mcg P.O. daily; increase by 12.5 to 25 mcg q 1 to 2 weeks until satisfactory response occurs. Usual maintenance dosage is 25 to 50 mcg daily.
*Patients older than age 65 and children:* 5 mcg daily; increase by 5 mcg daily q 1 to 2 weeks.
➤ **T₃ suppression test to differentiate hyperthyroidism from euthyroidism**
*Adults:* 75 to 100 mcg P.O. daily for 7 days.

### I.V. ADMINISTRATION
• Give repeat doses 4 to 12 hours apart.

### ACTION
Not clearly defined. Enhances oxygen consumption by most tissues of the body; increases the basal metabolic rate and the metabolism of carbohydrates, lipids, and proteins.

| Route | Onset | Peak | Duration |
|-------|-------|------|----------|
| P.O. | Unknown | 2-3 days | 3 days |
| I.V. | Unknown | Unknown | Unknown |

### ADVERSE REACTIONS
**CNS:** *nervousness, insomnia, tremor,* headache.
**CV:** *tachycardia,* **arrhythmias,** angina, **cardiac decompensation and collapse.**
**GI:** diarrhea, vomiting.
**GU:** menstrual irregularities.
**Metabolic:** weight loss.
**Musculoskeletal:** accelerated bone maturation in infants and children.
**Skin:** skin reactions, diaphoresis.
**Other:** heat intolerance.

### INTERACTIONS
**Drug-drug.** *Beta blockers:* May reduce beta blocker effects. Monitor patient for clinical effect.
*Cholestyramine, colestipol:* May impair liothyronine absorption. Separate doses by 4 to 5 hours.

---

*Digoxin:* May decrease glycoside effects. Monitor patient for clinical effect.

*Insulin, oral antidiabetics:* First thyroid replacement therapy may increase insulin or oral hypoglycemic requirements. Monitor glucose level. Dosage adjustments may be needed.

*Oral anticoagulants:* May alter PT. Monitor PT and INR. Dosage adjustments may be needed.

*Sympathomimetics such as epinephrine:* May increase risk of coronary insufficiency. Monitor patient closely.

*Theophylline:* May decrease theophylline clearance in hypothyroidism; clearance may return to normal when euthyroid state is achieved. Monitor theophylline level.

**Drug-herb.** *Lemon balm:* May have antithyroid effects; may inhibit thyroid-stimulating hormone. Discourage use together.

**EFFECTS ON LAB TEST RESULTS**
● May decrease thyroid function test result values.
● May alter results of liothyronine, protein-bound iodine, and radioactive [131]I uptake studies.

**CONTRAINDICATIONS & CAUTIONS**
● Contraindicated in patients hypersensitive to drug and in those with acute MI uncomplicated by hypothyroidism, untreated thyrotoxicosis, or uncorrected adrenal insufficiency.
● Use cautiously in elderly patients and in those with angina pectoris, hypertension, other CV disorders, renal insufficiency, or ischemia.
● Use cautiously in patients with diabetes mellitus, diabetes insipidus, or myxedema and during rapid replacement in those with arteriosclerosis.

**NURSING CONSIDERATIONS**
● Watch for angina, coronary occlusion, or CVA in patients with arteriosclerosis who are receiving rapid replacement. In patients with coronary artery disease who must receive thyroid hormones, watch for possible coronary insufficiency.
● *Alert:* Levothyroxine is usually the preferred drug for thyroid hormone replacement therapy. Liothyronine may be used when a rapid-onset or a rapidly reversible

drug is desirable, or in patients with impaired peripheral conversion of levothyroxine to liothyronine.
● Long-term therapy causes bone loss in premenopausal and postmenopausal women. Consider a basal bone density measurement and monitor closely for osteoporosis.
● Regulation of liothyronine dosage is difficult.
● Thyroid hormone replacement requirements are about 25% lower in patients older than age 60 than in young adults.
● Monitor pulse and blood pressure.
● When changing from levothyroxine to liothyronine, stop levothyroxine and start liothyronine at a low dosage. Increase dosage in small increments after residual effects of levothyroxine have disappeared. When changing from liothyronine to levothyroxine, start levothyroxine several days before stopping liothyronine to avoid relapse.
● When switching from I.V. to P.O. therapy, gradually increase I.V. dose while starting P.O. dose.
● Patients taking liothyronine who need [131]I uptake studies done must stop drug 7 to 10 days before test.
● *Alert:* Don't confuse levothyroxine with liothyronine or liotrix. Don't confuse Cytomel with Cytotec.
● *Alert:* Don't give injection I.M. or S.C.

**PATIENT TEACHING**
● Teach patient importance of compliance. Tell him to take thyroid hormones at same time each day, preferably before breakfast, to maintain constant hormone levels and help prevent insomnia.
● Make sure patient understands that replacement therapy is usually for a lifetime. Drug should never be stopped unless directed by prescriber.
● Advise patient who has achieved a stable response not to change brands.
● Warn patient (especially elderly patient) to notify prescriber at once about chest pain, palpitations, sweating, nervousness, or other signals of overdose or aggravated CV disease.
● Tell patient to report unusual bleeding and bruising.
● Advise diabetic patients to monitor blood sugars closely.

---

Reactions may be *common*, uncommon, *life-threatening*, or **COMMON AND LIFE-THREATENING**.

• Tell patient not to take OTC or other prescription medications without first consulting his prescriber.

## liotrix
Thyrolar†

*Pregnancy risk category A*

### AVAILABLE FORMS
*Tablets:* levothyroxine sodium 12.5 mcg and liothyronine sodium 3.1 mcg (Thyrolar-1/4); levothyroxine sodium 25 mcg and liothyronine sodium 6.25 mcg (Thyrolar-1/2); levothyroxine sodium 50 mcg and liothyronine sodium 12.5 mcg (Thyrolar-1); levothyroxine sodium 100 mcg and liothyronine sodium 25 mcg (Thyrolar-2); levothyroxine sodium 150 mcg and liothyronine sodium 37.5 mcg (Thyrolar-3)

### INDICATIONS & DOSAGES
➤ **Hypothyroidism**
Dosages are expressed in thyroid equivalents and must be individualized to approximate the deficit in patient's thyroid secretion.
*Adults:* Initially, a single daily dose of Thyrolar-1/4 or Thyrolar-1/2. Adjust dosage at 2-week intervals.

### ACTION
Not clearly defined. Stimulates metabolism of all body tissues by accelerating the rate of cellular oxidation and provides both $T_3$ and $T_4$ to the tissues.

| Route | Onset | Peak | Duration |
|-------|-------|------|----------|
| P.O. | Unknown | Unknown | Unknown |

### ADVERSE REACTIONS
**CNS:** *nervousness, insomnia, tremor,* headache.
**CV:** *tachycardia,* **arrhythmias,** angina pectoris, **cardiac decompensation and collapse.**
**GI:** diarrhea, vomiting.
**GU:** menstrual irregularities.
**Metabolic:** weight loss.
**Musculoskeletal:** accelerated rate of bone maturation in infants and children.
**Skin:** allergic skin reactions, diaphoresis.
**Other:** heat intolerance.

### INTERACTIONS
**Drug-drug.** *Beta blockers:* May reduce beta blocker effects. Monitor patient for clinical effect.
*Cholestyramine, colestipol:* May impair liotrix absorption. Separate doses by 4 to 5 hours.
*Digoxin:* May decrease glycoside effects. Monitor patient for clinical effect.
*Fosphenytoin, phenytoin:* May release free thyroid. Monitor patient for tachycardia.
*Insulin, oral antidiabetics:* May alter glucose level. Monitor glucose level. Dosage adjustments may be needed.
*Oral anticoagulants:* May alter PT. Monitor PT and INR. Dosage adjustments may be needed.
*Sympathomimetics such as epinephrine:* May increase risk of coronary insufficiency. Monitor patient closely.
*Theophylline:* May decrease theophylline clearance in hypothyroidism; clearance may return to normal when euthyroid state is achieved. Monitor theophylline level.
**Drug-herb.** *Lemon balm:* May have antithyroid effects; may inhibit thyroid-stimulating hormone. Discourage use together.

### EFFECTS ON LAB TEST RESULTS
• May decrease thyroid function test result values.

### CONTRAINDICATIONS & CAUTIONS
• Contraindicated in patients hypersensitive to drug and in those with acute MI uncomplicated by hypothyroidism, untreated thyrotoxicosis, or uncorrected adrenal insufficiency.
• Use cautiously in elderly patients and in those with angina pectoris, hypertension, other CV disorders, renal insufficiency, or ischemia.
• Use cautiously in patients with diabetes mellitus, diabetes insipidus, or myxedema and during rapid replacement in those with arteriosclerosis.

### NURSING CONSIDERATIONS
• Watch for angina, coronary occlusion, or CVA in patients with arteriosclerosis who are receiving rapid replacement.
• In patients with coronary artery disease who must receive thyroid hormones, watch carefully for possible coronary in-

sufficiency. Also watch carefully during surgery because arrhythmias may arise.
• Thyroid hormone replacement requirements are about 25% lower in patients older than age 60 than in young adults.
• Monitor pulse and blood pressure.
• Long-term therapy causes bone loss in premenopausal and postmenopausal women. Consider a basal bone density measurement and monitor closely for osteoporosis.
• Patients taking liotrix who need [131]I uptake studies done must stop drug 7 to 10 days before test. Results of liothyronine, protein-bound iodine, and radioactive [131]I uptake studies may be altered.
• *Alert:* Don't confuse Thyrolar with thyroid or Synthroid; don't confuse liotrix with levothyroxine or liothyronine.

## PATIENT TEACHING
• Teach patient importance of compliance. He should take thyroid hormones at same time each day, preferably before breakfast, to maintain constant hormone levels and help prevent insomnia.
• Tell patient that drug should never be stopped unless directed by prescriber.
• Warn patient (especially elderly patient) to notify prescriber at once about chest pain, palpitations, sweating, nervousness, or other signs of overdose or aggravated CV disease.
• Tell patient to report unusual bleeding and bruising.
• Advise patient not to take OTC or other prescription medications without first consulting his prescriber.

---

## thyroid, desiccated
Armour Thyroid

*Pregnancy risk category A*

---

## AVAILABLE FORMS
*Tablets:* 15 mg, 30 mg, 60 mg, 90 mg, 120 mg, 180 mg, 240 mg, 300 mg

## INDICATIONS & DOSAGES
➤ **Mild hypothyroidism**
*Adults:* Initially, 60 mg P.O. daily, increased by 60 mg q 30 days until desired response occurs. Usual maintenance dose is 60 to 120 mg daily as single dose.

*Elderly patients:* Start at lower dose.
➤ **Severe hypothyroidism**
*Adults:* Initially, 15 mg P.O. daily; increased by 30 mg daily after 2 weeks, and 2 weeks later increased to 60 mg daily. After 2 months, increased to 120 mg daily if response is still inadequate.
*Patients older than age 65:* 7.5 to 15 mg daily. May double dose q 6 to 8 weeks until desired result is obtained.
➤ **Congenital or severe hypothyroidism in children**
*Children older than age 12:* 1.2 to 1.8 mg/kg daily P.O.
*Children ages 6 to 12:* 2.4 to 3 mg/kg daily P.O.
*Children ages 1 to 5:* 3 to 3.6 mg/kg daily P.O.
*Children ages 6 months to 1 year:* 3.6 to 4.8 mg/kg daily P.O.
*Children younger than 6 months:* 4.8 to 6 mg/kg daily P.O.
*Adjust-a-dose:* In patients with long-term disease, other endocrine diseases, severe hypothyroidism, or CV disease, start at lower dose.

## ACTION
Not clearly defined. Stimulates metabolism of all body tissues by accelerating the rate of cellular oxidation.

| Route | Onset | Peak | Duration |
|-------|-------|------|----------|
| P.O. | Unknown | Unknown | Unknown |

## ADVERSE REACTIONS
**CNS:** *nervousness, insomnia,* tremor, headache.
**CV:** *tachycardia,* **arrhythmias,** angina pectoris, **cardiac decompensation and collapse.**
**GI:** diarrhea, vomiting.
**GU:** menstrual irregularities.
**Metabolic:** weight loss.
**Musculoskeletal:** accelerated rate of bone maturation in infants and children.
**Skin:** allergic skin reactions, diaphoresis.
**Other:** heat intolerance.

## INTERACTIONS
**Drug-drug.** *Beta blockers:* May reduce beta blocker effects. Monitor patient for clinical effect.
*Cholestyramine:* May impair thyroid absorption. Separate doses by 4 to 5 hours.

---

*Digoxin:* May decrease glycoside effects. Monitor patient for clinical effect.

*Insulin, oral antidiabetics:* May alter glucose level. Monitor glucose level and adjust dosage as needed.

*Oral anticoagulants:* May alter PT. Monitor PT and INR. Adjust dosage as needed.

*Sympathomimetics, such as epinephrine:* May increase risk of coronary insufficiency. Monitor patient closely.

*Theophylline:* May decrease theophylline clearance in hypothyroidism; clearance may return to normal when euthyroid state is achieved. Monitor theophylline level.

**Drug-herb.** *Lemon balm:* May have antithyroid effects; may inhibit thyroid-stimulating hormone. Discourage use together.

## EFFECTS ON LAB TEST RESULTS
• May decrease thyroid function test result values.

## CONTRAINDICATIONS & CAUTIONS
• Contraindicated in patients hypersensitive to drug and in those with acute MI uncomplicated by hypothyroidism, untreated thyrotoxicosis, or uncorrected adrenal insufficiency.
• Use cautiously in elderly patients and in those with angina pectoris, hypertension, other CV disorders, renal insufficiency, or ischemia.
• Use cautiously in patients with myxedema, diabetes mellitus, or diabetes insipidus.

## NURSING CONSIDERATIONS
• Check for coronary insufficiency in patients with coronary artery disease.
• Thyroid hormone replacement requirements are about 25% lower in patients older than age 60 than in young adults.
• Monitor pulse and blood pressure.
• Reduce dose if angina occurs.
• Long-term therapy causes bone loss in premenopausal and postmenopausal women. Consider a basal bone density measurement and monitor closely for osteoporosis.
• In children, treatment is guided by sleeping pulse rate and basal morning temperature.
• Thyroid hormones alter thyroid function test results. Results of liothyronine,

protein-bound iodine, and radioactive $^{131}$I uptake studies may be altered.
• Patient must stop thyroid hormones 7 to 10 days before undergoing $^{131}$I studies.
• *Alert:* Don't confuse thyroid with Thyrolar.

## PATIENT TEACHING
• Tell patient to take thyroid hormones at same time each day, preferably before breakfast, to maintain constant hormone levels and help prevent insomnia.
• Tell patient the drug should never be stopped unless directed by prescriber.
• Advise patient who has achieved stable response not to change brands.
• Warn patient (especially elderly patient) to notify prescriber at once about chest pain, palpitations, or other signs of overdose or aggravated CV disease.
• Tell patient to report unusual bleeding and bruising.
• Advise patient not to take OTC or other prescription medications without first consulting his prescriber.

**methimazole**
**potassium iodide**
**propylthiouracil**
**radioactive iodine**

### COMBINATION PRODUCTS
None.

---

### methimazole
Tapazole

*Pregnancy risk category D*

### AVAILABLE FORMS
*Tablets:* 5 mg, 10 mg

### INDICATIONS & DOSAGES
➤ **Hyperthyroidism**
*Adults:* If mild, 15 mg P.O. daily. If moderately severe, 30 to 40 mg daily. If severe, 60 mg daily. Daily amount is divided into three equal doses and given at 8-hour intervals. Maintenance dosage is 5 to 30 mg daily.
*Children:* 0.4 mg/kg P.O. in three divided doses daily. Maintenance dosage is 0.2 mg/kg in divided doses daily.

### ACTION
Inhibits oxidation of iodine in thyroid gland, blocking ability of iodine to combine with tyrosine to form $T_4$. Also may prevent coupling of monoiodotyrosine and diiodotyrosine to form $T_4$ and $T_3$.

| Route | Onset | Peak | Duration |
|-------|-------|------|----------|
| P.O. | Rapid | 30-60 min | Unknown |

### ADVERSE REACTIONS
**CNS:** headache, drowsiness, vertigo, paresthesia, neuritis, neuropathies, CNS stimulation, depression, fever.
**GI:** diarrhea, nausea, vomiting, salivary gland enlargement, loss of taste, epigastric distress.
**GU:** nephritis.
**Hematologic:** *agranulocytosis, leukopenia, thrombocytopenia, aplastic anemia.*

**Hepatic:** jaundice, hepatic dysfunction, *hepatitis.*
**Metabolic:** hypothyroidism.
**Musculoskeletal:** arthralgia, myalgia.
**Skin:** rash, urticaria, discoloration, pruritus, erythema nodosum, exfoliative dermatitis, lupuslike syndrome, abnormal hair loss.
**Other:** lymphadenopathy.

### INTERACTIONS
**Drug-drug.** *Aminophylline, oxtriphylline, theophylline:* May decrease clearance of these drugs. Dosage may need to be adjusted.
*Anticoagulants:* May alter dosage requirements. Monitor PT, PTT, and INR.
*Beta blockers:* Hyperthyroidism may increase beta blocker clearance. May need to reduce dosage of beta blocker when patient becomes euthyroid.
*Cardiac glycosides:* May increase cardiac glycoside level. Cardiac glycoside dosage may need to be reduced.
*Potassium iodide:* May decrease response to drug. Methimazole dosage may need to be increased.

### EFFECTS ON LAB TEST RESULTS
● May decrease hemoglobin and granulocyte, WBC, and platelet counts.
● May alter selenomethionine ($^{75}$Se) uptake by the pancreas and $^{123}$I or $^{131}$I uptake by the thyroid.

### CONTRAINDICATIONS & CAUTIONS
● Contraindicated in patients hypersensitive to drug and in breast-feeding women.
● Use cautiously in pregnant patients.

### NURSING CONSIDERATIONS
● Pregnant women may need less drug as pregnancy progresses. Monitor thyroid function studies closely. Thyroid hormone may be added to regimen. Drug may be stopped during last few weeks of pregnancy.
● Monitor CBC periodically to detect impending leukopenia, thrombocytopenia,

and agranulocytosis; also monitor hepatic function.
- **Alert:** Doses higher than 30 mg/day increase risk of agranulocytosis.
- **Alert:** Patients older than age 40 may have an increased risk of drug-induced agranulocytosis.
- Watch for evidence of hypothyroidism (mental depression; cold intolerance; hard, nonpitting edema); notify prescriber because patient may need dosage adjustment.
- **Alert:** Stop drug and notify prescriber if severe rash or enlarged cervical lymph nodes develop.
- **Alert:** Don't confuse methimazole with mebendazole or methazolamide.

### PATIENT TEACHING
- Tell patient to take drug with meals to reduce adverse GI reactions.
- Warn patient to report fever, sore throat, mouth sores, skin eruptions, anorexia, itching, right upper quadrant pain, yellow skin or eyes.
- Tell patient to ask prescriber about using iodized salt and eating shellfish, because the iodine in these products may make the drug less effective.
- Warn patient that drug may cause drowsiness; advise patient to use caution when operating machinery or a vehicle.
- Instruct patient to store drug in light-resistant container.
- Teach patient to watch for evidence of hypothyroidism (unexplained weight gain, fatigue, cold intolerance) and to notify prescriber if it arises.
- Tell woman not to use drug while breast-feeding.

## potassium iodide
Pima, saturated solution (SSKI), strong iodine solution (Lugol's solution), Thyro-Block

*Pregnancy risk category D*

### AVAILABLE FORMS
*Oral solution (Lugol's solution):* iodine 5% and potassium iodide 10%
*Oral solution (SSKI):* 1 g/ml
*Syrup:* 325 mg/5 ml
*Tablets:* 130 mg

### INDICATIONS & DOSAGES
➤ **To prepare for thyroidectomy**
*Adults and children:* 3 to 5 drops strong iodine solution P.O. t.i.d.; or 1 to 5 drops SSKI in water P.O. t.i.d. after meals for 10 days before surgery.
➤ **Thyrotoxic crisis**
*Adults and children:* 500 mg P.O. q 4 hours (about 10 drops of SSKI); or 1 ml of strong iodine solution t.i.d. Give at least 1 hour after the first dose of propylthiouracil or methimazole.
➤ **Radiation protectant for thyroid gland**
*Adults:* 130 mg P.O. daily for 10 days after radiation exposure. Start no later than 3 or 4 hours after acute exposure. Or, 3 ml Pima P.O. once daily 24 hours before and for 10 days after exposure.
*Children ages 3 to 18:* 65 mg P.O. daily for 10 days after exposure. Start no later than 3 or 4 hours after acute exposure.
*Children ages 1 to 18:* 2 ml Pima P.O. once daily 24 hours before and for 10 days after exposure.
*Infants and children up to age 1 year:* 1 ml Pima P.O. once daily 24 hours before and for 10 days after exposure.

### ACTION
Inhibits thyroid hormone formation, limits iodide transport into the thyroid gland, and blocks thyroid hormone release.

| Route | Onset | Peak | Duration |
|-------|-------|------|----------|
| P.O. | < 24 hr | 10-15 days | Unknown |

### ADVERSE REACTIONS
**CNS:** fever.
**EENT:** periorbital edema.
**GI:** diarrhea, inflammation of salivary glands, burning mouth and throat, sore teeth and gums, *metallic taste.*
**Metabolic:** *potassium toxicity.*
**Skin:** acneiform rash.
**Other:** hypersensitivity reactions.

### INTERACTIONS
**Drug-drug.** *ACE inhibitors, potassium-sparing diuretics:* May cause hyperkalemia. Avoid using together.
*Antithyroid drugs:* May increase hypothyroid or goitrogenic effects. Monitor patient closely.

*Lithium carbonate:* May cause hypothyroidism. Use together cautiously.

## EFFECTS ON LAB TEST RESULTS
● May increase potassium level.
● May alter thyroid function test results.

## CONTRAINDICATIONS & CAUTIONS
● Contraindicated in patients with tuberculosis, acute bronchitis, iodide hypersensitivity, or hyperkalemia. Some formulations
contain sulfites, which may precipitate allergic reactions in hypersensitive patients.
● Use cautiously in patients with hypo-
complementemic vasculitis, goiter, or autoimmune thyroid disease.

## NURSING CONSIDERATIONS
● Expect to give with other antithyroid
drugs.
● For thyrotoxicosis, first iodine dose is
given at least 1 hour after first dose of
propylthiouracil and methimazole.
● Dilute oral solution in water, milk, or
fruit juice, and give after meals to prevent
gastric irritation, hydrate patient, and
mask salty taste.
● Give iodides through straw to avoid
tooth discoloration.
● *Alert:* Earliest signs of delayed hypersensitivity reactions caused by iodides are irritation and swollen eyelids.
● Monitor patient for iodism, which can
cause metallic taste, burning in mouth and
throat, sore teeth and gums, increased salivation, coryza, sneezing, eye irritation
with swelling of eyelids, severe headache,
productive cough, GI irritation, diarrhea,
rash, or soreness of the pharynx, larynx,
and tonsils.
● Store in light-resistant container.

## PATIENT TEACHING
● Show patient how to mask salty taste of
oral solution. Tell him to take all forms of
drug after meals.
● *Alert:* Warn patient that sudden withdrawal may precipitate thyroid crisis.
● *Alert:* Teach patient signs and symptoms
of potassium toxicity, including confusion,
irregular heartbeat, numbness, tingling,
pain or weakness of hands or feet, and
tiredness.
● Tell patient to ask prescriber about using
iodized salt and eating shellfish. These

foods contain iodine and may alter drug's
effectiveness.
● Tell patient not to increase the amount of
potassium through diet.
● Tell patient to stop drug and notify prescriber if epigastric pain, rash, metallic
taste, nausea, or vomiting occurs.

## propylthiouracil (PTU)
Propyl-Thyracil†

*Pregnancy risk category D*

## AVAILABLE FORMS
*Tablets:* 50 mg, 100 mg†

## INDICATIONS & DOSAGES
➤ **Hyperthyroidism**
*Adults:* 300 to 450 mg P.O. daily in three
divided doses at 8-hour intervals; up to
1,200 mg daily has been used in severe
cases. Maintenance dosage varies but usually ranges from 100 to 150 mg daily to
t.i.d.
*Neonates and children:* 5 to 7 mg/kg P.O.
daily in divided doses t.i.d. Or, give according to ages shown below.
*Children older than age 10:* 100 mg P.O.
daily in divided doses t.i.d. Maintenance
dosage determined by patient response.
*Children ages 6 to 10:* 50 to 150 mg P.O.
daily in divided doses t.i.d. Maintenance
dosage determined by patient response.
➤ **Thyrotoxic crisis**
*Adults and children:* 200 mg P.O. q 4 to 6
hours on first day; once symptoms are fully controlled, gradually reduce dosage to
usual maintenance levels.

## ACTION
Inhibits oxidation of iodine in thyroid
gland, blocking ability of iodine to combine with tyrosine to form $T_4$, and may
prevent coupling of monoiodotyrosine and
diiodotyrosine to form $T_4$ and $T_3$.

| Route | Onset | Peak | Duration |
|---|---|---|---|
| P.O. | Unknown | 60-90 min | Unknown |

## ADVERSE REACTIONS
**CNS:** headache, drowsiness, vertigo,
paresthesia, neuritis, neuropathies, CNS
stimulation, depression, fever.
**CV:** vasculitis.

**EENT:** visual disturbances, loss of taste.
**GI:** diarrhea, *nausea, vomiting,* epigastric distress, salivary gland enlargement.
**GU:** nephritis.
**Hematologic:** *agranulocytosis, leukopenia, thrombocytopenia, aplastic anemia.*
**Hepatic:** jaundice, *hepatotoxicity.*
**Metabolic:** dose-related hypothyroidism.
**Musculoskeletal:** arthralgia, myalgia.
**Skin:** rash, urticaria, skin discoloration, pruritus, erythema nodosum, exfoliative dermatitis, lupuslike syndrome.
**Other:** lymphadenopathy.

## INTERACTIONS
**Drug-drug.** *Aminophylline, oxtriphylline, theophylline:* May decrease clearance of these drugs. Dosage may need to be adjusted.
*Anticoagulants:* May increase anticoagulant effects. Monitor PT and INR.
*Cardiac glycosides:* May increase glycoside level. Dosage may need to be reduced.
*Potassium iodide:* May decrease response to drug. Dosage of antithyroid drug may need to be increased.

## EFFECTS ON LAB TEST RESULTS
● May decrease hemoglobin and granulocyte, WBC, and platelet counts.

## CONTRAINDICATIONS & CAUTIONS
● Contraindicated in patients hypersensitive to drug and in breast-feeding women.
● Use cautiously in pregnant patients.

## NURSING CONSIDERATIONS
● Pregnant women may need less drug as pregnancy progresses. Monitor thyroid function studies closely. Thyroid hormone may be added to regimen. Drug may be stopped during last few weeks of pregnancy.
● *Alert:* Patients older than age 40 may have an increased risk of agranulocytosis.
● Give drug with meals to reduce adverse GI reactions.
● Watch for hypothyroidism (mental depression; cold intolerance; hard, nonpitting edema); adjust dosage.
● Monitor CBC periodically to detect impending leukopenia, thrombocytopenia, and agranulocytosis. PTU therapy alters $^{75}$Se levels and liothyronine uptake.

● *Alert:* Stop drug and notify prescriber if severe rash develops or cervical lymph nodes enlarge.
● Store drug in light-resistant container.

## PATIENT TEACHING
● Instruct patient to take drug with meals.
● Warn patient to report fever, sore throat, mouth sores, and skin eruptions.
● Tell patient to report unusual bleeding or bruising.
● Tell patient to ask prescriber about using iodized salt and eating shellfish. These foods contain iodine and may alter effectiveness of drug.
● Teach patient to watch for signs and symptoms of hypothyroidism (unexplained weight gain, fatigue, cold intolerance) and to notify prescriber if they occur.

# radioactive iodine (sodium iodide $^{131}$I)
Iodotope, Sodium Iodide $^{131}$I
Therapeutic

*Pregnancy risk category X*

## AVAILABLE FORMS
All radioactivity concentrations are determined at time of calibration.
**Iodotope**
*Capsules:* Radioactivity range 8 to 100 millicuries (mCi)/capsule
*Oral solution:* Radioactivity concentration 7.05 mCi/ml
**Sodium Iodide $^{131}$I Therapeutic**
*Capsules:* Radioactivity range 0.75 to 100 mCi/capsule
*Oral solution:* Radioactivity range 3.5 to 150 mCi/vial

## INDICATIONS & DOSAGES
➤ **Hyperthyroidism**
*Adults:* Usual dosage is 4 to 10 mCi P.O. Dosage is based on estimated weight of thyroid gland and thyroid uptake. Repeat treatment after 6 weeks, based on $T_4$ level.
➤ **Thyroid cancer**
*Adults:* Initially, 50 to 100 mCi P.O., with subsequent doses of 100 to 150 mCi. Dosage is based on estimated malignant thyroid tissue and metastatic tissue as determined by total body scan. Repeat treatment according to clinical status.

## ACTION
Limits thyroid hormone secretion by destroying thyroid tissue. Affinity of thyroid tissue for radioactive iodine facilitates uptake of drug by cancerous thyroid tissue that has metastasized to other sites in the body.

| Route | Onset | Peak | Duration |
|-------|-------|------|----------|
| P.O. | Unknown | 60-90 min | Unknown |

## ADVERSE REACTIONS
**CV:** chest pain, tachycardia.
**EENT:** *fullness in neck,* pain on swallowing, sore throat.
**Hematologic:** anemia, blood dyscrasia, *leukopenia, thrombocytopenia.*
**Metabolic:** hypothyroidism, radiation-induced thyroiditis.
**Respiratory:** cough.
**Skin:** rash, pruritus, urticaria, temporary thinning of hair.
**Other:** radiation sickness, allergic-type reactions.

## INTERACTIONS
**Drug-drug.** *Lithium carbonate:* May cause hypothyroidism. Use together with caution.

The following drugs may interfere with the action of $^{131}$I and should be withheld for the specified time before the $^{131}$I dose is given:
*Adrenocorticoids:* 1 week.
*Benzodiazepines:* 1 month.
*Cholecystographic drugs:* 6 to 9 months.
*Contrast media that contain iodine:* 1 to 2 months.
*Products containing iodine, including topical drugs, and vitamins:* 2 weeks.
*Salicylates:* 1 to 2 weeks.

## EFFECTS ON LAB TEST RESULTS
• May decrease $T_4$ and thyroid-stimulating hormone levels. May increase or decrease protein-bound iodine level.
• May decrease hemoglobin and WBC and platelet counts.
• May alter $^{131}$I thyroid uptake.

## CONTRAINDICATIONS & CAUTIONS
• Contraindicated during pregnancy (except to treat thyroid cancer) and in breast-feeding women.

## NURSING CONSIDERATIONS
• All antithyroid drugs and thyroid preparations must be stopped 1 week before $^{131}$I dose. If this isn't possible, patient may receive thyroid-stimulating hormone for 3 days before $^{131}$I dose. When treating women of childbearing age, give dose during menstruation or within 7 days afterward.
• After therapy for hyperthyroidism, patient shouldn't resume antithyroid drugs but should continue propranolol or other drugs used to treat symptoms of hyperthyroidism until onset of full $^{131}$I effect (usually 6 weeks).
• Monitor thyroid function by $T_4$ and thyroid-stimulating hormone levels.
• Institute full radiation precautions. Have patient use proper disposal methods when coughing and expectorating. After dose for hyperthyroidism, patient's urine and saliva are slightly radioactive for 24 hours; vomitus is highly radioactive for 6 to 8 hours.
• After dose for thyroid cancer, patient's urine, saliva, and perspiration are radioactive for 3 days. Isolate patient and observe these precautions: Don't allow pregnant personnel to care for patient; provide disposable eating utensils and linens; instruct patient to save urine in lead container for 24 to 48 hours; limit contact with patient to 30 minutes per shift per person on day 1, and increase time, as needed, to 1 hour on day 2 and longer on day 3.

## PATIENT TEACHING
• Tell patient to fast overnight before therapy and to drink as much fluid as possible for 48 hours afterward.
• Instruct patient about appropriate radiation exposure precautions to use after receiving drug.
• Warn patient who is discharged fewer than 7 days after $^{131}$I dose for thyroid cancer to avoid close contact with small children and not to sleep in same room with another person for 7 days after treatment.
• Teach patient the signs and symptoms of hypothyroidism (unexplained weight gain, fatigue, cold intolerance) and instruct him to notify prescriber if they occur.

---

Reactions may be *common,* uncommon, *life-threatening,* or COMMON AND LIFE-THREATENING.

**corticotropin**
**desmopressin acetate**
**leuprolide acetate**
(See Chapter 70, ANTINEOPLASTICS
THAT ALTER HORMONE BALANCE.)
**repository corticotropin**
**somatrem**
**somatropin**
**vasopressin**

**COMBINATION PRODUCTS**
None.

---

## corticotropin
## (adrenocorticotropic hormone [ACTH])
ACTH, Acthar

## repository corticotropin
ACTH-80, H.P. Acthar Gel

*Pregnancy risk category C*

**AVAILABLE FORMS**
*Injection:* 25-unit vial, 40-unit vial
*Repository injection:* 40 units/ml,
80 units/ml
*Suspension for depot injection:* 30 mg

**INDICATIONS & DOSAGES**
➤ **Diagnostic test of adrenocortical function**
*Adults:* 10 to 25 units in 500 ml of $D_5W$ I.V. over 8 hours, between blood samplings; or 40 units I.M. (repository) q 12 hours for 1 to 2 days.
Individual dosages vary with sensitivity of adrenal glands to stimulation and with specific disease. Infants and younger children need larger doses per kg than older children and adults.
➤ **Anti-inflammatory or immunosuppressant**
*Adults:* 20 units I.M. or S.C. q.i.d. Or, 40 to 80 units I.M. or S.C. q 24 to 72 hours (repository form). For an acute worsening of multiple sclerosis, 80 to 120 units (injection or repository) I.M. daily in divided doses for 2 to 3 weeks.

**I.V. ADMINISTRATION**
● Use only aqueous form for I.V. administration. Dilute in 500 ml $D_5W$, and infuse over 8 hours.
● Refrigerate reconstituted solution and use within 24 hours.

**ACTION**
By replacing the body's own tropic hormone, drug stimulates the adrenal cortex to secrete its entire spectrum of hormones.

| Route | Onset | Peak | Duration |
|---|---|---|---|
| I.V., I.M. | Rapid | 1 hr | 2-4 hr |
| I.M. (repository) | Unknown | Unknown | 3 days |
| S.C. | Unknown | Unknown | Unknown |

**ADVERSE REACTIONS**
**CNS:** *seizures, dizziness,* vertigo, *increased intracranial pressure with papilledema, pseudotumor cerebri.*
**CV:** hypertension, *heart failure,* necrotizing vasculitis, *shock.*
**EENT:** cataracts, glaucoma.
**GI:** peptic ulceration with perforation and hemorrhage, *pancreatitis,* abdominal distention, ulcerative esophagitis, nausea, vomiting.
**GU:** menstrual irregularities.
**Metabolic:** activation of latent diabetes mellitus, *sodium and fluid retention,* hypokalemic alkalosis.
**Musculoskeletal:** suppression of growth in children, muscle weakness, steroid myopathy, loss of muscle mass, osteoporosis, vertebral compression fractures.
**Respiratory:** pneumonia, *bronchospasm.*
**Skin:** impaired wound healing, thin fragile skin, petechiae, facial erythema, diaphoresis, acne, hyperpigmentation, allergic reactions, hirsutism, ecchymoses.
**Other:** cushingoid symptoms, abscess and septic infection, hypersensitivity reactions.

**INTERACTIONS**
**Drug-drug.** *Amphotericin B, potassium-sparing diuretics:* May increase risk of hypokalemia. Monitor potassium level.

---

*Anticonvulsants, barbiturates, rifampin:* May increase metabolism of corticotropin and decrease effectiveness. Watch for lack of effect.

*Antidiabetics:* May increase antidiabetic requirements because of intrinsic hyperglycemic activity of corticotropin. Monitor glucose level closely.

*Estrogens:* May increase cortisol effects. Dosage adjustments may be needed.

*NSAIDs, salicylates:* May increase risk of GI bleeding. Avoid using together.

*Oral anticoagulants:* May alter PT. Monitor PT and INR. Dosage adjustments may be needed.

*Vaccines:* May cause neurologic complications and lack of antibody response. Don't give with smallpox vaccine, and use extremely cautiously with other immunizations.

## EFFECTS ON LAB TEST RESULTS
● May increase glucose level. May decrease potassium and calcium levels.

## CONTRAINDICATIONS & CAUTIONS
● Contraindicated in patients hypersensitive to pork and pork products and in those with peptic ulcer, scleroderma, osteoporosis, systemic fungal infections, ocular herpes simplex, peptic ulceration, heart failure, hypertension, Cushing's syndrome, and adrenocortical hyperfunction or primary insufficiency. Also contraindicated after recent surgery.

● Use cautiously in pregnant women and women of childbearing age. Also, use cautiously in patients being immunized and in those with latent tuberculosis or tuberculin reactivity, hypothyroidism, cirrhosis, acute gouty arthritis, psychotic tendencies, renal insufficiency, diverticulitis, nonspecific ulcerative colitis, thromboembolic disorders, seizures, uncontrolled hypertension, or myasthenia gravis.

## NURSING CONSIDERATIONS
● *Alert:* Check product label to be certain medication is for I.V. use; corticotropin repository injection is for I.M. or S.C. use only, not for I.V. use.

● Verify adrenal responsiveness and test for hypersensitivity and allergic reactions before giving corticotropin.

● If giving gel, warm it to room temperature and draw into large needle. Replace needle (using 21G or 22G) and give slowly as deep I.M. injection.

● Corticotropin may mask signs of chronic disease and decrease host resistance and ability to localize infection.

● Note and record weight changes, fluid exchange, and resting blood pressures until minimal effective dosage is achieved.

● Watch neonates of corticotropin-treated mothers for signs of hypoadrenalism.

● In patients with diabetes, monitor glucose level more frequently.

● Unusual stress may require additional use of rapid-acting steroids. When possible, gradually reduce corticotropin dosage to lowest effective level to minimize induced adrenocortical insufficiency. Therapy can be restarted if stressful situation (trauma, surgery, severe illness) occurs shortly after drug is stopped.

● *Alert:* Don't confuse corticotropin with cosyntropin.

## PATIENT TEACHING
● Warn patient that injection is painful.

● Stress importance of informing all members of health care team about therapeutic use of drug because unusual stress may require additional use of rapidly acting steroids.

● Instruct patient how to handle troublesome adverse reactions, such as limiting sodium intake to reduce severity of swelling and increasing protein intake to combat nitrogen loss.

● Inform patient of need for close follow-up care.

● Advise patient not to stop therapy abruptly.

● Instruct patient to avoid people with varicella (chickenpox or shingles) infections.

● Tell patient to avoid alcohol, salicylates, and NSAIDs because of the increased risk of ulcers.

● Tell patient to report to prescriber symptoms of fluid retention, muscle weakness, abdominal pain, seizures, or headache.

● Tell patient to avoid vaccinations during therapy.

---

# desmopressin acetate
DDAVP, Minirin‡, Octostim‡,
Stimate

*Pregnancy risk category B*

## AVAILABLE FORMS
*Injection:* 4 mcg/ml, 15 mcg/ml
*Nasal solution:* 0.1 mg/ml, 1.5 mg/ml
*Tablets:* 0.1 mg, 0.2 mg

## INDICATIONS & DOSAGES
➤ **Nonnephrogenic diabetes insipidus, temporary polyuria, and polydipsia related to pituitary trauma**
*Adults and children older than age 12:*
0.1 to 0.4 ml intranasally daily in one to three doses. Most adults need 0.2 ml daily in two divided doses. Or, give 0.5 to 1 ml I.V. or S.C. daily, usually in two divided doses. Or, give 0.05 mg P.O. b.i.d.; adjust dosage to patient response. If patient previously received the drug intranasally, begin oral therapy 12 hours after last intranasal dose.
*Children ages 3 months to 12 years:*
0.05 to 0.3 ml intranasally daily in one or two doses.
➤ **Hemophilia A and von Willebrand's disease**
*Adults and children:* 0.3 mcg/kg diluted in normal saline solution and infused I.V. over 15 to 30 minutes. Repeat dose, if needed, as indicated by laboratory response and patient's condition. Or, 300 mcg (one spray in each nostril) of solution containing 1.5 mcg/ml. Dose of 150 mcg (one spray of solution containing 1.5 mg/ml into a single nostril) may be adequate for patients weighing less than 50 kg (110 lb). Give drug 2 hours before surgery.
➤ **Primary nocturnal enuresis**
*Children age 6 and older:* Initially, 20 mcg (0.2 ml) intranasally h.s. (10 mcg in each nostril). Adjust dosage based on response; maximum recommended dosage is 40 mcg daily. Or, initially 0.2 mg P.O. h.s., may adjust dose up to 0.6 mg to achieve desired response. For patients previously on intranasal DDAVP therapy, start tablet 24 hours after last intranasal dose in the nighttime.

## I.V. ADMINISTRATION
● For adults and children weighing more than 10 kg (22 lb), dilute with 50 ml sterile physiologic saline solution. For children weighing 10 kg or less, 10 ml of diluent is recommended.
● Inspect for particulate matter and discoloration before infusing drug.
● Monitor blood pressure and pulse during infusion.

## ACTION
Increases the permeability of renal tubular epithelium to adenosine monophosphate and water; the epithelium promotes reabsorption of water and produces a concentrated urine. Also increases factor VIII activity by releasing endogenous factor VIII from plasma storage sites.

| Route | Onset | Peak | Duration |
|---|---|---|---|
| P.O. | 1 hr | 1-1½ hr | 8-12 hr |
| I.V. | 15-30 min | Unknown | 4-12 hr |
| Intranasal | 1 hr | 1-5 hr | 8-12 hr |

## ADVERSE REACTIONS
**CNS:** headache.
**CV:** flushing, slight rise in blood pressure.
**EENT:** rhinitis, epistaxis, sore throat.
**GI:** nausea, abdominal cramps.
**GU:** vulvar pain.
**Respiratory:** cough.
**Skin:** local erythema, swelling, or burning after injection.

## INTERACTIONS
**Drug-drug.** *Carbamazepine, chlorpropamide:* May increase ADH; may increase effects of desmopressin. Avoid using together.
*Clofibrate:* May enhance and prolong effects of desmopressin. Monitor patient closely.
*Demeclocycline, epinephrine, heparin, lithium:* May increase risk of adverse effects. Monitor patient closely.
*Pressor agents:* May enhance pressor effects with large doses of desmopressin. Monitor patient closely.
**Drug-lifestyle.** *Alcohol use:* May increase risk of adverse effects. Discourage use together.

## EFFECTS ON LAB TEST RESULTS
None reported.

## CONTRAINDICATIONS & CAUTIONS
● Contraindicated in patients hypersensitive to drug and in those with type IIB von Willebrand's disease.
● Use cautiously in patients with coronary artery insufficiency, hypertensive CV disease, and conditions linked to fluid and electrolyte imbalances, such as cystic fibrosis, because these patients are susceptible to hyponatremia.
● It's unknown if drug appears in breast milk. Use cautiously in breast-feeding women.

## NURSING CONSIDERATIONS
● Morning and evening doses are adjusted separately for adequate diurnal rhythm of water turnover.
● Don't use desmopressin injection in patients with hemophilia A with factor VIII of up to 5% or severe von Willebrand's disease.
● Ensure nasal passages are intact, clean, and free of obstruction before giving intranasally.
● Intranasal use can cause changes in the nasal mucosa, resulting in erratic, unreliable absorption. Report worsening condition to prescriber, who may recommend injectable DDAVP.
● Adjust fluid intake to reduce risk of water intoxication and sodium depletion, especially in children or elderly patients.
● *Alert:* Overdose may cause oxytocic or vasopressor activity. Withhold drug and notify prescriber. Use furosemide if fluid retention is excessive.
● *Alert:* Don't confuse desmopressin with vasopressin.
● Nasal spray pump only delivers doses of 10 mcg DDAVP or 150 mcg Stimate. If doses other than those are required, use the nasal tube delivery system or injection.

## PATIENT TEACHING
● Instruct patient to clear nasal passages before giving drug.
● Instruct patient to press down four times to prime pump. Tell him to discard the bottle after 25 (150 mcg/spray) or 50 doses (10 mcg/spray), depending on the strength, because the amount left may be less than desired dose.
● Some patients may have trouble measuring and inhaling drug into nostrils. Teach patient and caregivers correct method of administration.
● Advise patient to report nasal congestion, allergic rhinitis, or upper respiratory tract infection to prescriber; dosage adjustment may be needed.
● Teach patient using S.C. desmopressin to rotate injection sites to prevent tissue damage.
● Warn patient to drink only enough water to satisfy thirst.
● Inform patient with hemophilia A or von Willebrand's disease that taking desmopressin may prevent hazards of using blood products.
● Advise patient to carry or wear medical identification indicating use of drug.

---

## somatrem
Protropin

*Pregnancy risk category C*

### AVAILABLE FORMS
*Injectable lyophilized powder:* 5-mg (about 15-IU) vial, 10-mg (about 30-IU) vial

### INDICATIONS & DOSAGES
➤ **Long-term treatment of children who have growth failure because of lack of adequate endogenous growth hormone (GH) secretion**
*Children (prepubertal):* Highly individualized; up to 0.1 mg/kg S.C. (preferred) or I.M. three times weekly. Don't exceed 0.3 mg/kg per week.

### ACTION
Purified GH of recombinant DNA origin that stimulates linear, skeletal muscle, and organ growth.

| Route | Onset | Peak | Duration |
|---|---|---|---|
| I.M., S.C. | Unknown | 3-5 hr | Unknown |

### ADVERSE REACTIONS
**Metabolic:** hypothyroidism, hyperglycemia.
**Other:** *antibodies to GH.*

### INTERACTIONS
**Drug-drug.** *Glucocorticoids:* May inhibit growth-promoting action of somatrem. Adjust glucocorticoid dosage, as needed.

## EFFECTS ON LAB TEST RESULTS
• May increase glucose level.
• May decrease $T_4$-binding capacity and radioactive uptake into the thyroid.

## CONTRAINDICATIONS & CAUTIONS
• Contraindicated in patients hypersensitive to benzyl alcohol and in those with epiphyseal closure or active neoplasia.
• Use cautiously in patients with hypothyroidism and in those whose GH deficiency is caused by an intracranial lesion.

## NURSING CONSIDERATIONS
• Check product's expiration date.
• To prepare solution, inject supplied bacteriostatic water for injection into vial containing drug. Then swirl vial gently until contents are completely dissolved. Don't shake vial.
• After reconstitution, make sure solution is clear. Don't inject solution if it's cloudy or contains particles.
• If prepared for other than neonatal use, store reconstituted drug in refrigerator; use within 14 days.
• *Alert:* Toxicity in neonates has occurred from exposure to benzyl alcohol used as a preservative. If drug is given to neonates, reconstitute immediately before use with sterile water for injection (without bacteriostat). Use vial once; then discard.
• Regular checkups are needed, including monitoring of height and blood and radiologic studies.
• Observe patient for evidence of glucose intolerance and hyperglycemia.
• Watch for slipped capital femoral epiphysis or progression of scoliosis in patients with rapid growth.
• Monitor periodic thyroid function tests for hypothyroidism; condition may need treatment with a thyroid hormone.
• Do funduscopic examination of patient for intracranial hypertension at start of therapy and periodically thereafter.
• *Alert:* Don't confuse somatrem with somatropin, Serostim, or sumatriptan.

## PATIENT TEACHING
• Reassure patient and caregivers that somatrem is pure and safe. Drug replaces pituitary-derived human GH, which was removed from the market in 1985 because of its link with a rare but fatal viral infection (Creutzfeldt-Jakob disease).
• Review evidence of hypothyroidism and hyperglycemia. Instruct patient and parents to report such evidence promptly.
• Instruct patient to report to prescriber headache, weakness, localized muscle pain, swelling, and limb, hip, or knee pain.

# somatropin
Genotropin, Genotropin Miniquick, Humatrope, Norditropin, Nutropin, Nutropin AQ, Nutropin Depot, Saizen, Serostim

*Pregnancy risk category C (B; Serostim)*

## AVAILABLE FORMS
*Genotropin injection:* 1.5 mg (about 4.5 IU/vial), 5.8 mg (about 17.4 IU/vial), 13.8 mg (about 41.4 IU/vial)
*Genotropin Miniquick injection:* 0.2 mg/vial, 0.4 mg/vial, 0.6 mg/vial, 0.8 mg/vial, 1 mg/vial, 1.2 mg/vial, 1.4 mg/vial, 1.6 mg/vial, 1.8 mg/vial, 2 mg/vial
*Humatrope injection:* 2 mg (about 6 IU/vial†), 5 mg (about 15 IU/vial), 6 mg (18 IU/cartridge), 12 mg (36 IU/cartridge), 24 mg (72 IU/cartridge)
*Norditropin injection:* 4 mg (about 12 IU/ml), 8 mg (about 24 IU/ml), 5 mg/1.5 ml cartridges, 10 mg/1.5 ml cartridges, 15 mg/1.5 ml cartridges
*Nutropin AQ injection:* 10 mg (about 30 IU/vial)
*Nutropin Depot injection:* 13.5 mg/vial, 18 mg/vial, 22.5 mg/vial
*Nutropin injection:* 5 mg (about 15 IU/vial), 10 mg (about 30 IU/vial)
*Saizen injection:* 5 mg (about 15 IU/vial)
*Serostim injection:* 4 mg (about 12 IU/vial), 5 mg (about 15 IU/vial), 6 mg (about 18 IU/vial)

## INDICATIONS & DOSAGES
➤ **Long-term treatment of growth failure in children with inadequate secretion of endogenous GH**
*Children:* 0.18 mg/kg Humatrope I.M. or S.C. weekly, divided equally and given on three alternate days, six times weekly or once daily. Or, 0.3 mg/kg Nutropin or Nutropin AQ S.C. weekly in daily divided

doses. Or, 0.06 mg/kg Saizen I.M. or S.C. three times weekly. Or, 0.024 to 0.034 mg/kg Norditropin S.C., six to seven times weekly. Or, 0.16 to 0.24 mg/kg Genotropin S.C. weekly, divided into five to seven doses. Or 1.5 mg/kg Nutropin Depot S.C. once monthly or 0.75 mg/kg S.C. twice monthly on the same days of each month.

➤ **Growth failure from chronic renal insufficiency up to time of renal transplantation**
*Children:* Up to 0.35 mg/kg/week Nutropin or Nutropin AQ S.C. divided into daily doses.

➤ **Long-term treatment of short stature caused by Turner's syndrome**
*Children:* Up to 0.375 mg/kg/week Humatrope, Nutropin, or Nutropin AQ S.C. divided into equal doses given three to seven times weekly.

➤ **Long-term treatment of growth failure in children with Prader-Willi syndrome (PWS) diagnosed by genetic testing**
*Children:* 0.24 mg/kg Genotropin S.C. weekly, divided into six to seven doses.

➤ **Replacement of endogenous GH in adult patients with GH deficiency**
*Adults:* Initially, not more than 0.006 mg/kg Genotropin, Humatrope, Nutropin, or Nutropin AQ S.C. daily. May be increased to maximum of 0.0125 mg/kg Humatrope daily.
Nutropin or Nutropin AQ dosages may be increased to maximum of 0.025 mg/kg daily in patients younger than age 35 or 0.0125 mg/kg daily in patients older than age 35. Or, starting dosages not exceeding 0.04 mg/kg Genotropin S.C. weekly, divided into six to seven doses, may be increased at 4- to 8-week intervals to a maximum dose of 0.08 mg/kg S.C. weekly, divided into six to seven doses.

➤ **AIDS wasting or cachexia**
*Adults and children weighing more than 55 kg (121 lb):* 6 mg Serostim S.C. h.s.
*Adults and children weighing 45 to 55 kg (99 to 121 lb):* 5 mg Serostim S.C. h.s.
*Adults and children weighing 35 to 45 kg (77 to 99 lb):* 4 mg Serostim S.C. h.s.
*Adults and children weighing less than 35 kg:* 0.1 mg/kg/day Serostim S.C. h.s.

➤ **Long-term treatment of growth failure in children born small for gestation-**al age (SGA) who don't achieve catch-up growth by age 2
*Children:* 0.48 mg/kg Genotropin S.C. weekly, divided into five to seven doses.

✳ **NEW INDICATION: Idiopathic short stature**
*Children:* Up to 0.37 mg/kg Humatrope S.C. weekly, divided into six to seven equal doses.

**ACTION**
Purified GH of recombinant DNA origin that stimulates skeletal, linear, muscle, and organ growth.

| Route | Onset | Peak | Duration |
|-------|-------|------|----------|
| I.M., S.C. | Unknown | 3-5 hr | 12-48 hr |

**ADVERSE REACTIONS**
**CNS:** headache, weakness.
**CV:** mild, transient edema.
**Hematologic:** *leukemia.*
**Metabolic:** mild hyperglycemia, hypothyroidism.
**Musculoskeletal:** localized muscle pain.
**Skin:** injection site pain.
**Other:** antibodies to GH.

**INTERACTIONS**
**Drug-drug.** *Corticotropin, corticosteroids:* Long-term use may inhibit growth response to GH. Monitor patient for lack of effect.

**EFFECTS ON LAB TEST RESULTS**
● May increase glucose, inorganic phosphorus, alkaline phosphatase, and parathyroid hormone levels.

**CONTRAINDICATIONS & CAUTIONS**
● Contraindicated in patients with closed epiphyses or an active underlying intracranial lesion. Humatrope shouldn't be reconstituted with supplied diluent for patients hypersensitive to either Metacresol or glycerin. Genotropin is also contraindicated in patients with Prader-Willi syndrome who are severely obese or have severe respiratory impairment.
● Use cautiously in children with hypothyroidism and in those whose GH deficiency is caused by an intracranial lesion.

**NURSING CONSIDERATIONS**
● Frequently examine children with hypothyroidism and those whose GH deficien-

cy is caused by an intracranial lesion for progression or recurrence of underlying disease.

• To prepare solution, inject supplied diluent into vial containing drug by aiming stream of liquid against wall of glass vial. Then swirl vial gently until contents are completely dissolved. Don't shake vial.

• After reconstitution, make sure solution is clear. Don't inject solution if it's cloudy or contains particles.

• Patients on dialysis need changes in drug administration schedule as follows: For hemodialysis, give drug before bedtime or 3 to 4 hours after dialysis. For long-term cycling peritoneal dialysis, give drug in the morning after completion of dialysis. For long-term ambulatory peritoneal dialysis, give drug in the evening at the time of the overnight exchange.

• Store reconstituted drug in refrigerator; use within 14 days.

• If patient develops sensitivity to diluent, reconstitute drug with sterile water for injection. When drug is reconstituted in this manner, use only one reconstituted dose per vial, refrigerate solution if it isn't used immediately after reconstitution, use reconstituted dose within 24 hours, and discard unused portion.

• **Alert:** Fatalities have occurred in patients with Prader-Willi syndrome who are morbidly obese and in those with a history of respiratory impairment, sleep apnea, or unidentified respiratory infection. Evaluate patients with Prader-Willi syndrome for sleep apnea and upper airway obstruction before starting treatment. Interrupt treatment if signs of upper airway obstruction occur.

• Monitor patient with Prader-Willi syndrome for signs of respiratory infection.

• Monitor child's height regularly. Regular checkups, including monitoring of blood and radiologic studies, also are needed.

• Monitor patient's glucose level regularly because GH may induce a state of insulin resistance.

• Excessive glucocorticoid therapy inhibits somatropin's growth-promoting effect. Patients with coexisting corticotropin deficiency should have their glucocorticoid replacement dosage carefully adjusted to avoid growth inhibition.

• Watch for slipped capital femoral epiphysis or progression of scoliosis in patients with rapid growth.

• Monitor results of periodic thyroid function tests for hypothyroidism; condition may need thyroid hormone treatment. Laboratory measurements of thyroid hormone may change.

• Do funduscopic examination of patient for intracranial hypertension when therapy starts and periodically during therapy.

• **Alert:** Don't confuse somatropin with somatrem or sumatriptan.

**PATIENT TEACHING**
• Inform parents that child with endocrine disorders (including GH deficiency) may have an increased risk of slipped capital epiphyses. Tell them to notify prescriber if they notice their child limping.

• Instruct patients with diabetes to monitor glucose level closely and report changes to prescriber.

• Stress importance of close follow-up care.

## vasopressin (ADH)
Pitressin

*Pregnancy risk category C*

**AVAILABLE FORMS**
*Injection:* 20 units/ml

**INDICATIONS & DOSAGES**
➤ **Nonnephrogenic, nonpsychogenic diabetes insipidus**
*Adults:* 5 to 10 units I.M. or S.C. b.i.d. to q.i.d., p.r.n. Or, intranasally (aqueous solution used as spray or applied to cotton balls) in individualized dosages, based on response.
*Children:* 2.5 to 10 units I.M. or S.C. b.i.d. to q.i.d., p.r.n. Or, intranasally (aqueous solution used as spray or applied to cotton balls) in individualized dosages.
➤ **To prevent and treat abdominal distention**
*Adults:* Initially, 5 units I.M.; give subsequent injections q 3 to 4 hours, increasing to 10 units if needed. Children may receive reduced dosages. Or, for adults, aqueous vasopressin 5 to 15 units S.C. at 2 hours before and again at 30 minutes be-

fore abdominal radiography or kidney
biopsy.

## ACTION
Increases permeability of the renal tubular
epithelium to adenosine monophosphate
and water; the epithelium promotes reabsorption of water and produces a concentrated urine.

| Route | Onset | Peak | Duration |
|-------|-------|------|----------|
| I.M., S.C., intranasal | 2-8 hr | Unknown | Unknown |

## ADVERSE REACTIONS
**CNS:** tremor, headache, vertigo.
**CV:** vasoconstriction, *arrhythmias, car-
diac arrest,* myocardial ischemia, circum-
oral pallor, decreased cardiac output, angi-
na in patients with vascular disease.
**GI:** abdominal cramps, nausea, vomiting,
flatulence.
**GU:** uterine cramps.
**Respiratory:** bronchoconstriction.
**Skin:** diaphoresis, cutaneous gangrene,
urticaria.
**Other:** water intoxication, *hypersensitivi-
ty reactions.*

## INTERACTIONS
**Drug-drug.** *Carbamazepine, chlorpropamide, clofibrate, fludrocortisone, tricyclic
antidepressant:* May increase antidiuretic
response. Use together cautiously.
*Demeclocycline, heparin, lithium, norepi-
nephrine:* May reduce antidiuretic activity.
Use together cautiously.
**Drug-lifestyle.** *Alcohol use:* May reduce
antidiuretic activity. Discourage use together.

## EFFECTS ON LAB TEST RESULTS
None reported.

## CONTRAINDICATIONS & CAUTIONS
• Contraindicated in patients with chronic
nephritis and nitrogen retention.
• Use cautiously in children, elderly patients, pregnant women, preoperative and
postoperative polyuric patients, and those
with seizure disorders, migraines, asthma,
CV disease, heart failure, renal disease,
goiter with cardiac complications, arteriosclerosis, or fluid overload.

## NURSING CONSIDERATIONS
• Monitor patient for hypersensitivity reactions, including urticaria, angioedema,
bronchoconstriction, and anaphylaxis.
• Synthetic desmopressin is sometimes
preferred because of its longer duration of
action and less frequent adverse reactions.
Desmopressin also is available commercially as a nasal solution.
• Drug may be used for transient polyuria
resulting from ADH deficiency related to
neurosurgery or head injury.
• Use minimum effective dose to reduce
adverse reactions.
• Give with 1 to 2 glasses of water to reduce adverse reactions and improve therapeutic response.
• Warm the vasopressin vial in your
hands, and mix until the hormone is distributed throughout the solution before administration.
• Monitor urine specific gravity and fluid
intake and output to aid evaluation of drug
effectiveness.
• To prevent possible seizures, coma, and
death, observe patient closely for early evidence of water intoxication, including
drowsiness, listlessness, headache, confusion, and weight gain.
• Monitor blood pressure of patient taking
vasopressin twice daily. Watch for excessively elevated blood pressure or lack of
response to drug, which may be indicated
by hypotension. Also, monitor weight
daily.
• *Alert:* Don't confuse vasopressin with
desmopressin.

## PATIENT TEACHING
• Instruct patient to rotate injection sites to
prevent tissue damage.
• Tell patient to report adverse reactions to
prescriber promptly.
• Tell patient to report drowsiness, listlessness, and headache to prescriber.
• Tell patient to avoid alcohol and OTC
medications unless approved by prescriber.
• Tell patient to restrict water intake.

---

Reactions may be *common,* uncommon, *life-threatening,* or COMMON AND LIFE-THREATENING.

**alendronate sodium**
**calcitonin (salmon)**
**calcitriol**
**pamidronate disodium**
**risedronate sodium**
**teriparatide**
**zoledronic acid**

**COMBINATION PRODUCTS**
None.

---

## alendronate sodium
Fosamax🖉

*Pregnancy risk category C*

### AVAILABLE FORMS
*Tablets:* 5 mg, 10 mg, 35 mg, 40 mg, 70 mg

### INDICATIONS & DOSAGES
➤ **Osteoporosis in postmenopausal women; to increase bone mass in men with osteoporosis**
*Adults:* 10 mg P.O. daily or 70-mg tablet P.O. once weekly.
➤ **Paget's disease of bone**
*Adults:* 40 mg P.O. daily for 6 months.
➤ **To prevent osteoporosis in postmenopausal women**
*Adults:* 5 mg P.O. daily or 35-mg tablet P.O. once weekly.
➤ **Glucocorticoid-induced osteoporosis in men and women receiving glucocorticoids in a daily dose equivalent to 7.5 mg or more of prednisone and who have low bone mineral density**
*Adults:* 5 mg P.O. daily. For postmenopausal women not receiving estrogen, recommended dose is 10 mg P.O. daily.

### ACTION
Suppresses osteoclast activity on newly formed resorption surfaces, which reduces bone turnover. Bone formation exceeds resorption at remodeling sites, leading to progressive gains in bone mass.

| Route | Onset | Peak | Duration |
|-------|-------|------|----------|
| P.O. | Unknown | Unknown | Unknown |

### ADVERSE REACTIONS
**CNS:** headache.
**GI:** abdominal pain, nausea, dyspepsia, constipation, diarrhea, flatulence, acid regurgitation, esophageal ulcer, vomiting, dysphagia, abdominal distention, gastritis, taste perversion.
**Musculoskeletal:** musculoskeletal pain.

### INTERACTIONS
**Drug-drug.** *Antacids, calcium supplements, many oral drugs:* May interfere with absorption of alendronate. Instruct patient to wait at least 30 minutes after taking alendronate before taking other drug orally.
*Aspirin, NSAIDs:* May increase risk of upper GI adverse reactions with drug doses greater than 10 mg/day. Monitor patient closely.
*Ranitidine (I.V. form):* May increase availability of alendronate. Reduce dosage, as needed.
**Drug-food.** *Any food:* May decrease absorption of drug. Advise patient to take with full glass of water at least 30 minutes before food, beverages, or ingestion of other drugs.

### EFFECTS ON LAB TEST RESULTS
● May decrease calcium and phosphate levels.

### CONTRAINDICATIONS & CAUTIONS
● Contraindicated in patients hypersensitive to drug and in those with hypocalcemia, severe renal insufficiency, or abnormalities of the esophagus that delay esophageal emptying.
● Use cautiously in patients with active upper GI problems (dysphagia, symptomatic esophageal diseases, gastritis, duodenitis, ulcers) or mild to moderate renal insufficiency.

---

## NURSING CONSIDERATIONS
• Correct hypocalcemia and other disturbances of mineral metabolism (such as vitamin D deficiency) before therapy begins.
• When used to treat osteoporosis, disease may be confirmed by findings of low bone mass on diagnostic studies or by history of osteoporotic fracture.
• When used to treat Paget's disease, drug is indicated for patients with alkaline phosphatase level at least two times upper limit of normal, for those who are symptomatic, and for those at risk for future complications from the disease.
• *Alert:* Give drug with 6 to 8 ounces of water at least 30 minutes before patient's first food or drink of the day, to facilitate delivery to the stomach. Don't allow patient to lie down for 30 minutes after taking drug.
• Monitor patient's calcium and phosphate levels throughout therapy.
• *Alert:* Don't confuse Fosamax with Flomax.

## PATIENT TEACHING
• Stress importance of taking tablet only with 6 to 8 ounces of water at least 30 minutes before ingesting anything else, including food, beverages, and other drugs. Tell patient that waiting longer than 30 minutes improves absorption.
• Warn patient not to lie down for at least 30 minutes after taking drug to facilitate delivery to stomach and to reduce risk of esophageal irritation.
• Advise patient to report adverse effects immediately, especially chest pain or difficulty swallowing.
• Advise patient to take supplemental calcium and vitamin D if dietary intake is inadequate.
• Tell patient about benefits of weight-bearing exercises in increasing bone mass. If applicable, explain importance of reducing or eliminating cigarette smoking and alcohol use.

# calcitonin (salmon)
Miacalcin, Salmonine

*Pregnancy risk category C*

## AVAILABLE FORMS
*Injection:* 200 IU/ml, 2-ml ampules
*Nasal spray:* 200 IU/activation in 2-ml bottle

## INDICATIONS & DOSAGES
➤ **Paget's disease of bone (osteitis deformans)**
*Adults:* Initially, 100 IU of calcitonin (salmon) daily I.M. or S.C. Maintenance dosage is 50 to 100 IU daily I.M. or S.C., every other day, or three times weekly.
➤ **Hypercalcemia**
*Adults:* 4 IU/kg of calcitonin (salmon) q 12 hours I.M. or S.C. If response is inadequate after 1 or 2 days, increase dosage to 8 IU/kg I.M. q 12 hours. If response remains unsatisfactory after 2 additional days, increase dosage to maximum of 8 IU/kg I.M. q 6 hours.
➤ **Postmenopausal osteoporosis**
*Adults:* 100 IU of calcitonin (salmon) daily I.M. or S.C. Or, 200 IU (one activation) of calcitonin (salmon) daily intranasally, alternating nostrils daily. Patient should receive adequate vitamin D and calcium supplements (1.5 g calcium carbonate and 400 units of vitamin D) daily.

## ACTION
Decreases osteoclastic activity by inhibiting osteocytic osteolysis; decreases mineral release and matrix or collagen breakdown in bone.

| Route | Onset | Peak | Duration |
|-------|-------|------|----------|
| I.M., S.C. | 15 min | 4 hr | 8-24 hr |
| Intranasal | Rapid | 30 min | 1 hr |

## ADVERSE REACTIONS
**CNS:** headache, weakness, dizziness, paresthesia.
**CV:** chest pressure, *facial flushing.*
**EENT:** eye pain, *nasal congestion, rhinitis.*
**GI:** *transient nausea,* unusual taste, diarrhea, anorexia, *vomiting,* epigastric discomfort, abdominal pain.

---

Reactions may be *common*, uncommon, *life-threatening*, or COMMON AND LIFE-THREATENING.

**GU:** *increased urinary frequency,* nocturia.

**Respiratory:** shortness of breath.

**Skin:** rash, pruritus of ear lobes, *inflammation at injection site.*

**Other:** hypersensitivity reactions, *anaphylaxis,* edema of feet, chills, tender palms and soles.

**INTERACTIONS**
None significant.

**EFFECTS ON LAB TEST RESULTS**
None reported.

**CONTRAINDICATIONS & CAUTIONS**
● Contraindicated in patients hypersensitive to salmon calcitonin.

**NURSING CONSIDERATIONS**
● Skin test is usually done before starting therapy.
● *Alert:* Systemic allergic reactions are possible because hormone is protein. Keep epinephrine nearby.
● Give at bedtime, when possible, to minimize nausea and vomiting.
● I.M. route is preferred if volume of dose to be given exceeds 2 ml.
● Use freshly reconstituted solution within 2 hours.
● *Alert:* Observe patient for signs of hypocalcemic tetany during therapy (muscle twitching, tetanic spasms, and seizures when hypocalcemia is severe).
● Monitor calcium level closely. Watch for symptoms of hypercalcemia relapse: bone pain, renal calculi, polyuria, anorexia, nausea, vomiting, thirst, constipation, lethargy, bradycardia, muscle hypotonicity, pathologic fracture, psychosis, and coma.
● Periodic examinations of urine sediment are recommended.
● Monitor periodic alkaline phosphatase and 24-hour urine hydroxyproline levels to evaluate drug effect.
● In Paget's disease, maximum reductions of alkaline phosphatase and urinary hydroxyproline excretion may take 6 to 24 months of continuous treatment.
● In patients with good first clinical response to calcitonin who have a relapse, expect to evaluate antibody response to the hormone protein.

● If symptoms have been relieved after 6 months, treatment may be stopped until symptoms or radiologic signs recur.
● Refrigerate calcitonin (salmon) at 36° to 46° F (2° to 8° C).
● *Alert:* Don't confuse calcitonin with calcifediol or calcitriol.

**PATIENT TEACHING**
● When drug is given for postmenopausal osteoporosis, remind patient to take adequate calcium and vitamin D supplements.
● Show home care patient and family member how to give drug. Tell them to do so at bedtime if only one dose is needed daily. If nasal spray is prescribed, tell patient to alternate nostrils daily.
● Advise patient to notify prescriber if significant nasal irritation or evidence of an allergic response occurs.
● Inform patient that facial flushing and warmth occur in 20% to 30% of patients within minutes of injection and usually last about 1 hour. Reassure patient that this is a transient effect.
● Tell patient that nausea and vomiting may occur at the onset of therapy.
● Tell patient to inform prescriber promptly if signs and symptoms of hypercalcemia occur. Inform patient that, if calcitonin loses its hypocalcemic activity, other drugs or increased dosages won't help.

# calcitriol (1,25-dihydroxy-cholecalciferol)
Calcijex, Rocaltrol

*Pregnancy risk category C*

**AVAILABLE FORMS**
*Capsules:* 0.25 mcg, 0.5 mcg
*Injection:* 1 mcg/ml, 2 mcg/ml
*Oral solution:* 1 mcg/ml

**INDICATIONS & DOSAGES**
➤ **Hypocalcemia in patients undergoing long-term dialysis**
*Adults:* Initially, 0.25 mcg P.O. daily; may increase by 0.25 mcg daily at 4- to 8-week intervals. Maintenance dosage is 0.5 to 3 mcg daily. Or, 0.5 mcg I.V. three times weekly about every other day. If response

to first dosage is inadequate, may increase by 0.25 to 0.5 mcg at 2- to 4-week intervals. Maintenance dosage is 0.5 to 3 mcg I.V. three times weekly.

➤ **Hypoparathyroidism, pseudohypoparathyroidism**
*Adults and children age 6 and older:* Initially, 0.25 mcg P.O. daily in the morning. Dosage may be increased at 2- to 4-week intervals. Maintenance dosage is 0.25 to 2 mcg P.O. daily.

➤ **Hypoparathyroidism**
*Children ages 1 to 5:* 0.25 to 0.75 mcg P.O. daily.

➤ **To manage secondary hyperparathyroidism and resulting metabolic bone disease in predialysis patients (with creatinine clearance of 15 to 55 ml/minute)**
*Adults and children age 3 and older:* Initially, 0.25 mcg P.O. daily. Dosage may be increased to 0.5 mcg/day if needed.
*Children younger than age 3:* Initially, 0.01 to 0.015 mcg/kg P.O. daily.

## I.V. ADMINISTRATION
● For hypocalcemic patients with chronic renal failure who are undergoing hemodialysis, give drug by rapid I.V. injection through catheter at end of hemodialysis session.

## ACTION
A vitamin D analogue that stimulates calcium absorption from the GI tract and promotes movement of calcium from bone to blood.

| Route | Onset | Peak | Duration |
|-------|-------|------|----------|
| P.O. | 2-6 hr | 3-6 hr | 3-5 days |
| I.V. | Immediate | Unknown | 3-5 days |

## ADVERSE REACTIONS
**CNS:** headache, somnolence, weakness, irritability.
**CV:** hypertension, *arrhythmias.*
**EENT:** conjunctivitis, photophobia, rhinorrhea.
**GI:** nausea, vomiting, constipation, polydipsia, *pancreatitis,* metallic taste, dry mouth, anorexia.
**GU:** polyuria, nocturia.
**Metabolic:** weight loss.
**Musculoskeletal:** bone and muscle pain.
**Skin:** pruritus.

**Other:** hyperthermia, nephrocalcinosis, decreased libido.

## INTERACTIONS
**Drug-drug.** *Cardiac glycosides:* May increase risk of arrhythmias. Avoid using together.
*Cholestyramine, colestipol, excessive use of mineral oil:* May decrease absorption of oral vitamin D analogues. Avoid using together.
*Corticosteroids:* May counteract vitamin D analogue effects. Avoid using together.
*Magnesium-containing antacids:* May cause hypermagnesemia, especially in patients with chronic renal failure. Avoid using together.
*Phenytoin, phenobarbital:* May inhibit calcitriol synthesis. Dose may need to be increased.
*Thiazides:* May cause hypercalcemia. Use together with caution.

## EFFECTS ON LAB TEST RESULTS
None reported.

## CONTRAINDICATIONS & CAUTIONS
● Contraindicated in patients with hypercalcemia or vitamin D toxicity. Withhold all preparations containing vitamin D.
● Use cautiously in patients receiving cardiac glycosides and in those with sarcoidosis or hyperparathyroidism.

## NURSING CONSIDERATIONS
● Monitor calcium level; multiplied by phosphate level, it shouldn't exceed 70. During adjustment, determine calcium level twice weekly. Stop and notify prescriber if hypercalcemia occurs, but resume after calcium level returns to normal. Patient should receive adequate daily intake of calcium. Observe for hypocalcemia, bone pain, and weakness before and during therapy.
● Vitamin D intoxication causes various adverse effects, including headache, somnolence, weakness, irritability, hypertension, arrhythmias, conjunctivitis, photophobia, rhinorrhea, nausea, vomiting, constipation, polydipsia, pancreatitis, metallic taste, dry mouth, anorexia, nephrocalcinosis, polyuria, nocturia, weight loss, bone and muscle pain, pruritus, hyperthermia, and decreased libido.

---

Reactions may be *common*, uncommon, *life-threatening*, or COMMON AND LIFE-THREATENING.

• Protect drug from heat and light.
• *Alert:* Don't confuse calcitriol with calcifediol or calcitonin.

## PATIENT TEACHING
• Tell patient to immediately report early symptoms of vitamin D intoxication: weakness, nausea, vomiting, dry mouth, constipation, muscle or bone pain, or metallic taste.
• Instruct patient to adhere to diet and calcium supplementation and to avoid unapproved OTC drugs and magnesium-containing antacids.
• *Alert:* Tell patient that drug mustn't be taken by anyone for whom it wasn't prescribed. It's the most potent form of vitamin D available.

## pamidronate disodium
Aredia

*Pregnancy risk category D*

## AVAILABLE FORMS
*Powder for injection:* 30-mg /vial, 90-mg/vial
*Solution for injection:* 3 mg/ml, 6 mg/ml, 9 mg/ml, in 10-ml vials

## INDICATIONS & DOSAGES
➤ **Moderate to severe hypercalcemia from cancer (with or without bone metastases)**
*Adults:* Dosage depends on severity of hypercalcemia. Correct calcium level for albumin. Corrected calcium (CCa) level is calculated using this formula:

$$\frac{CCa}{(mg/dl)} = \frac{serum}{calcium +} \frac{0.8 (4 - serum}{albumin)}$$

Patients with CCa levels of 12 to 13.5 mg/dl may receive 60 to 90 mg by I.V. infusion as a single dose over 2 to 24 hours. Patients with CCa levels greater than 13.5 mg/dl may receive 90 mg by I.V. infusion over 2 to 24 hours. Allow at least 7 days before retreatment to permit full response to first dose.
➤ **Moderate to severe Paget's disease**
*Adults:* 30 mg I.V. as a 4-hour infusion on 3 consecutive days for total dose of 90 mg. Repeat cycle, p.r.n.

➤ **Osteolytic bone metastases of breast cancer with standard antineoplastic therapy**
*Adults:* 90 mg I.V. infusion over 2 hours q 3 to 4 weeks.
➤ **Osteolytic bone lesions of multiple myeloma**
*Adults:* 90 mg I.V. over 4 hours once monthly.

## I.V. ADMINISTRATION
• Reconstitute drug with 10 ml of sterile water for injection. After drug is completely dissolved, add to 250 ml (2-hour infusion), 500 ml (4-hour infusion), or 1,000 ml (up to 24-hour infusion) of half-normal or normal saline solution for injection or $D_5W$.
• Don't mix with infusion solutions that contain calcium, such as Ringer's injection or lactated Ringer's injection. Visually inspect for precipitate before use.
• Infusions longer than 2 hours may reduce the risk for renal toxicity, particularly in patients with preexisting renal insufficiency.
• *Alert:* Give drug only by I.V. infusion. Injecting a bolus may cause nephropathy.
• Solution is stable for 24 hours at room temperature.
• Store reconstituted drug at 36° to 46° F (2° to 8° C).

## ACTION
An antihypercalcemic that inhibits resorption of bone. Adsorbs to hydroxyapatite crystals in bone and may directly block dissolution of calcium phosphate. Blocks mature osteoclast formation. Apparently doesn't inhibit bone formation or mineralization.

| Route | Onset | Peak | Duration |
|-------|-------|------|----------|
| I.V. | Unknown | Unknown | Unknown |

## ADVERSE REACTIONS
**CNS:** *seizures, fatigue,* somnolence, syncope, fever.
**CV:** *atrial fibrillation,* tachycardia, *hypertension, fluid overload.*
**GI:** *abdominal pain, anorexia, constipation, nausea, vomiting,* **GI hemorrhage.**
**GU:** renal dysfunction, *renal failure.*
**Hematologic:** *leukopenia, thrombocytopenia, anemia.*

**Metabolic:** hypophosphatemia, hypokalemia, hypomagnesemia, hypocalcemia.
**Skin:** *infusion-site reaction, pain at infusion site.*

**INTERACTIONS**
None significant.

**EFFECTS ON LAB TEST RESULTS**
● May increase creatinine level. May decrease phosphate, potassium, magnesium, and calcium levels.
● May decrease hemoglobin and WBC and platelet counts.

**CONTRAINDICATIONS & CAUTIONS**
● Contraindicated in patients hypersensitive to drug or other bisphosphonates, such as etidronate.
● Use with extreme caution, and consider risks versus benefits in patients with renal impairment.

**NURSING CONSIDERATIONS**
● Assess hydration status before treatment. Use drug only after patient has been vigorously hydrated with normal saline solution. In patients with mild to moderate hypercalcemia, hydration alone may be sufficient.
● Because drug can cause electrolyte disturbances, carefully monitor electrolyte levels, especially calcium, phosphate, and magnesium. Short-term administration of calcium may be needed in patients with severe hypocalcemia. Also monitor creatinine level, CBC and differential count, hemoglobin, and hematocrit.
● Carefully monitor patients with anemia, leukopenia, or thrombocytopenia during first 2 weeks of therapy.
● Monitor patient's temperature. Some patients experience an elevation of 1.8° F (1° C) for 24 to 48 hours after therapy.
● *Alert:* Because renal dysfunction may lead to renal failure, single doses of pamidronate shouldn't exceed 90 mg.
● Monitor creatinine level before each treatment.
● Patients treated for bone metastases who have renal dysfunction should have the dose withheld until renal function returns to baseline. Treatment of bone metastases in patients with severe renal impairment is not recommended. In other indications,

clinical judgment should determine whether the potential benefit outweighs the potential risk in such patients.
● It's unknown if drug appears in breast milk. Use cautiously in breast-feeding women.

**PATIENT TEACHING**
● Explain use and administration of drug to patient and family.
● Instruct patient to report adverse reactions promptly.
● Advise patient to alert her health care provider if she is pregnant or breast-feeding.

**risedronate sodium**
Actonel◆

*Pregnancy risk category C*

**AVAILABLE FORMS**
*Tablets:* 5 mg, 30 mg, 35 mg

**INDICATIONS & DOSAGES**
➤ **To prevent and treat postmenopausal osteoporosis**
*Adults:* 5-mg tablet P.O. once daily, or 35-mg tablet once weekly.
➤ **Glucocorticoid-induced osteoporosis in patients taking 7.5 mg or more of prednisone or equivalent glucocorticoid daily**
*Adults:* 5 mg P.O. daily.
➤ **Paget's disease**
*Adults:* 30 mg P.O. daily for 2 months. If relapse occurs or alkaline phosphatase level doesn't normalize, may retreat with same dose and duration 2 months or more after completing first treatment.
*Adjust-a-dose:* Drug isn't recommended for patients with creatinine clearance less than 30 ml/minute.

**ACTION**
Reverses the loss of bone mineral density in postmenopausal women by reducing bone turnover and bone resorption. In patients with Paget's disease, drug causes bone turnover to return to normal.

| Route | Onset | Peak | Duration |
|-------|-------|------|----------|
| P.O. | 1 hr | Unknown | Unknown |

## ADVERSE REACTIONS

**CNS:** asthenia, *headache,* depression, dizziness, insomnia, anxiety, neuralgia, vertigo, hypertonia, paresthesia, *pain.*
**CV:** *hypertension,* CV disorder, angina pectoris, chest pain, peripheral edema.
**EENT:** pharyngitis, rhinitis, sinusitis, cataract, conjunctivitis, otitis media, amblyopia, tinnitus.
**GI:** *nausea, diarrhea, abdominal pain,* flatulence, gastritis, rectal disorder, constipation.
**GU:** *UTI,* cystitis.
**Hematologic:** ecchymosis, anemia.
**Musculoskeletal:** *arthralgia,* neck pain, *back pain,* myalgia, bone pain, leg cramps, bursitis, tendon disorder.
**Respiratory:** dyspnea, pneumonia, bronchitis.
**Skin:** *rash,* pruritus, skin carcinoma.
**Other:** *infection,* tooth disorder.

## INTERACTIONS

**Drug-drug.** *Calcium supplements, antacids that contain calcium, magnesium, or aluminum:* May interfere with risedronate absorption. Advise patient to separate dosing times.
**Drug-food.** *Any food:* May interfere with risedronate absorption. Advise patient to take drug at least 30 minutes before first food or drink of the day (other than water).

## EFFECTS ON LAB TEST RESULTS

● May decrease calcium and phosphorus levels.

## CONTRAINDICATIONS & CAUTIONS

● Contraindicated in patients hypersensitive to any component of the product, in hypocalcemic patients, in patients with creatinine clearance less than 30 ml/minute, and in those who can't stand or sit upright for 30 minutes after administration.
● Use cautiously in patients with upper GI disorders such as dysphagia, esophagitis, and esophageal or gastric ulcers.

## NURSING CONSIDERATIONS

● Risk factors for the development of osteoporosis include family history, previous fracture, smoking, a decrease in bone mineral density below the premenopausal mean, a thin body frame, White or Asian race, and early menopause.
● *Alert:* Give drug with 6 to 8 ounces of water at least 30 minutes before patient's first food or drink of the day, to facilitate delivery to the stomach. Don't allow patient to lie down for 30 minutes after taking drug.
● Consider weight-bearing exercise along with cessation of smoking and alcohol consumption, as appropriate.
● *Alert:* Bisphosphonates have been linked to such GI disorders as dysphagia, esophagitis, and esophageal or gastric ulcers. Monitor patient for symptoms of esophageal disease (such as dysphagia, retrosternal pain, or severe persistent or worsening heartburn).
● Patients should receive supplemental calcium and vitamin D if dietary intake is inadequate. Because calcium supplements and drugs containing calcium, aluminum, or magnesium may interfere with risedronate absorption, separate dosing times.
● Store drug at 68° to 77° F (20° to 25° C).
● Bisphosphonates can interfere with bone-imaging agents.

## PATIENT TEACHING

● Explain that risedronate is used to replace bone lost because of certain disease processes.
● Caution patient about the importance of adhering to special dosing instructions.
● Tell patient to take drug at least 30 minutes before the first food or drink of the day other than water. Urge patient to take the drug with 6 to 8 ounces of water while sitting or standing. Warn patient against lying down for 30 minutes after taking risedronate.
● Tell patient not to chew or suck the tablet because doing so may irritate his mouth.
● Advise patient to contact prescriber immediately if he develops symptoms of esophageal disease (such as difficulty or pain when swallowing, retrosternal pain, or severe heartburn).
● Advise patient to take calcium and vitamin D if dietary intake is inadequate, but to take them at a different time than risedronate.
● Advise patient to stop smoking and drinking alcohol, as appropriate. Also, ad-

vise patient to perform weight-bearing exercise.
• Tell patient to store drug in a cool, dry place, at room temperature, and away from children.
• Urge patient to read the Patient Information Guide before starting therapy.
• Tell patient if he misses a dose of the 35-mg tablet, he should take 1 tablet on the morning after he remembers and return to taking 1 tablet once a week, as originally scheduled on his chosen day. Patient shouldn't take 2 tablets on the same day.

---

✳ *NEW DRUG*

## teriparatide (rDNA origin)
Forteo

*Pregnancy risk category C*

---

### AVAILABLE FORMS
*Injection:* 750 mcg/3 ml in a prefilled pen

### INDICATIONS & DOSAGES
➤ **Osteoporosis in postmenopausal women at high risk for fracture; primary or hypogonadal osteoporosis in men at high risk for fracture**
*Adults:* 20 mcg S.C. in thigh or abdominal wall once daily.

### ACTION
Promotes new bone formation, skeletal bone mass, and bone strength by regulating calcium and phosphorus metabolism in bones and kidneys.

| Route | Onset | Peak | Duration |
|-------|-------|------|----------|
| S.C. | Rapid | 30 min | 3 hr |

### ADVERSE REACTIONS
**CNS:** asthenia, depression, dizziness, headache, insomnia, syncope, vertigo.
**CV:** angina pectoris, hypertension, orthostatic hypotension.
**EENT:** pharyngitis, rhinitis.
**GI:** constipation, diarrhea, dyspepsia, nausea, tooth disorder, vomiting.
**Metabolic:** hypercalcemia.
**Musculoskeletal:** *arthralgia,* leg cramps.
**Respiratory:** dyspnea, increased cough, pneumonia.
**Skin:** rash, sweating.
**Other:** neck pain, *pain.*

### INTERACTIONS
**Drug-drug.** *Calcium supplements:* May increase urinary calcium excretion. Dosage may need adjustment.
*Digoxin:* Hypercalcemia may predispose patient to digitalis toxicity. Use together cautiously.

### EFFECTS ON LAB TEST RESULTS
• May increase calcium and uric acid levels. May decrease phosphorus level.
• May increase urinary calcium and phosphorus excretion.

### CONTRAINDICATIONS & CAUTIONS
• Contraindicated in patients hypersensitive to teriparatide or its components.
• Contraindicated in patients at increased risk for osteosarcoma, such as those with Paget's disease or unexplained alkaline phosphatase elevations, children, and patients who have had skeletal radiation; in patients with bone metastases, a history of skeletal malignancies, hypercalcemia, or metabolic bone diseases other than osteoporosis; and in patients with hypercalcemia.
• Use cautiously in patients with active or recent urolithiasis or hepatic, renal, or cardiac disease.

### NURSING CONSIDERATIONS
• *Alert:* Because of the risk of osteosarcoma, give drug only to patients for whom benefits outweigh risk.
• Don't continue therapy for longer than 2 years.
• If patient may have urolithiasis or hypercalciuria, measure urinary calcium excretion before treatment.
• Monitor patient for orthostatic hypotension, which may occur within 4 hours of dosing.
• Monitor calcium level. If persistent hypercalcemia develops, stop drug and evaluate possible cause.

### PATIENT TEACHING
• Instruct patient on proper use and disposal of prefilled pen.
• Tell patient not to share pen with others.
• Advise patient to sit or lie down if drug causes a fast heartbeat, light-headedness, or dizziness. Tell patient to report persistent or worsening symptoms.

---

Reactions may be *common,* uncommon, *life-threatening,* or COMMON AND LIFE-THREATENING.

• Urge patient to report persistent symptoms of hypercalcemia, which include nausea, vomiting, constipation, lethargy, and muscle weakness.

## zoledronic acid
Zometa

*Pregnancy risk category D*

### AVAILABLE FORMS
*Injection:* 4 mg/vial

### INDICATIONS & DOSAGES
➤ **Hypercalcemia caused by malignancy**
*Adults:* 4 mg by I.V. infusion over at least 15 minutes. If albumin-corrected calcium level doesn't return to normal, consider retreatment with 4 mg. Allow at least 7 days to pass before retreatment to allow a full response to the first dose.
*Adjust-a-dose:* The following guidelines are for patients who received zoledronic acid, have reduced renal function as a result, and must be retreated with the drug. If patient had a normal creatinine level before treatment and has an increase in creatinine level of 0.5 mg/dl within 2 weeks of the next dose, withhold drug until level is within 10% of baseline value. Likewise, if patient had an abnormal creatinine level before treatment and has an increase of 1 mg/dl within 2 weeks of the next dose, withhold drug until level is within 10% of baseline value.
➤ **Multiple myeloma and bone metastases of solid tumors in conjunction with standard antineoplastic therapy; prostate cancer that has progressed after treatment with at least one course of hormonal therapy**
*Adults:* 4 mg I.V. infused over 15 minutes q 3 or 4 weeks. Treatment may last 15 months for prostate cancer, 12 months for breast cancer and multiple myeloma, and 9 months for other solid tumors.
*Adjust-a-dose:* Withhold drug in patients with normal baseline creatinine level who have an increase of 0.5 mg/dl and in those with abnormal baseline creatinine level who have an increase of 1 mg/dl. Resume treatment only when creatinine level has returned to within 10% of baseline value.

### I.V. ADMINISTRATION
• Reconstitute by adding 5 ml of sterile water to each vial. The drug must be completely dissolved.
• Inspect solution to make sure there is no particulate matter or discoloration.
• Give drug as a single I.V. solution in a line separate from all other drugs.
• Withdraw 4 mg of drug and mix in 100 ml of normal saline solution or $D_5W$.
• *Alert:* Don't mix drug with calcium-containing solutions (such as lactated Ringer's solution).
• Give as I.V. infusion over at least 15 minutes.
• If drug not used immediately after reconstitution, refrigerate solution and give within 24 hours.

### ACTION
Inhibits bone resorption, probably by inhibiting osteoclast activity and osteoclastic resorption of mineralized bone and cartilage. Decreases calcium release induced by the stimulatory factors produced by tumors.

| Route | Onset | Peak | Duration |
|-------|-------|------|----------|
| I.V. | Unknown | Unknown | 7-28 days |

### ADVERSE REACTIONS
**Hypercalcemia trials**
**CNS:** headache, somnolence, *anxiety, confusion, agitation, insomnia, fever.*
**CV:** hypotension.
**GI:** *nausea, constipation, diarrhea, abdominal pain, vomiting,* anorexia, dysphagia.
**GU:** *decreased creatinine level, urinary infection, candidiasis.*
**Hematologic:** ANEMIA, *granulocytopenia, thrombocytopenia, pancytopenia.*
**Metabolic:** *decreased calcium, phosphate, and magnesium levels;* dehydration.
**Musculoskeletal:** *skeletal pain,* arthralgia.
**Respiratory:** *dyspnea, cough,* pleural effusion.
**Other:** *progression of cancer,* infection.
**Bone metastases trials**
**CNS:** *headache,* anxiety, *insomnia, depression, paresthesia, hypoesthesia, fatigue, weakness, dizziness, fever.*
**CV:** *hypotension, leg edema.*

**GI:** *nausea, constipation, diarrhea, abdominal pain, vomiting, anorexia, increased appetite.*
**GU:** *decreased creatinine level, urinary infection.*
**Hematologic:** *anemia, neutropenia.*
**Metabolic:** *decreased calcium, phosphate, and magnesium levels; dehydration; weight decrease.*
**Musculoskeletal:** *skeletal pain, arthralgia, myalgia, back pain.*
**Respiratory:** *dyspnea, cough.*
**Skin:** *alopecia, dermatitis.*
**Other:** PROGRESSION OF CANCER, *rigors,* infection.

## INTERACTIONS
**Drug-drug.** *Aminoglycosides, loop diuretics:* May have additive effects that lower calcium level. Use together cautiously, and monitor calcium level.
*Thalidomide:* May increase risk of renal dysfunction in multiple myeloma patients, Use together cautiously.

## EFFECTS ON LAB TEST RESULTS
• May increase creatinine level. May decrease calcium, phosphorus, magnesium, and potassium levels.
• May decrease hemoglobin, hematocrit, and RBC, WBC, and platelet counts.

## CONTRAINDICATIONS & CAUTIONS
• Contraindicated in patients hypersensitive to drug, other bisphosphonates, or ingredients in formulation.
• Contraindicated in patients with hypercalcemia of malignancy whose creatinine level is more than 4.5 mg/dl and in patients with bone metastases whose creatinine level is more than 3 mg/dl.
• Contraindicated in breast-feeding women.
• Use cautiously in patients with aspirin-sensitive asthma because other bisphosphonates have been linked to bronchoconstriction in aspirin-sensitive patients with asthma.
• Use cautiously in elderly patients.

## NURSING CONSIDERATIONS
• Make sure patient is adequately hydrated before giving drug; urine output should be about 2 L daily.

• Each vial also contains 220 mg mannitol and 24 mg sodium citrate.
• *Alert:* Because of the risk of a decline in renal function that could progress to renal failure, single doses shouldn't exceed 4 mg and infusion should last at least 15 minutes.
• No acute overdoses reported, but rapid infusion and high doses may increase risk of renal toxicity. Overdose may cause hypocalcemia, hypophosphatemia, and hypomagnesemia.
• Monitor calcium, phosphate, magnesium, and creatinine levels carefully after giving drug. Correct calcium, phosphorus, and magnesium level reductions by I.V. administration of calcium gluconate, potassium and sodium phosphate, and magnesium sulfate.
• Monitor renal function closely. Drug is excreted mainly through kidneys. The risk of adverse reactions may be greater in patients with impaired renal function; give drug to these patients only if benefits outweigh risks.
• Drug is used cautiously in elderly patients because of the greater likelihood of disease, additional drug therapy, and decreased hepatic, renal, or cardiac function.
• Give patients an oral calcium supplement of 500 mg and a multiple vitamin containing 400 IU of vitamin D daily.

## PATIENT TEACHING
• Review the use and administration of drug with patient and family.
• Instruct patient to report adverse effects promptly.
• Explain the importance of periodic laboratory tests to monitor therapy and renal function.
• Advise woman to alert prescriber if she is pregnant or breast-feeding.

acetazolamide
acetazolamide sodium
amiloride hydrochloride
bumetanide
ethacrynate sodium
ethacrynic acid
furosemide
hydrochlorothiazide
indapamide
mannitol
metolazone
spironolactone
torsemide
triamterene

## COMBINATION PRODUCTS

ALDACTAZIDE: spironolactone 25 mg and hydrochlorothiazide 25 mg; spironolactone 50 mg and hydrochlorothiazide 50 mg.
DYAZIDE, MAXZIDE-25 MG: triamterene 37.5 mg and hydrochlorothiazide 25 mg.
MAXZIDE: triamterene 75 mg and hydrochlorothiazide 50 mg.
MODURETIC: amiloride hydrochloride 5 mg and hydrochlorothiazide 50 mg.
ZIAC: bisoprolol fumarate 2.5 mg, 5 mg, or 10 mg and hydrochlorothiazide 6.25 mg.

---

## acetazolamide
Acetazolam†, Apo-Acetazolamide†, Dazamide, Diamox†, Diamox Sequels†

## acetazolamide sodium
Diamox†

*Pregnancy risk category C*

## AVAILABLE FORMS
**acetazolamide**
*Capsules (extended-release):* 500 mg
*Tablets:* 125 mg, 250 mg
**acetazolamide sodium**
*Injection:* 500-mg vial

## INDICATIONS & DOSAGES
➤ **Secondary glaucoma; preoperative treatment of acute angle-closure glaucoma**
*Adults:* 250 mg P.O. q 4 hours or 250 mg P.O. b.i.d. for short-term therapy. In acute cases, 500 mg P.O.; then 125 to 250 mg P.O. q 4 hours. To rapidly lower intraocular pressure, initially, 500 mg I.V.; may repeat in 2 to 4 hours, if needed, followed by 125 to 250 mg P.O. q 4 hours.
*Children:* 10 to 15 mg/kg P.O. daily in divided doses q 6 to 8 hours. For acute angle-closure glaucoma, 5 to 10 mg/kg I.V. q 6 hours.
➤ **Chronic open-angle glaucoma**
*Adults:* 250 mg to 1 g P.O. daily in divided doses q.i.d., or 500 mg (sustained-release) P.O. b.i.d.
➤ **To prevent or treat acute mountain sickness**
*Adults:* 500 mg to 1 g (regular or sustained-release) P.O. daily in divided doses q 12 hours. Start 24 to 48 hours before ascent and continue for 48 hours while at high altitude.
➤ **Adjunctive treatment of myoclonic, refractory, generalized tonic-clonic, absence, or mixed seizures**
*Adults and children:* 8 to 30 mg/kg P.O. daily in divided doses. For adults, optimum dosage range is 375 mg to 1 g daily. Usually given with other anticonvulsants.
➤ **Edema caused by heart failure; drug-induced edema**
*Adults:* 250 mg to 375 mg (5 mg/kg) P.O. daily in the morning. For best results, use every other day or 2 days on followed by 1 to 2 days off.
*Children:* 5 mg/kg or 150 mg/m² P.O. or I.V. daily in the morning.

## I.V. ADMINISTRATION
● Reconstitute drug in 500-mg vial with at least 5 ml of sterile water for injection. Use within 24 hours of reconstitution.
● Inject 100 to 500 mg/minute into a large vein using a 21G or 23G needle. Intermittent or continuous infusion isn't recommended.

---

## ACTION
Promotes renal excretion of sodium, potassium, bicarbonate, and water. As anticonvulsant, drug normalizes neuronal discharge. In mountain sickness, drug stimulates ventilation and increases cerebral blood flow; also reduces intraocular pressure.

| Route | Onset | Peak | Duration |
|-------|-------|------|----------|
| P.O. | 60-90 min | 1-4 hr | 8-12 hr |
| P.O. (extended-release) | 2 hr | 3-6 hr | 18-24 hr |
| I.V. | 2 min | 15 min | 4-5 hr |

## ADVERSE REACTIONS
**CNS:** drowsiness, paresthesia, confusion, depression, *seizures,* weakness.
**EENT:** transient myopia, hearing dysfunction, tinnitus.
**GI:** nausea, vomiting, anorexia, metallic taste, diarrhea, black tarry stools.
**GU:** polyuria, hematuria, crystalluria, glycosuria, phosphaturia, renal calculus.
**Hematologic:** *aplastic anemia,* hemolytic anemia, *leukopenia.*
**Metabolic:** hypokalemia, asymptomatic hyperuricemia, hyperchloremic acidosis.
**Skin:** rash, urticaria, *Stevens-Johnson syndrome,* pain at injection site.
**Other:** sterile abscesses.

## INTERACTIONS
**Drug-drug.** *Amphetamines, anticholinergics, mecamylamine, procainamide, quinidine:* May decrease renal clearance of these drugs, increasing toxicity. Monitor patient for toxicity.
*Cyclosporine:* May increase cyclosporine level, causing nephrotoxicity and neurotoxicity. Monitor patient for toxicity.
*Diflunisal:* May increase acetazolamide adverse effects; may significantly decrease intracranial pressure. Use together cautiously.
*Lithium:* May increase lithium excretion, decreasing its effectiveness. Monitor lithium level.
*Methenamine:* May reduce acetazolamide effectiveness. Avoid using together.
*Primidone:* May decrease serum and urine primidone levels. Monitor patient closely.
*Salicylates:* May cause accumulation and toxicity of acetazolamide, including CNS

depression and metabolic acidosis. Monitor patient for toxicity.
**Drug-lifestyle.** *Sun exposure:* May increase risk of photosensitivity reactions. Advise patient to avoid excessive sunlight exposure.

## EFFECTS ON LAB TEST RESULTS
- May increase uric acid level. May decrease potassium level.
- May decrease hemoglobin, WBC count, and thyroid iodine uptake.
- May cause false-positive urine protein test result.

## CONTRAINDICATIONS & CAUTIONS
- Contraindicated in patients hypersensitive to drug and in those with hyponatremia or hypokalemia, renal or hepatic disease or dysfunction, renal calculi, adrenal gland failure, hyperchloremic acidosis, or severe pulmonary obstruction.
- Contraindicated in those receiving long-term treatment for chronic noncongestive angle-closure glaucoma.
- Use cautiously in patients receiving other diuretics and in those with respiratory acidosis, emphysema, or chronic pulmonary disease.

## NURSING CONSIDERATIONS
- Cross-sensitivity between antibacterial sulfonamides and sulfonamide-derivative diuretics such as acetazolamide has been reported.
- If patient can't swallow oral form, pharmacist may make a suspension using crushed acetazolamide tablets in a highly flavored syrup, such as cherry, raspberry, or chocolate. Although concentrations up to 500 mg/5 ml are feasible, concentrations of 250 mg/5 ml are more palatable. Refrigeration improves palatability but doesn't improve stability. Suspensions are stable for 1 week.
- Monitor fluid intake and output, glucose, and electrolytes, especially potassium, bicarbonate, and chloride. When drug is used in diuretic therapy, consult prescriber and dietitian about providing a high-potassium diet.
- Monitor elderly patients closely because they are especially susceptible to excessive diuresis.

- Weigh patient daily. Rapid or excessive fluid loss causes weight loss and hypotension.
- Diuretic effect decreases when acidosis occurs but can be reestablished by withdrawing drug for several days and then restarting or by using intermittent administration schedules.
- Monitor patient for signs of hemolytic anemia (pallor, weakness, and palpitations).
- Drug may increase glucose level and cause glycosuria.
- *Alert:* Don't confuse acetazolamide with acetohexamide or acyclovir.

### PATIENT TEACHING
- Tell patient to take oral form with food to minimize GI upset.
- Caution patient not to perform hazardous activities if adverse CNS reactions occur.
- Instruct patient to avoid prolonged exposure to sunlight because drug may cause phototoxicity.
- Instruct patient to notify prescriber of any unusual bleeding, bruising, tingling, or tremors.

---

## amiloride hydrochloride
Midamor

*Pregnancy risk category B*

### AVAILABLE FORMS
*Tablets:* 5 mg

### INDICATIONS & DOSAGES
➤ **Hypertension; hypokalemia; edema from heart failure, usually in patients also taking thiazide or other potassium-wasting diuretics**
*Adults:* 5 mg P.O. daily, increased to 10 mg daily, if needed; then 15 mg. Maximum, 20 mg daily.
➤ **Lithium-induced polyuria ◆**
*Adults:* 10 to 20 mg P.O. daily.

### ACTION
A potassium-sparing diuretic that inhibits sodium reabsorption and potassium excretion in the distal tubules.

| Route | Onset | Peak | Duration |
|-------|-------|------|----------|
| P.O. | 2 hr | 6-10 hr | 24 hr |

### ADVERSE REACTIONS
**CNS:** fatigue, *headache,* weakness, dizziness, *encephalopathy.*
**CV:** orthostatic hypotension.
**GI:** *nausea, anorexia, diarrhea, vomiting,* abdominal pain, constipation, appetite changes.
**GU:** impotence.
**Hematologic:** *aplastic anemia, neutropenia.*
**Metabolic:** *hyperkalemia,* hyponatremia.
**Musculoskeletal:** muscle cramps.
**Respiratory:** dyspnea.

### INTERACTIONS
**Drug-drug.** *ACE inhibitors, indomethacin, potassium-sparing diuretics, potassium supplements:* May cause hyperkalemia. Monitor potassium level closely if using together.
*Digoxin:* May decrease clearance of digoxin. Monitor digoxin level.
*Lithium:* May decrease lithium clearance, increasing risk of lithium toxicity. Monitor lithium level.
*NSAIDs:* May decrease diuretic effectiveness. Avoid using together.
**Drug-herb.** *Licorice:* May increase risk of hypokalemia. Discourage use together.
**Drug-food.** *Foods high in potassium (such as bananas, oranges), salt substitutes containing potassium:* May cause hyperkalemia. Advise patient to choose diet carefully and to use low-potassium salt substitutes.

### EFFECTS ON LAB TEST RESULTS
- May increase BUN and potassium levels. May decrease sodium and liver enzyme levels.
- May decrease hemoglobin and neutrophil count.

### CONTRAINDICATIONS & CAUTIONS
- Contraindicated in patients hypersensitive to drug and in those with potassium level higher than 5.5 mEq/L, anuria, acute or chronic renal insufficiency, or diabetic nephropathy.
- Contraindicated in patients receiving potassium supplementation or other potassium-sparing diuretics, such as spironolactone and triamterene.
- Use cautiously in patients with diabetes mellitus, cardiopulmonary disease, or

---

severe, existing hepatic or renal insufficiency.
● Use cautiously in elderly or debilitated patients.

## NURSING CONSIDERATIONS
● To prevent nausea, give drug with meals.
● Monitor potassium level because of increased risk of hyperkalemia. Alert prescriber immediately if potassium level exceeds 5.5 mEq/L, and expect to stop drug.
● Drug causes severe hyperkalemia in diabetic patients after glucose tolerance testing; stop drug at least 3 days before testing.
● *Alert:* Don't confuse amiloride with amiodarone.

## PATIENT TEACHING
● Instruct patient to take drug with food to minimize GI upset.
● Advise patient to avoid sudden posture changes and to rise slowly to avoid dizziness upon standing quickly.
● Caution patient not to perform hazardous activities if adverse CNS reactions occur.
● To prevent serious hyperkalemia, warn patient to avoid eating too much potassium-rich food, potassium-containing salt substitutes, and potassium supplements.
● Advise patient to report signs of hyperkalemia: tingling, muscle weakness, fatigue, limb paralysis.
● Instruct patient to check with prescriber or pharmacist before taking new prescription or OTC drugs.

---

## bumetanide
Bumex✷, Burinex‡

*Pregnancy risk category C*

## AVAILABLE FORMS
*Injection:* 0.25 mg/ml
*Tablets:* 0.5 mg, 1 mg, 2 mg

## INDICATIONS & DOSAGES
➤ **Edema caused by heart failure or hepatic or renal disease**
*Adults:* 0.5 to 2 mg P.O. once daily. If diuretic response isn't adequate, a second or third dose may be given at 4- to 5-hour intervals. Maximum dose is 10 mg/day.

May be given parenterally if oral route isn't feasible. Usual first dose is 0.5 to 1 mg given I.V. or I.M. If response isn't adequate, a second or third dose may be given at 2- to 3-hour intervals. Maximum, 10 mg/day.

## I.V. ADMINISTRATION
● Give I.V. doses directly using a 21G or 23G needle over 1 to 2 minutes.
● For intermittent infusion, give diluted drug through an intermittent infusion device or piggyback into an I.V. line containing a free-flowing, compatible solution.
● Infuse at ordered rate.
● In patients with severe chronic renal insufficiency, a continuous infusion of 12 mg over 12 hours may be more effective and less toxic than intermittent bolus therapy.

## ACTION
A potent loop diuretic that inhibits sodium and chloride reabsorption at the ascending loop of Henle.

| Route | Onset | Peak | Duration |
|-------|-------|------|----------|
| P.O. | 30-60 min | 1-2 hr | 4-6 hr |
| I.V. | Within min | 15-30 min | 30-60 min |
| I.M. | 40 min | Unknown | 5-6 hr |

## ADVERSE REACTIONS
**CNS:** *weakness,* dizziness, headache, vertigo, pain.
**CV:** orthostatic hypotension, ECG changes, chest pain.
**EENT:** transient deafness, tinnitus.
**GI:** nausea, vomiting, upset stomach, dry mouth, diarrhea.
**GU:** premature ejaculation, difficulty maintaining erection, oliguria.
**Hematologic:** azotemia, *thrombocytopenia.*
**Metabolic:** volume depletion and dehydration; hypokalemia; hypochloremic alkalosis; hypomagnesemia; asymptomatic hyperuricemia.
**Musculoskeletal:** arthritic pain, muscle pain and tenderness.
**Skin:** rash, pruritus, diaphoresis.

## INTERACTIONS
**Drug-drug.** *Aminoglycoside antibiotics:* May increase ototoxicity. Use together cautiously.

---

*Antidiabetics:* May decrease hypoglycemic effects. Monitor glucose level.

*Antihypertensives:* May increase risk of hypotension. Use together cautiously.

*Cardiac glycosides:* May increase risk of digoxin toxicity from bumetanide-induced hypokalemia. Monitor potassium and digoxin levels.

*Chlorothiazide, chlorthalidone, hydrochlorothiazide, indapamide, metolazone:* May cause excessive diuretic response resulting in serious electrolyte abnormalities or dehydration. Adjust doses carefully, and monitor patient closely for excessive diuretic responses.

*Cisplatin:* May increase risk of ototoxicity. Monitor patient closely.

*Lithium:* May decrease lithium clearance, increasing risk of lithium toxicity. Monitor lithium level.

*Neuromuscular blockers:* May prolong neuromuscular blockade. Monitor patient closely.

*NSAIDs, probenecid:* May inhibit diuretic response. Use together cautiously.

*Other potassium-wasting drugs (such as amphotericin B, corticosteroids):* May increase risk of hypokalemia. Use together cautiously.

*Warfarin:* May increase anticoagulant effect. Use together cautiously.

**Drug-herb.** *Dandelion:* May interfere with diuretic activity. Discourage use together.

*Licorice:* May cause unexpected rapid potassium loss. Discourage use together.

**EFFECTS ON LAB TEST RESULTS**
● May increase AST, ALT, LDH, alkaline phosphatase, bilirubin, creatinine, urine urea, glucose, and cholesterol levels. May decrease potassium, magnesium, sodium, and calcium levels.
● May decrease platelet count. May increase or decrease WBC count.

**CONTRAINDICATIONS & CAUTIONS**
● Contraindicated in patients hypersensitive to drug or sulfonamides (possible cross-sensitivity) and in patients with anuria, hepatic coma, or severe electrolyte depletion.
● Use cautiously in patients with hepatic cirrhosis and ascites, in elderly patients, and in those with depressed renal function.

**NURSING CONSIDERATIONS**
● To prevent nocturia, give drug in the morning. If second dose is needed, give in early afternoon.
● Safest and most effective dosage schedule for control of edema is intermittent dosage given on alternate days or 3 to 4 days with 1 or 2 days off between cycles.
● Monitor fluid intake and output, weight, and electrolyte, BUN, creatinine, and carbon dioxide levels frequently.
● Watch for evidence of hypokalemia, such as muscle weakness and cramps. Instruct patient to report these symptoms.
● Consult prescriber and dietitian about a high-potassium diet. Foods rich in potassium include citrus fruits, tomatoes, bananas, dates, and apricots.
● Monitor glucose level in diabetic patients.
● Monitor uric acid level, especially in patients with history of gout.
● Monitor blood pressure and pulse rate during rapid diuresis. Bumetanide can lead to profound water and electrolyte depletion.
● If oliguria or azotemia develops or increases, prescriber may stop drug.
● Bumetanide can be safely used in patients allergic to furosemide; 1 mg of bumetanide equals 40 mg of furosemide.
● *Alert:* Don't confuse Bumex with Buprenex.

**PATIENT TEACHING**
● Instruct patient to take drug with food to minimize GI upset.
● Advise patient to take drug in morning to avoid nighttime urination; if second dose is needed, have him take it in early afternoon.
● Advise patient to avoid sudden posture changes and to rise slowly to avoid dizziness upon standing quickly.
● Instruct patient to notify prescriber about muscle weakness, cramps, nausea, or dizziness.
● Instruct patient to weigh himself daily to monitor fluid status.

---

## ethacrynate sodium
Edecrin Sodium

## ethacrynic acid
Edecril‡, Edecrin

*Pregnancy risk category B*

### AVAILABLE FORMS
**ethacrynate sodium**
*Injection:* 50 mg (with 62.5 mg of mannitol and 0.1 mg of thimerosal)
**ethacrynic acid**
*Tablets:* 25 mg, 50 mg

### INDICATIONS & DOSAGES
➤ **Acute pulmonary edema**
*Adults:* 50 mg or 0.5 to 1 mg/kg I.V. Usually only one dose is needed, although a second dose may be needed.
➤ **Edema**
*Adults:* 50 to 200 mg P.O. daily. May increase to 200 mg b.i.d. for desired effect.
*Children:* First dose is 25 mg P.O., increase cautiously by 25 mg daily until desired effect is achieved. Dosage for infants hasn't been established.
*Adjust-a-dose:* If added to an existing diuretic regimen, first dose is 25 mg and dosage adjustments are made in 25-mg increments.

### I.V. ADMINISTRATION
● Add to vial 50 ml of $D_5W$ or normal saline solution. Give slowly through tubing of running infusion over several minutes. Discard unused solution after 24 hours. Don't use cloudy or opalescent solutions.
● If more than one I.V. dose is needed, use a new injection site to avoid thrombophlebitis.
● Don't mix with whole blood or its derivatives.

### ACTION
A potent loop diuretic that inhibits sodium and chloride reabsorption at the proximal and distal tubules and the ascending loop of Henle.

| Route | Onset | Peak | Duration |
|-------|-------|------|----------|
| P.O. | 30 min | 2 hr | 6-8 hr |
| I.V. | 5 min | 15-30 min | 2 hr |

### ADVERSE REACTIONS
**CNS:** malaise, confusion, fatigue, vertigo, headache, nervousness, fever.
**CV:** orthostatic hypotension.
**EENT:** transient or permanent deafness with too-rapid I.V. injection, blurred vision, tinnitus, hearing loss.
**GI:** cramping, diarrhea, anorexia, nausea, vomiting, GI bleeding, *pancreatitis.*
**GU:** oliguria, hematuria, nocturia, polyuria, frequent urination.
**Hematologic:** *agranulocytosis, neutropenia, thrombocytopenia,* azotemia.
**Metabolic:** asymptomatic hyperuricemia, hypokalemia; hypochloremic alkalosis; fluid and electrolyte imbalances, including dilutional hyponatremia, hypocalcemia, and hypomagnesemia; hyperglycemia and impaired glucose tolerance; volume depletion and dehydration.
**Skin:** rash.
**Other:** chills.

### INTERACTIONS
**Drug-drug.** *Aminoglycoside antibiotics:* May increase ototoxic adverse reactions of both drugs. Use together cautiously.
*Antidiabetics:* May decrease hypoglycemic effects. Monitor glucose level.
*Antihypertensives:* May increase risk of hypotension. Use together cautiously.
*Cardiac glycosides:* May increase risk of digoxin toxicity from ethacrynate-induced hypokalemia. Monitor potassium and digoxin levels.
*Chlorothiazide, chlorthalidone, hydrochlorothiazide, indapamide, metolazone:* May cause excessive diuretic response resulting in serious electrolyte abnormalities or dehydration. Adjust doses carefully, and monitor patient closely for excessive diuretic responses.
*Cisplatin:* May increase risk of ototoxicity. Avoid using together.
*Lithium:* May decrease lithium clearance, increasing risk of lithium toxicity. Monitor lithium level.
*Neuromuscular blockers:* May enhance neuromuscular blockade. Monitor patient closely.
*NSAIDs:* May decrease diuretic effectiveness. Use together cautiously.
*Other potassium-wasting drugs (amphotericin B, corticosteroids):* May increase

risk of hypocalcemia. Use together cautiously.

*Probenecid:* May decrease diuretic effectiveness. Avoid using together.

*Warfarin:* May increase anticoagulant effect. Use together cautiously.

**Drug-herb.** *Dandelion:* May interfere with diuretic activity. Discourage use together.

*Licorice:* May cause unexpected rapid potassium loss. Discourage use together.

## EFFECTS ON LAB TEST RESULTS
● May increase glucose and uric acid levels. May decrease potassium, sodium, calcium, and magnesium levels.
● May decrease granulocyte, neutrophil, and platelet counts.

## CONTRAINDICATIONS & CAUTIONS
● Contraindicated in infants, patients hypersensitive to drug, and patients with anuria.
● Use cautiously in patients with electrolyte abnormalities or hepatic impairment.

## NURSING CONSIDERATIONS
● Give oral doses in the morning to prevent nocturia.
● Don't give I.M. or S.C. because of local pain and irritation.
● Monitor fluid intake and output, weight, blood pressure, and electrolyte levels.
● Watch for signs of hypokalemia, such as muscle weakness and cramps.
● Monitor glucose level in diabetic patients.
● Consult prescriber and dietitian about providing a high-potassium diet. Foods rich in potassium include citrus fruits, tomatoes, bananas, dates, and apricots. Potassium chloride and sodium supplements may be needed.
● Drug may increase risk of gastric hemorrhage caused by steroid treatment.
● Monitor elderly patients, who are especially susceptible to excessive diuresis.
● Monitor uric acid level, especially in patients with history of gout.
● *Alert:* Stop drug if patient has severe diarrhea. Patient shouldn't receive drug again after diarrhea has resolved.

## PATIENT TEACHING
● Instruct patient to take drug with food to minimize GI upset.
● Advise patient to take drug in morning to avoid nighttime urination; if second dose is needed, have him take it in early afternoon.
● Advise patient to avoid sudden posture changes and to rise slowly to avoid dizziness upon standing quickly.
● Tell patient to notify prescriber about muscle weakness, cramps, nausea, or dizziness.
● Caution patient not to perform hazardous activities if drug causes drowsiness.
● Advise diabetic patient to closely monitor glucose level.

---

# furosemide (frusemide†)
Apo-Furosemide†, Furoside†, Lasix*❤, Novosemide†, Uritol†

*Pregnancy risk category C*

## AVAILABLE FORMS
*Injection:* 10 mg/ml
*Oral solution:* 10 mg/ml, 40 mg/5 ml
*Tablets:* 20 mg, 40 mg, 80 mg, 500 mg†

## INDICATIONS & DOSAGES
➤ **Acute pulmonary edema**
*Adults:* 40 mg I.V. injected slowly over 1 to 2 minutes; then 80 mg I.V. in 60 to 90 minutes if needed.
➤ **Edema**
*Adults:* 20 to 80 mg P.O. daily in the morning, second dose in 6 to 8 hours; carefully adjusted up to 600 mg daily if needed. Or, 20 to 40 mg I.V. or I.M., increased by 20 mg q 2 hours until desired effect achieved.
*Infants and children:* 2 mg/kg P.O. daily, increased by 1 to 2 mg/kg in 6 to 8 hours if needed; carefully adjusted up to 6 mg/kg daily if needed.
➤ **Hypertension**
*Adults:* 40 mg P.O. b.i.d. Dosage adjusted based on response. May be used as adjunct to other antihypertensives if needed.

## I.V. ADMINISTRATION
● For direct injection, give over 1 to 2 minutes.

---

• For infusion, dilute with $D_5W$, normal saline solution, or lactated Ringer's solution, and infuse no more than 4 mg/minute to avoid ototoxicity. Use prepared infusion solution within 24 hours.

• Don't use discolored (yellow) injectable preparation.

## ACTION

A potent loop diuretic that inhibits sodium and chloride reabsorption at the proximal and distal tubules and the ascending loop of Henle.

| Route | Onset | Peak | Duration |
|-------|-------|------|----------|
| P.O. | 20-60 min | 1-2 hr | 6-8 hr |
| I.V. | 5 min | 30 min | 2 hr |

## ADVERSE REACTIONS

**CNS:** vertigo, headache, dizziness, paresthesia, weakness, restlessness, fever.
**CV:** orthostatic hypotension; thrombophlebitis with I.V. administration.
**EENT:** transient deafness, blurred or yellowed vision.
**GI:** abdominal discomfort and pain, diarrhea, anorexia, nausea, vomiting, constipation, *pancreatitis.*
**GU:** nocturia, polyuria, frequent urination, oliguria.
**Hematologic:** *agranulocytosis, leukopenia, thrombocytopenia,* azotemia, anemia, *aplastic anemia.*
**Hepatic:** hepatic dysfunction.
**Metabolic:** volume depletion and dehydration, asymptomatic hyperuricemia, impaired glucose tolerance, hypokalemia, hypochloremic alkalosis, hyperglycemia, and fluid and electrolyte imbalances, including dilutional hyponatremia, hypocalcemia, and hypomagnesemia.
**Musculoskeletal:** muscle spasm.
**Skin:** dermatitis, purpura, photosensitivity reactions, transient pain at I.M. injection site.
**Other:** gout.

## INTERACTIONS

**Drug-drug.** *Aminoglycoside antibiotics, cisplatin:* May increase ototoxicity. Use together cautiously.
*Amphotericin B, corticosteroids, corticotropin, metolazone:* May increase risk of hypokalemia. Monitor potassium level closely.

*Antidiabetics:* May decrease hypoglycemic effects. Monitor glucose level.
*Antihypertensives:* May increase risk of hypotension. Use together cautiously.
*Cardiac glycosides, neuromuscular blockers:* May increase toxicity of these drugs from furosemide-induced hypokalemia. Monitor potassium level.
*Chlorothiazide, chlorthalidone, hydrochlorothiazide, indapamide, metolazone:* May cause excessive diuretic response resulting in serious electrolyte abnormalities or dehydration. Adjust doses carefully, and monitor patient closely for excessive diuretic responses.
*Ethacrynic acid:* May increase risk of ototoxicity. Avoid using together.
*Lithium:* May decrease lithium excretion, resulting in lithium toxicity. Monitor lithium level.
*NSAIDs:* May inhibit diuretic response. Use together cautiously.
*Phenytoin:* May decrease diuretic effects of furosemide. Use together cautiously.
*Propanolol:* May increase propranolol level. Monitor patient closely.
*Salicylates:* May cause salicylate toxicity. Use together cautiously.
*Sucralfate:* May reduce diuretic and antihypertensive effect. Separate doses by 2 hours.
**Drug-herb.** *Aloe:* May increase drug effects. Discourage use together.
*Dandelion:* May interfere with diuretic activity. Discourage use together.
*Ginseng:* May decrease loop diuretic effect. Discourage use together.
*Licorice:* May cause unexpected rapid potassium loss. Discourage use together.
**Drug-lifestyle.** *Sun exposure:* May increase risk for photosensitivity reactions. Advise patient to avoid excessive sunlight exposure.

## EFFECTS ON LAB TEST RESULTS

• May increase glucose, cholesterol, and uric acid levels. May decrease potassium, sodium, calcium, and magnesium levels.
• May decrease hemoglobin and granulocyte, WBC, and platelet counts.

## CONTRAINDICATIONS & CAUTIONS

• Contraindicated in patients hypersensitive to drug and in those with anuria.

---

Reactions may be *common,* uncommon, *life-threatening,* or COMMON AND LIFE-THREATENING.

• Use cautiously in patients with hepatic cirrhosis and in those allergic to sulfonamides. Use furosemide during pregnancy only if potential benefits to mother clearly outweigh risks to fetus.

**NURSING CONSIDERATIONS**
• To prevent nocturia, give P.O. and I.M. preparations in the morning. Give second dose in early afternoon.
• *Alert:* Monitor weight, blood pressure, and pulse rate routinely with long-term use and during rapid diuresis. Furosemide can lead to profound water and electrolyte depletion.
• If oliguria or azotemia develops or increases, drug may need to be stopped.
• Monitor fluid intake and output and electrolyte, BUN, and carbon dioxide levels frequently.
• Watch for signs of hypokalemia, such as muscle weakness and cramps.
• Consult prescriber and dietitian about a high-potassium diet. Foods rich in potassium include citrus fruits, tomatoes, bananas, and dates.
• Monitor glucose level in diabetic patients.
• Furosemide may not be well absorbed orally in patient with severe heart failure. Drug may need to be given I.V. even if patient is taking other oral drugs.
• Monitor uric acid level, especially in patients with a history of gout.
• Monitor elderly patients, who are especially susceptible to excessive diuresis, because circulatory collapse and thromboembolic complications are possible.
• Store tablets in light-resistant container to prevent discoloration (doesn't affect potency). Refrigerate oral furosemide solution to ensure drug stability.
• *Alert:* Don't confuse furosemide with torsemide or Lasix with Lonox.

**PATIENT TEACHING**
• Advise patient to take drug with food to prevent GI upset, and to take drug in morning to prevent nighttime urination. If second dose is needed, tell patient to take it in early afternoon, 6 to 8 hours after morning dose.
• Inform patient of possible need for potassium or magnesium supplements.

• Instruct patient to stand slowly to prevent dizziness and to limit alcohol intake and strenuous exercise in hot weather to avoid worsening dizziness upon standing quickly.
• Advise patient to immediately report ringing in ears, severe abdominal pain, or sore throat and fever; these symptoms may indicate furosemide toxicity.
• *Alert:* Discourage patient taking furosemide at home from storing different types of drugs in the same container, increasing the risk of drug errors. The most popular strengths of furosemide and digoxin are white tablets about equal in size.
• Tell patient to check with prescriber or pharmacist before taking OTC drugs.
• Teach patient to avoid direct sunlight and to use protective clothing and a sunblock because of risk of photosensitivity reactions.

# hydrochlorothiazide
Apo-Hydro†, Dichlotride‡, Diuchlor H†, Esidrix, Ezide, HydroDIURIL⌀, Hydro-Par, Microzide, Neo-Codema†, Novo-Hydrazide†, Oretic, Urozide†

*Pregnancy risk category B*

**AVAILABLE FORMS**
*Capsules:* 12.5 mg
*Oral solution:* 50 mg/5 ml
*Tablets:* 25 mg, 50 mg, 100 mg

**INDICATIONS & DOSAGES**
➤ **Edema**
*Adults:* 25 to 100 mg P.O. daily or intermittently; up to 200 mg initially for several days until nonedematous weight is attained.
➤ **Hypertension**
*Adults:* 12.5 to 50 mg P.O. once daily. Increase or decrease daily dose based on blood pressure.
*Children ages 2 to 12:* 2.2 mg/kg or 60 mg/m$^2$ daily in two divided doses. Usual dosage range is 37.5 to 100 mg/day.
*Children ages 6 months to 2 years:* 2.2 mg/kg or 60 mg/m$^2$ daily in two divided doses. Usual dosage range is 12.5 to 37.5 mg/day.

*Children younger than age 6 months:* Up to 3.3 mg/kg P.O. daily in two divided doses.

## ACTION
A thiazide diuretic that increases sodium and water excretion by inhibiting sodium and chloride reabsorption in distal segment of the nephron.

| Route | Onset | Peak | Duration |
|-------|-------|------|----------|
| P.O. | 2 hr | 4-6 hr | 6-12 hr |

## ADVERSE REACTIONS
**CNS:** dizziness, vertigo, headache, paresthesia, weakness, restlessness.
**CV:** orthostatic hypotension, allergic myocarditis, vasculitis.
**GI:** anorexia, nausea, *pancreatitis,* epigastric distress, vomiting, abdominal pain, diarrhea, constipation.
**GU:** polyuria, frequent urination, *renal failure,* interstitial nephritis.
**Hematologic:** *aplastic anemia, agranulocytosis, leukopenia, thrombocytopenia,* hemolytic anemia.
**Hepatic:** jaundice.
**Metabolic:** asymptomatic hyperuricemia; hypokalemia; hyperglycemia and impaired glucose tolerance; fluid and electrolyte imbalances, including dilutional hyponatremia and hypochloremia; metabolic alkalosis; hypercalcemia; volume depletion and dehydration.
**Musculoskeletal:** muscle cramps.
**Respiratory:** *respiratory distress,* pneumonitis.
**Skin:** dermatitis, photosensitivity reactions, rash, purpura, alopecia.
**Other:** hypersensitivity reactions, gout, *anaphylactic reactions.*

## INTERACTIONS
**Drug-drug.** *Amphotericin B, corticosteroids:* May increase risk of hypokalemia. Monitor potassium level closely.
*Antidiabetics:* May decrease effectiveness of hypoglycemics; dosage adjustments may be needed. Monitor glucose level.
*Antihypertensives:* Has additive antihypertensive effect. Use together cautiously.
*Barbiturates, opiates:* May increase orthostatic hypotensive effect. Monitor patient closely.

*Bumetanide, ethacrynic acid, furosemide, torsemide:* May cause excessive diuretic response resulting in serious electrolyte abnormalities or dehydration. Adjust doses carefully, and monitor patient closely for excessive diuretic responses.
*Cardiac glycosides:* May increase risk of digoxin toxicity from hydrochlorothiazide-induced hypokalemia. Monitor potassium and digoxin levels.
*Cholestyramine, colestipol:* May decrease intestinal absorption of thiazides. Separate doses by 2 hours.
*Diazoxide:* May increase antihypertensive, hyperglycemic, and hyperuricemic effects. Use together cautiously.
*Lithium:* May decrease lithium excretion, increasing risk of lithium toxicity. Monitor lithium level.
*NSAIDs:* May increase risk of NSAID-induced renal failure. Monitor renal function closely.
**Drug-herb.** *Dandelion:* May interfere with diuretic activity. Discourage use together.
*Licorice:* May cause unexpected rapid potassium loss. Discourage use together.
**Drug-lifestyle.** *Alcohol use:* May increase orthostatic hypotensive effect. Discourage use together.

## EFFECTS ON LAB TEST RESULTS
• May increase glucose, cholesterol, triglyceride, calcium, and uric acid levels. May decrease potassium, sodium, and chloride levels.
• May decrease hemoglobin and granulocyte, WBC, and platelet counts.

## CONTRAINDICATIONS & CAUTIONS
• Contraindicated in patients with anuria and patients hypersensitive to other thiazides or other sulfonamide derivatives.
• Use cautiously in children and in patients with severe renal disease, impaired hepatic function, or progressive hepatic disease.

## NURSING CONSIDERATIONS
• To prevent nocturia, give drug in the morning.
• Monitor fluid intake and output, weight, blood pressure, and electrolyte levels.
• Watch for signs and symptoms of hypokalemia, such as muscle weakness

---

Reactions may be *common,* uncommon, *life-threatening,* or COMMON AND LIFE-THREATENING.

and cramps. Drug may be used with potassium-sparing diuretic to prevent potassium loss.
• Consult prescriber and dietitian about a high-potassium diet. Foods rich in potassium include citrus fruits, tomatoes, bananas, apricots, and dates.
• Monitor creatinine and BUN levels regularly. Cumulative effects of drug may occur with impaired renal function.
• Monitor uric acid level, especially in patients with history of gout.
• Monitor glucose level, especially in diabetic patients.
• Monitor elderly patients, who are especially susceptible to excessive diuresis.
• Stop thiazides and thiazide-like diuretics before parathyroid function tests.
• In patients with hypertension, therapeutic response may be delayed several weeks.

**PATIENT TEACHING**
• Instruct patient to take drug with food to minimize GI upset.
• Advise patient to take drug in morning to avoid nighttime urination; if second dose is needed, have him take it in early afternoon.
• Advise patient to avoid sudden posture changes and to rise slowly to avoid dizziness upon standing quickly.
• Encourage patient to use a sunblock to prevent photosensitivity reactions.
• Tell patient to check with prescriber or pharmacist before using OTC drugs.

---

## indapamide
Lozide†, Lozol, Natrilix‡

*Pregnancy risk category B*

**AVAILABLE FORMS**
*Tablets:* 1.25 mg, 2.5 mg

**INDICATIONS & DOSAGES**
➤ **Edema**
*Adults:* Initially, 2.5 mg P.O. daily in the morning. Increased to 5 mg daily after 1 week, if needed.
➤ **Hypertension**
*Adults:* Initially, 1.25 mg P.O. daily in the morning. Increased to 2.5 mg daily after 4 weeks, if needed. Increased to 5 mg daily after 4 more weeks, if needed.

**ACTION**
Unknown. A thiazide-like diuretic that probably inhibits sodium reabsorption in distal segment of nephron. Also has a direct vasodilating effect, possibly resulting from calcium channel–blocking action.

| Route | Onset | Peak | Duration |
|-------|-------|------|----------|
| P.O. | 1-2 hr | 2-5 hr | 18 hr |

**ADVERSE REACTIONS**
**CNS:** headache, nervousness, dizziness, light-headedness, weakness, vertigo, restlessness, drowsiness, fatigue, anxiety, depression, numbness of limbs, irritability, agitation.
**CV:** orthostatic hypotension, palpitations, PVCs, irregular heartbeat, vasculitis, flushing.
**EENT:** rhinorrhea.
**GI:** anorexia, nausea, epigastric distress, vomiting, abdominal pain, diarrhea, constipation.
**GU:** nocturia, polyuria, frequent urination, impotence.
**Metabolic:** asymptomatic hyperuricemia; fluid and electrolyte imbalances, including dilutional hyponatremia, hypochloremia, metabolic alkalosis, and hypokalemia; weight loss; volume depletion and dehydration; hyperglycemia.
**Musculoskeletal:** muscle cramps and spasms.
**Skin:** rash, pruritus, urticaria.
**Other:** gout.

**INTERACTIONS**
**Drug-drug.** *Amphotericin B, corticosteroids:* May increase risk of hypokalemia. Monitor potassium level closely.
*Antidiabetics:* May decrease hypoglycemic effectiveness. May need to adjust dosage. Monitor glucose level.
*Barbiturates, opiates:* May increase orthostasis. Monitor patient closely.
*Bumetanide, ethacrynic acid, furosemide, torsemide:* May cause excessive diuretic response resulting in serious electrolyte abnormalities or dehydration. Adjust doses carefully, and monitor patient closely for excessive diuretic responses.
*Cardiac glycosides:* May increase risk of digoxin toxicity from indapamide-induced hypokalemia. Monitor potassium and digoxin levels.

---

*Cholestyramine, colestipol:* May decrease absorption of thiazides. Separate doses by 2 hours.

*Diazoxide:* May increase antihypertensive, hyperglycemic, and hyperuricemic effects. Use together cautiously.

*Lithium:* May decrease lithium clearance that may increase lithium toxicity. Avoid using together.

*NSAIDs:* May increase risk of NSAID-induced renal failure. Monitor patient for signs and symptoms of renal failure.

**Drug-herb.** *Dandelion:* May interfere with diuretic activity. Discourage use together.

*Licorice:* May cause unexpected rapid potassium loss. Discourage use together.

**Drug-lifestyle.** *Alcohol:* May increase orthostatic hypotensive effect. Discourage use together.

### EFFECTS ON LAB TEST RESULTS
• May increase glucose, cholesterol, triglyceride, and uric acid levels. May decrease potassium, sodium, and chloride levels.

### CONTRAINDICATIONS & CAUTIONS
• Contraindicated in patients hypersensitive to other sulfonamide-derived drugs and in those with anuria.
• Use cautiously in patients with severe renal disease, impaired hepatic function, or progressive hepatic disease.

### NURSING CONSIDERATIONS
• To prevent nocturia, give drug in the morning.
• Monitor fluid intake and output, weight, blood pressure, and electrolyte levels.
• Watch for signs of hypokalemia, such as muscle weakness and cramps. Drug may be used with potassium-sparing diuretic to prevent potassium loss.
• Consult prescriber and dietitian about a high-potassium diet. Foods rich in potassium include citrus fruits, tomatoes, bananas, apricots, and dates.
• Monitor creatinine and BUN levels regularly. Cumulative effects of drug may occur in patients with impaired renal function.
• Monitor uric acid level, especially in patients with history of gout.

• Monitor glucose level, especially in diabetic patients.
• Monitor elderly patients, who are especially susceptible to excessive diuresis.
• Stop thiazides and thiazide-like diuretics before parathyroid function tests.
• Therapeutic response may be delayed several weeks in hypertensive patients.

### PATIENT TEACHING
• Instruct patient to take drug in morning to prevent nighttime urination.
• Tell patient to take drug with food to minimize GI upset.
• Advise patient to avoid sudden posture changes and to rise slowly to avoid dizziness upon standing quickly.

---

## mannitol
Osmitrol

*Pregnancy risk category C*

### AVAILABLE FORMS
*Injection:* 5%, 10%, 15%, 20%, 25%

### INDICATIONS & DOSAGES
➤ **Test dose for marked oliguria or suspected inadequate renal function**
*Adults and children older than age 12:*
200 mg/kg or 12.5 g as a 15% to 20% I.V. solution over 3 to 5 minutes. Response is adequate if 30 to 50 ml of urine/hour is excreted over 2 to 3 hours; if response is inadequate, a second test dose is given. If still no response after second dose, stop drug.

➤ **Oliguria**
*Adults and children older than age 12:*
50 to 100 g I.V. as a 15% to 25% solution over 90 minutes to several hours.

➤ **To prevent oliguria or acute renal failure**
*Adults and children older than age 12:*
50 to 100 g I.V. of a 5% to 25% solution. Determine exact concentration by fluid requirements.

➤ **To reduce intraocular or intracranial pressure**
*Adults and children older than age 12:*
1.5 to 2 g/kg as a 15% to 20% I.V. solution over 30 to 60 minutes. For maximum intraocular pressure reduction before surgery, give 60 to 90 minutes preoperatively.

➤ **Diuresis in drug intoxication**
*Adults and children older than age 12:* 5% to 10% solution continuously up to 200 g I.V., while maintaining 100 to 500 ml urine output/hour and a positive fluid balance.

➤ **Irrigating solution during transurethral resection of prostate gland**
*Adults:* 2.5% to 5% solution, p.r.n.

## I.V. ADMINISTRATION
● Give as intermittent or continuous infusion at prescribed rate, using an in-line filter and an infusion pump. Don't give as direct injection.
● Check I.V. line patency at infusion site before and during administration.
● Monitor patient for signs and symptoms of infiltration; if it occurs, watch for inflammation, edema, and necrosis.
● To redissolve crystallized solution (crystallization occurs at low temperatures or in concentrations higher than 15%), warm bottle or bag in a hot water bath and shake vigorously. Cool to body temperature before giving. Don't use solution with undissolved crystals.

## ACTION
Increases osmotic pressure of glomerular filtrate, inhibiting tubular reabsorption of water and electrolytes; drug elevates plasma osmolality, increasing water flow into extracellular fluid.

| Route | Onset | Peak | Duration |
|-------|-------|------|----------|
| I.V. | 30-60 min | Unknown | 3-8 hr |

## ADVERSE REACTIONS
**CNS:** *seizures,* dizziness, headache, fever.
**CV:** edema, thrombophlebitis, hypotension, hypertension, *heart failure,* tachycardia, angina-like chest pain, vascular overload.
**EENT:** blurred vision, rhinitis.
**GI:** thirst, dry mouth, nausea, vomiting, *diarrhea.*
**GU:** urine retention.
**Metabolic:** dehydration.
**Skin:** local pain, urticaria.
**Other:** chills.

## INTERACTIONS
**Drug-drug.** *Lithium:* May increase urinary excretion of lithium. Monitor lithium level closely.

## EFFECTS ON LAB TEST RESULTS
● May increase or decrease electrolyte levels.
● May interfere with tests for inorganic phosphorus or ethylene glycol level.

## CONTRAINDICATIONS & CAUTIONS
● Contraindicated in patients hypersensitive to drug.
● Contraindicated in patients with anuria, severe pulmonary congestion, frank pulmonary edema, severe heart failure, severe dehydration, metabolic edema, progressive renal disease or dysfunction, or active intracranial bleeding (except during craniotomy).

## NURSING CONSIDERATIONS
● Monitor vital signs, including central venous pressure and fluid intake and output hourly. Report increasing oliguria. Check weight, renal function, fluid balance, and serum and urine sodium and potassium levels daily.
● Use urinary catheter in comatose or incontinent patient because therapy is based on strict evaluation of fluid intake and output. If patient has urinary catheter, use an hourly urometer collection bag to evaluate output accurately and easily.
● Drug can be used to measure glomerular filtration rate.
● To relieve thirst, give frequent mouth care or fluids.
● Drug is commonly used in chemotherapy regimens to enhance diuresis of renally toxic drugs.
● Don't give electrolyte-free mannitol solutions with blood. If blood is given simultaneously, add at least 20 mEq of sodium chloride to each liter of mannitol solution to avoid pseudoagglutination.

## PATIENT TEACHING
● Tell patient that he may feel thirsty or have a dry mouth, and emphasize importance of drinking only the amount of fluids ordered.
● Instruct patient to promptly report adverse reactions and discomfort at I.V. site.

---

*Rapid onset*   †Canada   ‡Australia   ◇OTC   ◆Off-label use   ⊘Photoguide   *Liquid contains alcohol.

# metolazone
Mykrox, Zaroxolyn

*Pregnancy risk category B*

## AVAILABLE FORMS
*Tablets (extended-release):* 2.5 mg, 5 mg,
10 mg Zaroxolyn
*Tablets (prompt-release):* 0.5 mg Mykrox

## INDICATIONS & DOSAGES
➤ **Edema in heart failure or renal disease**
*Adults:* 5 to 20 mg (Zaroxolyn) P.O. daily.
➤ **Hypertension**
*Adults:* 2.5 to 5 mg (Zaroxolyn) P.O. daily.
Base maintenance dosage on blood pressure. Or, 0.5 mg (Mykrox) P.O. once daily
in morning, increased to 1 mg P.O. daily,
p.r.n.

## ACTION
Increases sodium and water excretion by
inhibiting sodium reabsorption in ascending loop of Henle.

| Route | Onset | Peak | Duration |
|-------|-------|------|----------|
| P.O.  | 1 hr  | 2-8 hr | 12-24 hr |

## ADVERSE REACTIONS
**CNS:** *dizziness,* headache, fatigue, vertigo, paresthesia, weakness, restlessness,
drowsiness, anxiety, depression, nervousness, blurred vision.
**CV:** orthostatic hypotension, palpitations,
vasculitis.
**GI:** anorexia, nausea, *pancreatitis,* epigastric distress, vomiting, abdominal pain, diarrhea, constipation, dry mouth.
**GU:** nocturia, polyuria, impotence.
**Hematologic:** *aplastic anemia, agranulocytosis, leukopenia,* purpura.
**Hepatic:** jaundice, *hepatitis.*
**Metabolic:** hyperglycemia and impaired
glucose tolerance; fluid and electrolyte
imbalances, including hypokalemia, hypomagnesemia, dilutional hyponatremia and
hypochloremia, metabolic alkalosis, and
hypercalcemia; volume depletion and dehydration.
**Musculoskeletal:** muscle cramps.
**Skin:** dermatitis, photosensitivity reactions, rash, pruritus, urticaria.

## INTERACTIONS
**Drug-drug.** *Amphotericin B, corticosteroids:* May increase risk of hypokalemia.
Monitor potassium level closely.
*Anticoagulants:* May affect hypoprothrombinemic response. Monitor PT and
INR.
*Antidiabetics:* May alter glucose level requiring dosage adjustment of antidiabetics. Monitor glucose level.
*Barbiturates, opiates:* May increase orthostatic hypotensive effect. Monitor patient
closely.
*Bumetanide, ethacrynic acid, furosemide,
torsemide:* May cause excessive diuretic
response resulting in serious electrolyte
abnormalities or dehydration. Adjust doses carefully, and monitor patient closely
for excessive diuretic responses.
*Cardiac glycosides:* May increase risk of
digoxin toxicity from metolazone-induced
hypokalemia. Monitor potassium and
digoxin levels.
*Cholestyramine, colestipol:* May decrease
intestinal absorption of thiazides. Separate
doses.
*Diazoxide:* May increase antihypertensive,
hyperglycemic, and hyperuricemic effects.
Use together cautiously.
*Lithium:* May decrease lithium clearance,
increasing risk of lithium toxicity. Monitor
lithium level.
*NSAIDs:* May increase risk of NSAID-
induced renal failure. Monitor patient for
signs of renal failure.
*Other antihypertensives:* May have additive effects. Use together cautiously.
**Drug-herb.** *Dandelion:* May interfere
with diuretic activity. Discourage use together.
*Licorice:* May cause unexpected rapid
potassium loss. Discourage use together.
**Drug-lifestyle.** *Alcohol use:* May increase
orthostatic hypotensive effect. Discourage
use together.
*Sun exposure:* May increase risk for photosensitivity reaction. Advise patient to
avoid excessive sunlight exposure.

## EFFECTS ON LAB TEST RESULTS
● May increase glucose, calcium, cholesterol, and triglyceride levels. May decrease potassium, sodium, magnesium,
and chloride levels.

---

Reactions may be *common,* uncommon, *life-threatening,* or COMMON AND LIFE-THREATENING.

• May decrease hemoglobin and granulocyte and WBC counts.

**CONTRAINDICATIONS & CAUTIONS**
• Contraindicated in patients hypersensitive to thiazides or other sulfonamide-derived drugs and in those with anuria, hepatic coma, or precoma.
• Use cautiously in patients with impaired renal or hepatic function.

**NURSING CONSIDERATIONS**
• To prevent nocturia, give drug in the morning.
• Mykrox (prompt-release) tablets are more rapidly and completely absorbed than other brands, mimicking an oral solution. Don't substitute.
• Monitor fluid intake and output, weight, blood pressure, and electrolyte levels.
• Watch for signs and symptoms of hypokalemia, such as muscle weakness and cramps. Drug may be used with potassium-sparing diuretic to prevent potassium loss.
• Consult prescriber and dietitian about a high-potassium diet. Foods rich in potassium include citrus fruits, tomatoes, bananas, dates, and apricots.
• Monitor glucose level, especially in diabetic patients.
• Monitor uric acid level, especially in patients with history of gout.
• Monitor elderly patients, who are especially susceptible to excessive diuresis.
• In hypertensive patients, therapeutic response may be delayed several weeks.
• Monitor blood pressure. If response is inadequate, another antihypertensive may be added.
• Metolazone and furosemide may be used together to enhance diuretic effect.
• Unlike thiazide diuretics, metolazone is effective in patients with decreased renal function.
• Stop thiazides and thiazide-like diuretics before parathyroid function tests.
• *Alert:* Don't confuse Zaroxolyn with Zarontin.

**PATIENT TEACHING**
• Tell patient to take drug in morning to prevent nighttime urination.

• Advise patient to avoid sudden posture changes and to rise slowly to avoid effects of dizziness upon standing quickly.
• Instruct patient to use a sunblock to prevent photosensitivity reactions.

## spironolactone
Aldactone, Novospiroton†, Spiractin‡

*Pregnancy risk category D*

**AVAILABLE FORMS**
*Tablets:* 25 mg, 50 mg, 100 mg

**INDICATIONS & DOSAGES**
➤ **Edema**
*Adults:* 25 to 200 mg P.O. daily or in two to four divided doses.
*Children:* 3.3 mg/kg P.O. daily or in divided doses.
➤ **Hypertension**
*Adults:* 50 to 100 mg P.O. daily or in divided doses.
*Children:* 1 to 2 mg/kg P.O. b.i.d.
➤ **Diuretic-induced hypokalemia**
*Adults:* 25 to 100 mg P.O. daily.
➤ **To detect primary hyperaldosteronism**
*Adults:* 400 mg P.O. daily for 4 days (short test) or 3 to 4 weeks (long test). If hypokalemia and hypertension are corrected, a presumptive diagnosis of primary hyperaldosteronism is made.
➤ **To manage primary hyperaldosteronism**
*Adults:* 100 to 400 mg P.O. daily. Use lowest effective dose.
➤ **Heart failure, as adjunct to ACE inhibitor or loop diuretic, with or without cardiac glycoside)** ◆
*Adults:* 12.5 to 25 mg P.O. daily. May increase to 50 mg daily after 8 weeks.
➤ **Hirsutism in women** ◆
*Adults:* 50 to 200 mg P.O. daily. Or, 50 mg P.O. b.i.d. days 4 to 21 of menstrual cycle.
➤ **Premenstrual syndrome** ◆
*Adults:* 25 mg P.O. q.i.d. starting on day 14 of the menstrual cycle.
➤ **Acne vulgaris** ◆
*Adults:* 100 mg P.O. daily.

---

*Rapid onset    †Canada    ‡Australia    ◇ OTC    ◆ Off-label use    ✐Photoguide    *Liquid contains alcohol.*

➤ **Familial male precocious puberty ◆**
*Adults:* 2 mg/kg spironolactone P.O. daily
with 20 to 40 mg/kg testolactone P.O. daily for at least 6 months.

## ACTION

Potassium-sparing diuretic; antagonizes
aldosterone in the distal tubules, increasing sodium and water excretion.

| Route | Onset | Peak | Duration |
|-------|-------|------|----------|
| P.O. | 1-2 days | 2-3 days | 2-3 days |

## ADVERSE REACTIONS

**CNS:** headache, drowsiness, lethargy,
confusion, ataxia.
**GI:** diarrhea, gastric bleeding, ulceration,
cramping, gastritis, vomiting.
**GU:** inability to maintain erection, menstrual disturbances.
**Hematologic:** *agranulocytosis.*
**Metabolic:** hyponatremia, *hyperkalemia,*
dehydration, mild acidosis.
**Skin:** urticaria, hirsutism, maculopapular
eruptions.
**Other:** gynecomastia, breast soreness,
drug fever, *anaphylaxis.*

## INTERACTIONS

**Drug-drug.** *ACE inhibitors, indomethacin, other potassium-sparing diuretics,
potassium supplements:* May increase risk
of hyperkalemia. Use together cautiously,
especially in patients with renal impairment.
*Anticoagulants:* May decrease anticoagulant effects. Monitor PT and INR.
*Aspirin:* May block diuretic effect of
spironolactone. Watch for diminished
spironolactone response.
*Digoxin:* May alter digoxin clearance, increasing risk of digoxin toxicity. Monitor
digoxin level.
**Drug-herb.** *Licorice:* May block ulcer-
healing and aldosterone-like effects of
licorice; increases risk of hypokalemia.
Discourage use together.
**Drug-food.** *Potassium-containing salt
substitutes, potassium-rich foods (such as
citrus fruits, tomatoes):* May increase risk
of hyperkalemia. Tell patient to use low-
potassium salt substitutes and to eat high-
potassium foods cautiously.

## EFFECTS ON LAB TEST RESULTS

● May increase BUN and potassium levels. May decrease sodium level.
● May decrease granulocyte count.
● May alter fluorometric determinations of
plasma and urinary 17-hydroxycorticos-
teroid levels.

## CONTRAINDICATIONS & CAUTIONS

● Contraindicated in patients hypersensitive to drug.
● Contraindicated in those with anuria,
acute or progressive renal insufficiency, or
hyperkalemia.
● Use cautiously in patients with fluid or
electrolyte imbalances, impaired renal
function, or hepatic disease.
● Use with extreme caution in pregnant
women.

## NURSING CONSIDERATIONS

● To enhance absorption, give drug with
meals.
● Protect drug from light.
● Monitor electrolyte levels, fluid intake
and output, weight, and blood pressure.
● Monitor elderly patients closely, who are
more susceptible to excessive diuresis.
● Inform laboratory that patient is taking
spironolactone because drug may interfere
with tests that measure digoxin level.
● Drug is less potent than thiazide and
loop diuretics and is useful as an adjunct
to other diuretic therapy. Diuretic effect is
delayed 2 to 3 days when used alone.
● Maximum antihypertensive response
may be delayed for up to 2 weeks.
● Watch for hyperchloremic metabolic acidosis, which may occur during therapy, especially in patients with hepatic cirrhosis.
● Breast cancer has been reported in some
patients taking spironolactone, although a
causal relationship hasn't been established.
● *Alert:* Don't confuse Aldactone with Aldactazide.

## PATIENT TEACHING

● Instruct patient to take drug in morning
to prevent nighttime urination. If second
dose is needed, tell him to take it with
food in early afternoon.
● *Alert:* To prevent serious hyperkalemia,
warn patient to avoid excessive ingestion
of potassium-rich foods (such as citrus

---

fruits, tomatoes, bananas, dates, and apricots), potassium-containing salt substitutes, and potassium supplements.
• Caution patient not to perform hazardous activities if adverse CNS reactions occur.
• Advise men about possible breast tenderness or breast enlargement.

## torsemide
Demadex

*Pregnancy risk category B*

### AVAILABLE FORMS
*Injection:* 10 mg/ml
*Tablets:* 5 mg, 10 mg, 20 mg, 100 mg

### INDICATIONS & DOSAGES
➤ **Diuresis in patients with heart failure**
*Adults:* Initially, 10 to 20 mg P.O. or I.V. once daily. If response is inadequate, double dose until desired effect is achieved. Maximum, 200 mg daily.
➤ **Diuresis in patients with chronic renal failure**
*Adults:* Initially, 20 mg P.O. or I.V. once daily. If response is inadequate, double dose until response is obtained. Maximum, 200 mg daily.
➤ **Diuresis in patients with hepatic cirrhosis**
*Adults:* Initially, 5 to 10 mg P.O. or I.V. once daily with an aldosterone antagonist or a potassium-sparing diuretic. If response is inadequate, double dose until desired effect is achieved. Maximum, 40 mg daily.
➤ **Hypertension**
*Adults:* Initially, 5 mg P.O. daily. Increased to 10 mg if needed and tolerated. Add another antihypertensive if response is still inadequate.

### I.V. ADMINISTRATION
• Inspect ampules for precipitate or discoloration before use.
• Drug may be given by direct injection over at least 2 minutes. Rapid injection may cause ototoxicity. Don't give more than 200 mg at a time.

### ACTION
A loop diuretic that enhances excretion of sodium, chloride, and water by acting on the ascending loop of Henle.

| Route | Onset | Peak | Duration |
|---|---|---|---|
| I.V. | 10 min | 1 hr | 6-8 hr |
| P.O. | 1 hr | 1-2 hr | 6-8 hr |

### ADVERSE REACTIONS
**CNS:** asthenia, dizziness, headache, nervousness, insomnia, syncope.
**CV:** ECG abnormalities, chest pain, edema, orthostatic hypotension.
**EENT:** rhinitis, sore throat.
**GI:** *excessive thirst,* diarrhea, constipation, nausea, dyspepsia, *hemorrhage.*
**GU:** excessive urination, impotence.
**Metabolic:** *electrolyte imbalances including hypokalemia and hypomagnesemia, dehydration,* hypochloremic alkalosis, hyperuricemia, hypercholesterolemia.
**Musculoskeletal:** arthralgia, myalgia.
**Respiratory:** cough.
**Skin:** rash.

### INTERACTIONS
**Drug-drug.** *Aminoglycoside antibiotics, cisplatin:* May increase ototoxicity. Use together cautiously.
*Amphotericin B, corticosteroids, metolazone:* May increase risk of hypokalemia. Monitor potassium level.
*Antidiabetics:* May decrease hypoglycemic effects. Monitor glucose level.
*Chlorothiazide, chlorthalidone, hydrochlorothiazide, indapamide, metolazone:* May cause excessive diuretic response, resulting in serious electrolyte abnormalities or dehydration. Adjust doses carefully, and monitor patient closely for excessive diuretic responses.
*Cholestyramine:* May decrease absorption of torsemide. Separate doses by at least 3 hours.
*Digoxin:* May decrease torsemide clearance. Use together cautiously.
*Indomethacin:* May decrease diuretic effectiveness in sodium-restricted patients. Avoid using together.
*Lithium:* May increase lithium level and cause toxicity. Use together cautiously and monitor lithium level.
*NSAIDs:* May increase nephrotoxicity of NSAIDs. Use together cautiously.

*Probenecid:* May decrease diuretic effectiveness. Avoid using together.
*Salicylates:* May decrease excretion, possibly leading to salicylate toxicity. Avoid using together.
*Spironolactone:* May decrease renal clearance of spironolactone. Use together cautiously.
**Drug-herb.** *Dandelion:* May interfere with diuretic activity. Discourage use together.
*Licorice:* May cause unexpected rapid potassium loss. Discourage use together.

**EFFECTS ON LAB TEST RESULTS**
● May increase BUN, creatinine, cholesterol, and uric acid levels. May decrease potassium and magnesium levels.

**CONTRAINDICATIONS & CAUTIONS**
● Contraindicated in patients hypersensitive to drug or other sulfonamide derivatives and in those with anuria.
● Use cautiously in patients with hepatic disease and related cirrhosis and ascites; sudden changes in fluid and electrolyte balance may precipitate hepatic coma in these patients.

**NURSING CONSIDERATIONS**
● To prevent nocturia, give drug in the morning.
● Monitor fluid intake and output, electrolyte levels, blood pressure, weight, and pulse rate during rapid diuresis and routinely with long-term use. Drug can cause profound diuresis and water and electrolyte depletion.
● Watch for signs of hypokalemia, such as muscle weakness and cramps.
● Consult prescriber and dietitian about providing a high-potassium diet. Foods rich in potassium include citrus fruits, tomatoes, bananas, dates, and apricots.
● Monitor elderly patients, who are especially susceptible to excessive diuresis with potential for circulatory collapse and thromboembolic complications.
● *Alert:* Don't confuse torsemide with furosemide.

**PATIENT TEACHING**
● Tell patient to take drug in morning to prevent nighttime urination.

● Advise patient to change positions slowly to prevent dizziness and to limit alcohol intake and strenuous exercise in hot weather to prevent dizziness.
● Advise patient to immediately report ringing in ears because it may indicate toxicity.
● Tell patient to check with prescriber or pharmacist before taking OTC drugs.

---

# triamterene
Dyrenium

*Pregnancy risk category B*

**AVAILABLE FORMS**
*Capsules:* 50 mg, 100 mg

**INDICATIONS & DOSAGES**
➤ **Edema**
*Adults:* Initially, 100 mg P.O. b.i.d. after meals. Maximum, 300 mg daily.

**ACTION**
A potassium-sparing diuretic that inhibits sodium reabsorption and potassium and hydrogen excretion by direct action on the distal tubules.

| Route | Onset | Peak | Duration |
|-------|-------|------|----------|
| P.O. | 2-4 hr | 6-8 hr | 12-16 hr |

**ADVERSE REACTIONS**
**CNS:** dizziness, weakness, fatigue, headache.
**CV:** hypotension.
**GI:** dry mouth, nausea, vomiting, diarrhea.
**GU:** interstitial nephritis, nephrolithiasis.
**Hematologic:** megaloblastic anemia related to low folic acid level, *thrombocytopenia, agranulocytosis.*
**Hepatic:** jaundice.
**Metabolic:** azotemia, *hyperkalemia,* hypokalemia, hyponatremia, hyperglycemia, acidosis.
**Musculoskeletal:** muscle cramps.
**Skin:** photosensitivity reactions, rash.
**Other:** *anaphylaxis.*

**INTERACTIONS**
**Drug-drug.** *ACE inhibitors, potassium supplements:* May increase risk of hyper-

kalemia. If used together, monitor potassium level.

*Amantadine:* May increase risk of amantadine toxicity. Avoid using together.

*Chlorpropamide:* May increase risk of hyponatremia. Monitor sodium level.

*Cimetidine:* May increase bioavailability and decrease renal clearance of triamterene. Monitor potassium level and blood pressure closely.

*Lithium:* May decrease lithium clearance, increasing risk of lithium toxicity. Monitor lithium level.

*NSAIDs:* May enhance risk of nephrotoxicity. Use together cautiously.

*Quinidine:* May interfere with some laboratory tests that measure quinidine level. Inform laboratory that patient is taking triamterene.

**Drug-herb.** *Licorice:* May increase risk of hypokalemia. Discourage use together.

**Drug-food.** *Potassium-containing salt substitutes, potassium-rich foods:* May increase risk of hyperkalemia. Use cautiously, and monitor potassium level.

**Drug-lifestyle.** *Sun exposure:* May increase risk for photosensitivity reactions. Advise patient to avoid excessive sunlight exposure.

## EFFECTS ON LAB TEST RESULTS
• May increase BUN, creatinine, glucose, and uric acid levels. May decrease sodium level. May increase or decrease potassium level.
• May decrease hemoglobin and granulocyte and platelet counts. May increase liver function test values.
• May interfere with enzyme assays that use fluorometry, such as quinidine determinations.

## CONTRAINDICATIONS & CAUTIONS
• Contraindicated in patients hypersensitive to drug and in those with anuria, severe or progressive renal disease or dysfunction, severe hepatic disease, or hyperkalemia.
• Use cautiously in elderly or debilitated patients and in those with hepatic impairment or diabetes mellitus.

## NURSING CONSIDERATIONS
• To minimize nausea, give drug after meals.

• Monitor blood pressure, uric acid, CBC, and glucose, BUN, and electrolyte levels.
• Watch for blood dyscrasia.
• To minimize excessive rebound potassium excretion, withdraw drug gradually.
• Drug is less potent than thiazides and loop diuretics and is useful as an adjunct to other diuretic therapy. It's usually used with potassium-wasting diuretics; full effect is delayed 2 to 3 days when used alone.
• *Alert:* Don't confuse triamterene with trimipramine.

## PATIENT TEACHING
• Tell patient to take drug after meals to minimize nausea.
• If a single daily dose is prescribed, instruct patient to take it in the morning to prevent nighttime urination.
• *Alert:* Warn patient that to prevent serious hyperkalemia, he should avoid excessive ingestion of potassium-rich foods (such as citrus fruits, tomatoes, bananas, dates, and apricots), potassium-containing salt substitutes, and potassium supplements
• Teach patient to avoid direct sunlight, wear protective clothing, and use sunblock to prevent photosensitivity reactions.
• Tell patient that urine may turn blue.

# 61

# Electrolytes and replacement solutions

calcium acetate
calcium carbonate
calcium chloride
calcium citrate
calcium glubionate
calcium gluconate
calcium lactate
calcium phosphate, dibasic
calcium phosphate, tribasic
magnesium chloride
magnesium sulfate
potassium acetate
potassium bicarbonate
potassium chloride
potassium gluconate
sodium chloride

**COMBINATION PRODUCTS**
CITRACAL +D: calcium 316.5 mg with 200 units cholecalciferol.
DICAL-D; DIOSTATE D: calcium 116.7 mg (as phosphate tribasic) with cholecalciferol 133 units.
DICAL-D WAFERS: calcium 232 mg (as phosphate tribasic) with cholecalciferol 200 units.
KLORVESS*: potassium and chloride 20 mEq each (from potassium chloride, potassium bicarbonate, and L-lysine monohydrochloride).
K-LYTE/CL: potassium 25 mEq, chloride 25 mEq (from potassium chloride, potassium bicarbonate, and lysine hydrochloride).
KOLYUM: potassium 20 mEq, chloride 3.4 mEq per 15 ml (from potassium gluconate and potassium chloride).
NEUTRA-PHOS: phosphorus 250 mg, sodium 164 mg, potassium 278 mg (from dibasic and monobasic sodium and potassium phosphate).
POSTURE-D: calcium 600 mg (as phosphate tribasic) with cholecalciferol 125 units.
TWIN-K: 15 ml supplies 20 mEq of potassium ions as a combination of potassium gluconate and potassium citrate.

## calcium acetate
PhosLo

## calcium carbonate
Apo-Cal†◇, Cal-Carb Forte, Cal Carb-HD◇, Calci-Chew◇, Calciday-667◇, Calci-Mix◇, Calcite 500†◇, Calcium 600◇, Calglycine◇, Cal-Plus◇, Calsan†◇, Caltrate 600◇, Chooz◇, Dicarbosil◇, Gencalc 600◇, Mallamint◇, Nephro-Calci◇, Nu-Cal†◇, Os-Cal†◇, Os-Cal 500◇, Os-Cal Chewable†◇, Oysco◇, Oysco 500 Chewable◇, Oyst-Cal 500◇, Oystercal 500◇, Oyster Shell Calcium-500◇, Rolaids Calcium Rich◇, Super Calcium 1200◇, Titralac◇, Tums◇, Tums E-X◇

## calcium chloride◇
Calciject†

## calcium citrate◇
Citracal◇, Citracal Liquitab†◇

## calcium glubionate
Calciquid, Calcium-Sandoz†, Neo-Calglucon

## calcium gluconate

## calcium lactate◇

## calcium phosphate, dibasic◇

## calcium phosphate, tribasic
Posture◇

*Pregnancy risk category C*

**AVAILABLE FORMS**
**calcium acetate**
Contains 253 mg or 12.7 mEq of elemental calcium/g
*Capsules:* 333.5 mg, 667 mg
*Tablets:* 667 mg

---

**calcium carbonate**
Contains 400 mg or 20 mEq of elemental calcium/g
*Capsules:* 1.25 g ◇
*Oral suspension:* 1.25 g/5 ml ◇
*Powder packets:* 6.5 g (2,400 mg calcium) per packet ◇
*Tablets:* 650 mg ◇, 1.25 g ◇, 1.5 g ◇
*Tablets (chewable):* 500 mg ◇, 625 mg ◇†, 750 mg ◇, 1 g ◇, 1.25 g ◇

**calcium chloride**
Contains 270 mg or 13.5 mEq of elemental calcium/g
*Injection:* 10% solution in 10-ml ampules, vials, and syringes

**calcium citrate**
Contains 211 mg or 10.6 mEq of elemental calcium/g
*Tablets:* 250 mg, 950 mg ◇
*Tablets (effervescent):* 2.376 g ◇

**calcium glubionate**
Contains 64 mg or 3.2 mEq elemental calcium/g
*Syrup:* 1.8 g/5 ml

**calcium gluconate**
Contains 90 mg or 4.5 mEq of elemental calcium/g
*Injection:* 10% solution in 10-ml ampules and vials, 10-ml or 50-ml vials
*Powder for oral suspension:* 3756 mg/15 ml
*Tablets:* 500 mg ◇, 650 mg ◇, 1 g ◇

**calcium lactate**
Contains 130 mg or 6.5 mEq of elemental calcium/g
*Capsules:* 500 mg
*Tablets:* 325 mg, 650 mg

**calcium phosphate, dibasic**
Contains 230 mg or 11.5 mEq of elemental calcium/g
*Tablets:* 500 mg ◇

**calcium phosphate, tribasic**
Contains 400 mg or 20 mEq of elemental calcium/g
*Tablets:* 300 mg ◇, 600 mg ◇

## INDICATIONS & DOSAGES
➤ **Hypocalcemic emergency**
*Adults:* 7 mEq to 14 mEq calcium I.V. May give as a 10% calcium gluconate solution, 2% to 10% calcium chloride solution.
*Children:* 1 mEq to 7 mEq calcium I.V.
*Infants:* Up to 1 mEq calcium I.V.

➤ **Hypocalcemic tetany**
*Adults:* 4.5 mEq to 16 mEq calcium I.V. Repeat until tetany is controlled.
*Children:* 0.5 to 0.7 mEq/kg calcium I.V. t.i.d. to q.i.d. until tetany is controlled.
*Neonates:* 2.4 mEq/kg calcium I.V. daily in divided doses.

➤ **Adjunctive treatment of cardiac arrest**
*Adults:* 0.027 to 0.054 mEq/kg calcium chloride I.V. or 2.3 mEq to 3.7 mEq calcium gluconate I.V.
*Children:* 0.27 mEq/kg calcium chloride I.V. Repeat in 10 minutes if needed; determine calcium levels before giving more doses.

➤ **Adjunctive treatment of magnesium intoxication**
*Adults:* Initially, 7 mEq I.V. Base subsequent doses on patient's response.

➤ **During exchange transfusions**
*Adults:* 1.35 mEq I.V. with each 100 ml citrated blood.
*Neonates:* 0.45 mEq I.V. after each 100 ml citrated blood.

➤ **Hyperphosphatemia**
*Adults:* 1,334 to 2,000 mg P.O. calcium acetate or 2 to 5.2 g calcium ion t.i.d. with meals. Most dialysis patients need 3 to 4 tablets with each meal.

➤ **Dietary supplement**
*Adults:* 500 mg to 2 g P.O. daily.

➤ **Hyperkalemia with secondary cardiac toxicity**
*Adults:* 2.25 mEq to 14 mEq I.V. Repeat dose after 1 to 2 minutes if needed.

## I.V. ADMINISTRATION
● Give calcium chloride only by I.V. route. When adding to parenteral solutions that contain other additives (especially phosphorus or phosphate), watch for precipitate. Use an in-line filter.
● When giving calcium gluconate as injection, give only by I.V. route.
● *Alert:* Calcium salts aren't interchangeable; verify preparation before use.
● Monitor ECG when giving calcium I.V. Stop and notify prescriber if patient complains of discomfort.
● *Alert:* Severe necrosis and tissue sloughing can occur after extravasation. Calcium gluconate is less irritating to veins and tissues than calcium chloride.

### Direct injection
● Warm solution to body temperature before administration.
● Give slowly through a small needle into a large vein or through an I.V. line containing a free-flowing, compatible solution at 1 ml/minute (1.5 mEq/minute) for calcium chloride, 2 ml/minute for calcium gluconate. Don't use scalp veins in children.
● After I.V. injection, patient should remain recumbent for 15 minutes.

### Intermittent infusion
● Infuse diluted solution through an I.V. line containing a compatible solution. Maximum of 200 mg/minute suggested for calcium gluconate.
● Drug will precipitate if given I.V. with sodium bicarbonate or other alkaline drugs.

### ACTION
Replaces calcium and maintains calcium level.

| Route | Onset | Peak | Duration |
|---|---|---|---|
| P.O. | Unknown | Unknown | Unknown |
| I.V., I.M. | Immediate | Immediate | 30 min-2 hr |

### ADVERSE REACTIONS
**CNS:** tingling sensations, sense of oppression or heat waves with I.V. use; syncope with rapid I.V. injection.
**CV:** mild drop in blood pressure, vasodilation, *bradycardia, arrhythmias, cardiac arrest with rapid I.V. injection.*
**GI:** irritation, *constipation,* chalky taste, hemorrhage, nausea, vomiting, thirst, abdominal pain.
**GU:** polyuria, renal calculi.
**Metabolic:** hypercalcemia.
**Skin:** local reactions, including burning, necrosis, tissue sloughing, cellulitis, soft-tissue calcification with I.M. use, pain, irritation at S.C. injection site.

### INTERACTIONS
**Drug-drug.** *Atenolol, fluoroquinolones, tetracyclines:* May decrease bioavailability of these drugs and calcium when oral preparations are taken together. Separate dosing times.
*Calcium channel blockers:* May decrease calcium effectiveness. Avoid using together.
*Cardiac glycosides:* May increase digoxin toxicity. Give calcium cautiously, if at all, to digitalized patients.
*Ciprofloxacin, gatifloxacin, levofloxacin, lomefloxacin, moxifloxacin, norfloxacin, ofloxacin:* May decrease effects of quinolone. Give calcium carbonate at least 6 hours before or 2 hours after the quinolone.
*Fosphenytoin, phenytoin:* Use together may decrease absorption of both drugs. Avoid using together, or monitor levels carefully.
*Sodium polystyrene sulfonate:* May cause metabolic acidosis in patients with renal disease. Avoid using together.
*Thiazide diuretics:* May cause hypercalcemia. Avoid using together.
**Drug-food.** *Foods containing oxalic acid (rhubarb, spinach), phytic acid (bran, whole-grain cereals), phosphorus (dairy products, milk):* May interfere with calcium absorption. Discourage use together.

### EFFECTS ON LAB TEST RESULTS
● May increase calcium level.

### CONTRAINDICATIONS & CAUTIONS
● Contraindicated in cancer patients with bone metastases and in patients with ventricular fibrillation, hypercalcemia, hypophosphatemia, or renal calculi.

### NURSING CONSIDERATIONS
● Use all calcium products with extreme caution in digitalized patients and patients with sarcoidosis and renal or cardiac disease. Use calcium chloride cautiously in patients with cor pulmonale, respiratory acidosis, or respiratory failure.
● Give I.M. injection in gluteal region in adults and in lateral thigh in infants. Use I.M. route only in emergencies when no I.V. route is available because of irritation of tissue by calcium salts.
● *Alert:* Make sure prescriber specifies form of calcium to be given; crash carts may contain both calcium gluconate and calcium chloride.
● Monitor calcium levels frequently. Hypercalcemia may result after large doses in chronic renal failure. Report abnormalities.
● Signs and symptoms of severe hypercalcemia may include stupor, confusion,

delirium, and coma. Signs and symptoms of mild hypercalcemia may include anorexia, nausea, and vomiting.
• To avoid constipation and bloating and to improve absorption, give calcium carbonate in divided doses.

**PATIENT TEACHING**
• Tell patient to take oral calcium 1 to 1½ hours after meals if GI upset occurs.
• Tell patient to take oral calcium with a full glass of water.
• Warn patient to avoid oxalic acid (in rhubarb and spinach), phytic acid (in bran and whole-grain cereals), and phosphorus (in dairy products) in the meal preceding calcium consumption; these substances may interfere with calcium absorption.
• Inform patient that some products may contain phenylalanine.

---

## magnesium chloride
Slow-Mag ◇

## magnesium sulfate

*Pregnancy risk category D*

## AVAILABLE FORMS
**magnesium chloride**
*Injection:* 20% in 50 ml vials
*Tablets (delayed-release):* 64 mg
**magnesium sulfate**
*Injectable solutions:* 10%, 12.5%, 50% in 2-ml, 5-ml, 10-ml, 20-ml, and 30-ml ampules, vials, and prefilled syringes

## INDICATIONS & DOSAGES
➤ **Mild hypomagnesemia**
*Adults:* 1 g I.V. by piggyback or I.M. q 6 hours for four doses, depending on magnesium level. Or, 3 g P.O. q 6 hours for four doses.
➤ **Symptomatic severe hypomagnesemia, with magnesium 0.8 mEq/L or less**
*Adults:* 2 to 5 g I.V. in 1 L of solution over 3 hours. Base subsequent doses on magnesium level.
➤ **Magnesium supplementation**
*Adults:* 64 mg (one tablet) P.O. t.i.d.

➤ **Magnesium supplementation in total parenteral nutrition (TPN)**
*Adults and children:* 4 to 24 mEq I.V. daily added to TPN solution.
*Infants:* 2 to 10 mEq I.V. daily added to TPN solution. Each 2 ml of 50% solution contains 1 g, or 8.12 mEq, magnesium sulfate.
➤ **Seizures**
*Adults:* 4 to 5 g magnesium sulfate 50% solution I.M. q 4 hours, p.r.n. Or 4 g of 10% to 20% magnesium sulfate solution I.V. at no more than 1.5 ml/minute of 10% solution. Or, for I.V. infusion, 4 to 5 g in 250 ml of $D_5W$ or sodium chloride, not exceeding 3 ml/minute.
*Children:* 20 to 40 mg/kg I.M. in a 20% solution. Repeat p.r.n.

## I.V. ADMINISTRATION
• Inject I.V. bolus dose slowly, using infusion pump for continuous infusion, if available, to avoid respiratory or cardiac arrest. Maximum infusion rate is 150 mg/minute. Rapid drip causes feeling of heat.
• *Alert:* When giving I.V. for severe hypomagnesemia, watch for respiratory depression and evidence of heart block. Respirations should exceed 16 breaths/minute before dose is given.
• Drug is incompatible with alkalis, including carbonates and bicarbonates. Precipitate may form if mixed with solutions containing alcohol, arsenates, barium, calcium, clindamycin, heavy metals, hydrocortisone sodium succinate, phosphates, polymyxin B sulfate, procaine, salicylates, or tartrates.

## ACTION
Replaces magnesium and maintains magnesium level; as an anticonvulsant, reduces muscle contractions by interfering with release of acetylcholine at myoneural junction.

| Route | Onset | Peak | Duration |
|-------|-------|------|----------|
| P.O. | Unknown | 4 hr | 4-6 hr |
| I.V. | Immediate | Unknown | 30 min |
| I.M. | 1 hr | Unknown | 3-4 hr |

## ADVERSE REACTIONS
**CNS:** toxicity, *weak or absent deep tendon reflexes,* flaccid paralysis, drowsiness, stupor.

**CV:** slow, weak pulse; *arrhythmias, hypotension, circulatory collapse,* flushing.
**GI:** diarrhea.
**Metabolic:** hypocalcemia.
**Respiratory:** *respiratory paralysis.*
**Skin:** diaphoresis.
**Other:** hypothermia.

**INTERACTIONS**
**Drug-drug.** *Alendronate, nitrofurantoin, penicillamine, fluoroquinolones, sodium polystyrene sulfonate, tetracyclines:* May decrease bioavailability with oral magnesium supplements. Separate doses by 2 to 3 hours.
*Cardiac glycosides:* May cause serious cardiac conduction changes. Use together with extreme caution.
*CNS depressants:* May have additive effect. Use together cautiously.
*Neuromuscular blockers:* May cause increased neuromuscular blockage. Use together cautiously.

**EFFECTS ON LAB TEST RESULTS**
• May increase magnesium levels. May decrease calcium levels.

**CONTRAINDICATIONS & CAUTIONS**
• Contraindicated in patients with myocardial damage or heart block and in pregnant women in actively progressing labor.
• Use parenteral magnesium with extreme caution in patients with impaired renal function.

**NURSING CONSIDERATIONS**
• Undiluted 50% solutions may be given by deep I.M. injection to adults. Dilute solutions to 20% or less for use in children.
• Keep I.V. calcium available to reverse magnesium intoxication.
• Test knee-jerk and patellar reflexes before each additional dose. If absent, notify prescriber and give no more magnesium until reflexes return; otherwise, patient may develop temporary respiratory failure and need cardiopulmonary resuscitation or I.V. administration of calcium.
• Check magnesium level after repeated doses.
• Monitor fluid intake and output. Output should be 100 ml or more during 4-hour period before dose.
• Monitor renal function.

• After giving to toxemic pregnant woman within 24 hours before delivery, watch neonate for signs and symptoms of magnesium toxicity, including neuromuscular and respiratory depression.

**PATIENT TEACHING**
• Explain use and administration of drug to patient and family.
• Tell patient to report adverse effects.

## potassium acetate

*Pregnancy risk category C*

**AVAILABLE FORMS**
*Injection:* 2 mEq/ml in 20-ml, 50-ml, and 100-ml vials; 4 mEq/ml in 50-ml vials

**INDICATIONS & DOSAGES**
➤ **Hypokalemia**
*Adults:* No more than 20 mEq/hour in concentration of 40 mEq/L or less. Total 24-hour dose shouldn't exceed 150 mEq (3 mEq/kg in children).
➤ **To prevent hypokalemia**
*Adults:* Dosage is individualized to patient's needs, not to exceed 150 mEq/day. Give as an additive to I.V. infusions. Usual dose is 20 mEq/L infused at no more than 20 mEq/hour.
*Children:* Individualized dose not to exceed 3 mEq/kg/day. Give as an additive to I.V. infusions.

**I.V. ADMINISTRATION**
• Use I.V. route only for life-threatening hypokalemia or when oral replacement isn't feasible.
• Give only by I.V. infusion, never I.V. push or I.M. Watch for pain and redness at infusion site. Large-bore needle reduces local irritation.
• *Alert:* Give slowly as diluted solution; potentially fatal hyperkalemia may result from too-rapid infusion.

**ACTION**
Replaces potassium and maintains potassium level.

| Route | Onset | Peak | Duration |
|-------|-------|------|----------|
| I.V. | Immediate | Immediate | Unknown |

## ADVERSE REACTIONS
**CNS:** paresthesia of limbs, listlessness, mental confusion, weakness or heaviness of legs, flaccid paralysis, pain, fever.
**CV:** hypotension, *arrhythmias, heart block,* ECG changes, *cardiac arrest.*
**GI:** nausea, vomiting, abdominal pain, diarrhea.
**Metabolic:** *hyperkalemia.*
**Respiratory:** *respiratory paralysis.*
**Skin:** redness at infusion site.

## INTERACTIONS
**Drug-drug.** *ACE inhibitors, digoxin, potassium-sparing diuretics:* May increase risk of hyperkalemia. Use together with extreme caution.

## EFFECTS ON LAB TEST RESULTS
• May increase potassium level.

## CONTRAINDICATIONS & CAUTIONS
• Contraindicated in patients with severe renal impairment with oliguria, anuria, or azotemia.
• Contraindicated in those with untreated Addison's disease, acute dehydration, heat cramps, hyperkalemia, hyperkalemic form of familial periodic paralysis, or conditions linked to extensive tissue breakdown.
• Use cautiously in patients with cardiac disease or renal impairment.

## NURSING CONSIDERATIONS
• During therapy, monitor ECG, renal function, fluid intake and output, and potassium, creatinine, and BUN levels. Never give potassium postoperatively until urine flow is established.
• Many adverse reactions may reflect hyperkalemia.
• *Alert:* Potassium preparations aren't interchangeable; verify preparation before use.

## PATIENT TEACHING
• Explain use and administration to patient and family.
• Tell patient to report adverse effects, especially pain at insertion site.

# potassium bicarbonate
K+Care ET, K-Lyte

*Pregnancy risk category C*

## AVAILABLE FORMS
*Tablets (effervescent):* 25 mEq

## INDICATIONS & DOSAGES
➤ **To prevent hypokalemia**
*Adults and children:* Initially, 25 mEq P.O. daily, in divided doses. Adjust dosage, p.r.n.
➤ **Hypokalemia**
*Adults and children:* 50 mEq to 100 mEq P.O. divided into two to four daily doses. Use I.V. potassium chloride when oral replacement isn't feasible. Don't exceed 150 mEq P.O. daily in adults and 3 mEq/kg daily P.O. in children.

## ACTION
Replaces potassium and maintains potassium level.

| Route | Onset | Peak | Duration |
|---|---|---|---|
| P.O. | Unknown | 4 hr | Unknown |

## ADVERSE REACTIONS
**CNS:** paresthesia of limbs, listlessness, confusion, weakness or heaviness of legs, flaccid paralysis.
**CV:** *arrhythmias,* ECG changes, hypotension, *heart block, cardiac arrest.*
**GI:** *nausea, vomiting, abdominal pain,* diarrhea.

## INTERACTIONS
**Drug-drug.** *ACE inhibitors, digoxin, potassium-sparing diuretics:* May cause hyperkalemia. Use with extreme caution.

## EFFECTS ON LAB TEST RESULTS
• May increase potassium level.

## CONTRAINDICATIONS & CAUTIONS
• Contraindicated in patients with severe renal impairment with oliguria, anuria, or azotemia; untreated Addison's disease; or acute dehydration, heat cramps, hyperkalemia, hyperkalemic form of familial periodic paralysis, or other conditions linked to extensive tissue breakdown.

• Use cautiously in patients with cardiac disease or renal impairment.

**NURSING CONSIDERATIONS**
• Dissolve potassium bicarbonate tablets completely in 4 to 8 ounces of cold water.
• Ask patient's flavor preference; available in lime, fruit punch, citrus, and orange flavors.
• Don't give potassium supplements postoperatively until urine flow has been established.
• *Alert:* Potassium preparations aren't interchangeable; verify preparation before use. Never switch potassium products without prescriber's order. Potassium chloride can't be given instead of potassium bicarbonate.
• Monitor fluid intake and output and BUN, potassium, and creatinine levels.

**PATIENT TEACHING**
• Tell patient to take drug with meals and sip slowly over 5 to 10 minutes.
• Tell patient to report adverse effects.
• Warn patient not to use salt substitutes at the same time, except with prescriber's permission.

---

**potassium chloride**
Apo-K\*, Cena-K, Gen-K, K+8, K-10\*, K+10, Kaochlor, Kaochlor S-F, Kaon-Cl, Kaon Cl-10, Kaon-Cl 20%, Kay Ciel, K+ Care, K-Dur 10, K-Dur 20✔, K-Lease, K-Lor, Klor-Con, Klor-Con 8, Klor-Con 10, Klor-Con/25, Klorvess, Klotrix, K·Lyte/Cl, K-Norm, K-Tab, K-vescent Potassium Chloride, Micro-K Extencaps, Micro-K 10 Extencaps, Micro-K LS, Potasalan, Rum-K, Slow-K, Ten-K

*Pregnancy risk category C*

---

**AVAILABLE FORMS**
*Capsules (controlled-release):* 8 mEq, 10 mEq
*Injection concentrate:* 1.5 mEq/ml, 2 mEq/ml
*Injection for I.V. infusion:* 0.1mEq/ml, 0.2 mEq/ml, 0.3 mEq/ml, 0.4 mEq/ml
*Oral liquid:* 20 mEq/15 ml, 30 mEq/ 15 ml, 40 mEq/15 ml
*Powder for oral administration:* 15 mEq/ packet, 20 mEq/packet, 25 mEq/packet
*Tablets (controlled-release):* 6.7 mEq, 8 mEq, 10 mEq, 20 mEq
*Tablets (extended-release):* 8 mEq, 10 mEq

**INDICATIONS & DOSAGES**
➤ **To prevent hypokalemia**
*Adults and children:* Initially, 20 mEq of potassium supplement P.O. daily, in divided doses. Adjust dosage, p.r.n., based on potassium levels.
➤ **Hypokalemia**
*Adults and children:* 40 to 100 mEq P.O. in two to four divided doses daily. Maximum dose of diluted I.V. potassium chloride is 40 mEq/L at 10 mEq/hour. Don't exceed 150 mEq daily in adults and 3 mEq/kg daily in children. Further doses are based on potassium levels and blood pH. Give I.V. potassium replacement only with monitoring of ECG and potassium level.
➤ **Severe hypokalemia**
*Adults and children:* Dilute potassium chloride in a suitable I.V. solution of less than 80 mEq/L, and give at no more than 40 mEq/hour.
Further doses are based on potassium level. Don't exceed 150 mEq I.V. daily in adults and 3 mEq/kg I.V. daily or 40 mEq/m² daily in children. Give I.V. potassium replacement only with monitoring of ECG and potassium level.
➤ **Acute MI ♦**
*Adults:* For high dose, 80 mEq/L at 1.5 ml/kg/hour for 24 hours with an I.V. infusion of 25% dextrose and 50 units/L regular insulin. For low dose, 40 mEq/L at 1 ml/kg/hour for 24 hours, with an I.V. infusion of 10% dextrose and 20 units/L regular insulin.

**I.V. ADMINISTRATION**
• Use I.V. route only when oral replacement isn't feasible or when hypokalemia is life threatening.
• *Alert:* Give by I.V. infusion only, never I.V. push or I.M. Give slowly as dilute solution; potentially fatal hyperkalemia may result from too-rapid infusion. Decrease I.V. rate if burning occurs during infusion.

---

## ACTION
Replaces potassium and maintains potassium level.

| Route | Onset | Peak | Duration |
|-------|-------|------|----------|
| P.O. | Unknown | Unknown | Unknown |
| I.V. | Immediate | Immediate | Unknown |

## ADVERSE REACTIONS
**CNS:** paresthesia of limbs, listlessness, confusion, weakness or heaviness of limbs, flaccid paralysis.
**CV:** *arrhythmias, heart block, cardiac arrest,* ECG changes, hypotension, *postinfusion phlebitis.*
**GI:** nausea, vomiting, abdominal pain, diarrhea.
**Metabolic:** *hyperkalemia.*
**Respiratory:** *respiratory paralysis.*

## INTERACTIONS
**Drug-drug.** *ACE inhibitors, digoxin, potassium-sparing diuretics:* May cause hyperkalemia. Use together with extreme caution.

## EFFECTS ON LAB TEST RESULTS
● May increase potassium level.

## CONTRAINDICATIONS & CAUTIONS
● Contraindicated in patients with severe renal impairment with oliguria, anuria, or azotemia; with untreated Addison's disease; or with acute dehydration, heat cramps, hyperkalemia, hyperkalemic form of familial periodic paralysis, or other conditions linked to extensive tissue breakdown.
● Use cautiously in patients with cardiac disease or renal impairment.

## NURSING CONSIDERATIONS
● *Alert:* Give oral potassium supplements with extreme caution because different forms deliver varying amounts of potassium. Never switch products without prescriber's order.
● *Alert:* Potassium preparations aren't interchangeable; verify preparation before use.
● Make sure powders are completely dissolved before giving.
● Enteric-coated tablets aren't recommended because of increased risk of GI bleeding and small-bowel ulcerations.

● Tablets in wax matrix sometimes lodge in the esophagus and cause ulceration in cardiac patients with esophageal compression from an enlarged left atrium. Use liquid form in such patients and in those with esophageal stasis or obstruction.
● Drug is commonly used orally with potassium-wasting diuretics to maintain potassium levels.
● Sugar-free liquid is available (Kaochlor S-F 10%); use if tablet or capsule passage is likely to be delayed, as in GI obstruction. Have patient sip slowly to minimize GI irritation.
● Don't crush sustained-release potassium products.
● Monitor ECG and electrolyte levels during therapy.
● Monitor renal function. Potassium shouldn't be given during immediate postoperative period until urine flow is established.
● Many adverse reactions may reflect hyperkalemia.

## PATIENT TEACHING
● Teach patient how to prepare (powders) and give drug form prescribed. Tell patient to take with or after meals with full glass of water or fruit juice to lessen GI distress.
● Teach patient signs and symptoms of hyperkalemia, and tell patient to notify prescriber if they occur.
● Tell patient to report discomfort at I.V. insertion site.
● Warn patient not to use salt substitutes concurrently, except with prescriber's permission.
● *Alert:* Patient should not be concerned if controlled-release tablets in a wax matrix appear in stool. The potassium has already been absorbed.

## potassium gluconate
Kaon, Kaylixir*, K-G Elixir*

*Pregnancy risk category C*

## AVAILABLE FORMS
*Elixir:* 20 mEq/15 ml*
*Tablets:* 500 mg (83 mg potassium), 595 mg (99 mg potassium)

## INDICATIONS & DOSAGES

➤ **To prevent hypokalemia**
*Adults and children:* Initially, 20 mEq of potassium supplement P.O. daily, in divided doses. Adjust dosage, p.r.n., based on potassium level.

➤ **Hypokalemia**
*Adults and children:* 40 mEq to 100 mEq P.O. divided into two to four daily doses. Use I.V. potassium chloride when oral replacement isn't feasible. Don't exceed 150 mEq P.O. daily in adults and 3 mEq/kg daily P.O. in children.

## ACTION

Replaces potassium and maintains intracellular and extracellular potassium levels.

| Route | Onset | Peak | Duration |
|-------|-------|------|----------|
| P.O. | Unknown | Unknown | 4 hr |

## ADVERSE REACTIONS

**CNS:** paresthesia of limbs, listlessness, confusion, weakness or heaviness of legs, flaccid paralysis.
**CV:** *arrhythmias,* ECG changes.
**GI:** *nausea, vomiting, abdominal pain,* diarrhea.

## INTERACTIONS

**Drug-drug.** *ACE inhibitors, digoxin, potassium-sparing diuretics:* May cause hyperkalemia. Use with extreme caution.

## EFFECTS ON LAB TEST RESULTS

● May increase potassium level.

## CONTRAINDICATIONS & CAUTIONS

● Contraindicated in patients with severe renal impairment with oliguria, anuria, or azotemia; untreated Addison's disease; or acute dehydration, heat cramps, hyperkalemia, hyperkalemic form of familial periodic paralysis, or other conditions linked to extensive tissue breakdown.
● Use cautiously in patients with cardiac disease or renal impairment.

## NURSING CONSIDERATIONS

● *Alert:* Give oral potassium supplements with extreme caution because different forms deliver varying amounts of potassium. Never switch products without prescriber's order.

● Don't give potassium supplements postoperatively until urine flow has been established.
● Monitor ECG, fluid intake and output, and BUN, potassium, and creatinine levels.

## PATIENT TEACHING

● Advise patient to sip liquid potassium slowly to minimize GI irritation. Also tell him to take drug with meals, with a full glass of water or fruit juice.
● Warn patient not to use potassium gluconate with a salt substitute, except with prescriber's permission.
● Teach patient signs and symptoms of hyperkalemia, and tell patient to notify prescriber if they occur.

---

## sodium chloride

*Pregnancy risk category C*

## AVAILABLE FORMS

*Injection:* Half-normal saline solution 25 ml, 50 ml, 150 ml, 250 ml, 500 ml, 1,000 ml; normal saline solution 2 ml, 3 ml, 5 ml, 10 ml, 20 ml, 25 ml, 30 ml, 50 ml, 100 ml, 150 ml, 250 ml, 500 ml, 1,000 ml; 3% sodium chloride solution 500 ml; 5% sodium chloride solution 500 ml; 14.6% sodium chloride solution 20 ml, 40 ml, 200 ml; 23.4% sodium chloride solution 30 ml, 50 ml, 100 ml, and 200 ml
*Tablets:* 650 mg, 1 g, 2.25 g
*Tablets (slow-release):* 600 mg

## INDICATIONS & DOSAGES

➤ **Fluid and electrolyte replacement in hyponatremia caused by electrolyte loss or in severe salt depletion**
*Adults:* Dosage is individualized; use 3% or 5% solution only with frequent electrolyte level determination and given only slow I.V. With 0.45% solution, 3% to 8% of body weight, according to deficiencies, over 18 to 24 hours; with 0.9% solution, 2% to 6% of body weight, according to deficiencies, over 18 to 24 hours.
➤ **Heat cramp caused by excessive perspiration**
*Adults:* 1 g P.O. with each glass of water.

---

## I.V. ADMINISTRATION
● *Alert:* Don't confuse concentrates (14.6%, 23.4%) available to add to parenteral nutrient solutions with normal saline solution for injection, and never give without diluting. Read labels carefully.
● *Alert:* Infuse 3% and 5% solutions slowly and cautiously to avoid pulmonary edema. Use only for critical situations, and observe patient continually. Infuse through central line if possible.
● *Alert:* Never use bacteriostatic sodium chloride injection in neonates.

## ACTION
Replaces sodium and chloride and maintains levels.

| Route | Onset | Peak | Duration |
|-------|-------|------|----------|
| P.O. | Unknown | Unknown | Unknown |
| I.V. | Immediate | Immediate | Unknown |

## ADVERSE REACTIONS
**CV:** *aggravation of heart failure,* thrombophlebitis, edema when given too rapidly or in excess.
**Metabolic:** hypernatremia, aggravation of existing metabolic acidosis with excessive infusion.
**Respiratory:** *pulmonary edema.*
**Skin:** local tenderness, tissue necrosis at injection site.
**Other:** abscess.

## INTERACTIONS
None significant.

## EFFECTS ON LAB TEST RESULTS
● May increase sodium level. May decrease potassium level.
● May cause electrolyte imbalance.

## CONTRAINDICATIONS & CAUTIONS
● Contraindicated in patients with conditions in which sodium and chloride administration is detrimental.
● Sodium chloride 3% and 5% injections contraindicated in patients with increased, normal, or only slightly decreased electrolyte levels.
● Use cautiously in elderly or postoperative patients and in patients with heart failure, circulatory insufficiency, renal dysfunction, or hypoproteinemia.

## NURSING CONSIDERATIONS
● Monitor electrolyte levels.

## PATIENT TEACHING
● Explain use and administration of drug to patient and family.
● Tell patient to report adverse reactions promptly.

# 62

# Acidifiers and alkalinizers

**sodium bicarbonate**
**sodium lactate**
**tromethamine**

**COMBINATION PRODUCTS**
None.

---

## sodium bicarbonate
Arm & Hammer Baking Soda ◇,
Bell/ans ◇, Neut, Soda Mint ◇ ♦

*Pregnancy risk category C*

### AVAILABLE FORMS
*Injection:* 4% (2.4 mEq/5 ml), 4.2%
(5 mEq/10 ml), 5% (297.5 mEq/500 ml),
7.5% (8.92 mEq/10 ml and 44.6 mEq/
50 ml), 8.4% (10 mEq/10 ml and 50 mEq/
50 ml)
*Tablets* ◇: 325 mg, 650 mg

### INDICATIONS & DOSAGES
➤ **Cardiac arrest**
*Adults:* 1 mEq/kg I.V. of 7.5% or 8.4% solution; then 0.5 mEq/kg I.V. q 10 minutes,
depending on arterial blood gas (ABG)
level. Base further dosages on results of
ABG analysis. If ABG level is unavailable, use 0.5 mEq/kg I.V. q 10 minutes until spontaneous circulation returns.
*Infants and children:* 1 mEq/kg (1 ml/kg
of 8.4% solution) I.V. slowly followed by
1 mEq/kg q 10 minutes of arrest. Don't
give more than 8 mEq/kg I.V. daily; a
4.2% solution may be preferred.
➤ **Metabolic acidosis**
*Adults and children:* Dosage depends on
blood carbon dioxide content, pH, and patient's condition; usually, 2 to 5 mEq/kg
I.V. infused over 4- to 8-hour period.
➤ **Systemic or urinary alkalinization**
*Adults:* Initially, 4 g P.O.; then 1 to 2 g q 6
hours.
*Children:* 84 to 840 mg/kg P.O. daily.
➤ **Antacid**
*Adults:* 300 mg to 2 g P.O. up to q.i.d. tak-
en with glass of water.

### I.V. ADMINISTRATION
● *Alert:* Sodium bicarbonate isn't routinely
recommended for use in cardiac arrest because it may produce a paradoxical acidosis from carbon dioxide production. It
shouldn't be routinely given during the
early stages of resuscitation unless acidosis is clearly present.
● Sodium bicarbonate 4% is usually used
for neutralizing certain I.V. drugs, such as
erythromycin. Consult pharmacist before
use.
● Drug may be added to other I.V. fluids.
Sodium bicarbonate inactivates such catecholamines as norepinephrine, dobutamine and dopamine, and forms precipitate
with calcium. Don't mix sodium bicarbonate with I.V. solutions of these drugs, and
flush I.V. line adequately.

### ACTION
Restores buffering capacity of the body
and neutralizes excess acid.

| Route | Onset | Peak | Duration |
|-------|-------|------|----------|
| P.O. | Unknown | Unknown | Unknown |
| I.V. | Immediate | Immediate | Unknown |

### ADVERSE REACTIONS
**CNS:** tetany.
**CV:** edema.
**GI:** gastric distention, belching, flatu-
lence.
**Metabolic:** hypokalemia, *metabolic alka-
losis*, hypernatremia, hyperosmolarity
with overdose.
**Skin:** pain and irritation at injection site.

### INTERACTIONS
**Drug-drug.** *Anorexiants, flecainide,
mecamylamine, methenamine, quinidine,
sympathomimetics:* May decrease renal
clearance of these drugs and increase risk
of toxicity. Monitor patient closely for toxicity.
*Chlorpropamide, lithium, methotrexate,
salicylates, tetracycline:* May increase
urine alkalinization, increase renal clearance of these drugs, and decrease effec-

---

tiveness. Monitor patient closely for effectiveness.

*Enteric-coated drugs:* May be released prematurely in stomach. Avoid using together.

*Ketoconazole:* May decrease absorption of ketoconazole. Separate administration times.

## EFFECTS ON LAB TEST RESULTS
• May increase sodium and lactate levels. May decrease potassium level.

## CONTRAINDICATIONS & CAUTIONS
• Contraindicated in patients with metabolic or respiratory alkalosis and in those with hypocalcemia in which alkalosis may produce tetany, hypertension, seizures, or heart failure. Also contraindicated in patients who are losing chlorides because of vomiting or continuous GI suction and in those receiving diuretics that produce hypochloremic alkalosis. Oral sodium bicarbonate is contraindicated for patients with acute ingestion of strong mineral acids.
• Use with extreme caution in patients with renal insufficiency, heart failure, or other edematous or sodium-retaining condition.

## NURSING CONSIDERATIONS
• To avoid risk of alkalosis, obtain blood pH, partial pressure of arterial oxygen, partial pressure of arterial carbon dioxide, and electrolyte levels. Keep prescriber informed of laboratory results.

## PATIENT TEACHING
• Tell patient not to take drug with milk because doing so may cause high levels of calcium in the blood, abnormally high alkalinity in tissues and fluids, or kidney stones.

---

## sodium lactate

*Pregnancy risk category NR*

## AVAILABLE FORMS
*Injection:* 1/6 M solution (167 mEq/L)

## INDICATIONS & DOSAGES
➤ **To alkalinize urine**
*Adults:* 30 ml/kg (1/6 M solution) I.V. daily, in divided doses.
➤ **Metabolic acidosis**
*Adults:* Dosage of 1/6 M solution depends on degree of bicarbonate deficit. A suggested formula follows:

$$\frac{60 - \text{plasma } CO_2}{} \times 0.8 \times \frac{\text{body weight}}{\text{in pounds}} = \frac{\text{Dose}}{\text{in ml}}$$

## I.V. ADMINISTRATION
• Add sodium lactate to other I.V. solutions or give as an isotonic 1/6 M solution. Drug is compatible with most common I.V. solutions.
• Don't mix with sodium bicarbonate; drugs are incompatible.
• Don't exceed I.V. infusion rate of 300 ml/hour.

## ACTION
Metabolizes to sodium bicarbonate, producing buffering effect.

| Route | Onset | Peak | Duration |
|-------|-------|------|----------|
| I.V. | Immediate | 1-2 hr | Unknown |

## ADVERSE REACTIONS
**CNS:** fever.
**CV:** thrombophlebitis at injection site.
**Metabolic:** *metabolic alkalosis*, hypernatremia, hyperosmolarity with overdose.
**Other:** infection.

## INTERACTIONS
None significant.

## EFFECTS ON LAB TEST RESULTS
• May increase sodium level.

## CONTRAINDICATIONS & CAUTIONS
• Contraindicated in patients with hypernatremia, severe acidosis, lactic acidosis, or conditions in which sodium administration is detrimental, such as heart failure or during corticosteroid administration.
• Use with extreme caution in patients with metabolic or respiratory alkalosis, severe hepatic or renal disease, heart failure, shock, hypoxia, or beriberi.

---

## NURSING CONSIDERATIONS
● Monitor electrolyte levels to avoid alkalosis.

## PATIENT TEACHING
● Explain use and administration of drug to patient and family.
● Tell patient to report adverse reactions to prescriber.

# tromethamine
Tham

*Pregnancy risk category C*

## AVAILABLE FORMS
*Injection:* 18 g/500 ml

## INDICATIONS & DOSAGES
➤ **Metabolic acidosis during cardiac bypass surgery or cardiac arrest**
*Adults:* Dosage depends on bicarbonate deficit. Calculate as follows:

$$\begin{array}{l}\text{Each ml}\\\text{of 0.3 M}\\\text{tromethamine}\\\text{solution}\\\text{needed}\end{array} = \begin{array}{l}\text{weight}\\\text{in kg}\end{array} \times \begin{array}{l}\text{bicarbonate}\\\text{deficit}\\\text{(mEq/L)}\end{array} \times 1.1$$

Base additional therapy on serial bicarbonate deficit determinations. Give over at least 1 hour; don't exceed 500 mg/kg per dose.
➤ **Acidosis during bypass surgery**
*Adults:* Average dose of 9 ml/kg (2.7 mEq/kg or 0.32 g/kg); total single dose of 500 ml (150 mEq or 18 g) is adequate for most adults. Don't exceed 500 mg/kg over less than 1 hour.

## I.V. ADMINISTRATION
● Give slowly either through 18G to 20G needle into largest antecubital vein or through indwelling I.V. catheter.
● If extravasation occurs, infiltrate area with 1% procaine.

## ACTION
Combines with hydrogen ions and associated acid anions; resulting salts are excreted. Also has osmotic diuretic effect.

| Route | Onset | Peak | Duration |
|---|---|---|---|
| I.V. | Immediate | Immediate | Unknown |

## ADVERSE REACTIONS
**CNS:** fever.
**Hepatic:** *hemorrhagic hepatic necrosis.*
**Metabolic:** *hypoglycemia, hyperkalemia with decreased urine output.*
**Respiratory:** *respiratory depression.*
**Other:** venospasm, I.V. thrombosis, inflammation, necrosis, sloughing if extravasation occurs.

## INTERACTIONS
None significant.

## EFFECTS ON LAB TEST RESULTS
● May increase potassium level. May decrease glucose level.

## CONTRAINDICATIONS & CAUTIONS
● Contraindicated in patients with anuria, uremia, or chronic respiratory acidosis; also contraindicated during pregnancy (except in acute, life-threatening situations).
● Use cautiously in patients with renal disease and poor urine output. Monitor ECG and potassium level.

## NURSING CONSIDERATIONS
● Determine blood pH, carbon dioxide tension, and bicarbonate, glucose, and electrolyte levels before, during, and after therapy.
● Have mechanical ventilation available for patients with respiratory acidosis.
● To prevent blood pH from rising above normal, be prepared to adjust dosage carefully.

## PATIENT TEACHING
● Explain use of drug to patient and family.
● Tell patient to report adverse reactions to prescriber.

# 63

## Hematinics

ferrous fumarate
ferrous gluconate
ferrous sulfate
ferrous sulfate, dried
iron dextran
iron sucrose injection
polysaccharide-iron complex
sodium ferric gluconate complex

### COMBINATION PRODUCTS
FERRO-SEQUELS ◇: ferrous fumarate 150 mg and docusate sodium 100 mg. Various iron products in combination with vitamins.

---

### ferrous fumarate
Femiron ◇, Feostat ◇, Hemocyte ◇, Ircon ◇, Nephro-Fer ◇, Novofumar†, Palafer†, Palafer Pediatric Drops†, Vitron-C

*Pregnancy risk category A*

### AVAILABLE FORMS
Each 100 mg of ferrous fumarate provides 33 mg of elemental iron.
*Drops:* 45 mg/0.6 ml ◇
*Oral suspension:* 100 mg/5 ml ◇
*Tablets:* 63 mg ◇, 200 mg ◇, 324 mg ◇, 325 mg ◇, 350 mg ◇
*Tablets (chewable):* 100 mg ◇

### INDICATIONS & DOSAGES
➤ **Iron deficiency**
*Adults:* 100 to 200 mg (2 to 3 mg/kg) P.O. elemental iron daily in three divided doses.
*Children age 2 to 12:* 50 to 100 mg (1 to 1.5 mg/kg) P.O. elemental iron daily in three or four divided doses.
*Children age 6 months to 2 years:* 3 to 6 mg/kg P.O. elemental iron daily in three divided doses.
*Infants younger than age 6 months:* 10 to 25 mg P.O. elemental iron daily in three or four divided doses.
➤ **As a supplement during pregnancy**
*Women:* 15 to 30 mg elemental iron P.O. daily during last two trimesters.

### ACTION
Provides elemental iron, an essential component in the formation of hemoglobin.

| Route | Onset | Peak | Duration |
|-------|-------|------|----------|
| P.O. | 4 days | 7-10 days | 2-4 mo |

### ADVERSE REACTIONS
**GI:** *nausea,* epigastric pain, vomiting, *constipation,* diarrhea, *black stools,* anorexia.
**Other:** temporarily stained teeth from suspension and drops.

### INTERACTIONS
**Drug-drug.** *Antacids, cholestyramine resin, cimetidine:* May decrease iron absorption. Separate doses by at least 2 hours.
*Chloramphenicol:* May delay response to iron therapy. Monitor patient.
*Fluoroquinolones, penicillamine, tetracyclines:* May decrease GI absorption of these drugs, possibly resulting in decreased levels or efficacy. Separate doses by 2 to 4 hours.
*Levodopa, methyldopa:* May decrease absorption and efficacy of levodopa and methyldopa. Watch for decreased effect of these drugs.
*L-Thyroxine:* May decrease L-thyroxine absorption. Separate doses by at least 2 hours. Monitor thyroid function.
*Vitamin C:* May increase iron absorption. Use together for therapeutic effect.
**Drug-herb.** *Black cohosh, chamomile, feverfew, gossypol, hawthorn, nettle, plantain, St. John's wort:* May decrease iron absorption. Discourage use together.
*Oregano:* May reduce iron absorption. Separate ingestion of oregano from ingestion of iron supplements or iron-containing foods by at least 2 hours.
**Drug-food.** *Cereals, cheese, coffee, eggs, milk, tea, whole-grain breads, yogurt:* May impair oral iron absorption. Discourage use together.

---

## EFFECTS ON LAB TEST RESULTS
• May yield false-positive guaiac test results. May decrease uptake of technetium 99m and interfere with skeletal imaging.

## CONTRAINDICATIONS & CAUTIONS
• Contraindicated in patients with primary hemochromatosis or hemosiderosis, hemolytic anemia (unless iron-deficiency anemia is also present), peptic ulcer disease, regional enteritis, or ulcerative colitis.
• Contraindicated in those receiving repeated blood transfusions.
• Use cautiously on long-term basis.

## NURSING CONSIDERATIONS
• GI upset may be related to dose.
• Between-meal doses are preferable, but drug can be given with some foods, although absorption may be decreased.
• Enteric-coated products reduce GI upset but also reduce amount of iron absorbed.
• Check for constipation; record color and amount of stools.
• *Alert:* Oral iron may turn stools black. Although this unabsorbed iron is harmless, it could mask presence of melena.
• Monitor hemoglobin, hematocrit, and reticulocyte count during therapy.
• Combination products such as Ferro-Sequels contain stool softeners, which help prevent constipation, a common adverse reaction.

## PATIENT TEACHING
• Tell patient to take tablets with juice (preferably orange juice) or water but not with milk or antacids.
• To avoid staining teeth, tell patient to take suspension with straw and place drops at back of throat.
• Caution patient not to crush tablets or chew extended-release forms.
• Advise patient not to substitute one iron salt for another; the amount of elemental iron may vary.
• *Alert:* Inform parents that as few as 3 or 4 tablets can cause serious poisoning in children.
• Advise patient to report constipation and change in stool color or consistency.

# ferrous gluconate
Fergon◊, Fertinic†, Novoferrogluc†

*Pregnancy risk category A*

## AVAILABLE FORMS
Each 100 mg of ferrous gluconate provides 11.6 mg of elemental iron.
*Tablets:* 240 mg◊, 325 mg◊

## INDICATIONS & DOSAGES
➤ **Iron deficiency**
*Adults:* 100 to 200 mg (2 to 3 mg/kg) P.O. elemental iron daily in three divided doses.
*Children ages 2 to 12:* 50 to 100 mg (1 to 1.5 mg/kg) P.O. elemental iron daily in three or four divided doses.
*Children ages 6 months to 2 years:* 3 to 6 mg/kg P.O. elemental iron daily in three divided doses.
*Infants younger than age 6 months:* 10 to 25 mg P.O. elemental iron daily in three or four divided doses.
➤ **As a supplement during pregnancy**
*Adults:* 15 to 30 mg elemental iron P.O. daily during last two trimesters.

## ACTION
Provides elemental iron, an essential component in the formation of hemoglobin.

| Route | Onset | Peak | Duration |
|---|---|---|---|
| P.O. | 4 days | 7-10 days | 2-4 mo |

## ADVERSE REACTIONS
**GI:** *nausea,* epigastric pain, vomiting, *constipation,* diarrhea, *black stools,* anorexia.

## INTERACTIONS
**Drug-drug.** *Antacids, cholestyramine resin, cimetidine:* May decrease iron absorption. Separate doses by at least 2 hours.
*Chloramphenicol:* Delays response to iron therapy. Monitor patient.
*Fluoroquinolones, penicillamine, tetracyclines:* May decrease GI absorption of these drugs, possibly resulting in decreased levels or efficacy. Separate doses by 2 to 4 hours.

*Levodopa, methyldopa:* May decrease absorption and efficacy of levodopa and methyldopa. Watch for decreased effect of these drugs.
*L-Thyroxine:* May decrease L-thyroxine absorption. Separate doses by at least 2 hours. Monitor thyroid function.
*Vitamin C:* May increase iron absorption. Use together for therapeutic effect.
**Drug-herb.** *Black cohosh, chamomile, feverfew, gossypol, hawthorn, nettle, plantain, St. John's wort:* May decrease iron absorption. Discourage use together.
*Oregano:* May reduce iron absorption. Tell patient to separate ingestion of oregano from ingestion of iron supplements or iron-containing foods by at least 2 hours.
**Drug-food.** *Cereals, cheese, coffee, eggs, milk, tea, whole-grain breads, yogurt:* May impair oral iron absorption. Discourage use together.

### EFFECTS ON LAB TEST RESULTS
• May yield false-positive guaiac test results. May decrease uptake of technetium 99m and interfere with skeletal imaging.

### CONTRAINDICATIONS & CAUTIONS
• Contraindicated in patients with peptic ulceration, regional enteritis, ulcerative colitis, hemosiderosis, primary hemochromatosis, or hemolytic anemia (unless an iron-deficiency anemia is also present) and in those receiving repeated blood transfusions.
• Use cautiously on long-term basis.

### NURSING CONSIDERATIONS
• GI upset may be related to dose.
• Between-meal doses are preferable, but drug can be given with some foods, although absorption may be decreased.
• Enteric-coated products reduce GI upset but also reduce amount of iron absorbed.
• Check for constipation; record color and amount of stools.
• *Alert:* Oral iron may turn stools black. Although this unabsorbed iron is harmless, it could mask melena.
• Monitor hemoglobin, hematocrit, and reticulocyte count during therapy.

### PATIENT TEACHING
• Tell patient to take tablets with juice (preferably orange juice) or water, but not with milk or antacids.
• *Alert:* Inform parents that as few as 3 or 4 tablets can cause serious iron poisoning in children.
• Caution patient not to substitute one iron salt for another because the amounts of elemental iron vary.
• Advise patient to report constipation and change in stool color or consistency.

## ferrous sulfate
Apo-Ferrous Sulfate†, ED-IN-SOL, Feosol*◊, Fer-Gen-Sol*◊, Fer-In-Sol *◊, Fer-Iron*◊

## ferrous sulfate, dried
Fe50 ◊, Feosol ◊, Feratab ◊, Novoferrosulfate†, PMS-Ferrous Sulfate†, Slow FE ◊

*Pregnancy risk category A*

### AVAILABLE FORMS
Each 100 mg of ferrous sulfate provides 20 mg of elemental iron, about 30 mg of elemental iron in ferrous sulfate dried products.
*Caplets (extended-release)* ◊ *:* 160 mg (dried)
*Drops* ◊ *:* 125 mg/ml
*Elixir* ◊ *:* 220 mg/5 ml* ◊
*Syrup* ◊ *:* 90 mg/5 ml
*Tablets* ◊ *:* 187 mg (dried), 200 mg (dried), 324 mg, 325 mg
*Tablets (slow-release)* ◊ *:* 160 mg (dried)

### INDICATIONS & DOSAGES
➤ **Iron deficiency**
*Adults:* 100 to 200 mg (2 to 3 mg/kg) P.O. elemental iron daily in three divided doses.
*Children age 2 to 12:* 50 to 100 mg (1 to 1.5 mg/kg) P.O. elemental iron daily in three or four divided doses.
*Children age 6 months to 2 years:* 3 to 6 mg/kg P.O. elemental iron daily in three divided doses.
*Infants younger than age 6 months:* 10 to 25 mg P.O. elemental iron daily in three or four divided doses.

➤ **As a supplement during pregnancy**
*Adults:* 15 to 30 mg elemental iron P.O.
daily during last two trimesters.

## ACTION
Provides elemental iron, an essential component in the formation of hemoglobin.

| Route | Onset | Peak | Duration |
|-------|-------|------|----------|
| P.O. | 4 days | 7-10 days | 2-4 mo |

## ADVERSE REACTIONS
**GI:** *nausea,* epigastric pain, vomiting,
*constipation, black stools,* diarrhea,
anorexia.
**Other:** temporarily stained teeth from liquid forms.

## INTERACTIONS
**Drug-drug.** *Antacids, cholestyramine
resin, cimetidine:* May decrease iron absorption. Separate doses if possible.
*Chloramphenicol:* May delay response to
iron therapy. Monitor patient.
*Fluoroquinolones, penicillamine, tetracyclines:* May decrease GI absorption of
these drugs, possibly resulting in decreased levels or efficacy. Separate doses
by 2 to 4 hours.
*Levodopa, methyldopa:* May decrease absorption and efficacy of levodopa and
methyldopa. Watch for decreased effect of
these drugs.
*L-Thyroxine:* May decrease L-thyroxine
absorption. Separate doses by at least 2
hours. Monitor thyroid function.
*Vitamin C:* May increase iron absorption.
Use together for therapeutic effect.
**Drug-herb.** *Black cohosh, chamomile,
feverfew, gossypol, hawthorn, nettle, plantain, St. John's wort:* May decrease iron
absorption. Discourage use together.
*Oregano:* May reduce iron absorption.
Tell patient to separate ingestion of
oregano from ingestion of iron supplements or iron-containing foods by at least
2 hours.
**Drug-food.** *Cereals, cheese, coffee, eggs,
milk, tea, whole-grain breads, yogurt:*
May impair oral iron absorption. Discourage use together.

## EFFECTS ON LAB TEST RESULTS
● May yield false-positive guaiac test results. May decrease uptake of technetium
99m and interfere with skeletal imaging.

## CONTRAINDICATIONS & CAUTIONS
● Contraindicated in patients with hemosiderosis, primary hemochromatosis, hemolytic anemia (unless iron-deficiency
anemia is also present), peptic ulceration,
ulcerative colitis, or regional enteritis and
in those receiving repeated blood transfusions.
● Use cautiously on long-term basis.

## NURSING CONSIDERATIONS
● GI upset may be related to dose.
● Between-meal doses are preferable.
Drug can be given with some foods, although absorption may be decreased.
● Enteric-coated products reduce GI upset
but also reduce amount of iron absorbed.
● *Alert:* Oral iron may turn stools black.
Although this unabsorbed iron is harmless, it could mask melena.
● Monitor hemoglobin, hematocrit, and
reticulocyte count during therapy.
● *Alert:* Don't confuse different iron salts;
elemental content may vary.

## PATIENT TEACHING
● Tell patient to take tablets with juice
(preferably orange juice) or water, but not
with milk or antacids.
● Instruct patient not to crush or chew
extended-release forms.
● *Alert:* Inform parents that as few as 3 to
4 tablets can cause serious iron poisoning
in children.
● Caution patient not to substitute one iron
salt for another because amounts of elemental iron vary.
● Advise patient to report constipation and
change in stool color or consistency.

## iron dextran
DexFerrum, InFeD

*Pregnancy risk category C*

## AVAILABLE FORMS
1 ml iron dextran provides 50 mg elemental iron.
*Injection:* 50 mg elemental iron/ml

## INDICATIONS & DOSAGES
➤ **Iron-deficiency anemia**
*Adults and children:* I.V. or I.M. test dose is needed before administration. Total dose is calculated using the following formula:

$$\text{Dose (ml)} = (\text{desired Hb} - \text{observed Hb}) \times \frac{0.0442}{\text{Weight in kg}} + (0.26 \times \text{Weight in kg})$$

*I.V.*
Inject 0.5-ml test dose over 30 seconds. If no reaction occurs in 1 hour, give remainder of therapeutic I.V. dose. Repeat therapeutic I.V. dose daily. Single daily dose shouldn't exceed 100 mg. Give slowly (1 ml/minute).
*I.M. (by Z-track method)*
Inject 0.5-ml test dose. If no reaction occurs in 1 hour, give remainder of dose. Daily dose should ordinarily not exceed 0.5 ml (25 mg) for infants weighing less than 5 kg (11 lb); 1 ml (50 mg) for those weighing less than 10 kg (22 lb); and 2 ml (100 mg) for heavier children and adults. Don't give iron dextran in the first 4 months of life.

## I.V. ADMINISTRATION
• Check hospital policy before giving I.V. Don't mix with other parenteral drug or nutritional solutions containing liquid emulsions.
• After completing I.V. dose, flush the vein with 10 ml of normal saline solution. Patient should rest for 15 to 30 minutes after I.V. administration.

## ACTION
Provides elemental iron, an essential component in the formation of hemoglobin.

| Route | Onset | Peak | Duration |
|-------|-------|------|----------|
| I.V. | Unknown | Unknown | Unknown |
| I.M. | 72 hr | Unknown | 3-4 wk |

## ADVERSE REACTIONS
**CNS:** headache, transitory paresthesia, dizziness, malaise, fever, chills.
**CV:** chest pain, tachycardia, *bradycardia, hypotensive reaction, peripheral vascular flushing.*
**GI:** nausea, anorexia.
**Musculoskeletal:** arthralgia, myalgia.
**Respiratory:** *bronchospasm,* dyspnea.

**Skin:** rash; urticaria; *soreness, inflammation, brown skin discoloration at I.M. injection site; local phlebitis at I.V. injection site;* sterile abscess; necrosis; atrophy.
**Other:** fibrosis, *anaphylaxis, delayed sensitivity reactions.*

## INTERACTIONS
None significant.

## EFFECTS ON LAB TEST RESULTS
• May cause false increase in bilirubin level and false decrease in calcium level. Use of more than 250 mg iron may color the serum brown. Iron dextran may alter measurement of iron level and total iron-binding capacity for up to 3 weeks; I.M. injection may cause dense areas of activity for 1 to 6 days on bone scans using technetium 99m diphosphonate.

## CONTRAINDICATIONS & CAUTIONS
• Contraindicated in patients hypersensitive to drug, in those with acute infectious renal disease, and in those with any anemia except iron-deficiency anemia.
• Use cautiously in patients who have serious hepatic impairment, rheumatoid arthritis, or other inflammatory diseases because these patients may be at higher risk for certain delays and reactions.
• Use cautiously in patients with history of significant allergies or asthma.

## NURSING CONSIDERATIONS
• Have epinephrine immediately available in event of acute hypersensitivity reaction.
• Don't give iron dextran with oral iron preparations.
• I.V. or I.M. injections of iron are advisable only for patients in whom oral administration is impossible or ineffective.
• For I.M. route, inject deeply into upper outer quadrant of buttock—never into arm or other exposed area—with a 2- to 3-inch 19G or 20G needle. Use Z-track method to avoid leakage into subcutaneous tissue and staining of skin. After drawing up drug, use a new sterile needle to give injection.
• Monitor hemoglobin, hematocrit, and reticulocyte count.

## PATIENT TEACHING
- Teach patient signs and symptoms of hypersensitivity and iron toxicity, and tell him to report them to prescriber.
- Inform patient that drug may stain skin.

---

## iron sucrose injection
Venofer

*Pregnancy risk category B*

---

### AVAILABLE FORMS
*Injection:* 20 mg/ml of elemental iron

### INDICATIONS & DOSAGES
➤ **Iron-deficiency anemia in patients undergoing long-term hemodialysis who are receiving supplemental erythropoietin therapy**
*Adults:* 100 mg (5 ml) of elemental iron I.V. directly in the dialysis line, either by slow injection at a rate of 1 ml/minute or by infusion over 15 minutes during the dialysis session one to three times a week to a total of 1,000 mg in 10 doses; repeat p.r.n.

### I.V. ADMINISTRATION
- For slow injection, give drug at a rate of 1 ml (20 mg elemental iron) undiluted solution per minute, not exceeding 1 vial (100 mg elemental iron) per injection.
- For infusion, dilute drug to a maximum of 100 ml in normal saline solution immediately before infusion and infuse at a rate of 100 mg elemental iron over at least 15 minutes.
- Don't mix with other drugs or add to parenteral nutrition solutions of I.V. infusion.
- Inspect drugs for particulate matter and discoloration before giving.

### ACTION
Exogenous source of iron that replenishes depleted body iron stores and is essential for hemoglobin synthesis.

| Route | Onset | Peak | Duration |
|-------|-------|------|----------|
| I.V. | Unknown | Unknown | Variable |

### ADVERSE REACTIONS
**CNS:** headache, asthenia, malaise, dizziness, fever.

**CV:** *heart failure,* hypotension, chest pain, hypertension, fluid retention.
**GI:** nausea, vomiting, diarrhea, abdominal pain, taste perversion.
**Musculoskeletal:** *leg cramps,* bone and muscle pain.
**Respiratory:** dyspnea, wheezing, pneumonia, cough.
**Skin:** rash, pruritus, application site reaction.
**Other:** accidental injury, pain, *sepsis, hypersensitivity reactions.*

### INTERACTIONS
**Drug-drug.** *Oral iron preparations:* May reduce absorption of oral iron preparations. Avoid using together.

### EFFECTS ON LAB TEST RESULTS
- May increase liver enzyme levels.

### CONTRAINDICATIONS & CAUTIONS
- Contraindicated in patients with hypersensitivity to drug or its components, evidence of iron overload, or anemia not caused by iron deficiency.
- Use cautiously in breast-feeding women.

### NURSING CONSIDERATIONS
- *Alert:* Rare but fatal hypersensitivity reactions characterized by anaphylactic shock, loss of consciousness, collapse, hypotension, dyspnea, or seizures may occur. Have epinephrine readily available.
- Mild to moderate hypersensitivity reactions, with wheezing, dyspnea, hypotension, rash, or pruritus, may occur.
- Giving drug by infusion may reduce the risk of hypotension.
- Transferrin saturation level increases rapidly after I.V. administration of iron sucrose. Obtain iron level 48 hours after I.V. administration.
- Monitor hematocrit, hemoglobin, and ferritin and transferrin saturation levels.
- Withhold dose in patient with signs and symptoms of iron overload.
- Keep dose selection in elderly patients conservative because of decreased hepatic, renal, or cardiac function; other disease; and other drug therapy.

### PATIENT TEACHING
- Instruct patient to notify prescriber if symptoms of overdose (headache, nausea,

---

Reactions may be *common,* uncommon, *life-threatening,* or COMMON AND LIFE-THREATENING.

dizziness, joint aches, tingling, or abdominal and muscle pain) or of allergic reaction (labored breathing, collapse, or loss of consciousness) occur.

## polysaccharide-iron complex
**Ferrex 150** ◇, **Hytinic** ◇, **Niferex*** ◇, **Niferex-150** ◇, **Nu-Iron*** ◇, **Nu-Iron 150** ◇

*Pregnancy risk category NR*

### AVAILABLE FORMS
*Capsules:* 150 mg
*Elixir:* 100 mg/5 ml
*Tablets:* 50 mg

### INDICATIONS & DOSAGES
➤ **Iron deficiency**
*Adults:* 100 to 200 mg (2 to 3 mg/kg) P.O. elemental iron daily in three divided doses.
*Children ages 2 to 12:* 50 to 100 mg (1 to 1.5 mg/kg) P.O. elemental iron daily in three or four divided doses.
*Children ages 6 months to 2 years:* 3 to 6 mg/kg P.O. elemental iron daily in three divided doses.
*Infants younger than age 6 months:* 10 to 25 mg P.O. elemental iron daily in three or four divided doses.
➤ **As a supplement during pregnancy**
*Women:* 15 to 30 mg elemental iron P.O. daily during last two trimesters.

### ACTION
Provides elemental iron, an essential component in the formation of hemoglobin.

| Route | Onset | Peak | Duration |
|-------|-------|------|----------|
| P.O. | Few days | 2-10 days | 2 mo |

### ADVERSE REACTIONS
**GI:** *nausea*, epigastric pain, vomiting, *constipation, black stools,* diarrhea, anorexia.
**Other:** temporarily stained teeth from liquid forms.

### INTERACTIONS
**Drug-drug.** *Antacids, cholestyramine resin, cimetidine:* May decrease iron absorption. Separate doses by 2 to 4 hours.
*Chloramphenicol:* May delay response to iron therapy. Monitor patient.
*Fluoroquinolones, levodopa, methyldopa, penicillamine, tetracyclines:* May decrease GI absorption of these drugs, possibly resulting in decreased levels or efficacy. Separate doses by 2 to 4 hours.
*Levothyroxine sodium:* May decrease levothyroxine efficacy, leading to hypothyroidism. Separate doses by 2 to 4 hours.
*Thyroid:* May inhibit thyroid hormone absorption. Separate doses by 2 hours.
*Vitamin C:* May increase iron absorption. Use together for therapeutic effect.
**Drug-herb.** *Black cohosh, chamomile, feverfew, gossypol, hawthorn, nettle, plantain, St. John's wort:* May decrease iron absorption. Discourage use together.
*Oregano:* May reduce iron absorption. Tell patient to separate ingestion of oregano from ingestion of iron supplements or iron-containing foods by at least 2 hours.
**Drug-food.** *Cereals, cheese, coffee, eggs, milk, tea, whole-grain breads, yogurt:* May impair oral iron absorption. Separate use by 2 to 4 hours.

### EFFECTS ON LAB TEST RESULTS
• May increase hemoglobin, hematocrit, and reticulocyte count.
• May yield false-positive guaiac test results. May decrease uptake of technetium 99m and interfere with skeletal imaging.

### CONTRAINDICATIONS & CAUTIONS
• Contraindicated in patients hypersensitive to drug or its ingredients and in those with hemochromatosis or hemosiderosis.

### NURSING CONSIDERATIONS
• *Alert:* Oral iron may turn stools black. Although this unabsorbed iron is harmless, it may mask melena.
• Monitor hemoglobin, hematocrit, and reticulocyte count.
• Although nausea, constipation, black stools, and epigastric pain are common adverse reactions to iron therapy, few, if any, occur with polysaccharide iron complex.
• Iron overload may decrease uptake of technetium 99m and thus interfere with skeletal imaging.

### PATIENT TEACHING
• Tell patient to take tablets with juice (preferably orange juice) or water, but not with milk or antacids.
• *Alert:* Inform parents that as few as 3 tablets can cause serious iron poisoning in children.
• Caution patient not to substitute one iron salt for another because the amounts of elemental iron vary.

---

## sodium ferric gluconate complex
Ferrlecit

*Pregnancy risk category B*

### AVAILABLE FORMS
*Injection:* 62.5 mg elemental iron (12.5 mg/ml) in 5-ml ampules

### INDICATIONS & DOSAGES
➤ **Iron-deficiency anemia in patients receiving long-term hemodialysis and supplemental erythropoietin**
*Adults:* Before starting therapeutic doses, give test dose of 2 ml sodium ferric gluconate complex (25 mg elemental iron) I.V. over 1 hour. If patient tolerates test dose, give therapeutic dose of 10 ml (125 mg elemental iron) I.V. over 1 hour. Most patients need minimum cumulative dose of 1 g elemental iron given at more than eight sequential dialysis treatments to achieve a favorable hemoglobin or hematocrit response.

### I.V. ADMINISTRATION
• Dilute test dose of sodium ferric gluconate complex in 50 ml normal saline solution and give over 1 hour. Dilute therapeutic doses of drug in 100 ml normal saline solution and give over 1 hour.
• Don't mix sodium ferric gluconate complex with other drugs or add to parenteral nutrition solutions for I.V. infusion. Use immediately after dilution in normal saline solution.
• *Alert:* Profound hypotension with flushing, light-headedness, malaise, fatigue, weakness, or severe chest, back, flank, or groin pain may occur after rapid I.V. administration of iron. These reactions aren't related to hypersensitivity reactions and

may result from too-rapid administration. Don't exceed recommended rate of administration (2.1 mg/minute). Monitor patient closely during infusion.

### ACTION
Restores total body iron content, which is critical for normal hemoglobin synthesis and oxygen transport.

| Route | Onset | Peak | Duration |
|-------|---------|---------|----------|
| I.V.  | Unknown | Unknown | Unknown |

### ADVERSE REACTIONS
**CNS:** asthenia, headache, fatigue, malaise, *dizziness,* paresthesia, agitation, insomnia, somnolence, syncope, pain, chills, fever.
**CV:** *hypotension, hypertension,* tachycardia, *bradycardia,* angina, chest pain, *MI,* edema, flushing.
**EENT:** conjunctivitis, abnormal vision, rhinitis.
**GI:** *nausea, vomiting, diarrhea,* rectal disorder, dyspepsia, eructation, flatulence, melena, abdominal pain.
**GU:** urinary tract infection.
**Hematologic:** anemia.
**Metabolic:** *hyperkalemia, hypoglycemia,* hypokalemia, hypervolemia.
**Musculoskeletal:** myalgia, arthralgia, back pain, arm pain, *cramps.*
**Respiratory:** *dyspnea,* coughing, upper respiratory tract infection, pneumonia, pulmonary edema.
**Skin:** pruritus, increased sweating, rash, *injection site reaction.*
**Other:** infection, rigors, flu syndrome, *sepsis, carcinoma,* hypersensitivity reactions, lymphadenopathy.

### INTERACTIONS
None significant.

### EFFECTS ON LAB TEST RESULTS
• May increase or decrease potassium level. May decrease glucose level.
• May decrease hemoglobin.

### CONTRAINDICATIONS & CAUTIONS
• Contraindicated in patients hypersensitive to drug or its components (such as benzyl alcohol) and in those with iron overload or anemias not related to iron deficiency.

---

Reactions may be *common,* uncommon, *life-threatening,* or COMMON AND LIFE-THREATENING.

• Use cautiously in elderly patients.

**NURSING CONSIDERATIONS**
• *Alert:* Dosage is expressed in milligrams of elemental iron.
• Drug shouldn't be given to patients with iron overload, which often occurs in hemoglobinopathies and other refractory anemias.
• *Alert:* Potentially life-threatening hypersensitivity reactions (with CV collapse, cardiac arrest, bronchospasm, oral or pharyngeal edema, dyspnea, angioedema, urticaria, or pruritus sometimes linked to pain and muscle spasm of chest or back) may occur during infusion. Have adequate supportive measures readily available. Monitor patient closely during infusion.
• Monitor hemoglobin, hematocrit, and ferritin and iron saturation levels.
• Some adverse reactions in hemodialysis patients may be related to dialysis itself or to chronic renal failure.
• Check with patient about other potential sources of iron, such as OTC iron preparations and iron-containing multiple vitamins with minerals.

**PATIENT TEACHING**
• Urge patient to notify prescriber immediately if abdominal pain, diarrhea, vomiting, drowsiness, or rapid breathing occurs. These symptoms may indicate iron poisoning.

# 64

## Anticoagulants

argatroban
bivalirudin
dalteparin sodium
enoxaparin sodium
fondaparinux sodium
heparin calcium
heparin sodium
tinzaparin sodium
warfarin sodium

**COMBINATION PRODUCTS**
None.

---

### argatroban

*Pregnancy risk category B*

**AVAILABLE FORMS**
*Injection:* 100 mg/ml

**INDICATIONS & DOSAGE**
➤ **To prevent or treat thrombosis in patients with heparin-induced thrombocytopenia**
*Adults:* 2 mcg/kg/minute, given as a continuous I.V. infusion; adjust dose until the steady-state aPTT is 1.5 to 3 times the initial baseline value, not to exceed 100 seconds; maximum dose 10 mcg/kg/minute.
*Adjust-a-dose:* For patients with moderate hepatic impairment, reduce first dose to 0.5 mcg/kg/minute, given as a continuous infusion. Monitor the aPTT closely and adjust dosage p.r.n.
➤ **Anticoagulation in patients with or at risk for heparin-induced thrombocytopenia during percutaneous coronary interventions (PCI)**
*Adults:* 350 mcg/kg I.V. bolus over 3 to 5 minutes. Start a continuous I.V. infusion at 25 mcg/kg/minute. Check activated clotting time (ACT) 5 to 10 minutes after the bolus dose is completed.
*Adjust-a-dose:* Use the following table to adjust the dosage.

| ACT | Additional I.V. bolus | Continuous I.V. infusion |
|---|---|---|
| < 300 sec | 150 mcg/kg | 30 mcg/kg/min* |
| 300-450 sec | None needed | 25 mcg/kg/min |
| > 450 sec | None needed | 15 mcg/kg/min* |

*Check ACT again after 5 to 10 minutes.

In case of dissection, impending abrupt closure, thrombus formation during the procedure, or inability to achieve or maintain an ACT exceeding 300 seconds, give an additional bolus of 150 mcg/kg and increase infusion rate to 40 mcg/kg/minute. Check ACT again after 5 to 10 minutes.

**I.V. ADMINISTRATION**
• Dilute in normal saline solution, $D_5W$, or lactated Ringer's injection to a final concentration of 1 mg/ml.
• Dilute each 2.5-ml vial 100-fold by mixing it with 250 ml of diluent.
• Mix the constituted solution by repeated inversion of the diluent bag for 1 minute.
• Prepared solutions are stable for up to 24 hours at 77° F (25° C). Don't expose to direct sunlight.

**ACTION**
Reversibly binds to the thrombin-active site and inhibits thrombin-catalyzed or -induced reactions: fibrin formation, coagulation factor V, VIII, and XIII activation, protein C activation, and platelet aggregation. May inhibit the action of free and clot-associated thrombin.

| Route | Onset | Peak | Duration |
|---|---|---|---|
| I.V. | Rapid | 1-3 hr | Duration of infusion |

**ADVERSE REACTIONS**
**CNS:** *cerebrovascular disorder, hemorrhage,* fever, pain.
**CV:** *atrial fibrillation, cardiac arrest,* hypotension, *ventricular tachycardia.*
**GI:** abdominal pain, diarrhea, *GI bleeding,* nausea, vomiting.

---

Reactions may be *common*, uncommon, *life-threatening*, or COMMON AND LIFE-THREATENING.

**GU:** abnormal renal function, groin bleeding, *hematuria,* UTI.
**Respiratory:** cough, dyspnea, pneumonia, hemoptysis.
**Other:** allergic reactions, brachial bleeding, infection, *sepsis.*

**INTERACTIONS**
**Drug-drug.** *Antiplatelet agents, heparin, thrombolytics:* May increase risk of intracranial bleeding. Avoid using together.
*Oral anticoagulants:* May prolong PT and INR and may increase risk of bleeding. Monitor patient closely.

**EFFECTS ON LAB TEST RESULTS**
• May decrease hemoglobin and hematocrit.

**CONTRAINDICATIONS & CAUTIONS**
• Contraindicated in patients who have overt major bleeding who are hypersensitive to drug or any of its components.
• Use cautiously in patients with hepatic disease or conditions that increase the risk of hemorrhage, such as severe hypertension.
• Use cautiously in patients who have just had lumbar puncture, spinal anesthesia, or major surgery, especially of the brain, spinal cord, or eye; patients with hematologic conditions causing increased bleeding tendencies, such as congenital or acquired bleeding disorders; and patients with GI ulcers or other lesions.

**NURSING CONSIDERATIONS**
• Stop all parenteral anticoagulants before giving argatroban. Giving argatroban with antiplatelets, thrombolytics, and other anticoagulants may increase risk of bleeding.
• Get results of baseline coagulation tests, platelets, hemoglobin, and hematocrit before starting therapy, and report any abnormalities to the prescriber.
• Check aPTT 2 hours after giving drug; dose adjustments may be required to get a targeted aPTT of 1.5 to 3 times the baseline, no longer than 100 seconds. Steady state is achieved 1 to 3 hours after starting argatroban.
• Draw blood for additional ACT about every 20 to 30 minutes during a prolonged PCI procedure.

• Patients receiving argatroban can hemorrhage from any site in the body. Any unexplained decrease in hematocrit or blood pressure or any other unexplained symptoms may signify a hemorrhagic event.
• To convert to oral anticoagulant therapy, give warfarin P.O. with argatroban at up to 2 mcg/kg/minute until the INR exceeds 4 on combined therapy. After argatroban is stopped, repeat the INR in 4 to 6 hours. If the repeat INR is less than the desired therapeutic range, resume the I.V. argatroban infusion. Repeat the procedure daily until the desired therapeutic range on warfarin alone is reached.
• It's unknown if drug appears in breast milk. Tell patient to either stop breast-feeding or stop treatment, taking into account the importance of the drug to the mother.
• **Alert:** Don't confuse argatroban with Aggrastat (tirofiban).

**PATIENT TEACHING**
• Tell patient that this drug can cause bleeding, and ask him to report any unusual bruising or bleeding (nosebleeds, bleeding gums) or tarry stools to the prescriber immediately.
• Advise patient to avoid activities that carry a risk of injury, and to use a soft toothbrush and an electric razor while receiving argatroban.
• Instruct patient to notify prescriber if he has wheezing, trouble breathing, or skin rash.
• Instruct patient to notify prescriber if she is pregnant, has recently delivered, or is breast-feeding.
• Tell patient to notify prescriber if he has GI ulcers or liver disease, or has had recent surgery, radiation treatment, falling episodes, or injury.

**bivalirudin**
Angiomax

*Pregnancy risk category B*

**AVAILABLE FORMS**
*Injection:* 250-mg vial

## INDICATIONS & DOSAGES
➤ **Unstable angina in patients undergoing percutaneous transluminal coronary angioplasty (PTCA)**
*Adults:* 1 mg/kg I.V. bolus just before PTCA; then begin 4-hour I.V. infusion at 2.5 mg/kg/hour. After first 4-hour infusion, give an additional I.V. infusion at a rate of 0.2 mg/kg/hour for up to 20 hours p.r.n. Give with 300 to 325 mg aspirin.
*Adjust-a-dose:* For patients with renal impairment, give normal bolus dose and adjust infusion dose according to creatinine clearance. For creatinine clearance 30 to 59 ml/minute, reduce dose by 20%. For creatinine clearance 10 to 29 ml/minute, reduce dose by 60%. For dialysis-dependent patients (off dialysis), reduce dose by 90%.

## I.V. ADMINISTRATION
● Reconstitute each 250-mg vial with 5 ml of sterile water for injection. Further dilute each reconstituted vial in 50 ml D₅W or normal saline solution to yield a final concentration of 5 mg/ml.
● To prepare low-rate infusion, further dilute each reconstituted vial in 500 ml D₅W or normal saline solution to yield a final concentration of 0.5 mg/ml.
● Don't mix other drugs with bivalirudin before or during administration.
● The prepared solution is stable for 24 hours at 36° to 46° F (2° to 8° C).

## ACTION
Drug binds specifically and rapidly to thrombin to produce an anticoagulant effect.

| Route | Onset | Peak | Duration |
|-------|-------|------|----------|
| I.V. | Rapid | Immediate | 1-2 hr |

## ADVERSE REACTIONS
**CNS:** anxiety, *headache,* insomnia, nervousness, fever, *pain.*
**CV:** *bradycardia,* hypertension, *hypotension.*
**GI:** abdominal pain, dyspepsia, *nausea,* vomiting.
**GU:** urine retention.
**Hematologic:** *severe, spontaneous bleeding* (cerebral, retroperitoneal, GU, GI).
**Musculoskeletal:** *back pain,* pelvic pain.
**Skin:** pain at injection site.

## INTERACTIONS
**Drug-drug.** *Glycoprotein IIb/IIIa inhibitors:* Safety and effectiveness not yet established. Avoid using together.
*Heparin, warfarin, other oral anticoagulants:* May increase risk of bleeding. Use together cautiously. Stop heparin at least 8 hours before giving bivalirudin.

## EFFECTS ON LAB TEST RESULTS
None reported.

## CONTRAINDICATIONS & CAUTIONS
● Contraindicated in patients hypersensitive to drug or its components and in those with active major bleeding. Avoid using in patients with unstable angina who aren't undergoing PTCA or in patients with other acute coronary syndromes.
● Use cautiously in patients with heparin-induced thrombocytopenia or heparin-induced thrombocytopenia-thrombosis syndrome, and in patients with diseases linked to increased risk of bleeding.
● It's unknown if drug appears in breast milk. Use cautiously in breast-feeding women.

## NURSING CONSIDERATIONS
● Don't give by I.M. route.
● Hemorrhage can occur at any site in the body in patients receiving bivalirudin. Consider a hemorrhagic event if unexplained decrease in hematocrit, decrease in blood pressure, or other unexplained symptom occurs.
● Monitor coagulation test results, hemoglobin, and hematocrit before starting therapy and periodically throughout therapy.
● Monitor venipuncture sites for bleeding, hematoma, or inflammation.
● Puncture-site hemorrhage and catheterization site hematoma may occur in more patients age 65 and older than in younger patients.

## PATIENT TEACHING
● Advise patient that drug can cause bleeding and tell him to report unusual bruising or bleeding (nosebleeds, bleeding gums) or tarry stools immediately.
● Counsel patient that drug is given with aspirin and caution him to avoid other

---

aspirin-containing drugs or NSAIDs while receiving bivalirudin.
● Advise patient to avoid activities that carry a risk of injury and instruct him to use a soft toothbrush and electric razor while on drug.

---

## dalteparin sodium
Fragmin

*Pregnancy risk category B*

### AVAILABLE FORMS
*Injection:* 2,500 antifactor Xa IU/0.2 ml syringe, 5,000 antifactor Xa IU/0.2 ml syringe, 10,000 antifactor Xa IU/ml in 9.5-ml vial

### INDICATIONS & DOSAGES
➤ **To prevent deep vein thrombosis (DVT) in patients undergoing abdominal surgery who are at risk for thromboembolic complications**
*Adults:* 2,500 IU S.C. daily, starting 1 to 2 hours before surgery and repeated once daily for 5 to 10 days postoperatively.
➤ **To prevent DVT in patients undergoing hip replacement surgery**
*Adults:* 2,500 IU S.C. within 2 hours before surgery and second dose 2,500 IU S.C. in the evening after surgery (at least 6 hours after first dose). If surgery is performed in the evening, omit second dose on day of surgery. Starting on first postoperative day, give 5,000 IU S.C. once daily for 5 to 10 days. Or, give 5,000 IU S.C. on the evening before surgery; then 5,000 IU S.C. once daily starting in the evening of surgery for 5 to 10 days postoperatively.
➤ **Unstable angina and non–Q-wave MI**
*Adults:* 120 IU/kg S.C. q 12 hours with aspirin P.O., unless contraindicated. Maximum dose, 10,000 IU. Treatment usually lasts 5 to 8 days.

### ACTION
A low–molecular-weight heparin derivative that enhances inhibition of factor Xa and thrombin by antithrombin.

| Route | Onset | Peak | Duration |
|-------|-------|------|----------|
| S.C. | Unknown | 4 hr | Unknown |

### ADVERSE REACTIONS
**CNS:** fever.
**Hematologic:** *thrombocytopenia, hemorrhage,* ecchymoses, bleeding complications.
**Skin:** pruritus, rash, *hematoma at injection site,* injection site pain.
**Other:** *anaphylaxis.*

### INTERACTIONS
**Drug-drug.** *Antiplatelet drugs, oral anticoagulants, thrombolytics:* May increase risk of bleeding. Use together cautiously.

### EFFECTS ON LAB TEST RESULTS
● May increase ALT and AST levels.
● May decrease platelet count.

### CONTRAINDICATIONS & CAUTIONS
● Contraindicated in patients hypersensitive to drug, heparin, or pork products; in those with active major bleeding; and in those with thrombocytopenia and antiplatelet antibodies in presence of drug.
● Use with extreme caution in patients with history of heparin-induced thrombocytopenia and in patients at increased risk for hemorrhage, such as those with severe uncontrolled hypertension, bacterial endocarditis, congenital or acquired bleeding disorders, active ulceration, angiodysplastic GI disease, or hemorrhagic CVA; also use with extreme caution shortly after brain, spinal, or ophthalmic surgery. Monitor vital signs.
● Use with caution in patients with bleeding diathesis, thrombocytopenia, platelet defects, severe hepatic or renal insufficiency, hypertensive or diabetic retinopathy, or recent GI bleeding.

### NURSING CONSIDERATIONS
● *Alert:* Patients receiving low–molecular-weight heparins or heparinoids who have epidural or spinal anesthesia or spinal puncture are at risk for developing epidural or spinal hematoma that can result in long-term paralysis. Risk increases with use of epidural catheters, drugs affecting hemostasis, or traumatic or repeated epidural or spinal punctures. Monitor these patients frequently for signs of neurologic impairment. Urgent treatment is needed.

---

- DVT is a risk factor in patients who are candidates for therapy, including those older than age 40, those who are obese, those undergoing surgery under general anesthesia lasting longer than 30 minutes, and those who have additional risk factors (such as malignancy or history of DVT or pulmonary embolism).
- Have patient sit or lie supine when giving drug. Give S.C. injection deeply. Injection sites include a U-shaped area around the navel, upper outer side of thigh, and upper outer quadrangle of buttock. Rotate sites daily. When area around the navel or thigh is used, use thumb and forefinger to lift up a fold of skin while giving injection. Insert the entire length of needle at a 45- to 90-degree angle.
- Never give drug I.M.
- Don't mix with other injections or infusions unless specific compatibility data support such mixing.
- Multidose vial shouldn't be used in pregnant women.
- **Alert:** Drug isn't interchangeable (unit for unit) with unfractionated heparin or other low–molecular-weight heparin.
- Periodic, routine CBC and fecal occult blood tests are recommended during therapy. Patients don't need regular monitoring of PT or activated PTT.
- Monitor patient closely for thrombocytopenia.
- Stop drug if a thromboembolic event occurs despite dalteparin prophylaxis. May use alternative therapy, or may have been inadequate dose.

**PATIENT TEACHING**
- Instruct patient and family to watch for and report signs of bleeding (bruising and blood in stools).
- Tell patient to avoid OTC drugs containing aspirin or other salicylates unless ordered by prescriber.

## enoxaparin sodium
Lovenox

*Pregnancy risk category B*

**AVAILABLE FORMS**
*Ampules:* 30 mg/0.3 ml

*Syringes (prefilled):* 30 mg/0.3 ml, 40 mg/0.4 ml
*Syringes (graduated prefilled):* 60 mg/0.6 ml, 80 mg/0.8 ml, 100 mg/ml, 120 mg/0.8 ml, 150 mg/ml
*Vial (multi-dose):* 300 mg/3 ml (contains 15 mg/mL of benzyl alcohol)

**INDICATIONS & DOSAGES**
➤ **To prevent pulmonary embolism and deep vein thrombosis (DVT) after hip or knee replacement surgery**
*Adults:* 30 mg S.C. q 12 hours for 7 to 10 days. Give initial dose between 12 and 24 hours postoperatively, provided hemostasis has been established. Continue treatment during postoperative period until risk of DVT has diminished. Hip replacement patients may receive 40 mg S.C. given 12 hours preoperatively. After initial phase of therapy, hip replacement patients should continue with 40 mg S.C. daily for 3 weeks.
➤ **To prevent pulmonary embolism and DVT after abdominal surgery**
*Adults:* 40 mg S.C. daily with initial dose 2 hours before surgery. Give subsequent dose, provided hemostasis has been established, 24 hours after initial preoperative dose and continue once daily for 7 to 10 days. Continue treatment during postoperative period until risk of DVT has diminished.
➤ **To prevent ischemic complications of unstable angina and non–Q-wave MI with oral aspirin therapy**
*Adults:* 1 mg/kg S.C. q 12 hours until clinical stabilization (minimum 2 days) with aspirin 100 to 325 mg P.O. once daily.
➤ **Inpatient treatment of acute DVT with and without pulmonary embolism when given with warfarin sodium**
*Adults:* 1 mg/kg S.C. q 12 hours; or, 1.5 mg/kg S.C. once daily (at same time daily) for 5 to 7 days until therapeutic oral anticoagulant effect (INR 2 to 3) has been achieved. Warfarin sodium therapy is usually started within 72 hours of enoxaparin injection.
➤ **Outpatient treatment of acute DVT without pulmonary embolism when given with warfarin sodium**
*Adults:* 1 mg/kg S.C. q 12 hours for 5 to 7 days until therapeutic oral anticoagulant effect (INR 2 to 3) has been achieved.

Warfarin sodium therapy is usually started within 72 hours of enoxaparin injection.

➤ **To prevent embolism in patients with acute illness who are at increased risk because of decreased mobility**

*Adults:* 40 mg once daily S.C. for 6 to 11 days. Treatment for up to 14 days has been well tolerated.

*Adjust-a-dose:* If patient weighs less than 45 kg (99 lb) or has a creatinine clearance of less than 30 ml/minute, decrease dose.

## ACTION

A low–molecular-weight heparin derivative that accelerates formation of antithrombin III–thrombin complex and deactivates thrombin, preventing conversion of fibrinogen to fibrin. Has a higher antifactor Xa–to–antifactor IIa activity ratio.

| Route | Onset | Peak | Duration |
|-------|-------|------|----------|
| S.C. | Unknown | 3-5 hr | 24 hr |

## ADVERSE REACTIONS

**CNS:** fever, pain.
**CV:** edema, peripheral edema.
**GI:** nausea.
**Hematologic:** hypochromic anemia, *thrombocytopenia, hemorrhage,* ecchymoses, bleeding complications.
**Skin:** irritation, pain, hematoma, and erythema at injection site; *rash; urticaria.*
**Other:** *angioedema, anaphylaxis.*

## INTERACTIONS

**Drug-drug.** *Anticoagulants, antiplatelet drugs, NSAIDs:* May increase risk of bleeding. Use together cautiously. Monitor PT and INR.

## EFFECTS ON LAB TEST RESULTS

● May increase ALT and AST levels.
● May decrease hemoglobin.

## CONTRAINDICATIONS & CAUTIONS

● Contraindicated in patients hypersensitive to drug, heparin, or pork products; in those with active major bleeding; and in those with thrombocytopenia and antiplatelet antibodies in presence of drug.
● Use with extreme caution in patients with history of heparin-induced thrombocytopenia, aneurysms, cerebrovascular hemorrhage, spinal or epidural punctures (as with anesthesia), uncontrolled hypertension, or threatened abortion.
● Use cautiously in elderly patients and in those with conditions that place them at increased risk for hemorrhage, such as bacterial endocarditis, congenital or acquired bleeding disorders, ulcer disease, angiodysplastic GI disease, hemorrhagic CVA, or recent spinal, eye, or brain surgery. Also, use cautiously in patients with regional or lumbar block anesthesia, blood dyscrasias, recent childbirth, pericarditis or pericardial effusion, renal insufficiency, or severe CNS trauma.

## NURSING CONSIDERATIONS

● The vascular access sheath for instrumentation should remain in place for 6 to 8 hours after a dose; give next dose no sooner than 6 to 8 hours after sheath removal. Monitor vital signs.
● The use of enoxaparin is not recommended for thromboprophylaxis in patients with prosthetic heart valves, because they may be at higher risk for thromboembolism.
● Monitor closely pregnant women receiving enoxaparin. Warn pregnant women and women of childbearing age about the potential hazard to the fetus and the mother if enoxaparin is given during pregnancy.
● There have been reports of congenital anomalies in infants born to women who received enoxaparin during pregnancy, including cerebral and limb anomalies, hypospadias, peripheral vascular malformation, fibrotic dysplasia, and cardiac defect.
● **Alert:** Patients receiving low–molecular-weight heparins or heparinoids who have epidural or spinal anesthesia or spinal puncture are at risk for developing epidural or spinal hematoma that can result in long-term paralysis. Risk increases with use of epidural catheters, drugs affecting hemostasis, or traumatic or repeated epidural or spinal punctures. Monitor these patients frequently for signs of neurologic impairment. Urgent treatment is needed.
● Draw blood to establish baseline coagulation parameters before therapy.
● Never give drug I.M.
● **Alert:** Don't try to expel the air bubble from the 30- or 40-mg prefilled syringes.

---

This may lead to loss of drug and an incorrect dosage administration.

• With patient lying down, give by deep S.C. injection, alternating doses between left and right anterolateral and posterolateral abdominal walls.

• Don't massage after S.C. injection. Watch for signs of bleeding at site. Rotate sites and keep record.

• Avoid excessive I.M. injections of other drugs to prevent or minimize hematomas. If possible, don't give I.M. injections at all.

• Monitor platelet counts regularly. Patients with normal coagulation won't need close monitoring of PT or PTT.

• Regularly inspect patient for bleeding gums, bruises on arms or legs, petechiae, nosebleeds, melena, tarry stools, hematuria, hematemesis.

• To treat severe overdose, give protamine sulfate (a heparin antagonist) by slow I.V. infusion at concentration of 1% to equal dose of drug injected.

• *Alert:* Enoxaparin isn't interchangeable with heparin or other low–molecular-weight heparins.

## PATIENT TEACHING

• Instruct patient and family to watch for signs of bleeding or abnormal bruising and to notify prescriber immediately if any occur.

• Tell patient to avoid OTC drugs containing aspirin or other salicylates unless ordered by prescriber.

---

## fondaparinux sodium
Arixtra

*Pregnancy risk category B*

### AVAILABLE FORMS
*Injection:* 2.5 mg/0.5 ml single-dose pre-filled syringe

### INDICATIONS & DOSAGES
➤ **To prevent deep vein thrombosis (DVT), which may lead to pulmonary embolism, in patients undergoing surgery for hip fracture, hip replacement, or knee replacement**
*Adults:* 2.5 mg S.C. once daily for 5 to 9 days; maximum 11 days. Give initial

dose after hemostasis is established, 6 to 8 hours after surgery. Giving the dose earlier than 6 hours after surgery increases the risk for major bleeding. In patients undergoing hip fracture surgery, an extended prophylaxis course of up to 24 additional days is recommended, and a total of 32 days (perioperative and extended prophylaxis) has been tolerated.

### ACTION
Fondaparinux binds to antithrombin III (AT-III) and potentiates by about 300 times, the natural neutralization of factor Xa by AT-III. Neutralization of factor Xa interrupts the coagulation cascade and thereby inhibits formation of thrombin and blood clots.

| Route | Onset | Peak | Duration |
|-------|-------|------|----------|
| S.C. | Unknown | 2-3 hr | Unknown |

### ADVERSE REACTIONS
**CNS:** *fever,* insomnia, dizziness, confusion, headache, pain.
**CV:** hypotension, edema.
**GI:** *nausea,* constipation, vomiting, diarrhea, dyspepsia.
**GU:** UTI, urinary retention.
**Hematologic:** *hemorrhage, anemia,* hematoma, *postoperative hemorrhage, thrombocytopenia.*
**Metabolic:** hypokalemia.
**Skin:** mild local irritation (injection site bleeding, rash, pruritus), bullous eruption, purpura, rash, increased wound drainage.

### INTERACTIONS
**Drug-drug.** *Drugs that increase risk of bleeding (NSAIDs, platelet inhibitors, anticoagulants):* May increase risk of hemorrhage. Stop use before starting fondaparinux. If drugs must be used together, monitor patient closely.

### EFFECTS ON LAB TEST RESULTS
• May increase AST, ALT, and bilirubin levels. May decrease potassium level.
• May decrease hemoglobin, hematocrit, and platelet count.

### CONTRAINDICATIONS & CAUTIONS
• Contraindicated in patients with creatinine clearance less than 30 ml/minute and

---

Reactions may be *common,* uncommon, *life-threatening,* or COMMON AND LIFE-THREATENING.

in those who are hypersensitive to the drug or weigh less than 50 kg (110 lb).
- Contraindicated in patients with active major bleeding, bacterial endocarditis, or thrombocytopenia with a positive test result for antiplatelet antibody after taking fondaparinux.
- Use with extreme caution in patients being treated with platelet inhibitors; in those at increased risk for bleeding, such as congenital or acquired bleeding disorders; in those with active ulcerative and angiodysplastic GI disease; in those with hemorrhagic stroke; or in patients shortly after brain, spinal, or ophthalmologic surgery.
- Use cautiously in patients who have had epidural or spinal anesthesia or spinal puncture; they are at increased risk for developing an epidural or spinal hematoma (which may cause paralysis).
- Use cautiously in elderly patients, in patients with creatinine clearance 30 to 50 ml/minute, and in those with a history of heparin-induced thrombocytopenia, a bleeding diathesis, uncontrolled arterial hypertension, history of recent GI ulceration, diabetic retinopathy, or hemorrhage.

**NURSING CONSIDERATIONS**
- Give by S.C. injection only, never I.M. Visually inspect the single-dose, prefilled syringe for particulate matter and discoloration before administration.
- Don't mix with other injections or infusions.
- Don't use interchangeably with heparin, low–molecular-weight heparins, or heparinoids.
- *Alert:* To avoid loss of drug, don't expel air bubble from the syringe.
- Give the drug S.C. in fatty tissue, rotating administration injection sites. If the drug has been properly injected, the needle will pull back into the syringe security sleeve and the white safety indicator will appear above the blue upper body. A soft click may be heard or felt when the syringe plunger is fully released. After injection of the syringe contents, the plunger automatically rises while the needle withdraws from the skin and retracts into the security sleeve. Don't recap the needle.
- *Alert:* Patients who have received epidural or spinal anesthesia are at increased risk

for developing an epidural or spinal hematoma, which may result in long-term or permanent paralysis. Monitor these patients closely for neurologic impairment.
- Monitor renal function periodically and stop drug in patients who develop unstable renal function or severe renal impairment while on therapy.
- Routinely assess patient for signs and symptoms of bleeding, and regularly monitor CBC, platelet count, creatinine level, and stool occult blood test results. Stop use if platelet count is less than 100,000/mm³.
- Anticoagulant effects may last for 2 to 4 days after stopping drug in patients with normal renal function.
- PT and activated PTT aren't suitable monitoring tests to measure fondaparinux activity. If unexpected changes in coagulation parameters or major bleeding occurs, stop drug.
- *Alert:* Don't confuse Arixtra (fondaparinux) with Bextra (valdecoxib).

**PATIENT TEACHING**
- Tell patient to report signs and symptoms of bleeding.
- Instruct patient to avoid OTC products that contain aspirin or other salicylates.
- Teach patient the correct technique of S.C. drug administration if patient is to self-administer.

---

**heparin calcium‡**
Uniparin-Ca‡

**heparin sodium**
Hepalean†, Heparin Leo†, Heparin Lock Flush Solution (with Tubex), Heparin Sodium Injection, Hep-Lock, Hep-Pak, Uniparin‡

*Pregnancy risk category C*

**AVAILABLE FORMS**
Products are derived from beef lung or pork intestinal mucosa.
**heparin calcium‡**
*Ampule:* 12,500 units/0.5 ml; 20,000 units/0.8 ml
*Syringe:* 5,000 units/0.2 ml
**heparin sodium**
*Carpuject:* 5,000 units/ml

*Premixed I.V. solutions:* 1,000 units in 500 ml of normal saline solution; 2,000 units in 1,000 ml of normal saline solution; 12,500 units in 250 ml of half-normal saline solution; 25,000 units in 250 ml of half-normal saline solution; 25,000 units in 500 ml of half-normal saline solution; 10,000 units in 100 ml of $D_5W$; 12,500 units in 250 ml of $D_5W$; 20,000 units in 500 ml of $D_5W$; 25,000 units in 250 ml $D_5W$; 25,000 units in 500 ml $D_5W$

*Syringes:* 1,000 units/ml, 2,500 units/ml, 5,000 units/ml, 7,500 units/ml, 10,000 units/ml, 20,000 units/ml

*Unit-dose vials:* 1,000 units/ml, 5,000 units/ml, 10,000 units/ml, 20,000 units/ml, 40,000 units/ml

*Vials:* 1,000 units/ml, 2,000 units/ml, 2,500 units/ml, 5,000 units/ml, 7,500 units/ml, 10,000 units/ml, 20,000 units/ml, 40,000 units/ml

**heparin sodium flush**
*Syringes:* 10 units/ml, 100 units/ml
*Vials:* 10 units/ml, 100 units/ml

## INDICATIONS & DOSAGES
Dosage is highly individualized depending on disease state, age, and renal and hepatic status.

➤ **Full-dose continuous I.V. infusion therapy for deep vein thrombosis (DVT), MI, pulmonary embolism**
*Adults:* Initially, 5,000 units by I.V. bolus; then 750 to 1,500 units/hour by I.V. infusion with pump. Titrate hourly rate based on PTT results (q 4 hours in the early stages of treatment).
*Children:* Initially, 50 units/kg I.V.; then 25 units/kg/hour or 20,000 units/m² daily by I.V. infusion pump. Titrate dosage based on PTT.

➤ **Full-dose S.C. therapy for DVT, MI, pulmonary embolism**
*Adults:* Initially, 5,000 units I.V. bolus and 10,000 to 20,000 units in a concentrated solution S.C.; then 8,000 to 10,000 units S.C. q 8 hours or 15,000 to 20,000 units in a concentrated solution q 12 hours.

➤ **Full-dose intermittent I.V. therapy for DVT, MI, pulmonary embolism**
*Adults:* Initially, 10,000 units by I.V. bolus; then titrated according to PTT, and 5,000 to 10,000 units I.V. q 4 to 6 hours.

*Children:* Initially, 100 units/kg by I.V. bolus; then 50 to 100 units/kg q 4 hours.

➤ **Fixed low-dose therapy for venous thrombosis, pulmonary embolism, atrial fibrillation with embolism, postoperative DVT, and prevention of embolism**
*Adults:* 5,000 units S.C. q 12 hours. In surgical patients, give first dose 1 to 2 hours before procedure; then 5,000 units S.C. q 8 to 12 hours for 5 to 7 days or until patient can walk.

➤ **Consumptive coagulopathy (such as disseminated intravascular coagulation)**
*Adults:* 50 to 100 units/kg by I.V. bolus or continuous I.V. infusion q 4 hours.
*Children:* 25 to 50 units/kg by I.V. bolus or continuous I.V. infusion q 4 hours. If no improvement within 4 to 8 hours, stop heparin.

➤ **Open-heart surgery**
*Adults:* For total body perfusion, 150 to 400 units/kg continuous I.V. infusion.

➤ **Patency maintenance of I.V. indwelling catheters**
*Adults:* 10 to 100 units I.V. flush. Use sufficient volume to fill device. Not intended for therapeutic use.

## I.V. ADMINISTRATION
• Give I.V. using infusion pump to provide maximum safety. Check constant I.V. infusions regularly, even when pumps are in good working order, to prevent overdose or underdose. Place notice above patient's bed to caution I.V. team or laboratory personnel to apply pressure dressings after taking blood.
• During intermittent I.V. therapy, always draw blood 30 minutes before next scheduled dose to avoid falsely elevated PTT. Blood for PTT may be drawn 4 hours after continuous I.V. heparin therapy starts. Blood for PTT should never be drawn from the I.V. tubing of the heparin infusion or from the infused vein, because falsely elevated PTT will result. Always draw blood from the opposite arm.
• Don't skip a dose or "catch up" with an I.V. solution containing heparin. If I.V. solution runs out, restart it as soon as possible, and reschedule bolus dose immediately. Monitor PTT.
• Concentrated heparin solutions (more than 100 units/ml) can irritate blood vessels.

• Never piggyback other drugs into an infusion line while heparin infusion is running. Never mix another drug and heparin in same syringe when giving a bolus.

## ACTION
Accelerates formation of antithrombin III–thrombin complex and deactivates thrombin, preventing conversion of fibrinogen to fibrin.

| Route | Onset | Peak | Duration |
|-------|-------|------|----------|
| I.V. | Immediate | Unknown | Variable |
| S.C. | 20-60 min | 2-4 hr | Variable |

## ADVERSE REACTIONS
**CNS:** fever.
**EENT:** rhinitis.
**Hematologic:** *hemorrhage, overly prolonged clotting time, thrombocytopenia.*
**Skin:** irritation, mild pain, hematoma, ulceration, cutaneous or S.C. necrosis, pruritus, urticaria.
**Other:** *white clot syndrome;* hypersensitivity reactions, including chills, *anaphylactoid reactions.*

## INTERACTIONS
**Drug-drug.** *Aspirin:* May increase risk of bleeding. Monitor coagulation studies and

hemophilia, thrombocytopenia, or hepatic disease with hypoprothrombinemia; suspected intracranial hemorrhage; suppurative thrombophlebitis; inaccessible ulcerative lesions (especially of GI tract) and open ulcerative wounds; extensive denudation of skin; ascorbic acid deficiency and other conditions that cause increased capillary permeability.
• Conditionally contraindicated during or after brain, eye, or spinal cord surgery; during spinal tap or spinal anesthesia; during continuous tube drainage of stomach or small intestine; and in subacute bacterial endocarditis, shock, advanced renal disease, threatened abortion, or severe hypertension.
• Use cautiously in women during menses or after childbirth and in patients with mild hepatic or renal disease, alcoholism, occupations with high risk of physical injury, or history of allergies, asthma, or GI ulcerations.

## NURSING CONSIDERATIONS
• Although heparin use is clearly hazardous in certain conditions, its risks and benefits must be evaluated.
• Draw blood to establish baseline coagulation parameters before therapy.
• When patient needs anticoagulation during pregnancy, most prescribers use heparin ... contain benzyl alcohol. Avoid using these products in neonates and pregnant women if possible.
• Drug requirements are higher in early phases of thrombogenic diseases and febrile states; they are lower when patient's condition stabilizes.
• Elderly patients should usually start at lower dosage.
• Check order and vial carefully; heparin comes in various concentrations.
• **Alert:** USP units and IU aren't equivalent for heparin.
• **Alert:** Heparin, low–molecular-weight heparins, and danaparoid aren't interchangeable.
• Give low-dose injections sequentially between iliac crests in lower abdomen deep into S.C. fat. Inject drug S.C. slowly into fat pad. Leave needle in place for 10 seconds after injection; then withdraw

orrhage. Monitor closely. May increase risk of hem-
**Drug-herb.** *Garlic, ginkgo, motherwort, red clover, white willow:* May increase risk of bleeding. Discourage use together.

**EFFECTS ON LAB TEST RESULTS**
• May increase ALT and AST levels.
• May increase INR, PT, and PTT. May decrease platelet count.
• Drug may cause false elevations in some tests for thyroxine level.

**CONTRAINDICATIONS & CAUTIONS**
• Contraindicated in patients hypersensitive to drug. Conditionally contraindicated in patients with active bleeding, blood dyscrasia, or bleeding tendencies, such as

*Rapid onset* †Canada ‡Australia ◇OTC ◆Off-label use ✐Photoguide *Liquid contains alcohol.

needle. Don't massage after S.C. injection, and watch for signs of bleeding at injection site. Alternate sites every 12 hours—right for morning, left for evening.
• Draw blood for PTT 4 to 6 hours after dose given by S.C. injection.
• Avoid excessive I.M. injections of other drugs to prevent or minimize hematomas. If possible, don't give I.M. injections at all.
• Measure PTT carefully and regularly. Anticoagulation is present when PTT values are 1½ to 2 times the control values.
• Monitor platelet count regularly. When new thrombosis accompanies thrombocytopenia (white clot syndrome), stop heparin.
• Regularly inspect patient for bleeding gums, bruises on arms or legs, petechiae, nosebleeds, melena, tarry stools, hematuria, and hematemesis.
• Monitor vital signs.
• *Alert:* To treat severe heparin calcium or sodium overdose, use protamine sulfate, a heparin antagonist. Dosage is based on the dose of heparin, its route of administration, and the time elapsed since it was given. Generally, 1 to 1.5 mg of protamine/100 units of heparin is given if only a few minutes have elapsed; 0.5 to 0.75 mg protamine/100 units heparin, if 30 to 60 minutes have elapsed; and 0.25 to 0.375 mg protamine/100 units heparin, if 2 hours or more have elapsed. Don't give more than 50 mg protamine.
• Abrupt withdrawal may cause increased coagulability; warfarin therapy usually overlaps heparin therapy for continuation of prophylaxis or treatment.

**PATIENT TEACHING**
• Instruct patient and family to watch for signs of bleeding or bruising and to notify prescriber immediately if any occur.
• Tell patient to avoid OTC drugs containing aspirin, other salicylates, or drugs that may interact with heparin unless ordered by prescriber.

## tinzaparin sodium
Innohep

*Pregnancy risk category B*

**AVAILABLE FORMS**
*Injection:* 20,000 anti-Xa IU/ml, in 2-ml vials

**INDICATIONS & DOSAGES**
➤ **Symptomatic deep vein thrombosis with or without pulmonary embolism with warfarin sodium**
*Adults:* 175 anti-Xa IU/kg of body weight S.C. once daily for at least 6 days and until patient is adequately anticoagulated with warfarin sodium (INR of at least 2) for 2 consecutive days. Start warfarin sodium therapy when appropriate, usually within 1 to 3 days of tinzaparin initiation. Volume of dose to be given may be calculated as follows:

$$\text{Patient weight} \times 0.00875 \text{ ml/kg} = \text{volume to be given in ml}$$

**ACTION**
A low–molecular-weight heparin that inhibits reactions that lead to blood clotting, including formation of fibrin clots. Also acts as a potent coinhibitor of several activated coagulation factors, especially factor ... of tissue ... may contribute ... fect.

| Route | Onset | Peak | Duration |
|-------|-------|------|----------|
| S.C. | 2-3 hr | 4-5 hr | 18-24 hr |

**ADVERSE REACTIONS**
**CNS:** headache, dizziness, insomnia, confusion, *cerebral or intracranial bleeding*, fever, pain.
**CV:** *arrhythmias*, chest pain, hypotension, hypertension, *MI, thromboembolism*, tachycardia, dependent edema, angina pectoris.
**EENT:** epistaxis, ocular hemorrhage.

Reactions may be common, uncommon, *life-threatening*, or COMMON AND LIFE-THREATENING.

**GI:** anorectal bleeding, constipation, flatulence, hematemesis, *GI hemorrhage,* nausea, vomiting, dyspepsia, retroperitoneal or intra-abdominal bleeding, melena.
**GU:** dysuria, hematuria, UTI, urine retention, *vaginal hemorrhage.*
**Hematologic:** *granulocytopenia, thrombocytopenia,* anemia, *agranulocytosis, pancytopenia, hemorrhage.*
**Musculoskeletal:** back pain, hemarthrosis.
**Respiratory:** pneumonia, respiratory disorder, dyspnea, *pulmonary embolism.*
**Skin:** bullous eruption, cellulitis, *injection site hematoma,* pruritus, purpura, rash, skin necrosis, wound hematoma, bullous eruption.
**Other:** hypersensitivity reaction, *spinal or epidural hematoma,* infection, impaired healing, *allergic reaction,* congenital anomaly, *fetal death,* fetal distress.

**INTERACTIONS**
**Drug-drug.** *Oral anticoagulants, platelet inhibitors (such as dextran, dipyridamole, NSAIDs, salicylates, sulfinpyrazone), thrombolytics:* May increase risk of bleeding. Use together cautiously. If drugs must be given together, monitor patient.

**EFFECTS ON LAB TEST RESULTS**
● May increase AST and ALT levels.
● May decrease hemoglobin and granulocyte, platelet, RBC, and WBC counts.

**CONTRAINDICATIONS & CAUTIONS**
● Contraindicated in patients hypersensitive to tinzaparin sodium or other low–molecular-weight heparins, heparin, sulfites, benzyl alcohol, or pork products. Also contraindicated in patients with active major bleeding and in those with history of heparin-induced thrombocytopenia.
● Use cautiously in patients with increased risk of hemorrhage, such as those with bacterial endocarditis; uncontrolled hypertension; diabetic retinopathy; congenital or acquired bleeding disorders, including hepatic failure and amyloidosis; GI ulceration; or hemorrhagic stroke. Also use cautiously in patients who have recently undergone brain, spinal, or ophthalmologic surgery, and in patients being treated with platelet inhibitors. Elderly patients

and patients with renal insufficiency may show reduced elimination of drug. Use drug with care in these patients.
● It's unknown if drug appears in breast milk. Use cautiously in breast-feeding women.

**NURSING CONSIDERATIONS**
● Drug isn't intended for I.M. or I.V. administration, nor should it be mixed with other injections or infusions.
● Don't interchange drug (unit to unit) with heparin or other low–molecular-weight heparins.
● When giving drug, have patient lie or sit down. Give by deep S.C. injection into abdominal wall. Introduce whole length of needle into skinfold held between thumb and forefinger. Make sure to hold skinfold throughout injection. Rotate injection sites between right and left anterolateral and posterolateral abdominal wall. To minimize bruising, don't rub injection site after administration.
● Use an appropriate calibrated syringe to ensure correct withdrawal of volume of drug from vials.
● Monitor platelet count during therapy. Stop drug if platelet count goes below 100,000/mm³.
● Periodically monitor CBC count and stool tests for occult blood during treatment.
● Drug may affect PT and INR levels. Patient also receiving warfarin should have blood for PT and INR drawn just before next scheduled dose of tinzaparin.
● Drug contains sodium metabisulfite, which may cause allergic reactions in susceptible people.
● *Alert:* When neuraxial anesthesia (epidural or spinal anesthesia) or spinal puncture is used, patient is at risk for developing spinal hematoma, which can result in long-term or permanent paralysis. Watch for signs and symptoms of neurologic impairment. Consider risk versus benefit of neuraxial intervention in patient being treated with low–molecular-weight heparins or heparinoids.
● If patient becomes pregnant while taking drug, warn her of potential hazards to fetus. Cases of gasping syndrome have occurred in premature infants when large

---

amounts of benzyl alcohol have been given.
• Store drug at room temperature.

**PATIENT TEACHING**
• Explain to patient importance of laboratory monitoring to ensure effectiveness of drugs while maintaining safety.
• Teach patient warning signs of bleeding and instruct him to report these signs immediately.
• Caution patient to use soft toothbrush and electric razor to prevent cuts and bruises.
• Instruct patient that warfarin therapy will be started when appropriate, within 1 to 3 days of tinzaparin administration. Explain importance of warfarin therapy and monitoring to ensure safety and efficacy.

---

# warfarin sodium
Coumadin✒, Warfilone†

*Pregnancy risk category X*

**AVAILABLE FORMS**
*Injection:* 2 mg/ml (powder)
*Tablets:* 1 mg, 2 mg, 2.5 mg, 3 mg, 4 mg, 5 mg, 6 mg, 7.5 mg, 10 mg

**INDICATIONS & DOSAGES**
➤ **Pulmonary embolism with deep vein thrombosis, MI, rheumatic heart disease with heart valve damage, prosthetic heart valves, chronic atrial fibrillation**
*Adults:* 2 to 5 mg P.O. daily for 2 to 4 days; then dosage based on daily PT and INR. Usual maintenance dosage is 2 to 10 mg P.O. daily; I.V. dosage is same as that used P.O.

**I.V. ADMINISTRATION**
• I.V. form may be ordered in rare instances when oral therapy can't be given. Reconstitute powder with 2.7 ml sterile water, or as instructed in manufacturer guidelines. Give I.V. as a slow bolus injection over 1 to 2 minutes into a peripheral vein.
• Because onset of action is delayed, heparin sodium is often given during first few days of treatment. When heparin is being given simultaneously, blood for PT and

INR shouldn't be drawn within 5 hours of intermittent I.V. heparin administration. However, blood for PT and INR may be drawn at any time during continuous heparin infusion.

**ACTION**
Inhibits vitamin K–dependent activation of clotting factors II, VII, IX, and X, formed in the liver.

| Route | Onset | Peak | Duration |
|-------|-------|------|----------|
| P.O. | 12 hr-3 days | Unknown | 2-5 days |
| I.V. | Unknown | Unknown | Unknown |

**ADVERSE REACTIONS**
**CNS:** headache, *fever.*
**GI:** anorexia, nausea, vomiting, cramps, *diarrhea,* mouth ulcerations, sore mouth, melena.
**GU:** hematuria, excessive menstrual bleeding.
**Hematologic:** *hemorrhage.*
**Hepatic:** *hepatitis,* jaundice.
**Skin:** dermatitis, urticaria, necrosis, gangrene, alopecia, *rash.*
**Other:** enhanced uric acid excretion.

**INTERACTIONS**
**Drug-drug.** *Acetaminophen:* May increase bleeding with long-term therapy (more than 2 weeks) at high doses (more than 2 g/day) of acetaminophen. Monitor patient very carefully.
*Allopurinol, amiodarone, anabolic steroids, antidepressants, antifungals, cephalosporins, chloramphenicol, cimetidine, danazol, diazoxide, diflunisal, disulfiram, erythromycin, ethacrynic acid, fluoroquinolones, glucagon, heparin, influenza virus vaccine, isoniazid, meclofenamate, methimazole, metronidazole, nalidixic acid, neomycin (oral), NSAIDs, omeprazole, pentoxifylline, propafenone, propoxyphene, propylthiouracil, quinidine, sulfinpyrazone, sulfonamides, tamoxifen, tetracyclines, thiazides, thrombolytics, thyroid drugs, vitamin E:* May increase PT and INR. Monitor patient carefully for bleeding. Reduce anticoagulant dosage as directed.
*Anticonvulsants:* May increase levels of phenytoin and phenobarbital. Monitor drug levels closely.

---

*Aspirin, NSAIDs, salicylates:* May increase PT and INR; ulcerogenic effects. Avoid using together.

*Barbiturates, carbamazepine, corticosteroids, corticotropin, dicloxacillin, ethchlorvynol, griseofulvin, haloperidol, meprobamate, mercaptopurine, nafcillin, oral contraceptives containing estrogen, rifampin, spironolactone, sucralfate, trazodone:* May decrease PT and INR with reduced anticoagulant effect. Monitor patient carefully.

*Chloral hydrate, hypolipidemics, propylthiouracil:* May increase or decrease PT and INR. Avoid using, if possible, and monitor patient carefully.

*Cholestyramine:* May decrease response when given too closely together. Give 6 hours after oral anticoagulants.

*Sulfonylureas (oral antidiabetics):* May increase hypoglycemic response. Monitor glucose levels.

**Drug-herb.** *Angelica:* May significantly prolong PT and INR when *Angelica sinensis* is given with warfarin. Discourage use together.

*Anise, arnica flower, asafoetida, bromelain, celery, chamomile, clove, Danshen, devil's claw, dong quai, fenugreek, feverfew, garlic, ginger, ginkgo, ginseng, horse chestnut, licorice, meadowsweet, motherwort, onion, papain, parsley, passion flower, quassia, red clover, reishi mushroom, rue, sweet clover, turmeric, white willow:* May increase risk of bleeding. Discourage use together.

*Coenzyme Q10, ginseng, St. John's wort:* May reduce action of drug. Ask patient about use of herbal remedies, and advise caution.

*Green tea:* May decrease anticoagulant effect caused by vitamin K content of green tea. Advise patient to minimize variable consumption of green tea and other foods or nutritional supplements containing vitamin K.

**Drug-food.** *Foods, multivitamins, or enteral products containing vitamin K:* May impair anticoagulation. Tell patient to maintain consistent daily intake of leafy green vegetables.

**Drug-lifestyle.** *Alcohol use:* May enhance anticoagulant effects. Tell patient to avoid large amounts of alcohol.

## EFFECTS ON LAB TEST RESULTS
● May increase ALT and AST levels.
● May increase INR, PT, and PTT.
● May falsely decrease theophylline level.

## CONTRAINDICATIONS & CAUTIONS
● Contraindicated in patients hypersensitive to drug and in those with bleeding from the GI, GU, or respiratory tract; aneurysm; cerebrovascular hemorrhage; severe or malignant hypertension; severe renal or hepatic disease; subacute bacterial endocarditis, pericarditis, or pericardial effusion; or blood dyscrasias or hemorrhagic tendencies.
● Contraindicated during pregnancy, threatened abortion, eclampsia, or preeclampsia, and after recent surgery involving large open areas, eye, brain, or spinal cord; recent prostatectomy; major regional lumbar block anesthesia, spinal puncture, or diagnostic or therapeutic invasive procedures.
● Avoid using in patients with a history of warfarin-induced necrosis; in unsupervised patients with senility, alcoholism, or psychosis; or in situations in which there are inadequate laboratory facilities for coagulation testing.
● Use cautiously in patients with diverticulitis, colitis, mild or moderate hypertension, or mild or moderate hepatic or renal disease; with drainage tubes in any orifice; with regional or lumbar block anesthesia; or in conditions that increase risk of hemorrhage.
● Use cautiously in breast-feeding women.

## NURSING CONSIDERATIONS
● Draw blood to establish baseline coagulation parameters before therapy.
● PT and INR determinations are essential for proper control.
● Give warfarin at same time daily. INR range for chronic atrial fibrillation is 2 to 3.
● I.M. administration isn't recommended.
● Regularly inspect patient for bleeding gums, bruises on arms or legs, petechiae, nosebleeds, melena, tarry stools, hematuria, and hematemesis.
● Check for unexpected bleeding in breast-fed infants of women on drug.

• *Alert:* Withhold drug and call prescriber at once in the event of fever or rash (signs of severe adverse reactions).
• Half-life of warfarin's anticoagulant effect is 36 to 44 hours. Effect can be neutralized by parenteral or oral vitamin K.
• Elderly patients and patients with renal or hepatic failure are especially sensitive to warfarin effect.

## PATIENT TEACHING

• Stress importance of complying with prescribed dosage and follow-up appointments. Tell patient to carry a card that identifies his increased risk of bleeding.
• Tell patient and family to watch for signs of bleeding or abnormal bruising and to call prescriber at once if they occur.
• Warn patient to avoid OTC products containing aspirin, other salicylates, or drugs that may interact with warfarin unless ordered by prescriber.
• Tell patient to consult a prescriber before using miconazole vaginal cream or suppositories. Abnormal bleeding and bruising have occurred.
• Instruct woman to notify prescriber if menstruation is heavier than usual; she may need dosage adjustment.
• Tell patient to use electric razor when shaving to avoid scratching skin, and to use a soft toothbrush.
• Tell patient to read food labels. Food, nutritional supplements, and multivitamins that contain vitamin K may impair anticoagulation.
• Tell patient to eat a daily, consistent diet of food and drinks containing vitamin K, because eating varied amounts may alter anticoagulant effects.

albumin 5%
albumin 25%
antihemophilic factor
anti-inhibitor coagulant complex
antithrombin III, human
factor IX complex
factor IX (human)
factor IX (recombinant)
plasma protein fractions

**COMBINATION PRODUCTS**
None.

## albumin 5%
Albuminar-5, Albunex, Albutein
5%, Buminate 5%, Plasbumin-5

## albumin 25%
Albuminar-25, Albutein 25%,
Buminate 25%, Plasbumin-25

*Pregnancy risk category C*

**AVAILABLE FORMS**
**albumin 5%**
*Injection:* 5-ml, 10-ml, 20-ml, 50-ml,
250-ml, 500-ml, 1,000-ml vials
**albumin 25%**
*Injection:* 20-ml, 50-ml, 100-ml vials

**INDICATIONS & DOSAGES**
➤ **Hypovolemic shock**
*Adults:* Initially, 500 to 750 ml of 5% solution by I.V. infusion, repeated q 30 minutes, p.r.n. As plasma volume approaches normal, rate of infusion of 5% solution shouldn't exceed 2 to 4 ml/minute. Or, 100 to 200 ml I.V. of 25% solution, repeated after 10 to 30 minutes, if needed. Dosage varies with patient's condition and response. As plasma volume approaches normal, rate of infusion of 25% solution shouldn't exceed 1 ml/minute.
*Children:* 12 to 20 ml of 5% solution/kg by I.V. infusion, repeated in 15 to 30 minutes if response is inadequate. Or, 2.5 to 5 ml I.V. of 25% solution/kg, repeated after 10 to 30 minutes, if needed.

➤ **Hypoproteinemia**
*Adults:* 200 to 300 ml of 25% albumin. Dosage varies with patient's condition and response. Rate of infusion shouldn't exceed 2 to 3 ml/minute.
➤ **Hyperbilirubinemia**
*Infants:* 1 g albumin (4 ml of 25%)/kg 1 to 2 hours before exchange transfusion.

**I.V. ADMINISTRATION**
● Make sure patient is properly hydrated before infusion.
● To minimize waste, take care when preparing and giving drug. This product is expensive, and supply shortages frequently occur.
● Avoid rapid I.V. infusion. Specific rate is based on patient's age, condition, and diagnosis. Albumin 5% is infused undiluted; albumin 25% may be infused undiluted or diluted with normal saline solution or $D_5W$ injection. Use solution promptly. Discard unused solution. Don't use cloudy or sediment-filled solutions. Make sure solution is a clear amber color.
● *Alert:* Don't give more than 250 g in 48 hours.

**ACTION**
Albumin 5% supplies colloid to the blood and expands plasma volume. Albumin 25% provides intravascular oncotic pressure in a 5:1 ratio, causing a fluid shift from interstitial spaces to the circulation and slightly increasing plasma protein level.

| Route | Onset | Peak | Duration |
|-------|-------|------|----------|
| I.V. | < 15 min | < 15 min | Several hr |

**ADVERSE REACTIONS**
**CNS:** headache, fever.
**CV:** *vascular overload after rapid infusion,* hypotension, tachycardia.
**GI:** increased salivation, nausea, vomiting.
**Musculoskeletal:** back pain.
**Respiratory:** altered respiration, dyspnea, pulmonary edema.

**Skin:** urticaria, rash.
**Other:** chills.

## INTERACTIONS
**Drug-drug.** *ACE inhibitors:* May increase risk of atypical reactions. Withhold ACE inhibitors 24 hours before giving albumin, if possible.

## EFFECTS ON LAB TEST RESULTS
• May increase albumin level.

## CONTRAINDICATIONS & CAUTIONS
• Contraindicated in patients hypersensitive to drug and in those with severe anemia, pulmonary edema, or cardiac failure.
• Use with extreme caution in patients with hypertension, low cardiac reserve, hypervolemia, pulmonary edema, or hypoalbuminemia with peripheral edema.

## NURSING CONSIDERATIONS
• Watch for hemorrhage or shock after surgery or injury. Rapid increase in blood pressure may cause bleeding from sites that aren't apparent at lower pressures.
• Monitor vital signs carefully.
• Watch for signs of vascular overload (heart failure or pulmonary edema).
• Monitor fluid intake and output; hemoglobin, hematocrit and protein and electrolyte levels during therapy.
• Follow storage instructions on bottle. Freezing may cause bottle to break.

## PATIENT TEACHING
• Explain use and administration of albumin to patient and family.
• Tell patient to report adverse reactions promptly.

---

## antihemophilic factor (AHF)
Helixate FS, Hemofil M, Hyate:C, Koate-DVI, Kogenate, Kogenate FS, Monoclate-P, Recombinate, ReFacto

*Pregnancy risk category C*

---

## AVAILABLE FORMS
*Injection:* Vials, with diluent; units specified on label

## INDICATIONS & DOSAGES
Drug provides hemostasis in factor VIII deficiency, hemophilia A. The specific dosage depends on the patient's weight, severity of hemorrhage, and presence of inhibitors. Mild bleeding episodes require a circulating factor VIII level of 20% to 40% of normal; moderate to major bleeding episodes and minor surgery, a level of 30% to 60% of normal; severe bleeding or major surgery, a level of 80% to 100% of normal. The following dosages provide guidelines. Refer to specific brand for actual dosing.

The dose (IU/kg) can be calculated by dividing the desired level (as a percent of normal) by 2. For example, if a peak level of 50% is the goal, divide 50 by 2 to get 25 IU/kg.

➤ **Mild bleeding in patients with hemophilia**
*Adults and children:* 10 to 20 IU/kg daily.
➤ **Moderate bleeding and minor surgery in patients with hemophilia**
*Adults and children:* Initially, 15 to 30 IU/kg, then repeat one dose at 12 to 24 hours if needed.
➤ **Severe bleeding and bleeding near vital organs in patients with hemophilia**
*Adults and children:* Initially, 40 to 50 IU/kg, then 20 to 25 IU/kg q 8 to 12 hours, p.r.n.
➤ **Major surgery in patients with hemophilia**
*Adults and children:* 50 IU/kg 1 hour before surgery, then repeat p.r.n. 6 to 12 hours after first dose. Maintain circulating factor levels at 30% of normal for 10 to 14 days after surgery.

## I.V. ADMINISTRATION
• Refrigerate concentrate until ready to use. Warm concentrate and diluent bottles to room temperature before reconstituting. To mix drug, gently roll vial between hands.
• Use reconstituted solution within 3 hours. Store away from heat and don't refrigerate. Refrigeration after reconstitution may cause active ingredient to precipitate. Don't shake or mix with other I.V. solutions. Filter solution before giving. Use plastic syringe; drug may bind to glass syringe.

---

● Give I.V. preparations at 2 ml/minute; may be given up to 10 ml/minute, depending on the preparation being used.
● Take baseline pulse rate before I.V. administration. If pulse rate increases significantly, reduce flow rate or stop administration.

## ACTION
Directly replaces deficient clotting factor.

| Route | Onset | Peak | Duration |
|-------|-------|------|----------|
| I.V. | Immediate | 1-2 hr | Unknown |

## ADVERSE REACTIONS
**CNS:** headache, somnolence, lethargy, dizziness, tingling asthenia, *fever.*
**CV:** tightness in chest, ***thrombosis.***
**GI:** nausea.
**Hematologic:** *hemolytic anemia, **thrombocytopenia.***
**Hepatic:** *risk of hepatitis B.*
**Respiratory:** wheezing.
**Skin:** *urticaria,* stinging at injection site.
**Other:** *chills,* hypersensitivity reactions, ***anaphylaxis, risk of HIV.***

## INTERACTIONS
None significant.

## EFFECTS ON LAB TEST RESULTS
● May decrease hemoglobin and platelet count.

## CONTRAINDICATIONS & CAUTIONS
● Monoclonally prepared AHF is contraindicated in patients hypersensitive to drug or murine (mouse) protein.
● Use cautiously in neonates, infants, and patients with hepatic disease because of their susceptibility to hepatitis, which may be transmitted in AHF.

## NURSING CONSIDERATIONS
● Monitor coagulation studies before therapy.
● Monitor patients with blood types A, B, and AB for possible hemolysis.
● Change in urine color to orange or red can signify a hemolytic reaction.
● Give hepatitis B vaccine before giving AHF.
● Don't give drug I.M. or S.C.
● Monitor vital signs regularly.

● Monitor coagulation studies frequently during therapy.
● Monitor patient for allergic reactions.
● Some patients develop inhibitors to factor VIII, resulting in decreased response to drug.
● Risk of hepatitis must be weighed against risk of patient not receiving drug.
● Because of manufacturing process, risk of HIV transmission is extremely low.

## PATIENT TEACHING
● Explain use and administration of AHF to patient and family.
● Advise patient to report adverse reactions promptly.
● Advise patient to carry or wear medical identification.
● Tell patient to notify prescriber if drug seems less effective; a change may signify the development of antibodies.

## anti-inhibitor coagulant complex
Autoplex T, Feiba VH Immuno

*Pregnancy risk category C*

## AVAILABLE FORMS
*Injection:* Number of units of factor VIII correctional activity indicated on label of vial

## INDICATIONS & DOSAGES
➤ **To prevent or control hemorrhagic episodes in some patients with hemophilia A in whom inhibitor antibodies to antihemophilic factor have developed; to manage bleeding in patients with acquired hemophilia who have spontaneously acquired inhibitors to factor VIII**
Drug controls hemorrhage in hemophilia A patients who have a factor VIII inhibitor level above 10 Bethesda units. Patients with a level of 2 to 10 Bethesda units may receive the drug if they have severe hemorrhage or respond poorly to factor VIII infusion.
 Dosage is highly individualized and varies among manufacturers. For Autoplex T, give 25 to 100 unit/kg I.V. depending on the severity of hemorrhage. If no hemostatic improvement occurs within 6 hours af-

ter first administration, repeat dosage. For Feiba VH Immuno, give 50 to 100 units/kg I.V. q 6 or 12 hours until patient shows signs of improvement. Maximum daily dose of Feiba VH Immuno is 200 unit/kg.

➤ **Joint hemorrhage**
*Adults and children:* 50 to 100 units Feiba VH Immuno/kg q 12 hours until patient's condition improves.

➤ **Mucous membrane hemorrhage**
*Adults and children:* 50 units Feiba VH Immuno/kg q 6 hours, increasing to 100 units/kg q 6 hours if hemorrhage continues. Maximum daily dose, 200 units/kg.

➤ **Soft-tissue hemorrhage**
*Adults and children:* 100 units Feiba VH Immuno/kg q 12 hours. Maximum daily dose, 200 units/kg.

➤ **Other severe hemorrhage**
*Adults and children:* 100 units Feiba VH Immuno/kg q 12 hours (occasionally, q 6 hours).

## I.V. ADMINISTRATION

● Warm drug and diluent to room temperature before reconstitution. Reconstitute according to manufacturer's directions. Use filter needle provided by manufacturer to withdraw reconstituted solution from vial into syringe; filter needle should then be replaced with a sterile injection needle for administration. Give as soon as possible. If drug is given as an I.V. infusion, administration set must contain a filter. Complete Autoplex T infusions within 1 hour after reconstitution; Feiba VH Immuno infusions, within 3 hours.

● Dosages of the two available products aren't equivalent.

● Individualize rate of administration based on patient's response. Autoplex T infusions may begin at 2 ml/minute; if well tolerated, infusion rate may be increased gradually to 10 ml/minute. Feiba VH Immuno infusion rate shouldn't exceed 2 units/kg/minute.

● *Alert:* If flushing, lethargy, headache, transient chest discomfort, or changes in blood pressure or pulse rate develop because of a rapid infusion, stop drug and notify prescriber. These symptoms usually disappear when infusion stops. The infusion may then be resumed at a slower rate.

## ACTION

Unknown. Efficacy may be related in part to presence of activated factors, which leads to more complete factor X activation with tissue factor, phospholipid, and ionic calcium and allows the coagulation process to proceed beyond those stages in which factor VIII is needed.

| Route | Onset | Peak | Duration |
|---|---|---|---|
| I.V. | 10-30 min | Unknown | Unknown |

## ADVERSE REACTIONS

**CNS:** headache, lethargy, fever.
**CV:** changes in blood pressure, flushing, *acute MI, thromboembolic events.*
**GI:** nausea, vomiting.
**Hematologic:** *DIC.*
**Hepatic:** *risk of hepatitis B.*
**Skin:** rash, urticaria.
**Other:** chills, hypersensitivity reactions, *anaphylaxis, risk of HIV infection.*

## INTERACTIONS

**Drug-drug.** *Antifibrinolytic drugs:* May alter effects of anti-inhibitor coagulant complex. Avoid using together.

## EFFECTS ON LAB TEST RESULTS

None reported.

## CONTRAINDICATIONS & CAUTIONS

● Contraindicated in patients with DIC or a normal coagulation mechanism, in those showing signs of fibrinolysis. Feiba VH Immuno is contraindicated in neonates.
● Use cautiously in patients with liver disease.
● Use Autoplex T cautiously in neonates.

## NURSING CONSIDERATIONS

● Give hepatitis B vaccine before giving drug.
● Keep epinephrine available to treat anaphylaxis.
● Feiba VH Immuno shouldn't be used in neonates, but Autoplex T can be used with caution.
● Monitor patient closely for hypersensitivity reactions.
● Monitor vital signs regularly, and report significant changes to prescriber.
● Observe patient closely for signs of thromboembolic events.

---

Reactions may be *common*, uncommon, *life-threatening*, or COMMON AND LIFE-THREATENING.

• Reassure patient that, because of manufacturing process, risk of HIV transmission is extremely low.

## PATIENT TEACHING
• Explain use and administration of anti-inhibitor coagulant complex to patient and family.
• Tell patient to report adverse reactions promptly.

---

## antithrombin III, human (AT-III, heparin cofactor I)
Thrombate III

*Pregnancy risk category B*

## AVAILABLE FORMS
*Injection:* 500 IU, 1,000 IU

## INDICATIONS & DOSAGES
➤ **Thromboembolism related to hereditary AT-III deficiency**
*Adults and children:* First dose is individualized to quantity needed to increase AT-III activity to 120% of normal activity as determined 20 minutes after administration. Usual dose is 50 to 100 IU/minute I.V., not to exceed 100 IU/minute. Dose is calculated based on anticipated 1.4 % increase in plasma AT-III activity produced by 1 IU/kg of body weight using the following formula:

$$\text{Dose required (IU)} = \frac{(\text{desired activity [\%]} - \text{baseline activity [\%]}) \times \text{weight (kg)}}{1.4}$$

Maintenance dose is individualized to quantity needed to increase AT-III activity to 80% of normal activity and is given at 24-hour intervals.

To calculate subsequent dosages, multiply desired AT-III activity (as percentage of normal) minus baseline AT-III activity (as percentage of normal) by body weight (in kg). Divide by actual increase in AT-III activity (as percentage) produced by 1 IU/kg as determined 20 minutes after first dose is given.

## I.V. ADMINISTRATION
• Bring solution to room temperature before using. Use solution within 3 hours of preparation.

• Reconstitute using 10 ml of sterile water (provided), normal saline solution, or $D_5W$. Don't shake vial. Withdraw the dissolved solution using the manufacturer-provided filter needle. Dilute further in same diluent solution if desired. Infuse over 10 to 20 minutes. Give I.V. only. Don't mix with other drugs or diluents.
• Store drug at 36° to 46° F (2° to 8° C) until reconstituted. Don't refrigerate after reconstitution.

## ACTION
Replaces AT-III in patients with hereditary AT-III deficiency, normalizing coagulation inhibition and inhibiting thromboembolism formation. Also deactivates plasmin (to lesser extent than clotting factor).

| Route | Onset | Peak | Duration |
|-------|-------|------|----------|
| I.V. | Immediate | Unknown | 4 days |

## ADVERSE REACTIONS
**CNS:** dizziness.
**CV:** vasodilation, lowered blood pressure, chest tightness.
**GI:** nausea, foul taste.
**GU:** diuresis.
**Other:** chills.

## INTERACTIONS
**Drug-drug.** *Heparin:* May increase anticoagulant effect of both drugs. Heparin dosage reduction may be needed.

## EFFECTS ON LAB TEST RESULTS
None reported.

## CONTRAINDICATIONS & CAUTIONS
• Use with extreme caution in children and neonates because safety and efficacy haven't been established.

## NURSING CONSIDERATIONS
• Prepared from pooled plasma from human donors, drug carries minimal risk of transmission of viruses, including hepatitis and HIV.
• Treatment usually lasts 2 to 8 days but may be prolonged in pregnancy or when used with surgery or immobilization.
• **Alert:** Because infants of parents with hereditary AT-III deficiency are at risk for sometimes-fatal neonatal thromboem-

---

bolism, expect to obtain AT-III level immediately after birth.
● Obtain AT-III activity level every 12 hours until dosage requirement has stabilized, and then daily immediately before dose. Functional assays are preferred because quantitative immunologic test results may be normal despite decreased AT-III activity.
● Watch for dyspnea and increased blood pressure, which may occur if administration rate is too rapid.
● One IU is equivalent to quantity of endogenous AT-III present in 1 ml of normal human plasma.
● Heparin binds to AT-III lysine-binding sites, increasing heparin efficacy.
● Drug isn't recommended for long-term prophylaxis of thrombotic episodes.

### PATIENT TEACHING
● Explain use and administration of AT-III to patient and parents.
● Instruct patient to report adverse reactions promptly.

# factor IX complex
Bebulin VH, Profilnine SD, Proplex T

# factor IX (human)
AlphaNine SD, Mononine

# factor IX (recombinant)
Benefix

*Pregnancy risk category C*

### AVAILABLE FORMS
*Injection:* Vials, with diluent; IU specified on label

### INDICATIONS & DOSAGES
➤ **Factor IX deficiency (hemophilia B [Christmas disease]), anticoagulant overdosage**
*Adults and children:* To calculate IU of factor IX needed, use the following equations:

*Human product*

$$1 \text{ IU/kg} \times \begin{array}{c} \text{body} \\ \text{weight} \\ \text{in kg} \end{array} \times \begin{array}{c} \text{percentage of} \\ \text{desired increase of} \\ \text{factor IX level.} \end{array}$$

*Recombinant product*

$$1.2 \text{ IU/kg} \times \begin{array}{c} \text{body} \\ \text{weight} \\ \text{in kg} \end{array} \times \begin{array}{c} \text{percentage of} \\ \text{desired increase of} \\ \text{factor IX level.} \end{array}$$

*Proplex T*

$$0.5 \text{ IU/kg} \times \begin{array}{c} \text{body} \\ \text{weight} \\ \text{in kg} \end{array} \times \begin{array}{c} \text{percentage of} \\ \text{desired increase of} \\ \text{factor IX level.} \end{array}$$

Infusion rates vary with product and patient comfort. Dosage is highly individualized, depending on degree of deficiency, level of factor IX desired, patient weight, and severity of bleeding.

### I.V. ADMINISTRATION
● Reconstitute according to manufacturer's directions with sterile water for injection for each vial of lyophilized drug. Keep refrigerated until ready to use; warm to room temperature before reconstituting. Use factor IX (human) within 3 hours after reconstitution. Factor IX complex is stable for 12 hours after reconstitution, although administration should begin within 3 hours of reconstitution.
● Don't shake, refrigerate, or mix with other I.V. solutions. Store away from heat.
● Filter before giving.
● Avoid rapid infusion. If tingling sensation, fever, chills, or headache develops, decrease flow rate and notify prescriber.

### ACTION
Directly replaces deficient clotting factor.

| Route | Onset | Peak | Duration |
|-------|-------|------|----------|
| I.V. | Immediate | 10-30 min | Unknown |

### ADVERSE REACTIONS
**CNS:** headache, *transient fever, chills.*
**CV:** *thromboembolic reactions, MI, DIC, pulmonary embolism,* changes in blood pressure, *flushing.*
**GI:** nausea, vomiting.
**Skin:** urticaria.
**Other:** *tingling.*

### INTERACTIONS
**Drug-drug.** *Aminocaproic acid:* May increase risk of thrombosis. Avoid using together.

### EFFECTS ON LAB TEST RESULTS
None reported.

---

Reactions may be *common,* uncommon, *life-threatening,* or COMMON AND LIFE-THREATENING.

## CONTRAINDICATIONS & CAUTIONS
• Mononine is contraindicated in patients hypersensitive to murine (mouse) protein.
• Use cautiously in neonates and infants because of susceptibility to hepatitis, which may be transmitted with factor IX complex.

## NURSING CONSIDERATIONS
• Give hepatitis B vaccine before giving factor IX complex.
• Observe patient for allergic reactions and monitor vital signs regularly.
• Observe patient closely for signs and symptoms of thromboembolic events.
• Risk of hepatitis must be weighed against risk of not receiving drug.
• Risk of HIV transmission is extremely low because of manufacturing process.

## PATIENT TEACHING
• Explain use and administration of factor IX to patient and family.
• Tell patient to report adverse reactions promptly and to stop using drug if they occur.
• Advise patient to report chest tightness, wheezing, respiratory distress, cough, or low blood pressure.

---

## plasma protein fractions
Plasmanate, Plasma-Plex, Plasmatein, Protenate

*Pregnancy risk category C*

---

## AVAILABLE FORMS
*Injection:* 5% solution in 50-ml, 250-ml, 500-ml vials

## INDICATIONS & DOSAGES
➤ **Shock**
*Adults:* Varies with patient's condition and response, but usual dose is 250 to 500 ml I.V. (12.5 to 25 g protein), usually no faster than 10 ml/minute.
*Infants and children:* 6.6 to 33 ml/kg (0.33 to 1.65 g/kg of protein) I.V., 5 to 10 ml/minute.
➤ **Hypoproteinemia**
*Adults:* 1,000 to 1,500 ml I.V. daily. Maximum infusion rate is 5 to 8 ml/minute.

## I.V. ADMINISTRATION
• Check expiration date before using.
• Don't use solutions that are cloudy, contain sediment, or have been frozen. Discard solutions in containers that have been open for longer than 4 hours because solution contains no preservatives.
• Don't infuse solutions containing amino acids or alcohol through same I.V. line; proteins may precipitate.
• If patient is dehydrated, give additional fluids either P.O. or I.V.
• Don't give more than 250 g or 5,000 ml in 48 hours.

## ACTION
Supplies colloid to the blood and expands plasma volume. Primary constituent is albumin.

| Route | Onset | Peak | Duration |
|-------|-------|------|----------|
| I.V. | Immediate | Immediate | Unknown |

## ADVERSE REACTIONS
**CNS:** headache, fever.
**CV:** hypotension, *vascular overload,* tachycardia, flushing.
**GI:** nausea, vomiting, hypersalivation.
**Musculoskeletal:** back pain.
**Respiratory:** dyspnea, *pulmonary edema.*
**Skin:** rash, erythema.
**Other:** chills.

## INTERACTIONS
None significant.

## EFFECTS ON LAB TEST RESULTS
None reported.

## CONTRAINDICATIONS & CAUTIONS
• Contraindicated in patients with severe anemia or heart failure and in those undergoing cardiac bypass.
• Use cautiously in patients with hepatic or renal failure, low cardiac reserve, or restricted sodium intake.

## NURSING CONSIDERATIONS
• Hypotension risk is greater when infusion rate exceeds 10 ml/minute.
• Monitor blood pressure. Be prepared to slow or stop infusion if hypotension suddenly occurs. Vital signs should return to normal gradually; assess them hourly.

---

*Rapid onset*  †Canada  ‡Australia  ◇OTC  ◆Off-label use  ✐Photoguide  *Liquid contains alcohol.

• Watch for signs of vascular overload (heart failure or pulmonary edema).
• *Alert:* Watch for hemorrhage or shock after surgery or injury. A rapid increase in blood pressure may cause bleeding from sites that isn't apparent at lower pressures.
• Report decreased urine output.
• Drug contains 130 to 160 mEq sodium/L.

## PATIENT TEACHING
• Explain use and administration of drug to patient and family.
• Tell patient to report adverse reactions promptly.

**alteplase**
**reteplase, recombinant**
**streptokinase**
**tenecteplase**
**urokinase**

**COMBINATION PRODUCTS**
None.

---

## alteplase (tissue plasminogen activator, recombinant; t-PA)
Actilyse‡, Activase, Cathflo Activase

*Pregnancy risk category C*

---

**AVAILABLE FORMS**
*Injection:* 50-mg (29 million–IU), 100-mg (58 million–IU) vials
*Injection (Cathflo Activase):* 2-mg single-patient vials

**INDICATIONS & DOSAGES**
➤ **Lysis of thrombi obstructing coronary arteries in acute MI**
*3-hour infusion*
*Adults:* 100 mg by I.V. infusion over 3 hours, as follows: 60 mg in first hour, of which 6 to 10 mg is given as a bolus over first 1 to 2 minutes. Then 20 mg/hour infused for 2 hours. Adults weighing less than 65 kg (143 lb) should receive 1.25 mg/kg in a similar fashion (60% in first hour, of which 10% is given as a bolus; then 20% of total dose per hour for 2 hours).
*Accelerated infusion*
*Adults weighing more than 67 kg (147 lb):* 100 mg total dose. Give 15 mg I.V. bolus over 1 to 2 minutes, followed by 50 mg infused over the next 30 minutes; then 35 mg infused over the next hour.
*Adults weighing 67 kg or less:* 15 mg I.V. bolus over 1 to 2 minutes, followed by 0.75 mg/kg, (not to exceed 50 mg) infused over the next 30 minutes; then 0.5 mg/kg (not to exceed 35 mg) infused over the next hour.

➤ **To manage acute massive pulmonary embolism**
*Adults:* 100 mg by I.V. infusion over 2 hours. Heparin begun at end of infusion when PTT or thrombin time returns to twice normal or less. Don't exceed 100-mg dose. Higher doses may increase risk of intracranial bleeding.
➤ **Acute ischemic CVA**
*Adults:* 0.9 mg/kg by I.V. infusion over 1 hour with 10% of total dose given as an initial I.V. bolus over 1 minute. Maximum total dose is 90 mg.
➤ **To restore function to central venous access devices**
*Cathflo Activase*
*Adults and children older than age 2:* For patients weighing more than 30 kg (66 lb), instill 2 mg in 2 ml sterile water into catheter. For patients weighing 10 kg (22 lb) to 30 kg, instill 110% of the internal lumen volume of the catheter, not to exceed 2 mg in 2 ml sterile water. After 30 minutes of dwell time, assess catheter function by aspirating blood. If function is restored, aspirate 4 to 5 ml of blood to remove drug and residual clot, and gently irrigate the catheter with normal saline solution. If catheter function isn't restored after 120 minutes, instill a second dose.
➤ **Lysis of arterial occlusion in a peripheral vessel or bypass graft ♦**
*Adults:* 0.05 to 0.1 mg/kg/hour infused intra-arterially for 1 to 8 hours.

**I.V. ADMINISTRATION**
● Give alteplase I.V. using a controlled infusion device.
● Reconstitute drug only with unpreserved sterile water for injection. (Check manufacturer's labeling for specific information.) Don't use 50-mg vial if vacuum isn't present; 100-mg vials don't have a vacuum. Reconstitute with large-bore (18G) needle, directing stream of sterile water at lyophilized cake. Don't shake. Slight foaming is common (allow foaming to settle before use), and solution should be clear or pale yellow.

---

• Drug may be given reconstituted (1 mg/ ml) or diluted with an equal volume of normal saline solution or $D_5W$ to make a 0.5-mg/ml solution. Adding other drugs to the infusion isn't recommended.

• Reconstitute solution immediately before administration; discard any unused portion after 8 hours.

**For Cathflo Activase**

• Reconstitute Cathflo Activase with 2.2 ml sterile water; dissolve completely into a colorless to pale yellow solution that yields a concentration of 1 mg/ml. Solutions are stable for up to 8 hours at room temperature.

• Assess the cause of catheter dysfunction before using alteplase. Some conditions that have occluded the catheter include catheter malposition, mechanical failure, constriction by a suture, and lipid deposits or drug precipitates within the catheter lumen. Don't try to suction because of the risk of damage to the vascular wall or collapse of soft-walled catheters.

• Don't use excessive pressure while instilling alteplase into the catheter, which could cause catheter rupture or expulsion of the clot into the circulation.

**ACTION**

Binds to fibrin in a thrombus and locally converts plasminogen to plasmin, which starts local fibrinolysis.

| Route | Onset | Peak | Duration |
|-------|-------|------|----------|
| I.V. | Unknown | Unknown | Unknown |

**ADVERSE REACTIONS**

**CNS:** fever, *cerebral hemorrhage.*
**CV:** hypotension, *arrhythmias,* edema.
**GI:** nausea, vomiting, *GI bleeding* (Cathflo Activase).
**Hematologic:** *spontaneous bleeding.*
**Other:** bleeding at puncture sites, *cholesterol embolization,* hypersensitivity reactions, *anaphylaxis; venous thrombosis, sepsis* (Cathflo Activase).

**INTERACTIONS**

**Drug-drug.** *Aspirin, coumadin anticoagulants, dipyridamole, drugs affecting platelet activity (abciximab), heparin:* May increase risk of bleeding. Monitor patient carefully.

*Nitroglycerin:* May decrease alteplase antigen level. Avoid using together. If use together is unavoidable, use the lowest effective dose of nitroglycerin.

**EFFECTS ON LAB TEST RESULTS**

• May alter coagulation and fibrinolytic test results.

**CONTRAINDICATIONS & CAUTIONS**

• Contraindicated in patients with active internal bleeding, intracranial neoplasm, arteriovenous malformation, aneurysm, severe uncontrolled hypertension, or history or current evidence of intracranial hemorrhage, suspicion of subarachnoid hemorrhage, or seizure at onset of CVA when used for acute ischemic CVA. Also contraindicated in patients with history of CVA, intraspinal or intracranial trauma or surgery within 2 months, or known bleeding diathesis.

• Use cautiously in patients having major surgery within 10 days (when bleeding is difficult to control because of its location); organ biopsy; trauma (including cardiopulmonary resuscitation); GI or GU bleeding; cerebrovascular disease; systolic pressure of 180 mm Hg or higher or diastolic pressure of 110 mm Hg or higher; mitral stenosis, atrial fibrillation, or other conditions that may lead to left heart thrombus; acute pericarditis or subacute bacterial endocarditis; hemostatic defects caused by hepatic or renal impairment; septic thrombophlebitis; or diabetic hemorrhagic retinopathy. Also use cautiously in patients receiving anticoagulants, in patients age 75 and older, and during pregnancy and the first 10 days postpartum.

**NURSING CONSIDERATIONS**

• *Alert:* When used for acute ischemic CVA, give drug within 3 hours after symptoms occur and only when intracranial bleeding has been ruled out.

• Addition of 150 to 200 units/ml aprotinin to blood sample may remedy interference with coagulation and fibrinolytic test results.

• Drug may be given to menstruating women.

• To recanalize occluded coronary arteries and improve heart function, begin treatment as soon as possible after symptoms start.

• Anticoagulant and antiplatelet therapy is commonly started during or after treatment, to decrease risk of another thrombosis.

• Monitor vital signs and neurologic status carefully. Keep patient on strict bed rest.

• Have antiarrhythmics readily available, and carefully monitor ECG. Coronary thrombolysis is linked with arrhythmias caused by reperfusion of ischemic myocardium. Such arrhythmias don't differ from those commonly linked with MI.

• Avoid invasive procedures during thrombolytic therapy. Closely monitor patient for signs of internal bleeding, and frequently check all puncture sites. Bleeding is the most common adverse effect and may occur internally and at external puncture sites.

• If uncontrollable bleeding occurs, stop infusion (and heparin) and notify prescriber.

**PATIENT TEACHING**

• Explain use and administration of drug to patient and family.

• Tell patient to report adverse reactions promptly.

---

## reteplase, recombinant
Retavase

*Pregnancy risk category C*

---

**AVAILABLE FORMS**
*Injection:* 10.4 units (18.1 mg)/vial. Supplied in a kit with components for reconstitution for two single-use vials.

**INDICATIONS & DOSAGES**
➤ **To manage acute MI**
*Adults:* Double-bolus injection of 10 + 10 units. Give each bolus I.V. over 2 minutes. If complications, such as serious bleeding or an anaphylactoid reaction, don't occur after first bolus, give second bolus 30 minutes after start of first one.

**I.V. ADMINISTRATION**
• Drug is given I.V. as a double-bolus injection. If bleeding or anaphylactoid reac-

tion occurs after first bolus, notify prescriber; second bolus may be withheld.

• Reconstitute drug according to manufacturer's instructions using items provided in kit and sterile water for injection, without preservatives. Make sure reconstituted solution is colorless; resulting concentration is 1 unit/ml. If foaming occurs, let vial stand for several minutes. Inspect for precipitation. Use within 4 hours of reconstitution; discard unused portions.

• Don't give with other I.V. drugs through same I.V. line. Note that heparin and reteplase are incompatible in solution.

**ACTION**
Enhances cleavage of plasminogen to generate plasmin, which leads to fibrinolysis.

| Route | Onset | Peak | Duration |
|-------|-------|------|----------|
| I.V. | Unknown | Unknown | Unknown |

**ADVERSE REACTIONS**
**CNS:** *intracranial hemorrhage.*
**CV:** *arrhythmias, cholesterol embolization, hemorrhage.*
**GI:** *hemorrhage.*
**GU:** hematuria.
**Hematologic:** *bleeding tendency,* anemia.
**Other:** bleeding at puncture sites, *hypersensitivity reaction.*

**INTERACTIONS**
**Drug-drug.** *Heparin, oral anticoagulants, platelet inhibitors (abciximab, aspirin, dipyridamole):* May increase risk of bleeding. Use together cautiously.

**EFFECTS ON LAB TEST RESULTS**
• May increase PT, PTT, and INR. May decrease hemoglobin.
• May alter coagulation study results.

**CONTRAINDICATIONS & CAUTIONS**
• Contraindicated in patients with active internal bleeding, known bleeding diathesis, history of CVA, recent intracranial or intraspinal surgery or trauma, severe uncontrolled hypertension, intracranial neoplasm, arteriovenous malformation, or aneurysm.
• Use cautiously in patients with previous puncture of noncompressible vessels; in those with recent (within 10 days) major surgery, obstetric delivery, organ biopsy,

GI or GU bleeding, or trauma; in those with cerebrovascular disease, systolic blood pressure 180 mm Hg or higher or diastolic pressure 110 mm Hg or higher, and conditions that may lead to left heart thrombus, including mitral stenosis, acute pericarditis, subacute bacterial endocarditis, and hemostatic defects; and in those with diabetic hemorrhagic retinopathy, septic thrombophlebitis, and other conditions in which bleeding would be difficult to manage. Also use cautiously in patients age 75 and older and in breast-feeding women.

**NURSING CONSIDERATIONS**
• Drug remains active in vitro and can lead to degradation of fibrinogen in sample, changing coagulation study results. Collect blood samples with phenylalanyl-L-prolyl-L-arginine chloromethylketone at 2-micromolar concentrations.
• Drug may be given to menstruating women.
• Carefully monitor ECG during treatment. Coronary thrombolysis may cause arrhythmias linked with reperfusion. Be prepared to treat bradycardia or ventricular irritability.
• Closely monitor patient for bleeding. Avoid I.M. injections, invasive procedures, and nonessential handling of patient. Bleeding is the most common adverse reaction and may occur internally or at external puncture sites. If local measures don't control serious bleeding, stop anticoagulant and notify prescriber. Withhold second bolus of reteplase.
• Use drug in pregnancy only if benefit to mother justifies risk to fetus.
• Safety and efficacy of drug in children haven't been established.
• Potency is expressed in units specific to reteplase and isn't comparable with other thrombolytic drugs.
• Avoid use of noncompressible pressure sites during therapy. If an arterial puncture is needed, use an arm vessel that can be compressed manually. Apply pressure for at least 30 minutes; then apply a pressure dressing. Check site frequently.

**PATIENT TEACHING**
• Explain use and administration of drug to patient and family.

• Tell patient to report adverse reactions immediately.

# streptokinase
Streptase

*Pregnancy risk category C*

**AVAILABLE FORMS**
*Injection:* 250,000 IU, 750,000 IU, 1,500,000 IU in vials for reconstitution

**INDICATIONS & DOSAGES**
➤ **Arteriovenous cannula occlusion**
*Adults:* 250,000 IU in 2 ml I.V. solution by I.V. pump infusion into each occluded limb of the cannula over 25 to 35 minutes. Clamp off cannula for 2 hours. Then aspirate contents of cannula, flush with normal saline solution, and reconnect.
➤ **Venous thrombosis, pulmonary embolism, arterial thrombosis, and embolism**
*Adults:* Loading dose is 250,000 IU by I.V. infusion over 30 minutes. Sustaining dose is 100,000 IU/hour I.V. infusion for 72 hours for deep vein thrombosis and 100,000 IU/hour over 24 to 72 hours by I.V. infusion pump for pulmonary embolism and arterial thrombosis or embolism.
➤ **Lysis of coronary artery thrombi following acute MI**
*Adults:* 1.5 million IU infused I.V. over 60 minutes.

**I.V. ADMINISTRATION**
• Reconstitute drug in each vial with 5 ml of normal saline solution for injection or $D_5W$ solution. Further dilute to 45 ml (if needed, total volume may be increased to 500 ml in a glass or 50 ml in a plastic container). Don't shake; roll gently to mix. Some flocculation may be present after reconstituting; discard if large amounts are present. Filter solution with 0.8-micron or larger filter. Use within 8 hours. Store powder at room temperature and refrigerate after reconstitution.
• *Alert:* Don't mix with other drugs or give other drugs through the same I.V. line.
• Heparin by continuous infusion is usually started within 1 to 4 hours after stopping streptokinase. Use infusion pump to

give heparin. Starting heparin 12 hours after intracoronary streptokinase may minimize bleeding risk.

## ACTION
Activates plasminogen in two steps: Plasminogen and streptokinase form a complex that exposes the plasminogen-activating site; plasminogen is then converted to plasmin by cleavage of the peptide bond, which leads to fibrinolysis.

| Route | Onset | Peak | Duration |
|-------|-------|------|----------|
| I.V. | Immediate | 20 min-2 hr | 4-24 hr |

## ADVERSE REACTIONS
**CNS:** polyradiculoneuropathy, headache, *fever.*
**CV: *reperfusion arrhythmias,*** hypotension, vasculitis, flushing.
**EENT:** periorbital edema.
**GI:** nausea.
**Hematologic: *bleeding;*** moderately decreased hematocrit.
**Respiratory:** minor breathing difficulty, ***bronchospasm, pulmonary edema.***
**Skin:** urticaria, pruritus.
**Other:** phlebitis at injection site, hypersensitivity reactions, ***anaphylaxis,*** delayed hypersensitivity reactions, ***angioedema.***

## INTERACTIONS
**Drug-drug.** *Anticoagulants:* May increase risk of bleeding. Monitor patient closely.
*Antifibrinolytic drugs:* Antifibrinolytic drugs such as aminocaproic acid may inhibit and reverse streptokinase activity. Avoid using together.
*Aspirin, dipyridamole, drugs affecting platelet activity, indomethacin, phenylbutazone:* May increase risk of bleeding. Monitor patient closely.

## EFFECTS ON LAB TEST RESULTS
• May increase PT, PTT, and INR. May decrease hematocrit.

## CONTRAINDICATIONS & CAUTIONS
• Contraindicated in patients with ulcerative wounds, active internal bleeding, recent CVA, recent trauma with possible internal injuries, visceral or intracranial malignant neoplasms, ulcerative colitis, diverticulitis, severe hypertension, acute or chronic hepatic or renal insufficiency,

uncontrolled hypocoagulation, chronic pulmonary disease with cavitation, subacute bacterial endocarditis or rheumatic valvular disease, previous severe allergic reaction to streptokinase, or recent cerebral embolism, thrombosis, or hemorrhage.
• Contraindicated within 10 days after intra-arterial diagnostic procedure or any surgery, including liver or kidney biopsy, lumbar puncture, thoracentesis, paracentesis, or extensive or multiple cutdowns.
• I.M. injections and other invasive procedures are contraindicated during streptokinase therapy.
• Use cautiously when treating arterial embolism that originates from left side of heart because of danger of cerebral infarction.

## NURSING CONSIDERATIONS
• Drug may be given to menstruating women.
• Only prescribers with experience managing thrombotic disease should use streptokinase. Give drug only where clinical and laboratory monitoring can be performed.
• Before using streptokinase to clear an occluded arteriovenous cannula, try flushing with heparinized saline solution.
• Keep aminocaproic acid available to treat bleeding, and keep corticosteroids available to treat allergic reactions.
• Before starting therapy, draw blood for coagulation studies, hematocrit, platelet count, and type and crossmatching. Rate of I.V. infusion depends on thrombin time and streptokinase resistance.
• To check for hypersensitivity reactions, give 100 IU intradermally; a wheal-and-flare response within 20 minutes means patient is probably allergic. Monitor vital signs frequently.
• If patient has had either a recent streptococcal infection or recent treatment with streptokinase, a higher loading dose may be needed. Consider alternative thrombolytics.
• Combined therapy with low-dose aspirin (162.5 mg) or dipyridamole has improved short- and long-term results.
• Monitor patient for excessive bleeding every 15 minutes for first hour, every 30 minutes for second through eighth

hours, and then every 4 hours. If bleeding is evident, stop therapy and notify prescriber. Pretreatment with heparin or drugs that affect platelets causes high risk of bleeding but may improve long-term results.

• Monitor pulse, color, and sensation of limbs every hour.

• Keep involved limb in straight alignment to prevent bleeding from infusion site.

• Avoid unnecessary handling of patient; pad side rails. Bruising is more likely during therapy.

• Keep a laboratory flow sheet on patient's chart to monitor PTT, PT, thrombin time, and hemoglobin level and hematocrit. Monitor vital signs and neurologic status.

• Avoid I.M. injection. Keep venipuncture sites to a minimum; use pressure dressing on puncture sites for at least 15 minutes.

• **Alert:** Watch for signs of hypersensitivity and notify prescriber immediately if any occur. Antihistamines or corticosteroids may be used to treat mild allergic reactions. If a severe reaction occurs, stop infusion immediately and notify prescriber.

• Thrombolytic therapy in patients with acute MI may decrease infarct size, improve ventricular function, and decrease risk of heart failure. For optimal effect, streptokinase must be given within 6 hours after symptoms start.

**PATIENT TEACHING**
• Explain use and administration of drug to patient and family.
• Tell patient to report adverse reactions promptly.

## tenecteplase
TNKase

*Pregnancy risk category C*

**AVAILABLE FORMS**
*Injection:* 50 mg

**INDICATIONS & DOSAGES**
➤ **Reduction of mortality from acute MI**
*Adults weighing 90 kg (198 lb) or more:* 50 mg (10 ml) by I.V. bolus over 5 seconds.

*Adults weighing 80 to 89 kg (176 to 196 lb):* 45 mg (9 ml) by I.V. bolus over 5 seconds.
*Adults weighing 70 to 79 kg (154 to 174 lb):* 40 mg (8 ml) by I.V. bolus over 5 seconds.
*Adults weighing 60 to 69 kg (132 to 152 lb):* 35 mg (7 ml) by I.V. bolus over 5 seconds.
*Adults weighing less than 60 kg (132 lb):* 30 mg (6 ml) by I.V. bolus over 5 seconds. Maximum dose is 50 mg.

**I.V. ADMINISTRATION**
• Use syringe prefilled with sterile water for injection, and inject the entire contents into drug vial.
• **Alert:** Gently swirl solution once mixed. Don't shake.
• Draw up the appropriate dose needed from the reconstituted vial with the syringe and discard any unused portion.
• Give drug immediately once reconstituted, or refrigerate and use within 8 hours.
• Visually inspect product for particulate matter before administration.
• Give the drug rapidly over 5 seconds.
• Don't give drug in the same I.V. line as dextrose. Flush dextrose-containing lines with normal saline solution before administration.
• Give tenecteplase by a designated line.

**ACTION**
A human tissue plasminogen activator that binds to fibrin and converts plasminogen to plasmin. The specificity to fibrin decreases systemic activation of plasminogen and the resulting breakdown of circulating fibrinogen.

| Route | Onset | Peak | Duration |
|-------|-------|------|----------|
| I.V. | Immediate | Immediate | Unknown |

**ADVERSE REACTIONS**
CNS: *CVA, intracranial hemorrhage.*
CV: *arrhythmias.*
EENT: pharyngeal bleeding, epistaxis.
GI: *GI bleeding.*
GU: hematuria.
Skin: *hematoma.*
Other: bleeding at puncture site, *hypersensitivity reactions.*

## INTERACTIONS
**Drug-drug.** *Anticoagulants (heparin, vitamin K antagonists), drugs that alter platelet function (acetylsalicylic acid, dipyridamole, glycoprotein IIb/IIIa inhibitors):* May increase risk of bleeding when used before, during, or after therapy with tenecteplase. Use together cautiously.

## EFFECTS ON LAB TEST RESULTS
• May increase PT, PTT, and INR. May decrease hemoglobin.

## CONTRAINDICATIONS & CAUTIONS
• Contraindicated in patients with an active internal bleed; history of CVA; intracranial or intraspinal surgery or trauma during previous 2 months; intracranial neoplasm, aneurysm, or arteriovenous malformation; severe uncontrolled hypertension; or bleeding diathesis.
• Use cautiously in patients who have had recent major surgery (such as coronary artery bypass graft), organ biopsy, obstetric delivery, or previous puncture of noncompressible vessels.
• Use cautiously in pregnant women, patients age 75 and older, and patients with recent trauma, recent GI or GU bleeding, high risk of left ventricular thrombus, acute pericarditis, systolic blood pressure 180 mm Hg or higher or diastolic pressure 110 mm Hg or higher, severe hepatic dysfunction, hemostatic defects, subacute bacterial endocarditis, septic thrombophlebitis, diabetic hemorrhagic retinopathy, or cerebrovascular disease.

## NURSING CONSIDERATIONS
• Begin therapy as soon as possible after onset of MI symptoms.
• Minimize arterial and venous punctures during treatment.
• Avoid noncompressible arterial punctures and internal jugular and subclavian venous punctures.
• Give heparin with tenecteplase but not in the same I.V. line.
• Monitor patient for bleeding. If serious bleeding occurs, stop heparin and antiplatelet drugs immediately.
• Use exact patient weight for dosing. An overestimation in patient weight can lead to significant increase in bleeding or intracerebral hemorrhage.

• Monitor ECG for reperfusion arrhythmias.
• Cholesterol embolism is rarely related to thrombolytic use, but it may be lethal. Signs and symptoms may include livedo reticularis ("purple toe" syndrome), acute renal failure, gangrenous digits, hypertension, pancreatitis, MI, cerebral infarction, spinal cord infarction, retinal artery occlusion, bowel infarction, and rhabdomyolysis.

## PATIENT TEACHING
• Advise patient about proper dental care to avoid excessive gum bleeding.
• Tell patient to report any adverse effects or excess bleeding immediately.
• Explain to patient and family about the use of tenecteplase.

---

# urokinase
Abbokinase

*Pregnancy risk category B*

## AVAILABLE FORMS
*Injection:* 250,000-IU vial

## INDICATIONS & DOSAGES
➤ **Lysis of acute massive pulmonary embolism and of pulmonary embolism with unstable hemodynamics**
*Adults:* For I.V. infusion *only* by constant infusion pump. For priming dose, give 4,400 IU/kg with normal saline solution or $D_5W$ solution, over 10 minutes, followed by 4,400 IU/kg/hour for 12 hours. Then give continuous I.V. infusion of heparin and oral anticoagulants.
➤ **Coronary artery thrombosis ♦**
*Adults:* After bolus dose of heparin ranging from 2,500 to 10,000 units, infuse 6,000 IU/minute into occluded artery for up to 2 hours. Average total dose is 500,000 IU. Start giving drug within 6 hours after symptoms start.
➤ **Venous catheter occlusion ♦**
*Adults:* Instill 5,000 IU into occluded line
➤ **Lysis of coronary artery thrombi in patients with acute MI ♦**
*Adults:* 2 to 3 million units over 45 to 90 minutes, with half or all of the dose given first as a rapid injection over 5 min-

utes and the remainder, if any, as a continuous infusion.

## I.V. ADMINISTRATION
● Reconstitute according to manufacturer's directions using sterile water for injection. Gently roll vial; don't shake. Don't use bacteriostatic water for injection to reconstitute; it contains preservatives. Dilute further with normal saline solution or $D_5W$ solution before infusion. Filter urokinase solutions through a 0.45-micron or smaller cellulose-membrane filter before administration. Discard unused solution. Total volume of fluid given by I.V. infusion shouldn't exceed 200 ml.
● Don't mix with other drugs. Give through separate I.V. line.
● Heparin by continuous infusion may be started concurrently or within 3 to 4 hours after urokinase has been stopped to prevent recurrent thrombosis.

## ACTION
Activates plasminogen to plasmin by directly cleaving peptide bonds at two different sites, causing fibrinolysis.

| Route | Onset | Peak | Duration |
|-------|-------|------|----------|
| I.V. | Immediate | 20 min-4 hr | 12-24 hr |

## ADVERSE REACTIONS
**CNS:** fever.
**CV:** reperfusion arrhythmias, tachycardia, transient hypotension or hypertension.
**GI:** nausea, vomiting.
**Hematologic:** bleeding.
**Respiratory:** bronchospasm, minor breathing difficulties.
**Skin:** phlebitis at injection site, rash.
**Other:** anaphylaxis, chills.

## INTERACTIONS
**Drug-drug.** *Anticoagulants:* May increase risk of bleeding. Monitor patient closely.
*Aspirin, dipyridamole, indomethacin, phenylbutazone, other drugs affecting platelet activity:* May increase risk of bleeding. Monitor patient.

## EFFECTS ON LAB TEST RESULTS
● May increase PT, PTT, and INR. May decrease hematocrit.

## CONTRAINDICATIONS & CAUTIONS
● Contraindicated in patients with active internal bleeding, history of CVA, aneurysm, arteriovenous malformation, known bleeding diathesis, recent trauma with possible internal injuries, visceral or intracranial malignancy, ulcerative colitis, diverticulitis, severe hypertension, hemostatic defects including those secondary to severe hepatic or renal insufficiency, uncontrolled hypocoagulation, chronic pulmonary disease with cavitation, subacute bacterial endocarditis or rheumatic valvular disease, and recent cerebral embolism, thrombosis, or hemorrhage
● Contraindicated within 10 days after intra-arterial diagnostic procedure or surgery (liver or kidney biopsy, lumbar puncture, thoracentesis, paracentesis, or extensive or multiple cutdowns) or within 2 months after intracranial or intraspinal surgery.
● Contraindicated during pregnancy or first 10 days postpartum.
● I.M. injections and other invasive procedures are contraindicated during urokinase therapy.

## NURSING CONSIDERATIONS
● Have typed and crossmatched RBCs, whole blood, plasma expanders (other than dextran), and aminocaproic acid available to treat bleeding. Keep corticosteroids, epinephrine, and antihistamines available to treat allergic reactions.
● Drug may be given to menstruating women.
● Only prescribers with extensive experience in thrombotic disease management should use urokinase and only in facilities where clinical and laboratory monitoring can be performed.
● Monitor patient for excessive bleeding every 15 minutes for first hour; every 30 minutes for second through eighth hours; then once every 4 hours. Pretreatment with drugs affecting platelets places patient at high risk of bleeding.
● Monitor pulse, color, and sensation of limbs every hour.
● Although risk of hypersensitivity reactions is low, monitor patient.
● Keep a laboratory flow sheet on patient's chart to monitor PTT, PT, thrombin time, hemoglobin level, and hematocrit.

---

Reactions may be *common*, uncommon, *life-threatening*, or COMMON AND LIFE-THREATENING.

...l neurologic sta-
...sure in legs, be-
...dge a clot.
... a minimum;
...cture sites for

...t alignment
...infusion site.
...ing is more likely during
..., avoid unnecessary handling of patient, and pad side rails.

• Rare reports of orolingual edema, urticaria, cholesterol embolization, and infusion reactions causing hypoxia, cyanosis, acidosis, and back pain have occurred in patients receiving this drug.

**PATIENT TEACHING**

• Explain use and administration of drug to patient and family.

• Instruct patient to report adverse reactions promptly.

busulfan
carboplatin
carmustine (BCNU)
chlorambucil
cisplatin carmustine
cyclophosphamide
ifosfamide
lomustine
mechlorethamine hydrochloride
melphalan
melphalan hydrochloride
oxaliplatin
thiotepa

**COMBINATION PRODUCTS**
None.

---

## busulfan
Busulfex, Myleran

*Pregnancy risk category D*

---

### AVAILABLE FORMS
*Injection:* 6 mg/ml
*Tablets:* 2 mg

### INDICATIONS & DOSAGES
➤ **Chronic myelocytic (granulocytic) leukemia**
*Adults:* 4 to 8 mg P.O. daily until WBC count falls to 15,000/mm³; drug stopped until WBC count rises to 50,000/mm³, and then resumed as before. Or, 4 to 8 mg P.O. daily until WBC count falls to 10,000 to 20,000/mm³; then reduce daily dose, p.r.n., to maintain WBC count at this level. Dosage is highly variable; range is 2 mg/week to 4 mg/day.
*Children:* 0.06 to 0.12 mg/kg/day or 1.8 to 4.6 mg/m²/day P.O.; adjust dosage to maintain WBC count at 20,000/mm³, but never below 10,000/mm³.
➤ **Allogenic hematopoietic stem cell transplantation in patients with chronic myelogenous leukemia**
*Adults:* 0.8 mg/kg I.V. q 6 hours for 4 days (a total of 16 doses). Give cyclophosphamide 60 mg/kg I.V. over 1 hour daily for

2 days beginning 6 hours after the 16th dose of busulfan injection.

### I.V. ADMINISTRATION
● Follow facility policy when preparing and handling drug. Label as a hazardous drug.
● Dilute drug in either $D_5W$ or normal saline solution to a final concentration of at least 0.5 mg/ml. Use the 5-micron nylon filter to withdraw the calculated volume from the ampule. A new needle should then be used to inject the drug into the I.V. bag or syringe. Invert several times to ensure mixing.
● Infuse over 2 hours through a central venous catheter using a controlled-infusion device. Flush the catheter line with 5 ml of $D_5W$ or normal saline solution before and after each infusion.
● Busulfan solutions are stable for 8 hours at room temperature, or 12 hours when diluted in normal saline solution and refrigerated. Infusions must be used and completed during these time frames.

### ACTION
Unknown. Thought to cross-link strands of cellular DNA and interfere with RNA transcription, causing an imbalance of growth that leads to cell death. Not specific to cell cycle.

| Route | Onset | Peak | Duration |
|-------|-------|------|----------|
| P.O. | 1-2 wk | Unknown | Unknown |
| I.V. | Unknown | Unknown | Unknown |

### ADVERSE REACTIONS
**CNS:** *fever, headache, asthenia, pain, insomnia, anxiety, dizziness, depression,* delirium, agitation, ***encephalopathy, confusion,*** hallucination, lethargy, somnolence, ***seizures.***
**CV:** *edema, chest pain, tachycardia, hypertension, hypotension,* ***thrombosis,*** *vasodilation, heart rhythm abnormalities,* cardiomegaly, ECG abnormalities, ***heart failure, pericardial effusion.***
**EENT:** *rhinitis, epistaxis, pharyngitis,* sinusitis, ear disorder, cataracts.

---

**GI:** *cheilosis (P.O.); nausea, stomatitis, mucositis, vomiting, anorexia, diarrhea, abdominal pain and enlargement, dyspepsia, constipation, dry mouth, rectal disorder,* pancreatitis.
**GU:** *dysuria, oliguria,* hematuria, hemorrhagic cystitis.
**Hematologic:** GRANULOCYTOPENIA, THROMBOCYTOPENIA, LEUKOPENIA, *anemia.*
**Hepatic:** *jaundice,* **hepatic necrosis,** hepatomegaly.
**Metabolic:** *hypomagnesemia, hyperglycemia, hypokalemia, hypocalcemia, hypervolemia, weight gain, hypophosphatemia,* hyponatremia.
**Musculoskeletal:** *back pain, myalgia, arthralgia.*
**Respiratory:** *lung disorder, cough, dyspnea,* **irreversible pulmonary fibrosis, alveolar hemorrhage,** asthma, atelectasis, pleural effusion hypoxia, hemoptysis.
**Skin:** *inflammation at injection site, rash, pruritus, alopecia,* exfoliative dermatitis, erythema nodosum, acne, skin discoloration, *hyperpigmentation,* anhidrosis.
**Other:** Addison-like wasting syndrome, gynecomastia (P.O.); *chills, allergic reaction,* **graft versus host disease, infection,** hiccup.

## INTERACTIONS
**Drug-drug.** *Acetaminophen:* May decrease busulfan clearance. Use together cautiously.
*Anticoagulants, aspirin:* May increase risk of bleeding. Avoid using together.
*Cyclophosphamide:* May increase risk of cardiac tamponade in patients with thalassemia. Monitor patient.
*Itraconazole:* May decrease busulfan clearance. Use together cautiously.
*Myelosuppressives:* May increase myelosuppression. Monitor patient.
*Other cytotoxic agents causing pulmonary injury:* May cause additive pulmonary toxicity. Avoid using together.
*Phenytoin:* May decrease busulfan level. Monitor busulfan level.
*Thioguanine:* May cause hepatotoxicity, esophageal varices, or portal hypertension. Use together cautiously.

## EFFECTS ON LAB TEST RESULTS
● May increase glucose, ALT, bilirubin, alkaline phosphatase, creatinine and BUN levels. May decrease magnesium, calcium, potassium, phosphorus, and sodium levels.
● May decrease hemoglobin and WBC and platelet counts.

## CONTRAINDICATIONS & CAUTIONS
● Contraindicated in patients with chronic myelogenous leukemia resistant to drug and in those with chronic lymphocytic or acute leukemia or in the blastic crisis of chronic myelogenous leukemia.
● Use cautiously in patients recently given other myelosuppressives or radiation treatment and in those with depressed neutrophil or platelet count. Because high-dose therapy has been linked to seizures, use cautiously in patients with history of head trauma or seizures and in those receiving other drugs that lower the seizure threshold.

## NURSING CONSIDERATIONS
● Give antiemetic before first dose of busulfan injection and then on a fixed schedule during therapy; give phenytoin to prevent seizures.
● Therapeutic effects are commonly accompanied by toxicity.
● To prevent bleeding, avoid all I.M. injections when platelet count is less than 50,000/mm³.
● Monitor patient response (increased appetite and sense of well-being, decreased total WBC count, reduced size of spleen), which usually begins in 1 to 2 weeks.
● Monitor for jaundice and liver function abnormalities in patients receiving high-dose busulfan.
● Anticipate possible blood transfusion during treatment because of cumulative anemia. Patients may receive injections of RBC colony-stimulating factor to promote RBC production and decrease the need for blood transfusions.
● *Alert:* Pulmonary fibrosis may occur as late as 8 months to 10 years after treatment with busulfan. (Average duration of therapy is 4 years.)

---

*Rapid onset*   †Canada   ‡Australia   ◇ OTC   ◆ Off-label use   🔊Photoguide   *Liquid contains alcohol.

## PATIENT TEACHING

• Advise patient to watch for signs of infection (fever, sore throat, fatigue) and bleeding (easy bruising, nosebleeds, bleeding gums, tarry stools). Tell patient to take temperature right.

• Instruct patient to report signs and symptoms of toxicity so dosage can be adjusted. Persistent cough and progressive labored breathing with liquid in the lungs, suggestive of pneumonia, may be caused by drug toxicity.

• Instruct patient to avoid OTC products containing aspirin and NSAIDs.

• Inform patient that drug may cause skin darkening.

• Advise women of childbearing age to avoid becoming pregnant during therapy. Recommend that she consult prescriber before becoming pregnant.

• Warn women to stop breast-feeding because of risk of toxicity to infant.

• Instruct patient to take drug on empty stomach to decrease nausea and vomiting.

• Because of risk of impotence and male sterility, advise man of childbearing potential about sperm banking before therapy begins.

---

## carboplatin
Paraplatin, Paraplatin-AQ†

*Pregnancy risk category D*

## AVAILABLE FORMS
*Injection:* 50-mg, 150-mg, 450-mg vials

## INDICATIONS & DOSAGES
➤ **Advanced ovarian cancer**
*Adults:* 360 mg/m² I.V. on day 1 q 4 weeks or 300 mg/m² when used with other chemotherapy drugs; doses shouldn't be repeated until platelet count exceeds 100,000/mm³ and neutrophil count exceeds 2,000/mm³. Subsequent doses are based on blood counts. Or, refer to package for formula dosing.
*Adjust-a-dose:* For renally impaired patients with creatinine clearance of 41 to 59 ml/minute, first dose is 250 mg/m²; if between 16 and 40 ml/minute, first dose is 200 mg/m². Drug isn't recommended for patients with creatinine clearance of 15 ml/minute or less.

## I.V. ADMINISTRATION

• *Alert:* Have epinephrine, corticosteroids, and antihistamines available when giving carboplatin because anaphylactoid reactions may occur within minutes of administration.

• *Alert:* Preparation and administration of parenteral form of drug may be mutagenic, teratogenic, or carcinogenic to staff. Follow institutional policy to reduce risks.

• Reconstitute with D₅W, normal saline solution, or sterile water for injection to yield 10 mg/ml. Add 5 ml of diluent to 50 mg vial, 15 ml of diluent to 150-mg vial, or 45 ml of diluent to 450-mg vial. Reconstituted drug can then be further diluted for infusion with normal saline solution or D₅W. A concentration as low as 0.5 mg/ml can be prepared. Give drug by continuous or intermittent infusion over at least 15 minutes.

• Don't use needles or I.V. administration sets containing aluminum to give carboplatin; precipitation and loss of potency may occur.

• Store unopened vials at room temperature. Once reconstituted and diluted as directed, drug is stable at room temperature for 8 hours. Because drug doesn't contain antibacterial preservatives, discard unused drug after 8 hours.

## ACTION
Unknown. Thought to cross-link strands of cellular DNA and interferes with RNA transcription, causing an imbalance of growth that leads to cell death. Not specific to cell cycle.

| Route | Onset | Peak | Duration |
|-------|-------|------|----------|
| I.V.  | Unknown | Unknown | Unknown |

## ADVERSE REACTIONS
**CNS:** *asthenia,* dizziness, confusion, **CVA,** peripheral neuropathy, central neurotoxicity, paresthesia.
**CV:** *heart failure, embolism.*
**EENT:** ototoxicity, visual disturbances.
**GI:** constipation, diarrhea, *nausea, vomiting,* mucositis, change in taste, stomatitis.
**Hematologic:** THROMBOCYTOPENIA, *leukopenia,* NEUTROPENIA, anemia, BONE MARROW SUPPRESSION.
**Skin:** alopecia.

---

Reactions may be *common,* uncommon, *life-threatening,* or COMMON AND LIFE-THREATENING.

**Other:** hypersensitivity reactions, *pain, anaphylaxis.*

## INTERACTIONS
**Drug-drug.** *Aspirin, NSAIDs:* May increase risk of bleeding. Avoid using together.
*Bone marrow suppressants, including radiation therapy:* May increase hematologic toxicity. Monitor CBC with differential closely.
*Nephrotoxic drugs, especially aminoglycosides and amphotericin B:* May enhance nephrotoxicity of carboplatin. Use together cautiously.

## EFFECTS ON LAB TEST RESULTS
● May increase BUN, creatinine, AST, and alkaline phosphatase levels. May decrease electrolyte levels.
● May decrease neutrophil, WBC, RBC, and platelet counts. May decrease hemoglobin and hematocrit.

## CONTRAINDICATIONS & CAUTIONS
● Contraindicated in patients with severe bone marrow suppression or bleeding or with history of hypersensitivity to cisplatin, platinum-containing compounds, or mannitol.

## NURSING CONSIDERATIONS
● Determine electrolyte, creatinine, and BUN levels, CBC, and creatinine clearance before first infusion and before each course of treatment.
● Monitor CBC and platelet count frequently during therapy and, when indicated, until recovery. WBC and platelet count nadirs usually occur by day 21. Levels usually return to baseline by day 28. Dose shouldn't be repeated unless platelet count exceeds 100,000/mm³.
● Bone marrow suppression may be more severe in patients with creatinine clearance below 60 ml/minute; dosage adjustments are recommended for such patients.
● *Alert:* Carefully check ordered dose against laboratory test results. Only one increase in dosage is recommended. Subsequent doses shouldn't exceed 125% of starting dose.
● Therapeutic effects are commonly accompanied by toxicity.

● Carboplatin has less nephrotoxicity and neurotoxicity than cisplatin, but it causes more severe myelosuppression.
● To prevent bleeding, avoid all I.M. injections when platelet count is below 50,000/mm³.
● Monitor vital signs during infusion.
● Give antiemetic to reduce nausea and vomiting.
● Anticipate blood transfusions during treatment because of cumulative anemia. Patient may receive injections of RBC colony-stimulating factor to promote cell production.
● Patients older than age 65 are at greater risk for neurotoxicity.
● *Alert:* Don't confuse carboplatin with cisplatin.

## PATIENT TEACHING
● Advise patient of most common adverse reactions: nausea, vomiting, bone marrow suppression, anemia, and reduction in blood platelets.
● Advise patient to watch for signs of infection (fever, sore throat, fatigue) and bleeding (easy bruising, nosebleeds, bleeding gums, tarry stools). Tell patient to take temperature daily.
● Instruct patient to avoid OTC products containing aspirin and NSAIDs.
● Advise women taking drug to stop breast-feeding because of risk of toxicity to infant.
● Because of risk of impotence, sterility, and menstruation cessation, counsel both men and women of childbearing age before starting therapy. Also recommend that women consult prescriber before becoming pregnant.

## carmustine (BCNU)
BiCNU, Gliadel Wafer

*Pregnancy risk category D*

## AVAILABLE FORMS
*Injection:* 100-mg vial (lyophilized), with a 3-ml vial of absolute alcohol supplied as a diluent
*Wafer:* 7.7 mg, for intracavitary use

---

## INDICATIONS & DOSAGES
➤ **Brain tumors, Hodgkin's disease, malignant lymphoma, multiple myeloma**

*Adults:* 150 to 200 mg/m² I.V. by slow infusion q 6 weeks; may be divided into daily injections of 75 to 100 mg/m² on two successive days; repeat dose q 6 weeks if platelet count is greater than 100,000/mm³ and WBC count is greater than 4,000/mm³.

*Adjust-a-dose:* Dosage is reduced by 30% when WBC nadir is 2,000 to 2,999/mm³ and platelet nadir is 25,000 to 74,999/mm³. Dosage is reduced by 50% when WBC nadir is less than 2,000/mm³ and platelet nadir is less than 25,000/mm³.

➤ **Adjunct to surgery to prolong survival in patients with recurrent glioblastoma multiforme for whom surgical resection is indicated**

*Adults:* 8 wafers placed in the resection cavity if size and shape of cavity allow. If 8 wafers can't be accommodated, use maximum number of wafers allowed. Or, 150 to 200 mg/m² I.V. by slow infusion as single dose, repeated q 6 to 8 weeks.

➤ **Cutaneous T-cell lymphoma (mycosis fungoides)** ◆

*Adults:* Apply 0.05% to 0.4% topical solution or ointment once or twice daily. Usual dose is 10 mg/day applied topically for 6 to 8 weeks. If response is inadequate, after a 6-week rest period, apply 20 mg/day topically for 30 days.

## I.V. ADMINISTRATION

● *Alert:* Preparation and administration of parenteral form of drug may be mutagenic, teratogenic, or carcinogenic to staff. Follow institutional policy to reduce risks. Manufacturer recommends wearing gloves when handling either form.

● To reconstitute, dissolve 100 mg of carmustine in 3 ml of absolute alcohol provided by manufacturer. Dilute solution with 27 ml of sterile water for injection. Resulting solution contains 3.3 mg of carmustine/ml in 10% alcohol. Dilute in normal saline solution or D₅W for I.V. infusion. Give at least 250 ml over 1 to 2 hours. To reduce pain on infusion, dilute further or slow infusion rate.

● Discard drug if powder liquefies or appears oily (decomposition has occurred).

● Give only in glass containers. Solution is unstable in plastic I.V. bags.

● Don't mix with other drugs during administration.

● Store reconstituted solution in refrigerator for 24 hours or at room temperature for 8 hours. May decompose at temperatures higher than 80° F (27° C).

## ACTION

Inhibits enzymatic reactions involved with DNA synthesis, cross-links strands of cellular DNA, and interferes with RNA transcription, causing an imbalance of growth that leads to cell death. Not specific to cell cycle.

| Route | Onset | Peak | Duration |
| --- | --- | --- | --- |
| I.V., intra-cavitary | Unknown | Unknown | Unknown |

## ADVERSE REACTIONS

**CNS:** ataxia, drowsiness, *brain edema, seizures.*
**EENT:** ocular toxicities.
**GI:** *nausea, vomiting, stomatitis.*
**GU:** *nephrotoxicity,* azotemia, *renal failure.*
**Hematologic:** *cumulative bone marrow suppression, leukopenia, thrombocytopenia, acute leukemia or bone marrow dysplasia,* anemia.
**Hepatic:** *hepatotoxicity.*
**Respiratory:** *pulmonary fibrosis.*
**Skin:** facial flushing, hyperpigmentation.
**Other:** *intense pain at infusion site from venous spasm, secondary malignancies.*

## INTERACTIONS

**Drug-drug.** *Anticoagulants, aspirin, NSAIDs:* May increase risk of bleeding. Avoid using together.
*Cimetidine:* May increase carmustine's bone marrow toxicity. Avoid using together.
*Digoxin, phenytoin:* May decrease levels of these drugs. Monitor patient.
*Mitomycin:* May increase corneal and conjunctival damage with high doses. Monitor patient.
*Myelosuppressives:* May increase myelosuppression. Monitor patient.

---

**EFFECTS ON LAB TEST RESULTS**
• May increase urine urea, AST, bilirubin, and alkaline phosphatase levels.
• May decrease hemoglobin and WBC and platelet counts.

**CONTRAINDICATIONS & CAUTIONS**
• Contraindicated in patients hypersensitive to drug.

**NURSING CONSIDERATIONS**
• Pulmonary toxicity appears to be dose-related and may occur 9 days to 15 years after treatment. Obtain pulmonary function tests before and during therapy.
• Bone marrow suppression is delayed with carmustine. Drug shouldn't be given more often than every 6 weeks.
• Give antiemetic before drug, to reduce nausea.
• Avoid contact with skin because carmustine causes a brown stain. If drug contacts skin, wash off thoroughly.
• Perform liver, renal function, and pulmonary function tests periodically.
• Monitor CBC with differential. The absolute neutrophil count may be used to better calculate the patient's immunosuppressive state.
• Monitor uric acid level. To prevent hyperuricemia with resulting uric acid nephropathy, allopurinol may be used with adequate hydration.
• Therapeutic effects are commonly accompanied by toxicity.
• Acute leukemia or bone marrow dysplasia may occur after long-term use.
• To prevent bleeding, avoid all I.M. injections when platelet count is less than 50,000/mm³.
• Anticipate blood transfusions during treatment because of cumulative anemia. Patient may receive injections of RBC colony-stimulating factor to promote cell production.
• Unopened foil pouches of wafer may be kept at ambient room temperature for a maximum of 6 hours.
• Wafers broken in half may be used; however, discard wafers broken into more than two pieces.

**PATIENT TEACHING**
• Advise patient about common adverse reactions to drug.

• Tell patient to watch for signs and symptoms of infection (fever, sore throat, fatigue) and bleeding (easy bruising, nosebleeds, bleeding gums, tarry stools). Tell him to take temperature daily.
• Instruct patient to avoid OTC products containing aspirin and NSAIDs.
• Advise women to stop breast-feeding during therapy because of possible risk of toxicity to infant.
• Caution woman of childbearing age to avoid becoming pregnant during therapy. Recommend that she consult prescriber before becoming pregnant.

## chlorambucil
Leukeran

*Pregnancy risk category D*

**AVAILABLE FORMS**
*Tablets:* 2 mg

**INDICATIONS & DOSAGES**
➤ **Chronic lymphocytic leukemia; malignant lymphomas, including lymphosarcoma, giant follicular lymphoma, and Hodgkin's disease**
*Adults:* 0.1 to 0.2 mg/kg P.O. daily for 3 to 6 weeks, then adjusted for maintenance (usually 4 to 10 mg daily); or, 3 to 6 mg/m² P.O. daily.
*Children:* 0.1 to 0.2 mg/kg P.O. or 4.5 mg/m² P.O. daily for 3 to 6 weeks.
*Adjust-a-dose:* Reduce first dose if given within 4 weeks after a full course of radiation therapy or myelosuppressive drugs, or if pretreatment leukocyte or platelet counts are depressed from bone marrow disease.
➤ **Macroglobulinemia ♦**
*Adults:* 2 to 10 mg P.O. daily for up to 9 years. Or, 8 mg/m² P.O. daily with prednisone for 10 days; repeat q 6 to 8 weeks p.r.n..
➤ **Nephrotic syndrome ♦**
*Children:* 0.1 to 0.2 mg/kg P.O. daily with prednisone for 8 to 12 weeks.
➤ **Intractable idiopathic uveitis, Behcet's syndrome ♦**
*Adults:* 6 to 12 mg or 0.1 to 0.2 mg/kg P.O. daily for at least 1 year.

## ACTION

Cross-links strands of cellular DNA and interferes with RNA transcription, causing an imbalance of growth that leads to cell death. Not specific to cell cycle.

| Route | Onset | Peak | Duration |
|-------|-------|------|----------|
| P.O. | Unknown | 1 hr | Unknown |

## ADVERSE REACTIONS

**CNS:** *seizures,* peripheral neuropathy, tremor, muscle twitching, confusion, agitation, ataxia, flaccid paresis.
**GI:** *nausea, vomiting,* stomatitis, diarrhea.
**GU:** *azoospermia, infertility,* sterile cystitis.
**Hematologic:** *neutropenia, bone marrow suppression, thrombocytopenia,* anemia, *myelosuppression.*
**Hepatic:** *hepatotoxicity.*
**Respiratory:** interstitial pneumonitis, *pulmonary fibrosis.*
**Skin:** rash, *erythema multiforme,* epidermal necrolysis, *Stevens-Johnson syndrome.*
**Other:** drug fever, hypersensitivity reactions, *secondary malignancies.*

## INTERACTIONS

**Drug-drug.** *Anticoagulants, aspirin:* May increase risk of bleeding. Avoid using together.
*Myelosuppressives:* May increase myelosuppression. Monitor patient.

## EFFECTS ON LAB TEST RESULTS

• May increase AST, alkaline phosphatase, and blood and urine uric acid levels.
• May decrease hemoglobin, neutrophil, platelet, WBC, granulocyte, and RBC counts.

## CONTRAINDICATIONS & CAUTIONS

• Contraindicated in patients with hypersensitivity or resistance to previous therapy. Patients hypersensitive to other alkylating drugs may also be hypersensitive to chlorambucil.
• Use cautiously in patients with history of head trauma or seizures and in patients receiving other drugs that lower the seizure threshold. Also use cautiously within 4 weeks of a full course of radiation or chemotherapy.

## NURSING CONSIDERATIONS

• Monitor CBC with differential.
• Monitor patient for neutropenia, which may not appear until after the third week of treatment. The neutrophil count may continue to decrease for up to 10 days after treatment ends.
• The absolute neutrophil count may be used to better calculate the patient's immunosuppressive state.
• Monitor uric acid level. To prevent hyperuricemia with resulting uric acid nephropathy, allopurinol may be used with adequate hydration.
• If WBC count falls below 2,000/mm$^3$ or granulocyte count falls below 1,000/mm$^3$, follow institutional policy for infection control in immunocompromised patients. Patients may receive injections of WBC colony-stimulating factor to increase WBC count recovery. Severe neutropenia is reversible up to cumulative dose of 6.5 mg/kg in a single course.
• Therapeutic effects are frequently accompanied by toxicity.
• To prevent bleeding, avoid all I.M. injections when platelet count is below 50,000/mm$^3$.
• Anticipate blood transfusions during treatment because of cumulative anemia. Patient may receive injections of RBC colony-stimulating factor to promote RBC production and decrease need for blood transfusions.

## PATIENT TEACHING

• Advise patient to watch for signs of infection (fever, sore throat, fatigue) and bleeding (easy bruising, nosebleeds, bleeding gums, tarry stools). Tell patient to take temperature daily.
• Instruct patient to avoid OTC products containing aspirin and NSAIDs.
• Tell women to stop breast-feeding during therapy because of risk of toxicity to infant.
• Advise women of childbearing age to avoid becoming pregnant during therapy and to notify prescriber immediately if pregnancy is suspected.

# cisplatin (CDDP, cis-platinum†)
Platinol AQ

*Pregnancy risk category D*

## AVAILABLE FORMS
*Injection:* 0.5 mg/ml†, 1 mg/ml

## INDICATIONS & DOSAGES
➤ **Adjunctive therapy in metastatic testicular cancer**
*Adults:* 20 mg/m² I.V. daily for 5 days. Repeat q 3 weeks for three or four cycles.
➤ **Adjunctive therapy in metastatic ovarian cancer**
*Adults:* 100 mg/m² I.V.; repeat q 4 weeks. Or, 50 to 100 mg/m² I.V. once q 3 to 4 weeks with cyclophosphamide.
➤ **Advanced bladder cancer**
*Adults:* 50 to 70 mg/m² I.V. q 3 to 4 weeks. Give 50 mg/m² q 4 weeks in patients who have received other antineoplastic drugs or radiation therapy.
➤ **Head and neck cancer** ◆
*Adults:* 80 to 120 mg/m² I.V. q 3 weeks or 50 mg/ m² I.V. on days 1 and 8 q 4 weeks. Doses of 50 to 120 mg/m² I.V. may be used in combination therapy.
➤ **Cervical cancer**
*Adults:* 40 to 75 mg/m² I.V. weekly or daily as monotherapy, in combination therapy, or with radiation therapy.
➤ **Non–small-cell lung cancer**
*Adults:* 75 to 100 mg/m² I.V. q 3 to 4 weeks in combination therapy.
➤ **Osteogenic sarcoma or neuroblastoma**
*Children:* 90 mg/m² I.V. q 3 weeks, or 30 mg/m² I.V. once weekly.
➤ **Recurrent brain tumor**
*Children:* 60 mg/m² I.V. daily for 2 consecutive days q 3 to 4 weeks.

## I.V. ADMINISTRATION
• *Alert:* Preparation and administration of parenteral form of drug may be mutagenic, teratogenic, or carcinogenic to staff. Follow institutional policy to reduce risks.
• Give mannitol or furosemide boluses or infusions before and during cisplatin infusion to maintain diuresis of 100 to 400 ml/hour during and for 24 hours after therapy.

• Hydrate patient with normal saline solution before giving drug. Maintain urine output of at least 100 ml/hour for 4 consecutive hours before therapy and for 24 hours after therapy.
• Reconstitute powder using sterile water for injection. Add 10 ml to 10-mg vial or 50 ml to 50-mg vial to make a solution containing 1 mg/ml. Further dilute with dextrose 5% in 0.3% sodium chloride injection or dextrose 5% in half-normal saline solution for injection. Solutions are stable for 20 hours at room temperature. Don't refrigerate.
• Infusions are most stable in chloride-containing solutions (such as normal or half-normal saline solution and 0.22% sodium chloride). Don't use $D_5W$ alone. The manufacturer recommends giving drug as an I.V. infusion in 2 L of dextrose 5% in half-normal saline solution or dextrose 5% in 0.33% sodium chloride solution with 37.5 g of mannitol over 6 to 8 hours.
• Don't use needles or I.V. administration sets that contain aluminum because they displace the platinum, causing loss of potency and formation of a black precipitate.
• Don't give drug through same I.V. line as mesna, sodium bicarbonate, or sodium thiosulfate, which inactivate cisplatin.
• To prevent hypokalemia, potassium chloride (10 to 20 mEq/L) is commonly added to I.V. fluids before and after cisplatin therapy. Magnesium sulfate may be added to prevent hypomagnesemia.

## ACTION
Unknown. Thought to cross-link strands of cellular DNA and interfere with RNA transcription, causing an imbalance of growth that leads to cell death. Not specific to cell cycle.

| Route | Onset | Peak | Duration |
|-------|-------|------|----------|
| I.V. | Unknown | Unknown | Several days |

## ADVERSE REACTIONS
**CNS:** *peripheral neuritis,* **seizures.**
**EENT:** *tinnitus, hearing loss, ototoxicity,* vestibular toxicity, optic neuritis, papilledema, cerebral blindness, blurred vision.
**GI:** loss of taste, *nausea, vomiting.*

**GU:** PROLONGED RENAL TOXICITY with repeated courses of therapy.
**Hematologic:** MYELOSUPPRESSION, *leukopenia, thrombocytopenia,* anemia.
**Metabolic:** *hypomagnesemia,* hypokalemia, hypocalcemia, hyponatremia, hypophosphatemia, hyperuricemia.
**Other:** *anaphylactoid reaction.*

### INTERACTIONS
**Drug-drug.** *Aminoglycosides:* May increase nephrotoxicity. Carefully monitor renal function studies.
*Aminoglycosides, bumetanide, ethacrynic acid, furosemide, torsemide:* May increase ototoxicity. Avoid using together, if possible.
*Aspirin, NSAIDs:* May increase risk of bleeding. Avoid using together.
*Fosphenytoin, phenytoin:* May decrease phenytoin and fosphenytoin levels. Monitor levels.
*Myelosuppressives:* May increase myelosuppression. Monitor patient.

### EFFECTS ON LAB TEST RESULTS
• May increase uric acid level. May decrease magnesium, potassium, calcium, sodium, and phosphate levels.
• May decrease hemoglobin and WBC and platelet counts.

### CONTRAINDICATIONS & CAUTIONS
• Contraindicated in patients hypersensitive to drug or other platinum-containing compounds and in those with severe renal disease, hearing impairment, or myelosuppression.
• Use cautiously in patients previously treated with radiation or cytotoxic drugs and in those with peripheral neuropathies; also use cautiously with other ototoxic and nephrotoxic drugs.

### NURSING CONSIDERATIONS
• Monitor CBC, electrolyte levels (especially potassium and magnesium), platelet count, and renal function studies before initial and subsequent doses.
• To detect hearing loss, obtain audiometry tests before initial and subsequent doses.
• Prehydration and mannitol diuresis may significantly reduce renal toxicity and ototoxicity.

• Therapeutic effects are frequently accompanied by toxicity.
• Check current protocol. Some prescribers use I.V. sodium thiosulfate or amifostine to minimize toxicity.
• Patients may experience vomiting 3 to 5 days after treatment, requiring prolonged antiemetic treatment. Some prescribers combine metoclopramide with dexamethasone and antihistamines, or ondansetron or granisetron with dexamethasone to control vomiting. Monitor intake and output. Continue I.V. hydration until patient can tolerate adequate oral intake.
• Renal toxicity is cumulative; renal function must return to normal before next dose can be given.
• Don't repeat dose unless platelet count is greater than 100,000/mm³, WBC count is greater than 4,000/mm³, creatinine level is less than 1.5 mg/dl, creatinine clearance is 50 ml/minute or more, and BUN level is less than 25 mg/dl.
• To prevent bleeding, avoid all I.M. injections when platelet count is less than 50,000/mm³.
• Anticipate need for blood transfusions during treatment because of cumulative anemia.
• *Alert:* Immediately give epinephrine, corticosteroids, or antihistamines for anaphylactoid reactions.
• Safety of drug in children hasn't been established.
• *Alert:* Don't confuse cisplatin with carboplatin; they aren't interchangeable.

### PATIENT TEACHING
• Advise patient to watch for signs and symptoms of infection (fever, sore throat, fatigue) and bleeding (easy bruising, nosebleeds, bleeding gums, tarry stools). Tell patient to take temperature daily.
• Tell patient to immediately report ringing in the ears or numbness in hands or feet.
• Instruct patient to avoid OTC products containing aspirin.
• Advise women to stop breast-feeding because of risk of toxicity to infant.
• Advise women of childbearing age to consult prescriber before becoming pregnant.

---

Reactions may be *common,* uncommon, *life-threatening,* or COMMON AND LIFE-THREATENING.

# cyclophosphamide
Cycloblastin‡, Cytoxan, Cytoxan
Lyophilized, Endoxan-Asta‡,
Neosar, Procytox†

*Pregnancy risk category D*

**AVAILABLE FORMS**
*Injection:* 100-mg, 200-mg, 500-mg, 1-g,
2-g vials
*Tablets:* 25 mg, 50 mg

**INDICATIONS & DOSAGES**
➤ **Breast and ovarian cancers,
Hodgkin's disease, chronic lymphocytic
leukemia, chronic myelocytic leukemia,
acute lymphoblastic leukemia, acute
myelocytic and monocytic leukemia,
neuroblastoma, retinoblastoma, malignant lymphoma, multiple myeloma,
mycosis fungoides, sarcoma**
*Adults:* Initially for induction, 40 to
50 mg/kg I.V. in divided doses over 2 to
5 days. Or, 10 to 15 mg/kg I.V. q 7 to
10 days, 3 to 5 mg/kg I.V. twice weekly,
or 1 to 5 mg/kg P.O. daily, based on patient tolerance.
*Children:* Initially for induction, 2 to
8 mg/kg or 60 to 250 mg/m² P.O. or I.V.
daily. Maintenance dose is 2 to 5 mg/kg
P.O. or 50 to 150 mg/m² P.O. twice
weekly.
Adjust subsequent doses according to evidence of antitumor activity or leukopenia.
➤ **Minimal-change nephrotic syndrome
in children**
*Children:* 2 to 3 mg/kg P.O. daily for 60 to
90 days.

**I.V. ADMINISTRATION**
● *Alert:* Preparation and administration of
parenteral form of drug may be mutagenic, teratogenic, or carcinogenic to staff.
Follow institutional policy to reduce risks.
● Reconstitute powder using sterile water
for injection or bacteriostatic water for
injection containing only parabens. For
the nonlyophilized product, add 5 ml to
100-mg vial, 10 ml to 200-mg vial, 25 ml
to 500-mg vial, 50 ml to 1-g vial, or
100 ml to 2-g vial to produce a solution
containing 20 mg/ml. Shake to dissolve;
this may take up to 6 minutes, and it may
be difficult to completely dissolve drug.

Lyophilized preparation is much easier to
reconstitute; check package insert for
quantity of diluent needed to reconstitute
drug.
● After reconstitution, give by direct I.V.
injection or infusion. For I.V. infusion, further dilute with D₅W, dextrose 5% in normal saline solution for injection, dextrose
5% in Ringer's injection, lactated Ringer's
injection, sodium lactate injection, or half-
normal saline solution for injection.
● Check reconstituted solution for small
particles. Filter solution if needed.
● Reconstituted solution is stable for 6
days if refrigerated, or 24 hours at room
temperature. However, use stored solutions cautiously because drug contains no
preservatives.

**ACTION**
Cross-links strands of cellular DNA and
interferes with RNA transcription, causing
an imbalance of growth that leads to cell
death. Not specific to cell cycle.

| Route | Onset | Peak | Duration |
|---|---|---|---|
| P.O. | Unknown | Unknown | Unknown |
| I.V. | Unknown | 2-3 hr | Unknown |

**ADVERSE REACTIONS**
**CV:** *cardiotoxicity with very high doses
and with doxorubicin,* flushing.
**GI:** anorexia, *nausea and vomiting,* ab-
dominal pain, stomatitis, mucositis.
**GU:** HEMORRHAGIC CYSTITIS, impaired
fertility.
**Hematologic:** *leukopenia, thrombocy-
topenia,* anemia.
**Hepatic:** *hepatotoxicity.*
**Metabolic:** hyperuricemia, SIADH.
**Respiratory:** *pulmonary fibrosis with
high doses.*
**Skin:** *reversible alopecia,* rash, pigmenta-
tion, nail changes, itching.
**Other:** *secondary malignant disease,
anaphylaxis,* hypersensitivity reactions.

**INTERACTIONS**
**Drug-drug.** *Allopurinol:* May increase
myelosuppression. Monitor toxicity.
*Anticoagulants:* May increase anticoagulant effect. Monitor for bleeding.
*Aspirin, NSAIDs:* May increase risk of
bleeding. Avoid using together.

*Barbiturates:* May increase pharmacologic effect and enhance cyclophosphamide toxicity from induction of hepatic enzymes. Monitor patient closely.

*Cardiotoxic drugs:* May increase adverse cardiac effects. Monitor toxicity.

*Chloramphenicol, corticosteroids:* May reduce activity of cyclophosphamide. Use together cautiously.

*Ciprofloxacin:* May decrease antimicrobial efficacy. Monitor for effect.

*Digoxin:* May decrease digoxin level. Monitor level closely.

*Myelosuppressives:* May increase myelosuppression. Monitor patient.

*Succinylcholine:* May prolong neuromuscular blockade. Avoid using together.

**EFFECTS ON LAB TEST RESULTS**
• May increase uric acid level. May decrease pseudocholinesterase level.
• May decrease hemoglobin and WBC, RBC, and platelet counts.
• May suppress positive reaction to *Candida,* mumps, *Trichophyton,* and tuberculin skin test. May cause a false-positive Papanicolaou test result.

**CONTRAINDICATIONS & CAUTIONS**
• Contraindicated in patients hypersensitive to drug and in those with severe bone marrow suppression.
• Use cautiously in patients with leukopenia, thrombocytopenia, malignant cell infiltration of bone marrow, or hepatic or renal disease and in those who have recently undergone radiation therapy or chemotherapy.

**NURSING CONSIDERATIONS**
• Don't give drug at bedtime; infrequent urination during the night may increase possibility of cystitis. If cystitis occurs, stop drug and notify prescriber. Cystitis can occur months after therapy ceases. Mesna may be given to reduce frequency and severity of bladder toxicity. Test urine for blood.
• Patients should receive adequate hydration before and after dose to decrease risk of cystitis.
• Use caution to ensure correct dose to decrease risk of cardiac toxicity.
• Monitor CBC and renal and liver function test results.

• Monitor patient closely for leukopenia (nadir between days 8 and 15, recovery in 17 to 28 days).
• Monitor uric acid level. To prevent hyperuricemia with resulting uric acid nephropathy, allopurinol may be used with adequate hydration.
• *Alert:* Monitor patient for cyclophosphamide toxicity (leukopenia, thrombocytopenia, cardiotoxicity) if patient's corticosteroid therapy is stopped.
• To prevent bleeding, avoid all I.M. injections when platelet count is less than 50,000/mm$^3$.
• Anticipate blood transfusions because of cumulative anemia. Patients may receive injections of RBC colony-stimulating factor to promote RBC production and decrease need for blood transfusions.
• Therapeutic effects are often accompanied by toxicity.
• Drug may be used to treat nononcologic disorders such as lupus, nephritis, and rheumatoid arthritis.

**PATIENT TEACHING**
• Warn patient that hair loss is likely to occur but that it's reversible.
• Advise patient to watch for signs and symptoms of infection (fever, sore throat, fatigue) and bleeding (easy bruising, nosebleeds, bleeding gums, tarry stools). Tell patient to take temperature daily.
• Instruct patient to avoid OTC products that contain aspirin.
• To minimize risk of hemorrhagic cystitis, encourage patient to urinate every 1 to 2 hours while awake and to drink at least 3 L of fluid daily. If patient is taking oral form of drug, instruct him to avoid taking it at bedtime because infrequent urination increases risk of cystitis.
• Advise both men and women to practice contraception during therapy and for 4 months afterward; drug may cause birth defects.
• Advise women taking drug to stop breast-feeding because of risk of toxicity to infant.
• Drug can cause irreversible sterility in both men and women. Counsel patients of childbearing potential before starting therapy. Also recommend that women consult prescriber before becoming pregnant.

---

# ifosfamide
Holoxan‡, Ifex

*Pregnancy risk category D*

## AVAILABLE FORMS
*Injection:* 1 g, 2 g†‡, 3 g

## INDICATIONS & DOSAGES
➤ **Testicular cancer**
*Adults:* 1.2 g/m$^2$/day I.V. for 5 consecutive days. Repeat treatment q 3 weeks or after patient recovers from hematologic toxicity.
➤ **Sarcomas ♦, small-cell lung cancer ♦, cervical cancer ♦, ovarian cancer ♦, uterine cancer ♦**
*Adults:* 1.2 to 2.5 g/m$^2$ I.V. daily for 3 to 5 days. Repeat cycle p.r.n. based on patient response.

## I.V. ADMINISTRATION
• *Alert:* Preparation and administration of parenteral form of drug may be mutagenic, teratogenic, or carcinogenic to staff. Follow institutional policy to reduce risks.
• Reconstitute each gram of drug with 20 ml of diluent to yield a solution of 50 mg/ml. Use sterile water for injection or bacteriostatic water for injection. Solutions may then be further diluted with sterile water, dextrose 2.5% or 5% in water, half-normal or normal saline solution for injection, dextrose 5% and normal saline solution for injection, or lactated Ringer's injection.
• Infuse each dose over at least 30 minutes.
• Give ifosfamide with a protective drug such as mesna to prevent hemorrhagic cystitis. Obtain urinalysis before each dose. If microscopic hematuria occurs, notify prescriber. Adjust dosage of concomitant mesna if needed. Adequate fluid intake (2 L/day, either P.O. or I.V.) is essential before, and 72 hours after, therapy.
• Ifosfamide and mesna are physically compatible and may be mixed in the same I.V. solution.
• Reconstituted solution is stable for 1 week at room temperature or 6 weeks if refrigerated. However, use solution within 6 hours if drug was reconstituted with

sterile water without a preservative (such as benzyl alcohol or parabens).

## ACTION
Cross-links strands of cellular DNA and interferes with RNA transcription, causing an imbalance of growth that leads to cell death. Not specific to cell cycle.

| Route | Onset | Peak | Duration |
|-------|-------|------|----------|
| I.V. | Unknown | Unknown | Unknown |

## ADVERSE REACTIONS
**CNS:** *somnolence, confusion,* **coma, seizures,** ataxia, hallucinations, depressive psychosis, dizziness, disorientation, cranial nerve dysfunction.
**GI:** *nausea, vomiting,* diarrhea.
**GU:** *hemorrhagic cystitis, hematuria,* **nephrotoxicity,** Fanconi's syndrome.
**Hematologic:** **leukopenia, thrombocytopenia, myelosuppression.**
**Hepatic:** **hepatotoxicity.**
**Metabolic:** *metabolic acidosis.*
**Skin:** *alopecia.*
**Other:** infection, phlebitis.

## INTERACTIONS
**Drug-drug.** *Anticoagulants, aspirin, NSAIDs:* May increase risk of bleeding. Avoid using together.
*Barbiturates, chloral hydrate, fosphenytoin, phenytoin:* May increase ifosfamide toxicity by inducing hepatic enzymes that hasten formation of toxic metabolites. Monitor patient closely.
*Corticosteroids:* May inhibit hepatic enzymes, reducing ifosfamide's effect. Monitor patient for increased ifosfamide toxicity if corticosteroid dosage is suddenly reduced or stopped.
*Cyclophosphamide:* May increase risk of cardiac tamponade in patients with thalassemia. Monitor patient closely during use.
*Myelosuppressives:* May enhance hematologic toxicity. Dosage adjustment may be needed.

## EFFECTS ON LAB TEST RESULTS
• May increase liver enzyme levels.
• May decrease WBC and platelet counts.

---

## CONTRAINDICATIONS & CAUTIONS

• Contraindicated in patients hypersensitive to drug and in those with severe bone marrow suppression.
• Use cautiously in patients with renal impairment or compromised bone marrow reserve as indicated by leukopenia, granulocytopenia, extensive bone marrow metastases, previous radiation therapy, or previous therapy with cytotoxic drugs.

## NURSING CONSIDERATIONS

• Give antiemetic before drug, to reduce nausea.
• Don't give drug at bedtime; infrequent urination during the night may increase possibility of cystitis. If cystitis develops, stop drug and notify prescriber.
• Bladder irrigation with normal saline solution may be done to treat cystitis.
• Monitor CBC and renal and liver function tests.
• To prevent bleeding, avoid all I.M. injections when platelet count is less than 50,000/mm³.
• Anticipate blood transfusions because of cumulative anemia. Patients may receive injections of RBC colony-stimulating factor to promote RBC production and decrease need for blood transfusions.
• Assess patient for mental status changes; dosage may have to be decreased.
• **Alert:** Don't confuse ifosfamide with cyclophosphamide.

## PATIENT TEACHING

• Remind patient to urinate frequently to minimize contact of drug and its metabolites with the lining of the bladder.
• Advise patient to watch for signs and symptoms of infection (fever, sore throat, fatigue) and bleeding (easy bruising, nosebleeds, bleeding gums, tarry stools). Tell patient to take temperature daily.
• Instruct patient to avoid OTC products that contain aspirin.
• Advise women to stop breast-feeding during therapy because of possible risk of toxicity to infant.
• Caution woman of childbearing age to avoid becoming pregnant during therapy. Recommend that she consult prescriber before becoming pregnant.

# lomustine (CCNU)
CeeNU

*Pregnancy risk category D*

## AVAILABLE FORMS

*Capsules:* 10 mg, 40 mg, 100 mg, dose pack (two 10-mg, two 40-mg, two 100-mg capsules)

## INDICATIONS & DOSAGES

➤ **Brain tumor, Hodgkin's disease**
*Adults and children:* 100 to 130 mg/m² P.O. as single dose q 6 weeks. Repeat doses shouldn't be given until WBC count exceeds 4,000/mm³ and platelet count is greater than 100,000/mm³.
*Adjust-a-dose:* Reduce dosage according to degree of bone marrow suppression or when used with other myelosuppressive drugs. Reduce dosage by 30% for WBC count nadir 2,000 to 2,999/mm³ and platelet count nadir 25,000 to 74,999/mm³; by 50% for WBC count nadir less than 2,000/mm³ and platelet count nadir less than 25,000/mm³.

## ACTION

Cross-links strands of cellular DNA and interferes with RNA transcription, causing an imbalance of growth that leads to cell death. Not specific to cell cycle.

| Route | Onset | Peak | Duration |
|-------|-------|------|----------|
| P.O. | Unknown | Unknown | Unknown |

## ADVERSE REACTIONS

**CNS:** disorientation, lethargy, ataxia.
**GI:** *nausea, vomiting,* stomatitis.
**GU:** *nephrotoxicity,* progressive azotemia, *renal failure,* amenorrhea, azoospermia.
**Hematologic:** *anemia, leukopenia, thrombocytopenia, bone marrow suppression.*
**Hepatic:** *hepatotoxicity.*
**Respiratory:** *pulmonary fibrosis.*
**Skin:** alopecia.
**Other:** *secondary malignant disease.*

## INTERACTIONS

**Drug-drug.** *Anticoagulants, aspirin, NSAIDs:* May increase risk of bleeding. Avoid using together.

---

Reactions may be *common,* uncommon, *life-threatening,* or **COMMON AND LIFE-THREATENING.**

*Myelosuppressives:* May increase myelosuppression. Monitor patient.

**EFFECTS ON LAB TEST RESULTS**
• May increase urine urea level.
• May decrease hemoglobin and WBC, RBC, and platelet counts.

**CONTRAINDICATIONS & CAUTIONS**
• Contraindicated in patients hypersensitive to drug.
• Use cautiously in patients with decreased platelet, WBC, or RBC counts and in those receiving other myelosuppressives.

**NURSING CONSIDERATIONS**
• Give antiemetic before drug, to reduce nausea.
• Give 2 to 4 hours after meals; drug will be more completely absorbed if taken when stomach is empty.
• Monitor CBC weekly. Usually not given more often than every 6 weeks; bone marrow toxicity is cumulative and delayed, usually occurring 4 to 6 weeks after drug administration.
• Periodically monitor liver function test results.
• To prevent bleeding, avoid all I.M. injections when platelet count is less than 50,000/mm³.
• Anticipate blood transfusions because of cumulative anemia. Patients may receive RBC colony-stimulating factor to promote RBC production and decrease need for blood transfusions.
• Therapeutic effects are commonly accompanied by toxicity.
• Store capsules at room temperature. Avoid exposure to moisture, and protect from temperatures greater than 104° F (40° C).

**PATIENT TEACHING**
• Advise patient to take capsules on an empty stomach, if possible.
• Advise patient to watch for signs and symptoms of infection (fever, sore throat, fatigue) and bleeding (easy bruising, nosebleeds, bleeding gums, tarry stools). Tell patient to take temperature daily.
• Instruct patient to avoid OTC products that contain aspirin or NSAIDs.

• Advise women to stop breast-feeding during therapy because of possible risk of toxicity to infant.
• Caution woman of childbearing age to avoid becoming pregnant during therapy. Recommend that she consult prescriber before becoming pregnant.

---

**mechlorethamine hydrochloride (nitrogen mustard)**
Mustargen

*Pregnancy risk category D*

**AVAILABLE FORMS**
*Injection:* 10-mg vials

**INDICATIONS & DOSAGES**
Dosage is based on patient response and degree of toxicity.
➤ **Hodgkin's disease**
*Adults and children:* 6 mg/m² daily on days 1 and 8 of 28-day cycle in combination with other antineoplastics, such as mechlorethamine-vincristine-procarbazine-prednisone (MOPP) regimen. Repeat dosage for six cycles.
*Adjust-a-dose:* Subsequent doses reduced by 50% in MOPP regimen when WBC count 3,000 to 3,999/mm³ and by 75% when WBC count 1,000 to 2,999/mm³, or platelet count is 50,000 to 100,000/mm³.
➤ **Polycythemia vera, chronic lymphocytic leukemia, chronic myelocytic leukemia, bronchogenic cancer**
*Adults and children:* 0.4 mg/kg as single dose or 0.1 to 0.2 mg/kg divided in two or four successive daily doses during each course of therapy.
➤ **Malignant effusions (pericardial, peritoneal, pleural)**
*Adults:* 0.4 mg/kg intracavitarily, although 0.2 mg/kg has been used intrapericardially.

**I.V. ADMINISTRATION**
• *Alert:* Preparation and administration of parenteral form of drug may be mutagenic, teratogenic, or carcinogenic to staff. Follow institutional policy to reduce risks.
• Reconstitute drug using 10 ml of sterile water for injection or normal saline solution for injection. Resulting solution con-

tains 1 mg/ml of mechlorethamine. Give by direct injection into a vein or into tubing of a free-flowing I.V. solution.

• Prepare immediately before infusion. Solution is very unstable. Visually inspect before using; make sure solution is colorless; use within 15 minutes, and discard unused solution.

• Dispose of equipment used in preparation and administration of mechlorethamine properly and according to institutional policy. Neutralize unused solution with an equal volume of 5% sodium bicarbonate and 5% sodium thiosulfate for 45 minutes.

• *Alert:* Make sure that I.V. solution doesn't infiltrate. Mechlorethamine is a potent vesicant. If extravasation occurs, apply cold compresses for 6 to 12 hours, and infiltrate area with isotonic sodium thiosulfate.

### ACTION
Cross-links strands of cellular DNA and interferes with RNA transcription, causing an imbalance of growth that leads to cell death. Not specific to cell cycle.

| Route | Onset | Peak | Duration |
|---|---|---|---|
| I.V., intra-cavitary | Few sec–few min | Unknown | Unknown |

### ADVERSE REACTIONS
**CNS:** weakness, vertigo, neurotoxicity.
**CV:** *thrombophlebitis.*
**EENT:** tinnitus, deafness with high doses.
**GI:** *nausea, vomiting, anorexia,* diarrhea, metallic taste.
**GU:** menstrual irregularities, impaired spermatogenesis.
**Hematologic:** *thrombocytopenia,* lymphocytopenia, *agranulocytosis,* mild anemia beginning in 2 to 3 weeks.
**Hepatic:** jaundice.
**Metabolic:** hyperuricemia.
**Skin:** *alopecia,* rash, sloughing, severe skin irritation with extravasation or contact.
**Other:** precipitation of herpes zoster, *anaphylaxis, secondary malignant disease.*

### INTERACTIONS
**Drug-drug.** *Anticoagulants, aspirin, NSAIDs:* May increase risk of bleeding. Avoid using together.
*Myelosuppressives:* May increase myelosuppression. Monitor patient.

### EFFECTS ON LAB TEST RESULTS
• May increase urine urea level.
• May decrease hemoglobin and granulocyte, lymphocyte, RBC, and platelet counts.

### CONTRAINDICATIONS & CAUTIONS
• Contraindicated in patients hypersensitive to drug and in those with infectious diseases.
• Use cautiously in patients with severe anemia or depressed neutrophil or platelet count. Also use cautiously in those who have recently undergone radiation therapy or chemotherapy. Monitor CBC.

### NURSING CONSIDERATIONS
• When given intracavitarily for sclerosing effect, dilute using up to 100 ml of normal saline solution for injection. Turn patient from side to side every 5 to 10 minutes for 1 hour to distribute drug.
• Monitor uric acid level. To prevent hyperuricemia with resulting uric acid or nephropathy, mechlorethamine may be used with adequate hydration.
• Therapeutic effects are commonly accompanied by toxicity.
• Neurotoxicity increases with dosage and patient age.
• To prevent bleeding, avoid all I.M. injections when platelet count is less than 50,000/mm$^3$.
• Monitor patient closely for bone marrow suppression (nadir of myelosuppression occurring between days 4 and 10 and lasting 10 to 21 days).
• Anticipate need for blood transfusions because of cumulative anemia. Patients may receive RBC colony-stimulating factor to promote RBC cell production and decrease need for blood transfusions.

### PATIENT TEACHING
• Advise patient to report any pain or burning at site of injection during or after administration.

---

• Advise patient to watch for signs and symptoms of infection (fever, sore throat, fatigue) and bleeding (easy bruising, nosebleeds, bleeding gums, tarry stools). Tell patient to take temperature daily.

• Tell patient that severe nausea and vomiting can occur.

• Instruct patient to avoid OTC products that contain aspirin or NSAIDs.

• Caution woman taking drug to stop breast-feeding because of risk of toxicity to infant.

• Advise women of childbearing age to consult prescriber before becoming pregnant.

• Tell patient about the risk of sterility.

---

## melphalan (L-phenylalanine mustard)
Alkeran

## melphalan hydrochloride
Alkeran

*Pregnancy risk category D*

### AVAILABLE FORMS
*Injection:* 50 mg
*Tablets (scored):* 2 mg

### INDICATIONS & DOSAGES
➤ **Multiple myeloma**
*Adults:* Initially, 6 mg P.O. daily for 2 to 3 weeks; then stop drug for up to 4 weeks or until WBC and platelet counts stop dropping and begin to rise again; maintenance dose is 2 mg daily. Or, 0.15 mg/kg P.O. daily for 7 days, or 0.25 mg/kg for 4 days; repeat q 4 to 6 weeks.
Or, give I.V. to patients who can't tolerate oral therapy, 16 mg/m² given by infusion over 15 to 20 minutes at 2-week intervals for four doses. After patient has recovered from toxicity, give drug at 4-week intervals.
*Adjust-a-dose:* For patients with renal insufficiency, reduce dosage by up to 50%.
➤ **Nonresectable advanced ovarian cancer**
*Adults:* 0.2 mg/kg P.O. daily for 5 days. Repeat q 4 to 6 weeks, depending on bone marrow recovery.

### I.V. ADMINISTRATION
• *Alert:* Preparation and administration of parenteral form of drug may be mutagenic, teratogenic, or carcinogenic to staff. Follow institutional policy to reduce risks.

• Because drug isn't stable in solution, reconstitute immediately before giving with the 10 ml of sterile diluent supplied by manufacturer. Shake vigorously until solution is clear. The resulting solution will contain 5 mg/ml of melphalan. Immediately dilute required dose in normal saline solution for injection to no more than 0.45 mg/ml. Give infusion over 15 to 20 minutes.

• Promptly dilute and give drug; reconstituted product begins to degrade within 30 minutes. After final dilution, nearly 1% of drug degrades every 10 minutes. Administration must be completed within 60 minutes of reconstitution.

• Don't refrigerate reconstituted product because precipitate will form.

### ACTION
Cross-links strands of cellular DNA and interferes with RNA transcription, causing an imbalance of growth that leads to cell death. Not specific to cell cycle.

| Route | Onset | Peak | Duration |
|---|---|---|---|
| P.O., I.V. | Unknown | Unknown | Unknown |

### ADVERSE REACTIONS
**CV:** hypotension, tachycardia, edema.
**GI:** nausea, vomiting, diarrhea, oral ulceration, stomatitis.
**Hematologic:** *thrombocytopenia, leukopenia, bone marrow suppression,* hemolytic anemia.
**Hepatic:** *hepatotoxicity.*
**Metabolic:** hyperuricemia.
**Respiratory:** *pneumonitis, pulmonary fibrosis,* dyspnea, *bronchospasm.*
**Skin:** pruritus, alopecia, urticaria, ulceration at injection site.
**Other:** *anaphylaxis,* hypersensitivity reactions.

### INTERACTIONS
**Drug-drug (I.V. melphalan only).** *Anticoagulants, aspirin, NSAIDs:* May increase risk of bleeding. Avoid using together.

---

*Carmustine:* May decrease threshold for pulmonary toxicity. Use together cautiously.

*Cimetidine:* May decrease melphalan concentrations. Monitor patient closely.

*Cisplatin:* May increase renal impairment causing decreased melphalan clearance. Monitor patient closely.

*Cyclosporine:* May cause severe renal failure. Monitor renal function closely.

*Interferon alfa:* May increase elimination of melphalan. Monitor patient closely.

*Myelosuppressives:* May increase myelosuppression. Monitor patient.

*Nalidixic acid:* May increase risk of severe hemorrhagic necrotic enterocolitis in children. Avoid using together.

*Vaccines:* May decrease effectiveness of killed virus vaccines and increase risk of toxicity from live virus vaccines. Postpone routine immunization for at least 3 months after last dose of melphalan.

**Drug-food.** *Any food:* May decrease oral drug absorption. Advise patient to take drug on empty stomach.

### EFFECTS ON LAB TEST RESULTS
• May increase urine urea level.
• May decrease hemoglobin and RBC, WBC, and platelet counts.

### CONTRAINDICATIONS & CAUTIONS
• Contraindicated in patients hypersensitive to drug and in those whose disease is resistant to drug. Patients hypersensitive to chlorambucil may have cross-sensitivity to melphalan.
• Contraindicated in patients with severe leukopenia, thrombocytopenia, or anemia and in those with chronic lymphocytic leukemia.
• Use cautiously in patients receiving radiation and chemotherapy.

### NURSING CONSIDERATIONS
• Dosage may need to be reduced in patients with renal impairment.
• Melphalan is drug of choice with prednisone in patients with multiple myeloma.
• Give oral form on empty stomach because food decreases drug absorption.
• Monitor uric acid level and CBC.
• To prevent bleeding, avoid all I.M. injections when platelet count is less than 50,000/mm³.

• Anticipate need for blood transfusions because of cumulative anemia. Patients may receive RBC colony-stimulating factor to promote RBC production and decrease need for blood transfusions.
• Anaphylaxis may occur. Keep antihistamines and steroids readily available to give if needed.
• *Alert:* Don't confuse melphalan with Mephyton.

### PATIENT TEACHING
• Advise patient to take tablets on empty stomach.
• Advise patient to watch for signs and symptoms of infection (fever, sore throat, fatigue) and bleeding (easy bruising, nosebleeds, bleeding gums, tarry stools). Tell patient to take temperature daily.
• Instruct patient to avoid OTC products that contain aspirin or NSAIDs.
• Caution woman taking drug to stop breast-feeding because of risk of toxicity to infant.
• Advise women of childbearing age to consult prescriber before becoming pregnant.

---

## oxaliplatin
Eloxatin, Eloxatine (EU)

*Pregnancy risk category D*

### AVAILABLE FORMS
*Injection:* 50- or 100-mg vials

### INDICATIONS & DOSAGES
➤ **Metastatic colon or rectal cancer that has recurred or progressed during or within 6 months of completion of first-line therapy with 5-fluorouracil (5-FU) and leucovorin and irinotecan**
*Adults:* On Day 1, give 85 mg/m² oxaliplatin I.V. in 250 to 500 ml $D_5W$ and leucovorin 200 mg/m² I.V. in $D_5W$, given simultaneously over 120 minutes, in separate bags using a Y-line, followed by 5-FU 400 mg/m² I.V. bolus given over 2 to 4 minutes, followed by 600 mg/m² 5-FU I.V. infusion in 500 ml $D_5W$ over 22 hours.

On Day 2, give 200 mg/m² leucovorin I.V. infusion over 120 minutes, followed by 400 mg/m² 5-FU I.V. bolus given over 2 to 4 minutes, followed by 600 mg/m²

5-FU I.V. infusion in 500 ml D$_5$W over 22 hours.

Repeat cycle q 2 weeks.

*Adjust-a-dose:* In patients with unresolved and persistent grade 2 neurosensory events, reduce dose to 65 mg/m$^2$. In those with persistent grade 3 neurosensory events, consider stopping drug. In patients recovering from grade 3 or 4 GI or hematologic events, reduce dose to 65 mg/m$^2$. Also reduce dose of 5-FU by 20%.

## I.V. ADMINISTRATION
● *Alert:* Preparation and administration of parenteral form of drug may be mutagenic, teratogenic, or carcinogenic to staff. Follow institutional policy to reduce risks.
● Reconstitute powder using sterile water for injection or D$_5$W. Add 10 ml to a 50-mg vial or 20 ml to a 100-mg vial, for a yield of 5 mg/ml. Never reconstitute with sodium chloride solution or other solution containing chloride.
● Reconstituted solutions must be further diluted in an infusion solution of 250 to 500 ml of D$_5$W.
● Visually inspect bag for particulate matter and discoloration before administration, and discard if present.
● Give oxaliplatin and leucovorin over 2 hours at the same time in separate bags, using a Y-line. Extend the infusion time to 6 hours to decrease acute toxicities.
● Don't use needles or I.V. administration sets that contain aluminum because they displace the platinum, causing loss of potency and formation of a black precipitate.
● Store unopened vials at room temperature. Reconstituted solutions are stable if refrigerated (36° to 46° F [2° to 8° C]) for up to 24 hours. After final dilution, solutions are stable for 6 hours at room temperature and up to 24 hours under refrigeration.
● Drug is incompatible with alkaline solutions or drugs such as 5-FU. Flush infusion line with D$_5$W before giving any other drugs simultaneously.

## ACTION
Exact mechanism of drug's antineoplastic action is unknown. Probably inhibits cell replication and transcription by forming platinum complexes that cross-link with DNA molecules. Not specific to cell cycle.

| Route | Onset | Peak | Duration |
|-------|---------|---------|----------|
| I.V. | Unknown | Unknown | Unknown |

## ADVERSE REACTIONS
**CNS:** *pain, peripheral neuropathy, fatigue, headache,* dizziness, *insomnia, fever.*
**CV:** chest pain, ***thromboembolism,*** *edema, flushing, peripheral edema.*
**EENT:** *rhinitis,* pharyngitis, epistaxis, abnormal lacrimation.
**GI:** *nausea, vomiting, diarrhea, stomatitis, abdominal pain, anorexia, constipation, dyspepsia, taste perversion,* gastroesophageal reflux, flatulence, mucositis.
**GU:** dysuria, hematuria.
**Hematologic:** FEBRILE NEUTROPENIA, *anemia,* LEUKOPENIA, THROMBOCYTOPENIA.
**Metabolic:** hypokalemia, dehydration.
**Musculoskeletal:** *back pain, arthralgia.*
**Respiratory:** *dyspnea, cough, upper respiratory tract infection,* hiccups, ***pulmonary toxicity.***
**Skin:** *injection site reaction,* rash, alopecia.
**Other:** ***anaphylaxis,*** *hand-foot syndrome, allergic reaction,* rigors.

## INTERACTIONS
**Drug-drug.** *Nephrotoxic drugs (such as gentamicin):* May decrease elimination of drug and increase levels. Monitor patient for signs and symptoms of toxicity.

## EFFECTS ON LAB TEST RESULTS
● May increase creatinine, bilirubin, AST, and ALT levels. May decrease potassium level.
● May decrease hemoglobin and neutrophil, WBC, and platelet counts.

## CONTRAINDICATIONS & CAUTIONS
● Contraindicated in patients allergic to drug or other platinum-containing compounds and in pregnant or breast-feeding patients.
● Use cautiously in patients with preexisting renal impairment or peripheral sensory neuropathy.

## NURSING CONSIDERATIONS
• Drug doesn't require patient prehydration.
• Give antiemetic with or without dexamethasone before drug to reduce nausea.
• Drug clearance is reduced in patients with renal impairment. Dosage adjustment for patients with renal impairment hasn't been established.
• Monitor CBC, platelet count, and liver and kidney function before each chemotherapy cycle.
• Monitor patient for hypersensitivity reactions, which may occur within minutes of administration.
• Monitor patient for injection site reaction. Extravasation may occur.
• Monitor patient for neuropathy and pulmonary toxicity. Peripheral neuropathy may be acute or persistent. Acute neuropathy is reversible; it occurs within 2 days of dosing and resolves within 14 days. Persistent peripheral neuropathy occurs more than 14 days after dosing and causes paresthesias, dysesthesias, hypoesthesias, and deficits in proprioception that can interfere with daily activities (such as walking or swallowing).
• Avoid ice and cold exposure during infusion of drug because cold temperatures can worsen acute neurologic symptoms. Cover patient with a blanket during infusion.
• Diarrhea, dehydration, hypokalemia, and fatigue may occur more frequently in elderly patients.

## PATIENT TEACHING
• Inform patient of potential adverse reactions.
• Tell patient to avoid exposure to cold or cold objects (such as cold drinks or ice cubes), which can bring on or worsen acute symptoms of peripheral neuropathy. Advise patient to have warm drinks, wear warm clothing, and cover any exposed skin (hands, face, and head). Have patient warm the air going into his lungs by wearing a scarf or ski cap. Have him wear gloves when touching cold objects (such as foods in the freezer, outside door handles, or mailbox).
• Tell patient to contact prescriber immediately if he has trouble breathing or experiences signs and symptoms of an allergic reaction, such as rash, hives, swelling of lips or tongue, or sudden cough.
• Tell patient to contact prescriber if fever, signs and symptoms of an infection, persistent vomiting, diarrhea, or signs and symptoms of dehydration (thirst, dry mouth, light-headedness, and decreased urination) occur.

---

# thiotepa (TESPA, triethylenethiophosphoramide, TSPA)
Thioplex

*Pregnancy risk category D*

## AVAILABLE FORMS
*Injection:* 15- and 30-mg vials

## INDICATIONS & DOSAGES
➤ **Breast and ovarian cancers, lymphoma, Hodgkin's disease**
*Adults and children older than age 12:* 0.3 to 0.4 mg/kg I.V. q 1 to 4 weeks or 0.2 mg/kg for 4 to 5 days at intervals of 2 to 4 weeks.
➤ **Bladder tumor**
*Adults and children older than age 12:* 30 to 60 mg in 30 to 60 ml of normal saline solution instilled in bladder for 2 hours once weekly for 4 weeks.
➤ **Neoplastic effusions**
*Adults and children older than age 12:* 0.6 to 0.8 mg/kg intracavitarily q 1 to 4 weeks.

## I.V. ADMINISTRATION
• *Alert:* Preparation and administration of parenteral form of drug may be mutagenic, teratogenic, or carcinogenic to staff. Follow institutional policy to reduce risks.
• Reconstitute with 1.5 ml of sterile water for injection in 15-mg vial or 3 ml in 30-mg vial to yield 10 mg/ml. Don't reconstitute with other solutions. Further dilute with normal saline solution for injection. If larger volume is desired, further dilute with sodium chloride solution, $D_5W$, dextrose 5% in normal saline solution for injection, Ringer's injection, or lactated Ringer's injection. Use solutions within 8 hours.

---

• If pain occurs at insertion site, dilute drug further or use a local anesthetic to reduce pain. Make sure drug doesn't infiltrate.

• Discard if solution appears grossly opaque or has a precipitate. Make sure solutions are clear to slightly opaque. To eliminate haze, filter solutions through a 0.22-micron filter before use.

• Refrigerate and protect dry powder from direct sunlight to avoid possible drug breakdown.

## ACTION
Cross-links strands of cellular DNA and interferes with RNA transcription, causing an imbalance of growth that leads to cell death. Not specific to cell cycle.

| Route | Onset | Peak | Duration |
|-------|-------|------|----------|
| I.V., intra-cavitary | Unknown | Unknown | Unknown |

## ADVERSE REACTIONS
**CNS:** headache, dizziness, fatigue, weakness, fever.
**EENT:** blurred vision, conjunctivitis.
**GI:** *nausea, vomiting,* abdominal pain, anorexia, stomatitis.
**GU:** amenorrhea, decreased spermatogenesis, dysuria, increased urine levels of uric acid, urine retention, hemorrhagic cystitis (with intravesicle administration).
**Hematologic:** *leukopenia, thrombocytopenia, neutropenia,* anemia.
**Metabolic:** hyperuricemia.
**Skin:** dermatitis, alopecia, pain at injection site.
**Other:** hypersensitivity reactions (including *anaphylaxis, laryngeal edema,* urticaria, rash)

## INTERACTIONS
**Drug-drug.** *Anticoagulants, aspirin, NSAIDs:* May increase risk of bleeding. Avoid using together.
*Myelosuppressives:* May increase myelosuppression. Monitor patient.
*Neuromuscular blockers:* May prolong muscular paralysis. Monitor patient.
*Other alkylating drugs, irradiation therapy:* May intensify toxicity rather than enhance therapeutic response. Avoid using together.

*Pancuronium, succinylcholine:* May increase apnea. Avoid using together.

## EFFECTS ON LAB TEST RESULTS
• May increase uric acid level. May decrease pseudocholinesterase level.
• May decrease hemoglobin and lymphocyte, platelet, WBC, RBC, and neutrophil counts.

## CONTRAINDICATIONS & CAUTIONS
• Contraindicated in patients hypersensitive to drug, in breast-feeding patients, and in those with severe bone marrow, hepatic, or renal dysfunction. Use in pregnant women only when benefits to mother outweigh risk of teratogenicity.
• Use cautiously in patients with mild bone marrow suppression and renal or hepatic dysfunction.

## NURSING CONSIDERATIONS
• For bladder instillation, dehydrate patient 8 to 10 hours before therapy. Instill drug into bladder by catheter; ask patient to retain solution for 2 hours. Volume may be reduced to 30 ml if discomfort is too great with 60 ml. Reposition patient every 15 minutes for maximum area contact.
• Monitor CBC weekly for at least 3 weeks after last dose.
• Stop drug and notify prescriber if patient's WBC count drops below 3,000/mm$^3$ or if platelet count falls below 150,000/mm$^3$. If WBC count falls below 2,000/mm$^3$ or granulocyte count falls below 1,000/mm$^3$, follow institutional policy for infection control in immunocompromised patients.
• Monitor uric acid level. To prevent hyperuricemia with resulting uric acid nephropathy, allopurinol may be used with adequate hydration.
• Therapeutic effects are commonly accompanied by toxicity.
• To prevent bleeding, avoid all I.M. injections when platelet count is below 50,000/mm$^3$.
• Anticipate blood transfusions because of cumulative anemia. Patient may need injections of RBC colony-stimulating factor to promote RBC production and decrease need for blood transfusions.

## PATIENT TEACHING

• Advise patient to watch for signs and symptoms of infection (fever, sore throat, fatigue) and bleeding (easy bruising, nosebleeds, bleeding gums, tarry stools). Tell patient to take temperature daily. Tell patient to report even mild infections.

• Instruct patient to avoid OTC products containing aspirin or NSAIDs.

• Advise women to stop breast-feeding during therapy because of risk of toxicity to infant.

• Caution woman of childbearing age to consult prescriber before becoming pregnant.

capecitabine
cytarabine
fludarabine phosphate
fluorouracil
gemcitabine hydrochloride
hydroxyurea
mercaptopurine
methotrexate
methotrexate sodium

**COMBINATION PRODUCTS**
None.

---

## capecitabine
Xeloda

*Pregnancy risk category D*

**AVAILABLE FORMS**
*Tablets:* 150 mg, 500 mg

**INDICATIONS & DOSAGES**
➤ **Metastatic breast cancer resistant to both paclitaxel and an anthracycline-containing chemotherapy regimen or resistant to paclitaxel in patients for whom further anthracycline therapy isn't indicated; first-line treatment of metastatic colorectal cancer when fluoropyrimidine therapy alone is preferred; metastatic breast cancer combined with docetaxel, after failure of anthracycline-containing chemotherapy**
*Adults:* 2,500 mg/m²/day P.O., in two divided doses, about 12 hours apart and after a meal, for 2 weeks, followed by a 1-week rest period; repeat q 3 weeks.
*Adjust-a-dose:* Follow National Cancer Institute of Canada (NCIC) Common Toxicity Criteria when adjusting dosage. Toxicity criteria relate to degrees of severity of diarrhea, nausea, vomiting, stomatitis, and hand-and-foot syndrome. Refer to drug package insert for specific toxicity definitions.

NCIC grade 1: Maintain dose level.
NCIC grade 2: At first appearance, stop treatment until resolved to grade 0 to 1; then restart at 100% of starting dose for next cycle. At second appearance, stop treatment until resolved to grade 0 to 1 and use 75% of starting dose for next cycle. At third appearance, stop treatment until resolved to grade 0 to 1 and use 50% of starting dose for next cycle. At fourth appearance, stop treatment permanently.

NCIC grade 3: At first appearance, stop treatment until resolved to grade 0 to 1 and use 75% of starting dose for next cycle. At second appearance, stop treatment until resolved to grade 0 to 1 and use 50% of starting dose for next cycle. At third appearance, stop treatment permanently.

NCIC grade 4: At first appearance, stop treatment permanently or until resolved to grade 0 to 1, and use 50% of starting dose for next cycle.

Reduce starting dose for patients with creatinine clearance 30 to 50 ml/minute to 75% of the starting dose.

**ACTION**
Converted to active 5-fluorouracil (5-FU), which changes to metabolites that cause cellular injury by interfering with DNA synthesis to inhibit cell division and with RNA processing and protein synthesis.

| Route | Onset | Peak | Duration |
|-------|-------|------|----------|
| P.O. | Unknown | 90-120 min | Unknown |

**ADVERSE REACTIONS**
**CNS:** dizziness, *fatigue,* headache, insomnia, *paresthesia, pyrexia.*
**CV:** edema, chest pain.
**EENT:** eye irritation, vision abnormality.
**GI:** *diarrhea, nausea, vomiting, stomatitis, abdominal pain, constipation, anorexia,* **intestinal obstruction,** *dyspepsia,* taste perversion.
**Hematologic:** NEUTROPENIA, THROMBO-CYTOPENIA, *anemia, lymphopenia.*
**Metabolic:** dehydration.
**Musculoskeletal:** myalgia, limb pain, back pain.
**Respiratory:** *dyspnea.*

**Skin:** *hand-and-foot syndrome, dermatitis,* nail disorder, alopecia.

## INTERACTIONS
**Drug-drug.** *Antacids containing aluminum hydroxide and magnesium hydroxide:* May increase exposure to capecitabine and its metabolites. Monitor patient.
*Leucovorin:* May increase cytotoxic effects of 5-FU with enhanced toxicity. Monitor patient carefully.
*Warfarin:* May decrease clearance of warfarin. Monitor PT and INR.

## EFFECTS ON LAB TEST RESULTS
• May increase bilirubin level.
• May decrease hemoglobin and WBC, platelet, and neutrophil counts.

## CONTRAINDICATIONS & CAUTIONS
• Contraindicated in patients hypersensitive to 5-FU and in those with severe renal impairment.
• Use cautiously in elderly patients and patients with history of coronary artery disease, mild to moderate hepatic dysfunction from liver metastases, hyperbilirubinemia, and renal insufficiency.
• Safety and efficacy of drug in patients age 18 or younger haven't been established.

## NURSING CONSIDERATIONS
• Patients older than age 80 may have a greater risk of adverse GI effects.
• Assess patient for severe diarrhea, and notify prescriber if it occurs. Give fluid and electrolyte replacement if patient becomes dehydrated. Drug may need to be immediately interrupted until diarrhea resolves or becomes less intense.
• Monitor patient for hand-and-foot syndrome (numbness, paresthesia, painless or painful swelling, erythema, desquamation, blistering, and severe pain of hands or feet), hyperbilirubinemia, and severe nausea. Drug therapy must be immediately adjusted. Hand-and-foot syndrome is staged from 1 to 4; drug may be stopped if severe or recurrent episodes occur.
• Hyperbilirubinemia may require stopping drug.
• **Alert:** Monitor patient carefully for toxicity, which may be managed by symptomatic treatment, dose interruptions, and dosage adjustments.

## PATIENT TEACHING
• Inform patient and caregiver about expected adverse effects of drug, especially nausea, vomiting, diarrhea, and hand-and-foot syndrome (pain, swelling or redness of hands or feet). Tell him that patient-specific dose adaptations during therapy are expected and needed.
• **Alert:** Instruct patient to stop taking drug and contact prescriber immediately if the following occur: diarrhea (more than four bowel movements daily or diarrhea at night), vomiting (two to five episodes in 24 hours), nausea, appetite loss or decrease in amount of food eaten each day, stomatitis (pain, redness, swelling or sores in mouth), hand-and-foot syndrome, temperature of 100.5° F (38° C) or higher, or other evidence of infection.
• Tell patient that most adverse effects improve within 2 to 3 days after stopping drug. If patient doesn't improve, tell him to contact prescriber.
• Tell patient how to take drug. Drug is usually taken for 14 days, followed by 7-day rest period (no drug), as a 21-day cycle. Prescriber determines number of treatment cycles.
• Instruct patient to take drug with water within 30 minutes after end of breakfast and dinner.
• If a combination of tablets is prescribed, teach patient importance of correctly identifying the tablets to avoid possible misdosing.
• For missed doses, instruct patient not to take the missed dose and not to double the next one. Instead, he should continue with regular dosing schedule and check with prescriber.
• Instruct patient to inform prescriber if he's taking folic acid.
• Advise woman of childbearing age to avoid becoming pregnant during therapy.
• Advise breast-feeding woman to stop breast-feeding during therapy.

# cytarabine (ara-C, cytosine arabinoside)
Cytosar†, Cytosar-U, Tarabine PFS

*Pregnancy risk category D*

## AVAILABLE FORMS
*Injection:* 20 mg/ml
*Powder for injection:* 100-mg, 500-mg, 1-g, 2-g vials

## INDICATIONS & DOSAGES
➤ **Acute nonlymphocytic leukemia, acute lymphocytic leukemia**
*Adults and children:* For single-agent therapy, 200 mg/m² daily by continuous I.V. infusion for 5 days at 2-week intervals. For combination therapy, 100 to 200 mg/m² I.V. daily by continuous I.V. infusion or in two or three divided doses by rapid I.V. injection or I.V. infusion for 5 to 10 days in a course of therapy or daily until remission is attained. For maintenance, 1 to 1.5 mg/kg I.M. or S.C. q 1 to 4 weeks.
➤ **Refractory acute leukemia; refractory non-Hodgkin's lymphoma** ♦
*Adults:* 3 g/m² I.V. over 1 to 3 hours q 12 hours for 4 to 12 doses. Repeat at 2- to 3-week intervals or after patient recovers from toxicity.
➤ **Meningeal leukemia**
*Adults and children:* Highly variable from 5 to 75 mg/m² intrathecally. Frequency also varies from once daily for 4 days to once q 2 to 7 days. The most frequently used dose is 30 mg/m² q 4 days until CSF fluid is normal; then one additional dose.

## I.V. ADMINISTRATION
● *Alert:* Preparation and administration of parenteral form of drug may be mutagenic, teratogenic, or carcinogenic to staff. Follow institutional policy to reduce risks.
● To reduce nausea, give antiemetic before giving drug. Nausea and vomiting are more frequent when large doses are given rapidly by I.V. push. These reactions are less frequent when given by infusion. Dizziness may occur with rapid infusion.
● Reconstitute drug using the provided diluent, which is bacteriostatic water for injection containing benzyl alcohol. Avoid this diluent when preparing drug for neonates or intrathecal use. Reconstitute drug in 100-mg vial with 5 ml of diluent or 500-mg vial with 10 ml of diluent. Reconstituted solution is stable for 48 hours. Discard cloudy reconstituted solution.
● For I.V. infusion, further dilute using normal saline solution for injection or D₅W.

## ACTION
Inhibits DNA synthesis.

| Route | Onset | Peak | Duration |
|---|---|---|---|
| I.V., I.M., intrathecal | Unknown | Unknown | Unknown |
| S.C. | Unknown | 20-60 min | Unknown |

## ADVERSE REACTIONS
**CNS:** neurotoxicity, malaise, dizziness, headache, cerebellar syndrome, *fever.*
**CV:** *thrombophlebitis,* edema.
**EENT:** conjunctivitis.
**GI:** *nausea, vomiting, diarrhea, anorexia, anal ulceration,* abdominal pain, oral ulcers in 5 to 10 days, projectile vomiting, bowel necrosis with high doses given rapid I.V.
**GU:** urine retention, renal dysfunction.
**Hematologic:** *leukopenia,* anemia, reticulocytopenia, *thrombocytopenia, megaloblastosis.*
**Hepatic:** *hepatotoxicity,* jaundice.
**Metabolic:** hyperuricemia.
**Musculoskeletal:** myalgia, bone pain.
**Respiratory:** pulmonary edema, shortness of breath, pulmonary hypersensitivity.
**Skin:** *rash,* pruritus, alopecia, freckling.
**Other:** flulike syndrome, infection, *anaphylaxis.*

## INTERACTIONS
**Drug-drug.** *Digoxin:* May decrease oral digoxin absorption. Monitor digoxin level closely. Digoxin oral liquid and liquid-filled capsules may not be affected.
*Flucytosine:* May decrease flucytosine activity. Avoid using together.
*Gentamicin:* May decrease activity against *Klebsiella pneumoniae.* Avoid using together.

---

## EFFECTS ON LAB TEST RESULTS
• May increase potassium, phosphorus, bilirubin, and uric acid levels.
• May increase megaloblast count. May decrease hemoglobin and WBC, RBC, platelet, and reticulocyte counts.

## CONTRAINDICATIONS & CAUTIONS
• Contraindicated in patients hypersensitive to drug.
• Use cautiously in patients with hepatic or renal compromise, gout, or myelosuppression.

## NURSING CONSIDERATIONS
• For intrathecal administration, use preservative-free normal saline solution. Add 5 ml to 100-mg vial or 10 ml to 500-mg vial. Use immediately after reconstitution. Discard unused drug.
• Monitor fluid intake and output carefully. Maintain high fluid intake and give allopurinol to avoid urate nephropathy in leukemia-induction therapy. Monitor uric acid level.
• Monitor hepatic and renal function studies and CBC.
• Therapy may be modified or stopped if granulocyte count is below 1,000/mm³ or platelet count is below 50,000/mm³.
• Corticosteroid eyedrops are prescribed to prevent drug-induced conjunctivitis.
• Provide diligent mouth care to help prevent stomatitis.
• **Alert:** Assess patient receiving high doses for neurotoxicity, which may first appear as nystagmus, but can progress to ataxia and cerebellar dysfunction.
• To prevent bleeding, avoid all I.M. injections when platelet count is below 50,000/mm³.
• Anticipate blood transfusions because of cumulative anemia. Patient may receive RBC colony-stimulating factors to promote RBC production and decrease need for blood transfusions.
• Therapeutic effects are frequently accompanied by toxicity.
• In leukopenia, initial WBC count nadir occurs 7 to 9 days after drug is stopped. A second, more severe nadir occurs 15 to 24 days after drug is stopped. In thrombocytopenia, platelet count nadir occurs on days 12 to 15.

## PATIENT TEACHING
• Instruct patient to watch for signs and symptoms of infection (fever, sore throat, fatigue) and bleeding (easy bruising, nosebleeds, bleeding gums, tarry stools). Tell patient to take temperature daily.
• Advise patient to report visual changes, blurred vision, or eye pain to prescriber.
• Advise breast-feeding woman to stop breast-feeding during therapy because of risk of toxicity to infant.
• Caution woman of childbearing age to consult prescriber before becoming pregnant because drug may harm fetus.

# fludarabine phosphate
Fludara

*Pregnancy risk category D*

## AVAILABLE FORMS
*Powder for injection:* 50 mg

## INDICATIONS & DOSAGES
➤ **B-cell chronic lymphocytic leukemia in patients with no or inadequate response to at least one standard alkylating drug regimen**
*Adults:* 25 mg/m² I.V. daily over 30 minutes for 5 consecutive days. Repeat cycle q 28 days.
**Adjust-a-dose:** In patients with creatinine clearance 30 to 70 ml/minute, decrease dose by 20%. Don't use drug in patients with clearance less than 30 ml/minute.

## I.V. ADMINISTRATION
• **Alert:** Preparation and administration of parenteral form of drug may be mutagenic, teratogenic, or carcinogenic to staff. Follow institutional policy to reduce risks.
• To prepare solution, add 2 ml of sterile water for injection to the solid cake of fludarabine. Dissolution should occur within 15 seconds; each milliliter will contain 25 mg of drug. Dilute further in 100 or 125 ml of D₅W or normal saline solution for injection. Use within 8 hours of reconstitution.
• Store drug in refrigerator at 36° to 46° F (2° to 8° C).

---

## ACTION
Unknown. An antineoplastic antimetabolite that may have multifaceted actions. After conversion to its active metabolite, fludarabine interferes with DNA synthesis by inhibiting DNA polymerase alpha, ribonucleotide reductase, and DNA primase.

| Route | Onset | Peak | Duration |
|-------|-------|------|----------|
| I.V. | 7-21 wk | Unknown | Unknown |

## ADVERSE REACTIONS
**CNS:** *fatigue, malaise, weakness, paresthesia,* peripheral neuropathy, *CVA,* headache, sleep disorder, depression, cerebellar syndrome, *transient ischemic attack,* agitation, *confusion, fever, coma.*
**CV:** *edema,* angina, phlebitis, *arrhythmias, heart failure, MI,* supraventricular tachycardia, *deep vein thrombosis, aneurysm, hemorrhage.*
**EENT:** *visual disturbances,* hearing loss, delayed blindness, sinusitis, pharyngitis, epistaxis.
**GI:** *nausea, vomiting, diarrhea,* constipation, *anorexia,* stomatitis, *GI bleeding,* esophagitis, mucositis.
**GU:** dysuria, *UTI,* urinary hesitancy, proteinuria, hematuria, *renal failure.*
**Hematologic:** *hemolytic anemia,* MYELOSUPPRESSION.
**Hepatic:** *liver failure,* cholelithiasis.
**Metabolic:** hypocalcemia, hyperkalemia, hyperglycemia, dehydration, hyperuricemia, hyperphosphatemia.
**Musculoskeletal:** *myalgia.*
**Respiratory:** *cough, pneumonia, dyspnea, upper respiratory tract infection,* allergic pneumonitis, hemoptysis, hypoxia, bronchitis.
**Skin:** *rash,* pruritus, alopecia, seborrhea, diaphoresis.
**Other:** *chills, pain,* tumor lysis syndrome, INFECTION, *anaphylaxis.*

## INTERACTIONS
**Drug-drug.** *Cytarabine:* May decrease metabolism of subsequently given fludarabine and inhibition of fludarabine activity. Monitor patient closely.
*Myelosuppressives:* May increase toxicity. Avoid using together, if possible.

*Pentostatin:* May increase risk of pulmonary toxicity, which can be fatal. Avoid using together.

## EFFECTS ON LAB TEST RESULTS
● May increase uric acid, glucose, potassium, and phosphate levels. May decrease calcium level.
● May decrease hemoglobin, WBC, platelets, and RBC count.

## CONTRAINDICATIONS & CAUTIONS
● Contraindicated in patients hypersensitive to drug or its components and in those with creatinine clearance less than 30 ml/minute.
● Use cautiously in patients with renal insufficiency.

## NURSING CONSIDERATIONS
● *Alert:* Monitor patient closely and expect modified dosage based on toxicity. Most toxic effects are dose-dependent. Advanced age, renal insufficiency, and bone marrow impairment may predispose patients to increased or excessive toxicity.
● *Alert:* Careful hematologic monitoring is needed, especially of neutrophil and platelet counts. Bone marrow suppression can be severe.
● To prevent bleeding, avoid all I.M. injections when platelet count is below 50,000/mm³.
● Anticipate blood transfusions because of cumulative anemia. Patients may receive RBC colony-stimulating factors to promote RBC production and decrease need for blood transfusions.
● Take preventive measures before starting drug treatment. Hyperuricemia, hypocalcemia, hyperkalemia, and renal failure may result from rapid lysis of tumor cells.
● *Alert:* Don't confuse fludarabine with floxuridine, fluorouracil, or flucytosine.

## PATIENT TEACHING
● Instruct patient to watch for signs and symptoms of infection (fever, sore throat, fatigue) and bleeding (easy bruising, nosebleeds, bleeding gums, tarry stools). Tell patient to take temperature daily.
● Advise woman of childbearing age to consult prescriber before becoming pregnant.

• Caution breast-feeding woman to stop breast-feeding during therapy because of risk of toxicity to infant.

---

## fluorouracil (5-fluorouracil, 5-FU)
Adrucil, Carac, Efudex, Fluoroplex

*Pregnancy risk category D (injection); X (topical form)*

### AVAILABLE FORMS
*Cream:* 1%, 5%
*Injection:* 50 mg/ml
*Topical solution:* 1%, 2%, 5%

### INDICATIONS & DOSAGES
➤ **Colon, rectal, breast, stomach, and pancreatic cancers**
*Adults:* Initially, 12 mg/kg I.V. daily for 4 days; if no toxicity, give 6 mg/kg on days 6, 8, 10, and 12; then give a single weekly maintenance dose of 10 to 15 mg/kg I.V. begun after toxicity (if any) from first course has subsided. (Recommended dosages are based on actual body weight unless patient is obese or retaining fluid.) Maximum single recommended dose is 800 mg/day.
➤ **Palliative treatment of advanced colorectal cancer**
*Adults:* 425 mg/m² I.V. daily for 5 consecutive days. Give with 20 mg/m² of leucovorin I.V. Repeat at 4-week intervals for two additional courses; then repeat at 4- to 5-week intervals if tolerated.
➤ **Early breast cancer**
*Adults:* 600 mg/m² I.V. on days 1 and 8 of each cycle, combined with cyclophosphamide 100 mg/m² on days 1 through 14 of each cycle and methotrexate 40 mg/m² on days 1 and 8 of each cycle. Repeat monthly for 6 to 12 months, allowing for a 2-week rest period between cycles. In adults older than age 60, first fluorouracil dose is 400 mg/m² and methotrexate dose is 30 mg/m².
➤ **Multiple actinic (solar) keratoses**
*Adults:* Apply Carac cream once daily for up to 4 weeks. Or apply Efudex or Fluoroplex cream or topical solution b.i.d. for 2 to 6 weeks.

➤ **Superficial basal cell carcinoma**
*Adults:* Apply 5% Efudex cream or topical solution b.i.d. Usual duration of treatment is 3 to 6 weeks; up to 12 weeks.

### I.V. ADMINISTRATION
• *Alert:* Preparation and administration of parenteral form of drug may be mutagenic, teratogenic, or carcinogenic to staff. Follow institutional policy to reduce risks.
• Give antiemetic before drug to reduce nausea.
• Drug may be given by direct injection without dilution. For I.V. infusion, drug may be diluted with D₅W, sterile water for injection, or normal saline solution for injection. Discard unused portion of vial after 1 hour.
• Don't use cloudy solution. If crystals form, redissolve by warming.
• Use plastic I.V. containers when giving continuous infusions. Solution is more stable in plastic I.V. bags than in glass bottles.
• Don't refrigerate fluorouracil. Protect drug from sunlight.

### ACTION
Thought to inhibit DNA and RNA synthesis.

| Route | Onset | Peak | Duration |
|---|---|---|---|
| I.V., topical | Unknown | Unknown | Unknown |

### ADVERSE REACTIONS
**CNS:** acute cerebellar syndrome, confusion, disorientation, euphoria, ataxia, headache, *weakness, malaise.*
**CV:** *myocardial ischemia,* angina, thrombophlebitis.
**EENT:** epistaxis, photophobia, lacrimation, lacrimal duct stenosis, nystagmus, visual changes, eye irritation.
**GI:** *stomatitis, GI ulcer, nausea, vomiting, diarrhea, anorexia, GI bleeding.*
**Hematologic:** *leukopenia, thrombocytopenia, agranulocytosis,* anemia.
**Skin:** *dermatitis, erythema, scaling, pruritus,* nail changes, pigmented palmar creases, erythematous contact dermatitis, desquamative rash of hands and feet, hand-and-foot syndrome with long-term use, photosensitivity, *reversible alopecia; pain, burning,* soreness, suppuration,

---

Reactions may be *common,* uncommon, *life-threatening,* or COMMON AND LIFE-THREATENING.

*swelling, dryness, erosion with topical use.*
**Other:** *anaphylaxis.*

## INTERACTIONS
**Drug-drug.** *Leucovorin calcium:* May increase cytotoxicity and toxicity of fluorouracil. Monitor patient closely.
**Drug-lifestyle.** *Sun exposure:* May cause photosensitivity reactions. Advise patient to avoid excessive sunlight exposure.

## EFFECTS ON LAB TEST RESULTS
• May increase alkaline phosphatase, AST, ALT, bilirubin, and lactate dehydrogenase levels. May decrease plasma albumin. May increase 5-hydroxyindoleacetic acid in urine.
• May decrease hemoglobin and WBC, RBC, platelet, and granulocyte counts.

## CONTRAINDICATIONS & CAUTIONS
• Contraindicated in patients hypersensitive to drug and in those with bone marrow suppression (WBC counts of 5,000/mm$^3$ or less or platelet counts of 100,000/mm$^3$ or less) or potentially serious infections.
• Contraindicated in patients in a poor nutritional state and those who have had major surgery within previous month.
• Topical formulations are contraindicated in pregnant women.
• Use cautiously in patients who have received high-dose pelvic radiation or alkylating drugs and in those with impaired hepatic or renal function or widespread neoplastic infiltration of bone marrow.

## NURSING CONSIDERATIONS
• Apply topical form cautiously near eyes, nose, and mouth.
• Avoid occlusive dressings with topical form because they increase risk of inflammatory reactions in adjacent normal skin.
• Apply topical form with a nonmetal applicator or suitable gloves. Wash hands immediately after handling topical form.
• The 1% topical strength is used on the face. Higher strengths, such as 5%, are used for thicker-skinned areas or resistant lesions, such as superficial basal cell carcinoma.

• Ingestion and systemic absorption of topical form may cause leukopenia, thrombocytopenia, stomatitis, diarrhea, or GI ulceration, bleeding, and hemorrhage. Application to large ulcerated areas may cause systemic toxicity.
• Watch for stomatitis or diarrhea (signs of toxicity). May use topical oral anesthetic to soothe lesions. Stop drug and notify prescriber if diarrhea occurs.
• Encourage diligent oral hygiene to prevent superinfection of denuded mucosa.
• Monitor WBC and platelet counts daily. Watch for ecchymoses, petechiae, easy bruising, and anemia.
• Monitor fluid intake and output, CBC, and renal and hepatic function tests.
• Long-term use of drug may cause erythematous, desquamative rash of the hands and feet, which may be treated with pyridoxine 50 to 150 mg P.O. daily for 5 to 7 days.
• Dermatologic adverse effects are reversible when drug is stopped.
• To prevent bleeding, avoid all I.M. injections when platelet count is below 50,000/mm$^3$.
• Anticipate blood transfusions because of cumulative anemia. Patient may receive injections of RBC colony-stimulating factors to promote RBC production and decrease need for blood transfusions.
• **Alert:** Fluorouracil toxicity may be delayed for 1 to 3 weeks.
• The WBC count nadir occurs 9 to 14 days after first dose; the platelet count nadir occurs in 7 to 14 days.
• **Alert:** Drug is sometimes ordered as 5-fluorouracil or 5-FU. The numeral 5 is part of drug name and shouldn't be confused with dosage units.
• **Alert:** Don't confuse fluorouracil with floxuridine, fludarabine, or flucytosine.

## PATIENT TEACHING
• Warn patient that hair loss may occur, but that it's reversible.
• Caution patient to avoid prolonged exposure to sunlight or ultraviolet light when topical form is used.
• Tell patient to use highly protective sunblock to avoid inflammatory skin irritation.
• Warn patient that topically treated area may be unsightly during therapy and for

several weeks afterward. Complete healing may take 1 or 2 months.
● Caution woman of childbearing age to consult prescriber before becoming pregnant.
● Advise breast-feeding woman to stop breast-feeding during therapy because of risk of toxicity to infant.

# gemcitabine hydrochloride
Gemzar

*Pregnancy risk category D*

## AVAILABLE FORMS
*Powder for injection:* 200-mg, 1-g vials

## INDICATIONS & DOSAGES
➤ **Locally advanced or metastatic adenocarcinoma of pancreas**
*Adults:* 1,000 mg/m² I.V. over 30 minutes once weekly for up to 7 weeks, unless toxicity occurs. Monitor CBC with differential and platelet count before giving each dose.
*Adjust-a-dose:* If bone marrow suppression is detected, adjust therapy. Give full dose if absolute granulocyte count (AGC) is 1,000/mm³ or more and platelet count is 100,000/mm³ or more. If AGC is 500 to 999/mm³ or platelet count is 50,000 to 99,999/mm³, give 75% of dose. Withhold dose if AGC is below 500/mm³ or platelet count is below 50,000/mm³. Treatment course of 7 weeks is followed by 1 week of rest. Subsequent dosage cycles consist of 1 infusion weekly for 3 of 4 consecutive weeks. Dosage adjustments for subsequent cycles are based on AGC and platelet count nadirs and degree of nonhematologic toxicity.
➤ **With cisplatin, first-line treatment of inoperable, locally advanced, or metastatic non–small-cell lung cancer**
*Adults:* For 4-week schedule, 1,000 mg/m² I.V. over 30 minutes on days 1, 8, and 15 of each 28-day cycle. Cisplatin 100 mg/m² on day 1 after gemcitabine infusion.
    For 3-week schedule, 1,250 mg/m² I.V. over 30 minutes on days 1 and 8 of each 21-day cycle. Cisplatin 100 mg/m² on day 1 after gemcitabine infusion.

## I.V. ADMINISTRATION
● *Alert:* Preparation and administration of parenteral form of drug may be mutagenic, teratogenic, or carcinogenic to staff. Follow institutional policy to reduce risks.
● To prepare solution, add 5 ml of unpreserved normal saline solution for injection to 200-mg vial or 25 ml of diluent to a 1-g vial. Shake to dissolve. Resulting concentration is 40 mg/ml; reconstitution at higher concentrations isn't recommended. May be further diluted with normal saline solution for injection to a concentration as low as 0.1 mg/ml, if needed. Make sure solution is clear to light straw-colored and free of particulates. It's stable for 24 hours at room temperature. Don't refrigerate reconstituted drug because crystallization may occur.
● Prolonging infusion time beyond 60 minutes or giving drug more frequently than once weekly may increase toxicity.

## ACTION
Cytotoxic and specific to cell cycle; inhibits DNA synthesis and blocks progression of cells through $G_1$/S-phase boundary.

| Route | Onset | Peak | Duration |
|-------|-------|------|----------|
| I.V. | Unknown | Unknown | Unknown |

## ADVERSE REACTIONS
**CNS:** *somnolence, paresthesia, pain, fever.*
**CV:** *edema, peripheral edema.*
**GI:** *stomatitis, nausea, vomiting, constipation, diarrhea.*
**GU:** *proteinuria, hematuria.*
**Hematologic:** *anemia,* **leukopenia, neutropenia, thrombocytopenia.**
**Hepatic:** **hepatotoxicity.**
**Respiratory:** *dyspnea,* **bronchospasm.**
**Skin:** *alopecia, rash,* pain at injection site.
**Other:** *flulike syndrome, infection.*

## INTERACTIONS
None significant.

## EFFECTS ON LAB TEST RESULTS
● May increase BUN, creatinine, ALT, and AST levels.
● May decrease hemoglobin and WBC, neutrophil, and platelet counts.

---

Reactions may be *common*, uncommon, *life-threatening*, or COMMON AND LIFE-THREATENING.

**CONTRAINDICATIONS & CAUTIONS**
- Contraindicated in patients hypersensitive to drug and in pregnant or breast-feeding women.
- Use cautiously in patients with renal or hepatic impairment.

**NURSING CONSIDERATIONS**
- Monitor patient closely. Expect dosage modification according to toxicity and degree of myelosuppression. Age, sex, and presence of renal impairment may predispose patient to toxicity.
- Carefully monitor hematologic values, especially of neutrophil and platelet counts.
- Obtain baseline and periodic renal and hepatic laboratory tests.
- Safety and effectiveness of drug in children haven't been determined.

**PATIENT TEACHING**
- Advise patient to watch for evidence of infection (fever, sore throat, fatigue) and bleeding (easy bruising, nosebleeds, bleeding gums, tarry stools). Tell patient to take temperature daily.
- Advise patient to promptly report flulike symptoms or breathing problems.
- Tell patient that adverse effects may continue after treatment ends.
- Caution woman of childbearing age to avoid pregnancy or breast-feeding during therapy.

---

# hydroxyurea
Droxia, Hydrea

*Pregnancy risk category D*

**AVAILABLE FORMS**
*Capsules:* 200 mg, 300 mg, 400 mg, 500 mg

**INDICATIONS & DOSAGES**
➤ **Melanoma; resistant chronic myelocytic leukemia; recurrent, metastatic, or inoperable ovarian cancer; head and neck cancers**
*Hydrea*
*Adults:* 80 mg/kg P.O. as single dose q 3 days; or 20 to 30 mg/kg P.O. as single daily dose.

➤ **To reduce frequency of painful crises and need for blood transfusions in adult patients with sickle-cell anemia with recurrent moderate to severe painful crises**
*Droxia*
*Adults:* 15 mg/kg P.O. once daily. If blood counts are in acceptable range, dose may be increased by 5 mg/kg/day q 12 weeks until maximum tolerated dose or 35 mg/kg/day has been reached. If blood counts are considered toxic, withhold drug until hematologic recovery occurs. Resume treatment after reducing dose by 2.5 mg/kg/day. Every 12 weeks, drug may then be adjusted up or down in 2.5-mg/kg/day increments until patient is at stable, nontoxic dose for 24 weeks.
➤ **To reduce platelet count and prevent thrombosis in patients with essential thrombocythemia ♦**
*Hydrea*
*Adults:* 15 mg/kg P.O. daily.
➤ **Refractory psoriasis ♦**
*Adults:* 0.5 to 1.5 g P.O. daily.

**ACTION**
Unknown. Thought to inhibit DNA synthesis.

| Route | Onset | Peak | Duration |
|-------|---------|------|----------|
| P.O. | Unknown | 2 hr | 24 hr |

**ADVERSE REACTIONS**
**CNS:** hallucinations, headache, dizziness, disorientation, *seizures,* malaise, fever.
**GI:** *anorexia, nausea, vomiting, diarrhea,* stomatitis, constipation.
**Hematologic:** *leukopenia, thrombocytopenia,* anemia, megaloblastosis, **bone marrow suppression.**
**Metabolic:** hyperuricemia, weight gain.
**Skin:** rash, itching, alopecia.
**Other:** chills.

**INTERACTIONS**
**Drug-drug.** *Cytotoxic drugs, radiation therapy:* May enhance toxicity of hydroxyurea. Use together cautiously.

**EFFECTS ON LAB TEST RESULTS**
- May increase BUN, creatinine, hepatic enzyme, and uric acid levels.
- May decrease hemoglobin and WBC, RBC, and platelet counts.

**CONTRAINDICATIONS & CAUTIONS**
● Contraindicated in patients hypersensitive to drug and in those with fewer than 2,500/mm$^3$ WBCs, fewer than 100,000/mm$^3$ platelets, or severe anemia.
● Use cautiously in patients with renal dysfunction.

**NURSING CONSIDERATIONS**
● Routinely measure BUN, uric acid, liver enzyme, and creatinine levels; monitor blood counts every 2 weeks.
● Acceptable blood counts during dosage adjustment are neutrophil count 2,500 cells/mm$^3$ or more; platelet count 95,000/mm$^3$ or more; hemoglobin more than 5.3 g/dl; and reticulocyte count (if hemoglobin is below 9 g/dl) more than 95,000/mm$^3$. Toxic levels are neutrophil count below 2,000 cells/mm$^3$, platelet count below 80,000/mm$^3$, hemoglobin less than 4.5 g/dl, and reticulocyte count (if hemoglobin is below 9 g/dl) below 80,000/mm$^3$.
● Hydroxyurea may dramatically lower the WBC count in 24 to 48 hours.
● Monitor fluid intake and output; keep patient hydrated.
● Allopurinol is used to treat or prevent tumor lysis syndrome.
● To prevent bleeding, avoid all I.M. injections when platelet count is below 50,000/mm$^3$.
● Anticipate need for blood transfusions because of cumulative anemia. Patient may receive injections of RBC colony-stimulating factors to promote RBC production and decrease need for blood transfusions.
● Dosage modification may be needed after chemotherapy or radiation therapy.
● Auditory and visual hallucinations and hematologic toxicity increase when renal function decreases.
● Drug crosses blood-brain barrier.
● Radiation therapy may increase risk or severity of GI distress or stomatitis.

**PATIENT TEACHING**
● Tell patient who can't swallow capsules that he may empty contents into water and take immediately. Patient should rinse mouth with water after taking drug this way. Inform patient that some inert material may not dissolve.
● Advise patient to watch for signs and symptoms of infection (fever, sore throat, fatigue) and bleeding (easy bruising, nosebleeds, bleeding gums, tarry stools). He also should take his temperature daily.
● Caution woman of childbearing age to consult prescriber before becoming pregnant.

# mercaptopurine
## (6-mercaptopurine, 6-MP)
Purinethol

*Pregnancy risk category D*

**AVAILABLE FORMS**
*Tablets (scored):* 50 mg

**INDICATIONS & DOSAGES**
➤ **Acute lymphoblastic leukemia, acute myeloblastic leukemia**
*Adults and children:* 2.5 mg/mg P.O. once daily (rounded to nearest 25 mg). May increase to 5 mg/kg daily after 4 weeks if no improvement.
After remission is attained, usual maintenance dose for adults and children is 1.5 to 2.5 mg/kg once daily.

**ACTION**
Inhibits RNA and DNA synthesis.

| Route | Onset | Peak | Duration |
|-------|---------|---------|----------|
| P.O. | Unknown | Unknown | Unknown |

**ADVERSE REACTIONS**
**GI:** nausea, vomiting, anorexia, painful oral ulcers, diarrhea, *pancreatitis,* GI ulceration.
**Hematologic:** *leukopenia, thrombocytopenia,* anemia.
**Hepatic:** *jaundice, hepatotoxicity.*
**Metabolic:** hyperuricemia.
**Skin:** rash, hyperpigmentation.

**INTERACTIONS**
**Drug-drug.** *Allopurinol:* Slows inactivation of mercaptopurine. Decrease mercaptopurine to 25% or 33% of normal dose.
*Co-trimoxazole:* May enhance bone marrow suppression; monitor CBC with differential carefully.

*Hepatotoxic drugs:* May enhance hepatotoxicity of mercaptopurine. Monitor patient for hepatotoxicity.

*Nondepolarizing neuromuscular blockers:* May antagonize muscle relaxant effect. Notify anesthesiologist that patient is receiving mercaptopurine.

*Warfarin:* May reduce or increase anticoagulant effect. Monitor PT and INR.

### EFFECTS ON LAB TEST RESULTS
● May increase uric acid, transaminase, alkaline phosphatase, and bilirubin levels.
● May decrease hemoglobin and WBC, RBC, and platelet counts.

### CONTRAINDICATIONS & CAUTIONS
● Contraindicated in patients whose disease has shown resistance to drug and in patients hypersensitive to the drug.

### NURSING CONSIDERATIONS
● Dosage modifications may be needed after chemotherapy or radiation therapy in patients with depressed neutrophil or platelet counts and in those with impaired hepatic or renal function.
● Drug is sometimes ordered as 6-mercaptopurine, or 6-MP. The numeral 6 is part of drug name and doesn't signify number of dosage units.
● Monitor CBC and transaminase, alkaline phosphatase, and bilirubin levels weekly during induction and monthly during maintenance.
● Leukopenia, thrombocytopenia, or anemia may persist for several days after drug is stopped.
● Observe for signs of bleeding and infection.
● Monitor fluid intake and output. Encourage adequate fluid intake (3 L daily).
● *Alert:* Watch for jaundice, clay-colored stools, and frothy, dark urine. Hepatic dysfunction is reversible when drug is stopped. If right-sided abdominal tenderness occurs, stop drug and notify prescriber.
● Monitor uric acid level. If allopurinol is ordered, use cautiously.
● To prevent bleeding, avoid all I.M. injections when platelet count is below 100,000/mm$^3$.
● Anticipate need for blood transfusions because of cumulative anemia. Patient may receive injections of RBC colony-stimulating factors to promote RBC production and decrease need for blood transfusions.
● GI adverse reactions are less common in children than in adults.

### PATIENT TEACHING
● Instruct patient to watch for signs and symptoms of infection (fever, sore throat, fatigue) and bleeding (easy bruising, nosebleeds, bleeding gums, tarry stools). Tell patient to take temperature daily.
● Caution woman of childbearing age to consult prescriber before becoming pregnant.
● Advise breast-feeding woman to stop breast-feeding during therapy because of risk of toxicity to infant.

## methotrexate (amethopterin, MTX)

## methotrexate sodium
Ledertrexate‡, Methoblastin‡, Methotrexate LPF, Rheumatrex, Trexall

*Pregnancy risk category X*

### AVAILABLE FORMS
*Injection:* 20-mg, 1,000-mg vials; lyophilized powder: 20mg, 1,000 mg vials, preservative-free solution: 2.5-mg/ml, 25-mg/ml vials
*Tablets (scored):* 2.5 mg, 5 mg, 7.5 mg, 10 mg‡, 15 mg

### INDICATIONS & DOSAGES
➤ **Trophoblastic tumors (choriocarcinoma, hydatidiform mole)**
*Adults:* 15 to 30 mg P.O. or I.M. daily for 5 days. Repeated after 1 or more weeks, based on response or toxicity. Number of courses is three to five, not to exceed five.
➤ **Acute lymphocytic leukemia**
*Adults and children:* 3.3 mg/m$^2$/day P.O., I.V., or I.M. for 4 to 6 weeks or until remission occurs; then 20 to 30 mg/m$^2$ P.O. or I.M. weekly in two divided doses or 2.5 mg/kg I.V. q 14 days.
➤ **Meningeal leukemia**
*Adults and children:* 12 mg/m$^2$ or less (maximum 15 mg) intrathecally q 2 to

5 days until CSF is normal; then one additional dose.

Or, for children, use dosages based on age:

*Children age 3 and older:* 12 mg intrathecally q 2 to 5 days.

*Children ages 2 to 3:* 10 mg intrathecally q 2 to 5 days.

*Children ages 1 to 2:* 8 mg intrathecally q 2 to 5 days.

*Children younger than age 1:* 6 mg intrathecally q 2 to 5 days.

➤ **Burkitt's lymphoma (stage I, II, or III)**

*Adults:* 10 to 25 mg P.O. daily for 4 to 8 days with 1-week rest intervals.

➤ **Lymphosarcoma (stage III)**

*Adults:* 0.625 to 2.5 mg/kg daily P.O., I.M., or I.V.

➤ **Osteosarcoma**

*Adults:* Initially, 12 g/m$^2$ I.V. as 4-hour infusion. Give subsequent doses 15 g/m$^2$ I.V. as 4-hour I.V. infusion at postoperative weeks 4, 5, 6, 7, 11, 12, 15, 16, 29, 30, 44, and 45. Give with leucovorin, 15 mg P.O. q 6 hours for 10 doses, beginning 24 hours after start of methotrexate infusion.

➤ **Breast cancer**

*Adults:* 40 mg/m$^2$ I.V. on days 1 and 8 of each cycle, combined with cyclophosphamide and fluorouracil.

*Adjust-a-dose:* In patients older than age 60, give 30 mg/m$^2$.

➤ **Mycosis fungoides**

*Adults:* 2.5 to 10 mg P.O. daily; or 50 mg I.M. weekly; or 25 mg I.M. twice weekly.

➤ **Psoriasis**

*Adults:* 10 to 25 mg P.O., I.M., or I.V. as single weekly dose; or 2.5 to 5 mg P.O. q 12 hours for three doses weekly. Dosage shouldn't exceed 30 mg/week.

➤ **Rheumatoid arthritis**

*Adults:* Initially, 7.5 mg P.O. weekly, either in single dose or divided as 2.5 mg P.O. q 12 hours for three doses once weekly. Dosage may be gradually increased to maximum of 20 mg weekly.

## I.V. ADMINISTRATION

● *Alert:* Preparation and administration of parenteral form of drug may be mutagenic, teratogenic, or carcinogenic to staff. Follow institutional policy to reduce risks.

● Dilution of drug depends on product, and infusion guidelines vary, depending on dose.

● Reconstitute solutions without preservatives immediately before use, and discard unused drug.

## ACTION

Reversibly binds to dihydrofolate reductase, blocking reduction of folic acid to tetrahydrofolate, a cofactor necessary for purine, protein, and DNA synthesis.

| Route | Onset | Peak | Duration |
|---|---|---|---|
| P.O. | Unknown | 1-2 hr | Unknown |
| I.V. | Immediate | Immediate | Unknown |
| I.M. | Unknown | 30 min-1 hr | Unknown |
| Intrathecal | Unknown | Unknown | Unknown |

## ADVERSE REACTIONS

**CNS:** *arachnoiditis within hours of intrathecal use,* subacute neurotoxicity possibly beginning a few weeks later, *leukoencephalopathy,* demyelination, malaise, fatigue, dizziness, headache, aphasia, hemiparesis, fever, drowsiness, *seizures.*

**EENT:** pharyngitis, blurred vision.

**GI:** gingivitis, *stomatitis, diarrhea,* abdominal distress, anorexia, GI ulceration and bleeding, enteritis, *nausea, vomiting.*

**GU:** nephropathy, *tubular necrosis, renal failure,* hematuria, menstrual dysfunction, defective spermatogenesis, infertility, abortion, cystitis.

**Hematologic:** *anemia, leukopenia, thrombocytopenia.*

**Hepatic:** *acute toxicity, chronic toxicity,* including cirrhosis and *hepatic fibrosis.*

**Metabolic:** diabetes, hyperuricemia.

**Musculoskeletal:** arthralgia, myalgia, osteoporosis in children on long-term therapy.

**Respiratory:** *pulmonary fibrosis; pulmonary interstitial infiltrates;* pneumonitis; dry, nonproductive cough.

**Skin:** *urticaria,* pruritus, hyperpigmentation, erythematous rashes, ecchymoses, rash, photosensitivity, alopecia, acne, psoriatic lesions aggravated by exposure to sun.

**Other:** chills, reduced resistance to infection, septicemia, *sudden death.*

---

Reactions may be *common*, uncommon, *life-threatening*, or COMMON AND LIFE-THREATENING.

## INTERACTIONS

**Drug-drug.** *Acyclovir:* Use with intrathecal methotrexate may cause neurologic abnormalities. Monitor patient closely.

*Digoxin:* May decrease digoxin level. Monitor digoxin level closely.

*Folic acid derivatives:* Antagonizes methotrexate effect. Avoid using together, except for leucovorin rescue with high-dose methotrexate therapy.

*Fosphenytoin, phenytoin:* May decrease phenytoin and fosphenytoin levels. Monitor drug levels closely.

*Hepatotoxic drugs:* May increase risk of hepatotoxicity. Monitor patient closely.

*NSAIDs, phenylbutazone, salicylates, sulfonamides:* May increase methotrexate toxicity. Avoid using together.

*Oral antibiotics:* May decrease absorption of methotrexate. Monitor patient closely.

*Penicillins, sulfonamides:* May increase methotrexate level. Monitor for methotrexate toxicity.

*Probenecid:* May impair excretion of methotrexate, causing increased level, effect, and toxicity of methotrexate. Monitor methotrexate level closely and adjust dosage accordingly.

*Procarbazine:* May increase risk of nephrotoxicity. Monitor patient closely.

*Theophylline:* May increase theophylline level. Monitor theophylline level closely.

*Thiopurines:* May increase levels of thiopurines. Monitor patient closely.

*Vaccines:* May make immunizations ineffective; may cause risk of disseminated infection with live virus vaccines. Defer immunization, if possible.

**Drug-food.** *Any food:* May delay absorption and reduce peak level of methotrexate. Instruct patient to take drug on an empty stomach.

**Drug-lifestyle.** *Alcohol use:* May increase hepatotoxicity. Discourage alcohol use.

*Sun exposure:* May cause photosensitivity reactions. Advise patient to avoid excessive sunlight exposure.

## EFFECTS ON LAB TEST RESULTS

• May increase uric acid level.

• May decrease hemoglobin and WBC, RBC, and platelet counts.

## CONTRAINDICATIONS & CAUTIONS

• Contraindicated in patients hypersensitive to drug and in those with psoriasis or rheumatoid arthritis who also have alcoholism, alcoholic liver, chronic liver disease, immunodeficiency syndromes, or blood dyscrasias. Also contraindicated in pregnant or breast-feeding women.

• Use cautiously and at modified dosage in patients with impaired hepatic or renal function, bone marrow suppression, aplasia, leukopenia, thrombocytopenia, or anemia. Also use cautiously in very young, elderly, or debilitated patients and in patients with infection, peptic ulceration, or ulcerative colitis.

## NURSING CONSIDERATIONS

• *Alert:* Methotrexate may be dosed daily or once weekly, depending on the disease. To avoid administration errors, be aware of which disease the patient has.

• Monitor pulmonary function tests periodically and fluid intake and output daily. Encourage fluid intake of 2 to 3 L daily.

• Monitor uric acid level.

• Methotrexate distributes readily into pleural effusions and other third-space compartments, such as ascites, leading to prolonged systemic level and potential for toxicity. Use drug cautiously in these patients.

• Methotrexate tablets may contain lactose. May give OTC lactose enzyme supplement.

• *Alert:* Alkalinize urine by giving sodium bicarbonate tablets or I.V. fluids containing sodium bicarbonate to prevent precipitation of drug, especially at high doses. Maintain urine pH above 7. Reduce dosage if BUN level is 20 to 30 mg/dl or creatinine level is 1.2 to 2 mg/dl. Stop drug and notify prescriber if BUN level exceeds 30 mg/dl or creatinine level is higher than 2 mg/dl.

• Use preservative-free formulation for intrathecal administration.

• Watch for increases in AST, ALT, and alkaline phosphatase levels, which may signal hepatic dysfunction.

• Drug may alter results of laboratory assay for folate, thus interfering with detection of folic acid deficiency.

• Watch for signs and symptoms of bleeding (especially GI) and infection.

---

*Rapid onset*   †Canada   ‡Australia   ◊OTC   ♦ Off-label use   ⦿Photoguide   *Liquid contains alcohol.

• To prevent bleeding, avoid all I.M. injections when platelet count is below 50,000/mm$^3$.

• Anticipate blood transfusions because of cumulative anemia. Patient may receive injections of RBC colony-stimulating factors to promote RBC production and decrease need for blood transfusions.

• Leucovorin rescue is needed with high-dose (over 100 mg) protocols and is started 24 hours after methotrexate therapy is begun. Leucovorin therapy is continued until methotrexate level is falls below 5 × 10$^{-8}$ M. Consult specialized references for specific recommendations for leucovorin dosing.

• Monitor methotrexate level and adjust leucovorin dose.

• The WBC and platelet count nadirs usually occur on day 7.

**PATIENT TEACHING**

• Advise patient to watch for signs and symptoms of infection (fever, sore throat, fatigue) and bleeding (easy bruising, nosebleeds, bleeding gums, tarry stools). Tell patient to take temperature daily.

• Teach and encourage diligent mouth care to reduce risk of superinfection in the mouth.

• Instruct patient how to take leucovorin. Stress the importance of taking medication as prescribed until instructed by prescriber to stop medication.

• Tell patient to use highly protective sunblock when exposed to sunlight.

• Warn patient to avoid conception during and immediately after therapy because of possible abortion or birth defects or problems.

• Advise breast-feeding woman to stop breast-feeding during therapy because of risk of toxicity to infant.

**bleomycin sulfate**
**daunorubicin citrate liposomal**
**daunorubicin hydrochloride**
**doxorubicin hydrochloride**
**doxorubicin hydrochloride**
  **liposomal**
**epirubicin hydrochloride**
**idarubicin hydrochloride**
**mitomycin**

**COMBINATION PRODUCTS**
None.

---

## bleomycin sulfate
Blenoxane

*Pregnancy risk category D*

---

### AVAILABLE FORMS
*Injection:* 15-unit vials, 30-unit vials

### INDICATIONS & DOSAGES
Dosages may vary. Check treatment proto-
col with prescriber.
➤ **Squamous cell carcinoma (head,
neck, skin, penis, cervix, and vulva),
non-Hodgkin's lymphoma, testicular
carcinoma**
*Adults:* 10 to 20 units/m² I.V., I.M., or
S.C. once or twice weekly to total of
400 units.
➤ **Hodgkin's disease**
*Adults:* 10 to 20 units/m² I.V., I.M., or
S.C. one or two times weekly. After 50%
response, maintenance dose is 1 unit I.V.
or I.M. daily or 5 units I.V. or I.M. weekly.
Total cumulative dose is 400 units.
➤ **Malignant pleural effusion**
*Adults:* 60 units given as single-dose bolus
intrapleural injection.

### I.V. ADMINISTRATION
• *Alert:* Preparation and administration of
parenteral form of drug may be mutagenic, teratogenic, or carcinogenic to staff.
Follow institutional policy to reduce risks.
• Reconstitute drug with 5 or 10 ml of
normal saline solution for injection to

equal 3 unit/ml solution. Drug may be giv-
en at this concentration over 10 minutes.
• Refrigerate unopened vials containing
dry powder. Use reconstituted solution
within 24 hours. Bleomycin may adsorb to
plastic I.V. bags. For prolonged infusions,
use glass containers.

### ACTION
Unknown. Thought to inhibit DNA synthesis and cause scission of single- and
double-stranded DNA. To a lesser extent,
inhibits RNA and protein synthesis.

| Route | Onset | Peak | Duration |
|-------|-------|------|----------|
| I.M. | Unknown | 30-60 min | Unknown |
| I.V., S.C. | Unknown | Unknown | Unknown |

### ADVERSE REACTIONS
**CNS:** fever.
**GI:** *stomatitis, anorexia, nausea, vomit-
ing,* diarrhea.
**Metabolic:** weight loss, hyperuricemia.
**Respiratory:** PNEUMONITIS, *pulmonary
fibrosis.*
**Skin:** *erythema, hyperpigmentation, acne,
rash, striae, skin tenderness, pruritus,
reversible alopecia,* hyperkeratosis, nail
changes.
**Other:** *chills,* **anaphylactoid reactions.**

### INTERACTIONS
**Drug-drug.** *Anesthesia:* May increase
oxygen requirements. Monitor patient
closely.
*Cardiac glycosides:* May decrease digoxin
level. Monitor digoxin level closely.
*Fosphenytoin, phenytoin:* May decrease
phenytoin and fosphenytoin levels. Monitor drug levels closely.

### EFFECTS ON LAB TEST RESULTS
• May increase uric acid level.

### CONTRAINDICATIONS & CAUTIONS
• Contraindicated in patients hypersensitive to drug.
• Use cautiously in patients with renal or
pulmonary impairment.

---

## NURSING CONSIDERATIONS

• Obtain pulmonary function tests. Stop drug if tests show a marked decline.

• *Alert:* Pulmonary toxicity appears to be dose-related, with an increase when total dose is more than 400 units. Give total doses of more than 400 units with caution.

• For intrapleural administration, dilute 60 units of drug in 50 to 100 ml normal saline solution for injection; drug is given through a thoracotomy tube.

• For I.M. use, dilute drug in 1 to 5 ml of sterile water for injection, bacteriostatic water for injection, or normal saline solution for injection.

• Monitor injection site for irritation.

• *Alert:* Adverse pulmonary reactions are more common in patients older than age 70. Pulmonary fibrosis is fatal in 1% of patients, especially when cumulative dosage exceeds 400 units. Also, pulmonary toxic adverse effects may be increased in patients receiving radiation therapy, patients with preexisting lung disease, and patients requiring $O_2$ therapy.

• Monitor chest X-ray and listen to lungs regularly.

• Obtain pulmonary function tests and chest X-rays before each course of therapy.

• If patient's condition requires sclerosis, drug may be instilled when chest tube drainage is 100 to 300 ml/24 hours before therapy; ideally, drainage should be less than 100 ml. After instillation, thoracotomy tube is clamped and patient is moved alternately from the supine to left and right lateral positions for the next 4 hours. The clamp is then removed and suction reestablished. Amount of time chest tube is left in place after sclerosis depends on patient's condition.

• Watch for fever, which may be treated with antipyretics. Fever usually occurs within 3 to 6 hours of administration.

• Watch for hypersensitivity reactions, which may be delayed for several hours, especially in patients with lymphoma. (Give test dose of 1 to 2 units before first two doses in these patients. If no reaction occurs, follow regular dosage.)

• Don't use adhesive dressings on skin.

## PATIENT TEACHING

• Warn patient that hair loss may occur, but that it's usually reversible.

• Tell patient to report adverse reactions promptly and to take infection-control and bleeding precautions.

• Instruct patient that, if he's to receive anesthesia, he must inform anesthesiologist of previous treatment with bleomycin. High oxygen levels inhaled during surgery may enhance pulmonary toxicity of drug.

---

## daunorubicin citrate liposomal
DaunoXome

*Pregnancy risk category D*

### AVAILABLE FORMS
*Injection:* 2 mg/ml (equivalent to 50 mg daunorubicin base)

### INDICATIONS & DOSAGES
➤ **First-line cytotoxic therapy for advanced HIV-related Kaposi's sarcoma**
*Adults:* 40 mg/m² I.V. over 60 minutes once q 2 weeks. Continue treatment until progressive disease become evident or until other complications of HIV infection preclude continuation of therapy.
*Adjust-a-dose:* For patients with impaired hepatic and renal function, reduce dosage as follows: if bilirubin level is 1.2 to 3 mg/dl, give three-fourths normal dose; if bilirubin or creatinine level exceeds 3 mg/dl, give one-half normal dose.

### I.V. ADMINISTRATION
• *Alert:* Preparation and administration of parenteral form of drug may be mutagenic, teratogenic, or carcinogenic to staff. Follow institutional policy to reduce risks.

• Dilute drug with $D_5W$ before use. Withdraw calculated volume of drug from vial and transfer into an equivalent amount of $D_5W$. Recommended concentration after dilution is 1 mg/ml.

• Don't mix daunorubicin citrate liposomal with bacteriostatic or other drugs, saline solution, or other solutions.

• After dilution, immediately give I.V. over 60 minutes. If unable to use immediately, refrigerate at 36° to 46° F (2° to 8° C) for up to 6 hours.

• Don't use in-line filters for I.V. infusion.

• *Alert:* A triad of back pain, flushing, and chest tightness may occur within first 5

---

Reactions may be *common,* uncommon, *life-threatening,* or COMMON AND LIFE-THREATENING.

minutes of infusion. These symptoms subside after infusion is stopped and usually don't recur when infusion is given at a slower rate.
• Monitor I.V. site closely and watch for irritation and infiltration; extravasation can cause tissue damage and necrosis. If extravasation occurs, stop I.V., apply ice, and notify prescriber.

## ACTION
Maximizes selectivity of daunorubicin for solid tumors in situ. After penetrating tumor, drug is released over time to exert antineoplastic activity by inhibiting DNA synthesis and DNA-dependent RNA synthesis through intercalation.

| Route | Onset | Peak | Duration |
|-------|-------|------|----------|
| I.V. | Unknown | Unknown | Unknown |

## ADVERSE REACTIONS
**CNS:** *headache, neuropathy,* depression, dizziness, syncope, insomnia, amnesia, anxiety, ataxia, confusion, *seizures,* hallucination, tremor, hypertonia, *meningitis, fatigue,* malaise, emotional lability, abnormal thinking, hyperkinesia, somnolence, abnormal gait, *fever.*
**CV:** *dose-related cardiomyopathy,* chest pain, hypertension, palpitations, *arrhythmias, pericardial effusion, pericardial tamponade, cardiac arrest,* angina pectoris, *pulmonary hypertension,* flushing, edema, tachycardia, *MI.*
**EENT:** *rhinitis,* stomatitis, sinusitis, abnormal vision, conjunctivitis, tinnitus, eye pain, deafness, earache.
**GI:** taste disturbances, dry mouth, gingival bleeding, *nausea, diarrhea, abdominal pain, vomiting, anorexia,* constipation, thirst, *GI hemorrhage,* gastritis, dysphagia, stomatitis, increased appetite, melena, hemorrhoids, tenesmus.
**GU:** dysuria, nocturia, polyuria.
**Hematologic:** NEUTROPENIA, THROMBOCYTOPENIA.
**Hepatic:** hepatomegaly.
**Metabolic:** dehydration.
**Musculoskeletal:** *rigors, back pain,* arthralgia, myalgia.
**Respiratory:** *cough, dyspnea,* hemoptysis, hiccups, pulmonary infiltration, increased sputum.

**Skin:** alopecia, pruritus, *increased sweating,* dry skin, seborrhea, folliculitis, injection site inflammation.
**Other:** splenomegaly, lymphadenopathy, tooth caries, *opportunistic infections,* allergic reactions, flulike symptoms.

## INTERACTIONS
None significant.

## EFFECTS ON LAB TEST RESULTS
• May decrease neutrophil and platelet counts.

## CONTRAINDICATIONS & CAUTIONS
• Contraindicated in patients who have experienced severe hypersensitivity reaction to drug or its components.
• Use cautiously in patients with myelosuppression, cardiac disease, previous radiotherapy encompassing the heart, previous anthracycline use (doxorubicin is 300 mg/m$^2$ or above), or hepatic or renal dysfunction.

## NURSING CONSIDERATIONS
• Liposomal daunorubicin is associated with less nausea, vomiting, alopecia, neutropenia, thrombocytopenia, and potentially less cardiotoxicity than conventional daunorubicin.
• Give only under supervision of prescriber specializing in cancer chemotherapy.
• Monitor cardiac function regularly. Assess patient before giving each dose because of risk of cardiac toxicity and heart failure. Determine left ventricular ejection fraction at total cumulative doses of 320 mg/m$^2$ and every 160 mg/m$^2$ thereafter. Total cumulative doses generally shouldn't exceed 550 mg/m$^2$.
• Careful hematologic monitoring is needed because severe myelosuppression may occur. Repeat blood counts and evaluate before giving each dose. Withhold treatment if absolute granulocyte count is below 750 cells/mm$^3$.
• Monitor patient closely for signs and symptoms of opportunistic infection, especially because patients with HIV infection are immunocompromised.
*Alert:* Don't confuse daunorubicin citrate liposomal with daunorubicin hydrochloride.

## PATIENT TEACHING
• Inform patient that hair loss may occur, but that it's usually reversible.
• Instruct patient to call prescriber if sore throat, fever, or other signs or symptoms of infection occur. Tell patient to avoid exposure to people with infections.
• Advise woman to report suspected or confirmed pregnancy during therapy.
• Tell patient to report back pain, flushing, or chest tightness during infusion.

# daunorubicin hydrochloride
Cerubidine

*Pregnancy risk category D*

## AVAILABLE FORMS
*Injection:* 20-mg and 50-mg vials

## INDICATIONS & DOSAGES
Dosages vary. Check treatment protocol with prescriber.
➤ **To induce remission in acute non-lymphocytic (myelogenous, monocytic, erythroid) leukemia**
*Adults age 60 and older:* In combination, 30 mg/m² per day I.V. on days 1, 2, and 3 of first course and on days 1 and 2 of subsequent courses with cytarabine infusions.
*Adults younger than age 60:* In combination, 45 mg/m² per day I.V. on days 1, 2, and 3 of first course and on days 1 and 2 of subsequent courses with cytarabine infusions.
➤ **To induce remission in acute lymphocytic leukemia (with combination therapy)**
*Adults:* 45 mg/m² per day I.V. on days 1, 2, and 3 of first course.
*Children age 2 and older:* 25 mg/m² I.V. on day 1 q week for up to 6 weeks, if needed.
*Children younger than age 2 or with body surface area less than 0.5 m²:* Dose based on body weight, not surface area.
*Adjust-a-dose:* For patients with impaired hepatic and renal function, reduce dosage as follows: If bilirubin level is 1.2 to 3 mg/dl, give three-fourths normal dose; if bilirubin or creatinine level exceeds 3 mg/dl, give one-half normal dose.

## I.V. ADMINISTRATION
• **Alert:** Preparation and administration of parenteral form of drug may be mutagenic, teratogenic, or carcinogenic to staff. Follow institutional policy to reduce risks.
• Reconstitute drug using 4 ml of sterile water for injection to produce a 5-mg/ml solution.
• Withdraw desired dose into syringe containing 10 to 15 ml of normal saline solution for injection. Inject over 2 to 3 minutes into tubing of a free-flowing I.V. solution of D₅W or normal saline solution for injection as a slow I.V. push.
• If extravasation occurs, stop I.V. infusion immediately, apply ice to area for 24 to 48 hours, and notify prescriber. Because drug is a vesicant, extravasation could cause severe tissue necrosis.
• **Alert:** Dexamethasone and heparin may form a precipitate when mixed with daunorubicin. Don't mix together.
• Optimally, use within 8 hours of preparation. Reconstituted solution is stable for 24 hours at room temperature, or 48 hours if refrigerated.

## ACTION
May interfere with DNA-dependent RNA synthesis by intercalation.

| Route | Onset | Peak | Duration |
|-------|-------|------|----------|
| I.V. | Unknown | Unknown | Unknown |

## ADVERSE REACTIONS
**CNS:** fever.
**CV:** IRREVERSIBLE CARDIOMYOPATHY, ECG changes.
**GI:** *nausea, vomiting,* diarrhea, stomatitis.
**GU:** red urine.
**Hematologic:** *bone marrow suppression.*
**Hepatic:** *hepatotoxicity.*
**Metabolic:** hyperuricemia.
**Skin:** rash, *reversible alopecia,* darkening or redness of previously irradiated areas; *severe cellulitis and tissue sloughing with drug extravasation,*
**Other:** *anaphylactoid reaction,* chills.

## INTERACTIONS
**Drug-drug.** *Doxorubicin:* May cause additive cardiotoxicity. Monitor patient for toxicity.

---

Reactions may be *common,* uncommon, *life-threatening,* or COMMON AND LIFE-THREATENING.

*Hepatotoxic drugs:* May increase risk of additive hepatotoxicity. Monitor hepatic function closely.

*Myelosuppressive drugs:* May increase risk of myelosuppression. Monitor patient closely.

## EFFECTS ON LAB TEST RESULTS
● May increase uric acid, AST, bilirubin, and alkaline phosphatase levels.
● May decrease hematocrit, hemoglobin, and WBC and platelet counts.

## CONTRAINDICATIONS & CAUTIONS
● Contraindicated in patients hypersensitive to the drug.
● Use cautiously in patients with myelosuppression or impaired cardiac, renal, or hepatic function.

## NURSING CONSIDERATIONS
● Take preventive measures (including adequate hydration) before starting treatment. Hyperuricemia may result from rapid lysis of leukemic cells. Allopurinol may be ordered.
● Perform cardiac function studies, including ECG and ejection fraction, before treatment and then periodically throughout therapy.
● Never give drug I.M. or S.C.
● *Alert:* Cumulative adult dosage is limited to 400 to 550 mg/m² (450 mg/m² when patient is also receiving or has received cyclophosphamide or radiation therapy to cardiac area).
● Therapeutic effects are commonly accompanied by toxicity.
● Monitor CBC and hepatic function tests; monitor ECG every month during therapy.
● Monitor pulse rate closely. Notify prescriber if light resting pulse rate (a sign of cardiac adverse reactions) occurs.
● *Alert:* Stop drug immediately and notify prescriber if signs of heart failure, cardiomyopathy, or arrhythmia develop.
● Watch for nausea and vomiting, which may last 24 to 48 hours.
● Anticipate need for blood transfusions to combat anemia. Patient may receive injected RBC colony-stimulating factor to promote RBC production and decrease need for blood transfusions.
● *Alert:* Reddish color of drug is similar to that of doxorubicin; don't confuse the two.

● Lowest blood counts occur 10 to 14 days after administration.
*Alert:* Don't confuse daunorubicin hydrochloride with daunorubicin citrate liposomal.

## PATIENT TEACHING
● Advise patient to report any pain or burning at site of injection during or after administration.
● Advise patient to watch for signs and symptoms of infection (fever, sore throat, fatigue) and bleeding (easy bruising, nosebleeds, bleeding gums, tarry stools) and to take temperature daily.
● Inform patient that red urine for 1 to 2 days is normal and doesn't indicate the presence of blood in urine.
● Advise patient that hair loss may occur, but that it's usually reversible.
● Caution woman of childbearing age to avoid becoming pregnant during therapy. Recommend that she consult prescriber before becoming pregnant.

# doxorubicin hydrochloride
Adriamycin‡, Adriamycin PFS, Adriamycin RDF, Rubex

*Pregnancy risk category D*

## AVAILABLE FORMS
*Injection (preservative-free):* 2 mg/ml
*Powder for injection:* 10-mg, 20-mg, 50-mg, 100-mg, 150-mg vials

## INDICATIONS & DOSAGES
Dosages vary. Check treatment protocol with prescriber.
➤ **Bladder, breast, lung, ovarian, stomach, and thyroid cancers; non-Hodgkin's disease; Hodgkin's disease; acute lymphoblastic and myeloblastic leukemia; Wilms' tumor; neuroblastoma; lymphoma; sarcoma**
*Adults:* 60 to 75 mg/m² I.V. as single dose q 3 weeks; or 30 mg/m² I.V. in single daily dose, days 1 to 3 of 4-week cycle. Or, 20 mg/m² I.V. once weekly. Maximum cumulative dose is 550 mg/m².
*Elderly patients:* May need reduced dosages.
*Adjust-a-dose:* Dosage may be reduced for patients with myelosuppression or im-

paired cardiac or liver function. Be prepared to decrease dosage if bilirubin level rises: Give 50% of dose when bilirubin level is 1.2 to 3 mg/100 ml; 25% when it's 3.1 to 5 mg/100 ml.

## I.V. ADMINISTRATION

• **Alert:** Preparation and administration of parenteral form of drug may be mutagenic, teratogenic, or carcinogenic to staff. Follow institutional policy to reduce risks.
• If drug leaks or spills, inactivate it with 5% sodium hypochlorite solution (household bleach).
• Reconstitute drug using preservative-free normal saline solution for injection. Add 5 ml to 10-mg vial, 10 ml to 20-mg vial, or 25 ml to 50-mg vial. Shake vial and allow drug to dissolve; final concentration will be 2 mg/ml. Give by direct injection into the tubing of a free-flowing I.V. solution containing $D_5W$ or normal saline solution for injection. Administration rate shouldn't be less than 3 minutes. Drug is a severe vesicant; if extravasation occurs, tissue necrosis may result.
• Don't place I.V. line over joints or in limbs with poor venous or lymphatic drainage. If extravasation occurs, stop I.V. infusion immediately, apply ice to area for 24 to 48 hours, and notify prescriber. Monitor area closely because extravasation may be progressive. Early consultation with a plastic surgeon may be advisable.
• If vein streaking occurs, slow administration rate. However, if welts appear, stop administration and notify prescriber.
• Some protocols give doxorubicin as a prolonged infusion, which requires central venous access.
• Refrigerated, reconstituted solution is stable for 48 hours; at room temperature, it's stable for 24 hours.

## ACTION

Exact mechanism unknown. May interfere with DNA-dependent RNA synthesis by intercalation.

| Route | Onset | Peak | Duration |
|-------|-------|------|----------|
| I.V. | Unknown | Unknown | Unknown |

## ADVERSE REACTIONS

**CNS:** fever.
**CV:** cardiac depression, *arrhythmias, acute left ventricular failure, irreversible cardiomyopathy.*
**EENT:** conjunctivitis.
**GI:** *nausea, vomiting,* diarrhea, *stomatitis,* esophagitis, anorexia.
**GU:** transient red urine.
**Hematologic:** *leukopenia, thrombocytopenia,* MYELOSUPPRESSION.
**Metabolic:** hyperuricemia.
**Skin:** *severe cellulitis and tissue sloughing with drug extravasation,* urticaria, facial flushing, *complete alopecia within 3 to 4 weeks,* hyperpigmentation of nail beds and dermal creases, radiation recall effect.
**Other:** chills, *anaphylaxis.*

## INTERACTIONS

**Drug-drug.** *Aminophylline, cephalothin, dexamethasone, fluorouracil, heparin, hydrocortisone:* May form a precipitate. Don't mix together.
*Calcium channel blockers:* May increase cardiotoxic effects. Monitor patient's ECG closely.
*Cyclosporine:* May increase doxorubicin concentration. Monitor patient for toxicity.
*Digoxin:* May decrease digoxin level. Monitor digoxin level closely.
*Fosphenytoin, phenytoin:* May decrease level of phenytoin or fosphenytoin. Monitor drug level.
*Paclitaxel:* May decrease doxorubicin clearance. Monitor patient for toxicity.
*Phenobarbital:* May increase doxorubicin clearance. Monitor patient closely.
*Streptozocin:* May increase and prolong doxorubicin level. Dosage may have to be adjusted.

## EFFECTS ON LAB TEST RESULTS

• May increase uric acid level.
• May decrease WBC and platelet counts.

## CONTRAINDICATIONS & CAUTIONS

• Contraindicated in patients with a history of sensitivity reactions to doxorubicin or its components. Contraindicated in patients with marked myelosuppression induced by previous treatment with other antitumor drugs or radiotherapy and in patients who have received a lifetime cumu-

lative dose of 550 mg/m² of doxorubicin
or daunorubicin.

## NURSING CONSIDERATIONS
• Perform cardiac function studies, including ECG and ejection fraction, before
treatment and then periodically throughout
therapy. Dexrazoxane may be given within
30 minutes of doxorubicin if the accumulated dose of doxorubicin has reached
300 mg/m².
• Take preventive measures, including adequate hydration of the patient, before
starting treatment. Hyperuricemia may result from rapid lysis of leukemic cells. Allopurinol may be ordered.
• Premedicate with antiemetic to reduce
nausea.
• If skin or mucosal contact occurs, immediately wash with soap and water.
• Never give drug I.M. or S.C.
• Dosage modification may be needed in
patients with myelosuppression or impaired cardiac or hepatic function, and in
elderly patients.
• Monitor CBC with differential and hepatic function tests; monitor ECG monthly
during therapy. If WBC count falls below
2,000/mm³ or granulocyte count falls below 1,000/mm³, follow institutional policy
for infection control in immunocompromised patients.
• Monitor ECG for changes such as sinus
tachycardia, T-wave flattening, ST-segment
depression, and voltage reduction.
• Leukopenia may occur during days 10 to
15, with recovery by day 21.
• Be prepared to stop drug or slow rate of
infusion, and notify prescriber if tachycardia develops.
• *Alert:* If signs of heart failure develop,
stop drug and notify prescriber. Heart failure can often be prevented by limiting cumulative dose to 550 mg/m² (400 mg/m²
when patient is also receiving or has received cyclophosphamide or radiation
therapy to cardiac area).
• Reddish color of drug is similar to that
of daunorubicin; don't confuse the two
drugs.
• Esophagitis is common in patients who
also have received radiation therapy.
• *Alert:* If patient has previously received
radiation therapy, he is susceptible to radiation recall effect.

*Alert:* Don't confuse doxorubicin with
doxorubicin liposomal.

## PATIENT TEACHING
• Advise patient to report any pain or
burning at site of injection during or after
administration.
• Advise patient to watch for signs and
symptoms of infection (fever, sore throat,
fatigue) and bleeding (easy bruising, nosebleeds, bleeding gums, tarry stools) and to
take temperature daily.
• Advise patient that orange to red urine
for 1 to 2 days is normal and doesn't indicate presence of blood.
• Inform patient that hair loss may occur,
but it's usually reversible. Hair may re-
grow 2 to 5 months after drug is stopped.

# doxorubicin hydrochloride liposomal
Doxil

*Pregnancy risk category D*

## AVAILABLE FORMS
*Injection:* 2 mg/ml

## INDICATIONS & DOSAGES
➤ **Metastatic ovarian carcinoma refractory to both paclitaxel- and platinum-
based chemotherapy regimens**
*Women:* 50 mg/m² (doxorubicin hydrochloride equivalent) I.V. at initial infusion
rate of 1 mg/minute once q 4 weeks for
minimum of 4 courses. Continue as long
as condition doesn't progress, patient
shows no evidence of cardiotoxicity, and
patient continues to tolerate treatment. If
no infusion-related adverse reactions are
observed, increase infusion rate to complete administration over 1 hour.
➤ **AIDS-related Kaposi's sarcoma
refractory to previous combination
chemotherapy and in patients intolerant of such therapy**
*Adults:* 20 mg/m² (doxorubicin hydrochloride equivalent) I.V. over 30 minutes
once every 3 weeks. Continue as long as
patient responds satisfactorily and tolerates treatment.
*Adjust-a-dose:* For patients with impaired
hepatic function, reduce dosage as follows: If bilirubin level is 1.2 to 3 mg/dl,

give one-half normal dose; if bilirubin level is more than 3 mg/dl, give one-fourth normal dose. Consult package insert for dose modifications for stomatitis, myelosuppression, and hand-foot syndrome.

## I.V. ADMINISTRATION

• Follow procedures for proper handling and disposal of antineoplastics.

• Dilute appropriate dose (to maximum of 90 mg) in 250 ml D₅W using aseptic technique. Refrigerate diluted solution at 36° to 46° F (2° to 8° C) and give within 24 hours.

• Carefully check label on I.V. bag before giving. Accidental substitution of doxorubicin hydrochloride liposomal for conventional doxorubicin hydrochloride has resulted in severe adverse reactions. The two products may not be substituted on a mg-per-mg basis.

• *Alert:* Don't use with in-line filters.

• Infuse over 30 to 60 minutes depending on dose. Monitor patient carefully during infusion. Acute infusion-related reactions (flushing, shortness of breath, facial swelling, headache, chills, back pain, tightness in chest or throat, and hypotension) may occur. Reactions resolve over several hours to a day once infusion is stopped, and may resolve when infusion rate is slowed.

• If signs or symptoms of extravasation occur, stop infusion immediately and restart in another vein. Applying ice over site of extravasation for about 30 minutes may help alleviate local reaction.

## ACTION

Consists of doxorubicin hydrochloride encapsulated in liposomes. Action possibly related to drug's ability to bind DNA and inhibit nucleic acid synthesis.

| Route | Onset | Peak | Duration |
|-------|-------|------|----------|
| I.V. | Unknown | Unknown | Unknown |

## ADVERSE REACTIONS

**CNS:** *asthenia,* paresthesia, headache, somnolence, dizziness, depression, insomnia, anxiety, malaise, emotional lability, fatigue, fever.

**CV:** chest pain, hypotension, tachycardia, peripheral edema, *cardiomyopathy, heart failure, arrhythmias,* pericardial effusion.

**EENT:** pharyngitis, rhinitis, conjunctivitis, retinitis, optic neuritis.

**GI:** *nausea, vomiting, constipation, anorexia, diarrhea,* abdominal pain, dyspepsia, oral candidiasis, enlarged abdomen, esophagitis, dysphagia, *stomatitis,* taste perversion, glossitis.

**GU:** albuminuria.

**Hematologic:** LEUKOPENIA, NEUTROPENIA, THROMBOCYTOPENIA, *anemia.*

**Hepatic:** hyperbilirubinemia.

**Metabolic:** dehydration, weight loss, hypocalcemia, hyperglycemia.

**Musculoskeletal:** myalgia, back pain.

**Respiratory:** dyspnea, increased cough, pneumonia.

**Skin:** *rash, alopecia,* dry skin, pruritus, skin discoloration, skin disorder, exfoliative dermatitis, sweating, *palmar-plantar erythrodysesthesia.*

**Other:** allergic reaction, chills, *herpes zoster,* infection, infusion-related reactions.

## INTERACTIONS

None reported. However, doxorubicin hydrochloride liposomal may interact with drugs known to affect the conventional formulation of doxorubicin hydrochloride.

## EFFECTS ON LAB TEST RESULTS

• May increase bilirubin and glucose levels. May decrease calcium level.

• May increase PT and INR. May decrease hemoglobin and WBC, neutrophil, and platelet counts.

## CONTRAINDICATIONS & CAUTIONS

• Contraindicated in patients hypersensitive to conventional formulation of doxorubicin hydrochloride or any component in the liposomal formulation.

• Contraindicated in patients with marked myelosuppression and those who have received a lifetime cumulative dose of 550 mg/m² (400 mg/m² in patients who have received radiotherapy to the mediastinal area or therapy with other cardiotoxic drugs such as cyclophosphamide).

• Use cautiously in patients who have received other anthracyclines.

## NURSING CONSIDERATIONS

• Consider previous or current therapy with related compounds such as daunorubicin when calculating total dose of drug

---

to be given. Heart failure and cardiomy-opathy may occur after stopping therapy.
• Give drug to patient with history of CV disease only when benefit outweighs risk to patient.
• Don't give I.M. or S.C.
• *Alert:* Monitor patient for signs and symptoms of palmar-plantar erythrodyses-thesia, hematologic toxicity, or stomatitis. These adverse reactions may be managed with dosage delays and adjustments.
• Evaluate patient's hepatic function before therapy, and adjust dosage accordingly.
• Drug exhibits pharmacokinetic proper-ties different from those of conventional doxorubicin hydrochloride and shouldn't be substituted on a mg-per-mg basis.
• Drug may potentiate toxicity of other an-tineoplastic therapies.
• Closely monitor cardiac function by en-domyocardial biopsy, echocardiography, or gated radionuclide scans. If results indi-cate possible cardiac injury, the benefit of continued therapy must be weighed against the risk of myocardial injury.
• Monitor CBC, including platelets, be-fore each dose and frequently throughout therapy. Leukopenia is usually transient. Persistent severe myelosuppression may result in superinfection or hemorrhage. Patient may need G-CSF (or GM-CSF) to support blood counts.

**PATIENT TEACHING**
• Tell patient to notify prescriber if he ex-periences signs and symptoms of hand-foot syndrome (such as tingling or burn-ing, redness, flaking, bothersome swelling, small blisters, or small sores on palms of hands or soles of feet).
• Advise patient to report signs and symp-toms of mouth inflammation (such as painful redness, swelling, or sores in mouth).
• Warn patient to avoid exposure to people with infections. Tell patient to report tem-perature of 100.5° F (38° C) or higher.
• Tell patient to report nausea, vomiting, tiredness, weakness, rash, or mild hair loss.
• Advise woman of childbearing age to avoid pregnancy during therapy.

# epirubicin hydrochloride
Ellence

*Pregnancy risk category D*

**AVAILABLE FORMS**
*Injection:* 2 mg/ml

**INDICATIONS & DOSAGES**
➤ **Adjuvant therapy in patients with evidence of axillary node tumor involve-ment after resection of primary breast cancer**
*Adults:* 100 to 120 mg/m² I.V. infusion over 3 to 5 minutes through a free-flowing I.V. solution on day 1 of each cycle, or divided equally in two doses on days 1 and 8 of each cycle; cycle repeated q 3 to 4 weeks for six cycles; used with regimens containing cyclophosphamide and fluo-rouracil.

Dosage modification after first cycle is based on toxicity. For patients with plate-let count nadir below 50,000/mm³, ab-solute neutrophil count (ANC) below 250/mm³, neutropenic fever, or grade 3 or 4 nonhematologic toxicity, reduce day 1 dose in subsequent cycles to 75% of day 1 dose given in current cycle. Delay day 1 therapy in subsequent cycles until platelet count is at least 100,000/mm³, ANC is at least 1,500/mm³, and nonhematologic tox-icities recover to grade 1.

For patients receiving divided doses (days 1 and 8), day 8 dose should be 75% of day 1 dose if platelet count is 75,000 to 100,000/mm³ and ANC is 1,000 to 1,499/mm³. If day 8 platelet count is below 75,000/mm³, ANC is below 1,000/mm³, or grade 3 or 4 nonhematologic toxicity has occurred, omit day 8 dose.
*Adjust-a-dose:* For patients with bone marrow dysfunction (heavily pretreated patients, patients with bone marrow de-pression, or those with neoplastic bone marrow infiltration), start at lower doses of 75 to 90 mg/m². For patients with he-patic dysfunction, if bilirubin is 1.2 to 3 mg/dl or AST is two to four times upper limit of normal, give one-half recom-mended starting dose. If bilirubin level is above 3 mg/dl or AST is more than four times upper limit of normal, give one-fourth recommended starting dose. For

patients with severe renal dysfunction (creatinine level over 5 mg/dl), consider lower doses.

## I.V. ADMINISTRATION
• Wear protective clothing (goggles, gown, disposable gloves) when handling drug.
• *Alert:* Drug is a vesicant. Never give I.M. or S.C. Always give through free-flowing I.V. solution of normal saline solution or D₅W over 3 to 5 minutes.
• Facial flushing and local erythematous streaking along vein may indicate excessively rapid administration.
• Avoid veins over joints or in limbs with compromised venous or lymphatic drainage.
• Immediately stop infusion if burning or stinging occurs, and restart in another vein.
• Avoid repeat injection into the same vein.
• Don't mix drug with heparin or fluorouracil because precipitation may result.
• Don't mix in same syringe with other drugs.
• Discard unused solution left in vial 24 hours after vial has been penetrated.

## ACTION
Exact mechanism unknown. Thought to form a complex with DNA by intercalation between nucleotide base pairs, thereby inhibiting DNA, RNA, and protein synthesis; DNA cleavage occurs, resulting in cytocidal activity. Drug may also interfere with replication and transcription of DNA and may generate cytotoxic free radicals.

| Route | Onset | Peak | Duration |
|-------|-------|------|----------|
| I.V. | Unknown | Unknown | Unknown |

## ADVERSE REACTIONS
**CNS:** *lethargy,* fever.
**CV:** ***cardiomyopathy, heart failure,*** hot flashes.
**EENT:** *conjunctivitis, keratitis.*
**GI:** *nausea, vomiting, diarrhea,* anorexia, mucositis.
**GU:** *amenorrhea,* red urine.
**Hematologic:** LEUKOPENIA, NEUTROPENIA, *febrile neutropenia,* anemia, THROMBOCYTOPENIA.
**Skin:** *alopecia,* rash, itch, skin changes, local toxicity.
**Other:** *infection.*

## INTERACTIONS
**Drug-drug.** *Calcium channel blockers, other cardioactive compounds:* May increase risk of heart failure. Monitor cardiac function closely.
*Cimetidine:* May increase epirubicin level by 50%. Avoid using together.
*Cytotoxic drugs:* May cause additive toxicities (especially hematologic and GI). Monitor patient closely.
*Radiation therapy:* May enhance effects. Monitor patient closely.

## EFFECTS ON LAB TEST RESULTS
• May decrease hemoglobin and WBC, neutrophil, and platelet counts.

## CONTRAINDICATIONS & CAUTIONS
• Contraindicated in patients hypersensitive to drug, other anthracyclines, or anthracenediones, and in patients with baseline neutrophil counts below 1,500 cells/mm³, severe myocardial insufficiency, recent MI, serious arrhythmias, or severe hepatic dysfunction. Also contraindicated in patients who have had previous treatment with anthracyclines to total cumulative doses.
• Use cautiously in patients with active or dormant cardiac disease, previous or current radiotherapy to mediastinal and pericardial areas, or previous therapy with other anthracyclines or anthracenediones; also use cautiously in patients receiving other cardiotoxic drugs.

## NURSING CONSIDERATIONS
• Give drug under supervision of prescriber experienced in cancer chemotherapy. Pregnant nurses shouldn't handle drug.
• Patients receiving 120 mg/m² of epirubicin should also receive prophylactic antibiotic therapy with co-trimoxazole or a fluoroquinolone.
• Antiemetics may be needed before epirubicin to reduce nausea and vomiting.
• Before therapy starts, obtain total bilirubin, AST, and creatinine levels; CBC including ANC; and left ventricular ejection fraction (LVEF).
• Monitor LVEF regularly during therapy. Stop drug at first sign of impaired cardiac function. Early signs of cardiac toxicity include sinus tachycardia, ECG abnormal-

---

Reactions may be *common,* uncommon, ***life-threatening,*** or COMMON AND LIFE-THREATENING.

ities, tachyarrhythmias, bradycardia, AV block, and bundle-branch block.
• Delayed cardiac toxicity may occur 2 to 3 months after treatment ends; indications include reduced LVEF and signs and symptoms of heart failure (tachycardia, dyspnea, pulmonary edema, dependent edema, hepatomegaly, ascites, pleural effusion, and gallop rhythm). Delayed cardiac toxicity depends on cumulative dose of epirubicin. Don't exceed cumulative dose of 900 mg/m$^2$.
• Obtain total and differential WBC, CBC, platelet counts, and liver function tests before and during each cycle of therapy.
• WBC nadir is usually reached 10 to 14 days after drug administration, and returns to normal by day 21.
• Monitor uric acid, potassium, calcium phosphate, and creatinine levels immediately after initial chemotherapy administration in patients susceptible to tumor lysis syndrome. Hydration, urine alkalinization, and prophylaxis with allopurinol may prevent hyperuricemia and minimize potential complications of tumor lysis syndrome.
• Administration of drug after previous radiation therapy may induce an inflammatory cell reaction at irradiation site.

## PATIENT TEACHING
• Advise patient to report any pain or burning at site of injection during or after administration.
• Advise patient to report nausea, vomiting, mouth inflammation, dehydration, fever, evidence of infection, or symptoms of heart failure (rapid heartbeat, labored breathing, swelling).
• Tell patient that urine will be reddish-pink for 1 to 2 days after treatment.
• Inform patient of risk of heart damage and treatment-related leukemia with use of drug.
• Advise men to use effective contraception during treatment.
• Advise women that irreversible cessation of menstruation or premature menopause may occur.
• Tell patient that hair usually regrows within 2 to 3 months after therapy stops.

# idarubicin hydrochloride
Idamycin, Idamycin PFS

*Pregnancy risk category D*

## AVAILABLE FORMS
*Injection:* 5 mg, 10 mg, 20 mg

## INDICATIONS & DOSAGES
Dosages vary. Check treatment protocol with prescriber.
➤ **Acute myeloid leukemia, including French-American-British (FAB) classifications M1 through M7, with other approved antileukemic drugs**
*Adults:* 12 mg/m$^2$ daily for 3 days by slow I.V. injection (over 10 to 15 minutes) with 100 mg/m$^2$ daily of cytarabine for 7 days by continuous I.V. infusion. Or, as a 25-mg/m$^2$ bolus (cytarabine); then 200 mg/m$^2$ daily (cytarabine) for 5 days by continuous infusion. A second course may be given, if needed.
*Adjust-a-dose:* If patient experiences severe mucositis, delay therapy until recovery is complete and reduce dosage by 25%. Reduce dosage in patients with hepatic or renal impairment. Don't give idarubicin if bilirubin level exceeds 5 mg/dl.

## I.V. ADMINISTRATION
• *Alert:* Preparation and administration of parenteral form of drug may be mutagenic, teratogenic, or carcinogenic to staff. Follow institutional policy to reduce risks.
• Reconstitute to final concentration of 1 mg/ml using normal saline solution for injection without preservatives. Add 5 ml to 5-mg vial, 10 ml to 10-mg vial, or 20 ml to 20-mg vial. Don't use bacteriostatic saline solution. Vial is under negative pressure.
• Give drug over 10 to 15 minutes into a free-flowing I.V. infusion of normal saline or D$_5$W solution running into a large vein.
• Drug is a vesicant; tissue necrosis may result. If extravasation occurs, stop infusion immediately and notify prescriber. Treat with intermittent ice packs—for one-half hour immediately, and then for one-half hour q.i.d. for 4 days.
• Reconstituted solutions are stable for 72 hours at 59° to 86° F (15° to 30° C);

7 days if refrigerated and protected from light. Label unused solutions with chemotherapy hazard label.

**ACTION**
Unknown. Probably inhibits nucleic acid synthesis by intercalation and interacts with the enzyme topoisomerase II. It's highly lipophilic, which results in an increased rate of cellular uptake.

| Route | Onset | Peak | Duration |
|-------|-------|------|----------|
| I.V. | Unknown | Few min | Unknown |

**ADVERSE REACTIONS**
**CNS:** *headache, changed mental status,* peripheral neuropathy, *seizures, fever.*
**CV:** *heart failure,* atrial fibrillation, chest pain, *MI,* asymptomatic decline in left ventricular ejection fraction, *myocardial insufficiency, arrhythmias,* HEMORRHAGE, *myocardial toxicity.*
**GI:** *nausea, vomiting, cramps, diarrhea,* mucositis.
**GU:** renal dysfunction, red urine.
**Hematologic:** *myelosuppression.*
**Hepatic:** changes in hepatic function.
**Metabolic:** hyperuricemia.
**Skin:** *alopecia, rash, urticaria, bullous erythrodermatous rash on palms and soles,* urticaria, erythema at previously irradiated sites, tissue necrosis if extravasation occurs.
**Other:** INFECTION, *hypersensitivity reactions.*

**INTERACTIONS**
**Drug-drug.** *Alkaline solutions, heparin:* Incompatible. Don't mix idarubicin with other drugs unless specific compatibility data are available.

**EFFECTS ON LAB TEST RESULTS**
• May increase uric acid level.
• May decrease hemoglobin, WBC, neutrophil and platelet counts.

**CONTRAINDICATIONS & CAUTIONS**
• Use with extreme caution in patients with bone marrow suppression induced by previous drug therapy or radiotherapy, impaired hepatic or renal function, previous treatment with anthracyclines or cardiotoxic drugs, or a cardiac condition.

**NURSING CONSIDERATIONS**
• Cardiotoxicity is the dose-limiting toxicity of drug.
• Take preventive measures, including adequate hydration, before starting treatment. Hyperuricemia may result from rapid lysis of leukemic cells. Allopurinol may be ordered.
• Assess patient for systemic infection and ensure that it's controlled before therapy begins.
• Give antiemetics to prevent or treat nausea and vomiting.
• Drug must never be given I.M. or S.C.
• Monitor hepatic and renal function tests and CBC frequently.
• To prevent bleeding, avoid all I.M. injections when platelet count is below 50,000/mm³.
• Anticipate need for blood transfusions to combat anemia. Patient may receive injections of RBC colony-stimulating factor to promote RBC production and decrease need for blood transfusions.
• Notify prescriber if signs or symptoms of heart failure occur.
• *Alert:* Don't confuse idarubicin with daunorubicin or doxorubicin.

**PATIENT TEACHING**
• Teach patient to recognize signs and symptoms of leakage of drug to surrounding tissue, and tell him to report them if they occur.
• Warn patient to watch for signs and symptoms of infection (fever, sore throat, fatigue) and bleeding (easy bruising, nosebleeds, bleeding gums, tarry stools).
• Advise patient that red urine for several days is normal and doesn't indicate presence of blood.
• Caution woman of childbearing age to avoid becoming pregnant during therapy. Recommend that she consult prescriber before becoming pregnant.

# mitomycin (mitomycin-C)
Mitozytrex, Mutamycin

*Pregnancy risk category NR*

**AVAILABLE FORMS**
*Injection:* 5-mg, 20-mg, 40-mg vials

## INDICATIONS & DOSAGES
Dosage and indications vary. Check treatment protocol with prescriber.
➤ **Disseminated adenocarcinoma of stomach or pancreas**
*Adults:* 10 to 20 mg/m$^2$ as an I.V. single dose. Repeat cycle after 6 to 8 weeks when WBC and platelet counts have returned to normal.
*Adjust-a-dose:* For patients with myelosuppression, if leukocytes are 2,000 to 2,999 /mm$^3$ and platelets are 25,000 to 74,999/mm$^3$, give 70% of initial dose. If leukocytes are less than 2,000/mm$^3$ and platelets are less than 25,000/mm$^3$, give 50% of initial dose.
➤ **Bladder cancer ♦**
*Adults:* 20 to 60 mg intravesically once weekly for 8 weeks.

## I.V. ADMINISTRATION
• *Alert:* Preparation and administration of parenteral form of drug may be mutagenic, teratogenic, or carcinogenic to staff. Follow institutional policy to reduce risks.
• Using sterile water for injection, reconstitute drug in 5-mg vials with 10 ml, 20-mg vials with 40 ml, and 40-mg vials with 80 ml.
• When reconstituted with sterile water, Mutamycin solution is stable for 14 days under refrigeration and 7 days at room temperature. When diluted, Mutamycin is stable in D$_5$W for 3 hours, normal saline solution for 12 hours, sodium lactate for 24 hours.
• When reconstituted with sterile water at a concentration of 0.5 mg/ml, Mitozytrex is stable for 14 days when refrigerated, or 7 days at room temperature. When diluted, Mitozytrex is stable in normal saline solution for 12 hours, sodium lactate for 24 hours.
• The combination of mitomycin (5 to 15 mg) and heparin (1,000 to 10,000 units) in 30 ml normal saline solution is stable for 48 hours (Mutamycin) and 48 hours (Mitozytrex) at room temperature.
• Give drug into the side arm of a free-flowing I.V.
• Avoid extravasation. Stop infusion immediately and notify prescriber if extravasation occurs because of potential for severe ulceration and necrosis.

## ACTION
Similar to an alkylating drug, cross-linking strands of DNA and causing an imbalance of cell growth, leading to cell death.

| Route | Onset | Peak | Duration |
|-------|-------|------|----------|
| I.V. | Unknown | Unknown | Unknown |

## ADVERSE REACTIONS
**CNS:** headache, neurologic abnormalities, confusion, drowsiness, fatigue, *fever.*
**EENT:** blurred vision.
**GI:** mucositis, *nausea, vomiting, anorexia, diarrhea, stomatitis.*
**GU:** *renal toxicity, hemolytic uremic syndrome.*
**Hematologic:** THROMBOCYTOPENIA, LEUKOPENIA, *microangiopathic hemolytic anemia.*
**Respiratory:** *interstitial pneumonitis,* pulmonary edema, dyspnea, nonproductive cough, *adult respiratory distress syndrome.*
**Skin:** cellulitis, induration, desquamation, pruritus, *pain at injection site, reversible alopecia,* purple bands on nails, rash, sloughing with extravasation.
**Other:** *septicemia,* ulceration, pain.

## INTERACTIONS
**Drug-drug.** *Vinca alkaloids:* May cause acute respiratory distress when given together. Monitor patient closely.

## EFFECTS ON LAB TEST RESULTS
• May increase BUN and creatinine levels.
• May decrease WBC and platelet count, and hemoglobin.

## CONTRAINDICATIONS & CAUTIONS
• Contraindicated in patients hypersensitive to drug and in those with thrombocytopenia, coagulation disorders, or an increased bleeding tendency from other causes.

## NURSING CONSIDERATIONS
• Never give drug I.M. or S.C.
• Continue CBC and blood studies at least 8 weeks after therapy stops. Leukopenia and thrombocytopenia are cumulative. If WBC count falls below 2,000/mm$^3$ or granulocyte count falls below 1,000/mm$^3$,

---

follow institutional policy for infection control in immunocompromised patients.
• To prevent bleeding, avoid all I.M. injections when platelet count is below 100,000/mm³.
• Anticipate need for blood transfusions to combat anemia. Patients may receive injections of RBC colony-stimulating factor to promote RBC production and decrease need for blood transfusions.
• Monitor patient for dyspnea with nonproductive cough; chest X-ray may show infiltrates.
• Monitor renal function tests.
• Leukopenia may occur up to 8 weeks after therapy and may be cumulative with successive doses.
• Hemolytic uremic syndrome is characterized by microangiopathic hemolytic anemia, thrombocytopenia, and renal failure.
• *Alert:* Don't confuse mitomycin with mithramycin.

**PATIENT TEACHING**
• Advise patient to report any pain or burning at site of injection during or after administration.
• Warn patient to watch for signs and symptoms of infection (fever, sore throat, fatigue) and bleeding (easy bruising, nosebleeds, bleeding gums, tarry stools). Tell patient to take temperature daily.
• Inform patient that hair loss may occur, but that it's usually reversible.

# 70

# Antineoplastics that alter hormone balance

anastrozole
estramustine phosphate sodium
exemestane
flutamide
fulvestrant
goserelin acetate
letrozole
leuprolide acetate
megestrol acetate
nilutamide
tamoxifen citrate
testolactone
toremifene citrate
triptorelin pamoate

**COMBINATION PRODUCTS**
None.

---

## anastrozole
Arimidex

*Pregnancy risk category D*

**AVAILABLE FORMS**
*Tablets:* 1 mg

**INDICATIONS & DOSAGES**
➤ **First-line treatment of postmeno-pausal women with hormone receptor–positive or hormone receptor–unknown locally advanced or metastatic breast cancer; advanced breast cancer in post-menopausal women with disease pro-gression after tamoxifen therapy; ad-junctive treatment of postmenopausal women with hormone receptor–positive early breast cancer**
*Adults:* 1 mg P.O. daily.

**ACTION**
A selective nonsteroidal aromatase inhibi-tor that significantly lowers estradiol lev-els, thereby inhibiting stimulation of breast cancer cell growth in postmeno-pausal women.

| Route | Onset | Peak | Duration |
|-------|-------|------|----------|
| P.O. | < 24 hr | Unknown | < 7 days |

**ADVERSE REACTIONS**
**CNS:** *headache, asthenia,* dizziness, de-pression, paresthesia, *pain.*
**CV:** chest pain, edema, ***thromboembolic disease,*** peripheral edema, *hot flashes.*
**EENT:** pharyngitis.
**GI:** *nausea,* vomiting, diarrhea, constipa-tion, abdominal pain, anorexia, dry mouth.
**GU:** vaginal hemorrhage, vaginal dryness, pelvic pain.
**Metabolic:** weight gain.
**Musculoskeletal:** bone pain, *back pain.*
**Respiratory:** dyspnea, increased cough.
**Skin:** alopecia, rash, sweating.

**INTERACTIONS**
None significant.

**EFFECTS ON LAB TEST RESULTS**
• May increase liver enzyme level.

**CONTRAINDICATIONS & CAUTIONS**
• Don't use in women who are or may be pregnant.
• Use cautiously in breast-feeding women.

**NURSING CONSIDERATIONS**
• Give drug under supervision of a pre-scriber experienced in use of anticancer drugs.
• Patients with hormone receptor–negative disease and patients who didn't respond to previous tamoxifen therapy rarely respond to anastrozole.
• For patients with advanced breast can-cer, continue anastrozole until tumor pro-gresses.

**PATIENT TEACHING**
• Instruct patient to report adverse reac-tions, especially difficulty breathing or chest pain.
• Tell patient to take medication at the same time each day.
• Stress need for follow-up care.
• Counsel woman of childbearing age about risks to pregnancy during therapy.

---

# estramustine phosphate sodium
Emcyt, Estracyt‡

*Pregnancy risk category X*

## AVAILABLE FORMS
*Capsules:* 140 mg

## INDICATIONS & DOSAGES
➤ **Palliative treatment of metastatic or progressive prostate cancer**
*Adults:* 10 to 16 mg/kg daily P.O. in three or four divided doses. Usual dose is 14 mg/kg daily. Continue therapy for up to 3 months and, if successful, maintain it as long as patient responds.

## ACTION
Unknown. A combination of estradiol and a nornitrogen mustard. This drug's uptake into prostate cancer cells is facilitated by the estrogen component. Once intracellular, it may have weak alkylating activity.

| Route | Onset | Peak | Duration |
|-------|-------|------|----------|
| P.O. | Unknown | Unknown | Unknown |

## ADVERSE REACTIONS
**CNS:** lethargy, insomnia, headache, anxiety, *CVA*.
**CV:** *MI,* edema, chest pain, ***thrombophlebitis, heart failure,*** edema, hypertension, flushing.
**GI:** *nausea, vomiting,* diarrhea, anorexia, flatulence, GI bleeding, thirst.
**Hematologic:** *leukopenia, thrombocytopenia, thrombosis.*
**Metabolic:** sodium and fluid retention.
**Musculoskeletal:** leg cramps.
**Respiratory:** *pulmonary embolism,* dyspnea.
**Skin:** rash, pruritus, dry skin, thinning of hair.
**Other:** decreased libido, *breast tenderness, painful gynecomastia.*

## INTERACTIONS
**Drug-drug.** *Calcium-containing drugs such as antacids:* May impair absorption of estramustine. Avoid using together.
**Drug-food.** *Calcium-rich foods, such as dairy products:* May impair absorption of estramustine. Discourage use together.

## EFFECTS ON LAB TEST RESULTS
● May increase AST, ALT, LDH, triglyceride, ceruloplasmin, cortisol, phospholipid, and prolactin levels. May decrease folate, pregnanediol, pyroxidine, and phosphate levels.
● May increase PT. May decrease glucose tolerance and WBC and platelet counts.

## CONTRAINDICATIONS & CAUTIONS
● Contraindicated in patients hypersensitive to estradiol or nitrogen mustard and in those with active thrombophlebitis or thromboembolic disorders, except when actual tumor mass is cause of thromboembolic phenomenon.
● Use cautiously in patients with history of thrombophlebitis, thromboembolic disorders, or cerebrovascular or coronary artery disease.
● Use cautiously in patients with impaired liver function.

## NURSING CONSIDERATIONS
● Monitor weight regularly in patients with history of thrombophlebitis, thromboembolic disorders, or cerebrovascular or coronary artery disease. Drug may worsen peripheral edema or heart failure.
● Monitor liver function periodically throughout therapy in patients with impaired liver function.
● Each 140-mg capsule contains 12.5 mg of sodium.
● Drug may increase blood pressure and decrease glucose level. Monitor periodically throughout therapy.
● Drug is a combination of estrogen estradiol and nitrogen mustard and may be effective in patients refractory to estrogen therapy alone.
● Patient may continue therapy as long as response is favorable. Some patients have taken drug for more than 3 years.
● Drug may increase norepinephrine-induced platelet aggregation and decrease response to the metyrapone test.
● Store capsules in refrigerator.

## PATIENT TEACHING
● Tell patient to take drug on an empty stomach (1 hour before or 2 hours after meals) and to avoid taking within 2 hours of dairy products.

---

Reactions may be *common,* uncommon, *life-threatening*, or **COMMON AND LIFE-THREATENING.**

• Because drug may harm fetus, advise patient and partner to use contraception if woman is of childbearing age.
• Instruct patient to store tablets in the refrigerator.

## exemestane
Aromasin

*Pregnancy risk category D*

### AVAILABLE FORMS
*Tablets:* 25 mg

### INDICATIONS & DOSAGES
➤ **Advanced breast cancer in postmenopausal women whose disease has progressed after treatment with tamoxifen**
*Adults:* 25 mg P.O. once daily after food.

### ACTION
A highly protein-bound, irreversible, steroidal aromatase inactivator that leads to reduced levels of circulating estrogens, thereby decreasing cell growth in estrogen-dependent breast cancer.

| Route | Onset | Peak | Duration |
|-------|-------|------|----------|
| P.O. | Unknown | 1 hr | 24 hr |

### ADVERSE REACTIONS
**CNS:** *depression, insomnia, anxiety, fatigue, pain,* dizziness, headache, paresthesia, generalized weakness, asthenia, confusion, hypoesthesia, fever.
**CV:** hypertension, edema, chest pain, *hot flashes.*
**EENT:** sinusitis, rhinitis, pharyngitis.
**GI:** *nausea,* vomiting, abdominal pain, anorexia, constipation, diarrhea, increased appetite, dyspepsia.
**GU:** UTI.
**Hematologic:** *lymphopenia.*
**Musculoskeletal:** pathologic fractures, arthritis, back pain, skeletal pain.
**Respiratory:** *dyspnea,* bronchitis, cough, upper respiratory tract infection.
**Skin:** rash, increased sweating, alopecia, itching.
**Other:** infection, flulike syndrome, lymphedema.

### INTERACTIONS
**Drug-drug.** *Drugs that induce CYP 3A4, estrogenic agents:* May decrease exemestane plasma level. Monitor patient closely.

### EFFECTS ON LAB TEST RESULTS
None reported.

### CONTRAINDICATIONS & CAUTIONS
• Contraindicated in patients hypersensitive to drug or its components.

### NURSING CONSIDERATIONS
• Use drug only in postmenopausal women. Pregnancy must be ruled out before starting drug therapy.
• Continue treatment until tumor progression is apparent.

### PATIENT TEACHING
• Direct patient to take drug after a meal.
• Tell patient that she may need to take drug for a long time.
• Advise patient to report adverse effects, especially fever or swelling of arms or legs.

## flutamide
Euflex†, Eulexin

*Pregnancy risk category D*

### AVAILABLE FORMS
*Capsules:* 125 mg, 250 mg†

### INDICATIONS & DOSAGES
➤ **Metastatic locally confined prostate cancer (stages B₂, C, D₂), combined with luteinizing hormone-releasing hormone analogues such as leuprolide acetate or goserelin**
*Adults:* 250 mg P.O. q 8 hours.

### ACTION
Inhibits androgen uptake or prevents binding of androgens in nucleus of cells in target tissues.

| Route | Onset | Peak | Duration |
|-------|-------|------|----------|
| P.O. | Unknown | 2 hr | Unknown |

**ADVERSE REACTIONS**
**CNS:** drowsiness, *encephalopathy,* confusion, depression, anxiety, nervousness, paresthesia.
**CV:** peripheral edema, hypertension, *hot flashes.*
**GI:** *diarrhea, nausea, vomiting,* anorexia.
**GU:** *impotence.*
**Hematologic:** anemia, *leukopenia, thrombocytopenia,* hemolytic anemia.
**Hepatic:** *hepatitis.*
**Skin:** rash, photosensitivity reactions.
**Other:** *loss of libido,* gynecomastia.

**INTERACTIONS**
**Drug-drug.** *Warfarin:* May increase PT. Monitor PT and INR.
**Drug-lifestyle.** *Sun exposure:* May cause photosensitivity reactions. Advise patient to avoid excessive sunlight exposure.

**EFFECTS ON LAB TEST RESULTS**
• May increase BUN, creatinine, and liver enzyme levels.
• May decrease hemoglobin and WBC and platelet counts.
• May alter pituitary-gonadal system tests during therapy and for 12 weeks thereafter.

**CONTRAINDICATIONS & CAUTIONS**
• Contraindicated in patients hypersensitive to drug and in those with severe liver dysfunction.

**NURSING CONSIDERATIONS**
• Monitor liver function tests and CBC periodically.
• Flutamide must be taken continuously with drug used for medical castration (such as leuprolide) to allow full benefit of therapy. Leuprolide suppresses testosterone production, whereas flutamide inhibits testosterone action at cellular level; together, they can impair growth of androgen-responsive tumors.

**PATIENT TEACHING**
• Advise patient not to stop drug without consulting prescriber.
• Instruct patient to report adverse reactions promptly, especially dark yellow or brown urine, vomiting, or yellowing of the eyes or skin.

---

# fulvestrant
Faslodex

*Pregnancy risk category D*

**AVAILABLE FORMS**
*Injection:* 50 mg/ml in 2.5-ml and 5-ml prefilled syringes

**INDICATIONS & DOSAGES**
➤ **Hormone receptor–positive metastatic breast cancer in postmenopausal women with disease progression after antiestrogen therapy**
*Adults:* 250 mg (one 5-ml syringe or two 2.5-ml syringes) by slow I.M. injection into buttocks once monthly.

**ACTION**
An estrogen-receptor antagonist. It competitively binds estrogen receptors and down-regulates estrogen-receptor protein in human breast cancer cells. It's effective in treating estrogen receptor–positive breast tumors.

| Route | Onset | Peak | Duration |
|-------|---------|--------|----------|
| I.M. | Unknown | 7 days | 1 mo |

**ADVERSE REACTIONS**
**CNS:** dizziness, *asthenia, headache,* insomnia, fever, paresthesia, depression, anxiety, *pain.*
**CV:** *hot flashes,* chest pain, peripheral edema.
**EENT:** *pharyngitis.*
**GI:** *nausea, vomiting, constipation, abdominal pain, diarrhea,* anorexia.
**GU:** UTI.
**Hematologic:** anemia.
**Musculoskeletal:** *bone pain, back pain, pelvic pain,* arthritis.
**Respiratory:** *dyspnea, cough.*
**Skin:** rash, *injection site pain,* sweating.
**Other:** accidental injury, flulike syndrome.

**INTERACTIONS**
None reported.

---

## EFFECTS ON LAB TEST RESULTS
• May decrease hemoglobin and hematocrit.

## CONTRAINDICATIONS & CAUTIONS
• Contraindicated in pregnant women and in patients allergic to drug or any of its components.
• Use cautiously in patients with moderate or severe hepatic impairment.

## NURSING CONSIDERATIONS
• Because drug is given I.M., don't use in patients with bleeding diatheses or thrombocytopenia, or in those taking anticoagulants.
• Make sure patient isn't pregnant before starting drug.
• Expel gas bubble from syringe before administration.
• *Alert:* If you are administering the 2.5-ml syringes, you must administer both syringes to give the full dose.

## PATIENT TEACHING
• Caution women of childbearing age to avoid pregnancy and to report suspected pregnancy immediately.
• Inform patient of the most common side effects, including pain at injection site, headache, GI symptoms, back pain, hot flashes, and sore throat.

---

## goserelin acetate
Zoladex

*Pregnancy risk category X (endometriosis and endometrial thinning); D (breast cancer)*

## AVAILABLE FORMS
*Implants:* 3.6 mg, 10.8 mg

## ACTION
A luteinizing hormone-releasing hormone (LH-RH) analogue that acts on the pituitary gland to decrease the release of follicle-stimulating hormone and LH, resulting in dramatically lowered levels of sex hormones (estrogen in women and testosterone in men).

| Route | Onset | Peak | Duration |
|-------|-------|------|----------|
| S.C. | Rapid | 30-60 min | Throughout therapy |

## INDICATIONS & DOSAGES
➤ **Endometriosis, including pain relief and lesion reduction; palliative treatment of advanced prostate cancer**
*Adults:* 3.6 mg S.C. q 28 days into upper abdominal wall. For endometriosis, maximum duration of therapy is 6 months. For prostate cancer, 10.8 mg S.C. into upper abdominal wall q 12 weeks.
➤ **Endometrial thinning before endometrial ablation**
*Adults:* 3.6 mg S.C. into upper abdominal wall. Give one or two depots, 4 weeks apart.
➤ **Palliative treatment of advanced breast cancer in premenopausal and perimenopausal women**
*Adults:* 3.6 mg S.C. q 28 days into upper abdominal wall.

## ADVERSE REACTIONS
**CNS:** lethargy, pain, dizziness, *insomnia,* anxiety, *depression, headache,* chills, *emotional lability, CVA, asthenia.*
**CV:** edema, *heart failure, arrhythmias, peripheral edema,* hypertension, *MI,* peripheral vascular disorder, chest pain, *hot flashes.*
**GI:** nausea, vomiting, diarrhea, constipation, ulcer, anorexia, abdominal pain.
**GU:** *sexual dysfunction, impotence, lower urinary tract symptoms,* renal insufficiency, urinary obstruction, *vaginitis,* UTI, *amenorrhea.*
**Hematologic:** anemia.
**Metabolic:** hypercalcemia, hyperglycemia, weight increase, gout.
**Musculoskeletal:** back pain, osteoporosis.
**Respiratory:** COPD, upper respiratory tract infection.
**Skin:** rash, *diaphoresis, acne, seborrhea,* hirsutism.
**Other:** breast swelling, pain, and tenderness, *changes in breast size, changes in libido, infection.*

## INTERACTIONS
None significant.

---

*Rapid onset*   †Canada   ‡Australia   ◇OTC   ◆Off-label use   ✐Photoguide   *Liquid contains alcohol.

## EFFECTS ON LAB TEST RESULTS
• May increase calcium and glucose levels.
• May decrease hemoglobin.

## CONTRAINDICATIONS & CAUTIONS
• Contraindicated in patients hypersensitive to LH-RH, LH-RH agonist analogues, or goserelin acetate. Also contraindicated in pregnant or breast-feeding women and in patients with obstructive uropathy or vertebral metastases. The 10.8-mg implant is contraindicated in women because data are insufficient to support reliable suppression of estradiol.
• Because use of drug is related to loss of bone mineral density in women, use cautiously in patients with risk factors for osteoporosis, such as family history of osteoporosis, chronic alcohol or tobacco abuse, or use of drugs such as corticosteroids or anticonvulsants that affect bone density.

## NURSING CONSIDERATIONS
• Before giving to women, rule out pregnancy.
• Never give by I.V. injection.
• Give drug into upper abdominal wall using aseptic technique. After cleaning area with an alcohol swab and injecting a local anesthetic, stretch patient's skin with one hand while grasping barrel of syringe with the other. Insert needle into the subcutaneous fat; then change direction of needle so that it parallels the abdominal wall. Push needle in until hub touches patient's skin; withdraw about 1 cm (this creates a gap for drug to be injected) before depressing plunger completely.
• To avoid need for a new syringe and injection site, don't aspirate after inserting needle. If needle penetrates a blood vessel, blood will appear in the syringe chamber. Withdraw needle, and inject elsewhere with a new syringe.
• *Alert:* Implant comes in a preloaded syringe. If package is damaged, don't use the syringe. Make sure drug is visible in the translucent chamber of the syringe.
• When used for prostate cancer, LH-RH analogues such as goserelin may initially worsen symptoms because drug first in-creases testosterone levels. Some patients may experience increased bone pain. Rarely, disease worsening (either spinal cord compression or ureteral obstruction) has occurred.
• When drug is used for endometrial thinning, surgery should be performed at 4 weeks if one depot is given. When two depots are given, surgery should be performed within 2 to 4 weeks after giving second depot.

## PATIENT TEACHING
• Advise patient to return every 28 days for a new implant. A delay of a couple of days is permissible.
• Tell patient that pain may worsen for first 30 days of treatment.
• Tell woman to use a nonhormonal form of contraception during treatment. Caution patient about significant risks to fetus.
• Urge woman to call prescriber if menstruation persists or if breakthrough bleeding occurs. Menstruation should stop during treatment.
• Inform woman that a delayed return of menstruation may occur after therapy ends. Persistent lack of menstruation is rare.

---

# letrozole
Femara

*Pregnancy risk category D*

---

## AVAILABLE FORMS
*Tablets:* 2.5 mg

## INDICATIONS & DOSAGES
➤ **Metastatic breast cancer in post-menopausal women with disease pro-gression after antiestrogen therapy (such as tamoxifen)**
*Adults:* 2.5 mg P.O. as single daily dose.
➤ **First-line treatment of hormone receptor–positive or hormone receptor–unknown, locally advanced, or metasta-tic breast cancer in postmenopausal women**
*Adults:* 2.5 mg P.O. once daily until tumor progression is evident.

---

## ACTION

A nonsteroidal competitive inhibitor of the aromatase enzyme system, which inhibits conversion of androgens to estrogens. Decreased estrogens lead to decreased tumor mass or delayed progression of tumor growth in some women.

| Route | Onset | Peak | Duration |
|-------|-------|------|----------|
| P.O. | Unknown | 2 days | Unknown |

## ADVERSE REACTIONS

**CNS:** headache, somnolence, dizziness, fatigue, mood changes.
**CV:** hypertension, *thromboembolism,* chest pain, edema, *hot flashes, MI.*
**GI:** *nausea,* vomiting, constipation, diarrhea, abdominal pain, anorexia.
**Metabolic:** hypercholesterolemia, weight gain.
**Musculoskeletal:** *bone pain, limb pain, back pain,* arthralgia.
**Respiratory:** dyspnea, cough.
**Skin:** rash, pruritus.
**Other:** viral infections, breast pain, alopecia, diaphoresis.

## INTERACTIONS
None significant.

## EFFECTS ON LAB TEST RESULTS
• May increase cholesterol level.

## CONTRAINDICATIONS & CAUTIONS
• Contraindicated in patients hypersensitive to drug or its components.
• Use cautiously in patients with severe liver impairment; dosage adjustment isn't needed in those with mild to moderate liver dysfunction.

## NURSING CONSIDERATIONS
• Dosage adjustment isn't needed in patients with creatinine clearance of 10 ml/minute or more.
• Food doesn't affect drug absorption.
• *Alert:* Don't confuse Femara (letrozole) with FemHRT (ethinyl estradiol and norethindrone acetate).

## PATIENT TEACHING
• Instruct patient to take drug exactly as prescribed.
• Tell patient to take drug with or without food.

• Inform patient about potential adverse reactions.

# leuprolide acetate
Eligard, Lucrin‡, Lupron, Lupron Depot, Lupron Depot-Ped, Lupron Depot-3 Month, Lupron Depot-4 Month, Lupron for Pediatric Use, Viadur

*Pregnancy risk category X*

## AVAILABLE FORMS
*Depot injection:* 3.75 mg, 7.5 mg, 11.25 mg, 15 mg, 22.5 mg, 30 mg
*Injection:* 1 mg/0.2 ml (5 mg/ml) in 2.8-ml multiple-dose vials
*Implant:* 72 mg

## INDICATIONS & DOSAGES
➤ **Advanced prostate cancer**
*Adults:* 1 mg S.C. (injection) daily. Or, 7.5 mg I.M. (depot injection) monthly. Or, 7.5 mg S.C. Eligard once monthly. Or, 22.5 mg I.M. q 3 months (depot injection). Or, 22.5 mg S.C. Eligard q 3 months. Or, 30 mg I.M. q 4 months (depot injection). Or, 30 mg S.C. (Eligard) q 4 months. Or, 72 mg (Viadur implant) inserted S.C. q. 12 months.
➤ **Endometriosis**
*Adults:* 3.75 mg I.M. (depot injection) as single injection once monthly for up to 6 months. Or, 11.25 mg I.M. q 3 months for up to 6 months.
➤ **Central precocious puberty**
*Children:* Initially, 0.3 mg/kg (minimum 7.5 mg) I.M. (depot injection) as single injection q 4 weeks. May increase in increments of 3.75 mg q 4 weeks, if needed. Stop drug before girl reaches age 11 or boy reaches age 12.
➤ **Anemia related to uterine fibroids (in combination with iron therapy)**
*Adults:* 3.75 mg I.M. (depot injection) once monthly for up to 3 consecutive months. Or 11.25 mg I.M. (depot injection) for 1 dose.

## ACTION
Initially stimulates but then inhibits release of follicle-stimulating hormone and

luteinizing hormone, resulting in testosterone and estrogen suppression.

| Route | Onset | Peak | Duration |
|-------|-------|------|----------|
| I.M., S.C. | < 2-4 wk | 1-2 mo | 60-90 days |
| Implant | Unknown | 4 hr | 12 mo |

## ADVERSE REACTIONS
**CNS:** *dizziness, depression, headache, pain,* insomnia, paresthesia, *asthenia.*
**CV: arrhythmias,** angina, **MI,** *peripheral edema,* ECG changes, hypotension, hypertension, murmur, *hot flashes.*
**GI:** *nausea, vomiting,* anorexia, constipation.
**GU:** *impotence, vaginitis,* urinary frequency, hematuria, UTI, *amenorrhea.*
**Hematologic:** anemia.
**Metabolic:** *weight gain or loss.*
**Musculoskeletal:** transient bone pain during first week of treatment, joint disorder, myalgia, neuromuscular disorder, bone loss.
**Respiratory:** dyspnea, sinus congestion, *pulmonary fibrosis.*
**Skin:** reactions at injection site, dermatitis, acne.
**Other:** gynecomastia, androgen-like effects.

## INTERACTIONS
None significant.

## EFFECTS ON LAB TEST RESULTS
● May increase BUN, creatinine, bilirubin, alkaline phosphatase, LDH, glucose, uric acid, albumin, calcium, and phosphorus levels.
● May decrease hemoglobin.
● Lab tests for pituitary-gonadal system may be misleading during therapy and for 12 weeks thereafter.

## CONTRAINDICATIONS & CAUTIONS
● Contraindicated in patients hypersensitive to drug or other gonadotropin-releasing hormone analogues, in women with undiagnosed vaginal bleeding, and in pregnant or breast-feeding women. The 30-mg depot injection is contraindicated in women. The Viadur implant is contraindicated in women and children.
● Use cautiously in patients hypersensitive to benzyl alcohol.

## NURSING CONSIDERATIONS
● Never give by I.V. injection.
● Give depot injections under medical supervision. Use supplied diluent to reconstitute drug (extra diluent is provided; discard remainder). Draw 1 ml into a syringe with a 22G needle. (When preparing Lupron Depot-3 Month 22.5 mg, use a 23G or larger needle.) Withdraw 1.5 ml from ampule for the 3-month formulation. Inject into vial; then shake well. Suspension will appear milky. Suspension is stable for 24 hours after reconstitution; it contains no bacteriostatic product. Use immediately.
● When using prefilled dual-chamber syringes, prepare for injection by screwing white plunger into end stopper until stopper begins to turn. Remove and discard tab around base of needle. Hold syringe upright and release diluent by slowly pushing plunger until first stopper is at blue line in middle of barrel. Gently shake syringe to form a uniform milky suspension. If particles adhere to stopper, tap syringe against your finger. Remove needle guard and advance plunger to expel air from syringe. Inject entire contents I.M. as with a normal injection.
● A fractional dose of drug formulated to give every 3 months isn't equivalent to same dose of once-a-month formulation.
● After the start of treatment for central precocious puberty, monitor patient response every 1 to 2 months with a gonadotropin-releasing hormone stimulation test and sex corticosteroid level determinations. Measure bone age for advancement every 6 to 12 months.
● During first few weeks of therapy, drug may increase signs and symptoms being treated (flare).

## PATIENT TEACHING
● Before starting child on treatment for central precocious puberty, make sure parents understand importance of continuous therapy.
● Carefully instruct patient who will give herself S.C. injection about proper administration techniques and advise her to use only the syringes provided by manufacturer.
● Advise patient that, if another syringe must be substituted, a low-dose insulin sy-

ringe (U-100, 0.5 ml) may be an appropriate choice but that needle gauge should be no smaller than 22G (except when using Lupron Depot-3 Month 22.5 mg).
• Instruct patient to store leuprolide acetate powder (depot) and diluent at room temperature. Refrigerate unopened vials of leuprolide acetate injection. Protect leuprolide acetate injection from heat and light.
• Inform patient with history of undesirable effects from other endocrine therapies that leuprolide is easier to tolerate.
• Reassure patient that adverse effects disappear after about 1 week. Explain that symptoms of prostate cancer or central precocious puberty may worsen at first.
• Advise patient to keep implant insertion site clean and dry for 24 hours after procedure and to avoid heavy physical activity until site has healed. Local insertion site reaction such as bruising, burning, itching, and pain may resolve within 2 weeks.
• Advise woman of childbearing age to use a nonhormonal form of contraception during treatment.

## megestrol acetate
Megace, Megace OS†, Megostat‡

*Pregnancy risk category D*

### AVAILABLE FORMS
*Oral suspension:* 40 mg/ml
*Tablets:* 20 mg, 40 mg

### INDICATIONS & DOSAGES
➤ **Breast cancer**
*Adults:* 40 mg P.O. q.i.d.
➤ **Endometrial cancer**
*Adults:* 40 to 320 mg P.O. daily in divided doses.
➤ **Anorexia, cachexia, or unexplained significant weight loss in patients with AIDS**
*Adults:* 800 mg P.O. (oral suspension) daily.
➤ **Anorexia or cachexia in patients with cancer ♦**
*Adults:* 480 to 600 mg P.O. daily.

### ACTION
A progestin that inhibits hormone-dependent tumor growth by inhibiting pituitary and adrenal steroidogenesis. Drug may also have direct cytotoxicity. Appetite-stimulating mechanism hasn't been established.

| Route | Onset | Peak | Duration |
|-------|-------|------|----------|
| P.O. | Unknown | 1-5 hr | Unknown |

### ADVERSE REACTIONS
**CV:** thrombophlebitis, *heart failure,* hypertension, *thromboembolism.*
**GI:** nausea, vomiting, diarrhea, flatulence, constipation, dry mouth, increased appetite.
**GU:** breakthrough menstrual bleeding, impotence, vaginal bleeding or discharge, UTI.
**Metabolic:** hyperglycemia, *weight gain.*
**Musculoskeletal:** carpal tunnel syndrome.
**Respiratory:** *pulmonary embolism,* dyspnea.
**Skin:** alopecia, rash.
**Other:** gynecomastia, tumor flare.

### INTERACTIONS
None significant.

### EFFECTS ON LAB TEST RESULTS
• May increase glucose level.

### CONTRAINDICATIONS & CAUTIONS
• Contraindicated in patients hypersensitive to drug. Also contraindicated as a diagnostic test for pregnancy.
• Use cautiously in patients with history of thrombophlebitis or thromboembolism.

### NURSING CONSIDERATIONS
• Glucose level may increase in diabetic patients.
• Drug is relatively nontoxic with a low risk of adverse effects.
• Two months is an adequate trial period in patients with cancer.

### PATIENT TEACHING
• Inform patient that therapeutic response isn't immediate.
• Advise breast-feeding woman to stop breast-feeding during therapy because of risk of toxicity to infant.
• Advise woman of childbearing age to use an effective form of contraception while receiving drug.

# nilutamide
Anandron†, Nilandron

*Pregnancy risk category C*

## AVAILABLE FORMS
*Tablets:* 50 mg, 100 mg†, 150 mg

## INDICATIONS & DOSAGES
➤ **Adjunct therapy with surgical castration for treatment of metastatic prostate cancer**
*Adults:* 300 mg P.O. once daily for 30 days; then 150 mg P.O. once daily thereafter.

## ACTION
A nonsteroidal antiandrogen that interacts with the androgen receptor and prevents normal androgenic response.

| Route | Onset | Peak | Duration |
|-------|-------|------|----------|
| P.O. | Unknown | Unknown | Unknown |

## ADVERSE REACTIONS
**CNS:** dizziness.
**CV:** hypertension, *hot flashes.*
**EENT:** *impaired adaptation to darkness,* photophobia, abnormal vision.
**GI:** nausea, constipation, diarrhea.
**GU:** UTI, impotence.
**Hematologic:** anemia.
**Hepatic:** *hepatitis.*
**Respiratory:** dyspnea, *interstitial pneumonitis.*
**Other:** *decreased libido.*

## INTERACTIONS
**Drug-drug.** *Phenytoin, theophylline, vitamin K antagonists:* May delay elimination and cause toxicity. Modify doses accordingly.
**Drug-lifestyle.** *Alcohol use:* May cause disulfiram-like reaction. Discourage use together.

## EFFECTS ON LAB TEST RESULTS
• May increase BUN, creatinine, glucose, AST, and ALT levels.
• May decrease hemoglobin and hematocrit.

## CONTRAINDICATIONS & CAUTIONS
• Contraindicated in patients hypersensitive to drug and in those with severe hepatic or respiratory disease.
• Safety and effectiveness of drug in children haven't been determined. Don't give drug to children.

## NURSING CONSIDERATIONS
• Drug is used with surgical castration; for maximum benefit, begin treatment on same day or day after surgery.
• Obtain baseline liver enzyme level, and repeat at 3-month intervals. Stop drug if transaminase level exceeds three times upper limit of normal.
• Obtain a baseline chest radiograph before therapy begins. Monitor patient (especially if Asian) for signs and symptoms of interstitial pneumonitis, and notify prescriber if they occur.

## PATIENT TEACHING
• Explain purpose of drug, how it's given, and importance of not stopping treatment without consulting prescriber.
• Tell patient to immediately report labored breathing or worsening of labored breathing.
• Inform patient about risk of developing hepatitis. Tell him to report nausea, vomiting, abdominal pain, or yellowed skin or eyes. Tell patient to avoid alcohol during therapy.
• Warn patient that visual disturbances, such as a delay in adaptation to darkness, may affect driving at night and in tunnels.
• Warn patient that drinking alcohol while taking drug may cause disulfiram-like reaction, causing facial flushing, malaise, and low blood pressure. Discourage alcohol use.
• Tell patient that drug may be taken with or without food.

# tamoxifen citrate
Nolvadex✐, Nolvadex-D‡, Novo-Tamoxifen†, Tamofen†, Tamonet†

*Pregnancy risk category D*

## AVAILABLE FORMS
*Tablets:* 10 mg, 20 mg
*Tablets (enteric-coated)†:* 10 mg, 20 mg

## INDICATIONS & DOSAGES

➤ **Advanced breast cancer in women and men**

*Adults:* 20 mg to 40 mg P.O. daily; divide doses greater than 20 mg per day b.i.d.

➤ **Adjunct treatment of breast cancer in women**

*Adults:* 20 mg to 40 mg P.O. daily for 5 years; divide doses greater than 20 mg per day b.i.d.

➤ **To reduce breast cancer occurrence in high-risk women**

*Adults:* 20 mg P.O. daily for 5 years.

➤ **Ductal carcinoma in situ (DCIS) after breast surgery and radiation**

*Adults:* 20 mg P.O. daily for 5 years.

➤ **McCune-Albright syndrome and precocious puberty** ◆

*Children ages 2 to 10:* 20 mg P.O. daily. Treat for up to 12 months.

➤ **To stimulate ovulation** ◆

*Adults:* 5 to 40 mg P.O. b.i.d. for 4 days.

➤ **Mastalgia** ◆

*Adults:* 10 mg P.O. daily for 10 months.

## ACTION

Exact neoplastic action unknown. Acts as a selective estrogen receptor modulator.

| Route | Onset | Peak | Duration |
|-------|-------|------|----------|
| P.O. | 1-several mo | Unknown | Several wk |

## ADVERSE REACTIONS

**CNS:** confusion, weakness, sleepiness, headache, ***stroke.***

**CV:** *fluid retention,* ***thromboembolism,*** *hot flashes.*

**EENT:** corneal changes, cataracts, retinopathy.

**GI:** *nausea, vomiting, diarrhea.*

**GU:** *vaginal discharge,* vaginal bleeding, *irregular menses, amenorrhea,* ***endometrial cancer, uterine sarcoma.***

**Hematologic:** *leukopenia,* ***thrombocytopenia.***

**Hepatic:** fatty liver, cholestasis, ***hepatic necrosis.***

**Metabolic:** *hypercalcemia, weight gain or loss.*

**Musculoskeletal:** brief worsening of pain from osseous metastases.

**Respiratory:** ***pulmonary embolism.***

**Skin:** *skin changes,* rash.

**Other:** temporary bone or tumor pain, alopecia.

## INTERACTIONS

**Drug-drug.** *Antacids:* May affect absorption of enteric-coated tablet. Separate dosing times by 2 hours.

*Bromocriptine:* May elevate tamoxifen level. Monitor patient closely.

*Coumadin-type anticoagulants:* May cause significant increase in anticoagulant effect. Monitor patient, PT, and INR closely.

*Cytotoxic agents:* May increase risk of thromboembolic events. Monitor patient.

*P450 3A4 inducers (such as rifampin):* May increase tamoxifen metabolism and lower drug levels. Monitor patient for clinical effects.

## EFFECTS ON LAB TEST RESULTS

• May increase BUN, calcium, $T_4$, and liver enzyme levels.

• May decrease WBC and platelet counts.

## CONTRAINDICATIONS & CAUTIONS

• Contraindicated in patients hypersensitive to drug. Also contraindicated as therapy to reduce risk of breast cancer in high-risk women who also need coumarin-type anticoagulant therapy or in women with history of deep vein thrombosis or pulmonary embolism.

• Use cautiously in patients with leukopenia or thrombocytopenia. Monitor CBC closely.

## NURSING CONSIDERATIONS

• Monitor lipid levels during long-term therapy in patients with hyperlipidemia.

• Monitor calcium level. At start of therapy, drug may compound hypercalcemia related to bone metastases.

• Patient should have baseline and periodic gynecologic examinations because of the small increased risk of endometrial cancer.

• Rule out pregnancy before treatment begins.

• Patient may initially experience worsening symptoms.

• Adverse reactions are usually minor and well tolerated.

• Variations on karyopyknotic index in vaginal smears and various degrees of estrogen effect on Papanicolaou smears may occur in postmenopausal patients.

• *Alert:* Women at high risk for breast cancer or who have DCIS taking tamoxifen to reduce risk may experience serious, life-threatening, or fatal endometrial cancer, uterine sarcoma, stroke, and pulmonary embolism. Prescriber should discuss with these patients the benefits of the drug versus the risks of these serious events. The benefits of tamoxifen outweigh its risks in women already diagnosed with breast cancer.

## PATIENT TEACHING
• Tell patient taking enteric-coated tablets (Nolvadex-D) to swallow them whole without crushing or chewing. Tell her not to take antacids within 2 hours of dose.
• Reassure patient that acute worsening of bone pain during therapy usually indicates drug will produce good response. Recommend analgesics to relieve pain.
• Strongly encourage woman who is taking or has taken tamoxifen to have regular gynecologic examinations because of increased risk of uterine cancer related to therapy.
• Encourage woman to have annual mammograms and breast examinations.
• Advise patient to use barrier form of contraception because short-term therapy induces ovulation in premenopausal patients.
• Instruct patient to report vaginal bleeding or changes in menstrual cycle.
• Caution woman of childbearing age to avoid becoming pregnant during therapy and first 2 months after stopping drug. Recommend that she consult prescriber before becoming pregnant.
• Advise patient that breast cancer risk assessment tools are available and that she should discuss her concerns with her prescriber.
• Tell patient to report symptoms of stroke (headache; vision changes; weakness of face, arm, or leg, especially on one side of the body; confusion; difficulty speaking or walking).
• Tell patients to report symptoms of pulmonary embolism (chest pain, difficulty breathing, rapid breathing, sweating, or fainting).

# testolactone
Teslac

*Pregnancy risk category C*
*Controlled substance schedule III*

## AVAILABLE FORMS
*Tablets:* 50 mg

## INDICATIONS & DOSAGES
➤ **Advanced premenopausal breast cancer in women whose ovarian function has been terminated; advanced postmenopausal breast cancer**
*Adults:* 250 mg P.O. q.i.d.

## ACTION
Exact antineoplastic action unknown. Appears to inhibit steroid aromatase activity and decrease estrone synthesis.

| Route | Onset | Peak | Duration |
|-------|-------|------|----------|
| P.O. | 6-12 wk | Unknown | Unknown |

## ADVERSE REACTIONS
**CNS:** paresthesia, peripheral neuropathy.
**CV:** increased blood pressure, edema.
**GI:** nausea, vomiting, diarrhea, anorexia, glossitis.
**Skin:** alopecia, erythema, nail changes.

## INTERACTIONS
**Drug-drug.** *Oral anticoagulants:* May increase pharmacologic effects. Monitor patient, PT, and INR carefully.

## EFFECTS ON LAB TEST RESULTS
• May increase calcium levels.

## CONTRAINDICATIONS & CAUTIONS
• Contraindicated in patients hypersensitive to drug and in men with breast cancer.

## NURSING CONSIDERATIONS
• Monitor fluid and electrolyte levels, especially calcium level.
• Force fluids to aid calcium excretion and encourage exercise to prevent hypercalcemia. Immobilized patients are susceptible to hypercalcemia.
• Higher-than-recommended doses may increase risk of remission in patients with visceral metastases.

---

Reactions may be *common*, uncommon, *life-threatening*, or COMMON AND LIFE-THREATENING.

• Estradiol levels measured by radioimmunoassay may be decreased.
• Although similar to testosterone, there are no androgenic effects.

## PATIENT TEACHING
• Inform patient that therapeutic response isn't immediate; 3 months is an adequate trial for drug.
• Tell patient to notify prescriber if numbness or tingling occurs in fingers, toes, or face.
• Advise patient to use contraception during therapy.

## toremifene citrate
Fareston

*Pregnancy risk category D*

## AVAILABLE FORMS
*Tablets:* 60 mg

## INDICATIONS & DOSAGES
➤ **Metastatic breast cancer in postmenopausal women with estrogen receptor–positive or estrogen receptor–unknown tumors**
*Adults:* 60 mg P.O. once daily. Continue until disease progresses.

## ACTION
A nonsteroidal triphenylethylene that exerts its antitumor effect by competing with estrogen for binding sites in the tumor. This blocks the growth-stimulating effects of endogenous estrogen in the tumor, causing an antiestrogenic effect.

| Route | Onset | Peak | Duration |
|-------|-------|------|----------|
| P.O. | Unknown | 3 hr | Unknown |

## ADVERSE REACTIONS
**CNS:** dizziness, fatigue, depression.
**CV:** edema, ***thromboembolism, heart failure, MI, pulmonary embolism,*** hot flashes.
**EENT:** visual disturbances, glaucoma, dry eyes, *cataracts.*
**GI:** *nausea,* vomiting.
**GU:** *vaginal discharge,* vaginal bleeding.
**Hepatic:** *hepatotoxicity.*
**Metabolic:** hypercalcemia.
**Skin:** *sweating.*

## INTERACTIONS
**Drug-drug.** *Calcium-elevating drugs such as hydrochlorothiazide:* May increase risk of hypercalcemia. Monitor calcium level closely.
*Coumadin-like anticoagulants such as warfarin:* May prolong PT and INR. Monitor PT and INR closely.
*Cytochrome P450 3A4 enzyme inducers (such as carbamazepine, phenobarbital, phenytoin):* May increase toremifene metabolism rate. Monitor patient closely.
*Cytochrome P450 3A4-6 enzyme inhibitors (such as erythromycin, ketoconazole):* May increase toremifene metabolism rate. Monitor patient closely.

## EFFECTS ON LAB TEST RESULTS
• May increase calcium and liver enzyme levels.

## CONTRAINDICATIONS & CAUTIONS
• Contraindicated in patients hypersensitive to drug. Also contraindicated in patients with a history of thromboembolic disease.

## NURSING CONSIDERATIONS
• Obtain periodic CBC, calcium levels, and liver function tests.
• Monitor calcium level closely during first weeks of treatment in patients with bone metastases because of increased risk of hypercalcemia.

## PATIENT TEACHING
• Instruct patient to take drug exactly as prescribed.
• Advise patient that doses may be taken without regard to meals.
• Warn patient not to stop therapy without consulting prescriber.
• Inform patient about vaginal bleeding and other adverse effects; tell her to notify prescriber if bleeding occurs.
• Warn patient that disease flare-up may occur during first weeks of therapy. Reassure her that this doesn't indicate treatment failure.
• Advise patient to report leg or chest pain, severe headache, visual changes, or shortness of breath.
• Counsel woman of childbearing age about risks of becoming pregnant during therapy.

## triptorelin pamoate
Trelstar Depot, Trelstar LA

*Pregnancy risk category X*

### AVAILABLE FORMS
*Injection:* 3.75 mg, 11.25 mg single-dose vials, and Debioclip single-dose delivery system

### INDICATIONS & DOSAGES
**Palliative treatment of advanced prostate cancer**
*Adults:* 3.75 mg I.M. Trelstar Depot given monthly as a single injection or 11.25 mg I.M. Trelstar LA given q 3 months as a single injection.

### ACTION
A potent inhibitor of gonadotropin secretion. After the first dose, levels of luteinizing hormone (LH), follicle-stimulating hormone (FSH), testosterone, and estradiol surge transiently. After long-term continuous administration, LH and FSH secretion steadily declines and testicular and ovarian steroidogenesis decreases. In men, testosterone declines to a level typically seen in surgically castrated men. As a result, tissues and functions that depend on these hormones become quiescent.

| Route | Onset | Peak | Duration |
|---|---|---|---|
| I.M. (Trelstar Depot) | 4 days | 2-4 wk | 1 mo |
| I.M. (Trelstar LA) | 2-5 days | 2-4 wk | 3 mo |

### ADVERSE REACTIONS
**CNS:** headache, dizziness, fatigue, insomnia, emotional lability, pain.
**CV:** hypertension, edema, *hot flashes.*
**GI:** diarrhea, vomiting, nausea.
**GU:** urinary retention, UTI, impotence.
**Hematologic:** anemia.
**Musculoskeletal:** *skeletal pain,* leg pain.
**Skin:** pruritus, injection site pain.
**Other:** breast pain, gynecomastia.

### INTERACTIONS
**Drug-drug.** *Hyperprolactinemic drugs:* May decrease pituitary gonadotropin-releasing hormone (GnRH) receptors. Avoid using together.

### EFFECTS ON LAB TEST RESULTS
● May increase liver enzymes and BUN and glucose levels; may transiently increase testosterone level.
● May decrease hemoglobin.
● May alter pituitary-gonadal function test results during and after therapy.

### CONTRAINDICATIONS & CAUTIONS
● Contraindicated in patients hypersensitive to triptorelin, its components, other luteinizing hormone–releasing hormone (LH-RH) agonists, or LH-RH. Contraindicated in women who are or may become pregnant during therapy. Use cautiously in patients with metastatic vertebral lesions or upper or lower urinary tract obstruction during the first few weeks of therapy.
● Patients with renal or hepatic impairment may retain the drug longer and have a twofold to fourfold higher exposure to the drug than young healthy men. The clinical consequence of this increase, as well as the potential need for dosage adjustment, are unknown.

### NURSING CONSIDERATIONS
● Give drug only under the supervision of prescriber.
● Reconstitute only with sterile water. Use no other diluent.
● Change the injection site periodically.
● Monitor testosterone and prostate specific antigen levels.
● Monitor patients with metastatic vertebral lesions or upper or lower urinary tract obstruction during the first few weeks of therapy.
● Initially, triptorelin causes a transient increase in testosterone levels. As a result, signs and symptoms of prostate cancer may worsen during the first few weeks of treatment.
● Patients may experience worsening of symptoms or onset of new symptoms, including bone pain, neuropathy, hematuria, or urethral or bladder outlet obstruction.
● Spinal cord compression may occur, which can lead to paralysis and possibly death. If spinal cord compression or renal impairment develops, give standard treatment. In extreme cases, immediate orchiectomy is considered.

• If patient has a hypersensitivity reaction, stop drug immediately and give supportive and symptomatic care.

• Diagnostic tests of pituitary-gonadal function conducted during and after therapy may be misleading.

**PATIENT TEACHING**

• Inform the patient about adverse reactions.

• Tell patient that symptoms may worsen during the first few weeks of therapy (such as bone pain, nerve inflammation, bloody urine, or obstructed urethral or bladder outlet)

• Inform patient that a blood test will be used to monitor response to therapy.

# 71

## Miscellaneous antineoplastics

alemtuzumab
arsenic trioxide
asparaginase
bacillus Calmette-Guérin (BCG),
   live intravesical
bexarotene
bortezomib
dacarbazine
docetaxel
etoposide
etoposide phosphate
gefitinib
gemtuzumab ozogamicin
ibritumomab tiuxetan
imatinib mesylate
irinotecan hydrochloride
mitoxantrone hydrochloride
paclitaxel
pegaspargase
procarbazine hydrochloride
rituximab
teniposide
topotecan hydrochloride
trastuzumab
vinblastine sulfate
vincristine sulfate
vinorelbine tartrate

**COMBINATION PRODUCTS**
None.

---

### alemtuzumab
Campath

*Pregnancy risk category C*

**AVAILABLE FORMS**
*Ampules:* 10 mg/ml, 3-ml ampules

**INDICATIONS & DOSAGES**
➤ **B-cell chronic lymphocytic leukemia in patients treated with alkylating drugs, in whom fludarabine therapy has failed**
*Adults:* Initially, 3 mg I.V. infusion over 2 hours daily; if tolerated (infusion-related toxicities are grade 2 or less), increase dosage to 10 mg daily and continue, as tolerated; then increase to 30 mg daily. As

maintenance, give 30 mg I.V. three times weekly on nonconsecutive days (such as Monday, Wednesday, Friday) for up to 12 weeks. Don't give single doses of more than 30 mg or weekly doses of more than 90 mg.
*Adjust-a-dose:* For patients with hematologic toxicity, see table.

| Hematologic toxicity | Dosage adjustment |
|---|---|
| First occurrence of absolute neutrophil count (ANC) < 250/mm³ or platelets ≤ 25,000/mm³ | Withhold therapy; resume at same dose when ANC ≥ 500/mm³ and platelets ≥ 50,000/mm³. If delay between doses is ≥ 7 days, start therapy at 3 mg; escalate to 10 mg, then 30 mg as tolerated. |
| Second occurrence of ANC < 250/mm³ or platelets ≤ 25,000/mm³ | Withhold therapy; when ANC ≥ 500/mm³ and platelets ≥ 50,000/mm³, resume at 10 mg. If delay between doses is ≥ 7 days, start therapy at 3 mg; escalate to 10 mg only. |
| Third occurrence of ANC < 250/mm³ or platelets ≤ 25,000/mm³ | Stop therapy. |
| For a decrease of ANC or platelet count ≤ 50% of baseline value in patients starting therapy with ANC ≤ 500/mm³ or platelet count ≤ 25,000/mm³ | Withhold therapy; when ANC and platelet count return to baseline, resume therapy. If delay between dosing is ≥ 7 days, start therapy at 3 mg, escalate to 10 mg, then 30 mg as tolerated. |

**I.V. ADMINISTRATION**
● Don't give as I.V. push or bolus.
● Premedicate with diphenhydramine 50 mg and acetaminophen 650 mg 30 minutes before infusion; give hydrocortisone 200 mg to decrease severe infusion-related events. Give anti-infective prophylaxis while patient is on therapy. TMP-sulfa DS b.i.d. three times a week and famciclovir (or equivalent) 250 mg b.i.d. have been used at beginning of alemtuzumab therapy. Continue for 2 months, or until CD4+

count is 200 cells/mm³ or more, whichever occurs later.

• Don't shake ampule before use. Withdraw the necessary amount of drug from the ampule and filter with a sterile, low protein-binding, 5-micron filter before dilution. Add to 100 ml normal saline solution or $D_5W$. Gently invert bag to mix solution. Infuse over 2 hours.

• Discard any unused portion of drug. Solutions may be stored at room temperature or refrigerated; protect solution from light. Diluted solutions must be used within 8 hours of preparation.

## ACTION
Proposed mechanism of action is antibody-dependent lysis of leukemic cells following cell-surface binding.

| Route | Onset | Peak | Duration |
|-------|-------|------|----------|
| I.V. | Unknown | Unknown | Unknown |

## ADVERSE REACTIONS
**CNS:** *insomnia,* depression, somnolence, *asthenia, headache, dysesthesia, dizziness, fatigue,* malaise, tremor, *fever, pain.*
**CV:** *edema, peripheral edema, chest pain, hypotension, hypertension, tachycardia,* **supraventricular tachycardia.**
**EENT:** epistaxis, rhinitis, *pharyngitis.*
**GI:** *anorexia, nausea, vomiting, diarrhea, stomatitis, ulcerative stomatitis, mucositis, abdominal pain, dyspepsia,* constipation.
**Hematologic:** NEUTROPENIA, *anemia,* **pancytopenia,** THROMBOCYTOPENIA, **purpura.**
**Musculoskeletal:** *skeletal pain, back pain, myalgias.*
**Respiratory:** *dyspnea, cough, bronchitis, pneumonitis,* **bronchospasm.**
**Skin:** *rash, urticaria, pruritus, increased sweating.*
**Other:** INFECTION, SEPSIS, *herpes simplex, rigors,* temperature change sensation, candidiasis.

## INTERACTIONS
None reported.

## EFFECTS ON LAB TEST RESULTS
• May decrease hemoglobin, hematocrit, and WBC, RBC, CD4+, platelet, neutrophil, and lymphocyte counts.

## CONTRAINDICATIONS & CAUTIONS
• Contraindicated in patients with active systemic infections, underlying immunodeficiency (such as HIV infection), or known type I hypersensitivity or anaphylactic reactions to alemtuzumab or its components.

## NURSING CONSIDERATIONS
• Start drug at low dose; escalate as tolerated.
• Monitor blood pressure and hypotensive symptoms during administration.
• Irradiate blood if transfusions are necessary to protect against graft vs. host disease. Monitor hematologic studies carefully.
• Don't exceed recommended doses.
• Don't give drug if patient has systemic infection at scheduled dose time.
• Don't immunize with live viral vaccines.
• Obtain CBC and platelet counts weekly during therapy and more frequently if worsening anemia, neutropenia, or thrombocytopenia occurs.
• Obtain CD4+ counts after treatment until CD4+ count is 200 cells/mm³ or higher.
• If therapy is interrupted for 7 days or longer, restart with gradual dose escalation.

## PATIENT TEACHING
• Tell patient to report immediately any infusion reactions, such as rigor, chills, fever, nausea, or vomiting.
• Advise patient that blood tests will be done during therapy to monitor for adverse effects.
• Advise patient to report immediately any signs or symptoms of infection.
• Safety and effectiveness in children haven't been established. Don't give drug to children.
• It's unknown whether drug appears in breast milk. Advise patient to stop breastfeeding during treatment and for at least 3 months after taking last dose of drug.

---

## arsenic trioxide
Trisenox

*Pregnancy risk category D*

### AVAILABLE FORMS
*Injection:* 1 mg/ml

### INDICATIONS & DOSAGES
➤ **Acute promyelocytic leukemia (APL) in patients who have relapsed or who are refractory to retinoid and anthracycline chemotherapy**
*Adults and children age 5 and older:* For induction phase, 0.15 mg/kg I.V. daily until bone marrow remission. Maximum 60 doses. For consolidation phase, 0.15 mg/kg I.V. daily for 25 doses over a period up to 5 weeks, beginning 3 to 6 weeks after completion of induction therapy.

### I.V. ADMINISTRATION
• Follow facility policy regarding preparation and handling of antineoplastics because the active ingredient is carcinogenic.
• Dilute with 100 to 250 ml of $D_5W$ or normal saline solution. After dilution, drug is stable for 24 hours at room temperature and for 48 hours if refrigerated.
• Give I.V. over 1 or 2 hours. Infusion time may be extended up to 4 hours if vasomotor reactions occur.
• Discard any remaining drug in the ampule. Don't mix arsenic trioxide with other medications.

### ACTION
Causes morphologic changes and DNA fragmentation, resulting in death of promyelocytic leukemic cells.

| Route | Onset | Peak | Duration |
|-------|-------|------|----------|
| I.V. | Unknown | Unknown | Unknown |

### ADVERSE REACTIONS
**CNS:** *headache, insomnia, paresthesia, dizziness,* tremor, **seizures,** somnolence, **coma,** anxiety, depression, agitation, confusion, *fatigue, weakness, fever, pain.*
**CV:** tachycardia, **PROLONGED QT INTERVAL, COMPLETE AV BLOCK,** *palpitations,* edema, chest pain, ECG abnormalities, hypotension, flushing, hypertension.
**EENT:** *eye irritation, epistaxis, blurred vision,* dry eye, earache, tinnitus, *sore throat, post nasal drip,* eyelid edema, sinusitis, nasopharyngitis, painful red eye.
**GI:** nausea, vomiting, diarrhea, anorexia, abdominal pain, constipation, loose stools, dyspepsia, oral blistering, fecal incontinence, **GI hemorrhage,** dry mouth, abdominal tenderness or distention, bloody diarrhea, oral candidiasis.
**GU:** **renal failure,** renal impairment, oliguria, incontinence, **vaginal hemorrhage,** intermenstrual bleeding.
**Hematologic:** leukocytosis, anemia, THROMBOCYTOPENIA, NEUTROPENIA, **disseminated intravascular coagulation, hemorrhage,** lymphadenopathy.
**Metabolic:** *hypokalemia, hypomagnesemia, hyperglycemia, hypocalcemia,* hypoglycemia, acidosis, *weight gain,* weight loss, **hyperkalemia.**
**Musculoskeletal:** *arthralgia, myalgia; bone, back, neck, and limb pain.*
**Respiratory:** *cough, dyspnea, hypoxia, pleural effusion, wheezing, decreased breath sounds, crepitations, rales,* hemoptysis, tachypnea, rhonchi, *upper respiratory tract infection.*
**Skin:** *dermatitis, pruritus, ecchymosis, dry skin, increased sweating,* night sweats, petechiae, hyperpigmentation, urticaria, skin lesions, local exfoliation, *pallor; erythema or edema at injection site.*
**Other:** *drug hypersensitivity,* rigor, lymphadenopathy, facial edema, *herpes simplex infection,* bacterial infection, herpes zoster, **sepsis,** APL DIFFERENTIATION SYNDROME.

### INTERACTIONS
**Drug-drug.** *Drugs that can lead to electrolyte abnormalities (diuretics or amphotericin B):* May increase risk of electrolyte abnormalities. Use together cautiously.
*Drugs that can prolong the QT interval, such as antiarrhythmics or thioridazine:* May further prolong QT interval. Use together cautiously and monitor ECG closely.
*Ziprasidone:* May increase the prolongation of the QT interval. Don't use together.

---

## EFFECTS ON LAB TEST RESULTS
• May increase ALT and AST levels. May decrease magnesium and calcium levels. May increase or decrease glucose and potassium levels.
• May increase WBC count. May decrease hemoglobin and neutrophil and platelet counts.

## CONTRAINDICATIONS & CAUTIONS
• Contraindicated in patients hypersensitive to arsenic.
• Use cautiously in patients with heart failure, renal failure, prolonged QT interval, conditions that result in hypokalemia or hypomagnesemia, or a history of torsades de pointes.

## NURSING CONSIDERATIONS
• Before starting drug, perform ECG; obtain potassium, calcium, magnesium, and creatinine levels; and correct electrolyte abnormalities.
• *Alert:* Arsenic trioxide can cause fatal arrhythmias and complete AV block.
• *Alert:* Arsenic trioxide has been linked to APL differentiation syndrome, characterized by fever, dyspnea, weight gain, pulmonary infiltrates, and pleural or pericardial effusions, with or without leukocytosis. This syndrome can be fatal and requires treatment with high-dose steroids.
• Monitor electrolytes and hematologic and coagulation profiles at least twice weekly during treatment. Keep potassium levels above 4 mEq/dl and magnesium levels above 1.8 mg/dl.
• Monitor patient for syncope and rapid or irregular heart rate. If these occur, stop drug, hospitalize patient, and monitor electrolytes and QTc interval. Drug may be restarted when electrolyte abnormalities are corrected and QTc interval falls below 460 msec.
• Monitor ECG at least weekly during therapy. Prolonged QTc interval commonly occurs between 1 and 5 weeks after infusion, and returns to baseline about 8 weeks after infusion. If QTc interval is higher than 500 msec at any time during therapy, assess patient closely and consider stopping drug.

## PATIENT TEACHING
• Tell patient to report fever, shortness of breath, or weight gain immediately.
• Caution woman of childbearing age to avoid becoming pregnant during therapy or to consult prescriber before becoming pregnant.
• Inform patient of the potential for serious adverse reactions in breast-feeding infants, and that patient should stop breast-feeding during therapy.
• Inform diabetic patient that drug may cause excessively high or low glucose levels, and instruct him to monitor glucose level closely.

---

## asparaginase
Elspar, Kidrolase†

*Pregnancy risk category C*

## AVAILABLE FORMS
*Injection:* 10,000-IU vial

## INDICATIONS & DOSAGES
➤ **Acute lymphocytic leukemia with other drugs**
*Adults and children:* 1,000 IU/kg I.V. daily for 10 days, injected over 30 minutes. Or, 6,000 IU/m² I.M. at intervals specified in protocol.
➤ **Sole induction drug for acute lymphocytic leukemia**
*Adults and children:* 200 IU/kg I.V. daily for 28 days.

## I.V. ADMINISTRATION
• *Alert:* Preparation and administration of parenteral form of drug may be mutagenic, teratogenic, or carcinogenic to staff. Follow institutional policy to reduce risks.
• Reconstitute drug with 5-ml of either sterile water for injection or saline solution for injection.
• Don't shake vial vigorously, or foaming may occur.
• Filtration through a 5-micron filter during administration removes gelatinous fiber-like particles that occasionally form, with no loss in drug potency.
• Give I.V. injection over 30 minutes through a running infusion of normal saline solution or $D_5W$ solution.

---

● Refrigerate unopened dry powder. Reconstituted solution is stable for 8 hours if refrigerated. Use only clear solutions.

## ACTION
Destroys the essential amino acid asparagine, which is needed for protein synthesis in acute lymphocytic leukemia, leading to death of the leukemic cell.

| Route | Onset | Peak | Duration |
|-------|-------|------|----------|
| I.V. | Immediate | Immediate | 23-33 days |
| I.M. | Unknown | 14-24 hr | 23-33 days |

## ADVERSE REACTIONS
**CNS:** confusion, drowsiness, depression, hallucinations, fatigue, agitation, headache, lethargy, somnolence, fever.
**GI:** *vomiting, anorexia, nausea,* cramps, stomatitis, **HEMORRHAGIC PANCREATITIS.**
**GU:** *azotemia, renal failure,* glycosuria, polyuria, uric acid nephropathy.
**Hematologic:** *anemia, hypofibrinogenemia,* depression of clotting factor synthesis, *leukopenia, DIC.*
**Hepatic:** *hepatotoxicity.*
**Metabolic:** weight loss, *hyperglycemia,* hyperuricemia, hyperammonemia, hypocalcemia.
**Skin:** *rash, urticaria.*
**Other:** **ANAPHYLAXIS,** chills, hypersensitivity reactions.

## INTERACTIONS
**Drug-drug.** *Methotrexate:* May decrease methotrexate effectiveness. Avoid using together, or give asparaginase after methotrexate.
*Prednisone:* May cause hyperglycemia. Monitor glucose level.
*Vincristine:* May increase neuropathy. Give asparaginase after vincristine, and monitor patient closely.

## EFFECTS ON LAB TEST RESULTS
● May increase BUN, AST, ALT, alkaline phosphatase, bilirubin, glucose, uric acid, and ammonia levels. May decrease calcium, serum albumin and cholesterol levels.
● May decrease hemoglobin, thyroid function test values, and WBC count.

## CONTRAINDICATIONS & CAUTIONS
● Contraindicated in patients hypersensitive to drug (unless desensitized) and in those with pancreatitis or history of pancreatitis.
● Use cautiously in patients with hepatic dysfunction. Drug should first be given in hospital setting under close supervision.

## NURSING CONSIDERATIONS
● Monitor blood and urine glucose levels before and during therapy. Watch for signs and symptoms of hyperglycemia.
● Start allopurinol before therapy begins to help prevent uric acid nephropathy.
● *Alert:* Risk of hypersensitivity increases with repeated doses. Perform an intradermal skin test before first dose and when drug is given after an interval of 1 week or more between doses. Give 2 IU asparaginase as intradermal injection. Observe site for at least 1 hour for erythema or a wheal, which indicates a positive response. Patient with negative skin test may still develop allergic reaction to drug. Desensitization may be needed before first treatment dose is given and with retreatment. One IU of drug may be ordered I.V. Dose is then doubled every 10 minutes, provided no reaction has occurred, until total amount given equals patient's total dose for that day.
● Drug shouldn't be used alone to induce remission unless combination therapy is inappropriate. Drug isn't recommended for maintenance therapy.
● For I.M. injection, reconstitute with 2 ml normal saline solution to the 10,000-IU vial. Refrigerate and use within 8 hours.
● Don't give more than 2 ml I.M. at one injection site.
● Don't use cloudy solutions.
● If drug touches skin or mucous membranes, wash with a generous amount of water for at least 15 minutes.
● Keep epinephrine, diphenhydramine, and I.V. corticosteroids available for treating anaphylaxis.
● Monitor CBC and bone marrow function tests.
● Obtain amylase and lipase levels to check pancreatic status. If levels are elevated, stop asparaginase.
● Help prevent occurrence of tumor lysis, which can result in uric acid nephropathy, by increasing fluid intake.
● Drug may affect clotting factor synthesis and cause hypofibrinogenemia, leading to

thrombosis or, more commonly, severe bleeding. Monitor patient and bleeding studies closely.

• Because of vomiting, give fluids parenterally for 24 hours or until oral fluids are tolerated.

• Some patients may become hypersensitive to asparaginase derived from cultures of *Escherichia coli. Erwinia asparaginase,* derived from cultures of *E. carotovora,* has been used in these patients without cross-sensitivity.

• Drug toxicity is more likely to occur in adults than in children.

• There are several protocols for use of this drug.

**PATIENT TEACHING**
• Tell patient to watch for signs of infection (fever, sore throat, fatigue) and bleeding (easy bruising, nosebleeds, bleeding gums, tarry stools). Tell patient to take temperature daily.

• Stress importance of maintaining adequate fluid intake to help prevent hyperuricemia. If adverse GI reactions prevent patient from drinking fluids, tell him to notify prescriber.

• Urge patient to immediately report severe headache, stomach pain with nausea or vomiting, or inability to move a limb.

• Advise patient to report signs of a hypersensitivity reaction, including rash, itching, chills, dizziness, chest tightness, or difficulty breathing.

---

**bacillus Calmette-Guérin (BCG), live intravesical**
PACIS, TheraCys, TICE BCG

*Pregnancy risk category C*

**AVAILABLE FORMS**
**PACIS**
*Powder for injection (lyophilized, preservative-free):* 120 mg/ampule
**TheraCys**
*Suspension (lyophilized) for bladder instillation:* 81 mg/vial
**TICE BCG**
*Suspension (lyophilized) for bladder instillation:* 50 mg/vial

**INDICATIONS & DOSAGES**
➤ **In situ carcinoma of the urinary bladder (primary and relapsed)**
*Adults:* One reconstituted and diluted vial, 81 mg, given intravesically once weekly for 6 weeks (induction); then additional treatments at 3, 6, 12, 18, and 24 months (TheraCys). Or, one bladder instillation (one ampule suspended in 50 ml of sterile, preservative-free saline solution) once weekly for 6 weeks; then once monthly for 6 to 12 months (TICE BCG). Or, instill 120 mg or 1 ampule intravesically into the bladder slowly by gravity flow, by catheter once weekly for 6 weeks. Schedule may be repeated if tumor remission isn't achieved and if clinical circumstances warrant (PACIS).

**ACTION**
Unknown. BCG vaccine is a live attenuated strain of *Mycobacterium bovis.* Instillation of the live bacterial suspension causes a local inflammatory response. Local infiltration of histiocytes and leukocytes is followed by a decrease in superficial tumors in the bladder.

| Route | Onset | Peak | Duration |
|---|---|---|---|
| Intravesical | Unknown | Unknown | Unknown |

**ADVERSE REACTIONS**
**CNS:** *malaise, fever.*
**GI:** nausea, vomiting, anorexia, diarrhea, abdominal pain.
**GU:** *bladder irritability, dysuria, urinary frequency, hematuria, cystitis, urinary urgency, nocturia,* urinary incontinence, urinary tract infection, urine retention, local pain.
**Musculoskeletal:** arthralgia, myalgia.
**Other:** hypersensitivity reactions, chills, *flulike syndrome.*

**INTERACTIONS**
**Drug-drug.** *Antituberculotics:* May attenuate response to BCG intravesical. Avoid using together.
*Bone marrow suppressants, immunosuppressants, radiation therapy:* May impair response to BCG intravesical by decreasing the immune response; may also increase the risk of osteomyelitis or disseminated BCG infection. Avoid using together.

---

**EFFECTS ON LAB TEST RESULTS**
None reported.

**CONTRAINDICATIONS & CAUTIONS**
• Contraindicated in immunocompromised patients, in those receiving immunosuppressive therapy, in asymptomatic carriers with a positive HIV serology, patients with active tuberculosis, and in those with urinary tract infection, gross hematuria, or fever of unknown origin. Also contraindicated in patients with stage TaG1 papillary tumors, unless they are judged to be at high risk of tumor recurrence.

**NURSING CONSIDERATIONS**
• Determine patient's reactivity to tuberculin before therapy. Tuberculin sensitivity may be rendered positive by BCG intravesical treatment.
• Drug shouldn't be handled by caregiver with immune deficiency.
• BCG intravesical shouldn't be given within 7 to 14 days of transurethral resection or biopsy. Fatal disseminated BCG infection has occurred after traumatic catheterization.
• Prepare product using sterile technique in a biocontainment hood. If preparation can't be performed in a biocontainment hood, person responsible for mixing the product should wear gloves, mask, and gown to avoid inhaling BCG organisms or contacting broken skin.
• To avoid cross-contamination, parenteral drugs shouldn't be prepared in areas where BCG has been in use.
• To prepare PACIS, add 1 ml of sterile diluent (preservative-free normal saline solution for injection) to 1 ampule of BCG to resuspend. Leave drug and diluent in contact for 1 minute. Then mix suspension by withdrawing it into syringe and expelling it gently back into ampule two or three times. Avoid creating foam; don't shake. Dilute the reconstituted product in another 49 ml of saline solution diluent, bringing the total volume to 50 ml.
• To give TheraCys, reconstitute only with 3 ml of provided diluent per vial just before use. Don't remove rubber stopper to prepare solution. Use immediately. Add contents of 3 reconstituted vials to 50 ml of sterile, preservative-free saline solution

(final volume, 53 ml). Insert a urethral catheter into bladder under aseptic conditions, drain bladder, and infuse 53 ml of prepared solution by gravity feed. Remove catheter and properly dispose of unused drug.
• Use suspensions immediately after preparation. Discard any prepared suspension after 2 hours.
• To give TICE BCG, use thermosetting plastic or sterile glass containers and syringes. Draw 1 ml of sterile, preservative-free saline solution into a 3-ml syringe. Add to 1 ampule of drug; gently expel back into ampule three times to ensure thorough mixing. Use immediately. Dispense cloudy suspension into top end of a catheter-tipped syringe that contains 49 ml of saline solution. Gently rotate syringe. Properly dispose of unused drug.
• Don't use reconstituted product if it has clumps that can't be dispersed with gentle shaking.
• Protect drug from exposure to direct or indirect sunlight.
• Handle drug and material used for instillation as infectious material because drug contains live, attenuated mycobacteria. Dispose of equipment (syringes, catheters, and containers) as biohazardous waste.
• Use strict aseptic technique to give drug to minimize trauma to GU tract and to prevent introduction of other contaminants.
• Notify prescriber if there is evidence of traumatic catheterization, and don't give drug. Subsequent treatment may resume after 1 week as if no interruption occurred.
• Carefully monitor patient's urinary status because drug causes an inflammatory response in the bladder.
• Closely monitor patient for evidence of systemic BCG infection. BCG infections are rarely detected by positive cultures. Withhold therapy if systemic infection is suspected (short-term high temperature over 103° F [39° C] or persistent temperature over 101° F [38° C] for longer than 2 days or with severe malaise). Contact an infectious disease specialist for initiation of fast-acting antituberculosis therapy.
• If fever is caused by infection, withhold drug until patient recovers.

---

• Drug isn't used as an immunizing product to prevent cancer or tuberculosis.
• Drug may cause hypersensitivity. Manage symptomatically.
• Patients with a small bladder capacity may experience increased local irritation with usual dose of BCG intravesical.
• Treat bladder irritation symptomatically with phenazopyridine, acetaminophen, and propantheline. Systemic hypersensitivity can be treated with diphenhydramine. To minimize risk of systemic infection, some prescribers give isoniazid for 3 days starting on first day of treatment.
• *Alert:* Don't confuse BCG intravesical with BCG vaccine.

## PATIENT TEACHING
• Tell patient to retain drug in bladder for 2 hours after instillation, if possible. For first hour, have patient lie 15 minutes prone, 15 minutes supine, and 15 minutes on each side; patient may spend second hour in sitting position.
• Advise patient to sit when voiding.
• Instruct patient to disinfect urine for 6 hours after instillation of drug. Tell him to pour undiluted household bleach (5% sodium hypochlorite solution) in equal volume to voided urine into the toilet bowl and wait 15 minutes before flushing.
• Tell patient to notify prescriber if symptoms worsen or if the following symptoms develop: blood in urine, fever and chills, frequent urge to urinate, painful urination, nausea, vomiting, joint pain, or rash.
• *Alert:* Warn patient that a cough that develops after therapy could indicate a life-threatening BCG infection. Tell him to report it immediately.
• Caution woman of childbearing age to avoid becoming pregnant or breast-feeding during therapy.

## bexarotene
Targretin

*Pregnancy risk category X*

## AVAILABLE FORMS
*Capsules:* 75 mg
*Topical gel:* 1%

## INDICATIONS & DOSAGES
➤ **Cutaneous T-cell lymphoma in patients refractory to at least one previous systemic therapy**
*Adults:* 300 mg/m$^2$ daily P.O. as a single dose with a meal. If no response after 8 weeks, increase to 400 mg/m$^2$ daily if first dose was tolerated.
*Adjust-a-dose:* Patients with hepatic insufficiency may need lower doses. If toxicity occurs, adjust dosage to 200 mg/m$^2$ daily and then to 100 mg/m$^2$ daily; or temporarily suspend drug. When toxicity is controlled, doses may be carefully readjusted upward.
➤ **Refractory cutaneous lesions in patients with cutaneous T-cell lymphoma (stage IA and IB)**
*Adults:* Initially, apply generously to affected areas every other day for first week; increase at weekly intervals to once daily, then b.i.d, then t.i.d., and finally q.i.d.

## ACTION
The exact mechanism of action in the treatment of cutaneous T-cell lymphoma is unknown. Bexarotene selectively binds and activates retinoid X receptor (RXR) subtypes. Once activated, these receptors function as transcription factors that regulate the expression of genes that control cellular differentiation and proliferation. Bexarotene inhibits the in vitro growth of some tumor cell lines of hematopoietic and squamous cell origin, and it induces in vivo tumor cell regression in some animal models.

| Route | Onset | Peak | Duration |
|---|---|---|---|
| P.O., Topical | Unknown | Unknown | Unknown |

## ADVERSE REACTIONS
**CNS:** *headache,* insomnia, *asthenia,* fatigue, syncope, depression, agitation, ataxia, *CVA,* confusion, dizziness, hyperesthesia, hypoesthesia, neuropathy, fever.
**CV:** *peripheral edema,* chest pain, hypertension, angina, **heart failure,** tachycardia.
**EENT:** cataracts, pharyngitis, rhinitis, dry eyes, conjunctivitis, ear pain, blepharitis, corneal lesion, keratitis, otitis externa, visual field defect.
**GI:** *nausea,* diarrhea, vomiting, anorexia, **pancreatitis,** abdominal pain, constipa-

tion, dry mouth, flatulence, colitis, dyspepsia, cheilitis, gastroenteritis, gingivitis, melena.

**GU:** albuminuria, hematuria, incontinence, urinary tract infection, urinary urgency, dysuria, abnormal kidney function.

**Hematologic:** *leukopenia,* anemia, eosinophilia, *hemorrhage,* thrombocythemia, lymphocytosis, *thrombocytopenia.*

**Hepatic:** *liver failure.*

**Metabolic:** *hyperlipidemia, hypothyroidism,* hyperglycemia, hypoproteinemia, hypocalcemia, hyponatremia, weight change.

**Musculoskeletal:** arthralgia, myalgia, back pain, bone pain, myasthenia, arthrosis.

**Respiratory:** pneumonia, dyspnea, hemoptysis, pleural effusion, bronchitis, cough, *pulmonary edema,* hypoxia.

**Skin:** *rash, dry skin,* exfoliative dermatitis, *alopecia, photosensitivity reaction,* pruritus, cellulitis, acne, skin ulcer, skin nodule; *contact dermatitis and skin disorder* (topical).

**Other:** *infection,* chills, flulike syndrome, breast pain, *sepsis.*

**INTERACTIONS**

**Drug-drug.** *Erythromycin, gemfibrozil, itraconazole, ketoconazole, other inhibitors of cytochrome P450 3A4:* May increase plasma bexarotene level. Avoid using together.

*Insulin, sulfonylureas, troglitazone:* May enhance hypoglycemic action of these drugs, resulting in hypoglycemia in patients with diabetes mellitus. Use together cautiously.

*Phenobarbital, phenytoin, rifampin, other inducers of cytochrome P450 3A4:* May decrease plasma bexarotene level. Avoid using together.

*Products containing DEET:* May increase DEET toxicity with topical gel preparation. Avoid using together.

*Vitamin A preparations:* May increase risk of vitamin A toxicity. Avoid vitamin A supplements.

**Drug-food.** *Any food:* May increase bexarotene absorption. Give drug with food.

*Grapefruit juice:* May inhibit cytochrome P450 3A4. Tell patient to avoid grapefruit juice during therapy.

**Drug-lifestyle.** *Sun exposure:* May cause photosensitivity reaction. Advise patient to avoid excessive sunlight exposure.

**EFFECTS ON LAB TEST RESULTS**

• May increase creatinine, LDH, AST, ALT, bilirubin, amylase, lipid, and glucose levels. May decrease protein, calcium, TSH, total $T_4$, and sodium levels.

• May increase eosinophil count. May decrease hemoglobin and WBC and lymphocyte counts. May increase or decrease platelet count.

• May increase CA-125 assay values in patients with ovarian cancer.

**CONTRAINDICATIONS & CAUTIONS**

• Contraindicated in pregnant women and patients hypersensitive to drug or its components. Drug isn't recommended for patients with risk factors for pancreatitis, such as previous pancreatitis, uncontrolled hyperlipidemia, excessive alcohol consumption, uncontrolled diabetes mellitus, or biliary tract disease. Also not recommended for patients taking drugs that increase triglyceride levels or who have pancreatic toxicity.

• Use cautiously in women of childbearing age, patients with hepatic insufficiency, and those hypersensitive to retinoids.

**NURSING CONSIDERATIONS**

• *Alert:* Woman of childbearing age should use effective contraception for at least 1 month before start of therapy, during therapy, and for at least 1 month after therapy ends. During therapy, she should use two reliable forms of contraception unless abstinence is the chosen method. Patient should have a negative pregnancy test within 1 week before starting therapy and monthly during therapy.

• Start therapy on the second or third day of a normal menstrual period.

• Men who are receiving therapy must wear condoms during sexual intercourse throughout and for at least 1 month after therapy if their sexual partners are pregnant or could become pregnant.

• Give no more than a 1-month supply of bexarotene to a woman of childbearing potential, so the results of pregnancy testing can be assessed regularly and so the patient can be reminded of the danger of birth defects if she becomes pregnant during therapy.

• Obtain total cholesterol, HDL cholesterol, and triglyceride levels at start of drug therapy, weekly until lipid response is established (2 to 4 weeks), and at 8-week intervals thereafter. Treat elevated triglyceride levels during therapy with antilipemic therapy and, if necessary, the dose of bexarotene reduced or suspended.

• Obtain baseline thyroid function tests and monitor them during treatment.

• Monitor WBC with differential at baseline and periodically during treatment.

• Monitor liver function test results at baseline and after 1, 2, and 4 weeks of treatment. If stable, monitor them every 8 weeks during treatment. Consider suspending treatment if results are three times the upper limit of normal.

• Obtain ophthalmologic evaluation for cataracts if patient has visual difficulties.

• With topical gel, you may see a response within 4 weeks; most patients require longer treatment.

**PATIENT TEACHING**
• Advise patient to minimize exposure to sunlight and artificial ultraviolet light and to take appropriate precautions.

• Teach patient that it may take several capsules to make the necessary dose and to take these capsules at the same time and with a meal.

• Teach women of childbearing potential the dangers of becoming pregnant while taking bexarotene and the need for non-hormonal contraception and monthly pregnancy tests during therapy. Contraception must continue for 1 month after discontinuation of therapy.

• Explain the need for obtaining baseline laboratory tests and for periodic monitoring of these tests.

• Tell patient to report any visual changes. For topical gel:
• Instruct patient to allow gel to dry before putting clothes on.

• Instruct patient to avoid the use of occlusive dressings.

• Tell patient not to apply drug to unaffected areas or mucosal areas.

✳ *NEW DRUG*

# bortezomib
Velcade

*Pregnancy risk category D*

**AVAILABLE FORMS**
*Powder for injection:* 3.5 mg

**INDICATIONS & DOSAGES**
➤ **Multiple myeloma still progressing after at least two therapies**
*Adults:* 1.3 mg/m² by I.V. bolus twice weekly for 2 weeks (days 1, 4, 8, and 11), followed by a 10-day rest period (days 12 through 21). This 3-week period is a treatment cycle.

***Adjust-a-dose:*** If patient develops grade 3 nonhematologic or grade 4 hematologic toxicity (excluding neuropathy), withhold drug. When toxicity has resolved, restart at a 25% reduced dose. If patient has neuropathic pain, peripheral neuropathy, or both, see the table below.

| Severity of neuropathy | Dosage |
|---|---|
| Grade 1 (paresthesias, loss of reflexes, or both) without pain or loss of function | No change. |
| Grade 1 with pain or grade 2 (function altered but not activities of daily living) | Reduce to 1 mg/m². |
| Grade 2 with pain or grade 3 (interference with activities of daily living) | Hold drug until toxicity resolves; then start at 0.7 mg/m² once weekly. |
| Grade 4 (permanent sensory loss that interferes with function) | Stop drug. |

**I.V. ADMINISTRATION**
• Use caution and aseptic technique when preparing and handling drug. Wear gloves and protective clothing to prevent skin contact.

• Reconstitute with 3.5 ml of normal saline solution. Give by I.V. bolus within 8 hours of reconstitution.

• Drug may be stored up to 3 hours in a syringe at 59° to 86° F (15° to 30° C), but total storage time for reconstituted solution must not exceed 8 hours under normal indoor lighting.

• Store unopened vials at a controlled room temperature, in original packaging, protected from light.

## ACTION
Disrupts intracellular homeostatic mechanisms by inhibiting the 26S proteosome, which regulates intracellular levels of certain proteins, thereby causing cells to die.

| Route | Onset | Peak | Duration |
|-------|-------|------|----------|
| I.V. | Unknown | Unknown | Unknown |

## ADVERSE REACTIONS
**CNS:** *anxiety, asthenia, dizziness, dysesthesia, fever, headache, insomnia, paresthesia, peripheral neuropathy, rigors.*
**CV:** *edema, hypotension.*
**EENT:** *blurred vision.*
**GI:** *abdominal pain, constipation, decreased appetite, diarrhea, dysgeusia, dyspepsia, nausea, vomiting.*
**Hematologic:** *anemia,* NEUTROPENIA, THROMBOCYTOPENIA.
**Musculoskeletal:** *arthralgia, back pain, bone pain, limb pain, muscle cramps, myalgia.*
**Respiratory:** *cough, dyspnea, pneumonia, upper respiratory tract infection.*
**Skin:** *rash, pruritus.*
**Other:** *dehydration, herpes zoster, pyrexia.*

## INTERACTIONS
**Drug-drug.** *Antihypertensives:* May cause hypotension. Monitor patient's blood pressure closely.
*Drugs linked to peripheral neuropathy, such as amiodarone, antivirals, isoniazid, nitrofurantoin, statins:* May worsen neuropathy. Use together cautiously.
*Inhibitors or inducers of cytochrome P450 3A4:* May increase risk of toxicity or may reduce drug's effects. Monitor patient closely.
*Oral antidiabetics:* May cause hypoglycemia or hyperglycemia. Monitor glucose level closely.

## EFFECTS ON LAB TEST RESULTS
• May decrease hemoglobin and neutrophil and platelet counts.

## CONTRAINDICATIONS & CAUTIONS
• Contraindicated in patients hypersensitive to bortezomib, boron, or mannitol.
• Use cautiously if patient is dehydrated, is receiving other drugs known to cause hypotension, or has a history of syncope. Use cautiously in patients with hepatic or renal impairment, and watch closely for evidence of toxicity.
• Safety and effectiveness haven't been established for pregnant patients. Advise women not to become pregnant during therapy.
• Safety and effectiveness haven't been established for children.

## NURSING CONSIDERATIONS
• Watch for evidence of neuropathy, such as a burning sensation, hyperesthesia, hypoesthesia, paresthesia, discomfort, or neuropathic pain.
• Patients who develop new or worsening peripheral neuropathy may need a change in bortezomib dose and schedule.
• Because experience with elderly patients is limited, watch carefully for adverse effects.
• Patient may need an antiemetic, antidiarrheal, or both because drug may cause nausea, vomiting, diarrhea, and constipation.
• Provide fluid and electrolyte replacement to prevent dehydration.
• Be prepared to adjust antihypertensive dosage, maintain hydration status, and give mineralocorticoids to manage orthostatic hypotension.
• *Alert:* Because thrombocytopenia is common, monitor patient's CBC and platelet counts carefully during treatment, especially on day 11.

## PATIENT TEACHING
• Tell patient to notify prescriber about new or worsening peripheral neuropathy.
• Urge women to use effective contraception and not to breast-feed during treatment.
• Teach patient how to avoid dehydration, and stress the need to tell prescriber about dizziness, light-headedness, or fainting spells.
• Tell patient to use caution when driving or performing other hazardous activities because drug may cause fatigue, dizzi-

ness, faintness, light-headedness, and doubled or blurred vision.

# dacarbazine (DTIC)
DTIC†, DTIC-Dome

*Pregnancy risk category C*

## AVAILABLE FORMS
*Injection:* 100-mg, 200-mg vials

## INDICATIONS & DOSAGES
➤ **Metastatic malignant melanoma**
*Adults:* 2 to 4.5 mg/kg I.V. daily for
10 days; repeated q 4 weeks, as tolerated.
Or 250 mg/m² I.V. daily for 5 days; repeated at 3-week intervals.
➤ **Hodgkin's disease**
*Adults:* 150 mg/m² I.V. daily (with other
drugs) for 5 days; repeated q 4 weeks. Or
375 mg/m² on first day of combination
regimen; repeated q 15 days.

## I.V. ADMINISTRATION
● *Alert:* Preparation and administration of
parenteral form of drug may be mutagenic, teratogenic, or carcinogenic to staff.
Follow institutional policy to reduce risks.
● Reconstitute drug using sterile water for
injection. Add 9.9 ml to 100-mg vial or
19.7 ml to 200-mg vial; resulting solution
will be colorless to clear yellow. For infusion, further dilute by using up to 250 ml
of normal saline solution or D₅W; infuse
over at least 15 to 30 minutes.
● Drug may be diluted further or given at a
slower infusion rate to decrease pain at insertion site.
● Watch for irritation and infiltration during infusion; extravasation can cause severe pain, tissue damage, and necrosis. If
I.V. solution infiltrates, stop immediately,
apply ice to area for 24 to 48 hours, and
notify prescriber.
● Reconstituted solutions in the vial are
stable for 8 hours at room temperature and
normal lighting conditions, or up to 3 days
if refrigerated. Further diluted solutions
are stable for 8 hours at normal room temperature and light, or up to 24 hours if refrigerated. If solution turns pink, discard
because it has decomposed.

## ACTION
Unknown. Probably cross-links strands of
cellular DNA and interferes with RNA
and protein synthesis. Not specific to cell
cycle.

| Route | Onset | Peak | Duration |
|-------|-------|------|----------|
| I.V. | Unknown | Unknown | Unknown |

## ADVERSE REACTIONS
**CNS:** facial paresthesia.
**GI:** *severe nausea and vomiting, anorexia,*
stomatitis.
**Hematologic:** *leukopenia, thrombocytopenia.*
**Skin:** phototoxicity, alopecia, rash, facial
flushing.
**Other:** tissue damage, *flulike syndrome,
anaphylaxis,* severe pain with infiltration
or a too-concentrated solution.

## INTERACTIONS
**Drug-lifestyle.** *Sun exposure:* May cause
photosensitivity reaction, especially during first 2 days of therapy. Advise patient
to avoid excessive sunlight exposure.

## EFFECTS ON LAB TEST RESULTS
● May increase BUN and liver enzyme
levels.
● May decrease WBC, RBC, and platelet
counts.

## CONTRAINDICATIONS & CAUTIONS
● Contraindicated in patients hypersensitive to drug.
● Use cautiously in patients with impaired
bone marrow function and those with severe renal or hepatic dysfunction.

## NURSING CONSIDERATIONS
● Give antiemetics before giving dacarbazine. Nausea and vomiting may subside
after several doses.
● To prevent bleeding, avoid all I.M. injections when platelet count is below
50,000/mm³.
● Anticipate need for blood transfusions to
combat anemia. Patient may receive injections of RBC colony-stimulating factors to
promote RBC production and decrease
need for blood transfusions.
● Therapeutic effects are commonly accompanied by toxicity. Monitor CBC and
platelet count.

• For Hodgkin's disease, drug is usually given with bleomycin, vinblastine, and doxorubicin.
• **Alert:** Don't confuse dacarbazine with Dicarbosil or procarbazine.

**PATIENT TEACHING**
• Tell patient to watch for evidence of infection (fever, sore throat, fatigue) and bleeding (easy bruising, nosebleeds, bleeding gums, tarry stools). Tell him to take temperature daily.
• Tell patient to avoid people with upper respiratory tract infections.
• Instruct patient to avoid OTC products that contain aspirin or NSAIDs.
• Advise patient to avoid sunlight and sunlamps for first 2 days after treatment.
• Reassure patient that flulike syndrome (fever, malaise, and muscle pain beginning 7 days after treatment ends and possibly lasting 7 to 21 days) may be treated with mild fever reducers, such as acetaminophen.
• Counsel woman to avoid pregnancy and breast-feeding during therapy.

## docetaxel
Taxotere

*Pregnancy risk category D*

**AVAILABLE FORMS**
*Injection:* 20 mg, 80 mg, in single-dose vials

**INDICATIONS & DOSAGES**
➤ **Locally advanced or metastatic breast cancer after failure of previous chemotherapy**
*Adults:* 60 to 100 mg/m² I.V. over 1 hour q 3 weeks.
**Adjust-a-dose:** In patients receiving 100 mg/m² who experience febrile neutropenia, neutrophil count of less than 500/mm³ for longer than 1 week, severe or cumulative cutaneous reactions, or severe peripheral neuropathy, reduce subsequent dose by 25%, to 75 mg/m². In patients who continue to experience reactions with decreased dose, either decrease it further to 55 mg/m² or stop drug.
➤ **Locally advanced or metastatic non–small-cell lung cancer after failure**

**of previous cisplatin-based chemotherapy**
*Adults:* 75 mg/m² I.V. over 1 hour q 3 weeks.
**Adjust-a-dose:** In patients who experience febrile neutropenia, neutrophil count of less than 500/mm³ for longer than 1 week, severe or cumulative cutaneous reactions, or severe peripheral neuropathy, withhold drug until toxicity resolves, then restart at 55 mg/m². In patients who develop grade 3 peripheral neuropathy or above, stop drug.
➤ **Unresectable, locally advanced, or metastatic non–small-cell lung cancer not previously treated with chemotherapy**
*Adults:* 75 mg/m² docetaxel I.V. over 1 hour, immediately followed by cisplatin 75 mg/m² I.V. over 30 to 60 minutes every 3 weeks.
**Adjust-a-dose:** In patients whose nadir of platelet count during the previous course of therapy is less than 25,000 cells/mm³, those with febrile neutropenia, and those with serious nonhematologic toxicities, decrease docetaxel dosage to 65 mg/m². For patients who require a further dose reduction, a dose of 50 mg/m² is recommended. For cisplatin dosage adjustments, see manufacturers' prescribing information.

**I.V. ADMINISTRATION**
• Wear gloves during drug preparation and administration. If solution contacts skin, wash immediately and thoroughly with soap and water. If drug contacts mucous membranes, flush thoroughly with water. Mark all waste materials with CHEMOTHERAPY HAZARD labels.
• Prepare and store infusion solutions in bottles (glass or polypropylene) or plastic bags, and give through polyethylene-lined administration sets. Give drug as 1-hour infusion; store unopened vials in refrigerator.
• Before giving drug, dilute using supplied diluent. Allow drug and diluent to stand at room temperature for 5 minutes before mixing. After adding all the diluent to drug vial, gently rotate vial for about 15 seconds. Allow solution to stand for a few minutes to enable foam to dissipate. All foam need not fully dissipate before proceeding to the next step.

• Prepare drug infusion solution by withdrawing needed amount of premixed solution from vial and injecting it into 250 ml normal saline solution or $D_5W$ to yield 0.3 to 0.74 mg/ml. Doses exceeding 200 mg need a larger volume of infusion solution to stay below 0.74 mg/ml of docetaxel. Mix infusion thoroughly by manual rotation.

• Discard solution if it isn't clear or it contains precipitates. Use infusion solution within 4 hours. The first diluted solution is stable for 8 hours.

## ACTION
Promotes formation and stabilization of nonfunctional microtubules. This prevents mitosis and leads to cell death.

| Route | Onset | Peak | Duration |
|-------|-------|------|----------|
| I.V. | Rapid | Unknown | Unknown |

## ADVERSE REACTIONS
**CNS:** *asthenia,* paresthesia, peripheral neuropathy.
**CV:** *fluid retention, peripheral edema,* hypotension, flushing, chest tightness.
**GI:** *stomatitis, nausea, vomiting, diarrhea.*
**Hematologic:** *anemia,* NEUTROPENIA, FEBRILE NEUTROPENIA, MYELOSUPPRESSION, LEUKOPENIA, THROMBOCYTOPENIA.
**Hepatic:** *hepatotoxicity.*
**Musculoskeletal:** *myalgia,* arthralgia, back pain.
**Respiratory:** dyspnea, *pulmonary edema.*
**Skin:** *alopecia,* skin eruptions, desquamation, nail pigmentation alterations, nail pain, rash, reaction at injection site.
**Other:** hypersensitivity reactions, *infection,* drug fever, chills, **death.**

## INTERACTIONS
**Drug-drug.** *Compounds that induce, inhibit, or are metabolized by cytochrome P450 3A4, such as cyclosporine, erythromycin, ketoconazole, troleandomycin:* May modify metabolism of docetaxel. Use together cautiously.

## EFFECTS ON LAB TEST RESULTS
• May increase ALT, AST, bilirubin, and alkaline phosphatase levels.
• May decrease hemoglobin and WBC and platelet counts.

## CONTRAINDICATIONS & CAUTIONS
• Contraindicated in patients severely hypersensitive to drug or to other formulations containing polysorbate 80 and in those with neutrophil counts below 1,500 cells/mm³.
• Don't give drug to patients with bilirubin levels exceeding upper limit of normal. Also, don't use drug in patients with ALT or AST levels above 1.5 times upper limit of normal and alkaline phosphatase levels over 2.5 times upper limit of normal or in patients with baseline neutrophil count less than 1,500/mm³.
• Safety and effectiveness in children haven't been established.

## NURSING CONSIDERATIONS
• Give oral corticosteroid such as dexamethasone 16 mg P.O. (8 mg b.i.d.) daily for 3 days starting 1 day before docetaxel administration, to reduce risk and severity of fluid retention and hypersensitivity reactions.
• Bone marrow toxicity is the most frequent and dose-limiting toxicity. Frequent blood count monitoring is needed during therapy.
• Monitor patient closely for hypersensitivity reactions, especially during first and second infusions.
• Contact between undiluted docetaxel concentrate and polyvinyl chloride equipment or devices isn't recommended.
• Fluid retention is dose-related and may be severe. Monitor patient closely.
• *Alert:* Don't confuse Taxotere with Taxol.

## PATIENT TEACHING
• Caution woman of childbearing age to avoid pregnancy or breast-feeding during therapy.
• Advise patient to report any pain or burning at site of injection during or after administration.
• Warn patient that hair loss occurs in almost 80% of patients but is reversible when treatment stops.
• Tell patient to report promptly sore throat, fever, or unusual bruising or bleeding, as well as signs and symptoms of fluid retention, such as swelling or shortness of breath.

---

# etoposide (VP-16, VP-16-213)
Toposar, VePesid

# etoposide phosphate
Etopophos

*Pregnancy risk category D*

## AVAILABLE FORMS
**etoposide**
*Capsules:* 50 mg
*Injection:* 20 mg/ml in 5-ml vials
**etoposide phosphate**
*Injection:* 119.3-mg vials equivalent to
100 mg etoposide

## INDICATIONS & DOSAGES
➤ **Testicular cancer**
*Adults:* 50 to 100 mg/m² daily I.V. on
5 consecutive days q 3 to 4 weeks. Or,
100 mg/m² daily I.V. on days 1, 3, and 5 q
3 to 4 weeks for three or four courses of
therapy.
➤ **Small-cell carcinoma of the lung**
*Adults:* 35 mg/m² daily I.V. for 4 days. Or,
50 mg/m² daily I.V. for 5 days. P.O. dose is
two times I.V. dose, rounded to nearest
50 mg.
*Adjust-a-dose:* For patients with creatine
clearance of 15 to 50 ml/minute, reduce
dose by 25%.
➤ **Kaposi's sarcoma** ♦
*Adults:* 150 mg/m² I.V. daily for 3 days q
4 weeks. Repeat p.r.n., based on response.

## I.V. ADMINISTRATION
● Dilute etoposide for infusion in either
$D_5W$ or normal saline solution to 0.2 or
0.4 mg/ml. Higher concentrations may
crystallize. Etoposide phosphate may be
given without further dilution or may be
diluted to as low as 0.1 mg/ml in either
$D_5W$ or normal saline solution.
● Etoposide diluted to 0.2 mg/ml is stable
for 96 hours at room temperature in plastic or glass unprotected from light; solutions diluted to 0.4 mg/ml are stable for
24 hours under same conditions. Diluted
solutions of etoposide phosphate are stable at room temperature or under refrigeration for 24 hours.
● Give etoposide by slow I.V. infusion
(over at least 30 minutes) to prevent severe

hypotension. Etoposide phosphate may be
given over 5 to 210 minutes.
● *Alert:* Monitor blood pressure every
15 minutes during infusion. Hypotension
can occur with too rapid an infusion. If
systolic pressure falls below 90 mm Hg,
stop infusion and notify prescriber.
● *Alert:* Preparation and administration of
parenteral form of drug may be mutagenic, teratogenic, or carcinogenic to staff.
Follow institutional policy to reduce risks.
● *Alert:* Don't confuse VePesid with
Versed.

## ACTION
Unknown. Inhibits topoisomerase II enzyme, which leads to inability to repair
DNA strand breaks. This ultimately leads
to cell death. Cell cycle specific to $G_2$ portion of cell cycle.

| Route | Onset | Peak | Duration |
|---|---|---|---|
| P.O., I.V. | Unknown | Unknown | Unknown |

## ADVERSE REACTIONS
**CNS:** peripheral neuropathy.
**CV:** hypotension.
**GI:** *nausea, vomiting, anorexia, diarrhea,*
abdominal pain, stomatitis.
**Hematologic:** *anemia, myelosuppression,*
LEUKOPENIA, THROMBOCYTOPENIA,
NEUTROPENIA.
**Hepatic:** *hepatotoxicity.*
**Skin:** *reversible alopecia,* rash.
**Other:** hypersensitivity reactions, *ana-
phylaxis.*

## INTERACTIONS
**Drug-drug.** *Phosphatase inhibitors, such
as levamisole hydrochloride:* May decrease etoposide effectiveness. Monitor
clinical effects.
*Warfarin:* May further prolong PT. Monitor PT and INR closely.

## EFFECTS ON LAB TEST RESULTS
● May decrease hemoglobin and WBC,
RBC, platelet, and neutrophil counts.

## CONTRAINDICATIONS & CAUTIONS
● Contraindicated in patients hypersensitive to drug.
● Use cautiously in patients who have had
cytotoxic or radiation therapy. Use cau-

tiously in patients with hepatic impairment.

**NURSING CONSIDERATIONS**
• Obtain baseline blood pressure before starting therapy.
• Anticipate need for antiemetics.
• Have diphenhydramine, hydrocortisone, epinephrine, and emergency equipment available to establish an airway in case anaphylaxis occurs.
• Store capsules in refrigerator.
• Monitor CBC. Watch for evidence of bone marrow suppression.
• Observe patient's mouth for signs of ulceration.
• To prevent bleeding, avoid all I.M. injections when platelet count is below 50,000/mm³.
• Anticipate need for blood transfusions to combat anemia. Patient may receive injections of RBC colony-stimulating factors to promote RBC production and decrease need for blood transfusions.
• Dose of etoposide phosphate is expressed as etoposide equivalents; 119.3 mg of etoposide phosphate is equivalent to 100 mg of etoposide.

**PATIENT TEACHING**
• Tell patient to watch for signs and symptoms of infection (fever, sore throat, fatigue) and bleeding (easy bruising, nosebleeds, bleeding gums, tarry stools). Tell patient to take temperature daily.
• Inform patient of need for frequent blood pressure readings during I.V. administration.
• Caution woman of childbearing age to avoid pregnancy and breast-feeding during therapy.

**✳ NEW DRUG**

# gefitinib
Iressa

*Pregnancy risk category D*

**AVAILABLE FORMS**
*Tablets:* 250 mg

**INDICATIONS & DOSAGES**
➤ **Locally advanced or metastatic non–small-cell lung cancer after platinum-**

**based and docetaxel chemotherapies have failed**
*Adults:* 250 mg P.O. once daily.
*Adjust-a-dose:* If patient takes a CYP3A4 enzyme inducer, gefitinib dosage may be increased to 500 mg daily.

**ACTION**
Inhibits cell growth and replication by binding to and blocking the intracellular enzyme (tyrosine kinase) of the epidermal growth factor receptor on the surface of many normal and cancer cells.

| Route | Onset | Peak | Duration |
|-------|---------|-------|----------|
| P.O. | Unknown | 3-7 hr | 48 hr |

**ADVERSE REACTIONS**
**CNS:** asthenia.
**CV:** peripheral edema.
**EENT:** amblyopia, conjunctivitis.
**GI:** anorexia, *diarrhea,* mouth ulcers, *nausea, vomiting,* weight loss.
**Respiratory:** *dyspnea, interstitial lung disease.*
**Skin:** *acne, dry skin,* pruritus, *rash.*

**INTERACTIONS**
**Drug-drug.** *Drugs that increase gastric pH, such as antacids, H₂ blockers, sodium bicarbonate, or ranitidine:* May reduce availability and efficacy of gefitinib. Monitor patient closely.
*Drugs that induce P450 CYP3A4, such as phenytoin and rifampin:* May decrease gefitinib level. If patient has no severe adverse reactions, gefitinib dosage may be increased to 500 mg daily.
*Drugs that inhibit P450 CYP3A4, such as itraconazole and ketoconazole:* May increase gefitinib level. Monitor patient closely, and adjust dosage as needed.
*Warfarin:* May increase INR and risk of bleeding. Monitor INR and patient closely.

**EFFECTS ON LAB TEST RESULTS**
• Increased AST, ALT, alkaline phosphatase, and bilirubin levels.

**CONTRAINDICATIONS & CAUTIONS**
• Contraindicated in patients hypersensitive to drug or its components.
• Give cautiously to patients with severe renal impairment.

• Drug may harm the fetus. Consider risks and benefits before giving drug to a pregnant woman. Because of potential harm to the infant, women should avoid breast-feeding during treatment.
• Safety and effectiveness in children haven't been established.

## NURSING CONSIDERATIONS
• *Alert:* Patients who develop acute dyspnea, cough, and a low-grade fever may have interstitial lung disease, and these effects may worsen quickly. Stop drug immediately. One-third of patients who develop this form of pulmonary toxicity die.
• Monitor liver function tests periodically during treatment.
• If patient takes warfarin, monitor PT and INR closely.
• Patients who have severe adverse GI or skin reactions may need to stop drug for up to 14 days; restart at 250 mg daily.
• Patients who develop ocular symptoms (eye pain; corneal erosion, sloughing, or ulceration; abnormal eyelash growth; ocular ischemia or hemorrhage) may need to stop taking the drug.

## PATIENT TEACHING
• Teach patient how to avoid dehydration.
• Tell patient to seek medical care immediately for severe or persistent diarrhea, nausea, anorexia, or vomiting; new or worsening pulmonary problems, such as shortness of breath or coughing; eye problems, such as irritation, pain, or altered vision; or a rash.
• Urge women of childbearing age to avoid becoming pregnant.
• Tell pregnant patient that drug may harm fetus.

---

# gemtuzumab ozogamicin
Mylotarg

*Pregnancy risk category D*

## AVAILABLE FORMS
*Powder for injection:* 5 mg

## INDICATIONS & DOSAGES
➤ CD33-positive acute myeloid leukemia patients who are in first relapse and aren't candidates for cytotoxic chemotherapy
*Adults age 60 and older:* 9 mg/m² I.V. over 2 hours q 14 days for a total of two doses. Premedicate with diphenhydramine 50 mg P.O. and acetaminophen 650 to 1,000 mg P.O. 1 hour before infusion.

## I.V. ADMINISTRATION
• Drug is light sensitive; protect from direct and indirect sunlight and unshielded fluorescent light during infusion preparation and administration.
• Reconstitute powder by adding 5 ml of sterile water for injection to yield solution containing 1 mg/ml. Gently swirl vial and inspect for any evidence of particulate matter.
• Give in 100 ml of normal saline solution for injection. Place the 100-ml I.V. bag into an ultraviolet protectant bag. Use the resulting drug solution in the I.V. bag immediately.
• A separate I.V. line equipped with a low protein-binding 1.2-micron terminal filter must be used for drug administration. May be infused by central or peripheral line.
• *Alert:* Don't give as a push or bolus.
• Reconstituted drug is stable for 8 hours if refrigerated.

## ACTION
Binds to the CD33 antigen on the surface of leukemic blasts, resulting in the formation of a complex that's internalized by the cell. The cytotoxic antibiotic is then released inside the cell, causing DNA double strand breaks and cell death.

| Route | Onset | Peak | Duration |
|-------|-------|------|----------|
| I.V. | Unknown | Unknown | Unknown |

## ADVERSE REACTIONS
**CNS:** *asthenia,* depression, *dizziness, headache, insomnia, pain, fever.*
**CV:** *hypertension, hypotension, tachycardia, peripheral edema.*
**EENT:** *epistaxis, pharyngitis, rhinitis.*
**GI:** enlarged abdomen, *abdominal pain, anorexia, constipation, diarrhea, dyspepsia, nausea, stomatitis, vomiting.*
**GU:** *hematuria,* **vaginal hemorrhage.**
**Hematologic:** *anemia,* HEMORRHAGE, LEUKOPENIA, NEUTROPENIA, NEUTROPENIC FEVER, THROMBOCYTOPENIA.

---

Reactions may be *common,* uncommon, *life-threatening,* or COMMON AND LIFE-THREATENING.

**Hepatic:** *hepatotoxicity.*
**Metabolic:** hyperglycemia, *hypokalemia, hypomagnesemia.*
**Musculoskeletal:** arthralgia, *back pain.*
**Respiratory:** *cough, dyspnea, hypoxia,* pneumonia.
**Skin:** ecchymoses, local reaction, petechiae, rash.
**Other:** *chills,* herpes simplex, SEPSIS.

### INTERACTIONS
None known.

### EFFECTS ON LAB TEST RESULTS
• May increase ALT, AST, LDH, and glucose levels. May decrease potassium and magnesium levels.
• May decrease hemoglobin and WBC, neutrophil, and platelet counts.

### CONTRAINDICATIONS & CAUTIONS
• Contraindicated in patients hypersensitive to drug or any of its components.
• Use cautiously in patients with hepatic impairment.

### NURSING CONSIDERATIONS
• Use drug only under the supervision of a clinician experienced in the use of cancer chemotherapeutics.
• Premedicate with diphenhydramine and acetaminophen. Additional doses of acetaminophen 650 to 1,000 mg P.O. can be given every 4 hours, as needed.
• Monitor vital signs during infusion and for 4 hours after infusion.
• Monitor postinfusion symptom complex of chills, fever, hypotension, hypertension, hyperglycemia, hypoxia, and dyspnea that may occur during first 24 hours after administration.
• *Alert:* Severe myelosuppression occurs in all patients given recommended dose of drug. Careful hematologic monitoring is required.
• Monitor electrolytes, hepatic function, CBC, and platelet counts during therapy.
• *Alert:* Cases of fatal hepatic reno-occlusive disease have been reported after treatment with gemtuzumab in association with subsequent chemotherapy.
• Tumor lysis syndrome may occur. Provide adequate hydration and treat with allopurinol to prevent hyperuricemia.

### PATIENT TEACHING
• Advise patient about postinfusion symptoms and instruct him to continue to take acetaminophen 650 to 1,000 mg every 4 hours, as needed.
• Urge patient to watch for signs of infection (fever, sore throat, fatigue) and bleeding (easy bruising, nosebleeds, bleeding gums, tarry stools). Tell patient to take temperature daily.
• Tell patient to avoid OTC products that contain aspirin.

---

## ibritumomab tiuxetan
Zevalin

*Pregnancy risk category D*

### AVAILABLE FORMS
*Injection:* 3.2 mg in kits containing four vials used to produce a single dose of In-111 or Y-90

### INDICATIONS & DOSAGES
➤ **Patients with relapsed or refractory low-grade, follicular, or transformed B-cell non-Hodgkin's lymphoma, including those with rituximab-refractory follicular non-Hodgkin's lymphoma**
*Adults:* **Day 1:** 250 mg/m² of rituximab by I.V. infusion, then 5 mCi (1.6 mg total antibody dose) of In-111 ibritumomab tiuxetan I.V. push over 10 minutes within 4 hours of completion of rituximab.

**Days 7 to 9:** 250 mg/m² of rituximab by I.V. infusion, followed by 0.4 mCi/kg of Y-90 ibritumomab tiuxetan I.V. push over 10 minutes within 4 hours of completion of rituximab. Maximum dose of Y-90 ibritumomab tiuxetan is 32 mCi (1,184 MBq).
*Adjust-a-dose:* In patients with mild thrombocytopenia (baseline platelet count between 100,000 and 149,000 cells/mm³), reduce Y-90 ibritumomab tiuxetan dose to 0.3 mCi/kg (11.1 MBq/kg).

### I.V. ADMINISTRATION
**For rituximab**
• Consider giving patient acetaminophen and diphenhydramine before each rituximab infusion.
• Give at an initial rate of 50 mg/hour.
• Don't mix or dilute with other drugs.

---

- If hypersensitivity or infusion-related events don't occur, increase infusion rate in 50-mg/hour increments every 30 minutes to a maximum of 400 mg/hour.
- If hypersensitivity or infusion-related event occurs, slow or stop infusion temporarily. Infusion can continue at one-half the previous rate as soon as symptoms improve.
- Start second infusion at a rate of 100 mg/hour (50 mg/hour if infusion-related event occurred during first administration) and increase rate by 100-mg/hour increments every 30 minutes to a maximum of 400 mg/hour, as tolerated.

**For radiolabeled ibritumomab tiuxetan**
- Measure dose with a suitable radioactivity calibration system immediately before administration.
- Use aseptic technique and precautions for handling radioactive materials.
- The drug vial contains a protein solution that may develop translucent particles. These particles are removed by filtration before administration.
- Follow manufacturer's directions for radiolabeling procedure.
- Procedures for preparing In-111 and Y-90 ibritumomab tiuxetan doses are different. Read directions carefully.
- Don't shake or agitate vial contents because this causes foaming and denaturation of the protein.
- Allow the reaction to occur at room temperature for 30 minutes. Allowing a longer or shorter reaction may result in inadequate labeling.
- Store at 36° to 46° F (2° to 8° C) until use.
- Give In-111 within 12 hours of radiolabeling.
- Give Y-90 within 8 hours of radiolabeling.
- The prescribed, measured, and given dose of Y-90 ibritumomab tiuxetan must not exceed the absolute maximum allowable dose of 32 mCi (1,184 MBq), regardless of patient's body weight.

## ACTION
Antineoplastic action: Drug binds to the CD20 antigen on B lymphocytes and induces apoptosis in CD20+ B-cell lines in vitro. The chelate tiuxetan, which tightly bonds In-111 or Y-90, is covalently linked to the amino groups of exposed lysines and arginines contained within the antibody. The beta emission from Y-90 causes cellular damage by forming free radicals in the target and neighboring cells.

| Route | Onset | Peak | Duration |
|---|---|---|---|
| I.V. | Unknown | Unknown | Unknown |

## ADVERSE REACTIONS
**CNS:** *asthenia, headache, dizziness,* insomnia, *fever, pain,* anxiety.
**CV:** hypotension, peripheral edema, flushing.
**EENT:** *throat irritation,* epistaxis, rhinitis.
**GI:** *abdominal pain, nausea, vomiting,* diarrhea, anorexia, abdominal enlargement, constipation, dyspepsia, **GI hemorrhage,** melena.
**Hematologic:** THROMBOCYTOPENIA, NEUTROPENIA, *anemia,* **pancytopenia.**
**Musculoskeletal:** back pain, arthralgia, myalgia.
**Respiratory:** *dyspnea, increased cough,* **bronchospasm, apnea.**
**Skin:** pruritus, rash, ecchymosis, urticaria, petechiae, sweating.
**Other:** *infection, chills,* **angioedema,** allergic reaction, tumor pain, secondary malignancies.

## INTERACTIONS
**Drug-drug.** *Drugs that interfere with platelet function or coagulation:* May increase risk of bleeding and hemorrhage. Use together cautiously and monitor patient frequently for thrombocytopenia.

## EFFECTS ON LAB TEST RESULTS
- May decrease hemoglobin, hematocrit, and neutrophil, RBC, WBC, and platelet counts.

## CONTRAINDICATIONS & CAUTIONS
- Contraindicated in patients with hypersensitivity or anaphylactic reactions to murine proteins or to any component of this product, including rituximab, yttrium chloride, and indium chloride. Also contraindicated in patients with at least 25% lymphoma marrow involvement or impaired bone marrow reserve and in those with a history of failed stem-cell collection.

• Use cautiously in patients with evidence of human antimouse antibodies and in those receiving live viral vaccines.

• Don't treat patients with platelet counts less than 100,000/mm³.

• If patient is or becomes pregnant while receiving this drug, inform her of the potential hazard to the fetus. Advise women of childbearing age to avoid becoming pregnant during therapy.

**NURSING CONSIDERATIONS**

• Only physicians and other professionals qualified by training and experienced in the safe use of radionuclides should give drug.

• Changing the ratio of any reactants in the radiolabeling process may adversely affect therapeutic results.

• The drug regimen may cause severe and potentially fatal infusion reactions, which typically occur during the first rituximab infusion with a time to onset of 30 to 120 minutes. Signs and symptoms include hypotension, angioedema, hypoxia, or bronchospasm; interruption of rituximab, In-111 ibritumomab tiuxetan, and Y-90 ibritumomab tiuxetan may be required.

• Keep drugs to treat hypersensitivity reactions available during administration.

• The dose of rituximab is lower when used as part of the ibritumomab tiuxetan regimen than when used alone.

• Don't give rituximab as I.V. push or bolus.

• Patient may be given acetaminophen and diphenhydramine before each rituximab infusion.

• Don't use In-111 and Y-90 without the rituximab pre-dose.

• Don't give Y-90 ibritumomab tiuxetan to patients with altered biodistribution as determined by imaging with In-111 ibritumomab tiuxetan.

• Monitor patient for cytopenia and its complications for up to 3 months after use of drug.

• The product contains albumin and carries a risk for transmission of viral diseases. A risk for transmission of Creutzfeldt-Jakob disease is considered extremely remote.

• Monitor CBC and platelet count weekly after ibritumomab tiuxetan therapy, and continue monitoring until levels recover.

Monitor more frequently in patients who develop severe cytopenia.

• Assess the biodistribution of In-111 ibritumomab tiuxetan per manufacturer's instructions at 2 to 24 hours and 48 to 72 hours after injection.

**PATIENT TEACHING**

• Warn patient of the adverse effects of the medication.

• Advise patient to report bleeding, fever, or signs and symptoms of infection.

• Explain to patient the importance of monitoring and follow-up for 3 months after treatment.

• Review standard radiation precautions for handling blood or body fluids.

---

## imatinib mesylate
Gleevec◆

*Pregnancy risk category D*

**AVAILABLE FORMS**
*Capsules:* 50 mg, 100 mg
*Tablets:* 100 mg, 400 mg

**INDICATIONS & DOSAGES**
➤ **Chronic myeloid leukemia (CML) in blast crisis, in accelerated phase, or in chronic phase after failure of alfa interferon therapy; newly diagnosed Philadelphia chromosome-positive chronic phase CML**
*Adults:* Chronic-phase CML: 400 mg P.O. daily as single dose with a meal and large glass of water. *Accelerated-phase CML or blast crisis:* 600 mg P.O. daily as single dose with a meal and large glass of water. Continue treatment as long as patient continues to benefit. May increase daily dose to 600 mg P.O. in chronic phase or to 800 mg P.O. (400 mg P.O. b.i.d.) in accelerated phase or blast crisis.

Consider dosage increases only if there is an absence of severe adverse reactions and absence of severe non–leukemia-related neutropenia or thrombocytopenia in the following circumstances: disease progression (at any time), failure to achieve a satisfactory hematologic response after at least 3 months of treatment, failure to achieve a cytogenetic response after 6 to 12 months of treatment, or loss of a previously achieved hematologic or cytogenetic response.

➤ **Kit (CD117)–positive unresectable or metastatic malignant GI stromal tumors (GIST)**
*Adults:* 400 or 600 mg P.O. daily.
➤ **Philadelphia chromosome–positive chronic phase CML in patients whose disease has recurred after stem cell transplant or who are resistant to interferon alfa therapy**
*Children age 3 and older:* 260 mg/m² daily P.O. as a single dose or divided into two doses. Have patient take with meal and large glass of water. May increase dosage to 340 mg/m² daily.

***Adjust-a-dose:*** For severe nonhematologic adverse reactions (severe hepatotoxicity or severe fluid retention), withhold drug until event has resolved; resume treatment as appropriate based on initial severity of event. For elevations in bilirubin level more than three times the institutional upper limit of normal (IULN) or liver transaminase levels more than five times IULN, withhold drug until bilirubin level returns to less than 1.5 IULN and transaminase levels to less than 2.5 IULN. May then resume drug at reduced daily dose. (Adults' dosages can be decreased from 400 mg to 300 mg or from 600 mg to 400 mg. Children's dosages can be decreased from 260 mg/m² daily to 200 mg/m² daily or from 340 mg/m² daily to 260 mg/m² daily.)

For hematologic adverse reactions in patients with chronic-phase CML, give starting dose 400 mg in adults or 260 mg/m² in children; in those with GIST, give starting dose 400 mg or 600 mg. If absolute neutrophil count (ANC) less than 1 × 10⁹/L or platelets less than 50 × 10⁹/L, or both, follow these steps.
1. Stop drug until ANC is 1.5 × 10⁹/L or greater and platelets are 75 × 10⁹/L or greater.
2. Resume treatment at original starting dose of 400 mg or 600 mg, or 260 mg/m² in children.
3. If recurrence of ANC less than 1 × 10⁹/L, and/or platelets less than 50 × 10⁹/L, repeat step 1 and resume drug at reduced dose (300 mg if starting dose was 400 mg; 400 mg if starting dose was

600 mg; or in children, 200 mg/m² if starting dose was 260 mg/m²).

In patients with accelerated phase CML and blast crisis, give starting dose 600 mg; if ANC less than 0.5 × 10⁹/L or platelets less than 10 × 10⁹/L, or both, after at least 1 month of treatment, follow these steps.
1. Check if cytopenia is related to leukemia via marrow aspirate or biopsy.
2. If cytopenia is unrelated to leukemia, reduce dose of drug to 400 mg.
3. If cytopenia persists 2 weeks, reduce further to 300 mg.
4. If cytopenia persists 4 weeks and is still unrelated to leukemia, stop Gleevec until ANC is 1 × 10⁹/L or greater and platelets are 20 × 10⁹/L or greater and then resume treatment at 300 mg.

## ACTION

Drug inhibits Bcr-Abl tyrosine kinase, which is the abnormal tyrosine kinase created by the Philadelphia chromosome abnormality in CML; in vivo, it inhibits tumor growth of Bcr-Abl transfected murine myeloid cells, as well as Bcr-Abl positive leukemia lines derived from CML patients in blast crisis.

| Route | Onset | Peak | Duration |
|-------|-------|------|----------|
| P.O. | Unknown | 2-4 hr | Unknown |

## ADVERSE REACTIONS

**CNS:** *headache,* CEREBRAL HEMORRHAGE, *fatigue, weakness, pyrexia.*
**CV:** *edema.*
**EENT:** *nasopharyngitis, epistaxis.*
**GI:** *anorexia, nausea, diarrhea, abdominal pain, constipation, vomiting, dyspepsia,* GI HEMORRHAGE.
**Hematologic:** HEMORRHAGE, NEUTROPENIA, THROMBOCYTOPENIA, *anemia.*
**Metabolic:** *hypokalemia,* weight increase.
**Musculoskeletal:** *myalgia, muscle cramps, musculoskeletal pain, arthralgia.*
**Respiratory:** *cough, dyspnea, pneumonia.*
**Skin:** *rash,* pruritus, *petechiae.*
**Other:** *night sweats.*

## INTERACTIONS

**Drug-drug.** *Acetaminophen:* May increase the risk of liver toxicity. Monitor patient closely.

---

Reactions may be *common,* uncommon, *life-threatening,* or COMMON AND LIFE-THREATENING.

*CYP3A4 inducers (carbamazepine, dexamethasone, phenobarbital, phenytoin, rifampin):* May increase metabolism and decreases imatinib levels. Use together cautiously.

*CYP3A4 inhibitors (clarithromycin, erythromycin, itraconazole, ketoconazole):* May decrease metabolism and may increase imatinib level. Monitor patient for toxicity.

*Dihydropyridine–calcium channel blockers, certain HMG-CoA reductase inhibitors (simvastatin), cyclosporine, pimozide, triazolo-benzodiazepines:* May increase levels of these drugs. Monitor patient for toxicity and obtain drug levels, if appropriate.

*Warfarin:* May alter metabolism of warfarin. Avoid using together; use standard heparin or a low molecular weight heparin.

**Drug-herb.** *St. John's wort:* May decrease imatinib effects. Discourage use together.

## EFFECTS ON LAB TEST RESULTS
● May increase creatinine, bilirubin, alkaline phosphatase, AST, and ALT levels. May decrease potassium level.
● May decrease hemoglobin and neutrophil and platelet counts.

## CONTRAINDICATIONS & CAUTIONS
● Contraindicated in patients hypersensitive to drug or its components.
● Use cautiously in patients with hepatic impairment.
● Safety and effectiveness in children younger than age 3 haven't been established.
● Elderly patients may have an increased incidence of edema when taking this drug.

## NURSING CONSIDERATIONS
● Monitor weight daily. Evaluate and treat unexpected rapid weight gain.
● Monitor patients closely for fluid retention, which can be severe.
● Monitor CBC weekly for first month, then decrease to biweekly for second month, and periodically thereafter.
● Because GI irritation is common, tell patient to take drug with food.
● Monitor liver function tests carefully because hepatotoxicity (occasionally severe) may occur; decrease dosage as needed.

● Although there are no data on long-term safety of this drug, monitor renal and liver toxicity and immunosuppression carefully.
● Consider dosage increases only if there are no severe adverse reactions or severe non–leukemia-related neutropenia or thrombocytopenia in the following circumstances: disease progression (at any time), failure to achieve a satisfactory hematologic response after at least 3 months of treatment, or loss of a previously achieved hematologic response.

## PATIENT TEACHING
● Tell patient to take drug with food and a large glass of water.
● Advise patient to report to prescriber any adverse effects, such as fluid retention.
● Advise patient to obtain periodic liver and kidney function tests and blood work to determine blood counts.
● Tell patient to avoid or restrict the use of acetaminophen in OTC or prescription products due to potential toxic effects on the liver.

# irinotecan hydrochloride
Camptosar

*Pregnancy risk category D*

## AVAILABLE FORMS
*Injection:* 100 mg/5-ml vial

## INDICATIONS & DOSAGES
➤ **Metastatic carcinoma of the colon or rectum that has recurred or progressed after fluorouracil (5-FU) therapy**
*Adults:* Initially, 125 mg/m$^2$ by I.V. infusion over 90 minutes once weekly for 4 weeks; then 2-week rest period. Thereafter, additional courses of treatment may be repeated q 6 weeks with 4 weeks on and 2 weeks off. Subsequent doses may be adjusted to low of 50 mg/m$^2$ or maximum of 150 mg/m$^2$ in 25- to 50-mg/m$^2$ increments based on patient's tolerance. Alternatively, 350 mg/m$^2$ by I.V. infusion over 90 minutes once q 3 weeks. Additional courses may continue indefinitely in patients who respond favorably and in those whose disease remains stable, provided intolerable toxicity doesn't occur.

*Elderly patients age 70 and older:*
300 mg/m$^2$ by I.V. infusion over 90 minutes once q 3 weeks.

***Adjust-a-dose:*** In patients who have received prior pelvic or abdominal radiation therapy, or who have a performance status of 2, give 300 mg/m$^2$ by I.V. infusion over 90 minutes once q 3 weeks.

➤ **First-line therapy for metastatic colorectal cancer with 5-fluorouracil (5-FU) and leucovorin**

*Regimen 1*

*Adults:* 125 mg/m$^2$ I.V. over 90 minutes on days 1, 8, 15, and 22; then leucovorin 20 mg/m$^2$ I.V. bolus on days 1, 8, 15, and 22 and 5-FU 500 mg/m$^2$ I.V. bolus on days 1, 8, 15, and 22. Courses are repeated q 6 weeks.

*Regimen 2*

*Adults:* 180 mg/m$^2$ I.V. over 90 minutes on days 1, 15, and 29; then leucovorin 200 mg/m$^2$ I.V. over 2 hours on days 1, 2, 15, 16, 29, and 30; then 5-FU 400 mg/m$^2$ I.V. bolus on days 1, 2, 15, 16, 29, and 30 and 5-FU 600 mg/m$^2$ I.V. infusion over 22 hours on days 1, 2, 15, 16, 29, and 30.

***Adjust-a-dose:*** See manufacturer's package insert for details on dosage adjustment.

## I.V. ADMINISTRATION

● Drug is packaged in a plastic blister to protect against inadvertent breakage and leakage. Inspect vial for damage and signs of leakage before removing blister.

● Store vial at 59° to 86° F (15° to 30° C). Protect from light.

● Premedicate patient with antiemetic drugs on day of treatment starting at least 30 minutes before giving irinotecan.

● Wear gloves while handling and preparing infusion solutions. If drug contacts skin, wash thoroughly with soap and water. If drug contacts mucous membranes, flush thoroughly with water.

● Irinotecan must be diluted in D$_5$W injection (preferred) or normal saline solution for injection before infusion. Final concentration range is 0.12 to 2.8 mg/ml.

● Irinotecan solution is stable for up to 24 hours at 77° F (25° C) and in ambient fluorescent lighting. Solutions diluted in D$_5$W, stored at 36° to 46° F (2° to 8° C), and protected from light are stable for 48 hours. However, because of possible microbial contamination during dilution,

use admixture within 24 hours if refrigerated or 6 hours if kept at room temperature. Refrigerating admixtures using normal saline solution isn't recommended because of low and sporadic risk of visible particulate. Don't freeze admixture because drug may precipitate.

● Don't add other drugs to irinotecan infusion.

● Watch for irritation and infiltration; extravasation can cause tissue damage and necrosis. If extravasation occurs, flush site with sterile water and apply ice. Notify prescriber.

## ACTION

A derivative of camptothecin. Camptothecins interact specifically with the enzyme topoisomerase I, which relieves torsional strain in DNA by inducing reversible single-strand breaks. Irinotecan and its active metabolite SN-38 bind to the topoisomerase I–DNA complex and prevent relegation of these single-strand breaks.

| Route | Onset | Peak | Duration |
|-------|-------|------|----------|
| I.V. | Unknown | 1 hr | Unknown |

## ADVERSE REACTIONS

**CNS:** *insomnia, dizziness, asthenia, headache,* akathisia, *fever, pain.*
**CV:** *vasodilation, edema,* orthostatic hypotension.
**EENT:** *rhinitis.*
**GI:** *diarrhea,* nausea, vomiting, anorexia, stomatitis, constipation, flatulence, dyspepsia; abdominal cramping, pain, and enlargement.
**Hematologic: leukopenia,** anemia, **neutropenia, thrombocytopenia.**
**Metabolic:** *weight loss, dehydration.*
**Musculoskeletal:** *back pain.*
**Respiratory:** *dyspnea, increased cough.*
**Skin:** *alopecia, sweating, rash.*
**Other:** *chills, infection.*

## INTERACTIONS

**Drug-drug.** *Dexamethasone:* May increase risk of irinotecan-induced lymphocytopenia. Monitor patient closely.
*Diuretics:* May increase risk of dehydration and electrolyte imbalance. Consider discontinuing diuretic during active periods of nausea and vomiting.

---

Reactions may be *common,* uncommon, *life-threatening,* or COMMON AND LIFE-THREATENING.

*Laxative use:* May increase risk of diarrhea. Avoid using together.

*Prochlorperazine:* May increase risk of akathisia. Monitor patient closely.

*Other antineoplastics:* May cause additive adverse effects, such as myelosuppression and diarrhea. Monitor patient closely.

**Drug-herb.** *St. John's wort:* May decrease blood levels of irinotecan by about 40%. Discourage use together.

### EFFECTS ON LAB TEST RESULTS
● May increase alkaline phosphatase, AST, and bilirubin levels.
● May decrease hemoglobin and WBC and neutrophil counts.

### CONTRAINDICATIONS & CAUTIONS
● Contraindicated in patients hypersensitive to drug.
● Safety and effectiveness of drug in children haven't been established.
● Use cautiously in elderly patients.

### NURSING CONSIDERATIONS
● Pelvic or abdominal irradiation may increase risk of severe myelosuppression. Avoid use of drug in patients undergoing irradiation.
● Diuretic may be withheld during therapy and periods of active vomiting or diarrhea to decrease risk of dehydration.
● Drug can induce severe diarrhea. Diarrhea occurring within 24 hours of administration may be preceded by diaphoresis and abdominal cramping and may be relieved by 0.25 to 1 mg atropine I.V., unless contraindicated. Diarrhea occurring more than 24 hours after drug administration may be prolonged, leading to dehydration and electrolyte imbalances; it may be life threatening.
● Treat late diarrhea (more than 24 hours after irinotecan administration) promptly with loperamide. Monitor patient for dehydration, electrolyte imbalance, or sepsis, and treat appropriately.
● Delay subsequent irinotecan treatments until normal bowel function returns for at least 24 hours without antidiarrhea medication. If grade 2, 3, or 4 late diarrhea occurs, decrease subsequent doses of irinotecan within the current cycle.
● Temporarily stop therapy if neutropenic fever occurs or if absolute neutrophil

count drops below 500/mm³. Reduce dosage, especially if WBC count is below 2,000/mm³, neutrophil count is below 1,000/mm³, hemoglobin level is below 8 g/dl, or platelet count is below 100,000/mm³.
● Routine administration of a colony-stimulating factor isn't needed but may be helpful in patients with significant neutropenia.
● Monitor WBC count with differential, hemoglobin level, and platelet count before each dose of irinotecan.

### PATIENT TEACHING
● Inform patient about risk of diarrhea and methods to treat it; tell him to avoid laxatives.
● Instruct patient to contact prescriber if any of the following occur: diarrhea for the first time during treatment; black or bloody stools; symptoms of dehydration such as light-headedness, dizziness, or faintness; inability to drink fluids due to nausea or vomiting; inability to control diarrhea within 24 hours; or fever or infection.
● Warn patient that hair loss may occur.
● Caution woman of childbearing age to avoid pregnancy or breast-feeding during therapy.

---

## mitoxantrone hydrochloride
Novantrone

*Pregnancy risk category D*

### AVAILABLE FORMS
*Injection:* 2 mg/ml in 10-ml, 12.5-ml, 15-ml vials

### INDICATIONS & DOSAGES
➤ **Combination initial therapy for acute nonlymphocytic leukemia**
*Adults:* Induction begins with 12 mg/m² I.V. daily on days 1 to 3, with 100 mg/m² daily of cytarabine on days 1 to 7. A second induction may be given if response isn't adequate. Maintenance therapy is 12 mg/m² on days 1 and 2, with cytarabine on days 1 to 5.
➤ **To reduce neurologic disability and frequency of relapse in chronic progres-**

sive, progressive relapsing, or worsening relapsing-remitting multiple sclerosis
*Adults:* 12 mg/m² I.V. over 5 to 15 minutes q 3 months.
✳ *NEW INDICATION:* Advanced hormone-refractory prostate cancer
*Adults:* 12 to 14 mg/m² as a short I.V. infusion q 21 days. Drug is given as an adjunct to corticosteroid therapy.

## I.V. ADMINISTRATION

● *Alert:* Preparation and administration of parenteral form of drug may be mutagenic, teratogenic, or carcinogenic to staff. Follow institutional policy to reduce risks.
● Dilute dose in at least 50 ml of normal saline solution for injection or D₅W injection. Give by direct injection into free-flowing I.V. line of normal saline solution or D₅W injection over at least 3 minutes, usually 15 to 30 minutes. Don't mix with other drugs.
● If extravasation occurs, stop infusion immediately and notify prescriber.
● Once vial is penetrated, undiluted solution may be stored at room temperature for 7 days, or 14 days in refrigerator. Don't freeze.
● Drug is physically incompatible with heparin. Don't mix.

## ACTION

Exact mechanism is unknown. Probably not specific to cell cycle. Reacts with DNA, producing cytotoxic effect.

| Route | Onset | Peak | Duration |
|-------|-------|------|----------|
| I.V. | Unknown | Unknown | Unknown |

## ADVERSE REACTIONS

**CNS:** *seizures,* headache, fever.
**CV:** *arrhythmias,* tachycardia, ECG abnormalities.
**EENT:** conjunctivitis, sinusitis.
**GI:** *bleeding, abdominal pain, diarrhea, nausea, mucositis, vomiting, stomatitis, constipation.*
**GU:** *renal failure, menstrual disorder, amenorrhea, UTI.*
**Hematologic:** *myelosuppression,* anemia.
**Hepatic:** jaundice.
**Metabolic:** hyperuricemia.
**Musculoskeletal:** back pain.
**Respiratory:** *dyspnea, cough, upper respiratory tract infection,* pneumonia.

**Skin:** *alopecia,* petechiae, ecchymoses, local irritation or phlebitis.
**Other:** *fungal infections,* **sepsis.**

## INTERACTIONS
None significant.

## EFFECTS ON LAB TEST RESULTS
● May increase ALT, AST, bilirubin, gamma-GT, and uric acid levels.
● May decrease hemoglobin, hematocrit, and leukocyte and granulocyte counts.

## CONTRAINDICATIONS & CAUTIONS
● Contraindicated in patients hypersensitive to drug.
● Use cautiously in patients with previous exposure to anthracyclines or other cardiotoxic drugs, previous radiation therapy to mediastinal area, or heart disease.

## NURSING CONSIDERATIONS
● Patients with significant myelosuppression shouldn't receive drug unless benefits outweigh risks.
● Give allopurinol. Uric acid nephropathy can be avoided by hydrating patient before and during therapy.
● Closely monitor hematologic and laboratory chemistry parameters.
● To prevent bleeding, avoid all I.M. injections if platelet count falls below 50,000/mm³.
● Anticipate need for blood transfusion to combat anemia. Patients may receive injections of RBC colony-stimulating factors to promote RBC production and decrease need for blood transfusions.
● Monitor left ventricular ejection fraction.
● Treat infections with antibiotics. Patients may receive injections of WBC colony-stimulating factors to promote cell growth and decrease risk of infection.
● If severe nonhematologic toxicity occurs during first course, delay second course until patient recovers.

## PATIENT TEACHING
● Advise patient to report any pain or burning at site of injection during or after administration.
● Tell patient that urine may appear blue-green within 24 hours after administration and that some bluish discoloration of the

---

Reactions may be *common,* uncommon, *life-threatening,* or **COMMON AND LIFE-THREATENING.**

whites of the eyes may occur. These effects aren't harmful and may persist during therapy.
• Advise patient to watch for signs and symptoms of bleeding and infection.
• Caution woman of childbearing age to avoid pregnancy during therapy. Recommend that she consult prescriber before becoming pregnant.

## paclitaxel
Onxol, Taxol

*Pregnancy risk category D*

### AVAILABLE FORMS
*Injection:* 30 mg/5 ml, 100 mg/16.7 ml

### INDICATIONS & DOSAGES
➤ **Second-line treatment of AIDS-related Kaposi's sarcoma (Taxol)**
*Adults:* 135 mg/m² I.V. over 3 hours q 3 weeks, or 100 mg/m² I.V. over 3 hours q 2 weeks.
*Adjust-a-dose:* Don't give drug if baseline or subsequent neutrophil counts are less than 1,000 cells/mm³. Reduce the doses of subsequent doses of Taxol by 20% for patients who experience severe neutropenia (neutrophil count < 500 cells/mm³ for 1 week or longer). Patient also may need reduction in dexamethasone premedication dose (10 mg P.O. instead of 20 mg P.O.) and start of a hematopoietic growth factor.
➤ **First-line and subsequent therapy for advanced ovarian cancer**
*Adults (previously untreated):* 175 mg/m² over 3 hours q 3 weeks, followed by cisplatin 75 mg/m²; or, 135 mg/m² over 24 hours, in combination with cisplatin 75 mg/m², q 3 weeks.
*Adults (previously treated):* 135 or 175 mg/m² I.V. over 3 hours q 3 weeks.
➤ **Breast cancer after failure of combination chemotherapy for metastatic disease or relapse within 6 months of adjuvant chemotherapy (previous therapy should've included an anthracycline unless clinically contraindicated); adjuvant treatment of node-positive breast cancer given sequentially to stan-**

**dard doxorubicin-containing combination chemotherapy**
*Adults:* 175 mg/m² I.V. over 3 hours q 3 weeks.
➤ **First treatment of advanced non–small-cell lung cancer for patients who aren't candidates for curative surgery or radiation (Taxol)**
*Adults:* 135 mg/m² I.V. infusion over 24 hours, followed by cisplatin 75 mg/m². Repeat cycle q 3 weeks.
*Adjust-a-dose:* Subsequent courses shouldn't be repeated until neutrophil count is at least 1,500 cells/mm³ and platelet count is at least 100,000 cells/mm³. Reduce the doses of subsequent doses of Taxol by 20% for patients who experience severe neutropenia (neutrophil less than 500 cells/mm³ for a week or longer) or severe peripheral neuropathy.
For patients with hepatic impairment, adjust doses for the first courses of therapy as follows:
For 24-hour infusion of Taxol, if transaminase levels are < 2 × ULN and bilirubin levels are ≤ 1.5 mg/dl, give 135 mg/m². If transaminase levels are 2 to < 10 × ULN and bilirubin levels are ≤ 1.5 mg/dl, give 100 mg/m². If transaminase levels are < 10 × ULN and bilirubin levels are 1.6 to 7.5 mg/dl, give 50 mg/m². If transaminase levels are ≥ 10 × ULN or bilirubin levels are > 7.5 mg/dl, don't use drug.
For 3-hour infusion of Taxol, if transaminase levels are < 10 × ULN and bilirubin levels are ≤ 1.25 × ULN, give 175 mg/m². If transaminase levels are < 10 × ULN and bilirubin levels are 1.26 to 2 × ULN, give 135 mg/m². If transaminase levels are < 10 × ULN and bilirubin levels are 2.01 to 5 × ULN, give 90 mg/m². If transaminase levels are ≥ 10 × ULN or bilirubin levels are > 5 × ULN, don't use drug.
For subsequent courses, base dosage adjustment on individual tolerance.

### I.V. ADMINISTRATION
• *Alert:* Preparation and administration of parenteral form of drug may be mutagenic, teratogenic, or carcinogenic to staff. Follow institutional policy to reduce risks.

Mark all waste materials with CHEMO-THERAPY HAZARD labels.

• Dilute concentrate before infusion. Compatible solutions include normal saline solution for injection, $D_5W$, 5% dextrose in normal saline solution for injection, and 5% dextrose in Ringer's lactate injection. Dilute to yield 0.3 to 1.2 mg/ml. Diluted solutions are stable for 24 hours at room temperature.

• Prepare and store infusion solutions in glass containers. Undiluted concentrate shouldn't contact polyvinyl chloride I.V. bags or tubing. Prepared solution may appear hazy. Store diluted solution in glass or polypropylene bottles, or use polypropylene or polyolefin bags. Give through polyethylene-lined administration sets, and use an in-line 0.22-micron filter.

• Watch for irritation and infiltration; extravasation can cause tissue damage and necrosis.

• Continuously monitor patient for 30 minutes after starting infusion. Continue close monitoring throughout infusion.

## ACTION

Prevents depolymerization of cellular microtubules, thus inhibiting normal reorganization of microtubule network needed for mitosis and other vital cellular functions.

| Route | Onset | Peak | Duration |
|-------|-------|------|----------|
| I.V. | Unknown | Unknown | Unknown |

## ADVERSE REACTIONS

**CNS:** *peripheral neuropathy, asthenia.*
**CV:** **bradycardia**, hypotension, abnormal ECG.
**GI:** *nausea, vomiting, diarrhea, mucositis.*
**Hematologic:** NEUTROPENIA, LEUKOPENIA, THROMBOCYTOPENIA, *anemia, bleeding.*
**Musculoskeletal:** *myalgia, arthralgia.*
**Skin:** *alopecia; cellulitis and phlebitis at injection site.*
**Other:** hypersensitivity reactions, ***anaphylaxis***, infections.

## INTERACTIONS

**Drug-drug.** *Carbamazepine, phenobarbital:* May increase metabolism and may decrease paclitaxel levels. Use together cautiously.
*Cisplatin:* May cause additive myelosuppressive effects. Give paclitaxel before cisplatin.
*Doxorubicin:* May increase plasma levels of doxorubicin and its active metabolite, doxorubicinol. Use together cautiously.
*Drugs that inhibit cytochrome P450, such as cyclosporine, dexamethasone, diazepam, etoposide, ketoconazole, quinidine, retinoic acid, teniposide, testosterone, verapamil, vincristine:* May increase paclitaxel level. Monitor patient for toxicity.

## EFFECTS ON LAB TEST RESULTS

• May increase alkaline phosphatase, AST, and triglyceride levels.
• May decrease hemoglobin and neutrophil, WBC, and platelet counts.

## CONTRAINDICATIONS & CAUTIONS

• Contraindicated in patients hypersensitive to drug or polyoxyethylated castor oil (a vehicle used in drug solution) and in those with baseline neutrophil counts below 1,500/mm³ or AIDS-related Kaposi's sarcoma with baseline neutrophil counts below 1,000/mm³.
• Use cautiously in patients with hepatic impairment.

## NURSING CONSIDERATIONS

• Some patients experience peripheral neuropathies, which may be cumulative and dose-related. Patients with severe symptoms may need dosage reduction.
• To reduce risk or severity of hypersensitivity, patients must receive pretreatment with corticosteroids, such as dexamethasone, and antihistamines. Both $H_1$-receptor antagonists, such as diphenhydramine, and $H_2$-receptor antagonists, such as cimetidine or ranitidine, may be used. Severe hypersensitivity reactions have occurred in as many as 2% of patients.
• Monitor blood counts often during therapy. Bone marrow toxicity is most common and dose-limiting toxicity. Packed RBC or platelet transfusions may be needed in severe cases. Institute bleeding precautions as appropriate.

---

• Patient may receive injections of RBC colony-stimulating factors to promote RBC production and decrease need for blood transfusions.

• Avoid all I.M. injections when platelet count is below 50,000/mm³.

• If patient develops significant cardiac conduction abnormalities, use appropriate therapy and continuous cardiac monitoring during therapy and subsequent infusions.

• *Alert:* Don't confuse paclitaxel with paroxetine; don't confuse Taxol with Paxil or Taxotere.

## PATIENT TEACHING

• Advise patient to report any pain or burning at site of injection during or after administration.

• Tell patient to watch for signs and symptoms of infection (fever, sore throat, fatigue) and bleeding (easy bruising, nosebleeds, bleeding gums, tarry stools). Tell patient to take temperature daily.

• Teach patient symptoms of peripheral neuropathy, such as a tingling or burning sensation or numbness in limbs, and advise her to report these symptoms immediately.

• Warn patient that reversible hair loss is common (up to 82% of patients).

• Caution woman of childbearing age to avoid becoming pregnant during therapy. Recommend that she consult prescriber before becoming pregnant.

## pegaspargase (PEG-L-asparaginase)
Oncaspar

*Pregnancy risk category C*

### AVAILABLE FORMS
*Injection:* 750 IU/ml

### INDICATIONS & DOSAGES
➤ **Acute lymphoblastic leukemia in patients who need L-asparaginase but have become hypersensitive to native forms of L-asparaginase**
*Adults and children with body surface area (BSA) of at least 0.6 m²:* 2,500 IU/m² I.V. or I.M. q 14 days.

*Children with BSA below 0.6 m²:* 82.5 IU/kg I.V. or I.M. q 14 days.

### I.V. ADMINISTRATION
• Don't give drug that has been frozen. Although its appearance may not change, its activity is destroyed after freezing.

• Avoid excessive agitation of drug; don't shake. Keep refrigerated at 36° to 46° F (2° to 8° C). Don't use if cloudy or contains precipitate. Don't use if stored at room temperature for longer than 48 hours. Don't freeze. Discard unused portions. Use only one dose per vial; don't reenter vial.

• Drug may be a contact irritant, and solution must be handled and given with care. Gloves are recommended. Avoid inhalation of vapors and contact with skin or mucous membranes, especially in the eyes. If contact occurs, wash with generous amounts of water for at least 15 minutes.

• When giving I.V., give over 1 to 2 hours in 100 ml of normal saline solution or D₅W injection through an infusion that is already running.

### ACTION
A modified version of the enzyme L-asparaginase that exerts cytotoxic effects by inactivating the amino acid asparagine. Asparagine is needed by tumor cells to synthesize proteins. Because the tumor cells can't synthesize their own asparagine, protein synthesis and, eventually, synthesis of DNA and RNA are inhibited.

| Route | Onset | Peak | Duration |
|-------|-------|------|----------|
| I.V., I.M. | Unknown | Unknown | Unknown |

### ADVERSE REACTIONS
**CNS:** *seizures,* headache, paresthesia, *status epilepticus,* somnolence, *coma,* mental status changes, dizziness, emotional lability, mood changes, parkinsonism, confusion, disorientation, fatigue, malaise.
**CV:** hypotension, tachycardia, chest pain, subacute bacterial endocarditis, hypertension, peripheral edema.
**EENT:** epistaxis.
**GI:** nausea, vomiting, abdominal pain, anorexia, diarrhea, constipation, indigestion, flatulence, mucositis, mouth tenderness, *pancreatitis,* severe colitis.

**GU:** increased urinary frequency, hematuria, proteinuria, severe hemorrhagic cystitis, renal dysfunction, *renal failure.*

**Hematologic:** *thrombosis, disseminated intravascular coagulation,* hemolytic anemia, *leukopenia; pancytopenia, agranulocytosis, thrombocytopenia,* easy bruising, *hemorrhage.*

**Hepatic:** jaundice, ascites, hypoalbuminemia, fatty changes in liver, *liver failure.*

**Metabolic:** hyperuricemia, hyponatremia, uric acid nephropathy, hypoproteinemia, weight loss, metabolic acidosis, hyperglycemia, *hypoglycemia.*

**Musculoskeletal:** arthralgia, myalgia, musculoskeletal pain, joint stiffness, cramps, pain in limbs.

**Respiratory:** cough, *bronchospasm,* upper respiratory tract infection.

**Skin:** urticaria, itching, alopecia, fever blister, purpura, hand whiteness, fungal changes, nail whiteness and ridging, erythema simplex, petechial rash, injection pain or reaction, localized edema, rash, erythema, ecchymoses.

**Other:** hypersensitivity reactions, night sweats, infection, *sepsis, septic shock, anaphylaxis.*

## INTERACTIONS

**Drug-drug.** *Aspirin, dipyridamole, heparin, NSAIDs, warfarin:* May cause imbalances in coagulation factors, predisposing patient to bleeding or thrombosis. Use together cautiously.

*Methotrexate:* During inhibition of protein synthesis and cell replication, pegaspargase may interfere with action of such drugs as methotrexate, which need cell replication for their lethal effects. Check patient for decreased effectiveness.

*Protein-bound drugs:* Depletion of proteins by pegaspargase may increase toxicity of other drugs that bind to proteins. Check for toxicity. Pegaspargase also may interfere with enzymatic detoxification of other drugs, particularly in the liver. Use together cautiously.

## EFFECTS ON LAB TEST RESULTS

● May increase BUN, creatinine, amylase, lipase, bilirubin, ALT, AST, uric acid, and ammonia levels. May decrease sodium and protein levels. May increase or decrease glucose levels.

● May increase PT, INR, PTT, and thromboplastin. May decrease antithrombin III, hemoglobin, and WBC, RBC, platelet, and granulocyte counts.

## CONTRAINDICATIONS & CAUTIONS

● Contraindicated in patients with pancreatitis or history of pancreatitis, in those who have had significant hemorrhagic events related to previous treatment with L-asparaginase, and in those with history of serious allergic reactions to drug, such as generalized urticaria, bronchospasm, laryngeal edema, hypotension, or other unacceptable adverse reactions.

● Use cautiously in patients with liver dysfunction; use only when clearly indicated in pregnant women.

## NURSING CONSIDERATIONS

● Use drug as sole induction drug only in patients refractory to other therapy, or when combined regimen using other chemotherapeutic drugs is inappropriate because of toxicity or other specific patient-related factors.

● Take preventive measures (including adequate hydration) before starting treatment. Hyperuricemia may result from rapid lysis of leukemic cells. Allopurinol may be ordered.

● I.M. route is preferred because it has the lowest risk of hepatotoxicity, coagulopathy, and GI and renal disorders.

● When giving I.M., limit volume given at a single injection site to 2 ml. If volume to be given exceeds 2 ml, use multiple injection sites.

● *Alert:* Monitor patient closely for hypersensitivity (including life-threatening anaphylaxis), especially those hypersensitive to other forms of L-asparaginase. As a routine precaution, keep patient under observation for 1 hour and have readily available resuscitation equipment and other drugs needed to treat anaphylaxis (such as epinephrine, oxygen, and I.V. corticosteroids). Moderate to life-threatening hypersensitivity requires stopping L-asparaginase.

● To assess effects of therapy, monitor patient's peripheral blood count and bone marrow. A drop in circulating lymphoblasts is often noted after therapy starts,

---

Reactions may be *common,* uncommon, *life-threatening,* or COMMON AND LIFE-THREATENING.

sometimes accompanied by a marked rise in uric acid level.
• Obtain frequent amylase and lipase determinations to detect pancreatitis. Monitor patient's glucose level during therapy to detect hyperglycemia.
• Monitor patient for liver dysfunction when drug is used with hepatotoxic chemotherapeutic drugs.
• Drug may affect several plasma proteins; monitoring of fibrinogen, PT, INR, and PTT may be indicated.

### PATIENT TEACHING
• Inform patient of risk of hypersensitivity reactions and importance of reporting them immediately.
• Tell patient not to take other drugs, including OTC preparations, until approved by prescriber because risk of bleeding is higher when pegaspargase is given with drugs such as aspirin. Pegaspargase may also increase toxicity of other drugs.
• Urge patient to report signs and symptoms of infection (fever, chills, and malaise); drug may suppress the immune system.
• Caution woman of childbearing age to avoid pregnancy and breast-feeding during therapy.

---

## procarbazine hydrochloride
Matulane, Natulan†

*Pregnancy risk category D*

### AVAILABLE FORMS
*Capsules:* 50 mg

### INDICATIONS & DOSAGES
➤ **Adjunct treatment of Hodgkin's disease (stages III and IV), other cancers using MOPP (nitrogen mustard, vincristine, procarbazine, prednisone) regimen**
*Adults:* 2 to 4 mg/kg P.O. daily in single dose or divided doses for first week. Then, 4 to 6 mg/kg daily until WBC count falls below 4,000/mm³, platelet count falls below 100,000/mm³, or maximum response is obtained. Maintenance dose is 1 to 2 mg/kg daily after bone marrow recovery. For MOPP regimen, 100 mg/m² daily P.O. for 14 days of 28-day cycle.

*Children:* 50 mg/m² P.O. daily for first week; then 100 mg/m² until response or toxicity occurs. Maintenance dose is 50 mg/m² P.O. daily after bone marrow recovery.

### ACTION
Unknown. Thought to inhibit DNA, RNA, and protein synthesis.

| Route | Onset | Peak | Duration |
|-------|-------|------|----------|
| P.O. | Unknown | Unknown | Unknown |

### ADVERSE REACTIONS
**CNS:** nervousness, depression, headache, dizziness, *coma*, insomnia, nightmares, paresthesia, neuropathy, *hallucinations*, confusion, syncope.
**CV:** hypotension, tachycardia, flushing.
**EENT:** retinal hemorrhage, nystagmus, photophobia.
**GI:** *nausea, vomiting,* abdominal pain, hematemesis, melena, anorexia, stomatitis, dry mouth, dysphagia, diarrhea, constipation.
**GU:** hematuria, urinary frequency, nocturia.
**Hematologic:** *bleeding tendency, thrombocytopenia, leukopenia, anemia,* hemolytic anemia, *pancytopenia,* eosinophilia.
**Hepatic:** *hepatotoxicity,* jaundice.
**Respiratory:** *pleural effusion,* cough, pneumonitis.
**Skin:** reversible alopecia, dermatitis, pruritus, rash, hyperpigmentation.
**Other:** gynecomastia, allergic reaction, herpes outbreak, *secondary malignancies.*

### INTERACTIONS
**Drug-drug.** *CNS depressants:* May cause additive depressant effects. Avoid using together.
*Digoxin:* May decrease digoxin levels. Monitor digoxin levels closely.
*Drugs high in tyramine, local anesthetics, MAO inhibitors, sympathomimetics, tricyclic antidepressants:* May cause tremor, palpitations, increased blood pressure. Monitor patient closely.
*Levodopa:* May cause sudden hypertensive crisis. Don't give within 2 to 4 weeks of procarbazine.
**Drug-food.** *Caffeine:* May result in arrhythmias, severe hypertension. Discourage caffeine intake.

*Foods high in tyramine (cheese, Chianti wine):* May cause tremor, palpitations, increased blood pressure. Monitor patient closely; advise him to avoid or limit intake.

**Drug-lifestyle.** *Alcohol use:* Mild disulfiram-like reaction may cause flushing, headache, nausea, and hypotension. Warn patient to avoid alcoholic beverages.

## EFFECTS ON LAB TEST RESULTS
● May increase eosinophil count. May decrease hemoglobin and platelet, WBC, and RBC counts.

## CONTRAINDICATIONS & CAUTIONS
● Contraindicated in patients hypersensitive to drug and in those with inadequate bone marrow reserve as shown by bone marrow aspiration.
● Use cautiously in patients with impaired hepatic or renal function.

## NURSING CONSIDERATIONS
● Monitor CBC and platelet counts.
● Bone marrow depression begins 2 to 8 weeks after the start of treatment.
● To prevent bleeding, avoid all I.M. injections when platelet count is below 50,000/mm³.
● Anticipate need for blood transfusions to combat anemia. Patients may receive injections of RBC colony-stimulating factors to promote RBC production and decrease need for blood transfusions.
● Stop drug if patient becomes confused or if paresthesia or other neuropathies develop. Notify prescriber.
● The manufacturer recommends that if radiation or chemotherapeutic agents known to have marrow-depressant activity have been used, give patient a 1 month interval without such therapy before beginning procarbazine therapy.

## PATIENT TEACHING
● To decrease nausea and vomiting, advise patient to take drug at bedtime and in divided doses.
● Tell patient to watch for signs of infection (fever, sore throat, fatigue) and bleeding (easy bruising, nosebleeds, bleeding gums, tarry stools). Tell patient to take temperature daily.

● Warn patient to avoid alcohol during therapy. Urge him to stop drug and check with prescriber immediately if, after drinking alcohol, he experiences a disulfiram-like reaction (chest pains, rapid or irregular heartbeat, severe headache, stiff neck).
● Instruct patient to avoid OTC medications that contain sympathomimetics. Also, tell him to avoid foods and drinks high in tyramine, such as wine, tea, coffee, cola, cheese, and bananas.
● Warn patient to avoid hazardous activities that require alertness and good motor coordination until CNS effects of drug are known.
● Caution woman of childbearing age to avoid becoming pregnant during therapy and to consult prescriber before becoming pregnant.

## rituximab
Rituxan

*Pregnancy risk category C*

### AVAILABLE FORMS
*Injection:* 10 mg/ml; 10-ml, 50-ml single-use, sterile vials

### INDICATIONS & DOSAGES
➤ **Relapsed or refractory low-grade or follicular, CD20-positive, B-cell non-Hodgkin's malignant lymphoma**
*Adults:* Initial therapy, 375 mg/m² I.V. infusion once weekly for 4 or 8 doses. Start first infusion at 50 mg/hour. If hypersensitivity or infusion-related events don't occur, increase rate in 50 mg/hour increments q 30 minutes to maximum of 400 mg/hour. Give subsequent infusions at initial rate of 100 mg/hour and increase by increments of 100 mg/hour q 30 minutes to maximum of 400 mg/hour as tolerated.

Retreatment for patients with progressive disease, 375 mg/m² I.V. infusion once weekly for 4 doses.

### I.V. ADMINISTRATION
● *Alert:* Drug must be given as I.V. infusion; don't give as I.V. push or bolus.
● Dilute to yield 1 to 4 mg/ml in bag of D₅W or normal saline solution. Gently invert bag to mix solution. Discard unused

portion left in vial. Diluted solutions are stable for 24 hours if refrigerated and for 12 hours at room temperature.
• Monitor patient's blood pressure closely during infusion. If hypotension, bronchospasm, or angioedema occurs, stop infusion and restart at a 50% rate reduction when symptoms resolve.
• Stop infusion if serious or life-threatening arrhythmias occur. Patients who develop clinically significant arrhythmias should undergo cardiac monitoring during and after subsequent infusions of rituximab.

## ACTION
A murine and human monoclonal antibody directed against CD20 antigen found on the surface of normal and malignant B lymphocytes. Binding to this antigen mediates the lysis of the B cells.

| Route | Onset | Peak | Duration |
|-------|-------|------|----------|
| I.V. | Variable | Variable | 6-12 mo |

## ADVERSE REACTIONS
**CNS:** dizziness, *asthenia, headache,* fatigue, paresthesia, malaise, agitation, insomnia, hypesthesia, hypertonia, nervousness, *fever,* pain, vertigo, somnolence.
**CV:** *hypotension, arrhythmias,* hypertension, peripheral edema, chest pain, tachycardia, *bradycardia,* flushing, edema.
**EENT:** sore throat, rhinitis, sinusitis, lacrimation disorder, conjunctivitis.
**GI:** *nausea,* vomiting, abdominal pain or enlargement, diarrhea, dyspepsia, anorexia, taste perversion.
**GU:** *acute renal failure.*
**Hematologic:** LEUKOPENIA, *thrombocytopenia, neutropenia,* anemia.
**Metabolic:** hyperglycemia, hypocalcemia, weight decrease.
**Musculoskeletal:** myalgia, back pain, arthritis.
**Respiratory:** *bronchospasm,* dyspnea, cough increase, bronchitis.
**Skin:** *pruritus, rash,* urticaria, *severe mucocutaneous reactions,* pain at injection site.
**Other:** ANGIOEDEMA, *chills, rigors,* tumor pain, tumor lysis syndrome, infection.

## INTERACTIONS
**Drug-drug.** *Cisplatin:* Use together may result in renal toxicity. Monitor renal function tests if used together.

## EFFECTS ON LAB TEST RESULTS
• May increase glucose and LDH levels. May decrease calcium level.
• May decrease hemoglobin and WBC, platelet, and neutrophil counts.

## CONTRAINDICATIONS & CAUTIONS
• Contraindicated in patients with type I hypersensitivity or anaphylactic reactions to murine proteins or components of rituximab.

## NURSING CONSIDERATIONS
• Monitor patient closely for signs and symptoms of hypersensitivity. Have drugs, such as epinephrine, antihistamines, and corticosteroids, available to immediately treat such a reaction. Premedicate with acetaminophen and diphenhydramine before each infusion.
• Severe mucocutaneous reactions (including toxic epidermal necrolysis [TEN], Stevens-Johnson syndrome, paraneoplastic pemphigus, and lichenoid or vesiculobullous dermatitis) have occurred in patients receiving rituximab ranging from 1 to 13 weeks after administration. Avoid further infusions and promptly start treatment of the skin reaction.
• Infusion-related reactions are most severe with the first infusion. Subsequent infusions are generally well tolerated.
• Obtain CBC at regular intervals and more frequently in patients who develop cytopenias.
• Protect vials from direct sunlight.

## PATIENT TEACHING
• Tell patient to report symptoms of hypersensitivity, such as itching, rash, chills, or rigor, during and after infusion.
• Urge patient to watch for signs and symptoms of infection (fever, sore throat, fatigue) and bleeding (easy bruising, nosebleeds, bleeding gums, tarry stools). Tell patient to take temperature daily.
• Advise breast-feeding women to stop breast-feeding until drug levels are undetectable.

---

# teniposide (VM-26)
Vumon

*Pregnancy risk category D*

## AVAILABLE FORMS
*Injection:* 10 mg/ml

## INDICATIONS & DOSAGES
➤ **Refractory childhood acute lymphoblastic leukemia**
*Children:* Optimum dosage hasn't been established. Dosages ranging from 165 to 250 mg/m² I.V. once or twice weekly for 4 to 8 weeks have been used. Usually given with other drugs.
*Adjust-a-dose:* Patients with both Down syndrome and leukemia are at higher risk for myelosuppression. Give first course of treatment at half the recommended dosage.

## I.V. ADMINISTRATION
● Dilute drug in either D₅W or normal saline solution for injection to 0.1, 0.2, 0.4, or 1 mg/ml. Don't agitate vigorously; precipitation may occur. Discard cloudy solutions. Prepare and store drug in glass containers. Infuse over at least 30 to 60 minutes to prevent hypotension.
● Don't mix with other drugs or solutions. Heparin solution can cause precipitation. Flush administration apparatus and catheters with D₅W or normal saline solution before and after infusion of drug.
● Ensure careful placement of I.V. catheter. Extravasation can cause local tissue necrosis or sloughing.
● Occlusion of catheters can occur (including those centrally placed), particularly during 24-hour infusions at 0.1 to 0.2 mg/ml. Monitor catheters carefully.
● Don't use a membrane-type in-line filter because diluent may dissolve it.
● Monitor blood pressure every 30 minutes during infusion. If systolic blood pressure falls below 90 mm Hg, stop infusion and notify prescriber.
● In normal saline solution or D₅W, concentrations of 0.1 to 0.4 mg/ml in glass containers are chemically stable for up to 24 hours at room temperature. Refrigeration isn't recommended. Give solutions

with a concentration of 1 mg/ml within 4 hours to reduce possible precipitation.
● **Alert:** Preparation and administration of parenteral form of drug may be mutagenic, teratogenic, or carcinogenic to staff. Follow institutional policy to reduce risks.
● Use non-DEHP (di[2-ethylhexyl] phthalate) containers and tubing for administration.

## ACTION
A phase-specific cytotoxic drug that acts in the late S or early G₂ phase of the cell cycle, thus preventing cells from entering mitosis.

| Route | Onset | Peak | Duration |
|-------|-------|------|----------|
| I.V. | Unknown | Unknown | Unknown |

## ADVERSE REACTIONS
**CNS:** fever.
**CV:** hypotension.
**GI:** *nausea, vomiting, mucositis, diarrhea.*
**Hematologic:** MYELOSUPPRESSION, LEUKOPENIA, NEUTROPENIA, THROMBOCYTOPENIA, anemia.
**Skin:** rash, alopecia; *extravasation at injection site.*
**Other:** *infection,* bleeding, hypersensitivity reactions, ***anaphylaxis,*** phlebitis.

## INTERACTIONS
**Drug-drug.** *Methotrexate:* May increase clearance and intracellular levels of methotrexate. Avoid using together.
*Sodium salicylate, sulfamethizole, tolbutamide:* May displace teniposide from protein-binding sites and increase toxicity. Avoid using together.

## EFFECTS ON LAB TEST RESULTS
● May decrease hemoglobin and WBC, platelet, and neutrophil levels.

## CONTRAINDICATIONS & CAUTIONS
● Contraindicated in patients hypersensitive to drug or to polyoxyethylated castor oil, an injection vehicle.

## NURSING CONSIDERATIONS
● Drug may be prescribed despite patient's history of hypersensitivity because therapeutic benefits outweigh risks. Treat such patients with antihistamines and cortico-

steroids before infusion begins, and observe continuously for first hour of infusion and at frequent intervals thereafter.
• Obtain baseline blood counts and renal and hepatic function tests.
• Monitor blood pressure before and during therapy. Hypotension can occur from rapid infusion.
• Have on hand diphenhydramine, hydrocortisone, epinephrine, and emergency equipment to establish an airway in case of anaphylaxis. Signs of hypersensitivity include chills, fever, urticaria, tachycardia, bronchospasm, dyspnea, hypotension, and flushing.
• Monitor blood counts and renal and hepatic function tests.

**PATIENT TEACHING**
• Advise patient to report any pain or burning at site of injection during or after administration.
• Tell patient to report signs and symptoms of infection (fever, sore throat, fatigue) and bleeding (easy bruising, nosebleeds, bleeding gums, tarry stools). Tell patient to take temperature daily.
• Caution woman of childbearing age to avoid becoming pregnant during therapy and to consult prescriber before becoming pregnant.

---

## topotecan hydrochloride
Hycamtin

*Pregnancy risk category D*

**AVAILABLE FORMS**
*Injection:* 4-mg single-dose vial

**INDICATIONS & DOSAGES**
➤ **Metastatic carcinoma of the ovary after failure of first or subsequent chemotherapy; small-cell lung cancer–sensitive disease after failure of first-line chemotherapy**
*Adults:* 1.5 mg/m² I.V. infusion given over 30 minutes daily for 5 consecutive days, starting on day 1 of a 21-day cycle. Give a minimum of four cycles.
*Adjust-a-dose:* For patients with creatinine clearance of 20 to 39 ml/minute, decrease dosage to 0.75 mg/m². If severe

neutropenia occurs, decrease dosage by 0.25 mg/m² for subsequent courses. Or, if severe neutropenia occurs, give granulocyte colony-stimulating factor after subsequent course (before resorting to dosage reduction) starting from day 6 of course (24 hours after completion of topotecan administration).

**I.V. ADMINISTRATION**
• Reconstitute each 4-mg vial with 4 ml sterile water for injection. Dilute appropriate volume of reconstituted solution in either normal saline solution or D₅W before administration.
• Because lyophilized dosage form contains no antibacterial preservative, use reconstituted product immediately.
• Protect unopened vials from light. Reconstituted drug stored at 68° to 77° F (20° to 25° C) and exposed to ambient lighting is stable for 24 hours.
• Inadvertent drug extravasation has been linked to mild local reactions, such as erythema and bruising.

**ACTION**
Relieves torsional strain in DNA by inducing reversible single-strand breaks. Binds to the topoisomerase I–DNA complex and prevents relegation of these single-strand breaks. Cytotoxicity of topotecan is thought to result from double-strand DNA damage produced during DNA synthesis when replication enzymes interact with the ternary complex formed by topotecan, topoisomerase I, and DNA.

| Route | Onset | Peak | Duration |
|-------|-------|------|----------|
| I.V. | Unknown | Unknown | Unknown |

**ADVERSE REACTIONS**
**CNS:** *fatigue, asthenia, headache, fever.*
**GI:** *nausea, vomiting, diarrhea, constipation, abdominal pain, stomatitis, anorexia.*
**Hematologic:** NEUTROPENIA, LEUKOPENIA, THROMBOCYTOPENIA, *anemia.*
**Hepatic:** *hepatotoxicity.*
**Musculoskeletal:** *back and skeletal pain.*
**Respiratory:** *dyspnea, coughing.*
**Skin:** *alopecia, rash.*
**Other:** *sepsis.*

## INTERACTIONS
**Drug-drug.** *Cisplatin:* May increase severity of myelosuppression. Use together with extreme caution.
*Granulocyte colony-stimulating factor:* May prolong duration of neutropenia. If granulocyte colony-stimulating factor is to be used, don't start it until day 6 of the course, 24 hours after completion of topotecan treatment.

## EFFECTS ON LAB TEST RESULTS
• May increase ALT, AST, and bilirubin levels.
• May decrease hemoglobin and WBC, platelet, and neutrophil counts.

## CONTRAINDICATIONS & CAUTIONS
• Contraindicated in patients hypersensitive to drug or its components and in those with severe bone marrow depression.
• Contraindicated in pregnant or breast-feeding women.
• Safety and effectiveness of drug in children haven't been established.

## NURSING CONSIDERATIONS
• *Alert:* Before first course of therapy is started, patient must have baseline neutrophil count over 1,500 cells/mm³ and platelet count over 100,000 cells/mm³.
• Prepare drug under vertical laminar flow hood; wear gloves and protective clothing. If drug solution contacts skin, wash immediately and thoroughly with soap and water. If mucous membranes are affected, flush areas thoroughly with water.
• Bone marrow suppression (primarily neutropenia) indicates toxic levels of topotecan. The nadir occurs at about 11 days. Neutropenia isn't cumulative over time.
• Duration of thrombocytopenia is about 5 days, with nadir at 15 days. The nadir for anemia is 15 days. Blood or platelet transfusions may be needed.
• Monitor peripheral blood cell counts frequently. Don't give subsequent courses of topotecan until neutrophil count recovers to more than 1,000 cells/mm³, platelet count recovers to more than 100,000 cells/mm³, and hemoglobin level recovers to more than 9 mg/dl (with transfusion, if needed).

• Patient may receive injections of WBC colony-stimulating factors to promote cell growth and decrease risk for infection.

## PATIENT TEACHING
• Urge patient to promptly report sore throat, fever, chills, or unusual bleeding or bruising.
• Caution woman of childbearing age to avoid pregnancy or breast-feeding during therapy.
• Teach patient and family about drug's adverse reactions and need for frequent monitoring of blood counts.

---

## trastuzumab
Herceptin

*Pregnancy risk category B*

## AVAILABLE FORMS
*Injection:* lyophilized sterile powder containing 440 mg per vial

## INDICATIONS & DOSAGES
➤ **Single-drug treatment of metastatic breast cancer in patients whose tumors overexpress the human epidermal growth factor receptor 2 (HER2) protein and who have received one or more chemotherapy regimens for their metastatic disease, or with paclitaxel for metastatic breast cancer in patients whose tumors overexpress the HER2 protein and who haven't received chemotherapy for their metastatic disease**
*Adults:* First loading dose is 4 mg/kg I.V. over 90 minutes. Maintenance dose is 2 mg/kg I.V. weekly as 30-minute I.V. infusion if first loading dose is well tolerated.

## I.V. ADMINISTRATION
• Don't give as an I.V. push or bolus.
• Reconstitute drug in each vial with 20 ml of bacteriostatic water for injection, 1.1% benzyl alcohol preserved, as supplied, to yield a multidose solution containing 21 mg/ml. Don't shake vial during reconstitution. Make sure reconstituted preparation is colorless to pale yellow and free of particulates. Immediately after re-

---

constitution, label vial with expiration 28 days from date of reconstitution.

• **Alert:** If patient is hypersensitive to benzyl alcohol, reconstitute drug with sterile water for injection, use immediately, and discard unused portion. Avoid use of other reconstitution diluents.

• Determine dose based on loading dose of 4 mg/kg or maintenance dose of 2 mg/kg. Calculate volume of 21-mg/ml solution and withdraw this amount from vial and add it to an infusion bag containing 250 ml of normal saline solution. Don't use D₅W or dextrose-containing solutions. Gently invert bag to mix solution.

• Infuse loading dose over 90 minutes. If well tolerated, infuse maintenance doses over 30 minutes.

• Don't mix or dilute with other drugs.

• Vials of drug are stable at 36° to 46° F (2° to 8° C) before reconstitution. Discard reconstituted solution after 28 days. Don't freeze drug that has been reconstituted. Store solution of drug diluted in normal saline solution for injection at 36° to 46° F (2° to 8° C) before use; it's stable for up to 24 hours.

## ACTION

A recombinant DNA-derived monoclonal antibody that selectively binds to HER2, inhibiting proliferation of human tumor cells that overexpress HER2.

| Route | Onset | Peak | Duration |
|-------|-------|------|----------|
| I.V. | Unknown | Unknown | Unknown |

## ADVERSE REACTIONS

**CNS:** depression, *dizziness, insomnia,* neuropathy, paresthesia, peripheral neuritis, *asthenia, headache, fever, pain.*
**CV: heart failure,** *peripheral edema,* tachycardia, hypotension.
**EENT:** *rhinitis, pharyngitis,* sinusitis.
**GI:** *anorexia, abdominal pain, diarrhea, nausea, vomiting.*
**GU:** UTI.
**Hematologic:** *leukopenia,* anemia.
**Musculoskeletal:** arthralgia, *back pain,* bone pain.
**Respiratory:** *dyspnea, increased cough.*
**Skin:** acne, *rash.*
**Other:** allergic reaction, herpes simplex, *chills, flulike syndrome,* infection, ANA-PHYLAXIS.

## INTERACTIONS

**Drug-drug.** *Anthracyclines, cyclophosphamide:* May increase cardiotoxicity. Use together very cautiously.

## EFFECTS ON LAB TEST RESULTS

• May decrease hemoglobin and WBC count.

## CONTRAINDICATIONS & CAUTIONS

• Contraindicated in patients hypersensitive to the drug.

• Use cautiously in elderly patients, in patients hypersensitive to drug or its components, and in those with cardiac dysfunction.

• Give drug with extreme caution in patients with pre-existing pulmonary compromise, symptomatic intrinsic pulmonary disease (such as asthma, COPD), or extensive tumor involvement of the lungs.

• Safety and effectiveness of drug in children haven't been established.

## NURSING CONSIDERATIONS

• Before beginning therapy, patient should undergo thorough baseline cardiac assessment, including history and physical examination and methods to identify risk of cardiotoxicity.

• Assess patient for signs and symptoms of cardiac dysfunction, especially if he is receiving drug with anthracyclines and cyclophosphamide.

• Check for dyspnea, increased cough, paroxysmal nocturnal dyspnea, peripheral edema, or S₃ gallop. Treatment may be stopped in patients who develop a significant decrease in left ventricular function.

• Monitor patient receiving both drug and chemotherapy closely for cardiac dysfunction or failure, anemia, leukopenia, diarrhea, and infection.

• Use drug only in patients with metastatic breast cancer whose tumors have HER2 protein overexpression.

• Check for first-infusion symptom complex, commonly consisting of chills or fever. Treat with acetaminophen, diphenhydramine, and meperidine (with or without reducing rate of infusion). Other signs or symptoms include nausea, vomiting, pain, rigors, headache, dizziness, dyspnea, hypotension, rash, and asthenia. These symptoms occur infrequently with subsequent infusions.

## PATIENT TEACHING
• Tell patient about risk of first-dose infusion-related adverse reactions.
• Urge patient to notify prescriber immediately if signs or symptoms of heart problems occur, such as shortness of breath, increased cough, or swelling in arms or legs. Tell patient that these effects can occur after infusion is complete.
• Instruct patient to report adverse effects to prescriber.
• Advise breast-feeding woman to stop breast-feeding during drug therapy and for 6 months after last dose of drug.

---

## vinblastine sulfate (VLB)
Velban, Velbe†‡

*Pregnancy risk category D*

### AVAILABLE FORMS
*Injection:* 10-mg vials (lyophilized powder), 1 mg/ml in 10-ml vials

### INDICATIONS & DOSAGES
➤ **Breast or testicular cancer, Hodgkin's disease and malignant lymphoma, choriocarcinoma, lymphosarcoma, mycosis fungoides, Kaposi's sarcoma, histiocytosis**
*Adults:* 3.7 mg/m² I.V. weekly. May increase to maximum dose of 18.5 mg/m² I.V. weekly based on response. Don't repeat dose if WBC count is below 4,000/mm³. Increase dosage at weekly intervals in increments of 1.8 mg/m² until desired therapeutic response is obtained, leukocyte count decreases to 3,000/mm³, or maximum weekly dose of 18.5 mg/m² is reached.
*Children:* First dose is 2.5 mg/m² I.V. weekly. Increase dosage by 1.25 mg/m² weekly until WBC count is below 3,000/mm³ or tumor response is seen. Maximum dose is 12.5 mg/m² I.V. weekly.
*Adjust-a-dose:* For patients with direct bilirubin over 3 mg/dl, reduce dose by 50%. For patients with recent exposure to radiation therapy or chemotherapy, single doses usually don't exceed 5.5 mg/m².

Once a dose is determined to produce a WBC count below 3,000/mm³, give maintenance doses of one increment less than this amount at weekly intervals.

### I.V. ADMINISTRATION
• *Alert:* Preparation and administration of parenteral form of drug may be mutagenic, teratogenic, or carcinogenic to staff. Follow institutional policy to reduce risks.
• *Alert:* Drug is fatal if given intrathecally; it's for I.V. use only.
• Inject drug directly into vein or tubing of running I.V. line over 1 minute. Drug is a vesicant; if extravasation occurs, stop infusion immediately and notify prescriber. The manufacturer recommends that moderate heat be applied to area of leakage. Local injection of hyaluronidase may help disperse drug. Moderate heat may be applied on and off every 2 hours for 24 hours, with local injection of hydrocortisone or normal saline solution.
• Reconstitute drug in 10-mg vial with 10 ml of saline solution for injection. Don't use other diluents. This yields 1 mg/ml. Protect solution from light. Drug reconstituted with diluent containing preservatives is stable for 28 days if refrigerated. Immediately discard any unused portion of solution reconstituted with diluent that doesn't contain preservatives.

### ACTION
Arrests mitosis in metaphase, blocking cell division.

| Route | Onset | Peak | Duration |
|-------|-------|------|----------|
| I.V. | Unknown | Unknown | Unknown |

### ADVERSE REACTIONS
**CNS:** depression, *paresthesia, peripheral neuropathy and neuritis, numbness,* headache, *CVA.*
**CV:** hypertension, *MI.*
**EENT:** pharyngitis.
**GI:** *nausea, vomiting,* bleeding ulcer, *constipation, ileus, anorexia,* diarrhea, abdominal pain, *stomatitis.*
**Hematologic:** anemia, **leukopenia, thrombocytopenia.**
**Metabolic:** hyperuricemia, *weight loss,* SIADH.

---

**Musculoskeletal:** *muscle pain and weakness,* jaw pain, *loss of deep tendon reflexes.*
**Respiratory:** *acute bronchospasm,* shortness of breath.
**Skin:** reversible alopecia, vesiculation; *irritation, phlebitis,* cellulitis, and necrosis with extravasation.

## INTERACTIONS
**Drug-drug.** *Erythromycin, itraconazole, other drugs that inhibit cytochrome P450 pathway:* May increase toxicity of vinblastine. Monitor patient closely for toxicity.
*Mitomycin:* May increase risk of bronchospasm and shortness of breath. Monitor patient's respiratory status.
*Ototoxic drugs such as platinum-containing antineoplastics:* May cause temporary or permanent hearing impairment. Monitor hearing function.
*Phenytoin:* May decrease plasma phenytoin level. Monitor phenytoin level closely.

## EFFECTS ON LAB TEST RESULTS
• May increase uric acid and bilirubin levels.
• May decrease hemoglobin and WBC and platelet counts.

## CONTRAINDICATIONS & CAUTIONS
• Contraindicated in patients with severe leukopenia or bacterial infection or in patients hypersensitive to the drug.
• Use cautiously in patients with hepatic dysfunction.

## NURSING CONSIDERATIONS
• To reduce nausea, give antiemetic before drug.
• Don't give drug into a limb with compromised circulation.
• *Alert:* After giving drug, check for development of life-threatening acute bronchospasm. If this occurs, notify prescriber immediately. Reaction is most likely to occur in patients who are also receiving mitomycin.
• Monitor patient for stomatitis. Stop drug if stomatitis occurs and notify prescriber.
• Assess bowel activity. Give laxatives as needed and ordered. Stool softeners may be used prophylactically.

• Dosage shouldn't be repeated more frequently than every 7 days or severe leukopenia will occur. Nadir occurs on days 4 to 10 and lasts another 7 to 14 days.
• Assess patient for numbness and tingling in hands and feet. Assess gait for early evidence of footdrop.
• Drug is less neurotoxic than vincristine.
• Anticipate a decrease in dosage by 50% if bilirubin levels exceed 3 mg/100 ml.
• Stop drugs known to cause urine retention for first few days after vinblastine therapy, particularly in elderly patients.
• *Alert:* Don't confuse vinblastine with vincristine, vindesine, or vinorelbine.

## PATIENT TEACHING
• Tell patient to report evidence of infection (fever, sore throat, fatigue) and bleeding (easy bruising, nosebleeds, bleeding gums, tarry stools). Tell patient to take temperature daily.
• Urge patient to report pain, swelling, burning, or any unusual feeling at injection site during infusion.
• Warn patient that hair loss may occur, but explain that it's usually reversible.
• Caution woman of childbearing age to avoid pregnancy during therapy.
• Tell patient that pain may occur in jaw and in organ containing tumor.

---

## vincristine sulfate (VCR)
Oncovin, Vincasar PFS

*Pregnancy risk category D*

### AVAILABLE FORMS
*Injection:* 1 mg/ml in 1-ml, 2-ml, 5-ml multidose vials; 1 mg/ml in 1-ml, 2-ml, 5-ml preservative-free vials

### INDICATIONS & DOSAGES
➤ **Acute lymphoblastic and other leukemias, Hodgkin's disease, malignant lymphoma, neuroblastoma, rhabdomyosarcoma, Wilms' tumor**
*Adults:* 0.4 to 1.4 mg/m$^2$ I.V. weekly. Maximum weekly dose is 2 mg.
*Children weighing more than 10 kg (22 lb):* 1.5 to 2 mg/m$^2$ I.V. weekly.
*Children weighing 10 kg and less or with body surface area less than 1 m$^2$:* Initially, 0.05 mg/kg I.V. weekly.

***Adjust-a-dose:*** For patients with direct bilirubin over 3 mg/dl, reduce dose by 50%.

## I.V. ADMINISTRATION
• ***Alert:*** Preparation and administration of parenteral form of drug may be mutagenic, teratogenic, or carcinogenic to staff. Follow institutional policy to reduce risks.
• Inject directly into vein or tubing of running I.V. line slowly over 1 minute. Vincristine is a vesicant; if it extravasates, stop infusion immediately and notify prescriber. Apply heat on and off every 2 hours for 24 hours.
• If protocol requires a continuous infusion of vincristine, a central line must be used.

## ACTION
Arrests mitosis in metaphase, blocking cell division.

| Route | Onset | Peak | Duration |
|-------|-------|------|----------|
| I.V. | Unknown | Unknown | Unknown |

## ADVERSE REACTIONS
**CNS:** *peripheral neuropathy,* sensory loss, *loss of deep tendon reflexes, paresthesia, wristdrop and footdrop, **seizures, coma,*** headache, ataxia, cranial nerve palsies, fever.
**CV:** hypotension, hypertension.
**EENT:** visual disturbances, blindness, diplopia, optic and extraocular neuropathy, ptosis, hoarseness, vocal cord paralysis, photophobia.
**GI:** diarrhea, *constipation, cramps,* ileus that mimics surgical abdomen, paralytic ileus, *nausea, vomiting,* anorexia, dysphagia, ***intestinal necrosis,*** stomatitis.
**GU:** urine retention, SIADH, dysuria, polyuria.
**Hematologic:** anemia, ***leukopenia, thrombocytopenia.***
**Metabolic:** weight loss, hyponatremia.
**Musculoskeletal:** *jaw pain, muscle weakness, cramps.*
**Respiratory:** ***acute bronchospasm,*** dyspnea.
**Skin:** rash, reversible alopecia, severe local reaction following extravasation, *phlebitis,* cellulitis at injection site.

## INTERACTIONS
**Drug-drug.** *Asparaginase:* May decrease hepatic clearance of vincristine. Use together also may result in additive neurotoxicity. Monitor patient for toxicity.
*Digoxin:* May decrease digoxin's effects. Monitor digoxin level.
*Mitomycin:* May increase frequency of bronchospasm and acute pulmonary reactions. Monitor patient's respiratory status.
*Ototoxic drugs:* May potentiate loss of hearing. Use together with caution.
*Phenytoin:* May reduce phenytoin level. Monitor phenytoin level closely.

## EFFECTS ON LAB TEST RESULTS
• May decrease sodium level. May increase uric acid level.
• May decrease hemoglobin and WBC and platelet counts.

## CONTRAINDICATIONS & CAUTIONS
• Contraindicated in patients hypersensitive to drug and in those with demyelinating form of Charcot-Marie-Tooth syndrome. Don't give to patients who are receiving radiation therapy through ports that include the liver.
• Use cautiously in patients with hepatic dysfunction, neuromuscular disease, or infection.

## NURSING CONSIDERATIONS
• Don't give 5-mg vial as a single dose. The 5-mg vials are for multiple-dose use.
• ***Alert:*** After giving drug, check for life-threatening acute bronchospasm. If this occurs, notify prescriber immediately. This reaction is most likely to occur in those also receiving mitomycin.
• Check for hyperuricemia, especially in patients with leukemia or lymphoma. Maintain hydration and give allopurinol to prevent uric acid nephropathy. Check for toxicity.
• Monitor fluid intake and output. Fluid restriction may be needed if SIADH develops.
• Because of risk of neurotoxicity, don't give drug more often than once weekly. Children are more resistant to neurotoxicity than adults. Neurotoxicity is dose-related and usually reversible. Some neurotoxicities may be permanent.

---

Reactions may be *common,* uncommon, *life-threatening,* or COMMON AND LIFE-THREATENING.

- Elderly patients and those with underlying neurologic disease may be more susceptible to neurotoxic effects.
- Check for depression of Achilles tendon reflex, numbness, tingling, footdrop or wristdrop, difficulty in walking, ataxia, and slapping gait. Also check ability to walk on heels. Support patient when walking.
- Monitor bowel function. Give stool softener, laxative, or water before giving dose. Constipation may be an early sign of neurotoxicity.
- All vials (1-mg, 2-mg, 5-mg) contain 1-mg/ml solution; refrigerate them.
- Stop drugs known to cause urine retention, particularly in elderly patients, for first few days after vincristine therapy.
- **Alert:** Drug is fatal if given intrathecally; it's for I.V. use only.
- **Alert:** Don't confuse vincristine with vinblastine or vindesine.

**PATIENT TEACHING**
- Advise patient to report any pain or burning at site of injection during or after administration.
- Tell patient to report evidence of infection (fever, sore throat, fatigue) and bleeding (easy bruising, nosebleeds, bleeding gums, tarry stools). Tell patient to take temperature daily.
- Warn patient that hair loss may occur, but explain that it's usually reversible.
- Caution woman of childbearing age to avoid becoming pregnant during therapy and to consult prescriber before becoming pregnant.

---

**vinorelbine tartrate**
Navelbine

*Pregnancy risk category D*

**AVAILABLE FORMS**
*Injection:* 10 mg/ml, 50 mg/5 ml

**INDICATIONS & DOSAGES**
➤ **Alone or as adjunct therapy with cisplatin for first-line treatment of ambulatory patients with nonresectable advanced non–small-cell lung cancer (NSCLC); alone or with cisplatin in**

**stage IV of NSCLC; with cisplatin in stage III of NSCLC**
*Adults:* 30 mg/m$^2$ I.V. weekly. In combination treatment, same dosage with 120 mg/m$^2$ of cisplatin given on days 1 and 29, then q 6 weeks.
*Adjust-a-dose:* If granulocyte count is 1,000 to 1,499 cells/mm$^3$, give 50% of dose. If less than 1,000 cells/mm$^3$, dose is withheld. If total bilirubin is 2.1 to 3 mg/dl, reduce dose by 50%; if more than 3 mg/dl, give 25% of dose.
➤ **Breast cancer ♦**
*Adults:* 20 to 30 mg/m$^2$ I.V. once weekly.

**I.V. ADMINISTRATION**
- Dilute drug before use to 1.5 to 3 mg/ml with D$_5$W or normal saline solution in a syringe. Or, dilute to 0.5 to 2 mg/ml in an I.V. bag. Give drug I.V. over 6 to 10 minutes into side port of a free-flowing I.V. line that is closest to I.V. bag; then flush with 75 to 125 ml or more of D$_5$W or normal saline solution.
- Drug may be stored for up to 24 hours at room temperature.
- Watch for irritation and infiltration when giving vinorelbine because drug can cause considerable irritation, localized tissue damage and necrosis, and thrombophlebitis. If extravasation occurs, stop drug immediately and inject remaining dose into a different vein; notify prescriber.

**ACTION**
A semisynthetic vinca alkaloid that exerts its primary antineoplastic effect by disrupting microtubule assembly, which in turn disrupts spindle formation and prevents mitosis.

| Route | Onset | Peak | Duration |
|-------|-------|------|----------|
| I.V. | Unknown | Unknown | Unknown |

**ADVERSE REACTIONS**
**CNS:** *peripheral neuropathy, asthenia, fatigue.*
**CV:** chest pain.
**GI:** *nausea, vomiting, anorexia, diarrhea, constipation, stomatitis.*
**Hematologic:** *bone marrow suppression, agranulocytosis,* LEUKOPENIA, *thrombocytopenia, anemia, granulocytopenia.*
**Hepatic:** hyperbilirubinemia.

---

**Musculoskeletal:** myalgia, arthralgia, jaw pain, loss of deep tendon reflexes.
**Respiratory:** dyspnea, shortness of breath.
**Skin:** *alopecia,* rash, *injection pain or reaction.*

## INTERACTIONS

**Drug-drug.** *Cisplatin:* May increase risk of bone marrow suppression when used with cisplatin. Monitor hematologic status closely.
*Cytochrome P450 inhibitors:* May decrease metabolism of vinorelbine. Monitor for increased adverse effects.
*Mitomycin:* May cause pulmonary reactions. Monitor respiratory status closely.

## EFFECTS ON LAB TEST RESULTS

• May increase bilirubin level.
• May increase liver function test values. May decrease hemoglobin and granulocyte, WBC, and platelet counts.

## CONTRAINDICATIONS & CAUTIONS

• Contraindicated in patients with pretreatment granulocyte counts below 1,000 cells/mm$^3$ and in patients hypersensitive to the drug.
• Use with extreme caution in patients whose bone marrow may have been compromised by previous exposure to radiation therapy or chemotherapy or whose bone marrow is still recovering from chemotherapy.
• Use cautiously in patients with hepatic impairment. Monitor liver enzyme levels.

## NURSING CONSIDERATIONS

• Check patient's granulocyte count before administration; make sure count is 1,000 cells/mm$^3$ or higher before giving drug. Withhold drug and notify prescriber if count is lower. Granulocyte nadirs occur between days 7 to 10.
• *Alert:* Drug is fatal if given intrathecally; it's for I.V. use only.
• Dosage adjustments are made according to hematologic toxicity or hepatic insufficiency, whichever results in the lower dosage. Expect dosage reduction of 50% if granulocyte count falls below 1,500 cells/mm$^3$ but is greater than 1,000 cells/mm$^3$. If three consecutive

doses are skipped because of agranulocytosis, don't resume vinorelbine therapy.
• Patient may receive injections of WBC colony-stimulating factors to promote cell growth and decrease risk of infection.
• Drug may be a contact irritant, and the solution must be handled and given with care. Gloves are recommended. Avoid inhalation of vapors and contact with skin or mucous membranes, especially those of the eyes. In case of contact, wash with generous amounts of water for at least 15 minutes.
• *Alert:* Monitor deep tendon reflexes; loss may represent cumulative toxicity.
• Monitor patient closely for hypersensitivity.
• As a guide to the effects of therapy, monitor patient's peripheral blood count and bone marrow.
• *Alert:* Don't confuse vinorelbine with vinblastine or vincristine.

## PATIENT TEACHING

• Advise patient to report any pain or burning at site of injection during or after administration.
• Instruct patient not to take other drugs, including OTC preparations, until approved by prescriber.
• Tell patient to report evidence of infection (fever, sore throat, fatigue) and bleeding (easy bruising, nosebleeds, bleeding gums, tarry stools). Tell him to take temperature daily.
• Advise patient to report increased shortness of breath, cough, abdominal pain, or constipation.
• Caution woman of childbearing age to avoid becoming pregnant during therapy.

---

Reactions may be *common,* uncommon, *life-threatening,* or COMMON AND LIFE-THREATENING.

adalimumab
alefacept
anakinra
azathioprine
basiliximab
cyclosporine
cyclosporine, modified
daclizumab
efalizumab
etanercept
infliximab
lymphocyte immune globulin
muromonab-CD3
mycophenolate mofetil
mycophenolate mofetil
  hydrochloride
sirolimus
tacrolimus

**COMBINATION PRODUCTS**
None.

❋ *NEW DRUG*

## adalimumab
Humira

*Pregnancy risk category B*

**AVAILABLE FORMS**
*Injection:* 40 mg/0.8 ml

**INDICATIONS & DOSAGES**
➤ **To reduce signs and symptoms and structural damage in patients with moderately to severely active rheumatoid arthritis and an inadequate response to one or more disease-modifying antirheumatic drugs**
*Adults:* 40 mg S.C. q other week. May increase to 40 mg q week if patient isn't taking methotrexate.

**ACTION**
A recombinant human IgG$_1$ monoclonal antibody that blocks human tumor necrosis factor (TNF)–alpha. TNF-alpha takes part in normal inflammatory and immune responses and in the inflammation and joint destruction of rheumatoid arthritis.

| Route | Onset | Peak | Duration |
|-------|-------|------|----------|
| S.C. | Variable | Variable | Unknown |

**ADVERSE REACTIONS**
**CNS:** headache.
**CV:** hypertension.
**EENT:** *sinusitis.*
**GI:** nausea, abdominal pain.
**GU:** urinary tract infection, hematuria.
**Metabolic:** hypercholesterolemia, hyperlipidemia.
**Musculoskeletal:** back pain.
**Respiratory:** *upper respiratory tract infection,* bronchitis.
**Skin:** *rash.*
**Other:** *injection site reactions (erythema, itching, hemorrhage, pain, swelling),* **malignancy,** flulike syndrome, *accidental injury,* allergic reactions.

**INTERACTIONS**
**Drug-drug.** *Live-virus vaccines:* May cause secondary transmission of infection from live-virus vaccines. Avoid using together.

**EFFECTS ON LAB TEST RESULTS**
● May increase cholesterol level.

**CONTRAINDICATIONS & CAUTIONS**
● Contraindicated in patients hypersensitive to adalimumab or its components, in immunosuppressed patients, or those with an active chronic or localized infection.
● Use cautiously in patients with a history of recurrent infection, patients with underlying conditions that predispose them to infections, or those who have lived in areas where tuberculosis and histoplasmosis are endemic.
● Use cautiously in patients with CNS-demyelinating disorders and in elderly patients because of their higher rate of infection and malignancies.
● Don't give adalimumab to pregnant women unless benefits outweigh risks. Because of the risk of serious adverse reactions, the patient should stop breast-feeding or stop using the drug.

• Safety and effectiveness in children haven't been established.

## NURSING CONSIDERATIONS

• Drug can be given alone or with methotrexate or other disease-modifying antirheumatic drugs.
• Give first dose under supervision of experienced prescriber.
• Evaluate patient for latent tuberculosis and, if present, start treatment before giving adalimumab.
• Serious infections and sepsis, including tuberculosis and invasive opportunistic fungal infections, may occur. If patient develops new infection during treatment, monitor closely.
• Stop drug if patient develops a severe infection, anaphylaxis, other serious allergic reaction, or evidence of a lupus-like syndrome.
• **Alert:** The needle cover contains latex and shouldn't be handled by those with latex sensitivity.

## PATIENT TEACHING

• Tell patient to report evidence of tuberculosis or infection.
• If appropriate, teach patient or caregiver how to give drug.
• Tell patient to rotate injection sites and to avoid tender, bruised, red, or hard skin.
• Teach patient to dispose of used vials, needles, and syringes properly and not in the household trash or recyclables.
• Tell patient to refrigerate adalimumab in its original container before use.

✳ NEW DRUG

# alefacept
Amevive

*Pregnancy risk category B*

## AVAILABLE FORMS

*Powder for I.V. injection:* 7.5-mg single-dose vial
*Powder for I.M. injection:* 15-mg single-dose vial

## INDICATIONS & DOSAGES

➤ **Moderate to severe chronic plaque psoriasis in candidates for systemic therapy or phototherapy**
*Adults:* 7.5 mg I.V. push over 5 seconds once weekly for 12 weeks or 15 mg I.M. once weekly for 12 weeks. Another 12-week course may be given if CD4+ T lymphocyte count is normal and at least 12 weeks have passed since the previous treatment.
*Adjust-a-dose:* Withhold dose if CD4+ T lymphocyte count is below 250 cells/mm³. Stop drug if CD4+ count remains below 250 cells/mm³ for 1 month.

## I.V. ADMINISTRATION

• Reconstitute 7.5-mg single-dose vial with 0.6 ml of supplied diluent to yield 7.5 mg/0.5 ml. Use only the diluent provided to reconstitute drug. Don't add other drugs to the reconstituted solution. Inject diluent slowly toward the side of the vial, and swirl vial gently. Don't shake or filter the resulting solution. Make sure reconstituted solution is clear and colorless to slightly yellow. Discard if discolored or cloudy. Use immediately or refrigerate and use within 4 hours.
• Give as I.V. bolus over 5 seconds.
• Prime infusion set with 3 ml of normal saline solution before giving drug, and flush it with 3 ml of normal saline solution after giving drug.
• Store powder at room temperature, protected from light.

## ACTION

An immunosuppressive protein that interferes with lymphocyte activation and reduces subsets of CD2+ T lymphocytes, which reduces circulating total CD4+ and CD8+ T lymphocyte counts.

| Route | Onset | Peak | Duration |
|---|---|---|---|
| I.V., I.M. | Unknown | Unknown | Unknown |

## ADVERSE REACTIONS

**CNS:** dizziness.
**CV:** *coronary artery disorder, MI.*
**EENT:** pharyngitis.
**GI:** nausea.
**Hematologic:** LYMPHOPENIA.
**Musculoskeletal:** myalgia.
**Respiratory:** cough.

---

Reactions may be *common,* uncommon, *life-threatening,* or COMMON AND LIFE-THREATENING.

**Skin:** pruritus; injection site *pain, inflammation,* bleeding, edema, or mass.
**Other:** *infection,* chills, *malignancy, hypersensitivity reaction,* accidental injury, antibody formation.

## INTERACTIONS
**Drug-drug.** *Immunosuppressants, phototherapy:* May increase risk of excessive immunosuppression. Avoid using together.

## EFFECTS ON LAB TEST RESULTS
● May decrease CD4+ and CD8+ T lymphocyte counts.

## CONTRAINDICATIONS & CAUTIONS
● Contraindicated in patients hypersensitive to drug or its components, in breast-feeding women, and in patients with a history of systemic malignancy or clinically important infection.
● Use cautiously in patients at high risk for malignancy, patients with chronic or recurrent infections, and pregnant patients. Give drug cautiously to elderly patients because of their increased rate of infection and malignancies.
● Safety and effectiveness in children haven't been established.

## NURSING CONSIDERATIONS
● Monitor CD4+ T lymphocyte count weekly for the 12-week course. Ensure that patient has normal CD4+ T lymphocyte count before starting therapy.
● Monitor patient carefully for evidence of infection or malignancy, and stop drug if it appears.
● For I.M. administration, reconstitute 15-mg vial of alefacept with 0.6 ml of supplied diluent.
● Rotate I.M. injection sites so that the new injection is given at least 1 inch away from the old site, and not in an area that is bruised, tender, or hard.
● Because effects on fetal development aren't known, give drug only if clearly needed. Enroll pregnant women receiving alefacept into the Biogen pregnancy registry by phoning 1-800-811-0104 so that drug effects can be studied.

## PATIENT TEACHING
● Tell patient about potential adverse reactions.

● Urge patient to report evidence of infection immediately.
● Tell patient that blood tests will be done regularly to monitor WBC counts.
● Tell patient to notify prescriber if she is or could be pregnant within 8 weeks of receiving drug.
● Advise patient to either stop breast-feeding or stop using the drug because of the risk of serious adverse reactions in the infant.

## anakinra
Kineret

*Pregnancy risk category B*

## AVAILABLE FORMS
*Injection:* 100 mg/ml in a prefilled glass syringe.

## INDICATIONS & DOSAGES
➤ **Moderately to severely active rheumatoid arthritis (RA) after one or more failures with disease-modifying antirheumatic drugs alone or combined**
*Adults:* 100 mg S.C. daily.

## ACTION
A recombinant, nonglycosylated form of the human interleukin-1 receptor antagonist (IL-1Ra). The level of naturally occurring IL-1Ra in synovium and synovial fluid from patients with RA isn't enough to compete with the elevated level of locally produced IL-1. Anakinra blocks the biological activity of IL-1 by competitively inhibiting IL-1 from binding to the interleukin-1 type receptor, which is expressed in various tissues and organs.

| Route | Onset | Peak | Duration |
|-------|-------|------|----------|
| S.C. | Unknown | 3-7 hr | Unknown |

## ADVERSE REACTIONS
**CNS:** *headache.*
**EENT:** sinusitis.
**GI:** abdominal pain, diarrhea, nausea.
**Hematologic:** *neutropenia,* eosinophilia.
**Respiratory:** *upper respiratory tract infection.*
**Skin:** *injection site reactions (erythema, ecchymosis, inflammation, pain).*

---

**Other:** *infection (cellulitis, pneumonia, bone and joint),* flulike symptoms.

## INTERACTIONS
**Drug-drug.** *Etanercept, other tumor necrosis factor (TNF)-blocking agents:* May increase risk of severe infection. Use together with caution.
*Vaccines:* May decrease effectiveness of vaccines or may increase risk of secondary transmission of infection with live vaccines. Avoid using together.

## EFFECTS ON LAB TEST RESULTS
• May increase eosinophil count. May decrease neutrophil, WBC, and platelet counts.

## CONTRAINDICATIONS & CAUTIONS
• Contraindicated in patients hypersensitive to *Escherichia coli*–derived proteins or any components of the product, or in patients with active infections.
• Use drug cautiously in elderly patients because they have a greater risk of infection and are more likely to have renal impairment.
• Use drug cautiously in immunosuppressed patients and in those with chronic infection.
• It's unknown whether drug appears in breast milk. Use cautiously in breast-feeding women.
• Safety and effectiveness in patients with juvenile rheumatoid arthritis haven't been established.

## NURSING CONSIDERATIONS
• Don't start treatment if patient has active infection.
• Obtain neutrophil count before treatment, monthly for the first 3 months of treatment, and then quarterly for up to 1 year.
• Inject entire contents of prefilled syringe.
• Monitor patient for infections and injection site reactions.
• Stop drug if patient develops a serious infection.
• Store drug in the refrigerator at 35° to 46° F (2° to 8°C). Don't freeze or shake.
• Protect drug from light.
• **Alert:** Don't confuse anakinra (Kineret) with amikacin (Amikin).

## PATIENT TEACHING
• Tell patient to store drug in refrigerator and not to freeze or expose to excessive heat. Advise letting drug come to room temperature before giving dose.
• Teach patient proper dosage and administration.
• Urge patient to rotate injection sites.
• Teach proper disposal of syringes in a puncture-resistant container. Also, caution patient not to reuse needles.
• Review signs and symptoms of allergic and other adverse reactions, especially signs of serious infections. Urge patient to contact prescriber if they arise.
• Inform patient that injection site reactions are common, usually mild, and typically last 14 to 28 days.
• Tell patient to avoid live-virus vaccines while taking anakinra.

# azathioprine
Azasan, Imuran, Thioprine‡

*Pregnancy risk category D*

## AVAILABLE FORMS
*Powder for injection:* 100 mg
*Tablets:* 25 mg, 50 mg, 75 mg, 100 mg

## INDICATIONS & DOSAGES
➤ **Immunosuppression in kidney transplantation**
*Adults:* Initially, 3 to 5 mg/kg P.O. or I.V. daily, usually beginning on day of transplantation. Maintained at 1 to 3 mg/kg daily based on patient response and tolerance.
**Adjust-a-dose:** Give drug in lower doses to patients with oliguria in the posttransplant period and in those with impaired renal function.
➤ **Severe, refractory rheumatoid arthritis**
*Adults:* Initially, 1 mg/kg P.O. as single dose or divided into two doses. Usual dose is 50 to 100 mg. If patient response isn't satisfactory after 6 to 8 weeks, dosage may be increased by 0.5 mg/kg daily to maximum of 2.5 mg/kg daily at 4-week intervals.

## I.V. ADMINISTRATION
- Reconstitute drug in 100-mg vial with 10 ml of sterile water for injection. Inspect for particles before use.
- Drug may be given by direct I.V. injection or further diluted in normal saline solution for injection or $D_5W$ solution and infused over 30 to 60 minutes.
- Use only in patients who can't tolerate oral drugs.

## ACTION
Unknown, but thought to cause variable alterations in antibody production.

| Route | Onset | Peak | Duration |
|-------|-------|------|----------|
| P.O., I.V. | Unknown | Unknown | Unknown |

## ADVERSE REACTIONS
**CNS:** fever.
**GI:** *nausea, vomiting,* anorexia, *pancreatitis,* steatorrhea, diarrhea, abdominal pain.
**Hematologic:** LEUKOPENIA, *myelosuppression,* macrocytic anemia, anemia, *pancytopenia,* THROMBOCYTOPENIA, *immunosuppression.*
**Hepatic:** *hepatotoxicity,* jaundice.
**Musculoskeletal:** arthralgia, myalgia.
**Skin:** rash, alopecia.
**Other:** *infections, increased risk of neoplasia.*

## INTERACTIONS
**Drug-drug.** *ACE inhibitors:* May cause severe leukopenia. Monitor patient closely.
*Allopurinol:* May impair inactivation of azathioprine. Decrease azathioprine to one-third to one-fourth normal dose.
*Co-trimoxazole and other drugs that interfere with myelopoiesis:* May cause severe leukopenia, especially in renal transplant patients. Use cautiously together.
*Cyclosporine:* May increase cyclosporine level. Monitor cyclosporine level closely.
*Warfarin:* May decrease action of warfarin. Monitor patient closely.

## EFFECTS ON LAB TEST RESULTS
- May increase AST, ALT, alkaline phosphatase, and bilirubin levels. May decrease uric acid level.
- May decrease hemoglobin and WBC, RBC, and platelet counts.

## CONTRAINDICATIONS & CAUTIONS
- Contraindicated in patients hypersensitive to drug or its components.
- Use cautiously in patients with hepatic or renal dysfunction.
- Benefits must be weighed against risk when giving to patient with systemic viral infection, such as chickenpox or herpes zoster.
- Patients with rheumatoid arthritis previously treated with alkylating drugs, such as cyclophosphamide, chlorambucil, or melphalan, may be at risk for tumor development if treated with azathioprine.

## NURSING CONSIDERATIONS
- Give drug after meals to minimize adverse GI effects.
- To prevent bleeding, avoid all I.M. injections when platelet count is below 100,000/mm³.
- Monitor CBC and platelet counts weekly for 1 month, then twice monthly. Notify prescriber if counts drop suddenly or become dangerously low. Drug may need to be temporarily withheld.
- Watch for early signs and symptoms of hepatotoxicity (such as clay-colored stools, dark urine, pruritus, and yellow skin and sclera) and for increased alkaline phosphatase, bilirubin, AST, and ALT levels.
- Therapeutic response usually occurs within 8 weeks.
- **Alert:** Don't confuse azathioprine with azidothymidine, Azulfidine, or azatadine.
- **Alert:** Don't confuse Imuran with Inderal.

## PATIENT TEACHING
- Warn patient to report even mild infections (colds, fever, sore throat, malaise), because drug is a potent immunosuppressant.
- Instruct patient to avoid conception during therapy and for 4 months after therapy stops.
- Warn patient that some hair thinning is possible.
- Tell patient taking drug for refractory rheumatoid arthritis that it may take up to 12 weeks to be effective.
- Advise patient to report unusual bleeding or bruising.

• Tell patient that drug may be taken with food to decrease nausea.

• Advise patient to use soft toothbrush and perform oral care cautiously.

## basiliximab
Simulect

*Pregnancy risk category B*

### AVAILABLE FORMS
*Injection:* 20-mg vials

### INDICATIONS & DOSAGES
➤ **To prevent acute organ rejection in patients receiving renal transplantation when used as part of an immunosuppressive regimen that includes cyclosporine and corticosteroids**
*Adults and children weighing 35 kg (77 lb) or more:* 20 mg I.V. given within 2 hours before transplant surgery and 20 mg I.V. given 4 days after transplantation.
*Children weighing less than 35 kg:* 10 mg I.V. given within 2 hours before transplant surgery and 10 mg I.V. given 4 days after transplantation.

### I.V. ADMINISTRATION
• Reconstitute with 5 ml sterile water for injection. Shake vial gently to dissolve powder. Dilute reconstituted solution to volume of 50 ml with normal saline solution or $D_5W$ for infusion. When mixing solution, gently invert bag to avoid foaming. Don't shake.
• Infuse over 20 to 30 minutes. Drug may be given as a bolus injection; however, this is associated with nausea, vomiting, pain, and local reactions. Don't add or infuse other drugs simultaneously through same I.V. line.
• Use reconstituted solution immediately; may be refrigerated at 36° to 46° F (2° to 8° C) for up to 24 hours or kept at room temperature for 4 hours.

### ACTION
Binds specifically to and blocks the interleukin (IL)–2 receptor alpha chain on the surface of activated T lymphocytes, inhibiting IL-2–mediated activation of lymphocytes, a critical pathway in the cellular immune response involved in allograft rejection.

| Route | Onset | Peak | Duration |
|-------|-------|------|----------|
| I.V. | Unknown | Immediate | Unknown |

### ADVERSE REACTIONS
**CNS:** agitation, anxiety, *asthenia,* depression, *dizziness, headache,* hypoesthesia, *insomnia,* neuropathy, paresthesia, *tremor, fever,* fatigue.
**CV:** angina pectoris, **arrhythmias,** atrial fibrillation, **heart failure,** chest pain, abnormal heart sounds, aggravated hypertension, *hypertension,* hypotension, tachycardia, *leg or peripheral edema,* generalized edema.
**EENT:** abnormal vision, cataract, conjunctivitis, *rhinitis, pharyngitis,* sinusitis.
**GI:** *abdominal pain, candidiasis, constipation, diarrhea, dyspepsia,* esophagitis, enlarged abdomen, flatulence, gastroenteritis, GI disorder, **GI hemorrhage,** gum hyperplasia, melena, *nausea,* ulcerative stomatitis, *vomiting.*
**GU:** abnormal renal function, albuminuria, bladder disorder, *dysuria,* frequent micturition, genital edema, hematuria, *increased nonprotein nitrogen,* oliguria, renal tubular necrosis, ureteral disorder, *UTI,* urinary retention, impotence.
**Hematologic:** *anemia,* hematoma, **hemorrhage,** polycythemia, purpura, **thrombocytopenia,** thrombosis.
**Metabolic:** *acidosis,* dehydration, diabetes mellitus, fluid overload, hypercalcemia, *hypercholesterolemia, hyperglycemia, hyperkalemia,* hyperlipemia, *hyperuricemia, hypocalcemia, hypokalemia,* hypomagnesemia, *hypophosphatemia,* hypoproteinemia, *weight gain.*
**Musculoskeletal:** arthralgia, arthropathy, *back pain,* bone fracture, cramps, hernia, *leg pain,* myalgia.
**Respiratory:** abnormal chest sounds, bronchitis, **bronchospasm,** cough, *dyspnea,* pneumonia, pulmonary disorder, **pulmonary edema,** *upper respiratory tract infection.*
**Skin:** *acne,* cyst, hypertrichosis, pruritus, rash, skin disorder or ulceration.
**Other:** accidental trauma, *viral infection,* infection, **sepsis,** *surgical wound complications,* herpes zoster, herpes simplex, *hypersensitivity reactions.*

---

Reactions may be *common,* uncommon, *life-threatening,* or COMMON AND LIFE-THREATENING.

## INTERACTIONS
None significant.

## EFFECTS ON LAB TEST RESULTS
• May increase calcium, cholesterol, glucose, lipids, and uric acid levels. May decrease magnesium, phosphorus, and protein levels. May increase or decrease potassium level.
• May increase RBC count. May decrease hemoglobin and platelet count.

## CONTRAINDICATIONS & CAUTIONS
• Contraindicated in patients hypersensitive to drug or its components.
• Use cautiously and only under supervision of prescriber qualified and experienced in immunosuppressive therapy and managing organ transplantation.
• Use cautiously in elderly patients.

## NURSING CONSIDERATIONS
• Severe acute hypersensitivity reactions can occur within 24 hours after administration. Make sure drugs for treating hypersensitivity reactions are readily available; withhold second dose if hypersensitivity reactions occur.
• Check for electrolyte imbalances and acidosis during drug therapy.
• Monitor patient's intake and output, vital signs, hemoglobin level, and hematocrit during therapy.
• Be alert for signs and symptoms of opportunistic infections during drug therapy.

## PATIENT TEACHING
• Inform patient of potential benefits of and risks related to immunosuppressive therapy, including decreased risk of graft loss or acute rejection.
• Advise patient that immunosuppressive therapy increases risk of developing infection. Tell him to report signs and symptoms of infection promptly.
• Inform woman of childbearing age to use effective contraception before therapy starts and for 4 months after therapy ends.
• Instruct patient to report adverse effects immediately.
• Explain that drug is used with cyclosporine and corticosteroids.

## cyclosporine
Neoral, Sandimmune, Sandimmun‡

## cyclosporine, modified
Gengraf

*Pregnancy risk category C*

## AVAILABLE FORMS
*Capsules:* 25 mg, 50 mg, 100 mg
*Capsules for microemulsion:* 25 mg, 50 mg, 100 mg
*Injection:* 50 mg/ml
*Oral solution:* 100 mg/ml

## INDICATIONS & DOSAGES
➤ **To prevent organ rejection in kidney, liver, or heart transplantation**
*Adults and children:* 15 mg/kg P.O. 4 to 12 hours before transplantation and continued daily for 1 to 2 weeks postoperatively. Then reduce dosage by 5% each week to maintenance level of 5 to 10 mg/kg daily. Or, 5 to 6 mg/kg I.V. concentrate 4 to 12 hours before transplantation given as a continuous infusion. Postoperatively, repeat dose daily until patient can tolerate P.O. forms.

For conversion from Sandimmune to Gengraf or Neoral, use same daily dose as previously used for Sandimmune. Monitor blood levels q 4 to 7 days after conversion, and monitor blood pressure and creatinine level q 2 weeks during the first 2 months.
➤ **Severe, active rheumatoid arthritis that hasn't adequately responded to methotrexate**
*Gengraf and Neoral*
*Adults:* 2.5 mg/kg daily P.O., taken b.i.d. as divided dose. Dosage may be increased by 0.5 to 0.75 mg/kg daily after 8 weeks and again after 12 weeks to a maximum of 4 mg/kg daily. If no response is seen after 16 weeks, stop therapy.
➤ **Psoriasis**
*Gengraf and Neoral*
*Adults:* 1.25 mg/kg P.O. b.i.d. for at least 4 weeks. Dosage may be increased by 0.5 mg/kg daily once every 2 weeks p.r.n. to a maximum dose of 4 mg/kg daily.
*Adjust-a-dose:* For patients with such adverse effects as hypertension, elevated creatinine level (30% above pretreatment lev-

el), or abnormal CBC and liver function test results, decrease dosage by 25% to 50%.

## I.V. ADMINISTRATION
• Give cyclosporine I.V. concentrate at one-third oral dose, and dilute before use.
• Dilute each ml of concentrate in 20 to 100 ml of $D_5W$ or normal saline solution for injection. Dilute immediately before use; infuse over 2 to 6 hours.
• I.V. administration is usually reserved for patients who can't tolerate oral drugs.
• Protect I.V. solution from light.

## ACTION
Unknown. Thought to inhibit proliferation and function of T lymphocytes and inhibit production and release of lymphokines.

| Route | Onset | Peak | Duration |
|-------|---------|------------|----------|
| P.O. | Unknown | 90 min-3 hr | Unknown |
| I.V. | Unknown | Unknown | Unknown |

## ADVERSE REACTIONS
**CNS:** *tremor, headache,* confusion, paresthesia.
**CV:** *hypertension,* flushing.
**EENT:** *gum hyperplasia,* sinusitis.
**GI:** *nausea, vomiting,* diarrhea, oral thrush, abdominal discomfort.
**GU:** NEPHROTOXICITY.
**Hematologic:** anemia, *leukopenia, thrombocytopenia.*
**Hepatic:** *hepatotoxicity.*
**Metabolic:** hyperglycemia.
**Skin:** *hirsutism,* acne.
**Other:** *infections, anaphylaxis,* gynecomastia.

## INTERACTIONS
**Drug-drug.** *Acyclovir, aminoglycosides, amphotericin B, cimetidine, co-trimoxazole, diclofenac, gentamicin, ketoconazole, melphalan, NSAIDs, ranitidine, sulfamethoxazole/trimethoprim, tacrolimus, tobramycin, vancomycin:* May increase risk of nephrotoxicity. Avoid using together.
*Allopurinol, bromocriptine, cimetidine, clarithromycin, danazol, diltiazem, erythromycin, fluconazole, imipenem-cilastatin, itraconazole, ketoconazole, methylprednisolone, metoclopramide, nicardipine, prednisolone, verapamil:*
May increase cyclosporine level. Monitor patient for increased toxicity.
*Azathioprine, corticosteroids, cyclophosphamide, verapamil:* May increase immunosuppression. Monitor patient closely.
*Carbamazepine, isoniazid, nafcillin, octreotide, phenobarbital, phenytoin, rifabutin, rifampin, ticlopidine:* May decrease immunosuppressant effect from low cyclosporine levels. Cyclosporine dosage may need to be increased.
*Digoxin, lovastatin, prednisolone:* May decrease clearance of these drugs. Use together cautiously.
*Mycophenolate mofetil:* May decrease mycophenolate level. Monitor patient closely when cyclosporine is either added or deleted from therapy.
*Potassium-sparing diuretics:* May induce hyperkalemia. Monitor patient closely.
*Sirolimus:* May increase sirolimus level. Take sirolimus at least 4 hours after cyclosporine dose. Monitor patient for increased adverse effects when used together.
*Vaccines:* May decrease immune response. Postpone routine immunization.
**Drug-herb.** *Alfalfa sprouts, astragalus, echinacea, licorice:* May interfere with immunosuppressive effect. Discourage use together.
*St. John's wort:* May reduce cyclosporine level, resulting in transplant failure. Discourage use together.
**Drug-food.** *Grapefruit and grapefruit juices:* May increase blood level and cause toxicity. Advise patient to avoid use of grapefruit products.
*High-fat meals:* May decrease Neoral absorption. Urge patient to take on empty stomach.

## EFFECTS ON LAB TEST RESULTS
• May increase BUN, creatinine, LDL, bilirubin, AST, ALT, and glucose levels.
• May decrease hemoglobin and WBC and platelet counts.

## CONTRAINDICATIONS & CAUTIONS
• Contraindicated in patients hypersensitive to drug or polyoxyethylated castor oil (found in injectable form).
• Contraindicated in patients with rheumatoid arthritis or psoriasis with abnormal

renal function, uncontrolled hypertension, or malignancies (Neoral or Gengraf).
• Psoriasis patients shouldn't receive psoralen plus ultraviolet A (PUVA) or ultraviolet B (UVB) therapy, methotrexate, other immunosuppressants, coal tar, or radiation (Neoral or Gengraf).

**NURSING CONSIDERATIONS**
• Cyclosporine can cause nephrotoxicity and hepatotoxicity.
• Neoral has greater bioavailability than Sandimmune. A lower dose of Neoral may be needed to provide similar blood levels achieved with Sandimmune. Monitor blood levels when switching patients between these two brands.
• Gengraf and Sandimmune aren't bioequivalent and can't be interchanged without prescriber supervision. Convert Gengraf to Sandimmune only with increased monitoring to prevent underdosing.
• Gengraf is bioequivalent to and interchangeable with Neoral capsules. Monitor levels when switching patients between these two products.
• Always give cyclosporine with adrenal corticosteroids.
• Use Neoral or Gengraf for treatment of rheumatoid arthritis or psoriasis.
• Before starting treatment in patients with rheumatoid arthritis, measure blood pressure at least twice and obtain two creatinine levels to estimate baseline. Evaluate blood pressure and creatinine every 2 weeks during first 3 months, then monthly if the patient is stable. Monitor blood pressure and creatinine level after an increase in NSAID dosage or introduction of a new NSAID. Monitor CBC and liver function tests monthly if patient also receives methotrexate. If hypertension occurs, decrease dosage of Gengraf or Neoral by 25% to 50%. If hypertension persists, decrease dosage further or control blood pressure with antihypertensives.
• For psoriasis patients, first measure blood pressure at least twice. Evaluate patient for occult infection and tumors initially and throughout treatment. Obtain baseline creatinine level (on two occasions), CBC, and BUN, magnesium, uric acid, potassium, and lipid levels. Evaluate creatinine and BUN levels every 2 weeks during first 3 months and then monthly

thereafter if patient is stable. If creatinine level is 25% above pretreatment levels, repeat creatinine measurement within 2 weeks. If creatinine level stays 25% to 50% above baseline, dosage is reduced by 25% to 50%. If at any time the creatinine level is 50% above baseline, reduce dosage by 25% to 50%. Stop therapy if creatinine level isn't reversed after two dosage modifications. Monitor creatinine level after increasing NSAID dose or starting a new NSAID. Evaluate blood pressure, CBC, and uric acid, potassium, lipid, and magnesium levels every 2 weeks for the first 3 months, then monthly if patient is stable, or more frequently when dosage adjustments are made. Reduce dosage by 25% to 50% for an abnormality of clinical concern.
• Improvement in psoriasis takes 12 to 16 weeks of therapy.
• Measure oral solution doses carefully in an oral syringe. To improve the taste of conventional oral solution, mix it with milk, chocolate milk, or orange juice. Oral solution for emulsion may be mixed with orange or apple juice (avoid grapefruit juice). Emulsion solution is less palatable when mixed with milk. Use a glass container to mix, and have patient drink at once. Don't rinse dosing syringe with water. If syringe is cleaned, it must be completely dry before reuse.
• Monitor elderly patient for renal impairment and hypertension.
• Monitor cyclosporine blood levels at regular intervals. Absorption of cyclosporine oral solution can be erratic.
• *Alert:* Don't confuse cyclosporine with cyclophosphamide or cycloserine.
• *Alert:* Don't confuse Sandimmune with Sandoglobulin or Sandostatin.

**PATIENT TEACHING**
• Encourage patient to take drug at same time each day, and teach him how to measure dosage and mask taste of oral solution, if prescribed. Tell him not to take cyclosporine with grapefruit juice.
• Instruct patient to fill glass with water after dose and drink it to make sure he consumes all of drug.
• Advise patient to take drug with meals if nausea occurs.

*Rapid onset*  †Canada  ‡Australia  ◇OTC  ◆Off-label use  ✐Photoguide  *Liquid contains alcohol.

• Advise patient to take Neoral or Gengraf on an empty stomach.
• Tell patient being treated for psoriasis that improvement may not occur until after 12 to 16 weeks of therapy.
• Stress that drug shouldn't be stopped without prescriber's approval.
• Explain to patient the importance of frequent laboratory monitoring while receiving therapy.
• Tell patient to avoid people with infections because drug lowers resistance to infection.
• Advise patient to perform careful oral care and to see a dentist regularly because drug can cause gum disease.
• Advise woman to use barrier contraception during therapy, not hormonal contraceptives. Advise her of the potential risk during pregnancy and the increased risk of tumors, high blood pressure, and kidney problems.
• Warn patient to wear protection in the sun and to avoid excessive sun exposure.

---

## daclizumab
Zenapax

*Pregnancy risk category C*

### AVAILABLE FORMS
*Injection:* 25 mg/5 ml

### INDICATIONS & DOSAGES
➤ **To prevent acute organ rejection in patients receiving renal transplants with an immunosuppressive regimen that includes cyclosporine and corticosteroids**
*Adults:* 1 mg/kg I.V. Standard course of therapy is five doses. Give first dose no more than 24 hours before transplantation; remaining four doses are given at 14-day intervals.

### I.V. ADMINISTRATION
• Don't use drug as direct I.V. injection.
• Dilute in 50 ml of sterile normal saline solution before giving. To avoid foaming, don't shake. Don't use if drug contains particulates or is discolored.
• Give over 15 minutes via a central or peripheral line. Don't add or infuse other drugs simultaneously through same I.V. line.
• Drug may be refrigerated at 36° to 46° F (2° to 8° C) for 24 hours, and is stable at room temperature for 4 hours. Discard solution if not used within 24 hours.

### ACTION
An interleukin (IL)-2 receptor antagonist that inhibits IL-2 binding to prevent IL-2–mediated activation of lymphocytes, a critical pathway in the cellular immune response against allografts. Once in circulation, drug impairs response of immune system to antigenic challenges.

| Route | Onset | Peak | Duration |
|-------|-------|------|----------|
| I.V. | Unknown | Unknown | Unknown |

### ADVERSE REACTIONS
**CNS:** tremor, headache, fever, dizziness, insomnia, generalized weakness, prickly sensation, fatigue, depression, anxiety.
**CV:** tachycardia, hypertension, hypotension, aggravated hypertension, edema, chest pain.
**EENT:** blurred vision, pharyngitis, rhinitis.
**GI:** constipation, nausea, diarrhea, vomiting, abdominal pain, dyspepsia, pyrosis, abdominal distention, epigastric pain, flatulence, gastritis, hemorrhoids.
**GU:** *oliguria,* dysuria, *renal tubular necrosis,* renal damage, urinary retention, hydronephrosis, urinary tract bleeding, urinary tract disorder, renal insufficiency.
**Hematologic:** lymphocele; platelet, bleeding, and clotting disorders.
**Metabolic:** diabetes mellitus, dehydration, fluid overload.
**Musculoskeletal:** musculoskeletal or back pain, arthralgia, myalgia, leg cramps.
**Respiratory:** dyspnea, coughing, atelectasis, congestion, *hypoxia,* crackles, abnormal breath sounds, pleural effusion, *pulmonary edema.*
**Skin:** acne, impaired wound healing without infection, pruritus, hirsutism, rash, night sweats, increased sweating.
**Other:** shivering, limb edema, pain.

### INTERACTIONS
None significant.

---

Reactions may be *common,* uncommon, *life-threatening,* or **COMMON AND LIFE-THREATENING.**

**EFFECTS ON LAB TEST RESULTS**
None reported.

**CONTRAINDICATIONS & CAUTIONS**
• Contraindicated in patients hypersensitive to drug or its components.
• Use cautiously and only under supervision of prescriber experienced in immunosuppressive therapy and management of organ transplantation.

**NURSING CONSIDERATIONS**
• Protect undiluted solution from direct light.
• Drug is used as part of an immunosuppressive regimen that includes corticosteroids and cyclosporine. Check patient for lipoproliferative disorders and opportunistic infections.
• Anaphylactoid reactions have been reported after administration of proteins. Keep immediately available drugs used to treat anaphylactic reactions.

**PATIENT TEACHING**
• Tell patient to consult prescriber before taking other drugs during therapy.
• Advise patient to practice infection prevention precautions.
• Inform patient that neither he nor any household member should receive vaccinations unless medically approved.
• Urge patient to immediately report wounds that fail to heal, unusual bruising or bleeding, or fever.
• Advise patient to drink plenty of fluids during drug therapy and to report painful urination, bloody urine, or decreased urine volume.
• Instruct woman of childbearing age to use effective contraception before therapy starts and to continue for 4 months after therapy stops.

**✳ NEW DRUG**

## efalizumab
Raptiva

*Pregnancy risk category C*

**AVAILABLE FORMS**
*Injection:* 125-mg single-use vial

**INDICATIONS & DOSAGES**
➤ **Chronic moderate to severe plaque psoriasis when systemic therapy or phototherapy is appropriate**
*Adults:* A single dose of 0.7 mg/kg S.C. followed by weekly doses of 1 mg/kg S.C., beginning 1 week after first dose. Maximum single dose, 200 mg.

**ACTION**
An immunosuppressant that binds to a leukocyte function antigen and decreases its expression, thus inhibiting the action of T lymphocytes at sites of inflammation, including psoriatic skin.

| Route | Onset | Peak | Duration |
|-------|-------|------|----------|
| S.C. | 1-2 days | Unknown | 25 days |

**ADVERSE REACTIONS**
**CNS:** *CVA,* fever, *headache, pain.*
**GI:** *nausea.*
**Musculoskeletal:** back pain, myalgia.
**Skin:** acne.
**Other:** *chills,* flulike syndrome, **hypersensitivity reaction,** *infection.*

**INTERACTIONS**
**Drug-drug.** *Other immunosuppressants:* May increase risk of infection and malignancy. Avoid using together.
*Vaccines:* May decrease or negate immune response to vaccine. Avoid using together.

**EFFECTS ON LAB TEST RESULTS**
• May increase alkaline phosphatase level.
• May increase lymphocyte and leukocyte counts. May decrease platelet count.

**CONTRAINDICATIONS & CAUTIONS**
• Contraindicated in patients hypersensitive to efalizumab or its components and in patients with significant infection.
• Use cautiously in patients with chronic infection or history of recurrent infection.
• Use cautiously in patients with history of or high risk for malignancy.
• It isn't known whether efalizumab appears in breast milk. Breast-feeding patients should consider stopping breast-feeding during therapy.

**NURSING CONSIDERATIONS**
• Reconstitute the drug immediately before use.

• To reconstitute, inject 1.3 ml of sterile water for injection into the vial. Swirl gently to dissolve the powder, which takes less than 5 minutes. Don't shake the vial.
• Don't use any other diluent besides sterile water, and use a vial only once.
• The reconstituted solution should be colorless to pale yellow and free of particulates. Don't use the solution if it contains particulates or is discolored.
• If not used immediately, the reconstituted solution may be stored at room temperature for up to 8 hours. Keep efalizumab powder refrigerated, and protect vials from light.
• Rotate injection sites.
• Don't add other drugs to reconstituted solution.
• Notify prescriber if patient develops a severe infection or malignancy is suspected.
• Watch for evidence of thrombocytopenia. Check patient's platelet count monthly during initial treatment and then every 3 months.
• Monitor patient for worsening of psoriasis during or after therapy.

## PATIENT TEACHING
• Tell patient to take the drug exactly as prescribed.
• Explain that platelet counts will be monitored during therapy.
• Urge patient to immediately report evidence of severe thrombocytopenia, such as bleeding gums, bruising, or petechiae.
• Tell patient to report weight changes because dose may need to be changed.
• Advise patient to report any infection or worsening psoriasis.
• Advise patient to hold off receiving vaccines during therapy because the immune response may be inadequate.
• Caution patient to immediately report pregnancy or suspected pregnancy.

## etanercept
Enbrel

*Pregnancy risk category B*

## AVAILABLE FORMS
*Injection:* 25-mg single-use vial

## INDICATIONS & DOSAGES
➤ **To reduce signs and symptoms of moderately to severely active polyarticular-course juvenile rheumatoid arthritis in patients whose response to one or more disease-modifying antirheumatic drugs has been inadequate**
*Children ages 4 to 17:* 0.4 mg/kg (up to maximum of 25 mg per dose) S.C. twice weekly, 72 to 96 hours apart. Or, 0.8 mg/kg (max 50 mg/week) S.C. once weekly.
➤ **Rheumatoid arthritis, psoriatic arthritis, ankylosing spondylitis**
*Adults:* 25 mg twice weekly S.C., 72 to 96 hours apart. Or, 50 mg S.C. once weekly. Methotrexate, glucocorticoids, salicylates, NSAIDs, or analgesics may be continued during treatment.

## ACTION
Binds specifically to tumor necrosis factor (TNF) and blocks its action with cell surface TNF receptors, reducing inflammatory and immune responses found in rheumatoid arthritis.

| Route | Onset | Peak | Duration |
|-------|-------|------|----------|
| S.C. | Unknown | 72 hr | Unknown |

## ADVERSE REACTIONS
**CNS:** asthenia, *headache,* dizziness.
**EENT:** *rhinitis,* pharyngitis, sinusitis.
**GI:** abdominal pain, dyspepsia.
**Respiratory:** *upper respiratory tract infections,* cough, respiratory disorder.
**Skin:** *injection site reaction,* rash.
**Other:** *infections,* malignancies.

## INTERACTIONS
**Drug-drug.** *Vaccines:* May affect normal immune response. Postpone live-virus vaccine until therapy stops.

## EFFECTS ON LAB TEST RESULTS
None reported.

## CONTRAINDICATIONS & CAUTIONS
• Contraindicated in patients hypersensitive to drug or its components and in those with sepsis. Live vaccines are contraindicated during drug therapy.
• Drug isn't indicated for use in children younger than age 4.
• Use cautiously in patients with underlying diseases that predispose them to infec-

---

tion, such as diabetes, heart failure, or history of active or chronic infections.
• Use caution when using in rheumatoid arthritis patients with pre-existing or recent onset of demyelinating disorders, including multiple sclerosis, myelitis, and optic neuritis.

## NURSING CONSIDERATIONS
• Methotrexate, glucocorticoids, salicylates, NSAIDs, or analgesics may be continued during treatment with etanercept.
• *Alert:* Anti-TNF therapies, including etanercept, may affect defenses against infection. Notify prescriber and stop therapy if serious infection occurs.
• *Alert:* Don't give live vaccines during therapy.
• If possible, bring patients with juvenile rheumatoid arthritis up-to-date with all immunizations before initiating treatment.
• Reconstitute aseptically with 1 ml of supplied sterile bacteriostatic water for injection (0.9% benzyl alcohol). Don't filter reconstituted solution during preparation or administration. Inject diluent slowly into vial. Minimize foaming by gently swirling during dissolution rather than shaking. Dissolution takes less than 5 minutes.
• Visually check solution for particulates and discoloration before use. Don't use solution if it's discolored or cloudy, or if it contains particulate matter.
• Don't add other drugs or diluents to reconstituted solution.
• Use reconstituted solution as soon as possible; may be refrigerated in vial for up to 6 hours at 36° to 46° F (2° to 8° C).
• Make injection sites at least 1 inch apart; never use areas where skin is tender, bruised, red, or hard. Recommended sites include the thigh, abdomen, and upper arm. Rotate sites regularly.
• Needle cover of diluent syringe contains dry natural rubber (latex) and shouldn't be handled by persons sensitive to latex.

## PATIENT TEACHING
• If patient will be giving drug, advise him about mixing and injection techniques, including rotation of injection sites.
• Instruct patient to use puncture-resistant container for disposal of needles and syringes.

• Tell patient that injection site reactions generally occur within first month of therapy and decrease thereafter.
• Inform patient of importance of avoiding live vaccine administration during therapy.
• Stress importance of alerting other health care providers of etanercept use.
• Instruct patient to promptly report signs and symptoms of infection to prescriber.
• Advise breast-feeding woman to stop breast-feeding during therapy.

# infliximab
Remicade

*Pregnancy risk category B*

## AVAILABLE FORMS
*Injection:* 100-mg vial

## INDICATIONS & DOSAGES
➤ **Reduction of signs and symptoms, and induction and maintenance of clinical remission in patients with moderately to severely active Crohn's disease who have had an inadequate response to conventional therapy; reduction in the number of draining enterocutaneous and rectovaginal fistulas and maintenance of fistula closure in patients with fistulizing Crohn's disease**
*Adults:* 5 mg/kg I.V. infusion (over a period of not less than 2 hours), given as an induction regimen at 0, 2, and 6 weeks, followed by a maintenance regimen of 5 mg/kg every 8 weeks thereafter. For patients who respond and then lose their response, consideration may be given to treatment with 10 mg/kg. Patients who don't respond by week 14 are unlikely to respond with continued dosing. In those patients, consider discontinuing infliximab.
➤ **In combination with methotrexate to reduce signs and symptoms, and to inhibit progression of structural damage and improve physical function in patients with moderately to severely active rheumatoid arthritis who have had an inadequate response to methotrexate**
*Adults:* 3 mg/kg I.V. infusion over a period of at least 2 hours. Give additional doses of 3 mg/kg at 2 and 6 weeks after first infusion and every 8 weeks thereafter. Dose

may be increased up to 10 mg/kg or doses may be given every 4 weeks if response is inadequate.

## I.V. ADMINISTRATION
• Reconstitute with 10 ml sterile water for injection, using syringe with 21G or smaller needle. Don't shake; gently swirl to dissolve powder. Make sure solution is colorless to light yellow and opalescent, and may develop a few translucent particles. Don't use if other types of particles develop or discoloration occurs. Use reconstituted drug immediately.
• Dilute total volume of reconstituted drug to 250 ml with normal saline solution for injection. Infusion concentration range is 0.4 to 4 mg/ml. Begin infusion within 3 hours of preparation and give over at least 2 hours.
• Don't infuse drug in same I.V. line with other drugs.

## ACTION
A monoclonal antibody that binds to human tumor necrosis factor (TNF)-alpha to neutralize its activity and inhibit its binding with receptors, thereby reducing the infiltration of inflammatory cells and TNF-alpha production in inflamed areas of the intestine.

| Route | Onset | Peak | Duration |
|-------|-------|------|----------|
| I.V. | Unknown | Unknown | Unknown |

## ADVERSE REACTIONS
**CNS:** *fever, headache, fatigue,* dizziness, malaise, insomnia, depression.
**CV:** *hypertension,* hypotension, tachycardia, chest pain, flushing.
**EENT:** *pharyngitis, rhinitis, sinusitis,* conjunctivitis.
**GI:** *nausea, abdominal pain,* vomiting, constipation, *dyspepsia, diarrhea,* flatulence, **intestinal obstruction,** oral pain, ulcerative stomatitis.
**GU:** dysuria, increased urinary frequency, *UTI.*
**Hematologic:** anemia, hematoma.
**Musculoskeletal:** myalgia, *arthralgia, back pain,* arthritis.
**Respiratory:** *upper respiratory tract infections,* bronchitis, *coughing,* dyspnea, respiratory tract allergic reaction.

**Skin:** *rash,* pruritus, candidiasis, acne, alopecia, eczema, erythema, erythematous rash, maculopapular rash, papular rash, dry skin, increased sweating, urticaria.
**Other:** toothache, flulike syndrome, ecchymosis, chills, pain, peripheral edema, hot flashes, abscess.

## INTERACTIONS
**Drug-drug.** *Vaccines:* May affect normal immune response. Postpone live-virus vaccine until therapy stops.

## EFFECTS ON LAB TEST RESULTS
• May increase liver enzyme level.
• May decrease hemoglobin and hematocrit.
• May cause false-positive antinuclear antibody test result.

## CONTRAINDICATIONS & CAUTIONS
• Contraindicated in patients hypersensitive to murine proteins or other components of drug and in those with congestive heart failure.
• Use cautiously in elderly patients and in patients with active infection or history of chronic or recurrent infections. In patients who have resided in regions where histoplasmosis is endemic, carefully consider the benefits and risks of infliximab therapy before starting therapy.

## NURSING CONSIDERATIONS
• *Alert:* Watch for infusion-related reactions, including fever, chills, pruritus, urticaria, dyspnea, hypotension, hypertension, and chest pain, during administration and for 2 hours afterward. If an infusion-related reaction occurs, stop drug, notify prescriber, and be prepared to give acetaminophen, antihistamines, corticosteroids, and epinephrine.
• Watch for development of lymphoma and infection. Patient with chronic Crohn's disease and long-term exposure to immunosuppressants is more likely to develop lymphoma and infection.
• Drug may affect normal immune responses. Patient may develop autoimmune antibodies and lupus-like syndrome; stop drug if this happens. Symptoms can be expected to resolve.

---

Reactions may be *common,* uncommon, *life-threatening,* or COMMON AND LIFE-THREATENING.

• Patient receiving infliximab may develop tuberculosis (frequently disseminated or extrapulmonary at clinical presentation), invasive fungal infections, and other opportunistic infections. These infections may be fatal.
• Evaluate patient for latent tuberculosis infection with a tuberculin skin test. Treat latent tuberculosis infection before starting therapy with infliximab.

## PATIENT TEACHING
• Tell patient about infusion-reaction symptoms and instruct him to report them.
• Inform patient of adverse effects that may occur after infusion, and instruct him to report them promptly.
• Tell breast-feeding woman to stop breast-feeding during therapy.
• Instruct patient to tell prescriber of drug use before receiving vaccines.

---

# lymphocyte immune globulin (antithymocyte globulin [equine], ATG, LIG)
Atgam

*Pregnancy risk category C*

## AVAILABLE FORMS
*Injection:* 50 mg of equine IgG/ml in 5-ml ampules

## INDICATIONS & DOSAGES
➤ **To prevent acute renal allograft rejection**
*Adults:* 15 mg/kg I.V. daily for 14 days; then alternate-day dosing for 14 days. Give first dose within 24 hours of transplantation.
*Children:* 5 to 25 mg/kg I.V. daily for 14 days; then alternate-day dosing for 14 days. Give first dose within 24 hours of transplantation.
➤ **Acute renal allograft rejection**
*Adults and children:* 10 to 15 mg/kg I.V. daily for 14 days. Additional alternate-day therapy to total of 21 doses can be given. Start therapy when rejection is diagnosed.
➤ **Aplastic anemia**
*Adults:* 10 to 20 mg/kg I.V. daily for 8 to 14 days. Additional alternate-day therapy to total of 21 doses can be given.

## I.V. ADMINISTRATION
• Dilute concentrated drug for injection before giving. Dilute required dose in 250 to 1,000 ml of half-normal or normal saline solution. Final concentration of drug shouldn't exceed 1 mg/ml. When adding ATG to infusion solution, make sure container is inverted so drug doesn't contact air inside container. Gently rotate or swirl container to mix contents; don't shake because this may cause excessive foaming or denature the drug protein. Infuse with an in-line filter with a pore size of 0.2 to 1 micron over at least 4 hours (most institutions use 4 to 8 hours) into a vascular shunt, arterial venous fistula, or high-flow central vein.
• Don't dilute ATG concentrate with dextrose solutions or solutions with a low salt concentration because a precipitate may form. Proteins in ATG can be denatured by air. ATG is unstable in acidic solutions.
• Don't use solutions that are older than 12 hours, including actual infusion time.
• Refrigerate at 35° to 47° F (2° to 8° C). ATG concentrate is heat-sensitive. Don't freeze. Allow diluted ATG to reach room temperature before infusion.

## ACTION
Unknown. Inhibits cell-mediated immune responses either by altering T-cell function or eliminating antigen-reactive T cells.

| Route | Onset | Peak | Duration |
|-------|-------|------|----------|
| I.V. | Immediate | 5 days | Unknown |

## ADVERSE REACTIONS
**CNS:** malaise, *seizures,* headache.
**CV:** *hypotension, chest pain,* thrombophlebitis, tachycardia, edema, iliac vein obstruction.
**EENT:** *laryngospasm.*
**GI:** *nausea, vomiting, diarrhea,* hiccups, epigastric pain, abdominal distention, stomatitis.
**GU:** renal artery stenosis.
**Hematologic:** LEUKOPENIA, THROMBOCYTOPENIA, hemolysis, *aplastic anemia.*
**Metabolic:** hyperglycemia.
**Musculoskeletal:** *arthralgia, myalgia.*
**Respiratory:** dyspnea, *pulmonary edema.*
**Skin:** *rash, pruritus, urticaria.*

---

**Other:** febrile reactions, hypersensitivity reactions, serum sickness, *anaphylaxis,* infections, night sweats, lymphadenopathy, chills.

**INTERACTIONS**
None significant.

**EFFECTS ON LAB TEST RESULTS**
• May increase liver enzyme and glucose levels.
• May decrease hemoglobin and WBC and platelet counts.

**CONTRAINDICATIONS & CAUTIONS**
• Contraindicated in patients hypersensitive to drug.
• Use cautiously in patients receiving additional immunosuppressive therapy (such as corticosteroids or azathioprine) because of increased risk of infection.

**NURSING CONSIDERATIONS**
• *Alert:* An intradermal skin test is recommended at least 1 hour before first dose. Give an intradermal dose of 0.1 ml of a 1:1,000 lymphocyte immune globulin along with a contralateral normal saline control. Marked local swelling or erythema larger than 10 mm indicates increased risk of severe systemic reaction such as anaphylaxis. Severe reactions to skin test, such as hypotension, tachycardia, dyspnea, generalized rash, or anaphylaxis, usually preclude further use of drug. Anaphylaxis has occurred in patients with negative skin tests.
• Monitor patient for hypotension, respiratory distress, and chest, flank, or back pain, which may indicate anaphylaxis or hemolysis.
• Keep airway adjuncts and anaphylaxis drugs at bedside during administration.
• Watch for signs and symptoms of infection, such as fever, sore throat, malaise.

**PATIENT TEACHING**
• Instruct patient to report adverse drug reactions promptly, especially signs and symptoms of infection (fever, sore throat, fatigue).
• Tell patient to immediately report discomfort at I.V. insertion site because drug can cause a chemical phlebitis.

• Advise woman of childbearing age to avoid pregnancy during therapy.

# muromonab-CD3
Orthoclone OKT3

*Pregnancy risk category C*

**AVAILABLE FORMS**
*Injection:* 1 mg/1 ml in 5-ml ampules

**INDICATIONS & DOSAGES**
➤ **Acute allograft rejection in renal transplant patients; in steroid-resistant hepatic or cardiac allograft rejection**
*Adults:* 5 mg I.V. daily for 10 to 14 days.
*Children:* Initially, 2.5 mg/day (if 30 kg or less) or 5 mg/day (if more than 30 kg) I.V. as a single bolus over less than 1 minute for 10 to 14 days. Daily dosage increases by 2.5-mg increments may be necessary to decrease CD3+ cells.

**I.V. ADMINISTRATION**
• Draw solution into syringe through low protein-binding 0.2- or 0.22-micron filter. Discard filter and attach needle for I.V. bolus injection.
• Give bolus over less than 1 minute.

**ACTION**
A murine monoclonal antibody that reacts in the T-lymphocyte membrane with a molecule (CD3) needed for antigen recognition. Depletes the blood of CD3+ T cells, which leads to restoration of allograft function and reversal of rejection.

| Route | Onset | Peak | Duration |
|-------|-------|------|----------|
| I.V. | Immediate | Unknown | 1 wk |

**ADVERSE REACTIONS**
**CNS:** *asthenia,* fatigue, lethargy, malaise, *fever,* **seizures,** dizziness, *headache, meningitis, tremor,* confusion, depression, nervousness, somnolence.
**CV:** vasodilation, **arrhythmia, bradycardia,** *hypertension, hypotension,* chest pain, *tachycardia,* vascular occlusion, *edema,* **cardiac arrest, shock, heart failure.**
**EENT:** photophobia, tinnitus.
**GI:** anorexia, *diarrhea, nausea,* abdominal pain, GI pain, *vomiting.*
**GU:** *renal dysfunction.*

---

Reactions may be *common,* uncommon, **life-threatening,** or COMMON AND LIFE-THREATENING.

**Hematologic:** anemia, *leukocytosis, leukopenia, thrombocytopenia,*
**Musculoskeletal:** arthralgia, myalgia.
**Respiratory:** *dyspnea,* hyperventilation, hypoxia, pneumonia, pulmonary edema, respiratory congestion, wheezing, *acute respiratory distress syndrome.*
**Skin:** diaphoresis, pruritus, *rash.*
**Other:** *chills,* pain in trunk area, *cytokine release syndrome, hypersensitivity reactions.*

### INTERACTIONS
**Drug-drug.** *Immunosuppressants:* May increase risk of infection. Use cautiously; consider reduced immunosuppressant dosage.
*Indomethacin:* May increase muromonab-CD3 levels with encephalopathy and other CNS effects. Monitor patient closely.
*Live-virus vaccines:* May increase replication and effects. Use with caution.

### EFFECTS ON LAB TEST RESULTS
• May increase BUN and creatinine levels.
• May cause abnormal urine cytologic study results.

### CONTRAINDICATIONS & CAUTIONS
• Contraindicated in patients hypersensitive to drug or other products of murine (mouse) origin, in those who have history of seizures or are predisposed to seizures, in pregnant or breast-feeding women, and in patients with uncontrolled hypertension. Also contraindicated in those who have antimurine antibody titers of 1:1,000 or more or fluid overload, as evidenced by chest radiograph or weight gain greater than 3% within the week before treatment.

### NURSING CONSIDERATIONS
• Obtain chest radiograph within 24 hours before starting drug treatment.
• Assess patient for signs and symptoms of fluid overload before treatment.
• Treatment should begin in facility equipped and staffed for cardiopulmonary resuscitation and where patient can be monitored closely.
• Most adverse reactions develop within 30 minutes to 6 hours after first dose.
• Before giving drug, give an antipyretic to help lower risk of expected pyrexia and chills. Treat temperature exceeding 100° F

(38° C) with antipyretics before drug administration, and evaluate risk of infection.
• *Alert:* Pretreatment with methylprednisolone 1 to 4 hours before first dose is recommended to reduce the severity of infusion reaction.
• Patients develop antibodies to muromonab-CD3 that can lead to loss of effectiveness and more severe adverse reactions if a second course of therapy is attempted. Therefore, some prescribers use drug for only a single course of treatment.

### PATIENT TEACHING
• Inform patient of expected adverse reactions.
• Reassure patient that reactions will diminish as treatment progresses.
• Tell patient to avoid people with infections because drug lowers resistance to infection.
• Advise woman to avoid pregnancy during therapy.

---

## mycophenolate mofetil
CellCept

## mycophenolate mofetil hydrochloride
CellCept Intravenous

*Pregnancy risk category C*

### AVAILABLE FORMS
**mycophenolate mofetil**
*Capsules:* 250 mg
*Tablets:* 500 mg
**mycophenolate mofetil hydrochloride**
*Injection:* 500 mg/vial

### INDICATIONS & DOSAGES
➤ **To prevent organ rejection in patients receiving allogenic renal transplants**
*Adults:* 1 g P.O. or I.V. b.i.d. with corticosteroids and cyclosporine.
*Adjust-a-dose:* For patients with severe chronic renal impairment outside of immediate posttransplant period, avoid doses above 1 g b.i.d. If neutropenia develops, interrupt or reduce dosing.

---

➤ **To prevent organ rejection in patients receiving allogenic cardiac transplant**
*Adults:* 1.5 g P.O. or I.V. b.i.d. with cyclosporine and corticosteroids.
➤ **To prevent organ rejection in patients receiving allogenic hepatic transplants**
*Adults:* 1 g I.V. b.i.d. over no less than 2 hours or 1.5 g P.O. b.i.d. with cyclosporine and corticosteroids.
*Adjust-a-dose:* If neutropenia develops, interrupt or reduce dosing.

## I.V. ADMINISTRATION
• Reconstitute CellCept Intravenous and dilute to 6 mg/ml using 14 ml of $D_5W$.
• Drug is incompatible with other I.V. solutions.
• Never give drug by rapid or bolus I.V. injection. Infuse drug over at least 2 hours.
• Use within 4 hours of reconstitution and dilution.

## ACTION
Inhibits proliferative response of T and B lymphocytes, suppresses antibody formation by B lymphocytes, and may inhibit recruitment of leukocytes into sites of inflammation and graft rejection.

| Route | Onset | Peak | Duration |
|-------|-------|------|----------|
| P.O. | Unknown | 30-75 min | 7-18 hr |
| I.V. | Unknown | Unknown | 10-17 hr |

## ADVERSE REACTIONS
**CNS:** *tremor,* insomnia, *fever,* dizziness, *headache, asthenia.*
**CV:** *chest pain, hypertension, edema.*
**EENT:** pharyngitis.
**GI:** *diarrhea, constipation, nausea, dyspepsia, vomiting, oral candidiasis, abdominal pain,* **hemorrhage.**
**GU:** *UTI, hematuria,* renal tubular necrosis.
**Hematologic:** *anemia,* LEUKOPENIA, THROMBOCYTOPENIA, hypochromic anemia, leukocytosis.
**Metabolic:** *hypercholesterolemia, hypophosphatemia, hypokalemia, hyperkalemia, hyperglycemia.*
**Musculoskeletal:** *back pain.*
**Respiratory:** *dyspnea, cough, infection,* bronchitis, pneumonia.
**Skin:** *acne,* rash.
**Other:** *pain, infection,* **sepsis,** *peripheral edema.*

## INTERACTIONS
**Drug-drug.** *Acyclovir, ganciclovir, other drugs that undergo renal tubular secretion:* May increase risk of toxicity for both drugs. Monitor patient closely.
*Antacids with magnesium and aluminum hydroxides:* May decrease mycophenolate absorption. Separate dosing times.
*Cholestyramine:* May interfere with enterohepatic recirculation, reducing mycophenolate bioavailability. Avoid using together.
*Phenytoin, theophylline:* May increase both drug levels. Monitor drug levels closely.
*Probenecid, salicylates:* May increase mycophenolate level. Monitor patient closely.

## EFFECTS ON LAB TEST RESULTS
• May increase cholesterol and glucose levels. May decrease phosphorus level. May increase or decrease potassium level.
• May decrease hemoglobin and platelet count. May increase or decrease WBC count.

## CONTRAINDICATIONS & CAUTIONS
• Contraindicated in patients hypersensitive to drug, its ingredients, or mycophenolic acid and in patients sensitive to polysorbate 80.
• Drug isn't recommended for use in pregnant women (unless benefits to mother outweigh risks to fetus) or in breast-feeding women.
• Safety and effectiveness of drug in children haven't been established.
• Use cautiously in patients with GI disorders.

## NURSING CONSIDERATIONS
• Start drug therapy within 24 hours after transplantation. Use I.V. form in patients unable to take oral forms.
• I.V. form can be given for up to 14 days; switch patient to capsules or tablets as soon as oral drugs can be tolerated.
• Avoid doses above 1 g b.i.d. after immediate posttransplant period in patients with severe chronic renal impairment.
• Because of potential teratogenic effects, don't open or crush capsule. Avoid inhaling powder in capsule or having it contact skin or mucous membranes. If such con-

---

tact occurs, wash thoroughly with soap and water, and rinse eyes with water.

**PATIENT TEACHING**
• Warn patient not to open or crush capsules, but to swallow them whole on an empty stomach.
• Stress importance of not interrupting or stopping therapy without first consulting prescriber.
• Tell woman to have a pregnancy test 1 week before therapy begins.
• Instruct woman of childbearing age to use two forms of contraception during therapy and for 6 weeks afterward, even with a history of infertility, unless a hysterectomy has been performed or abstinence is the chosen method. Tell her to notify prescriber immediately if she suspects pregnancy.
• Warn patient of the increased risk of lymphoma and other malignancies.

---

**sirolimus**
Rapamune

*Pregnancy risk category C*

**AVAILABLE FORMS**
*Oral solution:* 1 mg/ml
*Tablet:* 1 mg

**INDICATIONS & DOSAGES**
➤ **To prevent organ rejection in patients receiving renal transplants with cyclosporine and corticosteroids**
*Adults and adolescents:* Initially, 6 mg P.O. as one-time dose as soon as possible after transplantation; then maintenance dose of 2 mg P.O. once daily.
*Children age 13 and older weighing less than 40 kg (88 lb):* First dose is 3 mg/m$^2$ P.O. as one-time dose after transplantation; then 1 mg/m$^2$ P.O. once daily.
*Adjust-a-dose:* For patients with mild-to-moderate hepatic impairment, reduce maintenance dose by about one-third. It isn't necessary to reduce loading dose. Two to 4 months after transplantation in patients with low-to-moderate risk of graft rejection, taper off cyclosporine over 4 to 8 weeks. During the taper, adjust sirolimus dose q 1 to 2 weeks to obtain blood levels between 12 and 24 ng/ml. Base dosage ad-

justments in clinical status, tissue biopsies, and laboratory findings.
Maximum daily dose shouldn't exceed 40 mg. If a daily dose exceeds 40 mg due to a loading dose, give the loading dose over 2 days. Monitor trough concentrations at least 3 to 4 days after a loading dose.

**ACTION**
An immunosuppressant that inhibits T-lymphocyte activation and proliferation that occurs in response to antigenic and cytokine stimulation. Also inhibits antibody formation.

| Route | Onset | Peak | Duration |
|-------|-------|------|----------|
| P.O. | Unknown | 1-3 hr | Unknown |

**ADVERSE REACTIONS**
**CNS:** *headache, insomnia, tremor, anxiety, depression, asthenia,* malaise, *fever,* syncope, confusion, dizziness, emotional lability, hypertonia, hypesthesia, hypotonia, neuropathy, paresthesia, somnolence.
**CV:** *hypertension,* **heart failure, atrial fibrillation,** tachycardia, hypotension, *chest pain,* edema, **hemorrhage,** palpitations, peripheral vascular disorder, thrombophlebitis, thrombosis, vasodilatation, *peripheral edema.*
**EENT:** facial edema, *pharyngitis,* epistaxis, rhinitis, sinusitis, abnormal vision, cataract, conjunctivitis, deafness, ear pain, otitis media, tinnitus.
**GI:** *diarrhea, nausea, vomiting, constipation, abdominal pain, dyspepsia,* hernia, enlarged abdomen, ascites, peritonitis, anorexia, dysphagia, eructation, esophagitis, flatulence, gastritis, gastroenteritis, gingivitis, gum hyperplasia, ileus, mouth ulceration, oral candidiasis, stomatitis.
**GU:** dysuria, hematuria, albuminuria, **kidney tubular necrosis,** *UTI,* pelvic pain, glycosuria, bladder pain, hydronephrosis, impotence, kidney pain, nocturia, oliguria, pyuria, scrotal edema, testis disorder, **toxic nephropathy,** urinary frequency, urinary incontinence, urinary retention.
**Hematologic:** *anemia,* THROMBOCYTOPENIA, *leukopenia, thrombotic thrombocytopenia purpura,* ecchymosis, leukocytosis, polycythemia.
**Hepatic:** *hepatotoxicity, hepatic artery thrombosis.*

---

**Metabolic:** *hypercholesteremia, hyperlipidemia, hypokalemia, weight gain, hypophosphatemia, hyperkalemia,* hypervolemia, Cushing's syndrome, diabetes mellitus, acidosis, dehydration, hypercalcemia, hyperglycemia, hyperphosphatemia, hypocalcemia, ***hypoglycemia,*** hypomagnesemia, hyponatremia, weight loss.

**Musculoskeletal:** *back pain, arthralgia,* myalgia, arthrosis, bone necrosis, leg cramps, osteoporosis, tetany.

**Respiratory:** *dyspnea, cough, atelectasis, upper respiratory tract infection,* asthma, bronchitis, hypoxia, lung edema, pleural effusion, pneumonia, ***interstitial lung disease.***

**Skin:** *rash, acne,* hirsutism, fungal dermatitis, pruritus, skin hypertrophy, skin ulcer, sweating.

**Other:** *pain,* abscess, cellulitis, chills, flu syndrome, infection, ***sepsis,*** lymphadenopathy, lymphocele, abnormal healing including fascial dehiscence and anastomotic disruption (wound, vascular, airway, ureteral, biliary).

## INTERACTIONS

**Drug-drug.** *Aminoglycosides, amphotericin B, other nephrotoxic drugs:* May increase risk of nephrotoxicity. Use with caution.

*Bromocriptine, cimetidine, clarithromycin, clotrimazole, danazol, erythromycin, fluconazole, indinavir, itraconazole, metoclopramide, nicardipine, ritonavir, verapamil, other drugs that inhibit CYP 3A4:* May increase blood levels of sirolimus. Monitor sirolimus levels closely.

*Carbamazepine, phenobarbital, phenytoin, rifabutin, rifapentine, other drugs that induce CYP 3A4:* May decrease blood levels of sirolimus. Monitor patient closely.

*Cyclosporine:* May inhibit sirolimus metabolism. Sirolimus levels decrease when cyclosporine is stopped. Carefully increase sirolimus dose during cyclosporine taper to eventually be about fourfold higher.

*Diltiazem:* May increase sirolimus levels. Monitor sirolimus level, as needed.

*HMG-CoA reductase inhibitors or fibrates:* May increase risk of rhabdomyolysis with the combination of sirolimus and cyclosporine. Monitor patient closely.

*Ketoconazole:* May increase rate and extent of sirolimus absorption. Avoid using together.

*Live-virus vaccines (BCG; measles, mumps, rubella; oral polio; yellow fever; varicella; TY21a typhoid):* May reduce vaccine effectiveness. Avoid using together.

*Rifampin:* May decrease sirolimus level. Alternative therapy to rifampin may be prescribed.

**Drug-food.** *Grapefruit juice:* May decrease metabolism of sirolimus. Discourage use together.

**Drug-lifestyle.** *Sun exposure:* May increase risk of skin cancer. Tell patient to take precautions.

## EFFECTS ON LAB TEST RESULTS

• May increase BUN, creatinine, liver enzyme, cholesterol, and lipid levels. May decrease sodium and magnesium levels. May increase or decrease phosphate, potassium, glucose, and calcium levels.

• May increase RBC count. May decrease hemoglobin and platelet count. May increase or decrease WBC count.

## CONTRAINDICATIONS & CAUTIONS

• Contraindicated in patients hypersensitive to active drug, its derivatives, or components of product.

• Use cautiously in patients with hyperlipidemia and impaired liver or renal function.

• Safety and effectiveness of sirolimus as immunosuppressive therapy haven't been established in liver or lung transplant patients and such use isn't recommended.

## NURSING CONSIDERATIONS

• ***Alert:*** Use of sirolimus plus tacrolimus or cyclosporine was linked to an increase in hepatic artery thrombosis, leading to an excessive rate of death and graft loss in a liver transplant study. Most cases occurred within 30 days after transplant, and many of these patients had evidence of infection at or near the time of death.

• Only those experienced in immunosuppressive therapy and management of renal transplant patients should prescribe drug.

• Cases of bronchial anastomotic dehiscence, some fatal, have been reported in lung transplant recipients treated with sirolimus in combination with tacrolimus and corticosteroids.

• Use drug in regimen with cyclosporine and corticosteroids; have patient take drug 4 hours after cyclosporine dose.

• Cyclosporine withdrawal in patients with high-risk of graft rejection isn't recommended. This includes patients with Banff grade III acute rejection or vascular rejection before cyclosporine withdrawal, those who are dialysis-dependent, those with serum creatinine greater than 4.5 mg/dl, black patients, patients with re-transplants or multiorgan transplants, and patients with high panel of reactive antibodies.

• Patient should take drug consistently either with or without food.

• Dilute oral solution before use. After dilution, use immediately and discard oral solution syringe.

• When diluting oral solution, empty correct amount into glass or plastic (not Styrofoam) container holding at least ¼ cup (60 ml) of either water or orange juice. Don't use grapefruit juice or any other liquid. Stir vigorously and have patient drink immediately. Refill container with at least ½ cup (120 ml) of water or orange juice, stir again, and have patient drink all contents.

• After transplantation, give antimicrobial prophylaxis for *Pneumocystis carinii* for 1 year and for cytomegalovirus for 3 months.

• **Alert:** Patients taking drug are more susceptible to infection and lymphoma.

• Monitor renal function tests, because use with cyclosporine may cause creatinine level to increase. Adjustment of immuno-suppressive regimen may be needed.

• Monitor cholesterol and triglyceride levels. Treatment with lipid-lowering drugs during therapy isn't uncommon. If hyperlipidemia is detected, additional interventions, such as diet and exercise, should begin.

• Check for rhabdomyolysis.

• Monitor drug levels in patients age 13 and older who weigh less than 40 kg, patients with hepatic impairment, those also receiving drugs that induce or inhibit CYP 3A4, and patients in whom cyclosporine dosing is markedly reduced or stopped.

• A slight haze may develop during refrigeration. This doesn't affect potency of drug. If haze develops, bring to room temperature and shake until haze disappears.

• Store away from light, and refrigerate at 36° to 46° F (2° to 8° C). After opening bottle, use contents within 1 month. If needed, store bottles and pouches at room temperature (up to 77° F [25° C]) for several days. Drug may be kept in oral dosing syringe for 24 hours at room temperature.

## PATIENT TEACHING
• Tell patient how to properly store, dilute, and give drug.

• Advise woman of childbearing age about risks during pregnancy. Tell her to use effective contraception before and during therapy, and for 12 weeks after stopping therapy.

• Tell patient to take drug consistently with or without food to minimize absorption variability.

• Tell patient to take drug 4 hours after cyclosporine to avoid drug interactions.

• Advise patient to wash area with soap and water if drug solution touches skin or mucous membranes.

---

## tacrolimus (FK506)
Prograf

*Pregnancy risk category C*

### AVAILABLE FORMS
*Capsules:* 0.5 mg, 1 mg, 5 mg
*Injection:* 5 mg/ml

### INDICATIONS & DOSAGES
➤ **To prevent organ rejection in allogenic liver or kidney transplants**
*Adults:* 0.03 to 0.05 mg/kg daily I.V. as continuous infusion given no sooner than 6 hours after transplantation. Substitute P.O. therapy as soon as possible, with first oral dose given 8 to 12 hours after discontinuing I.V. infusion. Or, give P.O. dose within 24 hours of transplantation after renal function has recovered. Recommended first P.O. dosage for allogenic liver transplants is 0.1 to 0.15 mg/kg daily P.O. in two divided doses q 12 hours. Recommended first P.O. dosage for allogenic kidney transplants is 0.2 mg/kg daily in two

divided doses q 12 hours. Adjust dosages based on clinical response.
*Children:* Initially, 0.03 to 0.05 mg/kg daily I.V.; then 0.15 to 0.2 mg/kg daily P.O. on schedule similar to that of adults, adjusted p.r.n.
**Adjust-a-dose:** Give lowest recommended P.O. and I.V. dosages to patients with renal or hepatic impairment.

## I.V. ADMINISTRATION
● Dilute drug with normal saline solution for injection or $D_5W$ injection to 0.004 to 0.02 mg/ml before use. Store diluted infusion solution for up to 24 hours in glass or polyethylene containers. Don't store drug in a polyvinyl chloride container because of decreased stability and potential for extraction of phthalates.
● Monitor patient continuously during first 30 minutes of I.V. administration and frequently thereafter for signs and symptoms of anaphylaxis.

## ACTION
Exact mechanism unknown. Inhibits T-lymphocyte activation, which results in immunosuppression.

| Route | Onset | Peak | Duration |
|---|---|---|---|
| P.O., I.V. | Unknown | 1½-3 hr | Unknown |

## ADVERSE REACTIONS
**CNS:** *headache, tremor, insomnia, paresthesia, delirium,* **coma,** *fever, asthenia.*
**CV:** *hypertension, peripheral edema.*
**GI:** *diarrhea, nausea, vomiting, constipation, anorexia, abdominal pain, ascites.*
**GU:** *abnormal renal function, UTI, oliguria.*
**Hematologic:** *anemia, leukocytosis,* THROMBOCYTOPENIA.
**Metabolic:** *hyperkalemia, hypokalemia, hyperglycemia, hypomagnesemia.*
**Musculoskeletal:** *back pain.*
**Respiratory:** *pleural effusion, atelectasis, dyspnea.*
**Skin:** *pruritus, burning, rash, photosensitivity,* alopecia.
**Other:** *pain.*

## INTERACTIONS
**Drug-drug.** Bromocriptine, cimetidine, clarithromycin, clotrimazole, cyclosporine, danazol, diltiazem, erythromycin, fluconazole, itraconazole, ketoconazole, methylprednisolone, metoclopramide, nicardipine, verapamil: May increase tacrolimus level. Watch for adverse effects.
*Carbamazepine, phenobarbital, phenytoin, rifabutin, rifampin:* May decrease tacrolimus level. Monitor effectiveness of tacrolimus.
*Cyclosporine:* May increase risk of excess nephrotoxicity. Avoid using together.
*Immunosuppressants (except adrenal corticosteroids):* May oversuppress immune system. Monitor patient closely, especially during times of stress.
*Inducers of cytochrome P450 enzyme system:* May increase tacrolimus metabolism and decrease blood levels. Dosage adjustment may be needed.
*Inhibitors of cytochrome P450 enzyme system (phenobarbital, phenytoin, rifampin):* May decrease tacrolimus metabolism and increase blood level. Dosage adjustment may be needed.
*Live-virus vaccines:* May interfere with immune response to live-virus vaccines. Postpone routine immunizations.
*Nephrotoxic drugs (such as aminoglycosides, amphotericin B, cisplatin, cyclosporine):* May cause additive or synergistic effects. Monitor patient closely.
**Drug-food.** *Any food:* May inhibit drug absorption. Urge patient to take drug on empty stomach.
*Grapefruit juice:* May increase drug level. Discourage patient from taking together.

## EFFECTS ON LAB TEST RESULTS
● May increase BUN, creatinine, and glucose levels. May decrease magnesium level. May increase or decrease potassium level and cause abnormal liver function test values.
● May decrease hemoglobin, WBC and platelet counts.

## CONTRAINDICATIONS & CAUTIONS
● Contraindicated in patients hypersensitive to drug.
● I.V. form is contraindicated in patients hypersensitive to castor oil derivatives.

## NURSING CONSIDERATIONS
• *Alert:* Because of risk of anaphylaxis, use injection only in patients who can't take oral form.
• Keep epinephrine 1:1,000 and oxygen available to treat anaphylaxis.
• Children with normal renal and hepatic function may need higher dosages than adults.
• Patients with hepatic or renal dysfunction should receive lowest dosage possible.
• Expect to give adrenal corticosteroids with drug.
• Monitor patient for signs and symptoms of neurotoxicity and nephrotoxicity, especially if patient is receiving a high dose or has renal or hepatic dysfunction.
• Monitor patient for signs and symptoms of hyperkalemia, such as palpitations and muscle weakness or cramping. Obtain potassium levels regularly. Avoid potassium-sparing diuretics during drug therapy.
• Monitor patient's glucose level regularly. Also monitor patient for signs and symptoms of hyperglycemia, such as dizziness, confusion, and frequent urination. Treatment of hyperglycemia may be needed. Insulin-dependent posttransplant diabetes may occur; in some cases, it's reversible.
• Patient receiving drug is at increased risk for infections, lymphomas, and other malignant diseases.

## PATIENT TEACHING
• Advise patient to check with prescriber before taking other drugs during therapy.
• Urge patient to report adverse reactions promptly.
• Tell diabetic patient that glucose levels may increase.

## Vaccines and toxoids

BCG vaccine
cholera vaccine
diphtheria and tetanus toxoids
  and acellular pertussis vaccine
  adsorbed
diphtheria and tetanus toxoids,
  acellular pertussis adsorbed,
  hepatitis B (recombinant), and
  inactivated poliovirus vaccine
  combined
*Haemophilus* b conjugate
  vaccines
hepatitis A vaccine, inactivated
hepatitis B vaccine, recombinant
influenza virus vaccine live,
  intranasal
influenza virus vaccine, 2003-2004
  trivalent types A and B
  (purified surface antigen)
influenza virus vaccine, 2003-2004
  trivalent types A and B
  (subvirion or purified
  subvirion)
measles, mumps, and rubella
  virus vaccine, live
measles and rubella virus
  vaccine, live attenuated
measles virus vaccine, live
  attenuated
meningococcal polysaccharide
  vaccine
mumps virus vaccine, live
pneumococcal 7-valent conjugate
  vaccine (diphtheria $CRM_{197}$
  protein)
pneumococcal vaccine,
  polyvalent
poliovirus vaccine, inactivated
rabies vaccine, adsorbed
rabies vaccine, human diploid cell
rubella and mumps virus vaccine,
  live
rubella virus vaccine, live
  attenuated
smallpox vaccine, dried
tetanus toxoid, adsorbed
tetanus toxoid, fluid
varicella virus vaccine
yellow fever vaccine

### COMBINATION PRODUCTS
ActHIB/DTP: 10 mcg *Haemophilus* b
polyribosylribitol phosphate (PRP) conjugated to 24 mcg tetanus toxoid, 6.7 limit
flocculation (Lf) units diphtheria toxoid,
5 Lf units tetanus toxoid, and 4 units
whole-cell pertussis vaccine per 0.5 ml.
Comvax: 7.5 mcg *Haemophilus* b PRP,
125 mcg *Neisseria meningitidis* OMPC,
and 5 mcg hepatitis B surface antigen per
0.5 ml.
Tetramune: 10 mcg purified *Haemophilus* b saccharide and about 25 mcg
$CRM_{197}$ protein, 12.5 Lf units inactivated
diphtheria, 5 Lf units inactivated tetanus,
and 4 protective units pertussis per 0.5 ml.

---

### BCG vaccine
TICE BCG

*Pregnancy risk category C*

### AVAILABLE FORMS
*Percutaneous vaccine:* 1 to $8 \times 10^8$
colony-forming units (CFU)/vial (TICE
strain)

### INDICATIONS & DOSAGES
➤ **Tuberculosis (TB) exposure**
*Adults and children age 1 month and older:* 0.2 to 0.3 ml (percutaneous vaccine)
applied to clean skin; then apply multiple-puncture disk.
*Infants younger than age 1 month:* Reduce
dosage by 50% by using 2 ml of sterile
water without preservatives when reconstituting.

### ACTION
A live, attenuated bacterial vaccine prepared from *Mycobacterium bovis* that promotes active immunity to TB.

| Route | Onset | Peak | Duration |
|-------|-------|------|----------|
| Percutaneous | Unknown | Unknown | Unknown |

### ADVERSE REACTIONS
**Musculoskeletal:** osteomyelitis.

---

Reactions may be *common*, uncommon, *life-threatening*, or COMMON AND LIFE-THREATENING.

**Other:** lymphadenopathy, allergic reaction, *anaphylaxis.*

## INTERACTIONS
**Drug-drug.** *Immunosuppressants:* May reduce response to BCG vaccine. Avoid using together.
*Isoniazid, rifampin, streptomycin:* May inhibit multiplication of BCG. Avoid using together.

## EFFECTS ON LAB TEST RESULTS
None reported.

## CONTRAINDICATIONS & CAUTIONS
• Contraindicated in patients hypersensitive to vaccine. Contraindicated in patients with hypogammaglobulinemia, immunosuppression and a positive tuberculin reaction (when meant for use as immunoprophylactic after exposure to TB), fresh smallpox vaccinations, or burns. Also contraindicated in patients receiving corticosteroid therapy. Avoid use in pregnant patients.
• Use cautiously in patients with chronic skin disease.
• Safety and effectiveness in adults and children infected with HIV haven't been determined.

## NURSING CONSIDERATIONS
• Don't inject vaccine I.V., S.C., or I.D.
• Inject only into healthy skin.
• Obtain history of allergies and reaction to immunization.
• Keep epinephrine 1:1,000 available to treat anaphylaxis.
• Don't shake vial after reconstitution. Use within 2 hours.
• Don't give to febrile patients unless cause is known.
• For TICE BCG, add 1 ml of sterile diluent (preservative-free saline injection to 50-mg vial to resuspend. Leave drug and diluent in contact for 1 minute. Then mix suspension by withdrawing it into syringe and expelling it gently back into vial two or three times. Avoid producing foam; don't shake.
• Give vaccine using a multiple-puncture disc. Keep area dry for at least 24 hours after administration.
• Expect lesions in 10 to 14 days. Papules reach maximum diameter of 3 mm, then fade. Quicker results occur when the patient has tuberculosis.
• Allow at least 6 to 8 weeks between BCG and live-virus vaccines; give killed-virus vaccines 7 days before or 10 days after BCG.
• Vaccine is of no value as immunoprophylactic in patients with positive tuberculin test result.
• Tuberculin sensitivity may be rendered positive by BCG intravesical treatment. Determine patient's reactivity to tuberculin before therapy.
• Destroy live vaccine by autoclaving or treating with formaldehyde solution before disposal.

## PATIENT TEACHING
• Advise patient to have tuberculin skin test 2 to 3 months after BCG vaccination.
• Tell patient to report unusual signs and symptoms after vaccination, or signs of allergic reaction, including difficulty breathing, enlarged lymph nodes, or skin ulcer or lesion at injection site.
• Urge patient to keep site dry for 24 hours and not to expose area to others because live vaccine may infect them.

# cholera vaccine

*Pregnancy risk category C*

## AVAILABLE FORMS
*Injection:* Suspension of killed *Vibrio cholerae* (each ml contains 8 units of Inaba and Ogawa serotypes) in 1.5-ml and 20-ml vials

## INDICATIONS & DOSAGES
➤ **Primary immunization for persons traveling to areas where cholera is endemic or epidemic**
*I.M. or S.C. route*
*Adults and children older than age 10:* Two doses of 0.5 ml I.M. or S.C., 1 week to 1 month apart, before traveling in cholera area. Booster is 0.5 ml q 6 months, p.r.n.
*Children ages 5 to 10:* 0.3 ml I.M. or S.C. Give boosters of same dose q 6 months, p.r.n.

---

*Rapid onset*   †Canada   ‡Australia   ◇OTC   ♦ Off-label use   ⬭Photoguide   *Liquid contains alcohol.

*Children ages 6 months to 4 years:* 0.2 ml
I.M. or S.C. Give boosters of same dose q
6 months, p.r.n.
**I.D. route**
*Adults and children age 5 and older:* Two
doses of 0.2 ml I.D., 1 week to 1 month
apart, and q 6 months, p.r.n.

## ACTION
Promotes active immunity to cholera.

| Route | Onset | Peak | Duration |
|-------|-------|------|----------|
| I.M., S.C., I.D. | After 2nd dose | Unknown | 3-6 mo |

## ADVERSE REACTIONS
**CNS:** fever, headache, malaise.
**Skin:** *erythema, swelling, pain, induration
at injection site.*
**Other:** *anaphylaxis.*

## INTERACTIONS
**Drug-drug.** *Plague, typhoid, other vaccines with systemic adverse reactions:*
May increase toxicity. Avoid using together.
*Yellow fever vaccine:* Simultaneous use
may interfere with immune response to
both vaccines. Give 3 weeks apart.

## EFFECTS ON LAB TEST RESULTS
None reported.

## CONTRAINDICATIONS & CAUTIONS
• Contraindicated in those with acute illness or history of severe systemic reaction
or allergic response to vaccine.
• Contraindicated as I.M. injection in patients with thrombocytopenia or other coagulation disorders for which I.M. injection is contraindicated.

## NURSING CONSIDERATIONS
• Obtain history of allergies and reaction
to immunization.
• Keep epinephrine 1:1,000 available to
treat anaphylaxis.
• Shake vial vigorously before withdrawing each dose.
• Give vaccine I.M. in deltoid muscle in
adults and children older than age 3.
• I.M. and S.C. routes give higher levels
of protection in children younger than
age 5.

• Vaccine is about 50% effective in reducing clinical illness risk for 3 to 6 months.

## PATIENT TEACHING
• Advise patient that pain, hardening, and
swelling at injection site are common for
24 to 48 hours.
• Tell traveler to avoid food and water that
may be contaminated.
• Advise patient that malaise, headache,
and mild to moderate fever may persist for
1 to 2 days.

---

# diphtheria and tetanus toxoids
# and acellular pertussis
# vaccine adsorbed (DTaP)
Certiva, Daptacel, Infanrix,
Tripedia

*Pregnancy risk category C*

## AVAILABLE FORMS
*Injection:* 6.7 limit flocculation (Lf) units
diphtheria, 5 Lf units tetanus, and
46.8 mcg pertussis antigens per 0.5 ml
in single-dose and 7.5-ml vials; 15 Lf
units of diphtheria toxoid, 6 Lf units
tetanus toxoid, and 40 mcg pertussis toxoid per 0.5 ml in 7.5-ml vials; 15 Lf units
of diphtheria toxoid, 5 Lf units tetanus
toxoid, 10 mcg pertussis toxin, 5 mcg fila-
mentous hemagglutinin (FHA), 3 mcg
pertactin, 5 mcg fimbriae types 2 and
3 per 0.5 ml in 0.5- and 2.5-ml vials;
25 Lf units of diphtheria toxoid, 10 Lf
units tetanus toxoid, 25 mcg pertussis
toxin, 25 mcg FHA, 8 mcg pertactin per
0.5 ml in 0.5-ml vials

## INDICATIONS & DOSAGES
➤ **Primary immunization**
*Children ages 6 weeks to 7 years:* Give
0.5 ml I.M. 4 to 8 weeks apart for three
doses (6 to 8 weeks for Daptacel) and a
fourth dose at least 6 months after the
third dose.
➤ **Booster immunization**
If Tripedia was used for the first four doses, a fifth dose is recommended at age 4 to
6 before entering school. If the fourth
dose was given after age 4, a fifth dose
isn't needed.
    Certiva is recommended as a fourth
dose at ages 15 to 20 months in children

who received their first three doses as whole-cell diphtheria, tetanus, and pertussis (DTP) vaccine. A fifth dose is recommended at age 4 to 6 in children who received four doses of whole-cell DTP vaccine or three doses of whole-cell vaccine followed by one dose of DTaP, unless the fourth dose was given after the fourth birthday.

Infanrix is indicated as a fifth dose in children ages 4 to 6 before entering school in those who received at least one dose of whole-cell DTP vaccine, unless the fourth dose was given after the fourth birthday.

Daptacel may be given to complete the immunization series in children who have received at least one dose of whole-cell DTP vaccine.

## ACTION
Promotes active immunity to DTP by inducing production of antitoxins and antibodies.

| Route | Onset | Peak | Duration |
|-------|-------|------|----------|
| I.M. | 2 wk after last dose | Unknown | 10 yr |

## ADVERSE REACTIONS
**CNS:** *seizures,* fever, *drowsiness.*
**GI:** *anorexia,* vomiting.
**Skin:** *tenderness, redness, and swelling at injection site.*
**Other:** *hypersensitivity reactions, fretfulness,* irritability, crying longer than 1 hour.

## INTERACTIONS
**Drug-drug.** *Immunosuppressants:* May reduce response to DTP vaccine. Avoid using together.

## EFFECTS ON LAB TEST RESULTS
None reported.

## CONTRAINDICATIONS & CAUTIONS
• Contraindicated in adults or children older than age 7, immunosuppressed patients, those on corticosteroid therapy, and those with history of seizures.
• Pertussis component of vaccine is contraindicated in children who have preexisting neurologic disorders or who exhibited neurologic signs after previous injection. Give these children diphtheria and tetanus toxoids (DT) vaccine instead. Postpone

vaccination in patients with acute febrile illness.
• **Alert:** Give vaccine to patients age 7 and older only in special circumstances, never routinely.

## NURSING CONSIDERATIONS
• Children whose seizures are well controlled or who had an explainable single-episode seizure may receive the acellular vaccine.
• Obtain history of allergies and reaction to immunization, especially to pertussis vaccine.
• Keep epinephrine 1:1,000 available to treat anaphylaxis.
• If an immediate allergic reaction occurs after administration of the vaccine, withhold subsequent vaccination and refer patient to an allergist for evaluation. If a specific allergy can be documented, desensitization to tetanus toxoid may be warranted.
• Give only by deep I.M. injection, preferably in thigh or deltoid muscle. Don't give S.C.
• In infants, give I.M. injection in the anterolateral thigh.
• Vaccine may be given at same time as polio vaccine and, if indicated, when the patient receives vaccines against *Haemophilus influenzae* type b, measles, mumps, and rubella.
• Acellular vaccine may be linked to a lower risk of local pain and fever.
• **Alert:** DTP preparations usually aren't interchangeable. It's recommended to use the vaccine from the same manufacturer, if possible, for at least the first three doses.

## PATIENT TEACHING
• Explain risks and benefits of vaccine to parents before it's given.
• Tell parents to report systemic reactions promptly; remind them that local reactions are common. Acetaminophen in age-appropriate dosing will decrease occurrence of postvaccination fever in children susceptible to febrile seizure activity.
• Stress importance of keeping scheduled appointments for subsequent doses. Full immunization requires a series of injections.

---

**✳ NEW DRUG**

# diphtheria and tetanus toxoids, acellular pertussis adsorbed, hepatitis B (recombinant), and inactivated poliovirus vaccine combined
Pediarix

*Pregnancy risk category C*

## AVAILABLE FORMS
*Injection:* 0.5-ml single-dose vials and disposable, prefilled Tip-Lok syringes.

## INDICATIONS & DOSAGES
➤ **Active immunization**
*Children ages 6 weeks to 7 years:* Primary series is three 0.5-ml doses I.M. at 6- to 8-week intervals (preferably 8), usually starting at age 2 months. May be started at age 6 weeks.

## ACTION
Drug promotes active immunity to hepatitis B; poliomyelitis types 1, 2, and 3; diphtheria; tetanus; and pertussis by inducing antitoxin and antibody production.

| Route | Onset | Peak | Duration |
|-------|-------|------|----------|
| I.M. | Unknown | Unknown | Unknown |

## ADVERSE REACTIONS
**CNS:** *fever, fussiness, increased sleeping, restlessness, unusual cry.*
**GI:** *anorexia.*
**Skin:** *injection site reactions (pain, redness, swelling).*

## INTERACTIONS
**Drug-drug.** *Immunosuppressive therapies, such as alkylating agents, antimetabolites, corticosteroids, cytotoxic drugs, radiation:* May reduce immune response to the vaccine. If immunosuppressive therapy will end soon, postpone immunization until 3 months after immunosuppressive therapy; otherwise, vaccinate patient during immunosuppressive therapy, but expect that response may be inadequate.

## EFFECTS ON LAB TEST RESULTS
None reported.

## CONTRAINDICATIONS & CAUTIONS
● Contraindicated in patients hypersensitive to any component of the vaccine, including yeast, neomycin, and polymixin B.
● Contraindicated if a previous dose of vaccine or its components caused a serious allergic reaction.
● Contraindicated in patient with progressive neurologic disorder, including infantile spasms, uncontrolled epilepsy, progressive encephalopathy, or encephalopathy within 7 days of a previous dose of pertussis-containing vaccine that can't be attributed to another cause.
● Use cautiously in children with bleeding disorders, such as hemophilia or thrombocytopenia, and take steps to reduce the risk of hematoma after injection.
● Avoid giving drug to an infant younger than 6 weeks or a child age 7 or older. Avoid giving drug to a child receiving anticoagulant therapy unless the potential benefit outweighs the risk.
● Pediarix isn't indicated for adults.

## NURSING CONSIDERATIONS
● Inject vaccine into the anterolateral aspect of the thigh or the deltoid muscle of the upper arm. Don't inject in the gluteal area or any area that may contain a major nerve trunk.
● **Alert:** The tip cap and plunger of the needleless prefilled syringe contain latex and may cause allergic reactions in sensitive persons.
● Combined vaccine is more likely to cause fever than vaccines given separately.
● For children at high risk of seizures, give an antipyretic with vaccination and for 24 hours afterward to reduce risk of fever.
● Postpone vaccination if patient has a moderate or severe illness with or without fever.
● If patient has seizures within 3 days after being vaccinated, a temperature higher than 105° F (40.5° C), collapse or shock-like state, or persistent, inconsolable crying lasting 3 hours or more within 48 hours of the vaccine, postpone future doses of Pediarix or any vaccine containing pertussis until potential benefits and possible risks are reviewed.
● Interrupting the recommended schedule doesn't alter final immunity. The series

need not be started over, regardless of the time elapsed between doses.

• Don't give drug as a booster dose after the main three-dose series. Instead, give a DTaP vaccine at age 15 to 18 months (Infanrix, because its pertussis antigen components match those in Pediarix) and IPV at age 4 to 6.

**PATIENT TEACHING**

• Tell parent to expect some redness, soreness, swelling, and hardness at the injection site.

• Tell parent that a nodule may form at the injection site and may persist for several weeks.

• Recommend acetaminophen to relieve discomfort.

• Stress the importance of keeping scheduled appointments for subsequent doses.

---

## *Haemophilus* b conjugate vaccines

### *Haemophilus* b conjugate vaccine, diphtheria CRM$_{197}$ protein conjugate (HbOC)
HibTITER

### *Haemophilus* b conjugate vaccine, diphtheria toxoid conjugate (PRP-D)
Prohibit

### *Haemophilus* b conjugate vaccine, meningococcal protein conjugate (PRP-OMP)
Pedvaxhib

### *Haemophilus* b conjugate, tetanus toxoid conjugate (PRP-T)
ActHIB

*Pregnancy risk category C*

**AVAILABLE FORMS**
**Haemophilus b conjugate vaccine, diphtheria CRM$_{197}$ protein conjugate**
*Injection:* 10 mcg of purified *Haemophilus* b saccharide and about 25 mcg CRM$_{197}$ protein per 0.5 ml

**Haemophilus b conjugate vaccine, diphtheria toxoid conjugate**
*Injection:* 25 mcg of *Haemophilus influenzae* type B (HIB) capsular polysaccharide and 18 mcg of diphtheria toxoid protein per 0.5 ml
**Haemophilus b conjugate vaccine, meningococcal protein conjugate**
*Injection:* 7.5 mcg of *Haemophilus* b PRP and 125 mcg *Neisseria meningitidis* OMPC per 0.5 ml
*Powder for injection:* 15 mcg of *Haemophilus* b PRP, 250 mcg *N. meningitidis* OMPC per dose
*Haemophilus* b conjugate, tetanus toxoid conjugate
*Powder for injection:* 10 mcg *Haemophilus* b capsular polysaccharide, 24 mcg tetanus toxoid

**INDICATIONS & DOSAGES**
➤ **Immunization against HIB infection**
*Conjugate vaccine, diphtheria CRM$_{197}$ protein conjugate*
*Infants:* 0.5 ml I.M. at age 2 months. Repeat at 4 months and 6 months. Give booster dose at age 15 months.
*Previously unvaccinated children ages 15 months to 6 years:* 0.5 ml I.M. Booster dose isn't needed.
*Previously unvaccinated infants ages 12 to 14 months:* 0.5 ml I.M. Give booster dose at age 15 months (but no sooner than 2 months after first vaccination).
*Previously unvaccinated infants ages 7 to 11 months:* 0.5 ml I.M. Repeat in 2 months, for a total of two doses. Give booster dose at age 15 months (but no sooner than 2 months after last vaccination).
*Previously unvaccinated infants ages 2 to 6 months:* 0.5 ml I.M. Repeat in 2 months and again in 4 months for total of three doses. Give booster dose at age 15 months.
*Conjugate vaccine, diphtheria toxoid conjugate*
*Previously unvaccinated children ages 15 to 71 months:* 0.5 ml I.M. Booster dose isn't needed.
*Conjugate vaccine, meningococcal protein conjugate*
*Infants:* 0.5 ml I.M. at age 2 months. Repeat at 4 months. Give booster dose at age 12 months.

---

*Previously unvaccinated children ages 15 months to 6 years:* 0.5 ml I.M. Booster dose isn't needed.

Premature infants follow same schedule as full-term infants.

*Previously unvaccinated infants ages 12 to 14 months:* 0.5 ml I.M. Give booster dose at age 15 months (but no sooner than 2 months after first vaccination).

*Previously unvaccinated infants ages 7 to 11 months:* 0.5 ml I.M. Repeat in 2 months. Give booster dose at age 15 months (but no sooner than 2 months after last vaccination).

*Previously unvaccinated infants ages 2 to 6 months:* 0.5 ml I.M. Repeat in 2 months. Give booster dose at age 12 months.

*Conjugate vaccine, tetanus toxoid conjugate*

*Infants:* 0.5 ml I.M. at age 2 months. Repeat at 4 months and 6 months. Give booster dose at ages 15 to 18 months.

*Previously unvaccinated infants ages 7 to 11 months:* 0.5 ml I.M. Repeat in 2 months, for a total of two doses. Give booster dose at age 15 to 18 months.

*Previously unvaccinated infants ages 12 to 14 months:* 0.5 ml I.M. Repeat in 2 months, for a total of two doses.

## ACTION

Promotes active immunity to HIB; is a polymer of ribose, ribitol, and phosphate (PRP); and is linked by covalent bonds to highly antigenic substances, enabling the vaccine to promote an immune response in infants.

| Route | Onset | Peak | Duration |
|-------|-------|------|----------|
| I.M. | 2 wk after last dose | Unknown | Several yr |

## ADVERSE REACTIONS

**CNS:** fever.
**GI:** diarrhea, vomiting.
**Skin:** *erythema, pain at injection site.*
**Other:** *anaphylaxis,* crying.

## INTERACTIONS

**Drug-drug.** *Immunosuppressants:* May suppress antibody response to HIB vaccine. Postpone immunization.

## EFFECTS ON LAB TEST RESULTS

None reported.

## CONTRAINDICATIONS & CAUTIONS

● Contraindicated in patients hypersensitive to vaccine or its components and in those with acute illness.

## NURSING CONSIDERATIONS

● HIB is an important cause of meningitis in infants and preschool children.
● Immunization against HIB infection is recommended for children with HIV infections. Follow usual immunization schedule.
● Vaccine and DTP may be given simultaneously. A combination product is commercially available.
● Diphtheria toxoid conjugate vaccine (Prohibit) isn't recommended in children younger than age 15 months.
● Vaccine isn't routinely given to adults or children older than age 5 unless they're at high risk for infection (including patients with chronic conditions, such as functional asplenia, splenectomy, Hodgkin's disease, or sickle cell anemia).
● ActHIB reconstituted with diphtheria and tetanus toxoids and acellular pertussis vaccine adsorbed (DtaP; Tripedia) provides a combination containing antigens to diphtheria, tetanus, pertussis, and haemophilus b (TriHIBit). This combination can be used in children ages 15 to 18 months requiring both a fourth dose of DtaP and *Haemophilus* b vaccine. Don't use this combination for the first three primary doses or in children younger than age 15 months. Refer to manufacturer's instructions to reconstitute ActHIB with Tripedia.
● Keep epinephrine 1:1,000 available to treat anaphylaxis.
● Don't give vaccine I.D. or I.V.; give it only I.M.
● *Alert:* Don't give to febrile children.
● Give vaccine into anterolateral aspect of upper thigh in small children. Injections may be made into deltoid muscle of larger children if sufficient muscle is present.
● Drug may interfere with interpretation of antigen detection tests used to diagnose systemic HIB disease.

## PATIENT TEACHING

● Warn patient or parents that pain may occur at injection site.

---

Reactions may be *common,* uncommon, *life-threatening,* or COMMON AND LIFE-THREATENING.

• Tell patient or parents to notify prescriber if adverse reactions persist or become severe.

| Route | Onset | Peak | Duration |
|-------|-------|------|----------|
| I.M. | 1-15 days | Unknown | 6 mo |

# hepatitis A vaccine, inactivated
Havrix, Vaqta

*Pregnancy risk category C*

## AVAILABLE FORMS
**Havrix**
*Injection:* 360 ELISA units (ELU)/0.5 ml, 720 ELU/0.5 ml; 1,440 ELU/ml
**Vaqta**
*Injection:* 25 units/0.5 ml, 50 units/ml

## INDICATIONS & DOSAGES
➤ **Active immunization against hepatitis A virus**
*Adults:* 1,440 ELU Havrix or 50 units Vaqta I.M. as single dose. For booster dose, 1,440 ELU Havrix or 50 units Vaqta I.M. given 6 to 12 months after first dose. Booster recommended for prolonged immunity.
*Children ages 2 to 18:* 720 ELU Havrix or 25 units Vaqta I.M. as single dose. Then booster dose of 720 ELU Havrix or 25 units Vaqta I.M. given 6 to 12 months after first dose, or 360 ELU I.M. given 1 month apart and 360 ELU I.M. 6 to 12 months after primary course. Booster recommended for prolonged immunity.
➤ **To prevent hepatitis A in patients with chronic liver disease or clotting factor disorders and in food handlers**
*Adults:* 1,440 ELU Havrix I.M. as single dose. For booster dose, give 1,440 ELU Havrix I.M. 6 to 12 months after first dose. Booster recommended for prolonged immunity.
*Children ages 2 to 18:* 720 ELU Havrix I.M. as single dose. Then give booster dose of 720 ELU Havrix I.M. 6 to 12 months after first dose or two doses of 360 ELU I.M. 1 month apart and 360 ELU I.M. 6 to 12 months after primary course. Booster recommended for prolonged immunity.

## ACTION
Promotes active immunity to hepatitis A virus.

## ADVERSE REACTIONS
**CNS:** hypertonia, insomnia, *fever,* vertigo, *headache, fatigue, malaise, **seizures,*** encephalopathy, dizziness.
**EENT:** pharyngitis, photophobia.
**GI:** *anorexia, nausea,* abdominal pain, diarrhea, dysgeusia, vomiting.
**GU:** menstrual disorders.
**Musculoskeletal:** arthralgia, myalgia.
**Respiratory:** upper respiratory tract infections.
**Skin:** pruritus, rash, urticaria, *induration, redness, swelling,* hematoma, *injection site soreness,* jaundice.
**Other:** lymphadenopathy, ***anaphylaxis.***

## INTERACTIONS
**Drug-drug.** *Anticoagulants:* May increase risk of bleeding. Give I.M. injections cautiously.
*Immunosuppressants:* Antibody response may be suppressed in patients receiving immunosuppressive therapy. Monitor patient.

## EFFECTS ON LAB TEST RESULTS
• May increase CPK level.

## CONTRAINDICATIONS & CAUTIONS
• Contraindicated in patients hypersensitive to vaccine's components.
• Use cautiously in patients with thrombocytopenia or bleeding disorders and in those who are taking an anticoagulant because bleeding may occur after an I.M. injection.

## NURSING CONSIDERATIONS
• As with other vaccines, postpone hepatitis A vaccination, if possible, in patient with febrile illness.
• Keep epinephrine 1:1,000 available to treat anaphylaxis.
• If vaccine is given to immunosuppressed persons or those receiving immunosuppressants, expected immune response may not occur.
• Persons who should receive vaccine include people traveling to or living in areas endemic for hepatitis A (Africa, Asia [except Japan], the Mediterranean basin,

Eastern Europe, the Middle East, Central and South America, Mexico, and parts of the Caribbean), military personnel, native peoples of Alaska and the Americas, persons engaging in high-risk sexual activity, and users of illegal injectable drugs. Certain institutional workers, employees of child day-care centers, laboratory workers who handle live hepatitis A virus, and primate handlers also may benefit.

• For I.M. use, shake vial or syringe well before withdrawal. After it has been agitated thoroughly, vaccine is an opaque white suspension. Discard if it appears otherwise. No dilution or reconstitution is needed.

• Give as I.M. injection into the deltoid region in adults. Don't give in gluteal region; such injections may result in suboptimal response. Never inject I.V., S.C., or I.D.

## PATIENT TEACHING

• Inform patient that vaccine won't prevent hepatitis caused by other drugs or pathogens known to infect the liver.

• Warn patient about local adverse reactions. Tell him to report persistent or severe reactions promptly.

• Alert travelers to dangers of eating raw or undercooked shellfish or consuming food or drink in countries with poor hygienic conditions.

• Remind patient to return for second injection 6 to 12 months after the first.

# hepatitis B vaccine, recombinant
Engerix-B, Recombivax HB, Recombivax HB Dialysis Formulation

*Pregnancy risk category C*

## AVAILABLE FORMS

*Injection:* 5 mcg HBsAg/0.5 ml (Recombivax HB, pediatric and adolescent formulation with or without preservative); 10 mcg HBsAg/0.5 ml (Engerix-B, pediatric and adolescent formulation); 10 mcg HBsAg/ml (Recombivax HB, adult formulation); 20 mcg HBsAg/ml (Engerix-B, adult formulation); 40 mcg HBsAg/ml (Recombivax HB dialysis formulation)

## INDICATIONS & DOSAGES

➤ **Immunization against infection from all known subtypes of hepatitis B virus (HBV), primary preexposure prophylaxis against HBV, postexposure prophylaxis (when given with hepatitis B immune globulin)**

*Engerix-B*

*Adults age 20 and older:* Initially, 20 mcg I.M.; then second dose of 20 mcg I.M. after 30 days. A third dose of 20 mcg I.M. is given 6 months after the first dose.

*Adjust-a-dose:* For adults undergoing dialysis or receiving immunosuppressants, initially, 40 mcg I.M. (divided into two 20-mcg doses and given at different sites). Then second dose of 40 mcg I.M. in 30 days, a third dose after 2 months, and final dose of 40 mcg I.M. 6 months after first dose.

*Adolescents ages 11 to 19:* Initially, 10 mcg (pediatric and adolescent formulation) I.M.; then second dose of 10 mcg I.M. 30 days later. A third dose of 10 mcg I.M. is given 6 months after first dose. Or, 20 mcg (adult formulation) is given I.M.; then second dose of 20 mcg I.M. after 30 days. A third dose of 20 mcg I.M. is given 6 months after first dose.

*Neonates and children up to age 10:* Initially, 10 mcg I.M.; then second dose of 10 mcg I.M. after 30 days. A third dose of 10 mcg I.M. is given 6 months after first dose.

*Recombivax HB*

*Adults age 20 and older:* Initially, 10 mcg I.M.; then second dose of 10 mcg I.M. after 30 days. Give third dose of 10 mcg I.M. 6 months after first dose.

*Adjust-a-dose:* For adults undergoing dialysis, initially, 40 mcg I.M. (use dialysis formulation, which contains 40 mcg/ml); then second dose of 40 mcg I.M. in 30 days, and final dose of 40 mcg I.M. 6 months after first dose. A booster or revaccination may be indicated if anti-HBs level is below 10 mIU/ml 1 to 2 months after third dose.

*Infants, children, and adolescents from birth to age 19:* Initially, 5 mcg I.M.; then second dose of 5 mcg I.M. after 30 days. Give third dose of 5 mcg I.M. 6 months after first dose. Or, in adolescents ages 11 to 15, give 10 mcg (1 ml adult formulation) I.M.; then second dose of 10 mcg 4 to 6 months later.

*Infants born of HBsAg-positive mothers or mothers of unknown HbsAg status:* Initially, 5 mcg I.M.; then second dose of 5 mcg I.M. after 30 days. Give third dose of 5 mcg I.M. 6 months after first dose.

*Infants born of HBsAg-negative mothers:* Initially, 5 mcg I.M.; then second dose of 5 mcg I.M. after 30 days. Give third dose of 5 mcg I.M. 6 months after first dose.

*Note:* If the mother is found to be HbsAg positive within 7 days of delivery, also give the infant a dose of HBIG (0.5 ml) in the opposite anterolateral thigh.

➤ **Chronic hepatitis C infection**
*Engerix-B*
*Adults:* Initially, 20 mcg I.M.; then second dose of 20 mcg I.M. after 30 days. Give third dose of 20 mcg I.M. 6 months after first dose.

## ACTION
Promotes active immunity to hepatitis B.

| Route | Onset | Peak | Duration |
|-------|-------|------|----------|
| I.M. | 2 wk after last dose | Unknown | Years |

## ADVERSE REACTIONS
**CNS:** headache, fever, dizziness, insomnia, paresthesia, neuropathy, transient malaise.
**EENT:** pharyngitis.
**GI:** anorexia, diarrhea, nausea, vomiting.
**Musculoskeletal:** myalgia, arthralgia, neck stiffness.
**Skin:** local inflammation, *soreness at injection site,* pruritus.
**Other:** *anaphylaxis,* slight flulike syndrome.

## INTERACTIONS
**Drug-drug.** *Immunosuppressants:* May cause inadequate circulating antibody levels. May need larger than usual doses of hepatitis B vaccine (recombinant).

## EFFECTS ON LAB TEST RESULTS
None reported.

## CONTRAINDICATIONS & CAUTIONS
● Contraindicated in patients hypersensitive to yeast or components of vaccine; re-

combinant vaccines are derived from yeast cultures.
● Use cautiously in patients with serious, active infections or compromised cardiac or pulmonary status and in those for whom a febrile or systemic reaction could pose a risk.

## NURSING CONSIDERATIONS
● The American Academy of Pediatrics recommends hepatitis B vaccination for all neonates and encourages immunization for adolescents when resources allow.
● The Recombivax HB vaccine pediatric and adolescent formulation without preservatives may be used for persons for whom a thimerosal-free vaccine is recommended (such as infants up to age 6 months who may receive other vaccines containing thimerosal).
● Certain populations (neonates born to infected mothers, persons recently exposed to virus, and travelers to high-risk areas) may receive the four-dose regimen because it can induce immunity more quickly.
● Certain people are at increased risk for infection and should be considered for vaccine, including health care personnel (especially those working with dialysis patients, with high-risk patients and patient contacts who may be infected, in blood banks, in emergency medicine, or among populations in which infection is endemic [Indo-Chinese, native peoples of Alaska, and Haitian refugees]), certain military personnel, morticians and embalmers, sexually active homosexual men, prostitutes, prisoners, and users of illegal injectable drugs.
● Although anaphylaxis hasn't been reported, always keep epinephrine available when giving vaccine to counteract possible reaction.
● Thoroughly agitate vial just before giving to restore suspension.
● Inspect product for particulates or discoloration before giving. Make sure product is a slightly opaque white suspension. Discard if it appears otherwise.
● Give vaccine in deltoid muscle for adults and adolescents; give in anterolateral aspect of thigh for infants and young children. Never give I.V.

• Give S.C. in patients at risk for hemorrhage, such as hemophiliacs. Otherwise, don't use this route; it may lead to an increased occurrence or severity of local reactions.
• Recombinant hepatitis B vaccine isn't made with human plasma products.

## PATIENT TEACHING
• Warn patient or parents about local adverse reactions such as swelling or redness at injection site. Tell patient to report persistent or severe reactions promptly.
• Review immunization schedule with patient or parents; stress importance of completing series.

**✳ NEW DRUG**

# influenza virus vaccine live, intranasal
FluMist

*Pregnancy risk category C*

## AVAILABLE FORMS
*Intranasal spray:* 0.5 ml

## INDICATIONS & DOSAGES
➤ **Active immunization to prevent disease caused by influenza A and B viruses**
*Adults younger than age 50 and children older than age 9:* 0.5-ml intranasal dose (0.25 ml in each nostril) once each season.
*Children ages 5 through 8 not previously vaccinated with FluMist:* Two intranasal doses of 0.5 ml (0.25 ml in each nostril) 60 days apart for the first season.
*Children ages 5 through 8 previously vaccinated with FluMist:* 0.5-ml intranasal dose (0.25 ml in each nostril) once each season.

## ACTION
Induces antibodies to specific influenza strains, which may help prevent infection, speed recovery, or both.

| Route | Onset | Peak | Duration |
|---|---|---|---|
| Intranasal | Unknown | Unknown | Unknown |

## ADVERSE REACTIONS
**CNS:** fever, *headache, irritability, tiredness, weakness.*
**EENT:** *nasal congestion,* otitis media, *rhinitis,* sinusitis, *sore throat.*
**GI:** abdominal pain, diarrhea, vomiting.
**Musculoskeletal:** muscle aches.
**Respiratory:** *cough.*
**Other:** chills, *decreased activity.*

## INTERACTIONS
**Drug-drug.** *Antivirals active against influenza A virus, B virus, or both:* May interfere with vaccine. Wait at least 48 hours after antiviral therapy ends before giving vaccine. Wait at least 2 weeks after giving vaccine before starting antiviral therapy.
*Aspirin:* May cause Reye's syndrome in children and adolescents ages 5 to 17 when given with influenza vaccine. Discourage aspirin use in children.
*Immunosuppressants, such as alkylating drugs, antimetabolites, corticosteroids, radiation:* May increase risk of getting the flu. Avoid combining vaccine with immunosuppressants.

## EFFECTS ON LAB TEST RESULTS
• May cause nasopharyngeal secretions or swabs to be falsely positive for flu virus up to 3 weeks after vaccination.

## CONTRAINDICATIONS & CAUTIONS
• Contraindicated in patients hypersensitive to drug or its ingredients, including eggs or egg products, in children ages 5 to 17 who receive aspirin or products that contain aspirin because of the risk of Reye's syndrome, and in patients who may be immunosuppressed.
• Contraindicated in those with history of Guillain-Barré syndrome, asthma, or reactive airway disease.
• Safety and effectiveness in children younger than age 5 and adults age 50 and older haven't been established.

## NURSING CONSIDERATIONS
• *Alert:* Review patient's history for possible sensitivity to influenza vaccine components, including eggs and egg products.
• Have epinephrine injection (1:1,000) or compatible treatment readily available in case of acute anaphylactic reaction.

---

Reactions may be *common,* uncommon, *life-threatening,* or COMMON AND LIFE-THREATENING.

• Wait at least 72 hours after patient recovers from a febrile or respiratory illness before giving vaccine.
• Give vaccine before exposure to the influenza virus. Usually, influenza activity peaks in the United States between late December and early March.
• Annual revaccination may increase the likelihood of protection.
• Don't give vaccine with other vaccines.

## PATIENT TEACHING
• Inform parent that a child age 5 to 8 who hasn't received the vaccine before will need two doses about 60 days apart.
• Tell patient to avoid close (household) contact with immunocompromised or sick people for at least 21 days after vaccination.
• Urge patient or parent to report adverse effects to prescriber.
• Inform patient or parent that annual revaccination may increase the likelihood of protection.

## influenza virus vaccine, 2003-2004 trivalent types A & B (purified surface antigen)
Fluvirin

## influenza virus vaccine, 2003-2004 trivalent types A & B (subvirion or purified subvirion)
Fluogen, FluShield, Fluzone

*Pregnancy risk category C*

## AVAILABLE FORMS
*Injection (preservative-free):* 0.25-ml, 0.5-ml prefilled syringe
*Injection (containing preservative):* 0.5-ml prefilled syringe, 5-ml vial

## INDICATIONS & DOSAGES
➤ **Influenza prophylaxis**
*Adults and children age 9 and older:* 0.5 ml I.M. Only one dose is needed.
*Children ages 3 to 8:* 0.5 ml I.M. Repeat in 4 weeks unless child has been previously vaccinated.

*Children ages 6 to 35 months:* 0.25 ml I.M. Repeat in 4 weeks unless child has been previously vaccinated.

## ACTION
Promotes immunity to influenza by inducing production of antibodies.

| Route | Onset | Peak | Duration |
|-------|-------|------|----------|
| I.M. | 2-4 wk | Unknown | Unknown |

## ADVERSE REACTIONS
**CNS:** headache, fever, malaise.
**Musculoskeletal:** myalgia.
**Skin:** erythema, induration, *soreness at injection site.*
**Other:** *anaphylaxis.*

## INTERACTIONS
**Drug-drug.** *Immunosuppressants:* May reduce immune response to vaccine. Monitor patient closely.
*Theophylline, warfarin:* May impair clearance, causing increased levels of these drugs. Monitor patient closely.

## EFFECTS ON LAB TEST RESULTS
None reported.

## CONTRAINDICATIONS & CAUTIONS
• Contraindicated in patients hypersensitive to eggs or components of vaccine, including thimerosal.
• Postpone vaccination in patients with acute respiratory or other active infection and in those with active neurologic disorders.
• Use cautiously in patients with history of sulfite allergy.

## NURSING CONSIDERATIONS
• Fever and malaise occur most often in children and in others not exposed to influenza viruses. Severe reactions in adults are rare.
• Obtain history of allergies, especially to eggs, and reactions to immunizations.
• Keep epinephrine 1:1,000 available to treat anaphylaxis.
• Thoroughly shake vial just before giving to restore suspension.
• Give injections for adults and older children in deltoid muscle; give in anterolateral aspect of thigh for infants and children younger than age 3.

• Ideally, give vaccinations from October to mid-November because outbreaks of influenza typically don't occur until December. Don't give vaccine too early in season because antibody titers may begin to decline before flu season.

• Vaccines may be given to both children and adults throughout flu season, even as late as April.

• The American Academy of Pediatrics states that influenza vaccine can be given simultaneously (but at a different site and with a different syringe) with other routine vaccinations in children.

• *Alert:* Don't combine with or give within 3 days after whole-cell pertussis vaccine or combined diphtheria and tetanus toxoids and whole cell pertussis vaccine, adsorbed.

• Vaccine is considered safe in pregnant women. Don't postpone vaccination, regardless of stage of pregnancy, in patients who have high-risk conditions and who will be in first trimester of pregnancy when flu season begins.

• Immunodeficient patients may receive two doses 1 month apart; however, there is little evidence that booster doses improve immunogenic response to vaccine. Chemoprophylaxis with amantadine may be helpful.

• Vaccine is strongly recommended for anyone older than age 6 months, particularly patients with chronic disease, metabolic disorders, or medical conditions that put them at risk for complications from influenza; for health care workers (especially doctors, nurses, employees of nursing homes, volunteer workers, and other personnel in both hospital and outpatient settings); and for household members who may contact persons at high risk for medical complications of influenza. Also recommended for anyone who wishes to reduce chance of flu virus infection.

• Allergic reactions, which usually occur immediately, are extremely rare. Paralysis related to Guillain-Barré syndrome is rare and has been linked only to the 1976 vaccine.

• Don't use vaccine prepared for a previous influenza season to provide protection for current season.

• Although there's little information regarding influenza in persons with HIV, it's recommended that these patients receive vaccine. Patients with advanced disease may have a low response; there is no evidence that booster dose will improve immune response.

**PATIENT TEACHING**
• Advise patient about risks of vaccination compared with risks of influenza and its complications.

• Make sure patient understands that annual vaccination with current vaccine is needed because immunity to influenza decreases in year after injection.

• Explain that vaccine can't cause influenza. Fever, malaise, and muscle aches may begin 6 to 12 hours after vaccination and last 1 to 2 days. Such systemic reactions aren't common.

• Instruct patient to take appropriate acetaminophen dose for fever and apply ice compresses to injection site to minimize discomfort.

---

# measles, mumps, and rubella virus vaccine, live
M-M-R II

*Pregnancy risk category C*

**AVAILABLE FORMS**
*Injection:* Single-dose vial containing at least 1,000 tissue culture infective doses ($TCID_{50}$) of attenuated measles virus derived from Enders' attenuated Edmonston strain (grown in chick embryo culture), 20,000 $TCID_{50}$ of the Jeryl Lynn (B level) mumps strain (grown in chick embryo culture), and 1,000 $TCID_{50}$ of the Wistar RA 27/3 strain of rubella virus (propagated in human diploid cell culture) per 0.5-ml dose. Multidose vial available to institutions or government agencies.

**INDICATIONS & DOSAGES**
➤ **Routine immunization**
*Adults:* 0.5 ml S.C. Patients born after 1957 should receive two doses at least 1 month apart.
*Children:* 0.5 ml S.C. A two-dose schedule is recommended, with first dose given

---

at 15 months (12 months in high-risk areas) and second dose given either at ages 4 to 6 or 11 to 12.

## ACTION
Promotes immunity to measles, mumps, and rubella virus by inducing production of antibodies.

| Route | Onset | Peak | Duration |
|-------|-------|------|----------|
| S.C. | Unknown | Unknown | < 11 yr |

## ADVERSE REACTIONS
**CNS:** fever.
**GI:** diarrhea.
**Musculoskeletal:** arthritis, arthralgia.
**Skin:** rash, erythema at injection site, urticaria.
**Other:** regional lymphadenopathy, *anaphylaxis.*

## INTERACTIONS
**Drug-drug.** *Immune serum globulin, plasma, whole blood:* Antibodies in serum may interfere with immune response. Don't use vaccine within 3 to 11 months of these products, depending on dose of antibody or blood given.
*Immunosuppressants:* May decrease immune response to vaccine. Postpone immunization until immunosuppressant is stopped.

## EFFECTS ON LAB TEST RESULTS
• May temporarily decrease response to tuberculin skin testing.

## CONTRAINDICATIONS & CAUTIONS
• Contraindicated in immunosuppressed patients; in those with cancer, blood dyscrasia, gamma globulin disorders, fever, active untreated tuberculosis, or anaphylactic or anaphylactoid reactions to neomycin or eggs; in those receiving corticosteroid or radiation therapy; and in pregnant women.

## NURSING CONSIDERATIONS
• Obtain history of allergies, especially anaphylactic reactions to antibiotics, or reaction to immunization.
• Keep epinephrine 1:1,000 available to treat anaphylaxis.
• If skin test is needed, give it either before or simultaneously with vaccine.

• Use only diluent supplied. Discard vaccine 8 hours after reconstituting.
• Inject into outer aspect of upper arm with a 25G ⅝-inch needle. Don't give I.V.
• Refrigerate vaccine; protect from light. Solution may be used if red, pink, or yellow but must be clear.
• Risk of adverse effects is low (0.5% to 4%).
• Treat fever with antipyretics such as acetaminophen.
• Presence of maternal antibodies may prevent response in children younger than age 12 months.
• The Immunization Practices Advisory Committee recommends that colleges, other post–high school educational institutions, and medical institutions obtain documentation of receipt of two doses of vaccine after age 1 (or other evidence of immunity, such as infection, documented by prescriber). Combined measles, mumps, and rubella vaccine is preferred.
• *Alert:* The Centers for Disease Control and Prevention recommends that, during a measles outbreak in a health care facility, susceptible personnel exposed to measles virus (whether they received measles vaccine or immunoglobulin) avoid patient contact for days 5 through 21 after such exposure. If personnel become ill, they should avoid patient contact for at least 7 days after developing rash.

## PATIENT TEACHING
• Warn patient or parents about adverse reactions linked to vaccine.
• Review immunization schedule with parents, and stress importance of receiving second injection at the appropriate time to maintain immunization.
• Tell woman of childbearing age to use contraceptive measures until 3 months after immunization.
• Febrile seizures have rarely occurred in children after vaccination. Tell parents to treat and promptly report fever, especially in patient with family history of seizures.

## measles and rubella virus vaccine, live attenuated
M-R-Vax II

*Pregnancy risk category C*

### AVAILABLE FORMS
*Injection:* Single-dose vial containing not less than 1,000 tissue culture infective doses ($TCID_{50}$) per 0.5 ml of attenuated measles virus derived from Enders' attenuated Edmonston strain (grown in chick embryo culture); 1,000 $TCID_{50}$ of the Wistar RA 27/3 strain of rubella virus

### INDICATIONS & DOSAGES
➤ **Immunization**
*Adults and children age 15 months and older:* 0.5 ml (1,000 units) S.C.

### ACTION
Promotes immunity to measles and rubella virus by inducing production of antibodies.

| Route | Onset | Peak | Duration |
|-------|-------|------|----------|
| S.C. | Unknown | Unknown | < 11 yr |

### ADVERSE REACTIONS
**CNS:** fever.
**Musculoskeletal:** arthralgia.
**Skin:** rash, *burning and stinging at injection site.*
**Other:** lymphadenopathy, ***anaphylaxis.***

### INTERACTIONS
**Drug-drug.** *Immune serum globulin, plasma, whole blood:* Antibodies in serum may interfere with immune response. Don't use vaccine within 3 months of transfusion.
*Immunosuppressants:* May reduce immune response to vaccine. Postpone immunization until immunosuppressant is stopped.

### EFFECTS ON LAB TEST RESULTS
• May temporarily decrease response to tuberculin skin testing.

### CONTRAINDICATIONS & CAUTIONS
• Contraindicated in immunosuppressed patients; in those with cancer, blood dyscrasia, gamma globulin disorders,

fever, active untreated tuberculosis, or anaphylactic or anaphylactoid reactions to eggs or neomycin; in those receiving corticosteroid or radiation therapy; and in pregnant women.

### NURSING CONSIDERATIONS
• Obtain history of allergies, especially anaphylactic reactions to antibiotics.
• Keep epinephrine 1:1,000 available to treat anaphylaxis.
• If skin test is needed, give it either before or simultaneously with vaccine.
• Use only diluent supplied. Discard vaccine 8 hours after reconstituting.
• Inject into outer upper arm. Don't inject I.V.
• Store in refrigerator and protect from light. Make sure reconstituted solution is clear yellow.
• *Alert:* Don't give vaccine within 1 month of other live virus vaccines. Postpone immunization in patients with acute illness.
• Allow at least 3 weeks between BCG and rubella vaccines.

### PATIENT TEACHING
• Warn patient or parents about adverse reactions linked to vaccine.
• Caution woman of childbearing age to avoid pregnancy until 3 months after immunization.
• Advise use of fever-reducing drugs to control fever.

## measles virus vaccine, live attenuated
Attenuvax

*Pregnancy risk category C*

### AVAILABLE FORMS
*Injection:* Single-dose vial containing not less than 1,000 tissue culture infective doses ($TCID_{50}$) of measles virus derived from the more attenuated line of Enders' attenuated Edmonston strain (grown in chick embryo culture); available in 10- and 50-dose vials

### INDICATIONS & DOSAGES
➤ **Immunization**
*Adults and children age 15 months and older:* 0.5 ml (1,000 units) S.C. A two-

dose schedule is recommended, with first dose given at 15 months (12 months in high-risk areas) and second dose given at ages 4 to 6 or 11 to 12.

➤ **Measles outbreak control**

*Adults:* Revaccinate school personnel born in or after 1957 if they lack evidence of measles immunity. If outbreak is in a medical facility, revaccinate all workers born in or after 1957 if they lack evidence of immunity.

*Children:* If cases occur in children younger than age 1, vaccinate children as young as age 6 months. Revaccinate all students and siblings if they lack documentation of measles immunity.

## ACTION

Promotes immunity to measles virus by inducing production of antibodies.

| Route | Onset | Peak | Duration |
|-------|-------|------|----------|
| S.C. | Few days | Unknown | > 13 yr |

## ADVERSE REACTIONS

**CNS:** *febrile seizures in susceptible children,* fever.

**GI:** anorexia.

**Hematologic:** *leukopenia, thrombocytopenia.*

**Skin:** rash, erythema, swelling, tenderness at injection site.

**Other:** lymphadenopathy, *anaphylaxis.*

## INTERACTIONS

**Drug-drug.** *Immune serum globulin, plasma, whole blood:* Antibodies in serum may interfere with immune response. Don't use vaccine for at least 3 months after giving these products.

## EFFECTS ON LAB TEST RESULTS

• May decrease WBC and platelet counts.
• May temporarily decrease response to tuberculin skin testing.

## CONTRAINDICATIONS & CAUTIONS

• Contraindicated in pregnant women; in immunosuppressed patients; in patients with cancer, blood dyscrasia, gamma globulin disorders, fever, active untreated tuberculosis, or anaphylactic or anaphylactoid reactions to neomycin or eggs; and in patients receiving corticosteroid or radiation therapy.

• Don't give vaccine within 3 months of receiving blood or plasma transfusion or human immune serum globulin.

## NURSING CONSIDERATIONS

• Obtain history of allergies, especially anaphylactic reactions to antibiotics, or reaction to immunization. Postpone immunization in patients with acute illness or after giving blood or plasma.

• Keep epinephrine 1:1,000 available to treat anaphylaxis.

• If skin test is needed, give it either before or simultaneously with vaccine.

• Use only diluent supplied. Discard vaccine 8 hours after reconstituting.

• Don't give vaccine I.V.

• The Immunization Practices Advisory Committee recommends that colleges, other post–high school educational institutions, and medical institutions obtain documentation of receipt of two doses of vaccine after age 1 (or other evidence of immunity, such as infection, documented by prescriber). Combined measles, mumps, and rubella vaccine is preferred.

• *Alert:* The Centers for Disease Control and Prevention recommends that during a measles outbreak in a health care facility, susceptible personnel exposed to the measles virus (whether they received measles vaccine or immune globulin) avoid patient contact for days 5 through 21 after such exposure. If personnel become ill, they should avoid patient contact for at least 7 days after developing rash.

• If attenuated measles vaccine is given immediately after exposure to the disease, some protection may be provided. This level of protection is significantly increased if vaccine is given even a few days before exposure.

## PATIENT TEACHING

• Warn patient or parents about adverse reactions linked to vaccine.

• Review immunization schedule with patient or parents and stress importance of receiving second injection at appropriate time.

• Stress importance of avoiding pregnancy for 3 months after vaccination. Provide contraception information, if needed.

---

*Rapid onset*   †Canada   ‡Australia   ◇OTC   ♦ Off-label use   ✐Photoguide   *Liquid contains alcohol.

# meningococcal polysaccharide vaccine
Menomune-A/C/Y/W-135

*Pregnancy risk category C*

## AVAILABLE FORMS
*Injection:* 1-dose, 10-dose, and 50-dose vials with vial of diluent

## INDICATIONS & DOSAGES
➤ **To prevent meningococcal meningitis**
*Adults and children age 2 and older:*
0.5 ml S.C.

## ACTION
Promotes active immunity to meningitis.

| Route | Onset | Peak | Duration |
|-------|-------|------|----------|
| S.C. | Unknown | Unknown | 3 yr |

## ADVERSE REACTIONS
**CNS:** headache, fever, malaise.
**Musculoskeletal:** muscle cramps.
**Skin:** *pain, tenderness, erythema, induration at injection site.*
**Other:** chills, *anaphylaxis,* mild lymphadenopathy.

## INTERACTIONS
**Drug-drug.** *Immunosuppressants:* May reduce immune response to vaccine. Postpone immunization until 3 months after immunosuppressant therapy is stopped.

## EFFECTS ON LAB TEST RESULTS
None reported.

## CONTRAINDICATIONS & CAUTIONS
• Contraindicated in patients hypersensitive to thimerosal or other vaccine components; also contraindicated in pregnant women. Postpone vaccination in patients with acute illness.
• Don't give vaccine within 3 months of receiving blood or plasma transfusion or human immune serum globulin administration.

## NURSING CONSIDERATIONS
• Obtain history of allergies and reaction to immunization.
• Keep epinephrine 1:1,000 available to treat anaphylaxis.

• Don't give I.V., I.M., or I.D.
• Vaccine may be given with other immunizations and to immunocompromised patients.
• Routine vaccination isn't recommended. Reserve vaccine for persons at risk, such as those who live in or are traveling to epidemic or highly endemic areas, household or institutional contacts of meningococcal disease as an adjunct to appropriate antibiotic chemoprophylaxis, medical and laboratory personnel at risk for exposure to meningococcal disease, patients with terminal complement component deficiency, and those with anatomic or functional asplenia.
• Reconstitute vaccine only with supplied diluent.
• Some prescribers revaccinate children if they are at high risk and if they previously received vaccine before age 4.

## PATIENT TEACHING
• Warn patient or parents about adverse reactions linked to vaccine.
• Stress importance of avoiding pregnancy for 3 months after vaccination. Provide contraception information, if needed.
• Instruct patient to take correct acetaminophen dose to control fever.

# mumps virus vaccine, live
Mumpsvax

*Pregnancy risk category C*

## AVAILABLE FORMS
*Injection:* Single-dose vial containing not less than 20,000 tissue culture infective doses ($TCID_{50}$) of attenuated mumps virus derived from Jeryl Lynn mumps strain (grown in chick embryo culture) per 0.5 ml and vial of diluent; single-dose vial containing not less than 5,000 $TCID_{50}$ of the U.S. Reference Mumps Virus in each 0.5 ml

## INDICATIONS & DOSAGES
➤ **Immunization**
*Adults and children age 1 and older:*
0.5 ml (20,000 units) S.C.
    Not recommended in children younger than age 12 months; revaccinate children vaccinated before age 12 months.

### ACTION
Promotes active immunity to mumps.

| Route | Onset | Peak | Duration |
|-------|-------|------|----------|
| S.C. | Unknown | Unknown | > 15 yr |

### ADVERSE REACTIONS
**CNS:** *slight fever,* malaise.
**GI:** diarrhea.
**Skin:** rash, injection site reaction.
**Other:** *anaphylaxis,* mild allergic reactions, mild lymphadenopathy.

### INTERACTIONS
**Drug-drug.** *Immune serum globulin, plasma, whole blood:* Antibodies in serum may interfere with immune response. Don't use vaccine for at least 3 months after giving these products.

### EFFECTS ON LAB TEST RESULTS
• May temporarily decrease response to tuberculin skin test.

### CONTRAINDICATIONS & CAUTIONS
• Contraindicated in immunosuppressed patients; in those with cancer, blood dyscrasia, gamma globulin disorders, fever, untreated active tuberculosis, or anaphylactic or anaphylactoid reactions to neomycin or eggs; in those receiving corticosteroid or radiation therapy; and in pregnant women.
• Vaccine isn't recommended for infants younger than age 12 months because retained maternal mumps antibodies may interfere with immune response.
• Postpone use in patients with acute or febrile illness and for at least 3 months after transfusions or treatment with immune serum globulin.
• Don't give vaccine less than 1 month before or after immunization with other live virus vaccines.

### NURSING CONSIDERATIONS
• Obtain history of allergies, especially anaphylactic reactions to antibiotics, and reaction to immunization.
• Keep epinephrine 1:1,000 available to treat anaphylaxis.
• If skin test is needed, give it either before or simultaneously with vaccine.
• Use only diluent supplied. Discard vaccine 8 hours after reconstituting.

• Use a 25G ⅝-inch needle to inject.
• Don't give vaccine I.V.
• Refrigerate and protect from light. Reconstituted solution is clear yellow; don't use if discolored.
• Give to asymptomatic HIV-infected children.
• Don't use for delayed hypersensitivity (allergy) skin testing. Use mumps skin-test antigen, a killed viral product.

### PATIENT TEACHING
• Warn patient or parents about adverse reactions linked to vaccine.
• Stress importance of avoiding pregnancy for 3 months after vaccination. Provide contraception information, if needed.
• Tell patient to treat fever with fever-reducing drugs.

## pneumococcal 7-valent conjugate vaccine (diphtheria CRM$_{197}$ protein)
Prevnar

*Pregnancy risk category C*

### AVAILABLE FORMS
*Suspension for I.M. injection:* 0.5-ml vials

### INDICATIONS & DOSAGES
➤ **Active immunization of infants and toddlers against invasive disease caused by *Streptococcus pneumoniae* capsular serotypes 4, 6B, 9V, 14, 18C, 19F, and 23F; otitis media caused by serotypes of *S. pneumoniae***
*Ages 24 months through 9 years:* One dose.
*Previously unvaccinated older infants and children:* 0.5 ml I.M. according to the following schedules based on the age at the first dose.
*Ages 12 to 23 months:* Two doses at least 2 months apart.
*Ages 7 to 11 months:* Two doses at least 4 weeks apart, followed by a third dose given after the 1-year birthday and at least 2 months after the second dose.
*Infants and toddlers:* A total of four 0.5-ml doses, given I.M. at ages 2, 4, 6, and 12 to 15 months.

## ACTION
Promotes active immunity against invasive pneumococcal disease, including sepsis and meningitis, caused by the seven pneumococcal capsular serotypes included in the vaccine.

| Route | Onset | Peak | Duration |
|-------|-------|------|----------|
| I.M. | Unknown | Unknown | Unknown |

## ADVERSE REACTIONS
**CNS:** *drowsiness, irritability, fever, restless sleep.*
**GI:** *diarrhea, vomiting, decreased appetite.*
**Musculoskeletal:** interference with limb movement.
**Skin:** rash or urticaria, *injection site reactions including edema, erythema, induration, inflammation, skin discoloration, and tenderness.*
**Other:** hypersensitivity reactions.

## INTERACTIONS
**Drug-drug.** *Immunosuppressive drugs (antineoplastic drugs, corticosteroids):* May result in suboptimal active immunity. Monitor patient closely.

## EFFECTS ON LAB TEST RESULTS
None reported.

## CONTRAINDICATIONS & CAUTIONS
• Contraindicated in children who are allergic to any component of the vaccine, including diphtheria toxoid.
• Use with caution in patients with a history of latex allergy; product packaging contains dry natural rubber. Give vaccine cautiously to infants and children with thrombocytopenia or any coagulation disorder that would contraindicate I.M. injections.

## NURSING CONSIDERATIONS
• Vaccine won't protect against *S. pneumoniae* disease caused by serotypes unrelated to those in the vaccine or against other microorganisms that cause invasive infections such as bacteremia and meningitis or noninvasive infections such as otitis media.
• Postpone vaccination if the patient or parents report current or recent moderate to severe febrile illness because immunity may be impaired.
• Pneumococcal 7-valent conjugate vaccine isn't a substitute for routine diphtheria immunization or for 23-valent pneumococcal vaccine, when indicated.
• A reduced antibody response may occur in immunocompromised patients.
• Obtain a thorough allergy history, including any reactions to immunizations.
• Make sure epinephrine solution 1:1,000 and other necessary treatments are available to treat allergic reactions.
• If different sites and separate syringes are used, pneumococcal 7-valent conjugate vaccine may be given simultaneously with influenza, DTP, poliovirus, or *Haemophilus* b polysaccharide vaccines.
• Shake well to produce a uniform suspension. A nodule may form at injection site if vaccine isn't shaken.
• **Alert:** Don't inject I.V. Give by I.M. injection only, using the deltoid muscle or, in infants, the anterolateral thigh. Don't inject into or near a nerve or blood vessel.
• Refrigerate at 36° to 46° F (2° to 8° C). Don't freeze. Reconstitution or dilution is unnecessary.

## PATIENT TEACHING
• Provide patient or family with thorough information on the benefits and risks of immunization.
• Inform parent of the immunization schedule.
• Advise parent that the most common adverse effects occur within the first 3 days and include a mild fever, nausea, vomiting, diarrhea, irritability, decreased appetite, rash, and hives. Adverse effects at the injection site include pain, tenderness, redness, swelling, and inflammation.
• Tell parent to report any bothersome or persistent side effects.

# pneumococcal vaccine, polyvalent
Pneumovax 23

*Pregnancy risk category C*

## AVAILABLE FORMS
*Injection:* 25 mcg each of 23 polysaccharide isolates/0.5 ml

## INDICATIONS & DOSAGES
➤ **Pneumococcal immunization**
*Adults and children age 2 and older:*
0.5 ml I.M. or S.C.

## ACTION
Promotes active immunity to infections caused by *Streptococcus pneumoniae.*

| Route | Onset | Peak | Duration |
|-------|-------|------|----------|
| I.M., S.C. | 2-3 wk | Unknown | 5 yr |

## ADVERSE REACTIONS
**CNS:** slight fever.
**Musculoskeletal:** myalgia, arthralgia.
**Skin:** injection site rash, *injection site soreness,* severe local reaction caused by revaccination within 3 years.
**Other:** *anaphylaxis.*

## INTERACTIONS
**Drug-drug.** *Immunosuppressants:* May reduce immune response to vaccine. Postpone immunization until 3 months after immunosuppressant therapy is stopped.

## EFFECTS ON LAB TEST RESULTS
None reported.

## CONTRAINDICATIONS & CAUTIONS
• Contraindicated in patients hypersensitive to drug or its components (phenol) and in those with Hodgkin's disease who have received extensive chemotherapy or nodal irradiation.
• Postpone use in patients with acute respiratory distress syndrome.
• Vaccine isn't recommended for children younger than age 2.

## NURSING CONSIDERATIONS
• Vaccine is recommended for all adults older than age 65.
• Check immunization history to avoid revaccination within 3 years.
• Obtain history of allergies and reaction to immunization. Eggs and egg protein aren't used during the manufacture of vaccine; contains phenol as a preservative.
• Keep epinephrine 1:1,000 available to treat anaphylaxis.
• Inject in deltoid or midlateral thigh. Don't inject I.V or I.D.
• When splenectomy is being considered, give vaccine at least 2 weeks before procedure to ensure adequate antibody response. Vaccine may be less effective in splenectomized patients.
• Vaccine protects against 23 pneumococcal types, accounting for 90% of pneumococcal disease.
• Vaccine may be given to children age 2 and older to prevent pneumococcal otitis media, although the Centers for Disease Control and Prevention doesn't recommend otitis media as an indication for vaccine.
• Administration with influenza virus vaccine is safe and effective.

## PATIENT TEACHING
• Warn patient about adverse reactions linked to vaccine.
• Tell patient to treat fever with mild fever-reducing drugs and local site reaction with cold compresses.
• Warn patient with a skin rash related to low levels of platelets from unknown cause that there is a possibility of relapse 2 to 14 days after vaccination.

## poliovirus vaccine, inactivated (IPV)
IPOL

*Pregnancy risk category C*

## AVAILABLE FORMS
*0.5-ml prefilled syringe:* Mixture of three types of poliovirus (types 1, 2, and 3) grown in tissue culture.

## INDICATIONS & DOSAGES
➤ **Poliovirus immunization**
*Adults:* 0.5 ml S.C.; then second dose in 4 to 8 weeks. A third dose is given in 6 to 12 months.
*Children:* 0.5 ml S.C. at 2 and 4 months. A third dose is given at 15 to 18 months. Give a reinforcing dose of 0.5 ml S.C. before entry into school at ages 4 to 6.

## ACTION
Promotes immunity to poliomyelitis by inducing humoral antibodies and antibodies in the lymphatic tissue.

| Route | Onset | Peak | Duration |
|-------|-------|------|----------|
| S.C. | Unknown | Unknown | Yrs |

## ADVERSE REACTIONS
**CNS:** *fever,* sleepiness.
**GI:** decreased appetite.
**Skin:** injection site erythema, induration, *pain.*
**Other:** crying, hypersensitivity reaction.

## INTERACTIONS
**Drug-drug.** *Immune serum globulin, plasma, whole blood:* Antibodies in serum may interfere with immune response. Don't use vaccine within 3 months of transfusion.
*Immunosuppressants:* May reduce immune response to vaccine. Postpone immunization until immunosuppressant is stopped.

## EFFECTS ON LAB TEST RESULTS
None reported.

## CONTRAINDICATIONS & CAUTIONS
• Contraindicated in patients hypersensitive to neomycin, streptomycin, or polymyxin B and in neonates younger than age 6 weeks.

## NURSING CONSIDERATIONS
• Vaccine isn't effective in modifying or preventing existing or incubating poliomyelitis.
• Obtain history of allergies and reaction to immunization.
• If skin test is needed, give it either before or with vaccine.
• Keep epinephrine 1:1,000 available to treat anaphylaxis.
• Adults at high risk for exposure who have completed a primary course may receive another dose.
• Document manufacturer, lot number, date given, and name, address, and title of person giving vaccine on patient's record or log.
• Vaccine may temporarily decrease response to tuberculin skin test.

## PATIENT TEACHING
• Inform patient or parents about risks and benefits of vaccine before administration.
• Warn patient or parents about adverse reactions linked to vaccine.

# rabies vaccine, adsorbed

*Pregnancy risk category C*

## AVAILABLE FORMS
*Injection:* Single-dose 1-ml vial

## INDICATIONS & DOSAGES
➤ **Preexposure prophylaxis rabies immunization for persons in high-risk groups**
*Adults and children:* 1 ml I.M. at 0, 7, and 21 or 28 days for total of three injections. Check patients at increased risk for rabies q 6 months and give booster vaccination, 1 ml I.M, p.r.n., to maintain adequate serum titer.
➤ **To prevent postexposure rabies**
*Adults and children not previously vaccinated against rabies:* 20 IU/kg doses of human rabies immune globulin (HRIG) I.M. and five 1-ml injections of rabies vaccine, adsorbed I.M. given on days 0, 3, 7, 14, and 28.
*Adults and children previously vaccinated against rabies:* Two 1-ml injections of rabies vaccine, adsorbed I.M. given on days 0 and 3. Don't give HRIG.

## ACTION
Promotes active immunity to rabies.

| Route | Onset | Peak | Duration |
|-------|-------|------|----------|
| I.M. | Unknown | 2 wk after 3 doses | Unknown |

## ADVERSE REACTIONS
**CNS:** *headache, dizziness, slight fever, fatigue.*
**GI:** *abdominal pain, nausea.*
**Musculoskeletal:** *myalgia,* aching of injected muscle.
**Skin:** *transient pain, erythema, swelling, itching,* mild inflammatory reaction at injection site.
**Other:** reaction resembling serum sickness, ***anaphylaxis.***

## INTERACTIONS
**Drug-drug.** *Antimalarials, corticosteroids, immunosuppressants:* May decrease response to rabies vaccine. Avoid using together.

**EFFECTS ON LAB TEST RESULTS**
None reported.

**CONTRAINDICATIONS & CAUTIONS**
● Contraindicated in patients who have experienced life-threatening allergic reactions to previous injections of vaccine or to components of vaccine, including thimerosal.
● Use cautiously in patients hypersensitive to monkey-derived proteins, in those with history of non–life-threatening allergic reactions to previous injections of vaccine, and in children.

**NURSING CONSIDERATIONS**
● Keep epinephrine 1:1,000 available to treat anaphylaxis.
● Give as I.M. injection into deltoid region in adults and older children. For younger children, the midanterolateral aspect of the thigh also is acceptable. Don't use I.D. route. Avoid injecting vaccine near a peripheral nerve or into adipose or S.C. tissue.
● Vaccine is normally a light pink color because of presence of phenol red in suspension.
● *Alert:* If patient experiences serious adverse reaction to vaccine, report reaction promptly to local public health officials.
● *Alert:* Don't confuse vaccine with rabies immune globulin. Both drugs may be given in some situations.

**PATIENT TEACHING**
● Inform patient about adverse reactions linked to vaccine and importance of reporting serious adverse reactions.
● Warn patient not to perform hazardous activities if dizziness occurs.
● Advise proper fever-reducing drug dose for fever.
● Teach proper wound care and signs and symptoms of infection.

# rabies vaccine, human diploid cell (HDCV)
Imovax Rabies, Imovax Rabies I.D. Vaccine

*Pregnancy risk category C*

**AVAILABLE FORMS**
*I.M. injection:* 2.5 IU rabies antigen/ml, in single-dose vial with diluent
*I.D. injection:* 0.25 IU rabies antigen/dose

**INDICATIONS & DOSAGES**
➤ **Postexposure antirabies immunization**
*Adults and children:* Five 1-ml doses of HDCV I.M. First dose given as soon as possible after exposure; an additional dose given on each of days 3, 7, 14, and 28 after first dose. If no antibody response occurs after this primary series, booster dose is recommended.
➤ **Preexposure prophylaxis immunization for persons in high-risk groups**
*Adults and children:* Three 1-ml injections given I.M. First dose given on day 0 (first day of therapy), second dose on day 7, and third dose on day 21 or 28. Or, 0.1 ml I.D. on same dosage schedule.

**ACTION**
Promotes active immunity to rabies.

| Route | Onset | Peak | Duration |
|---|---|---|---|
| I.M., I.D. | 1 wk | 1-2 mo | > 2 yr |

**ADVERSE REACTIONS**
**CNS:** *headache, fever,* dizziness, *fatigue.*
**GI:** *nausea,* abdominal pain, diarrhea.
**Musculoskeletal:** muscle aches.
**Skin:** *injection site pain, erythema, swelling, itching.*
**Other:** *anaphylaxis,* serum sickness.

**INTERACTIONS**
**Drug-drug.** *Antimalarials, corticosteroids, immunosuppressants:* May decrease response to rabies vaccine. Avoid using together.

**EFFECTS ON LAB TEST RESULTS**
None reported.

## CONTRAINDICATIONS & CAUTIONS
• No contraindications reported for persons after exposure. An acute febrile illness contraindicates use of vaccine for persons previously exposed.
• Use cautiously in hypersensitive patients.

## NURSING CONSIDERATIONS
• Keep epinephrine 1:1,000 available to treat anaphylaxis.
• Use vaccine immediately after reconstitution.
• *Alert:* Don't use I.D. route for postexposure rabies vaccination.
• Alternative regimen of 0.1-ml doses given via the intradermal route is only for preexposure prophylaxis.
• Stop corticosteroid therapy during immunizing period unless therapy is essential for treatment of other conditions.
• Some patients who receive booster doses experience serum sickness–like hypersensitivity. These reactions usually respond to antihistamines.
• Report all serious reactions to the State Department of Health.
• *Alert:* Don't confuse vaccine with rabies immune globulin. Both drugs may be given in some situations.

## PATIENT TEACHING
• Inform patient about adverse reactions linked to vaccine. Tell patient to report persistent or severe reactions.
• Stress importance of receiving booster, if appropriate for patient.
• Tell patient to treat mild reaction with anti-inflammatory or fever-reducing drug at appropriate doses.

# rubella and mumps virus vaccine, live
Biavax II

*Pregnancy risk category C*

## AVAILABLE FORMS
*Injection:* Single-dose vial containing not less than 1,000 tissue culture infective doses (TCID$_{50}$) of Wistar RA 27/3 rubella virus (propagated in human diploid cell culture) and not less than 20,000 TCID$_{50}$ of Jeryl Lynn mumps strain (grown in chick embryo cell culture)

## INDICATIONS & DOSAGES
➤ **Rubella and mumps immunization**
*Adults and children age 1 and older:*
0.5 ml S.C.

## ACTION
Promotes immunity to rubella and mumps by inducing antibody production.

| Route | Onset | Peak | Duration |
|-------|-------|------|----------|
| S.C. | Unknown | Unknown | 10½ yr |

## ADVERSE REACTIONS
**CNS:** fever, polyneuritis.
**GI:** diarrhea.
**Musculoskeletal:** *arthritis, arthralgia.*
**Skin:** rash, pain, erythema, and induration at injection site; ***thrombocytopenic purpura;*** urticaria.
**Other:** *anaphylaxis,* lymphadenopathy.

## INTERACTIONS
**Drug-drug.** *Immune serum globulin, plasma, whole blood:* Antibodies in serum may interfere with immune response. Don't give vaccine for at least 3 months after use of these products.
*Immunosuppressants:* May reduce immune response to vaccine. Postpone immunization until immunosuppressant is stopped.

## EFFECTS ON LAB TEST RESULTS
• May temporarily decrease response to tuberculin skin test.

## CONTRAINDICATIONS & CAUTIONS
• Contraindicated in immunosuppressed patients; in those with cancer, blood dyscrasia, gamma globulin disorders, fever, active untreated tuberculosis, or history of anaphylaxis or anaphylactoid reactions to neomycin or eggs; in those receiving corticosteroid (except those receiving corticosteroids as replacement therapy) or radiation therapy; and in pregnant women.
• Postpone vaccination in patients with acute illness and after giving immune serum globulin, blood, or plasma.
• Allow an interval of at least 3 weeks between BCG and rubella vaccines.

## NURSING CONSIDERATIONS
• Obtain history of allergies, especially anaphylactic reaction to antibiotics, and reaction to immunization.

• Keep epinephrine 1:1,000 available to treat anaphylaxis.
• If skin test is needed, give it either before or with vaccine.
• Use only diluent supplied. Discard vaccine 8 hours after reconstituting.
• Inject into outer upper arm. Don't inject I.V.
• Document drug manufacturer, lot number, date, and name, address, and title of person giving dose on patient record or log.
• Patients born before 1956 are believed to have acquired natural immunity.

**PATIENT TEACHING**
• Inform patient about adverse reactions linked to vaccine.
• Stress importance of avoiding pregnancy for 3 months after vaccination. Provide contraception information, if needed.
• Inform women and girls older than age 12 about risk of self-limited joint pain or arthritis 2 to 4 weeks after vaccination.

---

## rubella virus vaccine, live attenuated (RA 27/3)
Meruvax II

*Pregnancy risk category C*

---

**AVAILABLE FORMS**
*Injection:* Single-dose vial containing not less than 1,000 tissue culture infective doses (TCID$_{50}$) of Wistar RA 27/3 strain of rubella virus (propagated in human diploid cell culture)

**INDICATIONS & DOSAGES**
➤ **Rubella immunization**
*Adults and children age 1 and older:*
0.5 ml or 1,000 units S.C.

**ACTION**
Promotes immunity to rubella by inducing production of antibodies.

| Route | Onset | Peak | Duration |
|-------|-------|------|----------|
| S.C. | 2-6 wk | Unknown | > 10 yr |

**ADVERSE REACTIONS**
**CNS:** fever, headache, malaise, polyneuritis.
**EENT:** sore throat.

**Musculoskeletal:** arthralgia, arthritis.
**Skin:** rash, pain, erythema, and induration at injection site; *thrombocytopenic purpura;* urticaria.
**Other:** *anaphylaxis,* lymphadenopathy.

**INTERACTIONS**
**Drug-drug.** *Immune serum globulin, plasma, whole blood:* Antibodies in serum may interfere with immune response. Don't give vaccine for at least 3 months after use of these products.
*Immunosuppressants, interferon:* May reduce immune response to vaccine. Postpone vaccine until immunosuppressant is stopped.

**EFFECTS ON LAB TEST RESULTS**
• May temporarily decrease response to tuberculin skin test.

**CONTRAINDICATIONS & CAUTIONS**
• Contraindicated in immunosuppressed patients; in patients with cancer, blood dyscrasia, gamma globulin disorders, fever, or active untreated tuberculosis; in patients hypersensitive to neomycin; in patients receiving corticosteroids (except those receiving corticosteroids as replacement therapy) or radiation therapy; and in pregnant women. Contraindicated in patients with AIDS or symptomatic HIV.
• Postpone immunization in patients with acute illness and after administration of human immune serum globulin, blood, or plasma.
• Allow at least 3 weeks between BCG and rubella vaccinations.

**NURSING CONSIDERATIONS**
• Obtain history of allergies and reaction to immunization.
• Keep epinephrine 1:1,000 available to treat anaphylaxis.
• If skin test is needed, give it either before or with vaccine.
• Use only diluent supplied. Discard vaccine 8 hours after reconstituting. Protect from light.
• Inject into outer upper arm. Don't inject vaccine I.V.
• Document drug manufacturer, lot number, date, and name, address, and title of person giving dose on patient record or log.

---

*Rapid onset*   †Canada   ‡Australia   ◇OTC   ♦Off-label use   ✏Photoguide   *Liquid contains alcohol.

## PATIENT TEACHING

• Inform patient about adverse reactions linked to vaccine.

• Stress importance of avoiding pregnancy for 3 months after vaccination. Provide contraception information, if needed.

• Tell patient to use correct dose of fever-reducing drug for treating fever.

✳ *NEW DRUG*

## smallpox vaccine, dried
Dryvax

*Pregnancy risk category C*

### AVAILABLE FORMS
*Injection:* About 100 million pock-forming units (pfu) per ml

### INDICATIONS & DOSAGES
**Active immunization against smallpox disease**
*Adults and children:* One drop of vaccine deposited over the deltoid or triceps muscle, followed by a multiple-puncture technique into the superficial layers of skin (two or three needle punctures for primary vaccination and 15 for revaccination).

### ACTION
Prevents smallpox by inducing production of antibodies to vaccinia virus.

| Route | Onset | Peak | Duration |
|-------|-------|------|----------|
| Multiple-puncture scarification | Unknown | Unknown | Unknown |

### ADVERSE REACTIONS
**CNS:** *fever.*
**Skin:** rash.
**Other:** accidental spread to another part of the body or to another person.

### INTERACTIONS
None reported.

### EFFECTS ON LAB TEST RESULTS
None reported.

### CONTRAINDICATIONS & CAUTIONS
**Nonemergency situations**
• Contraindicated in patients allergic to any component of the vaccine, including polymyxin B sulfate, dihydrostreptomycin sulfate, chlortetracycline hydrochloride, and neomycin sulfate; in infants younger than age 12 months.

• Contraindicated in patients or household contacts of patients with eczema, past history of eczema, or other exfoliative skin conditions; congenital or acquired immune system deficiencies, including HIV, leukemia, lymphomas, malignancy, organ transplantation, stem cell transplantation, agammaglobulinemia, and other malignant neoplasms affecting the bone marrow or lymphatic systems; of those receiving systemic corticosteroids, immunosuppressive drugs, or radiation; of women who are or may be pregnant, breast-feeding women, and elderly people.

• Contraindicated in patients with heart disease (such as cardiomyopathy, CHF, previous MI, history of angina, or evidence of coronary artery disease).

• Contraindicated in those who have three or more of these risk factors: hypertension, hypercholesterolemia, diabetes mellitus or hyperglycemia, smoking, or a first-degree relative with a heart condition before the age of 50.
**Emergency situations**
• For patients at high risk of exposure to smallpox, no contraindications exist for vaccination.

### NURSING CONSIDERATIONS
• Don't give I.M., I.V., or S.C.
• *Alert:* The vial stopper contains latex, which may cause hypersensitivity in patients with latex allergy.
• Give vaccination in the deltoid or posterior aspect of the arm over the triceps muscle.
• *Alert:* Rapidly make punctures into skin, and allow 15 to 20 seconds for blood to appear. After vaccination, blot off any vaccine remaining on skin at vaccination site with clean, dry gauze or cotton.
• Burn, boil, or autoclave all items that come in contact with the vaccine before their disposal.
• Inspect the site 6 to 8 days after vaccination to determine whether a major or equivocal reaction has occurred.
• Contact transmission of the virus can occur until the scab separates from the skin

---

Reactions may be *common,* uncommon, *life-threatening,* or COMMON AND LIFE-THREATENING.

lesion, usually 14 to 21 days after vaccination.

• Accidental inoculation of other sites is a common complication of the vaccine. The face, eyelid, nose, mouth, genitalia, and rectum are most frequently involved. Autoinoculation of the eye may cause blindness.

• Recently vaccinated health care workers should avoid contact with patients until the scab has separated from the skin at the vaccination site. If continued contact is essential and unavoidable, cover the vaccination site and maintain good hand-washing technique.

• Cardiac complications such as myopericarditis have occurred within 2 weeks of patients being vaccinated.

• The Centers for Disease Control and Prevention (CDC) can help diagnose and manage patients with suspected complications.

• Contact the Advisory Committee on Immunization Practices (ACIP), the Armed Forces, and the CDC for the most updated information and recommendations for use of the smallpox vaccine.

## PATIENT TEACHING

• Tell patient that although he should keep the vaccination site dry, he can still bathe the rest of the body.

• Advise patient that smallpox may be spread to another part of the body or to another person until the scab separates from the skin lesion (14 to 21 days after vaccination). Hand washing is essential for preventing inadvertent contact transmission of the virus.

• Tell patient to leave vaccination site uncovered or to cover it with a porous bandage, such as gauze, until the scab has separated and the underlying skin has healed. He shouldn't routinely use an occlusive bandage.

• Warn patient not to use salves or ointments on vaccination site.

• Instruct patient to seek immediate medical attention if he has chest pain, dyspnea, or other symptoms of cardiac disease in the first 2 weeks after vaccination.

• Instruct patient to place contaminated bandages in sealed plastic bags before trash disposal.

# tetanus toxoid, adsorbed

# tetanus toxoid, fluid

*Pregnancy risk category C*

## AVAILABLE FORMS
**tetanus toxoid, adsorbed**
*Injection:* 5 to 10 limit flocculation (Lf) units inactivated tetanus/0.5-ml dose, in 0.5-ml syringes and 5-ml vials
**tetanus toxoid, fluid**
*Injection:* 4 to 5 Lf units inactivated tetanus/0.5-ml dose, in 0.5-ml syringes and 7.5-ml vials

## INDICATIONS & DOSAGES
➤ **Primary immunization**
*Adults and children age 7 and older:*
0.5 ml (adsorbed) I.M. 4 to 8 weeks apart for two doses; then give third dose 6 to 12 months after second. Or, 0.5 ml (fluid) I.M. or S.C. 4 to 8 weeks apart for three doses; then give fourth dose of 0.5 ml 6 to 12 months after third dose.
*Children ages 6 weeks to 6 years:* Although use isn't recommended in children younger than age 7, the following dosage schedule may be used: 0.5 ml (adsorbed) I.M. at ages 2, 4, and 6 months. Give fourth dose at 15 to 18 months. Give fifth dose at ages 4 to 6, just before entry into school, if indicated. Diphtheria and tetanus toxoids and acellular pertussis vaccine adsorbed (DTaP) is recommended for active immunization in children younger than age 7.
➤ **Booster dose**
*Adults:* 0.5 ml I.M. at 10-year intervals.
➤ **Postexposure prophylaxis**
*Adults:* For a clean, minor wound, give emergency booster dose if more than 10 years have elapsed since last dose. For all other wounds, give booster dose if more than 5 years have elapsed since last dose.

## ACTION
Promotes immunity to tetanus by inducing antitoxin production.

| Route | Onset | Peak | Duration |
|---|---|---|---|
| I.M., S.C. | After 2 doses | Unknown | > 10 yr |

## ADVERSE REACTIONS
**CNS:** slight fever, headache, *seizures,* malaise, encephalopathy.
**CV:** tachycardia, hypotension, flushing.
**Musculoskeletal:** aches, pains.
**Skin:** erythema, induration, nodule at injection site; urticaria; pruritus.
**Other:** chills, *anaphylaxis.*

## INTERACTIONS
**Drug-drug.** *Chloramphenicol:* May interfere with response to tetanus toxoid. Watch patient for effect.
*Immunosuppressants, tetanus immune globulin:* May reduce immune response to vaccine. Postpone vaccine until 1 month after immunosuppressant is stopped.

## EFFECTS ON LAB TEST RESULTS
None reported.

## CONTRAINDICATIONS & CAUTIONS
• Contraindicated in immunosuppressed patients, in those with immunoglobulin abnormalities, and in those with severe hypersensitivity or neurologic reactions to toxoid or its ingredients. Contraindicated in patients with thrombocytopenia or other coagulation disorders that would contraindicate I.M. injection unless benefits outweigh risks.
• Use adsorbed form cautiously in infants or children with cerebral damage, neurologic disorders, or history of febrile seizures.
• Postpone vaccination in patients with acute illness and during polio outbreaks, except in emergencies.

## NURSING CONSIDERATIONS
• Obtain history of allergies and reaction to immunization.
• Determine date of last tetanus immunization.
• Keep epinephrine 1:1,000 available to treat anaphylaxis.
• Adsorbed form produces longer immunity. Fluid form provides quicker booster effect in patients actively immunized previously.
• Document manufacturer, lot number, date, and name, address, and title of person giving dose on patient record or log.

• **Alert:** Don't confuse drug with tetanus immune globulin, human. Both drugs may be given in some situations.

## PATIENT TEACHING
• Advise patient to avoid using hot or cold compresses at injection site; this may increase severity of local reaction.
• Instruct patient to report persistent or severe adverse reactions.
• Advise patient of proper fever-reducing drug dose for fever reaction.
• Tell patient that nodule at injection site may be present for a few weeks.

# varicella virus vaccine
Varivax

*Pregnancy risk category C*

## AVAILABLE FORMS
*Injection:* Single-dose vial containing 1,350 plague-forming units of Oka/Merck varicella virus (live)

## INDICATIONS & DOSAGES
➤ **To prevent varicella zoster (chickenpox) infections**
*Adults and children age 13 and older:* 0.5 ml S.C.; then second 0.5-ml dose 4 to 8 weeks later.
*Children ages 1 to 12:* 0.5 ml S.C.

## ACTION
Prevents chickenpox by inducing production of antibodies to varicella zoster virus.

| Route | Onset | Peak | Duration |
|-------|-------|------|----------|
| S.C. | 4-6 wk | Unknown | > 2 yr |

## ADVERSE REACTIONS
**CNS:** *fever.*
**Skin:** swelling, redness, pain, rash, varicella-like rash at injection site.
**Other:** *anaphylaxis,* herpes zoster, stiffness.

## INTERACTIONS
**Drug-drug.** *Blood products, immune globulin:* May inactivate vaccine. Don't give vaccine until at least 5 months after blood or plasma transfusions or administration of immune globulin or varicella zoster immune globulin.

---

*Immunosuppressants:* May cause severe reactions to live virus vaccines. Postpone routine vaccination.

*Salicylates:* Reye's syndrome has been reported after natural varicella infection. Avoid using salicylates for 6 weeks after varicella immunization.

**EFFECTS ON LAB TEST RESULTS**
None reported.

**CONTRAINDICATIONS & CAUTIONS**
• Contraindicated in patients hypersensitive to drug; in those with history of anaphylactoid reaction to neomycin; and in those with blood dyscrasia, leukemia, lymphomas, neoplasms affecting bone marrow or lymphatic system, or primary and acquired immunosuppressive states; and in those receiving immunosuppressants. Contraindicated in those with active untreated tuberculosis or any febrile illness or infection. Contraindicated in pregnant women.

**NURSING CONSIDERATIONS**
• To reconstitute vaccine, first withdraw 0.7 ml of diluent into syringe to be used for reconstitution. Inject all diluent in syringe into vial of lyophilized vaccine and gently agitate to mix thoroughly. Give immediately after reconstitution. Discard if not used within 30 minutes.
• Keep epinephrine available to treat anaphylaxis.
• Vaccine has been used safely and effectively with measles, mumps, and rubella vaccine.
• Document manufacturer, lot number, date, and name, address, and title of person giving dose on patient record or log.
• *Alert:* Vaccine contains live, attenuated virus. Vaccinated patients who develop rash may be able to transmit virus.

**PATIENT TEACHING**
• Inform patient or parents about adverse reactions linked to vaccine.
• Caution woman of childbearing age to report suspected pregnancy before administration.

• Instruct patient to avoid salicylates for 6 weeks after vaccination to prevent Reye's syndrome.
• Tell patient to avoid pregnancy for 3 months after vaccination.
• Warn patient to be careful after the injection to avoid close contact with susceptible high-risk people (such as pregnant women or immunocompromised persons).

## yellow fever vaccine
YF-Vax

*Pregnancy risk category C*

**AVAILABLE FORMS**
*Injection:* Live, attenuated 17D yellow fever virus in 1-, 5-, and 20-dose vials, with diluent; supplied only to centers authorized to issue yellow fever vaccination certificates

**ACTION**
Provides active immunity to yellow fever.

| Route | Onset | Peak | Duration |
|-------|-------|------|----------|
| S.C. | 7-10 days | 28 days | > 10 yr |

**INDICATIONS & DOSAGES**
➤ **Primary vaccination**
*Adults and children age 9 months and older:* 0.5 ml deep S.C.; booster is 0.5 ml S.C. q 10 years.
*Children ages 6 to 9 months:* Same dosage as above, if patient is traveling to areas of epidemic yellow fever.

**ADVERSE REACTIONS**
**CNS:** headache, *fever, malaise.*
**Musculoskeletal:** myalgia.
**Skin:** mild swelling, pain at injection site.
**Other:** *anaphylaxis.*

**INTERACTIONS**
**Drug-drug.** *Cholera vaccine:* May interfere with immune response to both yellow fever and cholera vaccines. Give 3 weeks apart.
*Immunosuppressants:* May increase viral replication and development of infection with yellow fever virus. Postpone vaccine until immunosuppressant is stopped.

## EFFECTS ON LAB TEST RESULTS
None reported.

## CONTRAINDICATIONS & CAUTIONS
• Contraindicated in immunosuppressed patients; in those with cancer, gamma globulin deficiency, or those hypersensitive to eggs; and in those receiving corticosteroid or radiation therapy. Contraindicated in pregnant women and in infants younger than age 6 months, except in high-risk areas.
• In patients who have received blood or plasma transfusions, wait 8 weeks before giving vaccine.
• Don't give yellow fever vaccine within 1 month of other live-virus vaccines.

## NURSING CONSIDERATIONS
• Obtain history of allergies, especially to eggs, and reactions to immunizations.
• Keep epinephrine 1:1,000 available to treat anaphylaxis.
• Reconstitute with unpreserved saline solution for injection (preservatives inactivate the yellow fever viruses).
• Keep vaccine frozen. Don't use unless shipping case contains some dry ice on arrival. Avoid vigorous shaking; carefully swirl mixture until suspension is uniform. Use within 1 hour after reconstituting. Discard remainder.
• Vaccine may be given with hepatitis B vaccine.

## PATIENT TEACHING
• Inform patient about adverse reactions linked to vaccine.
• Caution woman of childbearing age to report suspected pregnancy before administration.
• Advise patient to avoid insect bites by using sprays, repellents, protective clothing, and screens.

**black widow spider antivenin**
*Crotalidae* antivenin, polyvalent
**diphtheria antitoxin, equine**
*Micrurus fulvius* antivenin

### COMBINATION PRODUCTS
None.

---

## black widow spider antivenin
Antivenin *(Latrodectus mactans)*

*Pregnancy risk category C*

---

### AVAILABLE FORMS
*Injection:* Combination package–one vial
of antivenin (6,000-unit vial), one 2.5-ml
vial of diluent (sterile water for injection),
and one 1-ml vial of normal equine serum
(1:10 dilution) for sensitivity testing

### INDICATIONS & DOSAGES
➤ **Black widow spider bite**
*Adults and children:* 2.5 ml I.M. in anterolateral thigh. Second dose may be needed.
Test for sensitivity before giving drug with
0.02 ml of 1:10 antivenin in normal saline
solution. Evaluate result in 10 minutes.
For desensitization, use 1:10 and 1:100 dilutions of antivenin in normal saline solution for injection. I.V. route is preferred in
severe cases, in patients in shock, and in
patients younger than age 12.

### I.V. ADMINISTRATION
● Reconstitute antivenin with 2.5 ml of
diluent. Further dilute reconstituted solution in 10 to 50 ml normal saline solution
for injection and infuse over 15 minutes.
● Use reconstituted solutions within 48
hours; diluted solutions, within 12 hours.

### ACTION
Unknown.

| Route | Onset | Peak | Duration |
|-------|-------|------|----------|
| I.V. | Immediate | Unknown | Unknown |
| I.M. | Unknown | 2-3 days | Unknown |

### ADVERSE REACTIONS
**CNS:** *neurotoxicity.*
**Other:** hypersensitivity reactions, ***ana-
phylaxis,*** *serum sickness.*

### INTERACTIONS
**Drug-drug.** *Antihistamines:* May interfere
with sensitivity test results. Avoid using
together.

### EFFECTS ON LAB TEST RESULTS
None reported.

### CONTRAINDICATIONS & CAUTIONS
● Contraindicated in patients hypersensitive to drug or its components (horse
serum) when desensitization isn't feasible.

### NURSING CONSIDERATIONS
● Immobilize patient; splint the bitten limb
to prevent spread of venom.
● Obtain history of allergies, especially to
horses, and reaction to immunization.
Have epinephrine 1:1,000 available to
treat anaphylaxis.
● For best results, give antivenin as soon
as possible.
● Perform a skin or conjunctival test before administration.
● *Alert:* Give I.M. injection in anterolateral
thigh so that a tourniquet may be applied
if a systemic reaction occurs.
● Watch patient for 2 to 3 days. Venom is
neurotoxic and may cause respiratory
paralysis and seizures.
● Signs and symptoms usually subside in
1 to 3 hours.
● Refrigerate at 36° to 46° F (2° to 8° C).
● Discard if injection is frozen.

### PATIENT TEACHING
● Explain to patient and family how drug
will be given.
● Instruct patient to report adverse reactions promptly.
● Tell patient that serum sickness can occur 8 to 12 days after administration.

---

## *Crotalidae* antivenin, polyvalent

*Pregnancy risk category C*

### AVAILABLE FORMS
*Injection:* Combination package–one vial of lyophilized serum, one vial of diluent (10 ml of bacteriostatic water for injection), and one 1-ml vial of normal horse serum (diluted 1:10) for sensitivity testing

### INDICATIONS & DOSAGES
➤ **Crotalid (pit viper) bites**
*Adults and children:* Initially, 20 to 150 ml I.V., depending on severity of bite and patient response. For minimal envenomation: 20 to 40 ml I.V.; for moderate envenomation: 50 to 90 ml I.V.; for severe envenomation: 100 to 150 ml I.V. For a large amount of venom, more than 150 ml may be given I.V. directly into superficial vein. Subsequent doses are based on patient's response; may need another 10 to 50 ml if swelling progresses, systemic symptoms increase, or new signs and symptoms appear.

Test for sensitivity before giving drug. Give 0.02 to 0.03 ml of 1:10 dilution in normal saline solution I.D. Read results after 5 to 10 minutes. Watch carefully for delayed allergic reaction or relapse.

If sensitivity test result is positive, desensitize; prepare 1:10 and 1:100 dilutions of antivenin in normal saline solution for injection.
*Adjust-a-dose:* Children who have less resistance and less body fluid to dilute venom may need twice adult dose.

### I.V. ADMINISTRATION
● Reconstitute drug by adding 10 ml of supplied diluent. Further dilute to make a 1:1 to 1:10 solution using normal saline solution or D₅W. To avoid foaming, don't shake while mixing. Start by infusing 5 to 10 ml of diluted antivenin over 3 to 5 minutes; observe patient carefully. If no signs or symptoms of immediate systemic reaction occur, continue infusion.
● Use reconstituted solution within 48 hours and dilutions within 12 hours.

### ACTION
Neutralizes and binds venom of crotalids (pit vipers), including rattlesnakes, water moccasins, and copperheads.

| Route | Onset | Peak | Duration |
|-------|-------|------|----------|
| I.V. | Immediate | Unknown | Unknown |

### ADVERSE REACTIONS
**Musculoskeletal:** arthralgia.
**Skin:** erythema, urticaria.
**Other:** pain, hypersensitivity reactions, *anaphylaxis, serum sickness,* lymphadenopathy, fever.

### INTERACTIONS
**Drug-drug.** *Adrenergic blocking agents (including cardioselective beta adrenergic blocking agents):* May cause increased incidence and severity of anaphylaxis. Beta adrenergic blocking agents may also alter the effect of epinephrine and other adrenergic agents. Larger-than-normal doses of these drugs may be required for treatment of anaphylaxis.
*Antihistamines:* May increase toxicity of crotalid venoms. Avoid using together.

### EFFECTS ON LAB TEST RESULTS
None reported.

### CONTRAINDICATIONS & CAUTIONS
● Contraindicated in patients hypersensitive to drug or its components.
● Use drug cautiously. About 60% of patients treated with antivenin develop hypersensitivity.

### NURSING CONSIDERATIONS
● Immobilize patient immediately. Splint bitten limb.
● Obtain history of allergies, especially to horses, and reactions to immunizations. Have epinephrine 1:1,000 available in case of hypersensitivity reaction.
● *Alert:* Type and crossmatch blood as soon as possible; hemolysis from venom prevents accurate crossmatching.
● For best results, give antivenin as soon as possible, preferably within 4 hours of bite. In severe cases, can be given even after 24 hours have elapsed since the bite occurred.

• Give corticosteroids, as prescribed. If a large number of vials is given, serum sickness may result 5 to 24 days after infusion.
• Antivenin may be stored without refrigeration for 60 days, but it shouldn't be exposed to temperatures above 98.6° F (37° C).

**PATIENT TEACHING**
• Explain to patient and family that test dose will be given first to check for sensitivity to drug.
• Instruct patient to report adverse reactions promptly.

## diphtheria antitoxin, equine

*Pregnancy risk category C*

**AVAILABLE FORMS**
*Injection:* Not less than 500 units/ml in 10,000-unit and 20,000-unit vials

**INDICATIONS & DOSAGES**
➤ **Diphtheria prevention**
*Adults and children:* 5,000 to 10,000 units I.M.
➤ **Pharyngeal or laryngeal diphtheria lasting 48 hours**
*Adults and children:* 20,000 to 40,000 units I.M. or slow I.V. infusion.
➤ **Nasopharyngeal lesions**
*Adults and children:* 40,000 to 60,000 units I.M. or slow I.V. infusion.
➤ **Extensive disease lasting 3 or more days or disease with neck swelling**
*Adults and children:* 80,000 to 120,000 units by slow I.V. infusion.

**I.V. ADMINISTRATION**
• Dilute appropriate dose in $D_5W$ or normal saline solution to achieve a 1:20 dilution.
• Give solution by direct infusion at no more than 1 ml/minute.

**ACTION**
Binds with circulating toxin and prevents disease progression.

| Route | Onset | Peak | Duration |
|-------|-------|------|----------|
| I.V. | Immediate | Unknown | Unknown |
| I.M. | Unknown | 2 days | Unknown |

**ADVERSE REACTIONS**
**Skin:** erythema, urticaria.
**Other:** pain, hypersensitivity reactions, *anaphylaxis,* serum sickness.

**INTERACTIONS**
None significant.

**EFFECTS ON LAB TEST RESULTS**
None reported.

**CONTRAINDICATIONS & CAUTIONS**
• Contraindicated in patients hypersensitive to drug or its components.
• Use antitoxin with extreme caution in patients with history of allergic disorders.

**NURSING CONSIDERATIONS**
• Obtain history of allergies, especially to horses, and reactions to immunizations. Have epinephrine 1:1,000 available in case of anaphylaxis.
• Test for sensitivity before giving drug.
• *Alert:* If patient has signs or symptoms of diphtheria (sore throat, fever, tonsillar membrane), start therapy immediately, without waiting for culture reports.
• For storage, refrigerate antitoxin at 36° to 50° F (2° to 10° C). Before giving, warm to 90° to 95° F (32° to 35° C), never higher.
• Begin appropriate antimicrobial therapy.
• Monitor patient for serum sickness (urticaria, pruritus, fever, malaise, arthralgia), which may occur in 7 to 12 days.

**PATIENT TEACHING**
• Explain to patient and family that test dose will be given first to check for sensitivity to drug.
• Tell patient to report adverse reactions promptly.

## *Micrurus fulvius* antivenin

*Pregnancy risk category C*

**AVAILABLE FORMS**
*Injection:* Combination package with 10 ml of diluent

## INDICATIONS & DOSAGES
➤ **Eastern and Texas coral snake bite**
*Adults and children:* 30 to 50 ml or three to five vials slow I.V. through running I.V. of normal saline solution. Give 1 to 2 ml over 3 to 5 minutes; monitor patient closely for allergic reaction. If no signs or symptoms of allergic reaction develop, continue injection; 100 ml or more may be needed.

Test for sensitivity before giving drug. If sensitivity test result is positive, prepare to desensitize; prepare 1:10 and 1:100 dilutions of antivenin in normal saline solution for injection.

## I.V. ADMINISTRATION
• Reconstitute antivenin powder with diluent. Further dilute in normal saline solution to achieve a 1:1 to 1:10 dilution. Gently swirl solution to avoid foaming.
• Infuse first 1 to 2 ml over 3 to 5 minutes while closely monitoring patient. If no immediate systemic response occurs, continue infusion at maximum safe rate for I.V. fluid administration.
• Use reconstituted solution within 48 hours and dilutions within 12 hours.

## ACTION
Neutralizes and binds coral snake venom.

| Route | Onset | Peak | Duration |
|-------|-------|------|----------|
| I.V. | Immediate | Unknown | Unknown |

## ADVERSE REACTIONS
**CNS:** fever.
**Musculoskeletal:** arthralgia.
**Skin:** erythema, urticaria.
**Other:** pain, hypersensitivity reactions, *anaphylaxis,* lymphadenopathy.

## INTERACTIONS
None significant.

## EFFECTS ON LAB TEST RESULTS
None reported.

## CONTRAINDICATIONS & CAUTIONS
• Contraindicated in patients hypersensitive to drug or its components.

## NURSING CONSIDERATIONS
• *Alert:* Drug isn't effective for Sonoran or Arizona coral snake bites.

• Immobilize patient and splint bitten limb to prevent spread of venom.
• Obtain accurate patient history of allergies, especially to horses, and reactions to immunizations. Keep epinephrine 1:1,000 available to treat anaphylaxis.
• Give antivenin as soon as possible (before onset of neurotoxic signs), preferably within 4 hours of bite; treat asymptomatic patients because systemic symptoms usually develop later.
• Watch patient carefully for 24 hours. Venom is neurotoxic and may cause respiratory paralysis.
• Antivenin can be stored at room temperature for 10 days.

## PATIENT TEACHING
• Explain to patient and family that test dose will be given first to check for sensitivity to drug.
• Tell patient to report adverse reactions promptly.

cytomegalovirus immune
    globulin, intravenous
hepatitis B immune globulin,
    human
immune globulin intramuscular
immune globulin intravenous
rabies immune globulin, human
respiratory syncytial virus
    immune globulin intravenous,
    human
Rh$_o$(D) immune globulin, human
Rh$_o$(D) immune globulin
    intravenous, human
tetanus immune globulin,
    human
varicella zoster immune
    globulin

**COMBINATION PRODUCTS**
None.

## cytomegalovirus immune globulin (human), intravenous (CMV-IGIV)
CytoGam

*Pregnancy risk category C*

**AVAILABLE FORMS**
*Injection:* 2.5 g/50 ml†, 1 g/20 ml

**INDICATIONS & DOSAGES**
➤ **To attenuate primary CMV disease in seronegative kidney transplant recipients who receive a kidney from a CMV seropositive donor**
*Adults:* Give I.V. based on time after transplantation: within 72 hours, 150 mg/kg; 2 weeks after, 100 mg/kg; 4 weeks after, 100 mg/kg; 6 weeks after, 100 mg/kg; 8 weeks after, 100 mg/kg; 12 weeks after, 50 mg/kg; 16 weeks after, 50 mg/kg.

Give first dose at 15 mg/kg/hour. Increase infusion rate to 30 mg/kg/hour after 30 minutes if no adverse reactions occur, and then to 60 mg/kg/hour after another 30 minutes if no reactions occur. Volume shouldn't exceed 75 ml/hour. Subsequent doses may be given at 15 mg/kg/hour for 15 minutes, increasing q 15 minutes in a stepwise fashion to 60 mg/kg/hour.
➤ **To prevent CMV disease caused by lung, liver, pancreas, and heart transplants**
*Adults:* Used with ganciclovir in organ transplants from CMV seropositive donors into seronegative recipients. Maximum total dose per infusion is 150 mg/kg I.V. given as follows based on time after transplantation: within 72 hours, 150 mg/kg; 2 weeks after, 150 mg/kg; 4 weeks after, 150 mg/kg; 6 weeks after, 150 mg/kg; 8 weeks after, 150 mg/kg; 12 weeks after, 100 mg/kg; 16 weeks after, 100 mg/kg.

Give first dose at 15 mg/kg/hour. If no adverse reactions occur after 30 minutes, increase infusion rate to 30 mg/kg/hour. If no adverse reactions occur after another 30 minutes, increase rate to 60 mg/kg/hour (volume shouldn't exceed 75 ml/hour). Subsequent doses may be given at 15 mg/kg/hour for 15 minutes, increasing q 15 minutes in a stepwise fashion to maximum rate of 60 mg/kg/hour (volume shouldn't exceed 75 ml/hour). Monitor patient closely during and after each rate change.

**I.V. ADMINISTRATION**
● Remove tab portion of vial cap and clean rubber stopper with 70% alcohol or equivalent. To avoid foaming, don't shake vial. Inspect vial for clarity and particles.
● If possible, give through a separate I.V. line, using an infusion pump. Filters aren't needed. If unable to give through separate line, piggyback into line of normal saline solution for injection or into 5%, 10%, 20%, or 25% dextrose in water, with or without sodium chloride. Don't dilute more than 1:2 with any of these solutions.
● Begin infusion within 6 hours of entering vial; finish within 12 hours.

**ACTION**
Provides passive immunity by supplying a relatively high level of immunoglobulin G

antibodies against CMV. Increasing these antibody levels in CMV-exposed patients may attenuate or reduce risk of serious CMV disease.

| Route | Onset | Peak | Duration |
|-------|-------|------|----------|
| I.V. | Unknown | Unknown | Unknown |

### ADVERSE REACTIONS
**CNS:** fever, aseptic meningitis syndrome.
**CV:** hypotension, *flushing*.
**GI:** *nausea, vomiting*.
**Musculoskeletal:** muscle cramps, *back pain*.
**Respiratory:** *wheezing*.
**Other:** *anaphylaxis, chills*.

### INTERACTIONS
**Drug-drug.** *Live-virus vaccines:* May interfere with immune response to live-virus vaccines. Postpone vaccination for at least 3 months.

### EFFECTS ON LAB TEST RESULTS
None reported.

### CONTRAINDICATIONS & CAUTIONS
• Contraindicated in patients sensitive to other human immunoglobulin preparations or with selective immunoglobulin A deficiency.

### NURSING CONSIDERATIONS
• Monitor patient's vital signs closely before, during, and after infusion, and before and after increases in infusion rate.
• **Alert:** If anaphylaxis occurs or blood pressure drops, stop infusion, notify prescriber, and be prepared to give cardiopulmonary resuscitation and such drugs as diphenhydramine and epinephrine.
• Refrigerate drug at 36° to 46° F (2° to 8° C).

### PATIENT TEACHING
• Review drug therapy regimen with patient, and stress importance of compliance in follow-up visits.
• Instruct patient to report adverse reactions promptly.

# hepatitis B immune globulin, human
BayHep, HyperHep

*Pregnancy risk category C*

### AVAILABLE FORMS
*Injection:* 1-ml, 4-ml, 5-ml vials; 0.5-ml neonatal single-dose syringe

### INDICATIONS & DOSAGES
➤ **Hepatitis B exposure in high-risk patients**
*Adults and children:* 0.06 ml/kg (usual dose is 3 ml to 5 ml) I.M. within 7 days after exposure. Dose repeated 28 days after exposure if patient refuses hepatitis B vaccine.
*Neonates born to patients who test positive for hepatitis B surface antigen (HBsAg):* 0.5 ml I.M. within 12 hours of birth.

### ACTION
Provides passive immunity to hepatitis B.

| Route | Onset | Peak | Duration |
|-------|-------|------|----------|
| I.M. | 1-6 days | 3-11 days | 2 mo |

### ADVERSE REACTIONS
**Skin:** urticaria, *pain and tenderness at injection site*.
**Other:** *anaphylaxis, angioedema*.

### INTERACTIONS
**Drug-drug.** *Live-virus vaccines:* May interfere with response to live-virus vaccines. Postpone routine immunization for 3 months.

### EFFECTS ON LAB TEST RESULTS
None reported.

### CONTRAINDICATIONS & CAUTIONS
• Contraindicated in patients with history of anaphylactic reactions to immune serum.
• Give to patients with coagulation disorders or thrombocytopenia only if benefit outweighs risk.

### NURSING CONSIDERATIONS
• Obtain history of allergies and reactions to immunizations. Keep epinephrine 1:1,000 available.

• Inspect for discoloration or particulates. Make sure drug is clear, slightly amber, and moderately viscous.

• Inject into anterolateral thigh or deltoid muscle in older children and adults; inject into anterolateral thigh in neonates and children younger than age 3.

• For postexposure prophylaxis (such as after needlestick or direct contact), drug is usually given with hepatitis B vaccine.

• *Alert:* This immune globulin provides passive immunity; don't confuse with hepatitis B vaccine. Both drugs may be given at same time. Don't mix in the same syringe.

• *Alert:* Don't confuse HyperHep with Hyperstat or Hyper-Tet.

## PATIENT TEACHING

• Inform patient that pain and tenderness may occur at injection site.

• Tell patient to report signs and symptoms of hypersensitivity immediately.

---

## immune globulin intramuscular (gamma globulin, IG, IGIM)
BayGam

## immune globulin intravenous (IGIV)
Carimune, Gamimune N, Gammagard S/D, Gammar-P I.V., Gamunex, Iveegam EN, Panglobulin, Polygam S/D, Venoglobulin-S

*Pregnancy risk category C*

## AVAILABLE FORMS
**immune globulin intramuscular**
*Injection:* 2-ml, 10-ml vials (BayGam)
**immune globulin intravenous**
*Injection:* 5% and 10% in 10-ml, 50-ml, 100-ml, 200-ml vials and 5% in 250-ml vials (Gamimune N); 5%, 10% in 5-g, 10-g, 20-g vials (Venoglobulin-S)
*Powder for injection:* 1-g, 3-g, 6-g, 12-g vials (Carimune), 50 mg protein/ml in 2.5=g, 5-g, 10-g vials (Gammagard S/D); 1-g, 2.5-g, 5-g, 10-g vials (Gammar-P I.V.); 500-mg, 1-g, 2.5-g, 5-g vials (Iveegam EN); 6-g, 12-g vials (Panglobulin); 2.5-g, 5-g, 10-g vials (Polygam S/D)

*Solution for injection:* 1-g, 2.5-g, 5-g, 10-g, 20-g vials (Gamunex)

## INDICATIONS & DOSAGES
➤ **Primary immunodeficiency (IGIV)**
*Carimune, Panglobulin*
*Adults and children:* 200 mg/kg I.V. monthly. May increase dose to maximum of 300 mg/kg once monthly or give more frequently to produce desired effect.
*Gamimune N*
*Adults and children:* 100 to 200 mg/kg I.V. monthly. Maximum dosage is 400 mg/kg.
*Gammagard S/D*
*Adults and children:* 200 to 400 mg/kg I.V. once monthly. Minimum dose is 100 mg/kg once monthly.
*Gamunex*
*Adults and children:* 300 to 600 mg/kg I.V. q 3 to 4 weeks.
*Iveegam EN*
*Adults and children:* 200 mg/kg I.V. monthly. May increase dose to maximum of 800 mg/kg, or give more often than once monthly to produce desired effect.
*Polygam S/D*
*Adults and children:* 200 to 400 mg/kg I.V. once monthly. Minimum dose is 100 mg/kg once monthly.
➤ **Primary defective antibody synthesis such as agammaglobulinemia or hypogammaglobulinemia in patients at increased risk of infection**
*Gammar-P I.V.*
*Adults:* 200 to 400 mg/kg infused I.V. given q 3 to 4 weeks.
*Adolescents and children:* 200 mg/kg I.V. q 3 to 4 weeks. Adjust dosage according to clinical effect and to maintain IgG at desired level.
*Venoglobulin-S*
*Adults and children:* 200 mg/kg I.V. once monthly. May increase dose to 300 to 400 mg/kg, or give more often than once monthly if adequate IgG levels haven't been achieved.
➤ **Idiopathic thrombocytopenic purpura (IGIV)**
*Carimune, Panglobulin*
*Adults and children:* 400 mg/kg I.V. daily for 2 to 5 consecutive days. Maximum dosage is 1 g/kg/day.

---

### Gamimune N
*Adults and children:* 400 mg/kg 5% or
10% solution I.V. for 2 to 5 consecutive
days; or 1,000 mg/kg 5% or 10% solution
I.V. for 1 to 2 consecutive days with maintenance dose of 5% or 10% solution at
400 to 1,000 mg/kg I.V. single infusion to
maintain platelet count > 30,000/mm³.

### Gammagard S/D, Polygam S/D
*Adults and children:* 1 g/kg I.V. Additional
doses depend on response. Up to three
doses may be given on alternate days if
needed.

### Gamunex
*Adults and children:* 1,000 mg/kg I.V.
daily for 2 consecutive days. If adequate
increase in platelet count occurs after first
dose, second dose may be withheld. Or,
400 mg/kg I.V. daily for 5 consecutive
days. Total dosage is 2 g/kg.

### Venoglobulin-S
*Adults and children:* Maximum of
2,000 mg/kg I.V. divided over 5 or fewer
days. Maintenance dose is 1,000 mg/kg
I.V. p.r.n. to maintain platelet counts of
30,000/mm³ in children and 20,000/mm³
in adults, or to prevent bleeding episodes.
➤ **Bone marrow transplant (IGIV)**
### Gamimune N
*Adults older than age 20:* 500 mg/kg 5%
or 10% solution I.V. on days 7 and 2 before transplantation; then weekly until
90 days after transplantation.
➤ **B-cell chronic lymphocytic leukemia
(IGIV)**
*Adults:* 400 mg/kg Gammagard S/D or
Polygam S/D I.V. q 3 to 4 weeks.
➤ **To prevent coronary artery
aneurysms in patients with Kawasaki
syndrome (IGIV)**
*Note:* Combine with aspirin therapy and
start within 10 days of fever.
### Iveegam EN, Venoglobulin-S 5% or 10%
*Adults and children:* 2,000 mg/kg I.V. over
10 to 12 hours. Additional dose may be
given.
### Gammagard S/D
*Adults and children:* Single 1 g/kg dose.
➤ **Alternative dosing with Iveegam EN
or Gammagard S/D**
*Adults and children:* 400 mg/kg/day for
4 consecutive days.
➤ **Pediatric HIV infection (IGIV)**
*Children:* 400 mg/kg Gamimune N 5% or
10% solution I.V. q 28 days.

➤ **Hepatitis A exposure (IGIM)**
*Adults and children:* 0.02 ml/kg I.M. as
soon as possible after exposure. Up to
0.06 ml/kg may be given for prolonged or
intense exposure.
➤ **Measles exposure (IGIM)**
*Adults and children:* 0.2 to 0.25 ml/kg
I.M. within 6 days after exposure.
➤ **Postexposure prophylaxis of measles
(IGIM)**
*Immunocompromised children age 12
months or older:* 0.5 ml/kg I.M. within
6 days after exposure (maximum 15 ml).
➤ **Chickenpox exposure (IGIM)** ◆
*Adults and children:* 0.6 to 1.2 ml/kg I.M.
as soon as exposed.
➤ **Rubella exposure in first trimester
pregnancy (IGIM)** ◆
*Women:* 0.55 ml/kg I.M. as soon as possi-
ble after exposure (within 72 hours).

### I.V. ADMINISTRATION
● Before use, refrigerate Gamimune N and
Iveegan EN at 36° to 46° F (2° to 8° C).
Before reconstitution, store Gammagard
S/D, Gammar-P I.V., Polygam S/D, and
Venoglobulin-S at room temperature, not
to exceed 77° F (25° C). Before reconstitution, store Carimune and Panglobulin at
room temperature, below 86° F (30° C).
● Don't mix with other drugs or I.V. fluids.
● Most adverse reactions are related to a
rapid infusion rate. If adverse reactions
occur, decrease infusion rate or stop infusion until reaction subsides. Resume infusion at a rate that patient can tolerate.
● After reconstitution, Gammagard S/D
and Polygam S/D contain about 50 mg of
protein/ml for 5% solution or 100 mg of
protein per ml for 10% solution, and both
contain no less than 90% IgG. Gamimune
N contains 50 mg of protein/ml or 100 mg
of protein per ml for 10% solution, and
both contain no less than 98% IgG;
Gammar-P I.V. and Iveegam EN contain
50 mg of IgG/ml; Carimune and Panglobulin contain no less than 96% IgG;
Venoglobulin-S contains about 50 mg of
protein/ml for 5% solution or 100 mg of
protein per ml for 10% solution, and both
contain no less than 99% IgG.
### Carimune, Panglobulin
● Use 15-micron in-line filter when giving.
Reconstitute with normal saline solution,
D₅W, or sterile water. Infusion rate is

---

Reactions may be *common*, uncommon, *life-threatening*, or COMMON AND LIFE-THREATENING.

0.5 to 1 ml/minute for 3% solution. After 15 to 30 minutes, increase rate to 1.5 to 2.5 ml/minute.

**Gamimune N**
● Gamimune N 5% and 10% are incompatible with saline solutions; they may be diluted with $D_5W$, if needed. Start infusion at 0.01 to 0.02 ml/kg/minute for 30 minutes. If no problems, slowly increase rate to maximum of 0.08 ml/kg/minute.

**Gammagard S/D, Polygam S/D**
● Reconstitute according to package directions using sterile water for injection as diluent and the transfer device provided to prepare a solution containing 50 mg of protein per ml for 5% immune globulin solution or 100 mg of protein per ml for 10% immune globulin solution. Warm powder and sterile water for injection to room temperature before reconstitution. Give no more than 2 hours after reconstitution.
● Infuse with administration set provided or with 15-micron in-line filter. Begin infusion at 0.5 ml/kg/hour and increase to maximum of 4 ml/kg/hour. Patients who tolerate 5% concentration at 4 ml/kg/hour can be switched to 10% concentration at 0.5 ml/kg/hour and increased to 8 ml/kg/hour, if tolerated.

**Gammar-P I.V.**
● Reconstitute with sterile water for injection diluent provided. Warm powder and diluent to room temperature before reconstitution. After adding diluent, keep vial in upright position and undisturbed for 5 minutes. Gently swirl vial after 5 minutes. Don't shake. Dissolution may take up to 20 minutes. Start infusion within 3 hours of reconstituting.
● Use 15-micron in-line filter when giving. Start infusion at 0.01 ml/kg/minute and increase to 0.02 ml/kg/minute after 15 to 30 minutes, if tolerated. Maximum infusion rate is 0.06 ml/kg/minute.

**Gamunex**
● Incompatible with saline solutions. Compatible with $D_5W$, if needed.
● Infuse I.V. at a rate of 0.01 ml/kg/minute for first 30 minutes. If no problems, rate can be slowly increased to maximum of 0.08 ml/kg/minute.
● Store vials at 36° to 46° F (2° to 8° C). During first 18 months from the date of manufacture, vials may be stored for up to

5 months at room temperatures not exceeding 77° F (25° C), but then must be used immediately or discarded. Don't freeze vials.

**Iveegam EN**
● Reconstitute Iveegam with sterile water for injection diluent provided. Use 15-micron in-line filter when giving drug. Infusion rate is 1 to 2 ml/minute for 5% solution.

**Venoglobulin-S**
● Begin infusion at 0.01 to 0.02 ml/kg/minute for 30 minutes; then increase 5% solutions to a rate less than 0.08 ml/kg/minute and 10% solutions to a rate less than 0.05 ml/kg/minute, if tolerated.

**ACTION**
Provides passive immunity by increasing antibody titer. The primary component is immunoglobulin G. The mechanism for treating idiopathic thrombocytopenic purpura is unknown.

| Route | Onset | Peak | Duration |
|-------|-------|------|----------|
| I.V. | Immediate | Immediate | Unknown |
| I.M. | Unknown | 2-5 hr | Unknown |

**ADVERSE REACTIONS**
**CNS:** headache, fever, faintness, malaise, *severe headache requiring hospitalization.*
**CV:** chest pain, MI, congestive cardiac failure.
**GI:** nausea, vomiting.
**Musculoskeletal:** hip pain, chest pain, chest tightness, muscle stiffness at injection site.
**Respiratory:** dyspnea, *pulmonary embolism, transfusion related acute lung injury.*
**Skin:** urticaria; pain, erythema.
**Other:** *anaphylaxis,* chills.

**INTERACTIONS**
**Drug-drug.** *Live-virus vaccines:* Length of time to wait before giving live-virus vaccinations varies with dose of immune globulin given. Refer to recommendations by American Academy of Pediatrics.

**EFFECTS ON LAB TEST RESULTS**
None reported.

---

**CONTRAINDICATIONS & CAUTIONS**
• Contraindicated in patients hypersensitive to drug or its components.
• IGIV administration may be linked to thrombotic events. Use IGIV cautiously in patients with a history of CV disease or thrombotic episodes.

**NURSING CONSIDERATIONS**
• Obtain history of allergies and reactions to immunizations. Keep epinephrine 1:1,000 available to treat anaphylaxis.
• If risk of a thrombotic event is possible, make sure infusion concentration is no more than 5% and start infusion rate no faster than 0.5 ml/kg body weight per hour. Advance rate slowly only if well tolerated, to a maximum rate of 4 ml/kg body weight per hour.
• When giving I.M., use gluteal region. Divide doses larger than 10 ml and inject into several muscle sites to reduce pain and discomfort.
• Give drug soon after reconstitution.
• Don't give immune globulin for prophylaxis against hepatitis A if 6 weeks or more have elapsed since exposure or onset of clinical illness.

**PATIENT TEACHING**
• Explain to patient and family how drug will be given.
• Tell patient that local reactions may occur at injection site. Instruct him to notify prescriber promptly if adverse reactions persist or become severe.
• Inform patient of possible need to have therapy more than once monthly to maintain appropriate immunoglobulin G levels.

# rabies immune globulin, human
Hyperab, Imogam Rabies-HT

*Pregnancy risk category C*

**AVAILABLE FORMS**
*Injection:* 150 IU/ml in 2-ml, 10-ml vials

**INDICATIONS & DOSAGES**
➤ **Rabies exposure**
*Adults and children:* 20 IU/kg I.M. at time of first dose of rabies vaccine. Half of

dose is used to infiltrate wound area; remainder is given I.M. in a different site.

**ACTION**
Provides passive immunity to rabies.

| Route | Onset | Peak | Duration |
|-------|-------|------|----------|
| I.M. | 24 hr | Unknown | Unknown |

**ADVERSE REACTIONS**
**CNS:** slight fever.
**GU:** *nephrotic syndrome.*
**Skin:** *rash;* pain, redness, and induration at injection site.
**Other:** *anaphylaxis, angioedema.*

**INTERACTIONS**
**Drug-drug.** *Live-virus vaccines (measles, mumps, polio, or rubella):* May interfere with response to vaccine. Postpone immunization, if possible.

**EFFECTS ON LAB TEST RESULTS**
None reported.

**CONTRAINDICATIONS & CAUTIONS**
• No known contraindications.
• Use with caution in patients hypersensitive to thimerosal or history of systemic allergic reactions to human immunoglobulin preparations; also use cautiously in those with immunoglobulin A deficiency.

**NURSING CONSIDERATIONS**
• Obtain history of animal bites, allergies, and reactions to immunizations. Have epinephrine 1:1,000 ready to treat anaphylaxis.
• Ask patient when last tetanus immunization was received; many prescribers order a booster at this time.
• Use only with rabies vaccine and immediate local treatment of wound. Don't give rabies vaccine and rabies immune globulin in same syringe or at same site. Give as soon as possible after exposure or through day 7. After day 8, antibody response to culture vaccine has occurred.
• Don't give live-virus vaccines within 3 months of rabies immune globulin.
• Don't give more than 5 ml I.M. at one injection site; divide I.M. doses over 5 ml; give at different sites.
• Give large volumes (5 ml) in adults only. Use upper outer quadrant of gluteal area.

• *Alert:* This immune serum provides passive immunity. Don't confuse with rabies vaccine, a suspension of killed microorganisms that confers active immunity. The two drugs are often used together prophylactically after exposure to rabid animals.
• Clean wound thoroughly with soap and water; this is the best prophylaxis against rabies.

**PATIENT TEACHING**
• Inform patient that local reactions may occur at injection site. Instruct him to notify prescriber promptly if reactions persist or become severe.
• Tell patient that a tetanus shot also may be needed.
• Instruct patient in wound care.

---

## respiratory syncytial virus immune globulin intravenous, human (RSV-IGIV)
RespiGam

*Pregnancy risk category C*

**AVAILABLE FORMS**
*Injection:* 50 mg ± 10 mg/ml in 20-ml, 50-ml single-use vial

**INDICATIONS & DOSAGES**
➤ **To prevent serious lower respiratory tract infections from RSV in children with bronchopulmonary dysplasia (BPD) or history of premature birth (35 weeks' gestation or less)**
*Premature infants and children younger than age 2:* Single infusion monthly. Give 1.5 ml/kg/hour I.V. for 15 minutes; then, if condition allows higher rate, increase to 3 ml/kg/hour for 15 minutes and then to maximum of 6 ml/kg/hour until infusion ends. Maximum recommended total dose per monthly infusion is 750 mg/kg.

**I.V. ADMINISTRATION**
• Drug doesn't contain a preservative. Enter single-use vial only once; don't shake; avoid foaming. Begin infusion within 6 hours and end within 12 hours after vial is entered. Don't use if solution is turbid. Give through I.V. line using a constant infusion pump. Don't predilute drug before infusion. Although filters aren't needed for

infusion, an in-line filter with pore size larger than 15 microns may be used. Give drug separately from other drugs.
• Adhere to infusion rate guidelines; most adverse reactions may be related to rate used. Slower rates may be indicated in especially ill children with BPD.
• Assess cardiopulmonary status and vital signs before beginning infusion, before each rate increase, and every 30 minutes thereafter until 30 minutes after completion of infusion.
• *Alert:* If patient develops hypotension, anaphylaxis, or severe allergic reaction, stop infusion and give epinephrine 1:1,000. Patients with selective immunoglobulin A deficiency can develop antibodies to immunoglobulin A and have anaphylactic or allergic reactions to subsequent administration of blood products containing immunoglobulin A, including RSV-IGIV.

**ACTION**
Provides passive immunity to RSV.

| Route | Onset | Peak | Duration |
|-------|-------|------|----------|
| I.V. | Unknown | Unknown | > 1 mo |

**ADVERSE REACTIONS**
**CNS:** fever, dizziness, anxiety.
**CV:** tachycardia, hypertension, palpitations, chest tightness, flushing.
**GI:** vomiting, diarrhea, gastroenteritis, abdominal cramps.
**Metabolic:** fluid overload.
**Musculoskeletal:** myalgia, arthralgia.
**Respiratory:** respiratory distress, wheezing, crackles, hypoxia, tachypnea, dyspnea.
**Skin:** rash, pruritus, inflammation at injection site.
**Other:** overdose effect; hypersensitivity reactions including *anaphylaxis, angioneurotic edema.*

**INTERACTIONS**
**Drug-drug.** *Live-virus vaccines (such as mumps, rubella, and especially measles):* May interfere with response. If such vaccines are given during or within 10 months after RSV-IGIV, reimmunization is recommended, if appropriate.

---

*Rapid onset* †Canada ‡Australia ◇OTC ◆ Off-label use ✐Photoguide *Liquid contains alcohol.

**EFFECTS ON LAB TEST RESULTS**
None reported.

**CONTRAINDICATIONS & CAUTIONS**
• Contraindicated in patients severely hypersensitive to drug or other human immunoglobulin and selective immunoglobulin A deficiency.
• Children with fluid overload shouldn't receive drug.

**NURSING CONSIDERATIONS**
• Give first dose before RSV season (November to April) begins; give subsequent doses monthly throughout RSV season to maintain protection. Children with RSV should continue to receive monthly doses for duration of RSV season.
• Watch patient closely for signs and symptoms of fluid overload. Children with BPD may be more prone to this condition. Report increases in heart rate, respiratory rate, retractions, or crackles. Keep available a loop diuretic, such as furosemide or bumetanide.

**PATIENT TEACHING**
• Explain to parents importance of child receiving drug monthly throughout RSV season, even if he is already infected.
• Teach parents how drug is given and which adverse reactions are related to administration. Tell parents to report all adverse reactions promptly.

---

# Rh$_0$(D) immune globulin, human
BayRho-D Full Dose, BayRho-D Mini-Dose, MICRhoGAM, RhoGAM

# Rh$_0$(D) immune globulin intravenous, human

*Pregnancy risk category C*

**AVAILABLE FORMS**
**Rh$_0$(D) immune globulin, human**
*Injection:* 300 mcg of Rh$_0$(D) immune globulin/vial (standard dose); 50 mcg of Rh$_0$(D) immune globulin/vial (microdose)
**Rh$_0$(D) immune globulin I.V., human**
*Injection:* 120 mcg, 300 mcg

**INDICATIONS & DOSAGES**
➤ **Rh exposure after abortion, miscarriage, ectopic pregnancy, or childbirth**
*Rho(D) immune globulin, human*
*Adults:* Transfusion unit or blood bank determines fetal packed RBC volume entering patient's blood; one vial is given I.M. if fetal packed RBC volume is less than 15 ml. More than one vial I.M. may be needed if severe fetomaternal hemorrhage occurs; must be given within 72 hours after delivery or miscarriage.
➤ **To prevent Rh antibody formation after abortion or miscarriage**
*Adults:* Consult transfusion unit or blood bank. One microdose vial I.M. will suppress immune reaction to 2.5 ml Rh$_0$(D)-positive RBCs. Ideally, give within 3 hours, but may be given up to 72 hours after abortion or miscarriage.
➤ **Rh exposure after abortion, amniocentesis after 34 weeks' gestation, or other manipulations past 34 weeks' gestation with increased risk of Rh isoimmunization**
*Rho(D) immune globulin I.V., human*
*Adults:* 120 mcg I.V. or I.M.; must be given within 72 hours after delivery, miscarriage, or manipulation.
➤ **Pregnancy**
*Adults:* 300 mcg I.V. or I.M. at 28 weeks' gestation. If given early in pregnancy, give additional doses at 12-week intervals to maintain adequate levels of passively acquired anti-Rh antibodies. Then, within 72 hours of delivery, give 120 mcg I.M. or I.V. If 72 hours have elapsed, give drug as soon as possible, up to 28 days.
➤ **Transfusion accidents**
*Adults:* 600 mcg I.V. q 8 hours or 1,200 mcg I.M. q 12 hours until total dose given. Total dose depends on volume of packed RBCs or whole blood infused. Consult blood bank or transfusion unit at once; must be given within 72 hours.
➤ **Idiopathic thrombocytopenic purpura in Rh$_0$(D) antigen-positive adults**
*Adults:* Initially, 50 mcg/kg I.V. If hemoglobin is less than 10 g/dl, reduce first dose to 25 to 40 mcg/kg. First dose may be given as single dose or divided into two doses and given on separate days. Then, 25 to 60 mcg/kg I.V. may be given p.r.n. to elevate platelet counts with specific dosage that is determined individually.

---

Reactions may be *common*, uncommon, ***life-threatening***, or **COMMON AND LIFE-THREATENING**.

## I.V. ADMINISTRATION
- Reconstitute only with normal saline solution.
- Reconstitute drug in vials containing 600 or 1,500 units with 2.5 ml of normal saline solution and vials containing 5,000 units with 8.5 ml of normal saline solution.
- Slowly inject diluent onto the outside wall of vial and gently swirl vial until lyophilized pellet is dissolved. Don't shake vial.
- Give injection over 3 to 5 minutes.
- Don't give with other products.

## ACTION
Suppresses the active antibody response and formation of anti-$Rh_0$(D) antibodies in $Rh_0$(D)-negative, $D^u$-negative persons exposed to Rh-positive blood. $Rh_0$(D) immune globulin I.V. may form complexes with RBCs, blocking platelet destruction in adults who are $Rh_0$(D) antigen-positive. Mechanism of action isn't completely known.

| Route | Onset | Peak | Duration |
|---|---|---|---|
| I.V., I.M. | Unknown | Unknown | Unknown |

## ADVERSE REACTIONS
**CNS:** slight fever.
**Skin:** discomfort at injection site.
**Other:** *anaphylaxis.*

## INTERACTIONS
**Drug-drug.** *Live-virus vaccines:* May interfere with response. Postpone immunization for 3 months, if possible.

## EFFECTS ON LAB TEST RESULTS
None reported.

## CONTRAINDICATIONS & CAUTIONS
- Contraindicated in $Rh_0$(D)-positive or $D^u$-positive patients and in those previously immunized to $Rh_0$(D) blood factor. Contraindicated in patients with anaphylactic or severe systemic reaction to human globulin.
- Use extreme caution when giving drug to patients with immunoglobulin A deficiency.

## NURSING CONSIDERATIONS
- Patients with immunoglobulin A deficiency may develop immunoglobulin A antibodies and have an anaphylactic reaction; prescriber must weigh benefits of treatment against risk of hypersensitivity reactions before giving.
- Obtain history of allergies and reactions to immunizations. Keep epinephrine 1:1,000 ready to treat anaphylaxis.
- *Alert:* Immediately after delivery, send a sample of neonate's cord blood to laboratory for typing and crossmatching. Confirm if mother is $Rh_0$(D)-negative and $D^u$-negative. Give drug to mother only if infant is $Rh_0$(D)- or $D^u$-positive. Administration must occur within 72 hours of delivery.
- This immune serum provides passive immunity to patient exposed to $Rh_0$(D)-positive fetal blood during pregnancy and prevents formation of maternal antibodies (active immunity), which would endanger future $Rh_0$(D)-positive pregnancies.
- Postpone vaccination with live-virus vaccines for 3 months after administration of $Rh_0$(D) immune globulin.
- Minidose preparations are recommended for patient undergoing abortion or miscarriage up to 12 weeks' gestation unless she is $Rh_0$(D)-positive or $D^u$-positive or has Rh antibodies, or unless the father or fetus is Rh-negative.

## PATIENT TEACHING
- Explain how drug protects future $Rh_0$(D)-positive fetuses if used because of pregnancy, or explain other use, if indicated.
- Warn patient about adverse reactions related to drug.
- Reassure patient receiving this drug that there's no risk of HIV transmission.

# tetanus immune globulin, human
BayTet

*Pregnancy risk category C*

## AVAILABLE FORMS
*Injection:* 250-unit vial or syringe

## INDICATIONS & DOSAGES
➤ **Postexposure prevention of tetanus after injury, in patients whose immunization is incomplete or unknown**
*Adults and children:* 250 units deep I.M. injection.
➤ **Tetanus**
*Adults and children:* Single doses of 3,000 to 6,000 units I.M. have been used. Optimal dosage schedules haven't been established.

## ACTION
Provides passive immunity to tetanus.

| Route | Onset | Peak | Duration |
|-------|-------|------|----------|
| I.M. | Unknown | 2-3 days | 4 wk |

## ADVERSE REACTIONS
**CNS:** slight fever.
**GU:** *nephrotic syndrome.*
**Musculoskeletal:** stiffness.
**Skin:** erythema at injection site.
**Other:** pain, hypersensitivity reactions, *anaphylaxis, angioedema.*

## INTERACTIONS
**Drug-drug.** *Live-virus vaccines:* May interfere with response. Postpone administration of live-virus vaccines for 3 months after giving tetanus immune globulin.

## EFFECTS ON LAB TEST RESULTS
None reported.

## CONTRAINDICATIONS & CAUTIONS
• Contraindicated in patients with thrombocytopenia or other coagulation disorders that would contraindicate I.M. injection unless benefits outweigh risks.
• Use cautiously in patients with history of previous systemic allergic reactions after giving human immunoglobulin preparations and in those allergic to thimerosal.

## NURSING CONSIDERATIONS
• Obtain history of injury, tetanus immunizations, last tetanus toxoid injection, allergies, and reactions to immunizations. Keep epinephrine 1:1,000 available to treat hypersensitivity reaction.
• Don't give I.V. or I.D. Don't give in gluteal area.
• Tetanus immune globulin is used only if wound is more than 24 hours old or patient has had fewer than two tetanus toxoid injections.
• Thoroughly clean wound and remove all foreign matter.
• *Alert:* Don't confuse drug with tetanus toxoid. Tetanus immune globulin isn't a substitute for tetanus toxoid, which should be given at same time to produce active immunization. Don't give at same site as toxoid.
• Antibodies remain at effective levels for about 4 weeks, several times the duration of equine antitetanus antibodies, thereby protecting patients for incubation period of most tetanus cases.
• Don't give live-virus vaccines for 3 months after giving tetanus immune globulin.
• *Alert:* Don't confuse Hyper-Tet with HyperHep or Hyperstat.

## PATIENT TEACHING
• Warn patient about local adverse reactions related to drug.
• Instruct patient to report serious adverse reactions promptly.
• Advise patient to complete full series of tetanus immunizations.
• Instruct patient to take acetaminophen to reduce fever and to apply cool compresses at injection site for comfort.

# varicella zoster immune globulin (VZIG)

*Pregnancy risk category C*

## AVAILABLE FORMS
*Injection:* 10% to 18% solution of the globulin fraction of human plasma containing 125 units of varicella zoster virus antibody (volume is about 2.5 ml or less)

## INDICATIONS & DOSAGES
➤ **Passive immunization of susceptible immunodeficient patients after exposure to varicella (chickenpox or herpes zoster)**
*Adults and children weighing more than 40 kg (88 lb):* 625 units I.M.
*Children weighing 29.9 to 40 kg (66 to 88 lb):* 500 units I.M.
*Children weighing 19.9 to 30 kg (44 to 66 lb):* 375 units I.M.

*Children weighing 10 to 20 kg (22 to 44 lb):* 250 units I.M.
*Children weighing up to 10 kg (22 lb):* 125 units I.M.

## ACTION
Provides passive immunity to varicella zoster virus in immunodeficient patients.

| Route | Onset | Peak | Duration |
|-------|-------|------|----------|
| I.M. | Unknown | Unknown | 1 mo |

## ADVERSE REACTIONS
**CNS:** headache, malaise.
**GI:** GI distress.
**Respiratory:** respiratory distress.
**Skin:** discomfort at injection site, rash.
**Other:** *anaphylaxis.*

## INTERACTIONS
**Drug-drug.** *Live-virus vaccines:* May interfere with response. Postpone vaccination for 3 months after administration of VZIG.

## EFFECTS ON LAB TEST RESULTS
None reported.

## CONTRAINDICATIONS & CAUTIONS
• Contraindicated in patients with thrombocytopenia or history of severe reaction to human immune serum globulin or thimerosal; also contraindicated during pregnancy.

## NURSING CONSIDERATIONS
• Obtain accurate patient history of allergies and reactions to immunizations. Keep epinephrine 1:1,000 ready to treat anaphylaxis.
• For maximum benefit, give as soon as possible after presumed exposure. Drug may be of benefit when given as late as 96 hours after exposure.
• Give only by deep I.M. injection into a large muscle such as gluteal muscle. Never give I.V.
• Don't give in divided doses.
• Although usually restricted to children younger than age 15, VZIG may be given to adolescents and adults, if needed.
• VZIG isn't recommended for patients who aren't immunosuppressed.

• *Alert:* VZIG provides passive immunity; don't confuse with varicella vaccine. Don't use these two drugs together.
• Drug isn't commercially distributed and is available only from 20 regional United States distribution centers. These centers will distribute to Canada and overseas. Contact the Massachusetts Public Health Biologic Laboratories or the CDC at (800) 232-2522 for more information.

## PATIENT TEACHING
• Warn patient about local adverse reactions caused by the drug.
• Instruct patient to report serious adverse reactions to prescriber promptly.
• Suggest use of acetaminophen to reduce fever and cool compresses at injection site for comfort.

## Biological response modifiers

darbepoetin alfa
epoetin alfa
filgrastim
glatiramer acetate for injection
interferon alfacon-1
interferon alfa-2a, recombinant
  (rIFN-A)
interferon alfa-2b, recombinant
  (IFN-alpha 2)
interferon beta-1a
interferon beta-1b, recombinant
interferon gamma-1b
leflunomide
oprelvekin
pegfilgrastim
peginterferon alfa-2a
peginterferon alfa-2b
sargramostim

**COMBINATION PRODUCTS**
None.

---

### darbepoetin alfa
Aranesp

*Pregnancy risk category C*

**AVAILABLE FORMS**
*Injection:* 25 mcg/ml, 40 mcg/ml, 60 mcg/
ml, and 100 mcg/ml single-dose vials,
polysorbate solution; 25 mcg/ml, 40 mcg/
ml, 60 mcg/ml, and 100 mcg/ml single-
dose vials, albumin solution

**INDICATIONS & DOSAGES**
➤ **Anemia from chronic renal failure**
*Adults:* 0.45 mcg/kg I.V. or S.C. once
weekly. Adjust doses so that hemoglobin
doesn't exceed 12 g/dl. Don't increase
dose more often than once a month. In patients converting from epoetin alfa, base
starting dose on the previous epoetin alfa
dose (see table).

| Previous epoetin alfa dose (mcg/wk) | Darbepoetin alfa dose (units/wk) |
|---|---|
| < 2,500 | 6.25 |
| 2,500-4,999 | 12.5 |
| 5,000-10,999 | 25 |
| 11,000-17,999 | 40 |
| 18,000-33,999 | 60 |
| 34,000-89,999 | 100 |
| ≥ 90,000 | 200 |

Give darbepoetin alfa less often than
epoetin alfa. If patient was receiving epoetin alfa two to three times weekly, give
darbepoetin alfa once weekly. If patient
was receiving epoetin alfa once weekly,
give darbepoetin alfa once q 2 weeks.
*Adjust-a-dose:* If increasing hemoglobin
approaches 12 g/dl, reduce dose by 25%.
If hemoglobin continues to increase, withhold dose until hemoglobin begins to decrease; then restart therapy at a dose 25%
below the previous dose. If hemoglobin
increases more than 1 g/dl over 2 weeks,
decrease dose by 25%. If hemoglobin increases less than 1 g/dl over 4 weeks and
iron stores are adequate, increase dose by
25% of previous dose. Make further increases at 4-week intervals until target hemoglobin is reached.
    Patients who don't need dialysis may
need lower maintenance doses.
➤ **Anemia from chemotherapy in patients with nonmyeloid malignancies**
*Adults:* 2.25 mcg/kg S.C. weekly.
*Adjust-a-dose:* If hemoglobin increases
less than 1 g/dl after 6 weeks of therapy,
increase dose up to 4.5 mcg/kg. If hemoglobin increases by more than 1 g/dl in a
2-week period or if hemoglobin exceeds
12 g/dl, reduce dose by about 25%. If hemoglobin exceeds 13 g/dl, withhold drug
until hemoglobin drops to 12 g/dl. Therapy can then be restarted at a dose about
25% below the previous dose.

**I.V. ADMINISTRATION**
● Give undiluted by I.V. injection.

• Don't shake. Shaking can denature the drug.
• Don't mix with other drugs or solutions.
• Single-dose vials contain no preservatives; don't pool unused portions.
• Don't use if drug contains particles or is discolored.

## ACTION

Mimics effects of erythropoietin. Functions as a growth factor and as a differentiating factor, enhancing RBC production.

| Route | Onset | Peak | Duration |
|-------|---------|---------|----------|
| I.V. | Unknown | Unknown | 21 hr |
| S.C. | Unknown | 34 hr | 49 hr |

## ADVERSE REACTIONS

**CNS:** *headache, fever, dizziness, fatigue,* asthenia, *seizures.*
**CV:** *hypertension, hypotension,* CARDIAC ARRHYTHMIA, CARDIAC ARREST, *angina,* **heart failure, thrombosis,** *edema,* chest pain, **acute MI.**
**GI:** *diarrhea, vomiting, nausea, abdominal pain, constipation.*
**Metabolic:** dehydration.
**Musculoskeletal:** *myalgia, arthralgia, limb pain,* back pain.
**Respiratory:** *upper respiratory tract infection, dyspnea, cough,* bronchitis, pneumonia, **pulmonary embolism.**
**Skin:** pruritus, rash.
**Other:** *infection,* fluid overload, flulike symptoms, **hemorrhage at access site.**

## INTERACTIONS
None reported.

## EFFECTS ON LAB TEST RESULTS
None reported.

## CONTRAINDICATIONS & CAUTIONS
• Contraindicated in patients hypersensitive to the drug or its components and in those with uncontrolled hypertension.
• Safety and effectiveness haven't been established in patients with underlying hematologic disease, such as hemolytic anemia, sickle cell anemia, thalassemia or porphyria. Use with caution.

## NURSING CONSIDERATIONS
• Some patients have been treated successfully with a S.C. dose given once every 2 weeks.
• Hemoglobin may not increase until 2 to 6 weeks after starting therapy.
• Darbepoetin alfa may increase the risk of CV events. Control blood pressure and monitor carefully.
• **Alert:** Monitor hemoglobin weekly until stabilized. Don't exceed the target of 12 g/dl.
• Monitor renal function and electrolytes in predialysis patients.
• Monitor iron status before and during treatment. Provide supplemental iron in patients whose ferritin is less than 100 mcg/L and transferrin saturation is less than 20%.
• Patients who are marginally dialyzed may need adjustments in dialysis prescriptions.
• There is a potential for serious allergic reactions, including skin rash and urticaria. If an anaphylactic reaction occurs, stop the drug and give appropriate therapy.
• Store drug in the refrigerator; don't freeze. Protect drug from light.
• **Alert:** Decrease dosage if hemoglobin increases 1g/dl in any 2-week period.

## PATIENT TEACHING
• Instruct patients on proper administration and use and disposal of needles.
• Advise patient of possible side effects and allergic reactions.
• Inform patient of the need for frequent monitoring of blood pressure and hemoglobin; stress compliance with his treatment for high blood pressure.
• Instruct patient how to take drug correctly at home, including how to dispose of supplies properly.

---

## epoetin alfa (erythropoietin)
Epogen, Procrit

*Pregnancy risk category C*

## AVAILABLE FORMS
*Injection:* 2,000 units/ml, 3,000 units/ml, 4,000 units/ml, 10,000 units/ml; multidose vials of 10,000 units/ml, 20,000 units/ml

---

## INDICATIONS & DOSAGES

➤ **Anemia from reduced production of endogenous erythropoietin caused by end-stage renal disease**

*Adults:* Dosage is individualized. Starting dose is 50 to 100 units/kg I.V. three times weekly. Nondialysis patients with chronic renal failure or patients receiving continuous peritoneal dialysis may receive drug by S.C. injection or I.V. Maintenance dosage is highly individualized.

*Adjust-a-dose:* Reduce dosage when target hematocrit is reached or if hematocrit rises more than 4 points in 2 weeks. Increase dosage if hematocrit doesn't increase by 5 to 6 points after 8 weeks of therapy.

➤ **Adjunctive treatment of HIV-infected patients with anemia from zidovudine therapy**

*Adults:* 100 units/kg I.V. or S.C. three times weekly for 8 weeks or until target hemoglobin level is reached. If response isn't satisfactory after 8 weeks, increase dosage by 50 to 100 units/kg I.V. or S.C. three times weekly. After 4 to 8 weeks, further increase dosage in increments of 50 to 100 units/kg three times weekly, up to maximum of 300 units/kg I.V. or S.C. three times weekly.

➤ **Anemia from cancer chemotherapy**

*Adults:* 150 units/kg S.C. three times weekly for 8 weeks or until target hemoglobin level is reached. If response isn't satisfactory after 8 weeks, increase dosage up to 300 units/kg S.C. three times weekly.

*Adjust-a-dose:* If hematocrit exceeds 40%, withhold drug until hematocrit falls to 36%.

➤ **Reduce need for allogenic blood transfusion in anemic patients scheduled to have elective, noncardiac, non-vascular surgery**

*Adults:* 300 units/kg daily S.C. daily for 10 days before surgery, on day of surgery, and for 4 days after surgery. Or, 600 units/kg S.C. in once-weekly doses (21, 14, and 7 days before surgery), plus one-fourth dose on day of surgery.

➤ **Anemia in pediatric patients with chronic renal failure who are having dialysis**

*Infants and children ages 1 month to 16 years:* 50 units/kg I.V. or S.C. three times weekly. Maintenance dosage is highly individualized to maintain hematocrit level within target range.

*Adjust-a-dose:* Reduce dosage when target hematocrit level is reached or if hematocrit level rises more than 4 points within a 2-week period. Increase dosage if hematocrit level doesn't rise by 5 to 6 points after 8 weeks of therapy and is below target range.

## I.V. ADMINISTRATION

● Give by direct injection without dilution. Solution contains no preservatives. Discard unused portion. Don't mix with other drugs. Don't shake.

● Drug may be given via the venous return line of dialysis tubing after dialysis to eliminate need for additional I.V. access.

● To prevent adherence to tubing, inject drug while blood is still in I.V. line, and follow with a normal saline solution flush.

## ACTION

Mimics effects of erythropoietin. Functions as a growth factor and as a differentiating factor, enhancing RBC production.

| Route | Onset | Peak | Duration |
|-------|-------|------|----------|
| I.V. | Immediate | Immediate | Unknown |
| S.C. | Unknown | 5-24 hr | Unknown |

## ADVERSE REACTIONS

**CNS:** *headache, **seizures,** paresthesia, fatigue, dizziness, asthenia.*
**CV:** *hypertension, edema,* increased clotting of arteriovenous grafts.
**GI:** *nausea, vomiting, diarrhea.*
**Metabolic:** hyperuricemia, ***hyperkalemia,*** hyperphosphatemia.
**Musculoskeletal:** *arthralgia.*
**Respiratory:** *cough, shortness of breath.*
**Skin:** *rash, injection site reactions,* urticaria.
**Other:** *pyrexia.*

## INTERACTIONS

None significant.

## EFFECTS ON LAB TEST RESULTS

● May increase BUN, creatinine, uric acid, potassium, and phosphate levels.

## CONTRAINDICATIONS & CAUTIONS

● Contraindicated in patients hypersensitive to products derived from mammal

---

Reactions may be *common,* uncommon, ***life-threatening,*** or **COMMON AND LIFE-THREATENING.**

cells or albumin (human) and in those with uncontrolled hypertension.
• Use cautiously in breast-feeding women.

**NURSING CONSIDERATIONS**
• Monitor blood pressure before therapy. Up to 80% of patients with chronic renal failure have hypertension. Blood pressure may rise, especially when hematocrit is increasing in the early part of therapy.
• If hematocrit is increasing and approaching 36%, reduce dosage to maintain target hematocrit range. If hematocrit remains unchanged after reducing dosage, withhold dose temporarily until hematocrit decreases.
• When used in HIV-infected patients, be prepared to individualize dosage based on response. Dosage recommendations are for patients with endogenous erythropoietin levels of 500 units/L or less and cumulative zidovudine doses of 4.2 g/week or less.
• Patient treated with epoetin alfa may need additional heparin to prevent clotting during dialysis treatments.
• Monitor blood count. Hematocrit may rise and cause excessive clotting. Renal function, uric acid, and potassium levels may rise.
• Institute diet restrictions or drug therapy to control blood pressure. Reduce dosage in patients who exhibit rapid rise in hematocrit (more than 4 points in a 2-week period), to prevent hypertension.
• Patient's response to epoetin alfa depends on amount of endogenous erythropoietin in the plasma. Patients with levels of 500 units/L or more usually have transfusion-dependent anemia and probably won't respond to drug. Those with levels below 500 units/L usually respond well.
• Patient should receive adequate iron supplementation beginning no later than when epoetin alfa treatment starts and continuing throughout therapy. Patient also may need vitamin $B_{12}$ and folic acid.
• **Alert:** Don't confuse Epogen with Neupogen.

**PATIENT TEACHING**
• Inform patient that pain or discomfort in limbs (long bones) and pelvis, and coldness and sweating aren't uncommon after injection (usually occurring within 2 hours). Symptoms may last for 12 hours and then disappear.
• Advise patient that blood specimens will be drawn weekly for blood counts and that dosage adjustments may be made based on results.
• Advise patient to avoid driving or operating heavy machinery at start of therapy. There may be a relationship between excessively rapid hematocrit rise and seizures.
• Tell patient to monitor blood pressure at home and to adhere to dietary restrictions.
• Instruct patient to check that syringes used to give drug are in tenths-of-milliliter increments.

---

## filgrastim (G-CSF; granulocyte-colony stimulating factor)
Neupogen

*Pregnancy risk category C*

---

**AVAILABLE FORMS**
*Injection:* 300 mcg/ml

**INDICATIONS & DOSAGES**
➤ **To decrease risk of infection in patients with nonmyeloid malignant disease receiving myelosuppressive antineoplastics**
*Adults and children:* 5 mcg/kg daily I.V. or S.C. as single dose given no sooner than 24 hours after cytotoxic chemotherapy. Doses may be increased in increments of 5 mcg/kg for each chemotherapy cycle depending on duration and severity of the nadir of absolute neutrophil count (ANC).
➤ **To decrease risk of infection in patients with nonmyeloid malignant disease receiving myelosuppressive antineoplastics followed by bone marrow transplantation**
*Adults and children:* 10 mcg/kg daily I.V. infusion of 4 or 24 hours or as continuous 24-hour S.C. infusion at least 24 hours after cytotoxic chemotherapy and bone marrow infusion. Adjust subsequent dosages based on neutrophil response.
*Adjust-a-dose:* For patients with ANC over 1,000/mm³ for 3 consecutive days, reduce dosage to 5 mcg/kg daily; if ANC

remains over 1,000/mm³ for 3 more consecutive days, stop drug. If ANC decreases to below 1,000/mm³, resume therapy at 5 mcg/kg daily.

➤ **Congenital neutropenia**
*Adults:* 6 mcg/kg S.C. b.i.d. Adjust dosage based on patient response.
**Adjust-a-dose:** For patients with a persistently elevated ANC (above 10,000/mm³), reduce dosage, as directed.

➤ **Idiopathic or cyclic neutropenia**
*Adults:* 5 mcg/kg S.C. daily. Adjust dosage based on patient response.

➤ **Peripheral blood progenitor cell collection and therapy in cancer patients**
*Adults:* 10 mcg/kg S.C. daily. Give 4 days before leukapheresis and continue until last leukapheresis.
**Adjust-a-dose:** Patients with WBC count over 100,000/mm³ may need dosage adjustment.

➤ **To reduce the risk of bacterial infection in patients with HIV ◆**
*Adults and adolescents:* 5 to 10 mcg/kg S.C. once daily for 2 to 4 weeks.

## I.V. ADMINISTRATION
● Dilute in 50 to 100 ml of D₅W and give by intermittent infusion over 15 to 60 minutes or continuous infusion over 24 hours.
● Don't dilute with normal saline solution. Dilution to yield less than 5 mcg/ml isn't recommended.
● If drug yield is 5 to 15 mcg/ml, add albumin at a concentration of 2 mg/ml (0.2%) to minimize binding of drug to plastic containers or tubing.

## ACTION
A glycoprotein that stimulates proliferation and differentiation of hematopoietic cells. Is specific for neutrophils.

| Route | Onset     | Peak   | Duration  |
|-------|-----------|--------|-----------|
| I.V.  | 5-60 min  | 24 hr  | 1-7 days  |
| S.C.  | 5-60 min  | 2-8 hr | 1-7 days  |

## ADVERSE REACTIONS
**CNS:** *fever,* headache, weakness, *fatigue.*
**CV:** *MI, arrhythmias,* chest pain, hypotension.
**GI:** *nausea, vomiting, diarrhea, mucositis,* stomatitis, constipation.
**Hematologic:** *thrombocytopenia,* leukocytosis.

**Metabolic:** hyperuricemia.
**Musculoskeletal:** *bone pain.*
**Respiratory:** dyspnea, cough.
**Skin:** *alopecia,* rash, cutaneous vasculitis.
**Other:** hypersensitivity reactions.

## INTERACTIONS
**Drug-drug.** *Chemotherapeutic drugs:* Rapidly dividing myeloid cells may be sensitive to cytotoxic drugs. Don't use within 24 hours before or after a dose of one of these drugs.

## EFFECTS ON LAB TEST RESULTS
● May increase creatinine, uric acid, alkaline phosphatase, and LDH levels.
● May increase WBC count and decrease platelet count.

## CONTRAINDICATIONS & CAUTIONS
● Contraindicated in patients hypersensitive to drug or its components or to proteins derived from *Escherichia coli.*
● Use cautiously in breast-feeding women.

## NURSING CONSIDERATIONS
● Obtain baseline CBC and platelet count before therapy.
● Once a dose is withdrawn, don't reuse vial. Discard unused portion. Vials are for single-dose use and contain no preservatives.
● Obtain CBC and platelet count two to three times weekly during therapy. Patients who receive drug also may receive high doses of chemotherapy, which may increase risk of toxicities.
● A transiently increased neutrophil count is common 1 or 2 days after therapy starts. Give daily for up to 2 weeks or until ANC has returned to 10,000/mm³ after the expected chemotherapy-induced neutrophil nadir.
● *Alert:* Don't confuse Neupogen with Epogen or Neumega.

## PATIENT TEACHING
● If patient will give drug, teach him how to do so and how to dispose of used needles, syringes, drug containers, and unused medicine.
● Instruct patient to report persistent or serious adverse reactions promptly.

## glatiramer acetate for injection (formerly copolymer 1)
Copaxone

*Pregnancy risk category B*

### AVAILABLE FORMS
*Injection:* 20 mg lyophilized glatiramer acetate and 40 mg mannitol, USP, in a single-use 2-ml vial; 1-ml vial of sterile water for injection is included for reconstitution

### INDICATIONS & DOSAGES
➤ **Reduce frequency of relapse in patients with relapsing-remitting multiple sclerosis**
*Adults:* 20 mg S.C. daily.

### ACTION
Unknown. Thought to act by modifying immune processes responsible for the pathogenesis of multiple sclerosis.

| Route | Onset | Peak | Duration |
|-------|-------|------|----------|
| S.C. | Unknown | Unknown | Unknown |

### ADVERSE REACTIONS
**CNS:** abnormal dreams, fever, agitation, *anxiety, asthenia,* confusion, emotional lability, migraine, nervousness, speech disorder, stupor, tremor, vertigo, syncope.
**CV:** *chest pain,* hypertension, *palpitations, vasodilation,* tachycardia.
**EENT:** ear pain, eye disorder, laryngismus, *rhinitis,* nystagmus.
**GI:** anorexia, bowel urgency, *diarrhea,* gastroenteritis, GI disorder, *nausea,* oral candidiasis, salivary gland enlargement, ulcerative stomatitis, vomiting.
**GU:** amenorrhea, dysmenorrhea, hematuria, impotence, menorrhagia, abnormal Papanicolaou smear, *urinary urgency,* vaginal candidiasis, **vaginal hemorrhage.**
**Hematologic:** ecchymosis, *lymphadenopathy.*
**Metabolic:** weight gain.
**Musculoskeletal:** *arthralgia, back pain,* neck pain, foot drop, *hypertonia.*
**Respiratory:** bronchitis, *dyspnea,* hyperventilation.
**Skin:** eczema, erythema, *pruritus, rash, injection site reaction* or hemorrhage, skin atrophy, nodule, *diaphoresis,* urticaria, warts.
**Other:** bacterial infection, herpes simplex and zoster, chills, cyst, dental caries, peripheral and facial edema, *flulike syndrome, infection, pain.*

### INTERACTIONS
None significant.

### EFFECTS ON LAB TEST RESULTS
None reported.

### CONTRAINDICATIONS & CAUTIONS
● Contraindicated in patients hypersensitive to drug or mannitol.

### NURSING CONSIDERATIONS
● Give drug only by S.C. injection.
● Store drug in refrigerator (36° to 46° F [2° to 8° C]); diluent can be kept at room temperature.
● Swirl lyophilized material and diluent gently and let stand at room temperature until completely dissolved, about 5 minutes.
● Use immediately after reconstitution because drug doesn't contain preservatives; discard unused drug. Use diluent provided for reconstitution.
● Immediate postinjection reactions have occurred in some patients with multiple sclerosis; symptoms include flushing, chest pain, palpitations, anxiety, dyspnea, constriction of the throat, and urticaria. They typically are transient and self-limiting and don't need specific treatment. Onset of postinjection reaction may occur several months after treatment starts, and patients may have more than one episode.
● Some patients have experienced at least one episode of transient chest pain, which usually begins at least 1 month after treatment starts; it isn't accompanied by other signs or symptoms and doesn't appear to be clinically important.
● *Alert:* Don't confuse Copaxone with Compazine.

### PATIENT TEACHING
● Instruct patient how to reconstitute and self-inject drug. Supervise first injection.
● Explain need for aseptic self-injection techniques and warn patient against reuse of needles and syringes. Periodically re-

---

view proper disposal of needles, syringes, drug containers, and unused drug.
• Tell patient to notify prescriber about planned, suspected, or known pregnancy.
• Tell woman to notify prescriber if she is breast-feeding.
• Advise patient not to change drug or dosing schedule or to stop drug without medical approval.
• Tell patient to notify prescriber immediately if dizziness, hives, profuse sweating, chest pain, difficulty breathing, or if severe pain occurs after drug injection.

---

## interferon alfacon-1
Infergen

*Pregnancy risk category C*

### AVAILABLE FORMS
*Injection:* 9 mcg/0.3-ml, 15 mcg/0.5-ml vials

### INDICATIONS & DOSAGES
➤ **Chronic hepatitis C viral infection in patients with compensated liver disease**
*Adults:* 9 mcg S.C. three times weekly for 24 weeks; for patients who don't respond or who relapse, 15 mcg S.C. three times weekly for 6 months.
*Adjust-a-dose:* For patients intolerant to higher doses, dose may be reduced to 7.5 mcg. Don't give doses below 7.5 mcg because decreased efficacy may result.

### ACTION
Type-I interferons induce genetic-mediated biological responses that include antiviral, antiproliferative, and immunomodulatory effects and regulation of cytokine expression.

| Route | Onset | Peak | Duration |
|-------|-------|------|----------|
| S.C. | Unknown | 24-36 hr | Unknown |

### ADVERSE REACTIONS
**CNS:** *headache, insomnia, dizziness, paresthesia, amnesia, nervousness, depression, anxiety, emotional lability,* confusion, agitation, **suicidal ideation,** *malaise.*
**CV:** hypertension, tachycardia, palpitations.

**EENT:** *retinal hemorrhages,* loss of visual acuity or visual field, conjunctivitis, tinnitus, ear pain, *pharyngitis, sinusitis, rhinitis,* epistaxis.
**GI:** *abdominal pain, nausea, diarrhea,* taste perversion, *anorexia, dyspepsia, vomiting,* constipation, flatulence, hemorrhoids, decreased saliva.
**GU:** dysmenorrhea, vaginitis.
**Hematologic:** *granulocytopenia,* **leukopenia, thrombocytopenia,** ecchymosis, lymphadenopathy, lymphocytosis.
**Metabolic:** hypothyroidism.
**Respiratory:** *infection, cough, congestion,* dyspnea, bronchitis.
**Skin:** *alopecia, pruritus, rash,* dry skin, pain, *erythema* at injection site.
**Other:** toothache, decreased libido, **hypersensitivity reactions,** body pain, *flulike symptoms.*

### INTERACTIONS
**Drug-drug.** *Drugs metabolized by cytochrome P450:* May alter drug levels. Monitor changes in levels of these drugs.
*Myelosuppressives:* No studies have been conducted; however, use cautiously with interferon alfacon-1. Monitor CBC and therapeutic or toxic levels of drugs taken together with interferon alfacon-1.

### EFFECTS ON LAB TEST RESULTS
• May increase triglyceride and TSH levels. May decrease $T_4$ levels.
• May increase PT and INR. May decrease granulocyte, WBC, and platelet counts.

### CONTRAINDICATIONS & CAUTIONS
• Contraindicated in patients hypersensitive to alpha interferons, to *Escherichia coli*-derived products, or to any component of product. Also contraindicated in patients with history of severe psychiatric disorders, autoimmune hepatitis, or decompensated hepatic disease.
• Use with caution in patients with history of cardiac disease and other autoimmune or endocrine disorders, in those with abnormally low peripheral blood cell counts, and in those receiving drugs known to cause myelosuppression.

### NURSING CONSIDERATIONS
• Depression and suicidal behavior have been linked to drug.

---

• Perform the following laboratory tests before therapy, 2 weeks after it starts, and periodically during therapy: CBC with platelets, creatinine, albumin, bilirubin, TSH, and $T_4$.

• *Alert:* If hypersensitivity reaction occurs, stop drug immediately and treat. Premedication with acetaminophen or ibuprofen may decrease adverse effects.

• Allow at least 48 hours to elapse between doses.

• Dosages and adverse reactions vary among different subtypes of drug. Don't use different subtypes in a single treatment regimen.

• Store drug in refrigerator at 36° to 46° F (2° to 8° C); don't freeze. Injection may be allowed to reach room temperature just before use. Avoid vigorous shaking. Discard unused portion.

## PATIENT TEACHING

• If drug is to be used at home, instruct patient on appropriate use, dosage, and administration. Give the patient information leaflet available from the manufacturer to the patient. Also teach patient proper disposal procedures for needles, syringes, drug containers, and unused drug.

• Instruct patient not to reuse needles or syringes or reenter vial.

• Tell patient to discard all syringes and needles in a puncture-resistant container.

• Urge patient not to use vial that is discolored or contains particulates.

• Tell patient that nonnarcotic analgesics and bedtime administration may be used to prevent or lessen flulike symptoms (headache, fever, malaise, muscle pain) related to therapy.

• Instruct patient to immediately report symptoms of depression.

## interferon alfa-2a, recombinant (rIFN-A)
Roferon-A

*Pregnancy risk category C*

## AVAILABLE FORMS
*Injection:* 3, 6, 9, 36 million IU/single-use vial; 9, 18 million IU/multidose vial
*Sterile powder for injection:* 18 million IU/vial with diluent

## INDICATIONS & DOSAGES
➤ **Chronic hepatitis C**
*Adults:* 3 million IU three times a week I.M. or S.C. for 12 months (48 to 52 weeks). Or, induction dose of 6 million IU three times weekly for the first 3 months (12 weeks) followed by 3 million IU three times weekly for 9 months (36 weeks). If no response after 3 months, stop therapy. Retreatment with either 3 or 6 million IU three times weekly for 6 to 12 months may be considered.

➤ **Hairy cell leukemia**
*Adults:* For induction, 3 million IU I.M. or S.C. daily for 16 to 24 weeks. For maintenance, 3 million IU I.M. or S.C. three times weekly.

➤ **AIDS-related Kaposi's sarcoma**
*Adults:* For induction, 36 million IU I.M. or S.C. daily for 10 to 12 weeks. For maintenance, 36 million IU I.M. or S.C. three times weekly. Doses may begin at 3 million IU and escalated upward every 3 days until patient is given 36 million IU daily in order to decrease toxicity.

➤ **Philadelphia chromosome–positive chronic myelogenous leukemia**
*Adults:* Initially, 3 million IU I.M. or S.C. daily for 3 days; then 6 million IU for 3 days; then 9 million IU for duration of treatment.
*Children:* 2.5 to 5 million IU/m² I.M. daily.

## ACTION
Unknown. Appears to involve direct antiproliferative action against tumor or viral cells to inhibit replication and modulation of host immune response by enhancing phagocytic activity of macrophages and augmenting specific cytotoxicity of lymphocytes for target cells.

| Route | Onset | Peak | Duration |
|-------|---------|---------|----------|
| I.M. | Unknown | 2-12 hr | Unknown |
| S.C. | Unknown | 3-12 hr | Unknown |

## ADVERSE REACTIONS
**CNS:** *dizziness, confusion,* paresthesia, numbness, lethargy, *depression, decreased mental status,* forgetfulness, *coma,* nervousness, insomnia, sedation, apathy, anxiety, irritability, fatigue, vertigo, gait disturbances, incoordination, syncope.

**CV:** hypotension, chest pain, *arrhythmias,* palpitations, *heart failure,* hypertension, edema, *MI,* flushing.

**EENT:** *dryness or inflammation of the oropharynx,* rhinorrhea, sinusitis, conjunctivitis, earache, eye irritation.

**GI:** *anorexia, nausea, diarrhea, vomiting,* abdominal fullness, *abdominal pain,* flatulence, constipation, hypermotility, gastric distress, excessive salivation, *change in taste.*

**GU:** transient impotence.

**Hematologic:** LEUKOPENIA, THROMBO-CYTOPENIA, *anemia*

**Hepatic:** *hepatitis.*

**Metabolic:** *weight loss,* hypercalcemia, hyperphosphatemia.

**Respiratory:** cyanosis, cough, dyspnea.

**Skin:** *rash,* dryness, pruritus, *partial alopecia,* urticaria, diaphoresis, *inflammation at injection site.*

**Other:** *flulike syndrome,* night sweats, hot flashes.

**INTERACTIONS**
**Drug-drug.** *Aminophylline, theophylline:* May reduce theophylline clearance. Monitor serum level.

*Aspirin:* May increase risk of GI bleeding. Avoid using together.

*CNS depressants:* May increase CNS effects. Avoid using together.

*Live-virus vaccines:* May increase risk of adverse reactions and may decrease antibody response. Avoid using together.

*Drugs with neurotoxic, hematotoxic, cardiotoxic effects:* May increase the toxic effects of these drugs. Monitor patient for increased adverse effects.

**Drug-lifestyle.** *Alcohol use:* May increase risk of GI bleeding. Discourage patient from use during therapy.

**EFFECTS ON LAB TEST RESULTS**
• May increase calcium, phosphate, AST, ALT, alkaline phosphatase, LDH, and fasting glucose levels.
• May increase PT, INR, and PTT. May decrease hemoglobin, hematocrit, WBC, and platelet counts.

**CONTRAINDICATIONS & CAUTIONS**
• Contraindicated in patients hypersensitive to drug, murine (mouse) immunoglobulin, or other drug components. Also contraindicated in patients with history of autoimmune hepatitis or history of autoimmune disease, severe visceral AIDS-related Kaposi's sarcoma, neonates (injection contains benzyl alcohol), immunocompromised transplant patients, and severe depression or suicidal behavior.
• Use cautiously in patients with severe hepatic or renal function impairment, seizure disorders, compromised CNS function, cardiac disease, or myelosuppression.
• **Alert:** Neurotoxicity and cardiotoxicity are more common in elderly patients, especially those with underlying CNS or cardiac impairment.

**NURSING CONSIDERATIONS**
• **Alert:** Alpha interferons cause or aggravate fatal or life-threatening neuropsychiatric, autoimmune, ischemic, and infectious disorders. Monitor patient closely with periodic clinical and laboratory evaluations. Withdraw patients with persistently severe or worsening signs or symptoms of these conditions from therapy.
• Obtain allergy history. Drug contains phenol as a preservative and albumin as a stabilizer.
• Use S.C. administration route in patients whose platelet count is below 50,000/mm³.
• Give drug at bedtime to minimize daytime drowsiness.
• Ensure patient is well hydrated, especially during first stages of treatment.
• At beginning of therapy, assess patient for flulike signs and symptoms, which tend to diminish with continued therapy. Premedicate patient with acetaminophen to minimize signs and symptoms.
• Monitor patient for CNS adverse reactions, such as decreased mental status and dizziness, during therapy.
• Depression and suicidal behavior have been linked to treatment.
• Monitor CBC with differential, platelet count, blood chemistry and electrolyte studies, and liver function tests. If patient has cardiac disorder or advanced stages of cancer, monitor ECG.
• For patients who develop thrombocytopenia, exercise extreme care in performing invasive procedures; inspect injection site and skin frequently for bruising; limit

---

Reactions may be *common,* uncommon, *life-threatening,* or COMMON AND LIFE-THREATENING.

frequency of I.M. injections; test urine, emesis fluid, stool, and secretions for occult blood.
• *Alert:* Different brands of interferon may not be equivalent and may need different dosages.
• Severe adverse reactions may need dosage reduction to one-half or discontinuation of drug until reactions subside.
• Use with blood dyscrasia-causing drugs, bone marrow suppressant, or radiation therapy may increase bone marrow suppression. Dosage may need to be reduced.
• Keep drug refrigerated. Don't freeze.

## PATIENT TEACHING
• Advise patient that laboratory tests will be performed before and periodically during therapy.
• Teach patient proper oral hygiene during treatment because the bone marrow suppressant effects of interferon may lead to microbial infection, delayed healing, and bleeding gums. Drug also may decrease salivary flow.
• Stress need to follow prescriber's instructions about taking and recording temperature and how and when to take acetaminophen.
• Advise patient to check with prescriber for instructions after missing dose.
• Tell patient that drug may cause temporary partial hair loss; hair should return when drug is withdrawn.
• If patient will be giving drug to himself, teach him how to prepare and give it and how to dispose of used needles, syringes, containers, and unused drug.
• Instruct patient not to take aspirin or alcohol because use together increases risk of GI bleeding.
• Instruct patient not to change brands of interferon without medical consultation.
• Warn patient against performing tasks that require mental alertness.
• Advise patient to immediately report signs and symptoms of depression.

# interferon alfa-2b, recombinant (IFN-alpha 2)
Intron A

*Pregnancy risk category C*

## AVAILABLE FORMS
*Injection:* 3, 5 million IU/0.5-ml vial; 1, 10 million IU/1-ml vial; 18 million IU/3.8-ml vial; 25 million IU/3.2-ml vial
*Powder for injection:* 3, 5, 10, 18, 25, 50 million IU/vial with diluent

## INDICATIONS & DOSAGES
➤ **Hairy cell leukemia**
*Adults:* 2 million IU/m² I.M. or S.C., three times weekly for 6 months or more.
➤ **Condylomata acuminata (genital or venereal warts)**
*Adults:* 1 million IU for each lesion intralesionally three times weekly for 3 weeks.
➤ **AIDS-related Kaposi's sarcoma**
*Adults:* 30 million IU/m² S.C. or I.M. three times weekly. Maintain dose unless disease progresses rapidly or intolerance occurs.
➤ **Chronic hepatitis B**
*Adults:* 30 to 35 million IU weekly I.M. or S.C., given as 5 million IU daily or 10 million IU three times weekly for 16 weeks.
*Children ages 1 to 17:* 3 million IU/m² S.C. three times weekly for first week; then increase to 6 million IU/m² S.C. three times weekly (maximum is 10 million IU three times weekly) for total of 16 to 24 weeks.
➤ **Chronic hepatitis C**
*Adults:* 3 million IU I.M. or S.C. three times weekly. In patients tolerating therapy with normalization of ALT at 16 weeks of therapy, continue for 18 to 24 months. In patients who haven't normalized the ALT, consider stopping therapy.
➤ **Adjunct to surgical treatment in patients with malignant melanoma who are asymptomatic after surgery but at high risk for systemic recurrence for up to 8 weeks after surgery**
*Adults:* Initially, 20 million IU/m² by I.V. infusion 5 consecutive days weekly for 4 weeks; then maintenance dose of 10 million IU/m² S.C. three times weekly for

48 weeks. If adverse effects occur, stop therapy until they abate, then resume therapy at 50% of the previous dose. If intolerance persists, stop therapy.

➤ **First treatment of clinically aggressive follicular non-Hodgkin's lymphoma in conjunction with chemotherapy containing anthracycline**

*Adults:* 5 million IU S.C. three times weekly for up to 18 months.

## I.V. ADMINISTRATION

● Prepare infusion solution immediately before use.

● Based on desired dose, reconstitute appropriate vial strength of drug with diluent provided. Withdraw dose and inject into a 100-ml bag of normal saline solution. Final yield of drug shouldn't be less than 10 million IU/100 ml.

● Infuse over 20 minutes.

## ACTION

Unknown. Appears to involve direct antiproliferative action against tumor or viral cells to inhibit replication and modulation of host immune response by enhancing phagocytic activity of macrophages and augmenting specific cytotoxicity of lymphocytes for target cells.

| Route | Onset | Peak | Duration |
|---|---|---|---|
| I.M., S.C. | Unknown | 3-12 hr | 16 hr |
| I.V. | Unknown | 15-60 min | 4 hr |

## ADVERSE REACTIONS

**CNS:** *dizziness, confusion, paresthesia,* lethargy, *depression, difficulty in thinking or concentrating, insomnia,* anxiety, *fatigue, hypoesthesia, amnesia,* nervousness, *somnolence,* weakness, *malaise, asthenia,* **suicidal ideation.**
**CV:** hypotension, *chest pain,* flushing, tachycardia, **bradycardia,** angina, **arrhythmia, cardiac failure,** hypertension, angina.
**EENT:** visual disturbances, hearing disorders, pharyngitis, *nasal congestion, sinusitis,* rhinitis, stye.
**GI:** *anorexia, nausea, diarrhea, vomiting,* abdominal pain, *dyspepsia,* constipation, loose stools, eructation, *dry mouth,* dysgeusia, stomatitis, gingivitis.
**GU:** transient impotence.

**Hematologic:** *leukopenia; thrombocytopenia;* anemia.
**Metabolic:** hypercalcemia, hyperphosphatemia.
**Musculoskeletal:** *arthralgia, back pain.*
**Respiratory:** *dyspnea, coughing,* **pulmonary embolism.**
**Skin:** *rash, dryness, pruritus, alopecia,* candidiasis, dermatitis, *increased diaphoresis.*
**Other:** *flulike syndrome, rigors,* gynecomastia.

## INTERACTIONS

**Drug-drug.** *Aminophylline, theophylline:* May reduce theophylline clearance. Monitor theophylline level.
*CNS depressants:* May increase CNS effects. Avoid using together.
*Live-virus vaccines:* May increase adverse reactions to vaccine or decrease antibody response. Postpone immunization.
*Zidovudine:* May cause synergistic adverse effects (higher risk of neutropenia). Carefully monitor WBC count.

## EFFECTS ON LAB TEST RESULTS

● May increase calcium, phosphate, AST, ALT, LDH, alkaline phosphatase, and fasting glucose levels.
● May increase PT, INR, and PTT. May decrease hemoglobin and WBC and platelet counts.

## CONTRAINDICATIONS & CAUTIONS

● Contraindicated in patients hypersensitive to drug or its components.
● Use cautiously in patients with history of CV disease, pulmonary disease, diabetes mellitus, coagulation disorders, and severe myelosuppression.
● Depression and suicidal behavior have been linked to drug use; patients with psychotic disorders, especially depression, shouldn't continue drug treatment.
● *Alert:* Neurotoxicity and cardiotoxicity are more common in elderly patients, especially those with underlying CNS or cardiac impairment.

## NURSING CONSIDERATIONS

● *Alert:* Alpha interferons cause or aggravate fatal or life-threatening neuropsychiatric, autoimmune, ischemic, and infectious disorders. Monitor patients closely

---

Reactions may be *common,* uncommon, *life-threatening,* or **COMMON AND LIFE-THREATENING.**

with periodic clinical and laboratory evaluations. Withdraw patients with persistently severe or worsening signs or symptoms
of these conditions from therapy.
• Use S.C. administration route in
patients whose platelet count is below
50,000/mm³.
• Give drug at bedtime to minimize daytime drowsiness.
• When giving interferon for condylomata
acuminata, use only 10 million-IU vial
because dilution of other strengths needed
for intralesional use results in a hypertonic
solution. Don't reconstitute drug in 10
million-IU vial with more than 1 ml of
diluent. Use tuberculin or similar syringe
and 25G to 30G needle. Don't inject too
deeply beneath lesion or too superficially.
As many as five lesions can be treated at
one time. To ease discomfort, give in
evening with acetaminophen.
• Ensure patient is well hydrated, especially at beginning of treatment.
• At start of treatment, monitor patient for
flulike signs and symptoms, which tend to
diminish with continued therapy. Premedicate patient with acetaminophen to minimize these symptoms.
• Periodically check for adverse CNS reactions, such as decreased mental status
and dizziness, during therapy.
• Monitor CBC with differential, platelet
count, blood chemistry and electrolyte
studies, and liver function tests. Monitor
ECG if patient has cardiac disorder or advanced stages of cancer.
• For patients who develop thrombocytopenia, exercise extreme care in performing invasive procedures; inspect injection
site and skin frequently for signs and
symptoms of bruising; limit frequency of
I.M. injections; test urine, emesis fluid,
stool, and secretions for occult blood.
• Severe adverse reactions may need
dosage reduction to one-half or discontinuation of drug until reactions subside.
• Use with blood dyscrasia-causing drugs,
bone marrow suppressants, or radiation
therapy may increase bone marrow suppression. Dosage reduction may be
needed.
• In treatment of condylomata acuminata,
maximum response usually occurs 4 to
8 weeks after therapy starts. If results
aren't satisfactory after 12 to 16 weeks, a

second course may be instituted. Patients
with 6 to 10 condylomata may receive a
second course of treatment; patients with
more than 10 condylomata may receive
additional courses.

**PATIENT TEACHING**
• Advise patient to avoid contact with persons with viral illness; patient is at increased risk for infection during therapy.
• Advise patient that laboratory tests will
be performed before and periodically during therapy.
• Teach patient proper oral hygiene during
treatment because bone marrow suppressant effects of interferon may lead to microbial infection, delayed healing, and
bleeding gums. Drug also may decrease
salivary flow.
• Advise patient to check with prescriber
for instructions after missing a dose.
• Stress need to follow prescriber's instructions about taking and recording temperature and how and when to take acetaminophen.
• If patient will give drug to himself, teach
him how to prepare injection and use disposable syringe. Give him information on
drug stability.
• Tell patient that drug may cause temporary partial hair loss; hair should return after drug is withdrawn.
• Advise patient to notify prescriber if
signs or symptoms of depression occur.

---

## interferon beta-1a
Avonex, Rebif

*Pregnancy risk category C*

**AVAILABLE FORMS**
**Avonex**
*Lyophilized powder for injection:* 33 mcg
(6.6 million IU)
*Prefilled syringe:* 30 mcg
**Rebif**
*Parenteral:* 22 mcg (6 million IU) and
44 mcg (12 million IU) per 0.5-ml pre-
filled syringe

**INDICATIONS & DOSAGES**
➤ **Slow accumulation of physical disability and decrease frequency of clini-**

---

*Rapid onset   †Canada   ‡Australia   ◇OTC   ◆Off-label use   ⦿Photoguide   *Liquid contains alcohol.*

cal worsening in patients with relapsing forms of multiple sclerosis (MS)

*Adults age 18 and older:* 30 mcg Avonex I.M. once weekly. Or, initially, 8.8 mcg Rebif S.C. three times weekly for 2 weeks, then increase dose to 22 mcg three times weekly for another 2 weeks. Then increase to a maintenance dose of 44 mcg S.C. three times weekly.

*Adjust-a-dose:* For Rebif, in patients with leukopenia or elevated liver function test values (ALT greater than five times upper limit of normal), reduce dosage by 20% to 50% until toxicity is resolved. Stop treatment if jaundice or other signs of hepatic injury occur.

✳ *NEW INDICATION:* **First MS attack if brain magnetic resonance imaging shows abnormalities consistent with MS**
*Adults:* 30 mcg I.M. once weekly (Avonex).

## ACTION

Exact mechanism unknown. Interacts with specific cell receptors found on the surface of human cells. Binding of these receptors induces the expression of a number of interferon-induced gene products believed to mediate the biological actions of interferon beta-1a.

| Route | Onset | Peak | Duration |
|-------|-------|------|----------|
| I.M. | Unknown | 3-15 hr | Unknown |

## ADVERSE REACTIONS

**CNS:** *headache, sleep difficulty, dizziness, fever,* syncope, **suicidal tendency, depression, suicidal ideation or attempt,** *fatigue,* hypertonia, abnormal coordination, **seizures,** speech disorder, ataxia, *asthenia,* malaise.
**CV:** chest pain, vasodilation.
**EENT:** *abnormal vision,* otitis media, decreased hearing, *sinusitis.*
**GI:** *nausea, diarrhea, dyspepsia,* anorexia, *abdominal pain,* dry mouth.
**GU:** ovarian cyst, vaginitis, increased urinary frequency, urinary incontinence.
**Hematologic:** anemia, *leukopenia, lymphadenopathy, thrombocytopenia, pancytopenia.*
**Hepatic:** abnormal hepatic function, bilirubinemia, autoimmune hepatitis, hepatic injury, *hepatitis.*

**Metabolic:** hyperthyroidism, hypothyroidism.
**Musculoskeletal:** *muscle ache,* muscle spasm, arthralgia, *back pain, skeletal pain.*
**Respiratory:** *upper respiratory tract infection,* dyspnea.
**Skin:** ecchymosis at injection site, *injection site reaction,* urticaria, alopecia, nevus.
**Other:** *flulike syndrome, pain, chills, infection,* herpes zoster, herpes simplex, neutralizing antibodies, **hypersensitivity reactions.**

## INTERACTIONS

**Drug-lifestyle.** *Sun exposure:* May cause photosensitivity reactions. Advise patient to take precautions against sun exposure.

## EFFECTS ON LAB TEST RESULTS

• May increase liver function enzyme level. May increase or decrease thyroid function test levels.
• May increase eosinophil count. May decrease hemoglobin, hematocrit, and WBC and platelet counts.

## CONTRAINDICATIONS & CAUTIONS

• Contraindicated in patients hypersensitive to natural or recombinant interferon beta, human albumin, or other components of drug.
• Use cautiously in patients with depression, seizure disorders, or severe cardiac conditions.
• It's unknown if drug appears in breast milk; a breast-feeding woman must either stop breast-feeding or stop drug.
• Safety and effectiveness of drug in chronic progressive multiple sclerosis or in children younger than age 18 haven't been established.

## NURSING CONSIDERATIONS

• Monitor patient closely for depression and suicidal ideation. It isn't known if these symptoms are related to the underlying neurologic basis of multiple sclerosis or to interferon beta-1a.
• Monitor WBC count, platelet count, and blood chemistries, including liver function tests.
• To reconstitute drug, inject 1.1 ml of supplied diluent (sterile water for injec-

tion) into vial and gently swirl to dissolve drug. Don't shake.

• Use drug as soon as possible but may be used within 6 hours after being reconstituted if stored at 36° to 46° F (2° to 8° C).

• Rotate sites of injection.

• After administration of each dose, discard any remaining product in the syringe.

• Give analgesics or antipyretics to decrease flulike symptoms.

• Store Rebif in the refrigerator between 36° to 46° F (2° to 8° C). Don't freeze. Rebif may also be stored at or below 77° F (25° C) for up to 30 days and away from heat and light.

• Store Avonex prefilled syringes in the refrigerator at 36° to 46° F (2° to 8° C). Once removed from refrigerator, warm to room temperature (about 30 minutes) and use within 12 hours. Don't use external heat sources such as hot water to warm syringe, or expose to high temperatures. Don't freeze. Protect from light.

## PATIENT TEACHING

• Teach patient and family member how to reconstitute drug and give I.M.

• Caution patient not to change dosage or schedule of administration. If a dose is missed, tell him to take it as soon as he remembers. The regular schedule may then be resumed. Don't give two injections within 2 days of each other.

• Show patient how to store drug.

• Inform patient that flulike signs and symptoms, such as fever, fatigue, muscle aches, headache, chills, and joint pain, aren't uncommon at start of therapy. Acetaminophen 650 mg P.O. may be taken immediately before injection and for another 24 hours after each injection, to lessen severity of flulike signs and symptoms.

• Advise patient to report depression, suicidal thoughts, or other adverse reactions.

• Instruct patient to keep syringes and needles away from children. Also, instruct him not to reuse needles or syringes and to discard them in a syringe-disposal unit.

• Caution woman of childbearing age not to become pregnant during therapy because of the risk of spontaneous abortion. If pregnancy occurs, instruct patient to notify prescriber immediately and to stop drug.

• Advise patient to use sunscreen and avoid sun exposure while taking drug because photosensitivity may occur.

• Tell patient to store Rebif in the refrigerator between 36° to 46° F (2° to 8° C). Don't freeze. Rebif may also be stored at or below 77° F (25° C) for up to 30 days and away from heat and light.

## interferon beta-1b, recombinant
Betaseron

*Pregnancy risk category C*

### AVAILABLE FORMS
*Powder for injection:* 9.6 million IU (0.3 mg)

### INDICATIONS & DOSAGES
➤ **Reduce frequency of worsening in patients with relapsing-remitting multiple sclerosis**
*Adults:* 8 million IU (0.25 mg) S.C. every other day.

### ACTION
A naturally occurring antiviral and immunoregulatory drug derived from human fibroblasts. Attaches to membrane receptors and causes cellular changes, including increased protein synthesis.

| Route | Onset | Peak | Duration |
|-------|-------|------|----------|
| S.C. | Unknown | 1-8 hr | Unknown |

### ADVERSE REACTIONS
**CNS:** depression, anxiety, emotional lability, depersonalization, *suicidal tendencies,* confusion, somnolence, *hypertonia, asthenia, migraine, seizures, headache,* dizziness.

**CV:** palpitations, hypertension, tachycardia, peripheral vascular disorder, *hemorrhage.*

**EENT:** laryngitis, *sinusitis, conjunctivitis,* abnormal vision.

**GI:** *diarrhea, constipation, abdominal pain, vomiting.*

**GU:** *menstrual bleeding or spotting, early or delayed menses, fewer days of menstrual flow, menorrhagia.*

**Musculoskeletal:** *myasthenia.*

**Respiratory:** dyspnea.

**Skin:** *inflammation, pain, necrosis at injection site, diaphoresis,* alopecia.
**Other:** breast pain, *flulike syndrome, pelvic pain, lymphadenopathy, pain,* generalized edema.

## INTERACTIONS
None significant.

## EFFECTS ON LAB TEST RESULTS
• May increase ALT and bilirubin levels.
• May decrease WBC and neutrophil counts.

## CONTRAINDICATIONS & CAUTIONS
• Contraindicated in patients hypersensitive to interferon beta, human albumin, or components of drug.
• Use cautiously in women of childbearing age. Evidence is inconclusive about teratogenic effects, but drug may be an abortifacient.

## NURSING CONSIDERATIONS
• To reconstitute, inject 1.2 ml of supplied diluent (half normal saline solution for injection) into vial and gently swirl to dissolve drug. Don't shake. Reconstituted solution will contain 8 million IU (0.25 mg)/ ml. Discard vial that contains particulates or discolored solution.
• Inject immediately after preparation.
• New formulation is stored at room temperature. After reconstitution, if not used immediately, drug may be refrigerated for up to 3 hours.
• Rotate injection sites to minimize local reactions and observe site for necrosis.
• Monitor patient for signs of depression.

## PATIENT TEACHING
• Warn woman of childbearing age about dangers to fetus. If pregnancy occurs during therapy, tell her to notify prescriber and stop taking drug.
• Teach patient how to perform S.C. injections, including solution preparation, aseptic technique, injection site rotation, and equipment disposal. Periodically reevaluate patient's technique.
• Tell patient to take drug at bedtime to minimize mild flulike signs and symptoms that commonly occur.
• Advise patient to report suicidal thoughts or depression.

• Urge patient to immediately report signs or symptoms of tissue death at injection site.

# interferon gamma-1b
Actimmune

*Pregnancy risk category C*

## AVAILABLE FORMS
*Injection:* 100 mcg (2 million IU)/0.5-ml vial

## INDICATIONS & DOSAGES
➤ **Chronic granulomatous disease, severe malignant osteopetrosis**
*Adults with body surface area (BSA) greater than 0.5 m²:* 50 mcg/m² (1 million IU/m²) S.C. three times weekly, preferably h.s., in deltoid or anterior thigh muscle.
*Adults with a BSA 0.5 m² or less:* 1.5 mcg/ kg S.C. three times weekly.

## ACTION
Interleukin-type lymphokine. Has potent phagocyte-activating properties and increases the oxidative metabolism of tissue macrophages.

| Route | Onset | Peak | Duration |
|-------|-------|------|----------|
| S.C. | Unknown | 7 hr | Unknown |

## ADVERSE REACTIONS
**CNS:** *fatigue,* decreased mental status, gait disturbance, dizziness.
**GI:** *nausea, vomiting, diarrhea,* abdominal pain.
**GU:** proteinuria.
**Hematologic:** *neutropenia, thrombocytopenia.*
**Metabolic:** weight loss.
**Musculoskeletal:** back pain.
**Skin:** *erythema and tenderness at injection site, rash.*
**Other:** *flulike syndrome.*

## INTERACTIONS
**Drug-drug.** *Myelosuppressives:* May increase myelosuppression. Monitor patient closely.
*Zidovudine:* May increase levels of zidovudine. Adjust dosage when used together.

## EFFECTS ON LAB TEST RESULTS
• May increase liver enzyme level.
• May decrease neutrophil and platelet counts.

## CONTRAINDICATIONS & CAUTIONS
• Contraindicated in patients hypersensitive to drug or to genetically engineered products derived from *Escherichia coli*.
• Use cautiously in patients with cardiac disease, including arrhythmias, ischemia, or heart failure. The flulike syndrome commonly seen with high doses of drug can worsen these conditions.
• Use cautiously in patients with compromised CNS function or seizure disorders. CNS adverse reactions that may occur at high doses of drug can worsen these conditions.

## NURSING CONSIDERATIONS
• *Alert:* The drug's activity is expressed in international units (1 million IU/50 mcg). This is equal to what was previously expressed as units (1.5 million U/50 mcg).
• Use myelosuppressives together with caution.
• Premedicate patient with acetaminophen to minimize signs and symptoms at start of therapy; these tend to diminish with continued therapy.
• Before beginning therapy and at 3-month intervals, monitor CBC, platelets, renal and hepatic function tests, and urinalysis.
• Discard unused drug. Each vial is for single-dose use only and doesn't contain a preservative.

## PATIENT TEACHING
• If patient will give drug to himself, teach him how to give it and how to dispose of used needles, syringes, containers, and unused drug.
• Instruct patient how to manage flulike signs and symptoms (fever, fatigue, muscle aches, headache, chills, joint pain) that commonly occur.
• Advise use of acetaminophen.

# leflunomide
Arava

*Pregnancy risk category X*

## AVAILABLE FORMS
*Tablets:* 10 mg, 20 mg, 100 mg

## INDICATIONS & DOSAGES
➤ **In patients with active rheumatoid arthritis, to reduce signs and symptoms and to slow structural damage as shown by erosions and joint space narrowing on radiograph**
*Adults:* 100 mg P.O. q 24 hours for 3 days; then 20 mg (maximum daily dose) P.O. q 24 hours. Dose may be decreased to 10 mg daily if higher dose isn't well tolerated.

## ACTION
An immunomodulatory drug that inhibits dihydroorotate dehydrogenase, an enzyme involved in pyrimidine synthesis, and that has antiproliferative activity and anti-inflammatory effects.

| Route | Onset | Peak | Duration |
|-------|-------|------|----------|
| P.O. | Unknown | 6-12 hr | Unknown |

## ADVERSE REACTIONS
**CNS:** asthenia, dizziness, fever, headache, paresthesia, malaise, migraine, sleep disorder, vertigo, neuritis, anxiety, depression, insomnia, neuralgia.
**CV:** angina pectoris, *hypertension,* chest pain, palpitations, tachycardia, vasculitis, vasodilation, varicose veins, peripheral edema.
**EENT:** pharyngitis, rhinitis, sinusitis, epistaxis, blurred vision, cataracts, conjunctivitis, eye disorder.
**GI:** mouth ulcer, oral candidiasis, gingivitis, enlarged salivary glands, stomatitis, dry mouth, taste perversion, anorexia, *diarrhea,* dyspepsia, gastroenteritis, nausea, abdominal pain, vomiting, cholelithiasis, colitis, constipation, esophagitis, flatulence, gastritis, melena.
**GU:** UTI, albuminuria, cystitis, dysuria, hematuria, menstrual disorder, pelvic pain, vaginal candidiasis, prostate disorder, urinary frequency.
**Hematologic:** anemia.

**Hepatic:** *hepatotoxicity.*
**Metabolic:** diabetes mellitus, hyperglycemia, hyperthyroidism, hypokalemia, hyperlipidemia, weight loss.
**Musculoskeletal:** arthralgia, arthrosis, back pain, bursitis, muscle cramps, myalgia, bone necrosis, bone pain, leg cramps, joint disorder, neck pain, synovitis, tendon rupture, tenosynovitis.
**Respiratory:** bronchitis, increased cough, pneumonia, *respiratory infection,* asthma, dyspnea, lung disorder.
**Skin:** *alopecia,* eczema, pruritus, *rash,* dry skin, acne, contact dermatitis, fungal dermatitis, hair discoloration, hematoma, nail disorder, skin nodule, subcutaneous nodule, maculopapular rash, skin disorder, skin discoloration, skin ulcer.
**Other:** tooth disorder, allergic reaction, flulike syndrome, injury or accident, pain, abscess, cyst, hernia, increased sweating, ecchymoses, herpes simplex, herpes zoster.

**INTERACTIONS**
**Drug-drug.** *Charcoal, cholestyramine:* May decrease leflunomide levels. Sometimes used for this effect in overdose.
*Methotrexate, other hepatotoxic drugs:* May increase risk of hepatotoxicity. Monitor liver enzymes.
*NSAIDs (diclofenac, ibuprofen):* May increase levels of NSAIDs. Clinical significance is unknown.
*Rifampin:* May increase active leflunomide metabolite level. Use together cautiously.
*Tolbutamide:* May increase tolbutamide level. Clinical significance is unknown.

**EFFECTS ON LAB TEST RESULTS**
● May increase AST, ALT, glucose, lipid, and CK levels. May decrease potassium level.

**CONTRAINDICATIONS & CAUTIONS**
● Contraindicated in patients hypersensitive to drug or its components and in women who are or may become pregnant or who are breast-feeding.
● Drug isn't recommended for patients with hepatic insufficiency, hepatitis B or C, severe immunodeficiency, bone marrow dysplasia, or severe uncontrolled infec-

tions; in patients younger than age 18; or in men attempting to father a child.
● Use cautiously in patients with renal insufficiency.

**NURSING CONSIDERATIONS**
● Vaccination with live vaccines isn't recommended. Consider the long half-life of drug when contemplating administration of a live vaccine after stopping drug treatment.
● *Alert:* Men planning to father a child should stop drug therapy and follow recommended leflunomide removal protocol (cholestyramine 8 g, P.O. t.i.d. for 11 days). In addition to cholestyramine, verify drug levels are less than 0.02 mg/L by two separate tests at least 14 days apart. If level is greater than 0.02 mg/L, consider additional cholestyramine treatment.
● Risk of malignancy, particularly lymphoproliferative disorders, is increased with use of some immunosuppressants, including leflunomide.
● Monitor liver enzyme levels (ALT and AST) before starting therapy and monthly thereafter until stable. Frequency can then be decreased based on clinical situation.

**PATIENT TEACHING**
● Explain need and frequency of required blood tests and monitoring.
● Instruct patient to use birth control during course of treatment and until it has been determined that drug is no longer active.
● Warn patient to immediately notify prescriber if signs or symptoms of pregnancy occur (such as late menstrual periods or breast tenderness).
● Advise breast-feeding woman to stop breast-feeding during therapy.
● Inform patient that aspirin, other NSAIDs, and low-dose corticosteroids may be continued during treatment.

---

**oprelvekin**
Neumega

*Pregnancy risk category C*

**AVAILABLE FORMS**
*Injection:* 5-mg single-dose vial with diluent

## INDICATIONS & DOSAGES
➤ **To prevent severe thrombocytopenia and reduce need for platelet transfusions after myelosuppressive chemotherapy with nonmyeloid malignancies**
*Adults:* 50 mcg/kg as single daily S.C. injection until post-nadir platelet count is ≥ 50,000 cells/mm³. Treatment beyond 21 days per course isn't recommended.

## ACTION
A thrombopoietic growth factor that directly stimulates proliferation of hematopoietic stem cells and megakaryocyte progenitor cells. Also induces megakaryocyte maturation, resulting in increased platelet production.

| Route | Onset | Peak | Duration |
|-------|-------|------|----------|
| S.C. | Unknown | 3-5 hr | Unknown |

## ADVERSE REACTIONS
**CNS:** *asthenia, headache, insomnia, dizziness,* paresthesia, *syncope.*
**CV:** *tachycardia, palpitations,* ATRIAL FLUTTER OR FIBRILLATION, *edema.*
**EENT:** blurred vision, *conjunctival injection,* eye hemorrhage, pharyngitis.
**GI:** *oral candidiasis, nausea, vomiting, diarrhea.*
**Hematologic:** anemia.
**Metabolic:** dehydration, hypocalcemia.
**Respiratory:** dyspnea, cough, pleural effusions.
**Skin:** *rash,* skin discoloration, exfoliative dermatitis.

## INTERACTIONS
**Drug-drug.** *Diuretics, ifosfamide:* May cause severe hypokalemia resulting in death in patients receiving these drugs together with oprelvekin. Use with extreme caution.

## EFFECTS ON LAB TEST RESULTS
• May decrease calcium level.
• May decrease hemoglobin and hematocrit.

## CONTRAINDICATIONS & CAUTIONS
• Contraindicated in patients hypersensitive to drug or its components.
• Use drug cautiously in patients with heart failure because of fluid retention.

## NURSING CONSIDERATIONS
• Give S.C. in the abdomen, thigh, hip, or upper arm. Don't inject I.D. or intravascularly.
• Dosing should begin 6 to 24 hours after completion of chemotherapy and end at least 2 days before starting next planned cycle of chemotherapy.
• Reconstitute each single-dose vial with 1 ml of supplied diluent. Avoid excessive or vigorous agitation. Discard unused portions.
• Use reconstituted drug within 3 hours.
• Store drug and diluent in refrigerator until ready to use. Don't freeze.
• Closely monitor fluid and electrolyte status in patients receiving long-term diuretic therapy.
• Obtain a CBC before chemotherapy and at regular intervals during drug therapy.
• Fluid retention can be severe; monitor patient closely.

## PATIENT TEACHING
• Instruct patient about appropriate preparation and administration of drug if he is to self-administer at home.
• Warn patient about potential adverse reactions. Tell him to report any occurrence.
• Tell patient to keep drug refrigerated and not to reconstitute until just before use.
• Urge patient to call prescriber immediately if swelling, rapid heart beat, or difficulty breathing occurs.
• Tell patient to report signs and symptoms of increased bleeding or bruising.

---

# pegfilgrastim
Neulasta

*Pregnancy risk category C*

## AVAILABLE FORMS
*Injection:* 6-mg/0.6-ml single-use, preservative-free, prefilled syringes

## INDICATIONS & DOSAGES
➤ **To reduce frequency of infection in patients with nonmyeloid malignancies receiving myelosuppressive anticancer drugs that may cause febrile neutropenia**
*Adults:* 6 mg S.C. once per chemotherapy cycle. Don't give in the period between

---

14 days before and 24 hours after administration of cytotoxic chemotherapy.

## ACTION

Binds cell receptors to stimulate proliferation, differentiation, commitment, and end-cell function of neutrophils. Pegfilgrastim and filgrastim have the same mechanism of action. Pegfilgrastim has a reduced renal clearance and a longer half-life than filgrastim.

| Route | Onset | Peak | Duration |
|-------|-------|------|----------|
| S.C. | Unknown | Unknown | Unknown |

## ADVERSE REACTIONS

**CNS:** *dizziness, headache, fatigue, insomnia, fever.*
**GI:** *nausea, diarrhea, vomiting, constipation, anorexia, taste perversion, dyspepsia, abdominal pain, stomatitis, mucositis.*
**Hematologic:** GRANULOCYTOPENIA, NEUTROPENIC FEVER.
**Musculoskeletal:** *skeletal pain, generalized weakness, arthralgia, myalgia, bone pain.*
**Respiratory:** *acute respiratory distress syndrome (ARDS).*
**Skin:** *alopecia.*
**Other:** *peripheral edema,* **splenic rupture.**

## INTERACTIONS

**Drug-drug.** *Lithium:* May increase the release of neutrophils. Monitor neutrophil counts closely.

## EFFECTS ON LAB TEST RESULTS

• May increase LDH, alkaline phosphatase, and uric acid levels.
• May decrease granulocyte count.

## CONTRAINDICATIONS & CAUTIONS

• Contraindicated in patients hypersensitive to *Escherichia coli*–derived proteins, filgrastim, or any component of the drug. Don't use for peripheral blood progenitor cell mobilization.
• Use cautiously in patients with sickle cell disease, those receiving chemotherapy causing delayed myelosuppression, or those receiving radiation therapy.

• Infants, children, and adolescents weighing less than 45 kg (99 lb) shouldn't receive the 6-mg single-use syringe dose. Safety and effectiveness in children haven't been established.

## NURSING CONSIDERATIONS

• **Alert:** Splenic rupture has occurred rarely with filgrastim use. Evaluate patient who experiences signs or symptoms of left upper abdominal or shoulder pain for an enlarged spleen or splenic rupture.
• Obtain CBC and platelet count before therapy.
• Monitor patient's hemoglobin, hematocrit, CBC, and platelet count, as well as LDH, alkaline phosphatase, and uric acid levels during therapy.
• Monitor patient for allergic-type reactions, including anaphylaxis, skin rash, and urticaria, which can occur with first or subsequent treatment.
• Evaluate patient with fever, lung infiltrates, or respiratory distress for ARDS. If ARDS develops, notify prescriber.
• Keep patient with sickle cell disease well hydrated, and monitor him for symptoms of sickle cell crisis.
• Pegfilgrastim may act as a growth factor for tumors.

## PATIENT TEACHING

• Inform patient of the potential side effects of the drug.
• Tell patient to report signs and symptoms of allergic reactions, left upper abdominal or shoulder pain, fever, or breathing problems.
• Tell patient with sickle cell disease to keep drinking fluids and report signs or symptoms of sickle cell crisis.
• Instruct patient or caregiver how to give drug if it's to be given at home.

# peginterferon alfa-2a
Pegasys

*Pregnancy risk category C*

## AVAILABLE FORMS

*Injection:* 180 mcg/1 ml single-dose vials

## INDICATIONS & DOSAGES
➤ **Chronic hepatitis C with compensated hepatic disease in patients not previously treated with interferon alfa**
*Adults:* 180 mcg S.C. in abdomen or thigh, once weekly for 48 weeks.
*Adjust-a-dose:* For patients who experience moderate adverse reactions, decrease dose to 135 mcg S.C. once a week; for severe adverse reactions, decrease to 90 mcg S.C. once a week.

For patients who experience hematologic reactions, if the neutrophil count is less than 750 cells/mm³, reduce dose to 135 mcg S.C. once a week; if the absolute neutrophil count (ANC) is less than 500 cells/mm³, stop drug until ANC exceeds 1,000 cells/mm³ and restart at 90 mcg S.C. once a week. If platelet count is less than 50,000 cells/mm³, reduce dose to 90 mcg S.C. once a week; stop drug if platelet count drops below 25,000 cells/mm³.

In patients with end-stage renal disease requiring hemodialysis, decrease dose to 135 mcg S.C. once a week. In patients with ALT increases above baseline, decrease dose to 90 mcg S.C. once a week.

## ACTION
Causes reversible decreases in leukocyte and platelet counts, partially through stimulation of production of effector proteins in vitro.

| Route | Onset | Peak | Duration |
|-------|-------|------|----------|
| S.C. | Unknown | 3-4 days | < 1 wk |

## ADVERSE REACTIONS
**CNS:** *fatigue,* asthenia, *headache, insomnia, dizziness,* concentration impairment, memory impairment, *depression, irritability,* anxiety.
**GI:** *nausea, diarrhea, abdominal pain,* vomiting, dry mouth, *anorexia.*
**Hematologic:** NEUTROPENIA, *thrombocytopenia.*
**Musculoskeletal:** *myalgia, arthralgia,* back pain.
**Skin:** *alopecia, pruritus,* increased sweating, dermatitis, rash.
**Other:** *pain, pyrexia, rigors, injection site reaction.*

## INTERACTIONS
**Drug-drug.** *Theophylline:* May increase theophylline level. Monitor theophylline level and adjust dosage as needed.

## EFFECTS ON LAB TEST RESULTS
• May increase ALT level.
• May decrease hemoglobin, hematocrit, ANC, and WBC and platelet counts. May increase or decrease thyroid function test values.

## CONTRAINDICATIONS & CAUTIONS
• Contraindicated in patients hypersensitive to interferon alfa-2a or any components of formulation. Contraindicated in patients with autoimmune hepatitis or decompensated liver disease before or during treatment with drug and in neonates and infants. Contraindicated in patients who have failed to respond to other alfa interferon treatments, in organ transplant recipients with hepatitis C, and in patients with hepatitis C who have been infected simultaneously with HIV or hepatitis B.
• Use cautiously in patients with a history of depression. Use cautiously in patients with baseline neutrophil counts less than 1,500 cells/mm³, baseline platelet counts less than 90,000 cells/mm³, or baseline hemoglobin less than 10 g/dl. Also use cautiously in patients with creatinine clearance less than 50 ml/minute. Use cautiously in patients with preexisting cardiac disease or hypertension, thyroid disease, autoimmune disorders, pulmonary disorders, colitis, pancreatitis, and ophthalmologic disorders. Use cautiously in elderly patients because they may be at increased risk for adverse reactions.
• **Alert:** Drug may cause an abortion in a pregnant woman. Use in pregnant patient only if benefit outweighs risk.

## NURSING CONSIDERATIONS
• Monitor patient for neuropsychiatric reactions, including depression and suicidal ideation. These symptoms may occur in patients without previous psychiatric illness. If severe depression occurs, stop drug and start psychiatric treatment.
• Obtain CBC before treatment and monitor counts routinely during therapy. Stop

drug in patients who develop severe decrease in neutrophil or platelet counts.
• Stop drug if uncontrollable thyroid disease, hyperglycemia, hypoglycemia, or diabetes mellitus occurs during treatment.
• If persistent or unexplained pulmonary infiltrates or pulmonary dysfunction occur, stop drug.
• Stop drug if signs and symptoms of colitis occur, such as abdominal pain, bloody diarrhea, and fever. Symptoms should resolve within 1 to 3 weeks.
• Stop drug if signs and symptoms of pancreatitis occur, including fever, malaise, and abdominal pain.
• Obtain baseline eye examination and periodically monitor eye exams during treatment. Stop drug if new or worsening eye disorders occur.
• Monitor patient with impaired renal function for interferon toxicity.
• Use in women of childbearing potential only when effective contraception is being used.

**PATIENT TEACHING**
• Teach patient proper way to give drug and dispose of needles and syringes.
• Tell patient to immediately report depression or suicidal ideation.
• Tell patient to report signs and symptoms of pancreatitis, colitis, eye disorders, or respiratory disorders.
• Advise patient to avoid driving or operating machinery if he feels dizzy, tired, confused, or sleepy.

---

**peginterferon alfa-2b**
PEG-Intron

*Pregnancy risk category C*

---

**AVAILABLE FORMS**
*Injection:* 100 mcg/ml, 160 mcg/ml, 240 mcg/ml, 300 mcg/ml

**INDICATIONS & DOSAGES**
➤ **Chronic hepatitis C in patients not previously treated with interferon alfa**
Give S.C. once weekly for 48 weeks on same day each week; first dose based on weight:

*Adults weighing 137 to 160 kg (302 to 353 lb):* 150 mcg (0.5 ml) of 300-mcg/ml strength.
*Adults weighing 107 to 136 kg (236 to 300 lb):* 120 mcg (0.5 ml) of 240-mcg/ml strength.
*Adults weighing 89 to 106 kg (196 to 234 lb):* 96 mcg (0.4 ml) of 240-mcg/ml strength.
*Adults weighing 73 to 88 kg (161 to 194 lb):* 80 mcg (0.5 ml) of 160-mcg/ml strength.
*Adults weighing 57 to 72 kg (126 to 159 lb):* 64 mcg (0.4 ml) of 160-mcg/ml strength.
*Adults weighing 46 to 56 kg (101 to 123 lb):* 50 mcg (0.5 ml) of 100-mcg/ml strength.
*Adults weighing 37 to 45 kg (82 to 99 lb):* 40 mcg (0.4 ml) of 100-mcg/ml strength.
✳ *NEW INDICATION:* **Chronic hepatitis C in patients not previously treated with interferon alfa, combined with ribavirin**
*Adults:* Give 1.5 mcg/kg S.C. once weekly for 48 weeks on same day q week; first dose based on weight:
*Adults weighing more than 85 kg (more than 187 lb):* 150 mcg (0.5 ml) of 300-mcg/ml strength.
*Adults weighing 76 to 85 kg (167 to 187 lb):* 120 mcg (0.5 ml) of 240 mcg-mcg/ml strength.
*Adults weighing 61 to 75 kg (134 to 165 lb):* 96 mcg (0.4 ml) of 240 mcg-mcg/ml strength.
*Adults weighing 51 to 60 kg (112 to 132 lb):* 80 mcg (0.5 ml) of 160-mcg/ml strength.
*Adults weighing 40 to 50 kg (88 to 110 lb):* 64 mcg (0.4 ml) of 160-mcg/ml strength.
*Adults weighing less than 40 kg (less than 88 lb):* 50 mcg (0.5 ml) of 100-mcg/ml strength.
*Adjust-a-dose:* Decrease peginterferon alfa-2 dose by 50% in patients with WBCs less than 1,500/mm³, neutrophils less than 750/mm³, or platelets less than 80,000/mm³. Oral ribavirin dose can be continued. If hemoglobin is less than 10 g/dl, reduce oral ribavirin dose by 200 mg. Stop both drugs if hemoglobin is less than 8.5 g/dl, WBCs less than 1,000/mm³, neutrophils less than

---

500/mm³, or platelets less than
50,000/mm³.

If patient develops mild depression,
continue peginterferon alfa-2b, but evaluate patient once weekly. If moderate depression, reduce peginterferon alfa-2b
dose by 50% for 4 to 8 weeks and evaluate
patient q week. If symptoms improve and
remain stable for 4 weeks, continue at
present dose or resume previous dose. If
severe depression, stop peginterferon
alfa-2b.

For patients with preexisting stable CV
disease, decrease peginterferon alfa-2b
dose by 50% and ribavirin dosage by
200 mg daily if hemoglobin drops more
than 2 g/dl in any 4-week period. Stop
both drugs if hemoglobin goes below
12 g/dl after 4 weeks of reduced dosages.

## ACTION
Binds to specific membrane receptors on
the cell surface, initiating induction of certain enzymes, suppression of cell proliferation, and immunomodulating activities
and inhibition of virus replication in virus-
infected cells. Increases levels of effector
proteins and body temperature, and decreases leukocyte and platelet counts.

| Route | Onset | Peak | Duration |
|-------|-------|------|----------|
| S.C. | Unknown | 15-44 hr | Unknown |

## ADVERSE REACTIONS
**CNS:** *dizziness,* hypertonia, *fever, depres-
sion, insomnia, anxiety, emotional lability,
irritability, headache, fatigue,* malaise,
**suicidal behavior.**
**CV:** flushing.
**EENT:** *pharyngitis,* sinusitis.
**GI:** *nausea, anorexia, diarrhea, abdomi-
nal pain,* vomiting, dyspepsia, right upper
quadrant pain.
**Hematologic:** *neutropenia, thrombocy-
topenia.*
**Hepatic:** hepatomegaly.
**Metabolic:** hypothyroidism, hyperthyroid-
ism, *weight loss.*
**Musculoskeletal:** *musculoskeletal pain.*
**Respiratory:** cough.
**Skin:** *alopecia, pruritus, dry skin, rash,
injection site inflammation or reaction, in-
creased sweating,* injection site pain.
**Other:** *viral infection, flulike symptoms,
rigors.*

## INTERACTIONS
None reported.

## EFFECTS ON LAB TEST RESULTS
• May increase ALT level. May increase
or decrease TSH level.
• May decrease neutrophil and platelet
counts.

## CONTRAINDICATIONS & CAUTIONS
• Contraindicated in patients hypersensitive to drug or any of its components, in
patients with autoimmune hepatitis or decompensated liver disease, in those with
diabetes or thyroid disorders that can't be
controlled with medication, in patients
who have failed to respond to other alfa
interferon treatment or have had an organ
transplant, and in those with HIV or hepatitis B virus (HBV).
• Use cautiously in patients with psychiatric disorders, diabetes mellitus, CV disease, creatinine clearance less than 50 ml/
minute, pulmonary infiltrates, pulmonary
function impairment, or autoimmune, ischemic, or infectious disorders.

## NURSING CONSIDERATIONS
• *Alert:* Alfa interferons cause or aggravate fatal or life-threatening neuropsychiatric, autoimmune, ischemic, and infectious disorders. Monitor patients closely
with periodic clinical and laboratory evaluations. Withdraw patient with persistently severe or worsening signs or symptoms
of these conditions from therapy. In many
but not all cases, these disorders resolve
after stopping PEG-Intron therapy.
• Drug may cause or aggravate hypothyroidism, hyperthyroidism, or diabetes.
• Perform ECG on patient with history of
MI or arrhythmias before starting drug.
• Start treatment in patient who is well hydrated.
• Monitor patient with history of MI or arrhythmias closely for hypotension, arrhythmias, tachycardia, cardiomyopathy,
and signs and symptoms of MI.
• Monitor patient for depression and other
mental health disorders. If symptoms are
severe, stop drug and refer patient for psychiatric care.
• Monitor patient for signs and symptoms
of colitis, such as abdominal pain, bloody
diarrhea, and fever. Stop drug if colitis oc-

curs. Symptoms should resolve within 1 to 3 weeks after stopping drug.

• Monitor patient for signs and symptoms of pancreatitis or hypersensitivity reactions, and stop drug if these occur.

• Monitor patient with pulmonary disease for dyspnea, pulmonary infiltrates, pneumonitis, and pneumonia.

• Have eye examination done in patient with diabetes or hypertension before starting drug. Retinal hemorrhages, cotton-wool spots, and retinal artery or vein obstruction may occur.

• Monitor patient with renal disease for signs and symptoms of toxicity.

• Monitor CBC count, platelets, and AST, ALT, bilirubin, and TSH levels before starting drug and periodically during treatment.

• Notify prescriber if severe neutropenia or thrombocytopenia occurs.

## PATIENT TEACHING

• Teach patient the appropriate use of the drug and the benefits and risks of treatment. Tell patient that adverse reactions may continue for several months after treatment is stopped.

• Tell patient to immediately report symptoms of depression or suicidal thoughts.

• Instruct patient on importance of proper disposal of needles and syringes and caution him against reuse of old needles and syringes.

• Tell patient that drug won't prevent transmission of hepatitis C virus (HCV) to others and may not cure hepatitis C or prevent cirrhosis, liver failure, or liver cancer that may result from HCV infection.

• Advise patient that laboratory tests are needed before starting therapy and periodically thereafter.

• Tell patient to take drug at bedtime and to use fever-reducing drugs to decrease risk of flulike signs and symptoms.

• Inform breast-feeding patient of the potential for adverse reactions in infants. Tell her to either stop using drug or stop breast-feeding.

# sargramostim (GM-CSF; granulocyte macrophage-colony stimulating factor)
Leukine

*Pregnancy risk category C*

## AVAILABLE FORMS
*Powder for injection:* 250 mcg, 500 mcg
*Solution:* 500 mcg/ml

## INDICATIONS & DOSAGES
➤ **Accelerate hematopoietic reconstitution after autologous bone marrow transplantation in patients with malignant lymphoma or acute lymphoblastic leukemia or during autologous bone marrow transplantation in patients with Hodgkin's disease**
*Adults:* 250 mcg/m$^2$ daily for 21 consecutive days given as 2-hour I.V. infusion beginning 2 to 4 hours after bone marrow transplantation.
➤ **Bone marrow transplantation failure or engraftment delay**
*Adults:* 250 mcg/m$^2$ daily for 14 days as 2-hour I.V. infusion. Dose may be repeated after 7 days of no therapy. If engraftment still hasn't occurred, a third course of 500 mcg/m$^2$ daily I.V. for 14 days may be attempted after another therapy-free 7 days.
*Adjust-a-dose:* Stimulation of marrow precursors may result in rapid rise of WBC count. If blast cells appear or increase to 10% or more of WBC count or if the underlying disease progresses, stop therapy. If absolute neutrophil count is above 20,000/mm$^3$ or if platelet count is above 50,000/mm$^3$, temporarily stop drug or reduce dose by 50%.

## I.V. ADMINISTRATION
• Reconstitute with 1 ml of sterile water for injection. Direct stream of sterile water against side of vial and gently swirl contents to minimize foaming. Avoid excessive or vigorous agitation or shaking.

• Dilute in normal saline solution. If drug yield is below 10 mcg/ml, add human albumin at final concentration of 0.1% to saline solution before adding sargramostim to prevent adsorption to components of the delivery system. To yield 0.1%

human albumin, add 1 mg human albumin/1 ml saline solution (dilute 1 ml of 5% human albumin in 50 ml of saline solution).
• Give as soon as possible after mixing and no later than 6 hours after reconstituting.
• Don't add other drugs to infusion solution or use in-line filter.

## ACTION
Drug induces cellular responses by binding to specific receptors on cell surfaces of target cells.

| Route | Onset | Peak | Duration |
|-------|-------|------|----------|
| I.V., S.C. | 15 min | 2-4 hr | Unknown |

## ADVERSE REACTIONS
**CNS:** *malaise, fever, CNS disorders, asthenia.*
**CV:** *blood dyscrasias, edema,* **supraventricular arrhythmias,** pericardial effusion.
**GI:** *nausea, vomiting, diarrhea, anorexia,* **hemorrhage,** *GI disorders, stomatitis.*
**GU:** *urinary tract disorder,* abnormal kidney function.
**Hepatic:** *liver damage.*
**Respiratory:** *dyspnea, lung disorders,* pleural effusion.
**Skin:** *alopecia, rash.*
**Other:** *mucous membrane disorder, peripheral edema,* SEPSIS.

## INTERACTIONS
**Drug-drug.** *Corticosteroids, lithium:* May increase myeloproliferative effects of sargramostim. Use cautiously together.

## EFFECTS ON LAB TEST RESULTS
• May increase BUN, creatinine, AST, ALT, alkaline phosphatase, bilirubin, glucose, and cholesterol levels. May decrease calcium and albumin levels.

## CONTRAINDICATIONS & CAUTIONS
• Contraindicated in patients hypersensitive to drug or its components or to yeast-derived products and in those with excessive leukemic myeloid blasts in bone marrow or peripheral blood.
• Use cautiously in patients with cardiac disease, hypoxia, fluid retention, pulmonary infiltrates, heart failure, or impaired

renal or hepatic function because these conditions may be worsened.

## NURSING CONSIDERATIONS
• Anticipate reducing dose by 50% or temporarily stopping drug if severe adverse reactions occur; notify prescriber. Therapy may be resumed when reactions abate. Transient rash and local reactions at injection site may occur.
• Don't give within 24 hours of last dose of chemotherapy or within 12 hours of last dose of radiotherapy because rapidly dividing progenitor cells may be sensitive to these cytotoxic therapies and drug would be ineffective.
• Monitor CBC with differential, including examination for presence of blast cells, biweekly.
• Drug accelerates myeloid recovery in patients receiving bone marrow that is either unpurged or purged by anti-B cell monoclonal antibodies more than in those who receive bone marrow that is chemically purged.
• Drug may produce a limited response in transplant patients who have received extensive radiotherapy or who have received other myelotoxic drugs.
• Drug can act as a growth factor for any tumor type, particularly myeloid malignant disease.

## PATIENT TEACHING
• Review administration schedule with patient and caregivers, and address their concerns.
• Urge patient to report adverse reactions promptly.

**ciprofloxacin hydrochloride**
**erythromycin**
**gatifloxacin**
**gentamicin sulfate**
**moxifloxacin hydrochloride**
**ofloxacin 0.3%**
**sulfacetamide sodium 1%**
**sulfacetamide sodium 10%**
**sulfacetamide sodium 15%**
**sulfacetamide sodium 30%**
**tobramycin**
**vidarabine**

## COMBINATION PRODUCTS

AK-POLY-BAC: polymyxin B sulfate 10,000 units and bacitracin zinc 500 units.

BLEPHAMIDE STERILE OPHTHALMIC OINTMENT: sulfacetamide sodium 10% and prednisolone acetate 0.2%.

AK-Spore Ophthalmic Ointment: polymyxin B sulfate 10,000 units, neomycin sulfate 3.5 mg, and bacitracin zinc 400 units/g.

AK-Spore Ophthalmic Solution: polymyxin B sulfate 10,000 units, neomycin sulfate 1.75 mg, and gramicidin 0.025 mg.

CETAPRED OINTMENT: sulfacetamide sodium 10% and prednisolone acetate 0.25%.

CORTISPORIN OPHTHALMIC OINTMENT: polymyxin B sulfate 10,000 units, bacitracin zinc 400 units, neomycin sulfate 0.35%, and hydrocortisone 1%.

CORTISPORIN OPHTHALMIC SUSPENSION: polymyxin B sulfate 10,000 units, neomycin sulfate 0.35%, and hydrocortisone 1%.

ISOPTO CETAPRED: sulfacetamide sodium 10% and prednisolone acetate 0.25%.

MAXITROL OINTMENT/OPHTHALMIC SUSPENSION: dexamethasone 0.1%, neomycin sulfate 0.35%, and polymyxin B sulfate 10,000 units.

METIMYD OPHTHALMIC OINTMENT/SUSPENSION: sulfacetamide sodium 10% and prednisolone acetate 0.5%.

NEOSPORIN OPHTHALMIC OINTMENT: polymyxin B sulfate 10,000 units, neomycin sulfate 3.5 mg, and bacitracin zinc 400 units/g.

NEOSPORIN OPHTHALMIC SOLUTION: polymyxin B sulfate 10,000 units, neomycin sulfate 1.75 mg, and gramicidin 0.025 mg.

POLYSPORIN OPHTHALMIC OINTMENT: polymyxin B sulfate 10,000 units and bacitracin zinc 500 units.

POLYTRIM OPHTHALMIC: trimethoprim sulfate 1 mg and polymyxin B sulfate 10,000 units/ml.

PRED-G S.O.P.: prednisolone acetate 0.6% and gentamicin sulfate equivalent to gentamicin base 0.3%.

Terak with Polymyxin B Sulfate Ophthalmic Ointment: polymyxin B sulfate 10,000 units and oxytetracycline hydrochloride 5 mg/g.

TOBRADEX: dexamethasone 0.1% and tobramycin 0.3%.

VASOCIDIN OPHTHALMIC OINTMENT: sulfacetamide sodium 10% and prednisolone acetate 0.5%.

VASOCIDIN OPHTHALMIC SOLUTION: sulfacetamide sodium 10% and prednisolone phosphate 0.25%.

VASOSULF: sulfacetamide sodium 15% and phenylephrine hydrochloride 0.125%.

---

## ciprofloxacin hydrochloride
Ciloxan

*Pregnancy risk category C*

### AVAILABLE FORMS
*Ophthalmic solution:* 0.3% (base) in 2.5-ml and 5-ml containers

### INDICATIONS & DOSAGES
➤ **Corneal ulcers caused by *Pseudomonas aeruginosa, Staphylococcus aureus, Staphylococcus epidermidis, Streptococcus pneumoniae,* and possibly *Serratia marcescens* and *Streptococcus viridans***
*Adults and children older than age 12:*
Two drops in affected eye q 15 minutes for first 6 hours; then 2 drops q 30 minutes for remainder of first day. On day 2, two drops hourly. On days 3 to 14, 2 drops q 4 hours.

---

➤ **Bacterial conjunctivitis caused by** *Haemophilus influenzae,* **S. aureus, S. epidermidis,** **and possibly** *S. pneumoniae*
*Adults and children older than age 12:*
One or 2 drops into conjunctival sac of affected eye q 2 hours while awake for first 2 days. Then, 1 or 2 drops q 4 hours while awake for next 5 days.

## ACTION
Inhibits bacterial DNA gyrase, an enzyme needed for bacterial replication.

| Route | Onset | Peak | Duration |
|---|---|---|---|
| Ophthalmic | Unknown | Unknown | Unknown |

## ADVERSE REACTIONS
**EENT:** *local burning or discomfort, white crystalline precipitate in superficial portion of corneal defect in patients with corneal ulcers,* margin crusting, crystals or scales, foreign body sensation, itching, conjunctival hyperemia, allergic reactions.
**GI:** bad or bitter taste in mouth.

## INTERACTIONS
None significant.

## EFFECTS ON LAB TEST RESULTS
None reported.

## CONTRAINDICATIONS & CAUTIONS
• Contraindicated in patients hypersensitive to ciprofloxacin or other fluoroquinolone antibiotics.
• It's unknown if drug appears in breast milk after application to eye; however, ciprofloxacin given systemically has appeared in breast milk. Use cautiously in breast-feeding women.

## NURSING CONSIDERATIONS
• *Alert:* Stop drug at first sign of hypersensitivity, such as rash, and notify prescriber. Serious hypersensitivity reactions, including anaphylaxis, may occur in patients receiving systemic fluoroquinolone therapy.
• A topical overdose may be flushed from eyes with warm tap water.
• If corneal epithelium is still compromised after 14 days of treatment, continue therapy.
• Institute appropriate therapy if superinfection occurs. Prolonged use may result

in overgrowth of nonsusceptible organisms, including fungi.
• *Alert:* Don't confuse Ciloxan with Cytoxan or cinoxacin.

## PATIENT TEACHING
• Tell patient to clean eye area of excessive discharge before instilling.
• Teach patient how to instill drops. Advise him to wash hands before and after using solution and not to touch tip of dropper to eye or surrounding tissues.
• Instruct patient to apply light finger pressure on lacrimal sac for 1 minute after drops are instilled.
• Advise patient that drug may cause temporary blurring of vision or stinging after administration. If these symptoms become pronounced or worsen, contact prescriber.
• Tell patient to avoid wearing contacts while treating bacterial conjunctivitis. If approved by prescriber, tell patient to wait at least 15 minutes after instilling drops before inserting contact lenses.
• Tell patient not to share drug, washcloths, or towels with family members and to notify prescriber if anyone develops same signs or symptoms.
• Stress importance of compliance with recommended therapy.

---

## erythromycin
## Ilotycin

*Pregnancy risk category B*

## AVAILABLE FORMS
*Ophthalmic ointment:* 0.5%

## INDICATIONS & DOSAGES
➤ **Acute and chronic conjunctivitis, other eye infections**
*Adults and children:* Apply a ribbon of ointment about 1 cm long directly to infected eye up to six times daily, depending on severity of infection.
➤ **Chlamydial ophthalmic infections (trachoma)**
*Adults and children:* Apply small amount to each eye b.i.d. for 2 months or b.i.d. on first 5 days of each month for 6 months.

➤ **To prevent ophthalmia neonatorum caused by *Neisseria gonorrhoeae* or *Chlamydia trachomatis***
*Neonates:* Apply a ribbon of ointment about 1 cm long in lower conjunctival sac of each eye shortly after birth.

## ACTION
Inhibits protein synthesis; usually bacteriostatic, but may be bactericidal in high concentrations or against highly susceptible organisms.

| Route | Onset | Peak | Duration |
|---|---|---|---|
| Ophthalmic | Unknown | Unknown | Unknown |

## ADVERSE REACTIONS
**EENT:** slowed corneal wound healing, blurred vision, itching and burning eyes.
**Skin:** urticaria, dermatitis.
**Other:** overgrowth of nonsusceptible organisms with long-term use.

## INTERACTIONS
None significant.

## EFFECTS ON LAB TEST RESULTS
• May interfere with fluorometric determinations of urinary catecholamines.

## CONTRAINDICATIONS & CAUTIONS
• Contraindicated in patients hypersensitive to drug.
• Use cautiously in breast-feeding women.

## NURSING CONSIDERATIONS
• To prevent ophthalmia neonatorum, apply ointment no later than 1 hour after birth. Drug is used in neonates born either vaginally or by cesarean section. Gently massage eyelids for 1 minute to spread ointment.
• Use drug only when sensitivity studies show it's effective against infecting organisms; don't use in infections of unknown cause.
• Store drug at room temperature in tightly closed, light-resistant container.

## PATIENT TEACHING
• Tell patient to clean eye area of excessive discharge before application.
• Teach patient how to apply drug. Advise him to wash hands before and after applying ointment, and warn him not to touch

tip of applicator to eye or surrounding tissue.
• Tell patient that vision may be blurred for a few minutes after applying ointment.
• Advise patient to watch for and report signs and symptoms of sensitivity (itching lids, redness, swelling, or constant burning).
• Tell patient not to share drug, washcloths, or towels with family members and to notify prescriber if anyone develops same signs or symptoms.
• Stress importance of compliance with recommended therapy.

✳ *NEW DRUG*

# gatifloxacin
Zymar

*Pregnancy risk category C*

## AVAILABLE FORMS
*Solution:* 0.3% in 2.5-ml and 5-ml bottles

## INDICATIONS & DOSAGES
➤ **Bacterial conjunctivitis**
*Adults and children age 1 and older:* Instill 1 drop into affected eye q 2 hours while patient is awake, up to eight times daily for 2 days. Then instill 1 drop up to q.i.d. for 5 more days.

## ACTION
Antibiotic. Inhibits DNA gyrase and topoisomerase, preventing cell replication and division.

| Route | Onset | Peak | Duration |
|---|---|---|---|
| Ophthalmic | Unknown | Unknown | Unknown |

## ADVERSE REACTIONS
**CNS:** headache.
**EENT:** chemosis, conjunctival hemorrhage, *conjunctival irritation,* discharge, dry eyes, eye irritation, eyelid edema, *increased lacrimation, keratitis,* pain, *papillary conjunctivitis,* red eyes, reduced visual acuity.
**GI:** taste disturbance.

## INTERACTIONS
None reported.

---

Reactions may be *common,* uncommon, *life-threatening,* or COMMON AND LIFE-THREATENING.

**EFFECTS ON LAB TEST RESULTS**
None reported.

**CONTRAINDICATIONS & CAUTIONS**
• Contraindicated in patients hypersensitive to drug, quinolones, or their components.
• Use cautiously in pregnant or breastfeeding women.

**NURSING CONSIDERATIONS**
• Don't inject solution subconjunctivally or into the anterior chamber of the eye.
• Systemic gatifloxacin has caused serious hypersensitivity reactions. If allergic reaction occurs, stop drug and treat symptoms.
• Monitor patient for superinfection.

**PATIENT TEACHING**
• Urge patient to immediately stop drug and seek medical treatment if evidence of a serious allergic reaction develops, such as itching, rash, swelling of the face or throat, or difficulty breathing.
• Tell patient not to wear contact lenses during treatment.
• Warn patient to avoid touching the applicator tip to anything, including eyes and fingers.
• Teach patient that prolonged use may encourage infections with nonsusceptible bacteria.

---

**gentamicin sulfate**
Garamycin, Genoptic, Gentacidin, Gentak

*Pregnancy risk category C*

**AVAILABLE FORMS**
*Ophthalmic ointment:* 0.3% (base)
*Ophthalmic solution:* 0.3% (base)

**INDICATIONS & DOSAGES**
➤ **External ocular infections (conjunctivitis, keratoconjunctivitis, corneal ulcers, blepharitis, blepharoconjunctivitis, meibomianitis, and dacryocystitis) caused by susceptible organisms, especially *Pseudomonas aeruginosa, Proteus, Klebsiella pneumoniae, Escherichia coli,* and other gram-negative organisms**
*Adults and children:* 1 to 2 drops in eye q 4 hours. In severe infections, up to 2 drops

q hour. Or, apply ointment to lower conjunctival sac b.i.d. or t.i.d.

**ACTION**
Unknown. Thought to inhibit protein synthesis; is usually bactericidal.

| Route | Onset | Peak | Duration |
|-------|-------|------|----------|
| Ophthalmic | Unknown | Unknown | Unknown |

**ADVERSE REACTIONS**
**EENT:** burning, stinging, or blurred vision with ointment, transient irritation from solution, conjunctival hyperemia.
**Other:** overgrowth of nonsusceptible organisms with long-term use.

**INTERACTIONS**
None significant.

**EFFECTS ON LAB TEST RESULTS**
None reported.

**CONTRAINDICATIONS & CAUTIONS**
• Contraindicated in patients hypersensitive to drug.
• Use cautiously in patients with history of sensitivity to aminoglycosides because cross-sensitivity may occur.

**NURSING CONSIDERATIONS**
• Obtain culture before giving drug. Therapy may begin before culture results are known.
• If ophthalmic gentamicin is given together with systemic gentamicin, monitor gentamicin level.
• Systemic absorption from excessive use may cause toxicities.
• Solution isn't for injection into conjunctiva or anterior chamber of eye.
• Store drug away from heat.

**PATIENT TEACHING**
• Tell patient to clean eye area of excessive discharge before instilling drug.
• Teach patient how to instill drops or apply ointment. Advise him to wash hands before and after applying ointment or solution and not to touch tip of dropper or tube to eye or surrounding tissues.
• Instruct patient to apply light finger pressure on lacrimal sac for 1 minute after drops are instilled.

---

• Instruct patient to stop drug and notify prescriber if signs and symptoms of sensitivity (itching lids, swelling, or constant burning) occur.
• Advise patient not to share drug, washcloths, or towels with family members and to notify prescriber if anyone develops same signs or symptoms.
• Tell patient that vision may be blurred for few minutes after application of ointment.
• *Alert:* Stress importance of following recommended therapy. *Pseudomonas* infections can cause complete vision loss within 24 hours if infection isn't controlled.

✳ NEW DRUG

## moxifloxacin hydrochloride
Vigamox

*Pregnancy risk category C*

### AVAILABLE FORMS
*Solution:* 0.5%

### INDICATIONS & DOSAGES
➤ **Bacterial conjunctivitis**
*Adults and children age 1 and older:* 1 drop into affected eye t.i.d. for 7 days.

### ACTION
Antibiotic. Inhibits DNA gyrase and topoisomerase, preventing cell replication and division.

| Route | Onset | Peak | Duration |
|---|---|---|---|
| Ophthalmic | Unknown | Unknown | Unknown |

### ADVERSE REACTIONS
**CNS:** fever.
**EENT:** conjunctivitis; dry eyes; increased lacrimation; keratitis; ocular discomfort, pain, and pruritus; otitis media; pharyngitis; reduced visual acuity; rhinitis; subconjunctival hemorrhage.
**Respiratory:** increased cough.
**Skin:** rash.
**Other:** infection.

### INTERACTIONS
None reported.

### EFFECTS ON LAB TEST RESULTS
None reported.

### CONTRAINDICATIONS & CAUTIONS
• Contraindicated in patients hypersensitive to moxifloxacin, fluoroquinolones, or their components.
• Use cautiously in pregnant or breast-feeding women.

### NURSING CONSIDERATIONS
• Don't inject solution subconjunctivally or into anterior chamber of the eye.
• Systemic moxifloxacin has caused serious hypersensitivity reactions. If allergic reaction occurs, stop drug and treat symptoms.
• Monitor patient for superinfection.

### PATIENT TEACHING
• Tell patient to stop drug and seek medical treatment immediately if evidence of hypersensitivity reaction develops, such as itching, rash, swelling of the face or throat, or difficulty breathing.
• Tell patient not to wear contact lenses during treatment.
• Instruct patient not to touch dropper tip to anything, including eyes and fingers.

## ofloxacin 0.3%
Ocuflox

*Pregnancy risk category C*

### AVAILABLE FORMS
*Ophthalmic solution:* 0.3% in 1-ml, 5-ml, and 10-ml solution

### INDICATIONS & DOSAGES
➤ **Conjunctivitis caused by *Staphylococcus aureus, Staphylococcus epidermidis, Streptococcus pneumoniae, Enterobacter cloacae, Haemophilus influenzae, Proteus mirabilis,* and *Pseudomonas aeruginosa***
*Adults and children older than age 1:* 1 to 2 drops in conjunctival sac q 2 to 4 hours daily while patient is awake, for first 2 days; then q.i.d. for up to 5 additional days.
➤ **Bacterial corneal ulcer caused by *S. aureus, S. epidermidis, S. pneumoniae, P. aeruginosa, Serratia marcescens,* and *Propionibacterium acnes***
*Adults and children older than age 1:* 1 to 2 drops q 30 minutes while patient is

awake and 1 to 2 drops 4 to 6 hours after he goes to bed on days 1 and 2. Days 3 to 7, 1 to 2 drops hourly while patient is awake. Days 7 to 9, 1 to 2 drops q.i.d.

## ACTION
Bactericidal. Inhibits bacterial DNA gyrase, an enzyme needed for bacterial replication.

| Route | Onset | Peak | Duration |
|---|---|---|---|
| Ophthalmic | Unknown | Unknown | Unknown |

## ADVERSE REACTIONS
**EENT:** *transient ocular burning or discomfort,* stinging, redness, itching, photophobia, lacrimation, eye dryness, eye pain, chemical conjunctivitis or keratitis, periocular or facial edema.

## INTERACTIONS
None significant.

## EFFECTS ON LAB TEST RESULTS
None reported.

## CONTRAINDICATIONS & CAUTIONS
• Contraindicated in patients hypersensitive to ofloxacin, other fluoroquinolones, or other components of drug and in breast-feeding women.

## NURSING CONSIDERATIONS
• *Alert:* Don't inject drug into conjunctiva or introduce directly into anterior chamber of eye.
• Stop drug if improvement doesn't occur within 7 days. Prolonged use may result in overgrowth of nonsusceptible organisms, including fungi.
• *Alert:* Don't confuse Ocuflox with Ocufen.

## PATIENT TEACHING
• If an allergic reaction occurs, tell patient to stop drug and notify prescriber. Serious acute hypersensitivity reactions may need emergency treatment.
• Tell patient to clean excessive discharge from eye area before application.
• Teach patient how to instill drops. Advise him to wash hands before and after instilling solution, and warn him not to touch tip of dropper to eye or surrounding tissue.

• Advise patient to apply light finger pressure on lacrimal sac for 1 minute after drug instillation.
• Tell patient not to share drug, washcloths, or towels with family members and to notify prescriber if anyone develops same signs or symptoms.
• Stress importance of compliance with recommended therapy.
• Warn patient not to use leftover drug for new eye infection.
• Remind patient to discard drug when it's no longer needed.

---

**sulfacetamide sodium 1%**
Sulster

**sulfacetamide sodium 10%**
AK-Sulf, Bleph-10, Cetamide, OcuSulf-10, Sodium Sulamyd Ophthalmic, Storz Sulf, Sulf-10 Ophthalmic

**sulfacetamide sodium 15%**
Isopto-Cetamide Ophthalmic

**sulfacetamide sodium 30%**
Sodium Sulamyd Ophthalmic

*Pregnancy risk category C*

## AVAILABLE FORMS
*Ophthalmic ointment:* 10%
*Ophthalmic solution:* 1%, 10%, 15%, 30%

## INDICATIONS & DOSAGES
➤ **Inclusion conjunctivitis, corneal ulcers, chlamydial infection**
*Adults and children:* 1 to 2 drops of 10% solution into lower conjunctival sac q 2 to 3 hours during day, less often at night. Or, 1 to 2 drops of 15% solution instilled into lower conjunctival sac q 1 to 2 hours initially. Increase interval as condition responds. Or, instill 1 drop of 30% solution into lower conjunctival sac q 2 hours. Apply 0.5 inch of 10% ointment into conjunctival sac t.i.d. to q.i.d. and h.s. Ointment may be used at night along with drops during the day.
➤ **Trachoma**
*Adults and children:* 2 drops of 30% solution into lower conjunctival sac q 2 hours with systemic sulfonamide or tetracycline.

➤ **Steroid-responsive inflammatory ocular conditions for which a corticosteroid is indicated and where superficial bacterial ocular infection or a risk of bacterial ocular infection exists**
*Adults and children older than age 6:*
2 drops of 1% solution in eye q 4 hours. Dose may be reduced but don't stop therapy abruptly.

## ACTION
Bacteriostatic, although it may be bactericidal in high concentrations. Prevents uptake of PABA, a metabolite of bacterial folic acid synthesis.

| Route | Onset | Peak | Duration |
|---|---|---|---|
| Ophthalmic | Unknown | Unknown | Unknown |

## ADVERSE REACTIONS
**EENT:** slowed corneal wound healing with ointment, pain on instillation of eyedrops, headache or brow pain, photophobia, periorbital edema, eye itching, burning.
**Other:** overgrowth of nonsusceptible organisms.

## INTERACTIONS
**Drug-drug.** *Gentamicin (ophthalmic):*
May cause in vitro antagonism. Avoid using together.
*Local anesthetics (procaine, tetracaine), PABA derivatives:* May decrease sulfacetamide sodium action. Wait 30 minutes to 1 hour after instilling anesthetic or PABA derivative before instilling sulfacetamide.
*Silver preparations:* May cause precipitate formation. Avoid using together.
**Drug-lifestyle.** *Sun exposure:* May cause photophobia. Advise patient to avoid excessive sunlight exposure.

## EFFECTS ON LAB TEST RESULTS
None reported.

## CONTRAINDICATIONS & CAUTIONS
● Contraindicated in patients hypersensitive to sulfonamides and children younger than age 2 months. Contraindicated in epithelial herpes simplex keratitis, vaccinia, varicella, and many other viral diseases of the cornea and conjunctiva; in mycobacterial or fungal diseases of ocular structures;

and after uncomplicated removal of a corneal foreign body (corticosteroid combinations).

## NURSING CONSIDERATIONS
● Drug is often used with oral tetracycline in treating trachoma and inclusion conjunctivitis.
● Store drug away from heat in tightly closed, light-resistant container.

## PATIENT TEACHING
● Tell patient to clean excessive discharge from eye area before application.
● Teach patient how to instill drops or apply ointment. Advise him to wash hands before and after applying ointment or solution and not to touch tip of dropper to eye or surrounding tissues.
● Instruct patient to apply light finger pressure on lacrimal sac for 1 minute after drops are instilled.
● Warn patient that eyedrops burn slightly.
● Advise patient to watch for and report signs and symptoms of sensitivity (itching lids, swelling, or constant burning).
● Tell patient to wait at least 5 minutes before instilling other eyedrops.
● Warn patient that solution may stain clothing.
● Tell patient to minimize sensitivity to sunlight by wearing sunglasses and avoiding prolonged exposure to sunlight.
● Advise patient not to use discolored solution.
● Tell patient not to share drug, washcloths, or towels with family members and to notify prescriber if anyone develops same signs or symptoms.
● Stress importance of compliance with recommended therapy.
● Advise patient to alert prescriber if no improvement occurs.

---

# tobramycin
AKTob, Defy, Tobrex

*Pregnancy risk category B*

## AVAILABLE FORMS
*Ophthalmic ointment:* 0.3%
*Ophthalmic solution:* 0.3%

---

## INDICATIONS & DOSAGES
➤ **External ocular infections by susceptible bacteria**
*Adults and children:* In mild to moderate infections, instill 1 or 2 drops into affected eye q 4 hours, or apply thin strip (1 cm long) of ointment q 8 to 12 hours. In severe infections, instill 2 drops into infected eye q 30 to 60 minutes until condition improves; then reduce frequency. Or, apply thin strip (1 cm long) of ointment q 3 to 4 hours until improvement; then reduce frequency to b.i.d to t.i.d.

## ACTION
Unknown. Thought to inhibit protein synthesis; usually bactericidal.

| Route | Onset | Peak | Duration |
|---|---|---|---|
| Ophthalmic | Unknown | Unknown | Unknown |

## ADVERSE REACTIONS
**EENT:** burning or stinging on instillation, lid itching or swelling, conjunctival erythema, blurred vision with ointment, increased lacrimation.

## INTERACTIONS
None significant.

## EFFECTS ON LAB TEST RESULTS
None reported.

## CONTRAINDICATIONS & CAUTIONS
• Contraindicated in patients hypersensitive to drug or other aminoglycosides.

## NURSING CONSIDERATIONS
• When two different ophthalmic solutions are used, allow at least 5 minutes between instillations.
• *Alert:* Tobramycin ophthalmic solution isn't for injection.
• If topical ocular tobramycin is given with systemic tobramycin, carefully monitor levels.
• Prolonged use may result in overgrowth of nonsusceptible organisms, including fungi.
• *Alert:* Don't confuse tobramycin with Trobicin, or Tobrex with Tobradex.

## PATIENT TEACHING
• Tell patient to clean excessive discharge from eye area before application.
• Teach patient how to instill drops or apply ointment. Advise him to wash hands before and after applying and to avoid touching tip of dropper to eye or surrounding tissue.
• Instruct patient to apply light finger pressure on lacrimal sac for 1 minute after drops are instilled.
• Advise patient to watch for itching lids, swelling, or constant burning. Tell him to stop drug and notify prescriber if these signs and symptoms develop.
• Tell patient not to share drug, washcloths, or towels with family members and to notify prescriber if anyone develops same signs or symptoms.
• Stress importance of compliance with recommended therapy.

# vidarabine
Vira-A

*Pregnancy risk category C*

## AVAILABLE FORMS
*Ophthalmic ointment:* 3% in 3.5-g tube (equivalent to 2.8% vidarabine)

## INDICATIONS & DOSAGES
➤ **Acute keratoconjunctivitis, superficial keratitis, and recurrent epithelial keratitis caused by herpes simplex I and II**
*Adults and children:* 1 cm of ointment into lower conjunctival sac five times daily at 3-hour intervals. If there are no signs of improvement after 7 days, or if complete reepithelialization hasn't occurred in 21 days, consider other forms of therapy. Some severe cases may need longer treatment. After reepithelialization has occurred, treat for an additional 5 to 7 days at reduced frequency (such as b.i.d.) to prevent recurrence.

## ACTION
Unknown. Thought to interfere with DNA synthesis.

| Route | Onset | Peak | Duration |
|---|---|---|---|
| Ophthalmic | Unknown | Unknown | Unknown |

## ADVERSE REACTIONS
**EENT:** temporary burning, itching, mild irritation, pain, lacrimation, foreign body sensation, conjunctival infection, punctal occlusion, sensitivity, superficial punctate keratitis, photophobia.

## INTERACTIONS
None significant.

## EFFECTS ON LAB TEST RESULTS
None reported.

## CONTRAINDICATIONS & CAUTIONS
• Contraindicated in patients hypersensitive to drug.

## NURSING CONSIDERATIONS
• Use corticosteroids cautiously and monitor patient closely. Continue drug therapy for several days after corticosteroid therapy.
• Drug isn't effective against RNA virus, adenoviral ocular infections, or bacterial, fungal, or chlamydial infections.
• Store drug in tightly closed, light-resistant container.
• *Alert:* Don't confuse vidarabine with cytarabine.

## PATIENT TEACHING
• Tell patient to clean excessive discharge from eye area before application.
• Teach patient how to apply drug. Advise him to wash hands before and after applying ointment and to avoid touching tip of tube to eye or surrounding tissue.
• Instruct patient to apply light finger pressure on lacrimal sac for 1 minute after drops are instilled.
• Explain that ointment may produce a temporary visual haze.
• Advise patient to watch for signs of sensitivity, such as itching lids, swelling, or constant burning. Tell patient who develops such signs and symptoms to stop drug and notify prescriber immediately.
• Tell patient to minimize sensitivity to sunlight by wearing sunglasses and avoiding prolonged exposure to sunlight.
• Tell patient not to share drug, washcloths, or towels with family members and to notify prescriber if anyone develops same signs or symptoms.

• Stress importance of compliance with recommended therapy.
• Advise patient to notify prescriber if his condition doesn't improve or worsens after 7 days; alert prescriber if there's a decrease in vision, or if burning or irritation of eye occurs.

---

**dexamethasone**
**dexamethasone sodium**
   **phosphate**
**diclofenac sodium**
**fluorometholone**
**flurbiprofen sodium**
**ketorolac tromethamine**
**prednisolone acetate**
**prednisolone sodium phosphate**

**COMBINATION PRODUCTS**
Corticosteroids for ophthalmic use are commonly used with antibiotics and sulfonamides. See Chapter 77, Ophthalmic anti-infectives.

---

**dexamethasone**
Maxidex

**dexamethasone sodium phosphate**
AK-Dex, Decadron

*Pregnancy risk category C*

---

**AVAILABLE FORMS**
**dexamethasone**
*Maxidex*
*Ophthalmic suspension:* 0.1%
**dexamethasone sodium phosphate**
*Decadron*
*Ophthalmic solution:* 0.1%
*AK-Dex*
*Ophthalmic ointment:* 0.05%
*Ophthalmic solution:* 0.1%

**INDICATIONS & DOSAGES**
➤ **Uveitis; iridocyclitis; inflammatory conditions of eyelids, conjunctiva, cornea, anterior segment of globe; corneal injury from chemical or thermal burns, or penetration of foreign bodies; allergic conjunctivitis; suppression of graft rejection after keratoplasty**
*Adults and children:* 1 to 2 drops of suspension or solution or 1.25 to 2.5 cm of ointment into conjunctival sac. In severe disease, give drops q 1 to 2 hours, tapering to end as condition improves. In mild conditions, give drops up to four to six times daily or apply ointment t.i.d. or q.i.d. As condition improves, taper dosage to b.i.d.; then once daily. Treatment may extend from a few days to several weeks.

**ACTION**
Exerts anti-inflammatory action; suppresses edema, fibrin deposition, capillary dilation, leukocyte migration, capillary proliferation, and collagen deposition.

| Route | Onset | Peak | Duration |
|-------|-------|------|----------|
| Ophthalmic | Unknown | Unknown | Unknown |

**ADVERSE REACTIONS**
**EENT:** increased intraocular pressure; thinning of cornea; interference with corneal wound healing; increased susceptibility to viral or fungal corneal infection; corneal ulceration; glaucoma worsening, cataracts, defects in visual acuity and visual field, optic nerve damage with excessive or long-term use; mild blurred vision; burning, stinging, or redness of eyes; dry eyes; discharge; discomfort; ocular pain; foreign body sensation; photophobia.
**Other:** systemic effects, adrenal suppression with excessive or long-term use.

**INTERACTIONS**
None significant.

**EFFECTS ON LAB TEST RESULTS**
None reported.

**CONTRAINDICATIONS & CAUTIONS**
• Contraindicated in patients hypersensitive to any component of drug.
• Contraindicated in those with ocular tuberculosis or acute superficial herpes simplex (dendritic keratitis), vaccinia, varicella, or other fungal or viral diseases of cornea and conjunctiva; in patients with acute, purulent, untreated infections of eye; and in those who have had uncomplicated removal of superficial corneal foreign body.

---

• Use cautiously in patients with corneal abrasions that may be infected (especially with herpes).
• Use cautiously in patients with glaucoma (any form) because intraocular pressure may increase. Dosage of glaucoma drugs may need to be increased to compensate.
• Safe use in pregnant and breast-feeding women hasn't been established.

**NURSING CONSIDERATIONS**
• Drug isn't for long-term use.
• Watch for corneal ulceration; may require stopping drug.
• Corneal viral and fungal infections may be worsened by corticosteroid application.
• *Alert:* Don't confuse dexamethasone with desoximetasone.
• *Alert:* Don't confuse Maxidex with Maxzide.

**PATIENT TEACHING**
• Tell patient to shake suspension well before use.
• Teach patient how to instill drops or apply ointment. Advise him to wash hands before and after applying ointment or solution, and warn him not to touch tip of dropper to eye or surrounding tissue.
• Tell patient to apply light finger pressure on lacrimal sac for 1 minute after instillation.
• Advise patient that he may use eye pad with ointment.
• Warn patient not to use leftover drug for new eye inflammation; doing so may cause serious problems.
• *Alert:* Warn patient to call prescriber immediately and to stop drug if visual acuity changes or visual field diminishes.
• Tell patient not to share drug, washcloths, or towels with family members and to notify prescriber if anyone develops same signs or symptoms.
• Stress importance of compliance with recommended therapy.
• Tell patient who wears contact lenses to check with prescriber before using lenses again.

# diclofenac sodium
Voltaren Ophthalmic

*Pregnancy risk category B*

**AVAILABLE FORMS**
*Ophthalmic solution:* 0.1%

**INDICATIONS & DOSAGES**
➤ **Postoperative inflammation following removal of cataract**
*Adults:* 1 drop in conjunctival sac q.i.d., beginning 24 hours after surgery and continuing throughout first 2 weeks of postoperative period.
➤ **Corneal refractive surgery**
*Adults:* 1 to 2 drops to operative eye 1 hour before surgery. Within 15 minutes after surgery, instill 1 to 2 drops into operative eye. Then 1 drop q.i.d. beginning 4 to 6 hours after surgery up to 3 days.

**ACTION**
Unknown. Thought to inhibit the enzyme cyclooxygenase, which is essential in biosynthesis of prostaglandins. Prostaglandins may be mediators of certain kinds of intraocular inflammation.

| Route | Onset | Peak | Duration |
|---|---|---|---|
| Ophthalmic | Unknown | Unknown | Unknown |

**ADVERSE REACTIONS**
**EENT:** *transient stinging and burning, increased intraocular pressure, keratitis,* anterior chamber reaction, ocular allergy, increased bleeding of ocular tissues, including hyphemas with ocular surgery.
**GI:** nausea, vomiting.
**Other:** viral infection.

**INTERACTIONS**
None significant.

**EFFECTS ON LAB TEST RESULTS**
None reported.

**CONTRAINDICATIONS & CAUTIONS**
• Contraindicated in patients hypersensitive to any component of drug and in those wearing soft contact lenses. Because of known effects of prostaglandin-inhibiting drugs on fetal CV system (clo-

sure of ductus arteriosus), avoid use of drug during late pregnancy.
• Use cautiously in patients hypersensitive to acetylsalicylic acid, phenylacetic acid derivatives, and other NSAIDs; potential for cross-sensitivity exists.
• Use cautiously in surgical patients with known bleeding tendencies and in those receiving drugs that may prolong bleeding time.

### NURSING CONSIDERATIONS
• Drug may slow or delay healing.
• Most cases of increased intraocular pressure have occurred postoperatively and before drug administration.
• *Alert:* Don't confuse diclofenac with Diflucan or Duphalac.
• *Alert:* Don't confuse Voltaren with Verelan.

### PATIENT TEACHING
• Teach patient how to instill drops. Advise him to wash hands before and after instilling solution and not to touch tip of dropper to eye or surrounding tissue.
• Advise patient to apply light finger pressure on lacrimal sac for 1 minute after instilling drops.
• Stress importance of compliance with recommended therapy.
• Warn patient not to use leftover drug for new eye inflammation.
• Remind patient to discard drug when no longer needed.

---

## fluorometholone
Flarex, Fluor-Op, FML Forte, FML Liquifilm Ophthalmic, FML S.O.P.

*Pregnancy risk category C*

### AVAILABLE FORMS
*Ophthalmic ointment:* 0.1%
*Ophthalmic suspension:* 0.1%, 0.25%

### INDICATIONS & DOSAGES
➤ **Inflammatory and allergic conditions of cornea, conjunctiva, sclera, anterior uvea**
*Adults and children:* 1 to 2 drops in conjunctival sac b.i.d. to q.i.d. May be given q 2 hours during first 1 to 2 days, if needed. Or, apply 1.25-cm ribbon of ointment to

conjunctival sac q 4 hours, decreased to once daily to t.i.d. as inflammation subsides.

### ACTION
Exerts anti-inflammatory action. Suppresses edema, fibrin deposition, capillary dilation, leukocyte migration, capillary proliferation, and collagen deposition.

| Route | Onset | Peak | Duration |
|---|---|---|---|
| Ophthalmic | Unknown | Unknown | Unknown |

### ADVERSE REACTIONS
**EENT:** increased intraocular pressure, thinning of cornea, interference with corneal wound healing, corneal ulceration, increased susceptibility to viral or fungal corneal infections, glaucoma worsening, discharge, discomfort, ocular pain, foreign body sensation, cataracts, decreased visual acuity, diminished visual field, optic nerve damage with excessive or long-term use.
**Other:** systemic effects, adrenal suppression with excessive or long-term use.

### INTERACTIONS
None significant.

### EFFECTS ON LAB TEST RESULTS
None reported.

### CONTRAINDICATIONS & CAUTIONS
• Contraindicated in patients with vaccinia, varicella, acute superficial herpes simplex (dendritic keratitis), other fungal or viral eye diseases, ocular tuberculosis, or acute, purulent, untreated eye infections.
• Use cautiously in patients with corneal abrasions that may be contaminated (especially with herpes).
• Safety and efficacy of drug in children younger than age 2 haven't been established.

### NURSING CONSIDERATIONS
• Duration of treatment may range from a few days to several weeks; however, avoid long-term use. Monitor intraocular pressure.
• Drug is less likely to cause increased intraocular pressure with extended use than other ophthalmic anti-inflammatory drugs (except medrysone).

---

• In chronic conditions, withdraw treatment by gradually decreasing frequency of applications.

**PATIENT TEACHING**
• Teach patient how to instill drops or apply ointment. Advise him to wash hands before and after applying ointment or solution, and warn him not to touch tip of dropper to eye or surrounding tissue.
• Advise patient to apply light finger pressure on lacrimal sac for 1 minute after instillation.
• Urge patient to call prescriber immediately and to stop drug if visual acuity decreases or visual field diminishes.
• Tell patient not to share drug, washcloths, or towels with family members and to notify prescriber if anyone develops same signs or symptoms.
• Warn patient not to use leftover drug for new eye inflammation; it may cause serious problems.
• Advise patient to consult prescriber if no improvement after 2 days. Don't stop treatment prematurely.
• Tell patient to shake container well before use.
• Tell patient to store drug in tightly covered, light-resistant container.

---

**flurbiprofen sodium**
Ocufen

*Pregnancy risk category C*

**AVAILABLE FORMS**
*Ophthalmic solution:* 0.03%

**INDICATIONS & DOSAGES**
➤ **To inhibit intraoperative miosis**
*Adults:* Instill 1 drop into affected eye about q 30 minutes, beginning 2 hours before surgery; give total of 4 drops.

**ACTION**
Unknown. An NSAID thought to inhibit the cyclooxygenase enzyme essential in biosynthesis of prostaglandins.

| Route | Onset | Peak | Duration |
|-------|-------|------|----------|
| Ophthalmic | Unknown | Unknown | Unknown |

**ADVERSE REACTIONS**
**EENT:** transient burning and stinging on instillation, ocular irritation; increased bleeding tendency of ocular tissues in conjunction with ocular surgery.

**INTERACTIONS**
**Drug-drug.** *Acetylcholine, carbachol:* May be rendered ineffective. Avoid using together.
*Anticoagulants:* May increase risk of bleeding if significant systemic absorption occurs. Monitor patient closely for bleeding.

**EFFECTS ON LAB TEST RESULTS**
None reported.

**CONTRAINDICATIONS & CAUTIONS**
• Contraindicated in patients hypersensitive to drug. Safe use in pregnant and breast-feeding women hasn't been established.
• Use cautiously in patients who may be allergic to aspirin and other NSAIDs.
• Use cautiously in patients with bleeding tendencies and in those receiving drugs that may prolong clotting times.

**NURSING CONSIDERATIONS**
• Wound healing may be delayed with drug use.
• *Alert:* Don't confuse Ocufen with Ocuflox.

**PATIENT TEACHING**
• Advise patient to alert prescriber immediately if visual acuity decreases or visual field diminishes.
• Urge patient to take drug as prescribed.
• Tell patient to report excessive bleeding or bruising.

---

**ketorolac tromethamine**
Acular, Acular LS

*Pregnancy risk category C*

**AVAILABLE FORMS**
**Acular**
*Ophthalmic solution:* 0.5%
**Acular LS**
*Ophthalmic solution:* 0.4%

---

## INDICATIONS & DOSAGES
➤ **Relief from ocular itching caused by seasonal allergic conjunctivitis**
*Adults:* 1 drop into conjunctival sac in each eye q.i.d.
➤ **Postoperative inflammation in patients who have undergone cataract extraction**
*Adults:* 1 drop to affected eye q.i.d. beginning 24 hours after cataract surgery and continuing through first 2 weeks of postoperative period.
✷ *NEW INDICATION:* **Reduce ocular pain, burning, and stinging after corneal refractive surgery (Acular LS)**
*Adults and children age 3 and older:* 1 drop q.i.d. to affected eye, p.r.n., for up to 4 days after surgery.

## ACTION
Unknown. An NSAID thought to inhibit the action of cyclooxygenase, an enzyme responsible for prostaglandin synthesis. Prostaglandins mediate the inflammatory response and also cause miosis.

| Route | Onset | Peak | Duration |
|-------|-------|------|----------|
| Ophthalmic | Unknown | Unknown | Unknown |

## ADVERSE REACTIONS
**CNS:** headache (Acular LS).
**EENT:** *transient stinging and burning on instillation,* superficial keratitis, superficial ocular infections, ocular irritation, ocular pain, corneal edema, iritis, ocular inflammation (Acular); conjunctival hyperemia, corneal infiltrates, ocular edema and ocular pain (Acular LS).
**Other:** hypersensitivity reactions.

## INTERACTIONS
None significant.

## EFFECTS ON LAB TEST RESULTS
None reported.

## CONTRAINDICATIONS & CAUTIONS
• Contraindicated in patients hypersensitive to components of drug and in those wearing soft contact lenses.
• Use cautiously in patients with bleeding disorders or those hypersensitive to other NSAIDs or aspirin. Use cautiously in breast-feeding women.

## NURSING CONSIDERATIONS
• Store drug away from heat in a dark, tightly closed container and protect from freezing.
• *Alert:* Don't confuse Acular with Acthar.

## PATIENT TEACHING
• Teach patient how to instill drops. Advise him to wash hands before and after instilling solution, and warn him not to touch tip of dropper to eye or surrounding tissue.
• Advise patient to apply light finger pressure on lacrimal sac for 1 minute after instillation.
• Stress importance of compliance with recommended therapy.
• Tell patient not to instill drops while wearing contact lenses.
• Advise patient to report excessive bleeding or bruising to prescriber.
• Remind patient to discard drug when it's no longer needed.

# prednisolone acetate (suspension)
Econopred Ophthalmic, Econopred Plus Ophthalmic, Pred Forte, Pred Mild Ophthalmic

# prednisolone sodium phosphate (solution)
AK-Pred, Inflamase Forte, Inflamase Mild, Predsol Eye Drops‡

*Pregnancy risk category C*

## AVAILABLE FORMS
**prednisolone acetate**
*Ophthalmic suspension:* 0.12%, 0.125%, 1%
**prednisolone sodium phosphate**
*Ophthalmic solution:* 0.125%, 1%

## INDICATIONS & DOSAGES
➤ **Inflammation of palpebral and bulbar conjunctiva, cornea, and anterior segment of globe**
*Adults and children:* Instill 1 to 2 drops into eye. In severe conditions, may be used hourly, tapering to end as inflammation subsides. In mild or moderate inflammation or when a favorable response is at-

tained in severe conditions, dosage may be reduced to 1 or 2 drops q 3 to 12 hours.

## ACTION
Exerts anti-inflammatory action. Suppresses edema, fibrin deposition, capillary dilation, leukocyte migration, capillary proliferation, and collagen deposition.

| Route | Onset | Peak | Duration |
|---|---|---|---|
| Ophthalmic | Unknown | Unknown | Unknown |

## ADVERSE REACTIONS
**EENT:** increased intraocular pressure, thinning of cornea, interference with corneal wound healing, increased susceptibility to viral or fungal corneal infection, corneal ulceration, discharge, discomfort, foreign body sensation, glaucoma worsening, cataracts, visual acuity and visual field defects, optic nerve damage with excessive or long-term use.
**Other:** systemic effects, adrenal suppression with excessive or long-term use.

## INTERACTIONS
None significant.

## EFFECTS ON LAB TEST RESULTS
None reported.

## CONTRAINDICATIONS & CAUTIONS
• Contraindicated in patients with acute, untreated, purulent ocular infections; acute superficial herpes simplex (dendritic keratitis); vaccinia, varicella, or other viral or fungal eye diseases; or ocular tuberculosis.
• Use cautiously in patients with corneal abrasions that may be contaminated (especially with herpes).

## NURSING CONSIDERATIONS
• Shake suspension and check dosage before giving to ensure correct strength. Store in tightly covered container.
• **Alert:** Don't confuse prednisolone with prednisone.

## PATIENT TEACHING
• Teach patient how to instill drops. Advise him to wash hands before and after instillation, and warn him not to touch tip of dropper to eye or surrounding area.

• Advise patient to apply light finger pressure on lacrimal sac for 1 minute after instillation.
• Tell patient on long-term therapy to have frequent tests of intraocular pressure.
• Tell patient not to share drug, washcloths, or towels with family members and to notify prescriber if anyone develops same signs or symptoms.
• Stress importance of compliance with recommended therapy.
• Tell patient to notify prescriber if improvement doesn't occur within several days or if pain, itching, or swelling of eye occurs.
• Warn patient not to use leftover drug for new eye inflammation because serious problems may occur.

**acetylcholine chloride**
**carbachol**
**pilocarpine hydrochloride**
**pilocarpine nitrate**

### COMBINATION PRODUCTS
E-PILO: epinephrine bitartrate 1% and pilocarpine hydrochloride 1%, 2%, 3%, 4%, or 6%.

---

## acetylcholine chloride
Miochol-E

*Pregnancy risk category NR*

### AVAILABLE FORMS
*Ophthalmic injection:* 1%

### INDICATIONS & DOSAGES
➤ **Anterior segment surgery**
*Adults and children:* Before or after securing sutures, prescriber gently instills 0.5 to 2 ml into anterior chamber.

### ACTION
A cholinergic that causes contraction of the sphincter muscles of the iris, resulting in miosis. That produces ciliary spasm, deepening of the anterior chamber, and vasodilation of conjunctival vessels of the outflow tract.

| Route | Onset | Peak | Duration |
|---|---|---|---|
| Ophthalmic | Immediate | Unknown | 10 min |

### ADVERSE REACTIONS
**CV:** *bradycardia,* hypotension, flushing.
**EENT:** corneal edema, clouding, decompensation.
**Respiratory:** breathing difficulties.
**Other:** diaphoresis.

### INTERACTIONS
None significant.

### EFFECTS ON LAB TEST RESULTS
None reported.

### CONTRAINDICATIONS & CAUTIONS
● Contraindicated in patients hypersensitive to drug or its components.

### NURSING CONSIDERATIONS
● Reconstitute immediately before using, shaking vial gently until clear solution is obtained.
● Discard unused solution.
● Don't gas-sterilize vial. Ethylene oxide may produce formic acid. Watch for signs and symptoms of hypotension and bradycardia if this occurs.
● *Alert:* Don't confuse acetylcholine with acetylcysteine.

### PATIENT TEACHING
● Inform patient about need for drug during surgical procedure; answer questions and address concerns.
● Instruct patient to immediately report breathing difficulties.

---

## carbachol (intraocular)
Miostat

## carbachol (topical)
Carboptic, Isopto Carbachol

*Pregnancy risk category C*

### AVAILABLE FORMS
*Intraocular injection:* 0.01%
*Topical ophthalmic solution:* 0.75%, 1.5%, 2.25%, 3%

### INDICATIONS & DOSAGES
➤ **To produce pupillary miosis in ocular surgery**
*Adults:* Before or after securing sutures, prescriber gently instills 0.5 ml (intraocular form) into anterior chamber.
➤ **Glaucoma**
*Adults:* 1 to 2 drops (topical form) instilled up to t.i.d.

### ACTION
A cholinergic that causes contraction of the sphincter muscles of the iris, resulting

---

in miosis. That produces ciliary spasm, deepening of the anterior chamber, and vasodilation of conjunctival vessels of the outflow tract.

| Route | Onset | Peak | Duration |
|---|---|---|---|
| Intraocular | Secs | 2-5 min | 24-48 hr |
| Ophthalmic (topical) | 10-20 min | Unknown | 4-8 hr |

## ADVERSE REACTIONS
**CNS:** headache.
**CV:** syncope, *cardiac arrhythmia,* flushing, hypotension.
**EENT:** spasm of eye accommodation, conjunctival vasodilation, eye and brow pain, *transient stinging and burning,* corneal clouding, bullous keratopathy, salivation, iritis, retinal detachment, ciliary and conjunctival injection; salivation.
**GI:** GI cramps, vomiting, diarrhea, epigastric distress.
**GU:** tightness in bladder, frequent urge to urinate.
**Respiratory:** asthma.
**Other:** diaphoresis.

## INTERACTIONS
**Drug-drug.** *Pilocarpine:* May cause additive effects. Use together cautiously.

## EFFECTS ON LAB TEST RESULTS
None reported.

## CONTRAINDICATIONS & CAUTIONS
• Contraindicated in patients hypersensitive to drug and in those with conditions in which cholinergic effects, such as constriction, are undesirable (acute iritis, some forms of secondary glaucoma, pupillary block glaucoma, or acute inflammatory disease of the anterior chamber).
• Use cautiously in patients with acute heart failure, bronchial asthma, peptic ulcer, hyperthyroidism, GI spasm, Parkinson's disease, and urinary tract obstruction.

## NURSING CONSIDERATIONS
• In case of toxicity, give atropine parenterally.
• Drug is used in open-angle glaucoma, especially when patients are resistant or allergic to pilocarpine hydrochloride or nitrate.

• *Alert:* Patients with dark eyes (hazel or brown irises) may need stronger solutions or more frequent instillation because eye pigment may absorb drug.
• If tolerance to drug develops, prescriber may switch to another miotic for a short time.

## PATIENT TEACHING
• Teach patient how to instill drug. Advise him to wash hands before and after instillation and to apply light finger pressure on lacrimal sac for 1 minute after drops are instilled. Warn him not to exceed recommended dosage.
• Warn patient to avoid hazardous activities, such as operating machinery or driving, until temporary blurring subsides. Reassure patient that blurred vision usually diminishes with prolonged use.
• Tell glaucoma patient that long-term use may be needed. Stress compliance. Tell him to remain under medical supervision for periodic tests of intraocular pressure.
• Warn patient to use caution during night driving and while performing other hazardous activities in reduced light.

# pilocarpine hydrochloride
Adsorbocarpine, Akarpine, Isopto Carpine, Miocarpine†, Pilocar, Pilopine HS, Pilopt‡, Pilostat

# pilocarpine nitrate
Pilagan Liquifilm

*Pregnancy risk category C*

## AVAILABLE FORMS
**pilocarpine hydrochloride**
*Ophthalmic gel:* 4%
*Ophthalmic solution:* 0.25%, 0.5%, 1%, 2%, 3%, 4%, 5%, 6%, 8%, 10%
**pilocarpine nitrate**
*Ophthalmic solution:* 1%, 2%, 4%

## INDICATIONS & DOSAGES
➤ **Primary open-angle glaucoma**
*Adults and children:* Instill 1 to 2 drops up to q.i.d. or apply 1-cm ribbon of 4% gel h.s.

---

Reactions may be *common,* uncommon, *life-threatening,* or COMMON AND LIFE-THREATENING.

➤ **Emergency treatment of acute angle-closure glaucoma**
*Adults and children:* Instill 1 drop of 2% solution q 5 to 10 minutes for three to six doses; then 1 drop q 1 to 3 hours until pressure is controlled.

➤ **Mydriasis caused by mydriatic or cycloplegic drugs**
*Adults and children:* 1 drop of 1% solution.

## ACTION

A cholinergic that causes contraction of iris sphincter muscles, resulting in miosis, and that produces ciliary spasm, deepening of the anterior chamber, and vasodilation of conjunctival vessels of the outflow tract.

| Route | Onset | Peak | Duration |
|-------|-------|------|----------|
| Ophthalmic | 10-30 min | 30-85 min | 4-8 hr |

## ADVERSE REACTIONS

**CV:** hypertension, tachycardia.
**EENT:** periorbital or supraorbital headache, *myopia,* ciliary spasm, *blurred vision,* conjunctival irritation, transient stinging and burning, keratitis, lens opacity, retinal detachment, lacrimation, changes in visual field, *brow pain,* salivation.
**GI:** nausea, vomiting, diarrhea.
**Respiratory:** bronchiolar spasm, *pulmonary edema.*
**Other:** diaphoresis.

## INTERACTIONS

**Drug-drug.** *Carbachol, echothiophate:* May cause additive effects. Avoid using together.
*Cyclopentolate, ophthalmic belladonna alkaloids such as atropine, scopolamine:* May decrease pilocarpine antiglaucoma effectiveness and may block mydriatic effects of these drugs. Avoid using together.
*Phenylephrine:* May decrease dilation by phenylephrine. Avoid using together.

## EFFECTS ON LAB TEST RESULTS

None reported.

## CONTRAINDICATIONS & CAUTIONS

• Contraindicated in patients hypersensitive to drug and in conditions in which cholinergic effects, such as constriction, are undesirable (acute iritis, some forms of secondary glaucoma, pupillary block glaucoma, or acute inflammatory disease of the anterior chamber).
• Use cautiously in patients with acute cardiac failure, bronchial asthma, peptic ulcer, hyperthyroidism, GI spasm, urinary tract obstruction, and Parkinson's disease.

## NURSING CONSIDERATIONS

• Monitor vital signs.
• *Alert:* Patients with dark eyes (hazel or brown irises) may need stronger solutions or more frequent instillation because eye pigment may absorb drug.

## PATIENT TEACHING

• Instruct patient to apply gel at bedtime because it will blur vision. Warn him to avoid hazardous activities, such as operating machinery or driving, until temporary blurring subsides.
• Teach patient how to instill drug. Advise him to wash hands before and after instillation and to apply light finger pressure on lacrimal sac for 1 minute after drops are instilled. Warn patient not to touch applicator tip to eye or surrounding tissue.
• Warn patient that transient brow pain and nearsightedness are common at first but usually disappear in 10 to 14 days.
• Advise patient to wear or carry medical identification at all times during therapy.

**atropine sulfate**
**cyclopentolate hydrochloride**
**epinephrine hydrochloride**
**epinephryl borate**
**homatropine hydrobromide**
**phenylephrine hydrochloride**
**scopolamine hydrobromide**

### COMBINATION PRODUCTS
CYCLOMYDRIL OPHTHALMIC: cyclopentolate hydrochloride 0.2% and phenylephrine hydrochloride 1%.
MUROCOLL-2: scopolamine hydrobromide 0.3% and phenylephrine hydrochloride 10%.
ZINCFRIN ◊: phenylephrine hydrochloride 0.12% and zinc sulfate 0.25%.

---

### atropine sulfate
Atropine 1, Atropisol, Atropt‡,
Isopto Atropine

*Pregnancy risk category C*

---

### AVAILABLE FORMS
*Ophthalmic ointment:* 1%
*Ophthalmic solution:* 0.5%, 1%, 2%

### INDICATIONS & DOSAGES
➤ **Acute iritis, uveitis**
*Adults:* Instill 1 to 2 drops up to q.i.d. or apply small strip of ointment to conjunctival sac up to t.i.d.
*Children:* 1 to 2 drops of 0.5% solution up to t.i.d. or small strip of ointment applied to conjunctival sac up to t.i.d.
➤ **Cycloplegic refraction**
*Adults:* 1 to 2 drops of 1% solution 1 hour before refraction.
*Children:* 1 to 2 drops of 0.5% solution in each eye b.i.d. for 1 to 3 days before eye examination and 1 hour before refraction.

### ACTION
A potent mydriatic and cycloplegic whose anticholinergic action leaves the pupil under unopposed adrenergic influence, causing it to dilate.

| Route | Onset | Peak | Duration |
|-------|-------|------|----------|
| Ophthalmic | Unknown | 30 min-3 hr | 7-10 days |

### ADVERSE REACTIONS
**CNS:** confusion, somnolence, headache.
**CV:** tachycardia.
**EENT:** ocular congestion with long-term use, conjunctivitis, contact dermatitis of eye, ocular edema, *blurred vision,* eye dryness, photophobia, increased intraocular pressure (IOP), transient stinging and burning, irritation, hyperemia.
**GI:** dry mouth, abdominal distention in infants.
**Skin:** dryness.

### INTERACTIONS
**Drug-lifestyle.** *Sun exposure:* May cause photophobia. Advise patient to wear sunglasses.

### EFFECTS ON LAB TEST RESULTS
None reported.

### CONTRAINDICATIONS & CAUTIONS
● Contraindicated in patients hypersensitive to drug or belladonna alkaloids and in those with glaucoma or adhesions between the iris and lens. Don't use atropine in infants age 3 months or younger because of possible link between cycloplegia and development of amblyopia.
● Use cautiously in elderly patients and in others who may have increased IOP. Excessive use in children or in certain susceptible patients, including those with spastic paralysis, brain damage, or Down syndrome, may produce systemic symptoms of atropine poisoning.

### NURSING CONSIDERATIONS
● *Alert:* Treat drops and ointment as poison (not for internal use); signs of poisoning are disorientation and confusion. Antidote of choice is physostigmine salicylate I.V. or I.M.
● Watch patient for signs and symptoms of glaucoma, including increased IOP, ocular

---

pain, headache, and progressive blurring of vision; notify prescriber if they occur.
● *Alert:* Don't confuse Atropisol with Aplisol.

**PATIENT TEACHING**
● Teach patient how to instill atropine. Advise him to wash hands before and after instillation and to apply light finger pressure on lacrimal sac for 1 minute after instillation. Warn patient not to touch tip of dropper or tube to eye or surrounding tissue.
● Warn patient to avoid hazardous activities, such as operating machinery or driving, until temporary blurring subsides.
● Advise patient to ease photophobia by wearing dark glasses or staying out of bright light.

---

## cyclopentolate hydrochloride
AK-Pentolate, Cyclogyl, Pentolair

*Pregnancy risk category C*

---

**AVAILABLE FORMS**
*Ophthalmic solution:* 0.5%, 1%, 2%

**INDICATIONS & DOSAGES**
➤ **Diagnostic procedures requiring mydriasis and cycloplegia**
*Adults:* 1 or 2 drops of 0.5%, 1%, or 2% solution into each eye; then 1 or 2 drops in 5 to 10 minutes, if needed.
*Children:* 1 drop of 0.5%, 1%, or 2% solution into each eye; then 1 drop of 0.5% or 1% solution in 5 to 10 minutes, if needed.

**ACTION**
A potent mydriatic and cycloplegic whose anticholinergic action leaves the pupil under unopposed adrenergic influence, causing it to dilate.

| Route | Onset | Peak | Duration |
|-------|-------|------|----------|
| Ophthalmic | Rapid | 30-75 min | 6-24 hr |

**ADVERSE REACTIONS**
**CNS:** irritability, confusion, somnolence, hallucinations, ataxia, *seizures,* behavioral disturbances in children.
**CV:** tachycardia.

**EENT:** eye burning on instillation, blurred vision, eye dryness, *photophobia,* ocular congestion, contact dermatitis in eye, conjunctivitis, increased intraocular pressure (IOP), transient stinging and burning, irritation, hyperemia.
**GU:** urine retention.
**Skin:** dryness.

**INTERACTIONS**
**Drug-drug.** *Carbachol, pilocarpine:* May counteract mydriatic effect. Avoid using together.
*Long-acting cholinergic antiglaucoma drugs:* May inhibit miotic actions. Avoid using together.
**Drug-lifestyle.** *Sun exposure:* May cause photophobia. Advise patient to wear sunglasses.

**EFFECTS ON LAB TEST RESULTS**
None reported.

**CONTRAINDICATIONS & CAUTIONS**
● Contraindicated in patients hypersensitive to drug or belladonna alkaloids and in those with glaucoma or adhesions between the iris and lens.
● Use with extreme caution in infants and young children.
● Don't use the combination product containing 1% phenylephrine hydrochloride in infants younger than age 1 because of risk of severe hypertension.
● Use cautiously in elderly patients and in those who may have increased IOP.

**NURSING CONSIDERATIONS**
● Drug is superior to homatropine hydrobromide and has a shorter duration of action. Physostigmine is antidote of choice.

**PATIENT TEACHING**
● Teach patient how to instill drug. Advise him to wash hands before and after instillation and to apply light finger pressure on lacrimal sac for 1 minute after instillation. Warn him not to touch tip of dropper to eye or surrounding tissue and that drug will burn when instilled.
● Warn patient to avoid hazardous activities, such as operating machinery or driving, until temporary blurring subsides.
● Advise patient to ease photophobia by wearing dark glasses.

---

## epinephrine hydrochloride
Epifrin, Glaucon

## epinephryl borate
Epinal

*Pregnancy risk category C*

### AVAILABLE FORMS
**epinephrine hydrochloride**
*Ophthalmic solution:* 0.1%, 0.5%, 1%, 2%
**epinephryl borate**
*Ophthalmic solution:* 0.5%, 1%

### INDICATIONS & DOSAGES
➤ **Open-angle glaucoma**
*Adults:* 1 or 2 drops of 1% or 2% solution
once daily or b.i.d. Adjust dosage based on
tonometric readings.

### ACTION
An adrenergic that dilates the pupil by
contracting the dilator muscle.

| Route | Onset | Peak | Duration |
|-------|-------|------|----------|
| Ophthalmic | 1 hr | 4-8 hr | 24 hr |

### ADVERSE REACTIONS
**CNS:** brow ache, headache, lightheadedness.
**CV:** palpitations, tachycardia, *arrhythmias,* hypertension.
**EENT:** corneal or conjunctival pigmentation; corneal edema with long-term use;
follicular hypertrophy; chemosis; conjunctivitis; iritis; hyperemic conjunctiva; eye
stinging, burning, tearing on instillation;
eye pain; allergic lid reaction; ocular irritation.
**Skin:** maculopapular rash.

### INTERACTIONS
**Drug-drug.** *Antihistamines (dexchlor-
pheniramine, diphenhydramine), tricyclic
antidepressants:* May increase cardiac
effects of epinephrine. Monitor patient
closely.
*Beta blockers, osmotic drugs, systemic
carbonic anhydrase inhibitors, topical
miotics:* May cause additive lowering of
intraocular pressure. Use together cautiously.
*Cardiac glycosides:* May increase risk of
arrhythmias. Monitor patient closely.

*Cyclopropane, halogenated hydrocarbons:*
May cause arrhythmias, tachycardia. Use
together cautiously, if at all.
*Local or systemic sympathomimetics:* May
have additive toxic effects. Avoid using together.
*MAO inhibitors:* May exaggerate adrenergic effects. Adjust dosage of epinephrine
carefully.

### EFFECTS ON LAB TEST RESULTS
● May increase BUN and glucose levels.
● May interfere with urinary cate-
cholamine test results.

### CONTRAINDICATIONS & CAUTIONS
● Contraindicated in patients hypersensitive to drug or sulfites and in those with
hypertensive CV disease or coronary
artery disease. Contraindicated in patients
with aphakia, in those with angle-closure
glaucoma, and in those the nature of
whose glaucoma hasn't been established.
● Use cautiously in elderly patients and in
those with diabetes mellitus, hypertension,
Parkinson's disease, hyperthyroidism, cardiac disease, cerebral arteriosclerosis, or
bronchial asthma.

### NURSING CONSIDERATIONS
● Drug can be injected into anterior chamber to produce rapid mydriasis during
cataract removal or can be used to control
local bleeding during surgery.
● *Alert:* The hydrochloride and borate formulations aren't interchangeable.
● Monitor blood pressure and other vital
signs.
● *Alert:* Don't confuse epinephrine with
ephedrine, or Glaucon with glucagon.

### PATIENT TEACHING
● Teach patient how to instill drug. Advise
him to wash hands before and after instillation and to apply light finger pressure on
lacrimal sac for 1 minute after drops are
instilled. Warn him not to touch tip of
dropper to eye or surrounding tissue.
● Urge patient to immediately report any
decrease in visual acuity.
● Advise patient not to use drug while
wearing soft contact lenses because lenses
may discolor.
● Tell patient not to use darkened solution.

---

Reactions may be *common,* uncommon, *life-threatening,* or **COMMON AND LIFE-THREATENING.**

# homatropine hydrobromide
Isopto Homatropine, Minims
Homatropine†

*Pregnancy risk category C*

**AVAILABLE FORMS**
*Ophthalmic solution:* 2%, 5%

**INDICATIONS & DOSAGES**
➤ **Cycloplegic refraction**
*Adults and children:* 1 to 2 drops into each
eye; if needed, repeat in 5 to 10 minutes
for two or three doses.
➤ **Uveitis**
*Adults and children:* 1 to 2 drops into each
eye q 3 to 4 hours.

**ACTION**
An anticholinergic that leaves the pupil
under unopposed adrenergic influence,
causing it to dilate.

| Route | Onset | Peak | Duration |
|---|---|---|---|
| Ophthalmic | Rapid | 40-60 min | 1-3 days |

**ADVERSE REACTIONS**
**CNS:** confusion, headache, somnolence,
edema.
**CV:** tachycardia.
**EENT:** eye irritation, *blurred vision, pho-
tophobia,* increased intraocular pressure
(IOP), transient stinging and burning, con-
junctivitis, vascular congestion.
**GI:** dry mouth.
**Skin:** dryness, rash.

**INTERACTIONS**
**Drug-lifestyle.** *Sun exposure:* May cause
photophobia. Advise patient to wear sunglasses.

**EFFECTS ON LAB TEST RESULTS**
None reported.

**CONTRAINDICATIONS & CAUTIONS**
● Contraindicated in patients hypersensitive to drug or other belladonna alkaloids
such as atropine and in those with glaucoma or adhesions between the iris and lens.
● Use cautiously in elderly patients, in
those in whom increased IOP may be en-
countered, and in those with cardiac disease or hypertension.

● Use only 2% solution in children.

**NURSING CONSIDERATIONS**
● Larger doses may be needed in patients
with heavily pigmented irises.
● *Alert:* Homatropine is similar to atropine
but weaker, with a shorter duration of action. Drug may produce signs or symptoms of atropine poisoning, such as severe
mouth dryness or tachycardia.

**PATIENT TEACHING**
● Teach patient how to instill drug. Advise
him to wash hands before and after instillation and to apply light finger pressure on
lacrimal sac for 1 minute after drops are
instilled.
● Warn patient not to touch tip of dropper
to eye or surrounding tissue.
● Caution patient to avoid hazardous activities, such as operating machinery or driving, until temporary blurring subsides.
● Instruct patient to ease sensitivity to sunlight by wearing dark glasses.
● Advise patient to wear or carry medical
identification during therapy.

# phenylephrine hydrochloride
AK-Dilate, AK-Nefrin
Ophthalmic ◇, Isopto Frin ◇,
Mydfrin, Neo-Synephrine,
Phenoptic, Prefrin Liquifilm ◇,
Relief ◇

*Pregnancy risk category C*

**AVAILABLE FORMS**
*Ophthalmic solution:* 0.12%, 2.5%, 10%

**INDICATIONS & DOSAGES**
➤ **Mydriasis without cycloplegia**
*Adults and children:* Instill 1 drop of 2.5%
or 10% solution before examination. May
repeat in 1 hour, p.r.n. May need to apply
topical anesthetic before use to prevent
stinging and dilution from lacrimation.
➤ **Mydriasis and vasoconstriction**
*Adults and adolescents:* 1 drop of 2.5% or
10% solution.
*Children:* 1 drop of 2.5% solution.
➤ **Chronic mydriasis**
*Adults and adolescents:* 1 drop of 2.5% or
10% solution b.i.d. or t.i.d.

*Children:* Instill 1 drop of 2.5% solution b.i.d. or t.i.d.
➤ **Posterior synechia (adhesion of iris)**
*Adults and children:* Instill 1 drop of 2.5% or 10% solution. Don't use 10% concentration in infants.
➤ **Minor eye irritations**
*Adults and children:* 1 or 2 drops of the 0.12% solution in affected eye up to q.i.d., p.r.n.

## ACTION
An adrenergic that dilates the pupil by contracting the dilator muscle.

| Route | Onset | Peak | Duration |
|-------|-------|------|----------|
| Ophthalmic | Rapid | 10-90 min | 3-7 hr |

## ADVERSE REACTIONS
**CNS:** brow ache, headache.
**CV:** *hypertension* with 10% solution, tachycardia, palpitations, PVCs, *MI.*
**EENT:** transient eye burning or stinging on instillation, blurred vision, increased intraocular pressure, keratitis, lacrimation, reactive hyperemia of eye, allergic conjunctivitis, rebound miosis.
**Skin:** pallor, dermatitis, diaphoresis.
**Other:** trembling.

## INTERACTIONS
**Drug-drug.** *Atropine (topical), cyclopentolate, homatropine, scopolamine:* May increase pupil dilation. Use together cautiously.
*Beta blockers, MAO inhibitors:* May cause arrhythmias because of increased pressor effect. Use together cautiously.
*Guanethidine:* May increase mydriatic and pressor effects of phenylephrine. Use together cautiously.
*Levodopa:* May reduce mydriatic effect of phenylephrine. Use together cautiously.
*Tricyclic antidepressants:* May increase cardiac effects of epinephrine. Use together cautiously.
**Drug-lifestyle.** *Sun exposure:* May cause photophobia. Advise patient to wear sunglasses.

## EFFECTS ON LAB TEST RESULTS
● May lower intraocular pressure in normal eyes or in open-angle glaucoma; may cause false-normal tonometry readings.

## CONTRAINDICATIONS & CAUTIONS
● Contraindicated in patients hypersensitive to drug; also contraindicated in those with angle-closure glaucoma and in those who wear soft contact lenses.
● Use cautiously in patients with marked hypertension, cardiac disorders, advanced arteriosclerotic changes, type 1 diabetes, or hyperthyroidism; in children with low body weight; and in elderly patients.

## NURSING CONSIDERATIONS
● Systemic adverse reactions are least likely with 0.12% and 2.5% solutions and most likely with 10% solution.
● *Alert:* Don't confuse Mydfrin with Midrin.

## PATIENT TEACHING
● Teach patient how to instill drug. Advise him to wash hands before and after instillation and to apply light finger pressure on lacrimal sac for 1 minute after drops are instilled. Warn him not to touch tip of dropper to eye or surrounding tissue.
● Warn patient not to exceed recommended dosage because systemic effects can result. Monitor blood pressure and pulse rate.
● Tell patient not to use brown solution or solution that contains precipitate.
● Warn patient to avoid hazardous activities, such as operating machinery or driving, until temporary blurring subsides.
● Advise patient to contact prescriber if condition persists longer than 12 hours after stopping drug.
● Advise patient to ease photophobia by wearing dark glasses.

## scopolamine hydrobromide
Isopto Hyoscine

*Pregnancy risk category NR*

## AVAILABLE FORMS
*Ophthalmic solution:* 0.25%

## INDICATIONS & DOSAGES
➤ **Cycloplegic refraction**
*Adults:* Instill 1 to 2 drops of 0.25% solution 1 hour before refraction.
*Children:* Instill 1 drop of 0.25% solution b.i.d. for 2 days before refraction.

> **Iritis, uveitis**
*Adults:* Instill 1 to 2 drops of 0.25% solution once daily to q.i.d.
*Children:* Instill 1 drop of 0.25% solution once daily to q.i.d.

## ACTION
An anticholinergic that leaves the pupil under unopposed adrenergic influence, causing it to dilate.

| Route | Onset | Peak | Duration |
|---|---|---|---|
| Ophthalmic | Rapid | 15-45 min | < 1 wk |

## ADVERSE REACTIONS
**CNS:** confusion, delirium, somnolence, acute psychotic reactions, headache, hallucinations.
**CV:** tachycardia, edema.
**EENT:** ocular congestion with prolonged use, conjunctivitis, *blurred vision,* eye dryness, increased intraocular pressure, *photophobia,* transient stinging and burning.
**GI:** dry mouth.
**Skin:** dryness, contact dermatitis.

## INTERACTIONS
**Drug-lifestyle.** *Sun exposure:* May cause photophobia. Advise patient to wear sunglasses.

## EFFECTS ON LAB TEST RESULTS
None reported.

## CONTRAINDICATIONS & CAUTIONS
• Contraindicated in patients hypersensitive to drug and in those with shallow anterior chamber, angle-closure glaucoma, or adhesions between the iris and lens; also contraindicated in children with previous severe systemic reaction to atropine.
• Use cautiously in patients with cardiac disease and in elderly patients.
• Use with extreme caution in infants and small children.

## NURSING CONSIDERATIONS
• Observe patients closely for adverse CNS effects such as disorientation and delirium.
• Drug may be used in patients sensitive to atropine because it's faster acting and has a shorter duration of action and fewer adverse reactions.

## PATIENT TEACHING
• Teach patient how to instill drug. Advise him to wash hands before and after instillation and to apply light finger pressure on lacrimal sac for 1 minute after drops are instilled. Warn him to avoid touching tip of dropper to eye or surrounding tissue.
• Warn patient to avoid hazardous activities, such as operating machinery or driving, until temporary blurring subsides.
• Advise patient to ease sun sensitivity by wearing dark glasses.
• Instruct patient to wear or carry medical identification at all times during therapy.

# 81

## Ophthalmic vasoconstrictors

**naphazoline hydrochloride**
**oxymetazoline hydrochloride**
**tetrahydrozoline hydrochloride**

### COMBINATION PRODUCTS
OPCON-A OPHTHALMIC SOLUTION ◊:
naphazoline hydrochloride 0.027% and
pheniramine maleate 0.315%.

---

### naphazoline hydrochloride
AK-Con, Albalon Liquifilm,
Allerest‡ ◊, Allergy Drops ◊, Clear
Eyes ◊, Comfort Eye Drops ◊,
Degest 2, Nafazair, Naphcon ◊,
Naphcon Forte, Optazine‡,
VasoClear ◊, Vasocon Regular,
20/20 Eye Drops ◊

*Pregnancy risk category C*

---

### AVAILABLE FORMS
*Ophthalmic solution:* 0.012% ◊,
0.02% ◊, 0.03% ◊, 0.1%

### INDICATIONS & DOSAGES
➤ **Ocular congestion, irritation, itching**
*Adults:* Instill 1 drop of 0.1% solution q
3 to 4 hours or 1 drop of 0.012% to 0.03%
solution up to q.i.d.

### ACTION
Unknown. Thought to cause vasoconstriction by local adrenergic action on the
blood vessels of the conjunctiva.

| Route | Onset | Peak | Duration |
|-------|-------|------|----------|
| Ophthalmic | 10 min | Unknown | 2-6 hr |

### ADVERSE REACTIONS
**CNS:** headache, dizziness, nervousness,
weakness.
**EENT:** transient eye stinging, pupillary
dilation, eye irritation, photophobia,
blurred vision, increased intraocular pressure, keratitis, lacrimation.
**GI:** nausea.
**Skin:** diaphoresis.

### INTERACTIONS
**Drug-drug.** *Anesthetics:* Cyclopropane
and halothane may sensitize the myocardium to sympathomimetics; local anesthetics may increase the absorption of topical
drugs. Monitor patient for increased adverse effects.
*Beta blockers:* May cause more systemic
adverse effects. Monitor patient for adverse systemic effects.
*MAO inhibitors, maprotiline, tricyclic
antidepressants:* May cause hypertensive
crisis if naphazoline is systemically absorbed. Use together cautiously.

### EFFECTS ON LAB TEST RESULTS
None reported.

### CONTRAINDICATIONS & CAUTIONS
● Contraindicated in patients hypersensitive to drug's ingredients and in those with
acute angle-closure glaucoma. Use of
0.1% solution is contraindicated in infants
and small children.
● Use cautiously in patients with hyperthyroidism, cardiac disease, hypertension, or
diabetes mellitus.

### NURSING CONSIDERATIONS
● Drug is most widely used ocular decon-
gestant.
● Store drug in tightly closed container.

### PATIENT TEACHING
● Teach patient how to instill drug. Advise
him to wash hands before and after instillation and to apply light finger pressure on
lacrimal sac for 1 minute after drops are
instilled. Warn him not to touch tip of
dropper to eye or surrounding tissue.
● Warn patient not to exceed recommended dosage. Rebound congestion and
conjunctivitis may occur with frequent or
prolonged use.
● Tell patient to notify prescriber if sun
sensitivity, blurred vision, pain, or lid
swelling develops.
● Instruct patient not to use OTC preparations longer than 72 hours without consulting prescriber.

Reactions may be *common*, uncommon, *life-threatening*, or **COMMON AND LIFE-THREATENING**.

# oxymetazoline hydrochloride
OcuClear ◇ , Visine L.R. ◇

*Pregnancy risk category C*

## AVAILABLE FORMS
*Ophthalmic solution:* 0.025%

## INDICATIONS & DOSAGES
➤ **Relief from eye redness caused by minor eye irritation**
*Adults and children age 6 and older:* Instill 1 to 2 drops in affected eye q 6 hours, p.r.n.

## ACTION
A direct-acting sympathomimetic amine that acts on alpha-adrenergic receptors in the arterioles of the conjunctiva to produce vasoconstriction, resulting in decreased conjunctival congestion.

| Route | Onset | Peak | Duration |
|-------|-------|------|----------|
| Ophthalmic | 5 min | Unknown | 6 hr |

## ADVERSE REACTIONS
**CNS:** headache, light-headedness, nervousness, insomnia.
**CV:** palpitations, tachycardia, irregular heartbeat.
**EENT:** *transient stinging on first instillation,* blurred vision, keratitis, lacrimation, increased intraocular pressure, reactive hyperemia with excessive doses or prolonged use.
**Other:** trembling.

## INTERACTIONS
**Drug-drug.** *Anesthetics:* Cyclopropane and halothane may sensitize the myocardium to sympathomimetics; local anesthetics may increase the absorption of topical drugs. Monitor patient for increased adverse effects.
*Beta blockers:* May cause more systemic adverse effects. Monitor patient for adverse systemic effects.
*MAO inhibitors, maprotiline, tricyclic antidepressants:* If significant systemic absorption of oxymetazoline occurs, use together may increase pressor effect of oxymetazoline. Avoid using together.

## EFFECTS ON LAB TEST RESULTS
None reported.

## CONTRAINDICATIONS & CAUTIONS
• Contraindicated in patients hypersensitive to drug or its components and in those with angle-closure glaucoma.
• Use cautiously in patients with hyperthyroidism, cardiac disease, hypertension, and eye disease, infection, or injury.

## NURSING CONSIDERATIONS
• Don't use if solution has become cloudy or changes color.
• *Alert:* Don't confuse Visine with Visken.

## PATIENT TEACHING
• Teach patient how to instill drops. Advise him to wash hands before and after instillation, and warn him not to touch tip of dropper to eye or surrounding tissue.
• Instruct patient to apply light finger pressure on lacrimal sac for 1 minute after drug instillation.
• Advise patient to stop drug and consult prescriber if eye pain occurs, if vision changes, or if redness or irritation continues, worsens, or lasts for longer than 72 hours.

# tetrahydrozoline hydrochloride
Collyrium Fresh ◇ , Eyesine ◇ , Geneye ◇ , Murine Plus ◇ , Optigene 3 ◇ , Tetrasine ◇ , Visine Moisturizing ◇

*Pregnancy risk category C*

## AVAILABLE FORMS
*Ophthalmic solution:* 0.05% ◇

## INDICATIONS & DOSAGES
➤ **Conjunctival congestion, irritation, and allergic conditions**
*Adults and children older than age 2:* Instill 1 to 2 drops of 0.05% solution up to q.i.d. or as directed by prescriber.

## ACTION
Unknown. Thought to cause vasoconstriction by local adrenergic action on the blood vessels of the conjunctiva.

| Route | Onset | Peak | Duration |
|-------|-------|------|----------|
| Ophthalmic | Few min | Unknown | 1-4 hr |

## ADVERSE REACTIONS
**CNS:** headache, drowsiness, insomnia, dizziness, tremor.
**CV:** *arrhythmias.*
**EENT:** transient eye stinging, pupillary dilation, increased intraocular pressure, keratitis, lacrimation, eye irritation.

## INTERACTIONS
**Drug-drug.** *Anesthetics:* Cyclopropane and halothane may sensitize the myocardium to sympathomimetics; local anesthetics may increase the absorption of topical drugs. Monitor patient for increased adverse effects.
*Beta blockers:* May cause more systemic adverse effects. Monitor patient for adverse systemic effects.
*Guanethidine, MAO inhibitors, tricyclic antidepressants:* May cause hypertensive crisis if tetrahydrozoline is systemically absorbed. Avoid using together.

## EFFECTS ON LAB TEST RESULTS
None reported.

## CONTRAINDICATIONS & CAUTIONS
• Contraindicated in patients hypersensitive to drug or its components and in those with angle-closure glaucoma or other serious eye disease.
• Use cautiously in patients with hyperthyroidism, heart disease, hypertension, or diabetes mellitus.

## NURSING CONSIDERATIONS
• Rebound congestion may occur with frequent or prolonged use.
• *Alert:* Don't confuse Visine with Visken.

## PATIENT TEACHING
• Teach patient how to instill drug. Advise him to wash hands before and after instillation and to apply light finger pressure on lacrimal sac for 1 minute after drops are instilled. Warn him not to touch tip of dropper to eye or surrounding tissue.
• Warn patient not to exceed recommended dosage.
• Tell patient to stop drug and notify prescriber if redness or irritation persists or increases or if no relief occurs within 2 days.
• Warn patient not to share ophthalmic drugs.

---

Reactions may be *common*, uncommon, *life-threatening*, or COMMON AND LIFE-THREATENING.

**azelastine hydrochloride**
**betaxolol hydrochloride**
**bimatoprost**
**brimonidine tartrate**
**carteolol hydrochloride**
**dorzolamide hydrochloride**
**epinastine hydrochloride**
**ketotifen fumarate**
**latanoprost**
**levobunolol hydrochloride**
**sodium chloride, hypertonic**
**timolol maleate**
**travoprost**
**unoprostone isopropyl**

**COMBINATION PRODUCTS**
None.

---

## azelastine hydrochloride
Optivar

*Pregnancy risk category C*

**AVAILABLE FORMS**
*Ophthalmic solution:* 0.05%

**INDICATIONS & DOSAGES**
➤ **Itching of the eye with allergic conjunctivitis**
*Adults and children age 3 and older:* Instill 1 drop into affected eye b.i.d.

**ACTION**
Inhibits the release of histamine and other mediators from cells involved in the allergic response.

| Route | Onset | Peak | Duration |
|-------|-------|------|----------|
| Ophthalmic | 3 min | Unknown | 8 hr |

**ADVERSE REACTIONS**
**CNS:** fatigue, *headache.*
**EENT:** *transient eye burning or stinging, bitter taste,* conjunctivitis, eye pain, pharyngitis, rhinitis, temporary blurring.
**Respiratory:** asthma, dyspnea.
**Skin:** pruritus.
**Other:** flulike syndrome.

**INTERACTIONS**
None reported.

**EFFECTS ON LAB TEST RESULTS**
None reported.

**CONTRAINDICATIONS & CAUTIONS**
● Contraindicated in patients hypersensitive to any of drug's components.
● Contraindicated for irritation related to contact lenses.

**NURSING CONSIDERATIONS**
● Drug is for ophthalmic use only. Don't inject or give orally.
● Soft contacts may absorb the preservative benzalkonium.

**PATIENT TEACHING**
● Instruct patient not to touch any surface, eyelid, or surrounding areas with tip of dropper.
● Tell patient to keep bottle tightly closed when not in use.
● Advise patient not to wear contact lens if eye is red.
● Warn patient that soft contact lenses may absorb the preservative benzalkonium.
● Instruct patient who wears soft contact lenses and whose eyes aren't red to wait at least 10 minutes after instilling drug before inserting contact lenses.

---

## betaxolol hydrochloride
Betoptic, Betoptic S

*Pregnancy risk category C*

**AVAILABLE FORMS**
*Ophthalmic solution:* 0.5%
*Ophthalmic suspension:* 0.25%

**INDICATIONS & DOSAGES**
➤ **Chronic open-angle glaucoma, ocular hypertension**
*Adults:* Instill 1 or 2 drops of 0.5% solution or 0.25% suspension b.i.d.

---

## ACTION

Unknown. A cardioselective beta blocker that reduces aqueous formation and may increase outflow of aqueous humor.

| Route | Onset | Peak | Duration |
|---|---|---|---|
| Ophthalmic | 30-60 min | 2 hr | > 12 hr |

## ADVERSE REACTIONS

**CNS:** insomnia, *CVA,* depressive neurosis.
**CV:** *arrhythmias, heart block, heart failure,* palpitations.
**EENT:** *eye stinging on instillation causing brief discomfort,* photophobia, erythema, itching, keratitis, occasional tearing.
**Respiratory:** asthma, *bronchospasm.*

## INTERACTIONS

**Drug-drug.** *Calcium channel blockers:* May cause AV conduction disturbances, ventricular failure, and hypotension if significant systemic absorption occurs. Monitor patient closely.
*Cardiac glycosides:* May cause excessive bradycardia. Patient may need ECG monitoring if significant systemic absorption occurs.
*Dipivefrin, ophthalmic epinephrine:* May produce mydriasis. Use together cautiously.
*Inhaled hydrocarbon anesthetics:* May prolong severe hypotension if significant systemic absorption occurs. Tell anesthesiologist that patient is receiving ophthalmic betaxolol.
*Insulin, oral antidiabetics:* May cause hypoglycemia or hyperglycemia if significant systemic absorption occurs. May need to adjust dosage of antidiabetics.
*Phenothiazines:* May have additive hypotensive effects; may increase risk of adverse effects if significant systemic absorption occurs. Monitor patient closely.
*Prazosin:* May increase risk of orthostatic hypotension in early phases of use together. Assist patient to stand slowly until effects are known.
*Reserpine:* May cause excessive beta blockade. Monitor patient closely.
*Systemic beta blockers:* May have additive effects. Monitor patient closely.
*Verapamil:* May increase effects of both drugs. Monitor cardiac function closely and decrease dosages as necessary.

**Drug-lifestyle.** *Cocaine use:* May inhibit betaxolol's effects. Tell patient about this interaction.
*Sun exposure:* May cause photophobia. Advise patient to wear sunglasses.

## EFFECTS ON LAB TEST RESULTS

None reported.

## CONTRAINDICATIONS & CAUTIONS

• Contraindicated in patients hypersensitive to drug and in those with sinus bradycardia, greater than first-degree AV block, cardiogenic shock, or overt heart failure.
• Use cautiously in patients with restricted pulmonary function, diabetes mellitus, hyperthyroidism, or history of heart failure.

## NURSING CONSIDERATIONS

• Stabilization of intraocular pressure (IOP)–lowering response may take a few weeks. Determine IOP after 4 weeks of treatment.

## PATIENT TEACHING

• Teach patient how to instill drug. Advise him to wash hands before and after instillation and to apply light finger pressure on lacrimal sac for 1 minute after instilling drug. Warn him not to touch tip of dropper to eye or surrounding tissue. Tell him to shake suspension well before instilling.
• Encourage patient to comply with b.i.d. regimen.
• Tell patient to remove contact lenses before instilling drug. Lenses may be reinserted about 15 minutes after using drops.
• Advise patient to ease sun sensitivity by wearing sunglasses.
• Tell patient to avoid using other eye products with drug.

# bimatoprost
Lumigan

*Pregnancy risk category C*

## AVAILABLE FORMS

*Ophthalmic solution:* 0.03%

## INDICATIONS & DOSAGES

➤ **Increased intraocular pressure (IOP) in patients with open-angle glaucoma or ocular hypertension who can't toler-**

**ate or are unresponsive to other IOP-lowering drugs**
*Adults:* Instill 1 drop in conjunctival sac of affected eye once daily in the evening.

**ACTION**
Synthetic analogue of prostaglandin with ocular hypotensive activity, which selectively mimics the effects of naturally occurring prostaglandins. Drug is believed to lower IOP by increasing outflow of aqueous humor.

| Route | Onset | Peak | Duration |
|-------|-------|------|----------|
| Ophthalmic | 4 hr | 8-12 hr | Unknown |

**ADVERSE REACTIONS**
**CNS:** headache, asthenia.
**EENT:** *conjunctival hyperemia, growth of eyelashes, ocular pruritus,* ocular dryness, visual disturbance, ocular burning, foreign body sensation, eye pain, pigmentation of the periocular skin, blepharitis, cataract, superficial punctate keratitis, eyelid erythema, ocular irritation, eyelash darkening, eye discharge, tearing, photophobia, allergic conjunctivitis, asthenopia, increase in iris pigmentation, conjunctival edema.
**Respiratory:** *upper respiratory tract infection.*
**Skin:** hirsutism.
**Other:** *infection.*

**INTERACTIONS**
**Drug-herb.** *Areca, jaborandi:* May have additive IOP-lowering effects. Discourage use together.

**EFFECTS ON LAB TEST RESULTS**
• May cause abnormal liver function test values.

**CONTRAINDICATIONS & CAUTIONS**
• Contraindicated in patients hypersensitive to bimatoprost, benzalkonium chloride, or other ingredients in product.
• Contraindicated in patients with angle-closure glaucoma or inflammatory or neovascular glaucoma.
• Use cautiously in patients with renal or hepatic impairment.
• Use cautiously in patients with active intraocular inflammation (iritis, uveitis), aphakic patients, and pseudophakic pa-

tients with torn posterior lens capsule, and in patients at risk for macular edema.

**NURSING CONSIDERATIONS**
• Temporary or permanent increased pigmentation of iris and eyelid, as well as increased pigmentation and growth of eyelashes, may occur.
• Patient should remove contact lenses before using solution. Lenses may be reinserted 15 minutes after administration.
• If more than one ophthalmic drug is being used, give drugs at least 5 minutes apart.
• Store drug in original container between 59° and 77° F (15° and 25° C).

**PATIENT TEACHING**
• Tell patient receiving treatment in only one eye about potential for increased brown pigmentation of iris, eyelid skin darkening, and increased length, thickness, pigmentation, or number of lashes in treated eye.
• Teach patient how to instill drops, and advise him to wash hands before and after instilling solution. Warn him not to touch tip of dropper to eye or surrounding tissue.
• If eye trauma or infection occurs or if eye surgery is needed, tell patient to seek medical advice before continuing to use multidose container.
• Advise patient to immediately report eye inflammation or lid reactions.
• Advise patient to apply light pressure on lacrimal sac for 1 minute after instillation to minimize systemic absorption of drug.
• Tell patient to remove contact lenses before using solution and that lenses may be reinserted 15 minutes after administration.
• If patient is using more than one ophthalmic drug, tell him to apply them at least 5 minutes apart.
• Stress importance of compliance with recommended therapy.

---

**brimonidine tartrate**
Alphagan P

*Pregnancy risk category B*

**AVAILABLE FORMS**
*Ophthalmic solution:* 0.15% in 5-,10-, or 15-ml bottles

---

## INDICATIONS & DOSAGES
➤ **To reduce intraocular pressure (IOP) in open-angle glaucoma or ocular hypertension**
*Adults:* 1 drop in affected eye t.i.d., about 8 hours apart.

## ACTION
A selective alpha$_2$-adrenergic agonist that reduces aqueous humor production and increases uveoscleral outflow.

| Route | Onset | Peak | Duration |
|-------|-------|------|----------|
| Ophthalmic | Unknown | 30 min–2½ hr | Unknown |

## ADVERSE REACTIONS
**CNS:** asthenia, dizziness, headache.
**CV:** hypertension.
**EENT:** *ocular hyperemia, allergic conjunctivitis,* allergic reaction, *pruritus,* burning, stinging, follicular conjunctivitis, abnormal vision, blepharitis, conjunctival edema or hemorrhage, conjunctivitis, increased tearing, dryness, pain, eyelid edema or erythema, foreign body sensation, pharyngitis, rhinitis, sinus infection, sinusitis, photophobia, superficial punctate keratopathy, visual field defect, vitreous floaters, worsened visual acuity.
**GI:** oral dryness, dyspepsia.
**Respiratory:** bronchitis, cough, dyspnea.
**Skin:** rash.
**Other:** flulike syndrome.

## INTERACTIONS
**Drug-drug.** *Antihypertensives, beta blockers, cardiac glycosides:* May further decrease blood pressure or pulse. Monitor vital signs.
*CNS depressants:* May increase effects. Use cautiously together.
*MAO inhibitors:* May increase effects. Avoid use together.
*Tricyclic antidepressants:* May interfere with brimonidine's IOP-lowering effects. Use cautiously together.
**Drug-lifestyle.** *Alcohol use:* May increase CNS depressant effect. Urge patient to avoid alcohol.

## EFFECTS ON LAB TEST RESULTS
None reported.

## CONTRAINDICATIONS & CAUTIONS
● Contraindicated in patients hypersensitive to drug or benzalkonium chloride and in those receiving MAO inhibitor therapy.
● Use cautiously in patients with CV disease, cerebral or coronary insufficiency, hepatic or renal impairment, depression, Raynaud's phenomenon, orthostatic hypotension, or thromboangiitis obliterans.

## NURSING CONSIDERATIONS
● Monitor IOP because drug effect may reverse after first month of therapy.

## PATIENT TEACHING
● Tell patient to wait at least 15 minutes after instilling drug before wearing soft contact lenses.
● Caution patient to avoid hazardous activities because of risk of decreased mental alertness, fatigue, or drowsiness.
● Advise patient to avoid alcohol.

# carteolol hydrochloride
Ocupress

*Pregnancy risk category C*

## AVAILABLE FORMS
*Ophthalmic solution:* 1%

## INDICATIONS & DOSAGES
➤ **Chronic open-angle glaucoma, intraocular hypertension**
*Adults:* 1 drop into conjunctival sac of affected eye b.i.d.

## ACTION
Exact mechanism unknown. A nonselective beta blocker that reduces intraocular pressure (IOP) by decreasing aqueous humor production.

| Route | Onset | Peak | Duration |
|-------|-------|------|----------|
| Ophthalmic | Unknown | 2 hr | 12 hr |

## ADVERSE REACTIONS
**CNS:** headache, dizziness, insomnia, asthenia.
**CV:** *bradycardia,* hypotension, *arrhythmias,* palpitations.
**EENT:** *transient eye irritation, burning, tearing, conjunctival hyperemia, ocular*

*edema,* blurred and cloudy vision, photophobia, decreased night vision, ptosis, blepharoconjunctivitis, abnormal corneal staining, corneal sensitivity, sinusitis.
**GI:** taste perversion.
**Respiratory:** dyspnea.

### INTERACTIONS

**Drug-drug.** *Aminophylline, theophylline:* May act antagonistically, reducing the effects of one or both drugs. Elimination of theophylline may also be reduced. Monitor theophylline levels and patient closely.
*Catecholamine-depleting drugs such as reserpine, oral beta blockers:* May cause additive effects and development of hypotension or bradycardia. Monitor patient closely; monitor vital signs.
*Epinephrine:* May cause an initial hypertensive episode followed by bradycardia. Stop beta blocker 3 days before anticipated epinephrine use. Monitor patient closely.
*Insulin:* May mask symptoms of hypoglycemia as a result of beta blockade (such as tachycardia). Use together with extreme caution in patients with diabetes.
*Prazosin:* May increase risk of orthostatic hypotension in early phases of use together. Assist patient to stand slowly until effects are known.
*Verapamil:* May increase effects of both drugs. Monitor cardiac function closely and decrease dosages as necessary.
**Drug-lifestyle.** *Sun exposure:* May cause photophobia. Advise patient to wear sunglasses.

### EFFECTS ON LAB TEST RESULTS
None reported.

### CONTRAINDICATIONS & CAUTIONS
• Contraindicated in patients hypersensitive to drug or its components and in those with bronchial asthma, severe COPD, sinus bradycardia, second- or third-degree AV block, overt cardiac failure, or cardiogenic shock.
• Use cautiously in patients hypersensitive to other beta blockers; in those with nonallergic bronchospastic disease, diabetes mellitus, hyperthyroidism, or decreased pulmonary function; and in breast-feeding women.

### NURSING CONSIDERATIONS
• Monitor vital signs.
• *Alert:* Stop drug at first sign of cardiac failure, and notify prescriber.

### PATIENT TEACHING
• If patient is using more than one topical ophthalmic drug, tell him to apply them at least 10 minutes apart.
• Teach patient how to instill drops. Advise him to wash hands before and after instillation, and warn him not to touch tip of dropper to eye or surrounding tissue.
• Advise patient to apply light finger pressure on lacrimal sac for 1 minute after drug instillation to minimize systemic absorption.
• Tell patient to remove contact lenses before instilling drug.
• Instruct patient to keep bottle tightly closed when not in use and to protect it from light.
• Tell patient that drug is a beta blocker and, although given topically, has the potential to be absorbed systemically.
• Inform patient that adverse reactions from beta blockers can occur with topical administration. Advise him to stop drug and notify prescriber immediately if signs or symptoms of serious adverse reactions or hypersensitivity occur.
• Advise patient to monitor heart rate and blood pressure closely and to report slow heart rate to prescriber.
• Stress importance of compliance with recommended therapy.
• Advise patient to ease sun sensitivity by wearing sunglasses.

## dorzolamide hydrochloride
Trusopt

*Pregnancy risk category C*

### AVAILABLE FORMS
*Ophthalmic solution:* 2%

### INDICATIONS & DOSAGES
➤ **Increased intraocular pressure (IOP) in patients with ocular hypertension or open-angle glaucoma**
*Adults:* 1 drop into conjunctival sac of affected eye t.i.d.

## ACTION
Inhibits carbonic anhydrase in the ciliary processes of the eye, which decreases aqueous humor secretion, presumably by slowing the formation of bicarbonate ions. This reduces sodium and fluid transport, reducing IOP.

| Route | Onset | Peak | Duration |
|-------|-------|------|----------|
| Ophthalmic | Unknown | Unknown | Unknown |

## ADVERSE REACTIONS
**CNS:** headache, asthenia, fatigue.
**EENT:** *ocular burning, stinging, and discomfort; superficial punctate keratitis; ocular allergic reaction; blurred vision; lacrimation; dryness; photophobia;* iridocyclitis.
**GI:** nausea, *bitter taste.*
**GU:** urolithiasis.
**Skin:** rash.

## INTERACTIONS
**Drug-drug.** *Oral carbonic anhydrase inhibitors:* May cause additive effects. Avoid using together.

## EFFECTS ON LAB TEST RESULTS
None reported.

## CONTRAINDICATIONS & CAUTIONS
• Contraindicated in patients hypersensitive to drug or its components.
• Use cautiously in patients with hepatic or renal impairment.

## NURSING CONSIDERATIONS
• If more than one topical ophthalmic drug is used, give drugs at least 10 minutes apart.

## PATIENT TEACHING
• Teach patient how to instill drops. Advise him to wash hands before and after instillation, and warn him not to touch tip of dropper to eye or surrounding tissue.
• Tell patient that drug is a sulfonamide and, although it's given topically, it can be absorbed systemically. Advise patient to apply light finger pressure on lacrimal sac for 1 minute after drug instillation to minimize systemic absorption.
• Tell patient that adverse reactions may occur with topical administration. Tell him to stop drug and notify prescriber immedi-

ately if signs or symptoms of serious adverse reactions or hypersensitivity occur.
• Advise patient to stop drug and notify prescriber if adverse reactions occur, particularly eye inflammation and eyelid reactions.
• Tell patient not to wear soft contact lenses during therapy.
• Stress importance of compliance with recommended therapy.

❋ *NEW DRUG*

# epinastine hydrochloride
Elestat

*Pregnancy risk category C*

## AVAILABLE FORMS
*Ophthalmic solution:* 0.05% in 5- and 10-ml bottles

## INDICATIONS & DOSAGES
➤ **To prevent itching from allergic conjunctivitis**
*Adults and children age 3 and older:* Instill 1 drop into each eye b.i.d. Continue treatment as long as allergen is present, even if symptoms resolve.

## ACTION
Antagonizes $H_1$-receptors and stabilizes mast cells to inhibit release of mediators from cells involved in hypersensitivity reactions, thus temporarily preventing eye itching.

| Route | Onset | Peak | Duration |
|-------|-------|------|----------|
| Ophthalmic | Immediate | Unknown | 8 hr |

## ADVERSE REACTIONS
**CNS:** headache
**EENT:** burning eyes, hyperemia, increased lymph nodes near eyes, *cold symptoms,* pharyngitis, pruritus, rhinitis, sinusitis.
**Respiratory:** increased cough, *upper respiratory tract infection.*

## INTERACTIONS
None reported.

## EFFECTS ON LAB TEST RESULTS
None reported.

---

Reactions may be *common*, uncommon, *life-threatening*, or COMMON AND LIFE-THREATENING.

**CONTRAINDICATIONS & CAUTIONS**
• Contraindicated in patients hypersensitive to drug or its components.
• Contraindicated for irritation related to contact lenses.
• Use cautiously in pregnant or breast-feeding women.
• Safety and effectiveness haven't been established in children younger than age 3.

**NURSING CONSIDERATIONS**
• Drug is for ophthalmic use only. Don't inject or give orally.
• Monitor patient for signs and symptoms of infection.
• Soft contact lenses may absorb the preservative benzalkonium.

**PATIENT TEACHING**
• Teach patient proper instillation technique. Instruct him not to touch any surface, eyelid, or surrounding areas with tip of dropper.
• Caution patient not to use drops to treat contact lens–related eye irritation and not to wear contact lenses if eyes are red.
• Warn patient that soft contact lenses may absorb the preservative benzalkonium.
• Advise patient to report adverse reactions to drug.
• Tell patient to keep bottle tightly closed when not in use.
• Instruct patient who wears soft contact lenses and whose eyes aren't red to wait at least 10 minutes after instilling drug before inserting contact lenses.

---

**ketotifen fumarate**
Zaditor

*Pregnancy risk category C*

**AVAILABLE FORMS**
*Ophthalmic solution:* 0.025%

**INDICATIONS & DOSAGES**
➤ **To temporarily prevent eye itching from allergic conjunctivitis**
*Adults and children age 4 and older:* Instill 1 drop in affected eye q 8 to 12 hours.

**ACTION**
Stabilizes mast cells to inhibit release of mediators involved in hypersensitivity re-

actions and blocks action of histamine at the $H_1$ receptor, temporarily preventing itching of the eye.

| Route | Onset | Peak | Duration |
|-------|-------|------|----------|
| Ophthalmic | Within min | Unknown | Unknown |

**ADVERSE REACTIONS**
**CNS:** *headache.*
**EENT:** *conjunctival infection, rhinitis,* ocular allergic reactions, burning or stinging of eyes, conjunctivitis, eye discharge, dry eyes, eye pain, eyelid disorder, itching of eyes, keratitis, lacrimation disorder, mydriasis, photophobia, ocular rash, pharyngitis.
**Other:** flulike syndrome.

**INTERACTIONS**
None significant.

**EFFECTS ON LAB TEST RESULTS**
None reported.

**CONTRAINDICATIONS & CAUTIONS**
• Contraindicated in patients hypersensitive to components of drug.
• Contraindicated for irritation related to contact lenses.

**NURSING CONSIDERATIONS**
• Drug is for ophthalmic use only. Don't inject or give orally.
• Drug isn't indicated for irritation related to contact lenses.
• Soft contact lenses may absorb the preservative benzalkonium. Contact lenses shouldn't be inserted until 10 minutes after drug is instilled.
• To prevent contaminating dropper tip and solution, don't touch eyelids or surrounding areas with dropper tip of bottle.

**PATIENT TEACHING**
• Teach patient the proper technique for instilling drops.
• Advise patient not to wear contact lens if eye is red. Warn him not to use drug to treat contact lens–related irritation.
• Instruct patient who wears soft contact lenses and whose eyes aren't red to wait at least 10 minutes after instilling drug before inserting contact lenses.
• Advise patient to report adverse reactions.

• Advise patient to keep bottle tightly closed when not in use.

---

## latanoprost
Xalatan

*Pregnancy risk category C*

### AVAILABLE FORMS
*Ophthalmic solution:* 0.005% (50 mcg/ml)

### INDICATIONS & DOSAGES
➤ **First-line treatment of increased intraocular pressure (IOP) in patients with ocular hypertension or open-angle glaucoma**
*Adults:* Instill 1 drop in conjunctival sac of affected eyes once daily h.s.

### ACTION
A prostaglandin $F_2$ alpha-analogue believed to increase outflow of aqueous humor, thereby lowering IOP.

| Route | Onset | Peak | Duration |
|-------|-------|------|----------|
| Ophthalmic | 3-4 hr | 8-12 hr | Unknown |

### ADVERSE REACTIONS
**CV:** angina pectoris.
**EENT:** *blurred vision, burning, stinging,* conjunctival hyperemia, *foreign body sensation, itching, increased brown pigmentation of the iris,* dry eye, punctate epithelial keratopathy, lid crusting or edema, lid discomfort, excessive tearing, eye pain, photophobia, eyelash changes.
**Musculoskeletal:** muscle, joint, or back pain.
**Respiratory:** upper respiratory tract infection.
**Skin:** rash, allergic skin reaction.
**Other:** cold, flulike syndrome.

### INTERACTIONS
**Drug-drug.** *Eyedrops that contain thimerosal:* May cause precipitation of eyedrops. Give at least 5 minutes apart.

### EFFECTS ON LAB TEST RESULTS
None reported.

### CONTRAINDICATIONS & CAUTIONS
• Contraindicated in patients hypersensitive to drug, benzalkonium chloride, or other components of drug.
• Use cautiously in patients with impaired renal or hepatic function.
• It's unknown whether drug appears in breast milk; use cautiously in breast-feeding women.
• Safety and efficacy of drug in children haven't been established.

### NURSING CONSIDERATIONS
• Don't give drug while patient is wearing contact lenses.
• Giving drug more frequently than recommended may decrease its IOP-lowering effects.
• Drug may gradually change eye color, increasing amount of brown pigment in iris. This change in iris color occurs slowly and may not be noticeable for months or years. Increased pigmentation may be permanent.
• To avoid ocular infections, don't allow tip of dispenser to contact eye or surrounding tissue. Serious damage to eye and subsequent vision loss may be caused by contaminated solutions.

### PATIENT TEACHING
• Inform patient of risk that iris color may change in treated eye.
• Teach patient how to instill drops, and advise him to wash hands before and after instilling solution. Warn him not to touch tip of dropper to eye or surrounding tissue.
• Advise patient to apply light finger pressure on lacrimal sac for 1 minute after instillation to minimize systemic absorption.
• Instruct patient to report reactions in the eye, especially eye inflammation and lid reactions.
• Tell patient who wears contact lenses to remove them before instilling solution and not to reinsert the lenses until 15 minutes have elapsed.
• If patient is using more than one topical ophthalmic drug, tell him to apply them at least 5 minutes apart.
• If patient develops another eye condition (such as trauma or infection) or needs eye surgery, advise him to contact prescriber

---

Reactions may be *common*, uncommon, *life-threatening*, or **COMMON AND LIFE-THREATENING**.

about continued use of multidose container.
• Stress importance of compliance with recommended therapy.

---

## levobunolol hydrochloride
AKBeta, Betagan

*Pregnancy risk category C*

### AVAILABLE FORMS
*Ophthalmic solution:* 0.25%, 0.5%

### INDICATIONS & DOSAGES
➤ **Chronic open-angle glaucoma, ocular hypertension**
*Adults:* 1 to 2 drops once daily (0.5%) or b.i.d. (0.25%).

### ACTION
Unknown. A nonselective beta blocker thought to reduce formation, and possibly increase outflow, of aqueous humor.

| Route | Onset | Peak | Duration |
|-------|-------|------|----------|
| Ophthalmic | 1 hr | 2-6 hr | 24 hr |

### ADVERSE REACTIONS
**CNS:** headache, depression, insomnia, *syncope.*
**CV:** slight reduction in resting heart rate, *hypotension,* **bradycardia, heart failure.**
**EENT:** *transient eye stinging and burning,* tearing, erythema, itching, keratitis, corneal punctate staining, photophobia, decreased corneal sensitivity, blepharoconjunctivitis.
**GI:** nausea.
**Respiratory:** *bronchospasm.*
**Skin:** urticaria.

### INTERACTIONS
**Drug-drug.** *Dipivefrin, epinephrine, systemically administered carbonic anhydrase inhibitors, topical miotics:* May further reduce intraocular pressure (IOP). Use together cautiously.
*Metoprolol, propranolol, other oral beta blockers:* May increase ocular and systemic effects. Use together cautiously.
*Reserpine, other catecholamine-depleting drugs:* May increase hypotensive and

bradycardiac effects. Monitor blood pressure and heart rate closely.
**Drug-lifestyle.** *Sun exposure:* May cause photophobia. Advise patient to wear sunglasses.

### EFFECTS ON LAB TEST RESULTS
None reported.

### CONTRAINDICATIONS & CAUTIONS
• Contraindicated in patients hypersensitive to drug and in those with bronchial asthma, sinus bradycardia, second- or third-degree AV block, cardiac failure, cardiogenic shock, or history of bronchial asthma or severe COPD.
• Use cautiously in patients with chronic bronchitis, emphysema, diabetes mellitus, hyperthyroidism, or myasthenia gravis.
• Safe use in pregnant or breast-feeding women hasn't been established.

### NURSING CONSIDERATIONS
• Don't let tip of dropper touch patient's eye or surrounding tissue.

### PATIENT TEACHING
• Teach patient how to instill drug. Advise him to wash hands before and after instillation and to apply light finger pressure on lacrimal sac for 1 minute after drops are instilled.
• Warn patient not to touch tip of dropper to eye or surrounding tissue.
• Advise elderly patient to report shortness of breath, chest pain, or heart irregularities to prescriber. Drug may be absorbed systemically and produce signs and symptoms of beta blockade.
• Advise patient to wear or carry medical identification at all times during therapy.

---

## sodium chloride, hypertonic
Adsorbonac, AK-NaCl, Muro 128, Muroptic-5

*Pregnancy risk category NR*

### AVAILABLE FORMS
*Ophthalmic ointment:* 5%
*Ophthalmic solution:* 2%, 5%

---

## INDICATIONS & DOSAGES
➤ **To temporarily relieve corneal edema**
*Adults and children:* Apply 1 to 2 drops of solution or ¼ inch (6 mm) of ointment q 3 to 4 hours.

## ACTION
An osmotic that removes excess fluid from cornea.

| Route | Onset | Peak | Duration |
|---|---|---|---|
| Ophthalmic | Unknown | Unknown | Unknown |

## ADVERSE REACTIONS
**EENT:** slight eye stinging.
**Other:** hypersensitivity reactions.

## INTERACTIONS
None significant.

## EFFECTS ON LAB TEST RESULTS
None reported.

## CONTRAINDICATIONS & CAUTIONS
• Contraindicated in patients hypersensitive to drug or its components.

## NURSING CONSIDERATIONS
• Drug is for ophthalmic use only. Don't inject or give orally.
• Check expiration date before use.

## PATIENT TEACHING
• Teach patient how to instill drug. Advise him to wash hands before and after instillation and to apply light finger pressure on lacrimal sac for 1 minute after drops are instilled. Warn patient not to touch dropper to eye or surrounding tissue.
• Tell patient to prevent caking on dropper bottle tip by putting a few drops of sterile irrigation solution inside bottle cap.
• Warn patient that ointment may cause blurred vision.
• If patient experiences severe headache, pain, rapid change in vision, acute redness of eyes, sudden appearance of floating spots, pain on exposure to light, or double vision, tell him to stop drug and notify prescriber.
• Advise patient to store drug in tightly closed container.

# timolol maleate
Betimol, Timoptic, Timoptic-XE

*Pregnancy risk category C*

## AVAILABLE FORMS
*Ophthalmic gel:* 0.25%, 0.5%
*Ophthalmic solution:* 0.25%, 0.5%

## INDICATIONS & DOSAGES
➤ **To reduce intraocular pressure (IOP) in ocular hypertension or open-angle glaucoma**
*Adults:* Initially, 1 drop of 0.25% solution in each affected eye b.i.d.; maintenance dosage is 1 drop once daily. If no response, instill 1 drop of 0.5% solution in each affected eye b.i.d. If IOP is controlled, reduce dosage to 1 drop daily. Or, 1 drop of gel in each affected eye once daily.

## ACTION
Unknown. A beta blocker thought to reduce formation, and possibly increase outflow, of aqueous humor.

| Route | Onset | Peak | Duration |
|---|---|---|---|
| Ophthalmic | 30 min | 1-2 hr | 12-24 hr |

## ADVERSE REACTIONS
**CNS:** *CVA*, depression, fatigue, dizziness, lethargy, hallucinations, confusion, *syncope.*
**CV:** slight reduction in resting heart rate, **arrhythmia, cardiac arrest, heart block,** palpitations, *hypotension,* **bradycardia, heart failure.**
**EENT:** minor eye irritation, conjunctivitis, blepharitis, keratitis, visual disturbances, diplopia, ptosis, decreased corneal sensitivity with long-term use.
**Metabolic:** hyperglycemia, hyperuricemia.
**Respiratory:** *bronchospasm in patients with history of asthma.*

## INTERACTIONS
**Drug-drug.** *Aminophylline, theophylline:* May act antagonistically, reducing effects of one or both drugs. Elimination of theophylline may also be reduced. Monitor theophylline levels and patient closely.

---

Reactions may be *common*, uncommon, *life-threatening*, or COMMON AND LIFE-THREATENING.

*Calcium channel blockers, cardiac glyco-sides, quinidine:* May increase risk of adverse cardiac effects if significant amounts of timolol are systemically absorbed. Use together cautiously.

*Cimetidine:* May increase pharmacologic effects of beta blocker. Consider another $H_2$ agonist or decrease dose of beta blocker.

*Epinephrine:* May cause an initial hypertensive episode followed by bradycardia. Stop beta blocker 3 days before anticipated epinephrine use. Monitor patient closely.

*Insulin:* May mask symptoms of hypoglycemia (such as tachycardia) as a result of beta blockade. Use together with extreme caution in patients with diabetes.

*Oral beta blockers:* May increase ocular and systemic effects. Use together cautiously.

*Prazosin:* May increase risk of orthostatic hypotension in early phases of use together. Assist patient to stand slowly until effects are known.

*Reserpine, other catecholamine-depleting drugs:* May increase hypotensive and bradycardia-induced effects. Avoid using together.

*Verapamil:* May increase effects of both drugs. Monitor cardiac function closely and decrease dosages as necessary.

**EFFECTS ON LAB TEST RESULTS**
● May increase BUN, potassium, glucose, and uric acid levels.

**CONTRAINDICATIONS & CAUTIONS**
● Contraindicated in patients hypersensitive to drug and in those with bronchial asthma, sinus bradycardia, second- or third-degree AV block, cardiac failure, cardiogenic shock, or history of bronchial asthma or severe COPD.
● Use cautiously in patients with nonallergic bronchospasm, chronic bronchitis, emphysema, diabetes mellitus, hyperthyroidism, or cerebrovascular insufficiency.

**NURSING CONSIDERATIONS**
● Give other ophthalmic drugs at least 10 minutes before giving gel form of drug.
● Monitor diabetic patients carefully. Systemic beta-blocking effects can mask some signs and symptoms of hypoglycemia.
● Some patients may need a few weeks of treatment to stabilize pressure-lowering response. Determine IOP after 4 weeks of treatment.
● Drug can be used safely in patients with glaucoma who wear conventional poly-methylmethacrylate (PMMA) hard contact lenses.
● *Alert:* Don't confuse timolol with atenolol, or Timoptic with Viroptic.

**PATIENT TEACHING**
● Teach patient how to instill drops. Advise him to wash hands before and after instillation and to apply light finger pressure on lacrimal sac for 1 minute after drops are instilled. Warn patient not to touch tip of dropper to eye or surrounding tissue.
● Instruct patient using gel to invert container and shake once before each use. Also tell him to use other ophthalmic drugs at least 10 minutes before applying gel.
● Tell patient to instill drug without contact lenses in place. Lenses may be reinserted about 15 minutes after drug use.
● Advise patient to monitor pulse rate and report slow rate to prescriber. Drug may be absorbed systemically and produce signs and symptoms of beta blockade.
● Tell patient to report difficulty breathing or chest pain to prescriber.

---

**travoprost**
Travatan

*Pregnancy risk category C*

**AVAILABLE FORMS**
*Ophthalmic solution:* 0.004%

**INDICATIONS & DOSAGES**
➤ **To reduce intraocular pressure (IOP) in patients with open-angle glaucoma or ocular hypertension who can't tolerate or who respond inadequately to other IOP-lowering drugs**
*Adults:* 1 drop in conjunctival sac of affected eye once daily h.s.

---

## ACTION

Unknown. Thought to reduce IOP by increasing uveoscleral outflow.

| Route | Onset | Peak | Duration |
|-------|-------|------|----------|
| Ophthalmic | Unknown | 30 min | Unknown |

## ADVERSE REACTIONS

**CNS:** anxiety, depression, headache, pain.
**CV:** angina pectoris, *bradycardia*, chest pain, hypertension, hypotension.
**EENT:** *ocular hyperemia, decreased visual acuity, eye discomfort, foreign body sensation, eye pain, eye pruritus,* conjunctival hyperemia, abnormal vision, blepharitis, blurred vision, cataract, conjunctivitis, dry eye, eye disorder, iris discoloration, keratitis, lid margin crusting, photophobia, subconjunctival hemorrhage, tearing, sinusitis.
**GI:** dyspepsia, GI disorder.
**GU:** prostate disorder, urinary incontinence, UTI.
**Metabolic:** hypercholesterolemia.
**Musculoskeletal:** arthritis, back pain.
**Respiratory:** bronchitis.
**Other:** accidental injury, cold syndrome, infection.

## INTERACTIONS

**Drug-herb.** *Areca, jaborandi:* May increase effects. Discourage use together.

## EFFECTS ON LAB TEST RESULTS

● May increase cholesterol level.

## CONTRAINDICATIONS & CAUTIONS

● Contraindicated in patients hypersensitive to travoprost, benzalkonium chloride, or other drug components; in pregnant women or women trying to become pregnant; and in those with angle-closure, inflammatory, or neovascular glaucoma.
● Use cautiously in patients with renal or hepatic impairment, active intraocular inflammation (iritis, uveitis), or risk factors for macular edema.
● Use cautiously in aphakic patients and pseudophakic patients with a torn posterior lens capsule.

## NURSING CONSIDERATIONS

● Temporary or permanent increased pigmentation of the iris and eyelid may occur as well as increased pigmentation and growth of eyelashes.
● Patient should remove contact lenses before instilling drug and reinsert them 15 minutes after administration.
● If using more than one ophthalmic drug, give the drugs at least 5 minutes apart.
● Store drug between 36° and 77° F (2° and 25° C).
● If a pregnant woman or a woman attempting to become pregnant accidentally comes in contact with drug, thoroughly cleanse the exposed area with soap and water immediately.

## PATIENT TEACHING

● Teach patient how to instill drops, and advise him to wash hands before and after instilling solution. Warn him not to touch tip of dropper to eye or surrounding tissue.
● Advise patient to apply light finger pressure on lacrimal sac for 1 minute after instillation to minimize systemic absorption of drug.
● Tell patient to remove contact lenses before administration and explain that he can reinsert them 15 minutes afterward.
● Tell patient receiving treatment in only one eye about potential for increased iris pigmentation, eyelid darkening, and increased length, thickness, pigmentation, or number of lashes in the treated eye.
● If eye trauma or infection occurs or if eye surgery is needed, advise patient to seek medical advice before continuing to use the multidose container.
● Advise patient to immediately report eye inflammation or lid reactions.
● If patient is using more than one ophthalmic drug, tell him to apply them at least 5 minutes apart.
● Stress importance of compliance with recommended therapy.
● Tell patient to discard container within 6 weeks of removing it from the sealed pouch.
● If a pregnant woman or a woman attempting to become pregnant accidentally comes in contact with drug, tell her to thoroughly cleanse the exposed area with soap and water immediately.

# unoprostone isopropyl
Rescula

*Pregnancy risk category C*

## AVAILABLE FORMS
*Ophthalmic solution:* 0.15% (1.5 mg/ml)

## INDICATIONS & DOSAGES
➤ **To reduce intraocular pressure (IOP) in patients with open-angle glaucoma or ocular hypertension who can't tolerate or who respond inadequately to other IOP-lowering drugs**
*Adults:* Instill 1 drop in affected eye b.i.d.

## ACTION
Unknown. Thought to reduce elevated IOP by increasing outflow of aqueous humor.

| Route | Onset | Peak | Duration |
|-------|-------|------|----------|
| Ophthalmic | Unknown | Unknown | Unknown |

## ADVERSE REACTIONS
**CNS:** dizziness, headache, insomnia.
**CV:** hypertension.
**EENT:** abnormal vision, blepharitis, cataracts, conjunctivitis, corneal lesion, *dry eyes,* eye discharge, *eye burning or stinging, eye itching, eye redness,* eye discomfort, eye irritation, eye hemorrhage, decreased length of eyelashes, *increased length of eyelashes,* eyelid disorder, foreign body sensation, keratitis, lacrimal disorder, pharyngitis, photophobia, rhinitis, sinusitis, vitreous disorder.
**Metabolic:** diabetes mellitus.
**Musculoskeletal:** back pain.
**Respiratory:** bronchitis, increased cough.
**Other:** accidental injury, ***allergic reaction,*** flulike syndrome, pain.

## INTERACTIONS
None reported.

## EFFECTS ON LAB TEST RESULTS
None reported.

## CONTRAINDICATIONS & CAUTIONS
• Contraindicated in patients hypersensitive to unoprostone isopropyl, benzalkonium chloride, or other components of product.

• Use cautiously in patients with active intraocular inflammation (uveitis) or angle-closure, inflammatory, or neovascular glaucoma.
• Use cautiously in patients with renal or hepatic impairment.

## NURSING CONSIDERATIONS
• Don't give to patient wearing contact lenses because product contains benzalkonium chloride, which may be absorbed by the contact lenses.
• Patient should remove contact lenses before instilling drug and reinsert them 15 minutes after administration.
• Avoid touching tip of dropper to eye to avoid infection.
• Serious eye damage and blindness may result from using contaminated solutions.
• If using more than one ophthalmic drug, give the drugs at least 5 minutes apart.
• Store at 36° to 77° F (2° to 25° C).

## PATIENT TEACHING
• Instruct patient to report side effects, especially eye inflammation or eyelid reactions.
• Tell patient to remove contact lenses before instilling drops and then wait 15 minutes before reinserting them.
• Instruct patient to avoid touching tip of container to eye because tip could become contaminated, possibly causing an eye infection. Tell him that serious eye damage and blindness may result from using contaminated solutions.
• If eye trauma or infection occurs or if ocular surgery is needed, tell patient to consult prescriber about continued use of multidose container.
• Tell patient that drug can be used with other eye medications but that it's important to separate administration times by 5 minutes.
• Tell patient that drug may permanently change eye color. Change may be gradual, over months to years.
• Warn patient not to use drug if he's allergic to it, to benzalkonium chloride, or to other ingredients in this product.
• Instruct woman to notify prescriber if she's breast-feeding or becomes pregnant while taking drug.

---

*Rapid onset*    †Canada    ‡Australia    ◊OTC    ♦ Off-label use    ✏Photoguide    *Liquid contains alcohol.

**boric acid**
**chloramphenicol**
**triethanolamine polypeptide**
    **oleate-condensate**

**COMBINATION PRODUCTS**
None.

---

## boric acid
Auro-Dri ◇, Dri/Ear ◇, Ear-Dry ◇

*Pregnancy risk category NR*

**AVAILABLE FORMS**
*Otic solution:* 2.75% boric acid in iso-propyl alcohol

**INDICATIONS & DOSAGES**
➤ **External ear canal infection**
*Adults and children:* 3 to 8 drops into ear canal t.i.d. or q.i.d.; plug with cotton.

**ACTION**
A weak bacteriostatic that inhibits or destroys bacteria in the ear canal. Also a fungistatic.

| Route | Onset | Peak | Duration |
|-------|---------|---------|----------|
| Otic | Unknown | Unknown | Unknown |

**ADVERSE REACTIONS**
**EENT:** ear irritation or itching.
**Skin:** urticaria.
**Other:** overgrowth of nonsusceptible organisms.

**INTERACTIONS**
None significant.

**EFFECTS ON LAB TEST RESULTS**
None reported.

**CONTRAINDICATIONS & CAUTIONS**
• Contraindicated in patients with perforated eardrum or excoriated membranes.

**NURSING CONSIDERATIONS**
• Monitor patient for signs and symptoms of superinfection.

**PATIENT TEACHING**
• Show patient or caregiver how to give drug.
• To prevent reinfection, warn patient not to touch ear with dropper.
• Tell patient to always moisten cotton plug with drug.

---

## chloramphenicol
Chloromycetin Otic

*Pregnancy risk category NR*

**AVAILABLE FORMS**
*Otic solution:* 0.5%

**INDICATIONS & DOSAGES**
➤ **External ear canal infection**
*Adults and children:* 2 to 3 drops into ear canal t.i.d.

**ACTION**
Inhibits or destroys bacteria in ear canal.

| Route | Onset | Peak | Duration |
|-------|---------|---------|----------|
| Otic | Unknown | Unknown | Unknown |

**ADVERSE REACTIONS**
**EENT:** ear itching or burning.
**GU:** hemoglobinuria.
**Hematologic:** *bone marrow depression,* bone marrow hypoplasia, *aplastic anemia.*
**Metabolic:** lactic acidosis.
**Skin:** pruritus, urticaria.
**Other:** overgrowth of nonsusceptible organisms.

**INTERACTIONS**
None significant.

**EFFECTS ON LAB TEST RESULTS**
• May decrease hemoglobin.

**CONTRAINDICATIONS & CAUTIONS**
• Contraindicated in patients hypersensitive to drug or its components and in those with perforated eardrum.

---

Reactions may be *common*, uncommon, *life-threatening*, or COMMON AND LIFE-THREATENING.

## NURSING CONSIDERATIONS
• Obtain history of drug use and reactions.
• Monitor patient for signs and symptoms of superinfection. Avoid prolonged use.
• Reculture persistent drainage.
• Monitor patient for sore throat (early sign of toxicity).
• *Alert:* Don't confuse Chloromycetin with chlorambucil.

## PATIENT TEACHING
• Show patient or caregiver how to give drug.
• To avoid reinfection, warn patient not to touch ear with dropper.

---

# triethanolamine polypeptide oleate-condensate
Cerumenex

*Pregnancy risk category NR*

## AVAILABLE FORMS
*Otic solution:* 10% in 6- or 12-ml bottles with droppers

## INDICATIONS & DOSAGES
➤ **Impacted cerumen**
*Adults and children:* Fill ear canal with solution and insert cotton plug. After 15 to 30 minutes, flush with warm water.

## ACTION
A ceruminolytic that emulsifies and disperses accumulated cerumen.

| Route | Onset | Peak | Duration |
|-------|-------|------|----------|
| Otic | Unknown | Unknown | 15-30 min |

## ADVERSE REACTIONS
**EENT:** ear erythema or itching.
**Skin:** severe eczema.

## INTERACTIONS
None significant.

## EFFECTS ON LAB TEST RESULTS
None reported.

## CONTRAINDICATIONS & CAUTIONS
• Contraindicated in patients with perforated eardrum, otitis media, or otitis externa.

## NURSING CONSIDERATIONS
• *Alert:* If hypersensitivity is suspected, apply patch test. Place 1 drop of drug on patient's inner forearm; cover with bandage. Read results in 24 hours. If reaction occurs, drug shouldn't be used.
• *Alert:* Ototoxicity may occur if drug enters middle ear.

## PATIENT TEACHING
• Teach patient to moisten cotton plug with drug before insertion, leave cotton in place for a maximum of 30 minutes, and flush ear gently with warm water using a rubber bulb syringe.
• Tell patient not to use drops more often than prescribed.
• Warn patient that drug is for use only in the ears.
• Advise patient to stop drug and contact prescriber immediately if adverse reactions occur.
• Tell patient to keep container tightly closed and away from moisture.

**beclomethasone dipropionate
budesonide
epinephrine hydrochloride
flunisolide
fluticasone propionate
naphazoline hydrochloride
oxymetazoline hydrochloride
phenylephrine hydrochloride
tetrahydrozoline hydrochloride
triamcinolone acetonide**

### COMBINATION PRODUCTS
4-WAY FAST ACTING ORIGINAL ◊ :
phenylephrine hydrochloride 0.5%, naphazoline hydrochloride 0.05%, and pyrilamine maleate 0.2%.

---

### beclomethasone dipropionate
Beconase, Beconase AQ,
Vancenase, Vancenase AQ,
Vancenase Pockethaler

*Pregnancy risk category C*

### AVAILABLE FORMS
*Nasal aerosol:* 42 mcg/metered spray,
50 mcg/metered spray‡
*Nasal spray:* 42 mcg/metered spray,
50 mcg/metered spray‡, 84 mcg/metered
spray

### INDICATIONS & DOSAGES
➤ **To relieve symptoms of seasonal or
perennial rhinitis, to prevent nasal
polyp recurrence after surgical removal**
*Adults and children older than age 12:*
1 or 2 sprays in each nostril b.i.d., t.i.d., or
q.i.d.
*Children ages 6 to 12:* 1 spray into each
nostril t.i.d.

### ACTION
A corticosteroid that may reduce nasal inflammation by inhibiting mediators of inflammation.

| Route | Onset | Peak | Duration |
|-------|-------|------|----------|
| Nasal | 5-7 days | 3 wk | Unknown |

### ADVERSE REACTIONS
**CNS:** headache.
**EENT:** *mild, transient nasal burning and
stinging;* nasal congestion; sneezing; dryness; epistaxis; nasopharyngeal fungal infections.

### INTERACTIONS
None significant.

### EFFECTS ON LAB TEST RESULTS
None reported.

### CONTRAINDICATIONS & CAUTIONS
• Contraindicated in patients hypersensitive
to drug and in those with untreated localized infection involving the nasal mucosa.
• Use cautiously, if at all, in patients with
active or quiescent respiratory tract tuberculous infections or untreated fungal, bacterial, or systemic viral or ocular herpes
simplex infections.
• Use cautiously in patients who have recently had nasal septal ulcers, nasal surgery, or trauma until wound healing has
occurred.

### NURSING CONSIDERATIONS
• Observe patient for fungal infections.
• Drug isn't effective for acute exacerba-
tions of rhinitis. Decongestants or antihis-
tamines may be needed.
• *Alert:* Don't confuse Vancenase with
Vanceril.

### PATIENT TEACHING
• Advise patient to pump nasal spray three
or four times before first use.
• To instill, instruct patient to blow nose to
clear nasal passages, shake container, tilt
head slightly forward, and insert nozzle
into nostril, pointing away from septum.
Tell him to hold other nostril closed and
inhale gently while spraying, hold breath
for a few seconds, and exhale through the
mouth. Next, have him shake container
and repeat in other nostril.
• Tell patient to pump nasal spray once or
twice before first use each day. He should
clean the cap and nosepiece of the activa-

---

tor in warm water every day, then allow them to air-dry.
- Advise patient to use drug regularly, as prescribed, because its effectiveness depends on regular use.
- Explain that unlike decongestants, drug doesn't work right away. Most patients notice improvement within a few days, but some may need 2 to 3 weeks.
- Warn patient not to exceed recommended dosage because of risk of hypothalamic-pituitary-adrenal axis suppression.
- Tell patient to notify prescriber if signs and symptoms don't improve within 3 weeks or if nasal irritation persists.
- Teach patient good nasal and oral hygiene.

## budesonide
Rhinocort Aqua

*Pregnancy risk category C*

### AVAILABLE FORMS
*Nasal spray:* 32 mcg/metered spray

### INDICATIONS & DOSAGES
➤ **Symptoms of seasonal or perennial allergic rhinitis**
*Adults and children age 6 and older:*
1 spray in each nostril once daily. Maximum recommended dose for adults and children 12 and older is 4 sprays per nostril once daily (256 mcg daily). Maximum recommended dose for children 6 to 12 is 2 sprays per nostril once daily (128 mcg daily).

### ACTION
Unknown. A corticosteroid that may reduce nasal inflammation by inhibiting mediators of inflammation.

| Route | Onset | Peak | Duration |
|-------|-------|------|----------|
| Nasal | 10 hr | 2 wk | Unknown |

### ADVERSE REACTIONS
**CNS:** headache, nervousness.
**EENT:** *nasal irritation, epistaxis, pharyngitis,* reduced sense of smell, nasal pain, hoarseness.
**GI:** bad taste, dry mouth, dyspepsia, nausea.

**Respiratory:** *cough,* candidiasis, wheezing, dyspnea.
**Skin:** facial edema, rash, pruritus, contact dermatitis.
**Other:** hypersensitivity reactions.

### INTERACTIONS
None significant.

### EFFECTS ON LAB TEST RESULTS
None reported.

### CONTRAINDICATIONS & CAUTIONS
- Contraindicated in patients hypersensitive to drug or its components and in those who have had recent septal ulcers, nasal surgery, or nasal trauma until total healing has occurred.
- Contraindicated in those with untreated localized nasal mucosa infections.
- Use cautiously in patients with tuberculous infections, ocular herpes simplex, or untreated fungal, bacterial, or systemic viral infections.

### NURSING CONSIDERATIONS
- Systemic effects of corticosteroid therapy may occur if recommended daily dose is exceeded.

### PATIENT TEACHING
- Tell patient to avoid exposure to chickenpox or measles.
- To instill drug, instruct patient to shake container before use, blow nose to clear nasal passages, and tilt head slightly forward and insert nozzle into nostril, pointing away from septum. Tell him to hold other nostril closed and inhale gently while spraying. Next, have him shake container and repeat in other nostril.
- Advise patient not to freeze, break, incinerate, or store canister in extreme heat; contents are under pressure.
- Advise patient to store canister with valve upward.
- Warn patient not to exceed prescribed dosage or use drug for long periods because of risk of hypothalamic-pituitary-adrenal axis suppression.
- Tell patient to notify prescriber if signs or symptoms don't improve or worsen in 3 weeks.
- Teach patient good nasal and oral hygiene.

• Tell patient to use drug within 6 months of opening the protective aluminum pouch.
• Instruct patient not to share drug because this could spread infection.

• Caution patient not to share product to prevent spread of infection.
• Tell patient not to exceed recommended dosage and to use only when needed.

## epinephrine hydrochloride
Adrenalin Chloride

*Pregnancy risk category NR*

**AVAILABLE FORMS**
*Nasal solution:* 0.1%

**INDICATIONS & DOSAGES**
➤ **Nasal congestion, local superficial bleeding**
*Adults and children age 6 and older:* Instill 1 or 2 drops of solution into each nostril.

**ACTION**
Causes local vasoconstriction of dilated arterioles, reducing blood flow and nasal congestion.

| Route | Onset | Peak | Duration |
|-------|-------|------|----------|
| Nasal | 5 min | Unknown | 1 hr |

**ADVERSE REACTIONS**
**CNS:** nervousness, excitation.
**CV:** *tachycardia.*
**EENT:** rebound nasal congestion, slight stinging on application.

**INTERACTIONS**
None significant.

**EFFECTS ON LAB TEST RESULTS**
None reported.

**CONTRAINDICATIONS & CAUTIONS**
• Contraindicated in patients hypersensitive to drug.
• Use cautiously in patients with hyperthyroidism, coronary artery disease, hypertension, or diabetes mellitus.

**NURSING CONSIDERATIONS**
• Monitor heart rate.
• *Alert:* Don't confuse epinephrine with ephedrine.

**PATIENT TEACHING**
• Teach patient how to instill nose drops.

## flunisolide
Nasalide, Nasarel, Rhinalar†

*Pregnancy risk category C*

**AVAILABLE FORMS**
*Nasal inhalant:* 25 mcg/metered spray, 200 doses/bottle†
*Nasal solution:* 0.25 mg/ml in pump spray bottle (25 mcg/spray)

**INDICATIONS & DOSAGES**
➤ **Symptoms of seasonal or perennial rhinitis**
*Adults:* Starting dose is 2 sprays (50 mcg) in each nostril b.i.d. Total daily dose is 200 mcg. If needed, dosage may be increased to 2 sprays in each nostril t.i.d. Maximum total daily dose is 8 sprays in each nostril (400 mcg daily).
*Children ages 6 to 14:* Starting dose is 1 spray (25 mcg) in each nostril t.i.d. or 2 sprays (50 mcg) in each nostril b.i.d. Total daily dose is 150 to 200 mcg. Maximum total daily dose is 4 sprays in each nostril (200 mcg daily).

**ACTION**
Exact mechanism unknown. Decreases nasal inflammation, mainly by stabilizing leukocyte lysosomal membranes.

| Route | Onset | Peak | Duration |
|-------|-------|------|----------|
| Nasal | Unknown | Unknown | Unknown |

**ADVERSE REACTIONS**
**CNS:** headache.
**EENT:** *mild, transient nasal burning and stinging;* nasal congestion; nasopharyngeal fungal infection; dryness; sneezing; epistaxis; watery eyes.
**GI:** nausea, vomiting.

**INTERACTIONS**
None significant.

**EFFECTS ON LAB TEST RESULTS**
None reported.

---

Reactions may be *common,* uncommon, *life-threatening,* or COMMON AND LIFE-THREATENING.

## CONTRAINDICATIONS & CAUTIONS
• Contraindicated in patients hypersensitive to drug and in those with untreated localized infection involving nasal mucosa.
• Use cautiously, if at all, in patients with active or quiescent respiratory tract tuberculous infections or untreated fungal, bacterial, or systemic viral or ocular herpes simplex infections. Also use cautiously in patients who have recently had nasal septal ulcers, nasal surgery, or nasal trauma.

## NURSING CONSIDERATIONS
• Drug isn't effective for acute exacerbations of rhinitis. Decongestants or antihistamines may be needed.
• *Alert:* Don't confuse flunisolide with fluocinonide, fluticasone, or Flumadine.

## PATIENT TEACHING
• Tell patient to avoid exposure to chickenpox or measles.
• To instill drug, instruct patient to shake container before use, blow nose to clear nasal passages, tilt head slightly forward, and insert nozzle into nostril, pointing away from septum. Tell him to hold other nostril closed and inhale gently while spraying. Have him repeat procedure in other nostril. Tell him to clean nosepiece with warm water daily.
• Explain that drug doesn't work right away. Most patients notice improvement within a few days, but some may need 2 to 3 weeks.
• Advise patient to use drug regularly, as prescribed.
• Warn patient not to exceed recommended dosage to avoid hypothalamic-pituitary-adrenal axis suppression.
• Tell patient to stop drug and notify prescriber if signs and symptoms don't diminish in 3 weeks or if nasal irritation persists.

## fluticasone propionate
Flonase

*Pregnancy risk category C*

## AVAILABLE FORMS
*Nasal spray:* 50 mcg/metered spray (16-g bottles)

## INDICATIONS & DOSAGES
➤ **To manage nasal symptoms of seasonal and perennial allergic and nonallergic rhinitis**
*Adults:* 2 sprays (100 mcg) in each nostril once daily or 1 spray b.i.d. Reduce dosage to 1 spray in each nostril once daily for maintenance therapy. Or, for seasonal allergic rhinitis, 2 sprays in each nostril once daily as needed for symptom control, although greater symptom control may be achieved with regular use.
*Adolescents and children age 4 and older:* Initially, 1 spray (50 mcg) in each nostril once daily. If patient doesn't respond, increase to 2 sprays in each nostril daily. Once adequate control is achieved, decrease dose to 1 spray in each nostril daily. Maximum dose is 2 sprays in each nostril daily.

## ACTION
Exact mechanism unknown. Corticosteroid is thought to decrease nasal inflammation.

| Route | Onset | Peak | Duration |
|-------|-------|------|----------|
| Nasal | Unknown | Unknown | Unknown |

## ADVERSE REACTIONS
**CNS:** headache.
**EENT:** epistaxis, nasal burning, blood in nasal mucus, pharyngitis, nasal irritation.

## INTERACTIONS
None significant.

## EFFECTS ON LAB TEST RESULTS
None reported.

## CONTRAINDICATIONS & CAUTIONS
• Contraindicated in patients hypersensitive to drug or its components and in those with untreated local infections of the nasal mucosa.
• Contraindicated in patients with recent nasal septal ulcers, nasal surgery, or nasal trauma until healing is complete.
• Use cautiously, if at all, in patients with active or quiescent tuberculous infections; glaucoma; untreated fungal, bacterial, or systemic viral infections; or ocular herpes simplex.

---

• Use cautiously in patients already receiving systemic corticosteroids and in breast-feeding women.

**NURSING CONSIDERATIONS**
• Although rare, immediate hypersensitivity reaction or contact dermatitis may occur after intranasal administration.

**PATIENT TEACHING**
• Urge patient to read instruction sheet before using drug for first time.
• To instill drug, tell patient to shake container gently before use, blow nose to clear nasal passages, tilt head slightly forward, and insert nozzle into nostril, pointing away from septum. Tell him to hold other nostril closed and inhale gently while spraying. Next, have patient shake container and repeat procedure in other nostril. Tell him to rinse nozzle when done.
• *Alert:* Stress importance of adhering to a schedule for instillation because drug effectiveness depends on regular use. Caution patient that exceeding recommended dosage could lead to hyperadrenocorticism, hypothalamic-pituitary-adrenal axis suppression, or growth suppression in children and teenagers.
• Tell patient to notify prescriber if signs and symptoms don't improve or condition worsens.
• Warn patient to avoid exposure to chickenpox and measles and, if exposed, to obtain medical advice.
• Instruct patient to watch for and report signs and symptoms of nasal infection.
• Tell patient that sugarless gum, hard candy, and water help relieve dry mouth.

---

## naphazoline hydrochloride
Privine ◇

*Pregnancy risk category NR*

**AVAILABLE FORMS**
*Nasal spray:* 0.05% solution
*Nose drops:* 0.05% solution

**INDICATIONS & DOSAGES**
➤ **Nasal congestion**
*Adults and children age 12 and older:* 1 or 2 drops or sprays in each nostril at least 6 hours apart.

**ACTION**
Causes local vasoconstriction of dilated arterioles, reducing blood flow and nasal congestion.

| Route | Onset | Peak | Duration |
|-------|-------|------|----------|
| Nasal | 10 min | Unknown | 2-6 hr |

**ADVERSE REACTIONS**
**CNS:** restlessness, anxiety, headache.
**EENT:** rebound nasal congestion, sneezing, stinging, dryness of mucosa.
**Other:** systemic effects in children.

**INTERACTIONS**
None significant.

**EFFECTS ON LAB TEST RESULTS**
None reported.

**CONTRAINDICATIONS & CAUTIONS**
• Contraindicated in patients hypersensitive to drug.
• Use cautiously in patients with hyperthyroidism, heart disease, hypertension, or diabetes mellitus and in those who have difficulty urinating because of enlargement of prostate gland.

**NURSING CONSIDERATIONS**
• Don't give to children younger than age 12 unless directed by prescriber.

**PATIENT TEACHING**
• Teach patient how to use drug. For nose drops, instruct patient to tilt head back as far as possible, instill drops, then lean head forward while inhaling; then repeat procedure for other nostril. For nasal spray, have patient hold spray container and head upright and then point the adapter tip toward the inflamed nostril. Advise patient to hold the opposite nostril closed while pumping the drug. Tell patient not to shake container.
• Caution patient not to share product to prevent spread of infection.
• Warn patient not to exceed recommended dosage.
• Tell patient not to use drug for longer than 2 to 3 days because rebound congestion may develop.
• Instruct patient to call prescriber if nasal congestion persists after 5 days.

---

Reactions may be *common*, uncommon, *life-threatening*, or COMMON AND LIFE-THREATENING.

# oxymetazoline hydrochloride
Afrin◇, Allerest 12 Hour Nasal Spray◇, Chlorphed-LA◇, Dristan 12 Hour Nasal◇, Drixine Nasal‡, Duramist Plus 12 Hour◇, Duration◇, Genasal◇, Neo-Synephrine 12 Hour Spray◇, Nostrilla◇, NTZ Long Acting Nasal◇, Sinarest 12 Hour◇

*Pregnancy risk category NR*

## AVAILABLE FORMS
*Nasal solution:* 0.05%◇

## INDICATIONS & DOSAGES
➤ **Nasal congestion**
*Adults and children age 6 and older:* 2 to 3 drops or sprays of 0.05% solution in each nostril b.i.d.

## ACTION
Unknown. Thought to cause local vasoconstriction of dilated arterioles, reducing blood flow and nasal congestion.

| Route | Onset | Peak | Duration |
|-------|-------|------|----------|
| Nasal | 5-10 min | 6 hr | < 12 hr |

## ADVERSE REACTIONS
**CNS:** headache, anxiety, restlessness, dizziness, insomnia.
**CV:** palpitations, *CV collapse,* hypertension.
**EENT:** rebound nasal congestion or irritation, dryness of nose and throat, increased nasal discharge, stinging, sneezing.
**Other:** systemic effects in children.

## INTERACTIONS
None significant.

## EFFECTS ON LAB TEST RESULTS
None reported.

## CONTRAINDICATIONS & CAUTIONS
• Contraindicated in patients hypersensitive to drug and in children younger than age 6.
• Use cautiously in patients with hyperthyroidism, cardiac disease, hypertension, or diabetes mellitus.
• Use cautiously in those with difficulty urinating because of an enlarged prostate.

## NURSING CONSIDERATIONS
• Monitor patient for rebound congestion or systemic effects.
• Don't give to children younger than age 6.

## PATIENT TEACHING
• Teach patient how to use drug. Tell him to hold head upright to minimize swallowing of drug and to sniff spray briskly.
• Caution patient not to share drug because this could spread infection.
• Tell patient not to exceed recommended dosage and to use only when needed.
• Inform patient that prolonged use may result in rebound congestion.
• *Alert:* Warn patient that excessive use may cause slow or rapid heart rate, high blood pressure, dizziness, and weakness.

# phenylephrine hydrochloride
Alconefrin Nasal Drops 12◇, Alconefrin Nasal Drops 25◇, Alconefrin Nasal Drops 50◇, Doktors◇, Duration◇, Little Noses Gentle Formula◇, Neo-Synephrine◇, Nostril◇, Rhinall◇, Rhinall-10 Children's Flavored Nose Drops◇, Sinex◇

*Pregnancy risk category NR*

## AVAILABLE FORMS
*Nasal solution:* 0.125%, 0.25%, 0.5%, 1%

## INDICATIONS & DOSAGES
➤ **Nasal congestion**
*Adults and children age 12 and older:* 2 to 3 drops or 1 to 2 sprays in each nostril q 4 hours, p.r.n. Don't use for longer than 3 to 5 days.
*Children ages 6 to 12:* 2 to 3 drops or 1 to 2 sprays of 0.25% solution in each nostril q 4 hours, p.r.n.
*Children ages 2 to 6:* 2 to 3 drops of 0.125% solution q 4 hours, p.r.n.

## ACTION
Causes local vasoconstriction of dilated arterioles, reducing blood flow and nasal congestion.

| Route | Onset | Peak | Duration |
|-------|-------|------|----------|
| Nasal | Rapid | Unknown | 30 min-4 hr |

**ADVERSE REACTIONS**
**CNS:** headache, tremor, dizziness, nervousness.
**CV:** *palpitations, tachycardia,* PVCs, hypertension, pallor.
**EENT:** transient burning or stinging, dryness of nasal mucosa, rebound nasal congestion.
**GI:** nausea.

**INTERACTIONS**
None significant.

**EFFECTS ON LAB TEST RESULTS**
None reported.

**CONTRAINDICATIONS & CAUTIONS**
• Contraindicated in patients hypersensitive to drug.
• Use cautiously in patients with hyperthyroidism, marked hypertension, type 1 diabetes mellitus, cardiac disease, or advanced arteriosclerotic changes; in children with low body weight; and in elderly patients.

**NURSING CONSIDERATIONS**
• Monitor patient for systemic adverse effects.
• Don't use in children younger than age 2.

**PATIENT TEACHING**
• Teach patient how to use drug. Tell him to hold head upright to minimize swallowing of drug and to sniff spray briskly.
• Caution patient not to share drug because this could spread infection.
• Tell patient not to exceed recommended dosage and to use only when needed.
• Advise patient to contact prescriber if signs and symptoms persist longer than 3 days.
• Inform patient that prolonged use may result in rebound congestion.

---

# tetrahydrozoline hydrochloride
Tyzine, Tyzine Pediatric

*Pregnancy risk category C*

**AVAILABLE FORMS**
*Nasal solution:* 0.05%, 0.1%

**INDICATIONS & DOSAGES**
➤ **Nasal congestion**
*Adults and children older than age 6:* 2 to 4 drops or 3 to 4 sprays of 0.1% solution in each nostril no more than q 3 hours, p.r.n.
*Children ages 2 to 6:* 2 to 3 drops of 0.05% solution in each nostril no more than q 3 hours, p.r.n.

**ACTION**
Unknown. Thought to cause local vasoconstriction of dilated arterioles, reducing blood flow and nasal congestion.

| Route | Onset | Peak | Duration |
|-------|-------|------|----------|
| Nasal | Few min | Unknown | 4-8 hr |

**ADVERSE REACTIONS**
**EENT:** transient burning or stinging, sneezing, rebound nasal congestion.

**INTERACTIONS**
None significant.

**EFFECTS ON LAB TEST RESULTS**
None reported.

**CONTRAINDICATIONS & CAUTIONS**
• Contraindicated in patients hypersensitive to drug and in children younger than age 2. The 0.1% solution is contraindicated in children younger than age 6.
• Use cautiously in patients with hyperthyroidism, hypertension, or diabetes mellitus.

**NURSING CONSIDERATIONS**
• Drug should be used for only 3 to 5 days.

**PATIENT TEACHING**
• Teach patient how to use drug. Tell him to hold head upright to minimize swallowing of drug and to sniff spray briskly.
• Caution patient not to share drug because this could spread infection.
• Tell patient not to exceed recommended dosage and to use only as needed for 3 to 5 days.

---

## triamcinolone acetonide
Nasacort AQ

*Pregnancy risk category C*

### AVAILABLE FORMS
*Nasal spray pump:* 55 mcg/spray

### INDICATIONS & DOSAGES
➤ **Rhinitis, allergic disorders, inflammatory conditions**
*Adults and children 12 years and older:*
2 sprays in each nostril daily; may decrease to 1 spray in each nostril daily for allergic disorders.
*Children ages 6 to 11:* 1 spray in each nostril daily. Maximum dosage is 2 sprays in each nostril daily.

### ACTION
Unknown. A glucocorticoid with anti-inflammatory properties.

| Route | Onset | Peak | Duration |
|-------|-------|------|----------|
| Nasal | 12 hr | 3-4 days | Unknown |

### ADVERSE REACTIONS
**CNS:** *headache.*
**EENT:** *nasal irritation,* dry mucous membranes, nasal and sinus congestion, irritation, burning, stinging, throat discomfort, sneezing, epistaxis.

### INTERACTIONS
None significant.

### EFFECTS ON LAB TEST RESULTS
None reported.

### CONTRAINDICATIONS & CAUTIONS
• Contraindicated in patients hypersensitive to drug or its components and in those with untreated mucosal infection.
• Use with caution, if at all, in patients with active or quiescent tuberculous infection of respiratory tract and in patients with untreated fungal, bacterial, or systemic viral infection or ocular herpes simplex.
• Use cautiously in patients already receiving systemic corticosteroids because of increased likelihood of hypothalamic-pituitary-adrenal axis suppression.
• Use cautiously in breast-feeding women and in those with recent nasal septal ulcers, nasal surgery, or trauma because drug may inhibit wound healing.

### NURSING CONSIDERATIONS
• *Alert:* Excessive doses may cause signs and symptoms of hyperadrenocorticism and adrenal axis suppression; stop drug slowly.
• *Alert:* Don't confuse triamcinolone with Triaminicin.

### PATIENT TEACHING
• Urge patient to read patient instruction sheet contained in each package before using drug for first time.
• To instill, instruct patient to shake container before use, blow nose to clear nasal passages, tilt head slightly forward, and insert nozzle into nostril, pointing away from septum. Tell him to hold other nostril closed and inhale gently while spraying. Next, have patient shake container and repeat procedure in other nostril.
• Instruct patient to avoid getting aerosol in eyes. If this occurs, tell him to rinse with copious amounts of cool tap water.
• Stress importance of using drug on a regular schedule because its effectiveness depends on regular use. Warn patient not to exceed prescribed dosage because serious adverse reactions can occur.
• Tell patient to notify prescriber if signs and symptoms don't diminish or if condition worsens in 2 to 3 weeks.
• Warn patient to avoid exposure to chickenpox or measles and, if exposed, to notify prescriber.
• Instruct patient to watch for and report signs and symptoms of nasal infection. Drug may need to be stopped and appropriate local therapy given.

## Local anti-infectives

acyclovir
azelaic acid cream
clindamycin phosphate
clotrimazole
docosanol
econazole nitrate
erythromycin
gentamicin sulfate
ketoconazole
metronidazole
miconazole nitrate
mupirocin
neomycin sulfate
nitrofurazone
nystatin
silver sulfadiazine
terbinafine hydrochloride
terconazole
tolnaftate

### COMBINATION PRODUCTS

BENZAMYCIN: erythromycin 3% and benzoyl peroxide 5%.
LANABIOTIC ◊: polymyxin B sulfate
10,000 units, neomycin sulfate 3.5 mg/g,
bacitracin 500 units, and lidocaine
40 mg/g.
LOTRISONE: clotrimazole 1% and betamethasone dipropionate 0.05%.
MYCITRACIN ◊: polymyxin B sulfate
5,000 units, bacitracin 500 units, and
neomycin sulfate 3.5 mg/g.
MYCOLOG-II: triamcinolone acetonide
0.1% and nystatin 100,000 units/g.
NEOSPORIN CREAM ◊: polymyxin B sulfate 10,000 units and neomycin sulfate
3.5 mg/g.
NEOSPORIN OINTMENT ◊: polymyxin B
sulfate 5,000 units, bacitracin zinc
400 units, and neomycin sulfate 3.5 mg/g.
POLYSPORIN OPHTHALMIC OINTMENT ◊:
polymyxin B sulfate 10,000 units and bacitracin zinc 500 units/g.

## acyclovir
Avirax†, Zovirax

*Pregnancy risk category B*

### AVAILABLE FORMS
*Ointment:* 5%
*Cream:* 5% in 2-g tubes

### INDICATIONS & DOSAGES
➤ **Initial herpes genitalis; limited,
non–life-threatening mucocutaneous
herpes simplex virus infections in immunocompromised patients**
*Adults and children 12 years and older:*
Cover all lesions q 3 hours six times daily
for 7 days. Although dose varies depending on total lesion area, use about ½-inch
(1.3-cm) ribbon of ointment on each 4-
inch (10-cm) square of surface area.
✱ *NEW INDICATION:* **Recurrent herpes
labialis (cold sores)**
*Adults and children 12 years and older:*
Apply cream five times daily for 4 days.
Start therapy as early as possible after
signs and symptoms start.

### ACTION
Inhibits herpes simplex and varicella-
zoster viral DNA synthesis by inhibiting
viral DNA polymerase action.

| Route | Onset | Peak | Duration |
|-------|-------|------|----------|
| Topical | Unknown | Unknown | Unknown |

### ADVERSE REACTIONS
None significant.

### INTERACTIONS
None significant.

### EFFECTS ON LAB TEST RESULTS
None reported.

### CONTRAINDICATIONS & CAUTIONS
• Contraindicated in patients hypersensitive to drug and patients with chemical intolerance to drug.

## NURSING CONSIDERATIONS
• Start therapy as early as possible after signs or symptoms begin.
• Apply drug with a finger cot or rubber glove to prevent autoinoculation of other body sites and transmission of infection to other persons.
• All lesions must be thoroughly covered.
• Drug is for cutaneous use only; don't apply to eye.
• Drug isn't a cure for herpes, but it helps improve signs and symptoms.

## PATIENT TEACHING
• Teach patient that virus transmission can occur during treatment.
• Tell patient that there may be some discomfort with application.
• Stress importance of compliance for successful therapy.
• Teach patient that therapy should begin as soon as signs and symptoms appear.
• Tell patient to notify prescriber if adverse reactions occur.
• Instruct patient to store drug in a dry place at 59° to 77° F (15° to 25° C).

---

# azelaic acid cream
Azelex, Finacea, Finevin

*Pregnancy risk category B*

---

## AVAILABLE FORMS
*Cream:* 20%
*Gel:* 15%

## INDICATIONS & DOSAGES
➤ **Mild to moderate inflammatory acne vulgaris**
*Adults:* Apply thin film and gently but thoroughly massage into affected areas b.i.d., in morning and evening.
✳ **NEW INDICATION: Mild to moderate rosacea**
*Adults:* Apply thin film of Finacea and gently but thoroughly massage into affected areas b.i.d., in morning and evening.

## ACTION
Unknown. May inhibit microbial cellular protein synthesis.

| Route | Onset | Peak | Duration |
|---|---|---|---|
| Topical | Unknown | Unknown | Unknown |

## ADVERSE REACTIONS
**Skin:** pruritus, burning, stinging, tingling, dermatitis, peeling, erythema.
**Other:** allergic reaction.
**Finacea only**
**Respiratory:** worsening of asthma.
**Skin:** pruritus, *burning, stinging, tingling,* dermatitis, scaling, erythema, irritation, edema, acne.

## INTERACTIONS
None significant.

## EFFECTS ON LAB TEST RESULTS
None reported.

## CONTRAINDICATIONS & CAUTIONS
• Contraindicated in patients hypersensitive to drug or its components.
• Use cautiously in pregnant or breast-feeding women.

## NURSING CONSIDERATIONS
• Monitor patient for early signs and symptoms of hypopigmentation, especially patient with dark complexion.
• If sensitivity or severe irritation occurs, notify prescriber, who may stop drug and order appropriate treatment.
• Avoid using occlusive dressings.

## PATIENT TEACHING
• Instruct patient to wash and pat dry affected areas before applying drug and to wash hands well after application. Warn him not to apply occlusive dressings or wrappings to affected areas.
• Warn patient that skin irritation may occur, usually at start of therapy, if drug is applied to broken or inflamed skin. Tell him to notify prescriber if irritation persists.
• Advise patient to keep drug away from mouth, eyes, and other mucous membranes. If contact occurs, tell him to rinse thoroughly with water and to notify prescriber if irritation persists.
• Advise patient to report abnormal changes in skin color.
• Urge patient to use drug for full treatment period. In most patients with inflammatory lesions, improvement occurs in 1 to 2 months.
• Warn patients with rosacea to avoid foods and beverages that may cause flush-

ing, such as spicy foods, hot food or drinks, and alcohol.
• Instruct patient to store drug at 59° to 86° F (15° to 30° C) and protect it from freezing.

## clindamycin phosphate
Cleocin, Cleocin T, Clinda-Derm, Clindets, C/T/S

*Pregnancy risk category B*

### AVAILABLE FORMS
*Gel:* 1%
*Lotion:* 1%
*Pledget:* 1%*
*Topical solution:* 1%*
*Vaginal cream:* 2%
*Vaginal suppositories:* 100 mg

### INDICATIONS & DOSAGES
➤ **Inflammatory acne vulgaris**
*Adults and adolescents:* Apply to skin b.i.d., morning and evening.
➤ **Bacterial vaginosis**
*Adults:* 1 applicatorful intravaginally h.s. for 7 consecutive days or 1 suppository intravaginally h.s. for 3 consecutive days.

### ACTION
Bacteriostatic or bactericidal based on drug level and susceptibility of organism; suppresses growth of susceptible organisms in sebaceous glands by blocking protein synthesis.

| Route | Onset | Peak | Duration |
|-------|-------|------|----------|
| Topical, intravaginal | Unknown | Unknown | Unknown |

### ADVERSE REACTIONS
**GI:** GI upset, diarrhea, bloody diarrhea, abdominal pain, colitis including pseudomembranous colitis.
**GU:** *cervicitis, vaginitis,* Candida albicans overgrowth, *vulvar irritation.*
**Skin:** *dryness,* rash, *redness,* pruritus, swelling, irritation, contact dermatitis, burning.

### INTERACTIONS
**Drug-drug.** *Erythromycin:* May antagonize clindamycin's effect. Separate doses.

*Isotretinoin:* May cause cumulative dryness, resulting in excessive skin irritation. Use together cautiously.
*Neuromuscular blockers:* May increase action of neuromuscular blocker. Use together cautiously.
**Drug-lifestyle.** *Abrasive or medicated soaps or cleansers, acne products, or other preparations containing peeling drugs (benzoyl peroxide, resorcinol, salicylic acid, sulfur, tretinoin); alcohol-containing products (aftershave, cosmetics, perfumed toiletries, shaving creams or lotions); astringent soaps or cosmetics; medicated cosmetics or cover-ups:* May cause cumulative dryness, resulting in excessive skin irritation. Urge caution.

### EFFECTS ON LAB TEST RESULTS
• May increase liver enzyme levels.

### CONTRAINDICATIONS & CAUTIONS
• Contraindicated in patients hypersensitive to drug and in those with history of ulcerative colitis, regional enteritis, or antibiotic-related colitis.

### NURSING CONSIDERATIONS
• For treating acne, drug may be used with tretinoin or benzoyl peroxide as well as systemic antibiotics.
• Drug can cause excessive dryness.
• Monitor elderly patients for systemic effects.

### PATIENT TEACHING
• Tell patient to wash area with warm water and soap, rinse, pat dry, and wait 30 minutes after washing or shaving to apply.
• Warn patient to avoid excessive washing of area. Tell patient to cover entire affected area but to avoid contact with eyes, nose, mouth, and other mucous membranes.
• Instruct patient to use other prescribed acne medicines at a different time.
• Tell patient to use only as prescribed.
• Instruct patient to dab, not roll, applicator-tipped bottle. If tip becomes dry, patient should invert bottle and depress tip several times to moisten.
• Warn patient not to smoke while applying topical solution.

• For intravaginal application, make sure patient knows how to use applicators that come with drug.
• Advise patient to avoid sexual intercourse during intravaginal treatment.
• Instruct patient to notify prescriber immediately if abdominal pain or diarrhea occurs. Inform patient that antidiarrheal drug may worsen condition and should only be used as directed by prescriber.
• Tell patient to remove pledgets from foil before use.
• Advise patient to use pledgets only once, then discard. Also, more than 1 pledget may be used per application.
• Advise patient to complete entire course of therapy.

---

## clotrimazole
Canesten†, Cruex◇, Gyne-Lotrimin◇, Lotrimin, Lotrimin AF◇, Mycelex, Mycelex-7◇, Mycelex-G

*Pregnancy risk category B (C for lozenges)*

### AVAILABLE FORMS
*Combination pack:* Vaginal tablets 100 mg and vulvar cream 1%◇; vaginal tablets 200 mg and vulvar cream 1%◇
*Lozenges:* 10 mg
*Topical cream:* 1%
*Topical lotion:* 1%
*Topical solution:* 1%
*Vaginal cream:* 1%◇, 2%◇
*Vaginal suppositories:* 100 mg◇, 200 mg◇

### INDICATIONS & DOSAGES
➤ **Superficial fungal infections (tinea corporis, tinea cruris, tinea pedis, tinea versicolor, candidiasis)**
*Adults and children:* Apply thin film and massage into affected and surrounding area, morning and evening, for 2 to 4 weeks. If improvement doesn't occur after 4 weeks, reevaluate patient.
➤ **Vulvovaginal candidiasis**
*Adults:* One 100-mg vaginal suppository inserted daily h.s. for 7 consecutive days. Or, one 200-mg vaginal suppository h.s. for 3 days. Or, 1 applicatorful of vaginal cream daily h.s. for 7 days.

➤ **Oropharyngeal candidiasis**
*Adults and children age 3 and older:* Dissolve lozenge in mouth over 15 to 30 minutes five times daily for 14 consecutive days.
➤ **To prevent oropharyngeal candidiasis in patients immunocompromised by chemotherapy, radiotherapy, or corticosteroid therapy in the treatment of leukemia, solid tumors, or renal transplantation**
*Adults and children:* Dissolve lozenge in mouth over 15 to 30 minutes t.i.d. for duration of chemotherapy or until corticosteroid is reduced to maintenance levels.

### ACTION
Fungistatic or fungicidal, depending on level. Alters fungal cell wall permeability and produces osmotic instability.

| Route | Onset | Peak | Duration |
|---|---|---|---|
| P.O. | Unknown | Unknown | 3 hr |
| Topical, intravaginal | Unknown | Unknown | Unknown |

### ADVERSE REACTIONS
**GI:** lower abdominal cramps, nausea and vomiting with lozenges.
**GU:** *mild vaginal burning or irritation,* urinary frequency.
**Skin:** blistering, *erythema,* edema, pruritus, burning, stinging, peeling, urticaria, skin fissures, general irritation.

### INTERACTIONS
None significant.

### EFFECTS ON LAB TEST RESULTS
• May increase liver enzyme levels.

### CONTRAINDICATIONS & CAUTIONS
• Contraindicated in patients hypersensitive to drug.
• Contraindicated for ophthalmic use.

### NURSING CONSIDERATIONS
• Clean and dry area before applying drug.
• Watch for and report irritation or sensitivity; stop if irritation occurs, and notify prescriber.
• Improvement usually occurs within 1 week; if no improvement is seen within 4 weeks, review diagnosis.

---

*Rapid onset* †Canada ‡Australia ◇OTC ◆Off-label use ✐Photoguide *Liquid contains alcohol.

• *Alert:* Don't confuse clotrimazole with co-trimoxazole.

## PATIENT TEACHING
• Reassure patient that hypopigmentation from tinea versicolor does resolve gradually.
• Warn patient not to use occlusive wrappings or dressings.
• Warn patient to avoid drug contact with eyes.
• Caution patient that frequent or persistent yeast infections may suggest a more serious medical problem.
• Tell patient to refrain from sexual intercourse during intravaginal treatment.
• Warn patient that topical preparation may stain clothing.
• Tell patient that using a sanitary napkin protects clothing when using vaginal preparation.
• Stress need to continue use of vaginal preparations, as prescribed, even if menstruation begins.
• Tell patient with athlete's foot to change shoes and cotton socks daily and to dry between the toes after bathing.
• Tell patient to allow lozenges to dissolve in mouth; for maximum benefit, advise against chewing.
• Stress need to continue treatment for full course and to notify prescriber if no improvement occurs after 4 weeks.

## docosanol
Abreva ◇

*Pregnancy risk category B*

## AVAILABLE FORMS
*Cream:* 10% ◇

## INDICATIONS & DOSAGES
➤ **Recurrent oral and facial herpes simplex**
*Adults and children age 12 and older:* Apply topically five times daily, starting with first indication of an episode and continuing until lesion is healed. Rub in gently but completely.

## ACTION
Main mechanism appears to be inhibition of fusion between the cell's plasma membrane and the herpes simplex virus envelope, which blocks the entry and subsequent replication of the virus.

| Route | Onset | Peak | Duration |
|-------|-------|------|----------|
| Topical | Unknown | Unknown | Unknown |

## ADVERSE REACTIONS
**CNS:** *headache.*
**Skin:** reaction at application site.

## INTERACTIONS
None reported.

## EFFECTS ON LAB TEST RESULTS
None reported.

## CONTRAINDICATIONS & CAUTIONS
• Contraindicated in patients hypersensitive to drug or any of its components.
• It's unknown if drug appears in breast milk; use cautiously in breast-feeding patients.

## NURSING CONSIDERATIONS
• Use drug only to treat oral and facial herpes simplex lesions.
• Start treatment as early as possible after signs or symptoms begin.
• Continue treatment until the lesion has healed.

## PATIENT TEACHING
• Advise patient to start treatment as soon as signs or symptoms appear.
• Tell patient to use cream only on lips or face.
• Caution patient not to apply drug in or near the eyes because it may cause irritation.
• Tell patient to continue treatment until the lesion has healed.
• Notify patient that lesions are considered contagious until completely healed.
• Urge patient to notify prescriber if the condition gets worse.
• Caution woman to use drug during pregnancy only if clearly needed.
• Advise patient to store drug at room temperature and not to freeze it.
• Advise breast-feeding woman to use drug cautiously because it's unknown if it appears in breast milk.

Reactions may be *common*, uncommon, *life-threatening*, or COMMON AND LIFE-THREATENING.

## econazole nitrate
Ecostatin†, Spectazole

*Pregnancy risk category C*

### AVAILABLE FORMS
*Cream:* 1%

### INDICATIONS & DOSAGES
➤ **Tinea corporis, tinea cruris, tinea pedis, tinea versicolor**
*Adults and children:* Rub into affected areas daily for at least 2 weeks.
➤ **Cutaneous candidiasis**
*Adults and children:* Rub into affected areas b.i.d.

### ACTION
Fungistatic, but may be fungicidal depending on level. Appears to alter fungal cell wall permeability and produce osmotic instability.

| Route | Onset | Peak | Duration |
|-------|-------|------|----------|
| Topical | Unknown | Unknown | Unknown |

### ADVERSE REACTIONS
**Skin:** burning, pruritus, stinging, erythema.

### INTERACTIONS
**Drug-drug.** *Corticosteroids:* May inhibit antifungal activity against certain organisms. Monitor patient for clinical effect.

### EFFECTS ON LAB TEST RESULTS
None reported.

### CONTRAINDICATIONS & CAUTIONS
• Contraindicated in patients hypersensitive to drug or its components.

### NURSING CONSIDERATIONS
• Clean and dry affected area before applying.
• Don't use occlusive dressings.

### PATIENT TEACHING
• Tell patient to use drug for entire treatment period, even if signs and symptoms improve. Instruct him to notify prescriber if no improvement occurs after 2 weeks in fungal infection on hairless skin (tinea corporis), jock itch, or fungal skin infec-

tion (tinea versicolor), or after 4 weeks for athlete's foot.
• Reassure patient that lack of pigmentation from tinea versicolor resolves gradually.
• Tell patient to stop drug and notify prescriber if condition persists or worsens or if irritation occurs.
• Warn patient that drug may stain clothing.
• Tell patient with athlete's foot to change shoes and cotton socks daily and to dry between toes after bathing.
• Tell patient to keep drug out of eyes.

## erythromycin
Akne-mycin, A/T/S, Del-Mycin, Erycette, EryDerm, Erygel, Erymax, Ery-sol†, ETS†, Sans-Acne†, Staticin, T-Stat†

*Pregnancy risk category C (B for EryDerm, Erygel)*

### AVAILABLE FORMS
*Ointment:* 2%
*Pledgets:* 2%
*Topical gel:* 2%
*Topical solution:* 1.5%*, 2%*

### INDICATIONS & DOSAGES
➤ **Inflammatory acne vulgaris**
*Adults and children:* Apply to affected areas b.i.d., morning and evening.

### ACTION
Usually bacteriostatic, but may be bactericidal in high concentrations or against highly susceptible organisms. Disrupts protein synthesis in susceptible bacteria.

| Route | Onset | Peak | Duration |
|-------|-------|------|----------|
| Topical | Unknown | Unknown | Unknown |

### ADVERSE REACTIONS
**Skin:** sensitivity reactions, erythema, *burning, dryness, pruritus,* irritation, peeling, oily skin.

### INTERACTIONS
**Drug-drug.** *Clindamycin:* May antagonize clindamycin's effect. Separate doses.
*Isotretinoin:* May cause cumulative dryness, resulting in excessive skin irritation. Use together cautiously.

---

*Rapid onset* †Canada ‡Australia ◇OTC ♦Off-label use ⊘Photoguide *Liquid contains alcohol.

**Drug-lifestyle.** *Abrasive or medicated soaps or cleansers, acne products, or other preparations containing peeling drugs (benzoyl peroxide, resorcinol, salicylic acid, sulfur, tretinoin); alcohol-containing products (aftershave, cosmetics, perfumed toiletries, shaving creams or lotions); astringent soaps or cosmetics; medicated cosmetics or cover-ups:* May cause cumulative dryness, resulting in excessive skin irritation. Urge caution.

**EFFECTS ON LAB TEST RESULTS**
● Drug may interfere with fluorometric determinations of urinary catecholamines.

**CONTRAINDICATIONS & CAUTIONS**
● Contraindicated in patients hypersensitive to drug or its components.

**NURSING CONSIDERATIONS**
● Wash, rinse, and dry affected areas before application.
● Prolonged use may be needed when treating acne vulgaris, which may result in overgrowth of nonsusceptible organisms.

**PATIENT TEACHING**
● Advise patient to wash, rinse, and dry face thoroughly before each use.
● Advise patient to avoid use near eyes, nose, mouth, or other mucous membranes.
● Tell patient to wash hands after each application.
● Tell patient to stop using drug and notify prescriber if no improvement occurs or if condition worsens in 3 to 12 weeks.
● Advise patient not to share towels or washcloths.
● Instruct patient to use each pledget once, then discard.
● Caution patient to keep drug away from heat and open flame.

---

**gentamicin sulfate**
Garamycin, G-Myticin

*Pregnancy risk category C*

---

**AVAILABLE FORMS**
*Cream:* 0.1%
*Ointment:* 0.1%

**INDICATIONS & DOSAGES**
➤ **To treat or prevent superficial infections and superficial burns of the skin caused by susceptible bacteria**
*Adults and children older than age 1:* Rub in small amount gently t.i.d. or q.i.d., with or without gauze dressing.

**ACTION**
Exact mechanism unknown. An aminoglycoside that disrupts bacterial protein synthesis by binding to ribosomes.

| Route | Onset | Peak | Duration |
|-------|-------|------|----------|
| Topical | Unknown | Unknown | Unknown |

**ADVERSE REACTIONS**
**Skin:** minor skin irritation, photosensitivity, allergic contact dermatitis.

**INTERACTIONS**
None significant.

**EFFECTS ON LAB TEST RESULTS**
None reported.

**CONTRAINDICATIONS & CAUTIONS**
● Contraindicated in patients hypersensitive to drug or its components and in those who may have cross-sensitivity with other aminoglycosides such as neomycin.

**NURSING CONSIDERATIONS**
● *Alert:* Avoid use on large skin lesions or over a wide area because of possible systemic toxic effects.
● Restrict use of drug to selected patients; widespread use may lead to resistant organisms.
● Prolonged use may result in overgrowth of nonsusceptible organisms.

**PATIENT TEACHING**
● Tell patient to clean affected area and, to increase absorption, remove crusts of impetigo before applying drug.
● Instruct patient to store drug in cool place.
● Tell patient to stop using drug and notify prescriber immediately if no improvement occurs or if condition worsens.

---

Reactions may be *common*, uncommon, *life-threatening*, or COMMON AND LIFE-THREATENING.

# ketoconazole
Nizoral, Nizoral A-D ◇

*Pregnancy risk category C*

## AVAILABLE FORMS
*Cream:* 2%
*Shampoo:* 1% ◇, 2%

## INDICATIONS & DOSAGES
➤ **Tinea corporis, tinea cruris, tinea pedis, tinea versicolor from susceptible organisms; seborrheic dermatitis; cutaneous candidiasis**
*Adults:* Cover affected and immediate surrounding area daily for at least 2 weeks. For seborrheic dermatitis, apply b.i.d. for 4 weeks. Patients with tinea pedis need 6 weeks of treatment. When using shampoo, wet hair, lather, and massage for 1 minute. Leave drug on scalp for 3 minutes; then rinse and repeat. Shampoo twice weekly for 4 weeks, with at least 3 days between shampoos and then intermittently, p.r.n., to maintain control.

## ACTION
Unknown. An imidazole that probably inhibits yeast growth by altering the permeability of the cell membrane.

| Route | Onset | Peak | Duration |
|---|---|---|---|
| Topical | Unknown | Unknown | Unknown |

## ADVERSE REACTIONS
**Skin:** severe irritation, pruritus, and stinging with cream; increase in normal hair loss; irritation; abnormal hair texture; scalp pustules; pruritus, oiliness, or dryness of hair and scalp with shampoo use.

## INTERACTIONS
**Drug-drug.** *Topical corticosteroids:* May cause increased absorption of corticosteroid. Avoid using together.

## EFFECTS ON LAB TEST RESULTS
None reported.

## CONTRAINDICATIONS & CAUTIONS
• Contraindicated in patients hypersensitive to drug or its components.
• Use cautiously in breast-feeding women.

## NURSING CONSIDERATIONS
• Most patients show improvement soon after treatment begins.
• Treatment of tinea corporis or tinea cruris should continue for at least 2 weeks to reduce possibility of recurrence.
• **Alert:** Product contains sodium sulfite anhydrous, which may cause severe or life-threatening allergic reactions, including anaphylaxis, in patients with asthma.

## PATIENT TEACHING
• Tell patient to stop drug and notify prescriber if hypersensitivity reaction occurs.
• Advise patient to check with prescriber if condition worsens; drug may have to be stopped and diagnosis reevaluated.
• Tell patient to avoid using shampoo on scalp if skin is broken or inflamed.
• Warn patient that shampoo applied to permanent-waved hair removes curl.
• Warn patient to avoid drug contact with eyes.
• Tell patient to continue drug for intended duration of therapy, even if signs and symptoms improve soon after starting treatment.
• Tell patient not to store drug above room temperature (77° F [25° C]) and to protect from light.

---

# metronidazole
MetroCream, MetroGel, MetroGel Vaginal, MetroLotion, Noritate, Rosex

*Pregnancy risk category B*

## AVAILABLE FORMS
*Topical cream:* 0.75%, 1%
*Topical emulsion:* 0.75%
*Topical gel:* 0.75%
*Topical lotion:* 0.75%
*Vaginal gel:* 0.75%

## INDICATIONS & DOSAGES
➤ **Inflammatory papules and pustules of acne rosacea**
*Adults:* Apply thin film to affected area b.i.d., morning and evening. Frequency and duration of therapy are adjusted after response is seen. Results are usually noticed within 3 weeks.

---

➤ **Bacterial vaginosis**
*Adults:* 1 applicatorful intravaginally daily or b.i.d. for 5 days. For once-daily dosing, give h.s.

### ACTION
Unknown. May cause bactericidal effect by interacting with bacterial DNA. Drug is active against many anaerobic gram-negative bacilli, anaerobic gram-positive cocci, *Gardnerella vaginalis,* and *Campylobacter fetus.*

| Route | Onset | Peak | Duration |
|---|---|---|---|
| Topical | Unknown | Unknown | Unknown |
| Intravaginal | Unknown | 6-12 hr | Unknown |

### ADVERSE REACTIONS
**Topical forms**
**EENT:** lacrimation if applied around eyes.
**Skin:** rash, *transient redness, dryness, mild burning, stinging.*
**Vaginal form**
**CNS:** dizziness, headache.
**GI:** cramps, pain, nausea, diarrhea, constipation, metallic or bad taste in mouth, decreased appetite.
**GU:** *cervicitis, vaginitis,* perineal and vulvovaginal itching.
**Skin:** *transient redness, dryness, mild burning, stinging.*
**Other:** overgrowth of nonsusceptible organisms.

### INTERACTIONS
**Drug-drug.** *Disulfiram:* May cause disulfiram-like reaction. Avoid using together and wait 2 weeks after stopping disulfiram before starting metronidazole vaginal therapy.
*Lithium:* May increase lithium level. Monitor lithium level.
*Oral anticoagulants:* May increase anticoagulant effect. Monitor patient for adverse reactions.
**Drug-lifestyle.** *Alcohol use:* May cause disulfiram-like reaction. Discourage use together.

### EFFECTS ON LAB TEST RESULTS
• May interfere with AST, ALT, LDH, triglyceride, and glucose levels.
• May increase or decrease WBC count.

### CONTRAINDICATIONS & CAUTIONS
• Contraindicated in patients hypersensitive to drug or its ingredients, such as parabens, and other nitroimidazole derivatives.
• Use cautiously in patients with history or evidence of blood dyscrasia and in those with severe hepatic disease.
• Use vaginal gel cautiously in patients with history of CNS diseases. Oral form may cause seizures and peripheral neuropathy.

### NURSING CONSIDERATIONS
• Topical therapy hasn't been linked to adverse effects observed with parenteral or oral therapy, but some drug may be absorbed after topical use.
• Don't use vaginal gel in patients who have taken disulfiram within past 2 weeks.

### PATIENT TEACHING
• Instruct patient to avoid use of topical gel around eyes.
• Advise patient to clean area thoroughly before use and to wait 15 to 20 minutes after cleaning skin before applying drug to minimize risk of local irritation. Cosmetics may be used after applying drug.
• If local reactions occur, advise patient to apply drug less frequently or stop using it and notify prescriber.
• Advise patient to avoid sexual intercourse while using vaginal preparation.
• Caution patient to avoid alcohol while being treated with vaginal preparation.

---

## miconazole nitrate
Desenex◊ , Lotrimin AF◊ , Micatin◊ , Monistat-Derm, Monistat 3◊ , Monistat 7◊ , Ting◊ , Zeasorb-AF◊

*Pregnancy risk category C*

### AVAILABLE FORMS
*Aerosol powder:* 2%◊
*Aerosol spray:* 1%, 2%◊
*Lotion:* 2%◊
*Powder:* 2%◊
*Topical cream:* 2%◊
*Topical ointment:* 2%◊
*Topical solution:* 2%◊
*Vaginal cream:* 2%◊

---

Reactions may be *common*, uncommon, *life-threatening*, or COMMON AND LIFE-THREATENING.

*Vaginal suppositories:* 100 mg ◇,
200 mg ◇, 1,200 mg ◇

## INDICATIONS & DOSAGES
➤ **Tinea corporis, tinea cruris, tinea pedis, cutaneous candidiasis, common dermatophyte infections**
*Adults and children older than age 1:*
Apply sparingly b.i.d. for 2 to 4 weeks.
Powder or spray can be used liberally over affected area.
➤ **Tinea versicolor**
*Adults and children older than age 1:* Apply sparingly daily for 2 weeks.
➤ **Vulvovaginal candidiasis**
*Adults:* 1 applicatorful or 100-mg Monistat 7 suppository intravaginally h.s. for 7 days; repeat course, if needed. Or, 200-mg Monistat 3 suppository intravaginally h.s. for 3 days. Or, one 1,200-mg suppository intravaginally h.s. for 1 day. Or, apply topical cream sparingly to affected area b.i.d. for 7 days.

## ACTION
A fungicidal imidazole that disrupts fungal cell membrane permeability.

| Route | Onset | Peak | Duration |
|-------|-------|------|----------|
| Topical, intravaginal | Unknown | Unknown | Unknown |

## ADVERSE REACTIONS
**CNS:** headache.
**GU:** pelvic cramps; vulvovaginal burning, pruritus, and irritation with vaginal cream.
**Skin:** irritation, burning, maceration, allergic contact dermatitis.

## INTERACTIONS
None significant.

## EFFECTS ON LAB TEST RESULTS
None reported.

## CONTRAINDICATIONS & CAUTIONS
• Contraindicated in patients hypersensitive to drug or its components.

## NURSING CONSIDERATIONS
• Avoid using within 72 hours of certain intravaginal and latex products, such as condoms or vaginal contraceptive diaphragms because drug causes latex breakdown.

• Don't use occlusive dressings.
• Lotion is preferred in skinfolds.

## PATIENT TEACHING
• Advise patient that vaginal form of drug is for perineal or intravaginal use only and to keep drug out of eyes.
• Caution patient that frequent or persistent yeast infections may suggest a more serious medical problem.
• Tell patient to cautiously insert intravaginal form high into the vagina with applicator provided.
• *Alert:* Vaginal preparation shouldn't be used during first trimester of pregnancy. Advise patient to use vaginal preparation during pregnancy only if recommended by prescriber.
• Tell patient that drug may stain clothing.
• Warn patient to stop drug if sensitivity or chemical irritation occurs.
• Tell patient to use drug for full treatment period prescribed and to notify prescriber if signs and symptoms persist or worsen at end of therapy.
• Advise patient to avoid tampons and sexual intercourse during vaginal treatment.
• Instruct patient to apply sparingly in skinfolds and rub in well to prevent skin breakdown.
• Tell patient to store vaginal product between 59° and 86° F (15° and 30° C).

## mupirocin
Bactroban, Bactroban Cream, Bactroban Nasal

*Pregnancy risk category B*

## AVAILABLE FORMS
*Intranasal ointment:* 2%
*Topical cream:* 2%
*Topical ointment:* 2%

## INDICATIONS & DOSAGES
➤ **Impetigo**
*Adults and children:* Apply to affected areas t.i.d. for 1 to 2 weeks. Reevaluate patient in 3 to 5 days; may cover affected area with dressing.

➤ **Traumatic skin lesions infected with**
*Staphylococcus aureus* **or** *Streptococcus pyogenes*
*Adults and children:* Apply thin film t.i.d. for 10 days; may cover with gauze dressing, if needed. Reevaluate patient if improvement doesn't occur in 3 to 5 days.
➤ **To eradicate nasal colonization by methicillin-resistant** *S. aureus* **in adult patients and health care workers**
*Adults and children age 12 and older:* Divide ointment in single-use tube between nostrils (¼ tube per nostril) b.i.d. for 5 days. After application, close nostrils by pressing together and releasing sides of nose repeatedly for 1 minute to spread ointment throughout nares.

**ACTION**
Unknown. Thought to inhibit bacterial protein and RNA synthesis.

| Route | Onset | Peak | Duration |
|-------|-------|------|----------|
| Topical | Unknown | Unknown | Unknown |

**ADVERSE REACTIONS**
**CNS:** headache.
**EENT:** rhinitis, pharyngitis, burning or stinging with intranasal use.
**GI:** taste perversion, abdominal pain, ulcerative stomatitis.
**Respiratory:** upper respiratory tract congestion, cough with intranasal use.
**Skin:** burning, pruritus, stinging, rash, pain, erythema with topical use.

**INTERACTIONS**
*Chloramphenicol:* May interfere with the antibacterial action of mupirocin on RNA synthesis. Monitor patient for clinical effect.

**EFFECTS ON LAB TEST RESULTS**
None reported.

**CONTRAINDICATIONS & CAUTIONS**
• Contraindicated in patients hypersensitive to drug or its components.
• Use cautiously in patients with burns or impaired renal function because serious renal toxicity may occur.

**NURSING CONSIDERATIONS**
• Drug isn't for ophthalmic or internal use.

• Prolonged use may cause overgrowth of nonsusceptible bacteria and fungi.
• Local reactions appear to be caused by polyethylene glycol vehicle.
• Patient shouldn't use other nasal products with intranasal ointment.
• *Alert:* Don't confuse Bactroban with bacitracin.

**PATIENT TEACHING**
• Tell patient to notify prescriber immediately if condition doesn't improve or gets worse in 3 to 5 days.
• Tell patient not to use other nasal products with mupirocin.
• Warn patient about local adverse reactions related to drug use.
• Caution patient not to use cosmetics or other skin products on treated area.

---

**neomycin sulfate**
Myciguent ◊

*Pregnancy risk category C*

**AVAILABLE FORMS**
*Ointment:* 0.5% ◊

**INDICATIONS & DOSAGES**
➤ **To prevent or treat superficial bacterial infections**
*Adults and children:* Rub fingertip-size dose into affected area once daily to t.i.d.

**ACTION**
Unknown. Thought to disrupt bacterial protein synthesis by binding to bacterial ribosomes.

| Route | Onset | Peak | Duration |
|-------|-------|------|----------|
| Topical | Unknown | Unknown | Unknown |

**ADVERSE REACTIONS**
**CNS:** *neuromuscular blockade.*
**EENT:** *ototoxicity.*
**GU:** *nephrotoxicity.*
**Skin:** *rash, contact dermatitis,* urticaria.

**INTERACTIONS**
None significant.

**EFFECTS ON LAB TEST RESULTS**
None reported.

**CONTRAINDICATIONS & CAUTIONS**
• Contraindicated in patients hypersensitive to drug or its components.

**NURSING CONSIDERATIONS**
• Don't use more than once daily on burns covering more than 20% of body surface area.
• Prolonged use may result in overgrowth of nonsusceptible organisms.
• In products containing corticosteroids, use of occlusive dressings increases corticosteroid absorption and likelihood of systemic effects.
• Systemic absorption is enhanced on exposed or abraded areas.
• Watch for signs and symptoms of hypersensitivity and contact dermatitis.
• **Alert:** Watch for signs of ototoxicity with prolonged use.

**PATIENT TEACHING**
• Tell patient to stop drug and notify prescriber if condition doesn't improve or worsens.
• Tell patient to report adverse reactions, especially systemic reactions.
• Instruct patient not to use drug for longer than 1 week unless otherwise directed.

---

**nitrofurazone**
Furacin

*Pregnancy risk category C*

**AVAILABLE FORMS**
*Cream:* 0.2%
*Ointment:* 0.2% (soluble dressing)
*Topical solution:* 0.2%

**INDICATIONS & DOSAGES**
➤ **Adjunctive treatment of second- and third-degree burns (especially when resistance to other antibiotics and sulfonamides occurs); prevention of skin allograft rejection**
*Adults and children:* Apply directly to lesion daily or q few days, depending on severity of burn. Drug may also be applied to dressings used to cover affected area.

**ACTION**
Unknown. A broad-spectrum antibiotic that probably inhibits bacterial enzymes involved in carbohydrate metabolism.

| Route | Onset | Peak | Duration |
|---|---|---|---|
| Topical | Unknown | Unknown | Unknown |

**ADVERSE REACTIONS**
**Skin:** erythema, pruritus, burning, local edema, allergic contact dermatitis.

**INTERACTIONS**
None significant.

**EFFECTS ON LAB TEST RESULTS**
None reported.

**CONTRAINDICATIONS & CAUTIONS**
• Contraindicated in patients hypersensitive to drug.
• Use cautiously in patients with renal impairment.

**NURSING CONSIDERATIONS**
• In patients with renal impairment, use drug with caution and monitor creatinine levels regularly.
• Flush dressing with sterile normal saline solution to ease removal.
• Clean wound, as indicated by prescriber, before reapplying dressings.
• Use sterile application technique to prevent further wound contamination.
• When using wet dressing, protect skin around wound with zinc oxide ointment.
• Don't store dressings saturated with drug for longer than 24 hours.
• Drug may change color in light but still retains its potency.
• Discard cloudy solutions if warming to 131° to 140° F (55° to 60° C) doesn't restore clarity.
• Store solution in tight, light-resistant container (brown bottle). Avoid exposure to direct light, prolonged heat, and alkaline materials.

**PATIENT TEACHING**
• Tell patient to report irritation, sensitization, or infection.
• Explain all procedures to patient.
• Tell patient to notify prescriber if condition worsens.

---

● Tell patient to avoid drug contact with eyes.

---

## nystatin
Mycostatin, Nilstat, Nystex, Pedi-Dri

*Pregnancy risk category NR*

---

### AVAILABLE FORMS
*Cream:* 100,000 units/g
*Lozenges:* 200,000 units
*Ointment:* 100,000 units/g
*Oral suspension:* 100,000 units/ml
*Powder:* 100,000 units/g
*Vaginal tablets:* 100,000 units

### INDICATIONS & DOSAGES
➤ **Cutaneous and mucocutaneous infections caused by *Candida albicans***
*Adults and children:* Apply to affected area up to several times daily until healing is complete. Apply cream or ointment b.i.d. or as indicated; powder, b.i.d. or t.i.d.; lozenges, 1 or 2 four to five times daily until 48 hours after oral symptoms subside, but not longer than 14 days; suspension, 4 to 6 ml q.i.d. (one-half of dose in each side of mouth); retain dose as long as possible before swallowing.
➤ **Vulvovaginal candidiasis**
*Adults:* 1 vaginal tablet daily for 14 days.

### ACTION
Disrupts integrity of fungal cell wall, promoting osmotic instability.

| Route | Onset | Peak | Duration |
|---|---|---|---|
| P.O., topical intravaginal | Unknown | Unknown | Unknown |

### ADVERSE REACTIONS
**GI:** vomiting with vaginal tablet.
**Skin:** occasional contact dermatitis from preservatives in some forms.

### INTERACTIONS
None significant.

### EFFECTS ON LAB TEST RESULTS
None reported.

### CONTRAINDICATIONS & CAUTIONS
● Contraindicated in patients hypersensitive to drug or its components.

### NURSING CONSIDERATIONS
● Don't use occlusive dressings.
● Preparation doesn't stain skin or mucous membranes.
● Cream is recommended for skinfolds; powder, for moist areas; ointment, for dry areas.
● **Alert:** Don't confuse nystatin with Nitrostat.

### PATIENT TEACHING
● Show patient how to use vaginal tablets and tell her to continue using them during menstrual period.
● Tell patient to insert drug high in vagina (except during pregnancy) and to refrain from sexual intercourse during vaginal treatment.
● Instruct patient to refrigerate tablets.
● Tell patient to use drug for full prescribed period even if condition improves and to continue use for at least 2 days after symptoms subside (for oral therapy). Immunosuppressed patients may use drug on long-term basis.
● Warn patient to keep drug away from eyes.
● Instruct patient not to use occlusive dressings with skin application.
● Tell patient to dissolve oral lozenges slowly in mouth.
● Demonstrate and stress importance of proper oral hygiene, especially for denture wearers.

---

## silver sulfadiazine
Flamazine†, Silvadene, SSD, SSD AF, Thermazene

*Pregnancy risk category B*

---

### AVAILABLE FORMS
*Cream:* 1%

### INDICATIONS & DOSAGES
➤ **To prevent or treat wound infection in second- and third-degree burns**
*Adults:* Apply ¼-inch ribbon of cream to clean, debrided wound daily or b.i.d.

---

## ACTION
A broad-spectrum sulfonamide that acts on cell membrane and cell wall; it's bactericidal for many gram-positive and gram-negative organisms.

| Route | Onset | Peak | Duration |
|-------|-------|------|----------|
| Topical | Unknown | Unknown | Unknown |

## ADVERSE REACTIONS
**Hematologic:** *leukopenia.*
**Metabolic:** altered serum osmolality.
**Skin:** pain, burning, rash, pruritus, skin necrosis, *erythema multiforme,* skin discoloration.

## INTERACTIONS
**Drug-drug.** *Topical proteolytic enzymes:* May inactivate enzymes. Avoid using together.
**Drug-lifestyle.** *Sun exposure:* May cause photosensitivity. Advise patient to avoid excessive sun exposure.

## EFFECTS ON LAB TEST RESULTS
• May decrease WBC count.

## CONTRAINDICATIONS & CAUTIONS
• Contraindicated in patients hypersensitive to drug and in those with G6PD deficiency.
• Contraindicated in pregnant women at or near term and in premature or full-term neonates during first 2 months after birth. Drug may increase possibility of kernicterus.
• *Alert:* Use cautiously in patients hypersensitive to sulfonamides.

## NURSING CONSIDERATIONS
• Use sterile application technique to prevent wound contamination.
• Use drug only on affected areas. Keep these areas medicated at all times.
• Bathe patient daily, if possible.
• Inspect patient's skin daily, and note any changes. Notify prescriber if burning or excessive pain develops.
• Monitor sulfadiazine levels and renal function, and check urine for sulfa crystals in patients with extensive burns.
• Tell prescriber if hepatic or renal dysfunction occurs; drug may need to be stopped.

• Leukopenia usually resolves without intervention and doesn't always require stopping drug.
• Absorption of propylene glycol (contained in the cream) can interfere with serum osmolality.
• Discard darkened cream because drug is ineffective.

## PATIENT TEACHING
• Instruct patient to promptly report adverse reactions, especially burning or excessive pain with application.
• Inform patient of need for frequent blood and urine tests to watch for adverse effects.
• Tell patient that he may develop sensitivity to the sun.
• Tell patient to continue treatment until satisfactory healing occurs or until site is ready for grafting.

# terbinafine hydrochloride
Lamisil, Lamisil AT ◇

*Pregnancy risk category B*

## AVAILABLE FORMS
*Cream:* 1% ◇
*Spray:* 1% ◇

## INDICATIONS & DOSAGES
➤ **Athlete's foot**
*Adults and children age 12 and older:* Apply b.i.d. for 1 week.
➤ **Jock itch, ringworm**
*Adults and children age 12 and older:* Apply once daily for 1 week.

## ACTION
A fungicidal that selectively inhibits an early step in synthesis of sterols used by fungi for cell wall synthesis.

| Route | Onset | Peak | Duration |
|-------|-------|------|----------|
| Topical | Unknown | Unknown | Unknown |

## ADVERSE REACTIONS
**Skin:** irritation, pruritus.

## INTERACTIONS
None significant.

**EFFECTS ON LAB TEST RESULTS**
None reported.

**CONTRAINDICATIONS & CAUTIONS**
• Contraindicated in patients hypersensitive to drug or its components and in breast-feeding women.

**NURSING CONSIDERATIONS**
• Observe patient for 2 to 6 weeks after therapy is complete to determine whether treatment was successful; review diagnosis if condition persists.
• Drug isn't intended for oral, ophthalmic, or vaginal use.
• *Alert:* Don't confuse terbinafine with terfenadine or terbutaline.
• *Alert:* Don't confuse Lamisil with Lamictal.

**PATIENT TEACHING**
• Teach patient proper use of drug. Tell him to use only as directed for full recommended course, even if signs and symptoms disappear, and not to apply near eyes, mouth, or mucous membranes or to use occlusive dressings unless so directed.
• Tell patient to stop drug and contact prescriber if irritation or sensitivity develops.
• Tell patient to store drug between 41° and 86° F (5° and 30° C).

---

## terconazole
Terazol 3, Terazol 7

*Pregnancy risk category C*

---

**AVAILABLE FORMS**
*Vaginal cream:* 0.4%, 0.8%
*Vaginal suppositories:* 80 mg

**INDICATIONS & DOSAGES**
➤ **Vulvovaginal candidiasis**
*Adults:* 1 applicatorful of cream or 1 suppository inserted into vagina h.s.; 0.4% cream used for 7 consecutive days; 0.8% cream or 80-mg suppository for 3 consecutive days. Repeat course, if needed, after reconfirmation by smear or culture.

**ACTION**
Unknown. May increase fungal cell membrane permeability (*Candida* species only).

| Route | Onset | Peak | Duration |
|---|---|---|---|
| Intravaginal | Unknown | Unknown | Unknown |

**ADVERSE REACTIONS**
**CNS:** fever, *headache.*
**GI:** abdominal pain.
**GU:** dysmenorrhea, genital pain, vulvovaginal burning.
**Skin:** irritation, *pruritus,* photosensitivity.
**Other:** chills, body aches.

**INTERACTIONS**
None significant.

**EFFECTS ON LAB TEST RESULTS**
None reported.

**CONTRAINDICATIONS & CAUTIONS**
• Contraindicated in patients hypersensitive to drug or its inactive ingredients.

**NURSING CONSIDERATIONS**
• Therapeutic effect of drug is unaffected by menstruation or hormonal contraceptive use.
• *Alert:* Don't confuse terconazole with tioconazole.

**PATIENT TEACHING**
• Advise patient to continue treatment during menstrual period. However, tell her not to use tampons.
• Instruct patient to insert drug high in vagina (except during pregnancy).
• Tell patient to use drug for full treatment period prescribed. Explain how to prevent reinfection.
• Instruct patient to notify prescriber and stop drug if fever, chills, other flulike signs and symptoms, or sensitivity develops.
• Caution patient to refrain from sexual intercourse during treatment.
• Tell patient that drug base may react with latex, causing decreased effectiveness of condoms and diaphragms (for up to 72 hours after treatment is completed).
• Instruct patient to store drug at room temperature.

## tolnaftate

Absorbine Footcare ◇, Aftate for
Athlete's Foot ◇, Aftate for Jock
Itch ◇, Genaspor ◇, Quinsana
Plus ◇, Tinactin ◇, Ting ◇

*Pregnancy risk category C*

### AVAILABLE FORMS
*Aerosol liquid:* 1% (36% alcohol) ◇
*Aerosol powder:* 1% (14% alcohol) ◇
*Cream:* 1% ◇
*Gel:* 1% ◇
*Powder:* 1% ◇
*Pump spray liquid:* 1% (36% alcohol) ◇
*Topical solution:* 1% ◇

### INDICATIONS & DOSAGES
➤ **Superficial fungal infections of the
skin; infections caused by common
pathogenic fungi; tinea pedis, tinea
cruris, tinea corporis, tinea versicolor**
*Adults and children:* Apply ¼- to ½-inch
ribbon of cream or 2 to 3 drops of solution
to cover area; same amount of cream or
solution to cover toes and interdigital
webs; or gel, powder, or spray to cover affected area. Massage drug gently into skin
b.i.d. for 2 to 6 weeks.

### ACTION
Unknown, although it has been shown to
distort the hyphae and stunt mycelial
growth in susceptible fungi.

| Route | Onset | Peak | Duration |
|-------|-------|------|----------|
| Topical | Unknown | Unknown | Unknown |

### ADVERSE REACTIONS
**Skin:** irritation.

### INTERACTIONS
None significant.

### EFFECTS ON LAB TEST RESULTS
None reported.

### CONTRAINDICATIONS & CAUTIONS
• Contraindicated in patients hypersensitive to drug or its components.

### NURSING CONSIDERATIONS
• Drug isn't used to treat fungal infections
of hair or nails; tolnaftate is ineffective
against these fungi.
• Drug is odorless and greaseless; it won't
stain or discolor skin, hair, nails, or clothing.
• Powder or aerosol may be used inside
socks and shoes of persons susceptible to
tinea infections.
• Ointments, creams, and liquid are primarily used for treatment; powder and
aerosol are adjuncts unless infection is
very mild.
• *Alert:* Don't confuse tolnaftate with Tornalate.

### PATIENT TEACHING
• Teach patient to clean and dry area thoroughly before applying drug.
• Tell patient to use drug for full treatment
period prescribed, even if condition has
improved. Treatment should continue for
at least 2 weeks after signs and symptoms
have resolved.
• Advise patient to use only small amount
of cream or solution; treated area
shouldn't be wet with solution.
• Tell patient to stop drug and notify prescriber if no improvement occurs after
10 days or if condition worsens.
• Advise patient to wear shoes and cotton
socks that fit well and to change socks
daily.
• Tell patient to keep drug away from
eyes.

crotamiton
lindane
permethrin
pyrethrins

**COMBINATION PRODUCTS**
None.

---

## crotamiton
Eurax

*Pregnancy risk category C*

### AVAILABLE FORMS
*Cream:* 10%
*Lotion:* 10%

### INDICATIONS & DOSAGES
➤ **Parasitic infestation (scabies)**
*Adults:* Scrub entire body with soap and water. Remove scales or crusts. Then apply thin layer of cream over entire body, from chin down (with special attention to skinfolds, creases, interdigital spaces, and genital area). Apply second coat in 24 hours. Wait another 48 hours; then wash off. Repeat treatment in 7 to 10 days if mites reappear or new lesions develop.
➤ **Itching**
*Adults:* Apply locally, massaging gently into affected area until completely absorbed; repeat, p.r.n.

### ACTION
Unknown.

| Route | Onset | Peak | Duration |
|-------|-------|------|----------|
| Topical | Unknown | Unknown | Unknown |

### ADVERSE REACTIONS
**Skin:** *irritation*, allergic skin sensitivity.

### INTERACTIONS
None significant.

### EFFECTS ON LAB TEST RESULTS
None reported.

### CONTRAINDICATIONS & CAUTIONS
● Contraindicated in patients hypersensitive to drug or its components and in those whose skin is raw or inflamed.

### NURSING CONSIDERATIONS
● Estimate amount of cream needed per application; most patients tend to overuse scabicides. For most adults, a single tube of cream is enough for two applications.
● Don't apply drug to acutely inflamed or raw, weeping areas.
● Apply topical corticosteroids, as prescribed, if dermatitis develops from scratching.
● Make sure hospitalized patients are placed in isolation, with special linen-handling precautions, until treatment is completed.
● Monthly maintenance treatments may be needed in long-term care facilities where infestation is a problem.
● **Alert:** Don't confuse Eurax with Serax or Urex.
● Treat sexual contacts simultaneously.

### PATIENT TEACHING
● Tell patient or family member to shake product well before each use.
● Teach patient or family member how to apply drug. Tell patient not to apply to face, eyes, mucous membranes, or urethral opening. If accidental contact with eyes occurs, tell patient to flush with water and notify prescriber.
● Tell patient to stop using drug, wash it off skin, and notify prescriber immediately if skin irritation or hypersensitivity develops.
● Instruct patient to change all clothing and bed linens and launder them in hot cycle of washing machine or dry clean after drug is washed off body.
● Instruct patient to reapply drug if it's washed off during treatment time.
● Tell patient to warn other family members and sexual contacts about infestation.
● Reassure patient that although itching may continue for several weeks, it will stop; continued itching doesn't indicate that therapy is ineffective.

---

Reactions may be *common*, uncommon, *life-threatening*, or COMMON AND LIFE-THREATENING.

# lindane
GBH†, G-well, Kwellada†

*Pregnancy risk category B*

## AVAILABLE FORMS
*Cream:* 1%†
*Lotion:* 1%
*Shampoo:* 1%

## INDICATIONS & DOSAGES
➤ **Parasitic infestation (scabies, pediculosis)**
*Adults and children:* Centers for Disease Control and Prevention recommends not bathing before applying on skin. If patient does bathe, let skin dry and cool thoroughly before using. For scabies, apply thin layer of cream or lotion over entire skin surface from the neck down (with special attention to skinfolds, creases, interdigital spaces, and genital area) and rub in thoroughly; for pediculosis, apply thin layer of cream or lotion to hairy areas. After 8 to 12 hours, wash drug off. Repeat process in 1 week if mites reappear or new lesions develop.

Apply shampoo undiluted to dry hair and work into lather for 4 to 5 minutes; small amounts of water may increase lathering. Apply 30 ml of shampoo for short hair, 45 ml for medium-length hair, or 60 ml for long hair. Rinse thoroughly and rub dry with towel. Comb with a fine-tooth comb.
*Elderly patients:* May need to reduce dosage because of increased skin absorption.

## ACTION
Unclear. May inhibit neuronal membrane function in arthropods, causing neuronal hyperactivity, seizures, and death after penetrating the parasite's exoskeleton.

| Route | Onset | Peak | Duration |
|---|---|---|---|
| Topical | 190 min | Unknown | Unknown |

## ADVERSE REACTIONS
None reported.

## INTERACTIONS
**Drug-lifestyle.** *Oils:* May increase absorption of drug; if oil-based hair products are used, urge patient to wash and dry hair before using lindane.

## EFFECTS ON LAB TEST RESULTS
None reported.

## CONTRAINDICATIONS & CAUTIONS
• Contraindicated in patients hypersensitive to drug or its components, in those with seizure disorders, and in those with inflamed skin. Also contraindicated in premature infants.
• *Alert:* Use cautiously in infants, children, elderly patients, those with skin conditions other than lice infestation, and persons weighing less than 110 lb (50 kg); all are at greater risk of CNS toxicity, including seizures and death.

## NURSING CONSIDERATIONS
• Use lindane products only as second-line treatment of lice infestation or in patients who can't tolerate treatment with safer medications. Permethrin 1% cream rinse and pyrethrins with piperonyl butoxide are safer than lindane for the treatment of pubic lice.
• Apply topical corticosteroids or give oral antihistamines, as prescribed, for pruritus.
• Make sure that hospitalized patients are placed in isolation, with special linen-handling precautions, until treatment is completed.
• Intact skin absorbs 6% to 13% of drug. Absorption is increased if applied to face, scalp, axillae, neck, scrotum, or irritated or broken skin.
• Avoid contact of drug with eyes.
• When lindane is used appropriately, it's safe and effective. When overused, it can cause adverse reactions. Don't confuse prolonged itching with reinfestation.
• Treat sexual contacts simultaneously.

## PATIENT TEACHING
• Teach patient or family member how to give drug. Apply thin layer to cover body only once: 1 ounce is used for children younger than age 6 and 1 to 2 ounces for older children and adults. Drug shouldn't be left on for longer than 12 hours; remove drug thoroughly by washing.
• If patient bathes before application, tell him to let skin dry thoroughly and cool before applying drug.
• Inform patient that drug can be poisonous when misused. Warn patient not to apply to open areas, acutely inflamed skin, or to face, eyes, mucous membranes, or

urethral opening. If accidental contact with eyes occurs, advise patient to flush with water and notify prescriber.
• Tell patient to avoid inhaling vapors.
• Advise patient to wear gloves if applying on another person.
• Tell patient to wash drug off skin and to notify prescriber immediately if skin irritation or hypersensitivity develops.
• Discourage repeated use, which can lead to skin irritation, systemic toxicity, or seizures. Advise patient to repeat use only if live lice or nits are found after 1 week.
• Warn patient not to use other creams or oils during treatment because of potential for increased absorption.
• Instruct patient to change all clothing and bed linens and launder them in hot water or dry clean after drug is washed off body.
• After application for lice infestation, tell patient to use fine-tooth comb or tweezers to remove nits from hairy areas.
• Advise patient to use lindane shampoo to clean combs or brushes and to wash them thoroughly afterward. Warn patient not to use lindane routinely.
• Warn patient that itching may continue for several weeks after effective treatment, especially for scabies.
• Instruct patient to reapply drug if it's washed off during treatment time.
• Tell patient to warn other family members and sexual contacts about infestation.
• Advise patient to use product carefully and follow all directions. Overusing product will cause unwanted side effects. Tell him not to confuse prolonged itching with reinfestation.

---

# permethrin
Acticin, Elimite, Nix ◇

*Pregnancy risk category B*

## AVAILABLE FORMS
*Cream:* 5%
*Topical liquid (cream rinse):* 1%

## INDICATIONS & DOSAGES
➤ **Infestation with *Pediculus humanus capitis* (head louse) and its nits**
*Adults and children age 2 and older:* Use after hair has been washed with shampoo, rinsed with water, and towel-dried. Apply 25 to 50 ml of liquid to saturate hair and scalp. Allow drug to remain on hair for 10 minutes before rinsing off with water. Usually only one application is needed.
➤ **Infestation with *Sarcoptes scabiei***
*Adults and children age 2 months and older:* Thoroughly massage into the skin from the head to the soles. Treat infants on hairline, neck, scalp, temple, and forehead. Wash cream off after 8 to 14 hours.

## ACTION
Acts on parasites' nerve cells to disrupt the sodium channel current, causing parasitic paralysis.

| Route | Onset | Peak | Duration |
|-------|-------|------|----------|
| Topical | 10-15 min | Unknown | 10 days |

## ADVERSE REACTIONS
**Skin:** pruritus, *burning, stinging,* edema, tingling, scalp numbness or discomfort, mild erythema, scalp rash.

## INTERACTIONS
None significant.

## EFFECTS ON LAB TEST RESULTS
None reported.

## CONTRAINDICATIONS & CAUTIONS
• Contraindicated in patients hypersensitive to pyrethrins, chrysanthemums, or components of drug.

## NURSING CONSIDERATIONS
• Usually only one application is needed. Combing of nits isn't needed for effectiveness, but drug package supplies a fine-tooth comb for cosmetic use, as desired.
• Retreat for lice, as prescribed, if lice are observed 7 days after first application.
• Treat sexual contacts simultaneously.

## PATIENT TEACHING
• Explain that treatment may temporarily worsen signs and symptoms of head lice infestation, such as itching, redness, and swelling.
• Tell patient to disinfect headgear, comb and brush, scarves, coats, and bed linens by machine washing with hot water and machine drying for at least 20 minutes, using hot cycle. Tell him to seal nonwashable items in plastic bag for 2 weeks or spray

---

Reactions may be *common*, uncommon, *life-threatening*, or COMMON AND LIFE-THREATENING.

with product designed to eliminate lice and their nits.
• Warn patient not to use drug on eyes, eyelashes, eyebrows, nose, mouth, and mucous membranes.
• Tell patient to warn other family members and sexual contacts about infestation.

---

## pyrethrins
A-200, Barc ◇, Blue, End Lice, Pronto, Pyrinyl ◇, R & C, RID ◇, Tegrin-LT, Tisit ◇, Triple X

*Pregnancy risk category C*

---

### AVAILABLE FORMS
*Shampoo:* pyrethrins 0.2% and piperonyl butoxide 2%; pyrethrins 0.3% and piperonyl butoxide 3%; pyrethrins 0.33% and piperonyl butoxide 4%
*Shampoo and conditioner:* pyrethrins 0.33% and piperonyl butoxide technical 3.15%
*Topical gel:* pyrethrins 0.3% and piperonyl butoxide 3%
*Topical solution:* pyrethrins 0.18% and piperonyl butoxide 2%; pyrethrins 0.2%, piperonyl butoxide 2%, and deodorized kerosene 0.8%; pyrethrins 0.3% and piperonyl butoxide 3%; pyrethrins 0.3% and piperonyl butoxide 2%

### INDICATIONS & DOSAGES
➤ **Infestations of head, body, and pubic (crab) lice and their eggs**
*Adults and children:* Apply to hair, scalp, or other infested areas until entirely wet. Allow to remain for 10 minutes but no longer. Wash thoroughly with warm water and soap or shampoo. Remove dead lice and eggs with fine-tooth comb. Repeat treatment, if needed, in 7 to 10 days to kill newly hatched lice; not to exceed two applications within 24 hours.

### ACTION
Acts as contact poison that disrupts parasite's nervous system, causing paralysis and death of parasite.

| Route | Onset | Peak | Duration |
|---|---|---|---|
| Topical | Unknown | Unknown | Unknown |

### ADVERSE REACTIONS
**Skin:** *irritation with repeated use.*

### INTERACTIONS
None significant.

### EFFECTS ON LAB TEST RESULTS
None reported.

### CONTRAINDICATIONS & CAUTIONS
• Contraindicated in patients hypersensitive to drug, ragweed, or chrysanthemums.
• Use cautiously in infants and small children.

### NURSING CONSIDERATIONS
• Apply topical corticosteroids or give oral antihistamines, as prescribed, if dermatitis develops from scratching.
• Discard container by wrapping in several layers of newspaper.
• Inspect all family members daily for at least 2 weeks for infestation.
• Drug isn't effective against scabies.
• Treat sexual contacts simultaneously.

### PATIENT TEACHING
• Instruct patient not to apply to open areas, acutely inflamed skin, eyebrows, eyelashes, face, eyes, mucous membranes, or urethral opening. If accidental contact with eyes occurs, advise patient to flush with water and notify prescriber.
• Warn patient not to swallow or inhale vapors from the drug.
• Tell patient to stop using drug, wash it off skin, and notify prescriber immediately if skin irritation develops. All preparations contain petroleum distillates.
• Instruct patient to change and sterilize all clothing and bed linens after drug is washed off body. Tell him to disinfect washable items by machine washing in hot water and drying on hot cycle for at least 20 minutes. Other items can be dry cleaned and sealed in plastic bags for 2 weeks, or treated with products made for this purpose.
• Teach patient to remove dead parasites with a fine-tooth comb.
• Urge patient to warn other family members and sexual contacts about infestation.

---

*Rapid onset* †Canada ‡Australia ◇OTC ♦Off-label use ✐Photoguide *Liquid contains alcohol.

betamethasone dipropionate
betamethasone valerate
clobetasol propionate
desoximetasone
dexamethasone
dexamethasone sodium
    phosphate
fluocinolone acetonide
fluocinonide
flurandrenolide
fluticasone propionate
halcinonide
hydrocortisone
hydrocortisone acetate
hydrocortisone butyrate
hydrocortisone valerate
triamcinolone acetonide

### COMBINATION PRODUCTS
Corticosteroids for topical use are commonly combined with antibiotics and antifungals. (See Chapter 85, LOCAL ANTI-INFECTIVES.)

### betamethasone dipropionate
Alphatrex, Diprolene, Diprolene AF, Diprosone, Maxivate, Teladar

### betamethasone valerate
Betatrex, Beta-Val, Betnovate†‡, Luxiq, Psorion Cream, Valisone

*Pregnancy risk category C*

### AVAILABLE FORMS
betamethasone dipropionate
*Aerosol:* 0.1%
*Cream:* 0.05%
*Gel:* 0.05%
*Lotion:* 0.05%
*Ointment:* 0.05%
betamethasone valerate
*Cream:* 0.01%, 0.05%, 0.1%
*Foam:* 0.12%
*Lotion:* 0.1%
*Ointment:* 0.1%

### INDICATIONS & DOSAGES
➤ **Inflammation and pruritus from corticosteroid-responsive dermatoses**
*Adults and children older than age 12:*
Clean area; apply cream, ointment, lotion, aerosol spray, or gel sparingly. Dipropionate products are given once daily to b.i.d.; valerate products are given once daily to q.i.d. Maximum dose is 45 g/week for Diprolene cream and 50 ml/week for Diprolene lotion.
➤ **Inflammation and pruritus from corticosteroid-responsive dermatoses of scalp (valerate only)**
*Adults:* Gently massage small amounts of foam into affected scalp areas b.i.d., morning and evening, until control is achieved. If no improvement is seen in 2 weeks, reassess diagnosis.

### ACTION
Unclear. Diffuses across cell membranes to form complexes with specific cytoplasmic receptors. Exhibits anti-inflammatory, antipruritic, vasoconstrictive, and antiproliferative activity. Considered a group III (medium-potency) drug, according to vasoconstrictive properties.

| Route | Onset | Peak | Duration |
|---|---|---|---|
| Topical | Unknown | Unknown | Unknown |

### ADVERSE REACTIONS
**GU:** glycosuria with dipropionate.
**Metabolic:** hyperglycemia.
**Skin:** burning, pruritus, irritation, dryness, erythema, folliculitis, striae, acneiform eruptions, perioral dermatitis, hypopigmentation, hypertrichosis, allergic contact dermatitis, secondary infection, maceration, atrophy, miliaria with occlusive dressings.
**Other:** *hypothalamic-pituitary-adrenal axis suppression,* Cushing's syndrome.

### INTERACTIONS
None significant.

### EFFECTS ON LAB TEST RESULTS
● May increase glucose level.

**CONTRAINDICATIONS & CAUTIONS**
• Contraindicated in patients hypersensitive to corticosteroids.

**NURSING CONSIDERATIONS**
• Gently wash skin before applying. To prevent skin damage, rub in gently, leaving a thin coat. When treating hairy sites, part hair and apply directly to lesions.
• Avoid applying near eyes or mucous membranes or in ear canal, groin area, or axillae.
• Don't dispense foam directly into warm hands because foam will begin to melt upon contact.
• Because of alcohol content of vehicle, gel products may cause mild, transient stinging, especially when used on or near excoriated skin.
• For patients with eczematous dermatitis whose skin may be irritated by adhesive material, hold dressing in place with gauze, elastic bandages, stockings, or stockinette.
• *Alert:* Don't use occlusive dressings.
• If antifungal or antibiotic combined with corticosteroid fails to provide prompt improvement, stop corticosteroid until infection is controlled.
• Systemic absorption is likely with prolonged or extensive body surface treatment. Watch for symptoms.
• Avoid using plastic pants or tight-fitting diapers on treated areas in young children. Children may absorb larger amounts of drug and be more susceptible to systemic toxicity.
• Continue drug for a few days after lesions clear.
• *Alert:* Diprolene and Diprolene AF may not be replaced with generics because other products have different potencies.

**PATIENT TEACHING**
• Teach patient how to apply drug.
• Emphasize that drug is for external use only.
• Tell patient to wash hands after application.
• Tell patient to stop drug and report signs of systemic absorption, skin irritation or ulceration, hypersensitivity, or infection.
• Instruct patient not to use occlusive dressings.

• Discuss personal hygiene measures to reduce chance of infection.

## clobetasol propionate
Cormax, Dermovate†, Embeline E, Olux, Temovate

*Pregnancy risk category C*

**AVAILABLE FORMS**
*Cream:* 0.05%
*Foam:* 0.05%
*Gel:* 0.05%
*Ointment:* 0.05%
*Scalp application:* 0.05%*
*Solution:* 0.05%

**INDICATIONS & DOSAGES**
➤ **Inflammation and pruritus from corticosteroid-responsive dermatoses; short-term topical treatment of mild to moderate plaque-type psoriasis of non-scalp regions, excluding the face and intertriginous areas**
*Adults and children age 12 and older:*
Apply thin layer to affected skin areas b.i.d., morning and evening, for maximum of 14 days. Total dose shouldn't exceed 50 g of foam, cream, or ointment or 50 ml of lotion or solution weekly.
✱ *NEW INDICATION:* **Inflammation and pruritus of moderate to severe corticosteroid-responsive dermatoses of the scalp**
*Adults:* Apply to the affected scalp area b.i.d., morning and evening. Gently massage into affected scalp area until the foam disappears. Repeat until entire affected scalp area is treated. Limit treatment to 14 days, with no more than 50 g of foam weekly.

**ACTION**
Unclear. Diffuses across cell membranes to form complexes with specific cytoplasmic receptors. Exhibits anti-inflammatory, antipruritic, vasoconstrictive, and antiproliferative activity. Considered a very high-potency (group I) drug, according to vasoconstrictive properties.

| Route | Onset | Peak | Duration |
|---|---|---|---|
| Topical | Unknown | Unknown | Unknown |

**ADVERSE REACTIONS**
**GU:** glycosuria.
**Metabolic:** hyperglycemia.
**Skin:** burning, pruritus, irritation, dryness, erythema, folliculitis, perioral dermatitis, allergic contact dermatitis, hypopigmentation, hypertrichosis, acneiform eruptions.
**Other:** *hypothalamic-pituitary-adrenal axis suppression,* Cushing's syndrome.

**INTERACTIONS**
None significant.

**EFFECTS ON LAB TEST RESULTS**
● May increase glucose level.

**CONTRAINDICATIONS & CAUTIONS**
● Contraindicated in patients hypersensitive to corticosteroids and in those with primary scalp infections.

**NURSING CONSIDERATIONS**
● Gently wash skin before applying. To prevent skin damage, rub medication in gently and completely. When treating hairy sites, part hair and apply directly to lesions.
● Avoid applying near eyes or mucous membranes or in ear canal.
● *Alert:* Don't use occlusive dressings or bandages. Don't cover or wrap treated areas unless directed by prescriber.
● If antifungal or antibiotic combined with corticosteroid fails to provide prompt improvement, stop corticosteroid until infection is controlled.
● Stop drug and notify prescriber if skin infection, striae, or atrophy occurs.
● Hypothalamic-pituitary-adrenal axis suppression occurs at doses as low as 2 g/day.

**PATIENT TEACHING**
● Teach patient how to apply drug and to avoid contact with eyes.
● Tell patient to wash hands after application.
● Tell patient to stop drug and report signs of systemic absorption, skin irritation or ulceration, hypersensitivity, or infection.
● Warn patient to use drug for no longer than 14 consecutive days.
● Tell patient using the foam to invert can and dispense a small amount of Olux

foam (up to a golf-ball–size dollop) into the cap of the can, onto a saucer or other cool surface, or directly on the lesion, taking care to avoid contact with the eyes. Dispensing directly onto hands isn't recommended because the foam will melt immediately upon contact with warm skin. Tell him to move hair away from affected area of scalp so that foam can be applied to each affected area.
● Tell patient using foam that contents are flammable and under pressure, so he should avoid smoking during and immediately after application and keep can away from flames. Also tell him not to puncture or incinerate container.

---

**desoximetasone**
Topicort, Topicort LP

*Pregnancy risk category C*

**AVAILABLE FORMS**
*Cream:* 0.05%, 0.25%
*Gel:* 0.05%
*Ointment:* 0.25%

**INDICATIONS & DOSAGES**
➤ **Inflammation from corticosteroid-responsive dermatoses**
*Adults and children:* Clean area; apply sparingly b.i.d.

**ACTION**
Unclear. Diffuses across cell membranes to form complexes with specific cytoplasmic receptors. Exhibits anti-inflammatory, antipruritic, vasoconstrictive, and antiproliferative activity. Considered a medium-potency (group II to III) drug, according to vasoconstrictive properties.

| Route | Onset | Peak | Duration |
|-------|-------|------|----------|
| Topical | Unknown | Unknown | Unknown |

**ADVERSE REACTIONS**
**GU:** glycosuria.
**Metabolic:** hyperglycemia.
**Skin:** burning, pruritus, irritation, dryness, erythema, folliculitis, hypertrichosis, acneiform eruptions, perioral dermatitis, hypopigmentation, allergic contact dermatitis, *maceration, secondary infection,*

---

*atrophy, striae, miliaria with occlusive dressings.*
**Other:** *hypothalamic-pituitary-adrenal axis suppression,* Cushing's syndrome.

**INTERACTIONS**
None significant.

**EFFECTS ON LAB TEST RESULTS**
• May increase glucose level.

**CONTRAINDICATIONS & CAUTIONS**
• Contraindicated in patients hypersensitive to drug or its components.

**NURSING CONSIDERATIONS**
• Gently wash skin before applying. To prevent skin damage, rub in gently, leaving thin coat. When treating hairy sites, part hair and apply directly to lesions.
• Avoid applying near eyes, mucous membranes, or in ear canal.
• For patients with eczematous dermatitis whose skin may be irritated by adhesive material, hold dressing in place with gauze, elastic bandages, stockings, or stockinette.
• Change dressing as prescribed. Stop drug and notify prescriber if skin infection, striae, or atrophy occurs.
• If fever develops and occlusive dressing is in place, notify prescriber and remove occlusive dressing.
• If antifungal or antibiotic combined with corticosteroid fails to provide prompt improvement, stop corticosteroid until infection is controlled.
• Systemic absorption is likely with use of occlusive dressings, prolonged treatment, or extensive body surface treatment. Watch for symptoms.
• Avoid using plastic pants or tight-fitting diapers on treated areas in young children. Children may absorb larger amounts of drug and be more susceptible to systemic toxicity.
• Continue drug for a few days after lesions clear.
• Gel contains alcohol and may cause burning or irritation in open lesions.
• **Alert:** Don't confuse desoximetasone with dexamethasone.

**PATIENT TEACHING**
• Teach patient how to apply drug.

• If an occlusive dressing is ordered, advise patient to leave it in place for no longer than 12 hours each day and not to use the dressing on infected or weeping lesions.
• Tell patient to stop drug and report signs of systemic absorption, skin irritation or ulceration, hypersensitivity, or infection.

---

**dexamethasone**
Aeroseb-Dex, Decaspray

**dexamethasone sodium phosphate**
Decadron Phosphate

*Pregnancy risk category C*

**AVAILABLE FORMS**
**dexamethasone**
*Aerosol:* 0.01%, 0.04%
**dexamethasone sodium phosphate**
*Cream:* 0.1%

**INDICATIONS & DOSAGES**
➤ **Inflammation from corticosteroid-responsive dermatoses**
*Adults and children:* Clean area; apply cream or aerosol sparingly t.i.d. or q.i.d. For aerosol use on scalp, shake can well but gently, and apply to dry scalp after shampooing. Hold can upright or inverted and 6 inches (15 cm) away from area. Spray while moving container to all affected areas, which should take about 2 seconds. Don't massage drug into scalp or spray forehead or near eyes. When result is obtained, reduce dose gradually, then stop use.

**ACTION**
Unclear. Diffuses across cell membranes to form complexes with specific cytoplasmic receptors. Exhibits anti-inflammatory, antipruritic, vasoconstrictive, and antiproliferative activity. Considered a group IV (low-potency) drug, according to vasoconstrictive properties.

| Route | Onset | Peak | Duration |
|---|---|---|---|
| Topical | Unknown | Unknown | Unknown |

**ADVERSE REACTIONS**
**GU:** glycosuria.
**Metabolic:** hyperglycemia.
**Skin:** burning, pruritus, irritation, dryness, erythema, folliculitis, hypertrichosis, acneiform eruptions, perioral dermatitis, hypopigmentation, allergic contact dermatitis, *maceration, secondary infection, atrophy, striae, miliaria with occlusive dressings.*
**Other:** *hypothalamic-pituitary-adrenal axis suppression,* Cushing's syndrome, altered growth and development in children.

**INTERACTIONS**
None significant.

**EFFECTS ON LAB TEST RESULTS**
• May increase glucose level.

**CONTRAINDICATIONS & CAUTIONS**
• Contraindicated in patients hypersensitive to drug or its components.

**NURSING CONSIDERATIONS**
• Gently wash skin before applying. To prevent skin damage, rub cream in gently, leaving a thin coat. When treating hairy sites, part hair and apply directly to lesions.
• Avoid applying near eyes or mucous membranes or in ear canal, groin, or axillae.
• For patients with eczematous dermatitis whose skin may be irritated by adhesive material, hold dressing in place with gauze, stockings, or stockinette.
• Change dressing as prescribed. Stop drug and tell prescriber if skin infection, striae, or atrophy occurs.
• If an occlusive dressing has been applied and a fever develops, notify prescriber and remove dressing.
• When using aerosol around face, cover patient's eyes and warn against inhalation of spray. Aerosol preparation contains alcohol and may cause irritation or burning when used on open lesions. To avoid freezing tissues, don't spray longer than 1 to 2 seconds or from less than 6 inches (15 cm) away.
• If antifungal or antibiotic combined with corticosteroid fails to provide prompt im-

provement, stop corticosteroid until infection is controlled.
• Systemic absorption is likely with use of occlusive dressings, prolonged treatment, or extensive body surface treatment. Watch for symptoms.
• Avoid using plastic pants or tight-fitting diapers on treated areas in young children. Children may absorb larger amounts of drug and be more susceptible to systemic toxicity.
• Continue treatment for a few days after lesions clear.
• *Alert:* Don't confuse dexamethasone with desoximetasone.

**PATIENT TEACHING**
• Teach patient and family how to apply drug.
• If an occlusive dressing is ordered, advise patient to leave it in place for no longer than 12 hours each day and not to use the dressing on infected or weeping lesions.
• Tell patient to stop drug and report signs of systemic absorption, skin irritation or ulceration, hypersensitivity, or infection.
• Tell patient to avoid scratching.

# fluocinolone acetonide
Derma-Smoothe/FS, Fluonid, Flurosyn, FS Shampoo, Synalar, Synalar-HP

*Pregnancy risk category C*

**AVAILABLE FORMS**
*Cream:* 0.01%, 0.025%, 0.2%
*Oil:* 0.01%
*Ointment:* 0.025%
*Shampoo:* 0.01%
*Topical solution:* 0.01%

**INDICATIONS & DOSAGES**
➤ **Inflammation from corticosteroid-responsive dermatoses**
*Adults and children:* Clean area; apply product sparingly b.i.d. to q.i.d.

**ACTION**
Unclear. Diffuses across cell membranes to form complexes with specific cytoplasmic receptors. Exhibits anti-inflammatory, antipruritic, vasoconstrictive, and anti-

proliferative activity. Considered a low-potency (group IV to VI) drug, according to vasoconstrictive properties.

| Route | Onset | Peak | Duration |
|---|---|---|---|
| Topical | Unknown | Unknown | Unknown |

**ADVERSE REACTIONS**
**GU:** glycosuria.
**Metabolic:** hyperglycemia.
**Skin:** burning, pruritus, irritation, dryness, erythema, folliculitis, hypertrichosis, hypopigmentation, acneiform eruptions, perioral dermatitis, allergic contact dermatitis, *maceration, secondary infection, atrophy, striae, miliaria with occlusive dressings.*
**Other:** *hypothalamic-pituitary-adrenal axis suppression,* Cushing's syndrome.

**INTERACTIONS**
None significant.

**EFFECTS ON LAB TEST RESULTS**
● May increase glucose level.

**CONTRAINDICATIONS & CAUTIONS**
● Contraindicated in patients hypersensitive to drug or its components.

**NURSING CONSIDERATIONS**
● Gently wash skin before applying. To prevent skin damage, rub in gently, leaving a thin coat. When treating hairy sites, part hair and apply directly to lesions.
● Avoid application near eyes or mucous membranes; in axillae, groin, or rectal area; or in ear canal if eardrum is perforated.
● For patients with eczematous dermatitis whose skin may be irritated by adhesive material, hold dressing in place with gauze, elastic bandages, stockings, or stockinette.
● Change dressing as prescribed. Stop drug and notify prescriber if skin infection, striae, or atrophy occurs.
● If an occlusive dressing has been applied and a fever develops, notify prescriber and remove dressing.
● If antifungal or antibiotic combined with corticosteroid fails to provide prompt improvement, stop corticosteroid until infection is controlled.

● Systemic absorption is likely with use of occlusive dressings, prolonged treatment, or extensive body surface treatment. Watch for symptoms.
● Avoid using plastic pants or tight-fitting diapers on treated areas in young children. Children may absorb larger amounts of drug and be more susceptible to systemic toxicity.
● Fluonid solution on dry lesions may increase dryness, scaling, or pruritus; on denuded or fissured areas, it may cause burning or stinging. If these signs and symptoms persist and dermatitis hasn't improved, stop therapy and notify prescriber.
● *Alert:* Don't confuse fluocinolone with fluocinonide or fluticasone.

**PATIENT TEACHING**
● Teach patient or family how to apply drug using gloves or sterile applicator.
● Tell patient to wash hands after application.
● If an occlusive dressing is ordered, advise patient to leave it in place for no longer than 12 hours each day and not to use the dressing on infected or weeping lesions.
● Tell patient to stop using solution and notify prescriber if he develops signs of systemic absorption, skin irritation or ulceration, hypersensitivity, or infection.

---

**fluocinonide**
Fluonex, Lidex, Lidex-E

*Pregnancy risk category C*

---

**AVAILABLE FORMS**
*Cream:* 0.05%
*Gel:* 0.05%
*Ointment:* 0.05%
*Topical solution:* 0.05%

**INDICATIONS & DOSAGES**
➤ **Inflammation from corticosteroid-responsive dermatoses**
*Adults and children:* Clean area; apply cream, gel, ointment, or topical solution sparingly t.i.d. or q.i.d. In children, use lowest dosage that promotes healing.

## ACTION
Unclear. Diffuses across cell membranes to form complexes with specific cytoplasmic receptors. Exhibits anti-inflammatory, antipruritic, vasoconstrictive, and antiproliferative activity. Considered a high-potency (group II) drug, according to vasoconstrictive properties.

| Route | Onset | Peak | Duration |
|-------|-------|------|----------|
| Topical | Unknown | Unknown | Unknown |

## ADVERSE REACTIONS
**GU:** glycosuria.
**Metabolic:** hyperglycemia.
**Skin:** burning, pruritus, irritation, dryness, erythema, folliculitis, hypertrichosis, hypopigmentation, acneiform eruptions, perioral dermatitis, allergic contact dermatitis, *maceration, secondary infection, atrophy, striae, miliaria with occlusive dressings.*
**Other:** *hypothalamic-pituitary-adrenal axis suppression,* Cushing's syndrome.

## INTERACTIONS
None significant.

## EFFECTS ON LAB TEST RESULTS
● May increase glucose level.

## CONTRAINDICATIONS & CAUTIONS
● Contraindicated in patients hypersensitive to drug or its components.

## NURSING CONSIDERATIONS
● Gently wash skin before applying. To prevent skin damage, rub in gently, leaving a thin coat. When treating hairy sites, part hair and apply directly to lesion.
● Avoid applying near eyes, near mucous membranes, or in ear canal.
● For patients with eczematous dermatitis whose skin may be irritated by adhesive material, hold dressing in place with gauze, elastic bandages, stockings, or stockinette.
● Change dressing as prescribed. Stop drug and notify prescriber if skin infection, striae, or atrophy occurs.
● If an occlusive dressing has been applied and a fever develops, notify prescriber and remove dressing.
● If antifungal or antibiotic combined with corticosteroid fails to provide prompt improvement, stop corticosteroid until infection is controlled.
● Systemic absorption is likely with use of occlusive dressings, prolonged treatment, or extensive body surface treatment. Watch for symptoms.
● Avoid using plastic pants or tight-fitting diapers on treated areas in young children. Children may absorb larger amounts of drug and be more susceptible to systemic toxicity.
● Continue treatment for a few days after lesions clear.
● *Alert:* Don't confuse fluocinonide with fluocinolone or fluticasone.

## PATIENT TEACHING
● Teach patient and family how to apply drug using careful handwashing and gloves or sterile applicator.
● If an occlusive dressing is ordered, advise patient to leave it in place no more than 12 hours each day and not to use the dressing on infected or weeping lesions.
● Tell patient to stop drug and report signs of systemic absorption, skin irritation or ulceration, hypersensitivity, or infection.

# flurandrenolide
Cordran, Cordran SP, Drenison Tape†

*Pregnancy risk category C*

## AVAILABLE FORMS
*Cream:* 0.025%, 0.05%
*Lotion:* 0.05%
*Ointment:* 0.025%, 0.05%
*Tape:* 4 mcg/cm²

## INDICATIONS & DOSAGES
➤ **Inflammation and pruritus from corticosteroid-responsive dermatoses**
*Adults and children:* Clean area; apply cream, lotion, or ointment sparingly b.i.d. or t.i.d.
  Before applying Cordran tape, clean skin carefully, removing scales, crust, and dried exudate. Apply tape q 12 hours. Let skin dry for 1 hour before applying new tape. Shave or clip hair to allow good contact with skin and comfortable removal. If tape ends loosen prematurely, trim off and replace with fresh tape.

## ACTION
Unclear. Diffuses across cell membranes to form complexes with specific cytoplasmic receptors. Exhibits anti-inflammatory, antipruritic, vasoconstrictive, and antiproliferative activity. Considered a medium-potency (group III) drug, according to vasoconstrictive properties.

| Route | Onset | Peak | Duration |
|-------|-------|------|----------|
| Topical | Unknown | Unknown | Unknown |

## ADVERSE REACTIONS
**GU:** glycosuria.
**Metabolic:** hyperglycemia.
**Skin:** burning, pruritus, irritation, dryness, erythema, folliculitis, hypertrichosis, hypopigmentation, acneiform eruptions, allergic contact dermatitis, *maceration, secondary infection, atrophy, striae, miliaria with occlusive dressings,* purpura, stripping of epidermis, furunculosis with tape.
**Other:** *hypothalamic-pituitary-adrenal axis suppression,* Cushing's syndrome.

## INTERACTIONS
None significant.

## EFFECTS ON LAB TEST RESULTS
• May increase glucose level.

## CONTRAINDICATIONS & CAUTIONS
• Contraindicated in patients hypersensitive to drug or its components.

## NURSING CONSIDERATIONS
• Gently wash skin before applying. To prevent skin damage, rub in gently, leaving a thin coat. When treating hairy sites, part hair and apply directly to lesions.
• Avoid applying near eyes, near mucous membranes, or in ear canal.
• *Alert:* Don't use tape for exudative lesions or lesions in intertriginous areas.
• Don't tear Cordran tape; cut it with scissors. Make sure skin is dry for 1 hour before applying tape.
• For patients with eczematous dermatitis whose skin may be irritated by adhesive material, hold dressing in place with gauze, elastic bandages, stockings, or stockinette.
• Stop drug and tell prescriber if skin infection, striae, or atrophy occurs.
• Notify prescriber and remove occlusive dressing if fever develops.
• If antifungal or antibiotic combined with corticosteroid fails to provide prompt improvement, stop corticosteroid until infection is controlled.
• Systemic absorption is likely with use of occlusive dressings, prolonged treatment, or extensive body surface treatment. Watch for symptoms.
• Avoid using plastic pants or tight-fitting diapers on treated areas in young children. Children may absorb larger amounts of drug and be more susceptible to systemic toxicity.
• Continue treatment for a few days after lesions clear.

## PATIENT TEACHING
• Teach patient or family how to apply drug.
• Tell patient to wash hands after application.
• If an occlusive dressing is ordered, advise patient to leave it in place for no longer than 12 hours each day and not to use the dressing on infected or weeping lesions.
• Tell patient to stop drug and report signs of systemic absorption, skin irritation or ulceration, hypersensitivity, or infection.

# fluticasone propionate
Cutivate

*Pregnancy risk category C*

## AVAILABLE FORMS
*Cream:* 0.05%
*Ointment:* 0.005%

## INDICATIONS & DOSAGES
➤ **Inflammation and pruritus from corticosteroid-responsive dermatoses**
*Adults:* Apply sparingly to affected area b.i.d.; rub in gently and completely.
*Children age 3 months and older:* Apply a thin film (0.05%) to affected areas b.i.d. Rub in gently. Don't use for longer than 4 weeks.
➤ **Inflammation and pruritus from atopic dermatitis**
*Children age 3 months and older:* Apply thin film (0.05%) to affected areas once

daily or b.i.d. Rub in gently. Don't use for longer than 4 weeks.

### ACTION
Unclear. Diffuses across cell membranes to form complexes with specific cytoplasmic receptors. Exhibits anti-inflammatory, antipruritic, vasoconstrictive, and antiproliferative activity. Considered a medium-potency (group III) drug, according to vasoconstrictive properties.

| Route | Onset | Peak | Duration |
|-------|-------|------|----------|
| Topical | Rapid | Unknown | 10 hr |

### ADVERSE REACTIONS
**CNS:** light-headedness.
**GU:** glycosuria.
**Metabolic:** hyperglycemia.
**Skin:** urticaria, burning, hypertrichosis, pruritus, irritation, erythema.
**Other:** *hypothalamic-pituitary-adrenal axis suppression,* Cushing's syndrome.

### INTERACTIONS
None significant.

### EFFECTS ON LAB TEST RESULTS
• May increase glucose level.

### CONTRAINDICATIONS & CAUTIONS
• Contraindicated in patients hypersensitive to drug or its components and in those with viral, fungal, herpetic, or tubercular skin lesions.

### NURSING CONSIDERATIONS
• Don't mix drug with other bases or vehicles because doing so may affect potency.
• If adverse reactions occur, prescriber may order less potent drug.
• Stop drug if local irritation or systemic infection, absorption, or hypersensitivity occurs.
• Absorption of corticosteroid is increased when drug is applied to inflamed or damaged skin, eyelids, or scrotal area; it's lowest when applied to intact normal skin, palms of hands, or soles of feet.
• Don't use drug with an occlusive dressing or in diaper area.
• **Alert:** Don't confuse fluticasone with fluconazole.

### PATIENT TEACHING
• Teach patient or family member how to apply drug using gloves, sterile applicator, or after careful hand washing.
• Tell patient to wash hands after application.
• Tell patient to avoid prolonged use and contact with eyes. Warn him not to apply to face, in skin creases, or around eyes, genitals, underarms, or rectum.
• Instruct patient to notify prescriber if condition persists or worsens or if burning or irritation develops.

---

## halcinonide
Halog, Halog-E

*Pregnancy risk category C*

### AVAILABLE FORMS
*Cream:* 0.025%, 0.1%
*Ointment:* 0.1%
*Topical solution:* 0.1%

### INDICATIONS & DOSAGES
➤ **Inflammation from corticosteroid-responsive dermatoses**
*Adults and children:* Clean area; apply cream, ointment, or topical solution sparingly b.i.d. or t.i.d. Rub cream in gently.

### ACTION
Unclear. Diffuses across cell membranes to form complexes with cytoplasmic receptors. Exhibits anti-inflammatory, antipruritic, vasoconstrictive, and antiproliferative activity. Considered a high-potency (group II) drug, according to vasoconstrictive properties.

| Route | Onset | Peak | Duration |
|-------|-------|------|----------|
| Topical | Unknown | Unknown | Unknown |

### ADVERSE REACTIONS
**GU:** glycosuria.
**Metabolic:** hyperglycemia.
**Skin:** burning, pruritus, irritation, dryness, erythema, folliculitis, hypertrichosis, hypopigmentation, acneiform eruptions, allergic contact dermatitis, *maceration, secondary infection, atrophy, striae, miliaria with occlusive dressings.*
**Other:** *hypothalamic-pituitary-adrenal axis suppression,* Cushing's syndrome.

---

**INTERACTIONS**
None significant.

**EFFECTS ON LAB TEST RESULTS**
• May increase glucose level.

**CONTRAINDICATIONS & CAUTIONS**
• Contraindicated in patients hypersensitive to drug or its components.

**NURSING CONSIDERATIONS**
• Gently wash skin before applying. To prevent skin damage, rub in gently, leaving a thin coat. When treating hairy sites, part hair and apply directly to lesions.
• Avoid applying near eyes or mucous membranes or in ear canal, axillae, groin, or rectal area.
• Gently rub small amount of cream into lesion until it disappears. Reapply, leaving a thin coating on lesion, and cover with occlusive dressing, if ordered. Don't leave dressing in place for longer than 12 hours each day.
• Don't use occlusive dressings on infected or exudative lesions.
• For patients with eczematous dermatitis whose skin may be irritated by adhesive material, hold dressing in place with gauze, stockings, or stockinette.
• Stop drug and tell prescriber if skin infection, striae, or atrophy occurs.
• Good results have been obtained by applying occlusive dressings in the evening and removing them in the morning, providing 12-hour occlusion. Then reapply drug; don't apply occlusive dressings during the day.
• If an occlusive dressing has been applied and a fever develops, notify prescriber and remove dressing.
• If antifungal or antibiotic combined with corticosteroid fails to provide prompt improvement, stop corticosteroid until infection is controlled.
• Systemic absorption is especially likely with use of occlusive dressings, prolonged treatment, or extensive body surface treatment. Watch for symptoms.
• Avoid using plastic pants or tight-fitting diapers on treated areas in young children. Children may absorb larger amounts of drug and be more susceptible to systemic toxicity.

• Continue treatment for a few days after lesions clear.

**PATIENT TEACHING**
• Teach patient how to apply drug.
• If an occlusive dressing is ordered, advise patient to leave it in place for no longer than 12 hours each day and not to use the dressing on infected or weeping lesions.
• Tell patient to stop drug and report signs of systemic absorption, skin irritation or ulceration, hypersensitivity, or infection.

---

## hydrocortisone
Acticort 100, Aeroseb-HC, Ala-Cort, Ala-Scalp, Anusol-HC, Bactine Hydrocortisone◊, Cetacort, Cort-Dome, Cortisone-5◊, Cortisone-10◊, Delcort, Dermolate Anti-Itch◊, Dermtex HC◊, Hi-Cor 2.5, Hycort, Hydro-Tex, Hytone, LactiCare-HC, Penecort, Procort◊, Proctocort◊, Scalpicin◊, Synacort, Tegrin-HC◊, Texacort, T/Scalp

## hydrocortisone acetate
Anu-Med HC, Anusol HC-1◊, Caldecort (Maximum Strength), Cortaid◊, Cortamed†, Cortef Feminine Itch◊, Corticaine◊, Dermol HC, Gynecort◊, Hemril-HC Uniserts, Lanacort-5◊, Lanacort 10◊, ProctoCream-HC, ProctoFoam-HC

## hydrocortisone butyrate
Locoid

## hydrocortisone valerate
Westcort

*Pregnancy risk category C*

---

**AVAILABLE FORMS**
**hydrocortisone**
*Cream:* 0.5%◊, 1%◊, 2.5%
*Gel:* 1%
*Lotion:* 0.25%, 0.5%◊, 1%◊, 1%, 2%, 2.5%
*Ointment:* 0.5%◊, 1%◊, 2.5%
*Rectal cream:* 1%◊

---

*Rectal ointment:* 1%
*Spray:* 1% ◇
*Stick roll-on:* 1%
*Topical solution:* 1%
**hydrocortisone acetate**
*Cream:* 0.5% ◇, 1% ◇, 1%
*Ointment:* 0.5% ◇, 1% ◇
*Rectal foam:* 90 mg per application
*Suppositories:* 25 mg, 30 mg
**hydrocortisone butyrate**
*Cream:* 0.1%
*Ointment:* 0.1%
*Solution:* 0.1%
**hydrocortisone valerate**
*Cream:* 0.2%
*Ointment:* 0.2%

## INDICATIONS & DOSAGES
➤ **Inflammation and pruritus from corticosteroid-responsive dermatoses, adjunctive topical management of seborrheic dermatitis of scalp**
*Adults and children:* Clean area; apply cream, gel, lotion, ointment, or topical solution sparingly daily to q.i.d. Spray aerosol onto affected area daily to q.i.d. until acute phase is controlled; then reduce dosage to one to three times weekly, p.r.n. Children should receive lowest dose that provides positive results.
➤ **Inflammation from proctitis**
*Adults:* 1 applicatorful of rectal foam P.R. daily or b.i.d. for 2 to 3 weeks; then every other day, p.r.n. Enema is given once nightly for 21 days or until patient improves; may be used for 2 to 3 months if used every other night. Suppositories are inserted b.i.d. for 2 weeks.

## ACTION
Unclear. Diffuses across cell membranes to form complexes with specific cytoplasmic receptors. Exhibits anti-inflammatory, antipruritic, vasoconstrictive, and antiproliferative activity.

| Route | Onset | Peak | Duration |
|---|---|---|---|
| Topical, P.R. | Unknown | Unknown | Unknown |

## ADVERSE REACTIONS
**Topical use**
**GU:** glycosuria.
**Metabolic:** hyperglycemia.

**Skin:** burning, pruritus, irritation, dryness, erythema, folliculitis, hypertrichosis, hypopigmentation, acneiform eruptions, allergic contact dermatitis, *maceration, secondary infection, atrophy, striae, miliaria with occlusive dressings.*
**Other:** *hypothalamic-pituitary-adrenal axis suppression,* Cushing's syndrome.
**Rectal use**
**CNS:** *seizures, increased intracranial pressure,* vertigo, headache.
**CV:** hypertension.
**EENT:** cataracts, glaucoma.
**GI:** peptic ulcer, *pancreatitis,* abdominal distention.
**GU:** menstrual irregularities.
**Metabolic:** fluid or electrolyte disturbances, decreased carbohydrate tolerance.
**Musculoskeletal:** muscle weakness, osteoporosis, necrosis and fractures in bone.
**Skin:** impaired wound healing, fragile skin, petechiae, erythema, sweating.

## INTERACTIONS
None significant.

## EFFECTS ON LAB TEST RESULTS
● May increase glucose level.

## CONTRAINDICATIONS & CAUTIONS
● Contraindicated in patients hypersensitive to drug or its components.

## NURSING CONSIDERATIONS
● Gently wash skin before applying. To prevent skin damage, rub in gently, leaving a thin coat. When treating hairy sites, part hair and apply directly to lesions.
● Avoid applying near eyes or mucous membranes or in ear canal; may be safely used on face, groin, and armpits and under breasts.
● If an occlusive dressing is applied and a fever develops, notify prescriber and remove dressing.
● Change dressing as prescribed. Stop drug and tell prescriber if skin infection, striae, or atrophy occurs.
● When using aerosol near the face, cover patient's eyes and warn against inhaling spray. Aerosol contains alcohol and may cause irritation or burning when used on open lesions. Don't spray longer than 3 seconds or from closer than 6 inches (15 cm) to avoid freezing tissues. If spray

Reactions may be *common,* uncommon, *life-threatening,* or COMMON AND LIFE-THREATENING.

is applied to dry scalp after shampooing, drug need not be massaged into scalp.
• If antifungal or antibiotic combined with corticosteroid fails to provide prompt improvement, stop corticosteroid until infection is controlled.
• Systemic absorption is likely with use of occlusive dressings, prolonged treatment, or extensive body surface treatment. Watch for symptoms.
• Avoid using plastic pants or tight-fitting diapers on treated areas in young children. Children may absorb larger amounts of drug and be more susceptible to systemic toxicity.
• Continue treatment for a few days after lesions clear.
• Monitor patient for fluid or electrolyte disturbances (sodium and fluid retention, potassium loss, hypokalemic alkalosis, negative nitrogen balance from catabolism of protein).
• Drug may suppress skin reaction testing.
• *Alert:* Don't confuse hydrocortisone with hydroxychloroquine.

**PATIENT TEACHING**
• Teach patient or family member how to apply drug.
• Tell patient to wash hands after application.
• If an occlusive dressing is ordered, advise patient to leave it in place for no longer than 12 hours each day and not to use the dressing on infected or weeping lesions.
• Tell patient to stop drug and report signs of systemic absorption, skin irritation or ulceration, hypersensitivity, infection, or lack of improvement.
• Instruct patient to insert suppositories blunt end first after removing foil wrapper.
• For perianal application, instruct patient to place small amount of drug on a tissue and gently rub in.
• Tell patient to disassemble applicator or aerosol cap and clean with warm water after each use.

# triamcinolone acetonide
Aristocort, Aristocort A, Delta-Tritex, Flutex, Kenalog, Kenalone‡, Triacet, Triderm

*Pregnancy risk category C*

**AVAILABLE FORMS**
*Aerosol:* 0.2 mg/2-second spray
*Cream:* 0.02%‡, 0.025%, 0.1%, 0.5%
*Lotion:* 0.025%, 0.1%
*Ointment:* 0.02%‡, 0.025%, 0.1%, 0.5%
*Paste:* 0.1%

**INDICATIONS & DOSAGES**
➤ **Inflammation and pruritus from corticosteroid-responsive dermatoses**
*Adults and children:* Clean area; apply aerosol, cream, lotion, or ointment sparingly b.i.d. to q.i.d. Rub in lightly.
➤ **Inflammation from oral lesions**
*Adults and children:* Apply paste h.s. and, if needed, b.i.d. or t.i.d., preferably after meals. Apply small amount without rubbing; press to lesion in mouth until thin film develops.

**ACTION**
Unclear. Diffuses across cell membranes to form complexes with specific cytoplasmic receptors. Exhibits anti-inflammatory, antipruritic, vasoconstrictive, and antiproliferative activity. Considered a medium-potency (group III) drug, according to vasoconstrictive properties.

| Route | Onset | Peak | Duration |
|---|---|---|---|
| Topical | Several hr | Unknown | > 1 wk |

**ADVERSE REACTIONS**
**CV:** syncope.
**GU:** glycosuria.
**Metabolic:** hyperglycemia.
**Skin:** burning, pruritus, irritation, dryness, erythema, folliculitis, hypertrichosis, hypopigmentation, acneiform eruptions, perioral dermatitis, allergic contact dermatitis, *maceration, secondary infection, atrophy, striae, miliaria with occlusive dressings.*
**Other:** *hypothalamic-pituitary-adrenal axis suppression,* Cushing's syndrome.

---

## INTERACTIONS
None significant.

## EFFECTS ON LAB TEST RESULTS
● May increase glucose level.

## CONTRAINDICATIONS & CAUTIONS
● Contraindicated in patients hypersensitive to drug or its components.

## NURSING CONSIDERATIONS
● Gently wash skin before applying. To avoid skin damage, rub in gently, leaving a thin coat. When treating hairy sites, part hair and apply directly to lesions.
● Don't apply near eyes or in ear canal.
● Stop drug and tell prescriber if skin infection, striae, or atrophy occurs.
● When using aerosol near the face, cover patient's eyes and warn against inhaling spray. Aerosol contains alcohol and may cause irritation or burning when used on open lesions. Don't spray longer than 3 seconds or from closer than 6 inches (15 cm) to avoid freezing tissues.
● If antifungal or antibiotic combined with corticosteroid fails to provide prompt improvement, stop corticosteroid until infection is controlled.
● Systemic absorption is likely with the use of occlusive dressings, prolonged treatment, or extensive body surface treatment. Watch for symptoms.
● Avoid using plastic pants or tight-fitting diapers on treated areas in young children. Children may absorb larger amounts of drug and be more susceptible to systemic toxicity.
● *Alert:* Don't confuse triamcinolone with Triaminicin or Triaminicol.

## PATIENT TEACHING
● Teach patient or family member how to apply drug.
● If an occlusive dressing is ordered, advise patient to leave it in place for no longer than 12 hours each day and not to use the dressing on infected or weeping lesions.
● Tell patient to stop drug and report signs of systemic absorption, skin irritation or ulceration, hypersensitivity, infection, or lack of improvement.

---

Reactions may be *common*, uncommon, *life-threatening*, or COMMON AND LIFE-THREATENING.

# Vitamins and minerals

**vitamin A**
**vitamin B complex**
  **cyanocobalamin,**
    **hydroxocobalamin**
  **folic acid**
  **leucovorin calcium**
  **niacin**
  **niacinamide**
  **pyridoxine hydrochloride**
  **riboflavin**
  **thiamine hydrochloride**
**vitamin C**
**vitamin D**
  **cholecalciferol**
  **ergocalciferol**
**vitamin D analogue**
  **doxercalciferol**
  **paricalcitol**
**vitamin E**
**vitamin K analogue**
  **phytonadione**
**sodium fluoride**
**sodium fluoride, topical**
**trace elements**
  **chromium**
  **copper**
  **iodine**
  **manganese**
  **selenium**
  **zinc**

## COMBINATION PRODUCTS
**Vitamins**
B complex vitamins ◊
B complex vitamins with iron ◊
B complex with vitamin C ◊
B vitamin combinations ◊
Calcium and vitamin products ◊
Fluoride with vitamins ◊
Geriatric supplements with multivitamins and minerals ◊
Miscellaneous vitamins and minerals ◊
Multivitamins ◊
Multivitamins and minerals with hormones ◊
Multivitamins with B₁₂ ◊
Vitamin A and D combinations ◊
**Trace elements**
MULTIPLE TRACE ELEMENT NEONATAL: zinc sulfate 1.5 mg, copper sulfate 0.1 mg, manganese sulfate 0.025 mg, chromium chloride 0.85 mcg/ml.

MULTIPLE TRACE ELEMENT PEDIATRIC: zinc sulfate 0.5 mg, copper sulfate 0.1 mg, manganese sulfate 0.03 mg, and chromium chloride 1 mcg/ml.

MULTIPLE TRACE ELEMENT WITH SELENIUM: zinc sulfate 1 mg, copper sulfate 0.4 mg, manganese sulfate 0.1 mg, chromium chloride 4 mcg, and selenious acid 20 mcg/ml.

NEOTRACE-4: zinc sulfate 1.5 mg, copper sulfate 0.1 mg, manganese sulfate 0.025 mg, and chromium chloride 0.85 mcg/ml.

PEDTRACE-4: zinc sulfate 0.5 mg, copper sulfate 0.1 mg, manganese sulfate 0.025 mg, and chromium chloride 0.85 mcg/ml.

PTE-4: zinc sulfate 1 mg, copper sulfate 0.1 mg, manganese sulfate 0.025 mg, and chromium chloride 1 mcg/ml.

PTE-5: zinc sulfate 1 mg, copper sulfate 0.1 mg, manganese sulfate 0.025 mg, chromium chloride 1 mcg, and selenium (as selenious acid) 15 mcg/ml.

TRACE METALS ADDITIVE: zinc chloride 0.8 mg, copper chloride 0.2 mg, manganese chloride 0.16 mg, and chromium chloride 2 mcg/ml.

---

## vitamin A (retinol)
Aquasol A, Palmitate-A

*Pregnancy risk category A (if dose is under 800 mcg retinol equivalents); C (if dose exceeds 800 mcg retinol equivalents); X (for Aquasol)*

### AVAILABLE FORMS
*Capsules:* 10,000 IU ◊, 15,000 IU ◊, 25,000 IU
*Drops:* 30 ml with dropper (5,000 IU/0.1 ml, 50,000 IU/ml)
*Injection:* 2-ml vials (50,000 IU/ml with 0.5% chlorobutanol, polysorbate 80, butylated hydroxyanisole, butylated hydroxytoluene)
*Tablets:* 5,000 IU ◊, 10,000 IU

---

## INDICATIONS & DOSAGES
### ➤ RDA
*Men and boys older than age 11:*
1,000 mcg retinol equivalent (RE) or
3,330 IU.
*Women and girls older than age 11:*
800 mcg RE or 2,665 IU.
*Children ages 7 to 10:* 700 mcg RE or
2,330 IU.
*Children ages 4 to 6:* 500 mcg RE or
1,665 IU.
*Children ages 1 to 3:* 400 mcg RE or
1,330 IU.
*Neonates and infants younger than age 1:*
375 mcg RE or 1,238 IU.
*Pregnant women:* 800 mcg RE or
2,665 IU.
*Breast-feeding women (first 6 months):*
1,300 mcg RE or 4,330 IU.
*Breast-feeding women (second 6 months):*
1,200 mcg RE or 4,000 IU.
### ➤ Severe vitamin A deficiency
*Adults and children older than age 8:*
100,000 IU I.M. or 100,000 to 500,000 IU
P.O. for 3 days; then 50,000 IU P.O. or
I.M. for 2 weeks, followed by 10,000 to
20,000 IU P.O. for 2 months. Follow with
adequate dietary nutrition and RE vitamin
A supplements.
*Children age 8 and younger:* 5,000 to
15,000 IU I.M. daily for 10 days.
### ➤ Maintenance dose to prevent recurrence of vitamin A deficiency
*Children ages 1 to 8:* 5,000 to 10,000 IU
P.O. daily for 2 months; then adequate dietary nutrition and RE vitamin A supplements.

## ACTION
A coenzyme that stimulates retinal function, bone growth, reproduction, and integrity of epithelial and mucosal tissues.

| Route | Onset | Peak | Duration |
|-------|-------|------|----------|
| P.O. | Unknown | 3-5 hr | Unknown |
| I.M. | Unknown | Unknown | Unknown |

## ADVERSE REACTIONS
**CNS:** irritability, headache, ***increased intracranial pressure,*** fatigue, lethargy, malaise.
**EENT:** papilledema, exophthalmos.
**GI:** anorexia, epigastric pain, vomiting, polydipsia.
**GU:** hypomenorrhea, polyuria.

**Hepatic:** jaundice, hepatomegaly, ***cirrhosis.***
**Metabolic:** slow growth, hypercalcemia, weight loss.
**Musculoskeletal:** decalcification, periostitis, premature closure of epiphyses, migratory arthralgia, cortical thickening over the radius and tibia.
**Skin:** alopecia; dry, cracked, scaly skin; pruritus; lip fissures; erythema; inflamed tongue, lips, and gums; massive desquamation; increased pigmentation; night sweats.
**Other:** splenomegaly, ***anaphylactic shock.***

## INTERACTIONS
**Drug-drug.** *Cholestyramine resin, mineral oil:* May reduce GI absorption of fat-soluble vitamins. Avoid using together.
*Hormonal contraceptives:* May increase vitamin A level. Monitor patient closely.
*Isotretinoin, multivitamins containing vitamin A:* May increase risk of toxicity. Avoid using together.
*Neomycin (oral):* May decrease vitamin A absorption. Avoid using together.
*Orlistat:* May decrease absorption of fat-soluble vitamins. Separate doses by 2 hours.
*Warfarin:* May increase risk of bleeding with large doses of vitamin A. Monitor PT and INR closely.

## EFFECTS ON LAB TEST RESULTS
● May increase liver enzyme levels.

## CONTRAINDICATIONS & CAUTIONS
● Contraindicated orally in patients with malabsorption syndrome; if malabsorption is from inadequate bile secretion, oral route may be used together with bile salts (dehydrocholic acid).
● Contraindicated in patients hypersensitive to any ingredient in product and in those with hypervitaminosis A.
● I.V. route contraindicated except for special water-miscible forms intended for infusion with large parenteral volumes. I.V. push contraindicated (anaphylaxis or anaphylactoid reactions and death have resulted).
● Use cautiously in pregnant patients, avoiding doses exceeding 800 mcg RE.

## NURSING CONSIDERATIONS
● RDAs have been converted to REs. One RE has the activity of 1 mcg all-*trans* retinol, 6 mcg beta carotene.
● *Alert:* Give parenteral form by I.M. route or continuous I.V. infusion (that is, in total parenteral nutrition infusion). Never give as I.V. bolus.
● Assess patient's vitamin A intake from all sources. Consider dietary intake.
● Liquid products are available for nasogastric route. Preparation may be mixed with cereal or fruit juice.
● Vitamin may be given I.M. for malabsorption syndrome or when oral route isn't feasible.
● Adequate vitamin A absorption needs suitable dietary protein, fat, vitamin E, and zinc intake and bile secretion; give supplemental salts. Zinc supplements may be needed in patients receiving long-term total parenteral nutrition.
● Watch for adverse reactions if dosage is high. Monitor patient taking more than 25,000 IU daily for adverse effects. Adverse reactions usually occur only with doses that exceed physiologic requirement.
● Acute toxicity has resulted from single doses of 25,000 IU/kg of body weight; 350,000 IU in infants and over 2 million IU in adults have also caused acute toxicity. Doses that don't exceed RDA are usually nontoxic.
● Chronic toxicity in infants ages 3 to 6 months has resulted from doses of 18,500 IU daily for 1 to 3 months. In adults, chronic toxicity has resulted from doses of 50,000 IU daily for longer than 18 months, 500,000 IU daily for 2 months, and 1 million IU daily for 3 days.
● Watch for skin disorders, a symptom of chronic toxicity.
● Vitamin A therapy may falsely increase cholesterol and bilirubin levels.

## PATIENT TEACHING
● Warn patient not to take megadoses of vitamins without specific indications, to avoid toxicity.
● Stress that prescribed vitamins shouldn't be shared with others.
● Instruct patient to protect drug from light.
● Teach patient about good food sources of vitamin A, such as green and yellow

vegetables, cantaloupe, and liver (note that liver is also high in saturated fat).
● Advise patient that liquid product can be mixed with food, if desired.
● Tell patient to notify prescriber of signs of overdose (nausea, vomiting, appetite loss, malaise, dry and cracking skin and lips, irritability, hair loss, headache, visual disturbances, vertigo, bulging area on the top of the head [fontanels] in infants).

# vitamin B complex

## cyanocobalamin (vitamin $B_{12}$)
Crystamine, Crysti-12, Cyanocobalamin, Cyanoject, Cyomin, Rubramin PC

## hydroxocobalamin (vitamin $B_{12}$)
Hydro-Cobex, Hydro-Crysti-12, LA-12

*Pregnancy risk category A; C (if dose exceeds RDA)*

## AVAILABLE FORMS
**cyanocobalamin**
*Injection:* 100 mcg/ml, 1,000 mcg/ml
*Tablets:* 25 mcg ◊, 50 mcg ◊, 100 mcg ◊, 250 mcg ◊, 500 mcg ◊, 1,000 mcg ◊
**hydroxocobalamin**
*Injection:* 1,000 mcg/ml

## INDICATIONS & DOSAGES
➤ **RDA for cyanocobalamin**
*Adults and children age 11 and older:* 2 mcg.
*Children ages 7 to 10:* 1.4 mcg.
*Children ages 4 to 6:* 1 mcg.
*Children ages 1 to 3:* 0.7 mcg.
*Infants ages 6 months to 1 year:* 0.5 mcg.
*Neonates and infants younger than age 6 months:* 0.3 mcg.
*Pregnant women:* 2.2 mcg.
*Breast-feeding women:* 2.6 mcg.
➤ **Vitamin $B_{12}$ deficiency from inadequate diet, subtotal gastrectomy, or other condition, disorder, or disease, except malabsorption, related to pernicious anemia or other GI disease**
*Adults:* 30 mcg hydroxocobalamin I.M. daily for 5 to 10 days, depending on severity of deficiency. Maintenance dose is

100 to 200 mcg I.M. once monthly. For subsequent prophylaxis, advise adequate nutrition and daily RDA vitamin $B_{12}$ supplements.

*Children:* 1 to 5 mg hydroxocobalamin given over 2 or more weeks in doses of 100 mcg I.M., depending on severity of deficiency. Maintenance dose is 60 mcg/month I.M. For subsequent prophylaxis, advise adequate nutrition and daily RDA vitamin $B_{12}$ supplements.

➤ **Pernicious anemia or vitamin $B_{12}$ malabsorption**

*Adults:* Initially, 100 mcg cyanocobalamin I.M. or S.C. daily for 6 to 7 days; then 100 mcg I.M. or S.C. once monthly.
*Children:* 30 to 50 mcg I.M. or S.C. daily over 2 or more weeks; then 100 mcg I.M. or S.C. monthly for life.

➤ **Methylmalonicaciduria**

*Neonates:* 1,000 mcg cyanocobalamin I.M. daily.

➤ **Schilling test flushing dose**

*Adults and children:* 1,000 mcg hydroxocobalamin I.M. as single dose.

## ACTION

A coenzyme that stimulates metabolic function and is needed for cell replication, hematopoiesis, and nucleoprotein and myelin synthesis.

| Route | Onset | Peak | Duration |
|---|---|---|---|
| P.O., I.M. | Unknown | 1 hr | Unknown |
| S.C. | Unknown | 8-12 hr | Unknown |

## ADVERSE REACTIONS

**CV:** peripheral vascular thrombosis, *heart failure.*
**GI:** transient diarrhea.
**Respiratory:** pulmonary edema.
**Skin:** itching, transitory exanthema, urticaria.
**Other:** *anaphylaxis, anaphylactoid reactions with parenteral administration,* pain or burning at I.M. or S.C. injection sites.

## INTERACTIONS

**Drug-drug.** *Aminoglycosides, anticonvulsants, colchicine, extended-release potassium products, aminosalicylic acid, salts:* May cause malabsorption of vitamin $B_{12}$ from GI tract. Avoid using together.

*Ascorbic acid:* Large doses may destroy vitamin $B_{12}$ in GI tract. Separate doses by 1 hour.
*Chloramphenicol:* May decrease hematopoietic response to vitamin $B_{12}$. Monitor hematologic response and consider alternative anti-infectives.
**Drug-lifestyle.** *Alcohol use:* May cause malabsorption of vitamin $B_{12}$. Discourage use together.

## EFFECTS ON LAB TEST RESULTS
None reported.

## CONTRAINDICATIONS & CAUTIONS
● Contraindicated in patients hypersensitive to vitamin $B_{12}$ or cobalt and in those with early Leber's disease (hereditary optic nerve atrophy).
● Use cautiously in anemic patients with coexisting cardiac, pulmonary, or hypertensive disease. Also use cautiously in premature infants; product may contain benzyl alcohol, which may cause "gasping syndrome."

## NURSING CONSIDERATIONS
● Determine reticulocyte count, hematocrit, vitamin $B_{12}$, iron, and folate levels before beginning therapy.
● Obtain a sensitivity test history before administration. An intradermal test dose is recommended in patients with possible sensitivity.
● Vitamin $B_{12}$ may cause false-positive results for intrinsic factor antibodies, which are present in the blood of half of all patients with pernicious anemia. Methotrexate, pyrimethamine, and most anti-infectives invalidate diagnostic blood assays for vitamin $B_{12}$.
● *Alert:* Avoid I.V. administration because faster systemic elimination will reduce effectiveness of vitamin.
● Don't mix parenteral preparations in same syringe with other drugs.
● Drug is physically incompatible with dextrose solutions, alkaline or strongly acidic solutions, oxidizing or reducing agents, heavy metals, chlorpromazine, phytonadione, prochlorperazine, and other drugs.
● Hydroxocobalamin is approved for I.M. or deep S.C. use only. Its only advantage

over cyanocobalamin is its longer duration.
• Don't give large oral doses of vitamin $B_{12}$ routinely; drug is lost through excretion.
• Monitor patient for hypokalemia for first 48 hours, as anemia corrects itself. Give potassium supplement, as needed.
• Infection, tumors, or renal, hepatic, and other debilitating diseases may reduce therapeutic response.
• Deficiencies are more common in patients who are strict vegetarians and in their breast-fed infants.
• Vitamin $B_{12}$ deficiency may suppress symptoms of polycythemia vera.
• Protect vitamin $B_{12}$ from light. Don't refrigerate or freeze.

**PATIENT TEACHING**
• Stress need for patient with pernicious anemia to return for monthly injections. Although total body stores may last 3 to 6 years, anemia will recur if not treated monthly.
• Stress importance of follow-up visits and laboratory studies.
• Teach patient healthy dietary habits.
• Instruct patient not to take folic acid as a replacement for vitamin $B_{12}$; folic acid may ease blood-related symptoms of pernicious anemia, but neurologic complications will progress.

## folic acid (vitamin $B_9$)
Folvite, Novo-Folacid†

*Pregnancy risk category A*

**AVAILABLE FORMS**
*Injection:* 10-ml vials (5 mg/ml with 1.5% benzyl alcohol, 5 mg/ml with 1.5% benzyl alcohol and 0.2% ethylenediaminetetraacetic acid)
*Tablets:* 0.4 mg, 0.8 mg, 1 mg

**INDICATIONS & DOSAGES**
➤ **RDA**
*Adults and children age 14 and older:* 400 mcg.
*Children ages 9 to 13:* 300 mcg.
*Children ages 4 to 8:* 200 mcg.
*Children ages 1 to 3:* 150 mcg.
*Infants ages 6 months to 1 year:* 80 mcg

*Neonates and infants younger than age 6 months:* 65 mcg.
*Pregnant women:* 600 mcg.
*Breast-feeding women:* 500 mcg.
➤ **Megaloblastic or macrocytic anemia from folic acid or other nutritional deficiency, hepatic disease, alcoholism, intestinal obstruction, or excessive hemolysis**
*Adults and children age 4 and older:* 0.4 to 1 mg P.O., I.M., or S.C. daily. After anemia caused by folic acid deficiency is corrected, proper diet and RDA supplements are needed to prevent recurrence.
*Children younger than age 4:* Up to 0.3 mg P.O., I.M., or S.C. daily.
*Pregnant and breast-feeding women:* 0.8 mg P.O., I.M., or S.C. daily.
➤ **To prevent fetal neural tube defects during pregnancy**
*Adults:* 0.4 mg P.O. daily.
➤ **To prevent megaloblastic anemia during pregnancy to prevent fetal damage**
*Adults:* Up to 1 mg P.O., I.M., or S.C. daily throughout pregnancy.
➤ **Test for folic acid deficiency in patients with megaloblastic anemia without masking pernicious anemia**
*Adults and children:* 0.1 to 0.2 mg P.O. or I.M. for 10 days while maintaining a diet low in folate and vitamin $B_{12}$.
➤ **Tropical sprue**
*Adults:* 3 to 15 mg P.O. daily.

**ACTION**
Stimulates normal erythropoiesis and nucleoprotein synthesis.

| Route | Onset | Peak | Duration |
|---|---|---|---|
| P.O., I.M., S.C. | Unknown | 30-60 min | Unknown |

**ADVERSE REACTIONS**
**CNS:** altered sleep pattern, general malaise, difficulty concentrating, confusion, impaired judgment, irritability, hyperactivity.
**GI:** anorexia, nausea, flatulence, bitter taste.
**Respiratory:** *bronchospasm.*
**Skin:** allergic reactions including rash, pruritus, and erythema.

## INTERACTIONS
**Drug-drug.** *Aminosalicylic acid, chloramphenicol, hormonal contraceptives, methotrexate, sulfasalazine, trimethoprim:* May antagonize folic acid. Watch for decreased folic acid effect. Use together cautiously.
*Phenytoin:* May increase anticonvulsant metabolism, which decreases level of anticonvulsant. Monitor phenytoin level closely.

## EFFECTS ON LAB TEST RESULTS
• May decrease serum and RBC folate levels.

## CONTRAINDICATIONS & CAUTIONS
• Contraindicated in patients with undiagnosed anemia (it may mask pernicious anemia) and in those with vitamin $B_{12}$ deficiency.

## NURSING CONSIDERATIONS
• The U.S. Public Health Service recommends use of folic acid during pregnancy to decrease neural tube defects. In patients with a history of neural tube defects in pregnancy, increased folic acid intake for 1 month before and 3 months after conception is recommended.
• Patients with small-bowel resections and intestinal malabsorption may need parenteral administration.
• Most CNS and GI adverse reactions occur at higher doses, such as 15 mg daily for 1 month.
• Don't mix with other drugs in same syringe for I.M. injections.
• Protect drug from light and heat; store at room temperature.
• *Alert:* Don't confuse folic acid with folinic acid.

## PATIENT TEACHING
• Teach patient about proper nutrition to prevent recurrence of anemia.
• Stress importance of follow-up visits and laboratory studies.
• Teach patient about foods that contain folic acid: liver, oranges, whole wheat, broccoli, Brussels sprouts.

# leucovorin calcium (citrovorum factor, folinic acid)

*Pregnancy risk category C*

## AVAILABLE FORMS
*Injection:* 1-ml ampule (3 mg/ml with 0.9% benzyl alcohol); 10 mg/ml in 5-ml vial; 50-mg, 100-mg, 350-mg vials for reconstitution (contains no preservatives)
*Tablets:* 5 mg, 15 mg, 25 mg

## INDICATIONS & DOSAGES
➤ **Overdose of folic acid antagonist (methotrexate, trimethoprim, or pyrimethamine)**
*Adults and children:* I.M. or I.V. dose equivalent to weight of antagonist given. For methotrexate overdose, up to 75 mg I.V. infusion within 12 hours, followed by 12 mg I.M. q 6 hours for four doses. For adverse effects after average doses of methotrexate, 6 to 12 mg I.M. q 6 hours for four doses.
➤ **Leucovorin rescue after high methotrexate dose in treatment of malignant disease**
*Adults and children:* 10 mg/m² P.O., I.M., or I.V. q 6 hours until methotrexate level falls below $5 \times 10^{-8}$ M.
➤ **Megaloblastic anemia from congenital enzyme deficiency**
*Adults and children:* 3 to 6 mg I.M. daily.
➤ **Folate-deficient megaloblastic anemia**
*Adults and children:* Up to 1 mg I.M. daily. Duration of treatment depends on hematologic response.
➤ **To prevent hematologic toxicity from pyrimethamine or trimethoprim therapy**
*Adults and children:* 400 mcg to 5 mg I.M. with each dose of folic acid antagonist. Oral dosages of 10 to 35 mg once daily or 25 mg once weekly may also be used.
➤ **Hematologic toxicity from pyrimethamine or trimethoprim therapy**
*Adults and children:* 5 to 15 mg I.M. daily.
➤ **Palliative treatment of advanced colorectal cancer**
*Adults:* 20 mg/m² I.V.; then fluorouracil 425 mg/m² I.V. or 200 mg/m² I.V. (over

3 minutes or longer) followed by fluorouracil 370 mg/m² daily for 5 consecutive
days. Repeated at 4-week intervals for two
additional courses; then at intervals of 4 to
5 weeks, if tolerated.

### I.V. ADMINISTRATION
● When using powder for injection, reconstitute 50-mg vial with 5 ml, 100-mg vial
with 10 ml, or 350-mg vial with 17 ml of
sterile or bacteriostatic water for injection.
When doses exceed 10 mg/m², don't use
diluents containing benzyl alcohol.
● *Alert:* Don't exceed 160 mg/minute
when giving by I.V. infusion.
● Protect from light and heat and give reconstituted parenteral drug immediately.

### ACTION
A reduced form of folic acid that is readily
converted to other tetrahydrofolic acid derivatives.

| Route | Onset | Peak | Duration |
|-------|-------|------|----------|
| P.O. | 20-30 min | 2-3 hr | 3-6 hr |
| I.V. | 5 min | 10 min | 3-6 hr |
| I.M. | 10-20 min | < 1 hr | 3-6 hr |

### ADVERSE REACTIONS
**Skin:** urticaria.
**Other:** hypersensitivity reactions, *ana-
phylactoid reactions.*

### INTERACTIONS
**Drug-drug.** *Anticonvulsants:* May decrease effectiveness of these drugs. Monitor for seizure activity.
*Fluorouracil:* May increase fluorouracil
toxicity. Fluorouracil dose may need to be
reduced.
*Methotrexate:* High doses of leucovorin
may decrease efficacy of intrathecal
methotrexate. Monitor effects.

### EFFECTS ON LAB TEST RESULTS
None reported.

### CONTRAINDICATIONS & CAUTIONS
● Contraindicated in patients with pernicious anemia and other megaloblastic anemias secondary to lack of vitamin $B_{12}$.
Don't give leucovorin calcium intrathecally.
● In elderly or debilitated patients, use
combined leucovorin and fluorouracil

therapy with extreme caution because of
increased risk of severe GI toxicity.

### NURSING CONSIDERATIONS
● I.V. route is preferred in patients with GI
toxicity when doses exceed 25 mg.
● Drug may mask diagnosis of pernicious
anemia.
● Follow leucovorin rescue schedule and
protocol closely.
● Don't give leucovorin with systemic
methotrexate.
● *Alert:* Don't confuse leucovorin (folinic
acid) with folic acid.

### PATIENT TEACHING
● Explain need for drug to patient and
family, and answer any questions or concerns.
● Tell patient to report symptoms of hypersensitivity promptly.

---

# niacin (nicotinic acid, vitamin B₃)
Nia-Bid◊ , Niacor◊ , Niaspan,
Nicobid◊ , Nicotinex, Slo-Niacin◊

# niacinamide (nicotinamide)◊

*Pregnancy risk category A; C (if
dose exceeds RDA)*

---

### AVAILABLE FORMS
**niacin**
*Capsules (timed-release):* 125 mg◊ ,
250 mg◊ , 300 mg◊ , 400 mg◊ , 500 mg
*Elixir:* 50 mg/5 ml*◊
*Tablets:* 25 mg◊ , 50 mg◊ , 100 mg◊ ,
250 mg◊ , 500 mg
*Tablets (extended-release):* 250 mg◊ ,
375 mg◊ , 500 mg◊ , 750 mg◊ ,
1,000 mg◊
**niacinamide**
*Tablets:* 50 mg◊ , 100 mg◊ , 125 mg◊ ,
250 mg◊ , 500 mg◊

### INDICATIONS & DOSAGES
➤ **RDA**
*Pregnant women:* 18 mg.
*Breast-feeding women:* 17 mg.
*Healthy adult men and boys ages 14 to 18:*
16 mg.
*Healthy adult women and girls ages 14 to
18:* 14 mg.

*Children ages 9 to 13:* 12 mg.
*Children ages 4 to 8:* 8 mg.
*Children ages 1 to 3:* 6 mg.
*Infants ages 6 months to 1 year:* 4 mg.
*Neonates and infants younger than age 6 months:* 2 mg.
➤ **Pellagra**
*Adults:* 300 to 500 mg P.O. daily in divided doses.
*Children:* 100 to 300 mg P.O. daily in divided doses.
➤ **Hartnup disease**
*Adults:* 50 to 200 mg P.O. daily.
➤ **Niacin deficiency**
*Adults:* Up to 100 mg P.O. daily.
➤ **Hyperlipidemias, especially with hypercholesterolemia**
*Adults:* 250 mg P.O. daily h.s. Increase at 4- to 7-day intervals up to 1.5 to 2 g P.O. daily divided b.i.d. to t.i.d. Maximum 6 g daily. Or, 1 to 2 g extended-release tablets P.O. daily h.s.

## ACTION

Stimulates lipid metabolism, tissue respiration, and glycogenolysis; niacin decreases synthesis of LDL and inhibits lipolysis in adipose tissue.

| Route | Onset | Peak | Duration |
|-------|-------|------|----------|
| P.O. | Unknown | 45 min | Unknown |

## ADVERSE REACTIONS

**CV:** *excessive peripheral vasodilation, especially with niacin;* hypotension; atrial fibrillation; *arrhythmias; flushing.*
**EENT:** toxic amblyopia.
**GI:** *nausea, vomiting, diarrhea,* possible activation of peptic ulceration, epigastric or substernal pain.
**Hepatic:** *hepatic dysfunction.*
**Metabolic:** hyperglycemia, hyperuricemia.
**Skin:** pruritus, dryness, tingling, rash, hyperpigmentation.

## INTERACTIONS

**Drug-drug.** *Antihypertensives (ganglionic or sympathetic blockers):* May increase vasodilating effect, causing orthostatic hypotension. Use together cautiously and warn patient about orthostatic hypotension.

*Cholestyramine, colestipol:* May decrease bioavailability of extended-release products. Separate doses by 4 to 6 hours.
*Lovastatin (statin class):* May lead to rhabdomyolysis. Use together cautiously.
*Sulfinpyrazone:* May decrease uricosuric effects. Avoid using together.
**Drug-food.** *Hot drinks:* May increase flushing and pruritus. Urge patient not to take with hot liquids.
**Drug-lifestyle.** *Alcohol use:* May increase flushing and pruritus. Discourage use together.

## EFFECTS ON LAB TEST RESULTS

● May increase glucose, AST, ALT, and uric acid levels.

## CONTRAINDICATIONS & CAUTIONS

● Contraindicated in patients hypersensitive to drug and in those with hepatic dysfunction, active peptic ulcers, severe hypotension, or arterial hemorrhage.
● Use cautiously in patients with gallbladder disease, diabetes mellitus, or unstable angina and in patients with history of liver disease, peptic ulcer, allergy, gout, or significant alcohol intake.

## NURSING CONSIDERATIONS

● After symptoms of niacin deficiency subside, advise adequate nutrition and RDA supplements to prevent recurrence.
● Most reactions are dose-dependent.
● Drug may cause dose-related increase in glucose intolerance; carefully monitor glucose level in diabetic patients. Glycosuria may occur.
● Give niacin with meals to minimize adverse GI effects.
● Give 325 mg of aspirin P.O. 30 minutes before niacin dose, to help reduce flushing response to niacin.
● Extended-release niacin or niacinamide may prevent excessive flushing that occurs with large doses. However, extended-release niacin is linked to hepatic dysfunction, even at very low doses.
● Monitor hepatic function and glucose level early in therapy.
● *Alert:* Don't confuse Nicobid and Nicotinex with nicotine (Nicoderm, Nicotrol, Nicorette).

---

Reactions may be *common,* uncommon, *life-threatening,* or COMMON AND LIFE-THREATENING.

## PATIENT TEACHING
● Stress that niacin is a potent drug, not just a vitamin, and may cause serious adverse effects. Explain importance of adhering to therapy.
● Explain harmlessness of flushing syndrome. Tell patient that flushing and warmth may subside with continued use and that concurrent use of alcohol may increase flushing.
● Tell patient to take with food to minimize stomach upset.

---

## pyridoxine hydrochloride (vitamin B₆)
Nestrex◇, Rodex

*Pregnancy risk category A; C (if dose exceeds RDA)*

### AVAILABLE FORMS
*Injection:* 100 mg/ml
*Tablets:* 10 mg◇, 25 mg◇, 50 mg◇, 100 mg◇, 200 mg◇, 250 mg◇, 500 mg◇

### INDICATIONS & DOSAGES
➤ **RDA**
*Pregnant women:* 2.2 mg.
*Breast-feeding women:* 2.1 mg.
*Adults ages 19 to 50:* 1.3 mg
*Men age 51 and older:* 1.7 mg
*Women age 51 and older:* 1.5 mg
*Boys ages 14 to 19:* 1.3 mg.
*Girls ages 14 to 19:* 1.2 mg.
*Children ages 9 to 13:* 1 mg.
*Children ages 4 to 8:* 0.6 mg.
*Children ages 1 to 3:* 0.5 mg.
*Infants ages 6 months to 1 year:* 0.3 mg.
*Neonates and infants younger than age 6 months:* 0.1 mg.
➤ **Dietary vitamin B₆ deficiency**
*Adults:* 10 to 20 mg P.O., I.V., or I.M. daily for 3 weeks; then 2 to 5 mg daily as supplement to proper diet.
➤ **Seizures related to vitamin B₆ deficiency or dependency**
*Adults and children:* 100 mg I.V. or I.M. in single dose.

➤ **Vitamin B₆–responsive anemias or dependency syndrome (inborn errors of metabolism)**
*Adults:* Up to 500 mg P.O., I.V., or I.M. daily until symptoms subside; then 30 mg daily for life.
➤ **To prevent vitamin B₆ deficiency during drug therapy with isoniazid or penicillamine**
*Adults:* 10 to 50 mg P.O. daily.
➤ **To prevent seizures during cycloserine therapy**
*Adults:* 100 to 300 mg P.O. daily.
➤ **Antidote for isoniazid poisoning**
*Adults:* 4 g I.V.; then 1 g I.M. q 30 minutes until amount of pyridoxine given equals amount of isoniazid ingested.

### I.V. ADMINISTRATION
● Protect from light. Don't use solution if it contains a precipitate, although slight darkening is acceptable.
● Inject undiluted drug into I.V. line of free-flowing compatible solution. Or, infuse diluted drug over prescribed duration for intermittent infusion. Don't use for continuous infusion.
● *Alert:* Seizures may occur after large I.V. doses of this drug.

### ACTION
Acts as a coenzyme that stimulates various metabolic functions, including amino acid metabolism.

| Route | Onset | Peak | Duration |
|---|---|---|---|
| P.O., I.V., I.M. | Unknown | Unknown | Unknown |

### ADVERSE REACTIONS
**CNS:** paresthesia, unsteady gait, numbness, somnolence, *seizures,* headache.
**Skin:** photoallergic reaction.

### INTERACTIONS
**Drug-drug.** *Levodopa:* May decrease effectiveness of levodopa. Avoid using together. Pyridoxine has little to no effect on the combination drug levodopa and carbidopa.
*Phenobarbital, phenytoin:* May decrease anticonvulsant level, increasing risk of seizures. Avoid using together.

---

**Drug-lifestyle.** *Alcohol use:* May cause delirium and lactic acidosis. Discourage use together.

**EFFECTS ON LAB TEST RESULTS**
• May increase AST level. May decrease folic acid level.

**CONTRAINDICATIONS & CAUTIONS**
• Contraindicated in patients hypersensitive to drug.
• Don't use drug in patients with heart disease.

**NURSING CONSIDERATIONS**
• When used to treat isoniazid toxicity, expect to also give anticonvulsants.
• If sodium bicarbonate is needed to control acidosis in isoniazid toxicity, don't mix in same syringe with pyridoxine.
• Patients taking high doses (2 to 6 g/day) may have difficulty walking because of diminished proprioceptive and sensory function.
• Carefully monitor patient's diet. Excessive protein intake increases daily pyridoxine requirements.
• Long-term use of large doses may cause neurotoxicity.
• *Alert:* Don't confuse pyridoxine with pralidoxime or Pyridium.

**PATIENT TEACHING**
• Stress importance of compliance and of good nutrition if drug is prescribed for maintenance therapy to prevent recurrence of deficiency. Explain that pyridoxine with isoniazid has a specific therapeutic purpose and isn't just a vitamin.
• Advise patient taking levodopa alone to avoid multivitamins containing pyridoxine because of decreased levodopa effect.
• Warn patient that there may be burning at the injection site.

# riboflavin (vitamin B₂)◇

*Pregnancy risk category A; C (if dose exceeds RDA)*

**AVAILABLE FORMS**
*Tablets:* 25 mg ◇, 50 mg ◇, 100 mg ◇
*Tablets (sugar-free):* 50 mg ◇, 100 mg ◇

**INDICATIONS & DOSAGES**
➤ **RDA**
*Adult men:* 1.3 mg.
*Adult women:* 1.1 mg.
*Pregnant women:* 1.4 mg.
*Breast-feeding women:* 1.6 mg.
*Boys ages 14 to 19:* 1.3 mg.
*Girls ages 14 to 19:* 1 mg.
*Children ages 9 to 13:* 0.9 mg.
*Children ages 4 to 8:* 0.6 mg.
*Children ages 1 to 3:* 0.5 mg.
*Infants ages 6 months to 1 year:* 0.4 mg.
*Neonates and infants younger than age 6 months:* 0.3 mg.
➤ **Riboflavin deficiency or adjunct to thiamine treatment for polyneuritis or cheilosis secondary to pellagra**
*Adults and children older than age 12:* 5 to 30 mg P.O. daily, depending on severity.
*Children younger than age 12:* 3 to 10 mg P.O. daily, depending on severity.
   For maintenance, increase nutritional intake and supplement with vitamin B complex.

**ACTION**
Converts to two other coenzymes needed for normal tissue respiration. Drug is necessary for activation of pyridoxine.

| Route | Onset | Peak | Duration |
|-------|-------|------|----------|
| P.O. | Unknown | Unknown | Unknown |

**ADVERSE REACTIONS**
**GU:** bright yellow urine.

**INTERACTIONS**
**Drug-drug.** *Probenecid:* May reduce urinary excretion of riboflavin. Avoid using together.
*Propantheline, other anticholinergics:* May decrease rate and extent of absorption of riboflavin. Avoid using together.

**EFFECTS ON LAB TEST RESULTS**
None reported.

**CONTRAINDICATIONS & CAUTIONS**
No known contraindications.

**NURSING CONSIDERATIONS**
• Drug may be given I.V. or I.M. as a component of multiple vitamins.

• Riboflavin deficiency usually accompanies other vitamin B complex deficiencies; patient may need multivitamin therapy.
• Protect drug from air and light.
• *Alert:* Don't confuse riboflavin with ribavirin.

**PATIENT TEACHING**
• Tell patient to take drug with meals; food increases its absorption.
• Stress proper nutritional habits to prevent recurrence of deficiency.
• Inform patient that riboflavin usually causes bright yellow or orange discoloration of urine.

---

**thiamine hydrochloride
(vitamin B$_1$)**
Betamin‡, Beta-Sol‡

*Pregnancy risk category A; C (if dose exceeds RDA)*

**AVAILABLE FORMS**
*Elixir†:* 250 mcg/5 ml
*Injection:* 100 mg/ml
*Tablets:* 25 mg ◇, 50 mg ◇, 100 mg ◇, 250 mg ◇, 500 mg
*Tablets (enteric-coated):* 20 mg

**INDICATIONS & DOSAGES**
➤ **RDA**
*Adult men:* 1.2 mg.
*Adult women:* 1.1 mg.
*Pregnant women:* 1.4 mg.
*Breast-feeding women:* 1.5 mg.
*Boys ages 14 to 18:* 1.2 mg.
*Girls ages 14 to 18:* 1 mg.
*Children ages 9 to 13:* 0.9 mg.
*Children ages 4 to 8:* 0.6 mg.
*Children ages 1 to 3:* 0.5 mg.
*Infants ages 6 months to 1 year:* 0.3 mg.
*Neonates and infants younger than age 6 months:* 0.2 mg.
➤ **Beriberi**
*Adults:* Depending on severity, 5 to 30 mg I.M. t.i.d. for 2 weeks; then dietary correction and multivitamin supplement containing 5 to 30 mg thiamine daily for 1 month.
*Children:* Depending on severity, 10 to 25 mg I.V. or I.M. daily. For noncritically ill children, 10 to 50 mg P.O. daily in divided doses for several weeks with adequate diet.

➤ **Wet beriberi with myocardial failure**
*Adults and children:* 10 to 30 mg I.V. t.i.d.
➤ **Wernicke's encephalopathy**
*Adults:* Initially, 100 mg I.V.; then 50 to 100 mg I.V. or I.M. daily until patient is consuming a regular balanced diet.

**I.V. ADMINISTRATION**
• Dilute drug before use.
• *Alert:* Give large I.V. doses cautiously; give patient a skin test before therapy if he has history of hypersensitivity reactions. Have epinephrine available to treat anaphylaxis.
• Don't use drug with materials that yield alkaline solutions. Thiamine is unstable in alkaline solutions.

**ACTION**
Combines with adenosine triphosphate to form a coenzyme needed for carbohydrate metabolism.

| Route | Onset | Peak | Duration |
|---|---|---|---|
| P.O., I.V., I.M. | Unknown | Unknown | Unknown |

**ADVERSE REACTIONS**
**CNS:** restlessness, weakness.
**CV:** cyanosis, *CV collapse (with repeated I.V. injections).*
**EENT:** tightness of throat.
**GI:** nausea, *hemorrhage.*
**Respiratory:** pulmonary edema.
**Skin:** feeling of warmth, pruritus, urticaria, diaphoresis.
**Other:** *angioedema,* tenderness, induration after I.M. administration.

**INTERACTIONS**
**Drug-drug.** *Neuromuscular blockers:* May increase effects of these drugs. Monitor patient closely.

**EFFECTS ON LAB TEST RESULTS**
None reported.

**CONTRAINDICATIONS & CAUTIONS**
• Contraindicated in patients hypersensitive to thiamine products.

**NURSING CONSIDERATIONS**
• Use parenteral route only when use of oral route isn't feasible.

---

• Thiamine malabsorption is most likely in alcoholism, cirrhosis, and GI disease.
• Thiamine deficiency can occur after about 3 weeks of totally thiamine-free diet.
• Thiamine deficiency usually requires concurrent treatment for multiple deficiencies.
• Dosages over 30 mg t.i.d. may not be fully used. After tissue saturation with thiamine, drug is excreted in urine as pyrimidine.
• In Wernicke's encephalopathy, give thiamine before dextrose because dextrose increases thiamine requirement.
• *Alert:* Don't confuse thiamine with Thorazine.

## PATIENT TEACHING
• Inform breast-feeding woman that if beriberi occurs in infant, both she and her child should be treated with thiamine.
• Stress proper nutritional habits to prevent recurrence of deficiency.
• Instruct patient to protect oral doses from light.

## vitamin C (ascorbic acid)
Cebid Timecelles ◇, Cecon ◇, Cenolate ◇, Ce-Vi-Sol*, Dull-C ◇, Flavorcee ◇, N'ice w/Vitamin C Drops ◇, Vicks Vitamin C Drops ◇

*Pregnancy risk category A; C (if dose exceeds RDA)*

## AVAILABLE FORMS
*Capsules (timed-release):* 250 mg, 500 mg ◇
*Crystals:* 100 g (4 g/tsp) ◇, 500 g (4 g/tsp) ◇
*Injection:* 100 mg/ml, 222 mg/ml, 250 mg/ml, 500 mg/ml
*Lozenges:* 60 mg ◇
*Oral liquid:* 50 ml (35 mg/0.6 ml)* ◇
*Oral solution:* 100 mg/ml ◇
*Powder:* 100 g (4 g/tsp) ◇, 500 g (4 g/tsp) ◇
*Syrup:* 500 mg/5 ml ◇
*Tablets:* 25 mg ◇, 50 mg ◇, 100 mg ◇, 250 mg ◇, 500 mg ◇, 1,000 mg ◇
*Tablets (chewable):* 100 mg ◇, 250 mg ◇, 500 mg ◇, 1,000 mg ◇

*Tablets (timed-release):* 500 mg ◇, 1,000 mg ◇, 1,500 mg

## INDICATIONS & DOSAGES
➤ **RDA**
*Men age 19 and older:* 90 mg.
*Women age 19 and older:* 75 mg.
*Pregnant women:* 80 to 85 mg.
*Breast-feeding women:* 115 to 120 mg.
*Boys ages 14 to 18:* 75 mg.
*Girls ages 14 to 18:* 65 mg.
*Children ages 9 to 13:* 45 mg.
*Children ages 4 to 8:* 25 mg.
*Children ages 1 to 3:* 15 mg.
*Infants ages 7 months to 1 year:* 50 mg.
*Neonates and infants up to age 6 months:* 40 mg.
➤ **Frank and subclinical scurvy**
*Adults:* Depending on severity, 100 to 250 mg P.O., I.V., I.M., or S.C. daily; then 70 to 150 mg daily for maintenance.
*Children:* Depending on severity, 100 to 300 mg P.O., I.V., I.M., or S.C. daily; then at least 30 mg daily for maintenance.
➤ **Extensive burns, delayed fracture or wound healing, postoperative wound healing, severe febrile or chronic disease states**
*Adults:* 300 to 500 mg I.V., I.M., or S.C. daily for 7 to 10 days; 1 to 2 g daily for extensive burns.
*Children:* 100 to 200 mg P.O., I.V., I.M, or S.C. daily.
➤ **To prevent vitamin C deficiency in patients with poor nutritional habits or increased requirements**
*Adults:* 70 to 150 mg P.O., I.V., I.M., or S.C. daily.
*Pregnant and breast-feeding women:* At least 70 to 150 mg P.O., I.V., I.M., or S.C. daily.
*Children:* At least 40 mg P.O., I.V., I.M., or S.C. daily.
*Infants:* At least 35 mg P.O., I.V., I.M., or S.C. daily.
➤ **To acidify urine**
Adults: 4 to 12 g P.O. daily in divided doses.

## I.V. ADMINISTRATION
• Infuse cautiously in patients with renal insufficiency.
• *Alert:* Rapid infusion may cause faintness or dizziness.

### ACTION
Stimulates collagen formation and tissue repair; involved in oxidation-reduction reactions.

| Route | Onset | Peak | Duration |
|---|---|---|---|
| I.M., I.V. | Unknown | Unknown | Unknown |
| P.O., S.C. | Unknown | 2-3 hr | Unknown |

### ADVERSE REACTIONS
**CNS:** faintness, dizziness.
**GI:** diarrhea, heartburn, nausea, vomiting.
**GU:** acid urine, oxaluria, renal calculi.
**Other:** discomfort at injection site.

### INTERACTIONS
**Drug-drug.** *Aspirin (high doses):* May increase risk of salicylate toxicity. Monitor patient closely.
*Estrogen, hormonal contraceptives:* May increase estrogen level. Watch for adverse reactions.
*Oral iron supplements:* May increase iron absorption. Give together.
**Drug-herb.** *Bearberry:* May inactivate bearberry in urine. Tell patient to watch for effect.
**Drug-lifestyle.** *Smoking:* May increase metabolism of vitamin C. Tell patient to increase RDA by 35 mg daily.

### EFFECTS ON LAB TEST RESULTS
None reported.

### CONTRAINDICATIONS & CAUTIONS
• Contraindicated in patients with an allergy to tartrazine or sulfites. Large doses are contraindicated during pregnancy.

### NURSING CONSIDERATIONS
• When giving for urine acidification, check urine pH to ensure efficacy.
• Protect solution from light, and refrigerate ampules.

### PATIENT TEACHING
• For patient receiving vitamin C I.M., explain that I.M. route may promote better use of the vitamin by the body.
• Stress proper nutritional habits to prevent recurrence of deficiency.
• Inform patient that vitamin C is readily absorbed from citrus fruits, tomatoes, potatoes, and leafy vegetables.

• Advise smokers to increase intake of vitamin C.

## vitamin D

## cholecalciferol (vitamin D₃)
Delta-D ◊

## ergocalciferol (vitamin D₂)
Calciferol, Drisdol, Radiostol†

*Pregnancy risk category A; C (if dose exceeds RDA)*

### AVAILABLE FORMS
*Capsules:* 1.25 mg (50,000 IU)
*Injection:* 12.5 mg (500,000 IU)/ml
*Oral liquid:* 8,000 IU/ml in 60-ml dropper bottle ◊
*Tablets:* 1.25 mg (50,000 IU)

### INDICATIONS & DOSAGES
➤ **RDA for cholecalciferol**
*Adults older than age 70:* 600 IU.
*Adults ages 51 to 70:* 400 IU.
*Pregnant or breast-feeding women:* 200 IU.
*Children and adults up to age 50:* 200 IU.
➤ **Rickets and other vitamin D deficiency diseases, renal osteodystrophy**
*Adults:* Initially, 10,000 IU P.O. or I.M. daily, usually increased, based on response, to maximum of 500,000 IU daily.
*Children:* 1,500 to 5,000 IU P.O. or I.M. daily for 2 to 4 weeks; repeat after 2 weeks, if needed. Or, give single dose of 600,000 IU. After correction of deficiency, maintenance includes adequate diet and RDA supplements.
➤ **Hypoparathyroidism**
*Adults and children:* 25,000 to 200,000 IU P.O. or I.M. daily, with calcium supplement.
➤ **Familial hypophosphatemia**
*Adults:* 250 mcg to 1.5 mg P.O. daily with phosphate supplements.
*Children:* 1 to 2 mg P.O. daily with phosphorus supplement, increased in 250- to 500-mcg increments at 3- to 4-month intervals.

---

## ACTION

Promotes absorption and utilization of calcium and phosphate, helping to regulate calcium homeostasis.

| Route | Onset | Peak | Duration |
|---|---|---|---|
| P.O., I.M. | 2-14 hr | 4-12 hr | 2 days-6 mo |

## ADVERSE REACTIONS

Adverse reactions usually occur only in vitamin D toxicity.

**CNS:** headache, weakness, somnolence, overt psychosis, irritability.

**CV:** *calcification of soft tissues, including the heart;* hypertension; **arrhythmias.**

**EENT:** rhinorrhea, conjunctivitis (calcific), photophobia.

**GI:** anorexia, nausea, vomiting, constipation, dry mouth, metallic taste, polydipsia.

**GU:** polyuria, albuminuria, hypercalciuria, nocturia, **impaired renal function,** reversible azotemia.

**Metabolic:** hypercalcemia, hyperthermia, weight loss.

**Musculoskeletal:** bone and muscle pain, bone demineralization.

**Skin:** pruritus.

**Other:** decreased libido.

## INTERACTIONS

**Drug-drug.** *Antacids containing magnesium:* May cause hypermagnesemia, especially in patients with chronic renal failure. Monitor magnesium level.

*Cardiac glycosides:* May increase risk of arrhythmias. Monitor calcium level.

*Cholestyramine, colestipol, mineral oil:* May inhibit GI absorption of oral vitamin D. Separate doses. Use together cautiously.

*Corticosteroids:* May antagonize effect of vitamin D. Monitor vitamin D level closely.

*Orlistat:* May decrease GI absorption of vitamin D. Separate doses by 2 hours.

*Phenobarbital, phenytoin:* May increase vitamin D metabolism and decrease effectiveness. Monitor patient closely.

*Thiazide diuretics:* May cause hypercalcemia in patients with hypoparathyroidism. Monitor calcium level closely.

*Verapamil:* May cause atrial fibrillation because of increased calcium. Monitor calcium level closely.

## EFFECTS ON LAB TEST RESULTS

• May increase BUN, creatinine, AST, ALT, urine urea, calcium, and cholesterol levels.

## CONTRAINDICATIONS & CAUTIONS

• Contraindicated in patients with hypercalcemia, hypervitaminosis D, malabsorption syndrome, decreased renal function, or renal osteodystrophy with hyperphosphatemia.

• Use ergocalciferol with extreme caution, if at all, in patients with heart disease, renal calculi, or arteriosclerosis.

• Use cautiously in cardiac patients, especially those taking cardiac glycosides, and in patients with increased sensitivity to these drugs.

## NURSING CONSIDERATIONS

• Use I.M. injection of vitamin D dispersed in oil for patients unable to absorb oral form.

• **Alert:** Monitor patient's eating and bowel habits; dry mouth, nausea, vomiting, metallic taste, and constipation may be early signs of toxicity.

• Monitor serum and urine calcium, phosphorus, potassium, and urea levels when high therapeutic dosages are used.

• Doses of 60,000 IU/day can cause hypercalcemia. Hypercalcemia may require I.V. hydration and aggressive diuresis.

• Malabsorption from inadequate bile or hepatic dysfunction may require addition of exogenous bile salts to oral form.

• Patients with hyperphosphatemia need dietary phosphate restrictions and binding drugs to avoid metastatic calcifications and renal calculi.

• Mineral oil interferes with absorption of fat-soluble vitamins.

## PATIENT TEACHING

• Teach patient that vitamin D is needed to absorb calcium. Instruct patient to read labels for vitamin D content.

• Advise patient that vitamin D is fat soluble and that mineral oil interferes with absorption.

• Instruct patient to take only as directed, and stress the dangers of excessive doses of fat-soluble vitamins.

• Instruct patient taking vitamin D to restrict intake of antacids that contain magnesium.

---

Reactions may be *common,* uncommon, *life-threatening,* or COMMON AND LIFE-THREATENING.

• Instruct patient to notify prescriber if signs of toxicity occur, such as weakness, lethargy, headache, anorexia, weight loss, nausea, vomiting, abdominal cramps, diarrhea, constipation, vertigo, excess thirst, excess urine, dry mouth, or muscle or bone pain.

# vitamin D analogue

## doxercalciferol
Hectorol

*Pregnancy risk category B*

### AVAILABLE FORMS
*Capsules:* 2.5 mcg

### INDICATION & DOSAGES
➤ **To reduce elevated intact parathyroid hormone (PTH) levels in management of secondary hyperparathyroidism in patients undergoing long-term renal dialysis**
*Adults:* Initially, 10 mcg P.O. three times weekly at dialysis. Adjust dosage p.r.n. to lower intact PTH levels to 150 to 300 pg/ml. Dosage may be increased by 2.5 mcg at 8-week intervals if intact PTH level isn't decreased by 50% and fails to reach target range. Maximum dose is 20 mcg P.O. three times weekly. If intact PTH levels fall below 100 pg/ml, suspend drug for 1 week, then resume at dose at least 2.5 mcg lower than last given dose.

### ACTION
A vitamin D analogue that acts directly on the parathyroid glands to suppress PTH synthesis and secretion.

| Route | Onset | Peak | Duration |
|-------|-------|------|----------|
| P.O. | Unknown | 11-12 hr | Unknown |

### ADVERSE REACTIONS
**CNS:** *dizziness, headache, malaise,* sleep disorder.
**CV:** *bradycardia, edema.*
**GI:** anorexia, dyspepsia, *nausea, vomiting,* constipation.
**Metabolic:** weight gain or loss.
**Musculoskeletal:** arthralgia.
**Respiratory:** *dyspnea.*

**Skin:** pruritus.
**Other:** abscess.

### INTERACTIONS
**Drug-drug.** *Antacids containing magnesium:* May cause hypermagnesemia. Avoid using together.
*Cholestyramine, mineral oil:* May reduce intestinal absorption of doxercalciferol. Avoid using together.
*Glutethimide, phenobarbital, other enzyme inducers; phenytoin and other enzyme inhibitors:* May affect metabolism of doxercalciferol. Adjust dosage, as appropriate.
*Phosphate binders that contain calcium or don't contain aluminum:* May cause hypercalcemia or hyperphosphatemia and decrease effectiveness of doxercalciferol. Use together cautiously and adjust dosage of phosphate binders, as appropriate.
*Vitamin D supplements:* May cause additive effects and hypercalcemia. Avoid using together.

### EFFECTS ON LAB TEST RESULTS
None reported.

### CONTRAINDICATIONS & CAUTIONS
• Contraindicated in patients with recent history of hypercalcemia, hyperphosphatemia, or vitamin D toxicity.
• Use cautiously in patients with hepatic insufficiency.

### NURSING CONSIDERATIONS
• Monitor calcium, phosphorus, and intact PTH levels.
• Doxercalciferol is given with dialysis (about every other day). Dosing must be individualized and based on intact PTH levels, with monitoring of calcium and phosphorus levels before doxercalciferol therapy and weekly thereafter in the early phase of treatment.
• Management of secondary hyperparathyroidism may prevent bone disease in patients with renal failure.
• Calcium-based or non–aluminum-containing phosphate binders and a low-phosphate diet are used to control phosphorus levels in patients undergoing dialysis. Expect adjustments in dosages of doxercalciferol and concurrent therapies such as dietary phosphate binders to sus-

tain PTH suppression and maintain calcium and phosphorus levels within acceptable ranges.
• Progressive hypercalcemia secondary to vitamin D overdose may require emergency attention. Acute hypercalcemia may worsen arrhythmias and seizures and affect action of digoxin. Chronic hypercalcemia can lead to vascular and soft-tissue calcification.
• If hypercalcemia or hyperphosphatemia occurs or if the calcium-phosphorus product is > 70, immediately suspend administration until these values return to normal.

## PATIENT TEACHING
• Inform patient that dosage must be adjusted over several months to achieve satisfactory PTH suppression.
• Tell patient to follow instructions regarding calcium supplementation and to adhere to a low-phosphorus diet.
• Tell patient to obtain prescriber's approval before using OTC drugs, including antacids and vitamin products containing calcium or vitamin D.
• Inform patient that early signs and symptoms of hypercalcemia include weakness, headache, lethargy, nausea, vomiting, dry mouth, constipation, muscle pain, bone pain, and metallic taste. Late signs and symptoms include excess urination, excess thirst, appetite loss, weight loss, urination at night, eye inflammation, pancreatitis, sensitivity to the sun, mucus nasal discharge, itching, high body temperature, decreased sex drive, high blood pressure, and abnormal heart rhythms.

## paricalcitol
Zemplar

*Pregnancy risk category C*

### AVAILABLE FORMS
*Injection:* 5 mcg/ml

### INDICATIONS & DOSAGES
➤ **To prevent or treat secondary hyperparathyroidism and chronic renal failure**
*Adults:* 0.04 to 0.1 mcg/kg (2.8 to 7 mcg) I.V. no more frequently than every other day during dialysis. Doses as high as

0.24 mcg/kg (16.8 mcg) may be safely given. If satisfactory response isn't observed, dosage may be increased by 2 to 4 mcg at 2- to 4-week intervals.

### I.V. ADMINISTRATION
• Inspect drug for particulates and discoloration before use.
• Give drug only as an I.V. bolus. Discard unused portion.
• Store drug at a controlled room temperature (59° to 86° F [15° to 30° C]).

### ACTION
A synthetic vitamin D analogue that reduces parathyroid hormone (PTH) levels.

| Route | Onset | Peak | Duration |
|-------|-------|------|----------|
| I.V. | Immediate | Unknown | 15 hr |

### ADVERSE REACTIONS
**CNS:** fever, light-headedness, malaise.
**CV:** palpitations, edema.
**GI:** dry mouth, *GI bleeding, nausea,* vomiting.
**Respiratory:** pneumonia.
**Other:** chills, flulike syndrome, *sepsis.*

### INTERACTIONS
None significant.

### EFFECTS ON LAB TEST RESULTS
• May decrease total alkaline phosphatase level.

### CONTRAINDICATIONS & CAUTIONS
• Contraindicated in patients hypersensitive to drug or its ingredients and in those with evidence of vitamin D toxicity or hypercalcemia.
• Use cautiously in patients taking digitalis compounds. Patients taking digoxin are at greater risk for digitalis toxicity during drug therapy secondary to potential for hypercalcemia.

### NURSING CONSIDERATIONS
• Watch for ECG abnormalities.
• Monitor patient for symptoms of hypercalcemia, such as fatigue, muscle weakness, anorexia, depression, nausea, and constipation. Immediately notify prescriber if hypercalcemia is suspected.
• Monitor calcium and phosphorus levels twice weekly when dosage is being adjust-

ed, and then monitor monthly. Measure PTH level every 3 months during therapy.

• As PTH level decreases, paricalcitol dose may need to be decreased. Acute overdose of paricalcitol may cause hypercalcemia, which may require emergency attention.

• In patients with chronic renal failure, appropriate types of phosphate-binding compounds may be needed to control phosphorus levels, but avoid excessive use of aluminum-containing compounds.

**PATIENT TEACHING**

• Stress importance of adhering to a dietary regimen of calcium supplementation and phosphorus restriction during drug therapy.

• Caution against use of phosphate or vitamin D–related compounds during drug therapy.

• Explain need for frequent laboratory tests.

• Instruct patient with chronic renal failure to take phosphate-binding compounds as prescribed but to avoid excessive use of aluminum-containing compounds. Alert patient to early symptoms of excess calcium levels and vitamin D intoxication, such as weakness, headache, sleepiness, nausea, vomiting, dry mouth, constipation, muscle and bone pain, and metallic taste.

• Instruct patient to promptly report adverse reactions.

• Remind patient taking digoxin to watch for signs and symptoms of digitalis toxicity.

---

## vitamin E (tocopherols)
Aquasol E ◇, Aquavit-E ◇, d'Alpha E

*Pregnancy risk category A*

**AVAILABLE FORMS**
*Capsules:* 100 IU ◇, 200 IU ◇, 400 IU ◇, 600 IU ◇, 1,000 IU ◇
*Drops:* 15 IU/0.3 ml
*Liquid:* 15 IU/30 ml
*Tablets:* 100 IU ◇, 200 IU ◇, 400 IU ◇, 500 IU ◇, 600 IU ◇, 800 IU ◇, 1,000 IU ◇

**INDICATIONS & DOSAGES**
*Note:* RDAs for vitamin E have been converted to α-tocopherol equivalents (α-TE). One α-TE equals 1 mg of D-α tocopherol, or 1.49 IU.

➤ **RDA**
*Healthy adults and children ages 14 to 18:* 15 mg.
*Pregnant women:* 15 mg.
*Breast-feeding women:* 19 mg.
*Children ages 9 to 13:* 11 mg.
*Children ages 4 to 8:* 7 mg.
*Children ages 1 to 3:* 6 mg.
*Infants ages 6 months to 1 year:* 5 mg.
*Neonates and infants younger than age 6 months:* 4 mg.

➤ **Vitamin E deficiency in premature neonates and in patients with impaired fat absorption**
*Adults:* Depending on severity, 60 to 75 IU P.O. daily.
*Children:* 1 IU/kg daily.

**ACTION**
Unknown. Thought to act as an antioxidant and protect RBC membranes against hemolysis.

| Route | Onset | Peak | Duration |
|-------|-------|------|----------|
| P.O. | Unknown | Unknown | Unknown |

**ADVERSE REACTIONS**
None reported with recommended dosages.

**INTERACTIONS**
**Drug-drug.** *Cholestyramine, colestipol, mineral oil, orlistat:* Inhibits GI absorption of oral vitamin E. Separate doses. Use together cautiously.
*Iron:* Vitamin E may reduce hematologic response to iron therapy in children with iron-deficiency anemia. Monitor child's response to iron therapy.
*Oral anticoagulants:* May increase hypoprothrombinemic effects, possibly causing bleeding. Monitor patient closely.
*Vitamin K:* May antagonize effects of vitamin K when large doses of vitamin E are used. Avoid using together.

**EFFECTS ON LAB TEST RESULTS**
None reported.

---

**CONTRAINDICATIONS & CAUTIONS**
No known contraindications.

**NURSING CONSIDERATIONS**
• Monitor patient with liver or gallbladder disease for response to therapy. Adequate bile is essential for vitamin E absorption.
• Water-miscible forms are more completely absorbed in GI tract.
• Requirements increase with rise in dietary polyunsaturated acids.
• **Alert:** Don't give the drug I.V. (may cause death).
• Hypervitaminosis E symptoms include fatigue, weakness, nausea, headache, blurred vision, flatulence, and diarrhea.

**PATIENT TEACHING**
• Tell patient not to crush tablets or open capsules.
• Warn patient against taking megadoses, which can cause thrombophlebitis. Vitamin is fat soluble and may accumulate.
• Tell patient to store in dry, airtight container.

## vitamin K analogue

## phytonadione (vitamin K₁)
Mephyton

*Pregnancy risk category C*

**AVAILABLE FORMS**
*Injection (aqueous colloidal solution):*
2 mg/ml, 10 mg/ml
*Injection (aqueous dispersion):* 2 mg/ml, 10 mg/ml
*Tablets:* 5 mg

**INDICATIONS & DOSAGES**
➤ **RDA**
*Men age 19 and older:* 120 mcg.
*Women age 19 and older, including pregnant and breast-feeding women:* 90 mcg.
*Children ages 14 to 18:* 75 mcg.
*Children ages 9 to 13:* 60 mcg.
*Children ages 4 to 8:* 55 mcg.
*Children ages 1 to 3:* 30 mcg.
*Infants ages 7 months to 1 year:* 2.5 mcg.
*Neonates and infants younger than age 6 months:* 2 mcg.

➤ **Hypoprothrombinemia caused by vitamin K malabsorption, drug therapy, or excessive vitamin A dosage**
*Adults:* Depending on severity, 2.5 to 10 mg P.O., I.M., or S.C., repeated and increased up to 50 mg, if needed.
*Children:* 5 to 10 mg P.O. or parenterally.
*Infants:* 2 mg P.O. or parenterally.
➤ **Hypoprothrombinemia caused by effect of oral anticoagulants**
*Adults:* 2.5 to 10 mg P.O., I.M., or S.C. based on PT/INR, repeated if needed within 12 to 48 hours after oral dose or within 6 to 8 hours after parenteral dose. In emergency, 10 to 50 mg slow I.V. at rate not to exceed 1 mg/minute, repeated q 4 hours, p.r.n.
➤ **To prevent hemorrhagic disease of newborn**
*Neonates:* 0.5 to 1 mg I.M. within 1 hour after birth.
➤ **Hemorrhagic disease of newborn**
*Neonates:* 1 mg S.C. or I.M. Higher doses may be needed if mother has been receiving oral anticoagulants.
➤ **To prevent hypoprothrombinemia related to vitamin K deficiency in long-term parenteral nutrition**
*Adults:* 5 to 10 mg P.O. or I.M. weekly.
*Children:* 2 to 5 mg P.O. or I.M. weekly.
➤ **To prevent hypoprothrombinemia in infants receiving less than 0.1 mg/L vitamin K in breast milk or milk substitutes**
*Infants:* 1 mg I.M. monthly.

**I.V. ADMINISTRATION**
• **Alert:** I.V. use can cause death; use only when other routes of administration aren't feasible.
• Effects of I.V. injection are more rapid but shorter-lived than I.M. or S.C. injections.
• Dilute with normal saline solution for injection, D₅W, or 5% dextrose in normal saline solution for injection.
• Give I.V. by slow infusion over 2 to 3 hours. Don't exceed 1 mg/minute.
• Protect parenteral products from light. Wrap infusion container with aluminum foil or other dark cover.

## ACTION
An antihemorrhagic factor that promotes hepatic formation of active coagulation factors.

| Route | Onset | Peak | Duration |
|-------|-------|------|----------|
| I.V., I.M. | 1-2 hr | Unknown | Unknown |
| P.O., S.C. | 6-12 hr | Unknown | Unknown |

## ADVERSE REACTIONS
**CNS:** dizziness.
**CV:** flushing, transient hypotension after I.V. administration, rapid and weak pulse.
**Skin:** diaphoresis, erythema.
**Other:** *anaphylaxis or anaphylactoid reactions, usually after too-rapid I.V. administration;* pain, swelling, and hematoma at injection site.

## INTERACTIONS
**Drug-drug.** *Anticoagulants:* May cause temporary resistance to prothrombin-depressing anticoagulants, especially when larger doses of phytonadione are used. Monitor closely.
*Cholestyramine, mineral oil:* Inhibits GI absorption of oral vitamin K. Space doses. Use together cautiously.

## EFFECTS ON LAB TEST RESULTS
None reported.

## CONTRAINDICATIONS & CAUTIONS
• Contraindicated in patients hypersensitive to drug.

## NURSING CONSIDERATIONS
• Check brand name labels for administration route restrictions.
• For I.M. administration in adults and older children, give in upper outer quadrant of buttocks; for infants, give in anterolateral aspect of thigh or deltoid region. S.C. route is preferred to avoid hematoma formation.
• Allergic reactions may also occur after I.M. or S.C. use.
• Anticipate order for weekly addition of 5 to 10 mg of phytonadione to total parenteral nutrition solutions.
• Monitor PT or INR to determine dosage effectiveness.
• If severe bleeding occurs, don't delay other measures, such as administration of fresh frozen plasma or whole blood.

• Vitamin K doesn't reverse the anticoagulant effects of heparin.
• *Alert:* Watch for flushing, weakness, tachycardia, and hypotension; condition may progress to shock.
• Phytonadione therapy for hemorrhagic disease in infants causes fewer adverse reactions than other vitamin K analogues.

## PATIENT TEACHING
• Explain purpose of drug.
• Tell patient to avoid hazardous activities if dizziness occurs.
• Inform patient that drug is fat soluble; advise her to take drug only as prescribed to avoid accumulation.
• Teach patient that foods that provide vitamin K include cabbage, cauliflower, kale, spinach, fish, liver, eggs, meats, and dairy products.

---

## sodium fluoride
Fluor-A-Day†, Fluoritab, Fluorodex, Flura, Flura-Drops, Flura-Loz, Karidium, Luride, Luride Lozi-Tabs, Luride-SF Lozi-Tabs, Pediaflor, Pedi-Dent†, Pharmaflur, Pharmaflur df, Pharmaflur 1.1, Phos-Flur

## sodium fluoride, topical
ACT◇, Fluorigard◇, Fluorinse, Gel-Kam, Gel-Tin◇, Karigel, Karigel-N, Luride, Minute-Gel, MouthKote F/R◇, Point-Two, Prevident, Stop Gel◇, Thera-Flur, Thera-Flur-N

*Pregnancy risk category NR*

## AVAILABLE FORMS
**sodium fluoride**
*Drops:* 0.125 mg/drop, 0.25 mg/drop, 0.2 mg/ml, 0.5 mg/ml
*Lozenges:* 1 mg
*Tablets:* 1 mg
*Tablets (chewable):* 0.25 mg, 0.5 mg, 1 mg
**sodium fluoride, topical**
*Gel:* 0.1%, 0.5%, 1.2%, 1.23%
*Gel drops:* 0.5%
*Rinse:* 0.02%◇, 0.04%◇, 0.09%, 0.2%

---

## INDICATIONS & DOSAGES
### ➤ To prevent dental caries
*Adults and children older than age 6:* 5 to 10 ml of rinse or thin ribbon of gel applied to teeth with toothbrush or mouth trays for at least 1 minute h.s.

### *If fluoride ion level in drinking water is below 0.3 parts/million (ppm)*
*Children ages 6 to 16:* 1 mg P.O. daily.
*Children ages 3 to 5:* 0.5 mg P.O. daily.
*Infants and children ages 6 months to 2 years:* 0.25 mg P.O. daily.

### *If fluoride ion level in drinking water is 0.3 to 0.6 ppm*
*Children ages 6 to 16:* 0.5 mg P.O. daily.
*Children ages 3 to 5:* 0.25 mg P.O. daily.
### ➤ Osteoporosis ◆
*Adults:* Up to 60 mg P.O. daily in combination with calcium, vitamin D, or estrogen.

## ACTION
Stabilizes the apatite crystal of bone and teeth. Increases tooth resistance to acid breakdown.

| Route | Onset | Peak | Duration |
|-------|-------|------|----------|
| P.O. | Unknown | 30-60 min | Unknown |

## ADVERSE REACTIONS
**CNS:** headache, weakness.
**EENT:** staining of teeth.
**GI:** gastric distress.
**Other:** hypersensitivity reactions.

## INTERACTIONS
**Drug-drug.** *Aluminum hydroxide, calcium, iron, magnesium:* May decrease absorption. Separate doses.
**Drug-food.** *Dairy products:* Incompatibility may occur as a result of formation of calcium fluoride, which is poorly absorbed. Urge patient not to use together.

## EFFECTS ON LAB TEST RESULTS
None reported.

## CONTRAINDICATIONS & CAUTIONS
• Contraindicated in patients hypersensitive to fluoride and in those whose intake from drinking water exceeds 0.6 ppm.

## NURSING CONSIDERATIONS
• Give oral drops undiluted or mixed with fluids or food. Avoid simultaneous ingestion of dairy products.

• *Alert:* Chronic toxicity (fluorosis) may result from prolonged use of higher-than-recommended doses.

## PATIENT TEACHING
• Tell patient that tablets may be dissolved in mouth, chewed, or swallowed whole.
• Advise patient that topical rinses and gels shouldn't be swallowed by children younger than age 3 or used if water supply is fluoridated. Drug is most effective when used right after brushing teeth and just before bedtime. Tell patient to rinse around and between teeth for 1 minute; then spit out.
• Tell patient not to eat, drink, or rinse mouth for 30 minutes after application.
• Tell patient to dilute drops or rinses in plastic (not glass) containers.
• Advise patient to notify dentist if tooth mottling occurs.
• Instruct patient not to exceed recommended dosage.

# trace elements

## chromium (chromic chloride)
Chroma-Pak, Chromic Chloride

## copper (cupric sulfate)
Cupric Sulfate

## iodine (sodium iodide)
Iodopen

## manganese (manganese chloride, manganese sulfate)

## selenium (selenious acid)
Sele-Pak, Selepen

## zinc (zinc sulfate)
Zinca-Pak

*Pregnancy risk category C*

## AVAILABLE FORMS
**chromium**
*Injection:* 4 mcg/ml, 20 mcg/ml
**copper**
*Injection:* 0.4 mg/ml, 2 mg/ml
**iodine**
*Injection:* 100 mcg/ml

---

**manganese**
*Injection:* 0.1 mg/ml
**selenium**
*Injection:* 40 mcg/ml
**zinc**
*Injection:* 1 mg/ml, 5 mg/ml

## INDICATIONS & DOSAGES
➤ **To prevent individual trace element deficiencies in patients receiving long-term total parenteral nutrition (TPN)**
*chromium*
*Adults:* 10 to 15 mcg I.V. daily.
*Metabolically stable adults with intestinal fluid loss:* 20 mcg I.V. daily.
*Children:* 0.14 to 0.2 mcg/kg I.V. daily.
*copper*
*Adults:* 0.5 to 1.5 mg I.V. daily.
*Children:* 20 mcg/kg I.V. daily.
*iodine*
*Adults:* 1 to 2 mcg/kg I.V. daily.
*Pregnant and lactating women, children:* 2 to 3 mcg/kg I.V. daily.
*manganese*
*Adults:* 0.15 to 0.8 mg I.V. daily.
*Children:* 2 to 10 mcg/kg I.V. daily.
*selenium*
*Adults:* 20 to 40 mcg I.V. daily.
*Children:* 3 mcg/kg I.V. daily.
*zinc*
*Adults:* 2.5 to 4 mg I.V. daily. Add 2 mg daily for acute catabolic states.
*Full-term infants and children younger than age 5:* 100 mcg/kg I.V. daily.
*Premature infants weighing up to 3 kg (3.3 to 7 lb):* 300 mcg/kg I.V. daily.

## I.V. ADMINISTRATION
● Don't give undiluted because of potential for phlebitis.
● Cautiously infuse diluted solution through patent I.V. line over prescribed duration.

## ACTION
Participate in synthesis and stabilization of proteins and nucleic acids in subcellular and membrane transport systems.

| Route | Onset | Peak | Duration |
|-------|-------|------|----------|
| I.V. | Immediate | Immediate | Unknown |

## ADVERSE REACTIONS
**Other:** Hypersensitivity reactions to iodides.

## INTERACTIONS
None significant.

## EFFECTS ON LAB TEST RESULTS
None reported.

## CONTRAINDICATIONS & CAUTIONS
● Contraindicated in patients hypersensitive to iodine.

## NURSING CONSIDERATIONS
● Check levels of trace elements in patients who have received TPN for 2 months or longer. Give supplement, if ordered. Report low levels of these elements.
● Normal levels are 1 to 5 mcg/L chromium; 80 to 163 mcg/dl copper; 0.5 to 1.5 mcg/dl iodine; 6 to 12 mcg/dl manganese; 0.1 to 0.19 mcg/ml selenium; and 88 to 112 mcg/dl zinc.
● Solutions of trace elements are compounded by pharmacist for addition to TPN solutions according to various formulas.

## PATIENT TEACHING
● Explain need for zinc administration to patient and family.
● Tell patient to report signs of hypersensitivity promptly.
● Inform patient and family that trace elements are normally received from dietary intake and that, when patient begins eating well, supplements won't be needed.

---

amino acid infusions, crystalline
amino acid infusions in dextrose
amino acid infusions with
  electrolytes
amino acid infusions with
  electrolytes in dextrose
amino acid infusions for hepatic
  failure
amino acid infusions for high
  metabolic stress
amino acid infusions for renal
  failure
dextrose
fat emulsions

**COMBINATION PRODUCTS**
Various products contain dextrose or invert sugar in combination with electrolytes.

---

## amino acid infusions, crystalline
Aminosyn, Aminosyn II, Aminosyn-PF, Aminosyn-RF, FreAmine III, Novamine, Travasol, TrophAmine

## amino acid infusions in dextrose
Aminosyn II with Dextrose, Travasol in Dextrose

## amino acid infusions with electrolytes
Aminosyn with Electrolytes, Aminosyn II with Electrolytes, FreAmine III with Electrolytes, ProcalAmine with Electrolytes, Travasol with Electrolytes

## amino acid infusions with electrolytes in dextrose
Aminosyn II with Electrolytes in Dextrose, Travasol with Electrolytes in Dextrose

## amino acid infusions for hepatic failure
HepatAmine

## amino acid infusions for high metabolic stress
Aminosyn-HBC, BranchAmin, FreAmine HBC

## amino acid infusions for renal failure
Aminess, Aminosyn-RF, NephrAmine, RenAmin

*Pregnancy risk category C*

**AVAILABLE FORMS**
*Injection:* 250 ml, 500 ml, 1,000 ml, 2,000 ml containing amino acids in various concentrations
**amino acid infusions, crystalline**
*Aminosyn:* 3.5%, 5%, 7%, 8.5%, 10%
*Aminosyn II:* 3.5%, 5%, 7%, 8.5%, 10%, 15%
*Aminosyn-PF:* 7%, 10%
*Aminosyn-RF:* 5.2%
*FreAmine III:* 8.5%, 10%
*Novamine:* 11.4%, 15%
*Travasol:* 5.5%, 8.5%, 10%
*TrophAmine:* 6%, 10%
**amino acid infusions in dextrose**
*Aminosyn II:* 3.5% in 5% dextrose, 3.5% in 25% dextrose, 4.25% in 10% dextrose, 4.25% in 20% dextrose, 4.25% in 25% dextrose, 5% in 25% dextrose
*Travasol:* 2.75% in 5% dextrose, 2.75% in 10% dextrose, 2.75% in 25% dextrose, 4.25% in 5% dextrose, 4.25% in 10% dextrose, 4.25% in 25% dextrose
**amino acid infusions with electrolytes**
*Aminosyn:* 3.5%, 7%, 8.5%
*Aminosyn II:* 3.5%, 7%, 8.5%, 10%
*FreAmine III:* 3%, 8.5%
*ProcalAmine:* 3%
*Travasol:* 3.5%, 5.5%, 8.5%
**amino acid infusions with electrolytes in dextrose**
*Aminosyn II:* 3.5% with electrolytes in 5% dextrose, 3.5% with electrolytes in 25% dextrose, 4.25% with electrolytes in 10% dextrose, 4.25% with electrolytes in 20% dextrose, 4.25% with electrolytes in 25% dextrose

---

*Travasol:* 2.75% with electrolytes in 5%
dextrose, 2.75% with electrolytes in 10%
dextrose, 4.25% with electrolytes in 5%
dextrose, 4.25% with electrolytes in 10%
dextrose, 4.25% with electrolytes in 25%
dextrose
**amino acid infusions for hepatic failure**
*HepatAmine:* 8%
**amino acid infusions for high metabolic
stress**
*Aminosyn-HBC:* 7%
*BranchAmin:* 4%
*FreAmine HBC:* 6.9%
**amino acid infusions for renal failure**
*Aminess:* 5.2%
*Aminosyn-RF:* 5.2%
*NephrAmine:* 5.4%
*RenAmin:* 6.5%

**INDICATIONS & DOSAGES**
➤ **Total parenteral nutrition (TPN) in
patients who can't or won't eat**
*Adults:* 1 to 1.7 g/kg I.V. daily.
*Children weighing more than 10 kg
(22 lb):* 20 to 25 g I.V. daily for first
10 kg; then 1 to 1.25 g/kg I.V. daily for
each kg over 10 kg.
*Children weighing less than 10 kg:* 2 to
4 g/kg I.V. daily.
➤ **Nutritional support in patients with
cirrhosis, hepatitis, or hepatic encephalopathy**
*Adults:* 80 to 120 g of amino acids (12 to
18 g of nitrogen) I.V. daily of formulation
for hepatic failure.
➤ **Nutritional support in patients with
high metabolic stress**
*Adults:* 1.5 g/kg I.V. daily of formulation
for high metabolic stress.
➤ **Nutritional support in patients with
renal failure**
*Adults:* 0.6 to 0.8 g/kg I.V. daily of formulation for renal failure.
*Adjust-a-dose:* Patients receiving dialysis
may need 1 to 1.2 g/kg daily.

**I.V. ADMINISTRATION**
• Control infusion rate carefully with infusion pump. If infusion rate falls behind,
notify prescriber; don't increase rate to
catch up.
• *Alert:* Infuse amino acids only in I.V. fluids or TPN solution.
• Limit peripheral infusions to 2.5%
amino acids and dextrose 10%.

• Check infusion site frequently for erythema, inflammation, irritation, tissue
sloughing, necrosis, and phlebitis.

**ACTION**
Provides a substrate for protein synthesis
or increases conservation of existing body
protein.

| Route | Onset | Peak | Duration |
|---|---|---|---|
| I.V. | Immediate | Immediate | Unknown |

**ADVERSE REACTIONS**
**CNS:** fever.
**CV:** thrombophlebitis, edema, thrombosis,
flushing.
**GI:** nausea.
**GU:** glycosuria, osmotic diuresis.
**Metabolic:** *rebound hypoglycemia when
long-term infusions are abruptly stopped,*
hyperglycemia, metabolic acidosis, alkalosis, hypophosphatemia, *hyperosmolar hyperglycemic nonketotic syndrome,* hyperammonemia, electrolyte imbalances,
weight gain.
**Musculoskeletal:** osteoporosis.
**Other:** hypersensitivity reactions, tissue
sloughing at infusion site from extravasation, *catheter sepsis.*

**INTERACTIONS**
**Drug-drug.** *Tetracycline:* May reduce
protein-sparing effects of infused amino
acids because of its antianabolic activity.
Monitor patient.

**EFFECTS ON LAB TEST RESULTS**
• May increase ammonia and liver enzyme
levels. May decrease phosphate, magnesium, and potassium levels. May increase
or decrease glucose level.

**CONTRAINDICATIONS & CAUTIONS**
• Contraindicated in patients with anuria
and in those with inborn errors of amino
acid metabolism, such as maple syrup
urine disease and isovaleric acidemia.
• Standard amino acid formulations are
contraindicated in patients with severe renal failure or hepatic disease.
• Use with extreme caution in children
and neonates.
• Use cautiously in patients with renal or
hepatic impairment or failure or diabetes.

• Use cautiously in patients with cardiac disease or insufficiency; drug may cause circulatory overload.

## NURSING CONSIDERATIONS

• Patients with fluid restriction may tolerate only 1 to 2 L.
• When giving drug to diabetic patients, insulin requirements may be increased.
• Some products contain sulfites. Check contents before giving to patients with sulfite sensitivity.
• Obtain baseline electrolyte, glucose, BUN, calcium, and phosphorus levels before therapy; monitor these levels periodically throughout therapy.
• Safe and effective use of parenteral nutrition requires knowledge of nutrition and clinical expertise in recognizing and treating complications. Frequent evaluations of patient and laboratory studies are needed.
• Check fractional urine for glycosuria every 6 hours initially, then every 12 to 24 hours in stable patients. Abrupt onset of glycosuria may be an early sign of impending sepsis.
• Assess body temperature every 4 hours; elevation may indicate sepsis or infection.
• Watch for extraordinary electrolyte losses that may occur during nasogastric suction, vomiting, diarrhea, or drainage from GI fistula.
• If patient has chills, fever, or other signs of sepsis, replace I.V. tubing and bottle and send tubing and bottle to the laboratory to be cultured.
• *Alert:* Don't confuse Aminosyn with Amikacin.

## PATIENT TEACHING

• Explain need for supplement to patient and family, and answer any questions.
• Tell patient to report adverse reactions promptly.

---

## dextrose (d-glucose)

*Pregnancy risk category C*

## AVAILABLE FORMS

*Injection:* 3-ml ampule (10%); 10 ml (25%); 25 ml (5%); 50 ml (5% and 50% available in vial, ampule, and Bristoject); 70-ml pin-top vial (70% for additive use only); 100 ml (5%); 150 ml (5%); 250 ml (5%, 10%); 500 ml (5%, 10%, 20%, 30%, 40%, 50%, 60%, 70%); 650 ml (38.5%); 1,000 ml (2.5%, 5%, 10%, 20%, 30%, 40%, 50%, 60%, 70%); 2,000 ml (50%, 70%)

## INDICATIONS & DOSAGES

➤ **Fluid replacement and caloric supplementation in patients who can't maintain adequate oral intake or are restricted from doing so**
*Adults and children:* Dosage depends on fluid and caloric requirements. Peripheral I.V. infusion of 2.5%, 5%, or 10% solution or central I.V. infusion of 20% solution is used for minimal fluid needs. A 10% to 25% solution is used to treat acute hypoglycemia in neonate or older infant (2 ml/kg). A 50% solution is used to treat insulin-induced hypoglycemia (20 to 50 ml). Solutions of 10%, 20%, 30%, 40%, 50%, 60%, and 70% are diluted in admixtures, usually amino acid solutions, for total parenteral nutrition (TPN) given through a central vein.

## I.V. ADMINISTRATION

• Use infusion pump when giving with amino acids for TPN. Maximum rate is 0.8 g/kg/hour.
• *Alert:* Never infuse concentrated solutions rapidly. Rapid infusion may cause hyperglycemia and fluid shift.
• *Alert:* Use central veins to infuse dextrose solutions with concentrations above 10%.
• Check injection site frequently for irritation, tissue sloughing, necrosis, and phlebitis.

## ACTION

A simple water-soluble sugar that minimizes glyconeogenesis and promotes anabolism in patients whose oral caloric intake is limited.

| Route | Onset | Peak | Duration |
|-------|-------|------|----------|
| I.V. | Immediate | Immediate | Unknown |

## ADVERSE REACTIONS

**CNS:** fever, confusion, *unconsciousness in hyperosmolar hyperglycemic nonketotic syndrome.*

---

**CV:** *worsened hypertension and heart failure with fluid overload in susceptible patients;* phlebitis, venous sclerosis, and tissue necrosis with prolonged or concentrated infusions, especially when given peripherally.
**GU:** glycosuria, osmotic diuresis.
**Metabolic:** hyperglycemia, dehydration, and hyperosmolarity with rapid infusion of concentrated solution or prolonged infusion; hypoglycemia from rebound hyperinsulinemia with rapid termination of long-term infusions; hypervolemia; hypovolemia.
**Respiratory:** *pulmonary edema.*
**Skin:** sloughing and tissue necrosis if extravasation occurs with concentrated solutions.

## INTERACTIONS
**Drug-drug.** *Corticosteroids:* May cause salt and water retention and increase potassium excretion. Monitor glucose, sodium, and potassium levels.

## EFFECTS ON LAB TEST RESULTS
• May increase or decrease glucose level.

## CONTRAINDICATIONS & CAUTIONS
• Contraindicated in patients in diabetic coma while glucose level remains excessively high. Use of concentrated solutions contraindicated in patients with intracranial or intraspinal hemorrhage; in dehydrated patients with delirium tremens; and in patients with severe dehydration, anuria, diabetic coma, or glucose-galactose malabsorption syndrome. Also contraindicated in patients with known allergy to corn or corn products.
• Use cautiously in patients with cardiac or pulmonary disease, hypertension, renal insufficiency, urinary obstruction, or hypovolemia.

## NURSING CONSIDERATIONS
• **Alert:** Never stop hypertonic solutions abruptly. Have dextrose 10% in water available to treat hypoglycemia if rebound hyperinsulinemia occurs.
• Don't give concentrated solutions I.M. or S.C.
• Monitor glucose level carefully. Prolonged therapy with $D_5W$ can cause reduction of pancreatic insulin production and secretion.
• Check vital signs frequently. Report adverse reactions promptly.
• Monitor fluid intake and output and weight carefully. Watch closely for signs and symptoms of fluid overload.
• Monitor patient for signs of mental confusion.

## PATIENT TEACHING
• Explain need for supplement to patient and family, and answer any questions.
• Tell patient to report adverse reactions promptly.

# fat emulsions
Intralipid 10%, Intralipid 20%, Liposyn II 10%, Liposyn II 20%, Liposyn III 10%, Liposyn III 20%

*Pregnancy risk category C*

## AVAILABLE FORMS
*Injection:* 50 ml (10%, 20%), 100 ml (10%, 20%), 200 ml (10%, 20%), 250 ml (10%, 20%), 500 ml (10%, 20%)

## INDICATIONS & DOSAGES
➤ **Adjunct to total parenteral nutrition (TPN) to provide adequate source of calories**
*Adults:* 1 ml/minute I.V. for 15 to 30 minutes (10% emulsion) or 0.5 ml/minute I.V. for 15 to 30 minutes (20% emulsion). If no adverse reactions occur, increase rate to deliver 250 ml (20% Liposyn) or 500 ml (10% Liposyn; 10% or 20% Intralipid) over the first day; total daily dose shouldn't exceed 2.5 g/kg (10%) or 3 g/kg (20%).
*Children:* 0.1 ml/minute for 10 to 15 minutes (10% emulsion) or 0.05 ml/minute I.V. for 10 to 15 minutes (20% emulsion). If no adverse reactions occur, increase rate to deliver 1 g/kg over 4 hours; daily dose shouldn't exceed 3 g/kg. Equals up to 60% of daily caloric intake; protein-carbohydrate TPN should supply remaining 40%.
➤ **Fatty acid deficiency**
*Adults and children:* 8% to 10% of total caloric intake I.V.

➤ **To prevent fatty acid deficiency**
*Adults:* 500 ml Liposyn (10% emulsion)
I.V. twice weekly. Infuse initially at rate of
1 ml/minute for 30 minutes. Rate
shouldn't exceed 500 ml over 4 to 6 hours.
*Children:* 5 to 10 ml/kg Liposyn (10%
emulsion) I.V. daily. Infuse initially at rate
of 0.1 ml/minute for 30 minutes. Rate
shouldn't exceed 100 ml/hour.

## I.V. ADMINISTRATION
● *Alert:* Use an infusion pump to regulate
rate. Rapid infusion may cause fluid or fat
overloading.
● Don't use fat emulsion if it separates or
becomes oily.
● Drug may be mixed with amino acid solution, dextrose, electrolytes, and vitamins
in same I.V. container. Check with pharmacist for acceptable proportions and
compatibility information.
● Because lipids support bacterial growth,
change all I.V. tubing before each infusion. Check infusion site daily.
● Refrigeration of fat emulsion isn't needed unless it's part of an admixture.

## ACTION
Provides neutral triglycerides, predominantly unsaturated fatty acids; acts as a
source of calories and prevents fatty acid
deficiency. When substituted for dextrose
as a source of calories, fat emulsions decrease carbon dioxide production.

| Route | Onset | Peak | Duration |
|-------|-------|------|----------|
| I.V. | Immediate | Immediate | Unknown |

## ADVERSE REACTIONS
**Early reactions**
**CNS:** headache, sleepiness, dizziness,
fever.
**CV:** chest and back pains, flushing.
**EENT:** pressure over eyes.
**GI:** nausea, vomiting.
**Hematologic:** hypercoagulability.
**Respiratory:** dyspnea, cyanosis.
**Skin:** diaphoresis.
**Other:** hypersensitivity reactions, irrita-
tion at infusion site.
**Delayed reactions**
**CNS:** fever, *focal seizures.*
**Hematologic:** *thrombocytopenia, leuko-
penia,* leukocytosis.

**Hepatic:** hepatomegaly.
**Other:** splenomegaly.

## INTERACTIONS
None significant.

## EFFECTS ON LAB TEST RESULTS
● May increase lipid, bilirubin, and liver
enzyme levels.
● May decrease platelet count. May increase or decrease WBC count.

## CONTRAINDICATIONS & CAUTIONS
● Contraindicated in patients with severe
egg allergies, hyperlipidemia, lipid
nephrosis, or acute pancreatitis with hyperlipidemia.
● Use cautiously in patients with severe
hepatic or pulmonary disease, anemia, or
blood coagulation disorders including
thrombocytopenia, and in patients at risk
for fat embolism.
● Use cautiously in jaundiced or premature infants.

## NURSING CONSIDERATIONS
● Watch for adverse reactions, especially
during first half of infusion.
● Monitor lipid levels closely when patient
is receiving fat emulsion therapy. Lipemia
must clear between doses.
● Monitor hepatic function carefully in
long-term therapy.
● Check platelet count frequently in
neonates receiving fat emulsions I.V.
● Carefully monitor triglyceride levels and
free fatty acids in infants, especially premature and jaundiced infants.
● Available products differ mainly by their
fatty acid components.

## PATIENT TEACHING
● Explain need for fat emulsion therapy,
and answer any questions.
● Tell patient to report adverse reactions
promptly.

**allopurinol**
**colchicine**
**probenecid**
**sulfinpyrazone**

### COMBINATION PRODUCTS
COLBENEMID, PROBEN-C, PROBENECID
WITH COLCHICINE: probenecid 500 mg
and colchicine 0.5 mg.

---

## allopurinol
Aloprim, Apo-Allopurinol†,
Capurate‡, Zyloprim

*Pregnancy risk category C*

### AVAILABLE FORMS
*Capsules:* 100 mg‡, 300 mg‡
*Injection:* 500 mg/30-ml vial
*Tablets (scored):* 100 mg, 200 mg‡,
300 mg

### INDICATIONS & DOSAGES
➤ **Gout or hyperuricemia**
Dosage varies with severity of disease;
can be given as single dose or divided, but
doses greater than 300 mg should be divided.
*Adults:* Mild gout, 200 to 300 mg P.O.
daily; severe gout with large tophi, 400 to
600 mg P.O. daily. Maximum 800 mg
daily.
➤ **Hyperuricemia caused by malig-**
**nancies**
*Adults:* 200 to 400 mg/m² daily I.V. as a
single infusion or in equally divided doses
q 6, 8, or 12 hours. Maximum 600 mg daily.
*Children:* Initially, 200 mg/m² daily I.V. as
single infusion or in equally divided doses
q 6, 8, or 12 hours. Then titrate according
to uric acid levels. For children ages 6 to
10, give 300 mg P.O. daily or divided
t.i.d.; for children younger than age 6, give
50 mg P.O. t.i.d.
➤ **To prevent acute gout attacks**
*Adults:* 100 mg P.O. daily; increase at
weekly intervals by 100 mg without ex-

ceeding maximum dose (800 mg) until
uric acid falls to 6 mg/dl or less.
➤ **To prevent uric acid nephropathy**
**during cancer chemotherapy**
*Adults:* 600 to 800 mg P.O. daily for 2 to
3 days, with high fluid intake.
➤ **Recurrent calcium oxalate calculi**
*Adults:* 200 to 300 mg P.O. daily in single
or divided doses.
*Adjust-a-dose:* For renally impaired patients, 200 mg P.O. or I.V. daily if creatinine clearance is 10 to 20 ml/minute;
100 mg P.O. or I.V. daily if clearance is
less than 10 ml/minute; and 100 mg P.O.
or I.V. at extended intervals if clearance is
less than 3 ml/minute.

### I.V. ADMINISTRATION
• Dissolve contents of each 30-ml vial in
25 ml of sterile water for injection. Dilute
solution to desired concentration (no
greater than 6 mg/ml) with normal saline
solution for injection or $D_5W$. Don't use
solutions containing sodium bicarbonate.
• Refer to package insert for drugs that
are incompatible with allopurinol in solution.
• Store solution at 68° to 77° F (20° to
25° C) and use within 10 hours. Don't use
if particulates appear or discoloration occurs.

### ACTION
Reduces uric acid production by inhibiting
xanthine oxidase.

| Route | Onset | Peak | Duration |
|---|---|---|---|
| P.O. | Unknown | 30-120 hr | 1-2 wk |
| I.V. | Unknown | 30 min | Unknown |

### ADVERSE REACTIONS
**CNS:** fever, drowsiness, headache, paresthesia, peripheral neuropathy, neuritis.
**CV:** hypersensitivity vasculitis, necrotizing angiitis.
**EENT:** epistaxis.
**GI:** nausea, vomiting, diarrhea, abdominal
pain, gastritis, taste loss or perversion,
dyspepsia.

---

**GU:** *renal failure,* uremia.
**Hematologic:** *agranulocytosis,* anemia, *aplastic anemia, thrombocytopenia, leukopenia,* leukocytosis, eosinophilia.
**Hepatic:** *hepatitis, hepatic necrosis,* hepatomegaly, cholestatic jaundice.
**Musculoskeletal:** arthralgia, myopathy.
**Skin:** *rash;* exfoliative, urticarial, and purpuric lesions; *erythema multiforme;* severe furunculosis of nose; ichthyosis; alopecia; *toxic epidermal necrolysis.*
**Other:** ecchymoses, chills.

### INTERACTIONS
**Drug-drug.** *Amoxicillin, ampicillin:* May increase possibility of rash. Avoid using together.
*Anticoagulants:* May increase anticoagulant effect. Dosage may need to be adjusted.
*Antineoplastics:* May increase potential for bone marrow suppression. Monitor patient carefully.
*Chlorpropamide:* May increase hypoglycemic effect. Avoid using together.
*Diazoxide, diuretics, mecamylamine, pyrazinamide:* May increase uric acid level. Adjust dosage of allopurinol.
*Ethacrynic acid, thiazide diuretics:* May increase risk of allopurinol toxicity. Reduce dosage of allopurinol, and monitor renal function closely.
*Uricosurics:* May have additive effect. May be used to therapeutic advantage.
*Urine-acidifying drugs (ammonium chloride, ascorbic acid, potassium or sodium phosphate):* May increase possibility of kidney stone formation. Monitor patient carefully.
*Xanthines:* May increase theophylline level. Adjust dosage of theophylline, as needed.
**Drug-lifestyle.** *Alcohol use:* May increase uric acid level. Discourage use together.

### EFFECTS ON LAB TEST RESULTS
• May increase alkaline phosphatase, AST, and ALT levels.
• May increase eosinophil count. May decrease hemoglobin and granulocyte and platelet counts. May increase or decrease WBC count.

### CONTRAINDICATIONS & CAUTIONS
• Contraindicated in patients hypersensitive to drug and in those with idiopathic hemochromatosis.

### NURSING CONSIDERATIONS
• Monitor uric acid level to evaluate drug's effectiveness.
• Monitor fluid intake and output; daily urine output of at least 2 L and maintenance of neutral or slightly alkaline urine are desirable.
• Periodically monitor CBC and hepatic and renal function, especially at start of therapy.
• Optimal benefits may need 2 to 6 weeks of therapy. Because acute gout attacks may occur during this time, concurrent use of colchicine may be prescribed prophylactically.
• Don't restart drug in patients who have a severe reaction.
• *Alert:* Don't confuse Zyloprim with ZORprin.

### PATIENT TEACHING
• To minimize GI adverse reactions, tell patient to take drug with or immediately after meals.
• Encourage patient to drink plenty of fluids while taking drug unless otherwise contraindicated.
• Drug may cause drowsiness; tell patient not to drive or perform hazardous tasks requiring mental alertness until CNS effects of drug are known.
• If patient is taking allopurinol for recurrent calcium oxalate stones, advise him also to reduce his dietary intake of animal protein, sodium, refined sugars, oxalate-rich foods, and calcium.
• Tell patient to stop drug at first sign of rash, which may precede severe hypersensitivity or other adverse reactions. Rash is more common in patients taking diuretics and in those with renal disorders. Tell patient to report all adverse reactions.
• Advise patient to avoid alcohol during therapy.
• Teach patient importance of continuing drug even if asymptomatic.

# colchicine
Colgout‡

*Pregnancy risk category C (P.O.); D (I.V.)*

## AVAILABLE FORMS
*Injection:* 1 mg (⅟₆₀ grain)/2 ml
*Tablets:* 0.5 mg (⅟₁₂₀ grain), 0.6 mg (⅟₁₀₀ grain) as sugar-coated granules

## INDICATIONS & DOSAGES
➤ **To prevent acute gout attacks as prophylactic or maintenance therapy**
*Adults:* 0.5 or 0.6 mg P.O. daily. Patients who normally have one attack per year or fewer should receive drug only 3 to 4 days weekly; patients who have more than one attack per year should receive drug daily. In severe cases, 1 to 1.8 mg P.O. daily.
➤ **To prevent gout attacks in patients undergoing surgery**
*Adults:* 0.5 to 0.6 mg P.O. t.i.d. 3 days before and 3 days after surgery.
➤ **Acute gout, acute gouty arthritis**
*Adults:* Initially, 0.5 to 1.2 mg P.O.; then 0.5 to 1.2 mg q 1 to 2 hours until pain is relieved; nausea, vomiting, or diarrhea ensues; or maximum dose of 8 mg is reached. Wait 3 days before a second oral course to reduce cumulative toxicity. Or, 2 mg I.V.; then 0.5 mg I.V. q 6 hours if needed. (Some prescribers prefer to give a single I.V. injection of 3 mg.) Total I.V. dose over 24 hours (one course of treatment) shouldn't exceed 4 mg. Give no further colchicine (I.V. or P.O.) for at least 7 days.
*Adjust-a-dose:* If creatinine clearance is 10 to 50 ml/minute, reduce dose by 50%. Don't use in patients with creatinine clearance below 10 ml/minute. In patients with hepatic impairment, reduce dose by 50%.

## I.V. ADMINISTRATION
• Don't dilute colchicine injection with D₅W injection or other fluids that might change pH of colchicine solution.
• Give by slow I.V. push over 2 to 5 minutes.
• If lower concentration of colchicine injection is needed, dilute with normal saline solution or sterile water for injec-
tion and give over 2 to 5 minutes by direct injection.
• Preferably, inject into the tubing of a free-flowing I.V. solution.
• Don't inject if diluted solution becomes turbid.
• Monitor patient for extravasation because colchicine irritates tissues.

## ACTION
Unknown. As an antigout drug, probably decreases WBC motility, phagocytosis, and lactic acid production, decreasing urate crystal deposits and reducing inflammation. As an antiosteolytic, probably inhibits mitosis of osteoprogenitor cells and decreases osteoclast activity.

| Route | Onset | Peak | Duration |
|-------|-------|------|----------|
| P.O. | 12 hr | 30-120 min | Unknown |
| I.V. | 6-12 hr | Unknown | Unknown |

## ADVERSE REACTIONS
**CNS:** peripheral neuritis.
**GI:** *nausea, vomiting, abdominal pain, diarrhea.*
**GU:** reversible azoospermia.
**Hematologic:** *aplastic anemia, thrombocytopenia, agranulocytosis with long-term use,* nonthrombocytopenic purpura.
**Musculoskeletal:** myopathy.
**Skin:** alopecia, urticaria, dermatitis.
**Other:** severe local irritation if extravasation occurs, hypersensitivity reactions.

## INTERACTIONS
**Drug-drug.** *Vitamin B₁₂:* Impairs absorption of oral vitamin B₁₂. Avoid using together.
**Drug-lifestyle.** *Alcohol use:* May impair efficacy of colchicine prophylaxis. Discourage use together.

## EFFECTS ON LAB TEST RESULTS
• May increase alkaline phosphatase, AST, and ALT levels. May decrease carotene and cholesterol levels.
• May decrease hemoglobin and platelet and granulocyte counts.
• May cause false-positive urine RBC or urine hemoglobin test results.

## CONTRAINDICATIONS & CAUTIONS
• Contraindicated in patients hypersensitive to drug and in those with blood

dyscrasias, serious CV disease, renal disease, or GI disorders.
• Use cautiously in elderly or debilitated patients and in those with early signs of CV, renal, or GI disease.

## NURSING CONSIDERATIONS
• Obtain baseline laboratory test results, including CBC, before therapy and periodically throughout therapy.
• *Alert:* Don't give I.M. or S.C.; severe local irritation occurs.
• As maintenance therapy, give drug with meals to reduce GI effects. Drug may be used with uricosurics.
• Monitor fluid intake and output; keep output at 2 L daily.
• *Alert:* After full course of I.V. colchicine (4 mg), don't give colchicine by any route for at least 7 days. Colchicine is a toxic drug and death has resulted from overdose.
• First sign of acute overdose may be GI symptoms, followed by vascular damage, muscle weakness, and ascending paralysis. Delirium and seizures may occur without patient losing consciousness.
• Stop drug as soon as gout pain is relieved or at first sign of GI symptoms.

## PATIENT TEACHING
• Teach patient how to take drug, and tell him to drink extra fluids.
• Tell patient to report adverse reactions, especially signs of acute overdose (nausea, vomiting, abdominal pain, diarrhea, unusual bleeding, bruising, tiredness, weakness, numbness, or tingling).
• Advise patient to avoid using alcohol while taking drug.
• Tell patient with gout to limit intake of foods high in purine, such as anchovies, liver, sardines, kidneys, sweetbreads, peas, and lentils.

---

**probenecid**
Benuryl†

*Pregnancy risk category B*

---

## AVAILABLE FORMS
*Tablets:* 500 mg

## INDICATIONS & DOSAGES
➤ **Adjunct to penicillin therapy**
*Adults and children weighing more than 50 kg (111 lb):* 500 mg P.O. q.i.d.
*Children ages 2 to 14 or weighing 50 kg or less:* Initially, 25 mg/kg P.O.; then 40 mg/kg/day in divided doses q.i.d.
➤ **Gonorrhea**
*Adults:* Give 3.5 g ampicillin or 3 g amoxicillin P.O. along with 1 g probenecid P.O. Or, 1 g probenecid P.O. 30 minutes before 4.8 million units of aqueous penicillin G procaine I.M., injected at two different sites.
➤ **Hyperuricemia of gout, gouty arthritis**
*Adults:* 250 mg P.O. b.i.d. for first week; then 500 mg b.i.d., to maximum of 2 to 3 g daily. Review maintenance dose q 6 months and reduce by increments of 500 mg, if indicated.

## ACTION
Blocks renal tubular reabsorption of uric acid, increasing excretion, and inhibits active renal tubular secretion of many weak organic acids, such as penicillins and cephalosporins.

| Route | Onset | Peak | Duration |
|-------|-------|------|----------|
| P.O. | Unknown | 2-4 hr | Unknown |

## ADVERSE REACTIONS
**CNS:** fever, *headache,* dizziness.
**CV:** flushing.
**GI:** anorexia, nausea, vomiting, sore gums.
**GU:** urinary frequency, renal colic, nephrotic syndrome, costovertebral pain.
**Hematologic:** *hemolytic anemia,* anemia, *aplastic anemia.*
**Hepatic:** *hepatic necrosis.*
**Skin:** dermatitis, pruritus.
**Other:** worsening of gout, hypersensitivity reactions including *anaphylaxis.*

## INTERACTIONS
**Drug-drug.** *Acyclovir, cephalosporins, clofibrate, dapsone, ketamine, lorazepam, meclofenamate, penicillin, rifampin, sulfonamides, thiopental:* May increase levels of these drugs. Use together cautiously.
*Allopurinol:* May increase uric acid-lowering effects. May be used to therapeutic advantage.

*Methotrexate:* May impair excretion of methotrexate, causing increased level, effects, and toxicity of methotrexate. Monitor methotrexate level closely and adjust dosage accordingly.
*Nitrofurantoin:* May increase toxicity and reduce effectiveness of nitrofurantoin. Reduce probenecid dose.
*NSAIDs:* May increase NSAID toxicity. Avoid using together.
*Salicylates:* May inhibit uricosuric effect of probenecid, causing urate retention. Avoid using together.
*Sulfonylureas:* May increase hypoglycemic effect. Monitor glucose level closely. Dosage may need to be adjusted.
*Zidovudine:* May increase zidovudine level and toxicity symptoms. Monitor patient.
**Drug-lifestyle.** *Alcohol use:* May increase urate level. Discourage use together.

**EFFECTS ON LAB TEST RESULTS**
● May falsely elevate theophylline level.
● May decrease hemoglobin.

**CONTRAINDICATIONS & CAUTIONS**
● Contraindicated in patients hypersensitive to drug and in those with uric acid kidney stones or blood dyscrasias; also contraindicated in patients with an acute gout attack and in children younger than age 2.
● Use cautiously in patients with peptic ulcer or renal impairment.
● Use cautiously in patients with sulfa allergy because probenecid is a sulfonamide derivative.

**NURSING CONSIDERATIONS**
● To minimize GI distress, give drug with milk, food, or antacids. Continued disturbances might indicate need to reduce dosage.
● Force fluids to maintain minimum daily output of 2 to 3 L. Alkalinize urine with sodium bicarbonate or potassium citrate. These measures prevent hematuria, renal colic, urate stone development, and costovertebral pain.
● Don't start treating gout until acute attack subsides. Drug doesn't contain an analgesic or anti-inflammatory, and it's of no value during acute gout attacks.
● Monitor BUN and renal function test results periodically in long-term therapy.

● Drug is suitable for long-term use; no cumulative effects or tolerance have been reported.
● Drug is ineffective in patients with chronic renal insufficiency (glomerular filtration rate below 30 ml/minute).
● Drug may increase frequency, severity, and length of acute gout attacks during first 6 to 12 months of therapy. Prophylactic colchicine or another anti-inflammatory may be used during first 3 to 6 months.
● **Alert:** Don't confuse probenecid with Procanbid.

**PATIENT TEACHING**
● Instruct patient with gout to take drug regularly to prevent recurrence.
● Tell patient to visit prescriber regularly so that uric acid can be monitored and dosage adjusted, if needed. Lifelong therapy may be needed in patients with hyperuricemia.
● Advise patient with gout to avoid all drugs that contain aspirin, which may precipitate gout. Acetaminophen may be used for pain.
● Instruct patient to drink at least 6 to 8 glasses of water per day.
● Urge patient with gout to avoid alcohol; it increases urate level.
● Tell patient with gout to limit intake of foods high in purine, such as anchovies, liver, sardines, kidneys, sweetbreads, peas, and lentils. Also tell him to identify and avoid other foods that may trigger gout attacks.
● Instruct patient to take all medicine as prescribed when given with penicillin.

**sulfinpyrazone**
Anturan†, Anturane

*Pregnancy risk category NR*

**AVAILABLE FORMS**
*Capsules:* 200 mg
*Tablets:* 100 mg

**INDICATIONS & DOSAGES**
➤ **Intermittent or chronic gouty arthritis**
*Adults:* 200 to 400 mg P.O. b.i.d. first week; then 200 mg P.O. b.i.d. Maximum dose is 800 mg daily.

➤ **To decrease the incidence of sudden cardiac death 1 to 6 months after MI** ♦
*Adults:* 300 mg P.O. q.i.d.

## ACTION
A pyrazolone derivative that blocks renal tubular reabsorption of uric acid, increasing excretion, and inhibits platelet aggregation.

| Route | Onset | Peak | Duration |
|-------|-------|------|----------|
| P.O. | Unknown | 1-2 hr | 4-6 hr |

## ADVERSE REACTIONS
**GI:** *nausea, dyspepsia,* epigastric pain, reactivation of peptic ulcerations.
**Hematologic:** anemia, *leukopenia, agranulocytosis, thrombocytopenia, aplastic anemia.*
**Respiratory:** *bronchoconstriction in patients with aspirin-induced asthma.*
**Skin:** rash.

## INTERACTIONS
**Drug-drug.** *Aspirin, niacin, salicylates:* May inhibit uricosuric effect of sulfinpyrazone. Avoid using together.
*Oral anticoagulants:* May increase anticoagulant effect and risk of bleeding. Use together cautiously.
*Oral antidiabetics:* May increase effects of these drugs. Monitor glucose level.
*Probenecid:* May inhibit renal excretion of sulfinpyrazone. Use together cautiously.
*Theophylline, verapamil:* May increase clearance of these drugs. Use together cautiously.
**Drug-lifestyle.** *Alcohol use:* May decrease effectiveness. Discourage use together.

## EFFECTS ON LAB TEST RESULTS
• May increase BUN and creatinine level.
• May decrease hemoglobin and WBC, granulocyte, and platelet counts.

## CONTRAINDICATIONS & CAUTIONS
• Contraindicated in patients hypersensitive to pyrazole derivatives (including oxyphenbutazone and phenylbutazone) and in those with blood dyscrasias, active peptic ulcer, or symptoms of GI inflammation or ulceration.
• Use cautiously in patients with healed peptic ulcer and in pregnant women.

## NURSING CONSIDERATIONS
• Monitor BUN, CBC, and renal function studies periodically during long-term use.
• Monitor fluid intake and output closely. Therapy, especially at start, may lead to renal colic and formation of uric acid stones until acid levels are normal (about 6 mg/dl).
• Force fluids to maintain minimum daily output of 2 to 3 L. Alkalinize urine with sodium bicarbonate or other drug.
• Drug doesn't contain an analgesic or anti-inflammatory, and it's of no value during acute gout attacks.
• Drug may increase frequency, severity, and length of acute gout attacks during first 6 to 12 months of therapy. Prophylactic colchicine or another anti-inflammatory may be used during first 3 to 6 months.
• Lifelong therapy may be needed in patients with hyperuricemia.
• *Alert:* Don't confuse Anturane with Accutane, Artane, or Antabuse.

## PATIENT TEACHING
• Instruct patient and family that drug must be taken regularly, even during acute exacerbations.
• Tell patient to take drug with food, milk, or antacids to reduce GI upset.
• Tell patient to visit prescriber regularly so blood levels can be monitored and dosage adjusted, if needed.
• Warn patient with gout not to take aspirin-containing drugs because these may precipitate gout. Acetaminophen may be used for pain.
• Tell patient with gout to avoid foods high in purine, such as anchovies, liver, sardines, kidneys, sweetbreads, peas, and lentils, and to identify and avoid any other foods that may trigger gout attacks.
• Instruct patient to drink at least 10 to 12 glasses of fluid daily.
• Advise patient to avoid alcohol during therapy.
• Instruct patient to report unusual bleeding, bruising, or flulike symptoms.

---

**carboprost tromethamine**
**dinoprostone**
**methylergonovine maleate**
**mifepristone**
**oxytocin, synthetic injection**

**COMBINATION PRODUCTS**
None.

---

## carboprost tromethamine
Hemabate

*Pregnancy risk category C*

### AVAILABLE FORMS
*Injection:* 250 mcg/ml

### INDICATIONS & DOSAGES
➤ **To terminate pregnancy between weeks 13 and 20 of gestation**
*Adults:* Initially, 250 mcg deep I.M. Subsequent doses of 250 mcg given at intervals of 1½ to 3½ hours, depending on uterine response. Dosage may be increased in increments to 500 mcg if contractility is inadequate after several 250-mcg doses. Total dose shouldn't exceed 12 mg or continuous administration for more than 2 days.
➤ **Postpartum hemorrhage from uterine atony not managed by conventional methods**
*Adults:* 250 mcg by deep I.M. injection. Repeat doses q 15 to 90 minutes, p.r.n. Maximum total dose is 2 mg.

### ACTION
A prostaglandin that produces strong, prompt contractions of uterine smooth muscle, possibly mediated by calcium and cAMP.

| Route | Onset | Peak | Duration |
|-------|-------|------|----------|
| I.M. | Unknown | 15-60 min | 24 hr |

### ADVERSE REACTIONS
**CNS:** *fever,* headache, anxiety, paresthesia, syncope, weakness.

**CV:** chest pain, *arrhythmias,* flushing.
**EENT:** blurred vision, eye pain.
**GI:** *vomiting, diarrhea, nausea.*
**GU:** endometritis, *uterine rupture,* uterine or vaginal pain.
**Musculoskeletal:** backache, leg cramps.
**Respiratory:** coughing, wheezing.
**Skin:** rash, diaphoresis.
**Other:** breast tenderness, chills, hot flashes.

### INTERACTIONS
**Drug-drug.** *Other oxytocics:* May increase action. Avoid using together.

### EFFECTS ON LAB TEST RESULTS
None reported.

### CONTRAINDICATIONS & CAUTIONS
• Contraindicated in patients hypersensitive to drug and in those with acute pelvic inflammatory disease or active cardiac, pulmonary, renal, or hepatic disease.
• Use cautiously in patients with history of asthma, hypotension, hypertension, anemia, jaundice, or diabetes; and those with seizure disorders, previous uterine surgery, or CV, adrenal, renal, or hepatic disease.

### NURSING CONSIDERATIONS
• Unlike other prostaglandin abortifacients, drug is given by I.M. injection. Injectable form avoids risk of expelling vaginal suppositories if patient has profuse vaginal bleeding.
• Only trained personnel should give drug in a hospital setting.

### PATIENT TEACHING
• Explain use and administration of drug to patient and family.
• Instruct patient to report adverse reactions promptly.

---

*Rapid onset    †Canada    ‡Australia    ◇OTC    ◆Off-label use    ✐Photoguide    *Liquid contains alcohol.*

# dinoprostone
Cervidil, Prepidil, Prostin E2

*Pregnancy risk category C*

## AVAILABLE FORMS
*Endocervical gel:* 0.5 mg/application
(2.5-ml syringe)
*Vaginal insert:* 10 mg
*Vaginal suppositories:* 20 mg

## INDICATIONS & DOSAGES
➤ **To terminate second-trimester pregnancy; to evacuate uterus in missed abortion, intrauterine fetal death up to 28 weeks' gestation, or benign hydatidiform mole**
*Adults:* 20-mg suppository inserted high into posterior vaginal fornix; repeated q 3 to 5 hours until abortion is complete.
➤ **To ripen an unfavorable cervix in pregnant patients at or near term**
*Adults:* 0.5 mg endocervical gel intravaginally; if cervix remains unfavorable after 6 hours, repeat dose. Don't exceed 1.5 mg (three applications) within 24 hours. Or, 10-mg vaginal insert placed transversely in posterior vaginal fornix immediately after removing insert from foil. Take insert out when active labor begins or after 12 hours have passed, whichever occurs first.

## ACTION
A prostaglandin that produces strong, prompt contractions of uterine smooth muscle, possibly mediated by calcium and cAMP.

| Route | Onset | Peak | Duration |
|---|---|---|---|
| Intravaginal (gel) | 15-30 min | Unknown | Unknown |
| Intravaginal (insert) | Unknown | Unknown | Unknown |
| Intravaginal (suppository) | 10 min | Unknown | 2-6 hr |

## ADVERSE REACTIONS
**CNS:** *fever, headache, dizziness,* anxiety, paresthesia, weakness, syncope.
**CV:** chest pain, ***arrhythmias.***
**EENT:** blurred vision, eye pain.
**GI:** *nausea, vomiting, diarrhea.*
**GU:** vaginal pain, vaginitis, endometritis, uterine rupture.

**Musculoskeletal:** *nocturnal leg cramps,* backache, muscle cramps.
**Respiratory:** coughing, dyspnea.
**Skin:** rash, diaphoresis.
**Other:** breast tenderness, *shivering, chills,* hot flashes.

## INTERACTIONS
**Drug-drug.** *Other oxytocics:* May increase action. Avoid using together.
**Drug-lifestyle.** *Alcohol use:* May inhibit effectiveness of dinoprostone with high doses. Discourage use together.

## EFFECTS ON LAB TEST RESULTS
None reported.

## CONTRAINDICATIONS & CAUTIONS
• Gel form contraindicated in patients hypersensitive to prostaglandins or constituents of gel; in those for whom prolonged uterine contractions are undesirable; in those with placenta previa or unexplained vaginal bleeding during pregnancy; and in those for whom vaginal delivery isn't indicated (because of vasa previa or active genital herpes).
• Suppository form contraindicated in patients hypersensitive to drug, in those with acute pelvic inflammatory disease, and in those with active cardiac, pulmonary, renal, or hepatic disease.
• Insert form contraindicated in patients hypersensitive to drug, with evidence of fetal distress when delivery isn't imminent, with unexplained vaginal bleeding during pregnancy, or with evidence of marked fetal cephalopelvic disproportion; also contraindicated when oxytocics are contraindicated, when prolonged uterine contraction may be detrimental to fetal safety or uterine integrity, when membranes have ruptured, when patient is already receiving an oxytocic, and when patient is multipara with six or more previous term pregnancies.
• Insert gel cautiously in patients with asthma, renal or hepatic dysfunction, or ruptured membranes and in those with a history of asthma, glaucoma, or increased intraocular pressure.
• Use suppository form cautiously in patients with asthma, seizure disorders, anemia, diabetes, hypertension or hypotension, jaundice, scarred uterus, cervicitis,

---

acute vaginitis, or CV, renal, or hepatic disease.

## NURSING CONSIDERATIONS
• Give only when critical care facilities are available.
• For cervical ripening, have patient lie on her back; the cervix is examined using a speculum. A catheter provided with drug is used to insert gel into cervical canal just below level of the internal os.
• When giving gel form, don't try to give small amount of drug remaining in catheter.
• Patient should remain supine for 10 minutes after using gel.
• When using the vaginal insert, a minimal amount of water-soluble jelly may be used to aid insertion.
• Patient should remain supine for 2 hours after using vaginal insert. Remove insert on onset of active labor or 12 hours after insertion.
• Treat dinoprostone-induced fever with water sponging and increased fluid intake, not with aspirin.
• Check vaginal discharge regularly.
• Abortion should be complete within 30 hours when suppository form is used.

## PATIENT TEACHING
• Explain use and administration of drug to patient and family.
• Instruct patient to report adverse reactions promptly.

## methylergonovine maleate
Methergine

*Pregnancy risk category C*

### AVAILABLE FORMS
*Injection:* 0.2 mg/ml
*Tablets:* 0.2 mg

### INDICATIONS & DOSAGES
➤ **To prevent and treat postpartum hemorrhage caused by uterine atony or subinvolution**
*Adults:* 0.2 mg I.M. q 2 to 4 hours to a maximum of 5 doses. For excessive uterine bleeding or other emergencies, 0.2 mg I.V. over 1 minute while monitoring blood pressure and uterine contractions. After

first I.M. or I.V. dose, 0.2 mg P.O. q 6 to 8 hours for 2 to 7 days. Decrease dosage if severe cramping occurs.

### I.V. ADMINISTRATION
• *Alert:* Don't routinely give drug I.V. because of risk of severe hypertension and CVA.
• If drug must be given I.V., give slowly over at least 1 minute while carefully monitoring blood pressure.
• I.V. dose may be diluted to 5 ml with normal saline solution before use.
• Store I.V. solution below 46° F (8° C). Daily stock may be kept at room temperature for 60 to 90 days.

### ACTION
Increases motor activity of the uterus by direct stimulation of the smooth muscle, shortening the third stage of labor and reducing blood loss.

| Route | Onset | Peak | Duration |
|-------|-------|------|----------|
| P.O. | 5-10 min | 30 min | 3 hr |
| I.V. | Immediate | Unknown | 45 min |
| I.M. | 2-5 min | Unknown | 3 hr |

### ADVERSE REACTIONS
**CNS:** dizziness, headache, *seizures,* hallucinations, *CVA with I.V. use.*
**CV:** hypertension, transient chest pain, palpitations, hypotension, thrombophlebitis.
**EENT:** tinnitus, nasal congestion.
**GI:** *nausea, vomiting,* diarrhea, foul taste.
**GU:** hematuria.
**Musculoskeletal:** leg cramps.
**Respiratory:** dyspnea.
**Skin:** diaphoresis.

### INTERACTIONS
**Drug-drug.** *Dopamine, ergot alkaloids, I.V. oxytocin, regional anesthetics, vasoconstrictors:* May cause excessive vasoconstriction. Use together cautiously.

### EFFECTS ON LAB TEST RESULTS
• May decrease prolactin level.

### CONTRAINDICATIONS & CAUTIONS
• Contraindicated in pregnant patients, in patients sensitive to ergot preparations, and in patients with hypertension or toxemia.

• Use cautiously in patients with sepsis, obliterative vascular disease, or hepatic or renal disease.
• Use cautiously during last stage of labor.

## NURSING CONSIDERATIONS
• Monitor and record blood pressure, pulse rate, and uterine response; report sudden change in vital signs, frequent periods of uterine relaxation, and character and amount of vaginal bleeding.
• Monitor contractions, which may begin immediately. Contractions may continue for up to 45 minutes after I.V. use or for 3 hours or more after P.O. or I.M. use.
• Store tablets in tightly closed, light-resistant container. Discard if discolored.

## PATIENT TEACHING
• Explain use and administration of drug to patient and family.
• Instruct patient to report adverse reactions promptly.

---

## mifepristone
Mifeprex

*Pregnancy risk category NR*

## AVAILABLE FORMS
*Tablets:* 200 mg

## INDICATIONS & DOSAGES
➤ **To terminate intrauterine pregnancy during first 7 weeks**
*Adults:* 600 mg (three 200-mg tablets) P.O. as a single dose (considered day 1). On day 3, unless abortion is confirmed by clinical examination or ultrasonographic scan, give 400 mcg (two 200-mcg tablets) of misoprostol P.O.

## ACTION
Competitively interacts with progesterone at progesterone-receptor sites. Drug inhibits activity of endogenous and exogenous progesterone, resulting in termination of pregnancy.

| Route | Onset | Peak | Duration |
|-------|-------|------|----------|
| P.O. | Rapid | 90 min | 11 days |

## ADVERSE REACTIONS
**CNS:** fever, *headache, dizziness, fatigue,* insomnia, asthenia, anxiety, syncope.
**EENT:** sinusitis.
**GI:** *abdominal cramping, nausea, vomiting, diarrhea,* dyspepsia.
**GU:** vaginitis, *uterine cramping,* pelvic pain, ***uterine hemorrhage.***
**Hematologic:** anemia, leukorrhea.
**Musculoskeletal:** back pain, leg pain.
**Other:** rigors, viral infections.

## INTERACTIONS
**Drug-drug.** *Carbamazepine, dexamethasone, phenobarbital, phenytoin, rifampin:* May stimulate metabolism, reducing mifepristone level. Use together cautiously.
*Drugs that are CYP3A4 substrates and have narrow therapeutic ranges (general anesthetics):* May increase levels and prolong elimination of these drugs. Use together cautiously.
*Erythromycin, itraconazole, ketoconazole:* May inhibit metabolism and increase mifepristone level. Use together cautiously.
**Drug-herb.** *St. John's wort:* May stimulate metabolism, reducing mifepristone level. Discourage use together.
**Drug-food.** *Grapefruit juice:* May inhibit metabolism and increase mifepristone level. Discourage use together.

## EFFECTS ON LAB TEST RESULTS
• May decrease hemoglobin more than 2 g/dl.

## CONTRAINDICATIONS & CAUTIONS
• Contraindicated in patients allergic to mifepristone, misoprostol, or other prostaglandins; in those with confirmed or suspected ectopic pregnancy or undiagnosed adnexal mass; and in those with an intrauterine device (IUD) in place.
• Contraindicated in patients with chronic adrenal failure, inherited porphyrias, or hemorrhagic disorders, and in those on long-term corticosteroid therapy or taking anticoagulants.
• Don't use in patients without access to a medical facility equipped to provide emergency treatment of incomplete abortion, blood transfusions, and emergency resus-

---

Reactions may be *common*, uncommon, *life-threatening*, or COMMON AND LIFE-THREATENING.

citation from the first visit until discharged by the prescriber. Don't use in patient unable to understand effects of procedure or to comply with regimen.

• Use cautiously in patients with CV disease; hypertension; respiratory, renal, or hepatic disease; type 1 diabetes; or severe anemia.

• Use cautiously in heavy smokers, especially women older than age 35 who smoke 10 or more cigarettes per day, because drug's effects in these patients aren't known.

**NURSING CONSIDERATIONS**
• Drug is supplied only to prescribers who sign and return a Prescriber's Agreement. It's not available through pharmacies.

• For purposes of this treatment, pregnancy is dated from the first day of the last menstrual period in a presumed 28-day cycle with ovulation occurring at midcycle. Duration of pregnancy may be determined from menstrual history and clinical examination. Use ultrasonographic scan if duration of pregnancy is uncertain or if ectopic pregnancy is suspected.

• Patient must read the medication guide and sign the Patient Agreement before drug is given.

• *Alert:* If patient has an IUD in place, make sure that it is removed before treatment begins.

• For proper administration of mifepristone and misoprostol to terminate pregnancy, the patient must visit the prescriber three times. This treatment may be given only in a clinic, medical office, or hospital by or under the supervision of a prescriber able to assess the gestational age of an embryo and to diagnose an ectopic pregnancy. The prescriber must also be able to provide surgical intervention in case of incomplete abortion or severe bleeding, or have made plans to provide such care through others, and be able to ensure patient access to medical facilities equipped to provide blood transfusions and resuscitation, if needed.

• After taking misoprostol, patient may need medication for cramps or GI symptoms.

• Patient must return for a follow-up visit about 14 days after taking mifepristone to determine by clinical examination or ultrasound that pregnancy has been completely terminated and to assess the degree of bleeding. If the patient is still pregnant at this visit, the fetus is at risk for malformation resulting from the treatment. Surgical termination is recommended.

• Vaginal bleeding and uterine or abdominal cramping are expected effects of the drug. Vaginal bleeding or spotting occurs for about 9 to 16 days. Excessive bleeding may need treatment with vasoconstrictors, curettage, saline infusions, or blood transfusions. Persistence of heavy or moderate bleeding at the 14-day follow-up visit may indicate incomplete abortion.

• It's unknown if drug appears in breast milk. A breast-feeding woman should consult her prescriber to decide whether to discard her breast milk for a few days after taking drug.

• Store drug at controlled room temperature.

• *Alert:* Don't confuse mifepristone and misoprostol.

**PATIENT TEACHING**
• Give patient a copy of the medication guide and Patient Agreement. Review these with patient and allow her the chance to ask questions.

• Inform patient of importance of completing the treatment schedule and stress the necessity of returning for a follow-up visit about 14 days after taking mifepristone.

• Advise patient to expect vaginal bleeding, which may be heavy at times and accompanied by uterine cramping.

• Inform patient that vaginal bleeding isn't proof of a complete abortion and that she must return for follow-up visit to confirm the abortion has been completed.

• Tell patient that fetus may be harmed and that surgical termination may be needed if treatment fails.

• Supply patient with a name and telephone number to contact in case of emergency.

• Advise patient that she may become pregnant again as soon as termination of

---

*Rapid onset   †Canada   ‡Australia   ◇OTC   ◆Off-label use   ✐Photoguide   *Liquid contains alcohol.*

pregnancy is complete and before normal menstrual periods have returned.
• Inform patient of various contraception methods.

---

## oxytocin, synthetic injection
Pitocin

*Pregnancy risk category NR*

### AVAILABLE FORMS
*Injection:* 10 units/ml in 1-ml ampule, vial, or syringe

### INDICATIONS & DOSAGES
➤ **To induce or stimulate labor**
*Adults:* Initially, 10 units in 1,000 ml of $D_5W$ injection, lactated Ringer's, or normal saline solution I.V. infused at 1 to 2 milliunits/minute. Increase rate by 1 to 2 milliunits/minute at 15- to 30-minute intervals until normal contraction pattern is established. Decrease rate when labor is firmly established.
➤ **To reduce postpartum bleeding after expulsion of placenta**
*Adults:* 10 to 40 units in 1,000 ml of $D_5W$ injection, lactated Ringer's, or normal saline solution I.V. infused at rate needed to control bleeding, usually 20 to 40 milliunits/minute. Also, 10 units may be given I.M. after delivery of placenta.
➤ **Incomplete or inevitable abortion**
*Adults:* 10 units I.V. in 500 ml of normal saline solution, lactated Ringer's, or dextrose 5% in normal saline solution. Infuse at rate of 10 to 20 milliunits (20 to 40 gtt)/minute.

### I.V. ADMINISTRATION
• To induce or stimulate labor, dilute drug by adding 10 units to 1 L of normal saline, lactated Ringer's, or $D_5W$ solution.
• To produce intense uterine contractions and reduce postpartum bleeding, dilute drug by adding 10 units to 500 ml of normal saline, lactated Ringer's, or $D_5W$ solution.
• Don't give drug by I.V. bolus injection. Give drug only by piggyback infusion so that it may be stopped without interrupting I.V. line. Use an infusion pump.

### ACTION
Hormone that causes potent and selective stimulation of uterine and mammary gland smooth muscle.

| Route | Onset | Peak | Duration |
|-------|-------|------|----------|
| I.V. | Immediate | Unknown | 1 hr |
| I.M. | 3-5 min | Unknown | 2-3 hr |

### ADVERSE REACTIONS
**Maternal**
**CNS:** *subarachnoid hemorrhage, seizures, coma.*
**CV:** hypertension; increased heart rate, systemic venous return, and cardiac output; *arrhythmias.*
**GI:** nausea, vomiting.
**GU:** tetanic uterine contractions, *abruptio placentae,* impaired uterine blood flow, pelvic hematoma, increased uterine motility, *uterine rupture, postpartum hemorrhage.*
**Hematologic:** *afibrinogenemia possibly related to postpartum bleeding.*
**Other:** hypersensitivity reactions, *anaphylaxis, death from oxytocin-induced water intoxication.*
**Fetal**
**CNS:** *infant brain damage.*
**CV:** *bradycardia,* PVCs, *arrhythmias.*
**EENT:** neonatal retinal hemorrhage.
**Hepatic:** neonatal jaundice.
**Respiratory:** *anoxia, asphyxia.*
**Other:** *low Apgar scores at 5 minutes.*

### INTERACTIONS
**Drug-drug.** *Cyclopropane anesthetics:* May cause less pronounced bradycardia and hypotension. Use together cautiously.
*Thiopental anesthetics:* May delay induction. Use together cautiously.
*Vasoconstrictors:* May cause severe hypertension if oxytocin is given within 3 to 4 hours of vasoconstrictor in patient receiving caudal block anesthetic. Avoid using together.

### EFFECTS ON LAB TEST RESULTS
None reported.

### CONTRAINDICATIONS & CAUTIONS
• Contraindicated in patients hypersensitive to drug.
• Contraindicated when vaginal delivery isn't advised (placenta previa, vasa previa,

---

invasive cervical carcinoma, genital herpes), when cephalopelvic disproportion is present, or when delivery requires conversion, as in transverse lie.

• Contraindicated in fetal distress when delivery isn't imminent, in prematurity, in other obstetric emergencies, and in patients with severe toxemia or hypertonic uterine patterns.

• Use with extreme caution during first and second stages of labor because cervical laceration, uterine rupture, and maternal and fetal death have been reported.

• Use with extreme caution, if at all, in patients with invasive cervical cancer and in those with previous cervical or uterine surgery (including cesarean section), grand multiparity, uterine sepsis, traumatic delivery, or overdistended uterus.

## NURSING CONSIDERATIONS
• Drug isn't recommended for routine I.M. use, but 10 units may be given I.M. after delivery of placenta to control postpartum uterine bleeding.

• Never give oxytocin simultaneously by more than one route.

• Drug is used to induce or reinforce labor only when pelvis is known to be adequate, when vaginal delivery is indicated, when fetal maturity is assured, and when fetal position is favorable. Use drug only in hospital where critical care facilities and prescriber are immediately available.

• Monitor fluid intake and output. Antidiuretic effect may lead to fluid overload, seizures, and coma from water intoxication.

• Monitor and record uterine contractions, heart rate, blood pressure, intrauterine pressure, fetal heart rate, and character of blood loss every 15 minutes.

• Have 20% magnesium sulfate solution available to relax the myometrium.

• If contractions occur less than 2 minutes apart, exceed 50 mm, or last 90 seconds or longer, stop infusion, turn patient on her side, and notify prescriber.

• Drug doesn't cause fetal abnormalities when used as indicated.

• *Alert:* Don't confuse Pitocin with Pitressin.

## PATIENT TEACHING
• Explain use and administration of drug to patient and family.
• Instruct patient to report adverse reactions promptly.

flavoxate hydrochloride
oxybutynin chloride
phenazopyridine hydrochloride
tolterodine tartrate

### COMBINATION PRODUCTS
PYRIDIUM PLUS: phenazopyridine
150 mg, butabarbital 15 mg, hyoscyamine
0.3 mg

## flavoxate hydrochloride
Urispas

*Pregnancy risk category B*

### AVAILABLE FORMS
*Tablets:* 100 mg

### INDICATIONS & DOSAGES
➤ **Symptomatic relief of dysuria, urinary frequency and urgency, nocturia, incontinence, and suprapubic pain from urologic disorders**
*Adults and children older than age 12:*
100 to 200 mg P.O. t.i.d. to q.i.d. Dosage may be reduced with improvement of symptoms.

### ACTION
Produces a direct spasmolytic effect on urinary tract smooth muscles and provides some local anesthesia and analgesia.

| Route | Onset | Peak | Duration |
|-------|-------|------|----------|
| P.O. | Unknown | 2 hr | Unknown |

### ADVERSE REACTIONS
**CNS:** *confusion,* nervousness, dizziness, headache, drowsiness, vertigo, fever.
**CV:** tachycardia, palpitations.
**EENT:** *blurred vision,* disturbed eye accommodation, increased ocular tension.
**GI:** dry mouth, nausea, vomiting.
**GU:** dysuria.
**Hematologic:** eosinophilia, *leukopenia.*
**Skin:** urticaria, dermatoses.

### INTERACTIONS
**Drug-lifestyle.** *Exercise, hot weather:*
May precipitate heatstroke. Urge patient to use caution in hot weather.

### EFFECTS ON LAB TEST RESULTS
● May increase eosinophil count. May decrease WBC count.

### CONTRAINDICATIONS & CAUTIONS
● Contraindicated in patients with pyloric or duodenal obstruction, obstructive intestinal lesions or ileus, achalasia, GI hemorrhage, or obstructive uropathies of lower urinary tract.
● Safety and effectiveness of drug in children age 12 and younger are unknown.
● Use cautiously in patients who may have glaucoma and in pregnant or breast-feeding women.

### NURSING CONSIDERATIONS
● Check patient history for other drug use before giving drugs with anticholinergic adverse reactions. Such reactions may be intensified by flavoxate.
● *Alert:* Don't confuse Urispas with Urised.

### PATIENT TEACHING
● Warn patient to avoid hazardous activities, such as operating machinery or driving, until CNS effects of drug are known.
● Tell patient to contact prescriber if adverse reactions occur or if symptoms aren't diminished.
● Caution patient that using drug during very hot weather may precipitate fever or heatstroke because it suppresses diaphoresis.
● Tell patient drug may cause dry mouth or blurred vision.

# oxybutynin chloride
Ditropan, Ditropan XL, Oxytrol

*Pregnancy risk category B*

## AVAILABLE FORMS
*Syrup:* 5 g/5 ml
*Tablets:* 5 mg
*Tablets (extended-release):* 5 mg, 10 mg, 15 mg
*Transdermal patch:* 36-mg patch delivering 3.9 mg/day

## INDICATIONS & DOSAGES
➤ **Uninhibited or reflex neurogenic bladder**
*Adults:* 5 mg P.O. b.i.d. to t.i.d., to maximum of 5 mg q.i.d.
*Children older than age 5:* 5 mg P.O. b.i.d., to maximum of 5 mg t.i.d.
➤ **Overactive bladder**
*Adults:* Initially, 5 mg P.O. Ditropan XL once daily. Dosage adjustments may be made weekly in 5-mg increments, p.r.n., to maximum dose of 30 mg P.O. daily. Or, apply one patch twice weekly to dry, intact skin on the abdomen, hip, or buttock.

## ACTION
Produces a direct spasmolytic effect and an antimuscarinic (atropine-like) effect on urinary tract smooth muscles, increasing urinary bladder capacity, and provides some local anesthesia and analgesia.

| Route | Onset | Peak | Duration |
|---|---|---|---|
| P.O. | 30-60 min | 3-4 hr | 6-10 hr |
| P.O. (extended-release) | Unknown | 4-6 hr | 24 hr |
| Transdermal | 24-48 hr | Varies | 96 hr |

## ADVERSE REACTIONS
**CNS:** dizziness, insomnia, restlessness, hallucinations, asthenia, fever.
**CV:** *palpitations, tachycardia,* vasodilation.
**EENT:** mydriasis, cycloplegia, decreased lacrimation, amblyopia.
**GI:** nausea, vomiting, *dry mouth, constipation,* decreased GI motility.
**GU:** impotence, *urinary hesitancy, urine retention.*

**Skin:** rash, decreased diaphoresis.
**Other:** suppression of lactation.
**Transdermal patch**
**CNS:** fatigue, somnolence, headache.
**CV:** flushing.
**EENT:** abnormal vision.
**GI:** *dry mouth,* diarrhea, abdominal pain, nausea, flatulence.
**GU:** dysuria.
**Musculoskeletal:** back pain.
**Skin:** *pruritus,* erythema, vesicles, macules, rash, burning at injection site.

## INTERACTIONS
**Drug-drug.** *Anticholinergics:* May increase anticholinergic effects. Use together cautiously.
*Atenolol, digoxin:* May increase levels of these drugs. Monitor drug levels closely.
*CNS depressants:* May increase CNS effects. Use together cautiously.
*Haloperidol:* May decrease level of this drug. Monitor drug level closely.
**Drug-lifestyle.** *Alcohol use:* May increase CNS effects. Discourage use together.
*Exercise, hot weather:* May precipitate heatstroke. Urge patient to use caution in hot weather.

## EFFECTS ON LAB TEST RESULTS
None reported.

## CONTRAINDICATIONS & CAUTIONS
• Contraindicated in patients hypersensitive to drug or its components and in those with myasthenia gravis, GI obstruction, untreated angle-closure glaucoma, adynamic ileus, megacolon, severe colitis, ulcerative colitis when megacolon is present, urinary or gastric retention, or obstructive uropathy.
• Contraindicated in elderly or debilitated patients with intestinal atony and in hemorrhaging patients with unstable CV status.
• Use cautiously in elderly patients and in patients with autonomic neuropathy, reflux esophagitis, or hepatic or renal disease.
• Use extended-release form cautiously in patients with bladder outflow obstruction, gastric obstruction, ulcerative colitis, intestinal atony, myasthenia gravis, or gastroesophageal reflux and in those taking drugs that worsen esophagitis (bisphosphonates).

---

*Rapid onset*   †Canada   ‡Australia   ◇OTC   ♦Off-label use   ✐Photoguide   *Liquid contains alcohol.

• Use cautiously in patients with renal or hepatic disease and in pregnant or breast-feeding women.

NURSING CONSIDERATIONS
• Before giving drug, get confirmation of neurogenic bladder by cystometry and rule out partial intestinal obstruction in patients with diarrhea, especially those with colostomy or ileostomy.
• If patient has UTI, treat him with antibiotics.
• Drug may aggravate symptoms of hyperthyroidism, coronary artery disease, heart failure, arrhythmias, tachycardia, hypertension, or prostatic hyperplasia.
• Obtain periodic cystometry as directed to evaluate response to therapy.
• *Alert:* Don't confuse Ditropan with diazepam or Dithranol.

PATIENT TEACHING
• Warn patient to avoid hazardous activities, such as operating machinery or driving, until CNS effects of drug are known.
• Caution patient that using drug during very hot weather may precipitate fever or heatstroke because it suppresses diaphoresis.
• Tell patient to swallow Ditropan XL whole and not to chew or crush it.
• Instruct patient to measure syrup with a teaspoon.
• Advise patient to store drug in tightly closed container at 59° to 86° F (15° to 30° C).
• Instruct patient using transdermal patch to change patch twice a week and to choose a new application site with each new patch to avoid the same site within 7 days. Warn patient to only wear one patch at a time. Tell patient to dispose of old patches carefully in the trash in a manner that prevents accidental application or ingestion by children, pets, and others.
• Advise patient to avoid alcohol while taking drug.
• Tell patient that drug may cause dry mouth.

# phenazopyridine hydrochloride
Azo-Standard◊, Baridium◊, Geridium, Phenazo†, Prodium◊, Pyridiate, Pyridium, Urodine, Urogesic, UTI-Relief

*Pregnancy risk category B*

AVAILABLE FORMS
*Tablets:* 95 mg◊, 97.2 mg, 100 mg, 150 mg, 200 mg

INDICATIONS & DOSAGES
➤ **Pain with urinary tract irritation or infection**
*Adults:* 200 mg P.O. t.i.d. after meals for 2 days.
*Children ages 6 to 12:* 12 mg/kg P.O. daily in three equally divided doses after meals for 2 days.

ACTION
Exerts local anesthetic action on urinary mucosa through unknown mechanism.

| Route | Onset | Peak | Duration |
|-------|-------|------|----------|
| P.O. | Unknown | Unknown | Unknown |

ADVERSE REACTIONS
**CNS:** headache.
**EENT:** staining of contact lenses.
**GI:** nausea, GI disturbances.
**Hematologic:** hemolytic anemia, methemoglobinemia.
**Skin:** rash, pruritus.
**Other:** *anaphylactoid reactions.*

INTERACTIONS
None significant.

EFFECTS ON LAB TEST RESULTS
• May decrease hemoglobin.
• May alter Diastix or Chemstrip uG results and interfere with urinary ketone tests (Acetest or Ketostix).

CONTRAINDICATIONS & CAUTIONS
• Contraindicated in patients hypersensitive to drug and in those with glomerulonephritis, severe hepatitis, uremia, renal insufficiency, or pyelonephritis during pregnancy.

## NURSING CONSIDERATIONS
• When drug is used with an antibacterial, therapy shouldn't extend beyond 2 days.
• *Alert:* Don't confuse Pyridium with pyridoxine.

## PATIENT TEACHING
• Advise patient that taking drug with meals may minimize GI distress.
• Caution patient to stop drug and notify prescriber immediately if skin or sclera becomes yellow-tinged, which may indicate drug accumulation from impaired renal excretion.
• Inform patient that drug colors urine red or orange and may stain fabrics and contact lenses.
• Tell diabetic patient to use Clinitest for accurate urine glucose test results. Also tell patient that drug may interfere with urinary ketone tests (Acetest or Ketostix).
• Advise patient to notify prescriber if urinary tract pain persists. Tell him that drug shouldn't be used for long-term treatment.

---

## tolterodine tartrate
Detrol✐, Detrol LA

*Pregnancy risk category C*

## AVAILABLE FORMS
*Capsules (extended-release):* 2 mg, 4 mg
*Tablets:* 1 mg, 2 mg

## INDICATIONS & DOSAGES
➤ **Overactive bladder in patients with symptoms of urinary frequency, urgency, or urge incontinence**
*Adults:* 2-mg tablet P.O. b.i.d. or 4-mg extended-release capsule P.O. daily. Dose may be reduced to 1-mg tablet P.O. b.i.d. or 2-mg extended-release capsule P.O. daily, based on patient response and tolerance.
*Adjust-a-dose:* For patients with significantly reduced hepatic function or those taking a cytochrome P-450 inhibitor, 1-mg tablet P.O. b.i.d. or 2-mg extended-release capsule P.O. daily.

## ACTION
A competitive muscarinic receptor antagonist. Both urinary bladder contraction and salivation are mediated via cholinergic muscarinic receptors.

| Route | Onset | Peak | Duration |
|---|---|---|---|
| P.O. | Unknown | 1-2 hr | Unknown |
| P.O. (extended-release) | Unknown | 45-90 min | Unknown |

## ADVERSE REACTIONS
**CNS:** fatigue, paresthesia, vertigo, dizziness, *headache,* nervousness, somnolence.
**CV:** hypertension, chest pain.
**EENT:** abnormal vision, xerophthalmia, pharyngitis, rhinitis, sinusitis.
**GI:** *dry mouth,* abdominal pain, constipation, diarrhea, dyspepsia, flatulence, nausea, vomiting.
**GU:** dysuria, micturition frequency, urine retention, UTI.
**Metabolic:** weight gain.
**Musculoskeletal:** arthralgia, back pain.
**Respiratory:** bronchitis, coughing, upper respiratory tract infection.
**Skin:** pruritus, rash, erythema, dry skin.
**Other:** flulike syndrome, accidental injury, fungal infection, infection.

## INTERACTIONS
**Drug-drug.** *Antifungal drugs (itraconazole, ketoconazole, miconazole), cytochrome P-450 inhibitors (such as macrolide antibiotics clarithromycin and erythromycin):* May increase tolterodine level. Don't give more than 1-mg tablet b.i.d. or 2-mg extended-release capsule daily of tolterodine if used together.
*Fluoxetine:* May increase tolterodine level. Monitor patient. No dosage adjustment is needed.

## EFFECTS ON LAB TEST RESULTS
None reported.

## CONTRAINDICATIONS & CAUTIONS
• Contraindicated in patients hypersensitive to drug or its components and in those with uncontrolled angle-closure glaucoma or urine or gastric retention.
• Use cautiously in patients with significant bladder outflow obstruction, GI obstructive disorders (such as pyloric stenosis), controlled angle-closure glaucoma, and hepatic or renal impairment.

---

## NURSING CONSIDERATIONS
● Assess baseline bladder function and monitor therapeutic effects.

## PATIENT TEACHING
● Tell patient that sugarless gum, hard candy, or saliva substitute may help relieve dry mouth.
● Advise patient to avoid driving or other potentially hazardous activities until visual effects of drug are known.
● Advise breast-feeding woman to stop breast-feeding during therapy.
● Instruct patient to immediately report signs of infection, urine retention, or GI problems.
● Tell patient taking extended-release form to swallow capsule whole and take with liquids.

**auranofin**
**aurothioglucose**
**gold sodium thiomalate**

**COMBINATION PRODUCTS**
None.

---

**auranofin**
Ridaura

*Pregnancy risk category C*

**AVAILABLE FORMS**
*Capsules:* 3 mg

**INDICATIONS & DOSAGES**
➤ **Rheumatoid arthritis**
*Adults:* 6 mg P.O. daily, either as 3 mg b.i.d. or 6 mg once daily. After 6 months, may increase to 9 mg daily, given as 3 mg t.i.d.
*Children:* Initially, 0.1 mg/kg daily. Maintenance dose is 0.15 mg/kg daily; maximum dose is 0.2 mg/kg daily.

**ACTION**
Unknown. Anti-inflammatory effects probably result from inhibition of sulfhydryl systems, which alters cellular metabolism. May also alter enzyme function and immune response and suppress phagocytic activity.

| Route | Onset | Peak | Duration |
|-------|-------|------|----------|
| P.O. | Unknown | 2 hr | Unknown |

**ADVERSE REACTIONS**
**CNS:** confusion, hallucinations, *seizures.*
**EENT:** conjunctivitis.
**GI:** *diarrhea, abdominal pain, nausea, stomatitis,* glossitis, anorexia, metallic taste, dyspepsia, flatulence, constipation, dysgeusia, ulcerative colitis.
**GU:** proteinuria, hematuria, nephrotic syndrome, glomerulonephritis, *acute renal failure.*
**Hematologic:** *thrombocytopenia, aplastic anemia, agranulocytosis, leukopenia,* eosinophilia, anemia.

**Hepatic:** jaundice.
**Skin:** *rash, pruritus, dermatitis,* exfoliative dermatitis, urticaria, erythema, alopecia.

**INTERACTIONS**
**Drug-drug.** *Phenytoin:* May increase phenytoin blood levels. Watch for toxicity.

**EFFECTS ON LAB TEST RESULTS**
• May increase ALT, AST, and alkaline phosphatase levels.
• May increase eosinophil count. May decrease hemoglobin and platelet, granulocyte, and WBC counts.

**CONTRAINDICATIONS & CAUTIONS**
• Contraindicated in patients with history of severe gold toxicity or toxicity from previous exposure to other heavy metals and in those with necrotizing enterocolitis, pulmonary fibrosis, exfoliative dermatitis, bone marrow aplasia, or severe hematologic disorders. Also contraindicated in patients with urticaria, eczema, colitis, severe debilitation, hemorrhagic conditions, or systemic lupus erythematosus and in patients who have recently received radiation therapy. The manufacturer recommends avoiding use during pregnancy.
• Use cautiously with other drugs that cause blood dyscrasias. Also use cautiously in patients with rash, history of bone marrow depression, or renal, hepatic, or inflammatory bowel disease.

**NURSING CONSIDERATIONS**
• Monitor patient's platelet count monthly. Stop drug if platelet count falls below 100,000/mm³, if hemoglobin drops suddenly, if granulocyte count is less than 1,500/mm³, or if leukopenia (WBC count less than 4,000/mm³) or eosinophilia over 5% exists.
• *Alert:* Monitor patient's urinalysis results monthly. If proteinuria or hematuria is detected, stop drug because it can cause nephrotic syndrome or glomerulonephritis, and notify prescriber.

---

- Monitor renal and liver function test results.
- Warn women of childbearing potential about risks of drug therapy during pregnancy.

**PATIENT TEACHING**
- Encourage patient to take drug as prescribed.
- Tell patient to continue concomitant drug therapy if prescribed.
- Remind patient to see prescriber for monthly platelet counts.
- Suggest that patient have regular urinalysis.
- Tell patient to keep taking drug if mild diarrhea occurs but to immediately report blood in stool. Diarrhea is most common adverse reaction.
- Advise patient to report rash or other skin problems and to stop drug until reaction subsides. Itching may precede dermatitis; consider itchy skin eruptions during drug therapy to be a reaction until proven otherwise.
- Inform patient that inflammation of the mouth may be preceded by a metallic taste; tell him to notify prescriber if this occurs. Promote careful oral hygiene during therapy.
- Advise patient to report unusual bleeding or bruising.
- Inform patient that beneficial effect may be delayed as long as 3 months. If response is inadequate and maximum dose has been reached, expect prescriber to stop drug.
- Warn patient not to give drug to others. Auranofin is prescribed only for selected patients with rheumatoid arthritis.

---

**aurothioglucose**
Gold-50‡, Solganal

**gold sodium thiomalate**
Aurolate

*Pregnancy risk category C*

**AVAILABLE FORMS**
**aurothioglucose**
*Injection (suspension):* 50 mg/ml in sesame oil in 10-ml vial

**gold sodium thiomalate**
*Injection:* 50 mg/ml with benzyl alcohol in 2-ml and 10-ml vials

**INDICATIONS & DOSAGES**
➤ **Rheumatoid arthritis**
*aurothioglucose*
*Adults:* Initially, 10 mg I.M., followed by 25 mg q week for second and third doses. Then, 50 mg q week to total dose of 800 mg to 1 g. If condition improves and no toxicity occurs, continue 25 to 50 mg q 3 to 4 weeks indefinitely.
*Children ages 6 to 12:* One-fourth usual adult dose. Don't exceed 25 mg per dose.
*gold sodium thiomalate*
*Adults:* Initially, 10 mg I.M., followed by 25 mg in 1 week. Then, 25 to 50 mg q week to total dose of 1 g. If condition improves and no toxicity occurs, give 25 to 50 mg q 2 weeks for 2 to 20 weeks; then, 25 to 50 mg q 3 to 4 weeks as maintenance therapy. If relapse occurs, resume injections at weekly intervals.
*Children:* Initially, a test dose of 10 mg I.M.; then, 1 mg/kg I.M. weekly, not to exceed 50 mg for a single injection. Follow adult spacing of doses.

**ACTION**
Unknown. Anti-inflammatory effects probably result from inhibition of sulfhydryl systems, which alters cellular metabolism. May also alter enzyme function and immune response and suppress phagocytic activity.

| Route | Onset | Peak | Duration |
|-------|-------|------|----------|
| I.M. | Unknown | 3-6 hr | Unknown |

**ADVERSE REACTIONS**
**CNS:** confusion, hallucinations, *seizures.*
**CV:** *bradycardia,* hypotension.
**EENT:** corneal gold deposition, corneal ulcers.
**GI:** diarrhea, anorexia, abdominal cramps, nausea, vomiting, ulcerative enterocolitis, *metallic taste, stomatitis.*
**GU:** albuminuria, proteinuria, nephrotic syndrome, nephritis, acute tubular necrosis, hematuria, *acute renal failure.*
**Hematologic:** *thrombocytopenia, aplastic anemia, agranulocytosis, leukopenia,* eosinophilia, anemia.
**Hepatic:** *hepatitis,* jaundice.

---

**Skin:** photosensitivity reaction, *rash, dermatitis,* erythema, exfoliative dermatitis, diaphoresis.
**Other:** *anaphylaxis, angioedema.*

## INTERACTIONS
**Drug-lifestyle.** *Sun or ultraviolet light exposure:* May cause photosensitivity reaction. Advise patient to avoid excessive sunlight exposure.

## EFFECTS ON LAB TEST RESULTS
• May increase ALT, AST, and alkaline phosphatase levels.
• May increase eosinophil count. May decrease hemoglobin and platelet, granulocyte, and WBC counts.

## CONTRAINDICATIONS & CAUTIONS
• Contraindicated in patients hypersensitive to drug and in those with history of severe toxicity from previous exposure to gold or other heavy metals.
• Contraindicated in those who have recently received radiation therapy and in those with hepatitis, exfoliative dermatitis, severe uncontrollable diabetes, renal disease, hepatic dysfunction, uncontrolled heart failure, systemic lupus erythematosus, colitis, Sjögren's syndrome, urticaria, eczema, hemorrhagic conditions, or severe hematologic disorders.
• Use with extreme caution, if at all, in patients with rash, marked hypertension, compromised cerebral or CV circulation, or history of renal or hepatic disease, drug allergies, or blood dyscrasias.

## NURSING CONSIDERATIONS
• Warn women of childbearing potential about risks of gold therapy during pregnancy.
• *Alert:* Give drug I.M. only.
• Give drug only under constant supervision of prescriber thoroughly familiar with drug's toxicities and benefits.
• Immerse aurothioglucose vial in warm water; shake vigorously before injecting.
• Give I.M., preferably intragluteally. Drug is pale yellow; don't use if it darkens.
• When injecting gold sodium thiomalate, have patient lie down for 10 to 20 minutes to minimize hypotension.

• Watch for anaphylactoid reaction for 30 minutes after administration.
• *Alert:* Keep dimercaprol available to treat acute toxicity.
• Analyze urine for protein and sediment changes before each injection.
• Monitor CBC, including platelet count, before every second injection.
• Monitor platelet counts if patient develops purpura or ecchymoses.
• If adverse reactions are mild, some rheumatologists resume gold therapy after 2 to 3 weeks' rest.

## PATIENT TEACHING
• Inform patient that increased joint pain may occur for 1 to 2 days after injection but usually subsides.
• Advise patient to report rash or skin problems immediately and to stop drug until reaction subsides. Itching may precede skin inflammation; consider itchy skin eruptions during gold therapy to be a reaction until proven otherwise.
• Advise patient to report unusual bleeding or bruising.
• Instruct patient to report a metallic taste. Promote careful oral hygiene.
• Urge patient to avoid sunlight and artificial ultraviolet light, which may cause gray-blue skin pigmentation.
• Tell patient that benefits may not appear for 3 to 4 months.
• Stress need for medical follow-up.

## Miscellaneous antagonists and antidotes

activated charcoal
aminocaproic acid
digoxin immune Fab
dimercaprol
disulfiram
edetate calcium disodium
edetate disodium
flumazenil
naloxone hydrochloride
naltrexone hydrochloride
penicillamine
pralidoxime chloride
protamine sulfate
sodium polystyrene sulfonate
succimer

**COMBINATION PRODUCTS**
None.

---

### activated charcoal
Actidose ◊, Actidose-Aqua ◊,
Actidose with Sorbitol ◊,
CharcoAid ◊, CharcoAid 2000 ◊,
CharcoCaps ◊, Liqui-Char ◊

*Pregnancy risk category C*

**AVAILABLE FORMS**
*Capsules:* 260 mg ◊
*Granules:* 15 g
*Liquid:* 15 g, 50 g
*Oral suspension:* 15 g ◊, 30 g ◊, 50 g ◊
*Powder:* 15 g ◊, 30 g ◊, 40 g ◊, 120 g ◊, 240 g ◊
*Tablets:* 250 mg ◊

**INDICATIONS & DOSAGES**
➤ **Flatulence, dyspepsia**
*Adults:* 600 mg to 5 g P.O. as single dose or 0.975 to 3.9 g P.O. t.i.d. after meals.
➤ **Poisoning**
*Adults and children:* Initially, 1 to 2 g/kg (30 to 100 g) P.O. or 10 times the amount of poison ingested as a suspension in 120 to 240 ml (4 to 8 ounces) of water.

**ACTION**
An adsorbent that adheres to many drugs and chemicals, inhibiting their absorption from the GI tract.

| Route | Onset | Peak | Duration |
|-------|-------|------|----------|
| P.O. | Immediate | Unknown | Unknown |

**ADVERSE REACTIONS**
**GI:** *black stools,* nausea, constipation, *intestinal obstruction.*

**INTERACTIONS**
**Drug-drug.** *Acetaminophen, barbiturates, carbamazepine, digitoxin, digoxin, furosemide, glutethimide, hydantoins, methotrexate, nizatidine, phenothiazines, phenylbutazone, propoxyphene, salicylates, sulfonamides, sulfonylureas, tetracyclines, theophyllines, tricyclic antidepressants, valproic acid:* May reduce absorption of these drugs. Give charcoal at least 2 hours before or 1 hour after other drugs.
*Acetylcysteine, ipecac:* May inactivate these drugs. Give charcoal after vomiting has been induced by ipecac; remove charcoal by nasogastric tube before giving acetylcysteine.
**Drug-food.** *Milk, ice cream, sherbet:* May decrease adsorptive capacity of charcoal. Discourage use together.

**EFFECTS ON LAB TEST RESULTS**
None reported.

**CONTRAINDICATIONS & CAUTIONS**
No known contraindications.

**NURSING CONSIDERATIONS**
• Although there are no known contraindications, drug isn't effective for treating all acute poisonings.
• *Alert:* Drug is commonly used for treating poisoning or overdose with acetaminophen, aspirin, atropine, barbiturates, dextropropoxyphene, digoxin, poisonous mushrooms, oxalic acid, parathion, phenol, phenytoin, propantheline, propoxyphene, strychnine, or tricyclic antidepres-

sants. Check with poison control center for use in other types of poisonings or overdoses.

• Give after emesis is complete because activated charcoal absorbs and inactivates ipecac syrup.

• For maximal effect, give within 30 minutes after poison ingestion.

• Mix powder (most effective form) with tap water to consistency of thick syrup. Adding a small amount of fruit juice or flavoring makes mix more palatable. Don't mix with ice cream, milk, or sherbet because these decrease adsorptive capacity of activated charcoal.

• *Alert:* Don't aspirate or allow patient to aspirate charcoal powder; this has resulted in death.

• Give by large-bore nasogastric tube after lavage, if needed.

• If patient vomits shortly after administration, be prepared to repeat dose.

• Space doses at least 1 hour apart from other drugs if treatment is for indications other than poisoning.

• Follow treatment with stool softener or laxative to prevent constipation unless sorbitol is part of product ingredients. Preparations made with sorbitol have a laxative effect that lessens risk of severe constipation or fecal impaction.

• Don't use charcoal with sorbitol in fructose-intolerant patients or in children younger than age 1.

• *Alert:* Drug is ineffective for poisoning or overdose of cyanide, mineral acids, caustic alkalis, and organic solvents; it's not very effective for overdose of ethanol, lithium, methanol, and iron salts.

• *Alert:* Don't confuse Actidose with Actos.

## PATIENT TEACHING
• Explain use and administration of drug to patient (if awake) and family.

• Warn patient that stools will be black until all the charcoal has passed through the body.

• Instruct patient to drink 6 to 8 glasses of liquid per day because charcoal can cause constipation.

# aminocaproic acid
Amicar

*Pregnancy risk category C*

## AVAILABLE FORMS
*Injection:* 250 mg/ml
*Syrup:* 250 mg/ml
*Tablets:* 500 mg

## INDICATIONS & DOSAGES
➤ **Excessive bleeding resulting from hyperfibrinolysis**
*Adults:* Initially, 5 g P.O. or slow I.V. infusion; then 1 to 1.25 g hourly until bleeding is controlled. Maximum dose is 30 g daily.

## I.V. ADMINISTRATION
• Dilute solution with sterile water for injection, normal saline solution for injection, $D_5W$, or Ringer's injection.

• Infuse slowly. Arrhythmias may be precipitated by too-rapid infusion.

• Don't give by direct or intermittent injection.

• *Alert:* Don't give by bolus injection because of risk of hypotension, bradycardia, and arrhythmias.

## ACTION
Inhibits plasminogen activator substances and, to a lesser degree, blocks antiplasmin activity by inhibiting fibrinolysis.

| Route | Onset | Peak | Duration |
|-------|-------|------|----------|
| P.O. | 1 hr | 2 hr | Unknown |
| I.V. | 1 hr | Unknown | 3 hr |

## ADVERSE REACTIONS
**CNS:** dizziness, malaise, headache, delirium, *seizures,* hallucinations, weakness.
**CV:** hypotension, *bradycardia, arrhythmias.*
**EENT:** tinnitus, nasal congestion, conjunctival suffusion.
**GI:** nausea, cramps, diarrhea.
**GU:** *acute renal failure.*
**Hematologic:** generalized thrombosis.
**Musculoskeletal:** myopathy.
**Skin:** rash.

---

*Rapid onset*   †Canada   ‡Australia   ◇OTC   ◆Off-label use   ❡Photoguide   *Liquid contains alcohol.

### INTERACTIONS
**Drug-drug.** *Estrogens, hormonal contraceptives:* May increase probability of hypercoagulability. Use together cautiously.

### EFFECTS ON LAB TEST RESULTS
• May increase BUN, creatinine, CK, AST, and ALT levels.

### CONTRAINDICATIONS & CAUTIONS
• Contraindicated in patients with hematuria, active intravascular clotting, or DIC, unless used with heparin.
• Injectable form contraindicated in newborns.
• Use cautiously in patients with cardiac, hepatic, or renal disease.

### NURSING CONSIDERATIONS
• *Alert:* Monitor coagulation studies, along with heart rhythm and blood pressure. Notify prescriber of changes immediately.
• *Alert:* Don't confuse Amicar with Amikin.

### PATIENT TEACHING
• Explain use and administration of drug to patient and family.
• Instruct patient to report adverse reactions promptly.
• Monitor patient closely for response.

---

### digoxin immune Fab (ovine)
Digibind, DigiFab

*Pregnancy risk category C*

### AVAILABLE FORMS
*Injection:* 38-mg vial (Digibind), 40-mg vial (DigiFab)

### INDICATIONS & DOSAGES
➤ **Potentially life-threatening digitalis toxicity**
*Adults and children:* Base dosage on ingested amount or level of digoxin. When calculating amount of antidote, round up to the nearest whole number.

For digoxin tablets, calculate number of antidote vials as follows: multiply ingested amount by 0.8; then divide answer by 0.5. For example, if patient takes 25 tablets of 0.25 mg digoxin, the ingested amount is 6.25 mg. Multiply 6.25 mg by

0.8 and divide answer by 0.5 to obtain 10 vials of antidote.

For digoxin capsules, divide the ingested dose in mg by 0.5. For example, if patient takes 50 capsules of 0.2 mg, the ingested amount is 10 mg. Divide 10 mg by 0.5 to obtain 20 vials of antidote.

If digoxin level is known, determine the number of antidote vials as follows: multiply the digoxin level in nanograms per milliliter by patient's weight in kg, then divide by 100. For example, if digoxin level is 4 nanograms/ml, and patient weighs 60 kg, multiply together to obtain 240. Divide answer by 100 to obtain 2.4 vials; then round up to 3 vials.
➤ **Acute toxicity, or if estimated ingested amount or digoxin level is unknown**
*Adults and children:* Consider giving 10 vials of digoxin immune Fab and observing patient's response. Follow with another 10 vials if indicated. Dosage should be effective in most life-threatening cases in adults and children but may cause volume overload in young children.

### I.V. ADMINISTRATION
• Reconstitute drug immediately before use with 4 ml of sterile water for injection.
• For infusion, further dilute solution with normal saline solution.
• For children or other patients who need small doses, reconstitute 38-mg vial Digibind with 38 ml of normal saline solution to yield 1 mg/ml concentration; reconstitute 40-mg vial DigiFab with 40 ml of normal saline solution to yield 1 mg/ml concentration.
• Drug may be given by direct injection if cardiac arrest seems imminent. Or, dilute with normal saline solution for injection to an appropriate volume and give by intermittent infusion over 30 minutes.
• Infuse drug through a 0.22-micron membrane filter.
• Refrigerate powder for injection. Reconstituted solutions may be refrigerated for 4 hours.

### ACTION
Binds molecules of unbound digoxin and digitoxin, making them unavailable for binding at site of action on cells.

---

| Route | Onset | Peak | Duration |
|-------|-------|------|----------|
| I.V. | 30 min | End of infusion | 15-20 hr |

## ADVERSE REACTIONS
**CV:** *heart failure,* rapid ventricular rate, worsening low cardiac output.
**Metabolic:** hypokalemia.
**Other:** hypersensitivity reactions, *anaphylaxis.*

## INTERACTIONS
None significant.

## EFFECTS ON LAB TEST RESULTS
• May decrease potassium level.
• May interfere with digitalis immunoassay measurements until drug is cleared from the body (about 48 hours).

## CONTRAINDICATIONS & CAUTIONS
• Use cautiously in patients allergic to sheep proteins and in those who have previously received antibodies.

## NURSING CONSIDERATIONS
• In patients allergic to sheep proteins and in those who have previously received antibodies, skin testing is recommended because drug is derived from digoxin-specific antibody fragments obtained from immunized sheep.
• Drug is used for life-threatening overdose in patients with anaphylaxis, severe hypotension, or cardiac arrest and in those with ventricular arrhythmias (such as ventricular tachycardia or fibrillation), progressive bradycardia (such as severe sinus bradycardia), or second- or third-degree AV block not responsive to atropine.
• Heart failure and rapid ventricular rate may result by reversal of cardiac glycoside's therapeutic effects.
• Monitor potassium level closely.
• In most patients, signs of digitalis toxicity disappear within a few hours.

## PATIENT TEACHING
• Explain use and administration of drug to patient and family.
• Instruct patient to report adverse reactions promptly.

# dimercaprol
BAL in Oil

*Pregnancy risk category C*

## AVAILABLE FORMS
*Injection:* 100 mg/ml

## INDICATIONS & DOSAGES
➤ **Severe arsenic or gold poisoning**
*Adults and children:* 3 mg/kg deep I.M. q 4 hours for 2 days; then q.i.d. on third day; then b.i.d. for 10 days.
➤ **Mild arsenic or gold poisoning**
*Adults and children:* 2.5 mg/kg deep I.M. q.i.d. for 2 days; then b.i.d. on third day; then once daily for 10 days.
➤ **Mercury poisoning**
*Adults and children:* Initially, 5 mg/kg deep I.M.; then 2.5 mg/kg daily or b.i.d. for 10 days.
➤ **Acute lead encephalopathy or lead level greater than 100 mcg/ml**
*Adults and children:* 4 mg/kg deep I.M.; then q 4 hours with edetate calcium disodium for 2 to 7 days. Use separate sites. For less severe poisoning, reduce dose to 3 mg/kg after first dose.

## ACTION
Forms complexes with heavy metals to create chelates that are renally excreted.

| Route | Onset | Peak | Duration |
|-------|-------|------|----------|
| I.M. | Unknown | 30-60 min | 4 hr |

## ADVERSE REACTIONS
**CNS:** headache, *fever,* paresthesia, anxiety.
**CV:** *transient increase in blood pressure, tachycardia.*
**EENT:** blepharospasm, conjunctivitis, lacrimation, rhinorrhea.
**GI:** *nausea, vomiting,* excessive salivation, *abdominal pain, burning sensation in lips, mouth, and throat.*
**Musculoskeletal:** muscle pain or weakness.
**Other:** pain or tightness in throat, chest, or hands.

## INTERACTIONS
**Drug-drug.** *Iron:* May cause toxic metal complex. Take iron 24 hours after last dimercaprol dose.

**EFFECTS ON LAB TEST RESULTS**
• May block thyroid uptake of iodine 131, causing decreased values.

**CONTRAINDICATIONS & CAUTIONS**
• Contraindicated in patients with hepatic dysfunction (except postarsenical jaundice) or iron, cadmium, or selenium poisoning; also contraindicated in those allergic to peanuts.
• Don't use in pregnant patient except to treat life-threatening acute poisoning.
• Use cautiously in patients with hypertension, G6PD deficiency, or oliguria.

**NURSING CONSIDERATIONS**
• *Alert:* Don't give drug I.V.; give by deep I.M. route only.
• Don't let drug contact skin because it may cause a skin reaction.
• Drug has an unpleasant, garlicky odor.
• Solution with slight sediment is usable.
• Use antihistamine to prevent or relieve mild adverse reactions.
• Keep urine alkaline to prevent renal damage.

**PATIENT TEACHING**
• Explain use and administration of drug to patient and family.
• Instruct patient to report adverse reactions promptly.

---

# disulfiram
Antabuse

*Pregnancy risk category NR*

---

**AVAILABLE FORMS**
*Tablets:* 250 mg, 500 mg

**INDICATIONS & DOSAGES**
➤ **Adjunct to management of chronic alcoholism**
*Adults:* 250 to 500 mg P.O. as single dose in morning for 1 to 2 weeks or in evening if drowsiness occurs. Maintenance dosage is 125 to 500 mg P.O. daily (average 250 mg) until permanent self-control is established. Treatment may continue for months or years.

**ACTION**
Blocks oxidation of alcohol at the acetaldehyde stage. Excess acetaldehyde produces a highly unpleasant reaction in the presence of even small amounts of alcohol.

| Route | Onset | Peak | Duration |
|-------|-------|------|----------|
| P.O. | 1-2 hr | Unknown | 14 days |

**ADVERSE REACTIONS**
**CNS:** drowsiness, headache, fatigue, delirium, depression, neuritis, peripheral neuritis, polyneuritis, restlessness, psychotic reactions.
**EENT:** optic neuritis.
**GI:** metallic or garlicky aftertaste.
**GU:** impotence.
**Skin:** acneiform or allergic dermatitis, occasional eruptions.
**Other:** *disulfiram-like reaction precipitated by alcohol use.*

**INTERACTIONS**
**Drug-drug.** *Barbiturates:* May prolong duration of barbiturate effect. Closely monitor patient.
*CNS depressants:* May increase CNS depression. Use together cautiously.
*Coumarin anticoagulants:* May increase anticoagulant effect. Adjust dosage of anticoagulant.
*Isoniazid:* May cause ataxia or marked change in behavior. Avoid using together.
*Metronidazole:* May cause psychotic reaction. Avoid using together.
*Midazolam:* May increase levels of midazolam. Use together cautiously.
*Paraldehyde:* May cause toxic levels of acetaldehyde. Avoid using together.
*Phenytoin:* May increase toxic effects of phenytoin. Monitor phenytoin levels closely and adjust dose as necessary.
*Tricyclic antidepressants, especially amitriptyline:* May cause transient delirium. Closely monitor patient.
**Drug-herb.** *Herbal preparations containing alcohol:* May cause disulfiram-like reaction. Warn patient against using together. Alcohol reaction may occur as long as 2 weeks after single disulfiram dose.
**Drug-food.** *Caffeine:* May increase elimination half-life of caffeine. Tell patient to watch for effects.
**Drug-lifestyle.** *Alcohol use:* May cause disulfiram reaction including flushing,

tachycardia, bronchospasm, sweating, nausea, and vomiting, or death. Warn patient not to use products containing alcohol, including backrub preparations, cough syrups, liniments, and shaving lotion, or to drink alcoholic beverages.

## EFFECTS ON LAB TEST RESULTS
• May increase cholesterol level.

## CONTRAINDICATIONS & CAUTIONS
• Contraindicated in patients hypersensitive to disulfiram or other thiram derivatives used in pesticides and rubber vulcanization; in those with psychoses, myocardial disease, or coronary occlusion; in those receiving metronidazole, paraldehyde, alcohol, or alcohol-containing products; and in those experiencing alcohol intoxication or who have ingested alcohol in preceding 12 hours.
• Don't give drug during pregnancy.
• Use with caution in patients receiving concurrent phenytoin therapy and in those with diabetes mellitus, hypothyroidism, seizure disorder, cerebral damage, nephritis, or hepatic cirrhosis or insufficiency.

## NURSING CONSIDERATIONS
• Never give until patient has abstained from alcohol for at least 12 hours. He should clearly understand consequences of disulfiram therapy and give permission for its use. Use drug only in patients who are cooperative, well motivated, and receiving supportive psychiatric therapy.
• Complete physical examination and laboratory studies, including CBC, SMA-12, and transaminase level, should precede therapy and be repeated regularly.
• Disulfiram-like reaction may result from alcohol use, with flushing, throbbing headache, dyspnea, nausea, copious vomiting, diaphoresis, thirst, chest pain, palpitations, hyperventilation, hypotension, syncope, anxiety, weakness, blurred vision, confusion, and arthropathy.
• *Alert:* A severe disulfiram-like reaction can cause respiratory depression, CV collapse, arrhythmias, MI, acute heart failure, seizures, unconsciousness, and death.
• The longer the patient remains on the drug, the more sensitive he becomes to alcohol.

• *Alert:* Don't confuse Antabuse with Anturane.

## PATIENT TEACHING
• *Alert:* Caution patient's family that disulfiram should never be given to patient without his knowledge; severe reaction or death could result if patient drinks alcohol.
• Tell patient to wear or carry medical identification that identifies him as a disulfiram user.
• Mild reactions may occur in sensitive patient with blood alcohol levels of 5 to 10 mg/dl; symptoms are fully developed at 50 mg/dl; unconsciousness typically occurs at 125 to 150 mg/dl level. Reaction may last from 30 minutes to several hours or as long as alcohol remains in blood.
• Reassure patient that disulfiram-induced adverse reactions (unrelated to alcohol use), such as drowsiness, fatigue, impotence, headache, peripheral neuritis, and metallic or garlic taste, subside after about 2 weeks of therapy.
• Advise patient not to drink alcoholic beverages or use products containing alcohol, including topical preparations and mouthwash.
• Have patient verify content of OTC products with pharmacist before use.

---

# edetate calcium disodium
Calcium Disodium Versenate, Calcium EDTA

*Pregnancy risk category B*

## AVAILABLE FORMS
*Injection:* 200 mg/ml

## INDICATIONS & DOSAGES
➤ **Acute lead encephalopathy or lead levels greater than 70 mcg/dl**
*Adults and children:* 1 to 1.5 g/m² I.V. or I.M. daily in divided doses at 8- to 12-hour intervals for 5 days, usually with dimercaprol. A second course may be given after at least 2-day drug-free interval.
➤ **Lead poisoning without encephalopathy or asymptomatic with lead levels less than 70 mcg/dl**
*Children:* 1 g/m² I.V. or I.M. daily in divided doses for 5 days.

---

**I.V. ADMINISTRATION**
● Dilute the 5-ml ampule with 500 ml or 250 ml of $D_5W$ or normal saline solution for injection to 2 to 4 mg/ml, respectively.
● Infuse half of daily dose over 1 hour and rest of infusion at least 12 hours later. Or, give by slow infusion over at least 8 hours.

**ACTION**
Forms stable, soluble complexes with metals, particularly lead.

| Route | Onset | Peak | Duration |
|-------|-------|------|----------|
| I.V., I.M. | 1 hr | 24-48 hr | Unknown |

**ADVERSE REACTIONS**
**CNS:** fever, tremors, headache, paresthesia, malaise, fatigue.
**CV:** hypotension, rhythm irregularities.
**EENT:** histamine-like reactions (including sneezing, congestion, and lacrimation).
**GI:** cheilosis, nausea, vomiting, anorexia, excessive thirst.
**GU:** proteinuria, hematuria, *nephrotoxicity with renal tubular necrosis leading to fatal nephrosis.*
**Hematologic:** *transient bone marrow suppression,* anemia.
**Metabolic:** zinc deficiency, hypercalcemia.
**Musculoskeletal:** myalgia, arthralgia.
**Skin:** rash.
**Other:** pain at I.M. injection site, chills.

**INTERACTIONS**
**Drug-drug.** *Insulin:* May interfere with action of insulin by binding with zinc. Adjust insulin dosage as directed.

**EFFECTS ON LAB TEST RESULTS**
● May increase AST, ALT, and calcium levels.
● May decrease hemoglobin.

**CONTRAINDICATIONS & CAUTIONS**
● Contraindicated in patients with anuria, hepatitis, or acute renal disease.
● Use with caution in patients with mild renal disease. Expect dosages to be reduced.

**NURSING CONSIDERATIONS**
● Add procaine hydrochloride to I.M. solution to minimize pain. Watch for local reactions.

● **Alert:** Because rapid I.V. use may increase intracranial pressure, I.M. route may be preferred for treating lead encephalopathy.
● Although I.M. route may be preferred for children and patients with lead encephalopathy, most experts recommend I.V. infusion whenever possible.
● Monitor fluid intake and output, urinalysis, BUN level, and ECG daily.
● To avoid toxicity, use with dimercaprol; don't mix in same syringe.
● **Alert:** Don't confuse edetate calcium disodium with edetate disodium.

**PATIENT TEACHING**
● Explain use and administration of drug to patient and family.
● Tell patients with lead encephalopathy to avoid excess fluids.

**edetate disodium**
Disodium EDTA, Endrate

*Pregnancy risk category C*

**AVAILABLE FORMS**
*Injection:* 150 mg/ml

**INDICATIONS & DOSAGES**
➤ **Hypercalcemic crisis**
*Adults:* 50 mg/kg/day by slow I.V. infusion over at least 3 hours. Maximum dose is 3 g/day.
*Children:* 40 mg/kg/day by slow I.V. infusion over at least 3 hours. Maximum dose is 70 mg/kg/day.

**I.V. ADMINISTRATION**
● Dilute drug in 500 ml of $D_5W$ or normal saline solution and infuse over 3 or more hours.
● **Alert:** Avoid rapid I.V. infusion; profound hypocalcemia may occur, leading to tetany, seizures, arrhythmias, and respiratory arrest. Drug isn't recommended for direct or intermittent injection. Monitor patient for signs of extravasation.
● Record I.V. site used, and avoid repeated use of same site because doing so increases likelihood of thrombophlebitis.

**ACTION**
Chelates with metals such as calcium to form a stable, soluble complex.

Reactions may be *common,* uncommon, *life-threatening,* or COMMON AND LIFE-THREATENING.

| Route | Onset | Peak | Duration |
|-------|-------|------|----------|
| I.V. | Unknown | Unknown | Unknown |

## ADVERSE REACTIONS
**CNS:** circumoral paresthesia, numbness, headache.
**CV:** hypotension, thrombophlebitis.
**EENT:** erythema.
**GI:** nausea, vomiting, diarrhea.
**GU:** *nephrotoxicity with urinary urgency,* nocturia, dysuria, polyuria, proteinuria, renal insufficiency, *renal failure, tubular necrosis.*
**Metabolic:** severe hypocalcemia.
**Skin:** exfoliative dermatitis.
**Other:** pain at infusion site.

## INTERACTIONS
None significant.

## EFFECTS ON LAB TEST RESULTS
• May decrease calcium and magnesium levels.

## CONTRAINDICATIONS & CAUTIONS
• Contraindicated in patients hypersensitive to drug and in those with anuria, known or suspected hypocalcemia, significant renal disease, active or healed tubercular lesions, or history of seizures or intracranial lesions.
• Use cautiously in patients with limited cardiac reserve, heart failure, or hypokalemia.

## NURSING CONSIDERATIONS
• Keep I.V. calcium available to treat hypocalcemia.
• Keep patients in bed for 15 minutes after infusion to avoid effects of orthostatic hypotension. Monitor blood pressure closely.
• Monitor ECG and renal function tests frequently.
• Obtain calcium level after each dose.
• Don't use to treat lead toxicity; use edetate calcium disodium instead.
• *Alert:* Don't confuse edetate disodium with edetate calcium disodium.

## PATIENT TEACHING
• Explain use and administration of drug to patient and family.
• Instruct patient to report adverse reactions promptly.

# flumazenil
Romazicon

*Pregnancy risk category C*

## AVAILABLE FORMS
*Injection:* 0.1 mg/ml in 5- and 10-ml multiple-dose vials

## INDICATIONS & DOSAGES
➤ **Complete or partial reversal of sedative effects of benzodiazepines after anesthesia or conscious sedation**
*Adults:* Initially, 0.2 mg I.V. over 15 seconds. If patient doesn't reach desired level of consciousness after 45 seconds, repeat dose. Repeat at 1-minute intervals, if needed, until cumulative dose of 1 mg has been given (first dose plus four more doses). Most patients respond after 0.6 to 1 mg of drug. In case of resedation, dosage may be repeated after 20 minutes, but never give more than 1 mg at any one time or exceed 3 mg/hour.
*Children age 1 year and older:* 0.01 mg/kg I.V. over 15 seconds. If patient doesn't reach desired level of consciousness after 45 seconds, repeat dose. Repeat at 1-minute intervals, if needed, until cumulative dose of 0.05 mg/kg or 1 mg, whichever is lower, has been given (first dose plus four more doses).
➤ **Suspected benzodiazepine overdose**
*Adults:* Initially, 0.2 mg I.V. over 30 seconds. If patient doesn't reach desired level of consciousness after 30 seconds, give 0.3 mg over 30 seconds. If patient still doesn't respond adequately, give 0.5 mg over 30 seconds. Repeat 0.5-mg doses, p.r.n., at 1-minute intervals until cumulative dose of 3 mg has been given. Most patients with benzodiazepine overdose respond to cumulative doses between 1 and 3 mg; rarely, patients who respond partially after 3 mg may need additional doses, up to 5 mg total. If patient doesn't respond in 5 minutes after receiving 5 mg, sedation is unlikely to be caused by benzodiazepines. In case of resedation, dosage may be repeated after 20 minutes, but never give more than 1 mg at any one time or exceed 3 mg/hour.

## I.V. ADMINISTRATION
• Make sure airway is secure and patent.
• Inject drug into large vein through free-flowing I.V. line over 15 to 30 seconds to minimize pain at injection site. Compatible solutions include $D_5W$, lactated Ringer's injection, and normal saline solution.
• Store drug in vial until use. Drug is stable in a syringe for 24 hours.
• Monitor patient for signs of extravasation into perivascular tissues.

## ACTION
A benzodiazepine antagonist that competitively inhibits the actions of benzodiazepines on the gamma-aminobutyric acid–benzodiazepine receptor complex.

| Route | Onset | Peak | Duration |
|-------|-------|------|----------|
| I.V. | 1-2 min | 6-10 min | Variable |

## ADVERSE REACTIONS
**CNS:** *dizziness, abnormal or blurred vision, headache,* **seizures,** agitation, emotional lability, tremor, insomnia.
**CV:** *arrhythmias,* cutaneous vasodilation, palpitations.
**GI:** *nausea, vomiting.*
**Respiratory:** dyspnea, hyperventilation.
**Skin:** *diaphoresis.*
**Other:** *pain at injection site.*

## INTERACTIONS
**Drug-drug.** *Antidepressants, drugs that may cause seizures or arrhythmias:* May cause seizures or arrhythmias. Don't use flumazenil when overdose involves more than one drug, especially when seizures (from any cause) are likely to occur.

## EFFECTS ON LAB TEST RESULTS
None reported.

## CONTRAINDICATIONS & CAUTIONS
• Contraindicated in patients hypersensitive to flumazenil or benzodiazepines, in those who show evidence of serious tricyclic antidepressant overdose, and in those who have received benzodiazepines to treat a potentially life-threatening condition, such as status epilepticus.
• Use cautiously in patients with head injury, psychiatric disorders, or alcohol dependence.

• Use cautiously in patients at high risk for developing seizures and in those who have recently received multiple doses of a parenteral benzodiazepine, who display signs of seizure activity, or who may be at risk for benzodiazepine dependence, such as intensive care unit patients.

## NURSING CONSIDERATIONS
• Monitor patient closely for resedation that may occur after reversal of benzodiazepine effects because flumazenil's duration of action is shorter than that of all benzodiazepines. Duration of monitoring period depends on specific drug being reversed. Monitor patient closely after doses of long-acting benzodiazepines, such as diazepam, or after high doses of short-acting benzodiazepines, such as 10 mg of midazolam. In most cases, severe resedation is unlikely in patients who fail to show signs of resedation 2 hours after a 1-mg dose of flumazenil.

## PATIENT TEACHING
• Warn patient not to perform hazardous activities within 24 hours of procedure because of resedation risk.
• Tell patient to avoid alcohol, CNS depressants, and OTC drugs for 24 hours.
• Give family necessary instructions or provide patient with written instructions. Patient won't recall information given after the procedure; drug doesn't reverse amnesic effects of benzodiazepines.

---

# naloxone hydrochloride
Narcan

*Pregnancy risk category B*

## AVAILABLE FORMS
*Injection:* 0.02 mg/ml, 0.4 mg/ml, 1 mg/ml

## INDICATIONS & DOSAGES
➤ **Known or suspected narcotic-induced respiratory depression, including that caused by pentazocine and propoxyphene**
*Adults:* 0.4 to 2 mg I.V., I.M., or S.C., repeated q 2 to 3 minutes, p.r.n. If no response is observed after 10 mg has been given, question diagnosis of narcotic-induced toxicity.

---

*Children:* 0.01 mg/kg I.V.; then second dose of 0.1 mg/kg I.V., if needed. If I.V. route isn't available, drug may be given I.M. or S.C. in divided doses.
*Neonates:* 0.01 mg/kg I.V., I.M., or S.C. Repeat dose q 2 to 3 minutes, p.r.n.
➤ **Postoperative narcotic depression**
*Adults:* 0.1 to 0.2 mg I.V. q 2 to 3 minutes, p.r.n. Repeat dose within 1 to 2 hours, if needed.
*Children:* 0.005 to 0.01 mg I.V. repeated q 2 to 3 minutes, p.r.n.
*Neonates (asphyxia neonatorum):* 0.01 mg/ kg I.V. into umbilical vein. May be repeated q 2 to 3 minutes.

### I.V. ADMINISTRATION
• Be prepared to give continuous I.V. infusion to control adverse effects of epidural morphine.
• If 0.02 mg/ml isn't available, adult concentration (0.4 mg) can be diluted by mixing 0.5 ml with 9.5 ml of sterile water for injection to make neonatal concentration (0.02 mg/ml).
• Don't mix with drugs containing bisulfite, metabisulfite, long-chain or high–molecular-weight anions, or any solution with an alkaline pH.

### ACTION
Unknown. Thought to displace previously given narcotic analgesics from their receptors (competitive antagonism); drug has no pharmacologic activity of its own.

| Route | Onset | Peak | Duration |
|---|---|---|---|
| I.V. | 1-2 min | 5-15 min | Variable |
| I.M., S.C. | 2-5 min | 5-15 min | Variable |

### ADVERSE REACTIONS
**CNS:** tremors, *seizures.*
**CV:** tachycardia, hypertension with higher-than-recommended doses, hypotension, *ventricular fibrillation.*
**GI:** nausea, vomiting.
**Respiratory:** pulmonary edema.
**Skin:** diaphoresis.
**Other:** withdrawal symptoms in narcotic-dependent patients with higher-than-recommended doses.

### INTERACTIONS
None significant.

### EFFECTS ON LAB TEST RESULTS
None reported.

### CONTRAINDICATIONS & CAUTIONS
• Contraindicated in patients hypersensitive to drug.
• Use cautiously in patients with cardiac irritability or opiate addiction. Abrupt reversal of opiate-induced CNS depression may result in nausea, vomiting, diaphoresis, tachycardia, CNS excitement, and increased blood pressure.

### NURSING CONSIDERATIONS
• Duration of action of the narcotic may exceed that of naloxone, and patients may relapse into respiratory depression.
• Respiratory rate increases within 1 to 2 minutes.
• *Alert:* Drug is effective only in reversing respiratory depression caused by opiates, not against other drug-induced respiratory depression, including that caused by benzodiazepines.
• Patients who receive naloxone to reverse opioid-induced respiratory depression may exhibit tachypnea.
• Monitor respiratory depth and rate. Be prepared to provide oxygen, ventilation, and other resuscitation measures.
• *Alert:* Don't confuse naloxone with naltrexone.

### PATIENT TEACHING
• Inform family about use and administration of drug.
• Reassure family that patient will be monitored closely until effects of narcotic resolve.

### naltrexone hydrochloride
Depade, ReVia, Trexan

*Pregnancy risk category C*

### AVAILABLE FORMS
*Tablets:* 25 mg, 50 mg, 100 mg

### INDICATIONS & DOSAGES
➤ **Adjunct for maintenance of opioid-free state in detoxified persons**
*Adults:* Initially, 25 mg P.O. If no withdrawal signs occur within 1 hour, an additional 25 mg is given. Once patient has

been started on 50 mg q 24 hours, flexible maintenance schedule may be used. From 50 to 150 mg may be given daily, depending on schedule prescribed.
➤ **Alcohol dependence**
*Adults:* 50 mg P.O. once daily.

**ACTION**
Unknown. Probably reversibly blocks the subjective effects of opioids given I.V. by competitively occupying opiate receptors in the brain.

| Route | Onset | Peak | Duration |
|-------|-------|------|----------|
| P.O. | 15-30 min | 1 hr | 24 hr |

**ADVERSE REACTIONS**
**CNS:** *insomnia, anxiety, nervousness, headache,* depression, dizziness, fatigue, somnolence, ***suicidal ideation.***
**GI:** *nausea, vomiting,* anorexia, *abdominal pain,* constipation, increased thirst.
**GU:** delayed ejaculation, decreased potency.
**Hepatic:** *hepatotoxicity.*
**Musculoskeletal:** *muscle and joint pain.*
**Skin:** rash.
**Other:** chills.

**INTERACTIONS**
**Drug-drug.** *Opioid-containing products:* May decrease effect of opioid. Avoid using together.
*Thioridazine:* May increase somnolence and lethargy. Monitor patient closely.

**EFFECTS ON LAB TEST RESULTS**
● May increase AST, ALT, and LDH levels.
● May increase lymphocyte count.

**CONTRAINDICATIONS & CAUTIONS**
● Contraindicated in patients hypersensitive to drug, in those receiving opioid analgesics, in opioid-dependent patients, in patients in acute opioid withdrawal, and in those with positive urine screen for opioids or acute hepatitis or liver failure.
● Use cautiously in patients with mild hepatic disease or history of recent hepatic disease.

**NURSING CONSIDERATIONS**
● Treatment for opioid dependence shouldn't begin until patient receives naloxone challenge, a provocative test of

opioid dependence. If signs and symptoms of opioid withdrawal persist after naloxone challenge, don't give drug.
● Patient must be completely free from opioids before taking drug or severe withdrawal symptoms may occur. Patients who have been addicted to short-acting opioids, such as heroin and meperidine, must wait at least 7 days after last opioid dose before starting drug. Patients who have been addicted to longer-acting opioids such as methadone should wait at least 10 days.
● In an emergency, anticipate that patient receiving naltrexone may be given an opioid analgesic, but dose must be higher than usual to surmount naltrexone's effect. Watch for respiratory depression from the opioid; it may be longer and deeper.
● For patients expected to be noncompliant because of history of opioid dependence, be prepared to try a flexible maintenance dose regimen of 100 mg on Monday and Wednesday and 150 mg on Friday.
● Use drug only as part of a comprehensive rehabilitation program.
● ***Alert:*** Don't confuse naltrexone with naloxone.

**PATIENT TEACHING**
● Advise patient to wear or carry medical identification and to tell medical personnel that he takes naltrexone.
● Give patient names of nonopioid drugs that he can continue to take for pain, diarrhea, or cough.
● Tell patient to report adverse effects to prescriber immediately.

---

**penicillamine**
Cuprimine, Depen, D-Penamine‡

*Pregnancy risk category NR*

**AVAILABLE FORMS**
*Capsules:* 125 mg, 250 mg
*Tablets:* 125 mg‡, 250 mg

**INDICATIONS & DOSAGES**
➤ **Wilson's disease**
*Adults and children:* 250 mg P.O. q.i.d. on an empty stomach at least 60 minutes before any other drug, food, or milk, or 2

hours after meals. Adjust dosage to achieve urinary copper excretion of 0.5 to 1 mg daily.

➤ **Cystinuria**

*Adults:* 250 mg to 1 g P.O. q.i.d. on an empty stomach at least 60 minutes before any other drug, food, or milk, or 2 hours after meals. Adjust dosage to achieve urinary cystine excretion of less than 100 mg daily when renal calculi exist, or 100 to 200 mg daily when calculi don't exist. Maximum dose is 4 g daily.

*Children:* 30 mg/kg P.O. daily, divided q.i.d. at least 60 minutes before any other drug, food, or milk, or 2 hours after meals. Adjust dosage to achieve urinary cystine excretion of less than 100 mg daily when renal calculi exist, or 100 to 200 mg daily when calculi don't exist.

➤ **Rheumatoid arthritis**

*Adults:* Initially, 125 to 250 mg P.O. daily, with increases of 125 to 250 mg daily q 1 to 3 months, p.r.n. Maximum dose is 1.5 g daily.

## ACTION

Chelates heavy metals and may inhibit collagen formation. Mechanism unknown for rheumatoid arthritis.

| Route | Onset | Peak | Duration |
|-------|-------|------|----------|
| P.O. | Unknown | 1 hr | Unknown |

## ADVERSE REACTIONS

**EENT:** tinnitus, *optic neuritis.*

**GI:** *anorexia, epigastric pain, nausea, vomiting, diarrhea, loss of or altered taste perception, stomatitis.*

**GU:** nephrotic syndrome, glomerulo-nephritis, proteinuria, hematuria.

**Hematologic:** *leukopenia, eosinophilia, thrombocytopenia, monocytosis, agranulocytosis, aplastic anemia,* lupuslike syndrome.

**Hepatic:** *hepatotoxicity.*

**Metabolic:** *hypoglycemia.*

**Musculoskeletal:** *arthralgia.*

**Respiratory:** *pneumonitis.*

**Skin:** alopecia; friability, especially at pressure spots; wrinkling; erythema; urticaria; ecchymoses.

**Other:** myasthenia gravis syndrome with long-term use, allergic reactions, *lymphadenopathy.*

## INTERACTIONS

**Drug-drug.** *Antacids, oral iron:* May decrease effectiveness of penicillamine. Separate doses by at least 2 hours.

*Antimalarials, cytotoxic drugs, gold therapy, phenylbutazone:* May cause serious hematologic and renal reactions. Avoid using together.

*Digoxin:* May decrease digoxin level. Digoxin dose may need to be increased.

**Drug-food.** *Any food:* May delay and decrease absorption of drug. Tell patient to take drug 1 hour before or 2 hours after meals.

## EFFECTS ON LAB TEST RESULTS

• May decrease glucose level.

• May increase eosinophil count. May decrease hemoglobin and WBC, platelet, and granulocyte counts.

• May cause positive test results for antinuclear antibody with or without clinical systemic lupus-like syndrome.

## CONTRAINDICATIONS & CAUTIONS

• Contraindicated in breast-feeding women, in pregnant women who have cystinuria, in patients with penicillamine-related aplastic anemia or granulocytosis, and in those with rheumatoid arthritis or renal insufficiency.

• Use with caution, if at all, in patients hypersensitive to penicillin.

## NURSING CONSIDERATIONS

• Patients who have had a major toxic reaction to gold salt therapy may be at greater risk for serious adverse reactions.

• Patient should receive supplemental pyridoxine daily.

• If patient has a skin reaction, give antihistamines. Handle patient carefully to avoid skin damage.

• Monitor CBC and renal and hepatic function every 2 weeks for first 6 months; then monthly.

• Monitor urinalysis regularly for protein loss.

• *Alert:* Report rash and fever (important signs of toxicity) to prescriber immediately.

• Withhold drug and notify prescriber if WBC count falls below 3,500/mm³ or platelet count falls below 100,000/mm³. A progressive decline in platelet or WBC count in three successive blood tests may necessitate temporary cessation of therapy, even if such counts are within normal limits.

● *Alert:* Don't confuse penicillamine with penicillin, or Depen with Endep.

## PATIENT TEACHING
● Tell patient that therapeutic effect may be delayed up to 3 months in treatment of rheumatoid arthritis.
● Tell patient to take drug on an empty stomach, at least 1 hour before or 2 hours after meals, or 3 hours after the evening meal, and to maintain adequate fluid intake, especially at night.
● Advise patient to report early signs of granulocytopenia: fever, sore throat, chills, bruising, and prolonged bleeding time.
● Reassure patient that taste impairment usually resolves in 6 weeks without changes in dosage.

---

## pralidoxime chloride (2-PAM chloride, 2-pyridine-aldoxime methochloride)
Protopam Chloride

*Pregnancy risk category C*

## AVAILABLE FORMS
*Injection:* 1 g/20 ml in 20-ml vial without diluent or syringe; 600 mg/2 ml auto-injector, parenteral

## INDICATIONS & DOSAGES
➤ **Antidote for organophosphate poisoning**
*Adults:* 1 to 2 g in 100 ml of normal saline solution by I.V. infusion over 15 to 30 minutes. Repeat in 1 hour if muscle weakness persists. Additional doses may be given cautiously. I.M. or S.C. injection may be used if I.V. isn't feasible.
*Children:* 20 to 40 mg/kg I.V., given as for adults.
➤ **Cholinergic crisis in myasthenia gravis**
*Adults:* 1 to 2 g I.V.; then 250 mg I.V. q 5 minutes, p.r.n.

## I.V. ADMINISTRATION
● Reconstitute by adding 20 ml of sterile water for injection to vial containing 1 g

of drug. Further dilute by adding 100 ml of normal saline solution. Infuse over 15 to 30 minutes.
● If patient has pulmonary edema, give drug by slow I.V. push over 5 minutes. Don't exceed 200 mg/minute.
● *Alert:* If drug is infused too rapidly, tachycardia, laryngospasm, and muscle rigidity may result.

## ACTION
Reactivates cholinesterase inactivated by organophosphorus pesticides and related compounds, permitting degradation of accumulated acetylcholine and facilitating normal functioning of neuromuscular junctions.

| Route | Onset | Peak | Duration |
|-------|-------|------|----------|
| I.V. | Unknown | 5-15 min | Unknown |
| I.M. | Unknown | 10-20 min | Unknown |
| S.C. | Unknown | Unknown | Unknown |

## ADVERSE REACTIONS
**CNS:** dizziness, headache, drowsiness.
**CV:** tachycardia.
**EENT:** blurred vision, diplopia, impaired accommodation.
**GI:** nausea.
**Musculoskeletal:** muscle weakness.
**Respiratory:** hyperventilation.
**Other:** mild to moderate pain at injection site.

## INTERACTIONS
**Drug-drug.** *Barbiturates:* May increase anticholinesterases level. Use together cautiously to treat seizures.

## EFFECTS ON LAB TEST RESULTS
● May increase liver enzyme levels.

## CONTRAINDICATIONS & CAUTIONS
● Contraindicated in patients hypersensitive to drug.
● Use with caution in patients with myasthenia gravis (overdose may trigger myasthenic crisis) and in those with impaired renal function.

## NURSING CONSIDERATIONS
● Initially, remove secretions, maintain patent airway, and institute mechanical ventilation, if needed. After dermal exposure to organophosphate, remove patient's

---

clothing and wash his skin and hair with sodium bicarbonate, soap, water, and alcohol as soon as possible. A second washing may be needed. When washing patient, wear protective gloves and clothes to avoid exposure.

• Draw blood for cholinesterase level before giving drug.

• Use drug only in hospitalized patients; have respiratory and other supportive measures available. If possible, obtain accurate medical history and chronology of poisoning. Give drug as soon as possible after poisoning; treatment is most effective if started within 24 hours after exposure.

• To ameliorate muscarinic effects and block accumulation of acetylcholine associated with organophosphate poisoning, give atropine 2 to 4 mg I.V. with pralidoxime if cyanosis isn't present; if cyanosis is present, give atropine I.M. Give atropine every 5 to 10 minutes until signs of atropine toxicity (flushing, tachycardia, dry mouth, blurred vision, excitement, delirium, and hallucinations) appear; maintain atropinization for at least 48 hours.

• Observe patient for 48 to 72 hours if he ingested poison. Delayed absorption may occur from lower bowel. It's difficult to distinguish between toxic effects produced by atropine or organophosphate compounds and those resulting from pralidoxime.

• In patient with myasthenia gravis who is being treated for overdose of cholinergic drugs, watch for signs of rapid weakening. He can pass quickly from cholinergic crisis to myasthenic crisis and needs more cholinergic drugs to treat myasthenia. Keep edrophonium available for establishing differential diagnosis.

• Avoid use of aminophylline, morphine, phenothiazine-like tranquilizers, reserpine, succinylcholine, and theophylline in patients with organophosphate poisoning.

• Drug isn't effective against poisoning caused by phosphorus, inorganic phosphates, or organophosphates with no anticholinesterase activity.

• **Alert:** Don't confuse pralidoxime with pramoxine or pyridoxine.

**PATIENT TEACHING**
• Explain use and administration of drug to patient and family.
• Tell patient to report adverse effects.
• Caution patient treated for organophosphate poisoning to avoid contact with insecticides for several weeks.

---

## protamine sulfate

*Pregnancy risk category C*

**AVAILABLE FORMS**
*Injection:* 10 mg/ml

**INDICATIONS & DOSAGES**
➤ **Heparin overdose**
*Adults:* Base dosage on venous blood coagulation studies, usually 1 mg for each 90 to 115 units of heparin. Give by slow I.V. injection over 10 minutes in doses not to exceed 50 mg.

**I.V. ADMINISTRATION**
• Have emergency equipment available to treat anaphylaxis or severe hypotension.
• **Alert:** Give slowly by direct I.V. injection. Excessively rapid I.V. administration may cause acute hypotension, bradycardia, pulmonary hypertension, dyspnea, transient flushing, and feeling of warmth.

**ACTION**
A heparin antagonist that forms a physiologically inert complex with heparin sodium.

| Route | Onset | Peak | Duration |
|-------|-------|------|----------|
| I.V. | 30-60 sec | Unknown | 2 hr |

**ADVERSE REACTIONS**
**CNS:** lassitude.
**CV:** hypotension, *bradycardia, circulatory collapse,* transient flushing.
**GI:** nausea, vomiting.
**Respiratory:** dyspnea, pulmonary edema, *acute pulmonary hypertension.*
**Other:** feeling of warmth, *anaphylaxis, anaphylactoid reactions.*

**INTERACTIONS**
None significant.

---

**EFFECTS ON LAB TEST RESULTS**
None reported.

**CONTRAINDICATIONS & CAUTIONS**
• Contraindicated in patients hypersensitive to drug.

**NURSING CONSIDERATIONS**
• Base postoperative dose on coagulation studies, and repeat activated partial thromboplastin time 15 minutes after administration.
• Calculate dosage carefully. One milligram of protamine neutralizes 90 to 115 units of heparin, depending on salt (heparin calcium or heparin sodium) and source of heparin (beef or pork).
• Risk of hypersensitivity reaction increases in patients hypersensitive to fish; in vasectomized or infertile men; and in patients taking protamine-insulin products.
• Monitor patient continually.
• Watch for spontaneous bleeding (heparin rebound), especially in dialysis patients and in those who have undergone cardiac surgery.
• Protamine may act as an anticoagulant in very high doses.
• *Alert:* Don't confuse protamine with Protopam or protropin.

**PATIENT TEACHING**
• Explain use and administration of drug to patient and family.
• Tell patient to report adverse effects.

---

**sodium polystyrene sulfonate**
Kayexalate, Kionex, SPS

*Pregnancy risk category C*

**AVAILABLE FORMS**
*Powder:* 1-lb jar (3.5 g/tsp)
*Suspension:* 15 g/60 ml*

**INDICATIONS & DOSAGES**
➤ **Hyperkalemia**
*Adults:* 15 g P.O. daily to q.i.d. in water or sorbitol (3 to 4 ml/g of resin). Or, mix powder with appropriate medium—aqueous suspension or diet appropriate for renal failure—and instill through a nasogastric tube. Or, 30 to 50 g/dl of sorbitol q 6

hours as warm emulsion deep into sigmoid colon (20 cm).
*Children:* 1 g/kg of body weight/dose P.O. or P.R., p.r.n.

**ACTION**
A potassium-removing resin that exchanges sodium ions for potassium ions in the intestine: 1 g of sodium polystyrene sulfonate is exchanged for 0.5 to 1 mEq of potassium. The resin is then eliminated. Much of the exchange capacity is used for cations other than potassium (calcium and magnesium) and possibly for fats and proteins.

| Route | Onset | Peak | Duration |
|-------|-------|------|----------|
| P.O., P.R. | 2-12 hr | Unknown | Unknown |

**ADVERSE REACTIONS**
**GI:** *constipation,* fecal impaction, anorexia, gastric irritation, nausea, vomiting, *diarrhea with sorbitol emulsions.*
**Metabolic:** hypokalemia, hypocalcemia, hypomagnesemia, sodium retention.

**INTERACTIONS**
**Drug-drug.** *Antacids and laxatives (nonabsorbable cation-donating types, including magnesium hydroxide):* May cause systemic alkalosis and reduce potassium exchange capability. Avoid using together.

**EFFECTS ON LAB TEST RESULTS**
• May increase sodium level. May decrease potassium, calcium, and magnesium levels.

**CONTRAINDICATIONS & CAUTIONS**
• Contraindicated in patients hypersensitive to drug and in those with hypokalemia.
• Use cautiously in patients with severe heart failure, severe hypertension, or marked edema. Drug provides 100 mg of sodium per gram.

**NURSING CONSIDERATIONS**
• Don't heat resin; this impairs drug's effect. Mix resin only with water or sorbitol for P.O. administration. Never mix with orange juice (high potassium content) to disguise taste.
• Chill oral suspension for greater palatability.

---

Reactions may be *common*, uncommon, *life-threatening*, or COMMON AND LIFE-THREATENING.

• Oral administration is preferred because drug should remain in intestine for at least 30 minutes.
• If sorbitol is given, mix with resin suspension.
• Consider giving in solid form. Resin cookie and candy recipes are available; ask pharmacist or dietitian to supply.
• Premixed forms (SPS and others) are available. If preparing manually, mix polystyrene resin only with water or sorbitol for rectal use. Don't use mineral oil for P.R. administration to prevent impaction; ion exchange needs aqueous medium. Sorbitol content prevents impaction.
• Prepare P.R. dose at room temperature. Stir emulsion gently during administration.
• Use #28 French rubber tube for rectal dose; insert 20 cm into sigmoid colon. Tape tube in place. Or, consider an indwelling urinary catheter with a 30-ml balloon inflated distal to anal sphincter to aid in retention. This is especially helpful for patients with poor sphincter control. Use gravity flow. Drain returns constantly through Y-tube connection. Place patient in knee-chest position or with hips on pillow for a while if back leakage occurs.
• After P.R. administration, flush tubing with 50 to 100 ml of nonsodium fluid to ensure delivery of all drug. Flush rectum to remove resin.
• Prevent fecal impaction in elderly patients by giving resin P.R. Give cleansing enema before P.R. administration. Have patient retain enema for 6 to 10 hours if possible, but 30 to 60 minutes is acceptable.
• Watch for constipation with oral or nasogastric administration. Give 10 to 20 ml of 70% sorbitol syrup every 2 hours, as needed, to produce one or two watery stools daily.
• Monitor potassium level at least once daily. Treatment may result in potassium deficiency and is usually stopped when potassium is reduced to 4 or 5 mEq/L.
• Watch for signs of hypokalemia: irritability, confusion, arrhythmias, ECG changes, severe muscle weakness, or sometimes paralysis, and digitalis toxicity in digitalized patients.
• When hyperkalemia is severe, polystyrene resin alone isn't adequate for lowering potassium. Dextrose 50% with regular insulin I.V. push may also be given.
• Watch for symptoms of other electrolyte deficiencies (magnesium, calcium) because drug is nonselective. Monitor calcium in patients receiving sodium polystyrene therapy for more than 3 days. Supplementary calcium may be needed.
• Watch for sodium overload. Drug contains about 100 mg sodium per gram. About one-third of resin's sodium is retained.

**PATIENT TEACHING**
• Explain use and administration of drug to patient.
• Advise patient to report adverse reactions promptly.
• Teach patient about low-potassium diet.

## succimer
Chemet

*Pregnancy risk category C*

**AVAILABLE FORMS**
*Capsules:* 100 mg

**INDICATIONS & DOSAGES**
➤ **Lead poisoning in children with lead levels greater than 45 mcg/dl**
*Children:* Initially, 10 mg/kg or 350 mg/$m^2$ q 8 hours for 5 days. Because capsules come only in 100 mg, round dose to nearest 100 mg, as appropriate (see table). Then reduce frequency of administration to q 12 hours for an additional 2 weeks.

| Weight in kg (lb) | Dose (mg) |
|---|---|
| > 45 (> 100) | 500 |
| 35-44 (78-98) | 400 |
| 24-34 (53-76) | 300 |
| 16-23 (36-51) | 200 |
| 8-15 (18-33) | 100 |

**ACTION**
A chelating drug that forms water-soluble complexes with lead and increases its excretion in urine.

| Route | Onset | Peak | Duration |
|---|---|---|---|
| P.O. | Unknown | 1-2 hr | Unknown |

## ADVERSE REACTIONS

**CNS:** *drowsiness, dizziness, sensorimotor neuropathy, sleepiness, paresthesia, headache.*

**CV:** *arrhythmias.*

**EENT:** plugged ears, cloudy film in eyes, otitis media, watery eyes, sore throat, rhinorrhea, nasal congestion.

**GI:** *nausea, vomiting, diarrhea, anorexia, abdominal cramps, hemorrhoidal symptoms, metallic taste in mouth, loose stools.*

**GU:** decreased urination, difficult urination, proteinuria.

**Hematologic:** increased platelet count, intermittent eosinophilia, *neutropenia.*

**Musculoskeletal:** *leg, kneecap, back, stomach, rib, or flank pain.*

**Respiratory:** cough, head cold.

**Skin:** papular rash, herpetic rash, mucocutaneous eruptions, pruritus.

**Other:** *flulike syndrome,* candidiasis.

## INTERACTIONS

**Drug-drug.** *Other chelating drugs (such as calcium EDTA):* May cause unknown adverse effects. Separate administration times by 4 weeks.

## EFFECTS ON LAB TEST RESULTS

● May increase AST, ALT, alkaline phosphatase, and cholesterol levels.
● May increase eosinophil and platelet counts.
● May cause false-positive urine ketone results.

## CONTRAINDICATIONS & CAUTIONS

● Contraindicated in patients hypersensitive to drug.
● Use cautiously in patients with compromised renal function.

## NURSING CONSIDERATIONS

● Measure severity of poisoning by initial lead level and by rate and degree of rebound of lead level. Use severity as a guide for more frequent lead monitoring.
● Monitor patient at least once weekly for rebound lead levels. Elevated levels and associated symptoms may return rapidly after drug is stopped because of redistribution of lead from bone to soft tissues and blood.

● Monitor transaminase levels before and at least weekly during therapy. Transient mild elevations may occur.
● Course of treatment lasts 19 days and may be repeated if indicated by weekly monitoring of lead levels.
● Minimum of 2 weeks between courses is recommended unless high lead levels indicate need for immediate therapy.
● Don't give with other chelating drugs. Patient who has received edetate calcium disodium with or without dimercaprol may use succimer after a 4-week interval.
● Stop treatment if absolute neutrophil count is less than 1,200/mm³.

## PATIENT TEACHING

● Explain drug use and administration to parents and child. Stress importance of complying with frequent blood tests.
● Tell parents of young child who can't swallow capsules that capsule can be opened and its contents sprinkled on a small amount of soft food. Or, beads from capsule may be poured on a spoon and followed with flavored beverage.
● Tell parents to give child adequate fluids.
● Assist parents with identifying and removing sources of lead in child's environment. Chelation therapy isn't a substitute for preventing further exposure.
● Tell parents to notify prescriber if rash occurs. Tell them allergic or other mucocutaneous reactions may occur each time drug is used.

---

Reactions may be *common,* uncommon, *life-threatening,* or COMMON AND LIFE-THREATENING.

alfuzosin hydrochloride
alprostadil
amifostine
aprotinin
becaplermin
capsaicin
clomiphene citrate
diclofenac sodium (topical)
dihydroergotamine mesylate
dutasteride
eflornithine hydrochloride
finasteride
imiquimod
isotretinoin
mesna
minoxidil (topical)
nimodipine
orlistat
pimecrolimus
raloxifene hydrochloride
riluzole
sildenafil citrate
tacrolimus (topical)
tadalafil
tamsulosin hydrochloride
thalidomide
tretinoin
vardenafil hydrochloride

**COMBINATION PRODUCTS**
None.

✳ *NEW DRUG*

---

## alfuzosin hydrochloride
UroXatral✔

*Pregnancy risk category B*

**AVAILABLE FORMS**
*Tablets (extended-release):* 10 mg

**INDICATIONS & DOSAGES**
➤ **BPH**
*Adult men:* 10 mg P.O. immediately after same meal each day.

**ACTION**
Selectively blocks alpha receptors in the prostate, leading to relaxation of smooth muscles in the bladder neck and prostate, improving urine flow, and reducing symptoms of BPH.

| Route | Onset | Peak | Duration |
|-------|-------|------|----------|
| P.O. | Unknown | 8 hr | Unknown |

**ADVERSE REACTIONS**
**CNS:** dizziness, fatigue, headache, pain.
**EENT:** pharyngitis, sinusitis.
**GI:** abdominal pain, constipation, dyspepsia, nausea.
**GU:** impotence.
**Respiratory:** bronchitis, upper respiratory tract infection.

**INTERACTIONS**
**Drug-drug.** *Antihypertensives (diltiazem):* May cause hypotension. Monitor blood pressure, and use together cautiously.
*Atenolol:* May cause hypotension and reduce heart rate. Monitor blood pressure and heart rate for these effects.
*Cimetidine:* May increase alfuzosin level. Use together cautiously.
*CYP 3A4 inhibitors (itraconazole, ketoconazole, ritonavir):* May increase alfuzosin level. Avoid using together.

**EFFECTS ON LAB TEST RESULTS**
None reported.

**CONTRAINDICATIONS & CAUTIONS**
• Contraindicated in patients with Child-Pugh categories B and C and those hypersensitive to alfuzosin or its ingredients.
• Use cautiously in patients with severe renal insufficiency, congenital or acquired QT-interval prolongation, or symptomatic hypotension and hypotensive responses to other drugs.

**NURSING CONSIDERATIONS**
• Don't use alfuzosin to treat hypertension.
• Orthostatic hypotension may develop within a few hours after patient takes alfuzosin; it may not cause symptoms.
• Symptoms of BPH and prostate cancer are similar; rule out prostate cancer before starting therapy.

---

• Stop alfuzosin if angina pectoris develops or worsens.

**PATIENT TEACHING**
• Tell patient to take alfuzosin just after same meal each day.
• At start of therapy, warn patient about possible hypotension, and explain that it may cause dizziness. Caution patient against performing hazardous activities until he knows how the drug affects him.
• Tell patient to avoid situations in which he could be injured if he became light-headed or fainted.
• Warn patient not to crush or chew the tablets.

---

## alprostadil
Caverject, Edex, Muse

*Pregnancy risk category NR*

---

**AVAILABLE FORMS**
*Injection:* 5 mcg/ml, 10 mcg/ml, 20 mcg/ml, 40 mcg/ml after reconstitution
*Urogenital suppository:* 125 mcg, 250 mcg, 500 mcg, 1,000 mcg

**INDICATIONS & DOSAGES**
➤ **Erectile dysfunction of vasculogenic, psychogenic, or mixed causes**
*Injection*
*Adults:* Dosages are highly individualized; initially, inject 2.5 mcg intracavernously. If partial response occurs, give second dose of 2.5 mcg; then increase in increments of 5 to 10 mcg until patient achieves erection suitable for intercourse and lasting no longer than 1 hour. If patient doesn't respond to first dose, increase second dose to 7.5 mcg within 1 hour, then increase further in increments of 5 to 10 mcg until patient achieves suitable erection. Patient must remain in prescriber's office until complete detumescence occurs. Don't repeat procedure for at least 24 hours.
*Urogenital suppository*
*Adults:* Initially, 125 to 250 mcg, under supervision of prescriber. Adjust dosage p.r.n. until response is sufficient for sexual intercourse. Maximum of two administrations in 24 hours; maximum dose is 1,000 mcg.

➤ **Erectile dysfunction of neurogenic cause (spinal cord injury)**
*Adults:* Dosages are highly individualized; initially, inject 1.25 mcg intracavernously. If partial response occurs, give second dose of 1.25 mcg. Increase in increments of 2.5 mcg, to dose of 5 mcg; then increase in increments of 5 mcg until patient achieves erection suitable for intercourse and lasting no longer than 1 hour. If patient doesn't respond to first dose, give next higher dose within 1 hour. Patient must remain in prescriber's office until complete detumescence occurs. If there is a response, don't repeat procedure for at least 24 hours.

**ACTION**
A prostaglandin derivative that induces erection by relaxing trabecular smooth muscle and dilating cavernosal arteries. This leads to expansion of lacunar spaces and entrapment of blood by compressing venules against the tunica albuginea, a process referred to as the corporal veno-occlusive mechanism.

| Route | Onset | Peak | Duration |
|---|---|---|---|
| Intra-cavernous | 5-20 min | 5-20 min | 1-6 hr |
| Urogenital | 10 min | 16 min | 1 hr |

**ADVERSE REACTIONS**
**CNS:** headache, dizziness.
**CV:** hypertension, hypotension
**EENT:** sinusitis, nasal congestion.
**GU:** *penile pain;* prolonged erection; penile fibrosis, rash, or edema; prostatic disorder.
**Musculoskeletal:** back pain.
**Respiratory:** upper respiratory tract infection, cough.
**Skin:** injection site hematoma or ecchymosis.
**Other:** localized trauma or pain, flulike syndrome.

**INTERACTIONS**
**Drug-drug.** *Anticoagulants:* May increase risk of bleeding from intracavernosal injection site. Monitor patient closely.
*Cyclosporine:* May decrease cyclosporine level. Monitor cyclosporine level closely.
*Vasoactive drugs:* Safety and efficacy haven't been studied. Avoid using together.

---

**EFFECTS ON LAB TEST RESULTS**
None reported.

**CONTRAINDICATIONS & CAUTIONS**
• Contraindicated in patients hypersensitive to drug, in those with conditions predisposing them to priapism (sickle cell anemia or trait, multiple myeloma, leukemia) or penile deformation (angulation, cavernosal fibrosis, Peyronie's disease), in men with penile implants or for whom sexual activity is inadvisable or contraindicated, in women or children, and in sexual partners of pregnant women unless condoms are used.

**NURSING CONSIDERATIONS**
• Stop drug in patients who develop penile angulation, cavernosal fibrosis, or Peyronie's disease.

**PATIENT TEACHING**
• Teach patient how to prepare and give drug before he begins treatment at home. Stress importance of reading and following patient instructions in each package insert. Tell him to store unopened suppositories in refrigerator (36° to 46° F [2° to 8° C]) and store injection at or below room temperature (77° F [25° C]).
• Tell patient not to shake contents of reconstituted vial, and remind him that vial is designed for a single use. Tell him to discard vial if solution is discolored or contains precipitate.
• Instruct patient to urinate before inserting suppository because moisture makes it easier to insert drug in penis and will help dissolve it.
• Review administration and aseptic technique.
• Inform patient that he can expect an erection 5 to 20 minutes after administration, with a preferable duration of no more than 1 hour. If his erection lasts more than 6 hours, tell him to seek medical attention immediately.
• Remind patient to take drug as instructed (generally, no more than three times weekly, with at least 24 hours between each use). Warn him not to change dosage without consulting prescriber.
• Caution patient to use a condom if his sexual partner could be pregnant.

• Review possible adverse reactions. Tell patient to inspect his penis daily and to report redness, swelling, tenderness, curvature, excessive erection (priapism), unusual pain, nodules, or hard tissue.
• Urge patient not to reuse or share needles, syringes, or drug.
• Warn patient that drug doesn't protect against sexually transmitted diseases. Also, caution him that bleeding at injection site can increase risk of transmitting blood-borne diseases to his partner.
• Remind patient to keep regular follow-up appointments so prescriber can evaluate drug effectiveness and safety.

# amifostine
Ethyol

*Pregnancy risk category C*

**AVAILABLE FORMS**
*Injection:* 500 mg anhydrous base and 500 mg mannitol in 10-ml vial

**INDICATIONS & DOSAGES**
➤ **To reduce cumulative renal toxicity linked to repeated administration of cisplatin in patients with advanced ovarian cancer or non–small-cell lung cancer**
*Adults:* 910 mg/m² daily as a 15-minute I.V. infusion, starting 30 minutes before chemotherapy. If hypotension occurs and blood pressure doesn't return to normal within 5 minutes after stopping treatment, 740 mg/m² in subsequent cycles.
➤ **To reduce moderate to severe xerostomia in patients undergoing postoperative radiation treatment for head and neck cancer**
*Adults:* 200 mg/m² daily as 3-minute I.V. infusion, starting 15 to 30 minutes before standard fraction radiation therapy.

**I.V. ADMINISTRATION**
• Inspect vial for particulates and discoloration; discard drug if it's cloudy or precipitated.
• Reconstitute each single-dose vial with 9.7 ml of sterile normal saline injection. Other solutions aren't recommended.
• Drug can be prepared in polyvinyl chloride bags in concentrations of 5 to 40 mg/

---

*Rapid onset* †Canada ‡Australia ◇OTC ♦Off-label use ✐Photoguide *Liquid contains alcohol.

ml and has same stability as when it's re-constituted in single-use vial.

● Keep patient supine during infusion. Monitor blood pressure every 5 minutes. If hypotension occurs and requires interrupting therapy, notify prescriber and keep patient supine with legs elevated. Then give infusion of normal saline solution, using a separate I.V. line. If blood pressure returns to normal within 5 minutes and patient is asymptomatic, infusion may be restarted so full dose of drug can be given. If full dose can't be given, limit subsequent doses to 740 mg/m$^2$.

● Don't infuse for longer than 15 minutes; longer infusion has been linked to higher risk of adverse reactions.

● Reconstituted solution (500 mg amifostine/10 ml) is chemically stable for 5 hours at room temperature (about 77° F [25° C]) or 24 hours if refrigerated (36° to 46° F [2° to 8° C]).

## ACTION

Dephosphorylated by alkaline phosphatase in tissue to a pharmacologically active free thiol metabolite. Free thiol in normal tissues binds and detoxifies reactive metabolites of cisplatin, reducing the toxic effects of cisplatin on renal tissue. Free thiol can also act as a scavenger of free radicals that may be generated in tissues exposed to cisplatin.

| Route | Onset | Peak | Duration |
|-------|-------|------|----------|
| I.V. | 5-8 min | Unknown | Unknown |

## ADVERSE REACTIONS

**CNS:** dizziness, somnolence.
**CV:** *hypotension.*
**GI:** *nausea, vomiting.*
**Metabolic:** hypocalcemia.
**Respiratory:** hiccups, sneezing.
**Other:** flushing or feeling of warmth, chills or feeling of coldness, ***allergic reactions ranging from rash to rigors.***

## INTERACTIONS

**Drug-drug.** *Antihypertensives, other drugs that could increase hypotension:* May cause profound hypotension. Monitor patient closely.

## EFFECTS ON LAB TEST RESULTS

● May decrease calcium level.

## CONTRAINDICATIONS & CAUTIONS

● Contraindicated in patients hypersensitive to aminothiol compounds or mannitol.

● Contraindicated in patients who are hypotensive, dehydrated, or receiving antihypertensives that can't be stopped 24 hours before amifostine administration.

● Drug shouldn't be used in patients receiving chemotherapy for potentially curable malignancies (including certain malignancies of germ-cell origin), except for patients involved in clinical studies.

● Use cautiously in elderly patients and in patients with ischemic heart disease, arrhythmias, heart failure, or history of CVA or transient ischemic attacks.

● Use cautiously in patients for whom common adverse effects of nausea, vomiting, and hypotension may have serious consequences.

## NURSING CONSIDERATIONS

● If possible, stop antihypertensive therapy 24 hours before amifostine administration.

● Make sure patient is adequately hydrated before giving drug. Monitor patient's blood pressure before and immediately after infusion and periodically thereafter as clinically indicated.

● Give antiemetics, including dexamethasone 20 mg I.V. and a serotonin 5HT$_3$-receptor antagonist, before and with amifostine. Additional antiemetics may be needed, based on chemotherapeutic drugs given.

● Monitor patient's fluid balance if drug is used with highly emetogenic chemotherapeutic drugs.

● Monitor calcium level in patients at risk for hypocalcemia, such as those with nephrotic syndrome. If needed, give calcium supplements.

● Safety and effectiveness of drug in children haven't been established.

## PATIENT TEACHING

● Instruct patient to remain lying down throughout infusion.

● Advise patient not to breast-feed; it's unknown if drug appears in breast milk.

---

Reactions may be *common,* uncommon, *life-threatening,* or **COMMON AND LIFE-THREATENING.**

# aprotinin
Trasylol

*Pregnancy risk category B*

## AVAILABLE FORMS
*Injection:* 10,000 kallikrein inactivator units (KIU)/ml (1.4 mg/ml) in 100-ml and 200-ml vials

## INDICATIONS & DOSAGES
➤ **To reduce blood loss or the need for transfusion in patients undergoing coronary artery bypass grafts**
*Adults:* Initially, 10,000 KIU (1.4 mg) I.V. as test dose at least 10 minutes before loading dose. If no allergic reaction is evident, anesthesia may be induced while loading dose of 2 million KIU is given I.V. slowly over 20 to 30 minutes. When loading dose is complete, sternotomy may be performed. Before bypass is started, cardiopulmonary bypass circuit is primed with 2 million KIU of drug by replacing an aliquot of priming fluid with drug. A continuous infusion at 500,000 KIU/hour is then given I.V. until patient leaves operating room. This is known as high-dose regimen. Low-dose regimen is half the dosage of high-dose regimen (except for test dose).

## I.V. ADMINISTRATION
● Drug is incompatible with amino acids, corticosteroids, fat emulsions, heparin, and tetracyclines. Don't add other drugs to I.V. container and use separate I.V. line.
● Be prepared to give test dose, especially if patient has previously received drug because of a high risk of anaphylaxis. Pretreat with an antihistamine.
● Give all doses through a central line.
● Avoid rapid administration of large doses because of potential for hypotension and anaphylactic reactions.
● Store drug between 36° and 77° F (2° and 25° C). Protect drug from freezing.

## ACTION
A naturally occurring protease inhibitor that acts as a systemic hemostatic, decreasing bleeding and turnover of coagulation factors. Inhibits fibrinolysis by affecting kallikrein and plasmin, prevents triggering of the contact phase of the coagulation pathway, and increases the resistance of platelets to damage from mechanical injury and high plasmin levels that occur during cardiopulmonary bypass.

| Route | Onset | Peak | Duration |
|-------|-------|------|----------|
| I.V. | Unknown | Unknown | Unknown |

## ADVERSE REACTIONS
**CV:** fever, *cardiac arrest, heart failure, ventricular tachycardia, MI, heart block, atrial fibrillation, atrial flutter,* hypotension, supraventricular tachycardia.
**GU:** *nephrotoxicity, renal failure.*
**Metabolic:** acidosis, hypervolemia, hypokalemia, hyperglycemia.
**Respiratory:** pneumonia, respiratory disorder, apnea, asthma, dyspnea.
**Other:** hypersensitivity reactions, *anaphylaxis, shock, sepsis.*

## INTERACTIONS
**Drug-drug.** *Captopril:* May decrease hypotensive effects. Monitor patient closely.
*Fibrinolytic drugs:* May inhibit fibrinolytic effects. Avoid using together.
*Heparin:* May prolong activated clotting time. Monitor clotting time and PTT.

## EFFECTS ON LAB TEST RESULTS
● May increase AST, ALT, creatinine, and glucose levels. May decrease potassium level.
● May alter liver function test values.

## CONTRAINDICATIONS & CAUTIONS
● Contraindicated in patients hypersensitive to beef because drug is prepared from bovine lung.

## NURSING CONSIDERATIONS
● *Alert:* Use drug cautiously and monitor patient closely for hypersensitivity reaction. Patient may experience anaphylaxis after full therapeutic dose even if he remains asymptomatic after test dose. If symptoms of hypersensitivity (skin eruptions, itching, dyspnea, nausea, tachycardia) occur, stop infusion immediately, notify prescriber, and provide supportive treatment.
● Obtain history of possible allergies. Patients with history of allergies to drugs or other substances may be at higher risk for

---

*Rapid onset    †Canada    ‡Australia    ◇OTC    ◆ Off-label use    ⌀Photoguide    *Liquid contains alcohol.*

developing an allergic reaction to aprotinin.
• To avoid hypotension, make sure patient is supine when loading dose is given. Monitor blood pressure.
• Monitor laboratory studies, including liver function tests.
• Monitor patient for increased creatinine levels and other signs of nephrotoxicity. If nephrotoxicity occurs, it's usually mild and reversible.

### PATIENT TEACHING
• Explain use and administration of drug to patient and family.
• Reassure patient and family that patient will be monitored continuously throughout drug administration.

---

## becaplermin
Regranex Gel

*Pregnancy risk category C*

### AVAILABLE FORMS
*Gel:* 100 mcg/g in tubes of 2 g, 7.5 g, 15 g

### INDICATIONS & DOSAGES
➤ **Diabetic neuropathic ulcers of the leg that extend into the subcutaneous tissue or beyond and have adequate blood supply**
*Adults:* Apply 1/16-inch thick layer over entire wound surface daily. The following table shows the length of gel to apply in inches (or centimeters) based on tube size and wound size.

| Tube size | Inches | Centimeters |
|-----------|--------|-------------|
| 2 g | Ulcer length × ulcer width × 1.3 | Ulcer length × ulcer width ÷ 2 |
| 7.5, 15 g | Ulcer length × ulcer width × 0.6 | Ulcer length × ulcer width ÷ 4 |

### ACTION
Thought to promote chemotactic recruitment and proliferation of cells involved in wound repair and formation of new granulation tissue.

| Route | Onset | Peak | Duration |
|-------|-------|------|----------|
| Topical | Unknown | Unknown | Unknown |

### ADVERSE REACTIONS
**Musculoskeletal:** osteomyelitis.
**Skin:** erythematous rash.
**Other:** cellulitis, infection.

### INTERACTIONS
None significant.

### EFFECTS ON LAB TEST RESULTS
None reported.

### CONTRAINDICATIONS & CAUTIONS
• Contraindicated in patients hypersensitive to drug or its components (such as parabens or m-cresol) and in those with neoplasms at application site.
• Use cautiously in breast-feeding women.
• Safety and effectiveness of drug in children younger than age 16 haven't been established.

### NURSING CONSIDERATIONS
• *Alert:* Don't use drug on wounds that close by primary intention.
• Drug facilitates complete healing of diabetic ulcers when used as an adjunct to good ulcer care practices, which include initial sharp debridement, infection control, and pressure relief.
• Treatment efficacy hasn't been evaluated for diabetic neuropathic ulcers that don't extend through the dermis into subcutaneous tissue or for ischemic diabetic ulcers.
• To apply drug, calculate length of gel by measuring ulcer's greatest length and width, and use dosage formula. Squeeze calculated length of gel onto clean measuring surface such as waxed paper. Use cotton swab or other application aid to spread drug over entire ulcer area in a 1/16-inch thick continuous layer. Place a saline-moistened dressing over site and leave in place for about 12 hours. After 12 hours, remove dressing and rinse away residual gel with normal saline solution or water, and apply a fresh moist dressing, without becaplermin, for rest of day.
• Monitor wound size and healing; recalculate amount of drug to be applied at least once weekly. If ulcer doesn't decrease in size by about one-third after 10 weeks, or if complete healing hasn't occurred within 20 weeks, reassess treatment.

• Watch for application site reactions. Sensitization, or irritation caused by parabens or m-cresol, may occur.
• Drug is for external use only.

**PATIENT TEACHING**
• Instruct patient to wash hands thoroughly before applying gel.
• Advise patient not to touch tip of tube against ulcer or any other surfaces.
• Teach patient proper procedure for wound care, including applying gel and changing dressings.
• Stress need to keep area covered with a wet dressing at all times.
• Instruct patient to recap tube tightly after each use.
• Tell patient to store drug in refrigerator (36° to 46° F [2° to 8° C]).
• Instruct patient not to use drug after expiration date.

---

# capsaicin
Capsin ◇, Dolorac ◇, No Pain-HP ◇, Pain Doctor ◇ Pain-X ◇ Zostrix ◇ Zostrix-HP ◇

*Pregnancy risk category NR*

**AVAILABLE FORMS**
*Cream:* 0.025% (Zostrix), 0.075% (Zostrix HP), 0.25% (Dolorac)
*Gel:* 0.025%, 0.05%
*Lotion:* 0.025%, 0.075%
*Roll-on:* 0.075%

**INDICATIONS & DOSAGES**
➤ **Temporary relief from pain after herpes zoster infections; neuralgias, such as postoperative pain and painful diabetic neuropathy; pain from osteoarthritis or rheumatoid arthritis**
*Adults and children older than age 2:* Apply to affected areas no more than q.i.d.
➤ **Temporary relief from arthritis pain**
*Adults and children age 12 and older:* Apply thin film of Dolorac to affected area b.i.d.

**ACTION**
Unknown. May increase release of substance P, a principal neurotransmitter for pain, from peripheral type C sensory fibers to central neurons.

| Route | Onset | Peak | Duration |
|---|---|---|---|
| Topical | Unknown | Unknown | Unknown |

**ADVERSE REACTIONS**
**Respiratory:** cough, irritation.
**Skin:** redness, *stinging or burning on application.*

**INTERACTIONS**
None significant.

**EFFECTS ON LAB TEST RESULTS**
None reported.

**CONTRAINDICATIONS & CAUTIONS**
• Contraindicated in patients hypersensitive to drug.

**NURSING CONSIDERATIONS**
• Drug is for external use only.

**PATIENT TEACHING**
• Warn patient to avoid getting drug in eyes or on broken skin.
• Advise patient not to bandage area tightly after applying drug.
• Tell patient to wash hands after applying. If patient is using drug for arthritis of the hands, tell him to wait about 30 minutes after applying before he washes his hands.
• Inform patient that transient burning or stinging usually occurs at first treatment but decreases with cautious use. This effect persists in patients who use drug less often than three times daily.
• Tell patient to contact prescriber if symptoms persist beyond 2 to 4 weeks or resolve and shortly reappear.

---

# clomiphene citrate
Clomid, Milophene, Serophene

*Pregnancy risk category X*

**AVAILABLE FORMS**
*Tablets:* 50 mg

**INDICATIONS & DOSAGES**
➤ **To induce ovulation**
*Adults:* 50 mg P.O. daily for 5 days, starting on day 5 of menstrual cycle (first day of menstrual flow is day 1) if bleeding occurs, or at any time if patient hasn't

---

had recent uterine bleeding. If ovulation doesn't occur, may increase dose to 100 mg P.O. daily for 5 days as soon as 30 days after previous course. Repeat until conception occurs or until three courses of therapy are completed.

## ACTION

Unknown. Appears to stimulate release of follicle-stimulating hormone, luteinizing hormone, and pituitary gonadotropins, resulting in maturation of the ovarian follicle, ovulation, and development of the corpus luteum.

| Route | Onset | Peak | Duration |
|-------|-------|------|----------|
| P.O. | Unknown | Unknown | Unknown |

## ADVERSE REACTIONS

**CNS:** headache, restlessness, insomnia, dizziness, light-headedness, depression, fatigue.
**EENT:** blurred vision, diplopia, scotoma, photophobia.
**GI:** nausea, vomiting, bloating, distention.
**GU:** urinary frequency and polyuria, abnormal uterine bleeding, *ovarian enlargement,* ovarian cyst that regresses spontaneously when drug is stopped.
**Metabolic:** weight gain.
**Skin:** reversible alopecia, urticaria, rash, dermatitis.
**Other:** *hot flashes, breast discomfort.*

## INTERACTIONS
None significant.

## EFFECTS ON LAB TEST RESULTS
None reported.

## CONTRAINDICATIONS & CAUTIONS
● Contraindicated in pregnant patients and in those with undiagnosed abnormal genital bleeding, ovarian cyst not related to polycystic ovarian syndrome, hepatic disease or dysfunction, uncontrolled thyroid or adrenal dysfunction, or organic intracranial lesion (such as a pituitary tumor).

## NURSING CONSIDERATIONS
● Monitor patient closely because of potentially serious adverse reactions.
● Long-term cyclic therapy isn't recommended.

● *Alert:* Don't confuse clomiphene with clomipramine or clonidine. Don't confuse Serophene with Sarafem.

## PATIENT TEACHING
● Tell patient about the risk of multiple births, which increases with higher doses.
● Teach patient to take and chart basal body temperature to ascertain if ovulation has occurred.
● Reinforce importance of compliance with medication regimen.
● Reassure patient that ovulation typically occurs after first course of therapy. If pregnancy doesn't occur, therapy may be repeated twice.
● Advise patient to stop drug and contact prescriber immediately if pregnancy is suspected because drug may have teratogenic effect.
● *Alert:* Advise patient to stop drug and contact prescriber immediately if abdominal symptoms or pain occur; these symptoms may indicate ovarian enlargement or ovarian cyst. Also tell patient to immediately notify prescriber if signs and symptoms of impending visual toxicity occur, such as blurred vision, double vision, vision defect in one part of the eye (scotoma), or sensitivity to the sun.
● Warn patient to avoid hazardous activities, such as driving or operating machinery, until CNS effects are known. Drug may cause dizziness or visual disturbances.

---

# diclofenac sodium
Solaraze

*Pregnancy risk category B*

## AVAILABLE FORMS
*Topical gel:* 3% in 50-g tube

## INDICATIONS & DOSAGES
➤ **Actinic keratosis**
*Adults:* Apply gently to lesion b.i.d. for 60 to 90 days. Use enough gel to cover the lesion; for example, use 0.5 g of gel on a 5-cm × 5-cm lesion.

## ACTION
Unknown.

---

Reactions may be *common*, uncommon, *life-threatening*, or COMMON AND LIFE-THREATENING.

| Route | Onset | Peak | Duration |
|-------|-------|------|----------|
| Topical | Unknown | 4-12 hr | Unknown |

## ADVERSE REACTIONS
**CNS:** headache, pain, asthenia, migraine, hypokinesia, *paresthesia.*
**CV:** chest pain, hypertension.
**EENT:** sinusitis, pharyngitis, rhinitis, conjunctivitis, eye pain.
**GI:** diarrhea, dyspepsia, abdominal pain.
**GU:** hematuria, renal impairment.
**Hepatic:** liver impairment.
**Metabolic:** hypercholesterolemia, hyperglycemia.
**Musculoskeletal:** arthralgia, arthrosis, back pain, myalgia, neck pain.
**Respiratory:** asthma, dyspnea, pneumonia.
**Skin:** *reaction at application site, contact dermatitis, dry skin, pruritus, rash,* localized edema, *exfoliation,* acne, alopecia, *localized pain,* photosensitivity, skin carcinoma, skin ulcer.
**Other:** *anaphylaxis, flulike syndrome,* infection, allergic reaction.

## INTERACTIONS
**Drug-drug.** *Oral NSAIDs:* May increase drug effects. Minimize use together.
**Drug-lifestyle.** *Sun exposure:* May increase risk of photosensitivity reactions. Advise patient to avoid excessive sun exposure.

## EFFECTS ON LAB TEST RESULTS
• May increase phosphokinase, creatinine, glucose, AST, ALT, and cholesterol levels.

## CONTRAINDICATIONS & CAUTIONS
• Contraindicated in patients hypersensitive to diclofenac, benzyl alcohol, polyethylene glycol monomethyl ether 350, or hyaluronic acid.
• Use cautiously in patients with the aspirin triad; these patients are usually asthmatics who develop rhinitis, with or without nasal polyps, after taking aspirin or other NSAIDs.
• Use cautiously in patients with active GI bleeding or ulceration and in those with severe renal or hepatic impairment.
• It's unknown if drug appears in breast milk. Patient should either stop breast-feeding or stop treatment, taking into account importance of drug to mother.

## NURSING CONSIDERATIONS
• Don't apply to open wounds or broken skin.
• Avoid contact with eyes.
• Safety and effectiveness of sunscreens, cosmetics, or other topical medications used with drug are unknown.
• Complete healing or optimal therapeutic effect may not be seen until 30 days after therapy is complete.
• Reevaluate lesions that don't respond to therapy.
• Because of the risk of premature closure of the ductus arteriosus, avoid diclofenac in late pregnancy.

## PATIENT TEACHING
• Inform patient about risk of skin reactions (rash, itchiness, pain, irritation) at the application site. Urge patient to seek medical attention if adverse reactions persist or worsen.
• Encourage patient to minimize sun exposure during therapy. Explain that sunscreen may be helpful but that the safety of using sunscreen with diclofenac is unknown.
• Caution patient not to apply gel to open wounds or broken skin.
• Instruct patient to avoid contact with eyes.
• Instruct patient not to apply other topical drugs or cosmetics to affected area while using drug, unless directed.
• Tell patient to notify prescriber if she's pregnant or breast-feeding.

# dihydroergotamine mesylate
D.H.E. 45, Dihydergot‡,
Dihydroergotamine-Sandoz†,
Migranal

*Pregnancy risk category X*

## AVAILABLE FORMS
*Injection:* 1 mg/ml
*Intranasal solution:* 0.5 mg/metered spray (4 mg/ml)

## INDICATIONS & DOSAGES

➤ **Acute treatment of migraine headache with or without aura; acute cluster headache**

*Adults:* 1 mg I.M., S.C., or I.V., repeated q 1 to 2 hours, p.r.n., up to total of 2 mg I.V. or 3 mg I.M. or S.C. per 24 hours. Maximum, 6 mg weekly. Or, 1 spray into each nostril for total of 1 mg initially, repeated in 15 minutes for a total dose of 2 mg. Maximum, 4 mg weekly.

## I.V. ADMINISTRATION

● Protect ampules from heat and light. Discard if solution is discolored.
● Directly inject solution into the vein over 3 minutes. Continuous and intermittent infusions aren't recommended.

## ACTION

Causes peripheral vasoconstriction primarily by stimulating alpha receptors; may abort vascular headaches by direct vasoconstriction of dilated carotid artery bed with a decline in amplitude of pulsations. Also causes antagonistic effect of serotonin 5-HT$_2$ receptors.

| Route | Onset | Peak | Duration |
|---|---|---|---|
| I.V. | 5 min | 15 min | 8 hr |
| I.M. | 15-30 min | 30 min | 3-4 hr |
| Intranasal | Rapid | 30-60 min | Unknown |

## ADVERSE REACTIONS

**CV:** transient tachycardia or ***bradycardia,*** precordial distress and pain, increased arterial pressure.
**GI:** *nausea, vomiting,* diarrhea, dry mouth.
**GU:** uterine contractions.
**Musculoskeletal:** weakness in legs, muscle pain in arms and legs, numbness and tingling in fingers and toes.
**Skin:** itching.
**Other:** localized edema, injection site irritation.

## INTERACTIONS

**Drug-drug.** *CYP 3A4 inhibitors (azole antifungals, macrolides, protease inhibitors):* May cause life-threatening peripheral and cerebral ischemia. Avoid using together.
*Propranolol, other beta blockers:* May block natural pathway for vasodilation in patients receiving ergot alkaloids; may result in excessive vasoconstriction and cold

arms and legs. Monitor patient closely if used together.
*SSRIs:* May increase risk of weakness, hyperflexion, and incoordination. Monitor patient closely.
*Sumatriptan:* May have additive effect, increasing risk of coronary vasospasm. Separate doses by 24 hours.
*Vasoconstrictors:* May have additive effect, increasing risk of high blood pressure. Monitor blood pressure.
**Drug-lifestyle.** *Nicotine use:* May have additive effect, leading to vasoconstriction. Discourage use together.

## EFFECTS ON LAB TEST RESULTS

None reported.

## CONTRAINDICATIONS & CAUTIONS

● Contraindicated in patients hypersensitive to drug and in those with ischemic heart disease, coronary artery spasm including Prinzmetal's angina, hemiplegic or basilar migraine, peripheral and occlusive vascular disease, coronary artery disease, uncontrolled hypertension, severe hepatic or renal dysfunction, malnutrition, severe pruritus, or sepsis.
● Contraindicated in pregnant and breast-feeding patients and those taking concurrent CYP 3A4 inhibitors.

## NURSING CONSIDERATIONS

● Drug is most effective when used at first sign of migraine or soon after onset.
● Avoid prolonged use; don't exceed recommended dosage. Adjust to most effective minimal dosage for best results.
● Intranasal solution isn't intended for prolonged daily use.
● Give S.C. injection in thigh.
● *Alert:* Watch for ergotamine rebound, an increase in frequency and duration of headaches, which may occur when drug is stopped.

## PATIENT TEACHING

● Instruct patient to lie down and relax in a quiet, low-light environment after taking drug.
● Teach patient to pump nasal spray four times before use. Advise patient not to sniff or tilt head back after using spray.
● Advise patient to discard nasal spray applicator and opened ampule after 8 hours.

---

• Tell patient to report cold feeling in arms and legs or tingling in fingers and toes. Severe vasoconstriction may cause tissue damage. Keep arms and legs warm and give vasodilators.

• Help patient evaluate underlying causes of stress, which may precipitate attacks.

• Warn patient to notify prescriber if she's pregnant or plans to become pregnant.

## dutasteride
Avodart

*Pregnancy risk category X*

### AVAILABLE FORMS
*Capsules:* 0.5 mg

### INDICATIONS & DOSAGES
➤ **To improve the symptoms of BPH, reduce the risk of acute urine retention, and reduce the need for BPH-related surgery**
*Adults:* 0.5 mg P.O. once daily.

### ACTION
Inhibits conversion of testosterone to dihydrotestosterone (DHT). DHT is the androgen primarily responsible for the initial development and subsequent enlargement of the prostate gland.

| Route | Onset | Peak | Duration |
|-------|-------|------|----------|
| P.O. | Unknown | 2-3 hr | Unknown |

### ADVERSE REACTIONS
**GU:** impotence, decreased libido, ejaculation disorder.
**Other:** gynecomastia.

### INTERACTIONS
**Drug-drug.** *Cytochrome P-450 inhibitors (such as cimetidine, ciprofloxacin, diltiazem, ketoconazole, ritonavir, verapamil):* May increase dutasteride level. Use together cautiously.

### EFFECTS ON LAB TEST RESULTS
• May lower prostate-specific antigen (PSA) level.

### CONTRAINDICATIONS & CAUTIONS
• Contraindicated in women and children and in patients hypersensitive to dutasteride or its ingredients or to other 5-alpha-reductase inhibitors.

• Use cautiously in patients with hepatic disease and in those taking long-term potent cytochrome P-450 inhibitors.

### NURSING CONSIDERATIONS
• Because dutasteride may be absorbed through the skin, women who are or may become pregnant shouldn't handle the drug.

• If contact is made with leaking capsules, wash the contact area immediately with soap and water.

• Carefully monitor patients with a large residual urinary volume or severely diminished urinary flow, or both, for obstructive uropathy.

• Patients should wait at least 6 months after their last dose before donating blood.

• Establish a new baseline PSA level in men treated for 3 to 6 months and use it to assess potentially cancer-related changes in PSA.

• To interpret PSA values in men treated for 6 months or more, double the PSA value for comparison with normal values in untreated men.

### PATIENT TEACHING
• Tell patient to swallow the capsule whole.

• Inform patient that ejaculate volume may decrease but that sexual function should remain normal.

• Teach women who are pregnant or may become pregnant not to handle dutasteride. A male fetus exposed to dutasteride by the mother's swallowing or absorbing the drug through her skin may be born with abnormal sex organs.

• *Alert:* Tell patient not to donate blood for at least 6 months after final dose.

• Tell patient he'll need periodic blood tests to monitor therapeutic effects.

## eflornithine hydrochloride
Vaniqa

*Pregnancy risk category C*

### AVAILABLE FORMS
*Cream:* 13.9% in 30-g tube (single or double)

---

## INDICATIONS & DOSAGES
➤ **To reduce unwanted facial hair in women**

*Adults and children older than age 12:* Apply a thin layer to affected areas of the face and adjacent areas under chin; rub in thoroughly b.i.d., at least 8 hours apart. Don't wash area for at least 4 hours after application.

## ACTION
Thought to irreversibly inhibit skin enzyme ornithine decarboxylase activity. This inhibits cell division and synthesis, thereby slowing the rate of hair growth.

| Route | Onset | Peak | Duration |
|-------|-------|------|----------|
| Topical | Unknown | Unknown | Unknown |

## ADVERSE REACTIONS
**CNS:** headache, dizziness, asthenia, vertigo.
**GI:** dyspepsia, anorexia, nausea.
**Skin:** *acne, pseudofolliculitis barbae,* stinging or burning sensation, dry skin, pruritus, erythema, skin irritation, rash, alopecia, folliculitis, ingrown hair, facial edema.

## INTERACTIONS
No known interactions.

## EFFECTS ON LAB TEST RESULTS
None reported.

## CONTRAINDICATIONS & CAUTIONS
• Contraindicated in patients hypersensitive to drug or its components.
• It's unknown if drug appears in breast milk. Use cautiously in breast-feeding women.

## NURSING CONSIDERATIONS
• Limit application of the cream to the face and adjacent involved areas under the chin.
• Drug shouldn't cause contact sensitization, phototoxicity, or photosensitization reactions.
• If no improvement is seen after 6 months, stop treatment. Hair will return to normal about 8 weeks after stopping treatment.
• Store drug at 59° to 86° F (15° to 30° C).

## PATIENT TEACHING
• Tell patient that product is for external use only and to avoid getting into eyes, nose, or mouth. If drug gets into eyes, tell patient to rinse thoroughly with water and to contact her prescriber.
• Tell patient to avoid using on broken or abraded skin.
• Tell patient to apply a thin layer to affected areas of the face and adjacent involved areas under the chin and to rub thoroughly. Tell her not to wash treatment areas for at least 4 hours after application.
• Instruct patient to use product exactly as prescribed.
• Explain to patient that drug slows hair growth by inhibiting an enzyme in the hair follicle responsible for hair growth. Instruct her to continue current hair removal techniques of tweezing and plucking because drug won't permanently remove hair. Tell her to wait at least 5 minutes after hair removal to apply cream.
• Warn patient that results may occur in as few as 4 to 8 weeks but may take longer.
• Inform patient that she may use cosmetics or sunblocks after applying drug but that she should wait a few minutes to allow the cream to be absorbed.
• If adverse effects become bothersome, instruct patient to limit use to once a day. If adverse effects persist or if condition worsens, tell patient to stop drug and to consult prescriber.

# finasteride
Propecia, Proscar

*Pregnancy risk category X*

## AVAILABLE FORMS
*Tablets:* 1 mg, 5 mg

## INDICATIONS & DOSAGES
➤ **Male pattern hair loss (androgenetic alopecia) in men only**
*Adults:* 1 mg P.O. Propecia daily.
➤ **To improve symptoms of BPH and reduce risk of acute urine retention and need for surgery, including transurethral resection of prostate and prostatectomy**
*Adults:* 5 mg P.O. Proscar daily.

## ACTION
Inhibits corticosteroid 5-alpha-reductase, responsible for formation of potent androgen 5-alpha-dihydrotestosterone (DHT) from testosterone. Because DHT influences development of the prostate gland, decreasing DHT level in men should relieve the symptoms related to BPH. In male pattern baldness, the scalp contains miniaturized hair follicles and increased DHT level; drug decreases scalp DHT level in such cases.

| Route | Onset | Peak | Duration |
|---|---|---|---|
| P.O. | Unknown | 1-2 hr | 24 hr |

## ADVERSE REACTIONS
**GU:** impotence, decreased volume of ejaculate, decreased libido.

## INTERACTIONS
None significant.

## EFFECTS ON LAB TEST RESULTS
● May decrease prostate-specific antigen (PSA) levels.

## CONTRAINDICATIONS & CAUTIONS
● Contraindicated in patients hypersensitive to drug or to other 5-alpha-reductase inhibitors, such as dutasteride. Although drug isn't used in women or children, manufacturer indicates pregnancy as a contraindication.
● Use cautiously in patients with liver dysfunction.

## NURSING CONSIDERATIONS
● Before therapy, evaluate patient for conditions that mimic BPH, including hypotonic bladder, prostate cancer, infection, or stricture.
● Carefully monitor patients who have a large residual urine volume or severely diminished urine flow.
● Sustained increase in PSA levels could indicate noncompliance with therapy.
● A minimum of 6 months of therapy may be needed for treatment of BPH.

## PATIENT TEACHING
● Warn patient not to donate blood until at least 1 month after his final dose.
● Tell patient that drug may be taken without regard to meals.

● Warn woman who is or may become pregnant not to handle crushed tablets because of risk of adverse effects on male fetus.
● Inform patient that signs of improvement may require at least 3 months of daily use when drug is used to treat hair loss or at least 6 months when taken for BPH.
● Reassure patient that drug may decrease volume of ejaculate but doesn't impair normal sexual function

# imiquimod
Aldara

*Pregnancy risk category B*

## AVAILABLE FORMS
*Cream:* 5% in single-use packets containing 250 mg

## INDICATIONS & DOSAGES
➤ **External genital and perianal warts**
*Adults and adolescents age 12 and older:* Apply thin layer to affected area three times weekly before normal sleeping hours and leave on skin for 6 to 10 hours. Continue treatment until genital or perianal warts clear completely or maximum of 16 weeks.

## ACTION
Has no direct antiviral activity in cell culture. Drug induces mRNA-encoding cytokines including interferon-alfa at the treatment site.

| Route | Onset | Peak | Duration |
|---|---|---|---|
| Topical | Unknown | Unknown | Unknown |

## ADVERSE REACTIONS
**CNS:** headache.
**Musculoskeletal:** myalgia.
**Skin:** local itching, burning, pain, soreness, erythema, ulceration, edema, erosion, induration, flaking, excoriation.
**Other:** flulike symptoms, *fungal infection.*

## INTERACTIONS
None significant.

## EFFECTS ON LAB TEST RESULTS
None reported.

## CONTRAINDICATIONS & CAUTIONS
• Drug isn't recommended for treatment of urethral, intravaginal, cervical, rectal, or intra-anal human papillomavirus disease.
• Safety of drug in breast-feeding women is unknown.

## NURSING CONSIDERATIONS
• Don't use until genital or perianal tissue is healed from previous drug or surgical treatment.
• Patient usually experiences local skin reactions at site of application or surrounding areas. Use nonocclusive dressings, such as cotton gauze, or cotton undergarments in management of skin reactions. Patient's discomfort or severity of the local skin reaction may require a rest period of several days. Resume treatment once reaction subsides.
• Drug isn't a cure; new warts may develop during therapy.

## PATIENT TEACHING
• Advise patient that effect of cream on transmission of genital or perianal warts is unknown. New warts may develop during therapy; drug isn't a cure.
• Tell patient to use cream only as directed and to avoid contact with eyes.
• Tell patient to wash hands before and after applying cream.
• Advise patient to apply cream in thin layer over affected area and rub in until cream isn't visible. Advise patient to avoid excessive use of cream. Tell him not to occlude area after applying cream and to wash with mild soap and water 6 to 10 hours after application of cream.
• Advise patient that mild local skin reactions, such as redness, erosion, excoriation, flaking, and swelling at site of application or surrounding areas, are common. Tell him that most skin reactions are mild to moderate. Advise him to report severe skin reactions promptly.
• Instruct uncircumcised man being treated for warts under the foreskin to retract foreskin and clean area daily.
• Advise patient that drug can weaken condoms and vaginal diaphragms and that use together isn't recommended.
• Advise patient to avoid sexual contact while cream is on the skin.

• Tell patient to store drug at temperatures below 86° F (30° C) and to avoid freezing.

# isotretinoin
Accutane, Amnesteem, Claravis, Roaccutane‡, Sotret

*Pregnancy risk category X*

## AVAILABLE FORMS
*Capsules:* 10 mg, 20 mg, 40 mg

## INDICATIONS & DOSAGES
➤ **Severe recalcitrant nodular acne unresponsive to conventional therapy**
*Adults and adolescents:* 0.5 to 2 mg/kg P.O. daily in two divided doses with food for 15 to 20 weeks.

## ACTION
Unknown. Thought to normalize keratinization, reversibly decrease size of sebaceous glands, and alter composition of sebum to a less viscous form that is less likely to cause follicular plugging.

| Route | Onset | Peak | Duration |
|-------|-------|------|----------|
| P.O. | Unknown | 3 hr | Unknown |

## ADVERSE REACTIONS
**CNS:** *depression, psychosis, suicidal ideation or attempts, suicide, aggressive and violent behavior,* emotional instability, headache, fatigue, *pseudotumor cerebri.*
**EENT:** *conjunctivitis,* corneal deposits, dry eyes, visual disturbances, *epistaxis, drying of mucous membranes, dry nose,* hearing impairment (sometimes irreversible), decreased night vision.
**GI:** nonspecific GI symptoms, *nausea, vomiting,* anorexia, *abdominal pain, dry mouth,* gum bleeding and inflammation, *acute pancreatitis,* inflammatory bowel disease.
**Hematologic:** anemia, thrombocytosis, *increased erythrocyte sedimentation rate.*
**Hepatic:** *hepatitis.*
**Metabolic:** *hypertriglyceridemia,* hyperglycemia.
**Musculoskeletal:** skeletal hyperostosis, tendon and ligament calcification, premature epiphyseal closure, decreased bone mineral density and other bone abnormali-

ties, back pain, arthralgia, arthritis, tendinitis, ***rhabdomyolysis.***
**Skin:** *cheilosis, rash, dry skin, facial skin desquamation,* peeling of palms and toes, *petechiae, nail brittleness,* thinning of hair, skin infection, photosensitivity reaction, *cheilitis, pruritus, fragility.*

## INTERACTIONS
**Drug-drug.** *Corticosteroids:* May increase risk of osteoporosis. Use together cautiously.
*Medicated soaps, cleansers, and cover-ups; topical resorcinol peeling agents (benzoyl peroxide); alcohol-containing preparations:* May have cumulative drying effect. Use together cautiously.
*Micro-dosed progesterone oral contraceptives ("minipills") that don't contain estrogen:* May decrease effectiveness of contraceptive. Use alternative contraceptive methods.
*Phenytoin:* May increase risk of osteomalacia. Use together cautiously.
*Tetracyclines:* May increase risk of pseudotumor cerebri. Avoid using together.
*Vitamin A, products containing vitamin A:* May increase toxic effects of isotretinoin. Avoid using together.
**Drug-food.** *Any food:* May increase absorption of drug. Advise patient to take drug with milk, a meal, or shortly after a meal.
**Drug-lifestyle.** *Alcohol use:* May increase risk of hypertriglyceridemia. Discourage use together.
*Sun exposure:* May increase photosensitivity reaction. Advise patient to avoid excessive sunlight exposure.

## EFFECTS ON LAB TEST RESULTS
• May increase AST, ALT, alkaline phosphatase, triglyceride, glucose, and uric acid levels.
• May increase platelet count and erythrocyte sedimentation rate.

## CONTRAINDICATIONS & CAUTIONS
• Contraindicated in patients hypersensitive to parabens (which are used as preservatives), vitamin A, or other retinoids.
• Contraindicated in woman of childbearing potential, unless patient has had a negative serum pregnancy test within 2 weeks before beginning therapy, will begin drug

therapy on second or third day of next menstrual period, and will comply with stringent contraceptive measures for 1 month before therapy, during therapy, and for at least 1 month after therapy.
• Use cautiously in patients with a history of mental illness or a family history of psychiatric disorders, asthma, liver disease, diabetes, heart disease, osteoporosis, genetic predisposition for age-related osteoporosis, history of childhood osteoporosis, weak bones, anorexia nervosa, osteomalacia, or other disorders of bone metabolism.

## NURSING CONSIDERATIONS
• Before use, have patient read patient information and sign accompanying consent form.
• Patient must have negative results from two urine or serum pregnancy tests; one is performed in the office when the patient is qualified for therapy, the second on the second day of the next normal menstrual period or at least 11 days after the last unprotected act of sexual intercourse, whichever is later.
• Monitor baseline lipid studies, liver function tests, and pregnancy tests before therapy and at monthly intervals.
• Regularly monitor glucose level and CK levels in patients who participate in vigorous physical activity.
• Most adverse reactions occur at doses exceeding 1 mg/kg daily. Reactions are generally reversible when therapy is stopped or dosage is reduced.
• ***Alert:*** Screen patient who experiences headache, nausea and vomiting, or visual disturbances for papilledema. Signs and symptoms of pseudotumor cerebri require immediate discontinuation of drug and prompt neurologic intervention.
• ***Alert:*** Severe fetal abnormalities may occur if this drug is used during pregnancy.
• The FDA and drug manufacturer designed a program, System to Manage Accutane Related Teratogenicity (S.M.A.R.T.), to encourage the safe and appropriate use of drug, which can cause birth defects and fetal death if taken by a pregnant woman.
• If patient becomes pregnant during treatment, prescribers are encouraged to call Roche Medical Services at 1-800-526-

---

6367 or FDA (MedWatch) at 1-800-FDA-1088.

• A second course of therapy may begin 8 weeks after completion of the first course, if necessary. Improvements may continue after first course is complete.

• Patients may be at increased risk of bone fractures or injury when participating in sports with repetitive impact.

• Spontaneous reports of osteoporosis, osteopenia, bone fractures, and delayed healing of bone fractures have occurred in patients taking drug. To decrease this risk, don't exceed recommended doses and duration.

## PATIENT TEACHING

• Advise patient to take drug with or shortly after meals to facilitate absorption.

• Tell patient to immediately report visual disturbances and bone, muscle, or joint pain.

• Warn patient that contact lenses may feel uncomfortable during therapy.

• Warn patient against using abrasives, medicated soaps and cleansers, acne preparations containing peeling drugs, and topical products containing alcohol (including cosmetics, aftershave, cologne) because they may cause cumulative irritation or excessive drying of skin.

• Tell patient to avoid prolonged sun exposure and to use sunblock. Drug may have additive effect if used with other drugs that cause photosensitivity reaction.

• Advise patient of childbearing age to either abstain from sex or use two reliable forms of contraception simultaneously for 1 month before, during, and 1 month after treatment.

• Tell women that manufacturer will supply urine pregnancy tests for monthly testing during therapy.

• Warn patient that transient exacerbations may occur during therapy.

• Warn patient not to donate blood during therapy and for 1 month after stopping drug because drug could harm fetus of a pregnant recipient.

• Tell patient to report adverse reactions immediately, especially depression, suicidal thoughts, persistent headaches, and persistent GI pain.

## mesna
Mesnex

*Pregnancy risk category B*

## AVAILABLE FORMS
*Injection:* 100 mg/ml in 2- and 10-ml vials
*Tablets:* 400 mg

## INDICATIONS & DOSAGES
➤ **To prevent hemorrhagic cystitis in patients receiving ifosfamide**
*Adults:* Dosage varies with amount of ifosfamide given; calculated as 20% of ifosfamide dose at time of ifosfamide administration. Usual dose is 240 mg/m² as an I.V. bolus with administration of ifosfamide; repeated at 4 and 8 hours after administration of ifosfamide. Or, calculate daily dose as 100% of the ifosfamide dose. Give as a single bolus injection (20%), followed by two oral doses (40% each). Protocols that use 1.2 g/m² ifosfamide would use 240 mg/m² I.V. mesna at 0 hours, then 480 mg/m² P.O. at 2 and 6 hours.

## I.V. ADMINISTRATION
• Prepare I.V. solution by diluting commercially available ampules with $D_5W$, dextrose 5% and normal saline solution for injection, normal saline solution for injection, or lactated Ringer's solution to obtain final solution of 20 mg/ml.

• Although diluted solutions are stable for 24 hours at room temperature, they should be refrigerated and used within 6 hours. After opening ampule, discard any unused drug.

• Mesna and ifosfamide are compatible in same I.V. infusion.

• *Alert:* Mesna I.V. is incompatible with cisplatin; don't mix them.

## ACTION
Prevents ifosfamide-induced hemorrhagic cystitis by reacting with urotoxic ifosfamide metabolites.

| Route | Onset | Peak | Duration |
|-------|-------|------|----------|
| P.O. | Rapid | 4 hr | Unknown |
| I.V. | Rapid | Unknown | Unknown |

## ADVERSE REACTIONS
**CNS:** *fatigue, fever, asthenia,* dizziness, headache, somnolence, anxiety, confusion, insomnia.
**CV:** chest pain, edema, hypotension, tachycardia, flushing.
**GI:** *nausea, vomiting,* diarrhea, *constipation, anorexia, abdominal pain,* dyspepsia.
**GU:** hematuria.
**Hematologic:** *leukopenia, thrombocytopenia, anemia, granulocytopenia.*
**Metabolic:** hypokalemia, dehydration.
**Musculoskeletal:** back pain.
**Respiratory:** dyspnea, coughing, pneumonia.
**Skin:** alopecia, increased sweating, injection site reaction, pallor.
**Other:** allergy, pain.

## INTERACTIONS
None significant.

## EFFECTS ON LAB TEST RESULTS
● May decrease potassium level.
● May decrease hemoglobin, hematocrit, and WBC, platelet, and granulocyte counts.

## CONTRAINDICATIONS & CAUTIONS
● Contraindicated in patients hypersensitive to mesna or compounds containing thiol.

## NURSING CONSIDERATIONS
● Mesna isn't effective in preventing hematuria from other causes (such as thrombocytopenia).
● Because mesna is used with ifosfamide and other chemotherapeutic drugs, it's difficult to determine adverse reactions attributable solely to mesna.
● Although formulated to prevent hemorrhagic cystitis from ifosfamide, drug won't protect against other toxicities from drug therapy.
● Patients who vomit within 2 hours of taking P.O. mesna should repeat the dose or receive I.V. mesna.
● Monitor urine samples for hematuria daily. Monitor BUN and creatinine levels and intake and output.
● Drug contains benzyl alcohol, which has been linked to fatal gasping syndrome in premature infants.

## PATIENT TEACHING
● Explain to patient and family or other caregiver why drug is needed and how it's given.
● Instruct patient to report persistent or severe adverse reactions.
● Advise patient to promptly report blood in urine.

# minoxidil (topical)
Rogaine◇, Rogaine Extra Strength for Men◇, Rogaine for Women◇

*Pregnancy risk category C*

## AVAILABLE FORMS
*Topical solution:* 2%◇, 5%◇

## INDICATIONS & DOSAGES
➤ **Androgenetic alopecia**
*Adults:* 1 ml of solution applied to affected area b.i.d. Maximum daily dose is 2 ml.

## ACTION
Unknown. Stimulates hair growth, possibly by dilating arterial microcapillaries around hair follicles.

| Route | Onset | Peak | Duration |
|-------|-------|------|----------|
| Topical | Unknown | Unknown | Unknown |

## ADVERSE REACTIONS
**CNS:** headache, dizziness, faintness, light-headedness.
**CV:** edema, chest pain, hypertension, hypotension, palpitations, increased or decreased pulse rate.
**EENT:** sinusitis.
**GI:** diarrhea, nausea, vomiting.
**GU:** UTI, renal calculi, urethritis.
**Metabolic:** weight gain.
**Musculoskeletal:** back pain, tendinitis.
**Respiratory:** bronchitis, upper respiratory infection.
**Skin:** *irritant dermatitis,* allergic contact dermatitis, eczema, hypertrichosis, *local erythema, pruritus, dry skin or scalp, flaking,* worsening of hair loss.

## INTERACTIONS
**Drug-drug.** *Petroleum jelly, topical corticosteroids, topical retinoids, other drugs that may increase skin absorption:* May

increase risk of systemic effects of minox-idil. Avoid using together.

**EFFECTS ON LAB TEST RESULTS**
None reported.

**CONTRAINDICATIONS & CAUTIONS**
• Contraindicated in patients hypersensitive to drug or components of solution.
• Use cautiously in patients older than age 50 and in those with cardiac, renal, or hepatic disease.

**NURSING CONSIDERATIONS**
• Patient needs to have normal, healthy scalp before beginning therapy because absorption of drug through irritated skin may cause adverse systemic effects.
• Treatment will most likely succeed in patients with balding area smaller than 4 inches (10 cm) that developed within past 10 years.
• Don't use 5% solution in women.

**PATIENT TEACHING**
• Teach patient how to apply topical minoxidil. Tell him to dry hair and scalp thoroughly before application and not to apply drug to other body areas. Tell patient not to use drug on irritated or sunburned scalp or with other drugs on scalp. Tell him to thoroughly wash hands after application.
• Warn patient to avoid inhaling any spray or mist from drug and to avoid spraying around eyes, because solution contains alcohol and may be irritating.
• Inform patient that more frequent applications or using more than 2 ml/day won't increase hair growth but instead may increase adverse reactions. Tell patient not to double the dose for missed applications.
• Teach patient to monitor pulse rate and body weight.
• Advise patient that therapy will be prolonged and will continue for at least 4 months before clinical effects appear. Tell him that drug must be used daily for optimal results. About 40% of patients will experience moderate to dense hair growth.
• Tell patient that stopping drug may cause loss of new hair growth. New hair growth is usually fine and may be colorless, but will resemble existing hair after continued treatment.

# nimodipine
Nimotop

*Pregnancy risk category C*

**AVAILABLE FORMS**
*Capsules:* 30 mg

**INDICATIONS & DOSAGES**
➤ **To improve neurologic deficits after subarachnoid hemorrhage from ruptured congenital aneurysm**
*Adults:* 60 mg P.O. q 4 hours for 21 days. Begin therapy within 96 hours after subarachnoid hemorrhage.
*Adjust-a-dose:* For patients with hepatic failure, 30 mg P.O. q 4 hours for 21 days.

**ACTION**
Inhibits calcium ion influx across cardiac and smooth-muscle cells, decreasing myocardial contractility and oxygen demand; also dilates coronary and cerebral arteries and arterioles.

| Route | Onset | Peak | Duration |
|-------|-------|------|----------|
| P.O. | Unknown | 1 hr | Unknown |

**ADVERSE REACTIONS**
**CNS:** headache, psychic disturbances.
**CV:** hypotension, flushing, edema, tachycardia.
**GI:** nausea, diarrhea, abdominal discomfort.
**Musculoskeletal:** muscle cramps.
**Respiratory:** dyspnea, wheezing.
**Skin:** dermatitis, rash.

**INTERACTIONS**
**Drug-drug.** *Antihypertensives:* May increase hypotensive effect. Monitor blood pressure.
*Calcium channel blockers:* May increase CV effects. Monitor patient closely.
*Cimetidine:* May increase nimodipine bioavailability. Monitor patient for adverse effects.
**Drug-food.** *Any food:* May decrease absorption of nimodipine. Advise patient to take drug on empty stomach.

**EFFECTS ON LAB TEST RESULTS**
None reported.

**CONTRAINDICATIONS & CAUTIONS**
• Use cautiously in patients with hepatic failure.

**NURSING CONSIDERATIONS**
• Reserve drug for patients who are in good neurologic condition (for example, Hunt and Hess grades I to III).
• Monitor blood pressure and heart rate in all patients, especially at start of therapy.
• If patient can't swallow capsule, make a hole in each end of capsule with an 18G needle, and extract contents into syringe. Empty syringe into patient's nasogastric tube. Flush tube with 30 ml of normal saline solution.
• **Alert:** If using a needle to extract contents of capsule, make sure that drug isn't then given I.V. instead of P.O. Label the syringe "for oral use only" before withdrawing the contents of the capsule.

**PATIENT TEACHING**
• Explain use of drug and review administration schedule with patient and family. Stress importance of compliance for maximum drug effectiveness.
• Instruct patient to report persistent or severe adverse reactions promptly.
• Tell patient not to eat grapefruit or drink grapefruit juice while taking this drug.

---

**orlistat**
Xenical

*Pregnancy risk category B*

---

**AVAILABLE FORMS**
*Capsules:* 120 mg

**INDICATIONS & DOSAGES**
➤ **To manage obesity, including weight loss and weight maintenance with a reduced-calorie diet; to reduce risk of weight gain after previous weight loss**
*Adults:* 120 mg P.O. t.i.d. with or up to 1 hour after each main meal containing fat.

**ACTION**
A reversible lipase inhibitor that forms a bond with active site of gastric and pancreatic lipases, inactivating them. As a result, enzymes can't hydrolyze dietary triglycerides into absorbable free fatty acids and monoglycerides. The undigested triglycerides aren't absorbed, resulting in caloric deficit.

| Route | Onset | Peak | Duration |
|-------|-------|------|----------|
| P.O. | Unknown | Unknown | Unknown |

**ADVERSE REACTIONS**
**CNS:** *headache,* dizziness, fatigue, sleep disorder, anxiety, depression.
**CV:** pedal edema.
**EENT:** otitis.
**GI:** *flatus with discharge, fecal urgency, fatty or oily stool, oily spotting, increased defecation, abdominal pain,* fecal incontinence, nausea, infectious diarrhea, rectal pain, vomiting.
**GU:** menstrual irregularity, vaginitis, UTI.
**Musculoskeletal:** *back pain, leg pain,* arthritis, myalgia, joint disorder, tendinitis.
**Respiratory:** *influenza, upper respiratory tract infection,* lower respiratory tract infection.
**Skin:** rash, dry skin.
**Other:** tooth and gingival disorders.

**INTERACTIONS**
**Drug-drug.** *Cyclosporine:* May alter cyclosporine absorption with variations in dietary intake. Monitor patient's cyclosporine levels if used together.
*Fat-soluble vitamins (such as vitamins A and E and beta-carotene):* May decrease absorption of vitamins. Separate doses by 2 hours.
*Pravastatin:* May slightly increase pravastatin levels and lipid-lowering effects of drug. Monitor patient.
*Warfarin:* May change coagulation values. Monitor INR.

**EFFECTS ON LAB TEST RESULTS**
None reported.

**CONTRAINDICATIONS & CAUTIONS**
• Contraindicated in patients hypersensitive to drug or its components and in those with chronic malabsorption syndrome or cholestasis.
• Use cautiously in patients with history of hyperoxaluria or calcium oxalate nephrolithiasis or those at risk for anorexia nervosa or bulimia.
• Use cautiously in patients receiving cyclosporine therapy because of potential

---

changes in cyclosporine absorption related to variations in dietary intake.

## NURSING CONSIDERATIONS

- Exclude organic causes of obesity, such as hypothyroidism, before starting drug therapy.
- Drug is recommended for use in patients with an initial body mass index (BMI) of 30 kg/m$^2$ or more or those with a BMI of 27 kg/m$^2$ or more and other risk factors (such as hypertension, diabetes, or dyslipidemia).
- In diabetic patients, dosage of oral antidiabetic or insulin may need to be reduced because improved metabolic control may accompany weight loss.
- As with other weight-loss drugs, potential for misuse exists in certain patients (such as those with anorexia nervosa or bulimia).
- **Alert:** Don't confuse Xenical with Xeloda.

## PATIENT TEACHING

- Advise patient to follow a nutritionally balanced, reduced-calorie diet that derives only 30% of its calories from fat. Tell him to distribute daily intake of fat, carbohydrate, and protein over three main meals. If a meal is occasionally missed or contains no fat, tell patient that dose of drug can be omitted.
- Advise patient to adhere to dietary guidelines. GI effects may increase when patient takes drug with high-fat foods, specifically when more than 30% of total daily calories come from fat.
- Drug reduces absorption of some fat-soluble vitamins and beta-carotene. To ensure adequate nutrition, advise patient to take daily multivitamin supplements that contain fat-soluble vitamins at least 2 hours before or after administration of drug, such as at bedtime.
- Tell patient with diabetes that weight loss may improve his glycemic control, so dosage of his oral antidiabetic (such as sulfonylureas or metformin) or insulin may need to be reduced during drug therapy.
- Tell woman of childbearing age to inform prescriber if pregnancy or breast-feeding is planned during therapy.

# pimecrolimus
Elidel

*Pregnancy risk category C*

## AVAILABLE FORMS
*Cream:* 1% in tubes of 15 g, 30 g, and 100 g. Base contains benzyl alcohol, cetyl alcohol, oleyl alcohol, and stearyl alcohol.

## INDICATIONS & DOSAGES
➤ **Short- and intermittent long-term treatment of mild to moderate atopic dermatitis in nonimmunocompromised patients in whom the use of other conventional therapies is deemed inadvisable, or in patients with inadequate response to or intolerance of conventional therapies**
*Adults and children age 2 and older:* Apply a thin layer to the affected skin b.i.d. and rub in gently and completely.

## ACTION
Unknown. Drug inhibits T-cell activation by blocking the transcription of early cytokines. It also prevents the release of inflammatory cytokines and mediators from mast cells in vitro after stimulation by antigen and immunoglobulin E.

| Route | Onset | Peak | Duration |
|---|---|---|---|
| Topical | Unknown | Unknown | Unknown |

## ADVERSE REACTIONS
**CNS:** *headache, fever.*
**EENT:** *nasopharyngitis,* otitis media, sinusitis, pharyngitis, tonsillitis, eye infection, nasal congestion, rhinorrhea, sinus congestion, rhinitis, epistaxis, conjunctivitis, earache.
**GI:** gastroenteritis, abdominal pain, vomiting, diarrhea, nausea, constipation, loose stools.
**GU:** dysmenorrhea.
**Musculoskeletal:** back pain, arthralgias.
**Respiratory:** *upper respiratory tract infections,* pneumonia, *bronchitis, cough,* asthma, wheezing, dyspnea.
**Skin:** skin infections, impetigo, folliculitis, molluscum contagiosum, herpes simplex, varicella, papilloma, *application site reaction* (burning, irritation, erythema, pruritus), urticaria, acne.

---

Reactions may be *common,* uncommon, *life-threatening,* or COMMON AND LIFE-THREATENING.

**Other:** *influenza,* flulike illness, hypersensitivity, toothache, bacterial infection, staphylococcal infection, viral infection.

## INTERACTIONS
**Drug-drug.** *Cytochrome P-450 inhibitors (such as erythromycin, itraconazole, ketoconazole, fluconazole, calcium channel blockers):* May affect metabolism of pimecrolimus. Use together cautiously.
**Drug-lifestyle.** *Natural or artificial sunlight exposure:* May worsen atopic dermatitis. Avoid or minimize exposure.

## EFFECTS ON LAB TEST RESULTS
None reported.

## CONTRAINDICATIONS & CAUTIONS
• Contraindicated in patients hypersensitive to pimecrolimus or its components, in patients with Netherton's syndrome, or in immunocompromised patients.
• Contraindicated in patients with active cutaneous viral infections or clinically infected atopic dermatitis.
• Use cautiously in patients with varicella zoster virus infection, herpes simplex virus infection, or eczema herpeticum.
• Safety of use in pregnant patients hasn't been established.

## NURSING CONSIDERATIONS
• Drug may be used on all skin surfaces, including the head, neck, and intertriginous areas.
• Clear infections at treatment sites before using pimecrolimus.
• If symptoms persist longer than 6 weeks, reevaluate the patient.
• Don't use with occlusive dressing.
• May cause local symptoms such as skin burning. Most local reactions start within 1 to 5 days after treatment, are mild to moderately severe, and last no longer than 5 days.
• Monitor patient for lymphadenopathy. If lymphadenopathy occurs and its cause is unknown, or if the patient develops acute infectious mononucleosis, consider discontinuing drug.
• Drug use may cause papillomas or warts. Consider stopping drug if papillomas worsen or don't respond to conventional treatment.

• It's unknown if drug appears in breast milk. Serious adverse reactions may occur in breast-feeding infants exposed to pimecrolimus. Patient should either stop breast-feeding or stop treatment.

## PATIENT TEACHING
• Inform patient that this medication is for external use only and that he should use it as directed.
• Tell patient to report adverse reactions.
• Tell patient not to use with an occlusive dressing.
• Instruct patient to wash hands after application if hands aren't treated.
• Tell patient to stop therapy after signs and symptoms have resolved. If symptoms persist longer than 6 weeks, tell him to contact his prescriber.
• Tell patient to resume treatment at first signs of recurrence.
• Stress that patient should minimize or avoid exposure to natural or artificial sunlight (including tanning beds and UVA-UVB treatment) while using this drug.
• Tell patient to expect application site reactions but to notify his prescriber if reaction is severe or persists for longer than 1 week.

---

## raloxifene hydrochloride
Evista⌀

*Pregnancy risk category X*

### AVAILABLE FORMS
*Tablets:* 60 mg

### INDICATIONS & DOSAGES
➤ **To prevent or treat osteoporosis in postmenopausal women**
*Adults:* 60 mg P.O. once daily.

### ACTION
A selective estrogen receptor modulator that reduces resorption of bone and decreases overall bone turnover. These effects on bone are manifested as reductions in serum and urine levels of bone turnover markers and increases in bone mineral density.

| Route | Onset | Peak | Duration |
|-------|-------|------|----------|
| P.O. | Unknown | Unknown | 24 hr |

**ADVERSE REACTIONS**
**CNS:** depression, insomnia, fever, migraine.
**CV:** chest pain.
**EENT:** *sinusitis,* pharyngitis, laryngitis.
**GI:** nausea, dyspepsia, vomiting, flatulence, gastroenteritis, abdominal pain.
**GU:** vaginitis, UTI, cystitis, leukorrhea, endometrial disorder, vaginal bleeding.
**Metabolic:** weight gain.
**Musculoskeletal:** *arthralgia,* myalgia, arthritis, leg cramps.
**Respiratory:** increased cough, pneumonia.
**Skin:** rash, diaphoresis.
**Other:** breast pain, *infection, flulike syndrome, hot flashes,* peripheral edema.

**INTERACTIONS**
**Drug-drug.** *Cholestyramine:* May cause significant reduction in absorption of raloxifene. Avoid using together.
*Highly protein-bound drugs (such as clofibrate, diazepam, diazoxide, ibuprofen, indomethacin, naproxen):* May interfere with binding sites. Use together cautiously.
*Warfarin:* May cause a decrease in PT. Monitor PT and INR closely.

**EFFECTS ON LAB TEST RESULTS**
• May increase calcium, inorganic phosphate, total protein, albumin, hormone-binding globulin, and apolipoprotein A levels. May decrease total and LDL cholesterol levels and apolipoprotein B levels.

**CONTRAINDICATIONS & CAUTIONS**
• Contraindicated in women hypersensitive to drug or its components; in those with past or current venous thromboembolic events, including deep vein thrombosis, pulmonary embolism, and retinal vein thrombosis; in women who are pregnant, planning to get pregnant, or breastfeeding; and in children.
• Use cautiously in patients with severe hepatic impairment.
• Safety and efficacy of drug haven't been evaluated in men.

**NURSING CONSIDERATIONS**
• Watch for signs of blood clots. Greatest risk of thromboembolic events occurs during first 4 months of treatment.

• Stop drug at least 72 hours before prolonged immobilization and resume only after patient is fully mobilized.
• Report unexplained uterine bleeding; drug isn't known to cause endometrial proliferation.
• Watch for breast abnormalities; drug isn't known to cause an increased risk of breast cancer.
• Effect on bone mineral density beyond 2 years of drug treatment isn't known.
• Use with hormone replacement therapy or systemic estrogen hasn't been evaluated and isn't recommended.

**PATIENT TEACHING**
• Advise patient to avoid long periods of restricted movement (such as during traveling) because of increased risk of venous thromboembolic events.
• Inform patient that hot flashes or flushing may occur and that drug doesn't aid in reducing them.
• Instruct patient to practice other bone loss–prevention measures, including taking supplemental calcium and vitamin D if dietary intake is inadequate, performing weight-bearing exercises, and stopping alcohol consumption and smoking.
• Tell patient that drug may be taken without regard to food.
• Advise patient to report unexplained uterine bleeding or breast abnormalities during therapy.
• Explain adverse reactions and instruct patient to read patient package insert before starting therapy and each time prescription is renewed.

---

**riluzole**
Rilutek

*Pregnancy risk category C*

---

**AVAILABLE FORMS**
*Tablets:* 50 mg

**INDICATIONS & DOSAGES**
➤ **Amyotrophic lateral sclerosis**
*Adults:* 50 mg P.O. q 12 hours, taken on empty stomach.

---

## ACTION

May protect motor neurons from excitotoxic effects of glutamate by inhibiting glutamate release, inactivating some sodium channels, and interfering with transmitter binding.

| Route | Onset | Peak | Duration |
|-------|-------|------|----------|
| P.O. | Unknown | Unknown | Unknown |

## ADVERSE REACTIONS

**CNS:** headache, aggravation reaction, *asthenia,* hypertonia, depression, dizziness, insomnia, malaise, somnolence, vertigo, circumoral paresthesia.
**CV:** hypertension, tachycardia, palpitations, orthostatic hypotension.
**EENT:** rhinitis, sinusitis.
**GI:** abdominal pain, *nausea,* vomiting, dyspepsia, anorexia, diarrhea, flatulence, stomatitis, dry mouth, oral candidiasis.
**GU:** UTI, dysuria.
**Metabolic:** weight loss.
**Musculoskeletal:** back pain, arthralgia.
**Respiratory:** *decreased lung function,* increased cough.
**Skin:** pruritus, eczema, alopecia, exfoliative dermatitis.
**Other:** phlebitis, peripheral edema, tooth disorder.

## INTERACTIONS

**Drug-drug.** *Allopurinol, methyldopa, sulfasalazine:* May increase risk of hepatotoxicity. Monitor liver function closely.
*Cytochrome P-450 inducers (omeprazole, rifampin):* May increase riluzole elimination. Monitor for lack of effect.
*Cytochrome P-450 inhibitors (amitriptyline, caffeine, phenacetin, quinolones, theophylline):* May decrease riluzole elimination. Watch for adverse effects.
**Drug-food.** *Any food:* May decrease drug bioavailability. Advise patient to take drug 1 hour before or 2 hours after meals.
*Charcoal-broiled foods:* May increase elimination of drug. Discourage use together.
**Drug-lifestyle.** *Alcohol use:* May increase risk of hepatotoxicity. Discourage excessive use.
*Smoking:* May increase riluzole elimination. Discourage patient from smoking.

## EFFECTS ON LAB TEST RESULTS

● May increase AST, ALT, bilirubin, and GGT levels.

## CONTRAINDICATIONS & CAUTIONS

● Contraindicated in patients with history of severe hypersensitivity to drug or its components.
● Use cautiously in patients with hepatic or renal dysfunction, in elderly patients, and in women and Japanese patients (who may have lower metabolic capacity to eliminate drug than men and Caucasian patients, respectively).

## NURSING CONSIDERATIONS

● Elevations in baseline liver function studies (especially bilirubin) preclude drug use. Perform liver function studies periodically during therapy. In many patients, drug may increase aminotransferase level; if level exceeds five times upper limit of normal or if clinical jaundice develops, notify prescriber.
● Give drug at least 1 hour before or 2 hours after meals to avoid decreased bioavailability.

## PATIENT TEACHING

● Tell patient to take drug at same time each day. If a dose is missed, tell him to take next tablet when planned.
● Instruct patient to take drug on an empty stomach to facilitate full dose absorption.
● Instruct patient to report fever to prescriber, who may order a WBC count.
● Warn patient to avoid hazardous activities until CNS effects of drug are known and to limit alcohol use during therapy.
● Tell patient to store drug at room temperature, protect from bright light, and keep out of children's reach.

---

## sildenafil citrate
Viagra✐

*Pregnancy risk category B*

## AVAILABLE FORMS
*Tablets:* 25 mg, 50 mg, 100 mg

---

## INDICATIONS & DOSAGES
➤ **Erectile dysfunction**
*Adults younger than age 65:* 50 mg P.O., p.r.n., about 1 hour before sexual activity. Dosage range is 25 to 100 mg based on effectiveness and tolerance. Maximum is one dose daily.
*Elderly patients (age 65 and older):* 25 mg P.O., p.r.n., about 1 hour before sexual activity. Dosage may be adjusted based on patient response. Maximum is one dose daily.
***Adjust-a-dose:*** For adults with hepatic or severe renal impairment, 25 mg P.O. about 1 hour before sexual activity. Dosage may be adjusted based on patient response. Maximum is one dose daily.

## ACTION
Increases effect of nitric oxide by inhibiting phosphodiesterase type 5 ($PDE_5$), which is responsible for degradation of cyclic guanosine monophosphate (cGMP) in the corpus cavernosum. When sexual stimulation causes local release of nitric oxide, inhibition of $PDE_5$ by sildenafil causes increased levels of cGMP in the corpus cavernosum, resulting in smooth-muscle relaxation and inflow of blood to the corpus cavernosum.

| Route | Onset | Peak | Duration |
|-------|-------|------|----------|
| P.O. | 15-30 min | 30-120 min | 4 hr |

## ADVERSE REACTIONS
**CNS:** anxiety, *headache,* dizziness, ***seizures,*** somnolence, vertigo.
**CV:** ***MI, sudden cardiac death, ventricular arrhythmias, cerebrovascular hemorrhage, transient ischemic attack,*** hypotension, flushing.
**EENT:** diplopia, temporary vision loss, ocular redness or bloodshot appearance, increased intraocular pressure, retinal vascular disease, retinal bleeding, vitreous detachment or traction, paramacular edema, photophobia, altered color perception, blurred vision, burning, swelling, pressure, nasal congestion.
**GI:** *dyspepsia,* diarrhea.
**GU:** hematuria, prolonged erection, priapism, UTI.
**Musculoskeletal:** arthralgia, back pain.
**Respiratory:** respiratory tract infection.

**Skin:** rash.
**Other:** flulike syndrome.

## INTERACTIONS
**Drug-drug.** *Beta blockers, loop and potassium-sparing diuretics:* May increase sildenafil metabolite level. Monitor patient.
*Cytochrome P-450 inducers, rifampin:* May reduce sildenafil level. Monitor effect.
*Delavirdine, protease inhibitors:* May increase sildenafil level, increasing risk of adverse events, including hypotension, visual changes, and priapism. Reduce initial sildenafil dose to 25 mg.
*Hepatic isoenzyme inhibitors (such as cimetidine, erythromycin, itraconazole, ketoconazole):* May reduce sildenafil clearance. Avoid using together.
*Isosorbide, nitroglycerin:* May cause severe hypotension. Use of nitrates in any form with sildenafil is contraindicated.
**Drug-food.** *High-fat meal:* May reduce absorption rate and peak level of drug. Advise patient to take drug on empty stomach.
*Grapefruit:* May increase drug level, while delaying absorption. Advise patient to avoid use together.

## EFFECTS ON LAB TEST RESULTS
None reported.

## CONTRAINDICATIONS & CAUTIONS
• Contraindicated in patients hypersensitive to drug or its components and in those taking organic nitrates.
• Use cautiously in patients age 65 and older; in patients with hepatic or severe renal impairment, retinitis pigmentosa, bleeding disorders, or active peptic ulcer disease; in those who have suffered an MI, CVA, or life-threatening arrhythmia within last 6 months; in those with history of cardiac failure, coronary artery disease, uncontrolled high or low blood pressure, or anatomic deformation of the penis (such as angulation, cavernosal fibrosis, or Peyronie's disease); and in those with conditions that may predispose them to priapism (such as sickle cell anemia, multiple myeloma, leukemia).

---

Reactions may be *common,* uncommon, *life-threatening,* or COMMON AND LIFE-THREATENING.

## NURSING CONSIDERATIONS

• *Alert:* Drug increases risk of cardiac events. Systemic vasodilatory properties cause transient decreases in supine blood pressure and cardiac output (about 2 hours after ingestion). Patients with underlying CV disease are at increased risk for cardiac effects related to sexual activity.

• *Alert:* Serious CV events, including MI, sudden cardiac death, ventricular arrhythmias, cerebrovascular hemorrhage, transient ischemic attack, and hypertension, have been reported with drug use. Most, but not all, of these incidents involved CV risk factors. Many events occurred during or shortly after sexual activity; a few occurred shortly after drug use without sexual activity; and others occurred hours to days after drug use and sexual activity.

• Drug isn't indicated for use in newborns, children, or women.

## PATIENT TEACHING

• Advise patient that drug shouldn't be used with nitrates under any circumstances.

• Advise patient of potential cardiac risk of sexual activity, especially in presence of CV risk factors. Instruct patient to notify prescriber and refrain from further activity if such symptoms as chest pain, dizziness, or nausea occur when starting sexual activity.

• Warn patient that erections lasting longer than 4 hours and priapism (painful erections lasting longer than 6 hours) can occur, and tell him to report them immediately. Penile tissue damage and permanent loss of potency may result if priapism isn't treated immediately.

• Inform patient that drug doesn't protect against sexually transmitted diseases; advise patient to use protective measures such as condoms.

• Tell patient receiving HIV medications that he's at increased risk for sildenafil adverse events, including low blood pressure, visual changes, and priapism, and that he should promptly report such symptoms to his prescriber. Tell him not to exceed 25 mg of sildenafil in 48 hours.

• Instruct patient to take drug 30 minutes to 4 hours before sexual activity; maximum benefit can be expected less than 2 hours after ingestion.

• Advise patient that drug is most rapidly absorbed if taken on an empty stomach.

• Inform patient that impairment of color discrimination (blue, green) may occur and to avoid hazardous activities that rely on color discrimination.

• Instruct patient to notify prescriber of visual changes.

• Advise patient that drug is effective only in presence of sexual stimulation.

• Caution patient to take drug only as prescribed.

# tacrolimus (topical)
Protopic

*Pregnancy risk category C*

## AVAILABLE FORMS
*Ointment:* 0.03%, 0.1%

## INDICATION & DOSAGES
➤ **Moderate to severe atopic dermatitis in patients unresponsive to other therapies or unable to use other therapies because of potential risks**
*Adults:* Thin layer of 0.03% or 0.1% strength applied to affected areas b.i.d. and rubbed in completely. Continue for 1 week after affected area clears.
*Children age 2 and older:* Thin layer of 0.03% strength applied to affected areas b.i.d. and rubbed in completely. Continue for 1 week after affected area clears.

## ACTION
Unknown. Believed to act as an immune system modulator in the skin by inhibiting T-lymphocyte activation, which causes immunosuppression. Drug also inhibits the release of mediators from mast cells and basophils in skin.

| Route | Onset | Peak | Duration |
|-------|-------|------|----------|
| Topical | Unknown | Unknown | Unknown |

## ADVERSE REACTIONS
**CNS:** *headache,* hyperesthesia, asthenia, insomnia.
**CV:** peripheral edema.
**EENT:** *otitis media, pharyngitis,* rhinitis, sinusitis, conjunctivitis.
**GI:** diarrhea, vomiting, nausea, abdominal pain, gastroenteritis, dyspepsia.

---

*Rapid onset   †Canada   ‡Australia   ◊ OTC   ♦ Off-label use   ✐Photoguide   *Liquid contains alcohol.*

**GU:** dysmenorrhea.
**Musculoskeletal:** back pain, myalgia.
**Respiratory:** *increased cough, asthma,* pneumonia, bronchitis.
**Skin:** *burning, pruritus, erythema, infection, herpes simplex,* eczema herpeticum, pustular rash, *folliculitis,* urticaria, maculopapular rash, fungal dermatitis, acne, sunburn, tingling, benign skin neoplasm, vesiculobullous rash, dry skin, varicella zoster, herpes zoster, eczema, exfoliative dermatitis, contact dermatitis.
**Other:** *flulike symptoms, accidental injury, infection,* facial edema, alcohol intolerance, periodontal abscess, cyst, *allergic reaction, fever,* pain, lymphadenopathy.

### INTERACTIONS
**Drug-drug.** *Calcium channel blockers, cimetidine, CYP 3A4 inhibitors (erythromycin, itraconazole, ketoconazole, fluconazole):* May interfere with effects of tacrolimus. Use together cautiously.
**Drug-lifestyle.** *Sun exposure:* May cause phototoxicity. Advise patient to avoid excessive sunlight or artificial ultraviolet light exposure.

### EFFECTS ON LAB TEST RESULTS
None reported.

### CONTRAINDICATIONS & CAUTIONS
• Contraindicated in patients hypersensitive to tacrolimus.
• Don't use in patients with Netherton's syndrome or generalized erythroderma.

### NURSING CONSIDERATIONS
• Use drug only for short-term or intermittent long-term therapy.
• In patients with infected atopic dermatitis, clear infections at treatment site before using drug.
• Don't use with occlusive dressings.
• Use of this drug may increase the risk of varicella zoster, herpes simplex virus, and eczema herpeticum.
• Consider stopping drug in patients with lymphadenopathy, if cause is unknown or acute mononucleosis is diagnosed.
• Monitor all cases of lymphadenopathy until resolution.
• Local adverse effects are most common during the first few days of treatment.

• Use only the 0.03% ointment in children ages 2 to 15.

### PATIENT TEACHING
• Tell patient to wash hands before and after applying drug and to avoid applying drug to wet skin.
• Urge patient not to use bandages or other occlusive dressings.
• Tell patient not to bathe, shower, or swim immediately after application because doing so could wash the ointment off.
• Tell patient to continue treatment for 1 week after affected area clears.
• Advise patient to avoid or minimize exposure to natural or artificial sunlight.
• Caution patient not to use drug for any disorder other than that for which it was prescribed.
• Encourage patient to report adverse reactions.
• Tell patient to store the ointment at room temperature.

✳ *NEW DRUG*

## tadalafil
Cialis

*Pregnancy risk category B*

### AVAILABLE FORMS
*Tablets (film-coated):* 5 mg, 10 mg, 20 mg

### INDICATIONS & DOSAGES
➤ **Erectile dysfunction**
*Adults:* 10 mg P.O. as a single dose, p.r.n., before sexual activity. Range is 5 to 20 mg, based on effectiveness and tolerance. Maximum is one dose daily.
*Adjust-a-dose:* If creatinine clearance is 31 to 50 ml/minute, starting dosage is 5 mg once daily and maximum is 10 mg once q 48 hours. If clearance is 30 ml/minute or less, maximum is 5 mg once daily. Patients with Child-Pugh category A or B shouldn't exceed 10 mg daily. Patients taking potent cytochrome P-450 inhibitors (such as erythromycin, itraconazole, ketoconazole, and ritonavir) shouldn't exceed one 10-mg dose q 72 hours.

## ACTION
By preventing breakdown of cGMP by phosphodiesterase, drug increases cGMP levels, prolongs smooth muscle relaxation, and promotes blood flow into the corpus cavernosum.

| Route | Onset | Peak | Duration |
|-------|-------|------|----------|
| P.O. | Immediate | ½-6 hr | Unknown |

## ADVERSE REACTIONS
**CNS:** *headache.*
**CV:** flushing.
**EENT:** nasal congestion.
**GI:** *dyspepsia.*
**Musculoskeletal:** back pain, limb pain, myalgia.

## INTERACTIONS
**Drug-drug.** *Alpha blockers (except tamsulosin 0.4 mg daily), nitrates:* May enhance hypotensive effects. Use together is contraindicated.
*Potent cytochrome P-450 inhibitors (such as erythromycin, itraconazole, ketoconazole, ritonavir):* May increase tadalafil level. Patient shouldn't exceed a 10-mg dose q 72 hours.
*Rifampin and other cytochrome P-450 inducers:* May decrease tadalafil level. Monitor patient closely.
**Drug-food.** *Grapefruit:* May increase tadalafil level. Discourage use together.
**Drug-lifestyle.** *Alcohol use:* May increase risk of headache, dizziness, orthostatic hypotension, and increased heart rate. Discourage use together.

## EFFECTS ON LAB TEST RESULTS
None reported.

## CONTRAINDICATIONS & CAUTIONS
• Contraindicated in patients hypersensitive to drug or its components and in those taking nitrates or alpha-adrenergic blockers (other than tamsulosin 0.4 mg once daily).
• Drug isn't recommended for patients with Child-Pugh category C, unstable angina, angina that occurs during sexual intercourse, New York Health Association class II or greater heart failure within past 6 months, uncontrolled arrhythmias, hypotension (less than 90/50 mm Hg), uncontrolled hypertension (more than 170/100 mm Hg), stroke within past 6 months, or MI within past 90 days.
• Drug isn't recommended for patients whose cardiac status makes sexual activity inadvisable and for those with hereditary degenerative retinal disorders.
• Use cautiously in patients taking potent cytochrome P-450 inhibitors (such as erythromycin, itraconazole, ketoconazole, and ritonavir) and in patients with bleeding disorders, significant peptic ulceration, or renal or hepatic impairment.
• Use cautiously in patients with conditions predisposing them to priapism (such as sickle cell anemia, multiple myeloma, and leukemia), anatomical penis abnormalities, or left ventricular outflow obstruction.
• Use cautiously in elderly patients, who may be more sensitive to drug effects.

## NURSING CONSIDERATIONS
• **Alert:** Sexual activity may increase cardiac risk. Evaluate patient's cardiac risk before he starts taking drug.
• Before patient starts drug, assess for underlying causes of erectile dysfunction.
• Transient decreases in supine blood pressure may occur.
• Prolonged erections and priapism may occur.

## PATIENT TEACHING
• Warn patient that taking drug with nitrates could cause a serious drop in blood pressure, which increases the risk of heart attack or stroke.
• Tell patient to seek immediate medical attention if chest pain develops after taking the drug.
• Tell patient that drug doesn't protect against sexually transmitted diseases and that he should use protective measures.
• Urge patient to seek emergency medical care if his erection lasts more than 4 hours.
• Tell patient to take drug about 60 minutes before anticipated sexual activity. Explain that drug has no effect without sexual stimulation.
• Warn patient not to change dosage unless directed by prescriber.
• Caution patient against drinking large amounts of alcohol while taking drug.

## tamsulosin hydrochloride
Flomax

*Pregnancy risk category B*

### AVAILABLE FORMS
*Capsules:* 0.4 mg

### INDICATIONS & DOSAGES
➤ **BPH**
*Adults:* 0.4 mg P.O. once daily, given 30 minutes after same meal each day. If no response after 2 to 4 weeks, increase dosage to 0.8 mg P.O. once daily.

### ACTION
Selectively blocks alpha receptors in the prostate, leading to relaxation of smooth muscles in the bladder neck and prostate, improving urine flow, and reducing symptoms of BPH.

| Route | Onset | Peak | Duration |
|-------|-------|------|----------|
| P.O. | Unknown | 4-5 hr | 9-15 hr |

### ADVERSE REACTIONS
**CNS:** asthenia, *dizziness, headache,* insomnia, somnolence, syncope, vertigo.
**CV:** chest pain, orthostatic hypotension.
**EENT:** amblyopia, pharyngitis, *rhinitis,* sinusitis.
**GI:** diarrhea, nausea.
**GU:** decreased libido, abnormal ejaculation, priapism.
**Musculoskeletal:** back pain.
**Respiratory:** increased cough.
**Other:** *infection,* tooth disorder.

### INTERACTIONS
**Drug-drug.** *Alpha blockers:* May interact with tamsulosin. Avoid using together.
*Cimetidine:* May decrease tamsulosin clearance. Use together cautiously.

### EFFECTS ON LAB TEST RESULTS
None reported.

### CONTRAINDICATIONS & CAUTIONS
• Contraindicated in patients hypersensitive to drug or its components.

### NURSING CONSIDERATIONS
• Monitor patient for decreases in blood pressure.

• Symptoms of BPH and prostate cancer are similar; rule out prostate cancer before starting therapy.
• If treatment is interrupted for several days or more, restart therapy at 1 capsule daily.
• *Alert:* Don't confuse Flomax with Fosamax or Volmax.

### PATIENT TEACHING
• Instruct patient not to crush, chew, or open capsules.
• Tell patient to rise slowly from chair or bed when starting therapy and to avoid situations in which injury could occur as a result of fainting. Advise him that drug may cause sudden drop in blood pressure, especially after first dose or when changing doses.
• Instruct patient not to drive or perform hazardous tasks for 12 hours after first dose or changes in dose until response can be monitored.
• Tell patient to take drug about 30 minutes after same meal each day.

---

## thalidomide
Thalomid

*Pregnancy risk category X*

### AVAILABLE FORMS
*Capsules:* 50 mg

### INDICATIONS & DOSAGES
➤ **Cutaneous effects of moderate to severe erythema nodosum leprosum (ENL)**
*Adults and children age 12 and older:* 100 to 300 mg P.O. once daily, with water, preferably h.s. and at least 1 hour after the evening meal.
*Note:* If patient weighs less than 50 kg (111 lb), start dosing at lower end of range.
➤ **To prevent and suppress cutaneous effects of ENL recurrence**
*Adults and children age 12 and older:* Up to 400 mg P.O. daily h.s. or in divided doses, with water, at least 1 hour after meals.

---

## ACTION
Exact mechanism unknown. An immuno-modulatory drug.

| Route | Onset | Peak | Duration |
|-------|-------|------|----------|
| P.O. | Unknown | 3-6 hr | Unknown |

## ADVERSE REACTIONS
**CNS:** *asthenia, drowsiness, somnolence, dizziness,* peripheral neuropathy, *headache,* agitation, insomnia, malaise, nervousness, *paresthesia,* tremor, vertigo.
**CV:** orthostatic hypotension, ***bradycardia,*** peripheral edema.
**EENT:** pharyngitis, sinusitis.
**GI:** dry mouth, oral candidiasis, abdominal pain, anorexia, constipation, *diarrhea,* flatulence, *nausea.*
**GU:** albuminuria, *hematuria,* impotence.
**Hematologic: *neutropenia, increased HIV viral load,* anemia, LEUKOPENIA.**
**Musculoskeletal:** back pain, neck pain or rigidity.
**Skin:** acne, fungal dermatitis, nail disorder, pruritus, *maculopapular or other rash, sweating,* photosensitivity reaction.
**Other: *human teratogenicity,*** hypersensitivity reactions, facial edema, fever, chills, accidental injury, infection, *lymphadenopathy,* pain.

## INTERACTIONS
**Drug-drug.** *Barbiturates, chlorpromazine, reserpine:* May increase sedative activity. Use together cautiously.
*Drugs linked to peripheral neuropathy:* May increase risk of peripheral neuropathy. Use together cautiously.
*Drugs that may reduce efficacy of hormonal contraceptives (such as carbamazepine, griseofulvin, HIV-protease inhibitors, phenytoin, rifabutin, rifampin):* May cause thalidomide-induced teratogenicity if pregnancy occurs. Patient must be advised to use two other highly effective methods of contraception.
**Drug-food.** *Any food:* May decrease absorption of drug. Advise patient to take 1 hour after meals.
**Drug-lifestyle.** *Alcohol use:* May increase sedation. Discourage use together.

## EFFECTS ON LAB TEST RESULTS
• May increase AST, ALT, LDH, and lipid levels.

• May decrease hemoglobin and neutrophil and WBC counts.

## CONTRAINDICATIONS & CAUTIONS
• Contraindicated in patients hypersensitive to drug or its components; in pregnant women; and in those capable of becoming pregnant except when alternative therapies are inappropriate and patient meets all conditions listed in the System for Thalidomide Education and Prescribing Safety (S.T.E.P.S.) program.

## NURSING CONSIDERATIONS
• ***Alert:*** Give drug only if patient complies with all terms outlined in the S.T.E.P.S. program; drug may be prescribed and dispensed only by prescribers and pharmacists registered with the S.T.E.P.S. program.
• All sexually mature patients (men and women) capable of reproduction must meet rigid S.T.E.P.S. program requirements, including ability to understand and carry out instructions, ability and willingness to comply with mandatory contraceptive measures (use of at least two highly effective means of contraception), and written acknowledgment that they understand hazards of fetal exposure to drug and risk of contraceptive failure.
• Sexually mature women who haven't undergone a hysterectomy or who haven't been postmenopausal for at least 24 consecutive months (that is, who have had menses at some time in preceding 24 consecutive months) are considered to be women of childbearing potential even if they have a history of infertility.
• Perform mandatory pregnancy test within 24 hours before starting drug therapy in women of childbearing potential, then weekly during first month of therapy, then monthly for women with regular menstrual cycles. If menstrual cycles are irregular, pregnancy testing continues every 2 weeks during therapy. Retesting is performed if menstrual changes occur, including missed menses.
• Immediately report suspected fetal exposure to FDA (Medwatch) at 1-800-FDA-1088 and to manufacturer.
• Corticosteroids may be given together in patients with moderate to severe neuritis linked to severe ENL reaction. Corticoste-

---

*Rapid onset*   †Canada   ‡Australia   ◇ OTC   ♦ Off-label use   ✐Photoguide   *Liquid contains alcohol.

roids can be tapered and stopped when neuritis improves.

• Patient with history of requiring prolonged treatment to prevent recurrence of cutaneous ENL or who experiences flare during tapering, should use minimum effective dose. Attempt tapering every 3 to 6 months at dose reduction rate of 50 mg every 2 to 4 weeks.

• Obtain WBC count and differential before initiating therapy and periodically thereafter. Reevaluate patients with an absolute neutrophil count falling below 750/mm³ during treatment.

• Monitor patient for signs and symptoms of neuropathy at least once monthly during first 3 months of therapy, then periodically. Notify prescriber immediately if such symptoms as numbness, tingling, or pain in hands or feet occur.

• Viral load in HIV-positive patients may increase.

**PATIENT TEACHING**

• Warn patient of dangers of fetal exposure to any amount of thalidomide. Make sure patient understands and follows the S.T.E.P.S. program.

• Stress that blood and sperm donations are prohibited during therapy.

• Explain that at least two highly reliable means of contraception must be used simultaneously and continuously from at least 1 month before initiation to 1 month after completion of therapy.

• Instruct woman to report signs or symptoms of pregnancy immediately, even if her chances of becoming pregnant are minimal.

• Inform woman of childbearing potential of mandatory pregnancy testing schedule.

• Inform woman that drug must be stopped immediately if pregnancy occurs.

• Caution patient that it isn't known whether drug is present in ejaculate of men receiving thalidomide and that men receiving drug must always use a latex condom when engaging in sexual activity with women of childbearing potential.

• Advise patient to read package insert carefully.

• Instruct woman taking drugs that reduce the effect of hormonal contraceptives (such as carbamazepine, griseofulvin, HIV-protease inhibitors, phenytoin, ri-

fabutin, rifampin) to use two other effective means of contraception.

• Tell breast-feeding woman to stop breast-feeding during therapy.

• Stress importance of storing drug at room temperature, protected from light, and out of reach of children or others who may mistakenly take drug.

• Instruct patient to take drug only as prescribed.

• Caution patient against sharing drug with others, including those who also have a thalidomide prescription.

• Warn patient of potential for dizziness, especially when standing quickly; instruct him to change position slowly when rising.

• Inform patient that drug frequently causes drowsiness and lethargy. Advise him to avoid hazardous activities and alcohol or other drugs that might cause drowsiness.

• Tell patient to take drug at bedtime with glass of water, at least 1 hour after the evening meal.

• Teach patient signs and symptoms of peripheral neuropathy, and tell him to report their occurrence immediately.

• Tell patient to notify prescriber if hypersensitivity reactions, such as an inflamed rash, fever, rapid heartbeat, and low blood pressure, or other adverse reactions occur.

• Advise patient to use sunscreen because drug may cause sensitivity to the sun.

---

# tretinoin (retinoic acid, vitamin A acid)
Avita, Renova, Retin-A, Retin-A Micro, StieVA-A†

*Pregnancy risk category C*

**AVAILABLE FORMS**
*Cream:* 0.02%, 0.025%, 0.05%, 0.1%
*Gel:* 0.01%, 0.025%
*Microsphere gel:* 0.04%, 0.1%
*Solution:* 0.05%

**INDICATIONS & DOSAGES**
➤ **Acne vulgaris**
*Adults and children:* Clean affected area and lightly apply once daily h.s.
➤ **Adjunctive use in the mitigation of fine facial wrinkles in patients who use**

**comprehensive skin care and sunlight avoidance programs**
*Adults:* Apply a small, pearl-sized amount (¼-inch or 5 mm in diameter) to cover affected area lightly, once daily in the evening.

### ADVERSE REACTIONS
**Skin:** *feeling of warmth, slight stinging, local erythema, peeling,* chapping, swelling, blistering, crusting, temporary hyperpigmentation or hypopigmentation.

### ACTION
Inhibits comedones by increasing epidermal cell mitosis and turnover.

| Route | Onset | Peak | Duration |
|-------|-------|------|----------|
| Topical | Unknown | Unknown | Unknown |

### INTERACTIONS
**Drug-drug.** *Topical drugs containing benzoyl peroxide, resorcinol, salicylic acid, or sulfur:* May increase risk of skin irritation. Avoid using together.
*Topical minoxidil or photosensitizing drugs:* May increase risk of skin irritation. Avoid using together.
**Drug-lifestyle.** *Abrasive cleansers, medicated cosmetics, skin preparations containing alcohol:* May increase risk of skin irritation. Discourage use together.
*Sun exposure:* May increase photosensitivity reaction. Advise patient to avoid excessive sunlight exposure.

### EFFECTS ON LAB TEST RESULTS
None reported.

### CONTRAINDICATIONS & CAUTIONS
• Contraindicated in patients hypersensitive to drug or its components and in those with sunburn.
• Use cautiously in patients with eczema.

### NURSING CONSIDERATIONS
• Initially, drug may be applied every 2 to 3 days using a lower concentration to reduce irritation.
• Relapses generally occur within 3 to 6 weeks after therapy is stopped.
• *Alert:* Don't confuse tretinoin with trientine.

### PATIENT TEACHING
• Instruct patient to clean area thoroughly before application and to avoid getting drug in eyes, mouth, or mucous membranes.
• Tell patient to wash hands after application.
• Tell patient to wash face with mild soap no more than b.i.d. or t.i.d. Warn patient against using strong or medicated cosmetics, soaps, or other skin cleansers. Also advise him to avoid topical products containing alcohol, astringents, spices, and lime because they may interfere with drug's actions.
• Tell patient using drug for treatment of fine wrinkles to wait 20 minutes after washing face to apply drug, and to avoid washing face or applying another skin product or cosmetic for 1 hour after application.
• Tell patient that normal use of cosmetics is allowed.
• Advise patient not to stop drug if temporary worsening of inflammatory lesions occurs. If severe local irritation develops, advise patient to stop drug temporarily and notify prescriber. Dosage will be readjusted when application is resumed. Some redness and scaling are normal reactions.
• Warn patient that he may experience increased sensitivity to wind or cold temperatures.
• Instruct patient to minimize exposure to sunlight or ultraviolet rays during treatment. If he becomes sunburned, he should delay therapy until sunburn subsides. Tell patient who can't avoid exposure to sunlight to use SPF-15 sunblock and to wear protective clothing.
• Warn patient that he may have a temporary increase in lesions, which will improve in 2 to 3 weeks.

✳ *NEW DRUG*

### vardenafil hydrochloride
Levitra⟋

*Pregnancy risk category B*

### AVAILABLE FORMS
*Tablets (film-coated):* 2.5 mg, 5 mg, 10 mg, 20 mg

---

## INDICATIONS & DOSAGES

➤ **Erectile dysfunction**

*Adults:* 10 mg P.O. as a single dose, p.r.n., 1 hour before sexual activity. Dosage range is 5 to 20 mg, based on effectiveness and tolerance. Maximum, one dose daily.

*Adjust-a-dose:* For patients age 65 or older and those with Child-Pugh category B, first dose is 5 mg daily, p.r.n. Don't exceed 10 mg daily in patients with hepatic impairment.

## ACTION

Increases cGMP levels, prolongs smooth muscle relaxation, and promotes blood flow into the corpus cavernosum.

| Route | Onset | Peak | Duration |
|-------|-------|------|----------|
| P.O. | Immediate | 30-120 min | Unknown |

## ADVERSE REACTIONS

**CNS:** *headache,* dizziness.
**CV:** *flushing.*
**EENT:** rhinitis, sinusitis.
**GI:** dyspepsia, nausea.
**Musculoskeletal:** back pain.
**Other:** flulike syndrome.

## INTERACTIONS

**Drug-drug.** *Alpha blockers, nitrates:* May enhance hypotensive effects. Avoid using together.
*Antiarrhythmics of class Ia (quinidine, procainamide) and class III (amiodarone, sotalol):* May prolong QTc interval. Avoid using together.
*Erythromycin, indinavir, itraconazole, ketoconazole, ritonavir:* May increase vardenafil level. Reduce dose of vardenafil.
**Drug-food.** *High-fat meals:* May reduce peak level of drug. Discourage use with a high-fat meal.

## EFFECTS ON LAB TEST RESULTS

● May increase CK level.

## CONTRAINDICATIONS & CAUTIONS

● Contraindicated in patients hypersensitive to drug or its components and in those taking nitrates or alpha blockers.
● Contraindicated in patients with unstable angina, hypotension (systolic less than 90 mm Hg), uncontrolled hypertension (over 170/110 mm Hg), stroke, life-threatening arrhythmia, MI within past 6 months, severe cardiac failure, Child-Pugh category C, end-stage renal disease requiring dialysis, congenital QTc interval prolongation, or hereditary degenerative retinal disorders.
● Use cautiously in patients with bleeding disorders or significant peptic ulceration.
● Use cautiously in those with anatomical penis abnormalities or conditions that predispose patient to priapism (such as sickle cell anemia, multiple myeloma, or leukemia).

## NURSING CONSIDERATIONS

● *Alert:* Sexual activity may increase cardiac risk. Evaluate patient's cardiac risk before he starts taking drug.
● Before patient starts drug, assess for underlying causes of erectile dysfunction.
● Transient decreases in supine blood pressure may occur.
● Prolonged erections and priapism may occur.

## PATIENT TEACHING

● Tell patient that drug doesn't protect against sexually transmitted diseases and that he should use protective measures.
● Advise patient that drug is absorbed most rapidly if taken on an empty stomach.
● Tell patient to notify prescriber about visual changes.
● Urge patient to seek medical care if erection lasts more than 4 hours.
● Tell patient to take drug 60 minutes before anticipated sexual activity. Explain that drug has no effect without sexual stimulation.
● Warn patient not to change dosage unless directed by prescriber.

---

# Drugs that prolong the QTc interval

Changes in a patient's heart rate can affect the QT interval of his ECG. To account for variations in the degree to which the QT interval is affected, you can use a formula such as the one below. Such formulas let you determine the QTc interval, also called the corrected QT interval.

$$\frac{\text{QT interval}}{\sqrt{\text{R-R internal}}} = \text{QTc interval}$$

For men younger than age 55, a normal QTc interval is 350 to 430 msec; for wormen younger than age 55, a normal QTc interval is 350 to 450 msec.

A prolonged QTc interval may cause fatal arrhythmias, including ventricular tachycardia and torsades de pointes. The causes of a prolonged QTc interval include disorders such as hypokalemia, hypomagnesemia, renal failure, and heart failure. An abnormal QTc interval also may result from use of the following drugs.

amantadine
amiodarone
aripiprazole
arsenic trioxide
azithromycin
chloral hydrate
chlorpromazine
cisapride
clarithromycin
disopyramide
dofetilide
dolasetron
domperidone
droperidol
erythromycin
felbamate
flecainide
foscarnet
fosphenytoin
gatifloxacin
gemifloxacin
granisetron
halofantrine
haloperidol

ibutilide
indapamide
isradipine
levofloxacin
levomethadyl
lithium
mesoridazine
methadone
moexipril and hydrochlorothiazide
moxifloxacin
naratriptan
nicardipine
octreotide
ondansetron
pentamidine
pimozide
procainamide
quetiapine
quinidine
risperidone
salmeterol
sotalol
sparfloxacin
sumatriptan

tacrolimus
tamoxifen
thioridazine
tizanidine
venlafaxine
voriconazole
ziprasidone
zolmitriptan

# Adverse reactions misinterpreted as age-related changes

In elderly patients, adverse drug reactions can easily be misinterpreted as the typical signs and symptoms of aging. The table below, which shows possible adverse reactions for common drug classifications, can help you avoid such misinterpretations.

| Drug Classifications | Agitation | Anxiety | Arrhythmias | Ataxia | Changes in appetite | Confusion | Constipation | Depression |
|---|---|---|---|---|---|---|---|---|
| ACE inhibitors | | | | | | ● | ● | ● |
| Alpha₁ adrenergic blockers | | ● | | | | | ● | ● |
| Antianginals | ● | ● | ● | | | ● | | |
| Antiarrhythmics | | | ● | | | | ● | |
| Anticholinergics | ● | ● | ● | | | ● | ● | ● |
| Anticonvulsants | ● | | ● | ● | ● | ● | ● | ● |
| Antidepressants, tricyclic | ● | ● | ● | ● | ● | ● | ● | |
| Antidiabetics, oral | | | | | | | | |
| Antihistamines | | | | | | ● | ● | ● |
| Antilipemics | | | | | | | ● | |
| Antiparkinsonians | ● | ● | | ● | ● | ● | ● | ● |
| Antipsychotics | ● | ● | ● | ● | ● | ● | ● | ● |
| Barbiturates | ● | ● | ● | | | ● | | |
| Benzodiazepines | ● | | | ● | | ● | ● | ● |
| Beta blockers | | ● | ● | | | | | ● |
| Calcium channel blockers | | ● | ● | | | | ● | |
| Corticosteroids | ● | | | | | ● | | ● |
| Diuretics | | | | | | ● | | |
| NSAIDs | | ● | | | | ● | ● | ● |
| Opioids | ● | ● | | | | ● | ● | ● |
| Skeletal muscle relaxants | ● | ● | | ● | | ● | | ● |
| Thyroid hormones | | | ● | | ● | | | |

| Difficulty breathing | Disorientation | Dizziness | Drowsiness | Edema | Fatigue | Hypotension | Insomnia | Memory loss | Muscle weakness | Restlessness | Sexual dysfunction | Tremors | Urinary dysfunction | Visual changes |
|---|---|---|---|---|---|---|---|---|---|---|---|---|---|---|
|  |  | ● |  |  | ● | ● | ● |  |  |  | ● |  |  | ● |
|  |  | ● | ● | ● | ● | ● | ● |  |  |  | ● |  | ● | ● |
|  |  | ● |  | ● | ● | ● | ● |  |  | ● | ● |  | ● | ● |
| ● |  | ● |  |  | ● | ● |  |  |  |  |  |  |  |  |
|  | ● | ● | ● |  | ● | ● |  | ● | ● | ● |  |  | ● | ● |
| ● |  | ● | ● | ● | ● | ● | ● |  |  |  |  | ● | ● | ● |
| ● | ● | ● | ● |  | ● | ● | ● |  |  | ● | ● | ● | ● | ● |
|  |  | ● |  |  | ● |  |  |  |  |  |  |  |  |  |
|  | ● | ● | ● |  | ● |  |  |  |  |  |  | ● | ● | ● |
|  |  | ● |  |  | ● | ● |  |  | ● |  | ● |  | ● | ● |
|  | ● | ● | ● |  | ● | ● | ● |  | ● |  |  | ● | ● | ● |
|  |  | ● | ● |  | ● | ● | ● |  |  | ● | ● | ● | ● | ● |
| ● | ● |  | ● |  | ● | ● |  |  |  | ● |  |  |  |  |
| ● | ● | ● | ● |  | ● |  | ● | ● | ● |  |  | ● | ● | ● |
| ● |  | ● |  |  | ● | ● |  | ● |  |  | ● | ● | ● | ● |
| ● |  | ● |  | ● | ● | ● | ● |  |  |  | ● |  | ● | ● |
|  |  |  |  | ● | ● |  | ● |  | ● |  |  |  |  | ● |
|  |  | ● |  |  | ● | ● |  |  | ● |  |  |  | ● |  |
|  |  | ● | ● |  | ● |  | ● |  | ● |  |  |  |  | ● |
| ● | ● | ● | ● |  | ● | ● | ● | ● |  |  | ● | ● |  | ● |
|  |  | ● | ● |  | ● | ● | ● |  |  |  |  | ● |  |  |
|  |  |  |  |  |  | ● |  |  |  |  |  | ● |  |  |

# Herbal medicines

If your patient is taking an herbal medicine, ask him some general questions. For example, ask why he's taking the herb and how long he's been taking it. Find out if the condition he's trying to treat has been diagnosed. If so, is he taking or has he taken prescription or OTC drugs for the condition?

If your patient is taking a prescription or OTC drug as well as an herbal medicine, explain that drug-herb interactions can occur, and advise him to report any unusual signs or symptoms.

For more nursing considerations and patient-teaching information on specific herbal medicines, see the table below.

| Herb names and reported uses | Nursing considerations | Patient teaching |
|---|---|---|
| **ALOE**<br>• Cathartic<br>• Ease defecation<br>• Bowel evacuation<br>• Burns and skin irritation | • Aloe's laxative effects are apparent within 10 hours of ingestion.<br>• Monitor patient for signs of dehydration. Elderly patients are particularly at risk.<br>• Monitor electrolyte levels, especially potassium, after long-term use.<br>• If patient is using aloe topically, monitor wound for healing. | • Caution patient that if he delays seeking medical diagnosis and treatment, his condition could worsen.<br>• If patient is taking digoxin or another drug to control his heart rate, a diuretic, or a corticosteroid, warn him not to take aloe without consulting his health care provider.<br>• Advise patient to reduce dose if cramping occurs after a single dose and not to take aloe for longer than 1 to 2 weeks at a time without consulting his health care provider. |
| **ANGELICA**<br>• Diuretic<br>• Kidney and urinary, GI, respiratory tract conditions<br>• Rheumatic and neuralgic symptoms | • Monitor patient for persistent diarrhea, which may be a sign of something more serious.<br>• Monitor patient for dermatologic reactions.<br>• Photodermatosis is possible after contact with the plant juice or plant extract. | • Caution patient not to delay seeking medical treatment for symptoms that may be related to a serious medical condition.<br>• Advise patient not to take angelica if pregnant or if taking a gastric acid blocker or anticoagulant.<br>• Advise patient to notify his health care provider if he develops a rash. |
| **BITTER MELON**<br>• Diabetes symptoms<br>• GI disorders | • The juice of bitter melon has a bitter taste.<br>• The hypoglycemic effects of bitter melon are dose related, so dosage should be adjusted gradually.<br>• **ALERT:** Bitter melon seeds contain vicine, which may cause an acute condition characterized by headache, fever, abdominal pain, and coma. | • Advise patient not to use herb for longer than 4 weeks.<br>• Inform diabetic patient that herb may cause hypoglycemia.<br>• Tell patient to immediately report headache, fever, and abdominal pain. |
| **CAPSICUM**<br>• Rheumatic arthritis, osteoarthritis, postherpetic neuralgia, and diabetic neuropathy<br>• Personal defense spray | • Topical product shouldn't be used on broken or irritated skin or covered with a tight bandage.<br>• Adverse skin reactions to topically applied capsicum are treated by washing the area thoroughly with soap and water. Soaking the area in | • Advise against use during pregnancy or breast-feeding.<br>• If patient is using capsicum topically, instruct him to wash his hands before and immediately after applying it and to avoid contact with eyes. Advise contact lens wearer to wash |

| Herb names and reported uses | Nursing considerations | Patient teaching |
|---|---|---|
| **CAPSICUM** (continued)<br>• GI complaints<br>• Hypertension<br>• Weight loss | vegetable oil after washing provides a slower onset but longer duration of relief than cold water. Vinegar water irrigation is moderately successful. Rubbing alcohol may also help.<br>• EMLA, an emulsion of lidocaine and prilocaine, provides pain relief in about 1 hour to skin that has been severely irritated by capsicum.<br>• **ALERT:** Advise patient to avoid taking capsicum orally for longer than 2 days and then to avoid using again for 2 weeks.<br>• Topical application may take 1 to 2 weeks for maximum pain control. | his hands and to use gloves or an applicator if handling his lenses after applying capsicum.<br>• If patient is using capsicum topically, advise him not to use topical capsicum on broken or irritated skin and instruct him not to tightly bandage any area to which he has applied it.<br>• Advise patient to promptly contact his health care provider if his condition worsens or if symptoms persist for 2 to 4 weeks. |
| **CHAMOMILE**<br>• Diarrhea, flatulence, stomatitis, motion sickness<br>• Hemorrhagic cystitis<br>• Skin inflammation, wounds, burns<br>• Antibacterial, antiviral<br>• Sedation, relaxation | • **ALERT:** People sensitive to ragweed and chrysanthemums or other Compositae family members (arnica, yarrow, feverfew, tansy, artemisia) may be more susceptible to contact allergies and anaphylaxis. Patients with hay fever or bronchial asthma caused by pollens are more susceptible to anaphylactic reactions. | • Advise patient against use during pregnancy.<br>• If patient is taking an anticoagulant, advise him not to use chamomile because of possible enhanced anticoagulant effects.<br>• Advise patient that chamomile may enhance an allergic reaction or make existing symptoms worse in susceptible patients.<br>• Instruct parent not to give chamomile to any child before checking with a knowledgeable practitioner. |
| **CRANBERRY**<br>• Urinary tract infection (UTI)<br>• Kidney stones<br>• Asthma<br>• Fever | • Tinctures may contain up to 45% alcohol.<br>• Contrary to early investigations focusing on cranberry's ability to acidify the urine, its ability to prevent bacteria from adhering to the bladder wall seems to be more important in preventing UTIs.<br>• Cranberry is safe for use in pregnant and breast-feeding patients.<br>• When consumed regularly, cranberry may be effective in reducing the frequency of bacteriuria with pyuria in women with recurrent UTIs. | • Advise patient that an appropriate antibiotic is usually needed to treat an active UTI.<br>• If patient is using cranberry to prevent a UTI, advise him to notify his health care provider if signs or symptoms of a UTI appear.<br>• If patient has diabetes, inform him that cranberry juice contains sugar but that sugar-free cranberry supplements and juices are available.<br>• Only the unsweetened, unprocessed form of cranberry juice is effective in preventing bacteria from adhering to the bladder wall. |
| **ECHINACEA**<br>• Immune system stimulant<br>• Upper respiratory tract infection<br>• Abscesses, burns, eczema, skin ulcers<br>• Prevention of common cold, upper respiratory infections | • Daily dose depends on the preparation and potency but shouldn't exceed 8 weeks. Consult specific manufacturer's instructions for parenteral administration, if applicable.<br>• Echinacea is considered supportive treatment for infection; it shouldn't be used in place of antibiotic therapy.<br>• Echinacea is usally taken at the first sign of illness and continued for up to 14 days. Regular prophylactic use isn't recommended. | • Advise patient not to delay seeking appropriate medical evaluation for a prolonged illness.<br>• Advise patient that prolonged use may result in overstimulation of the immune system and possible immune suppression. Echinacea shouldn't be used longer than 14 days for supportive treatment of infection.<br>• The herb should be stored away from direct light. |

*(continued)*

| Herb names and reported uses | Nursing considerations | Patient teaching |
|---|---|---|
| **ECHINACEA** (continued) | • Herbalists recommend using liquid preparations because it's believed that echinacea functions in the mouth and should have direct contact with the lymph tissues at the back of the throat. | • Warn patients to keep all herbal products away from children and pets. |
| **EPHEDRA** • Respiratory tract diseases, mild bronchospasm • Asthma • CV stimulant • Chills, cough, cold, flu, fever, headache, edema, nasal congestion • Appetite suppressant • Venereal disease (North American species) | • Compounds containing ephedra have been linked to several deaths and more than 800 adverse effects, many of which appear to be dose related. • Monitor patient's pulse and blood pressure. • Ephedra shouldn't be used for more than 7 consecutive days because of the risk of anaphylaxis and dependence. • Patients with eating disorders may abuse this herb. • **ALERT:** Pills containing ephedra have been combined with other stimulants like caffeine and sold as "natural" stimulants in weight loss products. Deaths from overstimulation have been reported. • **ALERT:** Dosages high enough to produce psychoactive or hallucinogenic effects are toxic to the heart and shouldn't be used. • Signs and symptoms of toxic reaction include diaphoresis, dilated pupils, muscle spasms, fever, and cardiac and respiratory failure. • If overdose occurs, perform gastric lavage and administer activated charcoal. Treat spasms with diazepam, replace electrolytes with I.V. fluids, and prevent acidosis with sodium bicarbonate infusions. | • Advise patient not to use this herb in place of getting the proper medical evaluation for a prolonged illness. • **ALERT:** The FDA has banned the sale of dietary supplements containing ephedra because of unreasonable risk of injury or illness. • Advise patient with thyroid disease, hypertension, CV disease, or diabetes to avoid using ephedra. • Recommend standard pharmaceutical formulations of ephedrine or pseudoephedrine for those with a valid need for these compounds because preparations may differ in ephedrine alkaloid content by 130%. • Advise patient not to use ephedra at dosages that are purported to produce psychoactive or hallucinogenic effects because such dosages are toxic to the heart. • Advise patient to watch for adverse reactions, particularly chest pain, shortness of breath, palpitations, dizziness, and fainting. • Instruct patient to store ephedra away from direct light. • Warn patients to keep all herbal products away from children and pets. |
| **FEVERFEW** • Migraine headache • Rheumatoid arthritis • Asthma • Psoriasis • Menstrual cramps • Mouthwash • Abortifacient • Tranquilizer | • If patient is taking an anticoagulant, monitor appropriate coagulation values, such as INR, PTT, and PT. Also, observe patient for abnormal bleeding. • Rash or contact dermatitis may indicate sensitivity to feverfew. Patient should discontinue use immediately. • Abruptly stopping the herb may cause "postfeverfew syndrome," involving tension headaches, insomnia, joint stiffness and pain, and lethargy. | • Use during pregnancy isn't recommended. • Educate patient about the potential risk of abnormal bleeding when combining herb with an anticoagulant, such as warfarin or heparin, or an antiplatelet, such as aspirin or another NSAID. • Caution patient that a rash or abnormal skin alteration may indicate an allergy to feverfew. Instruct patient to stop taking the herb if a rash appears. |
| **FLAX** • Diarrhea • Constipation | • When flax is used internally, it should be taken with more than 5 oz of liquid per tablespoon of flaxseed. | • Warn patient not to treat chronic constipation or other GI disturbances or ophthalmic injury with flax before |

| Herb names and reported uses | Nursing considerations | Patient teaching |
|---|---|---|
| **FLAX** *(continued)* <br>• Diverticulitis <br>• Irritable bowel syndrome <br>• Externally as poultice for skin inflammation | • Cyanogenic glycosides may release cyanide; however, the body only metabolizes these to a certain extent. At therapeutic doses, flax doesn't elevate cyanide ion level. <br>• Although flax may decrease a patient's cholesterol level or increase bleeding time, it isn't necessary to monitor cholesterol level or platelet aggregation. | seeking appropriate medical evaluation because doing so may delay diagnosis of a potentially serious medical condition. <br>• Advise against use during pregnancy. <br>• Instruct patient to drink plenty of water when taking flaxseed. <br>• Instruct patient not to take any drug for at least 2 hours after taking flax. |
| **GARLIC** <br>• To decrease cholesterol and triglyceride levels <br>• To increase HDL cholesterol <br>• To help prevent atherosclerosis <br>• To decrease risk of GI tract cancers <br>• To decrease risk of stroke, heart attack <br>• To treat colds, coughs, fever, and sore throat | • Garlic isn't recommended for patients with diabetes, insomnia, pemphigus, organ transplants, or rheumatoid arthritis, or for postsurgical patients. <br>• Consuming excessive amounts of raw garlic increases the risk of adverse reactions. <br>• Monitor patient for signs and symptoms of bleeding. <br>• Garlic may lower glucose level. If patient is taking an antihyperglycemic, watch for signs and symptoms of hypoglycemia and monitor his glucose level. <br>• **ALERT:** Advise parents not to use garlic oil to treat inner ear infection in children. | • Advise patient not to delay seeking appropriate medical evaluation because doing so may delay diagnosis of a potentially serious medical condition. <br>• Advise patient to consume garlic in moderation, to minimize the risk of adverse reactions. <br>• Discourage heavy use of garlic before surgery. <br>• If patient is using garlic to lower his cholesterol levels, advise him to notify his health care provider and to have his cholesterol levels monitored. <br>• Advise patient that using garlic with anticoagulants may increase the risk of bleeding. <br>• If patient is using garlic as a topical antiseptic, avoid prolonged exposure to the skin because burns can occur. |
| **GINGER** <br>• Antiemetic <br>• To treat colic, flatulence, indigestion <br>• To treat hypercholesterolemia, burns, ulcers, depression, impotence, liver toxicity <br>• Anti-inflammatory, anti-arthritic <br>• Antispasmodic <br>• Antitumorigenic | • Adverse reactions are uncommon. <br>• Monitor patient for signs and symptoms of bleeding. If patient is taking an anticoagulant, monitor PTT, PT, and INR carefully. <br>• Use in pregnant patients is questionable, although small amounts used in cooking are safe. It's unknown if ginger appears in breast milk. <br>• Ginger may interfere with the intended therapeutic effect of conventional drugs. <br>• If overdose occurs, monitor patient for arrhythmias and CNS depression. | • If patient is pregnant, advise her to consult a knowledgeable practitioner before using ginger medicinally. <br>• Educate patients to look for signs and symptoms of bleeding, such as nosebleeds or excessive bruising. <br>• Warn patient to keep all herbal products away from children and pets. |
| **GINKGO** <br>• To manage cerebral insufficiency, dementia, and circulatory disorders <br>• To treat headaches, asthma, colitis, impotence, depression, altitude sickness, tinnitus, cochlear deafness, | • Ginkgo extracts are considered standardized if they contain 24% ginkgo flavonoid glycosides and 6% terpene lactones. <br>• Treatment should continue for at least 6 to 8 weeks, but therapy beyond 3 months isn't recommended. <br>• **ALERT:** Seizures have been reported in children after ingestion of more than 50 seeds. | • If patient is taking the herb for motion sickness, advise him to begin taking it 1 to 2 days before taking the trip and to continue taking it for the duration of his trip. <br>• Inform patient that the therapeutic and toxic components of ginkgo can vary significantly from product to product. Advise him to obtain his ginkgo from a reliable source. <br>*(continued)* |

| Herb names and reported uses | Nursing considerations | Patient teaching |
|---|---|---|
| **GINKGO** *(continued)* vertigo, premenstrual syndrome, macular degeneration, diabetic retinopathy, and allergies <br>• Adjunctive treatment for pancreatic cancer and schizophrenia | • Patients must be monitored for possible adverse reactions such as GI problems, headaches, dizziness, allergic reactions, and serious bleeding. <br>• Toxicity may cause atonia and adynamia. | • Warn patient to keep all herbal products away from children and pets. <br>• Advise patient to discontinue use at least 2 weeks before surgery. |
| **GINSENG, ASIAN** <br>• To manage fatigue and lack of concentration and to treat atherosclerosis, bleeding disorders, colitis, diabetes, depression, and cancer. <br>• To help recover health and strength after sickness or weakness | • The German Commission E doesn't recommend using ginseng for longer than 3 months. <br>• Ginseng may strengthen the body and increase resistance to disease. <br>• **ALERT:** Reports have circulated of a severe reaction known as the ginseng abuse syndrome in patients taking > 3 g/day for up to 2 years: Increased motor and cognitive activity with diarrhea, nervousness, insomnia, hypertension, edema, and skin eruptions. | • Inform patient that the therapeutic and toxic components of ginseng can vary significantly from product to product. Advise him to obtain his ginseng from a reliable source. |
| **GREEN TEA** <br>• To prevent cancer, hyperlipidemia, atherosclerosis, dental caries, headaches <br>• To treat wounds, skin disorders, stomach disorders, and infectious diarrhea <br>• CNS stimulant, mild diuretic, antibacterial, topical astringent | • Daily consumption should be limited to fewer than 5 cups, or the equivalent of 300 mg of caffeine, to avoid the adverse effects of caffeine. <br>• Prolonged high caffeine intake may cause restlessness, irritability, insomnia, palpitations, vertigo, headache, and adverse GI effects. <br>• The adverse GI effects of chlorogenic acid and tannin can be avoided if milk is added to the tea mixture. <br>• The tannin content in tea increases the longer it's left to brew; this increases the antidiarrheal properties of the tea. <br>• The first signs of a toxic reaction are vomiting and abdominal spasm. | • Advise patient that heavy consumption may be associated with esophageal cancer secondary to the tannin content in the mixture. <br>• Tell patient that the first signs of toxic reaction are vomiting and abdominal spasm. <br>• Tell patient that taking iron supplements or multivitamins with iron with green tea interferes with iron absorption. |
| **HAWTHORNE** <br>• To regulate blood pressure <br>• To treat atherosclerosis <br>• A cardiotonic and sedative <br>• Used in mild heart conditions | • High doses may cause hypotension and sedation. Monitor patient for CNS adverse effects, and monitor blood pressure. <br>• Hawthorne may interfere with digoxin's effects or serum monitoring. <br>• Observe patient closely for adverse reactions, especially adverse CNS reactions. | • Advise patient that when he fills a prescription, he should tell the pharmacist of any herb or dietary supplement he's taking. <br>• Advise patient to avoid use because of toxic adverse effects. <br>• Warn patient to keep all herbal products away from children and pets. |
| **HORSE CHESTNUT** <br>• To treat chronic venous insufficiency, varicose veins, leg pain, tiredness, tension, and leg swelling and edema | • **ALERT:** The nuts, seeds, twigs, sprouts, and leaves of horse chestnut are poisonous and can be lethal. <br>• Standardized formulations remove most of the toxins and standardize the amount of aescin. | • Inform patient that the FDA classifies horse chestnut as an unsafe herb and that deaths have occurred. <br>• Advise patient not to confuse horse chestnut with sweet chestnut, used as a food. |

| Herb names and reported uses | Nursing considerations | Patient teaching |
|---|---|---|
| **HORSE CHESTNUT** *(continued)* • To treat lymphedema, hemorrhoids, and enlarged prostate • Used as an analgesic, anticoagulant, antipyretic, astringent, expectorant, and tonic • To treat skin ulcers, phlebitis, leg cramps, cough, and diarrhea | • Signs and symptoms of toxicity include loss of coordination, salivation, hemolysis, headache, dilated pupils, muscle twitching, seizures, vomiting, diarrhea, depression, paralysis, respiratory and cardiac failure, and death. • Monitor patient for signs of toxicity. • Monitor glucose level in patients taking antidiabetics for hypoglycemia. | • Advise patient to keep the herb away from children. Consumption of amounts of leaves, twigs, and seeds equaling 1% of a child's weight may be lethal. |
| **KAVA** • To treat nervous anxiety, stress, and restlessness • To treat wound healing, headaches, seizure disorders, the common cold, respiratory tract infection, tuberculosis, and rheumatism • To treat urogenital infections, including chronic cystitis, venereal disease, uterine inflammation, menstrual problems, and vaginal prolapse • To treat skin diseases, including leprosy • Used as a poultice for intestinal problems, otitis, and abscesses | • Patient shouldn't use kava with conventional sedative-hypnotics, anxiolytics, MAO inhibitors, other psychopharmacologic drugs, levodopa, or antiplatelet drugs without first consulting a health care provider. • Use for longer than 3 months may be habit forming. • Kava can cause drowsiness and may impair motor reflexes. • Patients should avoid taking herb with alcohol because of increased risk of CNS depression and liver damage. • Periodic monitoring of liver function tests and CBC may be needed. • Toxic doses can cause progressive ataxia, muscle weakness, and ascending paralysis, all of which resolve when herb is stopped. Extreme use (more than 300 g per week) may increase GGT levels. | • Tell patient oral use is probably safe for 3 months or less, but use for longer than 3 months may be habit forming. • Warn patient to avoid taking herb with alcohol because of increased risk of CNS depression and liver damage. • **ALERT:** Tell patient that the FDA has reported kava is linked to liver problems including cirrhosis, hepatitis, and liver failure. Kava users should immediately contact their health care provider if their skin or eyes begin to yellow, or they experience severe itching, easy bruising, dark urine, or bloody vomit. |
| **MELATONIN** • To treat insomnia, jet lag, shift-work disorder, blind entrainment, immune system enhancement, tinnitus, depression, and benzodiazepine withdrawal • Cancer therapy adjuvant, antiaging product, contraceptive, and a prophylactic therapy for cluster headaches • Topically to protect skin against ultraviolet light | • Monitor patient for excessive daytime drowsiness. • May increase human growth hormone levels. | • Warn patient to avoid hazardous activities until full extent of CNS depressant effect is known. • If patient wishes to conceive, tell her that melatonin may have a contraceptive effect. However, herb shouldn't be used as birth control. • Although no chemical interactions have been reported in clinical studies, tell patient that melatonin may interfere with therapeutic effects of conventional drugs. • Warn patient about possible additive effects if taken with alcohol. • Advise patient not to use melatonin for prolonged periods because safety data aren't available. |
| **MILK THISTLE** • Dyspepsia, liver damage from chemicals, Amanita mushroom poisoning, supportive | • Mild allergic reactions may occur, especially in people allergic to members of the Astertaceae family, including ragweed, chrysanthemums, marigolds, and daisies. | • Warn patient not to take this herb while pregnant or breast-feeding. • Tell patient to stay alert for possible allergic reactions, especially if aller- |

*(continued)*

| Herb names and reported uses | Nursing considerations | Patient teaching |
|---|---|---|
| **MILK THISTLE** *(continued)* therapy for inflammatory liver disease and cirrhosis, loss of appetite, and gallbladder and spleen disorders <br>• Liver protectant | • Don't confuse milk thistle seeds or fruit with other parts of the plant or with blessed thistle. | gic to ragweed, chrysanthemums, marigolds, or daisies. <br>• Warn patient not to take herb for liver inflammation or cirrhosis before seeking appropriate medical evaluation because doing so may delay diagnosis of a potentially serious medical condition. |
| **NETTLE** <br>• To treat allergic rhinitis, osteoarthritis, rheumatoid arthritis, kidney stones, asthma, and BPH <br>• Diuretic, expectorant, general health tonic, blood builder and purifier, pain reliever and anti-inflammatory, and lung tonic for ex-smokers <br>• Used for eczema, hives, bursitis, tendinitis, laryngitis, sciatica, and premenstrual syndrome | • Nettle is reported to be an abortifacient and may affect the menstrual cycle. <br>• Allergic adverse effects from internal use are uncommon. | • Recommend caution if patient takes an antihypertensive or antidiabetic. <br>• Warn patient that external adverse effects result from skin contact and include burning and stinging that may persist for 12 hours or longer. <br>• Inform patient that capsules and extracts should be stored at room temperature, away from heat and direct light. <br>• Instruct women taking herb to notify health care provider about planned, suspected, or known pregnancy. <br>• Advise patient not to breast-feed while taking this herb. |
| **PASSION FLOWER** <br>• Sedative, hypnotic, analgesic, and antispasmodic, menstrual cramping, pain, or migraines <br>• Neuralgia, generalized seizures, hysteria, nervous agitation, and insomnia <br>• Topically for cuts and bruises | • Monitor patient for possible adverse CNS effects. <br>• No adverse effects have been observed with recommended doses. <br>• A disulfiram-like reaction may produce nausea, vomiting, flushing, headache, hypotension, tachycardia, ventricular arrhythmias, and shock leading to death. <br>• Patients with liver disease and alcoholics shouldn't use herbal products that contain alcohol. | • Because sedation is possible, caution patient to avoid hazardous activities. <br>• Warn patient not to take herb for chronic pain or insomnia before seeking medical attention because doing so may delay diagnosis of a potentially serious medical condition. <br>• Caution pregnant patients to avoid this herb. |
| **SAW PALMETTO** <br>• To treat symptoms of BPH and coughs and congestion from colds, bronchitis, or asthma <br>• Mild diuretic, urinary antiseptic, and astringent | • Herb should be used cautiously for conditions other than BPH because data about its effectiveness in other conditions are lacking. <br>• Obtain a baseline prostate-specific antigen (PSA) value before patient starts taking herb because it may cause a false-negative PSA result. <br>• Saw palmetto may not alter prostate size. <br>• Laboratory values didn't change significantly in clinical trials using dosages of 160 mg to 320 mg daily. | • Warn patient not to take herb for bladder or prostate problems before seeking medical attention because doing so could delay diagnosis of a potentially serious medical condition. <br>• Tell patient to take herb with food to minimize GI effects. <br>• Caution patient to promptly notify health care provider about new or worsened adverse effects. <br>• Warn women to avoid herb if planning pregnancy, if pregnant, or if breast-feeding. |
| **ST. JOHN'S WORT** <br>• To moderate depression, anxiety, sciatica, and viral infections, | • Recommended duration of therapy for depression is 4 to 6 weeks; if no improvement occurs, a different therapy should be considered. | • Instruct patient to consult a health care provider for a thorough medical evaluation before using St. John's wort. |

| Herb names and reported uses | Nursing considerations | Patient teaching |
|---|---|---|
| **ST. JOHN'S WORT** *(continued)* including herpes simplex virus, hepatitis C, influenza virus, murine cytomegalovirus, and poliovirus<br>• To treat bronchitis, asthma, gallbladder disease, nocturnal enuresis, gout, and rheumatism | • Monitor patient for response to herbal therapy, as evidenced by improved mood and lessened depression.<br>• By using standardized extracts, patient can better control the dosage. Clinical studies have used formulations of standardized 0.3% hypericin as well as hyperforin-stabilized version of the extract.<br>• Serotonin syndrome may cause dizziness, nausea, vomiting, headache, epigastric pain, anxiety, confusion, restlessness, and irritability.<br>• Because St. John's wort decreases the effect of certain prescription drugs, watch for signs of drug toxicity if patient stops using the herb. Drug dosage may need to be reduced.<br>• St. John's wort has mutagenic effects on sperm and egg cells. It shouldn't be used by pregnant patients, women planning pregnancy, or men wishing to father a child. | • If patient takes St. John's wort for mild to moderate depression, explain that several weeks may pass before effects occur. Tell patient that a new therapy may be needed if no improvement occurs in 4 to 6 weeks.<br>• Inform patient that St. John's wort interacts with many other prescription and OTC products and may reduce their effectiveness.<br>• Tell patient that St. John's wort may cause increased sensitivity to direct sunlight. Recommend protective clothing, sunscreen, and limited sun exposure.<br>• Inform patient that a sufficient wash-out period is needed after stopping an antidepressant before switching to St. John's wort.<br>• Tell patient to report adverse effects to a health care provider.<br>• Warn patient to keep all herbal products away from children and pets. |
| **TEA TREE OIL**<br>• Topically for contusions, inflammation, myalgia, burns, hemorrhoids, and vitiligo<br>• Gargle for tonsillitis and lotion for dermatoses | • Because of systemic toxicity, tea tree oil shouldn't be used internally.<br>• Essential oil should be used externally only after being diluted.<br>• Tea tree oil may cause burns or itching in tender areas and shouldn't be used around nose, eyes, and mouth.<br>• Pure (100%) essential tea tree oil is rarely used and only with close supervision by a health care provider. | • Explain that a few drops are sufficient in mouthwash, shampoo, or sitz bath.<br>• Caution patient not to apply oil to wounds or to skin that's dry or cracked.<br>• Warn patient to keep all herbal products away from children and pets. |

# Look-alike and sound-alike drug names

Watch out for the following drug names that resemble other drug names either in the way they're spelled or the way they sound.

abciximab and infliximab

acetazolamide and acetohexamide

acetylcholine and acetylcysteine

Aciphex and Aricept

Aggrastat and argatroban

albuterol and atenolol or Albutein

Aldactone and Aldactazide

Aldomet and Aldoril or Anzemet

alitretinoin and tretinoin

alprazolam and alprostadil

amantadine and rimantadine

Ambien and Amen

Amicar and Amikin

amiloride and amiodarone

aminophylline and amitriptyline or ampicillin

Aminosyn and Amikacin

amiodarone and amiloride

amitriptyline and nortriptyline or aminophylline

amlodipine and amiloride

amoxicillin and amoxapine

Anafranil and enalapril, nafarelin, or alfentanil

anakinra and amikacin

Anturane and Accutane or Artane

Anzemet and Aldomet

Apresoline and Apresazide

Aquasol A and AquaMEPHYTON

Aricept and Ascriptin

Asacol and Os-Cal

atenolol and timolol or albuterol

Atrovent and Alupent

Avinza and Invanz

baclofen and Bactroban

BCG intravesical and BCG vaccine

Benadryl and Bentyl or Benylin

Bentyl and Aventyl or Benadryl

benztropine and bromocriptine or brimonidine

Betagan and BetaGen or Betapen

Bumex and Buprenex

bupropion and buspirone

calcifediol and calcitriol

Carbatrol and carvedilol

carboplatin and cisplatin

Cardene and Cardura or codeine

Cardizem SR and Cardene SR

Cardura and Coumadin, K-Dur, Cardene, or Cordarone

Catapres and Cetapred or Combipres

Celebrex and Cerebyx or Celexa

Chloromycetin and chlorambucil

chlorpromazine and chlorpropamide

cimetidine and simethicone

clomiphene and clomipramine or clonidine

clonidine and quinidine or clomiphene

clorazepate and clofibrate

clotrimazole and co-trimoxazole

clozapine and Cloxapen, clofazimine, or Klonopin

codeine and Cardene, Lodine, or Cordran

corticotropin and cosyntropin

Cozaar and Zocor

cyclosporine and cycloserine

dacarbazine and Dicarbosil or procarbazine

Dantrium and Daraprim

Demerol and Demulen, Dymelor, or Temaril

desipramine and disopyramide or imipramine

desmopressin and vasopressin

desonide and Desogen or Desoxyn

dexamethasone and desoximetasone

Dexedrine and dextran or Excedrin

diazepam and diazoxide

diazoxide and Dyazide

diclofenac and Diflucan or Duphalac

dicyclomine and dyclonine or doxycycline

digoxin and doxepin or Desoxyn

Dilantin and Dilaudid

dimenhydrinate and diphenhydramine

Diprivan and Ditropan

dipyridamole and disopyramide

disopyramide and desipramine or dipyridamole

dobutamine and dopamine

doxapram and doxorubicin, doxepin, or doxazosin

doxycycline, and doxylamine or dicyclomine

d-penicillamine and penicillin

dronabinol and droperidol

DynaCirc and Dynacin

Eldepryl and enalapril

enalapril and Anafranil or Eldepryl

epinephrine and ephedrine or norepinephrine

Epogen and Neupogen

Estratab and Estratest

Ethmozine and Erythrocin

ethosuximide and methsuximide

etidronate and etretinate, etidocaine, or etomidate

Eurax and Serax or Urex

Femara and FemHRT

fentanyl and alfentanil

Flexeril and Floxin or Flaxedil

Flomax and Fosamax or Volmax

floxuridine and fludarabine or flucytosine

flunisolide and fluocinonide

fluorouracil and fludarabine, flucytosine, or floxuridine

fluoxetine and fluvoxamine or fluvastatin

fluticasone and fluconazole

folic acid and folinic acid

fosinopril and lisinopril

furosemide and torsemide

glimepiride and glyburide or glipizide

glucagon and Glaucon

guaifenesin and guanfacine

Haldol and Halcion or Halog

hydralazine and hydroxyzine

hydromorphone and morphine

hydroxyzine and hydroxyurea or hydralazine

HyperHep and Hyperstat or Hyper-Tet

Hyperstat and Nitrostat

idarubicin and daunorubicin or doxorubicin

ifosfamide and cyclophosphamide

imipramine and desipramine

Imodium and Ionamin

Inderal and Inderide, Isordil, Adderall, or Imuran

Isoptin and Intropin

Isordil and Isuprel or Inderal

K-Phos-Neutral and Neutra-Phos-K

Lamictal and Lamisil

lamotrigine and lamivudine

Lanoxin and Levoxyl or levothyroxine

Lantus and Lente

Leukeran and leucovorin

Levatol or Lipitor

levothyroxine and liothyronine or liotrix

Lithonate and Lithostat

Lithotabs and Lithobid or Lithostat

Lodine and codeine, iodine, or Iopidine

Lorabid and Lortab

lorazepam and alprazolam

Lotensin and Loniten or lovastatin

Luvox and Lasix

magnesium sulfate and manganese sulfate

Maxidex and Maxzide

melphalan and Mephyton

Mestinon and Mesantoin or Metatensin

metaproterenol and metoprolol or metipranolol

methimazole and mebendazole or methazolamide

methocarbamol and mephobarbital

methylprednisolone and medroxyprogesterone

methyltestosterone and medroxyprogesterone

metoprolol and metaproterenol or metolazone

Mevacor and Mivacron

Micronor and Micro-K or Micronase

Minocin and niacin or Mithracin

mitomycin and mithramycin

Monopril and Monurol

naloxone and naltrexone

Navane and Nubain or Norvasc

nelfinavir and nevirapine

Nicoderm and Nitro-Dur

Nicorette and Nordette

nifedipine and nimodipine or nicardipine

Nitro-Bid and Nicobid

nitroglycerine and nitroprusside

norepinephrine and epinephrine

Noroxin and Neurontin

nortriptyline and amitriptyline

Nubain and Navane

nystatin and Nitrostat

Ocuflox and Ocufen

olsalazine and olanzapine

opium tincture and camphorated opium tincture

oxaprozin and oxazepam

oxymorphone and oxymetholone

pancuronium and pipecuronium

Parlodel and pindolol

paroxetine and paclitaxel

Paxil and Doxil, paclitaxel, or Taxol

pemoline and Pelamine

penicillin G potassium and Polycillin, penicillamine, or other types of penicillin

pentobarbital and phenobarbital

pentostatin and pentosan

phentermine and phentolamine

phenytoin and mephenytoin

pindolol and Parlodel, Panadol, or Plendil

pioglitazone and rosiglitazone

Pitocin and Pitressin

Plendil and pindolol

pralidoxime and pramoxine or pyridoxine

Pravachol and Prevacid or propranolol

prednisolone and prednisone

Prilosec and Prozac, Prinivil, or Plendil

primidone and prednisone

Prinivil and Proventil or Prilosec

ProAmatine and protamine

probenecid and Procanbid

promethazine and promazine

propranolol and Pravachol

ProSom and Proscar, Prozac, or Psorcon

protamine and Protopam or Protropin

pyridoxine and pralidoxime or Pyridium

Questran and Quarzan

quinidine and quinine or clonidine

ranitidine and ritodrine or rimantadine

Reminyl and Robinul

Restoril and Vistaril

riboflavin and ribavirin

rifabutin and rifampin or rifapentine

Rifater and Rifadin or Rifamate

risperidone and reserpine

Ritalin and Rifadin

ritodrine and ranitidine

ritonavir and Retrovir

Sandimmune and Sandoglobulin or Sandostatin

saquinavir and saquinavir mesylate

Sarafem and Serophene

selegiline and Stelazine

Serentil and Serevent or Aventyl

Serzone and Seroquel

Sinequan and saquinavir

Solu-Cortef and Solu-Medrol

somatropin and somatrem or sumatriptan

sotalol and Stadol

streptozocin and streptomycin

sufentanil and alfentanil or fentanyl

sulfadiazine and sulfasalazine

sulfamethoxazole and sulfamethizole

sulfasalazine and sulfisoxazole, salsalate, or sulfadiazine

sumatriptan and somatropin

Survanta and Sufenta

Tegretol and Toradol

Tenex and Xanax, Entex, or Ten-K

terbutaline and tolbutamide or terbinafine

terconazole and tioconazole

Testoderm and Estraderm

testosterone and testolactone

thiamine and Thorazine

thioridazine and Thorazine

Tigan and Ticar

timolol and atenolol

Timoptic and Viroptic

tobramycin and Trobicin

Tobrex and Tobradex

tolnaftate and Tornalate

Toradol and Tegretol

Trental and Trendar or Trandate

triamcinolone and Triaminicin or Triaminicol

rifluoperazine and triflupromazine

trimipramine and triamterene or trimeprazine

Ultracet and Ultracef

Urispas and Urised

valacyclovir and valganciclovir

Vancenase and Vanceril

Vanceril and Vansil

Verelan and Vivarin, Ferralyn, or Virilon

Versed and VePesid

vidarabine and cytarabine

vinblastine and vincristine, vindesine, or vinorelbine

Volmax and Flomax

Voltaren and Ventolin or Verelan

Wellbutrin and Wellcovorin or Wellferon

Xanax and Zantac or Tenex

Xenical and Xeloda

Zarontin and Zaroxolyn

Zebeta and DiaBeta

Zestril and Zostrix

Zocor and Zoloft

Zofran and Zosyn, Zantac, or Zoloft

Zyprexa and Zyrtec

# Drugs that shouldn't be crushed

Many drug forms, such as slow-release, enteric-coated, encapsulated beads, wax-matrix, sublingual, and buccal forms, are made to release their active ingredients over a certain period of time or at preset points after administration. The disruptions caused by crushing these drug forms can dramatically affect the absorption rate and increase the risk of adverse reactions.

Other reasons not to crush these drug forms include such considerations as taste, tissue irritation, and unusual formulation—for example, a capsule within a capsule, a liquid within a capsule, or a multiple-compressed tablet. Avoid crushing the following drugs, listed by brand name, for the reasons noted beside them.

Accutane (irritant)
Aciphex (delayed release)
Adalat CC (sustained release)
Advicor (extended-release)
Aggrenox (extended release)
Allegra D (extended release)
Altocor (extended-release)
Amnesteem (irritant)
Arthrotec (delayed release)
Asacol (delayed release)
Augmentin XR (extended-release)
Avinza (extended-release)
Azulfidine EN-tabs (enteric coated)
Bellergal-S (slow release)
Biaxin XL (extended-release)
Bisacodyl (enteric coated)
Bontril Slow-Release (slow release)
Breonesin (liquid filled)
Brexin L.A. (slow release)
Bromfed (slow release)
Bromfed-PD (slow release)
Calan SR (sustained release)
Carbatrol (extended release)
Cardizem CD, LA, SR (slow release)
Cartia XT (extended-release)
Ceclor CD (slow release)
Ceftin (strong, persistent taste)
Charcoal Plus DS (enteric coated)
Chloral Hydrate (liquid within a capsule, taste)
Chlor-Trimeton Allergy 8-hour and 12-hour (slow release)
Choledyl SA (slow release)
Cipro XR (extended-release)
Claritin-D 12-hour (slow release)
Claritin-D 24-hour (slow release)

Colace (liquid within a capsule)
Colazal (granules within capsules must reach colon intact)
Colestid (protective coating)
Compazine Spansules (slow release)
Concerta (extended release)
Congess SR (sustained release)
Contac 12 Hour, Maximum Strength 12 Hour (slow release)
Cotazym-S (enteric coated)
Covera-HS (extended release)
Creon (enteric coated)
Cytovene (irritant)
Dallergy, Dallergy-Jr (slow release)
Deconamine SR (slow release)
Depakene (slow release, mucous membrane irritant)
Depakote (enteric coated)
Depakote ER (extended-release)
Desyrel (taste)
Dexedrine Spansule (slow release)
Diamox Sequels (slow release)
Dilacor XR (extended-release)
Dilatrate-SR (slow release)
Diltia XT (extended-release)
Dimetapp Extentabs (slow release)
Ditropan XL (slow release)
Dolobid (irritant)
Drisdol (liquid filled)
Dristan (protective coating)
Drixoral (slow release)
Dulcolax (enteric coated)
DynaCirc CR (slow release)
Easprin (enteric coated)
Ecotrin (enteric coated)
Ecotrin Maximum Strength (enteric coated)

E.E.S. 400 Filmtab (enteric coated)

Effexor XR (extended release)

Emend (hard gelatin capsule)

E-Mycin (enteric coated)

Entex LA (slow release)

Entex PSE (slow release)

Eryc (enteric coated)

Ery-Tab (enteric coated)

Erythrocin Stearate (enteric coated)

Erythromycin Base (enteric coated)

Eskalith CR (slow release)

Extendryl JR, SR (slow release)

Feldene (mucous membrane irritant)

Feosol (enteric coated)

Feratab (enteric coated)

Fergon (slow release)

Fero-Folic 500 (slow release)

Fero-Grad-500 (slow release)

Ferro-Sequel (slow release)

Feverall Children's Capsules, Sprinkle (taste)

Flomax (slow release)

Fumatinic (slow release)

Geocillin (taste)

Glucophage XR (extended-release)

Glucotrol XL (slow release)

Guaifed (slow release)

Guaifed-PD (slow release)

Guaifenex LA (slow release)

Guaifenex PSE (slow release)

Humibid DM, LA, Pediatric (slow release)

Hydergine LC (liquid within a capsule)

Hytakerol (liquid filled)

Iberet (slow release)

ICAPS Plus (slow release)

ICAPS Time Release (slow release)

Imdur (slow release)

Inderal LA (slow release)

Indocin SR (slow release)

InnoPran XL (extended-release)

Ionamin (slow release)

Isoptin SR (sustained release)

Isordil Sublingual (sublingual)

Isordil Tembids (slow release)

Isosorbide Dinitrate Sublingual (sublingual)

Kaon-Cl (slow release)

K-Dur (slow release)

Klor-Con (slow release)

Klotrix (slow release)

K-Tab (slow release)

Levbid (slow release)

Levsinex Timecaps (slow release)

Lithobid (slow release)

Macrobid (slow release)

Mestinon Timespans (slow release)

Metadate CD, ER (extended-release)

Methylin ER (extended release)

Micro-K Extencaps (slow release)

Motrin (taste)

MS Contin (slow release)

Mucinex (extended-release)

Naprelan (slow release)

Nexium (sustained release)

Niaspan (extended-release)

Nitroglyn (slow release)

Nitrong (slow release)

Nitrostat (sublingual)

Norflex (slow release)

Norpace CR (slow release)

Oramorph SR (slow release)

Oruvail (extended release)

OxyContin (slow release)

Pancrease (enteric coated)

Pancrease MT (enteric coated)

Paxil CR (controlled-release)

PCE (slow release)

Pentasa (controlled release)

Phazyme (slow release)

Phazyme 95 (slow release)

Phenytex (extended-release)

Plendil (slow release)

Prelu-2 (slow release)

Prevacid, Prevacid SoluTab (delayed release)

Prilosec (slow release)

Prilosec OTC (delayed-release)

Pro-Banthine (taste)

Procanbid (slow release)

Procardia (delayed absorption)

Procardia XL (slow release)

Protonix (delayed release)

Proventil Repetabs (slow release)

Prozac Weekly (slow release)

Quibron-T/SR (slow release)

Quinidex Extentabs (slow release)
Respaire SR (slow release)
Respbid (slow release)
Risperdal M-Tab (delayed-release)
Ritalin-LA, -SR (slow release)
Rondec-TR (slow release)
Sinemet CR (slow release)
Slo-bid Gyrocaps (slow release)
Slo-Niacin (slow release)
Slo-Phyllin GG, Gyrocaps (slow release)
Slow FE (slow release)
Slow-K (slow release)
Slow-Mag (slow release)
Sorbitrate (sublingual)
Sotret (irritant)
Sudafed 12 Hour (slow release)
Sustaire (slow release)
Tegretol-XR (extended release)
Ten-K (slow release)
Tenuate Dospan (slow release)
Tessalon Perles (slow release)
Theobid Duracaps (slow release)
Theochron (slow release)
Theoclear LA (slow release)
Theolair-SR (slow release)
Theo-Sav (slow release)
Theospan-SR (slow release)
Theo-24 (slow release)
Theovent (slow release)
Theo-X (slow release)
Thorazine Spansules (slow release)
Tiazac (sustained release)
Topamax (taste)
Toprol XL (extended release)
T-Phyl (slow release)
Trental (slow release)
Trinalin Repetabs (slow release)
Tylenol Extended Relief (slow release)
Uniphyl (slow release)
Vantin (taste)
Verelan, Verelan PM (slow release)
Volmax (slow release)
Voltaren (enteric coated)
Voltaren-XR (extended release)
Wellbutrin SR (sustained release)
Xanax XR (extended-release)

Zerit XR (extended-release)
Zomig-ZMT (delayed-release)
ZORprin (slow release)
Zyban (slow release)
Zyrtec-D 12 hour (extended-release)

# Therapeutic drug monitoring guidelines

| Drug | Laboratory test monitored | Therapeutic ranges of test |
|------|---------------------------|----------------------------|
| aminoglycoside antibiotics (amikacin, gentamicin, tobramycin) | Amikacin peak<br>Amikacin trough<br>Gentamicin, tobramycin peak<br>Gentamicin, tobramycin trough<br>Creatinine | 20-30 mcg/ml<br>1-8 mcg/ml<br>4-12 mcg/ml<br>< 2 mcg/ml<br>0.6-1.3 mg/dl |
| angiotensin-converting enzyme (ACE) inhibitors (benazepril, captopril, enalapril, enalaprilat, fosinopril, lisinopril, moexipril, quinapril, ramipril, trandolapril) | WBC with differential<br>Creatinine<br>BUN<br>Potassium | *****<br>0.6-1.3 mg/dl<br>5-20 mg/dl<br>3.5-5 mEq/L |
| amphotericin B | Creatinine<br>BUN<br>Electrolytes (especially potassium and magnesium)<br><br><br>Liver function<br>CBC with differential and platelets | 0.6-1.3 mg/dl<br>5-20 mg/dl<br>Potassium: 3.5-5 mEq/L<br>Magnesium: 1.5-2.5 mEq/L<br>Sodium: 135-145 mEq/L<br>Chloride: 98-106 mEq/L<br>*<br>***** |
| antibiotics | WBC with differential<br>Cultures and sensitivities | ***** |
| biguanides (metformin) | Creatinine<br>Fasting glucose<br>Glycosylated hemoglobin<br>CBC | 0.6-1.3 mg/dl<br>70-110 mg/dl<br>5.5%-8.5% of total hemoglobin<br>***** |
| carbamazepine | Carbamazepine<br>CBC with differential<br>Liver function<br>BUN<br>Platelet count | 4-12 mcg/ml<br>*****<br>*<br>5-20 mg/dl<br>150-450 × 10³/mm³ |
| clozapine | WBC with differential | ***** |
| corticosteroids (cortisone, hydrocortisone, prednisone, prednisolone, triamcinolone, methylprednisolone, dexamethasone, betamethasone) | Electrolytes (especially potassium)<br><br><br><br><br>Fasting glucose | Potassium: 3.5-5 mEq/L<br>Magnesium 1.7-2.1 mEq/L<br>Sodium 135-145 mEq/L<br>Chloride 98-106 mEq/L<br>Calcium 8.6-10 mg/dl<br>70-110 mg/dl |

Note: ***** For those areas marked with asterisks, the following values can be used:

Hemoglobin: Women: 12-16 g/dl
   Men: 14-18 g/dl
Hematocrit: Women: 37%-48%
   Men: 42%-52%
RBCs: 4-5.5 × 10⁶/mm³
WBCs: 5-10 × 10³/mm³

Differential: Neutrophils: 45%-74%
   Bands: 0%-8%
   Lymphocytes: 16%-45%
   Monocytes: 4%-10%
   Eosinophils: 0%-7%
   Basophils: 0%-2%

## Monitoring guidelines

Wait until the administration of the third dose to check drug levels. Obtain blood for peak level 30 minutes after I.V. infusion ends or 60 minutes after I.M. administration. For trough levels, draw blood just before next dose. Dosage may need to be adjusted accordingly. Recheck after three doses. Monitor creatinine and BUN levels and urine output for signs of decreasing renal function. Monitor urine for increased proteins, cells, casts.

Monitor WBC with differential before therapy, monthly during the first 3 to 6 months, then periodically for the first year. Monitor renal function and potassium level periodically.

Monitor creatinine, BUN, and electrolyte levels at least weekly during therapy. Also, regularly monitor blood counts and liver function test results during therapy.

Specimen cultures and sensitivities will determine the cause of the infection and the best treatment. Monitor WBC with differential weekly during therapy.

Check renal function and hematologic values before starting therapy and at least annually thereafter. If the patient has impaired renal function, don't use metformin because it may cause lactic acidosis. Monitor response to therapy by periodically evaluating fasting glucose and glycosylated hemoglobin levels. A patient's home monitoring of glucose levels helps monitor compliance and response.

Monitor blood counts and platelets before therapy, monthly during the first 2 months, then yearly. Liver function, BUN, and urinalysis should be checked before and periodically during therapy.

Obtain WBC with differential before starting therapy, weekly during therapy, and 4 weeks after stopping drug.

Monitor electrolyte and glucose levels regularly during long-term therapy.

*(continued)*

* For those areas marked with one asterisk, the following values can be used:

ALT: 7-56 units/L
AST: 5-40 units/L
Alkaline phosphatase: 17-142 units/L
LDH: 60-220 units/L
GGT: < 40 units/L
Total bilirubin: 0.2-1 mg/dl

| Drug | Laboratory test monitored | Therapeutic ranges of test |
|---|---|---|
| digoxin | Digoxin | 0.8-2 nanograms/ml |
| | Electrolytes (especially potassium, magnesium, and calcium) | Potassium: 3.5-5 mEq/L<br>Magnesium: 1.7-2.1 mEq/L<br>Sodium: 135-145 mEq/L<br>Chloride: 98-106 mEq/L<br>Calcium: 8.6-10 mg/dl |
| | Creatinine | 0.6-1.3 mg/dl |
| erythropoietin | Hematocrit | Women: 36%-48%<br>Men: 42%-52% |
| | Serum ferritin | 10-383 mg/ml |
| | Transferrin saturation | 220-400 mg/dl |
| | CBC with differential | ***** |
| | Platelet count | 150-450 × 10³/mm³ |
| ethosuximide | Ethosuximide | 40-100 mcg/ml |
| | Liver function | * |
| | CBC with differential | ***** |
| gemfibrozil | Lipids | Total cholesterol: < 200 mg/dl<br>LDL: < 130 mg/dl<br>HDL: Women: 40-75 mg/dl<br>Men: 37-70 mg/dl<br>Triglycerides: 10-160 mg/dl |
| | Liver function | * |
| | Serum glucose | 70-100 mg/dl |
| | CBC | ***** |
| heparin | Activated partial thromboplastin time (aPTT) | 1.5-2.5 times control |
| | Hematocrit | ***** |
| | Platelet count | 150-450 × 10³/mm³ |
| HMG-CoA reductase inhibitors (atorvastatin, fluvastatin, lovastatin, pravastatin, simvastatin) | Lipids | Total cholesterol: < 200 mg/dl<br>LDL: < 130 mg/dl<br>HDL: Women: 40-75 mg/dl<br>Men: 37-70 mg/dl<br>Triglycerides: 10-160 mg/dl |
| | Liver function | * |
| insulin | Fasting glucose | 70-110 mg/dl |
| | Glycosylated hemoglobin | 5.5%-8.5% of total hemoglobin |
| isotretinoin | Pregnancy test | negative |
| | Liver function | * |
| | Lipids | Total cholesterol: < 200 mg/dl<br>LDL: < 130 mg/dl<br>HDL: Women: 40-75 mg/dl<br>Men: 37-70 mg/dl<br>Triglycerides: 10-160 mg/dl |
| | CBC with differential | ***** |
| | Platelet count | 150-450 × 10³/mm³ |

Note: ***** For those areas marked with asterisks, the following values can be used:

Hemoglobin: Women: 12-16 g/dl
  Men: 14-18 g/dl
Hematocrit: Women: 37%-48%
  Men: 42%-52%
RBCs: 4-5.5 × 10⁶/mm³
WBCs: 5-10 × 10³/mm³

Differential: Neutrophils: 45%-74%
  Bands: 0%-8%
Lymphocytes: 16%-45%
Monocytes: 4%-10%
Eosinophils: 0%-7%
Basophils: 0%-2%

## Monitoring guidelines

Check digoxin levels just before the next dose or a minimum ≥ 6-8 hours after the last dose. To monitor maintenance therapy, check drug levels at least 1 to 2 weeks after therapy is initiated or changed. Make any adjustments in therapy based on entire clinical picture, not solely on drug levels. Also, check electrolyte levels and renal function periodically during therapy.

After therapy is initiated or changed, monitor the hematocrit twice weekly for 2 to 6 weeks until stabilized in the target range and a maintenance dose determined. Monitor hematocrit regularly thereafter.

Check drug level 8 to 10 days after therapy is initiated or changed. Periodically monitor CBC with differential, liver function tests, and urinalysis.

Therapy is usually withdrawn after 3 months if response is inadequate. Patient must be fasting to measure triglyceride levels. Periodically obtain blood counts during the first 12 months.

When drug is given by continuous I.V. infusion, check aPTT every 4 hours in the early stages of therapy, and daily thereafter. When drug is given by deep S.C. injection, check aPTT 4 to 6 hours after injection, and daily thereafter. Periodic platelet counts, hematocrits, and tests for occult blood in stool are recommended during therapy.

Perform liver function tests at baseline, 6 to 12 weeks after therapy is initiated or changed, and approximately every 6 months thereafter. If adequate response isn't achieved within 6 weeks, consider changing the therapy.

Monitor response to therapy by evaluating glucose and glycosylated hemoglobin levels. Glycosylated hemoglobin level is a good measure of long-term control. A patient's home monitoring of glucose levels helps measure compliance and response.

Use a serum or urine pregnancy test with a sensitivity of at least 25 mIU/ml. Perform one test before therapy and a second test during the first 5 days of the menstrual cycle before therapy begins or at least 11 days after the last unprotected act of sexual intercourse, whichever is later. Repeat pregnancy tests monthly. Obtain baseline liver function tests and lipid levels; repeat every 1 to 2 weeks until a response is established (usually 4 weeks).

*(continued)*

* For those areas marked with one asterisk, the following values can be used:

ALT: 7-56 units/L
AST: 5-40 units/L
Alkaline phosphatase: 17-142 units/L
LDH: 60-220 units/L
GGT: < 40 units/L
Total bilirubin: 0.2-1 mg/dl

| Drug | Laboratory test monitored | Therapeutic ranges of test |
|------|---------------------------|----------------------------|
| linezolid | CBC with differential | ***** |
| | Cultures and sensitivities | |
| | Platelet count | $150-450 \times 10^3/mm^3$ |
| | Liver function | * |
| | Amylase | 35-118 IU/L |
| | Lipase | 10-150 units/L |
| lithium | Lithium | 0.6-1.2 mEq/L |
| | Creatinine | 0.6-1.3 mg/dl |
| | CBC | ***** |
| | Electrolytes (especially potassium and sodium) | Potassium: 3.5-5 mEq/L |
| | | Magnesium: 1.7-2.1 mEq/L |
| | | Sodium: 135-145 mEq/L |
| | | Chloride: 98-106 mEq/L |
| | Fasting glucose | 70-110 mg/dl |
| | Thyroid function tests | TSH: 0.2-5.4 microunits/ml |
| | | $T_3$: 80-200 nanogram/dl |
| | | $T_4$: 5.4-11.5 mcg/dl |
| methotrexate | Methotrexate | Normal elimination: |
| | | ~ 10 micromol 24 hours postdose |
| | | ~ 1 micromol 48 hours postdose |
| | | < 0.2 micromol 72 hours postdose |
| | CBC with differential | ***** |
| | Platelet count | $150-450 \times 10^3/mm^3$ |
| | Liver function | * |
| | Creatinine | 0.6-1.3 mg/dl |
| non-nucleoside reverse transcriptase inhibitors (nevirapine, delavirdine, efavirenz) | Liver function | * |
| | CBC with differential and platelets | ***** |
| | Lipids (efavirenz) | Total cholesterol: < 200 mg/dl |
| | | LDL: < 130 mg/dl |
| | | HDL: Women: 40-75 mg/dl |
| | | Men: 37-70 mg/dl |
| | | Triglycerides: 10-160 mg/dl |
| | Amylase | 35-118 IU/L |
| phenytoin | Phenytoin | 10-20 mcg/ml |
| | CBC | ***** |
| procainamide | Procainamide | 3-10 mcg/ml (procainamide) |
| | N-acetylprocainamide (NAPA) | 10-30 mcg/ml (combined procainamide and NAPA) |
| | CBC | ***** |
| | Liver function | * |
| | ANA titer | Negative |

Note: ***** For those areas marked with asterisks, the following values can be used:

Hemoglobin: Women: 12-16 g/dl
    Men: 14-18 g/dl
Hematocrit: Women: 37%-48%
    Men: 42%-52%
RBCs: $4-5.5 \times 10^6/mm^3$
WBCs: $5-10 \times 10^3/mm^3$

Differential: Neutrophils: 45%-74%
    Bands: 0%-8%
    Lymphocytes: 16%-45%
    Monocytes: 4%-10%
    Eosinophils: 0%-7%
    Basophils: 0%-2%

## Monitoring guidelines

Obtain baseline CBC with differential and platelet count. Repeat weekly, especially if more than 2 weeks of therapy are received. Monitor liver function tests and amylase and lipase levels during therapy.

Checking lithium levels is crucial to the safe use of the drug. Obtain lithium levels immediately before next dose. Monitor levels twice weekly until stable. Once at steady state, levels should be checked weekly; when the patient is on the appropriate maintenance dose, levels should be checked every 2 to 3 months. Monitor creatinine, electrolyte, and fasting glucose levels; CBC; and thyroid function test results before therapy is initiated and periodically during therapy.

Monitor methotrexate levels according to dosing protocol. Monitor CBC with differential, platelet count, and liver and renal function test results more frequently when therapy is initiated or changed and when methotrexate levels may be elevated, such as when the patient is dehydrated.

Obtain baseline liver function tests and monitor closely during the first 12 weeks of therapy. Continue to monitor regularly during therapy. Check CBC with differential and platelet count before therapy and periodically during therapy. Monitor lipid levels during efavirenz therapy. Monitor amylase level during efavirenz and delavirdine therapy.

Monitor phenytoin levels immediately before next dose and 7 to 10 days after therapy is initiated or changed. Obtain a CBC at baseline and monthly early in therapy. Watch for toxic effects at therapeutic levels. Adjust the measured level for hypoalbuminemia or renal impairment, which can increase free drug levels.

Measure procainamide levels 6 to 12 hours after a continuous infusion is started or immediately before the next oral dose. Combined (procainamide and NAPA) levels can be used as an index of toxicity when renal impairment exists. Obtain CBC, liver function tests, and ANA titer periodically during longer-term therapy.

*(continued)*

---

* For those areas marked with one asterisk, the following values can be used:

ALT: 7-56 units/L
AST: 5-40 units/L
Alkaline phosphatase: 17-142 units/L
LDH: 60-220 units/L
GGT: < 40 units/L
Total bilirubin: 0.2-1 mg/dl

| Drug | Laboratory test monitored | Therapeutic ranges of test |
|------|---------------------------|----------------------------|
| quinidine | Quinidine<br>CBC<br>Liver function<br>Creatinine<br>Electrolytes (especially potassium) | 2-6 mcg/ml<br>*****<br>*<br>0.6-1.3 mg/dl<br>Potassium: 3.5-5 mEq/L<br>Magnesium: 1.7-2.1 mEq/L<br>Sodium: 135-145 mEq/L<br>Chloride: 98-106 mEq/L |
| sulfonylureas | Fasting glucose<br>Glycosylated hemoglobin | 70-110 mg/dl<br>4%-7% of total hemoglobin |
| theophylline | Theophylline | 10-20 mcg/ml |
| thiazolidinediones (rosiglitazone, pioglitazone) | Fasting glucose<br>Glycosylated hemoglobin<br>Liver function | 70-110 mg/dl<br>4%-7% of total hemoglobin<br>* |
| thyroid hormone | Thyroid function tests | TSH: 0.2-5.4 microunits/ml<br>$T_3$: 80-200 nanogram/dl<br>$T_4$: 5.4-11.5 mcg/dl |
| valproate sodium, valproic acid, divalproex sodium | Valproic acid<br>Liver function<br>Ammonia<br>PTT<br>BUN<br>Creatinine<br>CBC with differential<br>Platelet count | 50-100 mcg/ml<br>*<br>15-45 mcg/dl<br>10-14 seconds<br>5-20 mg/dl<br>0.6-1.3 mg/dl<br>*****<br>$150\text{-}450 \times 10^3/mm^3$ |
| vancomycin | Vancomycin<br><br>Creatinine | 20-40 mcg/ml (peak)<br>5-15 mcg/ml (trough)<br>0.6-1.3 mg/dl |
| warfarin | INR | For an acute MI, atrial fibrillation, treatment of pulmonary embolism, prevention of systemic embolism, tissue heart valves, valvular heart disease, or prophylaxis or treatment of venous thrombosis: 2-3<br>For mechanical prosthetic valves or recurrent systemic embolism: 3-4.5 |

Note: ***** For those areas marked with asterisks, the following values can be used:

Hemoglobin: Women: 12-16 g/dl
  Men: 14-18 g/dl
Hematocrit: Women: 37%-48%
  Men: 42%-52%
RBCs: $4\text{-}5.5 \times 10^6/mm^3$
WBCs: $5\text{-}10 \times 10^3/mm^3$

Differential: Neutrophils: 45%-74%
  Bands: 0%-8%
  Lymphocytes: 16%-45%
  Monocytes: 4%-10%
  Eosinophils: 0%-7%
  Basophils: 0%-2%

## Monitoring guidelines

Obtain levels immediately before next oral dose and 30 to 35 hours after therapy is initiated or changed. Periodically obtain blood counts, liver and kidney function test results, and electrolyte levels. With more specific assays, therapeutic levels are < 1 mcg/ml.

Monitor response to therapy by periodically evaluating fasting glucose and glycosylated hemoglobin levels. Patient should monitor glucose levels at home to help measure compliance and response.

Obtain theophylline levels immediately before next dose of sustained-release oral product and at least 2 days after therapy is initiated or changed.

Monitor response by evaluating fasting glucose and hemoglobin $A_{1c}$ levels. Obtain baseline liver function test results, and repeat tests periodically during therapy.

Monitor thyroid function test results every 2 to 3 weeks until appropriate maintenance dose is determined, and annually thereafter.

Monitor liver function test results, ammonia level, coagulation test results, renal function test results, CBC, and platelet count at baseline and periodically during therapy. Liver function test results should be closely monitored during the first 6 months.

Vancomycin levels may be checked with the third dose administered, at the earliest. Draw peak levels 1.5 to 2.5 hours after a 1-hour infusion or I.V. infusion is complete. Draw trough levels within 1 hour of the next dose administered. Renal function can be used to adjust dosing and intervals.

Check INR daily, beginning 3 days after therapy is initiated. Continue checking it until therapeutic goal is achieved, and monitor it periodically thereafter. Also, check levels 7 days after any change in warfarin dose or concomitant, potentially interacting therapy.

* For those areas marked with one asterisk, the following values can be used:

ALT: 7-56 units/L
AST: 5-40 units/L
Alkaline phosphatase: 17-142 units/L
LDH: 60-220 units/L
GGT: < 40 units/L
Total bilirubin: 0.2-1 mg/dl

# Combination drugs for pain management

Many common analgesics are combinations of two or more generic drugs. This table reviews common opioid analgesics.

| Trade names and controlled substance schedule (CSS) | Generic drugs | Indications and adult dosages |
|---|---|---|
| Aceta with Codeine, Tylenol with Codeine #3 *CSS III* | • acetaminophen 300 mg<br>• codeine phosphate 30 mg | For fever, mild to moderate pain. Give 1-2 tablets q 4 hours. Maximum, 12 tablets in 24 hours. |
| Alor 5/500, Azdone, Damason-P, Lortab ASA, Panesal *CSS III* | • aspirin 500 mg<br>• hydrocodone bitartrate 5 mg | For moderate to moderately severe pain. Give 1-2 tablets q 4 hours. Maximum, 8 tablets in 24 hours. |
| Anexsia 7.5/650, Lorcet Plus *CSS III* | • acetaminophen 650 mg<br>• hydrocodone bitartrate 7.5 mg | For arthralgia, bone pain, dental pain, headache, migraine, moderate pain. Give 1-2 tablets q 4 hours. Maximum, 6 tablets in 24 hours. |
| Anexsia 10/660, Vicodin HP *CSS III* | • acetaminophen 660 mg<br>• hydrocodone bitartrate 10 mg | For arthralgia, bone pain, dental pain, headache, migraine, moderate pain. Give 1 tablet q 4-6 hours. Maximum, 6 tablets in 24 hours. |
| Capital with Codeine, Tylenol with Codeine Elixir *CSS V* | • acetaminophen 120 mg<br>• codeine phosphate 12 mg/5 ml | For mild to moderate pain. Give 15 ml q 4 hours. |
| Darvocet-N 50 *CSS IV* | • acetaminophen 325 mg<br>• propoxyphene napsylate 50 mg | For mild to moderate pain. Give 1-2 tablets q 4 hours. Maximum, 12 tablets in 24 hours. |
| Darvocet-N 100, Propacet 100 *CSS IV* | • acetaminophen 650 mg<br>• propoxyphene napsylate 100 mg | For mild to moderate pain. Give 1 tablet q 4 hours. Maximum, 6 tablets in 24 hours. |
| Empirin with Codeine No. 3 *CSS III* | • aspirin 325 mg<br>• codeine phosphate 30 mg | For fever, mild to moderate pain. Give 1-2 tablets q 4 hours. Maximum, 12 tablets in 24 hours. |
| Empirin with Codeine No. 4 *CSS III* | • aspirin 325 mg<br>• codeine phosphate 60 mg | For fever, mild to moderate pain. Give 1 tablet q 4 hours. Maximum, 6 tablets in 24 hours. |
| Fioricet with Codeine *CSS III* | • acetaminophen 325 mg<br>• butalbital 50 mg<br>• caffeine 40 mg<br>• codeine phosphate 30 mg | For headache, mild to moderate pain. Give 1-2 capsules q 4 hours. Maximum, 6 capsules in 24 hours. |
| Fiorinal with Codeine *CSS III* | • aspirin 325 mg<br>• butalbital 50 mg<br>• caffeine 40 mg<br>• codeine phosphate 30 mg | For headache, mild to moderate pain. Give 1-2 tablets or capsules q 4 hours. Maximum, 6 tablets or capsules in 24 hours. |
| Lorcet 10/650 *CSS III* | • acetaminophen 650 mg<br>• hydrocodone bitartrate 10 mg | For moderate to moderately severe pain. Give 1 tablet q 4 hours. Maximum, 6 tablets in 24 hours. |

†Available in Canada only

| Trade names and controlled substance schedule (CSS) | Generic drugs | Indications and adult dosages |
|---|---|---|
| Lortab 2.5/500 *CSS III* | • acetaminophen 500 mg<br>• hydrocodone bitartrate 2.5 mg | For moderate to moderately severe pain. Give 1-2 tablets q 4 hours. Maximum, 8 tablets in 24 hours. |
| Lortab 5/500, Vicodin, Panacet 5/500, Lorcet HD, Anexsia 5/500 *CSS III* | • acetaminophen 500 mg<br>• hydrocodone bitartrate 5 mg | For moderate to moderately severe pain. Give 1-2 tablets q 4-6 hours. Maximum, 8 tablets in 24 hours. |
| Lortab 7.5/500 *CSS III* | • acetaminophen 500 mg<br>• hydrocodone bitartrate 7.5 mg | For moderate to moderately severe pain. Give 1 tablet q 4 hours. Maximum, 8 tablets in 24 hours. |
| Lortab 10/500 *CSS III* | • acetaminophen 500 mg<br>• hydrocodone bitartrate 10 mg | For moderate to moderately severe pain. Give 1 tablet q 4-6 hours. Maximum, 6 tablets in 24 hours. |
| Lortab Elixer *CSS III* | • acetaminophen 167 mg<br>• hydrocodone bitartrate 2.5 mg/5ml | For moderately severe pain. Give 15 ml q 4-6 hours. |
| Percocet 2.5/325 *CSS II* | • acetaminophen 325 mg<br>• oxycodone hydrochloride 2.5 mg | For moderate to moderately severe pain. Give 1-2 tablets q 4-6 hours. Maximum, 12 tablets in 24 hours. |
| Percocet 5/325, Roxicet *CSS II* | • acetaminophen 325 mg<br>• oxycodone hydrochloride 5 mg | For moderate to moderately severe pain. Give 1-2 tablets q 4 hours. Maximum, 12 tablets in 24 hours. |
| Percocet 7.5/500 *CSS II* | • acetaminophen 500 mg<br>• oxycodone hydrochloride 7.5 mg | For moderate to moderately severe pain. Give 1-2 tablets q 4-6 hours. Maximum, 8 tablets in 24 hours. |
| Percocet 10/650 *CSS II* | • acetaminophen 650 mg<br>• oxycodone hydrochloride 10 mg | For moderate to moderately severe pain. Give 1-2 tablets q 4-6 hours. Maximum, 6 tablets in 24 hours. |
| Percodan-Demi *CSS II* | • aspirin 325 mg<br>• oxycodone hydrochloride 2.25 mg<br>• oxycodone terephthalate 0.19 mg | For moderate to moderately severe pain. Give 1-2 tablets q 6 hours. Maximum, 8 tablets in 24 hours. |
| Percodan, Roxiprin *CSS II* | • aspirin 325 mg<br>• oxycodone hydrochloride 4.5 mg<br>• oxycodone terephthalate 0.38 mg | For moderate to moderately severe pain. Give 1 tablet q 6 hours. Maximum, 4 tablets in 24 hours. |
| Roxicet 5/500, Roxilox, Tylox *CSS II* | • acetaminophen 500 mg<br>• oxycodone hydrochloride 5 mg | For moderate to moderately severe pain. Give 1 tablet q 6 hours. |
| Roxicet Oral Solution *CSS II* | • acetaminophen 325 mg<br>• oxycodone hydrochloride 5 mg/5 ml | For moderate to moderately severe pain. Give 5-10 ml q 4-6 hours. Maximum, 60 ml in 24 hours. |
| Talacen *CSS IV* | • acetaminophen 650 mg<br>• pentazocine hydrochloride 25 mg | For mild to moderate pain. Give 1 tablet q 4 hours. Maximum, 6 tablets in 24 hours. |

*(continued)*

| Trade names and controlled substance schedule (CSS) | Generic drugs | Indications and adult dosages |
|---|---|---|
| Talwin Compound<br>*CSS IV* | • aspirin 325 mg<br>• pentazocine hydrochloride 12.5 mg | For moderate pain. Give 2 tablets q 6 hours. Maximum, 8 tablets in 24 hours. |
| Tylenol with Codeine No. 2<br>*CSS III* | • acetaminophen 300 mg<br>• codeine phosphate 15 mg | For fever, mild to moderate pain. Give 1-2 tablets q 4 hours. Maximum, 12 tablets in 24 hours. |
| Tylenol with Codeine No. 4<br>*CSS III* | • acetaminophen 300 mg<br>• codeine phosphate 60 mg | For fever, mild to moderate pain. Give 1 tablet q 4 hours. Maximum, 6 tablets in 24 hours. |
| Vicodin ES<br>*CSS III* | • acetaminophen 750 mg<br>• hydrocodone bitartrate 7.5 mg | For moderate to moderately severe pain. Give 1 tablet q 4-6 hours. Maximum, 5 tablets in 24 hours. |
| Wygesic<br>*CSS IV* | • acetaminophen 650 mg<br>• propoxyphene napsylate 65 mg | For mild to moderate pain. Give 1 tablet q 4 hours. Maximum, 6 tablets in 24 hours. |
| Zydone 5/400<br>*CSS III* | • acetaminophen 400 mg<br>• hydrocodone bitartrate 5 mg | For moderate to moderately severe pain. Give 1-2 tablets q 4-6 hours. Maximum, 8 tablets in 24 hours. |
| Zydone 7.5/400<br>*CSS III* | • acetaminophen 400 mg<br>• hydrocodone bitartrate 7.5 mg | For moderate to moderately severe pain. Give 1 tablet q 4-6 hours. Maximum, 6 tablets in 24 hours. |
| Zydone 10/400<br>*CSS III* | • acetaminophen 400 mg<br>• hydrocodone bitartrate 10 mg | For moderate to moderately severe pain. Give 1 tablet q 4-6 hours. Maximum, 6 tablets in 24 hours. |

# Infusion flow rates

The infusion flow rates are based on the concentrations shown at the top of each table. Be sure to check the label on the medication you're infusing to verify the correct infusion flow rate.

## Epinephrine infusion rates
Mix 1 mg in 250 ml (4 mcg/ml).

| Dose (mcg/min) | Infusion rate (ml/hr) |
|---|---|
| 1 | 15 |
| 2 | 30 |
| 3 | 45 |
| 4 | 60 |
| 5 | 75 |
| 6 | 90 |
| 7 | 105 |
| 8 | 120 |
| 9 | 135 |
| 10 | 150 |
| 15 | 225 |
| 20 | 300 |
| 25 | 375 |
| 30 | 450 |
| 35 | 525 |
| 40 | 600 |

## Isoproterenol infusion rates
Mix 1 mg in 250 ml (4 mcg/ml).

| Dose (mcg/min) | Infusion rate (ml/hr) |
|---|---|
| 0.5 | 8 |
| 1 | 15 |
| 2 | 30 |
| 3 | 45 |
| 4 | 60 |
| 5 | 75 |
| 6 | 90 |
| 7 | 105 |
| 8 | 120 |
| 9 | 135 |
| 10 | 150 |
| 15 | 225 |
| 20 | 300 |
| 25 | 375 |
| 30 | 450 |

## Nitroglycerin infusion rates
Determine the infusion rate in ml/hr using the ordered dose and the concentration of the drug solution.

| Dose (mcg/min) | 25 mg/250 ml (100 mcg/ml) | 50 mg/250 ml (200 mcg/ml) | 100 mg/250 ml (400 mcg/ml) |
|---|---|---|---|
| 5 | 3 | 2 | 1 |
| 10 | 6 | 3 | 2 |
| 20 | 12 | 6 | 3 |
| 30 | 18 | 9 | 5 |
| 40 | 24 | 12 | 6 |
| 50 | 30 | 15 | 8 |
| 60 | 36 | 18 | 9 |
| 70 | 42 | 21 | 10 |
| 80 | 48 | 24 | 12 |
| 90 | 54 | 27 | 14 |
| 100 | 60 | 30 | 15 |
| 150 | 90 | 45 | 23 |
| 200 | 120 | 60 | 30 |

*(continued)*

## Dobutamine infusion rates

Mix 250 mg in 250 ml of $D_5W$ (1,000 mcg/ml). Determine the infusion rate in ml/hr using the ordered dose and the patient's weight in pounds or kilograms.

| Dose (mcg/kg/min) | lb 88 | 99 | 110 | 121 | 132 | 143 | 154 | 165 | 176 | 187 | 198 | 209 | 220 | 231 | 242 |
|---|---|---|---|---|---|---|---|---|---|---|---|---|---|---|---|
| | kg 40 | 45 | 50 | 55 | 60 | 65 | 70 | 75 | 80 | 85 | 90 | 95 | 100 | 105 | 110 |
| 2.5 | 6 | 7 | 8 | 8 | 9 | 10 | 11 | 11 | 12 | 13 | 14 | 14 | 15 | 16 | 17 |
| 5 | 12 | 14 | 15 | 17 | 18 | 20 | 21 | 23 | 24 | 26 | 27 | 29 | 30 | 32 | 33 |
| 7.5 | 18 | 20 | 23 | 25 | 27 | 29 | 32 | 34 | 36 | 38 | 41 | 43 | 45 | 47 | 50 |
| 10 | 24 | 27 | 30 | 33 | 36 | 39 | 42 | 45 | 48 | 51 | 54 | 57 | 60 | 63 | 66 |
| 12.5 | 30 | 34 | 38 | 41 | 45 | 49 | 53 | 56 | 60 | 64 | 68 | 71 | 75 | 79 | 83 |
| 15 | 36 | 41 | 45 | 50 | 54 | 59 | 63 | 68 | 72 | 77 | 81 | 86 | 90 | 95 | 99 |
| 20 | 48 | 54 | 60 | 66 | 72 | 78 | 84 | 90 | 96 | 102 | 108 | 114 | 120 | 126 | 132 |
| 25 | 60 | 68 | 75 | 83 | 90 | 98 | 105 | 113 | 120 | 128 | 135 | 143 | 150 | 158 | 165 |
| 30 | 72 | 81 | 90 | 99 | 108 | 117 | 126 | 135 | 144 | 153 | 162 | 171 | 180 | 189 | 198 |
| 35 | 84 | 95 | 105 | 116 | 126 | 137 | 147 | 158 | 168 | 179 | 189 | 200 | 210 | 221 | 231 |
| 40 | 96 | 108 | 120 | 132 | 144 | 156 | 168 | 180 | 192 | 204 | 216 | 228 | 240 | 252 | 264 |

## Dopamine infusion rates

Mix 400 mg in 250 ml of $D_5W$ (1,600 mcg/ml). Determine the infusion rate in ml/hr using the ordered dose and the patient's weight in pounds or kilograms.

| Dose (mcg/kg/min) | lb 88 | 99 | 110 | 121 | 132 | 143 | 154 | 165 | 176 | 187 | 198 | 209 | 220 | 231 |
|---|---|---|---|---|---|---|---|---|---|---|---|---|---|---|
| | kg 40 | 45 | 50 | 55 | 60 | 65 | 70 | 75 | 80 | 85 | 90 | 95 | 100 | 105 |
| 2.5 | 4 | 4 | 5 | 5 | 6 | 6 | 7 | 7 | 8 | 8 | 8 | 9 | 9 | 10 |
| 5 | 8 | 8 | 9 | 10 | 11 | 12 | 13 | 14 | 15 | 16 | 17 | 18 | 19 | 20 |
| 7.5 | 11 | 13 | 14 | 15 | 17 | 18 | 20 | 21 | 23 | 24 | 25 | 27 | 28 | 30 |
| 10 | 15 | 17 | 19 | 21 | 23 | 24 | 26 | 28 | 30 | 32 | 34 | 36 | 38 | 39 |
| 12.5 | 19 | 21 | 23 | 26 | 28 | 30 | 33 | 35 | 38 | 40 | 42 | 45 | 47 | 49 |
| 15 | 23 | 25 | 28 | 31 | 34 | 37 | 39 | 42 | 45 | 48 | 51 | 53 | 56 | 59 |
| 20 | 30 | 34 | 38 | 41 | 45 | 49 | 53 | 56 | 60 | 64 | 68 | 71 | 75 | 79 |
| 25 | 38 | 42 | 47 | 52 | 56 | 61 | 66 | 70 | 75 | 80 | 84 | 89 | 94 | 98 |
| 30 | 45 | 51 | 56 | 62 | 67 | 73 | 79 | 84 | 90 | 96 | 101 | 107 | 113 | 118 |
| 35 | 53 | 59 | 66 | 72 | 79 | 85 | 92 | 98 | 105 | 112 | 118 | 125 | 131 | 138 |
| 40 | 60 | 68 | 75 | 83 | 90 | 98 | 105 | 113 | 120 | 128 | 135 | 143 | 150 | 158 |
| 45 | 68 | 76 | 84 | 93 | 101 | 110 | 118 | 127 | 135 | 143 | 152 | 160 | 169 | 177 |
| 50 | 75 | 84 | 94 | 103 | 113 | 122 | 131 | 141 | 150 | 159 | 169 | 178 | 188 | 197 |

## Nitroprusside infusion rates

Mix 50 mg in 250 ml of $D_5W$ (200 mcg/ml). Determine the infusion rate in ml/hr using the ordered dose and the patient's weight in pounds or kilograms.

| Dose (mcg/kg/min) | lb 88 kg 40 | 99 45 | 110 50 | 121 55 | 132 60 | 143 65 | 154 70 | 165 75 | 176 80 | 187 85 | 198 90 | 209 95 | 220 100 | 231 105 | 242 110 |
|---|---|---|---|---|---|---|---|---|---|---|---|---|---|---|---|
| 0.3 | 4 | 4 | 5 | 5 | 5 | 6 | 6 | 7 | 7 | 8 | 8 | 9 | 9 | 9 | 10 |
| 0.5 | 6 | 7 | 8 | 8 | 9 | 10 | 11 | 11 | 12 | 13 | 14 | 14 | 15 | 16 | 17 |
| 1 | 12 | 14 | 15 | 17 | 18 | 20 | 21 | 23 | 24 | 26 | 27 | 29 | 30 | 32 | 33 |
| 1.5 | 18 | 20 | 23 | 25 | 27 | 29 | 32 | 34 | 36 | 38 | 41 | 43 | 45 | 47 | 50 |
| 2 | 24 | 27 | 30 | 33 | 36 | 39 | 42 | 45 | 48 | 51 | 54 | 57 | 60 | 63 | 66 |
| 3 | 36 | 41 | 45 | 50 | 54 | 59 | 63 | 68 | 72 | 77 | 81 | 86 | 90 | 95 | 99 |
| 4 | 48 | 54 | 60 | 66 | 72 | 78 | 84 | 90 | 96 | 102 | 108 | 114 | 120 | 126 | 132 |
| 5 | 60 | 68 | 75 | 83 | 90 | 98 | 105 | 113 | 120 | 128 | 135 | 143 | 150 | 158 | 165 |
| 6 | 72 | 81 | 90 | 99 | 108 | 117 | 126 | 135 | 144 | 153 | 162 | 171 | 180 | 189 | 198 |
| 7 | 84 | 95 | 105 | 116 | 126 | 137 | 147 | 158 | 168 | 179 | 189 | 200 | 210 | 221 | 231 |
| 8 | 96 | 108 | 120 | 132 | 144 | 156 | 168 | 180 | 192 | 204 | 216 | 228 | 240 | 252 | 264 |
| 9 | 108 | 122 | 135 | 149 | 162 | 176 | 189 | 203 | 216 | 230 | 243 | 257 | 270 | 284 | 297 |
| 10 | 120 | 135 | 150 | 165 | 180 | 195 | 210 | 225 | 240 | 255 | 270 | 285 | 300 | 315 | 330 |

# Normal laboratory test values

Normal values may differ from laboratory to laboratory. Standard International units are abbreviated SI.

## Hematology
**Bleeding time**
*Template:* 3-6 min (SI, 3-6 m)
*Ivy:* 3-6 min (SI, 3-6 m)
*Duke:* 1-3 min (SI, 1-3 m)

**Fibrinogen, plasma**
200-400 mg/dl (SI, 2-4 g/L)

**Hematocrit**
*Men:* 42%-52% (SI, 0.42-0.52)
*Women:* 36%-48% (SI, 0.36-0.48)

**Hemoglobin, total**
*Men:* 14-17.4 g/dl (SI, 140-174 g/L)
*Women:* 12-16 g/dl (SI, 120-160 g/L)

**Activated partial thromboplastin time**
21-35 sec (SI, 21-35 sec)

**Platelet aggregation**
3-5 min (SI, 3-5 min)

**Platelet count**
140,000-400,000/mm$^3$ (SI, 140-400 × 10$^9$/L)

**Prothrombin time**
10-14 sec (SI, 10-14 sec); INR for patients on warfarin therapy, 2-3 (SI, 2-3) (those with prosthetic heart valve, 2.5-3.5 [SI, 2.5-3.5])

**Red blood cell count**
*Men:* 4.5-5.5 million/mm$^3$ (SI, 4.5-5.5 × 10$^{12}$/L) venous blood
*Women:* 4-5 million/mm$^3$ (SI, 4-5 × 10$^{12}$/L) venous blood

**Red blood cell indices**
*Mean corpuscular volume:* 82-98 femtoliters
*Mean corpuscular hemoglobin:* 26-34 picograms/cell
*Mean corpuscular hemoglobin concentration:* 31-37 g/dl

**Reticulocyte count**
0.5%-1.5% (SI, 0.005-0.025) of total RBC count

**White blood cell count**
4,500-10,500 cells/mm$^3$

**White blood cell differential, blood**
*Neutrophils:* 54%-75% (SI, 0.54-0.75)
*Lymphocytes:* 25%-40% (SI, 0.25-0.4)
*Monocytes:* 2%-8% (SI, 0.02-0.08)
*Eosinophils:* up to 4% (SI, up to 0.04)
*Basophils:* up to 1% (SI, up to 0.01)

## Blood chemistry
**Alanine aminotransferase**
*Adults:* 10-35 units/L (SI, 0.17-0.6 mu kat/L)
*Newborns:* 13-45 units/L (SI, 0.22-0.77 mu kat/L)

**Amylase, serum**
*Adults ≥ age 18:* 25-85 units/L (SI, 0.39-1.45 mu kat/L)

**Arterial blood gases**
*pH:* 7.35-7.45 (SI, 7.35-7.45)
*Paco$_2$:* 35-45 mm Hg (SI, 4.7-5.3 kPa)
*Pao$_2$:* 80-100 mm Hg (SI, 10.6-13.3 kPa)
*HCO$_3^-$:* 22-26 mEq/L (SI, 22-25 mmol/L)
*Sao$_2$:* 94%-100% (SI, 0.94-1.00)

**Aspartate aminotransferase**
*Men:* 14-20 units/L (SI, 0.23-0.33 mu kat/L)
*Women:* 7-34 units/L (SI, 0.12-0.58 mkat/L)

**Bilirubin, serum**
*Adults, total:* 0.2-1 mg/dl (SI, 3.5-17 micromol/L)
*Neonates, total:* 1-10 mg/dl (SI, 17-170 micromol/L)
*Neonates, unconjugated indirect:* 0-10 mg/dl (SI, 0-170 micromol/L)

**Blood urea nitrogen**
8-20 mg/dl (SI, 2.9-7.5 mmol/L)

**Calcium, serum**
*Adults:* 8.2-10.2 mg/dl (SI, 2.05-2.54 mmol/L)
*Children:* 8.6-11.2 mg/dl (SI, 2.15-2.79 mmol/L)

**Carbon dioxide, total blood**
22-26 mEq/L (SI, 22-26 mmol/L)

**Cholesterol, total serum**
*Men:* < 205 mg/dl (SI, < 5.30 mmol/L) (desirable)
*Women:* < 190 mg/dl (SI, < 4.90 mmol/L) (desirable)

**Creatine kinase, isoenzymes**
*CK-BB:* none
*CK-MB:* 0-7%
*CK-MM:* 96-100%

**Creatinine, serum**
*Adults:* 0.6-1.3 mg/dl (SI, 53-115 micro-mol/L)

**Glucose, plasma, fasting**
70-110 mg/dl (SI, 3.9-6.1 mmol/L)

**Glucose, plasma, 2-hour postprandial**
< 145 mg/dl (SI, < 8 mmol/L)

**Lactate dehydrogenase**
*Total:* 71-207 units/L in adults (SI, 1.2-3.52 mu kat/L)
*LD1:* 14%-26% (SI, 0.14-0.26)
*LD2:* 29%-39% (SI, 0.29-0.39)
*LD3:* 20%-26% (SI, 0.20-0.26)
*LD4:* 8%-16% (SI, 0.08-0.16)
*LD5:* 6%-16% (SI, 0.06-0.16)

**Lipase**
< 160 units/L (SI, < 2.72 mu kat/L)

**Magnesium, serum**
1.8-2.6 mg/dl (SI, 0.74-1.07 mmol/L)

**Phosphates, serum**
2.7-4.5 mg/dl (SI, 0.87-1.45 mmol/L)

**Potassium, serum**
3.8-5 mEq/L (SI, 3.5-5 mmol/L)

**Protein, serum**
*Total:* 6.3-8.3 g/dl (SI, 64-83 g/L)
*Albumin fraction:* 3.5-5 g/dl (SI, 35-50 g/L)

**Sodium, serum**
135-145 mEq/L (SI, 135-145 mmol/L)

**Triglycerides, serum**
*Men > age 20:* 40-180 mg/dl (SI, 0.11-2.01 mmol/L)
*Women > age 20:* 10-190 mg/dl (SI, 0.11-2.21 mmol/L)

**Uric acid, serum**
*Men:* 3.4-7 mg/dl (SI, 202-416 micro-mol/L)
*Women:* 2.3-6 mg/dl (SI, 143-357 micro-mol/L)

# Dialyzable drugs

The amount of a drug removed by dialysis differs among patients and depends on several factors, including the patient's condition, the drug's properties, length of dialysis and dialysate used, rate of blood flow or dwell time, and purpose of dialysis. This table indicates the effect of conventional hemodialysis on selected drugs.

| Drug | Level reduced by hemodialysis | Drug | Level reduced by hemodialysis |
|---|---|---|---|
| acetaminophen | Yes (may not influence toxicity) | cefoxitin | Yes |
| | | cefpodoxime | Yes |
| acetazolamide | No | ceftazidime | Yes |
| acyclovir | Yes | ceftibuten | Yes |
| allopurinol | Yes | ceftizoxime | Yes |
| alprazolam | No | ceftriaxone | No |
| amikacin | Yes | cefuroxime | Yes |
| amiodarone | No | cephalexin | Yes |
| amitriptyline | No | cephalothin | Yes |
| amlodipine | No | cephradine | Yes |
| amoxicillin | Yes | chloral hydrate | Yes |
| amoxicillin and clavulanate potassium | Yes | chlorambucil | No |
| | | chloramphenicol | Yes (very small amount) |
| amphotericin B | No | chlordiazepoxide | No |
| ampicillin | Yes | chloroquine | No |
| ampicillin and sulbactam sodium | Yes | chlorpheniramine | No |
| aprepitant | No | chlorpromazine | No |
| aspirin | Yes | chlorthalidone | No |
| atenolol | Yes | cimetidine | Yes |
| azathioprine | Yes | ciprofloxacin | Yes (only by 20%) |
| aztreonam | Yes | cisplatin | No |
| bretylium | Yes | clindamycin | No |
| captopril | Yes | clofibrate | No |
| carbamazepine | No | clonazepam | No |
| carbenicillin | Yes | clonidine | No |
| carmustine | No | clorazepate | No |
| cefaclor | Yes | cloxacillin | No |
| cefadroxil | Yes | codeine | No |
| cefamandole | Yes | colchicine | No |
| cefazolin | Yes | cortisone | No |
| cefepime | Yes | co-trimoxazole | Yes |
| cefoperazone | Yes | cyclophosphamide | Yes |
| cefotaxime | Yes | diazepam | No |
| cefotetan | Yes (only by 20%) | diazoxide | Yes |

| Drug | Level reduced by hemodialysis | Drug | Level reduced by hemodialysis |
|---|---|---|---|
| diclofenac | No | hydroxyzine | No |
| dicloxacillin | No | ibuprofen | No |
| didanosine | Yes | imipenem and cilastatin | Yes |
| digoxin | No | imipramine | No |
| diltiazem | No | indapamide | No |
| diphenhydramine | No | indomethacin | No |
| dipyridamole | No | insulin | No |
| disopyramide | Yes | irbesartan | No |
| doxazosin | No | iron dextran | No |
| doxepin | No | isoniazid | Yes |
| doxorubicin | No | isosorbide | Yes |
| doxycycline | No | isradipine | No |
| enalapril | Yes | kanamycin | Yes |
| erythromycin | Yes (only by 20%) | ketoconazole | No |
| ethacrynic acid | No | ketoprofen | Yes |
| ethambutol | Yes (only by 20%) | labetalol | No |
| ethosuximide | Yes | levofloxacin | No |
| famciclovir | Yes | lidocaine | No |
| famotidine | No | lisinopril | Yes |
| fenoprofen | No | lithium | Yes |
| flecainide | No | lomefloxacin | No |
| fluconazole | Yes | lomustine | No |
| flucytosine | Yes | loracarbef | Yes |
| fluorouracil | Yes | loratadine | No |
| fluoxetine | No | lorazepam | No |
| flurazepam | No | mechlorethamine | No |
| foscarnet | Yes | mefenamic acid | No |
| fosinopril | No | meperidine | No |
| furosemide | No | mercaptopurine | Yes |
| gabapentin | Yes | meropenem | Yes |
| ganciclovir | Yes | methadone | No |
| gemfibrozil | No | methicillin | No |
| gemifloxacin | Yes | methotrexate | Yes |
| gentamicin | Yes | methyldopa | Yes |
| glipizide | No | methylprednisolone | No |
| glyburide | No | metoclopramide | No |
| guanfacine | No | metolazone | No |
| haloperidol | No | metoprolol | No |
| heparin | No | metronidazole | Yes |
| hydralazine | No | mexiletine | Yes |
| hydrochlorothiazide | No | | (continued) |

| Drug | Level reduced by hemodialysis | Drug | Level reduced by hemodialysis |
|---|---|---|---|
| mezlocillin | Yes | procainamide | Yes |
| miconazole | No | promethazine | No |
| midazolam | No | propoxyphene | No |
| minocycline | No | propranolol | No |
| minoxidil | Yes | protriptyline | No |
| misoprostol | No | pyridoxine | Yes |
| morphine | No | quinapril | No |
| nabumetone | No | quinidine | Yes |
| nadolol | Yes | quinine | Yes |
| nafcillin | No | ranitidine | Yes |
| naproxen | No | rifampin | No |
| nelfinavir | Yes | rofecoxib | No |
| netilmicin | Yes | salsalate | Yes |
| nifedipine | No | sertraline | No |
| nimodipine | No | sotalol | Yes |
| nitazoxanide | No | stavudine | Yes |
| nitrofurantoin | Yes | streptomycin | Yes |
| nitroglycerin | No | sucralfate | No |
| nitroprusside | Yes | sulbactam | Yes |
| nizatidine | No | sulfamethoxazole | Yes |
| norfloxacin | No | sulindac | No |
| nortriptyline | No | tazobactam | Yes |
| ofloxacin | Yes | temazepam | No |
| olanzapine | No | theophylline | Yes |
| omeprazole | No | ticarcillin | Yes |
| oxacillin | No | ticarcillin and clavulanate | Yes |
| oxazepam | No | timolol | No |
| paroxetine | No | tobramycin | Yes |
| penicillin G | Yes | tocainide | Yes |
| pentamidine | No | tolbutamide | No |
| pentazocine | Yes | topiramate | Yes |
| perindopril | Yes | trazodone | No |
| phenobarbital | Yes | triazolam | No |
| phenylbutazone | No | trimethoprim | Yes |
| phenytoin | No | valacyclovir | Yes |
| piperacillin | Yes | valproic acid | No |
| piperacillin and tazobactam | Yes | valsartan | No |
| piroxicam | No | vancomycin | Yes |
| prazosin | No | verapamil | No |
| prednisone | No | warfarin | No |
| primidone | Yes | zolpidem | No |

# English-Spanish drug phrase translator

## Medication history

**Do you take any medications?**
– Prescription?
– Over-the-counter?
– Other?

**¿Toma Ud. medicamentos?**
– ¿De receta?
– ¿Sin necesidad de receta?
– ¿Otro?

**Which prescription medications do you take routinely?**
**Which over-the-counter medications do you take routinely?**
– How often do you take them?
– Once daily?
– Twice daily?
– Three times daily?
– Four times daily?
– More often?

**¿Qué medicamentos de receta toma Ud. por rutina?**
**¿Qué medicamentos que no necesitan receta toma Ud. por rutina?**
– ¿Con qué frecuencia los toma?
– ¿Una vez al día?
– ¿Dos veces al día?
– ¿Tres veces al día?
– ¿Cuátro veces al día?
– ¿Con más frecuencia?

**Why do you take these medications?**

**¿Por qué toma Ud. estos medicamentos?**

**What is the dosage for each medication?**

**¿Cuál es la dosis para cada uno de los medicamentos?**

**Are you allergic to any medications?**

**¿Está Ud. alérgico(a) a algúnos medicamentos?**

## Medication teaching

### PURPOSE OF THE MEDICATION
**This medication will:**
– elevate your blood pressure.
– improve circulation to your ____.

– lower your blood pressure.
– lower your blood sugar.
– make your heart rhythm more even.
– raise your blood sugar.
– reduce or prevent the formation of blood clots.
– remove fluid from your body.
– remove fluid from your feet, ankles, or legs.
– remove fluid from your lungs so that they work better.
– remove fluid from your pancreas so that it works better.
– kill the bacteria in your ____.
– slow down your heart rate.
– soften your bowel movements.
– speed up your heart rate.

**Este medicamento hará que:**
– su presión sanguínea suba.
– la circulación por (la región del cuerpo) mejore.
– su presión sanguínea baje.
– el nivel de azucar en la sangre baje.
– el ritmo del corazón sea más uniforme.
– su nivel de azucar en la sangre suba.
– se reduzca o evite la formación de coágulos de sangre.
– se le quite fluido en el cuerpo.
– se le quite fluido de los pies, tobillos o piernas.
– se le quite fluido de los pulmones para que funcionen mejor.
– se le quite fluido de la páncreas para que funcione mejor.
– destruir la bacteria de la ____.
– reducir el latir del corazón.
– ablandar sus evacuaciones.
– acelerar el latir del corazón.

– help your body to use insulin more efficiently.

**This medication will help you to:**
– breathe better.
– fight infections.
– relax.
– sleep.
– think more clearly.

**This medication will relieve or reduce:**

– the acid production in your stomach.
– anxiety.
– bladder spasms.
– burning in your stomach or chest.
– burning when you urinate.
– diarrhea.
– muscle cramps.
– nausea.
– pain in your _____.

**MEDICATION ADMINISTRATION**
**I would like to give you:**
– an injection.
– an I.V. medication.
– a liquid medication.
– a medicated cream or powder.
– a medication through your epidural
catheter.
– a medication through your rectum.
– a medication through your _____ tube.
– a medication under your tongue.
– some pill(s).
– a suppository.

**This is how you take this medication.**

**If you can't swallow this pill, I can get it in
another form.**

**If you can't swallow a pill, you can crush
it and mix it in soft food.**

**I need to mix this medication in juice or
water.**

**I need to give you this injection in your:**
– abdomen.
– buttocks.
– hip.
– outer arm.
– thigh.

– le ayudar a su cuerpo a usar la insulina
más eficazmente.

**Este medicamento le ayudará a Ud. a:**
– respirar con mayor facilidad.
– luchar contra infecciones.
– relajarse.
– dormir.
– pensar con mayor claridad.

**Este medicamento le aliviará o dis-
minuirá:**
– la producción de acido en el estómago.
– la angustia.
– espasmos en la vejiga.
– sensasión ardiente en el estómago o tórax.
– sensación ardiente al orinar.
– diarrea.
– espasmos en los músculos.
– nausea.
– dolor en la (el) _____.

**Quisiera darle a Ud. un(a):**
– inyección.
– medicamento por vía intravenosa.
– medicamento en forma líquida.
– medicamento en pomada o polvo.
– medicamento por el catéter epidural.

– medicamento por el recto.
– medicamento por su _____ tubo.
– medicamento debajo de la lengua.
– píldoras.
– supositorio.

**Así se toma este medicamento.**

**Si Ud. no puede tragarse esta píldora,
puede obtenerla en otra forma.**

**Si Ud. no se puede tragar la píldora, la
puede moler y mezclarla en un alimento
blando.**

**Tengo que mezclar este medicamento en
jugo (zumo) o agua.**

**Tengo que ponerle esta inyección:**
– en el abdomen.
– en las nalgas.
– en la cadera.
– en el brazo.
– en el muslo.

Some medications are coated with a special substance to protect your stomach from getting upset.

Algunos medicamentos están cubiertos con una sustancia especial para protegerle contra un trastorno estomacal.

**Do not chew:**
- enteric-coated pills.
- long-acting pills.
- capsules.
- sublingual medication.

**No masque Ud.:**
- píldoras con recubrimientoentérico.
- píldoras de efecto prolongado.
- cápsulas.
- medicamentos sublinguales.

**Ask your doctor or pharmacist whether you can:**
- mix your medication with food or fluids.
- take your medication with or without food.

**Pregúntele Ud. a su doctor o farmacéutico si debiera:**
- mezclar su medicamento con un alimento o con líquidos.
- tomar su medicamento con o sin alimento.

**You need to take your medication:**
- after meals.
- before meals.
- on an empty stomach.
- with meals or food.

**Ud. tiene que tomarse el medicamento:**
- después de las comidas.
- antes de las comidas.
- con el estómago vacío.
- con las comidas o con un alimento.

**SKIPPING DOSES**
**If you skip or miss a dose:**
- Take it as soon as you remember it.
- Wait until the next dose.
- Call the doctor if you are not sure.
- Do not take an extra dose.

**Si Ud. omite o se salta una dosis:**
- Tómesela encuanto se acuerde.
- Espérese hasta la siguiente dosis.
- Llame al doctor si Ud. no está seguro(a).
- No se tome una dosis extra.

**ADVERSE EFFECTS**
**Some common adverse effects of _____ are:**
- constipation
- diarrhea
- difficulty sleeping
- dry mouth
- fatigue
- headache
- itching
- light-headedness
- nausea
- poor appetite
- rash
- upset stomach
- weight loss or gain
- frequent urination.

**Unos efectos adversos comunes a __ __ son:**
- estreñimiento
- diarrea
- dificultad en dormir
- boca seca
- fatiga
- dolor de cabeza
- comezón (picazón)
- mareo
- nausea
- poco apetito
- erupción
- trastorno estomacal
- perdida o aumento de peso
- orinar con frecuencia.

**These adverse effects:**
- will go away after your body gets used to the medication.
- may persist as long as you take the medication.

**Estos efectos adversos:**
- desaparecerán una vez que su cuerpo se acostumbre al medicamento.
- puede continuar mientras Ud. tome el medicamento.

| | |
|---|---|
| If you have an adverse reaction to your medication, call your doctor right away. | Si Ud. tiene una reacción adversa a su medicamento, llame a su doctor inmediatamente. |

## OTHER CONCERNS

| | |
|---|---|
| Tell your doctor if you are pregnant or breast-feeding. | Dígale a su doctor si Ud. está ebarazada o si cría a los pechos. |
| While you are taking this medication, ask your doctor if: | Mientras Ud. tome este medicamento, pregúntele a su doctor si: |
| – you can safely take other over-the-counter medications. | – puede tomar otros medicamentos que no necesitan receta. |
| – you can drink alcoholic beverages. | – puede tomar bebidas alcohólicas. |
| – your medications interact with each other. | – sus medicamentos interaccionan uno con el otro. |

## STORING MEDICATION

| | |
|---|---|
| You should keep your medication: | Ud. debiera guardar sus medicamentos: |
| – in a cool, dry place. | – en un lugar fresco, seco. |
| – in the refrigerator. | – en el refrigerador. |
| – at room temperature. | – al tiempo. |
| – out of direct sunlight. | – fuera de la luz de sol. |
| – away from heat. | – lejos de la calefacción. |
| – away from children. | – lejos del alcance de los niños. |

## TEACHING A PATIENT TO GIVE A SUBCUTANEOUS INJECTION

| | |
|---|---|
| To give yourself an injection, follow these steps: | Así es como uno se pone una inyección a sí mismo(a): |
| – Draw up the medication. | – Saque el medicamento. |
| – Replace the cap carefully. | – Coloque de nuevo la tapa con cuidado. |
| – Decide where you are going to give the injection. | – Decida Ud. donde va a ponerse la inyección. |
| – Clean the skin area with alcohol. | – Limpie el área de la piel con alcohol. |
| – Gently pinch up a little skin over the area. | – Suavemente pellizque un poco de piel sobre el área. |
| – Using a dartlike motion, stab the needle into your skin. | – Con un movimiento rápido, penetre la aguja en su piel. |
| – Gently pull back on the plunger to see if there is any blood in the syringe. | – Con cuidado retire el émbolo para ver si hay sangre en la jeringa. |
| – Steadily push the medication into your skin. | – Constantemente empuje el medicamento dentro de su piel. |
| – Pull the needle out. | – Saque la aguja. |
| – Apply gentle pressure with the alcohol wipe. | – Ejerza presión suavemente con un limpión de alcohol. |
| – Dispose of the needle in a proper receptacle. | – Deshagase de la aguja en un recipiente apropiado. |

## INSULIN PREPARATION AND ADMINISTRATION

| | |
|---|---|
| The doctor has ordered insulin for you. | El doctor ha recetado insulina para Ud. |
| To draw up insulin, follow these steps: | Para extraer la insulina siga las siguientes pasos: |
| – Wipe the rubber top of the insulin bottle with alcohol. | – Limpie la tapa de hule (goma) de la botella de la insulina con alcohol. |
| – Remove the needle cap. | – Quítele el capuchón a la aguja. |

– Pull out the plunger until the end of the plunger in the barrel aligns with the number of units of insulin that you need.

– Push the needle through the rubber top of the insulin bottle.

– Inject the air into the bottle.

– Without removing the needle from the bottle, turn it upside down.

– Withdraw the plunger until the end of the plunger aligns with the number of units you need.

– Gently pull the needle out of the bottle.

**To mix insulin, follow these steps:**

– Wipe the rubber tops of the insulin bottles with alcohol.

– Gently roll the cloudy insulin between your palms.

– Remove the needle cap.

– Pull out the plunger until the end of the plunger in the barrel aligns with the number of units of NPH or Lente insulin that you need.

– Push the needle through the rubber top of the cloudy insulin bottle.

– Inject the air into the bottle.

– Remove the needle.

– Pull out the plunger until the end of the plunger in the barrel aligns with the number of units of clear regular insulin that you need.

– Push the needle through the rubber top of the clear insulin bottle.

– Inject the air into the bottle.

– Without removing the needle, turn the bottle upside down.

– Withdraw the plunger until it aligns with the number of units of clear regular insulin that you need.

– Gently pull the needle out of the bottle.

– Push the needle into the cloudy (NPH or Lente) insulin without injecting it into the bottle.

– Withdraw the plunger until you reach your total dosage of insulin in units (regular combined with NPH or Lente).

– We will practice again.

– Saque el émbolo hasta el otro extremo del émbolo en la cuba esté al nivel de la dosis de insulina (número de unidades) que Ud. necesita.

– Empuje la aguja por la tapa de hule (goma) de la botella de insulina.

– Inyecte el aire dentro de la botella.

– Sin sacar la aguja de la botella, póngala al revés.

– Retire el émbolo hasta que llegue la insulina al número de unidades que Ud. necesita.

– Retire Ud. la aguja de la botella suavemente.

**Para mezclar la insulina siga los siguientes pasos:**

– Limpie la tapa de hule (goma) de las botellas de insulina con alcohol.

– Suavemente mueva la insulina turbia entre las palmas de la mano.

– Retire el capuchón de la aguja.

– Saque el émbolo hasta que el otro extremo del émbolo en el barril esté al nivel con la dosis de insulina turbia (NPH o insulina Lente) (número de unidades) que Ud. necesita.

– Empuje la aguja por la tapa de goma (hule) de la botella de insulina turbia.

– Inyecte el aire dentro de la botella.

– Saque la aguja.

– Retire el émbolo hasta que el otro extremo del émbolo en el barril esté al nivel con la dosis de insulina clara (regular) (número de unidades) que Ud. necesita.

– Empuje Ud. la aguja por la tapa de goma de la botella de insulna clara.

– Inyecte el aire dentro de la botella.

– Sin sacar la aguja, vuelva la botella al revés.

– Retire el émbolo hasta que llegue a la dosis de insulina (regular) clara (número de unidades) que Ud. necesita.

– Suavemente saque Ud. la aguja de la botella.

– Empuje la aguja en la insulina turbia (NPH o insulina Lente) sin inyectarla dentro de la botella.

– Retire el émbolo hasta que llegue a su dosis total de insulina en unidades (regular y NPH/Lente conbinadas).

– Practicaremos juntos(as) otra vez.

## Home care phrases

| | |
|---|---|
| Wash your hands before touching medications. | Lávese Ud. las manos antes de tocar los medicamentos. |
| Check the medication bottle for name, dose, and frequency (how often it's supposed to be taken). | En el envase del medicamento verifique Ud. el nombre, la dosis y la frecuencia (con que frequencia se debe tomar). |
| Check the expiration date on all medications. | Verifique Ud. la fecha en la que el medicamento expira. |
| Store medications according to pharmacy instructions. | Guarde Ud. los medicamentos según las instrucciones de la farmacia. |
| Under adequate lighting, read medication labels carefully before taking doses. | Bajo luz adecuada, lea Ud. la etiqueta del medicamento con mucho cuidado antes de tomar las dosis. |
| Don't crush medication without first asking the doctor or pharmacist. | No machaque Ud. el medicamento sin antes preguntárselo al doctor o al farmacéutico. |
| Contact your doctor if a new or unexpected symptom or another problem appears. | Póngase Ud. en contacto con su doctor si un síntoma nuevo o inesperado u otros problemas aparecen. |
| Don't stop taking medication unless instructed by your doctor. | No deje Ud. de tomar el medicamento sólo que se lo ordene su doctor. |
| Discard outdated medications. | Deshágase Ud. de medicamentos caducos. |
| Never take someone else's medications. | Nunca tome Ud. los medicamentos de otra persona. |
| Keep a record of your current medications. | Apunte Ud. (tome nota de) sus medicamentos actuales. |

## General drug therapy phrases

### DRUG CLASSES

| | |
|---|---|
| Analgesic | Analgésico |
| Anesthetic | Anestético |
| Antacid | Antiácido |
| Antianginal agent | Agente antianginal |
| Antianxiety agent | Agente ansiolítico |
| Antiarrhythmic agent | Agente antiarrítmico |
| Antibiotic | Antibiótico |
| Anticancer agent | Agente anticarcinógeno |
| Anticoagulant | Anticoagulante |
| Anticonvulsant | Anticonvulsivante |
| Antidepressant | Antidepresivo |
| Antidiarrheal | Antidiarreico |
| Antifungal agent | Agente antifúngico |
| Antigout agent | Agente antigota |

| | |
|---|---|
| Antihistamine | Antihistamínico |
| Antihyperlipemic agent | Agente hiperlipémico |
| Antihypertensive agent | Agente antihipertenso |
| Anti-inflammatory agent | Agente antiinflamatorio |
| Antimalarial agent | Agente antimalárico |
| Antiparkinsonian agent | Agente antiparkinsoniano |
| Antipsychotic agent | Agente antipsicótico |
| Antipyretic | Antipirético |
| Antiseptic | Antiséptico |
| Antispasmodic | Antiespasmódico |
| Antithyroid agent | Agente antitiroideo |
| Antituberculosis agent | Agente antituberculoso |
| Antitussive agent | Agente antitusígeno |
| Antiviral agent | Agente antiviral |
| Appetite stimulant | Estimulante para el apetito |
| Appetite suppressant | Supresor de apetito |
| Bronchodilator | Broncodilatador |
| Decongestant | Descongestivo |
| Digestant | Digestivo (agente que estimula la digestión) |
| Diuretic | Diurético |
| Emetic | Emético |
| Fertility agent | Agente para la fertilidad |
| Hypnotic | Hipnótico |
| Insulin | Insulina |
| Laxative | Laxante |
| Muscle relaxant | Relajante de músculos |
| Oral contraceptive | Anticonceptivo oral |
| Oral hypoglycemic agent | Agente hipoglucémico oral |
| Sedative | Sedante |
| Steroid | Esteroide |
| Thyroid hormone | Hormona de la glándula tiroides |
| Vaccine | Vacuna |
| Vasodilator | Vasodilatador |
| Vitamin | Vitamina |

## PREPARATIONS

| | |
|---|---|
| Capsule | Cápsula |
| Cream | Pomada |
| Drops | Gotas |
| Elixir | Elixir |
| Inhaler | Inhalador |

| Injection | Inyección |
| Lotion | Loción |
| Lozenge | Pastilla |
| Powder | Polvo |
| Spray | Atomizador |
| Suppository | Supositorio |
| Suspension | Suspensión |
| Syrup | Jarabe |
| Tablet | Tableta |

## FREQUENCY

| Once daily | Una vez al día |
| Twice daily | Dos veces al día |
| Three times daily | Tres veces al día |
| Four times daily | Cuatro veces al día |
| In the morning | Por la mañana |
| With meals | Con las comidas |
| Before meals | Antes de las comidas |
| After meals | Después de las comidas |
| Before bedtime | Antes de acostarse |
| When you have_____ | Cuando Ud. tome_____ |
| Only when you need it | Sólo cuando lo necesite |
| Every four hours | Cada cuatro horas |
| Every six hours | Cada seis horas |
| Every eight hours | Cada ocho horas |

# Acknowledgments

We would like to thank the following companies for granting us permission to include their drugs in the full-color photoguide. We would also like to thank Facts and Comparisons for the use of their resources.

**Abbott Laboratories**
Biaxin®, Biaxin® XL, Depakote®, Depakote® Sprinkle, E-Mycin®, Ery-Tab®, Hytrin®, Isoptin® SR, Kaletra™, Synthroid®, Vicodin®, Vicodin ES®

**AstraZeneca LP**
Arimidex®, Crestor®, Nolvadex®, Prilosec®, Tenormin®, Toprol-XL®, Zestril®

**Aventis Pharmaceuticals**
Allegra®, DiaBeta®, Lasix®, Trental®

**Axcan Pharma**
Carafate®

**Bayer Corporation**
Cipro®, Levitra®

**Biovail Pharmaceuticals, Inc.**
Cardizem®, Cardizem® CD, Cardizem® LA, Cardizem® SR, Vasotec®

**Bristol-Myers Squibb Company**
BuSpar®, Capoten®, Cefzil®, Coumadin®, Desyrel®, Monopril®, Pravachol®, Reyataz®, Serzone®

**Elan Pharmaceuticals, Inc.**
Frova™

**Forest Pharmaceuticals, Inc.**
Celexa®, Lexapro™

**Gilead Sciences**
Viread®

**GlaxoSmithKline**
Copyright GlaxoSmithKline. Used with permission.
Amoxil®, Augmentin®, Augmentin® Chewable, Avandia®, Ceftin®, Combivir®, Compazine®, Coreg®, Imitrex®, Lanoxin®, Lotronex®, Paxil®, Relafen®, Retrovir®, Tagamet®, Wellbutrin®, Wellbutrin® SR, Zovirax®, Zyban®

**Janssen Pharmaceutica, Inc.**
Risperdal®, Risperdal M-Tab®

**King Pharmaceuticals, Inc.**
Levoxyl®

**Eli Lilly and Company**
Evista®, Prozac®, Strattera™

**Mallinckrodt, Inc.**
Pamelor®, Restoril®

**McNeil-PPC, Inc.**
Concerta®

**MedPointe Pharmaceuticals**
Soma®

**Merck & Co., Inc.**
Used with permission of Merck & Co., Inc.
Cozaar®, Crixivan®, Fosamax®, HydroDIURIL®, Mevacor®, Pepcid®, Prinivil®, Sinemet®, Sinemet CR®, Singulair®, Vioxx®, Zocor®

**Merck Sant**
An associate of Merck KGaA, Darmstadt, Germany.
Glucophage®, Glucophage® XR

**Merck/Schering-Plough Pharmaceuticals**
Used with permission of Merck/Schering-Plough Pharmaceuticals.
Zetia™

**Novartis Pharmaceuticals, Inc.**
Gleevec®, Lescol®, Lotensin®, Ritalin®, Ritalin SR®, Stalevo®

**Ortho-McNeil Pharmaceutical**
Floxin®, Levaquin®, Tylenol® with Codeine No. 3, Ultracet®

**Otsuka Pharmaceutical Company, Ltd.**
Abilify®

**Pfizer, Inc.**
Registered Trademarks of Pfizer Inc. All Rights Reserved. Courtesy of Pfizer Inc. Accupril®, Cardura®, Celebrex®, Diflucan®, Dilantin® Kapseals®, Glucotrol®, Glucotrol XL®, Lipitor®, Lopid®, Neurontin®, Nitrostat®, Norvasc®, Procardia®, Procardia XL®, Relpax®, Viagra®, Zantac®, Zithromax®, Zoloft®, Zyrtec®

**Pharmacia Corporation**
Registered Trademarks of Pharmacia Corporation, a Pfizer Inc. corporation. All Rights Reserved. Courtesy of Pfizer Inc. Bextra®, Calan®, Deltasone®, Demulen®, Detrol®, Medrol®, Micronase®, Motrin, Pletal®, Provera®, Xanax®

**Procter and Gamble Pharmaceuticals, Inc.**
Actonel®, Macrobid®

**Purdue Pharma L.P.**
OxyContin®

**Roche Laboratories, Inc.**
Bumex®, Klonopin®, Naprosyn®, Ticlid®, Valium®

**Sanofi-Synthelabo, Inc.**
Ambien®, Demerol®, UroXatral®

**Sankyo Pharma**
Benicar™

**Schering Corporation and Key Pharmaceuticals, Inc.**
Clarinex™, K-Dur®

**Schwarz Pharma**
Verelan®

**Tap Pharmaceuticals, Inc.**
Prevacid®

**UCB Pharmaceuticals, Inc.**
Lortab®

**Warner Chilcott Laboratories, Inc.**
Duricef, Eryc®, Estrace®, Ovcon® 35, Sarafem®

**Women First HealthCare, Inc.**
Bactrim DS®

**Wyeth Pharmaceuticals**
The appearance of these tablets and capsules is a trademark of Wyeth Pharmaceuticals, Philadelphia, Pa. Effexor®, Effexor® XR

The appearance of these tablets is a trademark of Wyeth Pharmaceuticals. Courtesy of Wyeth Pharmaceuticals division of Wyeth, Collegeville, Pa. Premarin®

The "C" design of these tablets is a registered trademark of Wyeth Pharmaceuticals, Philadelphia, Pa. Cordarone®

The appearance of these tablets and capsules is a registered trademark of Wyeth Pharmaceuticals, Philadelphia, Pa. Inderal®, Inderal® LA

The appearance of these tablets is a trademark of Wyeth Pharmaceuticals, Philadelphia, Pa. Phenergan®

# Index

---

t refers to a table; **boldface** refers to full-color photographs.

---

† refers to a table; **boldface** refers to full-color photographs.

---

t refers to a table; **boldface** refers to full-color photographs.